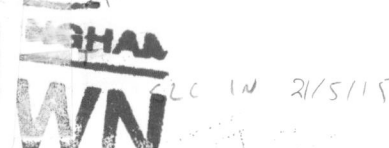

UNIV... W...GHAM

WN

D1422964

ROM THE LIBRAR

GLC IN 21/5/15

EIGHTH EDITION

Exercise Physiology

Nutrition, Energy, and Human Performance

EIGHTH EDITION

Exercise Physiology

Nutrition, Energy, and Human Performance

UNIVERSITY OF NOTTINGHAM
JAMES CAMERON-GIFFORD LIBRARY

William D. McArdle

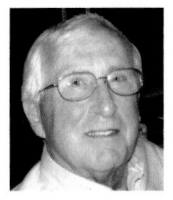

Professor Emeritus, Department of Family, Nutrition,
  and Exercise Science
Queens College of the City University of New York
Flushing, New York
Exercise Physiologist, Weight Watchers International

Frank I. Katch

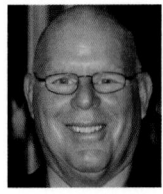

Instructor and Board Member
Certificate Program in Fitness Instruction
UCLA Extension, Los Angeles, California
Former Professor and Chair of Exercise Science
University of Massachusetts, Amherst, Massachusetts

Victor L. Katch

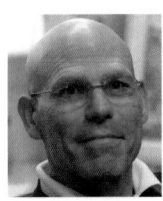

Professor of Movement Science
School of Kinesiology
Associate Professor, Pediatrics
School of Medicine
University of Michigan, Ann Arbor, Michigan

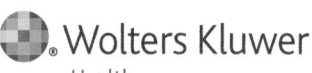
. Wolters Kluwer

Health

Philadelphia • Baltimore • New York • London
Buenos Aires • Hong Kong • Sydney • Tokyo

Acquisitions Editor: Emily Lupash
Supervisor, Product Development: Eve Malakoff-Klein
Marketing Manager: Shauna Kelley
Production Project Manager: David Orzechowski
Design Coordinator: Stephen Druding
Art Director: Jennifer Clements
Artist: Dragonfly Media Group
Compositor: SPi Global

Copyright © 2015, 2010, 2007, 2001, 1996, 1986, 1981
Wolters Kluwer Health | Lippincott Williams & Wilkins.

351 West Camden Street	**Two Commerce Square**
Baltimore, MD 21201	**2001 Market Street**
	Philadelphia, PA 19103

Selected photographs © 2008 by Fitness Technologies, Inc., Frank I. Katch, and Victor L. Katch. This material is protected by copyright. No photographs may be reproduced in any form or by any means without permission from the copyright holders.

All rights reserved. This book is protected by copyright. No part of this book may be reproduced or transmitted in any form or by any means, including as photocopies or scanned-in or other electronic copies, or utilized by any information storage and retrieval system without written permission from the copyright owner, except for brief quotations embodied in critical articles and reviews. Materials appearing in this book prepared by individuals as part of their official duties as U.S. government employees are not covered by the above-mentioned copyright. To request permission, please contact Wolters Kluwer Health |Lippincott Williams & Wilkins at permissions@lww.com.

Printed in China
1007409156

Not authorised for sale in United States, Canada, Australia, New Zealand, Puerto Rico, and United States Virgin Islands.

Disclaimer
Care has been taken to confirm the accuracy of the information presented and to describe generally accepted practices. However, the authors, editors, and publisher are not responsible for errors or omissions or for any consequences from application of the information in this book and make no warranty, expressed or implied, with respect to the currency, completeness, or accuracy of the contents of the publication. Application of this information in a particular situation remains the professional responsibility of the practitioner; the clinical treatments described and recommended may not be considered absolute and universal recommendations.

The authors, editors, and publisher have exerted every effort to ensure that drug selection and dosage set forth in this text are in accordance with the current recommendations and practice at the time of publication. However, in view of ongoing research, changes in government regulations, and the constant flow of information relating to drug therapy and drug reactions, the reader is urged to check the package insert for each drug for any change in indications and dosage and for added warnings and precautions. This is particularly important when the recommended agent is a new or infrequently employed drug.

Some drugs and medical devices presented in this publication have Food and Drug Administration (FDA) clearance for limited use in restricted research settings. It is the responsibility of the health care provider to ascertain the FDA status of each drug or device planned for use in his or her clinical practice.

To purchase additional copies of this book, call our customer service department at (800) 638-3030 or fax orders to (301) 223-2320. International customers should call (301) 223-2300. Visit Wolters Kluwer Health | Lippincott Williams & Wilkins online at www.lww.com.

9 8 7 6 5 4 3 2 1

To my wife Kathleen, my best friend and biggest supporter, and to the rest of the
"A team," whose lives give meaning to my own: my children, Theresa, Amy, Kevin,
and Jennifer; their spouses, Christian, Jeff, Nicole, and Andy;
and my grandchildren, Liam, Aidan, Dylan, Kelly Rose, Owen,
Henry, Kathleen (Kate), Grace, Elizabeth, Claire, Elise,
Charlotte, and Sophia.

—BILL McARDLE

To my wife and life partner Kerry for 44 years of love, patience, and support;
to my two sons, David and Kevin, for achieving the honorable in their
professional lives; to my daughter Ellen (and her husband Sean) for all
her success as a caring pediatrician and mom; and to my
one-year-old grandson pal, James Patrick. Life is good!

—FRANK KATCH

To those most important to me: my wife Heather, my daughters
Erika and Leslie, my son Jesse, and my grandkids
Ryan, Cameron, Ella, and Emery.

—VICTOR KATCH

Preface

Since the first edition of our textbook more than threee decades ago, knowledge concerning the physiologic effects of exercise in general and the body's unique and specific responses to training in particular has exploded. Tipton's search of the 1946 English literature for the terms *exercise* and *exertion* yielded 12 citations in 5 journals.[73] Tipton also cited a 1984 analysis by Booth, who reported that in 1962, the number of yearly citations of the term *exertion* increased to 128 in 51 journals, and by 1981, there were 655 citations to the word *exertion* in 224 journals. The graph on this page highlights the huge number of entries for the words *exercise* or *exertion* from a recent Internet search of *Index Medicus* (Medline) and for the years 2000 to December 3, 2013, using the NCBI database (www.ncbi.nlm.nih.gov/sites/entrez). In just a 4-year period since publication of our seventh edition, the number of citations increased by over 66,700 to 291,194, a 29.8% increase! Although we had thought that citation frequency was leveling off from 1986 to 1996, the rate of increase has instead steadily increased beyond our wildest expectations. Obviously, we misjudged how greatly exercise-related topics would affect scholarly productivity in biologic sciences research. With expanding interest in the role of exercise and physical activity in the allied health professions, the rate of citations devoted to these topics undoubtedly will continue to accelerate.

As graduate students in the late 1960s, we never imagined that interest in exercise physiology would increase so dramatically. New generations of scholars committed to studying the scientific basis of exercise had set to work. Some studied the physiologic mechanisms involved in adaptations to regular exercise; others evaluated individual differences in exercise and sports performance. Collectively, both approaches expanded knowledge in the growing field of exercise physiology. At our first scientific conference (American College of Sports Medicine [ACSM] in Las Vegas, 1967), still as graduate students, we rubbed elbows with the "giants" of the field, many of whom were themselves students of the leaders of their era. Several hundred ACSM members listened attentively as the superstars of exercise physiology and physical fitness (Erling Asmussen, Per-Olof Åstrand, Bruno Balke, Elsworth Buskirk, Thomas Cureton, Lars Hermansen, Steven Horvath, Henry Montoye, Bengt Saltin, and Charles Tipton) presented their research and fielded penetrating questions from an audience of young graduate students eager to devour the latest scientific information delivered by these "stars of our field."

Sitting under an open tent in the Nevada desert with one of the world's leading physiologists, Dr. David Bruce Dill (then age 74; profiled later in this book's introduction), we listened to his research assistant—a high school student— lecture about temperature regulation in the desert burro. Later, one of us (Frank Katch) sat next to a white-haired gentleman and chatted about his master's thesis project. Only later did an embarrassed Frank learn that this gentleman was Captain Albert R. Behnke, MD (1898–1993; ACSM Honor Award, 1976), the modern-day "father" of human body composition assessment whose crucial experiment in diving physiology established standards for decompression and use of mixed gases for deep dives.

Dr. Behnke's pioneering studies of hydrostatic weighing in 1942 (which Frank Katch put into practice with a swimming pool underwater weighing tank for his master of science thesis at the University of California, Santa Barbara, in 1966), the development of a reference man and reference woman model, and the creation of the somatogram based on anthropometric measurements

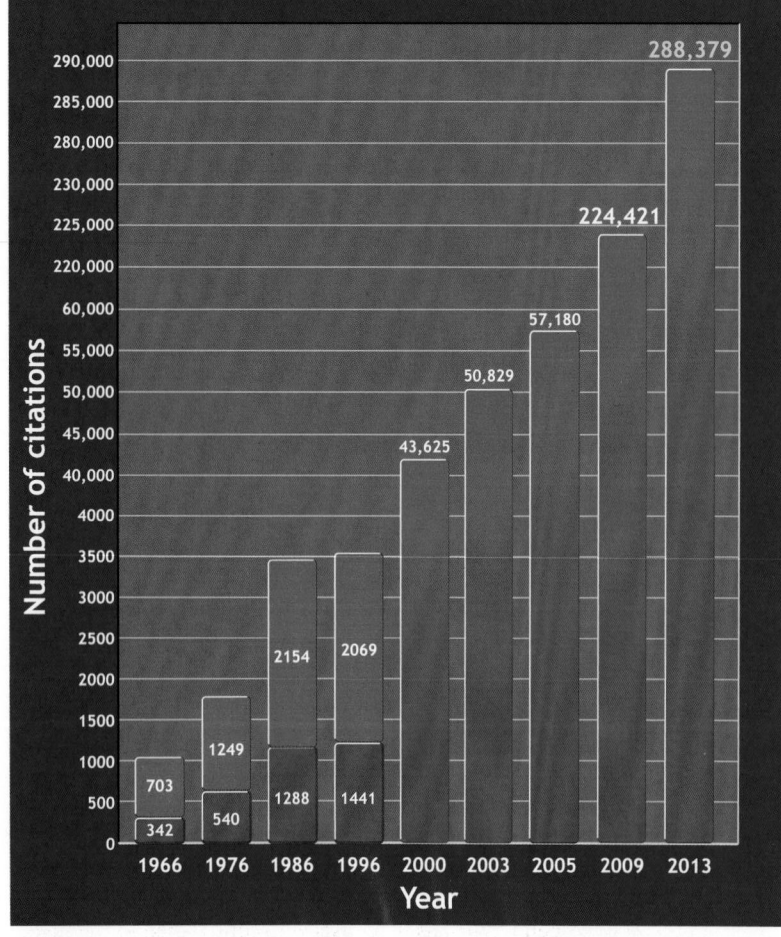

Exercise or *exertion* as a topic (*top bars*) and frequency of the word *exercise* appearing in a scientific journal (*bottom bars*) for the years 1966 to 2013 from Index Medicus. The last four columns used PubMed via an Internet search for citations with the terms *exercise* or *exertion*.

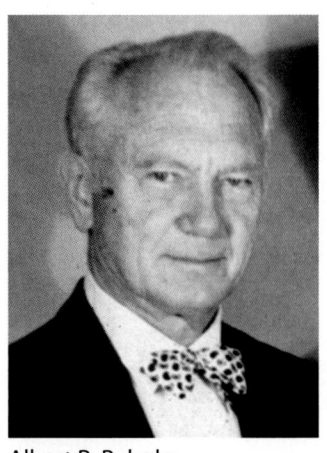

Albert R. Behnke

form the basis for much current work in body composition assessment.

That fortuitous meeting began a lasting personal and fulfilling professional friendship until Dr. Behnke's death in 1993. Over the years, the three of us were indeed fortunate to work with the very best scholars in our field. William McArdle studied for his PhD at the University of Michigan with Dr. Henry Montoye (charter member of ACSM; President of ACSM, 1962–1963; Citation Award, 1973) and Dr. John Faulkner (President of ACSM, 1971–1972; Citation Award, 1973; ACSM Honor Award, 1992). At the University of California, Berkeley, Victor Katch completed his master of science thesis under the supervision of Dr. Jack Wilmore (ACSM President, 1978–1979; Citation Award, 1984; first editor of *Exercise and Sport Science Reviews*, 1973–1974) and was a doctoral student of Dr. Franklin Henry (ACSM Honor Award, 1975; originator of the "Memory-Drum Concept" about the specificity of exercise; author of the seminal paper "Physical Education—an Academic Discipline," *JOHPER* 1964;35:32). Frank Katch completed his master of science under the supervision of thesis advisors Dr. Ernest Michael, Jr. (former PhD student of pioneer exercise physiologist–physical fitness scientist Dr. Thomas Kirk Cureton; ACSM Honor Award, 1969), and Dr. Barbara Drinkwater (President of ACSM, 1988–1989; ACSM Honor Award, 1996), and then completed doctoral studies at UC Berkeley with Professor Franklin Henry.

As the three of us reexamine those earlier times, we realize, like many of our colleagues, that our academic good fortunes prospered because our professors and mentors shared an unwavering commitment to study sport, exercise, and movement from a strong scientific and physiologic perspective. These scholars demonstrated why it was crucial that physical educators be well grounded in both the scientific basics and underlying concepts and principles of exercise physiology.

Moving Forward

As in the publication of the first edition of *Exercise Physiology: Energy, Nutrition, and Human Performance* in 1981, this eighth edition reflects our continued commitment to integrate the concepts and science of the different disciplines that contribute to a more comprehensive understanding and appreciation of modern-day exercise physiology. As in prior editions, we continue to believe that the exercise physiology discipline demands integration of study areas relevant to nutrition, exercise biochemistry and bioenergetics, physiology, medicine, exercise training and sports performance, and the health-related aspects of regular physical activity. All of these areas naturally and inexorably link within the fabric of what currently comprises the field called exercise physiology or, in deference to the early scholars in the field, the physiology of

exercise. As an example, proper nutrition links to good health, effective weight control, and optimal levels of physical activity and sports performance, while regular physical activity and exercise training provide an important means to control body weight and optimize one's overall health profile. We are encouraged that the medical establishment and government agencies continue to acknowledge (and now promote) regular physical activity as an important weapon in the armamentarium for prevention and rehabilitation of diverse disease states, including diabetes, obesity, cancer, and heart disease.

We are gratified with the small part we have played in the education of more than 400,000 undergraduate and graduate students who have used this text since the publication of the first edition in 1981. A source of great pride for us is that some of the first students enrolled in our classes that used this text have gone on to earn advanced degrees in the same or similar fields. This tradition of textbook adoption has now been passed down to their students, many of whom comprise the next generation of aspiring teachers, exercise specialists, and researchers. We are forever grateful to our former teachers and mentors for igniting a spark that has not diminished. We hope you will become as excited as we first were (and continue to be) in the science of exercise physiology and human performance.

We leave you with this apt quote in Latin attributed to prolific French author and astronomer Nicolas Camille Flammarion (1842 –1925): "Ad Veritatum Per Scientiam" (To Truth Through Science), inscribed in gold above the observatory and museum entrance to his Chateau at Juvisy-Sur-Orge outside of Paris.

ORGANIZATION

This eighth edition maintains an eight-section structure and an introductory section about the origins of exercise physiology. The concluding "On the Horizons" section and its chapter have changed from an addendum to a numbered chapter, reflective of molecular biology's place as an established part of exercise science.

The eighth edition also has undergone a complete art makeover. Most of the existing figures have been redrawn to provide consistency with newly created illustrations. Throughout the text, we have included Internet resources (URLs) to provide an expanded Web access to supplement student insights of relevant text material. The text continues the tradition of FYI (For Your Information) boxes that provide relatively short inserts of related information, current research, or interesting sidebars germane to the text's topic, ranging from "One-Minute Bouts of Intense Physical Activity Improves Fitness and Health" to "Consuming Excess Calories Produces Fat Gain Regardless of Nutrient Source."

FEATURES

This text's features have been specifically designed to help students facilitate learning. They include:

Introduction: A View of the Past. The text's introduction, "Exercise Physiology: Roots and Historical Perspectives," reflects our interest and respect for the earliest underpinnings of the field, and the direct and indirect contributions of the men and women physicians–scientists who contributed to the field.

Chapter Objectives. Each chapter opens with a comprehensive summary of learning goals, helping students to become familiar with the materials to be covered in a chapter.

Ancillaries at-a-Glance. A complete list of all electronic resources associated with a chapter makes accessing online materials easy; callouts in the text reinforce for students opportunities to broaden their knowledge beyond the pages of the text.

In a Practical Sense. Every chapter highlights practical applications about specific topic areas.

Integrative Questions. Open-ended questions encourage students to thoughtfully consider complex concepts without a single "correct" answer.

Expanded Art Program. The full-color art program continues to be an important feature of the textbook. Nearly every figure has been revised to make its textual and visual elements "pop," or altered to highlight important teaching points that reinforce text material. New figures have been added to chapters to enhance new and updated content, including the use of many new medical illustrations. A new table format clearly organizes essential data.

Up-Close and Personal Interviews. The text features nine contemporary scientists whose important research contributions and visionary leadership continue the tradition of the scientists of prior generations—Drs. Steven Blair, Frank Booth, Claude Bouchard, David Costill, Barbara Drinkwater, John Holloszy, Loring Rowell, Bengt Saltin, and Charles Tipton. These individuals merit recognition not only for expanding knowledge through their many scientific contributions, but also for elucidating mechanisms that underlie responses and adaptations to exercise and health enhancement. Each person has been placed within a section linked to his or her main scholarship interests, yet all of them span one or more sections in terms of scientific contributions.

thePoint Appendix C, available online at http://thepoint. lww.com/mkk8e, lists individual honors and awards for each of these distinguished and meritorious scientist–researchers.

The intimate insights from the "superstars" should inspire current exercise physiology students to actualize their potential, whether through accomplishments in graduate school, teaching, research, or numerous other exciting professional opportunities to achieve excellence.

References, Appendices, and Animations (available online). All references and appendices are available online at http://thepoint.lww.com/mkk8e. Appendices feature valuable information about nutritive values, energy expenditures, metabolic computations in open-circuit spirometry, and more.

Focus on Research (available online). Almost all chapters have a companion online Focus on Research, featuring a key research article from a renowned scientist. These well-designed studies illustrate, within a historical perspective, how "theory comes to life" via the dynamics of research.

NEW TO THE EIGHTH EDITION

The flow of information in this edition remains similar to prior editions. Components of the entire text have been upgraded to reflect current research findings related to the diverse areas of exercise physiology. We have revised almost every figure, and supplemented them with high-quality medical illustrations. We also have added new tables, and listed numerous new Web sites to provide readers access to the abundance of updated information available about the intricacies relevant to topic areas in exercise physiology. "On the Horizon" has been upgraded to a full section and chapter, reflecting the increasing importance of research in molecular biology on exercise physiology.

Our current reference list includes up-to-date research results gleaned from national and international journals related to specific topic areas. In selected chapters, "Additional References" provide a bibliography of articles that augment the materials already presented in the chapter. All references for a chapter are located online at http://thePoint.lww.com/ mkk8e. We hope you profit from and enjoy this continuation of our journey through the ever-expanding and maturing field of exercise physiology.

ANCILLARIES: THE TOTAL TEACHING PACKAGE

Exercise Physiology: Nutrition, Energy, and Human Performance, Eighth Edition includes additional resources for both instructors and students that are available on the book's companion Web sites at http://thePoint.lww.com/mkk8e.

Approved adopting instructors will be given access to the following resources:

- Animations illustrating the most important concepts in human physiology
- Test generator
- PowerPoint presentations: one set with lecture outlines, one set with images only
- Image bank of downloadable figures and tables in multiple formats
- Searchable full text online
- Blackboard, Angel, and Moodle LMS cartridges

Students

Students who purchase *Exercise Physiology: Nutrition, Energy, and Human Performance,* Eighth Edition have access to the following additional resources, accessible with the scratch-off code provided on this book's inside cover:

- Online interactive quiz bank with study and test options
- Animations
- References
- Appendixes
- Focus on Research article abstracts and analysis
- Featured information on microscope technologies, notable events in genetics, Nobel prizes, outstanding female scientists, and much more.

Ancillaries were prepared by the authors and by Jeff Woods (Professor of Kinesiology and Community Health, University of Illinois at Urbana–Champaign) and Lamia Scherzinger (Indiana University–Perdue University Indianapolis).

Acknowledgments

We wish to thank many individuals. First, to Dr. Loring Rowell for his constructive comments on the chapters related to pulmonary and cardiovascular dynamics during rest and exercise, particularly the sections related to the possible role of the venous system as an active vasculature. We thank Dr. Victor Convertino, U.S. Army Institute of Surgical Research at Fort Sam Houston, TX, for insightful comments and suggestions on the microgravity chapter, and Dr. Charles Tipton, Professor Emeritus, University of Arizona, Tuscon, AZ, for valuable comments and for providing new information about the historical development of the physiology of exercise, including material about the first textbook devoted to exercise and physiology in the 16th century, and physiology of exercise textbook used in the late 1800s and early 1900s.

Stephen Lee (Exercise Physiology Laboratory, Johnson Space Center, Houston, TX; www.nasa.gov/centers/johnson/slsd/about/divisions/hacd/laboratories/exercise-physiology.html) kindly supplied original NASA photos and documents, and Mission Specialist Astronaut Dr. Martin Fettman (Colorado State University, Ft. Collins, CO) provided an original slide of the rotating chair experiment he took during his Skylab 2 Mission. Dr. Helen Lane (Chief Nutritionist and Manager, University Research and Affairs, NASA Johnson Space Center, Houston, TX), provided prepublication documents and resource materials. Dr. Ron White, National Space Biomedical Research Institute Houston, TX, allowed us to use charts he helped to create from *Human Physiology in Space Teacher's Manual*. Dr. Susan Bloomfield (Bone Biology Laboratory, Texas A&M University, College Station, TX) kindly provided images of hind-limb suspension experiments from her lab. We sincerely appreciate the expertise of Drs. Frank Booth, University of Missouri, Columbia, MO; Kristin Steumple, Department of Health and Exercise Science at Gettysburg College, Gettysburg, PA; and Marvin Balouyt, Washtenaw Community College, Ann Arbor, MI, for their expert opinions and suggestions for improving the chapter on molecular biology. Hypoxico Inc. provided photos of the Hypoxico altitude tent. Mr. John Selby (www.hyperlite.co.uk) kindly provided timely information and photos of the portable, collapsible decompression chamber. Dr. Alex Knight, York University, United Kingdom, graciously provided information about molecular biology techniques he has pioneered (*in vitro* motility assay) and other information and a photograph about myosin, muscle, and single molecules. Yakl Freedman (www.dna2z.com) was supportive in supplying recent information about DNA and molecular biology. Sue Hilt of the American College of Sports Medicine, Indianapolis, IN, did a superb job of securing the text of the Citation and Honor Awards reproduced in Appendix C. Dr. James A. Freeman, Professor of English, University of Massachusetts, Amherst, unselfishly lent his know-how to make words sing in the introductory history MI. Dr. Barry Franklin, Beaumont Hospital, Detroit, MI, supplied original information about cardiac rehabilitation. The Trustees of Amherst College and Archival Library, Amherst, MA, gave permission to reproduce the photographs and materials of Dr. Hitchcock. Magnus Mueller from the University of Geisen, Germany, kindly provided the photo of Liebig's Geisen lab. We are grateful to marine artist Ron Scobie, ASMA (www.ronscobie-marineartist.com), for his kind permission to reproduce his rendering of the HMS *Beagle*. We thank Nancy Mullis for graciously providing the photo of Dr. Kary Mullis.

We are collectively indebted to the nine researchers/scholars who took time from their busy schedules to answer our interview questions and provide personal photos. Each of those individuals, in his or her own unique way, inspired the three of us in our careers by their work ethic, scientific excellence, and generosity of time and advice with colleagues and students. Over the years, we have had the good fortune to come to know these individuals both socially and in the academic arena. We are grateful for the opportunity to conduct the interviews because they provided insights about their personal lives previously unknown to us. We hope you too are as impressed as we are by all they have accomplished and returned to the profession.

We acknowledge our master's and senior honors students who worked in our labs for their projects, and contributed so much to our research and personal experiences: Pedro Alexander, Christos Balabinis, Margaret Ballantyne, Brandee Black, Michael Carpenter, Steven Christos, Roman Czula, Gwyn Danielson, Toni Denahan, Marty Dicker, Sadie Drumm, Peter Frykman, Scott Glickman, Marion Gurry, Carrie Hauser, Margie King, Peter LaChance, Jean Lett, Maria Likomitrou, Robert Martin, Cathi Moorehead, Susan Novitsky, Joan Perry, Sharon Purdy, Michelle Segar, Debra Spiak, Lorraine Turcotte, Lori Waiter, Stephen Westing, and Howard Zelaznik.

We also dedicate this edition to that special group of former students who earner doctoral degrees in physical education, exercise science, or medicine, and who have gone on to distingush themselves as teachers, practitioners, and researchers in the related areas of exercise physiology. These include Denise Agin, Stamitis Agiovlasitis, Doug Ballor, Dan Becque, Geroge Brooks, Barbara Campaigne, Ed Chaloupka, Ken Cohen, Edward Coyle, Dan Delio, Julia Chase Delio, Chris Dunbar, Patti Freedson, Roger Glaser, Ellen Glickman, Kati Haltiwinger, Everett Harmon, Jay Hoffman, Tibor Hortobagyi, Jie Kang, Mitch Kanter, Betsy Keller, Marliese Kimmerly, George Lesmses, Steve Lichtman, Charles Marks, Robert Mofatt, Laren Nau-White, Steve Ostrove, James Rimmer, Deborah Rinaldi, Stan Sady, Lapros Sidossis, Bob Spina, John Spring, Bill Thorland, Mike Toner, Laurel Trager-Mackinnon, Lorraine Turcotte, John Villanacci, Jonnis Vrabis, Nancy

Weiss, Art Weltman, Nancy Wessingeer, Stephen Westing, Anthony Wilcox, and Libnda Zwiren.

Finally, we would like to recognize the creative individuals at Wolters Kluwer who helped to shepherd this eighth edition through the various stages of production. We are particularly indebted to Eve Malakoff-Klein, our talented and superb Supervisor of Product Development, who continually provided much-needed support, patience, subtle urging, and excellence in organization and expertise in handling critical editing issues in bringing this edition to fruition in a timely manner. She clearly served in a highly professional manner as our advocate in issues related to the production process. We also gratefully acknowledge and appreciate the outstanding technical and creative expertise of Jennifer Clements, Art Director, for going well beyond the call of duty for insightful and creative contributions in revising the art in every chapter and dealing with our sometimes trivial requests. David Orzechowski, Production Project Manager, helped to translate the edited chapters into galley magic. Also, the talented artists at Dragonfly (www.dragonflymediagroup.com/) deserve recognition for their elegant medical illustration and artistic and technical expertise. Thank you so much Eve, Jen, Dave, and Dragonfly for a job exceptionally well done!

William D. McArdle
Sound Beach, NY

Frank I. Katch
Santa Barbara, CA

Victor L. Katch
Ann Arbor, MI

Contents

Introduction: A View of the Past

EXERCISE PHYSIOLOGY: ROOTS AND HISTORICAL PERSPECTIVES

Acknowledging all of the pioneers who created the field of exercise physiology is a difficult task in the span of an introduction to a textbook in this area. Indeed, it would be a herculean task to faithfully chronicle the rich history of exercise physiology from its origins in ancient Asia to the present. For this brief overview, we present a chronological historical tour regarding topics often not adequately developed in exercise physiology courses or their traditional textbooks. Along the way, we delve into events and people that have profoundly influenced the emerging field of exercise physiology—specifically the creation of science-based curriculum in colleges and universities at the turn of the 19th century, and the influential scientists who helped to create these early programs. It was the dogged insistence of the latter on innovation and experimental rigor that propelled desperate fields in medicine and the biological sciences to make rapid strides in creating new knowledge about how humans functioned during various modes and intensities of physical activity and the impact on humans of heat, cold, depth/pressure, altitude, and microgravity environmental stressors.

Our discussion begins with an acknowledgment of the ancient but tremendously influential Indian, Arabic, and prominent Greek physicians; we highlight some milestones (and ingenious experiments), including the many contributions from Sweden, Denmark, Norway, and Finland that fostered the study of sport and exercise as a respectable field of scientific inquiry. A treasure-trove of information about the early beginnings of exercise physiology in America was uncovered in the archives of Amherst College, Massachusetts, in an anatomy and physiology textbook (incorporating a student study guide) written by the first American father-and-son writing team. The father, Edward Hitchcock, was President of Amherst College; the son, Edward Hitchcock, Jr., an Amherst graduate and Harvard-trained physician, made detailed anthropometric and strength measurements of almost every student enrolled at Amherst College for almost three decades from 1861 to 1889. In 1891, much of what forms current college curricula in exercise physiology, including evaluation of body composition by anthropometry and muscular strength by dynamic measurements, began in the first physical education scientific laboratory at Harvard's University's prestigious Lawrence Scientific School (founded in 1847, and in 1906, absorbed into Harvard College and Graduate School of Arts and Letters). Even before the fortuitous creation of this science-oriented laboratory, another less formal but still tremendously influential factor affected the development of exercise physiology: the publication during the 19th century of American textbooks on anatomy and physiology, physiology, physiology and hygiene, and anthropometry. The availability of physiology texts allowed teachers and research scientists with an interest in physiology to offer formal coursework in these topics as they related to exercise and human movement. More than 45 textbooks published between 1801 and 1899 contained information about the muscular, circulatory, respiratory, nervous, and digestive systems—including the influence of exercise and its effects—and eventually shaped the content area of exercise physiology during the next century.

thePoint Appendix A, available online at http://thepoint. lww.com/mkk8e, provides several bibliographies of influential publications pertaining to anatomy and physiology, anthropometry, exercise and training, and exercise physiology.

Professor Roberta Park, distinguished UC Berkeley physical education, exercise science, and sport historian, chronicles the early contributions of many physicians and science-oriented physical educators who steadfastly believed that physical education (and medicine) should be grounded on a sound scientific foundation fueled by cutting-edge research.[53,54,56,58,60,61]

Well-documented historical chronologies and other contributions[8,9,55,57,59] provide context and foster appreciation for the scholars and educators who paved the way for the new generation of researchers; the early innovators developed new techniques and methodologies in the fields of health, fitness, sports performance, and physical activity that became essential components of the early exercise physiology core curriculum. Appendix A (online) lists additional influential texts from 1900 to 1947 dealing with exercise, training, and exercise physiology.[a]

IN THE BEGINNING: ORIGINS OF EXERCISE PHYSIOLOGY FROM ANCIENT GREECE TO AMERICA IN THE EARLY 1800S

Exercise physiology arose primarily in the civilizations of early Greece and Asia Minor, although the topics of exercise, sports, games, and health concerned even earlier civilizations. These included the Minoan and Mycenaean cultures; the great

---

[a]Buskirk[13] provides a bibliography of books and review articles on exercise, fitness, and exercise physiology from 1920 to 1979. Berryman[7] lists many textbooks and essays from the time of Hippocrates through the Civil War period in the United States.

biblical realms of David and Solomon; and the territories of Assyria, Babylonia, Media, and Persia, including the empires of Alexander the Great. Early references to sports, games, and health practices (personal hygiene, exercise, and training) were recorded by the ancient civilizations of Syria, Egypt, Macedonia, Arabia, Mesopotamia and Persia, India, and China. Tipton chronicles the doctrines and teachings of Sushruta, an Indian physician, teacher of aspiring medical students, and surgeon who practiced in the 5th century BC. Sushruta is remembered as the first plastic surgeon,[66] and as a scholar who produced the ancient treatise *Sushruta Samhita* 150 years before Hippocrates lived. Sushruta's compendium from 600 BC is housed in the Oxford University library, and a 1911 English translation in three volumes can be read online at **http://archive.org/stream/englishtranslati00susruoft#page/ n3/mode/2up**. He detailed 800 medical procedures, described 120 blunt and sharp surgical instruments, and penned detailed accounts of hundreds of medical conditions relating to various disease states and organ deficiencies (**www.faqs.org/health/ topics/50/Sushruta.html**), including the influence of different modes of exercise on human health and disease.[74] Tipton notes that Sushruta considered obesity a disease, and posited that a sedentary lifestyle contributed to obesity. The greatest influence on Western Civilization, however, came from the Greek physicians of antiquity—Herodicus (5th century BC), Hippocrates (460–377 BC), and Claudius Galenus or Galen (AD 131–201[b]).

Herodicus, a physician and athlete, strongly advocated proper diet in physical training. His early writings and devoted followers influenced the famous physician Hippocrates, considered to be the "father" of modern medicine, who first wrote about preventative medicine. Hippocrates is credited with producing 87 treatises on medicine—several on health and hygiene—during the influential Golden Age of Greece.[7,47] He espoused a profound understanding of human suffering, emphasizing a doctor's place at the patient's bedside. Today, physicians take either the classical or modern Hippocratic Oath (**www.nlm.nih. gov/hmd/greek/greek_oath.html**) based on Hippocrates' "Corpus Hippocratum."

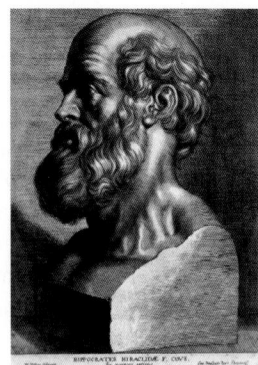

Hippocrates

Five centuries after Hippocrates, during the early decline of the Roman Empire, Galen emerged as perhaps the most well-known and influential physician that ever lived. The son of a wealthy architect, Galen was born in the city of Pergamos[c] and educated by scholars of the time. He began studying medicine at approximately age 16. During the next 50 years,

he implemented and enhanced current thinking about health and scientific hygiene, an area that some might consider "applied" exercise physiology. Throughout his life, Galen taught and practiced the "laws of health": breathe fresh air, eat proper foods, drink the right beverages, exercise, get adequate sleep, have a daily bowel movement, and control one's emotions.[7] A prolific writer, Galen produced at least 80 sophisticated treatises (and perhaps 500 essays) on numerous topics, many of which addressed human anatomy and physiology, nutrition, growth and development, the beneficial effects of exercise, the deleterious consequences of sedentary living, and a variety of diseases and their treatment including obesity. Sushruta's notions about obesity were undoubtedly influenced by Galen, who introduced the concept of *polisarkia* (now known as morbid obesity).[71] Galen proposed treatments commonly in use today—diet, exercise, and medications. One of the first "bench physiologists," Galen conducted original experiments in physiology, comparative anatomy, and medicine, and performed dissections of humans, goats, pigs, cows, horses, and elephants. As physician to the gladiators of Pergamos, Galen treated torn tendons and muscles ripped apart in combat with various surgical procedures he invented, including the procedure depicted in FIGURE I.1, a 1544 woodcut of shoulder surgery. Galen also formulated rehabilitation therapies and exercise regimens, including treatment for a dislocated shoulder. He followed the Hippocratic school of medicine that believed in logical science grounded in experimentation and observation.

Galen wrote detailed descriptions about the forms, kinds, and varieties of "swift" and vigorous exercises, including their proper quantity and duration. The following definition of exercise is from the first complete English translation by Green[27] of Hygiene (*De Sanitate Tuenda*, pp. 53–54; see TABLE I.1), Galen's insightful and detailed treatise on healthful living:

> To me it does not seem that all movement is exercise, but only when it is vigorous.... The criterion of vigorousness is change of respiration; those movements that do not alter the respiration are not called exercise. But if anyone is compelled by any movement to breathe more or less or faster, that movement becomes exercise from him. This therefore is what is commonly called exercise or gymnastics, from the gymnasium or public-place to which the inhabitants of a city come to anoint and rub themselves, to wrestle, throw the discus, or engage in some other sport.... The uses of exercise, I think are twofold, one for the evacuation of the excrements, the other for the production of good condition of the firm parts of the body.

During the early Greek period, the Hippocratic school of physicians devised ingenious methods to treat common maladies; these methods included procedures to reduce pain from

---

[b]According to Green, the dates for Galen's birth are estimates based on a notation Galen made when at age 38 he served as personal physician to the Roman emperors Marcus Aurelius and Lucius Verus.[27] Siegel's bibliography contains an excellent source for references to Galen.[62]

[c]An important city on the Mediterranean coast of Asia Minor, Pergamos influenced trade and commerce. From CE 152 to 156, Galen studied in Pergamos, renowned at the time for its library of 50,000 books (approximately one-fourth as many as in Alexandria, the greatest city for learning and education) and its famous medical center in the Temple of Asclepios (http://whc.unesco.org/en/list/491).

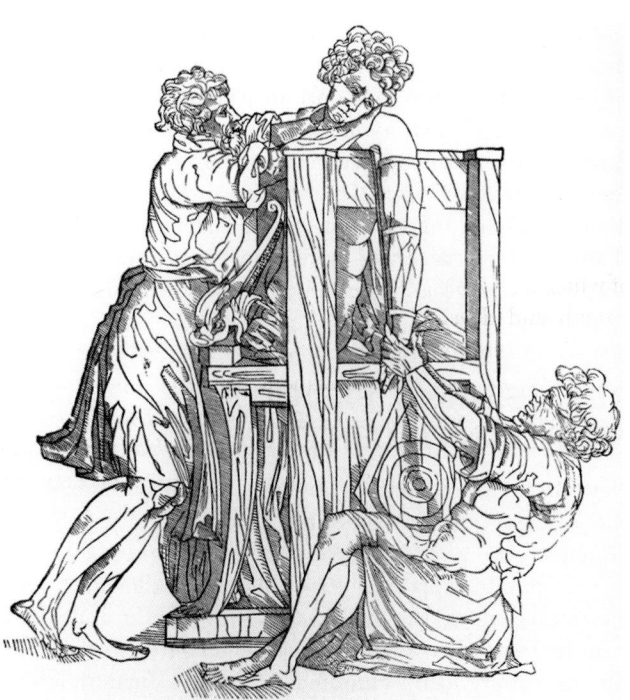

FIGURE I.1 • Woodcut by Renaissance artist Franceso Salviati (1510–1563) based on Galen's *De Fascius* from the first century BC. The woodcut showing shoulder surgery provides a direct link with Hippocratic surgical practice that continued through the Byzantine period.

dislocated lower lumbar vertebrae. The illustration from the 11th-century *Commentairies of Apollonius of Chitiron* on the Periarthron of Hippocrates (**FIG. I.2**) provided details about early Greek surgical "sports medicine" interventions to treat athletes and even the common citizen.

Most of the credit for modern-day medicine has been attributed to the early Greek physicians, but other influential physicians contributed to knowledge about physiology, particularly the pulmonary circulation. West, in an insightful review of the contribution of Arab physician Ibn al-Nafis (1213–1288),[75] points out that Ibn al-Nafis challenged the long-standing beliefs of Galen about how blood moved from the right to left sides of the heart, and also predicted the existence of capillaries 400 years before Malpighi's discovery of the pulmonary capillaries. The timeline in **FIGURE I.3** shows the period of the Islamic Golden Age of Medicine. During this interval, interspaced between the Galenic era in 200 AD to the late 1400s and early 1500s, many physicians, including Persian physician Ibn Sina (Avicenna [ca. 980–1037]: www.muslimphilosophy.com/sina/) contributed their knowledge to 200 books, including the influential *Shifa* (*The Book of Healing*) and *Al Qanun fi Tibb* (*The Canon of Medicine*) about bodily functions.[75]

The era of more "modern-day" exercise physiology includes the periods of Renaissance, Enlightenment, and Scientific Discovery in Europe. It was then that Galen's ideas affected the writings of the early physiologists, anatomists, doctors, and teachers of hygiene and health.[52,62,63] Significant contributions during this time period included those of da Vinci (1452–1519),

TABLE I.1 — Table of Contents for Books 1 and 2[a] of Galen's *De Sanitate Tuenda (Hygiene)*

Book 1 — The Art of Preserving Health

Chapter	Title
I	Introduction
II	The Nature and Sources of Growth and of Disease
III	Production and Elimination of Excrements
IV	Objectives and Hypothesis of Hygiene
V	Conditions and Constitutions
VI	Good Constitution: A Mean Between Extremes
VII	Hygiene of the Newborn
VIII	The Use and Value of Exercise
IX	Hygiene of Breast-Feeding
X	Hygiene of Bathing and Massage
XI	Hygiene of Beverages and Fresh Air
XII	Hygiene of the Second Seven Years
XIII	Causes and Prevention of Excrementary Retardation
XIV	Evacuation of Retained Excrements
XV	Summary of Book 1

Book 2 — Exercise and Massage

Chapter	Title
I	Standards of Hygiene Under Individual Conditions
II	Purposes, Time, and Methods of Exercise and Massage
III	Techniques and Varieties of Massage
IV	Theories of Theon and Hippocrates
V	Definitions of Various Terms
VI	Further Definitions About Massage
VII	Amount of Massage and Exercise
VIII	Forms, Kinds, and Varieties of Exercise
IX	Varieties of Vigorous Exercise
X	Varieties of Swift Exercises
XI	Effects, Exercises, Functions, and Movements
XII	Determination of Diet, Exercise, and Regime

[a]Book III. Apotherapy, Bathing, and Fatigue. Book IV. Forms and Treatment of Fatigue. Book V. Diagnosis, Treatment, and Prevention of Various Diseases. Book VI. Prophylaxis of Pathological Conditions.

Michael Servetus (1511–1564; discovered that blood passed through the pulmonary circulation without moving directly from the right to left ventricle), Realdus Columbus (1516–1559; student of Vesalius who developed concepts concerning pulmonary circulation and that the heart has two ventricles,

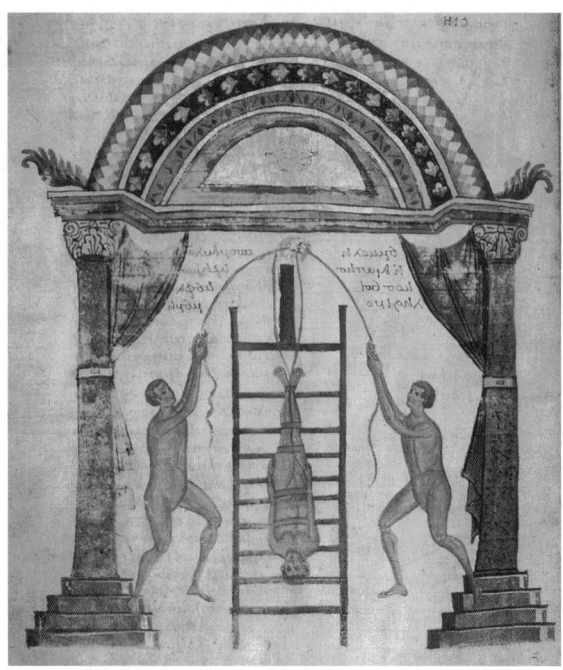

FIGURE I.2 • Ancient treatment for low-back pain, as illustrated in the Commentairies of Apollonius of Chitiron.

not three as postulated by the Galenic School), Andreas Vesalius (1514–1564), Santorio (1514–1564), and William Harvey (1578–1657). The contributions of da Vinci, Vesalius, Santorio, and Harvey are detailed later in this introduction.

Iin Venice in 1539, Italian physician Hieronymus Mercurialis (1530–1606) published *De Arte Gymnastica Apud Ancientes* (The Art of Gymnastics Among the Ancients). This text, heavily influenced by Galen and other early Greek

and Latin authors, profoundly affected subsequent writings about physical training and exercise (then called gymnastics) and health (hygiene), not only in Europe (influencing the Swedish and Danish gymnastic systems), but also in early America (the 19th-century gymnastic–hygiene movement). FIGURE I.4, redrawn from *De Arte Gymnastica*, acknowledges the early Greek influence of one of Galen's famous essays, "Exercise with the Small Ball," and his technical regimen of specific strengthening exercises (discus throwing and rope climbing).

RENAISSANCE PERIOD TO NINETEENTH CENTURY

New ideas formulated during the Renaissance exploded almost every concept inherited from antiquity. Johannes Gutenberg's (ca. 1400–1468 AD) printing press (the first to incorporate replaceable, movable type) allowed for the dissemination to the masses of both classic and newly acquired knowledge (www.ideafinder.com/history/inventors/gutenberg.htm). Hundreds of new text materials were created for the arts, history, geography, and the emerging sciences. New educational opportunities for the wealthy and privileged sprang up in universities and colleges throughout Europe (Angiers, Bologna, Cambridge, Cologne, Heidelberg, Lisbon, Montpellier, Naples, Oxford, Orleans, Padua, Paris, Pisa, Prague, Salamanca, Siena, Toulouse, Uppsala, Valencia). Art broke with past forms, emphasizing spatial perspective and realistic depictions of the human body (see Fig. I.4).

Although the supernatural still influenced discussions of physical phenomena, prior ideas grounded in religious dogma

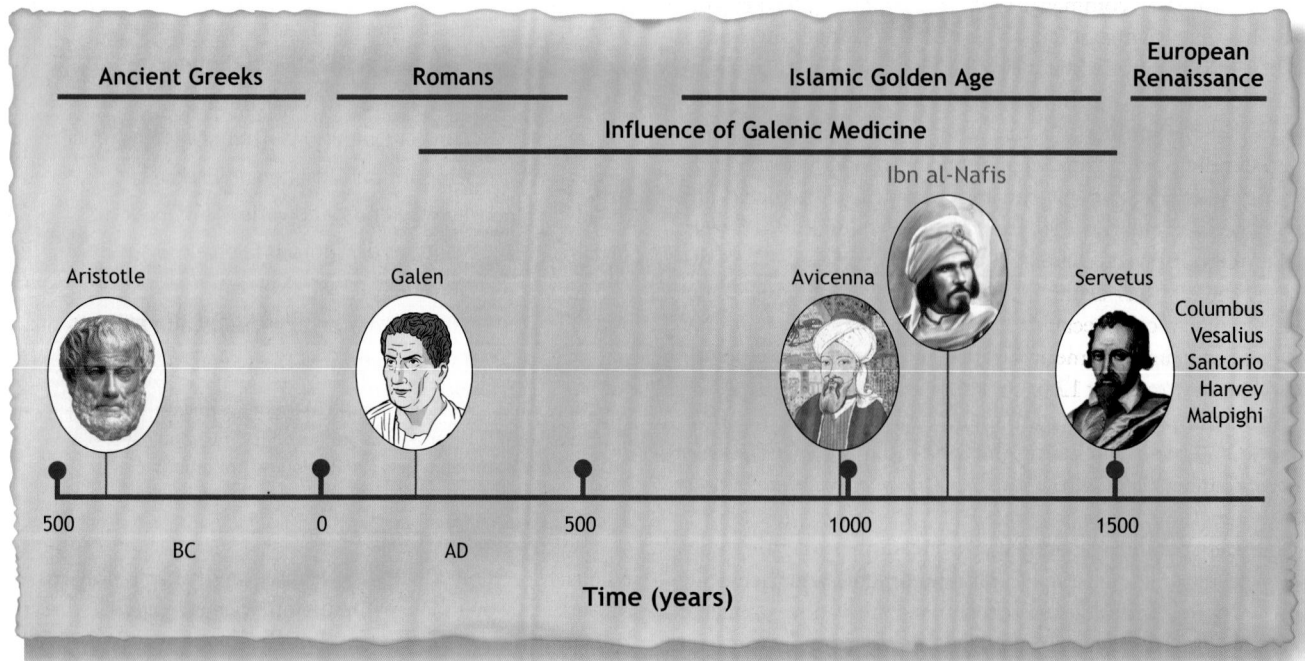

FIGURE I.3 • Timeline of the influence of Galenic medicine and the Islamic Golden Age.

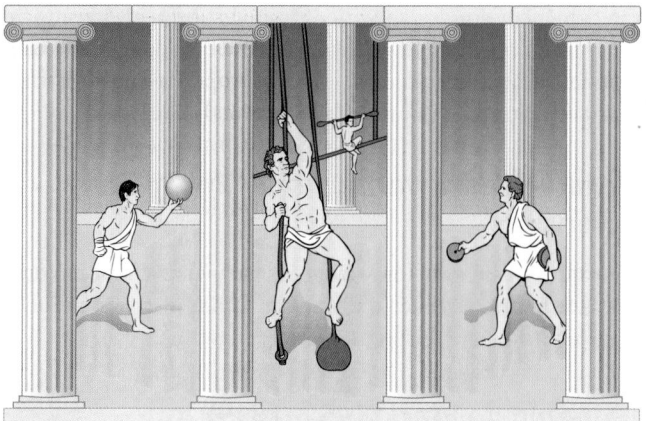

FIGURE I.4 • The early Greek influence of Galen's famous essay *Exercise with the Small Ball* and specific strengthening exercises (throwing the discus and rope climbing) appeared in Mercurialis's *De Arte Gumnastica*, a treatise about the many uses of exercise for preventative and therapeutic medical and health benefits. Mercurialis favored discus throwing to aid patients suffering from arthritis and to improve the strength of the trunk and arm muscles. He advocated rope climbing because it did not pose health problems, and he was a firm believer in walking (a mild pace was good for stimulating conversation, and a faster pace would stimulate appetite and help with digestion). He also believed that climbing mountains was good for those with leg problems, long jumping was desirable (but not for pregnant women), but tumbling and handsprings were not recommended because they would produce adverse effects from the intestines pushing against the diaphragm! The *three panels* above represent the exercises as they might have been performed during the time of Galen.

now expanded to scientific experimentation as a source of knowledge. For example, medicine had to confront the new diseases spread by commerce with distant lands. Plagues and epidemics decimated at least 25 million people throughout Europe in just 3 years (1348–1351; www.pegasplanet.com/articles/EuropeanBlackPlaque.htm). New towns and expanding populations in confined cities led to environmental pollution and pestilence, forcing authorities to cope with the problems of community sanitation and care for the sick and dying. Science had not yet uncovered the link between diseases and their insect and rat hosts.

As populations expanded throughout Europe and elsewhere, medical care became more important for all levels of society. Unfortunately, medical knowledge failed to keep pace with need. For roughly 12 centuries, with the exception of the Islamic physicians, few advances were made from those in Greek and Roman medicine. The writings of the early physicians had either been lost or preserved only in the Arab world. Thanks to the reverence given to classical authors, Hippocrates and Galen still dominated medical education until the end of the 15th century. Renaissance discoveries greatly modified these theories. New anatomists went beyond simplistic notions of four humors (fire, earth, water, air) and their qualities of hot, dry, cold, and wet as they discovered the complexities of circulatory, respiratory, and excretory mechanisms.[7,11]

Once rediscovered, these new ideas caused turmoil. The Vatican banned human dissections, yet a number of "progressive" medical schools continued to engage in such practices, usually sanctioning one or two cadavers a year or with official permission to perform an "anatomy" (the old name for a dissection) every 3 years. Performing autopsies helped physicians solve legal questions about a person's death, or determine cause of a disease. In the mid-1200s at the University of Bologna, every medical student had to attend one dissection each year, with 20 students assigned to a male cadaver and 30 students to a female cadaver. In 1442, the Rector of the University of Bologna required that cadavers used for an "anatomy" come from an area located at least 30 miles outside the city limits. The first sanctioned anatomical dissection in Paris, performed in public, took place in 1483.[45]

In Rembrandt's first major 1632 portrait commission, *The Anatomy Lesson of Dr. Nicholas Tulp* (**Fig. I.5**), medical students listen intensely (but without "hands-on" experience) to the renowned Dr. Tulp as he dissects the arm of a recently executed criminal. The pioneering efforts of Vesalius and Harvey made anatomic study a central focus of medical education, yet conflicted with the Catholic church's strictures against violation of the individual rights of the dead because of the doctrine concerning the eventual resurrection of each person's body. In fact, the Catholic church considered anatomic dissections a disfiguring violation of bodily integrity, despite the common practice of dismembering criminals as punishment. Nevertheless, the art of the period reflected close collaboration between artists and medical school physicians to portray anatomic dissections, essential for medical education, and to satisfy a public thirst for new information in the emerging fields of physiology and medicine.

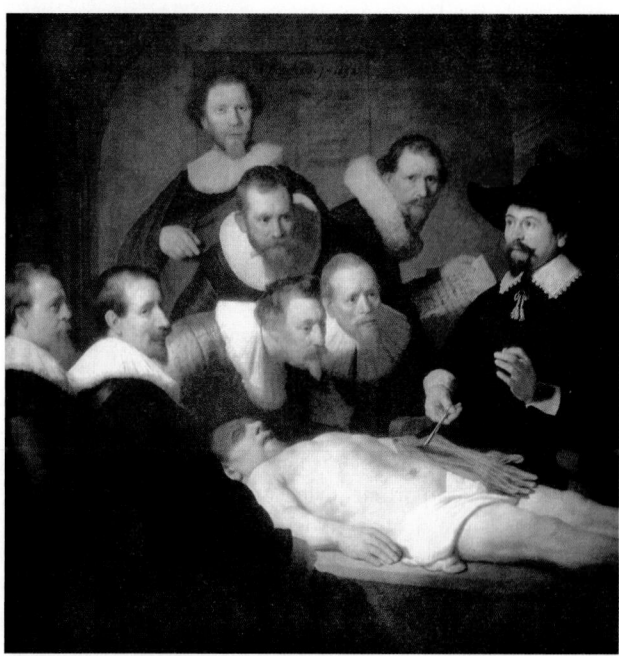

FIGURE I.5 • Rembrandt's 1632 *The Anatomy Lesson of Dr. Nicholas Tulp. (The Yorck Project: 10,000 Meisterwerke der Malerei.)*

In 1316, Mondino de Luzzio (ca. 1275–1326; http://lacytite.com/whatisit/anathomia/), a professor of anatomy at Bologna, published *Anathomia*, the first book of human anatomy. He based his teaching on human cadavers, not Greek and Latin authorities or studies of animals. The 1513 edition of *Anathomia* presented the same drawing of the heart with three ventricles as was in the original edition, a tribute to de Luzzio's accuracy in translation of the original inaccuracies! Certainly by the turn of the 15th century, anatomic dissections for postmortems were common in the medical schools of France and Italy; they paved the way for the Renaissance anatomists whose careful observations accelerated understanding of human form and function.

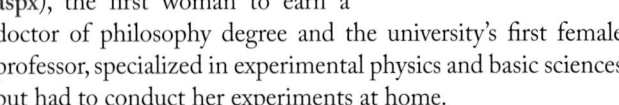

Early on, two women from the University of Bologna achieved distinction in the field of anatomy. Laura Caterina Bassi (1711–1778; www.sciencemuseum.org.uk/broughttolife/people/laurabassi.aspx), the first woman to earn a doctor of philosophy degree and the university's first female professor, specialized in experimental physics and basic sciences but had to conduct her experiments at home.

Professor Laura Bassi (Image courtesy National Library of Medicine)

Soon after, female scholars were allowed to teach in university classrooms. At the time, Bassi gave her yearly public lectures on topics related to physics (including electricity and hydraulics, correction distortion in telescopes, hydrometry, and relation between a flame and "stable air"). Anna Morandi Manzolini (1717–1774; www.timeshighereducation.co.uk/story.asp?storycode=415248), also a professor and chair of the Department of Anatomy at the University of Bologna, was an expert at creating wax models of internal organs and became the anatomy department's chief model maker.

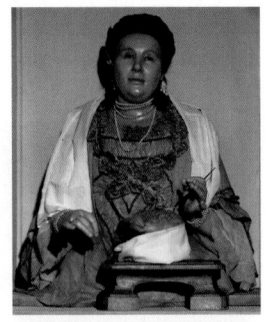

Professor Anna Manzolini (Erich Lessing/Art Resource, NY)

She produced an ear model that students took apart and reassembled to gain a better understanding of the ear's internal structures. Her wax and wood models of the abdomen and uterus were used didactically in the medical school for several hundred years. The wax self-portrait in the Museum of Human Anatomy at the University of Bologna (http://pacs.unica.it/cere/mono02_en.htm) shows Manzolini performing an anatomical dissection, clad in the traditional white lab coat, but also dressed in silks with diamonds and pearl jewelry—the manner expected of a woman of her high social and economic status.

Progress in understanding human anatomic form paved the way for specialists in physical culture and hygiene to design specific exercises to improve overall body strength, and the ever increasing popularity of training regimens to prepare for rowing, boxing, wrestling, competitive walking, and track and field activities and competitions. These specialist instructors were the early link to today's personal trainers.

Notable Achievements by European Scientists

An explosion of new knowledge in the physical and biologic sciences helped prepare the way for future discoveries about human physiology during rest and exercise.

Leonardo da Vinci (1452–1519)

Da Vinci dissected cadavers at the hospital of Santa Maria Nuova in Florence (www.lifeinthefastlane.com/2009/04/leonardo-da-vinci-first-anatomist/) and made detailed anatomic drawings.

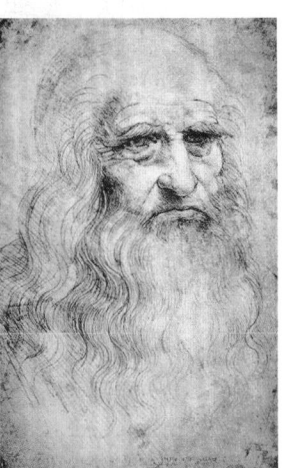

Da Vinci's achievements in anatomy include:

Leonardo Da Vinci self-portrait (c. 1512–1513)

1. Deduced the hierarchical structure of the nervous system, with the brain as a command center.
2. Deduced that the eye's retina, not the lens as previously believed, was sensitive to light. He dissected the fragile eye structures by inventing new dissection methods that included sectioning the eye after its proteins had been fixed by heating in egg whites.
3. Observed the lesions of atherosclerosis and their possible role in obstructing coronary arteries.
4. Identified the heart as a muscle "pump," and that the arterial pulse corresponded to ventricular contraction.
5. Developed a system to explain muscular movements by using an arrangement of wires. For example, he determined the mechanics of biceps brachii muscle and arm action. He explained elbow flexion and hand supination through the twisting action on the ulna. His detailed drawings with written explanations showed the full arm and its motions, including scapular function.
6. Deduced the equal contribution from the mother and father to the inherited characteristics of the fetus.

Accurate as his numerous and detailed sketches were (**FIG. I.6**), they still preserved Galenic ideas. Although he never saw the pores in the septum of the heart, he included them, believing they existed because Galen had "seen" them. Da Vinci first drew accurately the heart's inner structures and constructed models of valvular function that showed how the blood flowed in only one direction. This observation contradicted Galen's notion about the ebb and flow of blood between the heart's chambers. Da Vinci could not explain the role of

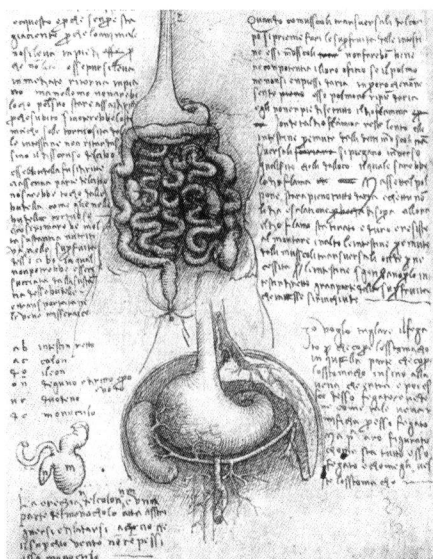

FIGURE I.6 • Anatomical sketch of stomach, intestines, kidney, and pancreas by Da Vinci.

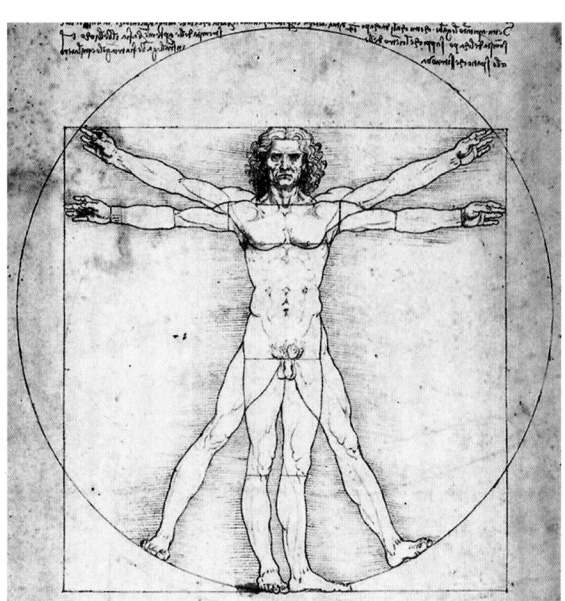

FIGURE I.7 • Da Vinci's *Vitruvian Man*.

the veins and arteries in blood flow to and from the heart. It would take another half-century for Harvey to discover that veins return blood to the heart, and only the arteries conduct blood from the heart to the periphery. Because many of Da Vinci's drawings were lost for nearly two centuries, they did not impact later anatomic research.

Da Vinci's work built on and led to discoveries by two fellow artists. Leon Battista Alberti (1404–1472; www.kirjasto.sci.fi/alberti.htm), an architect who perfected three-dimensional perspectives, which influenced Da Vinci's concepts of internal relationships. Da Vinci's drawings (while not published during his lifetime) no doubt inspired the incomparable Flemish anatomist Andreas Vesalius (1514–1564; www.evolution.berkeley.edu/evolibrary/article/history_02). These three exemplary Renaissance anatomists—Da Vinci, Alberti, and Vesalius—empowered physiologists to understand the systems of the body with technical accuracy, not theoretical or religious bias.

Albrecht Dürer (1471–1528)

Dürer, a German contemporary of Da Vinci (www.albrecht-durer.org), extended the Italian's concern for ideal dimensions as depicted in Da Vinci's famous "1513 Vitruvian Man" (**FIG I.7**) by illustrating age-related differences in body segment ratios formulated by 1st century BCE Roman architect Marcus Vitruvius Pollio (*De architectura libri decem* [*Ten books on architecture*]). Dürer created a canon of proportion, considering total height as unity. For example, in his schema, the length of the foot was one-sixth of this total, the head one-seventh, and the hand one-tenth. Relying on his artistic and printmaking skills rather than objective comparison, Dürer made the ratio of height between men and women as 17 to 18 (soon thereafter proved incorrect). Nonetheless, Dürer's work inspired Behnke in the 1950s to quantify body proportions relative to height into reference standards to evaluate body composition in men and women (see Chapter 28).

Michelangelo Buonarroti (1475–1564)

Michelangelo, like Da Vinci, was a superb anatomist (www.ncbi.nlm.nih.gov/pmc/articles/PMC1279184/). In his accurate drawings, body segments appear in proper proportion. His famous sculpture "David" clearly shows the veins, tendons, and muscles enclosing a realistic skeleton. His frescos on the ceiling of the Sistine Chapel (mv.vatican.va/3_EN/pages/CSN/CSN_Main.html) often exaggerate musculature; nevertheless they still convey a scientist's vision of the human body's proportions.

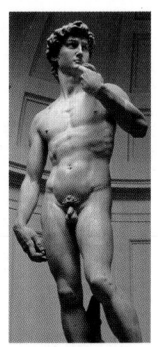

Michelangelo's "David"

Andreas Vesalius (1514–1564)

Belgian anatomist and physician Vesalius learned Galenic medicine in Paris, but after making careful human dissections, he rejected the Greek's ideas about bodily functions. At the start of his career, Vesalius authored books on anatomy, originally relying on Arabic texts, but then incorporating observations from his own dissections in addition to a self-portrait from *Fabrica* published at age 29 showing the anatomic details of an upper and lower right arm.

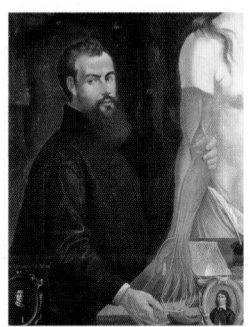

Portrait of Vesalius from his *De Humani Corporis Fabrica* (c. 1543) (Courtesy National Library of Medicine.)

His research culminated in the exquisitely illustrated text first published in Basel, Switzerland, in 1543, *De Humani Corporis Fabrica* (On the Fabric of the Human Body) (**FIG. I.8**).

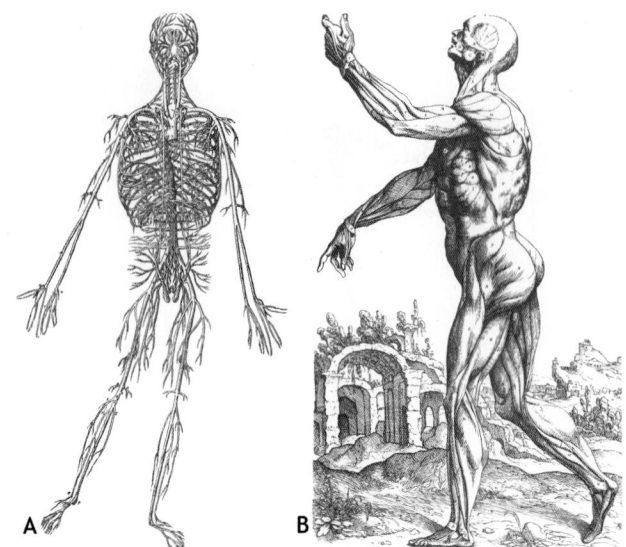

FIGURE I.8 • Vesalius's anatomic drawings. **(A)** Major nerves. **(B)** Muscular system in action. Note the graveyard crypts. (Courtesy National Library of Medicine.)

Many consider Vesalius's drawings and accompanying 200 woodcuts the best anatomical renderings ever made, ushering in the age of modern medicine (www.metmuseum. org/TOAH/HD/anat/ho_53.682.htm#). The same year, he published *Epitome*, a popular version of *De Fabrica* without Latin text (www.ncbi.nlm.nih.gov/pmc/articles/PMC1520217/).

Some physicians and clergymen became outraged, fearful that the new science was overturning Galen's time-honored speculations. Vesalius's treatise accurately rendered bones, muscles, nerves, internal organs, blood vessels (including veins for blood-letting, a popular technique to rid the body of diseases and toxins; medicalantiques.com/medical/Scarifications_and_Bleeder_Medical_Antiques.htm), and the brain, but he differed from Galenic tradition by ignoring what he could not see. His masterful detailed depiction of the muscular and skeletal architecture of the human body pared away one muscle layer at a time to reveal the hidden structures underneath.

Some of Vesalius's drawings contain curious inaccuracies. For example, he drew the inferior vena cava as a continuous vessel; inserted an extra muscle to move the eyeball; and added an extra neck muscle present only in apes. Despite these minor discrepancies, Vesalius clearly attempted to connect form with function. He showed that a muscle contracted when a longitudinal slice was made along the muscle's belly, but a transverse cut prevented contraction. Vesalius was one of the first to verify that nerves controlled muscles and stimulated movement. His two beautifully illustrated texts profoundly influenced medical education. Their intricate details about human structures demolished traditional theories about human anatomy and emboldened later researchers to explore circulation and metabolism unburdened by past misconceptions. The illuminating and detailed artwork of Vesalius hastened the subsequent important discoveries in physiology and the beginning of modern science.

Santorio Santorio (1561–1636)

A friend of Galileo and professor of medicine at Padua, Italy, Santorio invented innovative tools for his research (www.istrianet.org/istria/illustri/santorio/index.htm). He recorded changes in daily body temperature with the first air thermometer, crafted in 1612 as a temperature-measuring device. Accuracy was poor because scientists had not yet discovered the effects of differential air pressures on temperature. Santorio also measured pulse rate with Galileo's pulsilogium (pulsiometer; http://galileo.rice.edu/sci/instruments/pendulum.html). Ever inventive, Santorio, a pioneer physician in the science of physical measurement, intro-

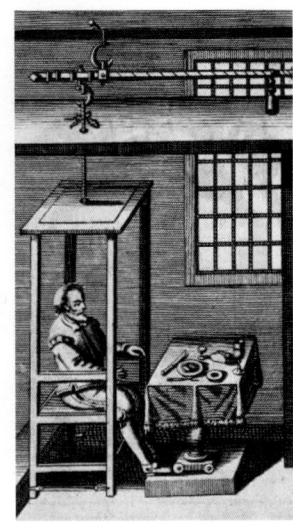

Santorio's scale. (Courtesy National Library of Medicine.)

duced quantitative experimentation into biological science in a treatise published in late 1602 or early 1603 (*Methodus vitandorum errorum omnium qui in arte medica contingent* [Methods to avoid errors in medical practice]). Santorio studied digestion and changes in metabolism by constructing a wooden frame that supported a chair, bed, and worktable. Suspended from the ceiling with scales, the frame recorded changes in body weight.

For 30 continuous years, Santorio slept, ate, worked, and made love in the weighing contraption to record how much his weight changed as he ate, fasted, or excreted. He coined the term "insensible perspiration" to account for differences in body weight because he believed that weight was gained or lost through the pores during respiration. Often depriving himself of food and drink, Santorio determined that the daily change in body mass approached 1.25 kg. Santorio's book of medical aphorisms, *De Medicina Statica Aphorismi* (1614), drew worldwide attention. Although this scientifically trained Italian instrument inventor did not explain the role of nutrition in weight gain or loss, Santorio nevertheless inspired later 18th-century researchers in metabolism by quantifying metabolic effects.

William Harvey (1578–1657)

William Harvey discovered that blood circulates continuously in one direction and, as Vesalius had done, overthrew 2000 years of medical dogma. Animal vivisection disproved the ancient supposition that blood moved from the right to left side of the heart through pores in the septum—pores that even Da Vinci and Vesalius had erroneously acknowledged. Harvey announced his discovery during a 3-day dissection–lecture on

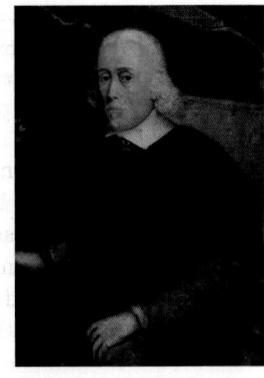

William Harvey

April 16, 1616, at the oldest medical institution in England—the Royal College of Physicians in London. Twelve years later, he published the details of his experiments in a 72-page monograph, *Exercitatio Anatomica de Motu Cordis et Sanguinis in Animalibus* (*An Anatomical Treatise on the Movement of the Heart and Blood in Animals*; www.bartleby.com/38/3/). Harvey was aware of the uniqueness of his contributions, and he penned these prescient thoughts in the introduction to his scientific masterpiece:

> At length, yielding to the requests of my friends, that all might be made participators in my labors, and partly moved by the envy of others, who, receiving my views with uncandid minds and understanding them indifferently, have essayed to traduce me publicly, I have moved to commit these things to the press, in order that all may be enabled to form an opinion both of me and my labours. This step I take all the more willingly, seeing that Hieronymus Fabricius of Aquapendente, although he has accurately and learnedly delineated almost every one of the several parts of animals in a special work, has left the heart alone untouched. Finally, if any use or benefit to this department of the republic of letters should accrue from my labours, it will, perhaps, be allowed that I have not lived idly.... So will it, perchance, be found with reference to the heart at this time; or others, at least, starting hence, with the way pointed out to them, advancing under the guidance of a happier genius, may make occasion to proceed more fortunately, and to inquire more accurately.

By combining the new technique of experimentation on living creatures with mathematical logic, Harvey deduced that contrary to conventional wisdom, blood flowed in only one direction—from the heart to the arteries and from the veins back to the heart. It then traversed to the lungs before completing a circuit and reentering the heart. Harvey publicly demonstrated the one-way flow of blood by placing a tourniquet around a man's upper arm that constricted arterial blood flow to the forearm and stopped the pulse (**Fig. I.9**). By loosening the tourniquet, Harvey allowed some blood into the veins. Applying pressure to specific veins forced blood from a peripheral segment where there was little pressure into the previously empty veins. Thus, Harvey proved that the heart pumped blood through a closed, unidirectional (circular) system, from arteries to veins and back to the heart. As he put it:

> It is proved by the structure of the heart that the blood is continuously transferred through the lungs into the aorta as by two clacks of a water bellows to raise water. It is proved by a ligature that there is a passage of blood from the arteries to the veins. It is therefore demonstrated that the continuous movement of the blood in a circle is brought about by the beat of the heart.[24]

Harvey's experiments with sheep proved mathematically that the mass of blood passing through the sheep's heart in a fixed time was greater than the body could produce—a conclusion identical to that concerning the human heart. Harvey reasoned that if a self-contained constant mass of blood exists, then the large circulation volumes would require a one-way, closed circulatory system. Harvey

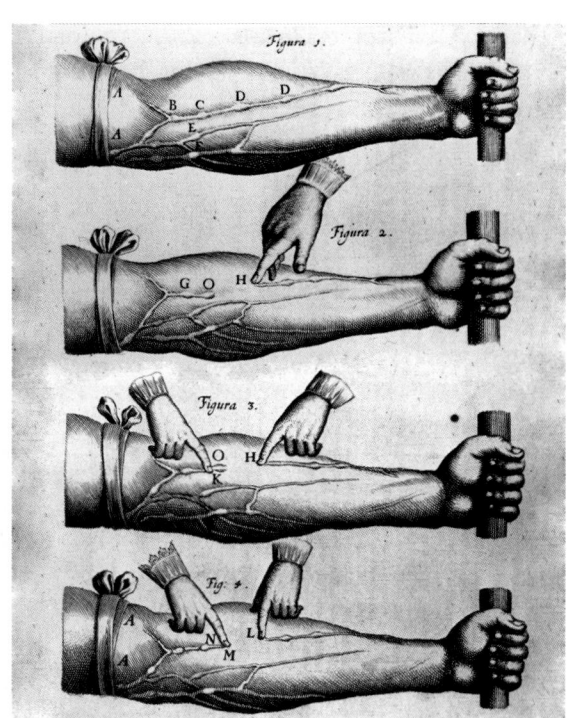

FIGURE I.9 • Harvey's famous illustration demonstrating the one-way flow of the circulation. (Courtesy National Library of Medicine.)

did not explain why the blood circulated, only that it did. However, he correctly postulated that circulation might distribute heat and nourishment throughout the body. Despite the validity of Harvey's observations, distinguished scientists publically and soundly criticized them. Jean Riolan (1577–1657), an ardent Galenist who chaired the anatomy and botany departments at the University of Paris in the 1640s, maintained that if anatomic findings differed from Galen's, then the body in question must be abnormal and the results faulty. Nevertheless, Harvey's epic discovery governed subsequent research on circulation and demolished 1500 years of rigid dogma.

Giovanni Alfonso Borelli (1608–1679)

Borelli, a protégé of Galileo and Benedetto Castelli (1578–1643) and a mathematician at the University of Pisa in Italy, used mathematical models to explain how muscles enabled animals to walk, fish to swim, and birds to fly. His ideas explaining how air entered and exited the lungs, though equally important, were less well known. Borelli's accomplished student, Marcello Malpighi (1628–1694; www.nndb.com/people/033/000095745/), described

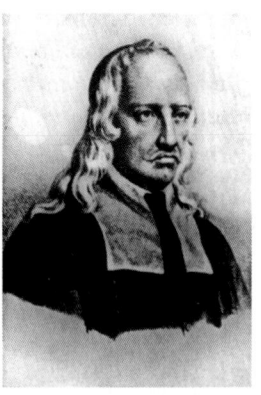

Giovanni Alfonso Borelli

blood flowing through microscopic structures (capillaries) around the lung's terminal air sacs (alveoli). Borelli observed that lungs filled with air because chest volume increased as the diaphragm moved downward. He concluded that air passed through the alveoli and into the blood, a sharp contrast to Galen's notion that air in the lungs cooled the heart, and an advance on Harvey's general observation concerning unidirectional blood flow.

Robert Boyle (1627–1691)

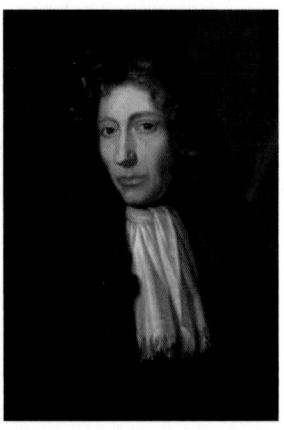

Working at Gresham College in London with his student Robert Hooke (1635–1703; www. ucmp.berkeley.edu/history/ hooke.html), Boyle devised experiments with a vacuum pump and bell jar to show that combustion and respiration required air. Boyle partially evacuated air from the jar containing a lit candle. The flame soon died. When he removed air from a jar containing a rodent or bird, it became unconscious; recirculating air back into the jar often revived the animal. Compressing the air produced the same results: animals and flames survived longer (www.woodrow.org/teachers/ci/1992/boyle.html).

Portrait of Robert Boyle by Johann Kerseboom, 1689

Boyle removed the diaphragm and ribs from a living dog and forced air into its lungs with a bellows. The experiment did not prove that air was essential for life, yet demonstrated that air pressure and volumes alternately contracted and expanded the lungs. He repeated the experiment, this time pricking the lungs so air could escape. Boyle kept the animal alive by forcing air into its lungs, proving that chest movement maintained airflow and disproving the earlier assertion that the lungs effected circulation.

Scientific societies and journals broadcasted these pioneering and insightful discoveries. Boyle belonged to the Royal Society of London (www.royalsociety.org/about-us/ history/), chartered in 1662 by King Charles II. Four years later in France, Louis XIV sponsored the Académie Royale des Sciences (the French Academy of Sciences was established to preserve French scientific research) so its staff could conduct and sponsor a variety of studies in physics, chemistry, medicine, agronomy, nutrition and metabolism, and exploratory expeditions to distant lands. Both societies established journals to disseminate information to scientists and an increasingly educated lay public fascinated by the quick pace of new discoveries.

Stephen Hales (1677–1761)

A renowned English plant physiologist and Fellow of the Royal Society (http://galileo.rice.edu/Catalog/NewFiles/ hales.html), Hales amassed facts from his experiments with

animals about blood pressure, the heart's capacity, and velocity of blood flow in *Vegetable Statics: Or, an Account of Some Statical Experiments on the Sap in Vegetables* (1727).

In this venerable text, Hales tells how water absorbed air when phosphorus and melted brimstone (sulfur) burned in a closed glass vessel

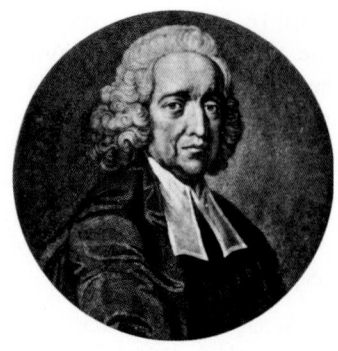

Stephen Hales (Courtesy National Library of Medicine)

(**Fig. I.10**) that shows the transfer of "air" released from substances burned in a closed vessel. Hales measured the volume of air either released or absorbed, and he demonstrated that air was a constituent of many common substances. His experiments proved that chemical changes occurred in solids and liquids during calcination (oxidation during combustion). Hales developed an idea suggested by Newton in 1713 that provided the first experimental evidence that the nervous system played a role in muscular contraction.

James Lind (1716–1794)

Trained in Edinburgh, Lind entered the British Navy as a Surgeon's Mate in 1739 (www.sportsci.org). During an extended trip in the English Channel in 1747 on the 50-gun, 960-ton H.M.S. *Salisbury* (www.ncbi.nlm. nih.gov/pmc/articles/ PMC539665/), Lind carried out a decisive experiment (the first planned, controlled clinical trial) that changed the course of naval medicine. He knew that scurvy often killed two thirds of a ship's crew. Their diet included 1 lb 4 oz of cheese biscuits daily, 2 lb of salt beef twice weekly, 2 oz of dried fish and butter thrice weekly, 8 oz of peas 4 days per week, and 1 gallon of beer daily. Deprived of vitamin C, sailors fell prey to scurvy ("the great sea plague"). By adding fresh fruit to their diet, Lind fortified their immune systems so that British sailors no

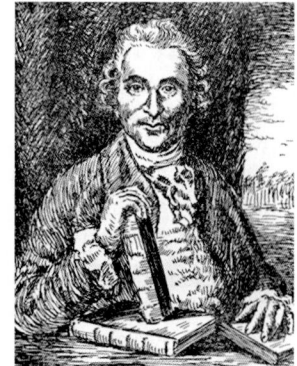

James Lind

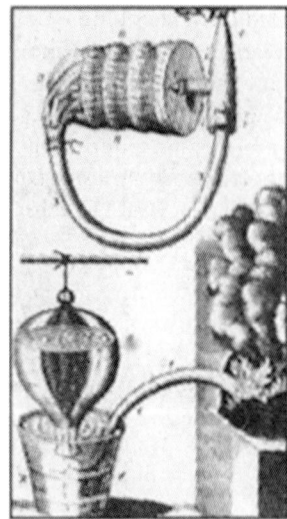

FIGURE I.10 • Hale's closed glass vessel experiment.

longer perished on extended voyages. From Lind's *Treatise on the Scurvy* (1753) comes the following poignant excerpt[38]:

> On the 20th of May, 1747, I selected 12 patients in the scurvy, on board the Salisbury at sea. Their cases were as similar as I could have them. They all in general had putrid gums, the spots and lassitude, with weakness of their knees…. The consequence was, that the most sudden and visible good effects were perceived from the use of oranges and lemons; one of those who had taken them, being at the end of 6 days fit for duty. The spots were not indeed at that time quite off his body, nor his gums sound; but without any other medicine than a gargle for his mouth he became quite healthy before we came into Plymouth which was on the 16th of June. The other was the best recovered in his condition; and being now pretty well, was appointed nurse to the rest of the sick…. Next to oranges, I thought the cyder had the best effects. It was indeed not very sound. However, those who had taken it, were in a fairer way of recovery than the others at the end of the fortnight, which was the length of time all these different courses were continued, except the oranges. The putrification of their gums, but especially their lassitude and weakness, were somewhat abated, and their appetite increased by it.

Lind published two books[72]: *An Essay on Preserving the Health of Seamen in the Royal Navy* (1757) and *Essay on Diseases Incidental to Europeans in Hot Climates* (1768). Easily available, his books were translated into German, French, and Dutch. Lind's landmark emphasis on the crucial importance of dietary supplements antedates modern practices. His treatment regimen defeated scurvy, but 50 years had to pass with many more lives lost before the British Admiralty required fresh citrus fruit on all ships (www.jameslindlibrary.org/illustrating/articles/james-lind-and-scurvy-1747-to-1795).

Joseph Black (1728–1799)

After graduating from the medical school in Edinburgh, Black became a professor of chemistry at Glasgow (www.chem.gla.ac.uk/~alanc/dept/black.htm). His *Experiments Upon Magnesia Alba, Quicklime, and Some Other Alcaline Substances* (1756) determined that air contained carbon dioxide gas. He observed that carbonate (lime) lost half its weight after burning. Black reasoned that removing air from lime treated

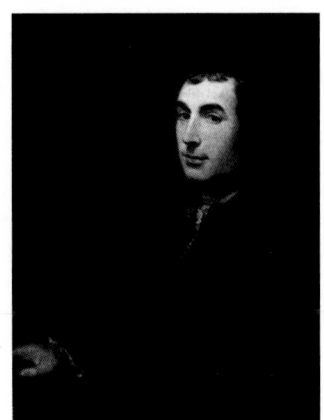

Joseph Black (Courtesy National Library of Medicine)

with acids produced a new substance he named "fixed air," or carbon dioxide ($CaCO_3 = CaO + CO_2$). Black's discovery that gas existed either freely or combined with other substances encouraged later, more refined experiments on the chemical composition of gases.

Joseph Priestley (1733–1804)

Although Priestley discovered oxygen by heating red oxide of mercury in a closed vessel, he stubbornly clung to the phlogiston theory that had misled other scientists (www.spartacus.schoolnet.co.uk/PRpriestley.htm). Dismissing Lavoisier's (1743–1794) proof that respiration produced carbon dioxide and water, Priestley continued to believe in an immaterial constituent (phlogiston) that supposedly escaped from substances upon

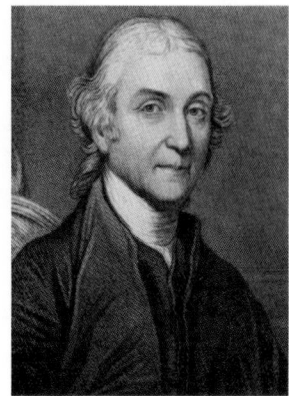

Joseph Priestly

burning. He lectured at the Royal Society about oxygen in 1772 and published *Observations on Different Kinds of Air* in 1773. Elated by his discovery, Priestley failed to grasp two facts that later research confirmed: (1) the body requires oxygen and (2) cellular respiration produces the end product carbon dioxide. **FIGURE I.11** depicts Priestly's London laboratory.

Karl Wilhelm Scheele (1742–1786)

In one of history's great coincidences, Scheele, a Swedish pharmacist, discovered oxygen independently of Priestley (www.britannica.com/EBchecked/topic/527125/Carl-Wilhelm-Scheele). Scheele noted that heating mercuric oxide released "fire-air" (oxygen); burning other substances in fire-air produced violent reactions. When different mixtures contacted air inside a sealed container, the air volume decreased by 25% and could not support combustion. Scheele named the gas that extinguished fire

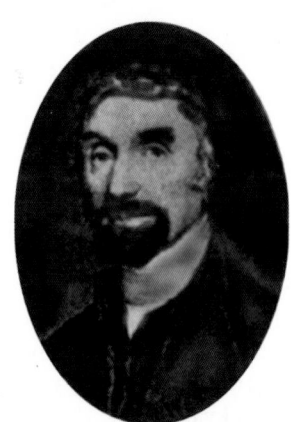

Carl Wilhelm Scheele (Artist J. Falander, Edgar Fahs Smith Collection, University of Pennsylvania Library)

"foul air." In a memorable experiment, he added two bees to a glass jar immersed in lime water containing fire-air (**FIG. I.12**). After a few days, the bees remained alive, but the level of lime water had risen in the bottle and become cloudy. Scheele concluded that fixed air replaced the fire-air to sustain the bees. At the end of 8 days, the bees died despite ample honey within the container. Scheele blamed their demise on phlogiston, which he felt was hostile to life. What Scheele

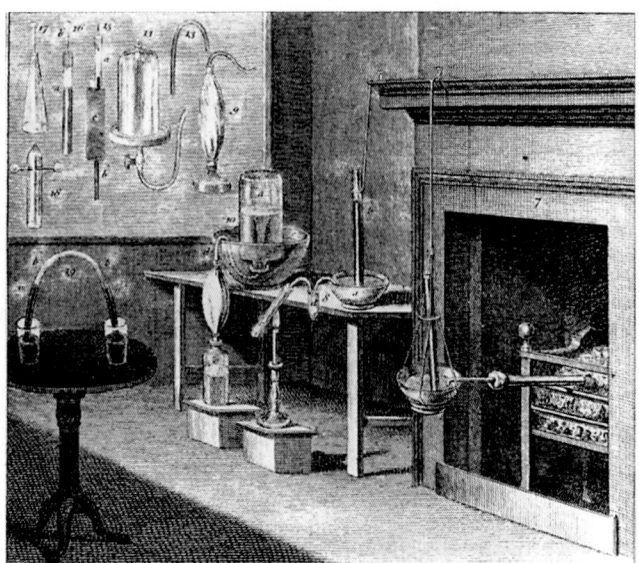

FIGURE I.11 • Priestley's London laboratory. (Edgar Fahs Smith Collection, University of Pennsylvania Library.)

called foul-air (phlogisticated air in Priestley's day) was later identified as nitrogen.

Just like Priestley, Scheele refused to accept Lavoisier's explanations concerning respiration. Although Scheele adhered to the phlogiston theory, he discovered, in addition to oxygen, chlorine, manganese, silicon, glycerol, silicon tetrafluoride, hydrofluoric acid, and copper arsenite (named Scheele's green in his honor). Scheele also experi-

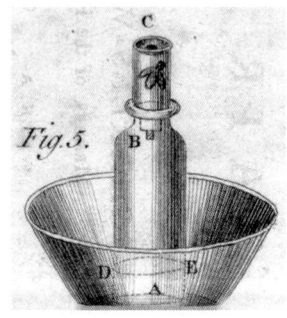

FIGURE I.12 • Scheele's instrument. (Edgar Fahs Smith Collection, University of Pennsylvania Library.)

mented with silver salts and how light influenced them (which became the basis of modern photography). He was the first and only student of pharmacy elected in 1775 into the prestigious Royal Swedish Academy of Sciences (founded by naturalist Carl Linnaeus [1707–1778] in 1739; www.kva.se/en/).

Henry Cavendish (1731–1810)

Cavendish and his contemporaries Black and Priestley began to identify the constituents of carbohydrates, lipids, and proteins (**www.nndb.com/people/030/000083778/**). *On Factitious Air* (1766) describes a highly flammable substance, later identified as hydrogen, that was liberated when acids combined with metals. *Experiments in Air* (1784) showed that "inflammable air" (hydrogen) combined with "deflogisticated air" (oxygen) produced water. Cavendish performed meticulous calculations using a sensitive torsion balance to measure the value of the gravitational constant G that allowed him

to compute the mass of the Earth (5.976×10^{24} kg). His work eventually played an important role in the development of the space sciences, especially modern rocketry and space exploration (see Chapter 27).

Antoine Laurent Lavoisier (1743–1794)

Lavoisier ushered in modern concepts of metabolism, nutrition, and exercise physiology (www.sportsci.org; http:// cti.itc.virginia.edu/~meg3c/ classes/tcc313/200Rprojs/ lavoisier2/home.html#history). His discoveries in respiration chemistry and human nutrition were as essential to these fields as Harvey's discoveries were to circulatory physiology and medicine. Lavoisier paved the way for studies of energy balance by recognizing for the first time that the elements car-

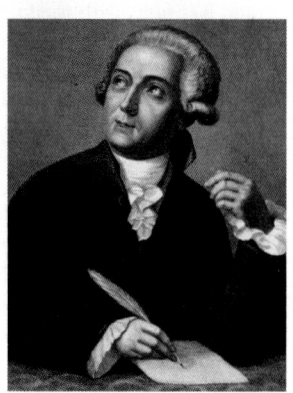

Antoine Laurent Lavoisier (Courtesy National Library of Medicine)

bon, hydrogen, nitrogen, and oxygen involved in metabolism neither appeared suddenly nor disappeared mysteriously. He supplied basic truths: only oxygen participates in animal respiration, and the "caloric" liberated during respiration is itself the source of the combustion. In the early 1770s, Lavoisier was the first person to conduct experiments on human respiration with his colleague, chemist Armand Séguin (1767–1835). They studied the influence of muscular work on metabolism. A contemporary painting shows the seated Séguin as he depresses a pedal while a copper mask captures the expired air (**FIG. I.13**). A physician takes Séguin's pulse to determine the separate effects of exercise and food consumption. (For several hours before the experiment, Séguin had abstained from food.) Resting energy metabolism without food in a cold environment increased by 10%; it increased 50% due solely to food, 200% with exercise, and 300% by combining food intake with exercise. According to Lusk,[44] Lavoisier told of his experiments in a letter written to a friend dated November 19, 1790, as follows:

The quantity of oxygen absorbed by a resting man at a temperature of 26°C is 1200 pouces de France (1 cubic pouce = 0.0198 L) hourly. (2) The quantity of oxygen required at a temperature of 12°C rises to 1400 pouces. (3) During the digestion of food the quantity of oxygen amounts to from 1800 to 1900 pouces. (4) During exercise 4000 pouces and over may be the quantity of oxygen absorbed.

These discoveries, fundamental to modern concepts of energy balance, could not protect Lavoisier from the intolerance of his revolutionary countrymen. The Jacobean tribunal beheaded him in 1794. Yet once more, thoughtless resistance to innovative science temporarily delayed the triumph of truth.

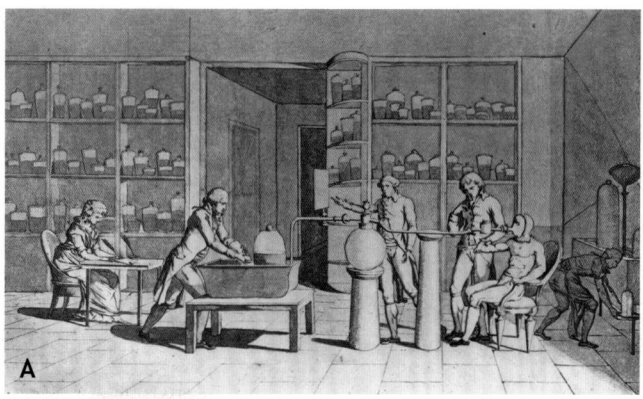
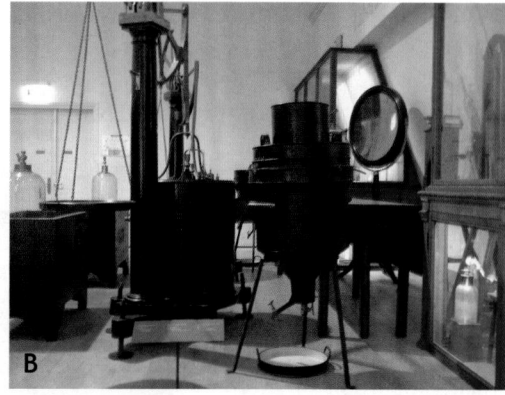

FIGURE I.13 • **(A)** Lavoisier supervises the first "true" exercise physiology experiment (heart rate and oxygen consumption measured as the seated subject at the right breathes through a copper pipe while pressing a foot pedal to increase external work). Sketched by Madame Lavoisier (sitting at the left taking notes). **(B)** The equipment of Lavoisier's laboratory from the mid-1700s can be viewed at Musee des Arts et Metiers in Paris, France, at 160 rue Reaumur. (Image © Frank Katch.)

Lazzaro Spallanzani (1729–1799)

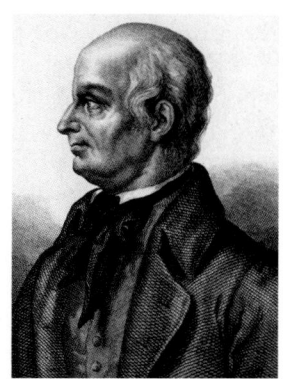

An accomplished Italian physiologist, Spallanzani debunked spontaneous generation as he studied fertilization and contraception in animals (www.whonamedit.com/doctor.cfm/2234.html). In a famous study of digestion, he refined regurgitation experiments similar to those of French entomologist and scientist René-Antoine Fercault de Réaumur (1683–1757; http://esapubs.org/bulletin/current/history_list/history21.pdf). Réaumur's *Digestion in Birds*

Lazzaro Spallanzani (Courtesy National Library of Medicine)

(1752) told how he recovered partially digested food from the gizzard of a kite. Spallanzani swallowed a sponge tied to the end of a string and then regurgitated it. He found that the sponge had absorbed a substance that dissolved bread and various animal tissues, thus indirectly observing how gastric juices function. His experiments with animals showed that the tissues of the heart, stomach, and liver consume oxygen and liberate carbon dioxide, even in creatures without lungs.

Spallanzani's idea that respiration and combustion took place within the tissues was novel and appeared posthumously in 1804. A century later, this phenomenon would be called *internal respiration*.[2]

Nineteenth Century Metabolism and Physiology

The untimely death of Lavoisier did not terminate fruitful research in nutrition and medicine. During the next half-century, scientists discovered the chemical composition of carbohydrates, lipids, and proteins and further clarified what we now term the energy balance equation.[14]

Claude Louis Berthollet (1748–1822)

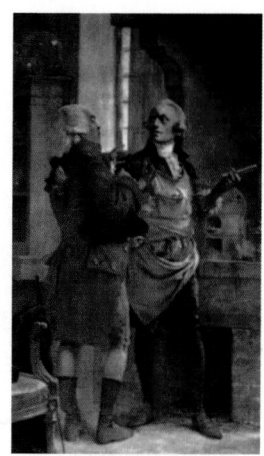

A French chemist and contemporary of Lavoisier, Berthollet identified the "volatile substances" associated with animal tissues. One of these "substances," nitrogen, was produced when ammonia gas burned in oxygen. Berthollet showed that normal tissues did not contain ammonia. He believed that hydrogen united with nitrogen during fermentation to produce ammonia. In 1865, Berthollet took exception to Lavoisier's ideas concerning the amount of heat liberated when the body oxidized an equal weight of carbohydrate or fat. According to Berthollet, "the quan-

Claude Louis Berthollet (in white lab coat)

tity of heat liberated in the incomplete oxidation of a substance equaled the difference between the total caloric value of the substance and that of the products formed." This established the foundation for the concept of metabolic efficiency—heat production above the actual heat required to produce work.

Joseph Louis Proust (1755–1826)

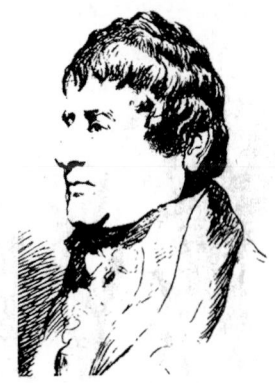

Proust proved that a pure substance isolated in the laboratory or found in nature would always contain the same elements in the same proportions. Known as the "Law of Definite Proportions," Proust's ideas about the chemical constancy of substances provided an important milestone for future nutritional explorers, helping them analyze the major

Joseph Louis Proust (Courtesy National Library of Medicine)

nutrients and calculate energy metabolism as measured by oxygen consumption.

Louis-Joseph Gay-Lussac (1778–1850)

In 1810, Gay-Lussac, a pupil of Berthollet, analyzed the chemical composition of 20 animal and vegetable substances (**www.nndb. com/people/885/000100585/**). He placed the vegetable substances into one of three categories depending on their proportion of hydrogen to oxygen atoms. One class of compounds he called saccharine, later identified as carbohydrate, was accepted by William Prout (1785–1850) in his classification of the three basic macronutrients.

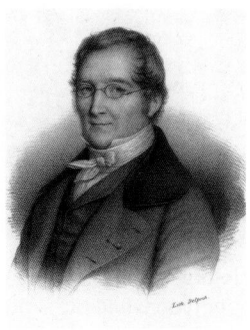
Louis-Joseph Gay-Lussac

William Prout (1785–1850)

Following up the studies of Lavoisier and Séguin on muscular activity and respiration, Prout, an Englishman, measured the carbon dioxide exhaled by men exercising to self-imposed fatigue (*Annals of Philosophy* 1813;2:328). Moderate exercise such as natural walking raised carbon dioxide production to an eventual plateau. This observation heralded the modern concept of steady-rate gas exchange kinetics in exercise. Prout could not determine the exact amount of carbon dioxide respired because no instrumentation existed to measure respiration rate, yet he nevertheless observed that carbon dioxide concentration in expired air decreased dramatically during fatiguing exercise (**www.jn.nutrition.org/ content/107/1/15.full.pdf**).

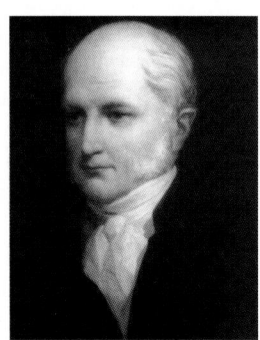
William Prout (© Royal College of Physicians of London)

François Magendie (1783–1855)

In 1821, Magendie founded the first journal for the study of experimental physiology (*Journal de Physiologie Expérimentale*), a field he literally created. The next year, he showed that anterior spinal nerve roots control motor activities and posterior roots control sensory functions.

Magendie's accomplishments were not limited to neural

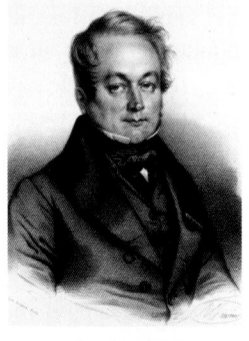
François Magendie (Courtesy National Library of Medicine)

physiology. Unlike others who claimed that the tissues derived their nitrogen from the air, Magendie argued that the food they consumed provided the nitrogen. To prove his point, he studied animals subsisting on nitrogen-free diets (**www. ncbi.nlm.nih.gov/pmc/articles/PMC1692468/pdf/medlib-histj00006-0055.pdf**).

William Beaumont (1785–1853)

One of the most fortuitous experiments in medicine began on June 6, 1822, at Fort Mackinac in upstate Michigan (**www.sportsci. org; www.james.com/beaumont/ dr_life.htm**). As fort surgeon, Beaumont tended the accidental shotgun wound that perforated the abdominal wall and stomach of a young French Canadian, Samata St. Martin, a voyageur for the American Fur Company.

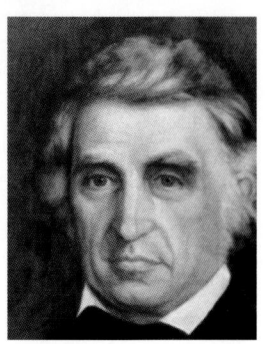
William Beaumont (Courtesy National Library of Medicine)

The wound healed after 10 months but continued to provide new insights concerning digestion. Part of the wound formed a small natural "valve" that led directly into the stomach. Beaumont turned St. Martin on his left side, depressing the valve, and then inserted a tube the size of a large quill 5 or 6 inches into the stomach. He began two kinds of experiments on the digestive processes from 1825 to 1833. First, he observed the fluids discharged by the stomach when different foods were eaten (*in vivo*); second, he extracted samples of the stomach's content and put them into glass tubes to determine the time required for "external" digestion (*in vitro*).

Beaumont revolutionized concepts about digestion. For centuries, the stomach was thought to produce heat that somehow "cooked" foods. Alternatively, the stomach was portrayed as a mill, a fermenting vat, or a stew pan.[d]

Beaumont published the first results of his experiments on St. Martin in the *Philadelphia Medical Recorder* in January 1825 and full details in his "Experiments and Observations on the Gastric Juice and the Physiology of Digestion" (1833).[24] Beaumont ends his treatise with a list of 51 inferences based on his 238 separate experiments. Although working away from the centers of medicine, Beaumont used findings culled from the writings of influential European scientists. Even with their information, he still obeyed the scientific method, basing all his inferences on direct experimentation. Beaumont concluded:

> Pure gastric juice, when taken directly out of the stomach of a healthy adult, unmixed with any other fluid, save a portion of the mucus of the stomach with which it is most commonly, and

---

[a] Jean Baptise van Helmont (1577–1644), a Flemish doctor, is credited as first to prescribe an alkaline cure for indigestion.[27] Observing the innards of birds, he reasoned that acid in the digestive tract could not alone decompose meats and that other substances ("ferments," now known as digestive enzymes) must break down food.

perhaps always combined, is a clear, transparent fluid; inodorous; a little saltish; and very perceptibly acid. Its taste, when applied to the tongue, is similar to thin mucilaginous water, slightly acidulated with muriatic acid. It is readily diffusible in water, wine or spirits; slightly effervesces with alkalis; and is an effectual solvent of the materia alimentaria. It possess the property of coagulating albumen, in an eminent degree; is powerfully antiseptic, checking the putrefaction of meat; and effectually restorative of healthy action, when applied to old, fetid sores, and foul, ulcerating surfaces.

Beaumont's accomplishment is even more remarkable because the United States, unlike England, France, and Germany, provided no research facilities for experimental medicine. Little was known about the physiology of digestion. Yet Beaumont, a "backwoods physiologist,"[14] inspired future studies of gastric emptying, intestinal absorption, electrolyte balance, rehydration, and nutritional supplementation with "sports drinks."

Michel Eugene Chevreul (1786–1889)

During his long life, Chevreul carried on a 200-year family tradition of studying chemistry and biology. His *Chemical Investigations of Fat* (1823) described different fatty acids (www.lipidlibrary.aocs.org/history/Chevreul/index.htm). In addition, he separated cholesterol from biliary fats, coined the term *margarine*, and was first to show that lard consisted of two main fats (a solid he called *stearine* and the other a liquid called *elaine*). Chevreul also demonstrated that sugar from a diabetic's urine resembled cane sugar.

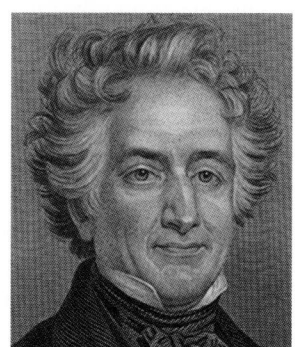

Michel Eugene Chevreul (Courtesy National Library of Medicine)

Jean Baptiste Boussingault (1802–1884)

Boussingault's studies of animal nutrition paralleled later studies of human nutrition (see, for example, jn.nutrition.org/content/84/1/1.full.pd). He calculated the effect of calcium, iron, and other nutrient intake (particularly nitrogen) on energy balance. His pioneering work among Columbians formed the basis for his recommendations that they receive iodine to counteract goiter. Boussingault also turned his attention to plants. He showed that the carbon within a plant

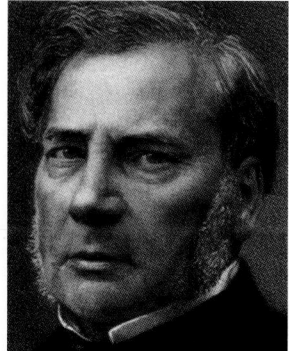

Jean Baptiste Boussingault (Courtesy National Library of Medicine)

came from atmospheric carbon dioxide. He also determined that a plant derived most of its nitrogen from the nitrates in the soil, not from the atmosphere, as previously believed.

Gerardus Johannis Mulder (1802–1880)

A professor of chemistry at Utrecht University, Netherlands, Mulder analyzed albuminous substances he named "proteine." He postulated a general protein radical identical in chemical composition to plant albumen, casein, animal fibrin, and albumen. This protein would contain substances other than nitrogen available only from plants. Because animals consume plants, substances from the plant kingdom, later called amino acids, served to build their tissues. Unfortunately, an influential German chemist, Justus von Liebig (1803–1873) attacked Mulder's theories about protein so vigorously that they fell out of favor.

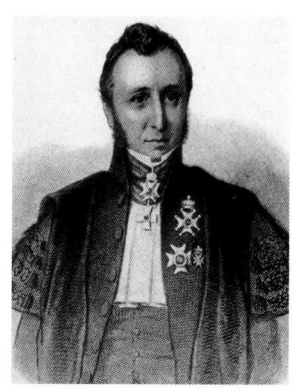

Gerardus Johannis Mulder (© Science Museum/Science & Society Picture Library)

Despite the academic controversy, Mulder strongly advocated society's role in promoting quality nutrition. He asked, "Is there a more important question for discussion than the nutrition of the human race?" Mulder urged people to observe the "golden mean" by eating neither too little nor too much food. He established minimum standards for his nation's food supply that he believed should be compatible with optimum health. In 1847, he gave these specific recommendations: laborers should consume 100 g of protein daily; those doing routine work about 60 g. He prescribed 500 g of carbohydrate as starch and included "some" fat without specifying an amount (www.encyclopedia.com/topic/Gerardus_Johannes_Mulder.aspx).

Justus von Liebig (1803–1873)

Embroiled in professional controversies, Liebig nevertheless established a large, modern chemistry laboratory that attracted numerous students (www.sportsci.org) (FIG. I.14). He developed unique equipment to analyze inorganic and organic substances. Liebig restudied protein compounds (alkaloids discovered by Mulder) and concluded that muscular exertion (by horses or humans) required mainly proteins, not just carbohydrates and fats. Liebig's

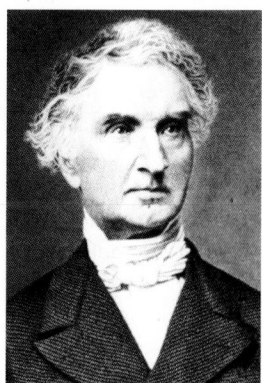

Justus von Liebig (Courtesy National Library of Medicine)

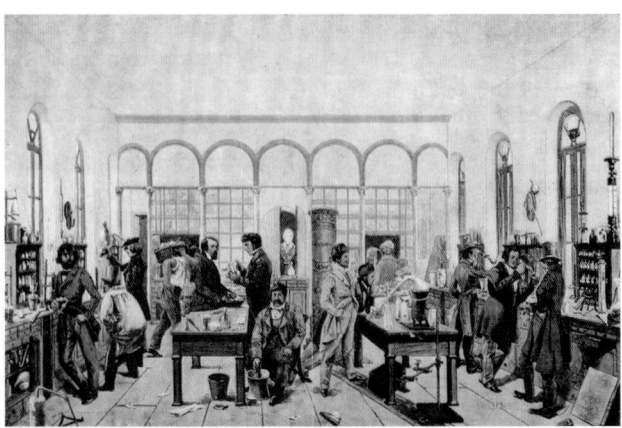

FIGURE I.14 • Hundreds of chemists trained at Liebig's Geisen laboratory, many achieving international reputations for pioneering discoveries in chemistry. (Photo courtesy of Magnus Mueller, Liebig Museum, Giessen, Germany.)

influential *Animal Chemistry* (1842) communicated his ideas about energy metabolism.

Liebig dominated chemistry; his theoretical pronouncements about the relation of dietary protein to muscular activity were usually accepted without critique by other scientists until the 1850s. Despite his pronouncements, Liebig never carried out a physiologic experiment or performed nitrogen balance studies on animals or humans. Liebig, ever so arrogant, demeaned physiologists, believing them incapable of commenting on his theoretic calculations unless they themselves achieved his level of expertise.

By midcentury, physiologist Adolf Fick (1829–1901) and chemist Johannes Wislicenus (1835–1903) challenged Liebig's dogma concerning protein's role in exercise. Their simple experiment measured changes in urinary nitrogen during a mountain climb. The protein that broke down could not have supplied all the energy for the hike (www.sportsci.org). The result discredited Liebig's principle assertion regarding the importance of protein metabolism in supplying energy for vigorous exercise.

Although erroneous, Liebig's notions about protein as a primary exercise fuel worked their way into popular writings. By the turn of the 20th century, an idea that survives today seemed unassailable: athletic prowess requires a large protein intake. He lent his name to two commercial products; *Liebig's Infant Food*, advertised as a replacement for breast milk, and *Liebig's Fleisch Extract* (meat extract) that supposedly conferred special benefits to the body. Liebig argued that consuming his extract and meat would help the body perform extra "work" to convert plant material into useful substances. Even today, fitness magazines tout protein supplements for peak performance with little except anecdotal confirmation. Whatever the merit of Liebig's claims, debate continues, building on the metabolic studies of W. O. Atwater (1844–1907), F. G. Benedict (1870–1957), and R. H. Chittenden (1856–1943) in the United States and M. Rubner (1854–1932) in Germany.[14]

Henri Victor Regnault (1810–1878)

With his colleague Jules Reiset, Henri Regnault, a professor of chemistry and physics at the University of Paris, used closed-circuit spirometry to determine the respiratory quotient (RQ; carbon dioxide ÷ oxygen) in dogs, insects, silkworms, earthworms, and frogs (1849). Animals were placed in a sealed, 45-L bell jar surrounded by a water jacket (**FIG. I.15**). A potash solution filtered the carbon dioxide gas produced during respiration. Water rising in a glass receptacle forced oxygen into the bell jar to replace the quantity consumed during energy metabolism. A thermometer recorded temperature, and a manometer measured variations in chamber pressure. For dogs, fowl, and rabbits deprived of food, the RQ was lower than when the same animals consumed meat. Regnault and Reiset reasoned that starving animals subsist on their own tissues. Foods never were completely destroyed during metabolism because urea and uric acid were recovered in the urine.

Regnault established relationships between different body sizes and metabolic rates. These ratios preceded the law of surface area and allometric scaling procedures now applied in kinesiology and the exercise sciences.

Claude Bernard (1813–1878)

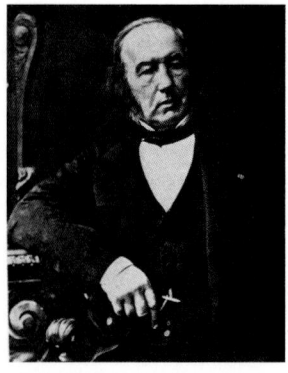

Claude Bernard

Bernard, typically acclaimed as the greatest physiologist of all time, succeeded Magendie as professor of medicine at the Collège de France (www. sportsci.org; www.claude-bernard.co.uk/page2.htm) (**FIG. I.16**). Bernard interned in medicine and surgery before serving as laboratory assistant (préparateur) to Magendie in 1839. Three years later, he followed Magendie to the Hôtel-Dieu (hospital) in Paris. For the next 35 years, Bernard discovered fundamental properties concerning physiology. He participated in the explosion of scientific knowledge in the midcentury. Bernard indicated his

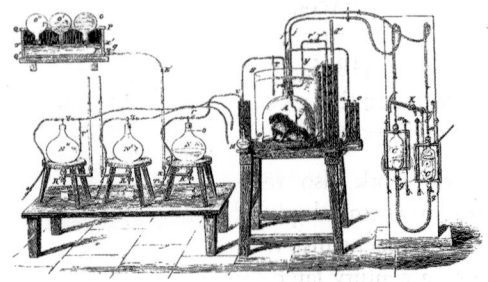

FIGURE I.15 • Regnault's closed-circuit spirometry experiment. (Courtesy Max Planck Institute for the History of Science, Berlin/Virtual Lab.; http:mpiwg-berlin.mpg/technology/data?id=tec205.)

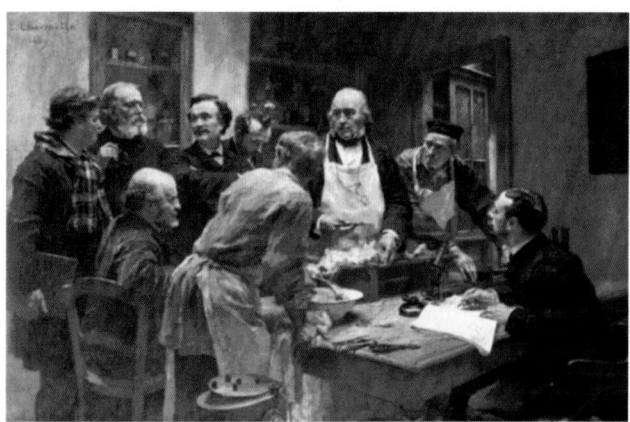

FIGURE I.16 • The Lesson of Claude Bernard, or Session at the Vivisection Laboratory, L'hermitte, Leon Augustine, Academie de Medicine, Paris, France, 1889. Students observing Bernard (white apron, no hat) perform a dissection as part of their medical training.

single-minded devotion to research by producing a doctorate thesis on gastric juice and its role in nutrition (*Du sac gastrique et de son rôle dans la nutrition*; 1843). Ten years later, he received the Doctorate in Natural Sciences for his study titled *Recherches sur une nouvelle fonction du foie, consideré comme organe producteur de matière sucrée chez l'homme et les ani-maux* (Research on a new function of the liver as a producer of sugar in man and animals). Before this seminal research, scientists assumed that only plants could synthesize sugar, and that sugar within animals must derive from ingested plant matter. Bernard disproved this notion by documenting the presence of sugar in the hepatic vein of a dog whose diet lacked carbohydrate.

Bernard's experiments that profoundly impacted medicine include:

1. Discovery of the role of the pancreatic secretion in the digestion of lipids (1848)
2. Discovery of a new function of the liver—the "internal secretion" of glucose into the blood (1848)
3. Induction of diabetes by puncture of the floor of the fourth ventricle (1849)
4. Discovery of the elevation of local skin temperature upon section of the cervical sympathetic nerve (1851)
5. Production of sugar by washed excised liver (1855) and the isolation of glycogen (1857)
6. Demonstration that curare specifically blocks motor nerve endings (1856)
7. Demonstration that carbon monoxide blocks the respiration of erythrocytes (1857)

Bernard's work also influenced other sciences.[24] His discoveries in chemical physiology spawned physiological chemistry and biochemistry, which in turn spawned molecular biology a century later. His contributions to regulatory physiology helped the next generation of scientists understand how metabolism and nutrition affected exercise. Bernard's influential *Introduction à l'étude de la médecine expérimentale* (*The Introduction to the Study of Experimental Medicine*,

1865) illustrates the self-control that enabled him to succeed despite external disturbances related to politics. Bernard urged researchers to vigorously observe, hypothesize, and then test their hypothesis. In the last third of the book, Bernard shares his strategies for verifying results. His disciplined approach remains valid, and exercise physiologists and their students would profit from reading this book (www.ncbi.nlm.nih.gov/pmc/articles/PMC195131/).

Edward Smith (1819–1874)

Edward Smith, physician, public health advocate, and social reformer, promoted better living conditions for Britain's lower class, including prisoners (www.sportsci.org). He believed prisoners were maltreated because they received no additional food while toiling on the exhausting "punitive treadmill." Smith had observed prisoners climbing up a treadwheel, whose steps resembled the side paddle wheels of a Victorian steamship. Prisoners climbed for 15 min, after which they were allowed a 15-min rest,

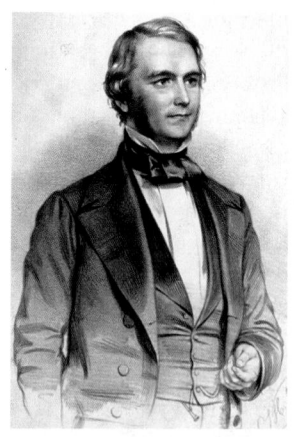

Edward Smith (Courtesy National Library of Medicine)

for a total of 4 hr of work three times a week. To overcome resistance from a sail on the prison roof attached to the treadwheel, each man traveled the equivalent of 1.43 miles up a steep hill.

Curious about this strenuous exercise, Smith conducted studies on himself. He constructed a closed-circuit apparatus (facemask with inspiratory and expiratory valves; **Fig. I.17**) to measure carbon dioxide production while climbing at Brixton prison.[24] He expired 19.6 more grams of carbon while climbing for 15 min and resting for 15 min than he expired while resting. Smith estimated that if he climbed and rested for 7.5 hr, his daily total carbon output would increase 66%. Smith analyzed the urine of four prisoners over a 3-wk period to show that urea output was related to the nitrogen content of the ingested foods, while carbon dioxide related more closely to exercise intensity.

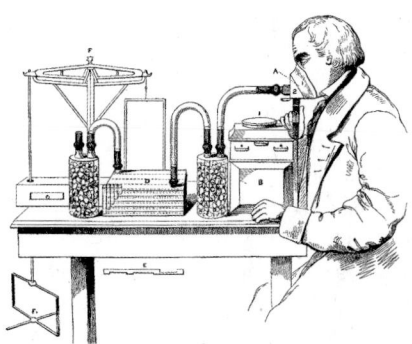

FIGURE I.17 • Edward Smith's apparatus. (Courtesy Max Planck Institute for the History of Science, Berlin/Virtual Lab; http://mpiwg-berlin.mpg/technology/data?id=tec2626.)

Smith inspired two German researchers to validate the prevailing idea that protein alone powered muscular contraction. Adolf Eugen Fick (1829–1901), a physiologist at the University of Zurich, and Johannes Wislicenus (1835–1903), a professor of chemistry at Zurich, questioned whether oxidation of protein or oxidation of carbohydrates and fats supplied energy for muscular work. In 1864, they climbed Mt. Faulhorn in the Swiss Alps. Prior to the climb, they eliminated protein from their diet, reasoning that nonprotein nutrients would have to supply them energy. They collected their urine before and immediately after the ascent and the following morning. They calculated the external energy equivalent of the 1956-m climb by multiplying body mass by the vertical distance. This external energy requirement exceeded protein catabolism reflected by nitrogen in the urine. Therefore, they concluded that the energy from protein breakdown hardly contributed to the exercise energy requirement. Again, these findings posed a serious challenge and decisive blow to Liebig's claim that protein served as the primary source of muscular power.

Health and Hygiene Influences in the United States

By the early 1800s in the United States, ideas about health and hygiene were strongly promoted by European science-oriented physicians and experimental anatomists and physiologists.[25,26] Prior to 1800, only 39 first edition American-authored medical books had been published, a few medical schools had been started in the 13 colonies (College of Philadelphia, 1765; Harvard Medical School 1782), seven medical societies existed (the New Jersey State Medical Society being the first in 1766[7,10]), and only one medical journal was available (*Medical Repository*, published in 1797; www.beckerexhibits.wustl.edu/rare/collections/periodicals.html). Outside of the United States, 176 medical journals were being published, but by 1850 the number in the United States had increased to 117.[70]

Medical journal publications in the United States had increased tremendously during the first half of the 19th century, concurrent with a steady growth in the number of scientific contributions, yet European influences still affected the thinking and practice of U.S. medicine.[49] This influence was particularly apparent in the "information explosion" that reached the public through books, magazines, newspapers, and traveling "health salesmen" who peddled an endless array of tonics, elixirs, and other products for purposes of optimizing health and curing disease. The "hot topics" of the early 19th century (also true today) included nutrition and dieting (slimming), general information concerning exercise, how to best develop overall fitness, training (or gymnastic) exercises for recreation and sport preparation, and all matters relating to personal health and hygiene.[27]By the middle of the 19th century, fledgling medical schools in the United States began to graduate their own students, many of whom assumed positions of leadership in the academic world and allied medical sciences. Interestingly, physicians had the opportunity either to teach in medical school and conduct research (and write textbooks) or become associated with departments of physical education and hygiene. There, they would oversee programs of physical training for students and athletes.[46]

Within this framework, we begin our discussion of the early physiology and exercise physiology pioneers with Austin Flint, Jr., MD, a respected physician, physiologist, and successful textbook author. His writings provided reliable information for those wishing to place their beliefs about exercise on a scientific footing.

the**Point** Appendix A, available online at http://thepoint. lww.com/mkk8e, provides several bibliographies of influential publications pertaining to anatomy and physiology, anthropometry, exercise and training, and exercise physiology, including those of Dr. Austin Flint.

Austin Flint, Jr., MD: American Physician-Physiologist

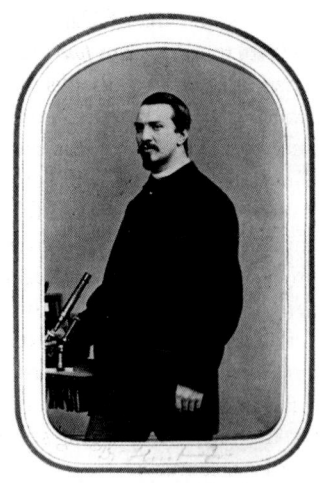

Austin Flint, Jr., MD (1836–1915), was one of the first influential American pioneer physician-scientists whose writings contributed significantly to the burgeoning literature in physiology. Flint served as a professor of physiology and physiological anatomy in the Bellevue Hospital Medical College of New York, and chaired the Department of Physiology and Microbiology from 1861 to 1897. In 1866, he published a series of five classic textbooks, the first titled *The Physiology of Man; Designed to Represent the Existing State of Physiological Science as Applied to the Functions of the Human Body. Vol. 1; Introduction; The Blood; Circulation; Respiration*. Eleven years later, Flint published *The Principles and Practice of Medicine*, a synthesis of his first five textbooks, which consisted of 987 pages of meticulously organized sections with supporting documentation. The text included 4 lithograph plates and 313 woodcuts of detailed anatomic illustrations of the body's major systems, along with important principles of physiology. In addition, there were illustrations of equipment used to record physiologic phenomena, such as Etienne-Jules Marey's (1830–1904) early cardiograph for registering the wave form and frequency of the pulse and a refinement of one of Marey's instruments, the sphygmograph, for making pulse measurements (**www.themitralvalve.org/mitralvalve/jean-baptiste-auguste-chauveau**)—the forerunner of modern cardiovascular instrumentation (**Fig. I.18**).

Austin Flint, Jr. (Courtesy National Library of Medicine)

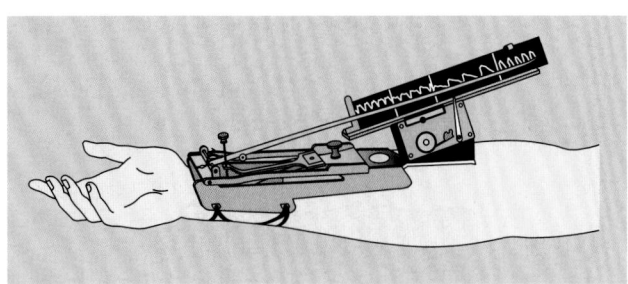

FIGURE I.18 • Marey's advanced sphygmograph, including portions of four original tracings of the pulse under different conditions. It was not until the next century in 1928 that Ernst P. Boas (1891–1955) and colleague Ernst F. Goldschmidt (cited in the 1932 Boas and Goldschmidt text *The Heart Rate*) reported on their human experiments with the first electronic cardiotachometer. (Goldschmidt had invented the pulse resonator for recording pulse rate in 1927.)

Dr. Flint, one of six generations of physicians spanning the years 1733 to 1955, was well trained in the scientific method. In 1858, he received the American Medical Association's prize for basic research on the heart, and his medical school thesis titled "The Phenomena of Capillary Circulation," was published in 1878 in the *American Journal of the Medical Sciences*. A characteristic of Flint's textbooks was his admiration for the work of other scholars. These included noted French physician Claude Bernard (1813–1878); the celebrated observations of Dr. William Beaumont; and William Harvey's momentous discoveries.

Dr. Flint was a careful writer. This was a refreshing approach, particularly because so many "authorities" in physical training, exercise, and hygiene in the United States and abroad were uninformed and unscientific about exercise and its possible role in health care. In his 1877 textbook, Flint wrote about many topics related to exercise. The following sample passages are quoted from Flint's 1877 book to present the flavor of the emerging science of exercise physiology in the late 19th century:

> It has been observed that the position of the body has a very marked influence upon the rapidity of the pulse. Experiments of a very interesting character have been made by Dr. Guy and others, with a view to determine the difference in the pulse in different postures. In the male, there is a difference of about ten beats between standing and sitting, and fifteen beats between standing and the recumbent posture. In the female, the variations with position are not so great. The average given by Dr. Guy is, for the male standing, 81; sitting, 71; lying, 66;-for the female: standing, 91; sitting, 84; lying, 80. This is given as the average of a large number of observations.
>
> *Influence of age and sex.* In both the male and female, observers have constantly found a great difference in the rapidity of the heart's action at different periods of life.
>
> *Influence of exercise, etc.* It is a fact generally admitted that muscular exertion increases the frequency of the pulsations of the heart; and the experiments just cited show that the difference in rapidity, which is by some attributed to change in posture (some positions, it is fancied, offering fewer obstacles to the current of blood than others), is mainly due to muscular exertion. Everyone knows, indeed, that the action of the heart is much more rapid after violent exertion, such as running, lifting, etc.
>
> Nearly all observers are agreed that there is a considerable increase in the exhalation of carbonic acid during and immediately following muscular exercise. In insects, Mr. Newport has found that a greater quantity is sometimes exhaled in an hour of violent agitation than in twenty-four hours of repose. In a drone, the exhalation in twenty-four hours was 0.30 of a cubic inch, and during violent muscular exertion the exhalation in one hour was 0.34. Lavoisier recognized the great influence of muscular activity upon the respiratory changes. In treating of the consumption of oxygen, we have quoted his observations on the relative quantities of air vitiated in repose and activity.

Through his textbooks, Austin Flint, Jr., influenced the first medically trained and scientifically oriented professor of physical education, Edward Hitchcock, Jr., MD. Hitchcock quoted Flint about the muscular system in his syllabus of Health Lectures, required reading for all students enrolled at Amherst College between 1861 and 1905.

The Amherst College Connection

Two physicians, father and son, pioneered the American sports science movement. Edward Hitchcock, DD, LLD (1793–1864), a professor of chemistry and natural history at Amherst College, also served as president of the college from 1845–1854. He convinced the college president in 1861 to allow his son Edward [(1828–1911); Amherst undergraduate (1849); Harvard medical degree (1853)] to assume the duties of his anatomy course. Subsequently, Edward Hitchcock, Jr., was officially appointed on August 15, 1861, as Professor of Hygiene and Physical Education with full academic rank in the Department of Physical Culture at an annual salary of $1000, a position he held almost continuously until 1911. This was the second such appointment in physical education to an American college in the United States.[e]

---

[e]Edward Hitchcock, Jr., is often accorded the distinction of being the first professor of physical education in the United States, whereas, in fact, John D. Hooker was first appointed to this position at Amherst College in 1860. Because of poor health, Hooker resigned in 1861, and Hitchcock was appointed in his place. The original idea of a Department of Physical Education with a professorship had been proposed in 1854 by William Agustus Stearns, DD, the fourth president of Amherst College, who considered physical education instruction essential for the health of the students and useful to prepare them physically, spiritually, and intellectually. Other institutions were slow to adopt this innovative concept; the next department of physical education in America was not created until 1879. In 1860, the Barrett Gymnasium at Amherst College was completed and served as the training facility where all students were required to perform systematic exercises for 30 min, 4 days a week. The gymnasium included a laboratory with scientific instruments (e.g., spirometer, strength and anthropometric equipment) and also a piano to provide rhythm during the exercises. Hitchcock reported to the Trustees that in his first year, he recorded the students' "vital statistics—including age, weight, height, size of chest and forearm, capacity of lungs, and some measure of muscular strength."

CHAPTER SECOND.

THE MOVING POWERS OF THE SYSTEM.—MYOLOGY, OR THE HISTORY OF THE MUSCLES.

DEFINITIONS AND DESCRIPTIONS.

228. Microscopic Structure of Muscle.—The Muscles, known as flesh or lean meat, compose a large part of the extremities, and the covering of the trunk. To the naked eye they appear to be fibrous, and, with the assistance of the microscope, these fibers are found to be bundles—called Fasciculi—of still smaller fibers, called Ultimate Fibers. These seem to be polygonal in form, and with an average diameter of $\frac{1}{400}$th of an inch in man, though in some of the lower animals their size is much less.

View of the stages of development of Muscular Fiber. 1, A Muscular Fiber of Animal life enclosed in its Sheath or Myolemma. 2, An Ultimate Fibril of the same. 3, A more highly magnified View of Fig. 1, showing the true nature of the Longitudinal Striæ, as well as the mode of formation of the Transverse Striæ. The Myolemma is here so thin as to permit the Ultimate Fibrils to be seen through it. 4, A Muscular Fibre of Organic life with two of its Nuclei; taken from the Urinary Bladder, and magnified 600 Diameters. 5, A Muscular Fibre of Organic life from the Stomach, magnified the same.

FIG. 120.

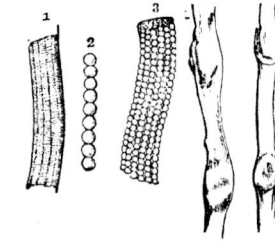

229. Fibrils.—The ultimate fibers are still further divisible into what are termed Fibrils. These have an average diameter of about $\frac{1}{10000}$th

228. What is lean meat? How does muscle appear to the naked eye? What are the three microscopic elements? Describe each. 229. What is the diameter of the Fibrils?

A

108   HITCHCOCK'S ANATOMY

FIG. 121.

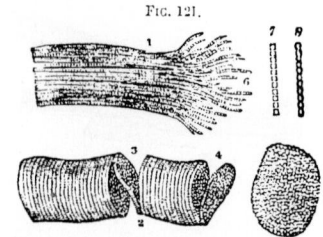

A View of the Fragments of Striped elementary Fibers, showing a cleavage in opposite directions—magnified 800 Diameters. 1, The Longitudinal Cleavage. 2, The Transverse Cleavage, the Longitudinal Lines being scarcely visible. 3, Incomplete Fracture, following the opposite surfaces of a Disc which stretches across the Interval and retains the two Fragments in connexion. The Edge and Surface of this Disc are seen to be minutely granular, the Granules corresponding in size to the thickness of the Disc and to the distance between the faint Longitudinal Lines. 4, Another Disc nearly detached. 5, A detached Disc more highly magnified, showing the Sarcous Elements. 6, Fibrillæ separated by violence from each other at the broken end of the Fiber. 7, 8, The two appearances commonly presented by the separated single Fibrillæ; more highly magnified, at 7 the spaces are rectangular, at 8 the borders are scalloped and the spaces bead-like.

of an inch, and number about 650 in each ultimate fiber. They are unprotected by any covering, while both the fasciculus and ultimate fiber are everywhere protected by a delicate sheath called the Sarcolemma.

FIG. 122.

Fibrils of Human Muscle.

230. Organic, or Unstriped, and Animal, or Striped Fibers.—All the muscles of the body are divided into two classes, according to their function. Those necessary for carrying on the vital functions, such as breathing and digestion, are called Organic, and those under the control of the will Animal Fibers. In addition to their use as a means of distinction, they may be known by their appearance under the micro-

What is the Sarcolemma? On what element of muscle is this wanting? 230. Give the two functional classes of the muscles.

B

FIGURE I.19 • Examples from the Hitchcocks' text on structure and function of muscles. (Reproduced from Hitchcock E, Hitchcock E Jr. Elementary anatomy and physiology for colleges, academies, and other schools. New York: Ivison, Phinney & Co., 1860:132, 137. Materials courtesy of Amherst College Archives and permission of the Trustees of Amherst College, 1995.)

The Hitchcocks geared their textbook to college physical education (Hitchcock E., Hitchcock E., Jr. *Elementary Anatomy and Physiology for Colleges, Academies, and Other Schools.* New York: Ivison, Phinney & Co., 1860; Edward Hitchcock, Sr., had previously published a textbook on hygiene in 1831). The Hitchcock and Hitchcock anatomy and physiology book predated Flint's anatomy and physiology text by 6 years. Topics covered were listed in numerical order by subject, and considerable attention was devoted to the physiology of species other than humans. The text included questions at the bottom of each page concerning the topics under consideration, making the textbook a "study guide" or "workbook," not an

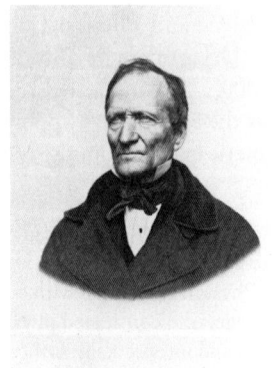

Dr. Edward Hitchcock
(1793–1864)

uncommon pedagogic feature (Cutter, 1848; see the bibliographies in Appendix A online). **FIGURE I.19** shows sample pages on muscle structure and function from the Hitchcock and Hitchcock text.

From 1865 to approximately 1905, Hitchcocks' syllabus of Health Lectures (a 38-page pamphlet titled *The Subjects and Statement of Facts Upon Personal Health Used for the Lectures Given to the Freshman Classes of Amherst College*) was part of the required curriculum. The topics included hygiene and physical education, with brief quotations about the topic, including a citation for the quote. In addition to quoting Austin Flint, Jr., regarding care of the muscles, "The condition of the muscular system is an almost

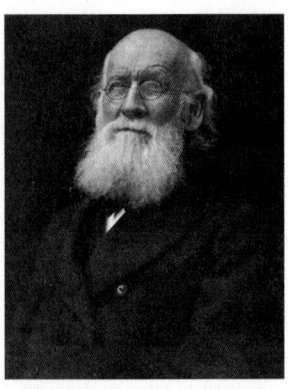

Dr. Edward Hitchcock, Jr., MD
(1828–1911)

unfailing evidence of the general state of the body," other quotations peppered each section of the pamphlet, some from well-known physiologists such as Englishman Thomas Henry Huxley (1825–1895: www.lexicorps.com/Huxley.htm) and Harvard's Henry Pickering Bowditch (1840–1911; cofounder of the American Physiological Society in 1887 and American editor of the *Journal of Physiology*; www.nasonline.org/publications/biographical-memoirs/memoir-pdfs/bowditch-henry-p.pdf). For example, with regard to physical education and hygiene, Huxley posited "The successful men in life are those who have stored up such physical health in youth that they can in an emergency work sixteen hours in a day without suffering from it." Concerning food and digestion, Bowditch stated: "A scientific or physiological diet for an adult, per day, is two pounds of bread, and three-quarters of a pound of lean meat," and in regard to tobacco use, "Tobacco is nearly as dangerous and deadly as alcohol, and a man with tobacco heart is as badly off as a drunkard." Other quotations were used for such tissues as skin. Dr. Dudley A. Sargent (1849–1924; pioneer Harvard physical educator; http://hul.harvard.edu/huarc/summersch/physed.html) told readers, "Wear dark clothes in winter and light in summer. Have three changes of underclothing—heavy flannels for winter, light flannels for spring and fall, lisle thread, silk or open cotton for summer."

Anthropometric Assessment of Body Build

During the years 1861 to 1888, Dr. Hitchcock, Jr., obtained 6 measures of segmental height, 23 girths, 6 breadths, 8 lengths, 8 measures of muscular strength, lung capacity, and pilosity (amount of hair on the body) from almost every student who attended Amherst College. From 1882 to 1888, according to Hitchcock, his standardization for measurement was improved based on the suggestions of Dr. W. T. Brigham of Boston and Dr. Dudley A. Sargent (Yale medical degree, 1878; assistant professor of physical training and director of Harvard's Hemenway Gymnasium).

In 1889, Dr. Hitchcock and his colleague in the Department of Physical Education and Hygiene, Hiram H. Seelye, MD (also served as college physician from 1884–1896), published a 37-page anthropometric manual that included five tables of anthropometric statistics of students from 1861 to 1891. This resource compendium provided detailed descriptions for taking measurements that also included eye testing and an examination of the lungs and heart before testing subjects for muscular strength. In the last section of the manual, Dr. Seelye wrote detailed instructions for using the various pieces of gymnasium apparatus for "enlarging and strengthening the neck, to remedy round or stooping shoulders, to increase the size of the chest and the capacity of the lungs, to strengthen and enlarge the arm, abdominal muscles, and weak back, and to enlarge and strengthen the thighs, calves, legs and ankles." The Hitchcock and Seelye manual, the first of its kind devoted to an analysis of anthropometric and strength data based on detailed measurements, influenced other departments of physical education in the United States (e.g., Yale, Harvard, Wellesley, Mt. Holyoke) to include anthropometric measurements as part of the physical education and hygiene curriculum.[f]

One reason for the early interest in anthropometric measurement was to demonstrate that engaging in daily, vigorous exercise produced desirable bodily results, particularly for muscular development. Although none of the early physical education scientists used statistics to evaluate the outcomes of exercise programs, it is instructive to apply modern methods of anthropometric analysis to the original data of Hitchcock on entering students at Amherst College in 1882 and on their graduation in 1886. FIGURE I.20 shows how the average student changed in anthropometric dimensions throughout 4 years of college in relation to Behnke's reference standards presented in Chapter 28. Note the dramatic increase in biceps girth and decreases in the nonmuscular abdomen and hip regions. Although data for a nonexercising "control" group of students were not available, these changes coincided with daily resistance training prescribed in the Hitchcock and Seelye *Anthropometric Manual*. This training used Indian club or barbell swinging exercises (FIG. I.21) and other strengthening modalities (horizontal bar, rope and ring exercises, parallel bar exercises, dipping machine, inclined presses with weights, pulley weights, and rowing machine workouts). The Hitchcock data presentation, a first of its kind initially reported in the *Anthropometric Manual* in March 1892, used "bodily stature" as the basis of comparison "from measurements of 1322

---

[f] Probably unknown to Hitchcock was the 1628 manuscript of the Flemish fencing instructor at the French Royal Court, Gerard Thibault, who studied optimal body proportions and success in fencing.[65] This early text, *L'Académie de l'Espée*, appeared at a time when important discoveries were being made by European scientists, particularly anatomists and physiologists, whose contributions played such an important role in laboratory experimentation and scientific inquiry. Had Hitchcock known about this early attempt to link anthropometric assessment with success in sport, the acceptance of anthropometry in the college curriculum might have been easier. Nevertheless, just 67 years after Hitchcock began taking anthropometric measurements at Amherst, and 37 years following the creation of Harvard's physical education scientific laboratory in 1891, anthropometric measurements were made of athletes at the 1928 Amsterdam Olympic Games. One of the athletes measured in Amsterdam, Ernst Jokl from South Africa, became a physician and then a professor of physical education at the University of Kentucky. Jokl was a charter member and founder of the American College of Sports Medicine. Thus, Hitchcock's visionary ideas about the importance of anthropometry finally caught on, and such assessment techniques are now used routinely in exercise physiology to assess physique status and the dynamics between physiology and performance. The more modern application of anthropometry is now known as *kinanthropometry*. This term, first defined at the International Congress of Physical Activity Sciences in conjunction with the 1976 Montreal Olympic Games,[64] was refined in 1980[65] as follows: "Kinanthropometry is the application of measurement to the study of human size, shape, proportion, composition, maturation, and gross function. Its purpose is to help us to understand human movement in the context of growth, exercise, performance, and nutrition. We see its essentially human-enobling purpose being achieved through applications in medicine, education, and government."

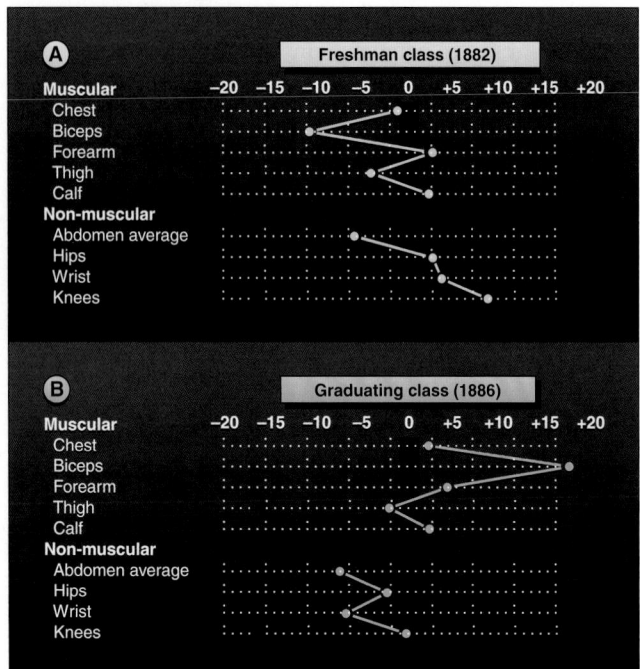

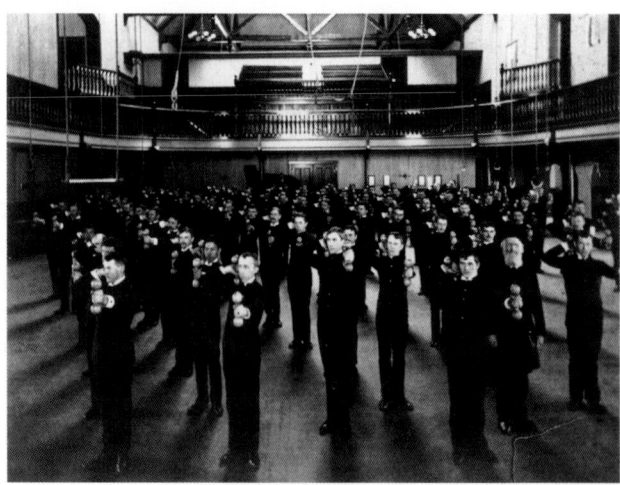

FIGURE I.21 • Dr. Edward Hitchcock, Jr. (second from right, with beard), observing the students perform barbell exercises in the Pratt Gymnasium of Amherst College. (Photo courtesy of Amherst College Archives and by permission of the Trustees of Amherst College, 1995.)

FIGURE 1.20 • Changes in selected girth measurements of Amherst College men over 4 years of college using Behnke's reference man standards (presented in Chapter 28). **(A)** The average body mass of the freshman class in 1882 was 59.1 kg (stature, 171.0 cm). **(B)** Four years later, average body mass increased 5.5 kg (11.3 lb) and stature increased by 7.4 cm (2.9 in).

students between 17 and 26 years of age. The strength tests are derived from 20,761 items." The Hitchcock anthropometric and strength studies were acknowledged in the first formal American textbook on anthropometry, published in 1896 by Jay W. Seaver, MD (1855–1915), physician and lecturer on personal hygiene at Yale University. TABLE I.2 presents a sample

TABLE I.2	Average and Best Anthropometric and Strength Records of Amherst College from 1861 to 1900 Inclusive					
	Average		**Maximal**			
Items[a]	**Metric**	**English**	**Metric**	**English**	**Held By**	**Date of Record**
Weight	61.2	134.9	113.7	250.6	K.R. Otis '03	Oct. 2, '99
Height	1725	67.9	1947	76.6	B. Matthews '99	Oct. 28, '95
Girth, head	572	22.5	630	24.8	W.H. Lewis '92	Feb '92
Girth, neck	349	13.7	420	16.5	D.R. Knight '01	Feb. '91
Girth, chest, repose	880	34.6	1140	44.9	K.R. Otis '03	Oct. 2, '99
Girth, belly	724	28.5	1017	40.1	G.H. Coleman '99	May '97
Girth, hips	893	35.1	1165	45.9	K.R. Otis '03	Oct. 2, '99
Girth, right thigh	517	20.3	745	29.3	K.R. Otis '03	Oct. 2, '99
Girth, right knee	361	14.2	460	18.1	K.R. Otis '03	Oct. 2, '99
Girth, right calf	359	14.1	452	17.8	K.R. Otis '03	Oct. 2, '99
Girth, upper-right arm	257	10.1	396	15.6	K.R. Otis '03	Oct. 2, '99
Girth, right forearm	267	10.5	327	12.8	K.R. Otis '03	Oct. 2, '99
Girth, right wrist	166	6.5	191	7.5	H.B. Haskell '94	April '92
Strength, chest, dip	6	–	45	–	H.W. Lane '95	March '95
Strength, chest, pull up	9	–	65	–	H.W. Seelye '79	Oct. '75
Strength, right forearm	41	90	86	189.6	A.J. Wyman '98	April '96
Strength, left forearm	38	84	73	160.9	A.J. Wyman '98	April '96

From Hitchcock E, et al. An anthropometric manual, 4th ed. Amherst, MA: Carpenter and Morehouse, 1900.
[a]Weight in kg or lb; height in. cm or in. girths in mm or in. strength in kg or lb.

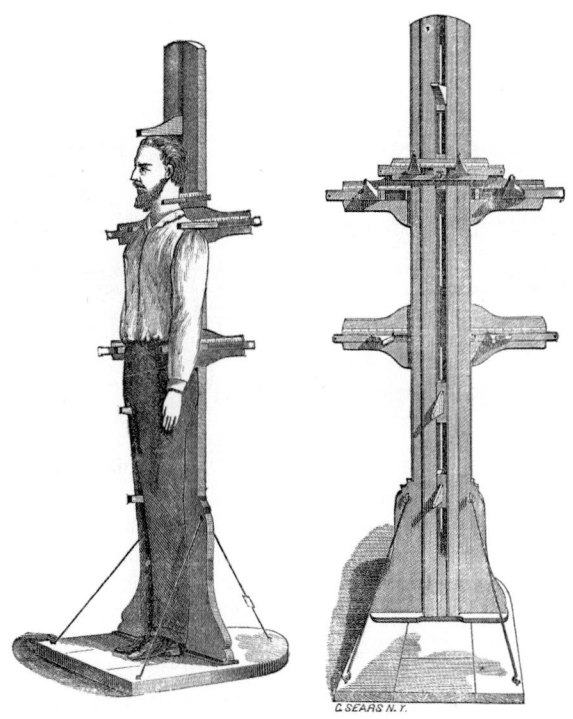

FIGURE I.22 • The andrometer, first used by the United States Sanitary Commission at numerous military installations along the Atlantic seaboard during the early 1860s, sized soldiers for clothing.

of the average and "best" anthropometric values at Amherst College from 1861 to 1900.

While Hitchcock was performing pioneering anthropometric studies at the college level, the military was making the first detailed anthropometric, spirometric, and muscular strength measurements on Civil War soldiers in the early 1860s, published in 1869 by Gould (see the bibliographies in Appendix A online). The specially trained military anthropometrists used a unique device, the *andrometer* (**Fig I.22**), to secure the physical dimensions to the nearest 1/10th of an inch of soldiers for purposes of fitting uniforms. The andrometer was originally devised in 1855 by a tailor in Edinburgh, Scotland, commissioned by the British government to determine the proper size for British soldiers' clothing. This device was set by special gauges to adjust "sliders" for measurement of total height; breadth of the neck, shoulders, and pelvis; and the length of the legs and height to the knees and crotch. Each examiner received

2 days of practice to perfect measurement technique before assignment to different military installations (e.g., Fort McHenry in Baltimore, Naval Rendezvous in New York City, Marine Barracks at the Brooklyn Navy Yard, and bases in South Carolina, Washington, D.C., Detroit, and New Orleans). Data were compiled on the actual and relative proportions of 15,781 men ("Whites, Blacks, Indians") between the ages of 16 and 45 years. These early investigations about muscular strength and body dimensions served as prototypical studies whose measurement techniques led the way to many later studies conducted in the military about muscular strength and human performance per se. Most laboratories in exercise physiology today include assessment procedures to evaluate aspects of muscular strength and body composition.[63,76]

Figure I.23A shows two views of the instrument used to evaluate muscular strength in the military studies; Figure I.23B shows the early spirometers used to evaluate pulmonary dimensions. The strength device predates the various strength-measuring instruments shown in **Figure I.24** used by Hitchcock (Amherst), Sargent (Harvard), and Seaver (Yale), as well as anthropometric measuring instruments used in their batteries of physical measurements. The *inset* shows the price list of some of the equipment from the 1889 and 1890 Hitchcock manuals on anthropometry. Note the progression in complexity of the early spirometers and strength devices used in the 1860 military studies (Fig. I.23), and the more "modern" equipment of the 1889–1905 period displayed in Figure I.24. **Figure I.25** includes three photographs (circa 1897–1901) of the strength-testing equipment (Kellogg's Universal Dynamometer) acquired by Dr. Hitchcock in 1897 to assess the strength of arms *(A)*; anterior trunk and forearm supinators *(B)*; and leg extensors, flexors, and adductors *(C)*.[g]

The First Exercise Physiology Laboratory and Degree Program in the United States

The first formal exercise physiology laboratory in the United States was established in 1891 at Harvard University and housed in a newly created Department of Anatomy, Physiology, and Physical Training at the Lawrence Scientific School.[25,44] Several instructors in the initial undergraduate BS degree program in Anatomy, Physiology, and Physical Training started at the same time were Harvard-trained

---

[g]According to Hitchcock and Selye's *Anthropometric Manual*, the device consisted "of a lever acting by means of a piston and cylinder on a column of mercury in a closed glass tube. Water keeps the oil in the cylinder from contact with the mercury and various attachments enable the different groups of muscles to be brought to bear on the lever. By means of this apparatus, the strength of most of the large muscles may be tested fairly objectively" (p. 25). In the photographs, note the attachment of the tube to each device. Interestingly, Hitchcock determined an individual's total strength as a composite of body weight multiplied by dip and pull tests, strength of the back, legs, and average of the forearms, and the lung strength. Hitchcock stated, "The *total strength* is purely an arbitrary, and relative, rather than an actual test of strength as its name would indicate. And while confessedly imperfect, it seems decidedly desirable that there should be some method of comparison which does not depend entirely on lifting a dead weight against gravity, or steel springs."

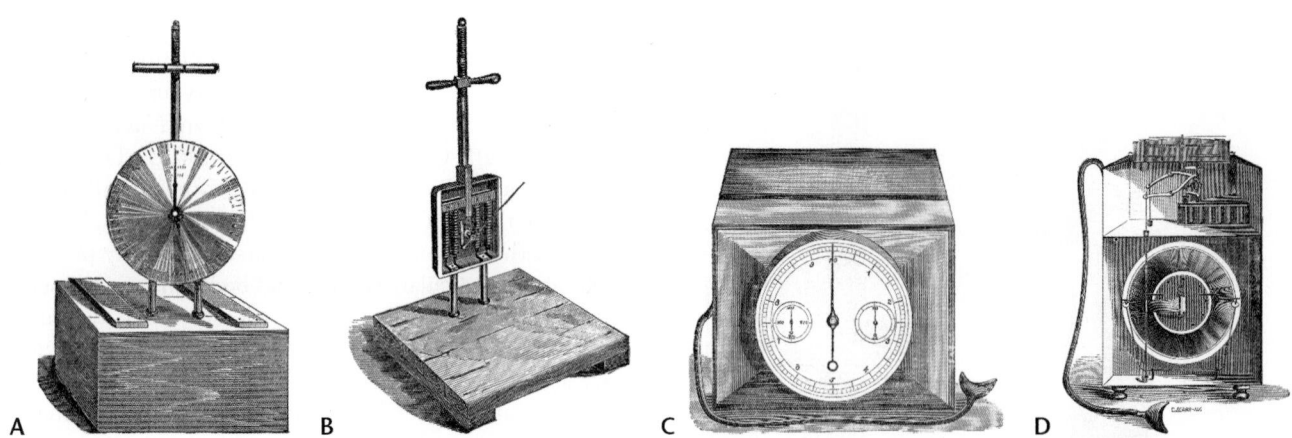

A   B   C   D

FIGURE I.23 • **(A** and **B)** Instrument used to evaluate muscular strength in the military studies of Gould in 1869. The illustration on the *left* shows the general look of the device, while the *right side* shows the internal arrangement without face-plate. Gould described the procedure for measuring muscular strength as follows: "The man stands upon the movable lid of the wooden packing box, to which the apparatus is firmly attached, and grasps with both hands the rounded extremities of a wooden bar, of convenient shape and adjustable in height. The handle is conveniently shaped for firm and easy grasp, its height well suited for application and the full muscular power, and the mechanism such as to afford results which are to all appearance very trustworthy." This was not the first dynamometer; Gould cites Regnier (no date given), who published a description of a dynamometer to measure the strength of Parisians; and Péron, who carried a dynamometer on an expedition to Australia. Other researchers in Europe had also used dynamometers to compare the muscular strength of men of different races. Figure 22.2C (in Chapter 22) shows the modern back-leg lift dynamometer still used for assessing muscular strength as part of physical fitness test procedures. **(C** and **D)** Spirometers (or dry gas meters), manufactured by the American Meter Company of Philadelphia, were used to measure vital capacity. According to Gould, the spirometers needed to be rugged "… to undergo the rough usage inseparable from transportation by army trains or on military railroads, which are in danger of being handled roughly at some unguarded moment by rude men …". The spirometers were graduated in cubic centimeters and were "furnished with a mouth-piece of convenient form, connected with the instrument by flexible tubing."

physicians; others—including Henry Pickering Bowditch, renowned professor of physiology who discovered the all-or-none principle of cardiac contraction and treppe, the staircase phenomenon of muscular contraction, and William T. Porter, also a distinguished physiologist in the Harvard Medical School—were respected for their rigorous scientific and laboratory training.

George Wells Fitz, MD: A Major Influence

An important influence in creating the new departmental major and recruiting top scientists as faculty in the Harvard

program was George Wells Fitz, MD (1860–1934). Fitz vociferously supported a strong, science-based curriculum in preparing the new breed of physical educators. The archival records show that the newly formed major was grounded in the basic sciences, including formal coursework in exercise physiology, zoology, morphology (animal and human), anthropometry, applied anatomy and animal

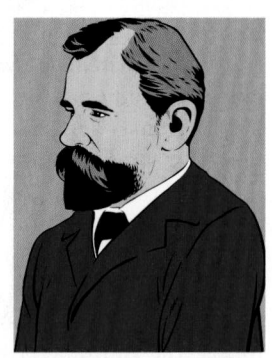

George Wells Fitz, MD

FIGURE I.24 • Anthropometric instruments used by Hitchcock, Seaver, and Sargent. Sargent, also an entrepreneur, constructed and sold specialized strength equipment used in his studies. **(A)** Metric graduated scale. **(B)** Height meter. **(C)** Sliding anthropometer. **(D)** Cloth tape measure, with an instrument made by the Narragansett Machine Co. at the suggestion of Dr. Gulick (head of the Department of Physical Training of the YMCA Training School, Springfield, MA) in 1887. The modern version of this tape, now sold as the "Gulick tape," was "for attachment to the end of a tape to indicate the proper tension, so that the pressure may be always alike." **(E)** Calipers for taking body depths. **(F)** Several types of hand dynamometers, including push holder and pull holder instruments. **(G)** Back and leg dynamometer, also used to measure the strength of the pectoral and "retractor" muscles of the shoulders. **(H)** Vital capacity spirometer and Hutchinson's wet spirometer. **(I)** Two stethoscopes. The soft rubber bell was used to "secure perfect coaptation to the surface of the chest." The Albion Stethoscope was preferred because it could be conveniently carried in the pocket. **(J)** Parallel bars for testing arm extensors during push-ups and testing of flexors in pull-ups. In special situations, physiology laboratories used Marey's cardiograph to record pulse, but the preferred instrument was a pneumatic kymograph (or sphygmograph; see Fig. 2). The *inset table* shows a price comparison for the testing equipment from the 1889 and 1890 Hitchcock manuals. Note the yearly variation in prices. (Inset courtesy of Amherst College Archives, reproduced by permission of the Trustees of Amherst College, 1995.)

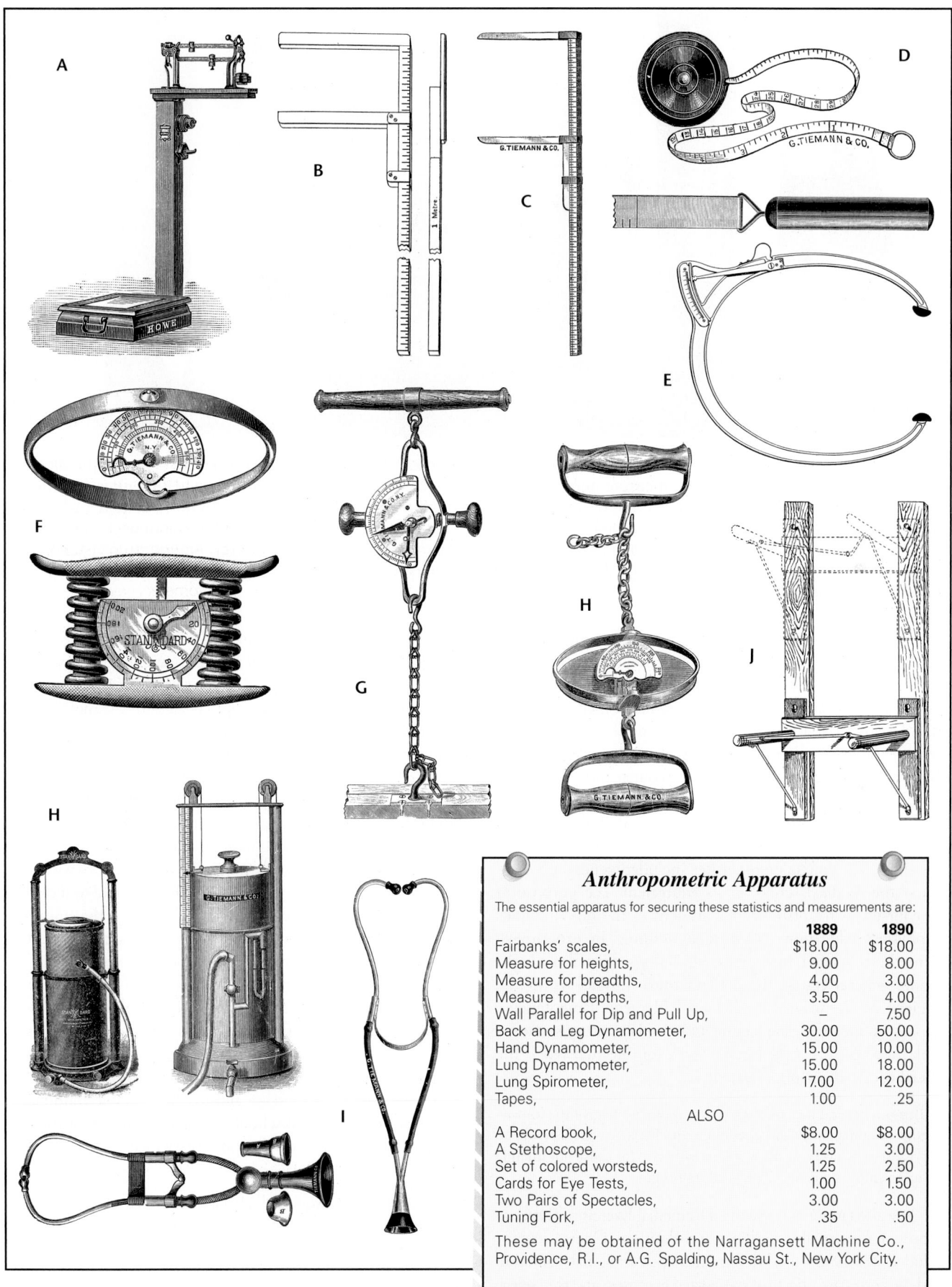

Anthropometric Apparatus

The essential apparatus for securing these statistics and measurements are:

	1889	1890
Fairbanks' scales,	$18.00	$18.00
Measure for heights,	9.00	8.00
Measure for breadths,	4.00	3.00
Measure for depths,	3.50	4.00
Wall Parallel for Dip and Pull Up,	–	7.50
Back and Leg Dynamometer,	30.00	50.00
Hand Dynamometer,	15.00	10.00
Lung Dynamometer,	15.00	18.00
Lung Spirometer,	17.00	12.00
Tapes,	1.00	.25
ALSO		
A Record book,	$8.00	$8.00
A Stethoscope,	1.25	3.00
Set of colored worsteds,	1.25	2.50
Cards for Eye Tests,	1.00	1.50
Two Pairs of Spectacles,	3.00	3.00
Tuning Fork,	.35	.50

These may be obtained of the Narragansett Machine Co., Providence, R.I., or A.G. Spalding, Nassau St., New York City.

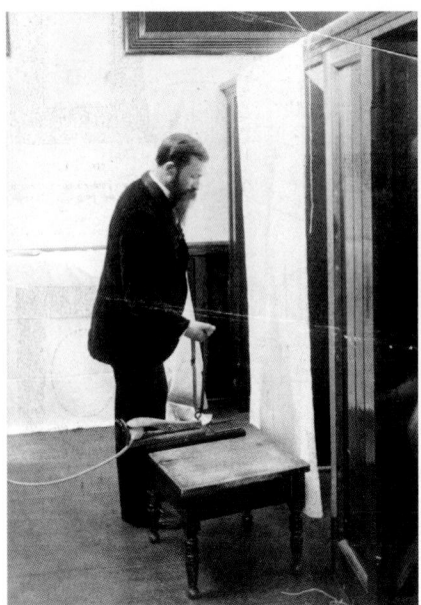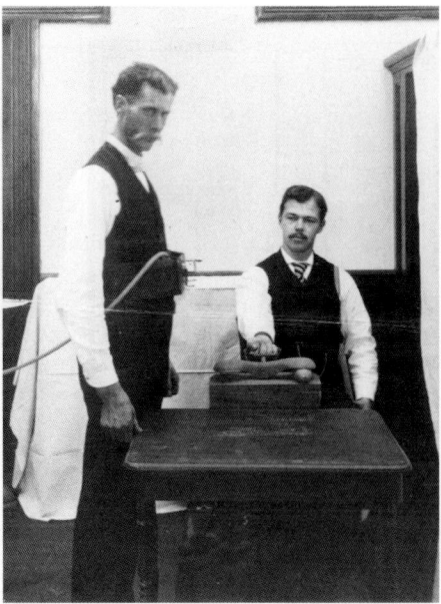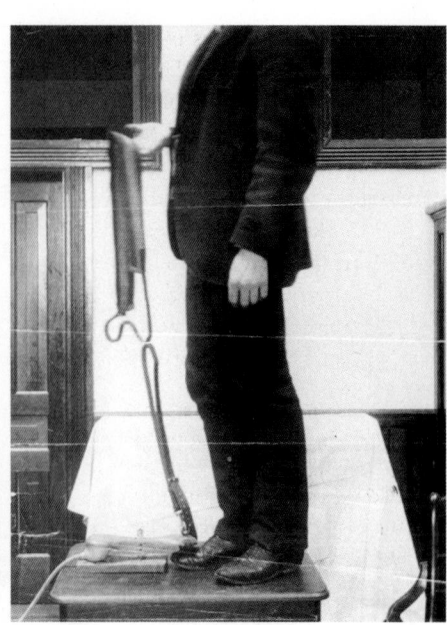

FIGURE I.25 • Kellogg's Universal Dynamometer acquired by Dr. Hitchcock to test the muscular strength of Amherst College students. From 1897 to 1900, strength measurements were taken on 328 freshmen, 111 sophomores, and 88 seniors, including retests of 58 individuals. Arm strength was measured bilaterally for the forearms and for the latissimus dorsi, deltoid, pectoral, and shoulder "retractor" muscles. Trunk measurements included the anterior trunk, and anterior and posterior neck. The leg measurements included the leg extensors and flexors and thigh adductors. (**Left**) "Arm pull." (**Center**) Anterior trunk (standing) and forearm supinators (sitting). (**Right**) Legs. (Photos courtesy of Amherst College Archives and by permission of the trustees of Amherst College, 1995.)

mechanics, medical chemistry, comparative anatomy, remedial exercises, physics, gymnastics and athletics, history of physical education, and English. Physical education students took general anatomy and physiology courses in the medical school; after 4 years of study, graduates could enroll as second-year medical students and graduate in 3 years with an MD degree. Dr. Fitz taught the *physiology of exercise* course; thus, we believe he was one of the first medically trained persons to formally teach such a course. It included experimental investigation and original work and thesis, including 6 hr a week of laboratory study. The course prerequisites included general physiology at the medical school or its equivalent. The purpose of the course was to introduce the student to the fundamentals of physical education and provide training in experimental methods related to exercise physiology. Fitz also taught a more general course titled Elementary Physiology of the Hygiene of Common Life, Personal Hygiene, Emergencies. The course included one lecture and one laboratory section a week for a year (or three times a week for one-half year). The official course description stated:

> This is a general introductory course intended to give the knowledge of human anatomy, physiology and hygiene which should be possessed by every student; it is suitable also for those not intending to study medicine or physical training.

Fitz also taught a course titled Remedial Exercises. The Correction of Abnormal Conditions and Positions. Course content included observations of deformities such as spinal curvature (and the corrective effects of specialized exercises) and the "selection and application of proper exercises, and in the diagnosis of cases when exercise is unsuitable." Several of Fitz's scientific publications dealt with spinal deformities; one study, published in the *Journal of Experimental Medicine* 1896;1(4) ("A Study of Types of Respiratory Movements") dealt with the mechanics of breathing. In addition to the remedial exercise course, students took a required course, *Applied Anatomy and Animal Mechanics. Action of Muscles in Different Exercises.* This thrice-weekly course, taught by Dr. Dudley Sargeant, was the forerunner of modern biomechanics courses. Its prerequisite was general anatomy at the medical school or its equivalent. Sargeant designed numerous exercise machines with pulleys and weights (www.ihpra.org/imagesa/sargentex.jpg), many of which he sold to individuals and schools, but not without the disdain of the university administration, which probably led to his unplanned separation from Harvard a few years after the last students graduated.

By the year 1900, nine men had graduated with bachelor of science degrees from the Department of Anatomy, Physiology, and Physical Training. The aim of the major was to prepare students to become directors of gymnasia or instructors in physical training, to provide students with the necessary knowledge about the science of exercise, and to offer suitable training for entrance to the medical school. The stated purpose of the new exercise physiology research laboratory was as follows:

> A large and well-equipped laboratory has been organized for the experimental study of the physiology of exercise. The object of this work is to exemplify the hygiene of the muscles, the conditions under which they act, the relation of their action to the body as a whole affecting blood supply and general hygienic conditions, and the effects of various exercises upon muscular growth and general health.

With the activities of the department in full operation, its outspoken and critical director was not afraid to speak his mind about academic topics. For example, Dr. Fitz reviewed a new physiology text (*American Text-Book of Physiology*, edited by William H. Howell, PhD, MD) in the March 1897 issue of the *American Physical Education Review* (Vol. II, No. 1, p. 56). The review praised Dr. Howell's collection of contributions from outstanding physiologists (such as Bowditch, Lee, Lusk, and Sewall), and attacked an 1888 French book by Lagrange that some writers consider the first important text in exercise physiology.[b] The following is Fitz's review:

> No one who is interested in the deeper problems of the physiology of exercise can afford to be without this book [referring to Howell's Physiology text], and it is to be hoped it may be used as a text-book in the normal schools of physical training. These schools have been forced to depend largely on Lagrange's "physiology of exercise" for the discussion of specific problems, or at least for the basis of such discussions. The only value Lagrange has, to my mind, is that he seldom gives any hint of the truth, and the student is forced to work out his own problems. This does very well in well-taught classes, but, Alas! for those schools and readers who take his statements as final in matters physiological. We have a conspicuous example of the disastrous consequences in Treve's contribution of the "Cyclopaedia of Hygiene on Physical Education," in which he quotes freely from Lagrange and rivals him in the absurdity of his conclusions.
>
> The time has surely come for a thoroughly scientific investigation of the physiological problems involved in physical exercise and the promulgation of the exact and absolute. It is not too much to hope that the use of the American Text-Book of Physiology by training schools and teachers, may aid to bring about this much needed consummation.

For unknown reasons, but coinciding with Fitz's untimely departure from Harvard in 1899,[i] the department changed its curricular emphasis (the term *physical training* was dropped from the department title), thus terminating at least temporarily this unique experiment in higher education.

One of the legacies of the Fitz-directed "Harvard experience" between 1891 and 1899 was the training it provided to the cadre of young scholars, who began their careers with a strong scientific basis in exercise and training and its relationship to health. Unfortunately, it would take another quarter century before the next generation of science-oriented physical educators (led not by physical educators but by such world-class physiologists as Nobel laureate A. V. Hill and 1963 ACSM Honor Award recipient David Bruce Dill) would once again exert a strong influence on the physical education curriculum.

Other individuals also contributed to the scientific explosion of new knowledge in exercise physiology. Russian-born research scientist Peter V. Karpovich (1896–1975; www.la84foundation.org/SportsLibrary/IGH/IGH0804/IGH0804c.pdf) directed the Physiological Research Laboratory at Springfield College in western Massachusettes for 40 years. His distinguished career included 150 published articles, book chapters, and monographs dealing with fitness and exercise (salient examples include the biomechanics of swimming, artificial respiration, caloric expenditure of physical activities, weightlifting and flexibility, warmup, and footwear studies). His influential textbook, *Physiology of Muscular Activity* (Philadelphia: W.B. Saunders, 3rd ed., 1948), first coauthored with Edward C. Schneider (1874–1954) in 1948 and then published under sole authorship in 1953, was translated into five languages and eight editions. It served to educate thousands of physical education students (including the authors of this textbook) on exercise physiology.

Karpovich also served as Chief of the Laboratory of Physical Fitness, School of Army Aviation Medicine, Army Air Force, Randolph Field, Texas from 1942 to 1945, and worked with the United States Army Quartermaster Research and Development Command in Natick, Massachusetts, on projects concerning soldiers' clothing and footwear (www.qmfound.com/quartermaster_research_development_command.htm). In 1966, he and son George received a patent for a rotary electrogoniometer to measure the degree of forearm rotation during arm movements—with subsequent publications using the apparatus applied to different limbs in humans and animals.

In May 1954, Karpovich and his wife Dr. Josephine L. Rathbone (1899–1989) (**Fig. I.26**), became founding members

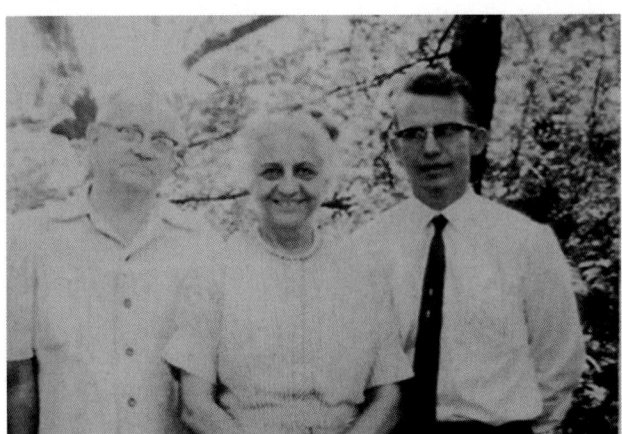

FIGURE I.26 • **(Left)** Peter V. Karpovich. Center. Wife Josephine Rathbone. **(Right)** Former graduate assistant Charles M. Tipton, 1964. (Photo courtesy of C. M. Tipton.)

---

[b]We disagree with Berryman's[6] assessment of the relative historical importance of the translation of the original Lagrange text. We give our reasons for this disagreement in a subsequent section, "First Textbook in Exercise Physiology: The Debate Continues."

[i]The reasons for Fitz's early departure from Harvard have been discussed in detail in Park's scholarly presentation of this topic.[50] His leaving was certainly unfortunate for the next generation of students of exercise physiology. In his 1909 textbook *Principles of Physiology and Hygiene* (New York: Henry Holt and Co.), the title page listed the following about Fitz's affiliation: Sometime Assistant Professor Physiology and Hygiene and Medical Visitor, Harvard University.

First Course in the Physiology of Exercise or in Exercise Physiology

Note: ACSM Honor Award winner Dr. Charles Tipton has been concerned about who taught the first college-/university-level course in exercise physiology, and when and where it was offered. Here are his written thoughts on the matter after spending time researching the question in the archives of both Harvard University and Springfield College. Tipton has previously written an historical perspective of our field (Tipton, CM. "Historical Perspective: Origin to Recognition." ACSM's Advanced Exercise Physiology. Baltimore: Lippincott Williams & Wilkins, 2006: 11–38.)

The first textbook devoted to exercise and physiology was written in Latin during 1553 by Spanish physician Cristóbal Méndez (1500–1561), entitled *Book of Bodily Exercise*.[1] In North America, the first time that the words "physiology of exercise" appeared in print was during 1855 in an article by physician William H. Byford (1817–1890). Byford lamented that physicians were indifferent to the health benefits of exercise while encouraging them to become better informed and to initiate research on the subject.[2] Although such physicians as Edward Hitchcock, Jr. (1828–1911), of Amherst College and Dudley A. Sargent (1849–1924) of Harvard University likely included physiology of exercise topics in their physical education courses, it was not until 1892–1893 or 1893–1894 that courses listed as the Physiology of Exercise were officially listed in an institutional Catalogue. In the 1892–1893 Catalogue of Harvard University, the Department of Anatomy, Physiology and Physical Training offered a formal course in Experimental Physiology, in which the Physiology of Exercise was listed as an integral component with physician George Wells Fitz (1896–1934) as the instructor.[3] During the 1893–1894 school year, senior students majoring in physical education at the International Young Men's Christian Association Training School in Springfield, Massachusetts, were enrolled in a Physiology of Exercise course with physician Luther Halsey Gulick, Jr. (1865–1928), responsible for the course.[4] However, there was no catalogue information concerning the semester when the course was taught. Although there is no official record of the assigned text for the Harvard students, it is known that at Springfield College, the required text for the Gulick course was the 1889 text of Fernand LaGrange translated from the French edition, titled, *The Physiology of Bodily Exercise*.[5]

Sources:
1. Méndez C. *The Book of Bodily Exercise (1553)*. Copyright Elizabeth Light. Baltimore: Waverly Press, 1960.
2. Byford WH. *On the Physiology of Exercise. AM J Med Sci* 1855;30:32.
3. *The Harvard University Catalogue, 1892–1893*. Cambridge, MA: Harvard University, 1892: 246–249.
4. *Ninth Catalogue of the International Young Men's Christian Association Training School*. Springfield, MA, 1893–1894.
5. LaGrange F. *Physiology of Bodily Exercise*. New York: D. Appleton, 1889.

of the American Federation of Sports Medicine (now the American College of Sports Medicine [ACSM; www.acsm.org]). Karpovich served as the fifth president of the ACSM (1961–1962). He trained a cadre of outstanding graduate students in exercise physiology who established their own productive laboratory research programs and service to the profession (e.g., Charles M. Tipton, ACSM President, 1974–1975; Howard Knuttgen, ACSM President, 1973–1974; Loring (Larry) Rowell, see "Interview with Dr. Loring B. Rowell").

Exercise Studies in Research Journals

Another notable event in the growth of exercise physiology occurred in 1898: the appearance of three articles dealing with physical activity in the first volume of the *American Journal of Physiology*.[j] This was followed in 1921 with the publication of the prestigious journal *Physiological Reviews* (physrev.physiology.org).

thePoint   Appendix A, available online at http://thepoint.lww.com/mkk8e, provides several bibliographies of influential publications pertaining to anatomy and physiology, anthropometry, exercise and training, and exercise physiology, and includes a list of the articles in this journal (and two from the *Annual Review of Physiology*), from the first review of the mechanisms of muscular contraction by A. V. Hill (www.sportsci.org) in 1922, to pioneer researcher in exercise physiology, physical medicine, and rehabilitation Professor Francis Hellebrandt's classic review of exercise in 1940 (www.secfac.wisc.edu/senate/2002/1007/1656(mem_res).pdf).

The German applied physiology publication *Internationale Zeitschrift fur angewandte Physiologie einschliesslich Arbeitsphysiologie* [1929–1973; now the *European Journal of Applied Physiology* (www.springerlink.com/content/1439-6319)], a significant journal for research in exercise physiology, published hundreds of research articles in numerous disciplines related to exercise physiology. The *Journal of Applied Physiology* (www.jap.physiology.org) first published in 1948. Its first volume contained the now-classic paper on ratio expressions of physiologic data with reference to body size and function by British child-growth and development researcher-pediatrician James M. Tanner, MD (1920-2010; *A History of the Study of Human Growth*, 1981), a must-read for exercise

---

[j]The originator of the *American Journal of Physiology* was physiologist William T. Porter of the St. Louis College of Medicine and Harvard Medical School, who remained editor until 1914.[12] Porter's research focused on cardiac physiology. The three articles in volume 1 concerned spontaneous physical activity in rodents and the influence of diet (C. C. Stewart, Department of Physiology, Clark University), neural control of muscular movement in dogs (R. H. Cunningham, College of Physicians and Surgeons, Columbia University), and perception of muscular fatigue and physical activity (J. C. Welch, Hull Physiological Laboratory, University of Chicago). As pointed out by Buskirk,[12] the next four volumes of the *American Journal of Physiology* (1898–1901) contained six additional articles about exercise physiology from experimental research laboratories at Harvard Medical School, the Massachusetts Institute of Technology, the University of Michigan, and the Johns Hopkins University.

physiologists. The journal *Medicine and Science in Sports* (now *Medicine and Science in Sports and Exercise* [www.journals.lww.com/acsm-msse/pages/default.aspx]).first published in 1969 with a goal of integrating the medical and physiologic aspects of the emerging fields of sports medicine and exercise science.

The First Textbook in Exercise Physiology: The Debate Continues

What was the first textbook in exercise physiology? Several recent exercise physiology texts give the distinction of being "first" to the English translation of Fernand Lagrange's book, *The Physiology of Bodily Exercise*, originally published in French in 1888.[6,73,76]

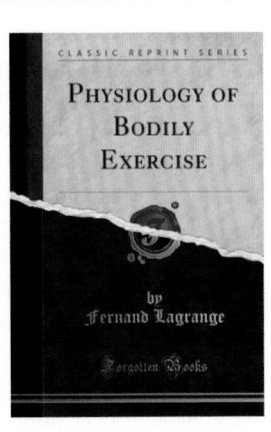

To deserve such historical recognition, we believe the work needs to meet the following three criteria:

1. Provide sound scientific rationale for major concepts
2. Provide summary information (based on experimentation) about important prior research in a particular topic area (e.g., contain scientific references to research in the area)
3. Provide sufficient "factual" information about a topic area to give it academic legitimacy

After reading the Lagrange book in its entirety, we came to the same conclusion as did George Wells Fitz in the early 1900s in a review of the text (see above). Specifically, it was a popular book about health and exercise with a "scientific" title. In our opinion, the book is *not* a legitimate "scientific" textbook of exercise physiology based on any reasonable criteria of the time. Despite Lagrange's assertion that the focus of his book assessed physiology applied to exercise and not hygiene and exercise, it is informed by a 19th-century hygienic perspective, not science. We believe Fitz would accept our evaluation.

Much information was available to Lagrange from existing European and American physiology textbooks about the digestive, muscular, circulatory, and respiratory systems, including some limited information on physical training,

hormones, basic nutrition, chemistry, and the biology of muscular contraction. Admittedly, this information was relatively scarce, but well-trained physiologists Austin Flint (profiled earlier), William H. Howell (1848–1896; first professor of physiology in the Johns Hopkins Medical School), John C. Dalton (1825–1889; first professor of physiology in America), and William B. Carpenter (1813–1885; textbook writer and experimentalist) had already produced high-quality textbooks that contained relatively detailed information about physiology in general, with some reference to muscular exercise.[49] We now understand why Fitz was so troubled by the Lagrange book. By comparison, the two-volume text by Howell, titled *An American Text-Book of Physiology*, was impressive; this edited volume contained articles from acknowledged American physiologists at the forefront of physiologic research. The Howell textbook represented a high-level physiology text even by today's standards. In his quest to provide the best possible science to teach his physical education and medical students, Fitz could not tolerate a book that did not live up to his expectations of excellence. In fact, the Lagrange book contained fewer than 20 reference citations, and most of these were ascribed to French research reports or were based on observations of friends performing exercise. This plethora of anecdotal reports must have given Fitz "fits."

Lagrange, an accomplished writer, wrote extensively on exercise. Despite the titles of several of his books,[k] Lagrange was not a scientist but probably a practicing "physical culturist." Bibliographic information about Lagrange is limited in the French and American archival records of the period—a further indication of his relative obscurity as a scholar of distinction. As far as we know, there have been no citations to his work in any physiology text or scientific article. For these reasons, we contend the Lagrange book does not qualify as the first exercise physiology textbook.[l]

Other Early Exercise Physiology Research Laboratories

The Nutrition Laboratory at the Carnegie Institute in Washington, D.C. (www.carnegiescience.edu/legacy/findingaids/CIW-Administration-Records.html), was created in 1904 to study nutrition and energy metabolism. The first research laboratories established in physical education in the United States to study exercise physiology were at George Williams

[k] The following books (including translations, editions, and pages) were published by Lagrange beginning in 1888: *Physiologie des Exercices du Corps*. Paris: Alcan, 1888, 372 pp. (6th ed., 1892); *L'Hygiene de l'Exercice Chez les Enfants et les Jeunes Gens*. Paris: Alcan, 1890, 312 pp. (4th ed., 1893; 6th ed., 1896; 7th ed, 1901; 8th ed., 1905); *Physiology of Bodily Exercise*. New York: D. Appleton, 1890, 395 pp.; *De l'Exercice Chez les Adultes*. Paris: Alcan, 1891, 367 pp. (2nd ed., 1892, 367 pp.; 4th ed., 1900, 367 pp.; Italian translation, *Fisiologia degli Esercizj del Corpo*. Milano: Dumolard, 1889; Hungarian translation, 1913); *La Medication par l'Exercice*. Paris: Alcan, 1894, 500 pp.

[l] Possible pre-1900 candidates for "first" exercise physiology textbook listed in Table 1 also include Combe's 1843 text *The Principles of Physiology Applied to the Preservation of Health, and to the Improvement of Physical and Mental Education* (read online at https://archive.org/stream/principlesofphys1835comb#page/n5/mode/2up); Hitchcock and Hitchcock's *Elementary Anatomy and Physiology for Colleges, Academies, and Other Schools* (1860; read online at https://archive.org/stream/0264002.nlm.nih.gov/0264002#page/n5/mode/2up); George Kolb's 1887 German monograph, translated into English in 1893 as *Physiology of Sport*; and the 1898 Martin text, *The Human Body. An Account of Its Structure and Activities and the Conditions of Its Healthy Working*.

College (1923), the University of Illinois (1925), and Spring-field College (1927). However, the real impact of laboratory research in exercise physiology (along with many other research specialties) occurred in 1927 with the creation of the 800-square foot Harvard Fatigue Laboratory in the basement of Morgan Hall of Harvard University's Business School.[36] During the next two decades, the outstanding work of this laboratory established the legitimacy of exercise physiology on its own merits as an important area of research and study.

Another exercise physiology laboratory started before World War II, the Laboratory of Physiological Hygiene, was created at the University of California, Berkeley in 1934. The syllabus for the Physiological Hygiene course (taught by professor Frank Lewis Kleeberger (1904–1993), the course was the precursor of contemporary exercise physiology courses) contained 12 laboratory experiments.[51] Several years later, Dr. Franklin M. Henry (1904–1993) assumed responsibility for the laboratory. Dr. Henry began publishing the results of different experiments in various physiology-oriented journals including the *Journal of Applied Physiology, Annals of Internal Medicine, Aviation Medicine, War Medicine,* and *Science*. Henry's first research project, published in 1938 as a faculty member in the Department of Physical Education, concerned the validity and reliability of the pulse–ratio test of cardiac efficiency;[29,30,31] a later paper dealt with predicting aviators' bends. Henry applied his training in experimental psychology to exercise physiology topics, including individual differences in the kinetics of the fast and slow components of the oxygen uptake and recovery curves during light- and moderate-cycle ergometer exercise; muscular strength; cardiorespiratory responses during steady-rate exercise; assessment of heavy-work fatigue; determinants of endurance performance; and neural control factors related to human motor performance (FIG. I.27).

Henry also is remembered for his experiments regarding specificity-generality of motor tasks and the "Memory-Drum Theory" of neuromotor reaction and physical performance (*J Mot Behav* 1986;18:77). Henry's seminal paper on "Physical Education as an Academic Discipline" (www.sph.umd.edu/KNES/IKE/Body/Papers/KNES/Henry-1978.pdf), paved the way for departments of physical education to change their emphasis to the science of physical activity that included in-depth study of exercise physiology, biomechanics, exercise biochemistry, motor control, and ergonomics. Henry's 1950 lab manual, *The Physiological Basis of Muscular Exercise*, was used by undergraduate and graduate students in the physiology of exercise course at UC Berkeley (*Res Q Exerc Sport* 1994;65:295).

Contributions of the Harvard Fatigue Laboratory (1927–1946)

Many of the great scientists of the 20th century with an interest in exercise were associated with the Harvard Fatigue Laboratory. This research facility was established by Lawrence J. Henderson, MD (1878–1942), renowned chemist and professor of biochemistry at the Harvard Medical School. The first

and only scientific director of the Fatigue Laboratory was David Bruce Dill (1891–1986; www.libraries.ucsd.edu/speccoll/testing/html/mss0517a.html), a Stanford PhD in physical chemistry. Dill changed his academic interest as a biochemist to an experimental physiologist while at the Fatigue Laboratory. He remained an influential driving force behind the laboratory's numerous scientific accomplishments.[20] His early academic association with Boston physician Arlen Vernon Bock (a stu-

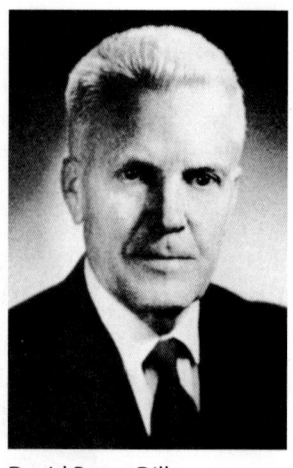

David Bruce Dill

dent of famous high-altitude physiologist Sir Joseph Barcroft [1872–1947] at the Cambridge Physiological Laboratory at Cambridge, England[5] [www.pdn.cam.ac.uk/doc/phys/; http://www.encyclopedia.com/doc/1G2-2830900266.html], and Dill's closest friend for 59 years) and contact with 1922 Nobel laureate Archibald Vivian (A. V.) Hill (for his discovery related to heat production in muscles) provided Dill with the confidence to successfully coordinate the research efforts of dozens of scholars from 15 different countries. A. V. Hill convinced Bock to write a third edition of Bainbridge's text *Physiology of Muscular Activity*. Bock, in turn, invited Dill to coauthor the book republished in 1931.[19]

Over a 20-year period, at least 352 research papers, numerous monographs,[37] and a book[20] were published in areas of basic and applied exercise physiology, including methodologic refinements concerned with blood chemistry analysis and simplified methods for analyzing the fractional concentrations of expired air.[18] Research at the Fatigue Laboratory before its demise[21] included many aspects of short-term responses and chronic physiologic adaptations to exercise under environmental stresses produced by exposure to altitude, heat, and cold (FIG. I.28).

Like the first exercise physiology laboratory established at Harvard's Lawrence Scientific School in 1892,[50] the Harvard Fatigue Laboratory demanded excellence in research and scholarship. Many of the scientists who had contact with the Fatigue Laboratory profoundly affected a new generation of exercise physiologists in the United States and abroad. Noteworthy were Ancel Keys (1904–2004), who established the Laboratory of Physiology and Physical Education (later renamed the Laboratory of Physiological Hygiene; www.cehd.umn.edu/kin/research/lphes/history.html) at the University of Minnesota, and Henry L. Taylor (1912–1983). Keys and Taylor were mentors to exercise physiologist Elsworth R. Buskirk (1925–2010), formerly at the National Institutes of Health and later the Noll Laboratory at Pennsylvania State University; Robert E. Johnson at the Human Environmental Unit at the University of Illinois; Sid Robinson (1902–1982; the first to receive a PhD from the Harvard Fatigue Laboratory) at Indiana University; Robert C. Darling (1908–1998) at the Department of Rehabilitation Medicine at Columbia

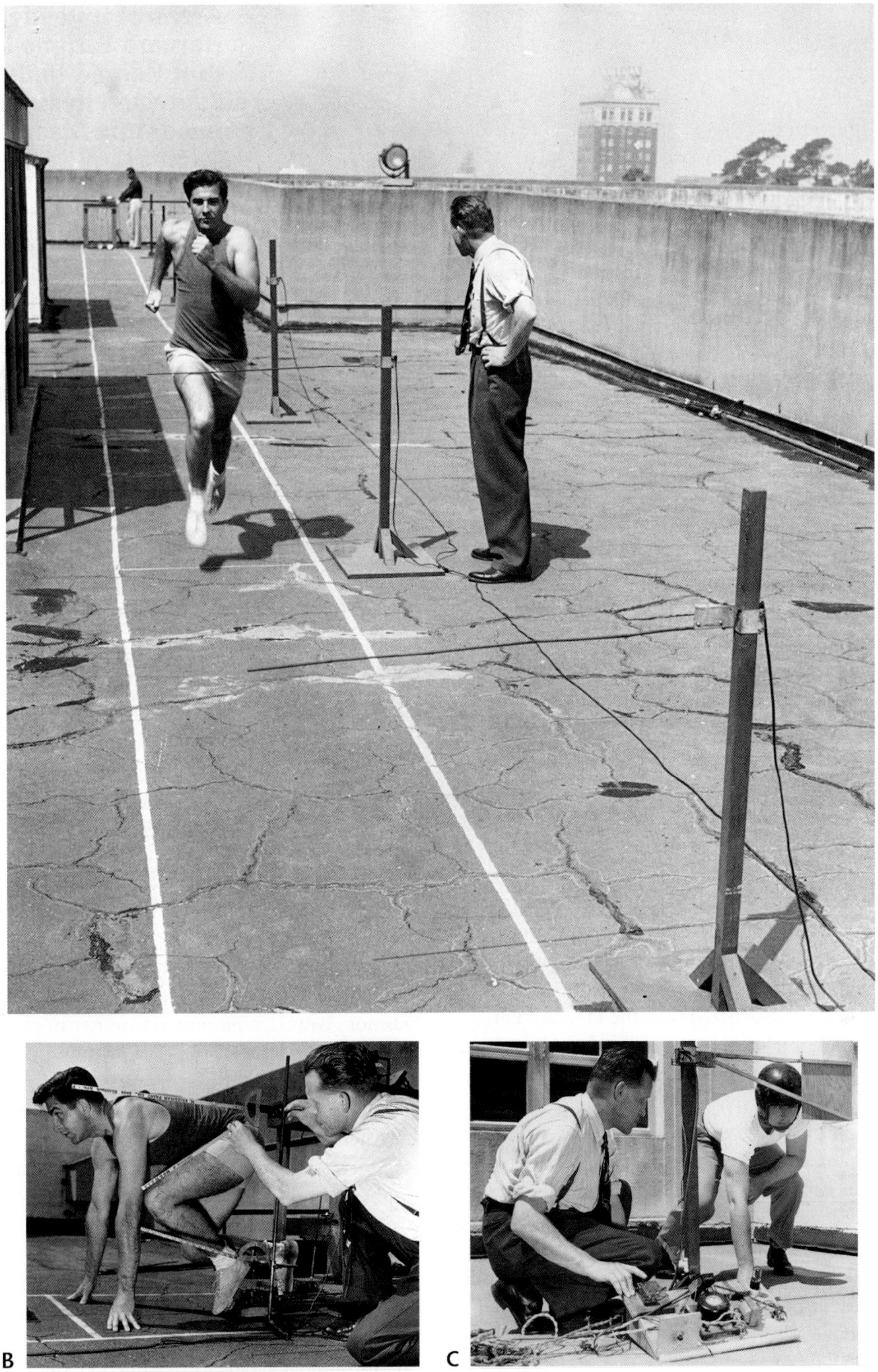

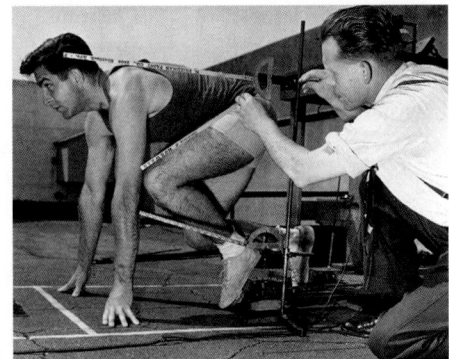

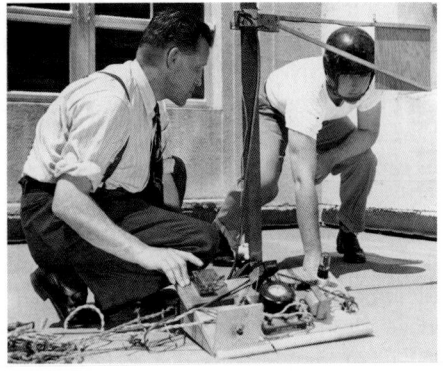

FIGURE I.27 • **(A)** Professor Franklin Henry supervising 50-yard sprints (at 5-yd intervals) on the roof of Harmon Gymnasium. Henry's study[31] was prompted by A. V. Hill's 1927 observations concerning the "viscosity" factor of muscular contraction that at first helped to explain the large decline in metabolic efficiency at fast rates of movement and that the oxygen requirement of running increased with the cube of speed. Henry verified that metabolic efficiency was not correlated with a muscle viscosity factor. **(B)** Henry making limb and trunk anthropometric measurements on a sprinter during continuous studies of the force-time characteristics of the sprint start[32] to further evaluate A. V. Hill's theoretical equation for the velocity of sprint running. **(C)** Henry recording the timing of the initial movements of blocking performance in football players.[48]

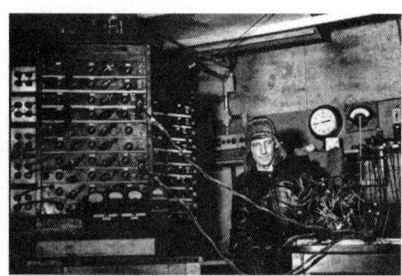

FIGURE I.28 • In 1944, researcher Donald Griffin tests the equipment he designed to assess heat distribution in gloves at −40°F. (From Folk, GE. The Harvard Fatigue Laboratory; contributions to World War II. *Adv Physiol Educ* 2010;34:119.) (www.advan.physiology.org/content/34/3/119.full.pdf+html)

University; Harwood S. Belding (1909–1973), who started the Environmental Physiology Laboratory at the University of Pittsburgh; C. Frank Consolazio (1924–1985) of the U.S. Army Medical Research and Nutrition Laboratory at Denver; Lucien Brouha (1899–1968), who headed the Fitness Research Unit at the University of Montreal and then went to the Dupont Chemical Company in Delaware; and Steven M. Horvath (1911–2007), who established the Institute of Environmental Stress at the University of California, Santa Barbara, where he worked with visiting scientists and mentored graduate students in the Departments of Biology and Ergonomics and Physical Education. After the Fatigue Laboratory was unfortunately forced to close in 1946, Dill continued as the deputy director of the U.S. Army Chemical Corps Medical Laboratory in Maryland from 1948 to 1961. Thereafter, he worked with Sid Robinson at Indiana University's physiology department. He then started the Desert Research Institute (www.dri.edu), where he studied the physiologic responses of men and animals to hot environments, a topic that culminated in a book on the subject.[22]

The group of scholars associated with the Harvard Fatigue Laboratory mentored the next generation of students who continue to make significant contributions to the field of exercise physiology. The monograph by Horvath and Horvath[36] and the chronology by Dill[21] are the best direct sources of historical information about the Harvard Fatigue Laboratory; recent studies have chronicled its research contributions.[23,67]

Exercise physiology continued to expand after the closing of the Fatigue Laboratory. Subsequent efforts probed the full range of physiologic functions. The depth and breadth of these early investigations, summarized in TABLE I.3, provides much of the current knowledge base for establishing exercise physiology as an academic field of study.

Research Methodology Textbook Focusing on Physiologic Research

In 1949, the Research Section of the Research Council of the Research Section of the American Association for Health, Physical Education, and Recreation (AAHPER; an outgrowth of the American Association for the Advancement of Physical Education created in 1885) sponsored publication of

TABLE I.3	Areas of Investigation at the Harvard Fatigue Laboratory that Helped to Establish Exercise Physiology as an Academic Discipline
1.	Specificity of the exercise prescription.
2.	Genetic components of an exercise response.
3.	Selectivity of the adaptive responses by diseased populations.
4.	Differentiation between central and peripheral adaptations.
5.	The existence of cellular thresholds.
6.	Actions of transmitters and the regulation of receptors.
7.	Feed-forward and feedback mechanisms that influence cardiorespiratory and metabolic control.
8.	Matching mechanisms between oxygen delivery and oxygen demand.
9.	The substrate utilization profile with and without dietary manipulations.
10.	Adaptive responses of cellular and molecular units.
11.	Mechanisms responsible for signal transduction.
12.	The behavior of lactate in cells.
13.	The plasticity of muscle fiber types.
14.	Motor functions of the spinal cord.
15.	The ability of hormonally deficient animals to respond to conditions of acute exercise and chronic disease.
16.	The hypoxemia of severe exercise.

From Tipton CM. Personal communication to F. Katch, June 12, 1995. From a presentation made to the American Physiological Society Meetings, 1995.

the first textbook devoted to research methodology in physical education.[1] Thomas Cureton, PhD (1901–1992; 1969 ACSM Honor Award), a pioneer researcher in physical fitness evaluation and director of the exercise physiology research laboratory, established at the University of Illinois in 1944, appointed Dr. Henry (UC Berkeley) to chair the committee to write the chapter on physiologic research methods. The other committee members were respected scientists in their own right and included the following: Anna Espenshade (1905–1973; PhD in psychology from UC Berkeley, specialist in motor development and motor performance during growth[58]); Pauline Hodgson (UC Berkeley PhD in physiology who did postdoctoral work at the Harvard Fatigue Laboratory); Peter V. Karpovich (originator of the Physiological Research Laboratory at Springfield College); Arthur H. Steinhaus, PhD (director of the research laboratory at George Williams College, one of the 11 founders of the American College of Sports Medicine and a research physiologist who authored an important review article [*Physiological Reviews*, 1933] about chronic effects of exercise); and distinguished Berkeley physiologist Hardin Jones, PhD (Donner Research Laboratory of Medical Physics at UC Berkeley).

The book chapter by this distinguished committee stands as a hallmark of research methodology in exercise physiology.

The 99 references, many of them key articles in this then-embryonic field, covered such exercise-related topics as the "heart and circulation, blood, urine and kidney function, work, lung ventilation, respiratory metabolism and energy exchange, and alveolar air."

Another masterful compendium of research methodologies published 14 years later, *Physiological Measurements of Metabolic Functions in Man*, by C. F. Consolazio and colleagues, provided complete details about specific measurements in exercise physiology.[18] Several sections in this book contained material previously published from the Harvard Fatigue Laboratory one year before its closing in 1946[35] and from another book dealing with metabolic methods published in 1951.[17]

THE NORDIC CONNECTION (DENMARK, SWEDEN, NORWAY, AND FINLAND)

Denmark and Sweden significantly impacted the history of physical education as an academic subject field. In 1800, Denmark was the first European country to include physical training (military-style gymnastics) as a requirement in the public school curriculum. Since that time, Danish and Swedish scientists have made outstanding contributions to research in both traditional physiology and exercise physiology.

Danish Influence

In 1909, the University of Copenhagen endowed the equivalent of a Chair in Anatomy, Physiology, and Theory of Gymnastics.[47] The first docent was Johannes Lindhard, MD (1870–1947). He later teamed with August Krogh (1874–1949; www.sportsci.org), Nobel Prize recipient specializing in physiological chemistry and research instrument design and

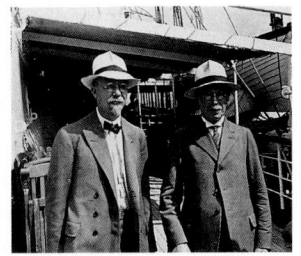

Professors August Krogh and Johannes Lindhard in the early 1930s

construction, to conduct many of the now classic experiments in exercise physiology (www.nobelprize.org/nobel_prizes/medicine/laureates/1920/krogh-bio.html). For example, Krogh and Lindhard investigated gas exchange in the lungs, pioneered studies of the relative contribution of fat and carbohydrate oxidation during exercise, measured the redistribution of blood flow during different exercise intensities, and measured cardiorespiratory dynamics in exercise (including cardiac output using nitrous oxide gas, a method described by a German researcher in 1770).

By 1910, Krogh and his wife Marie (a physician) had proven through a series of ingenious, decisive experiments[40–43]

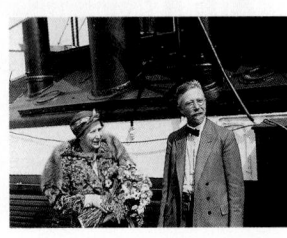

Marie and August Krogh

that diffusion was how pulmonary gas exchange occurred—not by secretion of oxygen from lung tissue into the blood during exercise and exposure to altitude, as postulated by Scottish physiologist Sir John Scott Haldane 1860–1936) and Englishman James Priestley.[28] By 1919, Krogh had published reports of a series of experiments (with three appearing in the *Journal of Physiology*, 1919) concerning the mechanism of oxygen diffusion and transport in skeletal muscles. The details of these early experiments are included in Krogh's 1936 textbook,[40] but he also was prolific in many other areas of science.[39–42] In 1920, Krogh received the Nobel Prize in Physiology or Medicine for discovering the mechanism of capillary control of blood flow in resting and exercising muscle (in frogs). To honor his prolific achievements (which included 300 scientific articles), the Institute for Physiologic Research in Copenhagen was named for him. We highly recommend the book by Schmidt-Nielsen that chronicles the incomparable contributions of August and Marie Krogh to science and exercise physiology.[68]

Three other Danish researcher-physiologists—Erling Asmussen (1907–1991; ACSM Citation Award, 1976 and ACSM Honor Award, 1979), Erik Hohwü-Christensen (1904–1996; ACSM Honor Award, 1981), and Marius Nielsen (1903–2000)—conducted pioneering studies in exercise physiology. These "three musketeers," as Krogh referred to them, published numerous research papers from the 1930s to the 1970s. Asmussen, initially an assistant in Lindhard's laboratory, became a productive researcher specializing in muscle fiber architecture and mechanics. He also

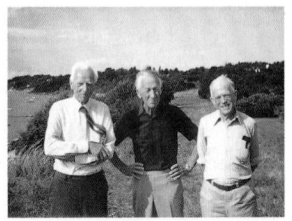

The "three musketeers," Drs. Erling Asmussen (left), Erik Hohwü-Christensen (center), and Marius Nielsen (right) (1988 photo).

published papers with Nielsen and Christensen as coauthors on many applied topics including muscular strength and performance, ventilatory and cardiovascular response to changes in posture and exercise intensity, maximum working capacity during arm and leg exercise, changes in oxidative response of muscle during exercise, comparisons of positive and negative work, hormonal and core temperature response during different intensities of exercise, and respiratory function in response to decreases in oxygen partial pressure. As evident in his classic review article of muscular exercise that cites many of his own studies (plus 75 references from other Scandinavian researchers)[2], Asmussen's grasp of the importance of the study of biologic functions during exercise is as relevant today as it was more than 45 years ago when the article was published. He clearly defines exercise physiology within the context of biologic science:

> The physiology of muscular exercise can be considered a purely descriptive science: it measures the extent to which the human organism can adapt itself to the stresses and strains of the environment and thus provides useful knowledge for athletes, trainers, industrial human engineers, clinicians, and workers in rehabilitation on the working capacity of humans and its limitations. But the physiology of muscular exercise is also part of the general biological science, physiology, which attempts to explain how the living

organism functions, by means of the chemical and physical laws that govern the inanimate world. Its important role in physiology lies in the fact that muscular exercise more than most other conditions, taxes the functions to their uttermost. Respiration, circulation, and heat regulation are only idling in the resting state. By following them through stages of increasing work intensities, a far better understanding of the resting condition is also achieved. Although the physiology of muscular exercise must be studied primarily in healthy subjects, the accumulated knowledge of how the organism responds to the stresses of exercise adds immensely to the understanding of how the organism adapts itself to disease or attempts to eliminate its effects by mobilizing its regulatory mechanisms.

Christensen became Lindhard's student in Copenhagen in 1925. Together with Krogh and Lindhard, Christensen published an important review article in 1936 that described physiologic dynamics during maximal exercise.[15] In his 1931 thesis, Christensen reported on studies of cardiac output with a modified Grollman acetylene method; body temperature and blood sugar concentration during heavy cycling exercise; comparisons of arm and leg exercise; and the effects of training. Together with Ové Hansen, he used oxygen consumption and the respiratory quotient to describe how diet, state of training, and exercise intensity and duration affected carbohydrate and fat use. Interestingly, the concept of "carbohydrate loading" was first discovered in 1939! Other notable studies included core temperature and blood glucose regulation during light-to-heavy fatiguing exercise at various ambient temperatures. A study by Christensen and Nielsen in 1942 used finger plethysmography to study regional blood flow (including skin temperature) during brief periods of constant-load cycle ergometer exercise.[15] Experiments published in 1936 by physician Olé Bang, inspired by his mentor Ejar Lundsgaard, described the fate of blood lactate during exercise of different intensities and durations.[4] The experiments of Christensen, Asmussen, Nielsen, and Hansen were conducted at the Laboratory for the Theory of Gymnastics at the University of Copenhagen. Today, the August Krogh Institute (www1.bio.ku.dk/english/) carries on the tradition of basic and applied research in exercise physiology. Since 1973, Swedish-trained scientist Bengt Saltin (1935-) (**Fig. I.29**) (the only Nordic researcher besides Erling Asmussen to receive the ACSM Citation Award [1980] and ACSM Honor Award [1990]; former student of Per-Olof Åstrand, discussed in the next section; see "Interview with Bengt Saltin," Section 4) has been a professor and continues his significant scientific studies as professor and director of the Copenhagen Muscle Research Centre at the University of Copenhagen in Denmark (www.cmrc.dk/people.htm).

Swedish Influence

Modern exercise physiology in Sweden can be traced to Per Henrik Ling (1776–1839) who in 1813 became the first director of Stockholm's Royal Central Institute of Gymnastics.[3] Ling, a specialist in fencing, developed a system of "medical gymnastics." This system, which became part of the school curriculum of Sweden in 1820, was based on his studies of anatomy and physiology.

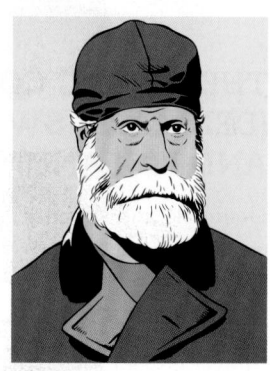

Hjalmar Ling

Ling's son Hjalmar also had a strong interest in medical gymnastics and physiology and anatomy, in part owing to his attendance at lectures by French physiologist Claude Bernard in Paris in 1854. Hjalmar Ling published a book on the kinesiology of body movements in 1866. As a result of the Lings' philosophy and influence, the physical educators who graduated from the Stockholm Central Institute were well schooled in the basic biologic sciences, in addition to being highly proficient in sports and games. Currently, the College of Physical Education (Gymnastik-Och Idrottshögskolan; www.gih.se/In-English/) and Department of Physiology in the Karolinska Institute Medical School in Stockholm continue to sponsor studies in exercise physiology and related disciplines (http://ki.se/?l=en).

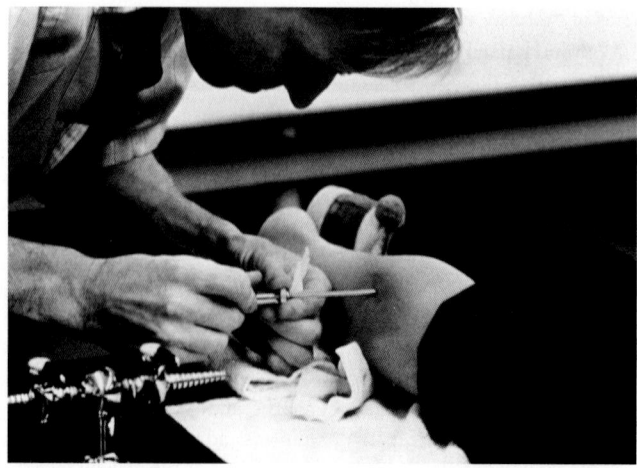

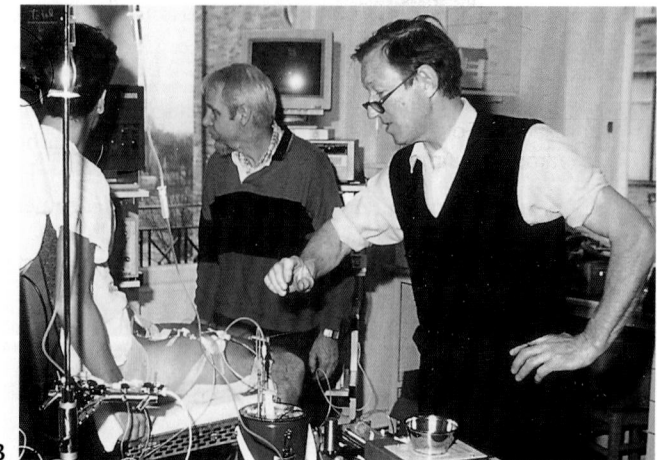

FIGURE I.29 • **(A)** Bengt Saltin taking muscle biopsy of gastrocnemius muscle. (Photo courtesy of Dr. David Costill.) **(B)** Saltin (hand on hip) during an experiment at the August Krogh Institute, Copenhagen. (Photo courtesy Per-Olof Åstrand.)

Per-Olof Åstrand, MD, PhD (1922–), is the most famous graduate of the College of Physical Education (1946); in 1952, he presented his thesis to the Karolinska Institute Medical School. Åstrand taught in the Department of Physiology in the College of Physical Education from 1946 to 1977. When the College of Physical Education became a department of the Karolinska Institute, Åstrand served as professor and department head from 1977 to 1987 (**FIG. I.30**). Christensen was Åstrand's mentor and supervised his doctoral dissertation, which included data on the physical working capacity of both sexes aged 4 to 33 years. This important study—along with collaborative studies with his wife Irma Ryhming—established a line of research that propelled Åstrand to the forefront of experimental exercise physiology for which he

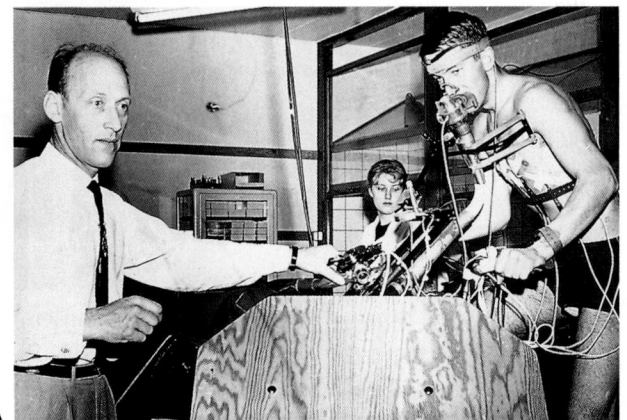

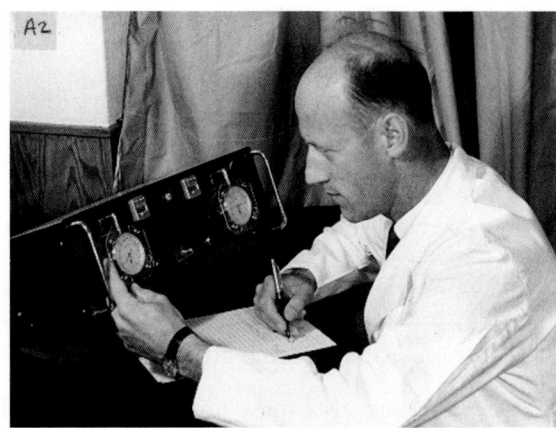

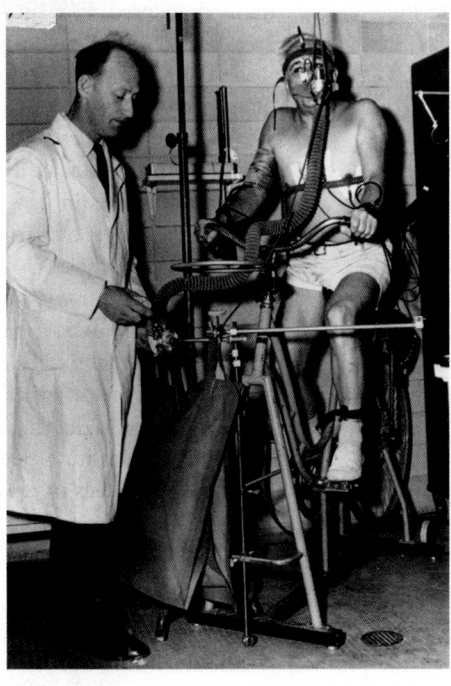

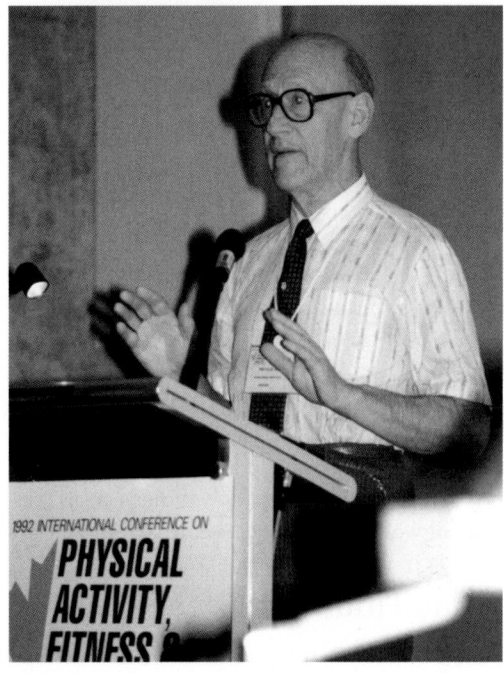

FIGURE I.30 • P-O. Åstrand, Department of Physiology. Karolinska Institute, Stockholm. **(A)** Measuring maximal performance of Johnny Nilsson, Olympic Gold Medal speed skater, 1964. **(B)** Maximal oxygen consumption measured during cycle ergometer exercise, 1958. **(C)** Laboratory experiment, 1955. **(D)** Invited lecture, 1992 International Conference on Physical Activity, Fitness and Health, Toronto.

---

[m] Personal communication to F. Katch, June 13, 1995, from Dr. Åstrand regarding his professional background. Recipient of five honorary doctorate degrees (Université de Grenoble [1968], University of Jyväskylä [1971], Institut Superieur d'Education Physique, Université Libre de Bruxelles [1987], Loughborough University of Technology [1991], and Aristoteles University of Thessaloniki [1992]). Åstrand is an honorary Fellow of nine international societies, a Fellow of the American Association for the Advancement of Science (for "outstanding career contributions to understanding of the physiology of muscular work and applications of this understanding"), and has received many awards and prizes for his outstanding scientific achievements, including the ACSM Honor Award in 1973. Åstrand served on a committee for awarding the Nobel Prize in physiology or medicine from 1977 to 1988 and is coauthor with Kaare Rodahl of *Textbook of Work Physiology* (3rd edition, 1986; translated in Chinese, French, Italian, Japanese, Korean, Portuguese, and Spanish). His English publications number about 200 (including book chapters, proceedings, a history of Scandinavian scientists in exercise physiology,[3] and monographs), and he has given invited lectures in approximately 50 countries and 150 different cities outside of Sweden. His classic 1974 pamphlet *Health and Fitness* has an estimated distribution of 15 to 20 million copies (about 3 million copies in Sweden)—unfortunately, all without personal royalty!

achieved worldwide fame.[m] Four papers published by Åstrand in 1960, with Christensen as one of the authors, stimulated further studies on the physiologic responses to intermittent exercise. Åstrand has mentored an impressive group of exercise physiologists, including such "superstars" as Bengt Saltin and Björn T. Ekblom.

Further evidence of their phenomenal international influence is seen in the number of times each is cited annually in the scientific literature: an average of 15,000 to 20,000 times *annually* from 1996 through April 2001.

thePoint   Appendix A, available online at http://thepoint. lww.com/mkk8e, provides several bibliographies of influential publications pertaining to anatomy and physiology, anthropometry, exercise and training, and exercise physiology, including a sampling of contributions to the exercise physiology literature by Åstrand and Saltin in books, book chapters, monographs, and research articles.

Two Swedish scientists at the Karolinska Institute, Drs. Jonas Bergström and Erik Hultman, performed important

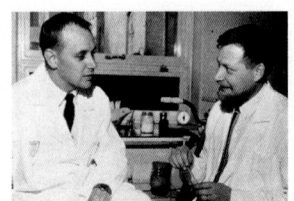

experiments with the needle biopsy procedure that have provided a new vista from which to study exercise physiology. With this procedure, it became relatively easy to conduct invasive studies of muscle under various exercise conditions, training, and nutritional status. Collaborative work with other Scan-

Drs. Jonas Bergström (left) and Eric Hultman, Karolinska Institute, mid-1960s

dinavian researchers (Saltin and Hultman from Sweden and Lars Hermanson from Norway) and leading researchers in the United States (e.g., Phillip Gollnick [1935–1991; Washington State University] and David Costill [1936-] [John and Janice Fisher Professor Emeritus of Exercise Science, Ball State University]) contributed a unique new dimension to the study of the physiology of muscular exercise.

Norwegian and Finnish Influence

The new generation of exercise physiologists trained in the late 1940s analyzed respiratory gases by means of a highly accurate sampling apparatus that measured relatively small quantities of carbon dioxide and oxygen in expired air. The method of analysis (and also the analyzer) was developed in 1947 by Norwegian scientist Per Scholander (1905–1980). A diagram of Scholander's micrometer gas analyzer[69] is presented in Chapter 8, Figure 8.7, along with its larger counterpart, the Haldane analyzer.

Another prominent Norwegian researcher was Lars A. Hermansen (1933–1984; ACSM Citation Award, 1985) from the Institute of Work Physiology, who died prematurely. Nevertheless, his many contributions include a classic 1969 article, "Anaerobic Energy Release," that appeared in the first volume of *Medicine and Science in Sports*.[33] Other papers included work with exercise physiologist K. Lange Andersen.[34]

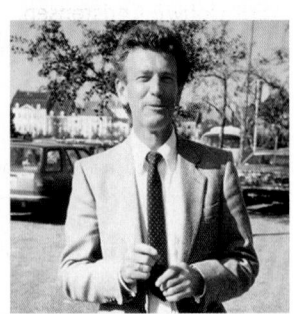

Lars A. Hermansen (1933–1984), Institute of Work Physiology, Oslo

In Finland, Martti Karvonen, MD, PhD (ACSM Honor Award, 1991; 1918–2009;), from the Physiology Department of the Institute of Occupational Health in Helsinki, is best known for a method to predict optimal exercise training heart rate, the so-called "Karvonen formula." He also conducted studies dealing with exercise performance and the role of exercise in longevity. In 1952, Lauri Pikhala, a physiologist, suggested that obesity was the consequence and not the cause of physical "unfitness." Ilkka Vuori, starting in the early 1970s, reported on hormone responses to exercise. Paavo Komi, Professor Emeritus from the Department of Biology of Physical Activity at the University of Jyväskylä, has been Finland's most prolific researcher, with numerous experiments published in the combined areas of exercise physiology and sport biomechanics. TABLE I.4 lists the Nordic researchers who have received the prestigious ACSM Honor Award or ACSM Citation Award.

OTHER CONTRIBUTORS TO THE KNOWLEDGE BASE IN EXERCISE PHYSIOLOGY

In addition to the distinguished American and Nordic applied scientists profiled earlier, there have been many other "giants" in the field of physiology and experimental science[n] who have made monumental contributions that indirectly added to the knowledge base in exercise physiology. The list includes:

---

[n]There are many excellent sources of information about the history of science and medicine, including the following: Bettman O. *A Pictorial History of Medicine*. Springfield, IL: Charles C Thomas, 1956; Clendening L. *Source Book of Medical History*. New York: Dover Publications/Henry Schuman, 1960; Coleman W. *Biology in the Nineteenth Century*. New York: Cambridge University Press, 1977; Franklin K. *A Short History of Physiology*, 2nd ed. London: Staples Press, 1949; Fye WB, *The Development of American Physiology. Scientific Medicine in the Nineteenth Century*. Baltimore: Johns Hopkins University Press, 1987; Guthrie D. A *History of Medicine*. London: T. Nelson & Sons, 1945; Haskins T. *Science and Enlightenment*. New York: Cambridge University Press, 1985; Holmes FL. *Lavoisier and the Chemistry of Life*. Madison: University of Wisconsin Press, 1985; Knight B. *Discovering the Human Body*. London: Bloomsbury Books; Lesch JE. *Science and Medicine in France. The Emergence of Experimental Physiology, 1790–1855*. Cambridge, MA: Harvard University Press, 1984; Vertinsky PA. *The Eternally Wounded Woman: Women, Exercise, and Doctors in the Late Nineteenth Century*. Urbana: University of Illinois Press; Walker K. *The Story of Medicine*. London: Arrow Books, 1954.

Nordic Researchers[a] Awarded the ACSM Honor Award and ACSM Citation Award

TABLE 1.4

ACSM Honor Award	ACSM Citation Award
Per-Olof Åstrand, 1973	Erling Asmussen, 1976
Erling Asmussen, 1979	Bengt Saltin, 1980
Erik Hohwü-Christensen, 1981	Lars A. Hermansen, 1985
Bengt Saltin, 1990	C. Gunnar Blomqvist, 1987
Martti J. Karvonen, 1991	

[a]Born and educated in a Nordic country.

Sir Joseph Barcroft (1872–1947). High-altitude research physiologist who pioneered fundamental work concerning the functions of hemoglobin, later confirmed by Nobel laureate August Krogh. Barcroft also performed experiments to determine how cold affected the central nervous system. For up to 1 hr, he would lie without clothing on a couch in subfreezing temperatures and record his subjective reactions.

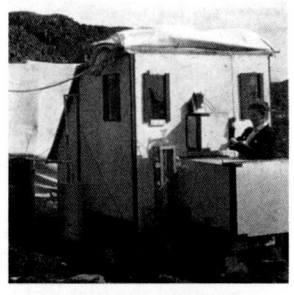

Marie Krogh collects data at Barcraft's high altitude experimental station to assess oxygen tension of gases

Christian Bohr (1855–1911). Professor of physiology in the medical school at the University of Copenhagen who mentored August Krogh, and father of nuclear physicist and Nobel laureate Niels Bohr. Bohr studied with Carl Ludwig in Leipzig in 1881 and 1883, publishing papers on the solubility of gases in various fluids,

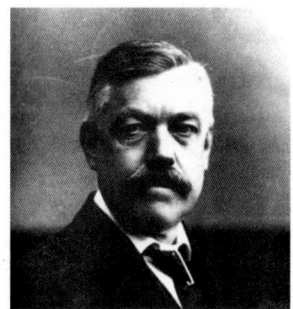

Christian Bohr

including oxygen absorption in distilled water and in solutions containing hemoglobin. Krogh's careful experiments using advanced instruments (microtonometer) disproved Bohr's secretion theory that both oxygen and carbon dioxide were secreted across the lung epithelium in opposite directions based on the time required for equalization of gas tension in blood and air.

John Scott Haldane (1860–1936; www.faqs.org/health/bios/55/John-Scott-Haldane.html). Conducted research in mine safety, investigating principally the action of dangerous gases (carbon monoxide), the use of rescue equipment, and the incidence of pulmonary disease. He devised a decompression apparatus for the safe ascent of deep-sea divers. The British Royal Navy and the United States Navy adopted tables

based on this work. In 1905, he discovered that carbon dioxide acted on the brain's respiratory center to regulate breathing. In 1911, he and several other physiologists organized an expedition to Pikes Peak, Colorado, to study the effects of low oxygen pressures at high altitudes. Haldane also showed that the reaction of oxyhemoglobin with ferricyanide rapidly and quantitatively released oxygen and formed methemoglobin. The amount of liberated oxygen could be accurately calculated

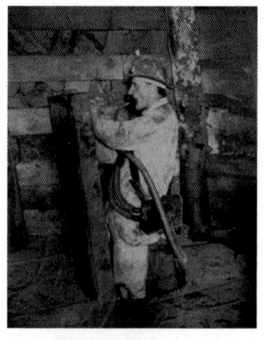

Haldane investigating carbon monoxide gas in an English coal mine at the turn of the 20th century

from the increased gas pressure in the closed reaction system at constant temperature and volume. Haldane devised a microtechnique to fractionate a sample of a mixed gas into its component gases (see Chapter 8). Haldane founded the *Journal of Hygiene.*

Otto Meyerhof (1884–1951; www.nobelprize.org/nobel_prizes/medicine/laureates/1922/meyerhof-bio.html). Meyerhof's experiments on the energy changes during cellular respiration led to discoveries on lactic acid related to muscular activity, research that led to the Nobel Prize (with A.V. Hill in 1923). In 1925, Meyerhof extracted from muscle the enzymes that convert glycogen to lactic acid. Subsequent research confirmed work

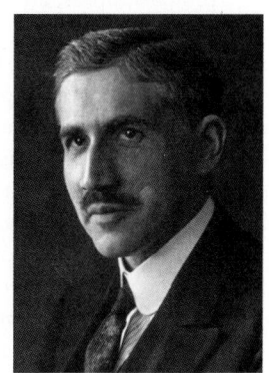

Otto Meyerhof (Courtesy National Library of Medicine)

done by Gustav Embden in 1933; together they discovered the pathway that converts glucose to lactic acid (the Embden-Meyerhof pathway).

Nathan Zuntz (1847–1920). Devised the first portable metabolic apparatus to assess respiratory exchange in animals and humans at different altitudes; proved that carbohydrates were precursors for lipid synthesis. He maintained that dietary lipids and carbohydrates should not be consumed equally for proper nutrition. He produced 430 articles concerning blood and blood gases, circulation, mechan-

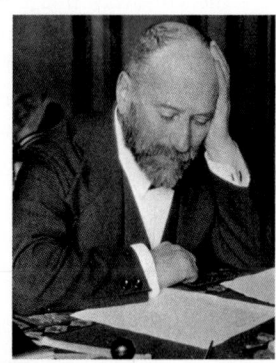

Nathan Zuntz (Courtesy National Library of Medicine)

ics and chemistry of respiration, general metabolism and metabolism of specific foods, energy metabolism and heat production, and digestion.

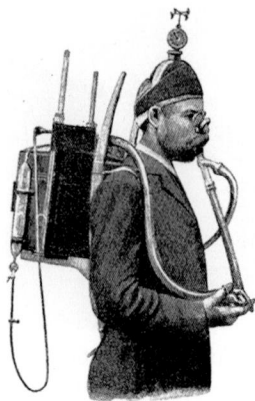

Zuntz tests his portable, closed-circuit spirometer, carried on his back. This device made it possible for the first time to measure O_2 consumed and CO_2 produced during ambulation. (Courtesy Max Planck Institute for the History of Science, Berlin/Virtual Lab; http://mpiwg-berlin.mpg/technology/data?id=tec1715.)

Carl von Voit (1831–1908; www.bookrags.com/biography/karl-von-voit-wsd/*)* and his student *Max Rubner (1854–1932)*. Discovered the isodynamic law and the calorific heat values of proteins, lipids, and carbohydrates; Rubner's surface area law states that resting heat production is proportional to body surface area and that consuming food

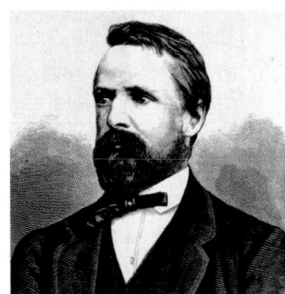

Carl von Voit (Courtesy National Library of Medicine)

increases heat production. Voit disproved Liebig's assertion that protein was a primary energy fuel by showing that protein breakdown does not increase in proportion to exercise duration or intensity.

Max Joseph von Pettenkofer (1818–1901). Perfected the respiration calorimeter (**Fig. I.31**) to study human and animal metabolism; discovered creatinine, an amino acid in urine. The top chamber of the figure below shows the entire calorimeter. The cut-away image shows a human experiment where fresh air was pumped into the sealed

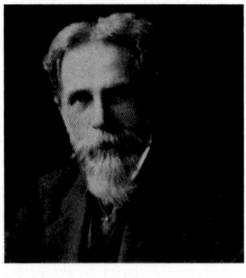

Max Joseph von Pettenkofer

chamber and vented air sampled for carbon dioxide.

Eduard F. W. Pflüger (1829–1910). First demonstrated that minute changes in the partial pressure of blood gases affect the rate of oxygen release across capillary membranes, thus proving that blood flow alone does not govern how tissues receive oxygen.

Wilbur Olin Atwater (1844–1907; www.sportsci.org*)*. Published data about the chemical composition of 2600 American foods currently used in databases of food composition. Also performed human calorimetric experiments and confirmed that the law of conservation of energy governs transformation of matter in the human body.

Russel Henry Chittenden (1856–1943; www.sportsci.org*)*. Refocused attention on the minimal protein requirement of humans while resting or exercising; concluded that no debilitation occurred if protein intake equaled $1.0 \text{ g} \cdot \text{kg}$ body mass^{-1} in either normal or athletic young men. Chittenden received the first PhD in physiological chemistry given by an American university. Some scholars[12] regard Chittenden as the father of biochemistry in the United States. He believed that physiological chemistry would provide basic tools for researchers to study important aspects of physiology and provided the impetus for incorporating biochemical analyses in exercise physiology.

Frederick Gowland Hopkins (1861–1947; www.sportsci.org*)*. Nobel Prize in 1929 for isolating and identifying the structure of the amino acid tryptophan. Hopkins collaborated with W. M. Fletcher (mentor to A. V. Hill) to study muscle chemistry. Their classic 1907 paper in experimental physiology used new methods to isolate lactic acid in muscle. Fletcher

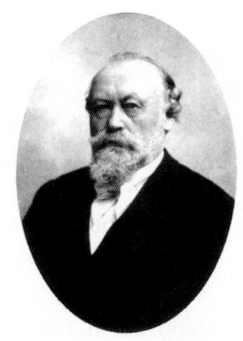

Edward F. W. Pflüger (Courtesy National Library of Medicine)

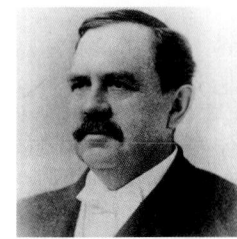

Wilbur Olin Atwater (Courtesy National Library of Medicine)

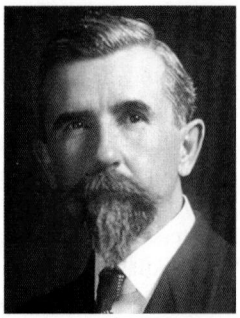

Russel Henry Chittenden (Courtesy National Library of Medicine)

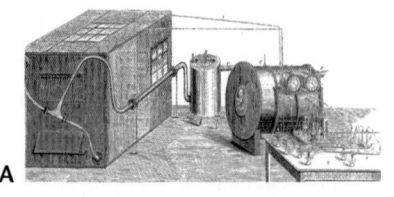
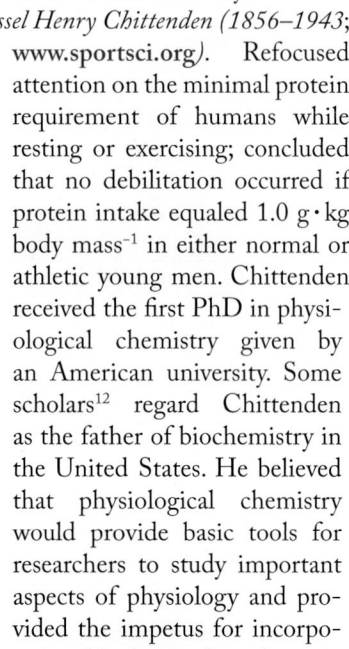
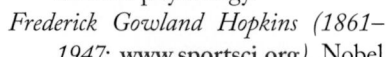

A   B

FIGURE I.31 • Human respiration calorimeter. (Courtesy Max Planck Institute for the History of Science, Berlin/Virtual Lab; http://mpiwg-berlin.mpg.de/technology/data?id=tec209.)

and Hopkins's chemical methods reduced the muscle's enzyme activity prior to analysis to isolate the reactions. They found that a muscle contracting under low oxygen conditions produced lactate at the expense of glycogen. Conversely, oxygen in muscle suppressed lactate formation. The researchers deduced that lactate forms from a nonoxidative (anaerobic) process during contraction; during recovery in a noncontracted state, an oxidative (aerobic) process removes lactate with oxygen present.

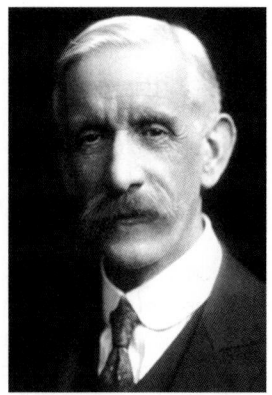

Frederick Gowland Hopkins (Courtesy National Library of Medicine)

Francis Gano Benedict (1870–1957; www.sportsci.org). Conducted exhaustive studies of energy metabolism in newborn infants, growing children and adolescents, starving persons, athletes, and vegetarians. Devised "metabolic standard tables" based on sex, age, height, and weight to compare energy metabolism in normals and patients. His last monograph, *Vital Energetics, A Study in Comparative Basal Metabolism* (Carnegie Institution Monograph no. 503, 1938), refers to many of his approximately 400 publications.

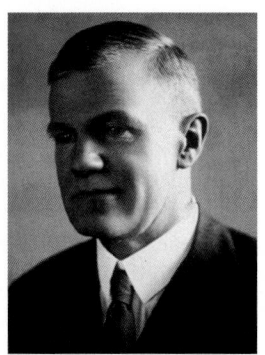

Francis Gano Benedict (Courtesy National Library of Medicine)

THE ROYAL SOCIETY OF LONDON

Arguably the oldest scientific society, founded in 1660 in England, the Royal Society of London began as a group of 12 physicians and philosophers who studied nature and the physical universe (the genesis of the natural sciences such as physics and astronomy) to advance discourse concerning the discoveries of new knowledge. The founders included Christopher Wren (1632–1723; astronomer, English architect who rebuilt 51 churches in London after the devastating fire of London in 1666) and Robert Boyle (1627–1691). Weekly meetings viewed experiments and discussed scientific topics of interest developed in England including continental Europe, most notably scientific advances in France. In 1662, King Charles II granted the organization its official charter, known formally in 1663 as The Royal Society of London for Improving Natural Knowledge or simply the Royal Society (http://royalsociety.org/about-us/history/) (**Fig. I.32**).

The society soon began publication of its journals (*The Philosophical Transactions*) the world's first devoted to science, published in March 1665, that included peer review,

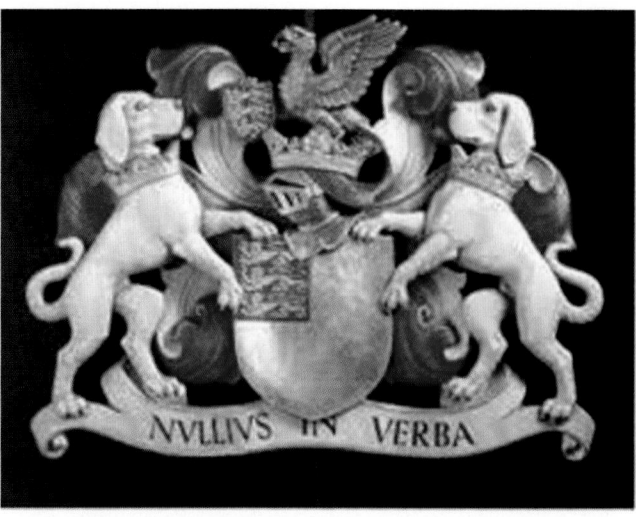

FIGURE I.32 • The Royal Society's motto "Nullius in verba" translates as "Take nobody's word for it," which expressed the members' desire to overcome the domination of aristocratic authority, and foster the appreciation of facts determined by experiment, not dogma, ritual, and personal opinion.

and currently deals with thematic issues. The *Proceedings of the Royal Society* includes *Series A* that publishes research related to mathematical, physical, and engineering sciences, and *Series B* that publishes research related to biology. Fellowship in the Society consists of the most eminent engineers, scientists, and technologists from the United Kingdom and British Commonwealth. Each year the Society elects 44 new Fellows, including 8 Foreign Members and up to 1 Honorary Member from about 700 proposed candidates. In 2012, there were 1450 Fellows and Foreign Members. The elite Society membership beginning in 1901 includes 80 Nobel Laureates. Within the domain relevant to exercise science, the Members include seven scientists we chronicle in this text, all winning the Nobel Prize in the category Physiology or Medicine (August Krogh, 1920; Otto Meyerhof, 1922; A.V. Hill, 1922; Frederick Hopkins, 1929; Hans Krebs, 1953; and James Watson and Maurice Wilkins, 1962).

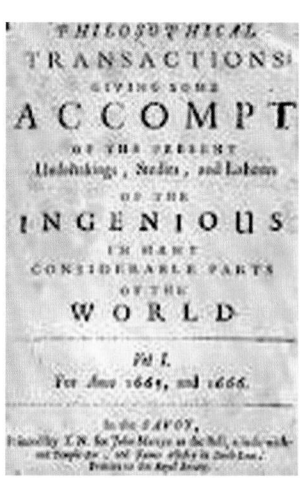

CONTRIBUTIONS OF WOMEN TO SCIENCE AT THE DAWN OF THE 20TH CENTURY

The triumphs and accomplishments during the evolution of exercise physiology reveal a glaring absence of credit to the contributions of women from the 1850s and continuing for the next 100 years. Many reasons explain this occurrence—but it was not from women's lack of interest in pursuing a career in the sciences. Rather, females who wished to stand with male colleagues found the going difficult. Opposition included hostility, ridicule, and professional discrimination, typically in chemistry, physics, and medicine, but also in related fields such as botany, biology, and mathematics. A few women did break through the almost exclusively male-dominated fields to make significant contributions despite such considerable hurdles. The leadership at the "top" of the scientific culture (college presidents, academic deans, curriculum and personnel committees, governing bodies, heads of departments, and review boards for grants and journals) subtly and directly repressed women's attempts to even enter some fields, let alone achieve parity with male scientists. Subtle discrimination included assignment to underequipped, understaffed, and substandard laboratory facilities; having to teach courses without proper university recognition; disallowing membership on graduate thesis or dissertation committees; and having a male colleague's name appear first (or only) on research publications, regardless of his involvement. Male "supervisors" typically presented the results of joint work at conferences and seminars when the woman clearly worked as the lead scientist. Direct suppression included outright refusal to hire women to teach at the university or college level. For those who were hired, many could not directly supervise graduate student research projects. Women also routinely experienced shameful inequity in salary received or were paid no salary as "assistants."

The Nobel Prize in the sciences, the most prestigious award for discoveries in physics, chemistry, and physiology or medicine, has honored 300 men but only 10 women since the award originated in 1901. The Karolinska Institute in Stockholm (http://ki.se/ki/jsp/polopoly.jsp?d=130&l=en) selects the Nobel laureates in physiology or medicine, and the Swedish Academy of Sciences awards the prizes in chemistry and physics. Considerable controversy has emerged over the years about the role of "infighting and politics" in the selection process. The difference in the gender-specific pool of outstanding scientists cannot adequately explain the disparity between male and female Nobel winners. Reading about the lives and times of the 10 female winners, including others who by all accounts probably deserved the honor, gives a better appreciation for the inequity. Each of the 10 female laureates and the other 3 world-class scientists listed here overcame huge "nonscientific" issues before achieving their eventual scientific triumphs.

1. Gerty Radnitz Cori (1896–1954); Biological chemistry
2. Marie Sklodowska Curie (1867–1934); Chemistry, physics
3. Irene Joliot-Curie (1897–1956); Chemistry
4. Barbara McClintock (1902–1992); Cytogenetics
5. Maria Goeppert Mayer (1906–1972); Physics
6. Rita Levi-Montalcini (1909–2012); Developmental neurology and physiology
7. Dorothy Crowfoot Hodgkin (1910–1994); x-ray crystallography and chemistry
8. Gertrude B. Elion (1918–1999); Chemistry
9. Rosalyn Sussman Yalow (1921–2011); Medicine
10. Christiane Nüsslein-Volhard (1942–); Developmental biology
11. Lise Meitner (1878–1968); Physics
12. Rosalind Franklin (1920–1958); Chemistry
13. Wu-Chien-Shiung Wu (1912–1997); Theoretical physics

thePoint Appendix B, "Scientific Contributions of 13 Outstanding Female Scientists," available online at http://thepoint.lww.com/mkk8e, provides details about the lives and times of the women listed above.

We hope the legacy of the exercise physiology pioneers discussed in this chapter inspires students to strive for excellence in their particular specialty. Successful scientists often must surmount many obstacles along the way to achieve success and recognition. They all shared common traits—an unyielding passion for science and uncompromising quest to explore new ground where others had not ventured. As you progress in your own careers, we hope that you too will experience the pure joy of discovering new truths in exercise physiology. Perhaps the achievements of women scientists from outside our field will serve as a gentle reminder to support the next generation of scientists from their accomplishments and passion for their field.

Summary

This introductory section on the historical development of exercise physiology illustrates that interest in exercise and health had its roots with the ancients. During the 2000 years that followed, the field we now call *exercise physiology* evolved from a symbiotic (albeit, sometimes rocky) relationship between the classically trained physicians, the academically based anatomists and physiologists, and a small cadre of physical educators who struggled to achieve their identity and academic credibility through research and experimentation in the basic and applied sciences. The physiologists used exercise to study the dynamics of human physiology, and the early physical educators often adapted the methodology and knowledge of physiology to study human responses to exercise.

Beginning in the mid-1850s in the United States, a small but slowly growing effort to raise standards for the scientific training of physical education and hygiene specialists primarily targeted teaching at the college and university level. The creation of the first exercise physiology laboratory at Harvard University in 1891 contributed to an already burgeoning knowledge explosion in basic physiology, primarily in Britain and throughout Europe. Originally, medically trained physiologists made the significant scientific advances in most of the subspecialties now included in the exercise physiology course curriculum. They studied oxygen metabolism, muscle structure and function, gas transport and exchange, mechanisms of circulatory dynamics, digestion, and neural control of voluntary and involuntary muscular activity.

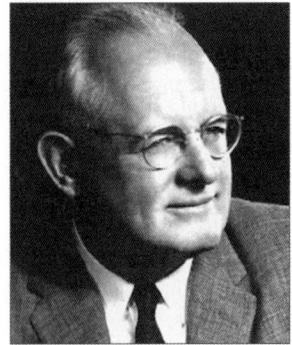

Thomas K. Cureton

The field of exercise physiology also owes a debt of gratitude to the pioneers of the physical fitness movement in the United States, spearheaded by Thomas K. Cureton (1901–1993). Cureton was one of the charter members of the American College of Sports Medicine (ACSM; 1969 recipient of the prestigious ACSM Honor Award) and a professor of physical education at the University of Illinois at Champaign. Cureton trained four generations of Master's and PhD degree students beginning in 1941 after an initial teaching period at Springfield College in Massachusetts that began in 1929.

Many of the graduates who were mentored by individuals such as T. K. Cureton assumed leadership positions as professors with teaching and research responsibilities in exercise physiology at numerous colleges and universities in the United States and throughout the world.

Although we have focused on the contributions of selected early American scientists and physical educators and their counterparts from the Nordic countries to the development of modern-day exercise physiology, we would be neglectful not to acknowledge the numerous contributions from many scholars in other countries. The group of foreign contributors, many still active researchers, includes but certainly is not limited to the following individuals: Roy Shephard, School of Physical and Health Education, University of Toronto (ACSM Citation Award, 1991; ACSM Honor Award, 2001; http://g-se.com/es/usuario/perfil/roy-j-shephard); Claude Bouchard, Pennington Biomedical Research "Center, Baton Rouge, LA (ACSM Citation Award, 1992; ACSM Honor Award, 2002; John W. Barton, Sr. Endowed Chair in Genetics and Nutrition); Oded Bar-Or (1937–2005), McMaster University, Hamilton, Ontario, Canada (ACSM Citation Award, 1997; ACSM President's Lecture); Rodolfo Margaria (1901–1983) and P. Cerretelli (1932–2008), Institute of Human Physiology, Medical School of the University of Milan; M. Ikai, School of Education, University of Japan; Wildor Holloman (1925–), Director of the Institute for Circulation, Research and Sports Medicine and L. Brauer and H. W. Knipping (1895-1984), Institute of Medicine, University of Cologne, Germany (in 1929, they described the "vita maxima," now called the maximal oxygen consumption); L. G. C. E. Pugh (1909–1994), Medical Research Council Laboratories, London; Z. I. Barbashova, Sechenov Institute of Evolutionary Physiology, Leningrad, USSR; Sir Cedric Stanton Hicks (1892–1976), Human Physiology Department, University of Adelaide, Australia; Otto Gustaf Edholm (1862–1950), National Institute for Medical Research, London; John Valentine George Andrew Durnin, Department of Physiology,

Glasgow University, Scotland; Lucien Brohua (1899–1968), Higher Institute of Physical Education, Faculty of Medicine of the State University of Liège, Belgium, and Harvard Fatigue Laboratory; Reginald Passmore (1910–1999), Department of Physiology, University of Edinburgh, Scotland; Ernst F. Jokl (1907–1997) [ACSM founder and charter member], Witwatersrand Technical College, Johannesburg, South Africa, and later the University of Kentucky; and C. H. Wyndham and N. B. Strydom, University of the Witwatersrand, South Africa. There were also many early German scientific contributions to exercise physiology and sports medicine.[35]

CONCLUDING COMMENT

One theme unites the history of exercise physiology: the value of mentoring by those visionaries who spent an extraordinary amount of their careers "infecting" students with love for hard science. These demanding but inspiring relationships developed researchers who, in turn, nurtured the next generation of productive scholars. This applies not only to the current group of exercise physiologists, but also to scholars of previous generations. Siegel[71] cites Payne,[62] who in 1896 wrote the following about Harvey's 1616 discovery of the mechanism of the circulation, acknowledging the discoveries of the past:

> No kind of knowledge has ever sprung into being without an antecedent, but is inseparably connected with what was known before…. We are led back to Aristotle and Galen as the real predecessors of Harvey in his work concerning the heart. It was the labors of the great school of Greek anatomists … that the problem though unsolved, was put in such a shape that the genius of Harvey was enabled to solve it…. The moral is, I think, that the influence of the past on the present is even more potent than we commonly suppose. In common and trivial things, we may ignore this connection; in what is of enduring worth we cannot.

We end our overview of the history of exercise physiology with a passage from *A Treatise on Physiology and Hygiene* (New York: Harper & Brothers 1868), a textbook written 146 years ago by John Call Dalton (1825–1889), MD, the first American-born professor of physiology at the College of Physicians and Surgeons in New York City. It shows how current themes in exercise physiology share a common bond with what was known and advocated at that time (the benefits of moderate physical activity, walking as an excellent exercise, the appropriate exercise intensity, the specificity of training, the importance of mental well-being). Even the "new" thoughts and ideas of Dalton penned in 1869 had their roots in antiquity—reinforcing to us the importance of maintaining a healthy respect for the importance of exercise in our daily lives.

> The natural force of the muscular system requires to be maintained by constant and regular exercise. If all of the muscles, or those of any particular part, be allowed to remain for a long time unused they diminish in size, grow softer, and finally become

sluggish and debilitated. By use and exercise, on the contrary, they maintain their vigor, continue plump and firm to the touch, and retain all the characters of their healthy organization. It is very important, therefore, that the muscles should be trained and exercised by sufficient daily use. Too much confinement by sedentary occupation, in study, or by simple indulgence in indolent habits, will certainly impair the strength of the body and injuriously affect the health. Every one who is in a healthy condition should provide for the free use of the muscles by at least two hours' exercise each day; and this exercise can not be neglected with impunity, any more than the due provision of clothing and food…. The muscular exercise of the body, in order to produce its proper effect, should be regular and moderate in degree. It will not do for any person to remain inactive during the greater part of the week, and then take an excessive amount of exercise on a single day…. It is only a uniform and healthy action of the parts that stimulates the muscles and provides for their nourishment and growth…. Walking is therefore one of the most useful kinds of exercise…. Running and leaping, being more violent should be used more sparingly…. The exact quantity of exercise to be taken is not precisely the same for different persons, but should be measured by its effect. It is always beneficial when it has fully employed the muscular powers without producing any sense of excessive fatigue or exhaustion…. In all cases, the exercise that is taken should be regular and uniform in degree, and should be repeated as nearly as possible for the same time every day.

As a student of exercise physiology, you are about to embark on an exciting journey into the world of human physiologic response and adaptation to physical activity. We hope our tour of the beginnings of exercise physiology inspires you in your studies to begin your own journey to new discoveries.

thePoint References are available online at http://thepoint.lww.com/mkk8e.

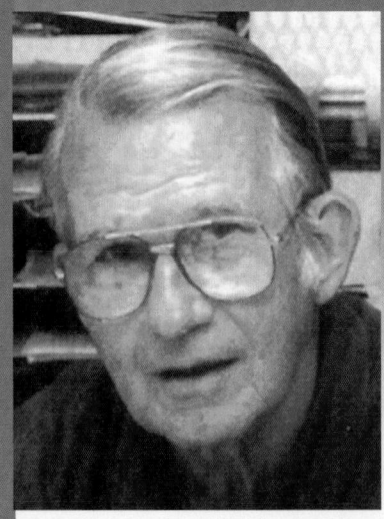

INTERVIEW WITH
Dr. Charles M. Tipton

Education: BA (Springfield College, Springfield, MA); MA, PhD in Physiology, with minors in Biochemistry and Anatomy (University of Illinois, Champaign).

Current Affiliation: Professor Emeritus of Physiology and Orthopaedic Surgery at the College of Medicine at the University of Arizona.

Honors, Awards, and ACSM Honor Award Statement of Contributions: See Appendix C, available online at http://thepoint.lww.com/mkk8e

Research Focus: The physiologic effects of short- and long-term exercise and their responsible mechanisms.

Memorable Publication: Tipton CM, et al. The influence of exercise, intensity, age, and medication on resting systolic blood pressure of SHR populations. *J Appl Physiol* 1983;55:1305.

What first inspired you to enter the exercise science field? What made you decide to pursue your degree and/or line of research?

➤ My experiences in athletics and as a Physical Fitness Instructor in an infantry division convinced me that I should secure an education on the G.I. Bill of Rights to be able to teach health and physical education while coaching in a rural high school. Once I realized that I did not enjoy my chosen career, I returned to the University of Illinois for more education in health education. To support a growing family, I secured a summer and part-time position as a 4-H Club Fitness Specialist who conducted fitness tests and clinics throughout the state of Illinois. When it became apparent that I had to have more physiology and biochemistry to explain what I was testing and advocating, I knew I had to be a physiologist with expertise in exercise physiology. So I transferred to the Physiology Department, and the rest is history.

What influences did your undergraduate education have on your final career choice?

➤ Very little. Although I had the late Peter V. Karpovich as my exercise physiology instructor at Springfield College, he did not stimulate, motivate, or encourage me to consider becoming one. My mindset was to teach and coach in a rural high school, and everything in the undergraduate curriculum or experience was to help me achieve that goal.

Who were the most influential people in your career, and why?

➤ The drive to learn and acquire more education was imprinted by my father, who had to leave school in the eighth grade to help support his family. Early in graduate school at the University of Illinois, I became interested in the physiological and biochemical foundations of physical fitness by the interesting and evangelical lectures of Dr. Thomas K. Cureton in the Physical Education Department and Director of the Physical Fitness Laboratory. However, my interest in physiological research and its scientific foundations was stimulated, developed, and perfected by Darl M. Hall, who was an intelligent critical and caring research scientist in the Illinois

Extension Service who had the responsibility of testing the fitness levels of 4-H Club members. Our discussions made me realize that functional explanations require in-depth scientific knowledge and encouraged me to transfer into the physiology department to secure such information. Once in physiology, I became exposed to the impressive intelligence and outstanding scholarship of Robert E. Johnson and to his example of the scientific attributes necessary to become a productive exercise physiologist. Inherent with this profile of recognition is the fact that without the love and support of my wife, Betty, and our four daughters, my transition to physiology and the survival of a poverty state would have never occurred.

What has been the most interesting/enjoyable aspect of your involvement in science? What was the least interesting/enjoyable aspect

➤ To me, the most interesting and stimulating aspect of exercise physiology was the planning, testing, and evaluation of a research hypotheses. The least enjoyable were the administrative aspects of supervising a laboratory and the constant search for funding of research ideas.

What are your most meaningful contributions to the field of exercise science, and why are they so important?

➤ There are two. The first requires the understanding that exercise science evolved from the discipline of physical education and includes exercise physiology. When I entered the profession in the 1950s, I lacked intellectual rigor and scientific knowledge. Consequently, my graduate years were spent securing an undergraduate education. Thus, my most meaningful and satisfying contribution to the field was the planning and implementation of a rigorous, science-based Ph.D. graduate program in exercise physiology at the University of Iowa, which served as a model for other departments of physical education to follow. It was important to me because it attracted many outstanding individuals to the University of Iowa who became dear friends and helped pave the way for exercise science to become an academic entity. As for influencing the most individuals, I would have to list our research pertaining to the Iowa Wrestling Studies and the search for a minimum wrestling weight. According to Caspersen,[1] our research findings and recommendations provided the foundation for the National Federation of State High School Association to require a certified minimal wrestling weight (7% fat) that involved 270,000 high school students.

What advice would you give to students who express an interest in pursuing a career in exercise science research?

➤ Research requires more than intellectual curiosity and infectious enthusiasm. It is an exciting occupation that demands hard work, while requiring an individual to be disciplined, dedicated, and honest. A future researcher must acquire an education that enables him/her to be well prepared in mathematics, the biological and physical sciences, and the ability to communicate by written and verbal means. Lastly, seek a mentor whose research interests you and one who is concerned about you as a future researcher and not as a contributor to their vitae.

What interests have you pursued outside of your professional career?

➤ Becoming a civil war "buff," enjoying the pleasures of dancing and listening to Dixieland jazz, exercising regularly, participating in road races, reading nonfiction, learning about poetry, being a member of a book club, watching televised sports, cheering for the Washington Redskins football team, and observing our grandchildren as they grow up.

Where do you see the exercise science field (particularly your area of greatest interest) heading in the next 20 years?

➤ It is my speculation that because of the genomic and molecular biology revolution, and the obesity and diabetes

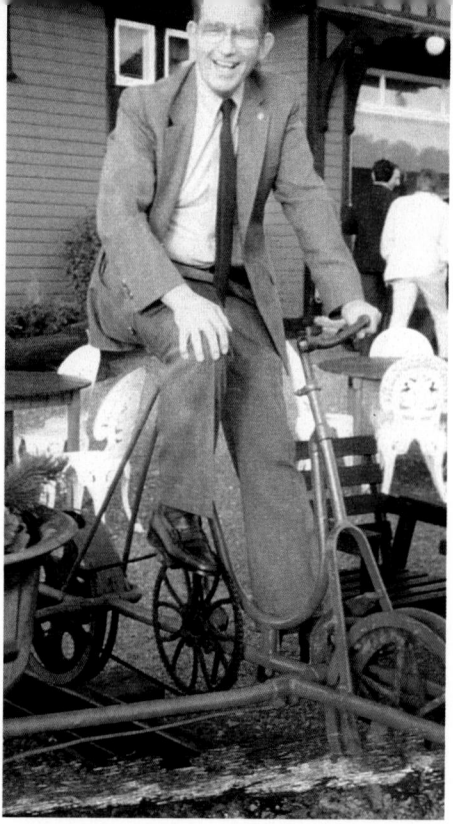

epidemics, the next 20 years will observe exercise physiologists addressing system diseases with molecular and genetic solutions. These solutions will be complex because the effects of acute and chronic exercise are a product of both genomic genetics and epigenetics. Consequently, future investigators must be thoroughly educated in these three sciences and the exercise response in normal and diseased populations.

You have the opportunity to give a "last lecture." Describe its primary focus.

➤ It would be titled "Exercise Physiology in the Last Frontier," and would pertain to what is known and unknown about exercising in a microgravity environment.

[1]Casperson, C. Dr. Charles M. Tipton selected as the 2012 recipient of the Clark W. Hetherington Award. *National Academy of Kinesiology Newsletter*. 34:15–17, 2012.

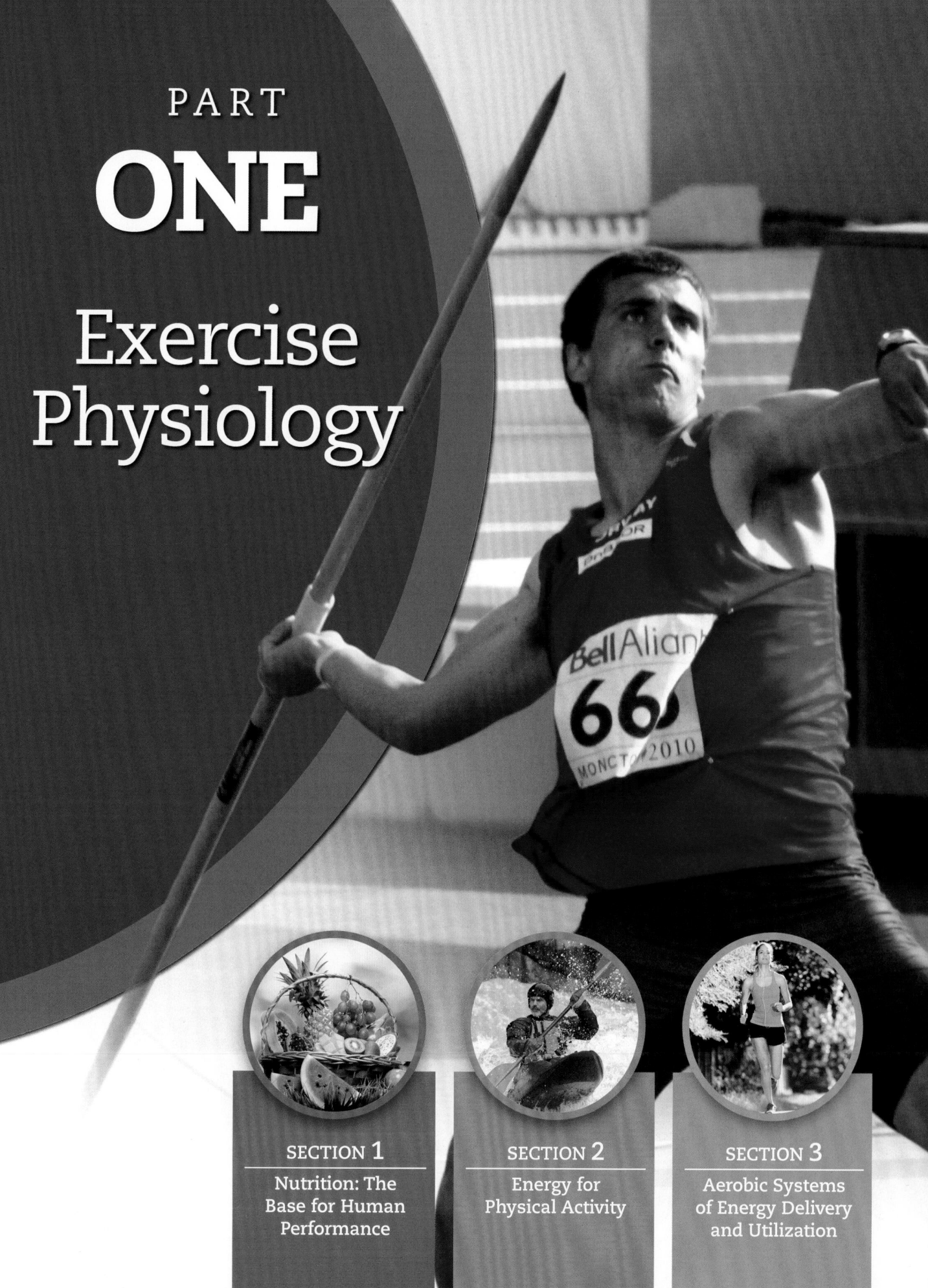

PART

ONE

Exercise Physiology

SECTION 1
Nutrition: The
Base for Human
Performance

SECTION 2
Energy for
Physical Activity

SECTION 3
Aerobic Systems
of Energy Delivery
and Utilization

Nutrition: The Base for Human Performance

OVERVIEW

Nutrition and exercise physiology share a natural linkage. Proper nutrition forms the foundation for physical performance; it provides the necessary fuel for biologic work and the chemicals for extracting and using the potential energy within this fuel. Nutrients from food also furnish essential elements to repair existing cells and synthesize new tissues.

Some have argued that a "well-balanced" diet readily provides adequate nutrients for physical activity and exercise, so in-depth nutrition knowledge would offer little value to exercise physiologists. We maintain, however, that the study of human movement, energy capacities, and performance highlight the relevance of energy sources and the role diverse nutrients play in energy release and transfer. With this knowledge and perspective, the exercise specialist can critically evaluate claims about special nutritional supplements, including dietary modifications, to enhance physical performance. Nutrients provide energy and regulate physiologic processes before, during, and following physical activity, so improved human performance often links with dietary modification. Too often, individuals devote considerable time and effort striving to optimize exercise performance, only to fall short because of inadequate, counterproductive, and sometimes harmful nutritional practices. The three chapters that follow present the six categories of nutrients—carbohydrates, lipids, proteins, vitamins, minerals, and water—and explore within the context of exercise physiology the following five questions related to nutrition:

What are nutrients?

Where are they found?

What are their functions?

What role do they play in physical activity?

How does optimal nutrition impact exercise performance and training responsiveness?

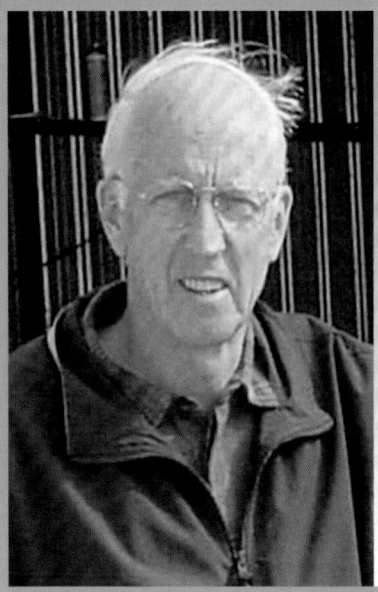

INTERVIEW WITH
Dr. David L. Costill

Education: BS (Ohio University, Athens, OH); MEd (Miami University, Oxford, OH); PhD (Physiology, Ohio State University, Columbus, OH)

Current Affiliation: Professor Emeritus, John and Janice Fisher Chair in Exercise Science, Ball State University, Muncie, IN

Honors, Awards, and ACSM Honor Award Statement of Contributions: See Appendix C, available online at http://thepoint.lww.com/mkk8e

Research Focus: My research interest was aimed at several areas: body fluid balance, carbohydrate metabolism in human muscle, thermal regulation during exercise, physiologic characteristics of runners and swimmers, aging distance runners, and changes in muscle fiber function during bed rest and space flight.

Memorable Publication: Costill DL, et al. Skeletal muscle enzymes and fiber composition in male and female track athletes. *J Appl Physiol* 1976;40:149.

What first inspired you to enter the exercise science field?

➤ Growing up in Ohio, I was always interested in biology and physiology, although I never thought of it in those terms. Even as an 8-year-old, I needed to know why animals differed and what made them work.

In college, I was more interested in anatomy and physiology than in physical education. But I was a poor student who was satisfied with taking all the activities classes and easy grades that I was able to attain. My primary interest was staying eligible for swimming. During my senior year at Ohio State University, I signed up for an independent study and was assigned a research project with 30 rats. The project never amounted to much, but I was left on my own and learned that the research process was challenging.

My first introduction to exercise physiology was as a graduate student at Miami University in Ohio. A faculty member (Fred Zeckman) in the Department of Zoology offered an exercise physiology class to about six students. Again, the class project involved data collection, a process I'd already found interesting. After teaching high school general science and biology for 3 years, as well as coaching three teams, I decided it was time to see if I could get the credentials to become a coach at a small college. I began working toward a doctorate in higher education. At the same time, I became close friends with Dick Bowers and Ed Fox, fellow graduate students who were majoring in exercise physiology under the direction of Dr. D. K. Mathews. It wasn't long before they persuaded me to switch over to work in the laboratory with them.

What influence did your undergraduate education have on your final career choice?

➤ It enabled me to get a degree and a teaching job. It was not until I had been teaching for several years that I identified what I really wanted to do. After one year at OSU, I moved to Cortland (State University of New York), where I coached cross-country track and swimming for 2 years. Although I enjoyed coaching, I just couldn't take the recruiting and continual exposure to 18-year-olds. So I decided to focus my energy on research. Exercise physiology gave me a chance to do research in an area that held numerous practical questions. My early studies with runners were a natural, considering the experience I'd had in coaching runners at Cortland. Interestingly, a few of those runners (e.g., Bob Fitts and Bob Gregor) have become well known in the exercise science field.

Who were the most influential people in your career, and why?

➤ Dr. Bob Bartels: Bob was my college swimming coach. First, he kept me on the freshman team, even though I was one of the least talented. There were moments during my senior year (as co-captain) when I'm sure he had second thoughts! Bob was also instrumental in getting me admitted to Miami University and OSU. Without his efforts, I'd probably still be teaching junior high science in Ohio.

Dr. David Bruce (D. B.) Dill: I worked with Bruce in the summer of 1968. His words of wisdom and advice headed me in the right direction.

Drs. Bengt Saltin and Phil Gollnick: Because I received my PhD after only one year at OSU, I had little research background and no postdoctoral experience. In 1972, I spent 6 months with Bengt and Phil in Bengt's laboratory in Stockholm. I learned a great deal working with them and the "gang" (Jan Karlsson, Björn Ekblom, E. H. Christensen, P. O. Åstrand, and others), which I consider to be my postdoctoral experience.

What has been the most interesting/enjoyable aspect of your involvement in science?

➤ Most interesting: Meeting people! The professional contact and friendships I had with other scientists (Charles Tipton, Skip Knuttgen, Jack Wilmore, Lars Hermansen, Harm Kuipers, Mark Hargreaves, Reggie Edgerton, Bill Fink, Clyde Williams, Per Blom, George Sheehan, astronauts from STS-78 flight, and others).

Most enjoyable: Following the success of my former students. Since I was a student with little talent but a good work ethic, I tended to recruit those types as graduate students. They were not always the ones with the high GPAs, but they were motivated and knew how to work. A number of them have become well known in our field, including Bill Evans, Ed Coyle, Mike Sherman, Mark Hargreaves, Bob Fitts, Bob Gregor, Paul Thompson, Carl Foster, Joe Houmard, Rick Sharp, Larry Armstrong, Rob Roberg, John Ivy, Hiro Tanaka, Mike Flynn, Scott and Todd Trappe, Abe Katz, Pete Van Handel, Darrell Neufer, Matt Hickey, and others.

One of the most enjoyable aspects of my research has been the opportunity to work with some very interesting subjects such as Bill Rogers, Steve Prefontaine, Alberto Salazar, Matt Biondi, Derek Clayton, Shella Young, Frank Shorter, Kenny Moore, and Ken Sparks.

What was the least interesting/enjoyable aspect?

➤ I have never liked writing books or chasing after grant money, but I knew that was essential to expand the laboratory and upgrade the facilities to continue to do research. Also, seeing students with great talent fail to live up to their full potential. Not every student achieved the level of success I expected, but their lives were often altered by events outside the laboratory. I always view my students as a part of my family, so when they had troubles and/or were unsuccessful, it was like watching my own kids struggle.

What advice would you give to students who express an interest in pursuing a career in exercise science research?

➤ There are six keys to success as a researcher: (1) Identify a worthy question. (2) Design a protocol that will give you the best possible answer. (3) Make sure the question is fundable; in other words, it must be a problem that an outside source is willing to support financially. (4) Be good at and enjoy collecting data. Precision in the laboratory is essential if you want to generate a clear answer to your question. (5) Be capable of reducing the data to an intelligible form and writing a clear/concise paper that is publishable in a creditable journal. (6) Be capable of presenting your research at scientific forums, as this helps to establish your scientific creditability.

What interests have you pursued outside of your professional career?

➤ Photography (1949–1955): I went to college to study photography (I won three national photo contests in high school) but switched to physical education during my sophomore year.

Distance running (1965–1982): I started running for fitness and eventually ran 16 marathons in the late 1970s and early 1980s. Knee injuries forced me back to swimming in 1982.

Masters Swimming (1982–present): After training for 6 months, Doc Counsilman, the famed Indiana University

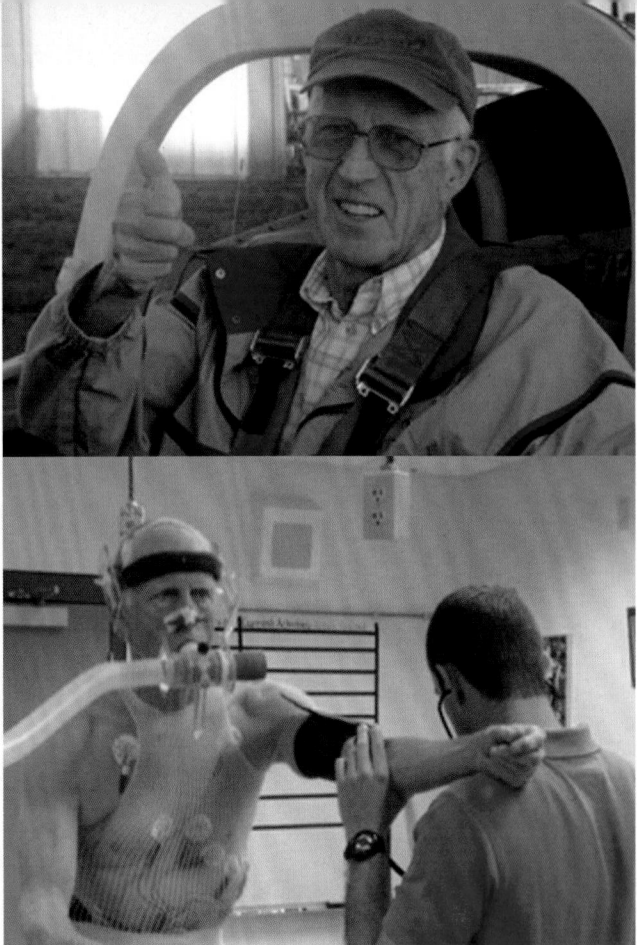

swim coach, talked me into entering a Masters meet, where he promptly beat me in a 500-yard freestyle event. My graduate students Rick Sharp and John Troup convinced me to "shave down" and compete in one more meet. Subsequently, I performed almost as well as I had in college, so I was hooked. At the age of 60 I could still beat my best college times and set six age-group national records.

I have two passions: aviation and auto restoration. I also enjoy fishing, camping, and canoeing. We have a cottage in northern Wisconsin where we spend as much time in the summer as possible. But I always like to come back to the small town of Muncie where there is no traffic, a nice house, a good airport, and all the University activities.

Where do you see the exercise physiology field heading in the next 20 years?

➤ This field has moved from whole body measurements (handgrip and vital capacity) to molecular biology (single muscle fiber physiology). To fully understand the physiology of exercise, the answers lie at the subcellular level. Students need solid training in chemistry and molecular biology to contribute to knowledge over the next 20 years.

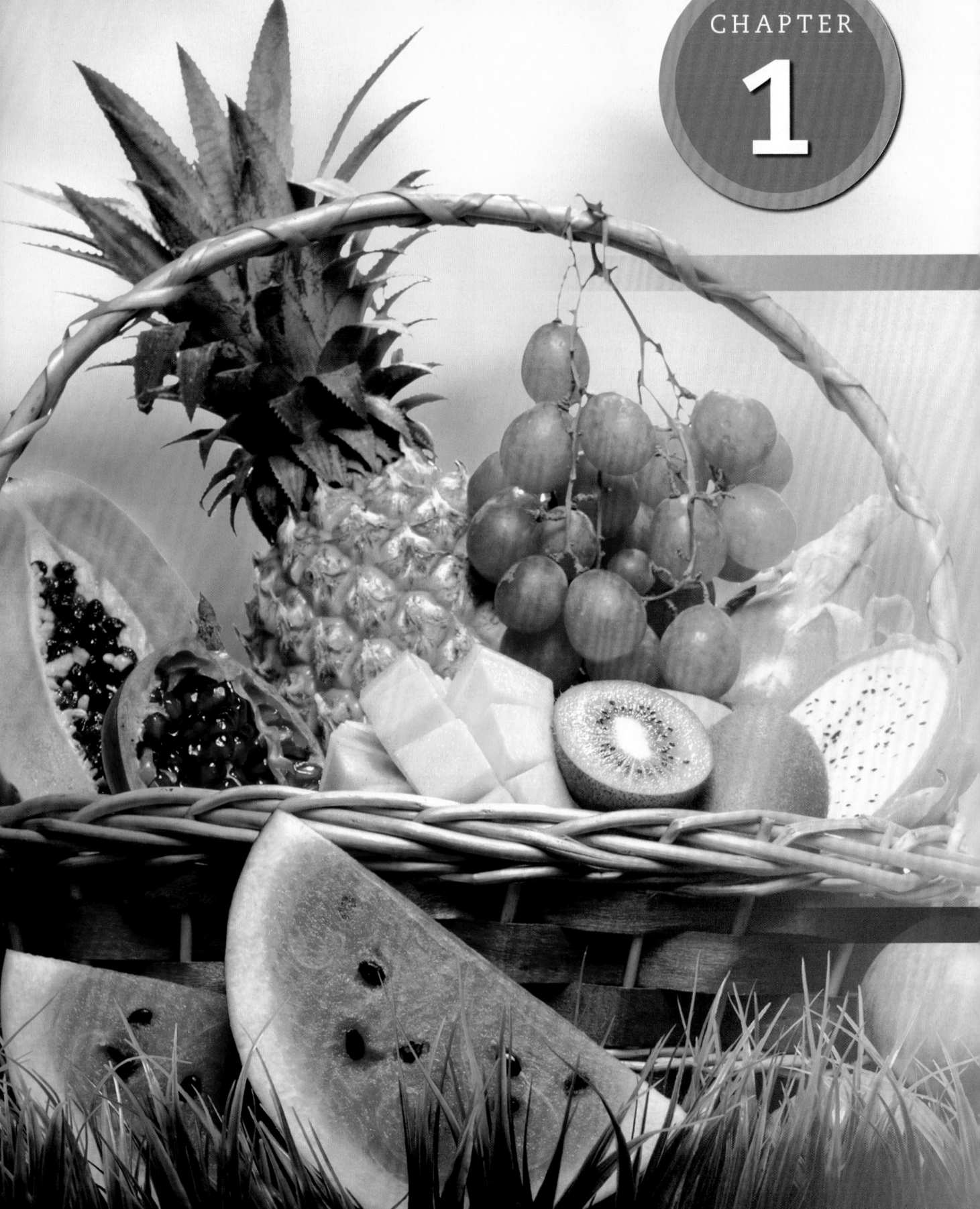

Carbohydrates, Lipids, and Proteins

CHAPTER OBJECTIVES

- Distinguish among monosaccharides, disaccharides, and polysaccharides
- Identify the two major classifications of dietary fiber and their roles in overall health
- Discuss physiologic responses to different dietary carbohydrates in the development of type 2 diabetes and obesity
- Quantify the amount, energy content, and distribution of carbohydrate within an average-sized man
- Summarize four major roles of carbohydrate in the body
- Outline the dynamics of carbohydrate metabolism during physical activities of various intensities and durations
- Contrast the speed of energy transfer from carbohydrate and fat combustion
- Discuss how diet affects muscle glycogen levels and endurance exercise performance
- For each of the diverse fatty acids (including trans- and omega-3 fatty acids), give an example of its food source, its physiologic functions, and its possible role in coronary heart disease
- List major characteristics of high- and low-density lipoprotein cholesterol and discuss the role of each in coronary heart disease
- Make prudent recommendations for dietary lipid intake, including cholesterol and types of fatty acids
- Quantify the amount, energy content, and distribution of fat within an average-sized woman
- Outline the dynamics of fat metabolism during physical activities of different intensities and durations
- Discuss how aerobic training affects fat and carbohydrate catabolism during exercise
- Explain how aerobic training affects fat-burning adaptations within skeletal muscle
- Define the terms *essential amino acid* and *nonessential amino acid* and give two food sources for each
- Discuss the advantages and potential limitations of a vegetarian diet in maintaining good health and a physically active lifestyle
- Outline the dynamics of protein metabolism during physical activities of various intensities and durations
- Provide a credible rationale for increasing protein intake above the Recommended Dietary Allowance (RDA) for individuals who perform strenuous endurance or resistance-exercise training
- Describe the alanine–glucose cycle and how the body uses amino acids for energy during exercise

ANCILLARIES 👁 at-a-Glance

Visit http://thePoint.lww.com/mkk8e to access the following resources.

- References: Chapter 1
- Appendix D: The Metric System and Conversion Constants in Exercise Physiology
- Interactive Question Bank
- Animation: Alanine–Glucose Cycle
- Animation: Condensation
- Animation: Digestion of Carbohydrate
- Animation: Fat Mobilization and Use
- Animation: General Digestion
- Animation: Glycogen Synthesis
- Animation: Hydrolysis
- Animation: Transamination
- Focus on Research: Protein and Exercise—How Much Is Enough?

The carbohydrate, lipid, and protein nutrients provide energy to maintain bodily functions during rest and physical activity. Aside from their role as biologic fuel, these nutrients, called **macronutrients**, preserve the structural and functional integrity of the organism. This chapter discusses each macronutrient's general structure, function, and dietary source. We emphasize their importance in sustaining physiologic function during physical activities of differing intensity and duration.

PART 1 CARBOHYDRATES

KINDS AND SOURCES OF CARBOHYDRATES

Atoms of carbon, hydrogen, and oxygen combine to form a basic carbohydrate (sugar) molecule in the general formula $(CH_2O)_n$, where *n* ranges from 3 to 7 carbon atoms with hydrogen and oxygen atoms attached by single bonds. Except for lactose and a small amount of glycogen from animal origin, plants provide the carbohydrate source in the human diet. Carbohydrates classify as monosaccharides, oligosaccharides, or polysaccharides. The number of simple sugars linked within each of these molecules distinguishes each carbohydrate form.

Monosaccharides

*The **monosaccharide** represents the basic unit of a carbohydrate.* Glucose, fructose, and galactose represent the three major monosaccharides.

Glucose, also called dextrose or blood sugar, consists of a 6-carbon (hexose) compound formed naturally in food or in the body through digestion of more complex carbohydrates. **Gluconeogenesis**, the body's process for making new sugar, occurs primarily in the liver from the carbon residues of other compounds (generally amino acids, but also glycerol, pyruvate, and lactate). After the small intestine absorbs glucose, it can follow one of three pathways:

1. Become available as an energy source for cellular metabolism
2. Form glycogen for storage in the liver and muscles
3. Convert to fat (triacylglycerol) for later use as energy

 See the animation "General Digestion" on http://thePoint.lww.com/mkk8e for a demonstration of this process.

FIGURE 1.1 illustrates glucose along with other carbohydrates formed in plants from photosynthesis. Glucose consists of 6 carbon, 12 hydrogen, and 6 oxygen atoms ($C_6H_{12}O_6$). Fructose and galactose, two other simple sugars with the same chemical formula as glucose, have a slightly different C-H-O linkage and are thus different substances with distinct biochemical characteristics.

Fructose (fruit sugar or levulose), the sweetest sugar, occurs in large amounts in fruits and honey. Fructose, like glucose, also serves as an energy source but usually rapidly moves directly from the digestive tract into the blood to primarily convert to fat but also glucose in the liver. **Galactose** does not exist freely in nature; rather, it combines with glucose to form milk sugar in the mammary glands of lactating animals. The body converts galactose to glucose for use in energy metabolism.

Oligosaccharides

Oligosaccharides form when 2 to 10 monosaccharides bond chemically. The major oligosaccharides, the **disaccharides**, or double sugars, form when two monosaccharide molecules combine. Monosaccharides and disaccharides collectively are called **simple sugars**.

What's in a Name?

Simple sugars are packaged commercially under a variety of names. This figure illustrates simple sugars with their percentage content of glucose and fructose.

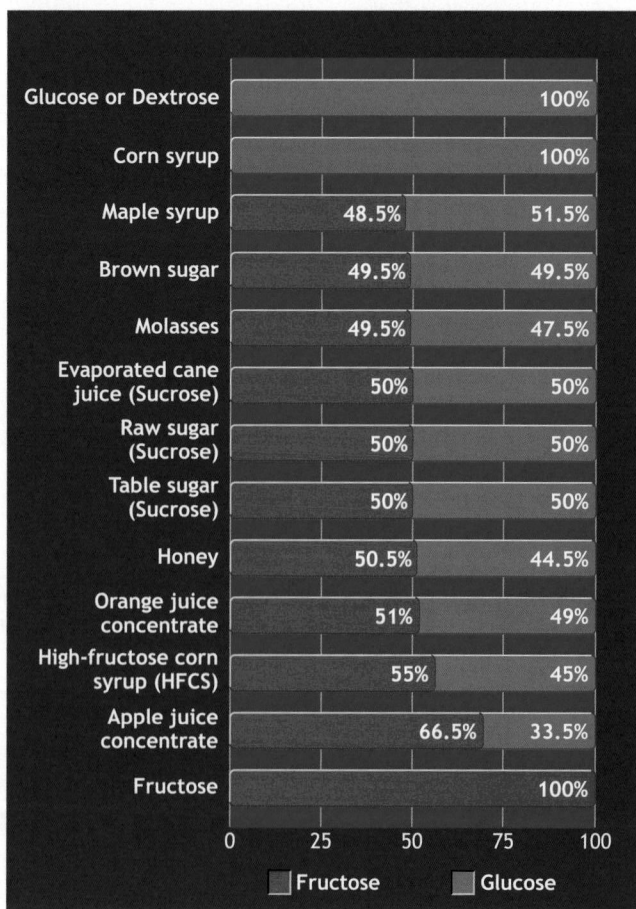

Source: US Department of Agriculture databases

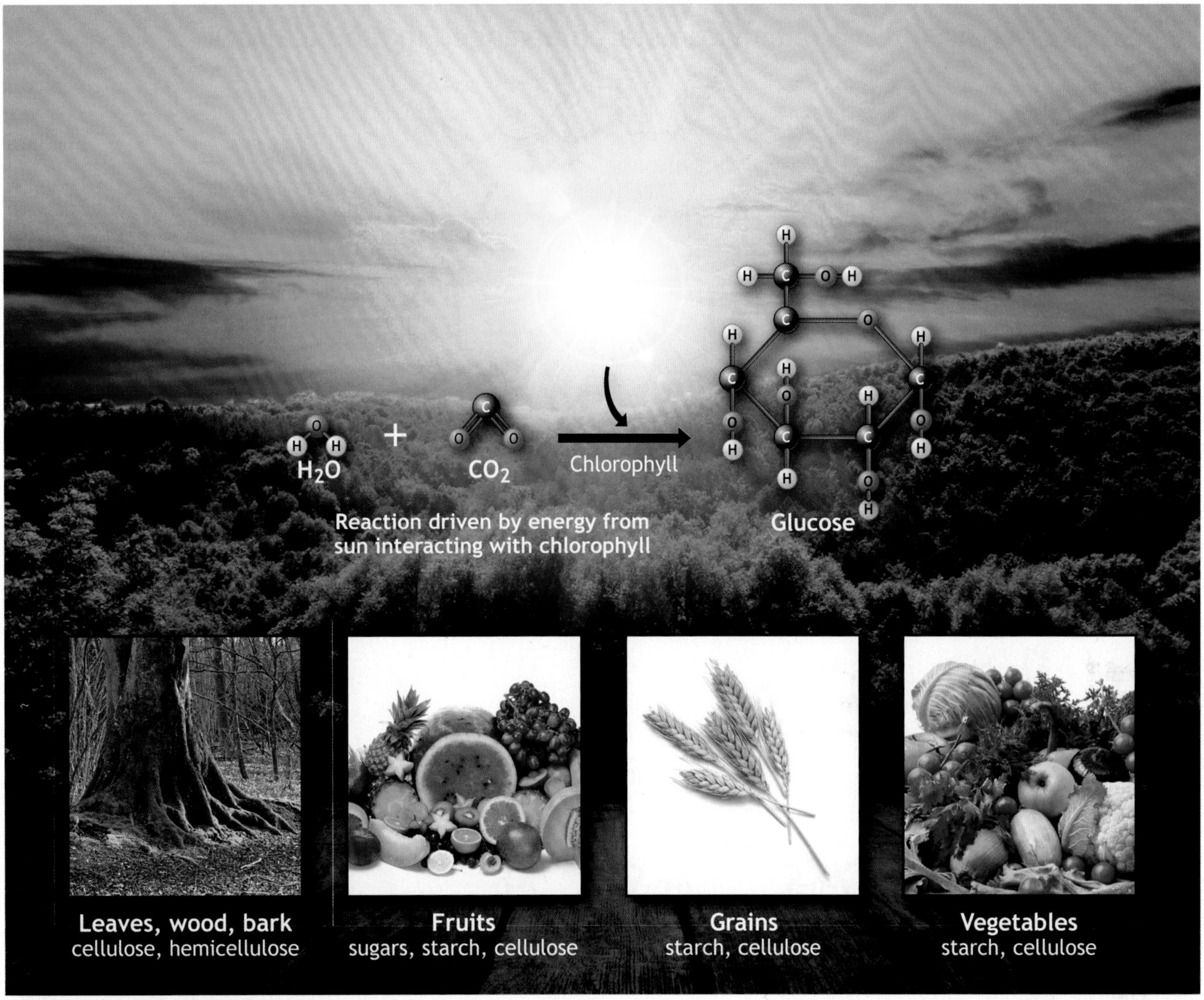

FIGURE 1.1 • Three-dimensional ring structure of the simple sugar glucose molecule formed during photosynthesis when energy from sunlight interacts with water, carbon dioxide, and the green pigment chlorophyll.

Disaccharides all contain glucose. The three principal disaccharides include:

- **Sucrose** (glucose + fructose), the most common dietary disaccharide, contributes up to 25% of the total calories consumed in the United States. It occurs naturally in most foods that contain carbohydrates, especially beet and cane sugar, brown sugar, sorghum, maple syrup, and honey.
- **Lactose** (glucose + galactose), a sugar *not* found in plants, exists in natural form only in milk as milk sugar. The least sweet of the disaccharides, lactose when artificially processed often becomes an ingredient in carbohydrate-rich, high-calorie liquid meals.
- **Maltose** (glucose + glucose) occurs in beer, breakfast cereals, and germinating seeds. Also called malt sugar, this sugar cleaves into two glucose molecules yet makes only a small contribution to the carbohydrate content of the diet.

See the animation "Digestion of Carbohydrate" on http://thePoint.lww.com/mkk8e for a demonstration of this process.

Polysaccharides

Polysaccharide describes the linkage of three or more (up to thousands) sugar molecules. Polysaccharides form during the chemical process of **dehydration synthesis**, a water-losing reaction that forms a more complex carbohydrate molecule. Plant and animal sources both contribute to these large chains of linked monosaccharides.

Plant Polysaccharides

Starch and fiber are the common forms of plant polysaccharides.

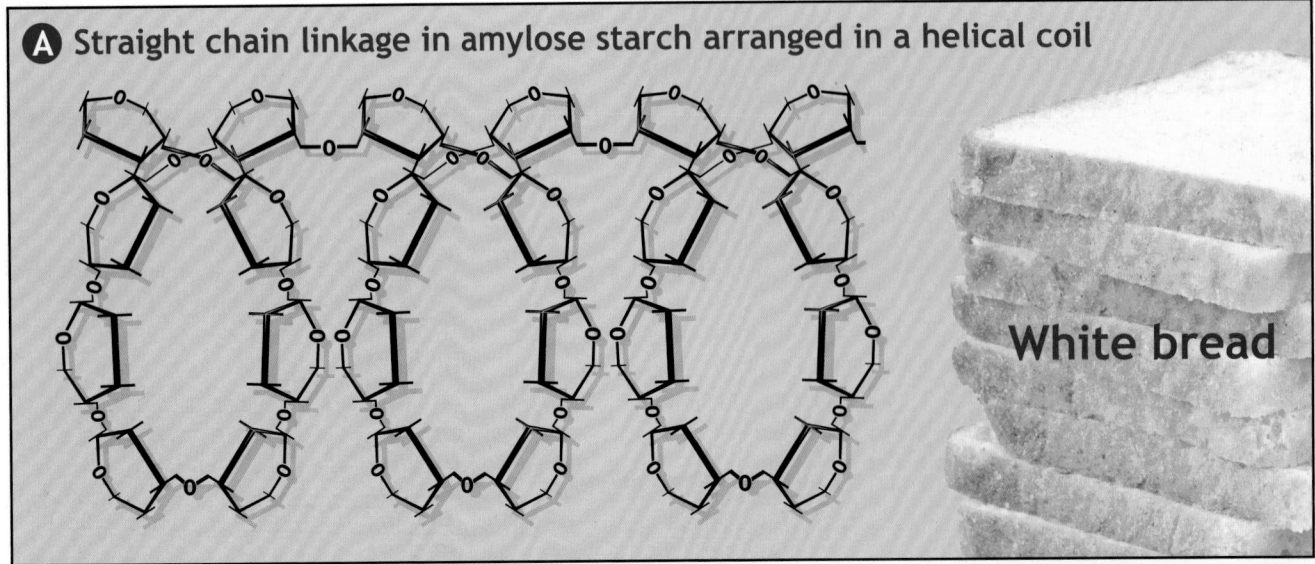

A Straight chain linkage in amylose starch arranged in a helical coil

White bread

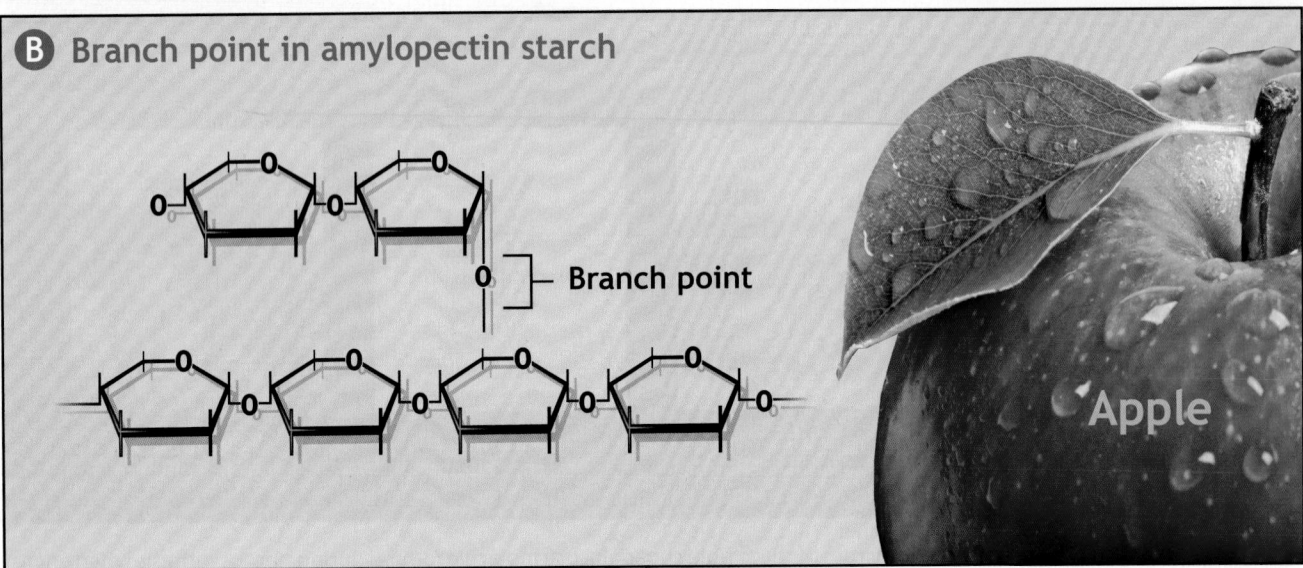

B Branch point in amylopectin starch

 Branch point

Apple

FIGURE 1.2 • The two forms of plant starch. **(A)** Straight-chain linkage with unbranched bonding of glucose residues (glycosidic linkages) in amylose. **(B)** Branch point in the highly branched amylopectin starch molecule. The amylopectin structure appears linear, but it exists as a helical coil. (Adapted with permission from McArdle WD, Katch FI, Katch VL. *Sports and Exercise Nutrition*, 4th ed. Philadelphia: Wolters Kluwer Health, 2013.)

Starch, the storage form of carbohydrate in plants, occurs in seeds, corn, and various grains of bread, cereal, pasta, and pastries. Starch exists in two forms (**Fig. 1.2**):

1. **Amylose**, a long straight chain of glucose units twisted into a helical coil
2. **Amylopectin**, a highly branched monosaccharide linkage

The relative proportion of each form of starch in a plant species determines the characteristics of the starch, including its "digestibility." *Starches with a relatively large amount of amylopectin digest and absorb rapidly, whereas starches with high amylose content break down (hydrolyze) at a slower rate.*

See the animation "Hydrolysis" on **http://thePoint. lww.com/mkk8e** for a demonstration of this process.

The term *complex carbohydrate* describes dietary starch, which represents the most important dietary source of carbohydrate in the typical U.S. diet, accounting for approximately 50% of the typical individual's total intake.

Fiber, classified as a nonstarch, structural polysaccharide, includes cellulose, the most abundant organic molecule on Earth. Fibrous materials resist chemical breakdown by human digestive enzymes, although a small portion ferments by action of bacteria in the large intestine and ultimately participates in metabolic reactions following intestinal absorption. *Fiber occurs exclusively in plants; it comprises the structure of leaves, stems, roots, seeds, and fruit coverings.*

Health Implications of Fiber Deficiency. Much of the interest in dietary fiber originates from studies that link high fiber intake, particularly whole-grain cereal fibers, with a lower occurrence of obesity, systemic inflammation, insulin resistance and type 2 diabetes, hypertension, the metabolic syndrome, digestive disorders, elevated blood cholesterol, colorectal cancer, and heart disease.[1,16,46,48,58]

Americans typically consume about 12 to 15 g of fiber daily, far short of the Food and Nutrition Board of the National Academy of Sciences (http://www.iom.edu/reports/2002/dietary-reference-intakes-for-energy-carbohydrate-fiber-fat-fatty-acids-cholesterol-protein-and-amino-acids.aspx) recommendations of 38 g for men and 25 g for women up to age 50, and 30 g for men and 21 g for women over age 50.[19]

thePoint Appendix D, available online at http://thepoint.lww.com/mkk8e, shows the relationship between metric units and U.S. units, including common expressions of work, energy, and power.

Fiber retains considerable water and gives "bulk" to the food residues in the intestinal tract. Fiber intake *modestly* reduces serum cholesterol in humans by lowering the low-density lipoprotein fraction of the cholesterol profile. Particularly effective are the **water-soluble,** mucilaginous fibers such as psyllium seed husk, β-glucan, pectin, and guar gum present in oats, beans, brown rice, peas, carrots, cornhusks, and many fruits.[31,78] Dietary fiber exerts no effect on high-density lipoproteins (see the section on *High-Density, Low-Density, and Very Low-Density Lipoproteins*).

TABLE 1.1	Recommended Daily Fiber Intake
Recommended Daily Fiber Intake (g)	
Children 1–3 y	19
Children 4–8 y	25
Boys 9–13 y	31
Boys 14–18 y	38
Girls 9–18 y	26
Men 19–50 y	38
Men 51 y and older	30
Women 19–50 y	25
Women 51 y and older	21

Adapted with permission from McArdle WD, Katch FI, Katch VL. *Sports and Exercise Nutrition*, 4th ed. Philadelphia: Wolters Kluwer Health, 2013, and US Department of Agriculture database.

The **water-insoluble** fibers cellulose, many hemicelluloses, and lignin and cellulose-rich products (wheat bran) do not lower cholesterol.

Heart disease and obesity protection may relate to dietary fiber's regulatory role in reducing insulin secretion by slowing nutrient absorption by the small intestine following food intake. Fiber consumption may also confer heart disease protection through beneficial effects on blood pressure, insulin sensitivity, and blood clotting characteristics.[43,79] On the negative side, excessive fiber intake inhibits intestinal absorption of the minerals calcium, phosphorus, and iron. *Present nutritional wisdom advocates a diet that contains 20 to 40 g of fiber (depending on age) per day (ratio of 3:1 for water-insoluble to soluble fiber).* TABLE 1.1 list the recommended daily fiber intake and TABLE 1.2 list the fiber content of some common foods.

TABLE 1.2	Fiber Content of Common Foods (Listed in Order of Total Fiber Content)			
Food	**Serving Size**	**Total Fiber (g)**	**Soluble Fiber (g)**	**Insoluble Fiber (g)**
100% bran cereal	1/2 cup	10.0	0.3	9.7
Peas	1/2 cup	5.2	2.0	3.2
Kidney beans	1/2 cup	4.5	0.5	4.0
Apple	1 small	3.9	2.3	1.6
Potato	1 small	3.8	2.2	1.6
Broccoli	1/2 cup	2.5	1.1	1.4
Strawberries	3/4 cup	2.4	0.9	1.5
Oats, whole	1/2 cup	1.6	0.5	1.1
Banana	1 small	1.3	0.6	0.7
Pasta	1/2 cup	1.0	0.2	0.8
Lettuce	1/2 cup	0.5	0.2	0.3
White rice	1/2 cup	0.5	0	0.5

Adapted with permission from McArdle WD, Katch FI, Katch VL. *Sports and Exercise Nutrition*, 4th ed. Philadelphia: Wolters Kluwer Health, 2013, and US Department of Agriculture database.

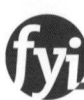
Added Sugar and the Blood Lipid Profile

Researchers divided 6113 participants in the long-running National Health and Nutrition Examination Survey (NHANES) into five groups based on the percentage of total calories consumed as added sugars. Groups ranged in added daily sugar intakes of less than 5% (three teaspoons of sugar) to 25% or more (46 teaspoons of sugar). Sugar intake varied inversely with the healthy levels of HDL cholesterol (58.7 mg·dL⁻¹ [deciliter or 100 mL] in the group consuming the least added sugar to 47.7 mg·dL⁻¹ in the group consuming the most) and directly with the unhealthy levels of triglycerides (105 mg·dL⁻¹ in the group consuming the least added sugar to 114 mg·dL⁻¹ in the group consuming the most). The research was not designed to show cause and effect, but it does argue for substituting the empty calories in sugars with foods containing a more nutritious package.

Source: Welsh JA, et al. Caloric sweetener consumption and dyslipidemia among US adults. *JAMA* 2010;303:1490.

Not All Carbohydrates Are Physiologically Equal. Digestion rates of different carbohydrate sources possibly explain the link between carbohydrate intake and diabetes and excess body fat. Foods containing dietary fiber slow carbohydrate digestion, minimizing surges in blood glucose. In contrast, low-fiber processed starches (and simple sugars in soft drinks) digest quickly and enter the blood at a relatively rapid rate (high glycemic index foods; see Chapter 3). The average American currently consumes 22 to 28 teaspoons of added sugars daily (equivalent to 350 to 440 empty calories)—mostly as high-fructose corn syrup and ordinary table sugar. The blood glucose surge after consuming refined, processed starch and simple sugar has three effects: it (1) stimulates overproduction of insulin by the pancreas to accentuate hyperinsulinemia, (2) elevates plasma triacylglycerol concentrations, and (3) accelerates fat synthesis. Consistently consuming high intakes of simple sugar reduces the body's sensitivity to insulin (i.e., peripheral tissues become more resistant to insulin's effects); this requires progressively more insulin to optimize blood sugar levels.[65] *Type 2 diabetes results when the pancreas cannot produce sufficient insulin to regulate blood glucose, causing it to rise.* Individuals should minimize sugary beverage intake, including fruit juices, to lower the risk of obesity, diabetes, heart disease, gout, and dental cavities. Light to moderate physical activity performed on a regular basis exerts a potent influence to improve insulin sensitivity, thereby reducing the insulin requirement for a given glucose uptake.[37] Chapter 20 discusses exercise, diabetes, and the associated risk of the metabolic syndrome.

Glycogen: The Animal Polysaccharide

Glycogen is the storage carbohydrate within mammalian muscle and liver. It forms as a large polysaccharide polymer synthesized from glucose in the process of **glycogenesis** (catalyzed by the enzyme **glycogen synthase**). Irregularly shaped, glycogen ranges from a few hundred to 30,000 glucose molecules linked together, much like a sausage link in a chain of sausages, with branch linkages for joining additional glucose units.

 See the animation "Glycogen Synthesis" on http://thePoint.lww.com/mkk8e for a demonstration of this process.

FIGURE 1.3 shows that glycogen biosynthesis involves adding individual glucose units to an existing glycogen polymer. Stage 4 of the figure shows an enlarged view of the chemical configuration of the glycogen molecule. Overall, glycogen synthesis is irreversible. Glycogen synthesis requires energy, as one adenosine triphosphate (ATP; stage 1) and one uridine triphosphate (UTP; stage 3) degrade during glucogenesis.

How Much Glycogen Does the Body Store? FIGURE 1.4 illustrates that a well-nourished 80-kg man stores approximately 500 g of carbohydrate. Of this, muscle glycogen accounts for the largest reserve (approximately 400 g), followed by 90 to 110 g as liver glycogen (highest concentration, representing 3 to 7% of the liver's weight), with only about 2 to 3 g as blood glucose. Each gram of either glycogen or glucose contains approximately 4 calories (kcal) of energy. This means that the average person stores about 2000 kcal as carbohydrate—enough total energy to power a 20-mile continuous run at high intensity.

The body stores comparatively little glycogen, so its quantity fluctuates considerably through dietary modifications. For example, a 24-hr fast or a low-carbohydrate, normal-calorie diet nearly depletes glycogen reserves. In contrast, maintaining a carbohydrate-rich diet for several days almost doubles the body's glycogen stores compared with levels attained with a typical, well-balanced diet. *The body's upper limit for glycogen storage averages about 15 g per kilogram (kg) of body mass, equivalent to 1050 g for a 70-kg (154 lb) male and 840 g for a 56-kg (124 lb) female.*

Several factors determine the rate and quantity of glycogen breakdown and resynthesis. During exercise, intramuscular glycogen provides the *major* carbohydrate energy source for active muscles. In addition, liver glycogen rapidly reconverts to glucose (regulated by a specific phosphatase enzyme) for release into the blood as an extramuscular glucose supply for exercise. The term **glycogenolysis** describes this reconversion of glycogen to glucose. Depletion of liver and muscle glycogen by dietary restriction of carbohydrates or intense exercise stimulates glucose synthesis. This occurs through gluconeogenic metabolic pathways from the structural components of other nutrients, particularly proteins.

Important Carbohydrate Conversions

Glucogenesis—glycogen synthesis from glucose (glucose → glycogen)

Gluconeogenesis—glucose synthesis largely from structural components of noncarbohydrate nutrients (protein → glucose)

Glycogenolysis—glucose formation from glycogen (glycogen → glucose)

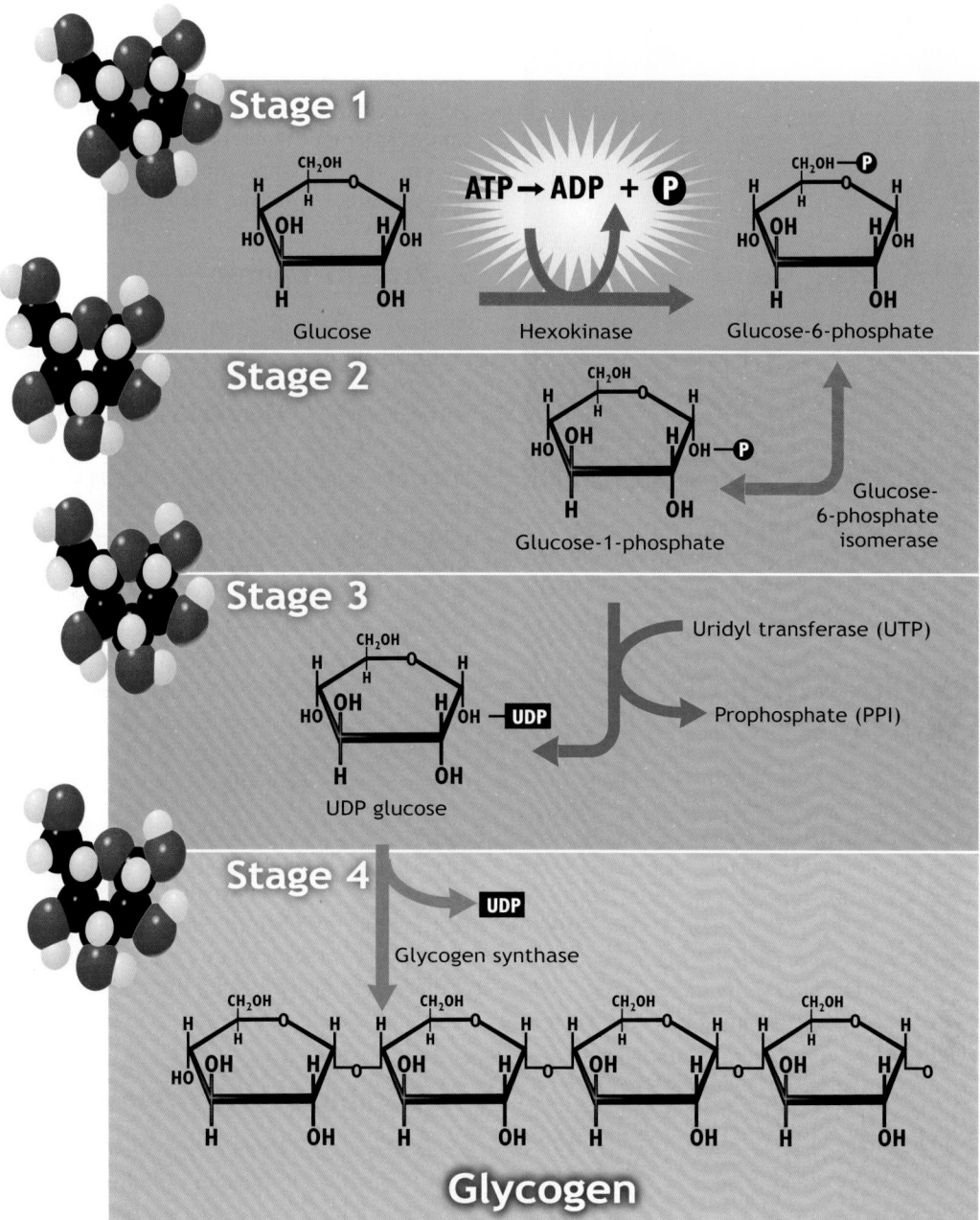

FIGURE 1.3 • Glycogen synthesis is a four-step process. *Stage 1*, ATP donates a phosphate to glucose to form glucose-6-phosphate. This reaction involves the enzyme hexokinase. *Stage 2*, Glucose-6-phosphate isomerizes to glucose-1-phosphate by the enzyme glucose-6-phosphate isomerase. *Stage 3*, The enzyme uridyl transferase reacts uridyl triphosphate (UTP) with glucose-1-phosphate to form uridine diphosphate (UDP)-glucose (a phosphate is released as UTP → UDP). *Stage 4*, UDP-glucose attaches to one end of an existing glycogen polymer chain. This forms a new bond (known as a glycoside bond) between the adjacent glucose units, with the concomitant release of UDP. For each glucose unit added, 2 moles of ATP converts to ADP and phosphate. (Adapted with permission from McArdle WD, Katch FI, Katch VL. *Sports and Exercise Nutrition*, 4th ed. Philadelphia: Wolters Kluwer Health, 2013.)

Hormones play a key role in regulating liver and muscle glycogen stores by controlling circulating blood sugar levels. Elevated blood sugar causes the beta (β) cells of the pancreas to secrete additional insulin; this facilitates cellular glucose uptake and inhibits further insulin secretion. This type of *feedback regulation* maintains blood glucose at an appropriate physiologic concentration. In contrast, when blood sugar falls below normal, the pancreas's alpha (α) cells secrete **glucagon** to normalize blood sugar concentration. Known as the "insulin antagonist" hormone (www.glucagon.com), glucagon elevates blood glucose by stimulating the liver's glycogenolytic and gluconeogenic pathways. Chapter 20 contains further discussion of hormonal regulation in exercise.

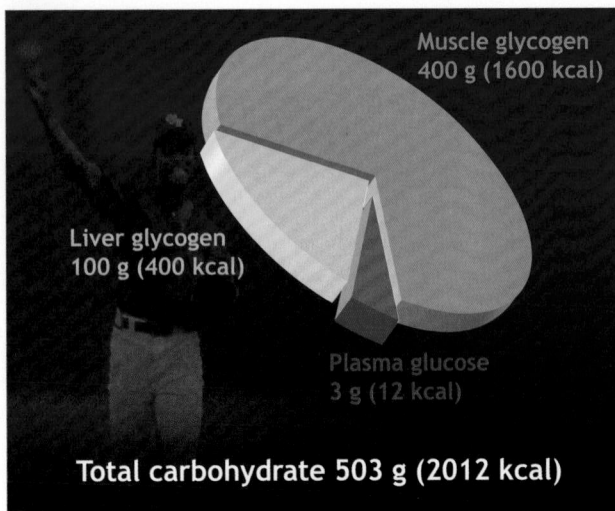

FIGURE 1.4 • Distribution of carbohydrate energy in an average 80-kg man. (Adapted with permission from McArdle WD, Katch FI, Katch VL. *Sports and Exercise Nutrition*, 4th ed. Philadelphia: Wolters Kluwer Health, 2013.)

RECOMMENDED INTAKE OF CARBOHYDRATES

Although there are no absolute minimum or maximum recommendations for total carbohydrate intake, a sedentary 70-kg person's daily carbohydrate intake typically amounts to about 300 g or between 40 and 50% of total calories. *For more physically active people and those involved in exercise training, carbohydrates should equal about 60% of daily calories or 400 to 600 g, predominantly as unrefined, fiber-rich fruits, grains, and vegetables. During periods of intense training, carbohydrate intake should increase to 70% of total calories consumed or approximately 8 to 10 g per kg of body mass.*

Nutritious dietary carbohydrate sources consist of fruits, grains, and vegetables, yet this does not represent the usual source of carbohydrate intake for all people. The typical American consumes about 50% of carbohydrate as simple sugars. This intake comes primarily from sugars in the form of sucrose and high-fructose corn syrup added in food processing. These sugars do not come in a nutrient-dense package characteristic of the sugar found naturally in fruits and vegetables.

ROLE OF CARBOHYDRATES IN THE BODY

Carbohydrates serve four important functions related to energy metabolism and exercise performance.

1. Energy Source

Carbohydrates primarily serve as an energy fuel, particularly during intense physical activity. Energy derived from the catabolism of bloodborne glucose and muscle glycogen powers the contractile elements of muscle and other forms of biologic work.

Sufficient daily carbohydrate intake for physically active individuals maintains the body's relatively limited glycogen stores. *Once cells reach their maximum capacity for glycogen storage, excess sugars convert to and store as fat.* The interconversion of macronutrients for energy storage explains how body fat can increase when dietary carbohydrate exceeds energy requirements, even if the diet contains little lipids.

2. Protein-Sparer

Adequate carbohydrate intake helps to preserve tissue protein. Normally, protein serves a vital role in tissue maintenance, repair, and growth, and to a considerably lesser degree, as a nutrient energy source. Depletion of glycogen reserves—readily occurring with starvation, reduced energy and/or carbohydrate intake, and prolonged, strenuous exercise—dramatically affects the metabolic mixture of fuels for energy. In addition to stimulating fat catabolism, glycogen depletion triggers glucose synthesis from the labile pool of amino acids (protein). This gluconeogenic conversion offers a metabolic option for augmenting carbohydrate availability (and maintaining plasma glucose levels) even with insufficient glycogen stores. The price paid strains the body's protein levels, particularly muscle protein. In the extreme, this reduces lean tissue mass and adds a solute load on the kidneys, forcing them to excrete the nitrogenous byproducts of protein breakdown.

 INTEGRATIVE QUESTION

Discuss the rationale for recommending adequate carbohydrate intake rather than an excess of protein to increase muscle mass through resistance training.

3. Metabolic Primer/Prevents Ketosis

Components of carbohydrate catabolism serve as "primer" substrate for fat oxidation. Insufficient carbohydrate breakdown—either through limitations in glucose transport into the cell (e.g., diabetes where insulin production wanes or insulin resistance increases) or glycogen depletion through inadequate diet or prolonged exercise—causes fat mobilization to exceed fat oxidation. The lack of adequate byproducts of glycogen catabolism produces incomplete fat breakdown with accumulation of **ketone bodies** (acetoacetate and β-hydroxybutyrate, acetone-like byproducts of incomplete fat breakdown). In excess, ketones increase body fluid acidity to produce a potentially harmful acid condition called **acidosis** or, specifically with regard to fat breakdown, **ketosis**. Chapter 6 continues the discussion of carbohydrate as a primer for fat catabolism.

4. Fuel for the Central Nervous System

The central nervous system requires an uninterrupted stream of carbohydrate for proper function. Under normal conditions, the brain metabolizes blood glucose almost exclusively as its fuel source. In poorly regulated diabetes, during starvation, or with a prolonged low-carbohydrate intake, the brain adapts after about 8 days and metabolizes larger amounts of fat (as ketones) for fuel. Chronic low-carbohydrate, high-fat diets also induce adaptations in skeletal muscle that increase fat use during low-to-moderate physical activity levels and spares muscle glycogen.

Blood sugar usually remains regulated within narrow limits for two main reasons:

1. Glucose serves as a primary fuel for nerve tissue metabolism
2. Glucose represents the sole energy source for red blood cells

At rest and during activity, liver glycogenolysis (glycogen-to-glucose conversion) maintains normal blood glucose levels, usually at $100 \text{ mg} \cdot \text{dL}^{-1}$. In prolonged activity such as marathon running (or similar duration intense activities), blood glucose concentration eventually falls below normal levels because liver glycogen depletes, while active muscle continues to catabolize the available blood glucose. Symptoms of clinically reduced blood glucose (**hypoglycemia**: $<45 \text{ mg glucose} \cdot \text{dL}^{-1}$ of blood) include weakness, hunger, mental confusion, and dizziness. This ultimately impairs exercise performance and can contribute to central nervous system fatigue associated with prolonged exercise. Sustained and profound hypoglycemia can trigger unconsciousness and produces irreversible brain damage.

CARBOHYDRATE DYNAMICS DURING PHYSICAL ACTIVITY

Biochemical and biopsy techniques (see Chapter 18) and labeled nutrient tracers assess the energy contribution of nutrients during physical activity. Such data indicate that two factors, intensity and duration of effort and the fitness and nutritional status of the exerciser, largely determine the fuel mixture during physical activity.[10,21]

The liver increases glucose release to active muscle as activity progresses from low to high intensity. Simultaneously, muscle glycogen supplies the predominant carbohydrate energy source during the early stages of exercise and as intensity increases.[26] Compared to fat and protein use, carbohydrate remains the preferential fuel in intense aerobic activity because it rapidly supplies energy as ATP (see Chapter 6) via oxidative processes. During anaerobic exercise that requires glycolysis (see Chapter 6), carbohydrate becomes the sole fuel for ATP resynthesis. Just 3 days of a diet with only 5% carbohydrate considerably depresses all-out exercise capacity.[41]

Carbohydrate availability in the metabolic mixture controls its use for energy. In turn, carbohydrate intake dramatically affects its availability. The concentration of blood glucose provides feedback regulation of the liver's glucose output; an increase in blood glucose inhibits hepatic glucose release during exercise.[29] Carbohydrate availability during exercise helps regulate fat mobilization and its use for energy.[11,13] For example, increasing carbohydrate oxidation by ingesting high-glycemic carbohydrates prior to exercise (with accompanying hyperglycemia and hyperinsulinemia) inhibits two processes:

1. Long-chain fatty acid oxidation by skeletal muscle
2. Free fatty acid (FFA) liberation from adipose tissue.

Adequate carbohydrate availability (and resulting increased catabolism) can inhibit transport of long-chain fatty acids into the mitochondria, thus controlling the metabolic mixture.

High-Intensity Exercise

Neural–humoral factors during intense exercise increase the output of epinephrine, norepinephrine, and glucagon and decrease insulin release. These hormonal responses activate **glycogen phosphorylase** (indirectly via activation of cyclic adenosine monophosphate, or cyclic AMP; see Chapter 20), the enzyme that facilitates glycogenolysis in the liver and active muscles. Think of glycogen phosphorylase as the controller of the glycogen–glucose interconversion to regulate circulating glucose concentration in the bloodstream. Because muscle glycogen provides energy without oxygen, it contributes considerable energy in the early minutes of exercise when oxygen use fails to meet oxygen demands. As exercise continues, bloodborne glucose increases its contribution as a metabolic fuel. For example, blood glucose may supply up to 30% of the total energy of vigorously active muscles, with the remaining carbohydrate energy supplied by muscle glycogen.

One hour of intense physical activity decreases liver glycogen by about 55%; a 2-hr strenuous workout almost depletes the glycogen of the liver and active muscles. FIGURE 1.5 illustrates that the muscles' uptake of circulating blood glucose increases sharply during the initial stage of cycling exercise and continues to increase as exercise continues. After 40 min, glucose uptake rises 7 to 20 times the uptake at rest, depending on exercise intensity. *The advantage of a selective dependence on carbohydrate metabolism during intense aerobic activity derives from its rate of energy transfer, which is twice that of fat*

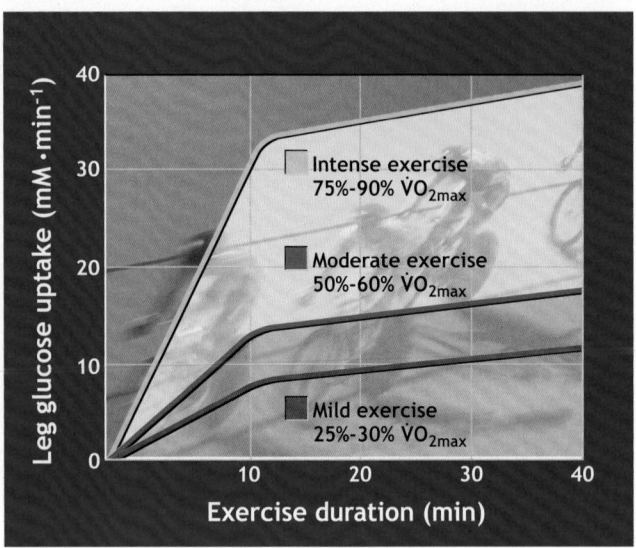

FIGURE 1.5 • Generalized response for blood glucose uptake by the leg muscles during cycling in relation to exercise duration and intensity. Exercise intensity is expressed as a percentage of $\dot{V}O_{2max}$.

or protein.[70] In addition, carbohydrate generates almost 6% more energy than fat per liter of oxygen consumed. Chapter 6 discusses in more detail the energy release from carbohydrate under anaerobic and aerobic conditions.

Moderate and Prolonged Exercise

Glycogen stored in active muscles supplies almost all of the energy in the initial transition from rest to moderate exercise. During the next 20 min, liver and muscle glycogen supply between 40 and 50% of the energy requirement, with the remainder provided by fat catabolism and a limited amount of protein. In essence, the nutrient mixture for energy depends on the *relative exercise intensity* (i.e., the percentage of one's maximum exercise capacity). During low-intensity physical activity, fat serves as the main energy substrate throughout exercise (see Fig. 1.17 later in the chapter). As exercise continues and muscle glycogen decreases, blood glucose becomes the major source of carbohydrate energy, while fat catabolism furnishes an increasingly greater percentage of the total energy. Eventually, the liver's glucose output fails to keep pace with glucose use by muscle, and plasma glucose concentration decreases. In such cases, circulating blood glucose may reach hypoglycemic

levels (symptoms of hypoglycemia usually do not occur until blood glucose concentration lowers to 2.8 to 3.0 mmol·L⁻¹ (50 to 54 mg·dL⁻¹).

Figure **1.6** depicts the metabolic profile during prolonged exercise in the glycogen-depleted and glycogen-loaded states. As submaximal activity progresses in the glycogen-depleted state, blood glucose levels fall and circulating fat, predominantly as free fatty acids or FFA, increases dramatically compared with exercise under glycogen-loaded conditions. Concurrently, the contribution of protein to the energy expenditure increases. Exercise intensity, expressed as percentage of maximum, also progressively decreases under the glycogen-depleted condition. At the end of 2 hr, an exerciser can only maintain about 50% of the initial exercise intensity. Reduced power output results directly from the relatively slow rate of aerobic energy release from fat oxidation, which now becomes the primary energy source. Any of the following seven potential rate-limiting metabolic processes that precede the citric acid cycle (see Chapter 6) could explain the relatively slower rate of fat oxidation compared with that of carbohydrate:

1. FFA mobilization from adipose tissue
2. FFA transport to skeletal muscle via circulation
3. FFA uptake by the muscle cell

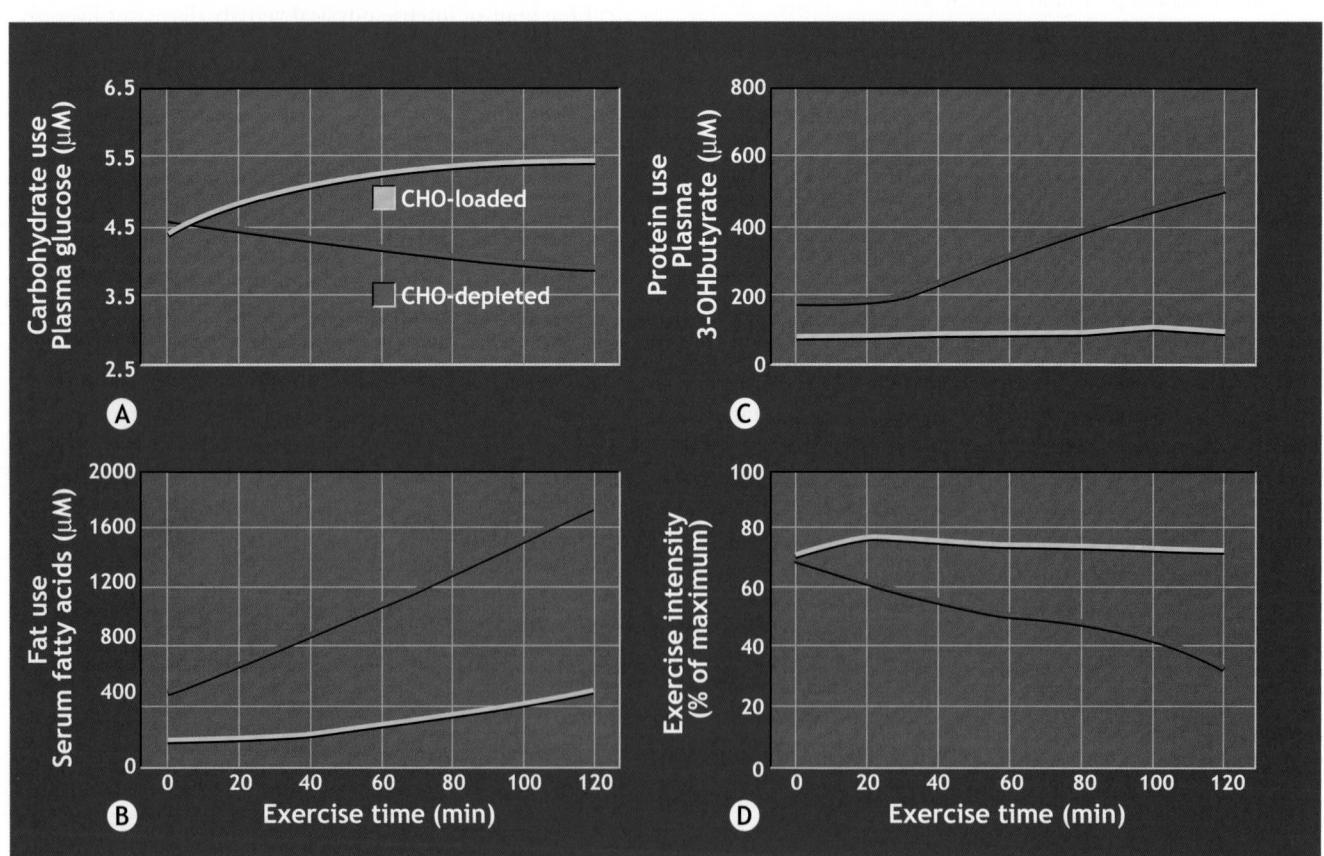

FIGURE 1.6 • Dynamics of nutrient metabolism during 2 hr of exercise in the glycogen-loaded and glycogen-depleted states. During exercise with limited carbohydrate availability, plasma glucose levels (**A**) progressively decrease, while fat metabolism (**B**) progressively increases compared with similar exercise when glycogen loaded. In addition, protein use for energy (**C**), as indicated by plasma levels of 3-OH butyrate, remains considerably higher with glycogen depletion. After 2 hr, exercise capacity (**D**) decreases to about 50% of the exercise level begun in the glycogen-depleted state. (Adapted with permission from Wagenmakers AJM, et al. Carbohydrate supplementation, glycogen depletion, and amino acid metabolism. *Am J Physiol* 1991;260:E883.)

4. FFA uptake by the muscle from triacylglycerols in chylomicrons and lipoproteins
5. Fatty acid mobilization from intramuscular triacylglycerols and cytoplasmic transport
6. Fatty acid transport into the mitochondria
7. Fatty acid oxidation within the mitochondria

Fatigue occurs when physical activity continues to the point that compromises the liver and muscle glycogen content. This occurs despite sufficient oxygen availability to muscle and an almost unlimited energy supply available from stored fat. Endurance athletes commonly refer to this sensation of fatigue as "bonking," or "**hitting the wall**." Because skeletal muscle lacks the phosphatase enzyme, which allows glucose exchange between cells, the relatively inactive muscles maintain their full glycogen content. What remains unclear is why muscle glycogen depletion coincides with the point of fatigue. The answer may relate to three factors:

1. Depressed availability of blood glucose for optimal central nervous system function
2. Muscle glycogen's role as a "primer" in fat breakdown
3. Slower rate of energy release from fat compared to carbohydrate breakdown

Effect of Diet on Muscle Glycogen Stores and Endurance

Diet composition profoundly affects glycogen reserves and subsequent exercise performance. In a classic experiment[3] illustrated in **FIGURE 1.7**, six subjects maintained normal caloric intake for 3 days but consumed most of their calories as lipid and 5% or less as carbohydrate (high-fat diet). In the second condition (normal diet), the 3-day diet contained the recommended daily percentages of carbohydrate, lipid, and protein. The third diet provided 82% of the calories as carbohydrates (high-carbohydrate diet). The glycogen content of the quadriceps femoris muscle, determined from needle biopsy specimens, averaged 0.63 g of glycogen per 100 g of wet muscle with the high-fat diet, 1.75 g for the normal diet, and 3.75 g for the high-carbohydrate diet.

Endurance capacity during cycling varied considerably, depending on what diet was consumed for 3 days before the exercise test. With the normal diet, exercise lasted an average of 114 min, whereas endurance averaged only 57 min with the high-fat diet. The high-carbohydrate diet improved endurance performance by more than three times that of the high-fat diet. Interestingly, the point of fatigue coincided with the same low level of muscle glycogen under the three diet conditions. These findings, complemented by the research of others,[20,24] conclusively demonstrate the importance of muscle glycogen to sustain intense physical activity lasting more than 1 hr.

A carbohydrate-deficient diet rapidly depletes muscle and liver glycogen and negatively affects performance in short-term anaerobic activity and prolonged intense aerobic activities. These observations apply particularly to individuals who modify their diets by reducing carbohydrate intake below recommended levels. Reliance on starvation diets or other extreme diet forms (e.g., high-fat, low-carbohydrate diets or "liquid-protein" diets) proves counterproductive to optimize exercise performance. Reliance on low-carbohydrate diets makes it particularly difficult from an energy supply standpoint to

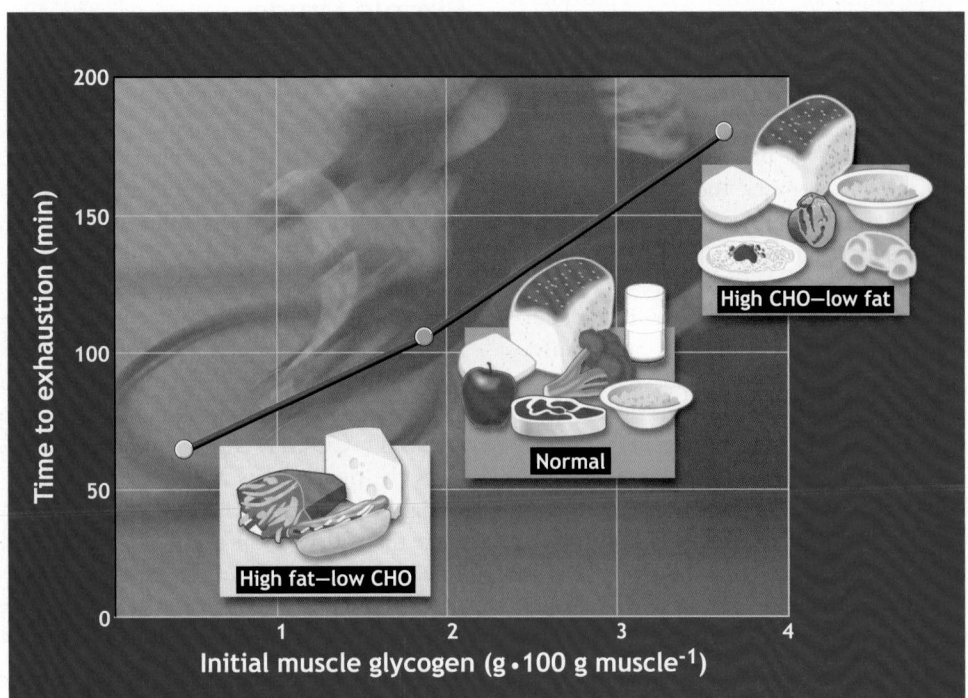

FIGURE 1.7 • Classic experiment illustrating the effects of a high-fat–low-carbohydrate (CHO) diet, a normal diet, and a high-carbohydrate–low-fat diet on the quadriceps femoris muscle's glycogen content and duration of endurance exercise on a bicycle ergometer. Endurance time with a high-carbohydrate diet is three times that on a low-carbohydrate diet. (Adapted with permission from Bergstrom J, et al. Diet, muscle glycogen and physical performance. *Acta Physiol Scand* 1967;71:140.)

engage regularly in longer-duration, vigorous physical activities. Chapter 3 discusses optimal provision for carbohydrate needs prior to, during, and in recovery from strenuous exercise.

Summary

1. Carbon, hydrogen, oxygen, and nitrogen represent the basic structural units for most of the body's bioactive substances. Carbon combined with oxygen and hydrogen form carbohydrates and lipids. Proteins form when combinations of carbon, oxygen, and hydrogen bind with nitrogen and minerals.

2. Simple sugars consist of chains of 3 to 7 carbon atoms, with hydrogen and oxygen in the ratio of 2:1. Glucose, the most common simple sugar, contains a 6-carbon chain as $C_6H_{12}O_6$.

3. Three major classifications of carbohydrates include monosaccharides (sugars such as glucose and fructose), oligosaccharides (disaccharides such as sucrose, lactose, and maltose), and polysaccharides that contain three or more simple sugars to create plant starch and fiber and glycogen (the large glucose polymer from the animal kingdom).

4. Glycogenolysis describes the reconversion of glycogen to glucose; gluconeogenesis refers to glucose synthesis, particularly from protein sources.

5. Americans consume 40 to 50% of total caloric intake as carbohydrates, typically as simple sugars and refined starches. Excess consumption of simple sugars and other rapidly absorbed carbohydrates may have negative health consequences.

6. Carbohydrate, stored in limited quantity in liver and muscle, serves four important functions. It (1) provides a major source of energy, (2) spares protein breakdown, (3) functions as a metabolic primer for fat catabolism, and (4) provides a required, uninterrupted fuel supply to the central nervous system.

7. Muscle glycogen provides the primary energy substrate (fuel) during anaerobic exercise. The body's glycogen stores (muscle glycogen and glucose from the liver) also contribute substantially to energy metabolism in longer-duration endurance-type activities.

8. Fat contributes about 50% of the energy requirement during light- and moderate-intensity exercise. Stored intramuscular fat and fat derived from adipocytes becomes important during prolonged exercise. In this situation, the fatty acid molecules (mainly as circulating FFAs) supply more than 80% of the exercise energy requirements.

9. A carbohydrate-deficient diet quickly depletes muscle and liver glycogen. This profoundly affects both all-out exercise capacity and the capacity to sustain intense aerobic exercise.

10. Individuals who train intensely should consume between 60 and 70% of daily calories as carbohydrates, predominantly in unrefined, complex form (400 to 800 g; 8 to 10 g per kg of body mass).

11. When muscles' supply of glycogen depletes, physical activity intensity decreases to a level determined by the body's ability to mobilize and oxidize fat.

PART 2 LIPIDS

THE NATURE OF LIPIDS

A lipid (from the Greek *lipos*, meaning "fat") molecule has the identical structural elements as carbohydrate but differs in its linkage and number of atoms. Specifically, the lipid's ratio of hydrogen to oxygen considerably exceeds that of carbohydrate. For example, the formula $C_{57}H_{110}O_6$ describes the common lipid stearin with an H:O ratio of 18.3:1. Recall for carbohydrate, the ratio remains constant at 2:1.

Lipid, the general term for a heterogeneous group of compounds, includes *oils*, *fats*, *waxes*, and *related compounds*. Oils become liquid at room temperature, whereas fats remain solid. Approximately 98% of dietary lipid exists as triacylglycerol (see next section), while about 90% of the body's total fat resides in the adipose tissue depots of the subcutaneous tissues.

KINDS AND SOURCES OF LIPIDS

Plants and animals contain lipids in long hydrocarbon chains. Lipids, generally greasy to the touch, remain insoluble in water but soluble in the nonpolar organic solvents acetone, ether, chloroform, and benzene. According to common classification, lipids belong to one of three main groups: simple lipids, compound lipids, and derived lipids.

Simple Lipids

The **simple lipids**, or "neutral fats," consist primarily of **triacylglycerols**—a term preferable to triglycerides among biochemists because it describes glycerol acylated by three fatty acids. The fats are "neutral" because at the pH of the cell they have no electrically charged groups. These completely nonpolar molecules have no affinity for water. Triacylglycerols constitute the major storage form of fat in fat cells (termed **adipocytes**). This molecule contains two different clusters of atoms. One cluster, **glycerol**, consists of a 3-carbon molecule that itself does not qualify as a lipid because of its high solubility in water. Three clusters of unbranched carbon-chained atoms, termed **fatty acids**, bond to the glycerol molecule. A carboxyl (–COOH) cluster at one end of the fatty acid chain gives the molecule its acidic characteristics. Fatty acids have straight hydrocarbon chains with as few as 4 carbon atoms or more than 20, with the most common chain lengths of 16 and 18 carbons.

The synthesis (**condensation**) of the triacylglycerol molecule produces three molecules of water. Conversely, during hydrolysis, when **lipase** enzymes cleave the molecule into its constituents, three molecules of water attach at the points where the fat molecule splits. **FIGURE 1.8** illustrates the basic structure of a **saturated fatty acid** and **unsaturated fatty acid** molecule. All lipid-containing foods consist of a mixture of different proportions of saturated and unsaturated fatty acids.

Ⓐ Saturated Fatty Acid

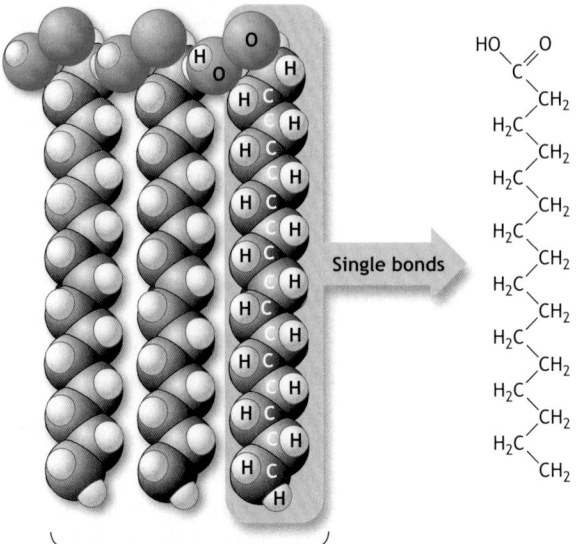

Single bonds →

Carbon atoms linked by single bonds enable close packing of these fatty acid chains

No double bonds; fatty acid chains fit close together

Ⓑ Unsaturated Fatty Acid

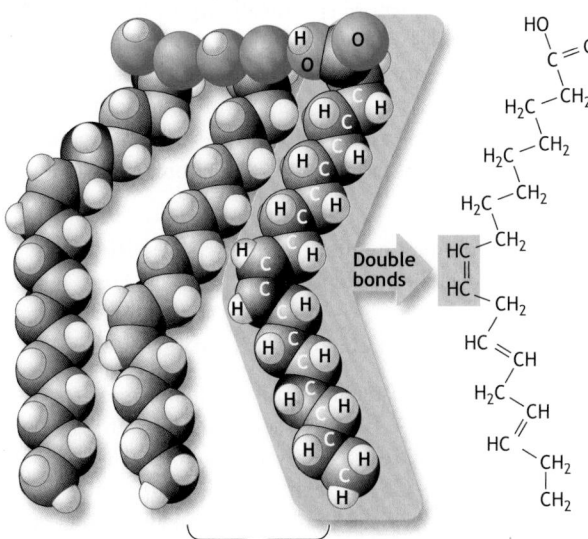

Double bonds →

Carbon atoms linked by double bonds increases distance between fatty acid chains

Double bonds present; fatty acid chains do not fit close together

FIGURE 1.8 • The presence or absence of double bonds between the carbon atoms is the major structural difference between saturated and unsaturated fatty acids. **(A)** The saturated fatty acid palmitic acid has no double bonds in its carbon chain and contains the maximum number of hydrogen atoms. Without double bonds, the three saturated fatty acid chains fit together closely to form a "hard" fat. **(B)** The three double bonds in linoleic acid, an unsaturated fatty acid, reduce the number of hydrogen atoms along the carbon chain. Insertion of double bonds into the carbon chain prevents close association of the fatty acids; this produces a "softer" fat, or an oil.

 Carbon Chains in Fatty Acids

Most naturally occurring fatty acids have an even number chain of carbon atoms that range from 4 to 28, often categorized as short to very long. Fatty acids undergo different metabolic fates depending on their chain length and degree of saturation.

- Short-chain fatty acids (SCFA) = <6 carbons (e.g., butyric, acetic, and caprylic acid) found in butter and some tropical fats.
- Medium-chain fatty acids (MCFA or MCT) = 6 to 12 carbons (e.g., lauric and capric acid) found in coconut oil, palm kernel oil, and breast milk.
- Long-chain fatty acids (LCFA) = 13 to 21 carbons (e.g., palmitic, oleic, and stearic acid) found in animals, fish, cocoa, seeds, nuts and vegetable oils.
- Very long chain fatty acids (VLCFA) = >22 carbons (cerotic acid) that are too long for metabolism in the mitochondria. These require breakdown by peroxisomes, the small vesicles around the cell that contain digestive enzymes for breaking down toxic materials.

SCFA and MCFAs diffuse directly from the GI tract into the portal vein without modification, and are readily available for use as energy substrate. LCFAs, in contrast, require bile salts for digestion and are incorporated into chylomicrons and transported through lymph for deposit as fat.

See the animation "Condensation" on **http://thePoint. lww.com/mkk8e** for a demonstration of this process.

A saturated fatty acid contains only single covalent bonds between carbon atoms; all of the remaining bonds attach to hydrogen. If the carbon within a fatty acid chain binds the maximum possible number of hydrogens, the fatty acid molecule is saturated with respect to hydrogen, and termed a saturated fatty acid.

Saturated fatty acids occur primarily in animal products—beef, lamb, pork, chicken, egg yolk, and dairy fats of cream, milk, butter, and cheese. Saturated fatty acids from the plant kingdom include coconut oil, palm oil, palm kernel oil—often called tropical oils—vegetable shortening, and hydrogenated margarine; commercially prepared cakes, pies, and cookies contain plentiful amounts of saturated fatty acids.

Unsaturated Fatty Acids

Unsaturated fatty acids contain one or more double bonds along their main carbon chain. Each double bond along the chain reduces the number of potential hydrogen-binding sites; the molecule, therefore, is unsaturated with respect to hydrogen. A **monounsaturated fatty acid** contains *one* double bond along the main carbon chain; examples include canola oil, olive oil, peanut oil, and the oil in almonds, pecans, and avocados. A **polyunsaturated fatty acid** contains *two or more* double bonds along the main carbon chain; safflower, sunflower, soybean, and corn oil serve as examples. **FIGURE 1.9** lists the saturated, monounsaturated, and polyunsaturated fatty acid content in

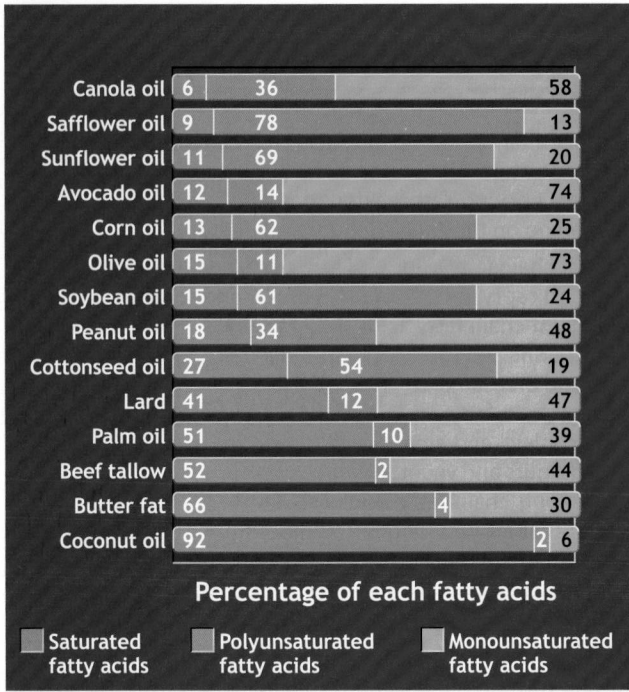

Percentage of each fatty acids

■ Saturated fatty acids	■ Polyunsaturated fatty acids	■ Monounsaturated fatty acids

Hidden fat percentage of total calories

Food	Fat %	Food	Fat %
Brazil nuts	67	Lamb roast	19
Walnuts	61	Avocado	16
Almonds	54	Ice cream	13
Peanuts	50	Herring	12
Sunflower seeds	47	Poached eggs	11
Pork sausage	44	Tuna, canned	8
Pork roast	30	Poultry, dark meat	7
Cheese	30	Oatmeal, dry	7
Bologna	28	Salmon	6
Beef roast	25	Whole milk	4
Ham, cured	22	Poultry, light meat	4
Hamburger	20	Shredded wheat cereal	2

FIGURE 1.9 • **Upper graph** shows the composition of diverse fatty acids (g per 100 g) in common lipid sources in the diet. **Lower table** shows the hidden total fat percentage of total calories in popular foods. (Data from Food Composition Tables, US Department of Agriculture; www.ndb.nal.usda.gov.)

common fats and oils (expressed in g per 100 g of the lipid). The inset table shows the hidden fat percentage in some popular foods. Several polyunsaturated fatty acids, most notably **linoleic acid** (an 18-carbon fatty acid with two double bonds present in cooking and salad oils), must originate from dietary sources because they serve as precursors of other fatty acids the body cannot synthesize and are termed **essential fatty acids**. Linoleic acid maintains the integrity of plasma membranes and sustains growth, reproduction, skin maintenance, and general body functioning. The heart-healthy omega-3 fatty acids found in fish also are polyunsaturated fats.

Fatty acids from plant sources generally remain unsaturated and liquefy at room temperature. In contrast, lipids containing longer carbon chains and more saturated fatty acids exist as solids at room temperature; those with shorter carbon chains and more

unsaturated fatty acids remain soft. Oils exist as liquids and contain unsaturated fatty acids. The chemical process of **hydrogenation** changes oils to semisolid fats by bubbling liquid hydrogen under pressure into vegetable oil. This reduces the unsaturated fatty acids' double bonds to single bonds so more hydrogens can attach to carbons along the chain. Firmer fat forms because adding hydrogen increases the lipid's melting temperature. Hydrogenated oil behaves like a saturated fat; the most common hydrogenated fats include lard substitutes and margarine.

Triacylglycerol Formation

FIGURE 1.10 outlines the sequence of reactions in triacylglycerol synthesis, a process termed **esterification**. Initially, a fatty acid substrate attached to coenzyme A forms fatty acyl-CoA, which then transfers to glycerol (as glycerol 3-phosphate). In subsequent reactions, two additional fatty acyl-CoAs link to the single glycerol backbone to form the composite triacylglycerol molecule. Triacylglycerol synthesis increases following a meal for two reasons: (1) food absorption increases blood levels of fatty acids and glucose and (2) relatively high levels of circulating insulin facilitate triacylglycerol synthesis.

Triacylglycerol Breakdown

The term *hydrolysis* (more specifically **lipolysis** when applied to lipids) describes triacylglycerol catabolism to yield glycerol and the energy-rich fatty acid molecules. **FIGURE 1.11** shows that lipolysis adds water in three distinct hydrolysis reactions, each catalyzed by hormone-sensitive lipase.[14] The mobilization of fatty acids via lipolysis predominates under four conditions:

1. Low-to-moderate–intensity physical activity
2. Low-calorie dieting or fasting
3. Cold stress
4. Prolonged exercise that depletes glycogen reserves

Triacylglycerol esterification and lipolysis occur in the cytosol of adipocytes. The fatty acids released during lipolysis can either reesterify to triacylglycerol following their conversion to a fatty acyl-CoA or exit from the adipocyte, enter the blood, and combine with the blood protein albumin for transport to tissues throughout the body. The term **free fatty acid (FFA)** describes this albumin–fatty acid combination.

Lipolysis also occurs in tissues other than adipocytes. Hydrolysis of dietary triacylglycerol occurs in the small intestine, catalyzed by pancreatic lipase; **lipoprotein lipase**, an enzyme located on the walls of capillaries, catalyzes the hydrolysis of the triacylglycerols carried by the blood's lipoproteins. Adjacent adipose tissue and muscle cells "take up" the fatty acids released by the action lipoprotein lipase; these fatty acids are resynthesized to triacylglycerol for energy storage.

Trans-Fatty Acids: Unwanted at Any Levels

***Trans*-fatty acids** derive from the partial hydrogenation of unsaturated corn, soybean, or sunflower oil. A *trans*-fatty acid

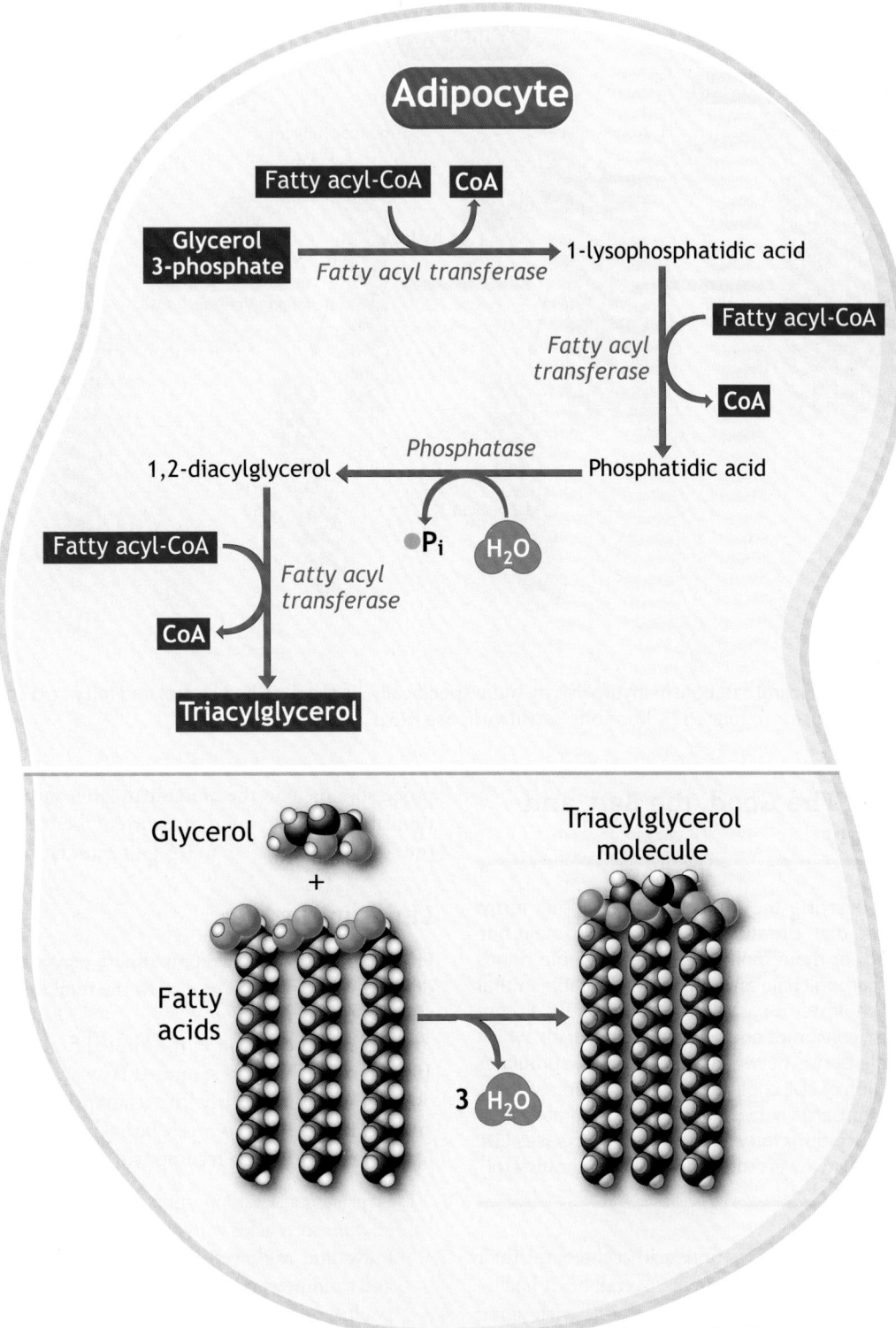

FIGURE 1.10 • Top. Triacylglycerol synthesis involves a series of reactions (dehydration synthesis) that link three fatty acid molecules to a single glycerol backbone. The **bottom** portion of the figure summarizes this linkage. (Adapted with permission from McArdle WD, Katch FI, Katch VL. *Sports and Exercise Nutrition*, 4th ed. Philadelphia: Wolters Kluwer Health, 2013.)

forms when one of the hydrogen atoms along the restructured carbon chain moves from its naturally occurring position (*cis* position) to the opposite side of the double bond that separates 2 carbon atoms (*trans* position). The richest *trans*-fat sources comprise vegetable shortenings, some margarines, and crackers, candies, cookies, snack foods, fried foods, baked goods, salad dressings, and other processed foods made with partially hydrogenated vegetable oils.

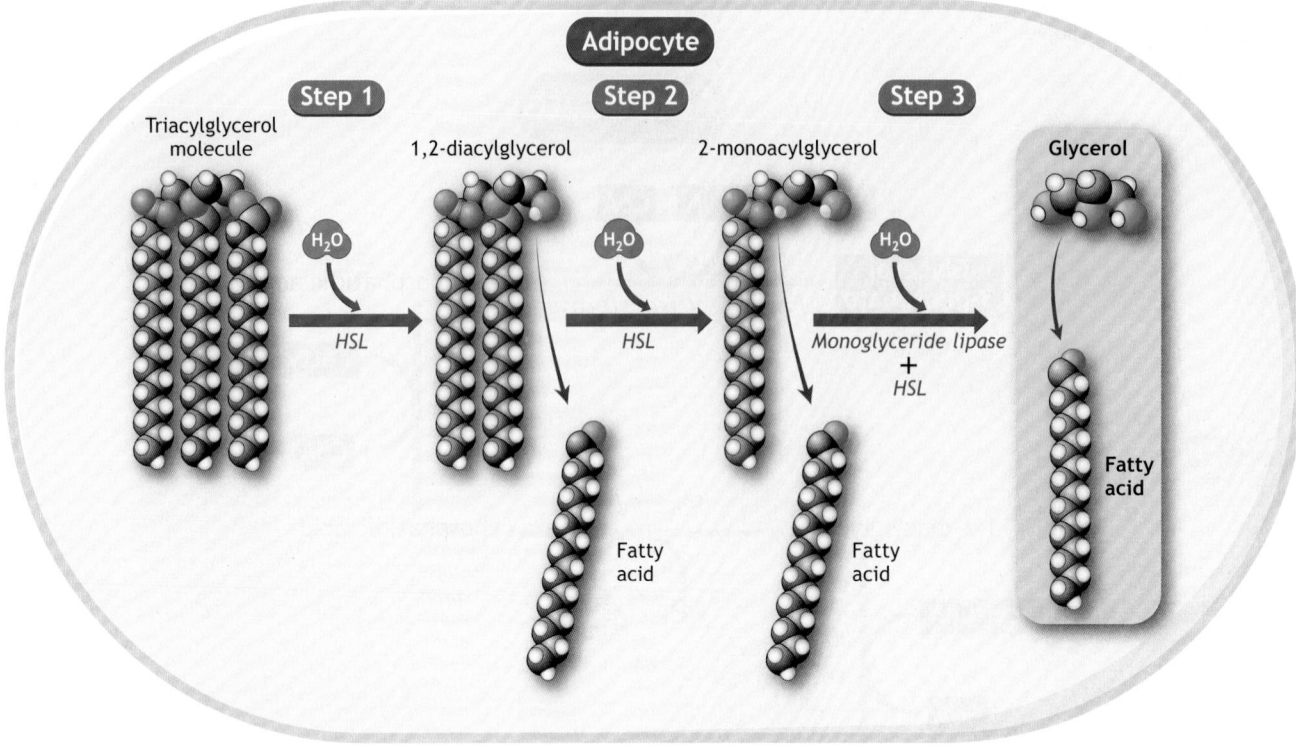

FIGURE 1.11 • Triacylglycerol catabolism (hydrolysis or, more specifically, lipolysis) to its glycerol and fatty acid components involves a three-step process regulated by hormone-sensitive lipase (HSL).

Lipids: The Good, the Bad, and the Ugly

Subjective terms describe the impact of the various forms of fatty acids in the diet. Unsaturated fatty acids contain one (monounsaturated) or more (polyunsaturated) double bonds along their main carbon chain and classify as desirable in that they lower blood cholesterol, particularly the harmful LDL cholesterol. In contrast, consumption of saturated fatty acids, which contain only single bonds between carbon atoms, stimulates the liver's production of LDL cholesterol. Even more disturbing, the consumption of partially hydrogenated unsaturated vegetable oils to produce *trans* fatty acids not only increases LDL concentrations but also lowers the beneficial HDL cholesterol.

Health concerns about *trans*-fatty acids centers on their detrimental effects on serum lipoproteins, overall heart health, and possible role in facilitating cognitive decline with aging in older adults.[5,45,47] A diet high in margarine and commercial baked goods (cookies, cakes, doughnuts, pies) and deep-fried foods prepared with hydrogenated vegetable oils increases low-density lipoprotein cholesterol concentration by a similar amount as a diet high in saturated fatty acids. Unlike saturated fats, hydrogenated oils also decrease the concentration of beneficial high-density lipoprotein cholesterol and adversely affect markers of inflammation and endothelial dysfunction.[38,49] In light of the strong evidence that *trans*-fatty acids place individuals at increased risk for heart disease,[76] the Food and Drug Administration (FDA; www.fda.gov) has mandated that food processors include the amount of *trans*-fatty acids on nutrition labels. Keep in mind that current food labeling rules allow products containing up to 0.5 g of *trans* fat to claim "zero."

Lipids in the Diet

FIGURE 1.12 displays the approximate percentage contribution of some common food groups to the total lipid content of the typical American diet.

The average person in the United States consumes about 15% of total calories as saturated fatty acids, the equivalent of over 23 kg (51 lbs) yearly. The relationship between saturated fatty acid intake and coronary heart disease risk has prompted health professionals to recommend two courses of action:

1. Replacing at least a portion of the saturated fatty acids and all *trans*-fatty acids with nonhydrogenated monounsaturated (olive and safflower) and polyunsaturated (soybean, corn, and sunflower) oils and replacing red meat and cheese with poultry and fish. Dietary recommendations that focus on selected nutrients, such as total fat or saturated fat, are often confusing, resulting in illogical dietary decisions that increase the potential for manipulation of nutrient targets by the food industry. For example, "low fat" associates with "low calorie," and "low saturated fat" is viewed as "healthy," when indeed for many products nothing could be further from the truth.

2. Balancing energy intake with regular physical activity to minimize weight gain (and associated increase in LDL, decrease in HDL, and increase in insulin resistance and blood pressure) and obtain the health benefits of regular exercise.

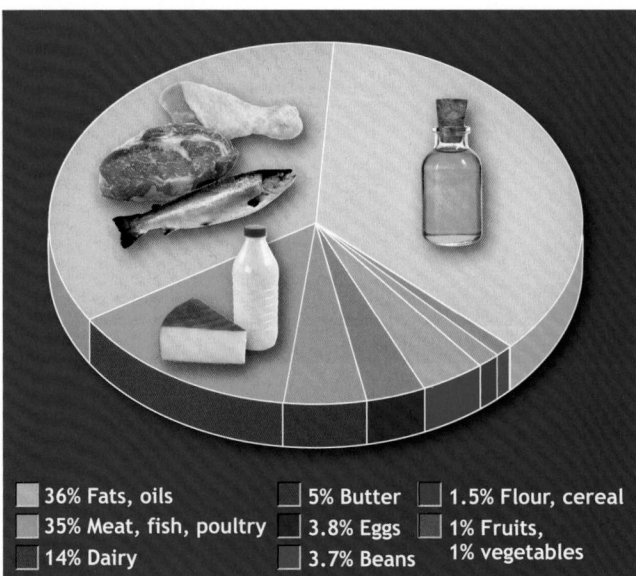

36% Fats, oils
35% Meat, fish, poultry
14% Dairy
5% Butter
3.8% Eggs
3.7% Beans
1.5% Flour, cereal
1% Fruits,
1% vegetables

FIGURE 1.12 • Contribution from the major food groups to the lipid content of the typical American diet.

From a health perspective, individuals should consume no more than 10% of total daily energy intake as saturated fatty acids (about 300 kcal, or 30 to 35 g for the average young adult male who consumes 3000 kcal daily).

Fish Oils. The health profiles and dietary patterns of Greenland Eskimos, who consume large quantities of lipids from fish, seal, and whale that are high in two essential long-chain polyunsaturated fatty acids, eicosapentaenoic acid and docosahexaenoic acid, show that these people have a low incidence of heart disease. These oils belong to the **omega-3 fatty acid** family (also termed *n*-3; the last double bond begins 3 carbons from the end carbon), and are found primarily in the oils of shellfish and cold-water herring, anchovies, sardines, salmon, mackerel, and sea mammals. Regular intake of fish (minimum two servings weekly, about 8 oz total) and possibly fish oil benefits the blood lipid profile, particularly plasma triacylglycerols[39]; overall heart disease risk and mortality rate (chance of ventricular fibrillation and sudden death)[15,34]; cognitive impairment or Alzheimer's disease[55,59]; inflammatory disease risk[80]; colon polyps in women[51]; and (for smokers) the risk of contracting chronic obstructive pulmonary disease.[62] One proposed mechanism for heart attack protection asserts that compounds in fish and their interactions help to prevent blood clot formation on arterial walls. They also may inhibit the growth of atherosclerotic plaques, reduce pulse pressure and total vascular resistance (increase arterial compliance), and stimulate endothelial-derived nitric oxide to facilitate myocardial perfusion (see Chapter 16).[53]

Compound Lipids

Compound lipids (triacylglycerol components combined with other chemicals) represent about 10% of the body's total fat content. One group of modified triacylglycerols, the **phospholipids**, contains one or more fatty acid molecules joined with a phosphorus-containing group and one of several nitrogen-containing molecules. These lipids form in all cells, with the liver synthesizing most of them. Phospholipids have four main functions:

1. Interacting with both water and lipid to modulate fluid movement across cell membranes
2. Maintaining the structural integrity of the cell
3. Playing an important role in blood clotting
4. Providing structural integrity to the insulating sheath that surrounds nerve fibers

Other compound lipids include **glycolipids** (fatty acids bound with carbohydrate and nitrogen) and water-soluble **lipoproteins** (protein spheres formed primarily in the liver when a protein molecule joins with either triacylglycerols or phospholipids). *Lipoproteins provide the major avenue for transporting lipids in the blood.* If blood lipids did not bind to protein, they literally would float to the top like cream in nonhomogenized fresh milk instead of dispersing throughout the vascular system.

High-Density, Low-Density, and Very Low-Density Lipoproteins

Lipoproteins categorize into types according to their size and density and whether they carry cholesterol or triacylglycerol. FIGURE **1.13** illustrates the general dynamics in the body of cholesterol and lipoproteins, including their transport among the small intestine, liver, and peripheral tissues. Four types of lipoproteins exist on the basis of gravitational density:

1. **Chylomicrons.** These form when emulsified lipid droplets (including long-chain triacylglycerols, phospholipids, and FFAs) leave the intestine and enter the lymphatic vessels. Normally, the liver metabolizes chylomicrons and sends them for storage in adipose tissue. Chylomicrons also transport the fat-soluble vitamins A, D, E, and K.
2. **High-density lipoproteins (HDLs).** Produced in the liver and small intestine, they contain the highest percentage of protein (about 50%) and the least total lipid (about 20%) and cholesterol (about 20%) of the lipoproteins.
3. **Very low-density lipoproteins (VLDLs).** These are degraded in the liver to produce **low-density lipoproteins** (**LDLs**; discussed below). VLDLs contain the highest percentage of lipid (95%), of which about 60% consists of triacylglycerol. VLDLs transport triacylglycerols to muscle and adipose tissue. Under the action of lipoprotein lipase, the VLDL molecule becomes a denser LDL molecule because it then contains fewer lipids. LDLs and VLDLs have the most lipid and fewest protein components.
4. **Low-density lipoproteins.** Commonly known as "bad" cholesterol (in contrast, HDL is known as "good" cholesterol), these normally carry from 60 to 80% of the total serum cholesterol and have the greatest affinity for cells of the arterial wall. LDL delivers cholesterol to arterial tissue where the LDL particles are (1) oxidized to alter their physiochemical properties and (2) taken up by macrophages inside the arterial wall to initiate atherosclerotic plaque development. LDL oxidation ultimately contributes to smooth muscle cell proliferation and other unfavorable cellular changes that damage and narrow arteries.

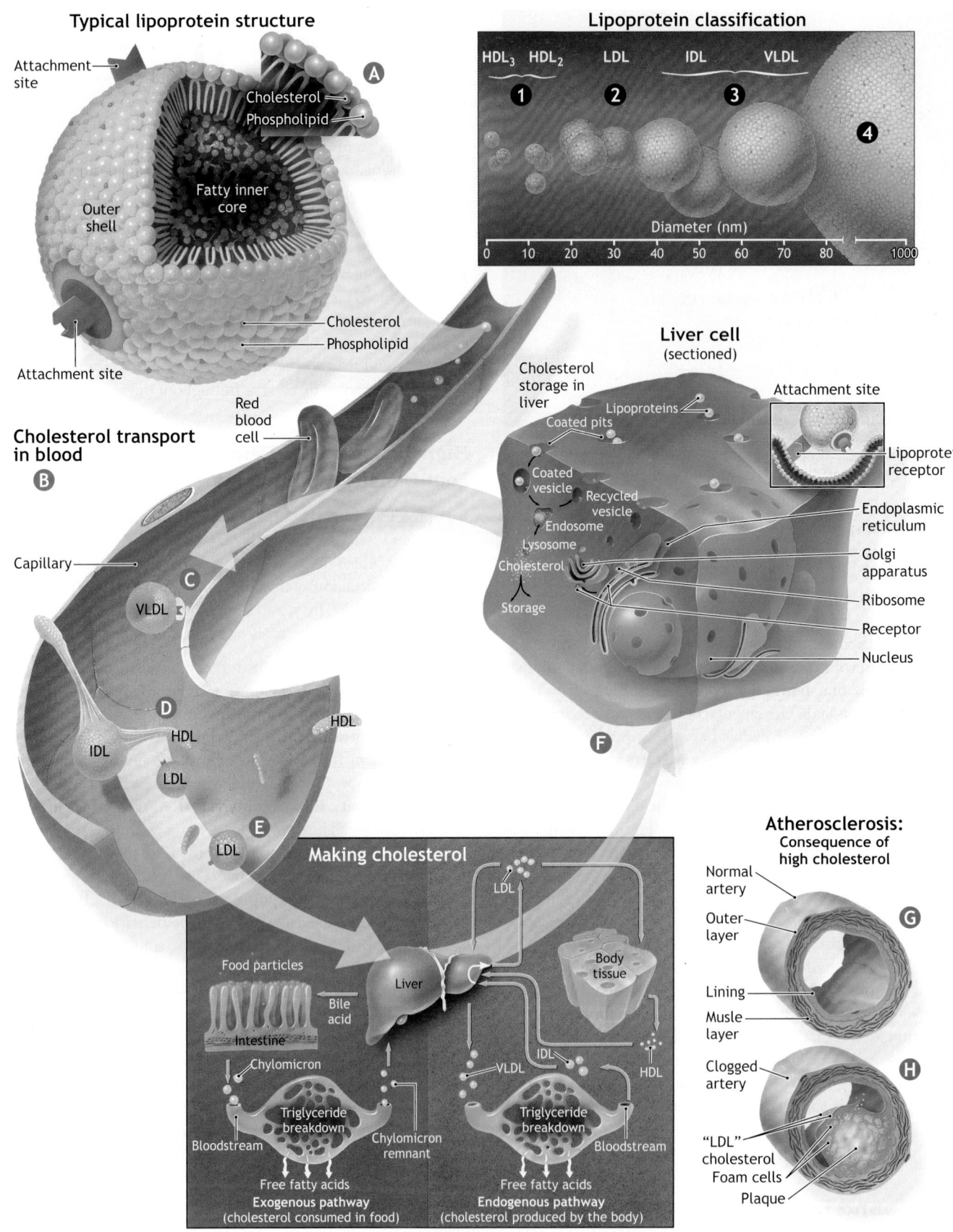

Typical lipoprotein structure

Attachment site

Cholesterol

Phospholipid

Fatty inner core

Outer shell

Attachment site

A

Cholesterol

Phospholipid

Lipoprotein classification

HDL₃ HDL₂   LDL   IDL   VLDL

1   2   3   4

Diameter (nm)

0   10   20   30   40   50   60   70   80   1000

Cholesterol transport in blood

B

Red blood cell

Capillary

C

VLDL

D

IDL

HDL

HDL

LDL

E

LDL

LDL

Liver cell (sectioned)

Cholesterol storage in liver

Coated pits

Coated vesicle

Endosome

Lysosome

Cholesterol

Storage

Lipoproteins

Recycled vesicle

Attachment site

Lipoprotein receptor

Endoplasmic reticulum

Golgi apparatus

Ribosome

Receptor

Nucleus

F

Making cholesterol

Food particles

Bile acid

Intestine

Chylomicron

Bloodstream

Triglyceride breakdown

Chylomicron remnant

Free fatty acids
Exogenous pathway
(cholesterol consumed in food)

Liver

LDL

Body tissue

IDL

VLDL

HDL

Triglyceride breakdown

Bloodstream

Free fatty acids
Endogenous pathway
(cholesterol produced by the body)

Atherosclerosis:
Consequence of high cholesterol

Normal artery

Outer layer

Lining

Musle layer

G

Clogged artery

"LDL" cholesterol

Foam cells

Plaque

H

HDL Versus LDL: A Health Perspective. Unlike LDL, HDL protects against heart disease. HDL acts as a scavenger in the **reverse transport of cholesterol** by removing it from the arterial wall and delivering it to the liver for incorporation into bile and subsequent excretion via the intestinal tract.

The amount of LDL and HDL and their specific ratios (e.g., HDL ÷ total cholesterol; LDL ÷ HDL) and subfractions provide more meaningful indicators of coronary artery disease risk than total cholesterol per se. Regular moderate- and high-intensity aerobic exercise and abstinence from cigarette smoking increase HDL, lower LDL, and favorably alter the LDL:HDL ratio.[36,42,64] We discuss these effects more fully in Chapter 31. An online computer program calculates the risk and the appropriate cholesterol levels for adults (www.nhlbi.nih.gov/guidelines/cholesterol/index.htm).

Derived Lipids

Simple and compound lipids form **derived lipids. Cholesterol**, the most widely known derived lipid, exists *only* in animal tissue. Cholesterol does not contain fatty acids but shares some of lipids' physical and chemical characteristics. For this reason, cholesterol is considered a lipid.

Cholesterol, widespread in the plasma membrane of all animal cells, originates either through the diet (*exogenous cholesterol*) or through cellular synthesis (*endogenous cholesterol*). More endogenous cholesterol forms with a diet high in saturated fatty acids and *trans*-fatty acids, which facilitate LDL cholesterol synthesis in the liver. The liver synthesizes about 70% of the body's cholesterol, but other tissues—including the walls of the arteries and intestines—also construct this compound.

Functions of Cholesterol

Cholesterol participates in many bodily functions; these include building plasma membranes and serving as a precursor in synthesizing vitamin D, adrenal gland hormones, and the sex hormones estrogen, androgen, and progesterone. Cholesterol furnishes a key component for bile (emulsifies lipids during digestion) synthesis and plays a crucial role in forming tissues, organs, and body structures during fetal development.

Egg yolk provides a rich source of cholesterol (average of about 186 mg per egg), as do red meats and organ meats (liver, kidney, and brain). Shellfish (particularly shrimp), dairy products (ice cream, cream cheese, butter, and whole milk), fast-food breakfasts, and processed meats contain relatively large amounts of cholesterol. *Foods from plants contain no cholesterol.*

Cholesterol and Coronary Heart Disease Risk

High levels of total serum cholesterol and the cholesterol-rich LDL molecule are powerful predictors of increased risk for coronary artery disease. These become particularly potent when combined with other risk factors of cigarette smoking, physical inactivity, excess body fat, and untreated hypertension.

A dietary cholesterol excess in "susceptible" individuals eventually produces **atherosclerosis,** a degenerative process that forms cholesterol-rich deposits (**plaque**) on the inner lining of the medium and larger arteries, causing them to narrow and eventually close. Reducing saturated fatty acid and cholesterol intake generally lowers serum cholesterol, yet for most people the effect remains modest.[63,75] Similarly, increasing dietary intake of monounsaturated and polyunsaturated fatty acids lowers blood cholesterol, particularly LDL cholesterol.[23,30,38] Chapter 31 presents specific recommended values for "desirable," "borderline," and "undesirable" plasma lipid and lipoprotein levels.

RECOMMENDED LIPID INTAKE

Recommendations for dietary lipid intake for physically active individuals generally follow prudent health-related recommendations for the general population. Although dietary lipid currently represents between 34 and 38% of total caloric intake in the United States, or about 50 kg (110 lb) of lipid consumed per person each year, current recommendations place intake between 20 and 35% depending on the type of lipid consumed. Rather than providing a precise number for daily cholesterol intake, the American Heart Association (AHA; www.americanheart.org) encourages Americans to focus more on replacing high-fat foods with fruits, vegetables, unrefined whole grains, fat-free and low-fat dairy products, fish, poultry, and lean meat.[35] Other components of the AHA guidelines include a focus on weight control and the addition of two weekly servings of fish high in omega-3 fatty acids. In addition to the AHA guidelines, a new line of research sounds a cautionary note on over-consuming omega-3 fatty acids because of increased risk of prostate cancer.[7] The analysis compared 834 men diagnosed with prostate cancer to a comparison group of 1393 men selected randomly from 35,000 study participants. Instead of finding a protective factor from

FIGURE 1.13 • Cholesterol dynamics in the body. **(A)** Lipoproteins are combined fat and protein particles that transport cholesterol throughout the body. **(B)** Lipoproteins transport cholesterol via the bloodstream. **(C)** The large VLDL particle attaches to the capillary lining where its cholesterol core is extracted. **(D)** The smaller IDL particle remains in the blood for transport back to the liver for removal. **(E)** LDL remains in the blood and travels back to the liver for removal. **(F)** An excess of cholesterol reduces the lipoprotein receptor number on the liver cell surface. **(G)** With normal blood cholesterol levels, arterial walls remain smooth and slippery. **(H)** High blood cholesterol levels concentrate cholesterol in arterial walls, thereby reducing blood flow. Lipoprotein Classification: 1, high density lipoprotein (HDL); 2, low density lipoprotein (LDL); 3, intermediate density lipoprotein (IDL) and very low density lipoprotein (VLDL); 4, chylomicron, dietary cholesterol and triacylglycerol particles absorbed by small intestine. (Adapted with permission from Anatomical Chart Company. © 2000 Anatomical Chart Company.)

the presence of omega-3 fatty acids in the blood, men with the highest blood levels had a 43% higher risk of developing prostate cancer, and 71% greater chance of developing a more fatal, high-grade form of prostate cancer.

The American Cancer Society (www.cancer.org) advocates a diet that contains only 20% of total calories from lipid to reduce risk of cancers of the colon and rectum, prostate, endometrium, and perhaps breast.

The main sources of dietary cholesterol include the same animal food sources rich in saturated fatty acids. Curtailing intake of these foods reduces preformed cholesterol intake and, more importantly, reduces intake of fatty acids known to stimulate endogenous cholesterol synthesis.

Reduce Saturated Fat and Cholesterol in the Diet

If You Eat This Food	To Reduce Fat, Substitute This Food
Egg	Egg whites or fat-free egg substitute
Cream cheese	Low-fat or fat-free cream cheese; blended low-fat cottage cheese or blended low-fat ricotta cheese
Cheeses	Part-skim milk cheeses
Sour cream	Low-fat or fat-free yogurt, low-fat cottage cheese blended with lemon juice
Cream/ whole milk	Nonfat milk; evaporated skim milk; nonfat buttermilk
Baking chocolate	Unsweetened cocoa powder

ROLE OF LIPID IN THE BODY

Four important functions of lipids in the body include:

1. Energy source and reserve
2. Protection of vital organs
3. Thermal insulation
4. Vitamin carrier and hunger suppressor

Energy Source and Reserve

Fat constitutes the ideal cellular fuel for three reasons:

1. It carries a large quantity of energy per unit weight.
2. It transports and stores easily.
3. It provides a ready source of energy.

Fat provides as much as 80 to 90% of the energy requirement of a well-nourished individual at rest. One gram of pure lipid contains about 9 kcal (38 kJ) of energy, more than twice the energy available to the body from an equal quantity of carbohydrate or protein. Recall that the synthesis of a

triacylglycerol molecule from glycerol and three fatty acid molecules produces three water molecules. In contrast, when glycogen forms from glucose, each gram of glycogen stores 2.7 g of water. *Fat exists as a relatively water-free, concentrated fuel, whereas glycogen remains hydrated and heavy relative to its energy content.*

 INTEGRATIVE QUESTION

What benefit derives from storing excess calories as fat in adipose tissue compared to storing an equivalent caloric excess as glycogen?

Fat and Energy Content of the Body. For young adults, approximately 15% of the body mass of males and 25% of females consists of fat. **Figure 1.14** illustrates the total mass (and energy content) of fat from various sources in an 80-kg man. The potential energy stored in the fat molecules of the adipose tissue translates to about 108,000 kcal (12,000 g body fat × 9.0 kcal·g^{-1}). A run from San Diego, California's football stadium to the convention center in downtown Seattle, Washington (assuming an energy expenditure of about 100 kcal per mile), would deplete the available energy from adipose tissue and intramuscular triacylglycerols and a small amount of plasma FFAs. Contrast this with the limited 2000-kcal reserve of stored carbohydrate that would provide energy for only a 20-mile run! Viewed from a different perspective, the body's energy reserves from carbohydrate could power intense running for about 1.6 hr, whereas exercise would continue for about 75 times longer or 120 hr using the body's fat reserves! Fat used as a fuel also "spares" protein to carry out its important functions of tissue synthesis and repair.

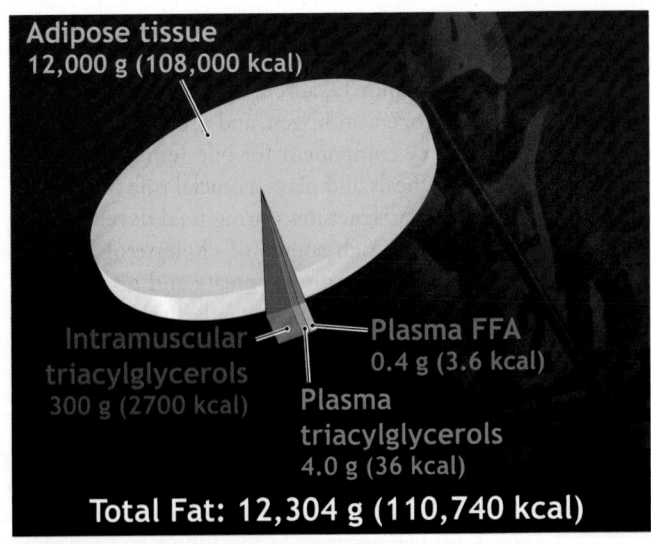

FIGURE 1.14 • Distribution of the quantity and energy stored as fat within an average 80-kg man. FFA, free fatty acids. (Adapted with permission from McArdle WD, Katch FI, Katch VL. *Sports and Exercise Nutrition*, 4th ed. Philadelphia: Wolters Kluwer Health, 2013.)

Protection of Vital Organs and Thermal Insulation

Up to 4% of the body's fat protects against trauma to vital organs (e.g., heart, liver, kidneys, spleen, brain, spinal cord). Fat stored just below the skin, called subcutaneous fat, provides insulation, permitting individuals to tolerate extreme cold.[68] A thicker layer of this insulatory fat benefits deep-sea divers, ocean and channel swimmers, or Arctic inhabitants. In contrast, excess body fat hinders temperature regulation during heat stress, most notably during sustained exercise in air, when the body's heat production can increase 20 times above resting levels. In this case, the insulatory shield from subcutaneous fat retards heat flow from the body.

For large-sized football linemen, excess fat storage provides additional cushioning to protect the participant from the sport's normal traumas. Nonetheless, any possible protective benefit must be weighed against the liability imposed by the "dead weight" of excess fat and its impact on energy expenditure, thermal regulation, and subsequent exercise performance.

Vitamin Carrier and Hunger Depressor

Consuming approximately 20 g of dietary fat daily provides a sufficient source and transport medium for the four fat-soluble vitamins A, D, E, and K. Severely reducing lipid intake depresses the body's level of these vitamins and ultimately may lead to vitamin deficiency. Dietary lipid also facilitates absorption of vitamin A precursors from nonlipid plant sources such as carrots and apricots. It takes about 3.5 hr after ingesting lipids for the stomach to empty them.

FAT DYNAMICS DURING PHYSICAL ACTIVITY

Intracellular and extracellular fat (FFAs, intramuscular triacylglycerols, and circulating plasma triacylglycerols bound to lipoproteins as VLDLs and chylomicrons) supply between 30 and 80% of the energy for physical activity, depending on nutritional and fitness status and exercise intensity and duration.[2,44] Increased blood flow through adipose tissue with exercise increases the release of FFAs for delivery to and use by muscle. The quantity of fat used for energy in light and moderate exercise is three times that compared to resting conditions. As activity becomes more intense (greater percentage of aerobic capacity), adipose tissue release of FFAs fails to increase much above resting levels, leading to a decrease in plasma FFAs. This in turn stimulates increased muscle glycogen use (see Fig. 1.17 later in the chapter).[61] The energy contribution from intramuscular triacylglycerols ranges between 15 and 35%, with endurance-trained athletes catabolizing the largest quantity and a substantial impairment in use among the obese and/or type 2 diabetics.[32,33,71] Long-term consumption of a high-fat diet induces enzymatic adaptations that enhance fat oxidation during submaximal exercise.[40,50] Unfortunately, this adaptation does not translate to improved exercise performance.

 See the animation "Fat Mobilization and Use" on http://thePoint.lww.com/mkk8e for a demonstration of this process.

The major energy for light-to-moderate exercise comes from fatty acids released from triacylglycerol storage sites and delivered to muscle as FFAs and intramuscular triacylglycerols. The start of exercise produces a transient initial drop in plasma FFA concentration because of increased FFA uptake by active muscles. An increased FFA release from adipose tissue follows (with concomitant suppression of triacylglycerol formation) owing to two factors:

1. Hormonal stimulation by the sympathetic nervous system
2. Decrease in plasma insulin levels

During moderate-intensity activity, approximately equal amounts of carbohydrate and fat supply energy. When physical activity continues at this level for more than 1 hr, fat catabolism gradually supplies a greater percentage of energy; this coincides with the progression of glycogen depletion. Carbohydrate availability also influences fat use for energy. With adequate glycogen reserves, carbohydrate becomes the preferred fuel during intense aerobic exercise because of its more rapid rate of catabolism. Toward the end of prolonged exercise (when glycogen reserves become nearly depleted), fat, mainly as circulating FFAs, supplies up to 80% of the total energy requirement. **Figure 1.15** illustrates the general

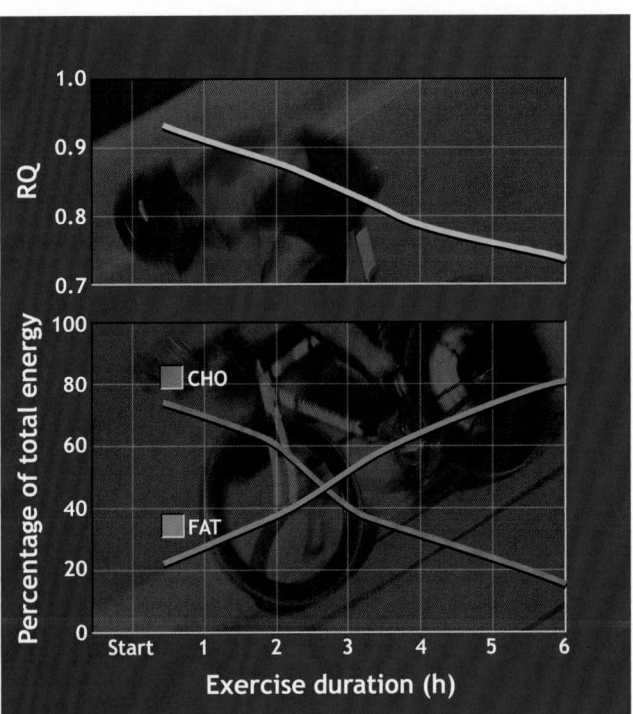

FIGURE 1.15 • The relationship between respiratory quotient (RQ) and substrate use during long-duration, submaximal exercise. (**Top**) Progressive reduction in RQ during 6 hr of continuous exercise. (**Bottom**) Percentage of energy derived from carbohydrate and fat. (Adapted with permission from Edwards HT, et al. Metabolic rate, blood sugar and utilization of carbohydrate. *Am J Physiol* 1934;108:203.)

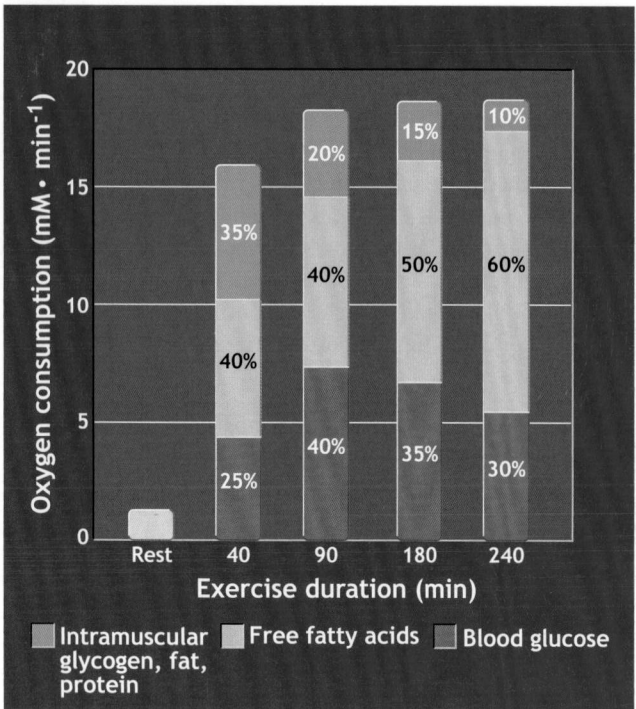

FIGURE 1.16 • Generalized percentage contribution of macronutrient catabolism in relation to oxygen consumption of the leg muscles during prolonged exercise.

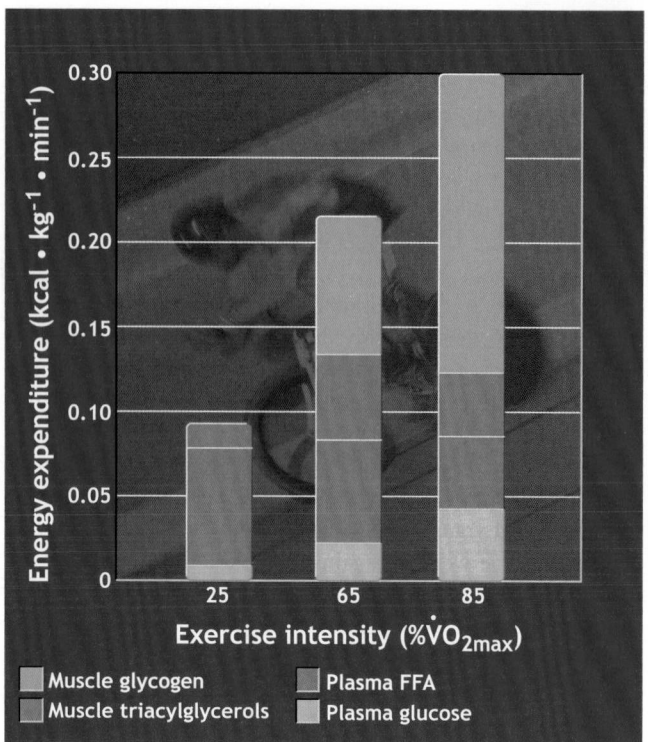

FIGURE 1.17 • Steady-state substrate use calculated using three isotopes and indirect calorimetry in trained men performing cycle ergometer exercise at 25, 65, and 85% of V̇O₂max. As exercise intensity increases, absolute use of glucose and muscle glycogen increases, whereas muscle triacylglycerol and plasma FFA use decreases. (Adapted with permission from Romijn JA, et al. Regulation of endogenous fat and carbohydrate metabolism in relation to exercise intensity and duration. *Am J Physiol* 1993;265:E380.)

response for substrate utilization during prolonged cycling exercise. Carbohydrate combustion (reflected by the RQ [respiratory quotient]; see Chapter 8) steadily declines during physical activity, with an associated increase in fat use. Toward the end of exercise, fat breakdown supplies nearly 85% of the total energy; it demonstrates fat oxidation's important role in providing energy during extended exercise with glycogen depletion.

The increase in fat catabolism during prolonged physical activity probably results from a small drop in blood sugar and decrease in insulin (a potent inhibitor of lipolysis), with a corresponding increase in glucagon output by the pancreas. Such responses ultimately reduce glucose catabolism and its potential inhibitory effect on long-chain fatty acid breakdown, further stimulating FFA liberation for energy. **FIGURE 1.16** reveals that FFA uptake by active muscle rises during hours 1 and 4 of moderate exercise. In the first hour, fat (including intramuscular fat) supplied about 50% of the energy; by the third hour, fat contributed up to 70% of the total energy requirement.

Exercise intensity governs fat's contribution to the metabolic mixture.[69,73] **FIGURE 1.17** illustrates the dynamics of fat use by trained men who exercised between 25 and 85% of their maximum aerobic metabolism. During light-to-moderate exercise (≤40% of maximum), fat provided the main energy source predominantly as plasma FFAs from adipose tissue depots. Increased exercise intensity produced an eventual *crossover* in the balance of fuel use—total energy from all sources of fat breakdown remained essentially unchanged. More intense exercise required added energy from blood glucose and muscle glycogen. Total energy from fats during

exercise at 85% of maximum did not differ from exercise at 25%. *Such data highlight the major role that carbohydrate, primarily muscle glycogen, plays as a preferential fuel for intense aerobic exercise.*

Exercise Training and Fat Use

Regular aerobic exercise profoundly improves long-chain fatty acid oxidation, particularly from triacylglycerols within active muscle during mild-to-moderate–intensity exercise.[4,26,72] **FIGURE 1.18** illustrates the percentage contribution of various energy substrates during 2 hr of moderate-intensity exercise in the trained and untrained state. For a total energy expenditure of about 1000 kcal, intramuscular triacylglycerol combustion supplied 25% of total energy expenditure before training; this increased to more than 40% following training. Energy from plasma FFA oxidation decreased from 18% pretraining to about 15% posttraining. Biopsy samples revealed a 41% reduction in muscle glycogen combustion in the trained state. This accounted for the overall decrease in total energy from all carbohydrate fuel sources (58% pretraining to 38% posttraining). The important point concerns the greater uptake of FFAs and concurrent conservation of glycogen reserves by the

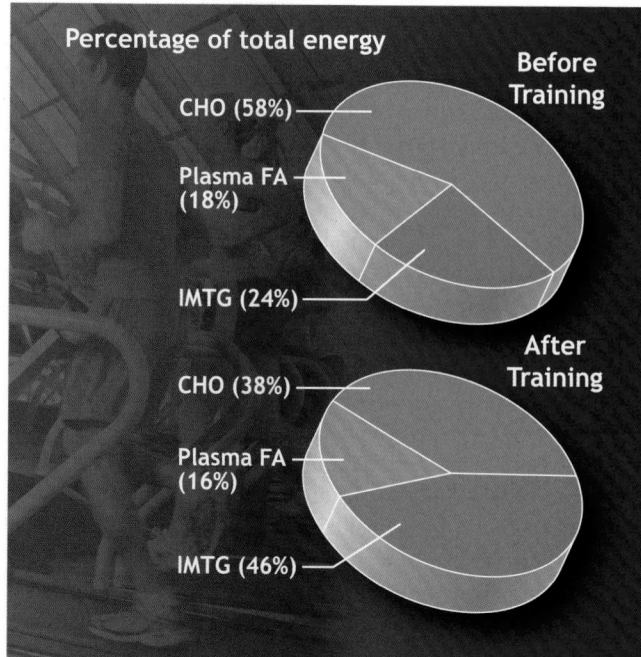

Percentage of total energy

Before Training

CHO (58%)

Plasma FA (18%)

IMTG (24%)

After Training

CHO (38%)

Plasma FA (16%)

IMTG (46%)

FIGURE 1.18 • Percentage of total energy derived from carbohydrate (CHO), intramuscular triacylglycerol (IMTG), and plasma fatty acid (FA) fuel sources during prolonged exercise (8.3 kcal·min⁻¹) before and after endurance training. (Adapted with permission from Martin WH III, et al. Effect of endurance training on plasma free fatty acid turnover and oxidation during exercise. *Am J Physiol* 1993;265:E708.)

trained than by untrained limbs at the same moderate absolute exercise level. Seven factors can impact training-induced increases in fat catabolism during physical activity:

1. Facilitated fatty acid mobilization from adipose tissue through increased rate of lipolysis within adipocytes
2. Proliferation of capillaries in trained muscle that increases the total number and density of these microvessels for energy substrate delivery
3. Improved transport of FFAs through the muscle fiber's plasma membrane
4. Increased fatty acid transport within the muscle cell, mediated by carnitine and carnitine acyltransferase
5. Increased size and number of mitochondria
6. Increased quantity of enzymes involved in β-oxidation, citric acid cycle metabolism, and the electron-transport chain within specifically trained muscle fibers
7. Maintenance of cellular integrity and function, which enhances endurance performance independent of conservation of glycogen reserves

Endurance athletes exercise at a higher absolute submaximal exercise level from an improved capacity for fat oxidation before experiencing the fatiguing effects of glycogen depletion. This adaptation does not sustain the level of aerobic metabolism generated when oxidizing glycogen for energy. Near-maximal sustained aerobic effort in well-nourished endurance athletes still requires almost total reliance on oxidation of stored glycogen for optimal performance.

 INTEGRATIVE QUESTION

Explain why a high level of daily physical activity requires regular carbohydrate intake. What "nonexercise" benefits occur from consuming a diet rich in unrefined, complex carbohydrates?

Summary

1. Lipids contain carbon, hydrogen, and oxygen atoms, but with a higher ratio of hydrogen to oxygen. The formula $C_{57}H_{110}O_6$ describes the lipid stearin. Lipid molecules consist of 1 glycerol molecule and 3 fatty acid molecules.
2. Lipids, synthesized by plants and animals, classify into one of three groups: simple lipids (glycerol plus three fatty acids), compound lipids (phospholipids, glycolipids, and lipoproteins) composed of simple lipids combined with other chemicals, and derived lipids such as cholesterol, synthesized from simple and compound lipids.
3. Saturated fatty acids contain as many hydrogen atoms as chemically possible; saturated describes this molecule with respect to hydrogen. Saturated fatty acids exist primarily in animal meat, egg yolk, dairy fats, and cheese. A large saturated fatty acid intake elevates blood cholesterol concentration and promotes coronary heart disease.
4. Unsaturated fatty acids contain fewer hydrogen atoms attached to the carbon chain. Unlike saturated fatty acids, double bonds connect carbon atoms; these fatty acids are either monounsaturated or polyunsaturated with respect to hydrogen. Increasing the diet's proportion of unsaturated fatty acids protects against coronary heart disease.
5. Lowering blood cholesterol (especially that carried by LDL cholesterol) provides significant heart disease protection.
6. Dietary lipid currently provides about 36% of total energy intake. Prudent recommendations suggest a level of 30% or less for dietary lipid, of which 70 to 80% should consist of unsaturated fatty acids.
7. Lipids provide the largest nutrient store of potential energy for biologic work. They also protect vital organs, provide insulation from the cold, and transport the four fat-soluble vitamins A, D, E, and K.
8. Fat contributes 50 to 70% of the energy requirement during light- and moderate-intensity physical activity. Stored fat (intramuscular and derived from adipocytes) plays an increasingly important role during prolonged exercise when acid molecules (mainly circulating FFAs) provide more than 80% of the exercise energy requirements.
9. Carbohydrate depletion reduces exercise intensity to a level determined by how well the body mobilizes and oxidizes fatty acids.
10. Aerobic training increases long-chain fatty acid oxidation during mild-to-moderate–intensity exercise, primarily fatty acids from triacylglycerols within active muscle.
11. Enhanced fat oxidation with training spares glycogen; this allows trained individuals to exercise at a higher absolute level of submaximal exercise before they experience the fatiguing effects of glycogen depletion.

PROTEINS

THE NATURE OF PROTEINS

Combinations of linked amino acids form proteins (from the Greek word meaning "of prime importance"). An average-sized adult contains between 10 and 12 kg of protein, with skeletal muscle containing the largest quantity of 6 to 8 kg or 60 to 75% of all proteins. Additionally, approximately 210 g of amino acids exist in free form, largely as glutamine, a key amino acid that serves as fuel for immune system cells. Humans typically ingest about 10 to 15% of their total calories as protein. During digestion, protein hydrolyzes to its amino acid constituents for absorption by the small intestine. The protein content of most adults remains remarkably stable and little amino acid "reserves" exist in the body. Amino acids not used to synthesize protein or other compounds (e.g., hormones) or not available for energy metabolism provide substrate for gluconeogenesis or convert to triacylglycerol for storage in adipocytes.

Structurally, proteins resemble carbohydrates and lipids because they contain atoms of carbon, oxygen, and hydrogen. Protein molecules also contain about 16% nitrogen, along with sulfur and occasionally phosphorus, cobalt, and iron. Just as glycogen forms from many simple glucose subunits linked together, the protein molecule polymerizes from its amino acid "building-block" constituents in numerous complex arrays. **Peptide bonds** link amino acids in chains that take on diverse forms and chemical combinations; two joined amino acids produce a **dipeptide**, and linking three amino acids produces a **tripeptide**. A **polypeptide** chain contains 50 to more than 1000 amino acids. A combination of more than 50 amino acids forms a **protein** of which humans can synthesize an array of different kinds. Single cells contain thousands of different protein molecules; some have a linear configuration, some are folded into complex shapes having three-dimensional properties. In total, approximately 50,000 different protein-containing compounds exist in the body. The biochemical functions and properties of each protein depend on the sequence of specific amino acids (this aspect is discussed more fully in the final chapter, "On the Horizon").

The 20 different amino acids required by the body each have a positively charged amine group at one end of the molecule and a negatively charged organic acid group at the other end. The **amine group** has two hydrogen atoms attached to nitrogen (NH_2), whereas the **organic acid group** (technically termed *carboxylic acid group*) contains 1 carbon atom, 2 oxygen atoms, and 1 hydrogen atom (COOH). The remainder of the amino acid, referred to as the **R group**, or **side chain**, takes on a variety of forms. *The R group's specific structure dictates the amino acid's particular characteristics.* **Figure 1.19** shows the four common features that constitute the general structure of all amino acids. The potential for combining the 20 amino acids produces an almost infinite number of possible proteins, depending on their amino acid combinations. For example, linking just three different amino acids could generate 20^3, or 8000, different proteins.

KINDS OF PROTEIN

The body cannot synthesize eight amino acids (nine in children and some older adults), so individuals must consume foods that contain them. These make up the **essential** (or indispensable) **amino acids**—isoleucine, leucine, lysine, methionine, phenylalanine, threonine, tryptophan, and valine. In addition, the body synthesizes cystine from methionine and tyrosine from phenylalanine. Infants cannot synthesize histidine, and children have reduced capability for synthesizing arginine. The body manufactures the remaining nine **nonessential amino acids.** The term *nonessential* does not indicate a lack of importance; rather, they are synthesized from other compounds already in the body at a rate that meets the body's needs for normal growth and tissue repair.

Animals and plants manufacture proteins that contain essential amino acids. An amino acid derived from an animal has no health or physiologic advantage over the same amino acid from vegetable origin. Plants synthesize amino acids by incorporating nitrogen from the soil (along with carbon, oxygen, and hydrogen from air and water). In contrast, animals have no broad capability for amino acid synthesis; instead, they consume most of their protein.

Synthesizing a specific protein requires the availability of appropriate amino acids. **Complete proteins** (sometimes referred to as higher-quality proteins) come from foods that contain all of the essential amino acids in the quantity and correct ratio to maintain nitrogen balance and to allow tissue growth and repair. An **incomplete protein** lacks one or more essential amino acids. A diet of incomplete protein eventually leads to protein malnutrition, whether or not the food sources contain an adequate *amount* of energy or protein.

Protein Sources

Sources of complete protein include eggs, milk, meat, fish, and poultry. Eggs provide the optimal mixture of essential amino acids among all food sources; hence, eggs receive the highest quality rating of 100 for comparison with other foods. **Table 1.3** rates some common sources of

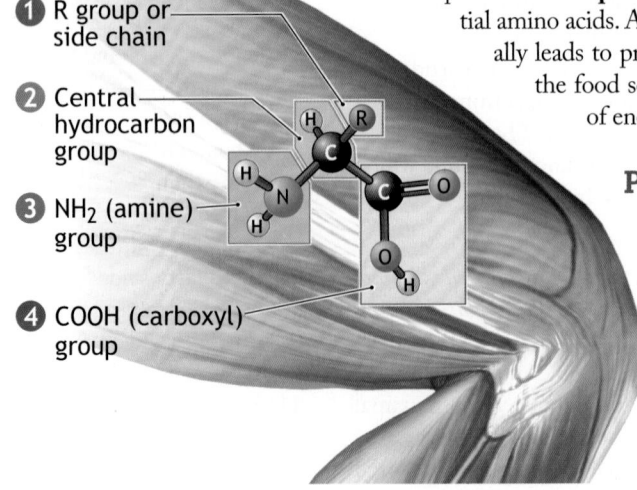

❶ R group or side chain

❷ Central hydrocarbon group

❸ NH_2 (amine) group

❹ COOH (carboxyl) group

FIGURE 1.19 • Four common features of amino acids.

TABLE 1.3	Common Sources of Dietary Protein Rated for Protein Quality	
Food		**Protein Rating**
Eggs		100
Fish		70
Lean beef		69
Cow's milk		60
Brown rice		57
White rice		56
Soybeans		57
Brewer's hash		45
Whole-grain wheat		44
Peanuts		43
Dry beans		34
White potato		34

protein in the diet while Table 1.4 provides good food sources of protein from animal, dairy, and plant categories. Reliance on animal sources for dietary protein accounts for the relatively high cholesterol and saturated fatty acid intake in the major industrialized nations.

With the exception of soy isolate proteins such as tofu, which provide all the essential amino acids, high-quality protein foods come from animal sources. Vegetables (lentils, dried beans and peas, nuts, and cereals) remain incomplete in one or

TABLE 1.4	Good Food Sources of Protein	
Food	**Serving Size**	**Protein (g)**
Animal		
Hamburger, cooked	4 oz	30
Tuna	3 oz	22
Turkey, light meat	4 oz	9
Egg, whole	1 large	6
Egg, white	1 large	4
Dairy		
Cottage cheese, regular	0.5 cup	15
Yogurt, low fat	8 oz	11
Cheese, regular (average for all types)	1 oz	8
Milk, skim	8 oz	8
Plant		
Chick peas	0.5 cup	20
Baked beans	1 cup	14
Tofu	3.5 oz	11
Lentils	0.5 cup	9
Pasta, dry	2 oz	7
Peanuts	1 oz	7
100% Whole wheat bread	2 slices	6
Peanut butter	1 Tbsp	4
Almonds, dry roasted	12	3

more essential amino acids making their proteins have a lower biologic value. It is not necessary to consume all of the essential amino acids in a single meal, as was once thought, as long as balance is maintained over a whole day. *Eating a variety of grains, fruits, and vegetables supplies all of the essential amino acids.*

The Vegan Approach

True vegetarians, or **vegans**, consume nutrients from only two sources—the plant kingdom and dietary supplements. Vegans constitute less than 4% of the U.S. population, yet between 5 and 7% of Americans consider themselves "almost" vegans. Nutritional diversity remains the key for these individuals. For example, a vegan diet contains all the essential amino acids if the recommended intake for protein (see next section) contains 60% of protein from grain products, 35% from legumes, and 5% from green leafy vegetables.

An increasing number of competitive and champion athletes consume diets consisting predominantly of nutrients from varied plant sources, including some dairy and meat products.[12,54] Vegetarian athletes often encounter difficulty in planning, selecting, and preparing nutritious meals with a proper amino acid mixture from only plant sources, without relying on supplementation. In contrast to diets that rely heavily on animal sources for protein, well-balanced vegetarian and vegetarian-type diets provide abundant carbohydrate so crucial in intense, prolonged training. Such diets contain little or no cholesterol but abundant fiber, and rich fruit and vegetable sources of diverse phytochemicals and antioxidant vitamins. A **lactovegetarian diet** provides milk and related products such as ice cream, cheese, and yogurt. The lactovegetarian approach minimizes the difficulty of consuming sufficient high-quality protein and increases the intake of calcium, phosphorus, and vitamin B_{12} (produced by bacteria in the digestive tract of animals). Adding an egg to the diet (**ovolactovegetarian diet**) ensures high-quality protein intake. Figure 1.20 displays the

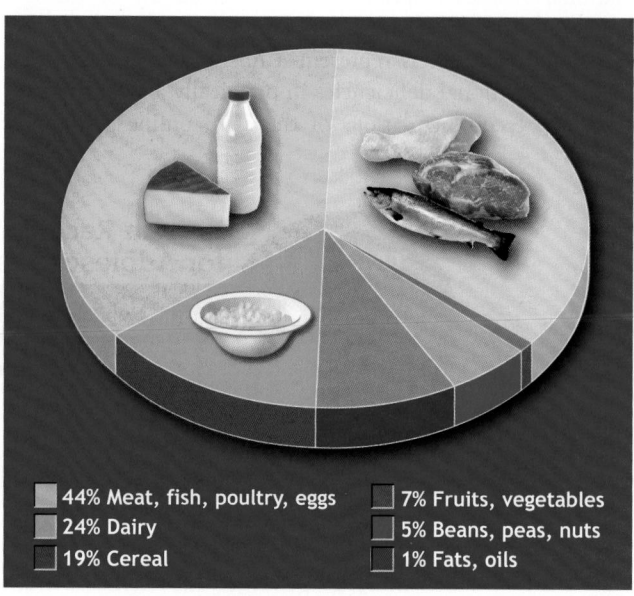

44% Meat, fish, poultry, eggs   7% Fruits, vegetables
24% Dairy   5% Beans, peas, nuts
19% Cereal   1% Fats, oils

FIGURE 1.20 • Contribution from the major food sources to the protein content of the typical American diet.

contribution of various food groups to the protein content of the American diet.

RECOMMENDED PROTEIN INTAKE

Despite the beliefs of many coaches, trainers, and athletes, little benefit accrues from consuming excessive protein. *Muscle mass does not increase simply by consuming high-protein foods.* The diets of elite endurance- and resistance-trained athletes often exceed two to three times the recommended intake, usually as meat. This occurs primarily for two reasons:

1. Athletes' diets normally emphasize high-protein foods, an idea from the late 19th century first promoted by German chemist Justus von Liebig (see this text's Introduction).
2. Caloric intake and energy output of athletes surpass those of sedentary counterparts.

If lean tissue synthesis resulted from all of the extra protein consumed by the typical athlete, then muscle mass would increase tremendously. For example, consuming an extra 100 g of protein (400 kcal) daily would translate to a daily 500 g (1.1 lb) increase in muscle mass. This obviously does not happen. Excessive dietary protein catabolizes directly for energy (following deamination) or recycles as components of other molecules including fat stored in subcutaneous depots. Excessive dietary protein intake can trigger harmful side effects, particularly strained liver and kidney function from elimination of urea.

The RDA: A Liberal Standard

The **Recommended Dietary Allowance (RDA)** for protein, vitamins, and minerals represents a standard for nutrient intake expressed as a daily average. These guidelines, initially developed in 1943 by the Food and Nutrition Board of the National Research Council/National Academy of Science (www.iom.edu/CMS/3708.aspx), have been revised periodically.[18] RDA levels represent a liberal yet safe excess to prevent nutritional deficiencies in practically all healthy persons. The recommendations of the 2013 online guidelines, (http://fnic.nal.usda.gov/fnic/interactiveDRI/; http://fnic.nal.usda.gov/dietary-guidance/dietary-reference-intakes/dri-tables) include 10 macronutrients, 15 vitamins, 21 minerals, and the calculation of body mass index, daily caloric needs, and recommended total water intake. The **Estimated Safe and Adequate Daily Dietary Intakes (ESADDIs)** recommendation for certain essential micronutrients (e.g., vitamins biotin and pantothenic acid and trace elements copper, manganese, fluoride, selenium, chromium, and molybdenum) required sufficient scientific data to formulate a range of intakes considered adequate and safe, yet insufficient for a precise RDA value. No RDA or ESADDI exists for sodium, potassium, and chlorine; instead, recommendations refer to a minimum requirement for health.

We emphasize that the RDA reflects nutritional needs of a *population* over a long time period; only laboratory measurements can assess a specific individual's requirement. Malnutrition occurs from cumulative weeks, months, and even years of inadequate nutrient intake. Someone who regularly consumes a diet that contains nutrients below the RDA standards may not become malnourished. *The RDA represents a probability statement for adequate nutrition; as nutrient intake falls below the RDA, the statistical probability for malnourishment increases for that person and the probability progressively increases with lower nutrient intake.* In Chapter 2, we discuss the **Dietary Reference Intakes** that represent the current set of standards for recommended intakes of nutrients and other food components.[17]

TABLE 1.5 lists the protein RDAs for adolescent and adult males and females. On average, 0.83 g of protein per kg body mass represents the recommended daily intake. To determine the protein requirement for men and women ages 18 to 65, multiply body mass in kg by 0.83. For a 90-kg man, total protein requirement equals 75 g (90 × 0.83). The protein RDA holds even for overweight persons; it includes a reserve of about 25% to account for individual differences in the protein requirement for about 97% of the population. Generally, the protein RDA (and the quantity of the required essential amino acids) decreases with age. In contrast, the protein RDA for infants and growing children equals 2.0 to 4.0 g per kg body mass. Pregnant

TABLE 1.5	Protein Recommended Dietary Allowance (RDA) for Adolescent and Adult Men and Women			
Recommended Amount	**Men**		**Women**	
	Adolescent	**Adult**	**Adolescent**	**Adult**
Grams of protein per kg body mass	0.9	0.8	0.9	0.8
Grams of protein per day based on average body mass[a]	59.0	56.0	50.0	44.0

[a]Average body mass based on a "reference" man and woman. For adolescents (ages 14–18), body mass averages 65.8 kg (145 lb) for males and 55.7 kg (123 lb) for females. For adult men, average mass equals 70 kg (154 lb); for adult women, mass averages 56.8 kg (125 lb).

women should increase total daily protein intake by 20 g, and nursing mothers should increase their intake by 10 g. *A 10% increase in the calculated protein requirement, particularly for a vegetarian-type diet, accounts for dietary fiber's effect in reducing the digestibility of many plant-based protein sources.* Stress, disease, and injury usually increase protein requirements.

Do Athletes Require a Larger Protein Intake?

Debate focuses on the need for a larger protein requirement for athletes that includes still-growing adolescent athletes, athletes involved in resistance-training programs that stimulate muscle growth and endurance-training programs that increase protein breakdown, and wrestlers and American football players subjected to recurring tissue microtrauma.[8,67] We present additional information about protein balance in exercise and training in subsequent sections of this chapter.

PROTEIN'S ROLE IN THE BODY

Blood plasma, visceral tissue, and muscle represent the three major sources of body protein. No "reservoirs" of this macronutrient exist; all protein contributes to tissue structures or exists as important constituents of metabolic, transport, and hormonal systems. Protein makes up between 12 and 15% of body mass, but the protein content of different cells varies considerably. A brain cell, for example, consists of about 10% protein, while red blood cells and muscle cells include up to 20% of their total weight as protein. The protein content of skeletal muscle can increase to varying degrees with the systematic application of resistance training.

Amino acids provide the major building blocks for synthesizing tissue. They also incorporate nitrogen into (1) coenzyme electron carriers nicotinamide adenine dinucleotide (NAD) and flavin adenine dinucleotide (FAD) (see Chapter 5), (2) heme components of hemoglobin and myoglobin compounds, (3) catecholamine hormones epinephrine and norepinephrine, and (4) the serotonin neurotransmitter. Amino acids activate vitamins that play a key role in metabolic and physiologic regulation. Tissue anabolism accounts for about one-third of the protein intake during rapid growth in infancy and childhood. As growth rate declines, so does the percentage of protein retained for anabolic processes.

Proteins serve as primary constituents for plasma membranes and internal cellular material. As the final chapter, "On the Horizon," discusses in some detail, the cell nucleus contains the genetically coded nucleic acid material deoxyribonucleic acid (DNA). DNA replicates itself before the cell divides to ensure that each new cell contains identical genetic material. It also provides the instructions or "master plan" for the cellular manufacture of all the body's proteins via its control over cytoplasmic ribonucleic acid (RNA). Collagenous structural proteins compose the hair, skin, nails, bones,

tendons, and ligaments. Globular proteins make up the nearly 2000 different enzymes that speed up chemical reactions and regulate the catabolism of nutrients for energy release. Blood plasma also contains the specialized proteins thrombin, fibrin, and fibrinogen required for blood clotting. Within red blood cells, the oxygen-carrying compound hemoglobin contains the large globin protein molecule. Proteins help to regulate the acid-base characteristics of bodily fluids. Buffering neutralizes excess acid metabolites formed during vigorous exercise. The structural proteins actin and myosin play the predominant role in muscle action as they slide past each other during movement.

DYNAMICS OF PROTEIN METABOLISM

Dietary protein's main contribution supplies amino acids to numerous anabolic processes. In addition, some protein is catabolized for energy. In well-nourished individuals at rest, protein catabolism contributes between 2 and 5% of the body's total energy requirement. During catabolism, protein first degrades into its component amino acids. The amino acid molecule then loses its nitrogen (amine group) in the liver (**deamination**) to form urea (H_2NCONH_2). The remaining deaminated amino acid either then converts to a new amino acid, converts to carbohydrate or fat, or catabolizes directly for energy. Urea formed in deamination, including some ammonia, leaves the body in solution as urine. Excessive protein catabolism promotes fluid loss because urea must dissolve in water for excretion.

Enzymes in muscle facilitate nitrogen removal from certain amino acids (usually a-keto acid or glutamate; **Fig. 1.21**), with nitrogen passed to other compounds in the reversible reactions of **transamination.** Transamination occurs when an

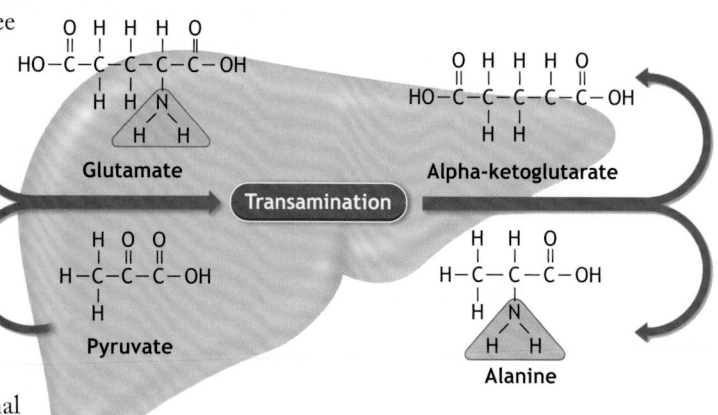

FIGURE 1.21 • Transamination provides for the intramuscular synthesis of amino acids from nonprotein sources. Enzyme action facilitates removal of an amine group from a donor amino acid for transfer to an acceptor, non-nitrogen-containing acid to form a new amino acid.

IN A PRACTICAL SENSE

Reading and Understanding the Food Label (Nutrition Panel)

The FDA and the Food Safety and Inspection Service (FSIS: www.fsis.gov) of the USDA issued new regulations concerning nutritional information about food labels to (1) help consumers choose more healthful diets and (2) offer an incentive to food companies to improve the nutritional qualities of their products. Also, the Nutrition Labeling and Education Act (NLEA) of 1990 (including 1993–1998 updates to the regulations) now requires food manufacturers to

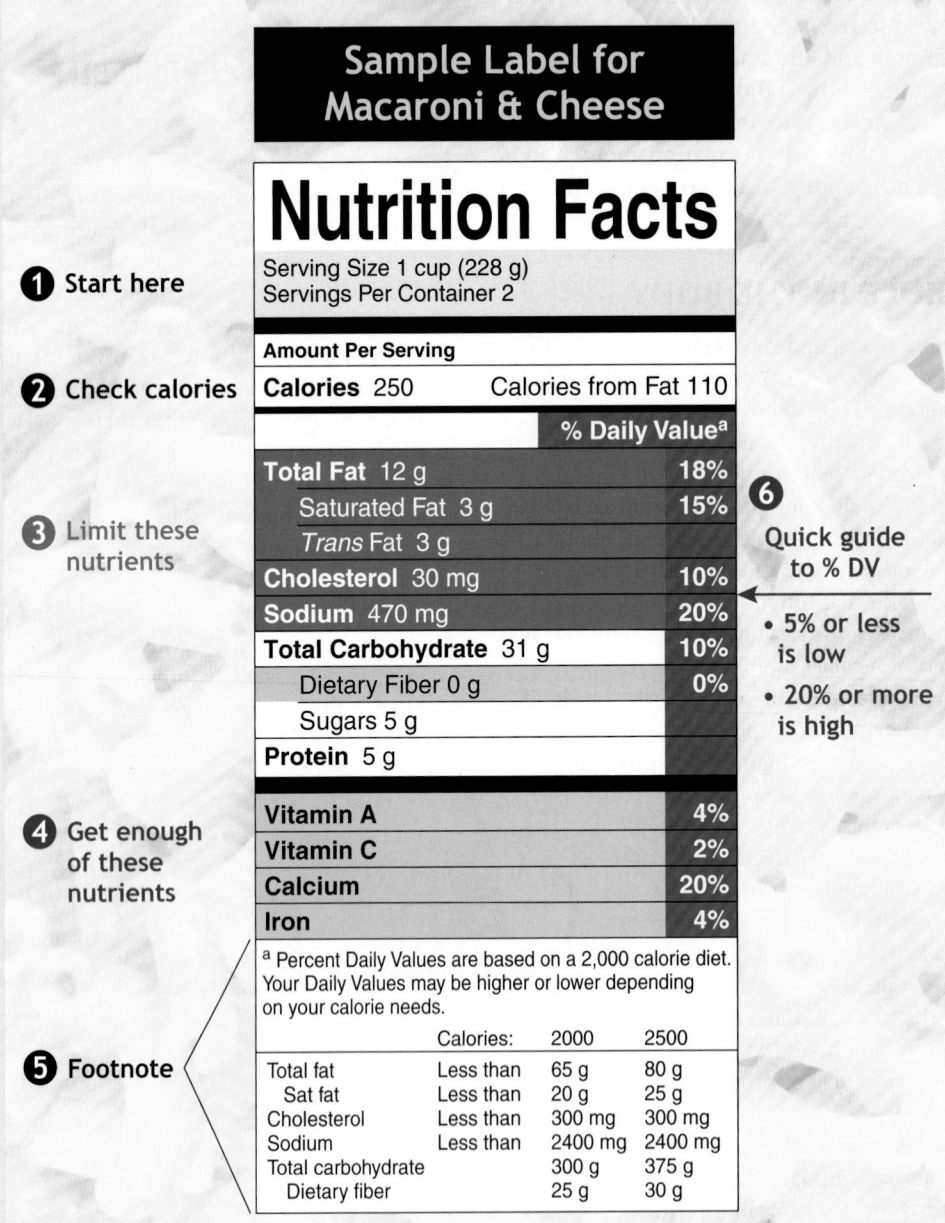

Reading the Nutrition Facts Panel. Food labels help one make informed choices. Foods that contain only a few of the nutrients required on the standard label have a shorter label format. What is on the label depends on what is in the food. Small- and medium-sized packages with limited label space also can use the short form. (Adapted with permission from McArdle WD, Katch FI, Katch VL. *Sports and Exercise Nutrition*, 4th ed. Philadelphia: Wolters Kluwer Health, 2013.)

IN A PRACTICAL SENSE *(continued)*

strictly adhere to regulations about what can and cannot be printed on food labels. The key provisions of food label reform include:

- Nutrition labeling for almost all foods to assist consumers in making more healthful food choices
- Information on the amount per serving of saturated fat, cholesterol, dietary fiber, and other nutrients considered of major health concern to consumers
- The amount of *trans* fatty acids on nutrition labels in light of mounting evidence that *trans* fatty acids increase heart disease risk
- Nutrient reference values, expressed as % Daily Values, to help consumers determine how a food fits into an overall daily diet
- Uniform definitions for terms that describe a food's nutrient content, such as "light," "low-fat," and "high-fiber," to ensure that such terms have the same meaning for any product on which they appear
- Substantiating claims about the relationship between a nutrient or food and a disease or health-related condition, such as calcium and osteoporosis, and fat and cancer
- Standardized serving sizes to make nutritional comparisons among similar products easier
- Declaration of total percentage of juice in juice drinks so consumers can determine a product's juice content
- Voluntary nutrition information for many raw foods

The food label must also list ingredients according to how much of the ingredient the food contains. In 2006, food makers were required to clearly state on food labels whether the product contained allergens such as milk, eggs, peanuts, wheat, soy, fish, shellfish, and tree nuts. The American Academy of Allergy Asthma & Immunology (**www.aaaai.org**) estimates that food allergies affect up to 2 million or 8% of the children in the United States.

NUTRITION PANEL TITLE

The food label displayed in the accompanying figure, entitled "Nutrition Facts," differs from the previous title (Nutrition Information Per Serving) and represents a more distinctive and easy-to-read label.

NUTRIENTS LISTED ON LABEL

The following information must be listed on all food labels:

- Calories from fat/calories from saturated fat
- Total fat
- Saturated fat, stearic acid, polyunsaturated fat, monounsaturated fat, *trans* fat
- Cholesterol
- Sodium
- Potassium
- Total carbohydrate
- Dietary fiber (soluble and insoluble fiber)
- Sugars (sugar alcohols)
- Other carbohydrates
- Protein
- Vitamins and minerals (for which RDIs have been established)

DEFINITIONS

The definitions for each of the nutrients listed on the label are as follows:

- **Total fat:** total lipid fatty acids expressed as triglycerides
- **Saturated fat:** the sum of all fatty acids containing no double bonds
- **Polyunsaturated fat:** *cis*, *cis*-methylene interrupted polyunsaturated fatty acids
- **Monounsaturated fat:** *cis*-monounsaturated fatty acids
- **Total carbohydrate:** amount calculated by subtraction of the sum of crude protein, total fat, moisture, and ash from the total weight of food
- **Sugars:** the sum of all free mono- and disaccharides
- **Other carbohydrate:** the difference between total carbohydrate and the sum of dietary fiber, sugars, and, when declared, sugar alcohol

---

amine group from a donor amino acid transfers to an acceptor acid to form a new amino acid. A specific transferase enzyme accelerates the transamination reaction. In muscle, transamination incorporates branched-chain amino acids (BCAAs; leucine, isoleucine, and valine) that generate branched-chain ketoacids (mediated by BCAA transferase). This allows amino acid formation from the non-nitrogen-carrying organic compound pyruvate formed in metabolism. In both deamination and transamination, the resulting carbon skeleton of the non-nitrogenous amino acid residue undergoes further degradation during energy metabolism.

 See the animation "Transamination" on **http://thePoint.lww.com/mkk8e** for a demonstration of this process.

 ### Fate of Amino Acids After Nitrogen Removal

After deamination, the remaining carbon skeletons of α-keto acids such as pyruvate, oxaloacetate, or α-ketoglutarate follow one of three diverse biochemical routes:

1. *Gluconeogenesis*—18 of the 20 amino acids serve as a source for glucose synthesis.
2. *Energy source*—The carbon skeletons oxidize for energy because they form intermediates in citric acid cycle metabolism or related molecules.
3. *Fat synthesis*—All amino acids provide a potential source of acetyl-CoA and thus furnish substrate to synthesize fatty acids.

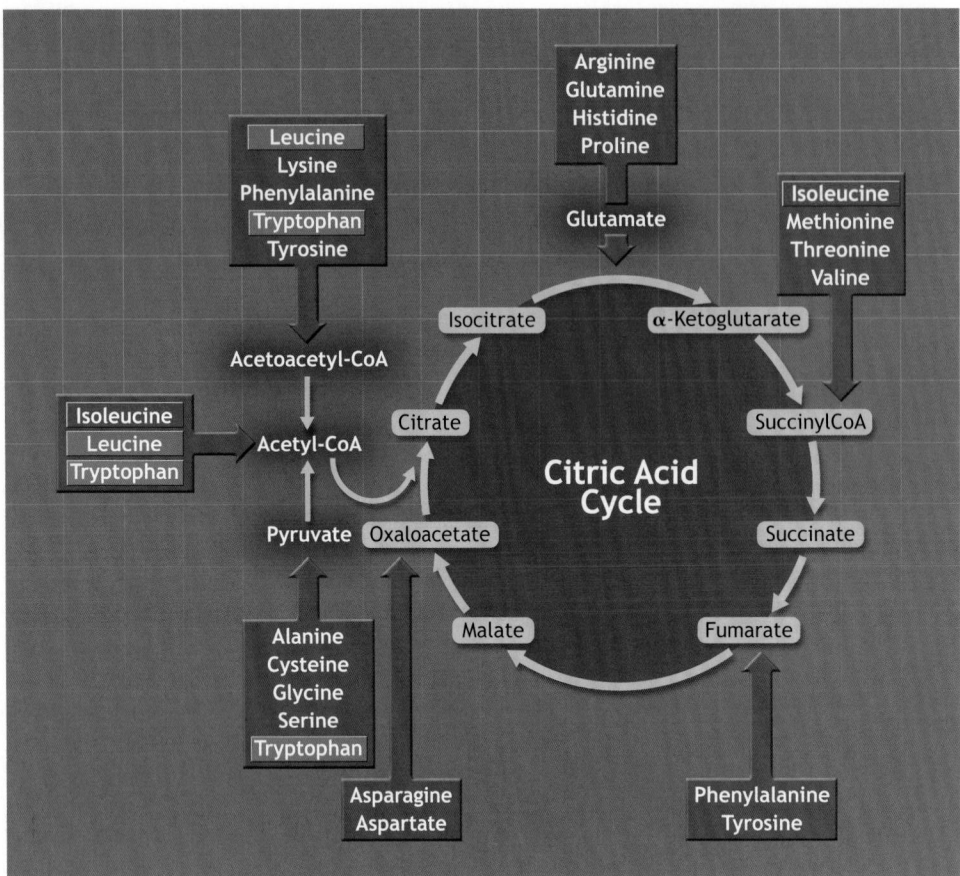

FIGURE 1.22 • Major metabolic pathways for amino acids following removal of the nitrogen group by deamination or transamination. Upon removal of their amine group, all amino acids form reactive citric acid cycle intermediates or related compounds. Some of the larger amino acid molecules (e.g., leucine, tryptophan, and isoleucine—colored green, aqua, and red, respectively) generate carbon-containing compounds that enter metabolic pathways at different sites.

FIGURE 1.22 shows the commonality of the carbon sources from amino acids and the major metabolic paths taken by the deaminated carbon skeletons.

NITROGEN BALANCE

Nitrogen balance occurs when nitrogen intake (protein) equals nitrogen excretion as follows:

$$\text{Nitrogen balance} = N_t - N_u - N_f - N_s = 0$$

where N_t = total nitrogen intake from food; N_u = nitrogen in urine; N_f = nitrogen in feces; and N_s = nitrogen in sweat.

In **positive nitrogen balance**, nitrogen intake exceeds nitrogen excretion to synthesize new tissues from the additional protein. With proper nutrition, positive nitrogen often occurs in:

1. Growing children
2. During pregnancy
3. In recovery from illness
4. During resistance-exercise training when muscle cells promote protein synthesis

The body does not develop a protein reserve as it does with fat storage in adipose tissue and storage of carbohydrate as muscle and liver glycogen. Nevertheless, individuals who consume the recommended protein intake have a higher content of muscle and liver protein than individuals fed too little protein. Also, muscle protein can be recruited for energy metabolism. In contrast, proteins in neural and connective tissues remain relatively "fixed" as cellular constituents and cannot be mobilized for energy without disrupting tissue functions.

Greater nitrogen output than intake, or **negative nitrogen balance**, indicates protein use for energy and possible encroachment on amino acids primarily from skeletal muscle. Interestingly, a negative nitrogen balance can occur even when protein intake exceeds the recommended standard if the body catabolizes protein from a lack of other energy nutrients. For example, an individual who participates regularly in intense training may consume adequate or excess protein but inadequate energy from carbohydrate or lipid. In this scenario, protein increasingly becomes an energy fuel, which creates a negative protein or nitrogen balance and a loss of lean tissue mass. The protein-sparing role of dietary carbohydrate and lipid previously discussed becomes important during tissue growth periods and the high-energy output and/or tissue synthesis requirements of intense training. A negative nitrogen balance can occur during diabetes, fever, burns, dieting, growth, steroid administration, and recovery from many illnesses. The greatest negative nitrogen balance takes place during starvation.

Protein breakdown increases only modestly with most modes and intensities of physical activity, yet muscle protein synthesis rises substantially following endurance- and resistance-type physical activities.[8,57] FIGURE 1.23 shows that muscle protein synthesis determined from labeled leucine incorporation into muscle increased between 10 and 80% within 4 hr following termination of aerobic exercise. It then remained elevated for at least 24 hr. Two factors justify reexamining protein intake recommendations for those involved in intense training:

1. Increased protein breakdown during long-term exercise and protracted training
2. Increased protein synthesis in recovery from physical activity

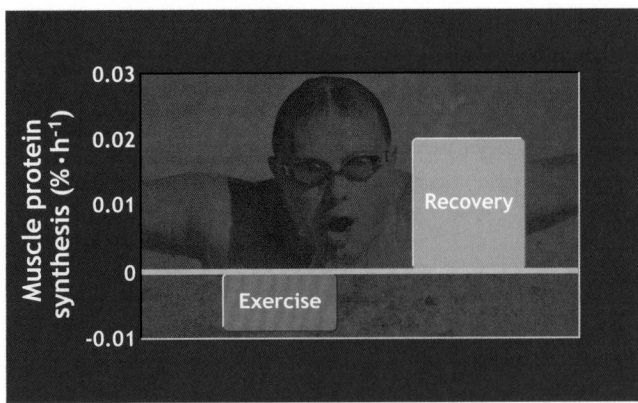

FIGURE 1.23 • Degradation of protein during exercise and stimulation of protein synthesis in recovery from aerobic exercise. Values refer to differences between the exercise group and the control group that received the same diet for each time interval. (Adapted with permission from Carraro F, et al. Whole body and plasma protein synthesis in exercise and recovery in human subjects. *Am J Physiol* 1990;258:E821.)

 INTEGRATIVE QUESTION

If muscle growth with resistance training occurs primarily from deposition of additional protein within the cell, discuss if consuming extra protein above the RDA facilitates muscle growth.

PROTEIN DYNAMICS DURING PHYSICAL ACTIVITY

Current understanding of protein dynamics during physical activity comes from studies that expanded the classic method of determining protein breakdown through urea excretion. For example, release of labeled CO_2 from amino acids injected or ingested increases during exercise in proportion to the metabolic rate.[74] As exercise progresses, the concentration of plasma urea also increases, coupled with a dramatic rise in nitrogen excretion in sweat, often without any change in urinary nitrogen excretion.[27,60] These observations account for prior conclusions concerning minimal protein breakdown during endurance exercise because the early studies only measured nitrogen in urine. The sweat mechanism serves an important role in excreting nitrogen from protein breakdown during physical acitivity (**Fig. 1.24**). Nonetheless, urea production may not reflect all aspects of protein breakdown because the oxidation of plasma and intracellular leucine—an essential BCAA—increases during moderate exercise independent of changes in urea production.[6,74]

Figure 1.24 also illustrates that protein use for energy reaches its highest level during exercise in the glycogen-depleted state. This emphasizes the important role of carbohydrate as a protein-sparer and indicates that carbohydrate availability affects the demand on protein "reserves" in physical activity. Protein breakdown and gluconeogenesis undoubtedly

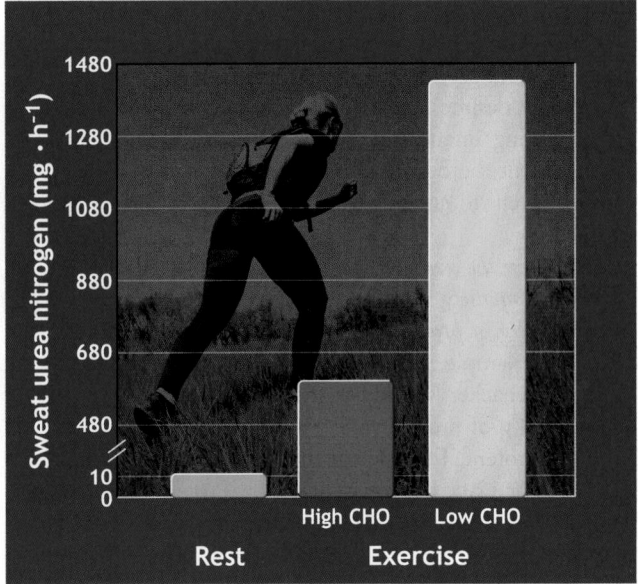

FIGURE 1.24 • Excretion of urea in sweat at rest and during exercise after carbohydrate loading (high CHO) and carbohydrate depletion (low CHO). The largest use of protein (as reflected by sweat urea) occurs when glycogen reserves are low. (Adapted with permission from Lemon PWR, Nagel F. Effects of exercise on protein and amino acid metabolism. *Med Sci Sports Exerc* 1981;13:141.)

play a role in endurance exercise or in frequent intense training when glycogen reserves diminish.

Increases in protein catabolism during endurance activities and intense training often mirror the metabolic mixture in acute starvation. With depleted glycogen reserves, gluconeogenesis from carbon skeletons of amino acids largely sustains the liver's glucose output. Augmented protein breakdown reflects the body's attempt to maintain blood glucose for central nervous system functioning. *Athletes in training should consume a high-carbohydrate diet with adequate energy to conserve muscle protein.* The increased protein use for energy and depressed protein synthesis during intense physical activity may partly explain why individuals who resistance-train to build muscle size generally refrain from glycogen-depleting endurance workouts to avoid the potential for muscle catabolism or "teardown."

Some Modification Required for Recommended Protein Intake

A continuing area of controversy concerns whether the initial increased protein demand when training begins creates a true long-term increase in protein requirement above the RDA. *A definitive answer remains elusive, but protein breakdown above the resting level does occur during endurance training and resistance training to a greater degree than previously believed.* Increased protein catabolism occurs to a greater extent when exercising with low carbohydrate reserves and/or low energy or protein intakes.[56] Unfortunately, research has not pinpointed protein requirements for individuals who train 4 to 6 hr daily by resistance exercise.

Their protein needs may average only slightly more than requirements for sedentary individuals (perhaps 1.0 to 1.2 g protein per kg of body mass). In addition, despite increased protein use for energy during intense training, adaptations may augment the body's efficiency in using dietary protein to enhance amino acid balance.

Based on the available evidence, athletes who train intensely should consume between 1.2 and 1.8 g of protein per kg of body mass daily. For example, a 220-pound (99.8-kg) middle linebacker would, at the upper end, require 180 g of protein (1.8×99.8), the equivalent of 6.3 oz of protein. The value at the lower end would equal 1.2×99.8 or 120 g of protein or 4.2 oz. Protein intake greater than the 1.8 g value offers no further advantage to athletes with regard to whole-body protein use.[22] This upper value falls within the range typically consumed by physically active men and women, obviating the need to consume supplementary protein.[12] With adequate protein intake, consuming animal sources of protein does not facilitate muscle strength or size gains with resistance training compared with protein intake from only plant sources.[28] Based on recommendations of the American College of Sports Medicine (www.acsm.org) and the American Dietetic Association (www.eatright.org), a reasonable daily protein intake for vegetarian athletes ranges between 1.3 and 1.8 g per kg of body weight.

 INTEGRATIVE QUESTION

Outline reasons why exercise physiologists debate the adequacy of the current protein RDA for individuals involved in intense exercise training.

The Alanine–Glucose Cycle

Some tissue proteins do not readily metabolize for energy, yet muscle proteins can provide energy for exercise.[9,25] For example, alanine *indirectly* participates in energy metabolism when the exercise energy demand increases; its release from active leg muscle increases proportionately to the severity of exercise.[77]

Active skeletal muscle synthesizes alanine during transamination from the glucose intermediate pyruvate with nitrogen derived in part from the amino acid leucine. The residual carbon fragment from the amino acid that formed alanine oxidizes for energy within skeletal muscle. The newly formed alanine leaves the muscle and enters the liver for deamination. Alanine's remaining carbon skeleton converts to glucose via gluconeogenesis and enters the blood for delivery to active muscle. **Figure 1.25** summarizes the sequence of the **alanine–glucose cycle** After 4 hr of continuous light exercise, the liver's output of alanine-derived glucose accounts for about 45% of

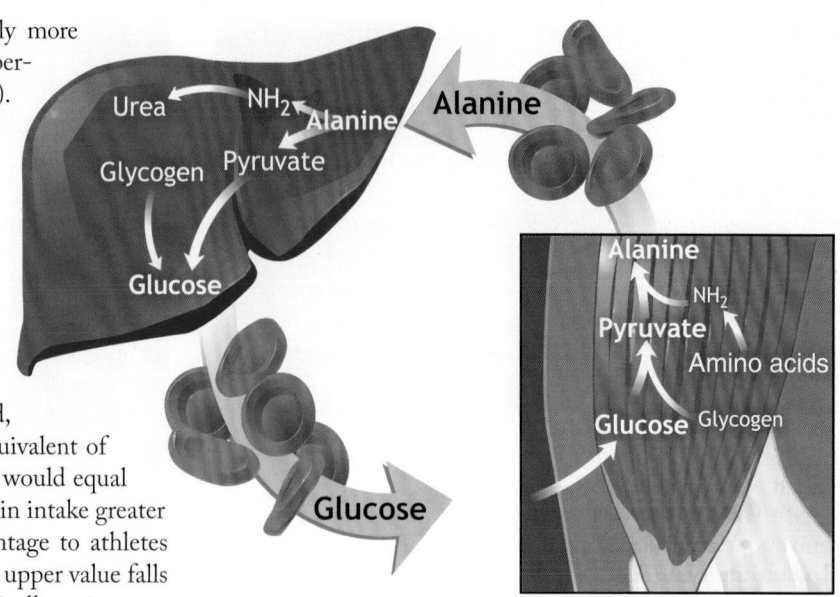

FIGURE 1.25 • The alanine–glucose cycle. Alanine, synthesized in muscle from glucose-derived pyruvate via transamination, enters the blood where the liver converts it to glucose and urea. Glucose release into the blood coincides with its subsequent delivery to the muscle for energy. During exercise, increased production and output of alanine from muscle helps to maintain blood glucose for nervous system and active muscle needs. Exercise training augments hepatic gluconeogenesis. (Reprinted with permission from Felig P, Wahren J. Amino acid metabolism in exercising man. *J Clin Invest* 1971;50:2703.)

the liver's total glucose release. *The alanine–glucose cycle generates from 10 to 15% of the total exercise energy requirement.* Regular exercise training enhances the liver's synthesis of glucose from the carbon skeletons of noncarbohydrate compounds.[66] This facilitates blood glucose homeostasis during prolonged physical activity.

 See the animation "Alanine–Glucose Cycle" on **http://thePoint.lww.com/mkk8e** for a demonstration of this process.

Summary

1. Proteins differ chemically from lipids and carbohydrates because they contain nitrogen in addition to sulfur, phosphorus, and iron.
2. Subunit amino acid structures form protein. The body requires 20 different amino acids, each containing an amine group (NH_2) and an organic acid group (carboxylic acid group; COOH). Amino acids contain a side chain (R group) that determines the amino acid's particular chemical characteristics.
3. The number of possible protein structures is enormous because of the tremendous number of combinations of 20 different amino acids.

4. Regular exercise training enhances the liver's synthesis of glucose from the carbon skeletons of noncarbohydrate compounds, particularly amino acids.

5. The body cannot synthesize 8 of the required 20 amino acids; these 8 essential amino acids must be consumed in the diet.

6. All animal and plant cells contain protein. Complete higher-quality proteins contain all the essential amino acids; incomplete lower-quality proteins represent the others. Examples of higher-quality, complete proteins include animal proteins in eggs, milk, cheese, meat, fish, and poultry.

7. Physically active people and competitive athletes can usually obtain the required nutrients predominantly from a broad array of plant sources.

8. Proteins provide the building blocks for synthesizing cellular material during anabolic processes. Their amino acids also contribute "carbon skeletons" for energy metabolism.

9. The Recommended Dietary Allowance (RDA) represents a liberal yet safe level of excess to meet the nutritional needs of practically all healthy persons. For adults, the protein RDA equals 0.83 g per kg of body mass.

10. Depleting carbohydrate reserves increases protein catabolism during exercise. Athletes who regularly train vigorously must maintain optimal levels of muscle and liver glycogen to minimize deterioration in athletic performance and a loss of muscle mass.

11. Protein serves as an energy fuel to a much greater extent than previously believed. This applies particularly to branched-chain amino acids oxidized in skeletal muscle rather than in the liver.

12. Reexamining the current protein RDA seems justified for athletes who engage in intense training. This examination must account for increased protein breakdown during exercise and augmented protein synthesis in recovery. Increasing protein intake to 1.2 to 1.8 g per kg body mass daily seems reasonable.

13. Proteins in neural and connective tissues generally do not participate in energy metabolism. The muscle-derived amino acid alanine plays a key role via gluconeogenesis in supporting carbohydrate availability during prolonged exercise. The alanine–glucose cycle accounts for up to 45% of the liver's release of glucose during long-duration exercise.

---

thePoint References are available online at **http://thepoint.lww.com/mkk8e.**

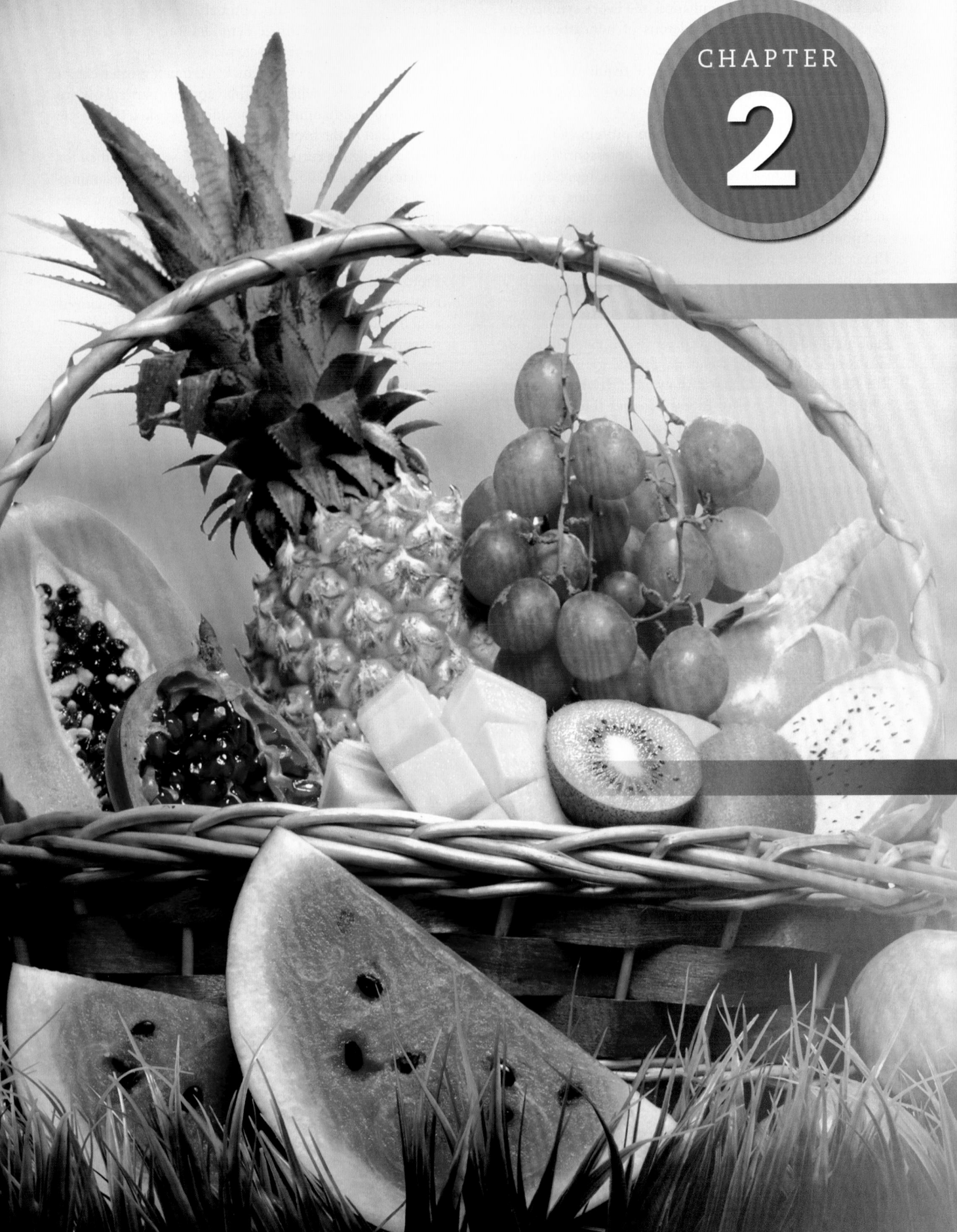

Vitamins, Minerals, and Water

CHAPTER OBJECTIVES

- List one function for each fat- and water-soluble vitamin and potential risks of their excess consumption

- Discuss how free radicals form in the body, particularly during physical activity, and the mechanisms to defend against oxidative stress

- Summarize the pros and cons of vitamin supplementation above the Recommended Dietary Allowance (RDA) for individuals engaged in intense physical training

- Summarize the effects of vitamin supplementation on exercise performance

- Outline three broad roles of minerals in the body

- Define the terms *osteoporosis*, *exercise-induced anemia*, and *sodium-induced hypertension*

- Describe how regular physical activity affects bone mass and the body's iron stores

- Present a possible explanation for "sports anemia"

- Outline factors related to the "female athlete triad"

- Summarize the pros and cons of mineral supplementation above the RDA for individuals involved in intense physical training

- List five functions of water in the body

- Quantify the volumes of the body's three water compartments

- List five predisposing factors to hyponatremia associated with prolonged exercise

ANCILLARIES ◉ *at-a-Glance*

Visit http://thePoint.lww.com/mkk8e to access the following resources.

- References: Chapter 2
- Interactive Question Bank
- Animation: Biologic Function of Vitamins
- Animation: Bone Growth
- Animation: Calcium in Muscles
- Animation: Renal Function
- Animation: Vitamin C as an Antioxidant
- Animation: Water Balance
- Focus on Research: Female Athletes with Osteoporosis

The effective regulation of all metabolic processes requires a delicate blending of food nutrients in the cell's watery medium. **Micronutrients**—small quantities of vitamins and minerals—play highly specific roles in facilitating energy transfer and tissue synthesis. The physically active person or competitive athlete need not consume vitamin and mineral supplements if they obtain proper nutrition from a variety of food sources. Such supplementation practices touted by advertising on radio, TV, and the print media, usually prove physiologically and economically wasteful. Consuming some micronutrients in excess poses a potential risk to health and safety.

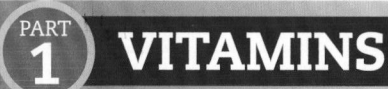

PART 1 VITAMINS

THE NATURE OF VITAMINS

Vitamins consist of different organic complexes required by the body in minute amounts. Vitamins have no particular chemical structure in common; they serve as accessory nutrients because they neither supply energy nor contribute substantially to the body's mass. With the exception of vitamin D, the body cannot manufacture vitamins. Instead, they must be supplied in the diet or through supplementation.

KINDS OF VITAMINS

Thirteen different vitamins have been isolated, analyzed, classified, synthesized, and assigned Recommended Dietary Allowances (RDAs). Vitamins are classified as **fat soluble**—A, D, E, and K—or **water soluble**—C and the B-complex vitamins: thiamine (B_1), riboflavin (B_2), pyridoxine (B_6), niacin (nicotinic acid), pantothenic acid, biotin, folic acid (folacin or folate, its active form in the body), and cobalamin (B_{12}).

Fat-Soluble Vitamins

Fat-soluble vitamins dissolve and remain in fatty tissues, obviating the need to ingest them daily. It may take years before "unhealthy" symptoms emerge that denote a fat-soluble vitamin deficiency. The liver stores vitamins A, D, and K, whereas vitamin E distributes throughout the body's fatty tissues. Dietary lipids provide the source of fat-soluble vitamins; these vitamins travel as part of lipoproteins in the lymph to the liver for dispersion to various tissues. Consuming a true "fat-free" diet would accelerate a fat-soluble vitamin insufficiency.

Fat-soluble vitamins should not be consumed in excess without medical supervision. Toxic reactions to excessive fat-soluble vitamin intake occur at a lower multiple of the RDA compared to water-soluble vitamins.

Water-Soluble Vitamins

Water-soluble vitamins act largely as **coenzymes**—small molecules combined with a larger protein compound called an apoenzyme to form an active enzyme that accelerates the interconversion of chemical compounds (see Chapter 5). Coenzymes participate directly in chemical reactions; after the reaction runs its course, coenzymes remain intact and participate in additional reactions. Water-soluble vitamins, similar to their fat-soluble counterparts, consist of atoms of carbon, hydrogen, and oxygen. They also contain nitrogen and metallic ions including iron, molybdenum, copper, sulfur, and cobalt.

Water-soluble vitamins disperse in bodily fluids without storage in tissues to any appreciable extent. Generally, an excess intake of water-soluble vitamins voids in the urine. Water-soluble vitamins exert their influence for 8 to 14 hr after ingestion; thereafter, their potency decreases in somewhat exponential fashion. For example, the half-life or time required to convert one-half of a reactant to a product of vitamin C averages approximately 30 min, whereas 9 to 18 days represents thiamine's half-life.

ROLE OF VITAMINS

FIGURE **2.1** summarizes the major biologic functions of vitamins. Vitamins contain no useful energy for the body; instead, they serve as essential links and regulators in metabolic reactions that release energy from food. Vitamins also control tissue synthesis and protect the integrity of the cells' plasma membrane. The water-soluble vitamins play important roles in energy metabolism. For example:

- Vitamin B_1 facilitates the conversion of pyruvate to acetyl-coenzyme A (CoA) in carbohydrate breakdown
- Niacin and vitamin B_2 regulate mitochondrial energy metabolism
- Vitamins B_6 and B_{12} catalyze protein synthesis
- Pantothenic acid, part of coenzyme A (CoA), participates in the aerobic breakdown of carbohydrate, fat, and protein macronutrients
- Vitamin C acts as a cofactor in enzymatic reactions, as a scavenger of free radicals in antioxidative processes, and as a component in hydroxylation reactions that provide connective tissue stability and wound healing

Vitamins participate repeatedly in metabolic reactions without degradation; the vitamin needs of physically active individuals do not exceed those of sedentary counterparts.

 See the animation "Biologic Function of Vitamins" on **http://thePoint.lww.com/mkk8e** for a demonstration of this process.

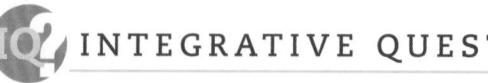 INTEGRATIVE QUESTION

If vitamins play such an important role in energy release, should athletes "supercharge" with vitamin supplements to enhance exercise performance and training responsiveness?

TABLE 2.1 lists the major bodily functions, dietary sources, and symptoms of a deficiency or excess for the water-soluble and fat-soluble vitamins. Well-balanced meals provide an adequate quantity of all vitamins, regardless of age and physical activity level. Indeed, individuals who expend considerable energy in physical activity generally need not consume special foods or supplements that increase vitamin intake above recommended levels. At high levels of daily physical activity, food intake generally increases to sustain the added energy requirements. Additional food through a variety of nutritious meals proportionately increases vitamin and mineral intakes.

Several exceptions for vitamin supplementation exist because of difficulty obtaining recommended amounts. For example, foods high in vitamin C and folic acid usually make up only a small part of most Americans' total caloric intake; the availability of such foods also varies by season. Also, different athletic groups have relatively low intakes of vitamins B_1 and B_6, two vitamins prevalent in fresh fruit, grains, and uncooked or steamed vegetables.[44,137] Vegans generally require vitamin B_{12} supplementation since it only exists in foods of animal origin.

DEFINING NUTRIENT NEEDS

Controversy surrounding the RDAs caused the Food and Nutrition Board of the Institute of Medicine (IOM) of the National Academies (www.iom.edu/CMS/3788.aspx) and scientific nutrition community to reexamine the usefulness of a single standard for specific nutrients. This process led the IOM (in cooperation with Canadian scientists) to develop the Dietary Reference Intakes (http://www.iom.edu/Activities/Nutrition/Summary-DRIs/DRI-Tables.aspx).

Dietary Reference Intakes

The **Dietary Reference Intakes (DRIs)** represent the umbrella term that encompasses the array of standards—RDAs, Estimated Average Requirements, Adequate Intakes, and the Tolerable Upper Intake Levels—for nutrient recommendations in planning and assessing diets for healthy persons.

Recommendations encompass not only daily intakes intended for health maintenance but also upper intake levels to reduce the likelihood of harm from excessive intake. The DRIs differ from their predecessor RDAs by focusing more on promoting health maintenance and risk reduction for nutrient-dependent diseases such as heart dysfunctions, diabetes, hypertension, osteoporosis, various cancers, and age-related macular degeneration. This contrasts with the traditional criterion of preventing the relatively rare deficiency diseases scurvy and beriberi. In addition to including values for energy, protein, and the micronutrients, the DRIs also provide the nutritionally important, but not essential, phytochemical compounds found in plants.

The DRI values also include recommendations that apply to gender and life stages of growth and development

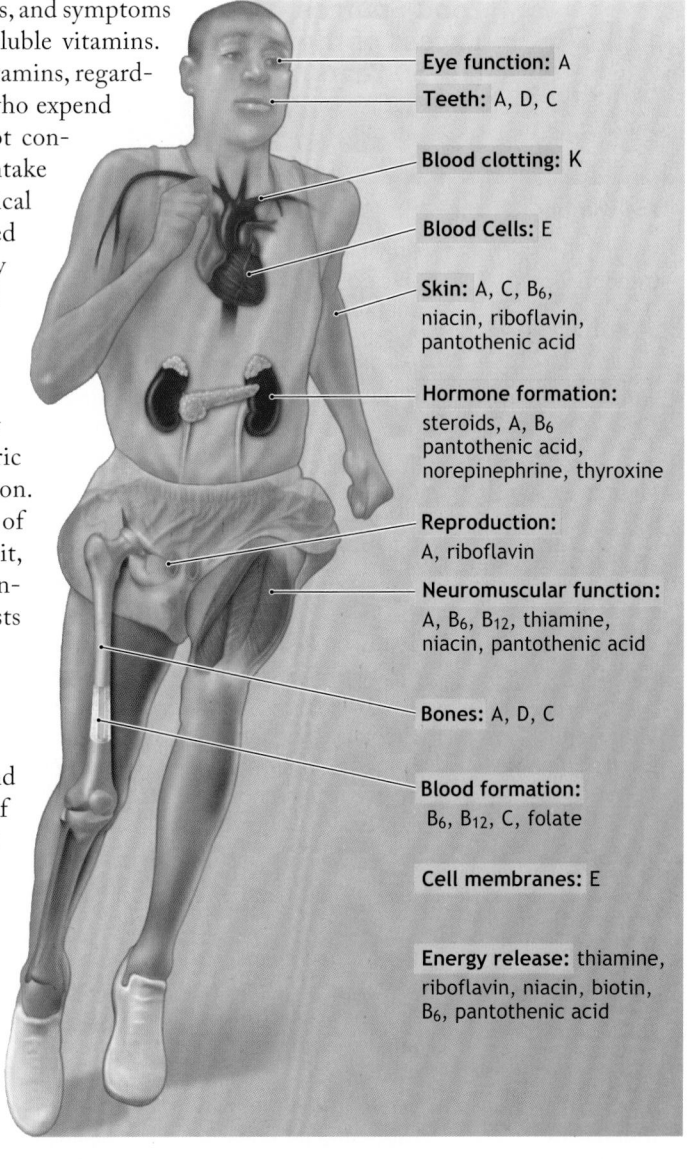

Eye function: A

Teeth: A, D, C

Blood clotting: K

Blood Cells: E

Skin: A, C, B_6, niacin, riboflavin, pantothenic acid

Hormone formation: steroids, A, B_6 pantothenic acid, norepinephrine, thyroxine

Reproduction: A, riboflavin

Neuromuscular function: A, B_6, B_{12}, thiamine, niacin, pantothenic acid

Bones: A, D, C

Blood formation: B_6, B_{12}, C, folate

Cell membranes: E

Energy release: thiamine, riboflavin, niacin, biotin, B_6, pantothenic acid

FIGURE 2.1 • Biologic functions of vitamins

based on age and, when appropriate, pregnancy and lactation. The following definitions apply to the four different sets of DRI values for the intake of nutrients and food components:

1. **Estimated Average Requirement (EAR):** Average level of daily nutrient intake to meet the requirement of one-half of the healthy individuals in a particular life-stage and gender group. The EAR provides a useful value to determine the prevalence of inadequate nutrient intake by the proportion of the population with intakes below this value.

2. **Recommended Dietary Allowance (RDA):** The average daily nutrient intake level sufficient to meet the requirement of about 97% of healthy individuals in a particular life-stage and gender group (**FIG. 2.2**). For most nutrients, this value represents the EAR *plus* 2 standard deviations of the requirement.

TABLE 2.1

Food Sources, Major Bodily Functions, and Symptoms of Deficiency or Excess of the Fat-Soluble and Water-Soluble Vitamins for Healthy Adults (19–50 Years)

Vitamin	Dietary Sources	Major Bodily Functions	Deficiency	Excess
Fat-soluble				
Vitamin A (retinol)	Provitamin A (β-carotene) widely distributed in green vegetables; retinol present in milk, butter, cheese, fortified margarine	Constituent of rhodopsin (visual pigment) Maintenance of epithelial tissues; role in mucopolysaccharide synthesis	Xerophthalmia (keratinization of ocular tissue), night blindness, permanent blindness	Headache, vomiting, peeling of skin, anorexia, swelling of long bones
Vitamin D	Cod-liver oil, eggs, dairy products, fortified milk and margarine	Promotes growth and mineralization of bones Increases absorption of calcium	Rickets (bone deformities) in children Osteomalacia in adults	Vomiting, diarrhea, loss of weight, kidney damage
Vitamin E (tocopherol)	Seeds, green leafy vegetables, margarine, shortening	Functions as an antioxidant to prevent cell damage	Possible anemia	Relatively nontoxic
Vitamin K (phylloquinone)	Green leafy vegetables; small amounts in cereals, fruits, and meats	Important in blood clotting (involved in formation of active prothrombin)	Conditioned deficiencies associated with severe bleeding; internal hemorrhages	Relatively nontoxic Synthetic forms at high doses may cause jaundice
Water-soluble				
Vitamin B$_1$ (thiamine)	Pork, organ meats, whole grains, nuts, legumes, milk, fruits, and vegetables	Coenzyme (thiamine prophosphate) in reactions involving the removal of carbon dioxide	Beriberi (peripheral nerve changes, edema, heart failure)	None reported
Vitamin B$_2$ (riboflavin)	Widely distributed in foods: meats, eggs, milk products, whole-grain and enriched cereal products, wheat germ, green leafy vegetables	Constituent of two flavin nucleotide coenzymes involved in energy metabolism (FAD and FMN)	Reddened lips, cracks at mouth corners (cheilosis), eye lesions	None reported
Niacin (nicotinic acid)	Liver, lean meats, poultry, grains, legumes, peanuts (can be formed from tryptophan)	Constituent of two coenzymes in oxidation reduction reactions (NAD and NADP)	Pellagra (skin and gastrointestinal lesions, nervous mental disorders)	Flushing, burning, and tingling around neck, face, and hands
Vitamin B$_6$ (pyridoxine)	Meats, fish, poultry, vegetables, whole grains, cereals, seeds	Coenzyme (pyridoxal phosphate) involved in amino acid and glycogen metabolism	Irritability, convulsions, muscular twitching, dermatitis, kidney stones	None reported
Pantothenic acid	Widely distributed in foods, meat, fish, poultry, milk products, legumes, whole grains	Constituent of coenzyme A, which plays a central role in energy metabolism	Fatigue, sleep disturbances, impaired coordination, nausea	None reported

| TABLE 2.1 | Food Sources, Major Bodily Functions, and Symptoms of Deficiency or Excess of the Fat-Soluble and Water-Soluble Vitamins for Healthy Adults (19–50 Years) *(Continued)* | | | |

Vitamin	Dietary Sources	Major Bodily Functions	Deficiency	Excess
Folate	Legumes, green vegetables, whole-wheat products, meats, eggs, milk products, liver	Coenzyme (reduced form) involved in transfer of single-carbon units in nucleic acid and amino acid metabolism	Anemia, gastrointestinal disturbances, diarrhea, red tongue	None reported
Vitamin B$_{12}$ (cobalamin)	Muscle meats, fish, eggs, dairy products (absent in plant foods)	Coenzyme involved in transfer of single-carbon units in nucleic acid metabolism	Pernicious anemia, neurologic disorders	None reported
Biotin	Legumes, vegetables, meats, liver, egg yolk, nuts	Coenzymes required for fat synthesis, amino acid metabolism, and glycogen (animal starch) formation	Fatigue, depression, nausea, dermatitis, muscle pain	None reported
Vitamin C (ascorbic acid)	Citrus fruits, tomatoes, green peppers, salad greens	Maintains intercellular matrix of cartilage, bone, and dentine; important in collagen synthesis	Scurvy (degeneration of skin, teeth, blood vessels, epithelial hemorrhages)	Relatively nontoxic Possibility of kidney stones

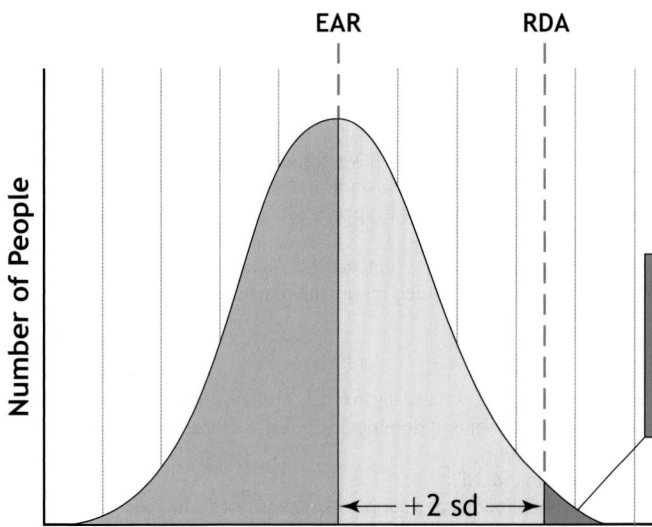

FIGURE 2.2 • Theoretical distribution of the number of persons adequately nourished by a given nutrient intake. The recommended dietary allowance (RDA) is set at an intake level that would meet the nutrient needs of 97% of the population (2 standard deviations [SD] above the mean). The Estimated Average Requirement (EAR) represents a nutrient intake value estimated to meet the requirements of half of the healthy individuals in a gender and life-stage group.

3. **Adequate Intake (AI):** Provides an assumed adequate nutritional goal when no RDA exists. It represents a recommended average daily nutrient intake level based on observed or experimentally determined approximations or estimates of nutrient intake by a group (or groups) of apparently healthy persons—used when an RDA cannot be determined. Intakes at or above the AI level indicate low risk.

4. **Tolerable Upper Intake Level (UL):** The highest average daily nutrient intake level likely to pose no risk of adverse health effects to almost all individuals in the specified gender and life-stage group of the general population. The potential risk of adverse effects increases as intake increases above the UL.

Although most individuals achieve the daily requirement without need for additional supplementation, the mineral iron represents an exception in that most pregnant women require supplements to obtain their increased daily requirement. TABLES 2.2 AND 2.3 present the RDA, AI, and UL values for vitamins.

Antioxidant Role of Vitamins

Most of the oxygen consumed within the mitochondria during energy metabolism combines with hydrogen to produce water. Nonetheless, 2 to 5% of oxygen normally forms the reactive oxygen- and nitrogen-containing free radicals superoxide

TABLE 2.2 Dietary Reference Intakes (DRIs): Recommended Vitamin Intakes

Life-Stage Group	Vitamin A (µg/d)[a]	Vitamin C (mg/d)	Vitamin D (µg/d)[b,c]	Vitamin E (mg/d)[d]	Vitamin K (µg/d)	Thiamin (mg/d)	Riboflavin (mg/d)	Niacin (mg/d)[e]	Vitamin B$_6$ (mg/d)	Folate (µg/d)[f]	Vitamin B$_{12}$ (µg/d)	Pantothenic Acid (mg/d)	Biotin (µg/d)	Choline (mg/d)[g]
Infants														
0–6 mo	400*	40*	5*	4*	2.0*	0.2*	0.3*	2*	0.1*	65*	0.4*	1.7*	5*	125*
7–12 mo	500*	50*	5*	5*	2.5*	0.3*	0.4*	4*	0.3*	80*	0.5*	1.8*	6*	150*
Children														
1–3 y	**300**	**15**	5*	**6**	30*	**0.5**	**0.5**	**6**	**0.5**	**150**	**0.9**	2*	8*	200*
4–8 y	**400**	**25**	5*	**7**	55*	**0.6**	**0.6**	**8**	**0.6**	**200**	**1.2**	3*	12*	250*
Males														
9–13 y	**600**	**45**	5*	**11**	60*	**0.9**	**0.9**	**12**	**1.0**	**300**	**1.8**	4*	20*	375*
14–18 y	**900**	**75**	5*	**15**	75*	**1.2**	**1.3**	**16**	**1.3**	**400**	**2.4**	5*	25*	550*
19–30 y	**900**	**90**	5*	**15**	120*	**1.2**	**1.3**	**16**	**1.3**	**400**	**2.4**	5*	30*	550*
31–50 y	**900**	**90**	5*	**15**	120*	**1.2**	**1.3**	**16**	**1.3**	**400**	**2.4**	5*	30*	550*
51–70 y	**900**	**90**	10*	**15**	120*	**1.2**	**1.3**	**16**	**1.7**	**400**	**2.4**[h]	5*	30*	550*
>70 y	**900**	**90**	15*	**15**	120*	**1.2**	**1.3**	**16**	**1.7**	**400**	**2.4**[h]	5*	30*	550*
Females														
9–13 y	**600**	**45**	5*	**11**	60*	**0.9**	**0.9**	**12**	**1.0**	**300**	**1.8**	4*	20*	375*
14–18 y	**700**	**65**	5*	**15**	75*	**1.0**	**1.0**	**14**	**1.2**	**400**[f]	**2.4**	5*	25*	400*
19–30 y	**700**	**75**	5*	**15**	90*	**1.1**	**1.1**	**14**	**1.3**	**400**[f]	**2.4**	5*	30*	425*
31–50 y	**700**	**75**	5*	**15**	90*	**1.1**	**1.1**	**14**	**1.3**	**400**[f]	**2.4**	5*	30*	425*
51–70 y	**700**	**75**	10*	**15**	90*	**1.1**	**1.1**	**14**	**1.5**	**400**	**2.4**[h]	5*	30*	425*
>70 y	**700**	**75**	15*	**15**	90*	**1.1**	**1.1**	**14**	**1.5**	**400**	**2.4**[h]	5*	30*	425*
Pregnancy[i,j]														
≤18 y	**750**	**80**	5*	**15**	75*	**1.4**	**1.4**	**18**	**1.9**	**600**[f]	**2.6**	6*	30*	450*
19–30 y	**770**	**85**	5*	**15**	90*	**1.4**	**1.4**	**18**	**1.9**	**600**[f]	**2.6**	6*	30*	450*
31–50 y	**770**	**85**	5*	**15**	90*	**1.4**	**1.4**	**18**	**1.9**	**600**[f]	**2.6**	6*	30*	450*
Lactation														
≤18 y	**1200**	**115**	5*	**19**	75*	**1.4**	**1.6**	**17**	**2.0**	**500**	**2.8**	7*	35*	550*
19–30 y	**1300**	**120**	5*	**19**	90*	**1.4**	**1.6**	**17**	**2.0**	**500**	**2.8**	7*	35*	550*
31–50 y	**1300**	**120**	5*	**19**	90*	**1.4**	**1.6**	**17**	**2.0**	**500**	**2.8**	7*	35*	550*

Note: This table (taken from the DRI reports, see **www.nap.edu**) presents Recommended Dietary Allowances (RDAs) in **bold type** and Adequate Intakes (AIs) in ordinary type followed by an asterisk (*). RDAs and AIs may both be used as goals for individual intake. RDAs are set to meet the needs of almost all (97–98%) individuals in a group. For healthy breastfed infants, the AI is the mean intake. The AI for other life-stage and gender groups is believed to cover the needs of all individuals in the group, but lack of data or uncertainty in the data prevent being able to specify with confidence the percentage of individuals covered by this intake.

[a]As retinol activity equivalents (RAEs). 1 RAE = 1 µg retinol, 12 µg β-carotene, 24 µg α-carotene, or 24 µg β-cryptoxanthin. To calculate RAEs from REs of provitamin A carotenoids in foods, divide the REs by 2. For preformed vitamin A in foods or supplements and for provitamin A carotenoids in supplements, 1 RE = 1 RAE.

[b]Calciferol. 1 µg calciferol = 40 IU vitamin D.

[c]In the absence of adequate exposure to sunlight.

[d]As α-tocopherol. α-Tocopherol includes *RRR*-α-tocopherol, the only form of α-tocopherol that occurs naturally in foods, and the 2R-stereoisometric forms of α-tocopherol (*RRR*-, *RSR*-, *RRS*-, and *RSS*-α-tocopherol) that occur in fortified foods and supplements. It does not include the 2S-stereoisometric forms of α-tocopherol (*SRR*-, *SSR*-, *SR*-, and *SSS*-α-tocopherol), also found in fortified foods and supplements.

[e]As niacin equivalents (NE). 1 mg of niacin = 60 mg of tryptophan; 0–6 mo = preformed niacin (not NE).

[f]As dietary folate equivalents (DFE). 1 DFE = 1 µg food folate = 0.6 µg of folic acid from fortified food or as a supplement consumed with food = 0.5 µg of a supplement taken on an empty stomach.

[g]AIs have been set for choline, yet there are few data to assess whether a dietary supply of choline is needed at all stages of the life cycle, and it may be that the choline requirement can be met by endogenous synthesis at some of these stages.

[h]Because 10–30% of older people may malabsorb food-bound B$_{12}$, it is advisable for those older than 50 y to meet their RDA mainly by consuming foods fortified with B$_{12}$ or a supplement containing B$_{12}$.

[i]In view of evidence linking folate intake with neural tube defects in the fetus, it is recommended that all women capable of becoming pregnant consume 400 µg from supplements or fortified foods in addition to intake of food folate from a varied diet.

[j]It is assumed that women will continue consuming 400 µg from supplements or fortified food until their pregnancy is confirmed and they enter prenatal care, which ordinarily occurs after the end of the periconceptional period—the critical time for formation of the neural tube.

Sources: Dietary Reference Intakes for Calcium, Phosphorus, Magnesium, Vitamin D, and Fluoride (1997); Dietary Reference Intakes for Thiamin, Riboflavin, Niacin, Vitamin B$_6$, Folate, Vitamin B$_{12}$, Pantothenic Acid, Biotin, and Choline (1998); Dietary Reference Intakes for Vitamin C, Vitamin E, Selenium, and Carotenoids (2000); and Dietary Reference Intakes for Vitamin A, Vitamin K, Arsenic, Boron, Chromium, Copper, Iodine, Iron, Manganese, Molybdenum, Nickel, Silicon, Vanadium, and Zinc (2001). These reports may be accessed via **www.nap.edu/catalog/dri**. © National Academy of Sciences. All rights reserved.

TABLE 2.3 — Dietary Reference Intakes (DRIs): Tolerable Upper Intake Levels (ULs[a])

Life-Stage Group	Vitamin A (μg/d)[b]	Vitamin C (mg/d)	Vitamin D (mg/d)	Vitamin E (mg/d)[c,d]	Vitamin K	Thiamin	Riboflavin	Niacin (mg/d)[d]	Vitamin B$_6$ (mg/d)[d]	Folate (μg/d)[d]	Vitamin B$_{12}$	Pantothenic Acid	Biotin	Choline (g/d)	Carotenoids[e]
Infants															
0–6 mo	600	ND[f]	25	ND	ND	ND	ND	ND	ND	ND	ND	ND	ND	ND	ND
7–12 mo	600	ND	25	ND	ND	ND	ND	ND	ND	ND	ND	ND	ND	ND	ND
Children															
1–3 y	600	400	50	200	ND	ND	ND	10	30	300	ND	ND	ND	1.0	ND
4–8 y	900	650	50	300	ND	ND	ND	15	40	400	ND	ND	ND	1.0	ND
Males, Females															
9–13 y	1700	1200	50	600	ND	ND	ND	20	60	600	ND	ND	ND	2.0	ND
14–18 y	2800	1800	50	800	ND	ND	ND	30	80	800	ND	ND	ND	3.0	ND
19–70 y	3000	2000	50	1000	ND	ND	ND	35	100	1000	ND	ND	ND	3.5	ND
>70 y	3000	2000	50	1000	ND	ND	ND	35	100	1000	ND	ND	ND	3.5	ND
Pregnancy[i,j]															
≤18 y	2800	1800	50	800	ND	ND	ND	30	80	800	ND	ND	ND	3.0	ND
19–50 y	3000	2000	50	1000	ND	ND	ND	35	100	1000	ND	ND	ND	3.5	ND
Lactation															
≤18 y	2800	1800	50	800	ND	ND	ND	30	80	800	ND	ND	ND	3.0	ND
19–50 y	3000	2000	50	1000	ND	ND	ND	35	100	1000	ND	ND	ND	3.5	ND

[a]UL = The maximum level of daily nutrient intake that is likely to pose no risk of adverse effects. Unless otherwise specified, the UL represents total intake from food, water, and supplements. Due to lack of suitable data, ULs could not be established for vitamin K, thiamin, riboflavin, vitamin B$_{12}$, pantothenic acid, biotin, or carotenoids. In the absence of ULs, extra caution may be warranted in consuming levels above recommended intakes.
[b]As preformed vitamin A only.
[c]As α-tocopherol; applies to any form of supplemental α-tocopherol.
[d]The ULs for vitamin E, niacin, and folate apply to synthetic forms obtained from supplements, fortified foods, or a combination of the two.
[e] β-carotene supplements are advised only to serve as a provitamin A source for individuals at risk of vitamin A deficiency.
[f]ND, not determinable due to lack of data of adverse effects in this age group and concern with regard to lack of ability to handle excess amounts. Source of intake should be from food only to prevent high levels of intake.
Sources: Dietary Reference Intakes for Calcium, Phosphorus, Magnesium, Vitamin D, and Fluoride (1997); Dietary Reference Intakes for Thiamin, Riboflavin, Niacin, Vitamin B$_6$, Folate, Vitamin B$_{12}$, Pantothenic Acid, Biotin, and Choline (1998); Dietary Reference Intakes for Vitamin C, Vitamin E, Selenium, and Carotenoids (2000); and Dietary Reference Intakes for Vitamin A, Vitamin K, Arsenic, Boron, Chromium, Copper, Iodine, Iron, Manganese, Molybdenum, Nickel, Silicon, Vanadium, and Zinc (2001). These reports may be accessed via **www.nap.edu/catalog/dri.** © National Academy of Sciences. All rights reserved.

(O_2^-), hydrogen peroxide (H_2O_2), hydroxyl (OH^-), and nitric oxide (NO), owing to electron "leakage" along the electron transport chain. *A free radical, a highly unstable, chemically reactive molecule or molecular fragment, contains at least one unpaired electron in its outer orbital or valence shell.* These same free radicals are produced by external heat and ionizing radiation and are carried in cigarette smoke, environmental pollutants, and even some medications. Once formed, free radicals interact with other compounds to create new free-radical molecules. The new molecules frequently damage the electron-dense cellular components' deoxyribonucleic acid (DNA) and lipid-rich cell membranes. By contrast, paired electrons within a molecule represent a far more stable electronic state.

Fortunately, cells possess enzymatic and nonenzymatic mechanisms that work in concert to immediately counter potential oxidative damage from a chemical and enzymatic mutagenic challenge. Antioxidants scavenge oxygen radicals or chemically eradicate them by reducing oxidized compounds. For example, when O_2^- forms, the enzyme superoxide dismutase catalyzes its dismutation to form hydrogen peroxide. This enzyme catalyzes the reaction of two identical molecules to produce two molecules in different states of oxidation as follows:

$$O_2^- + O_2^- \xrightarrow[\text{superoxide dismutase}]{2H^+} H_2O_2 + O_2$$

The hydrogen peroxide produced in this reaction breaks down further to water and oxygen in a reaction catalyzed by the widely distributed enzyme **catalase** as follows:

$$2H_2O_2 \xrightarrow[\text{catalase}]{} 2H_2O + O_2$$

See the animation "Vitamin C as an Antioxidant" on **http://thePoint.lww.com/mkk8e** for a demonstration of this process.

Protection from Disease

An accumulation of free radicals increases the potential for cellular damage, called **oxidative stress**, to biologically important substances through processes that add oxygen to cellular components. These substances include DNA, proteins, and lipid-containing structures, particularly the polyunsaturated fatty acid–rich bilayer membrane that isolates the cell from noxious toxins and carcinogens. Also, oxidative stress likely acts as a key regulator of cell signaling pathways that increase protein breakdown and muscle atrophy during prolonged periods of physical inactivity.[147] During unchecked oxidative stress, the plasma membrane's fatty acids deteriorate through a chain-reaction series of events termed **lipid peroxidation**. These reactions incorporate higher than normal amounts of oxygen into lipids, thereby increasing the vulnerability of the cell and its constituents. Free radicals facilitate peroxidation of low-density lipoprotein (LDL) cholesterol; this leads to cytotoxicity and enhanced coronary artery plaque formation.[96,161] Oxidative stress ultimately increases the likelihood of cellular deterioration associated with advanced aging, many diseases, and a general decline in central nervous system and immune functions.

The body has no way to stop oxygen reduction and free-radical production, but it does provide an elaborate natural defense against their damaging effects. This defense includes the antioxidant scavenger enzymes catalase, glutathione peroxidase, and superoxide dismutase, and metal-binding proteins called metalloenzymes.[74] In addition, the nutritive, nonenzymatic reducing agents selenium and vitamins A, C, and E and the vitamin A precursor β-carotene serve important protective functions.[19,50,68] These antioxidant chemicals protect the plasma membrane by reacting with and removing free radicals, thus quenching

 How Antioxidant Vitamins Serve to Neutralize Free Radicals

In the illustration below, vitamin C neutralizes a DNA-damaging free radical.

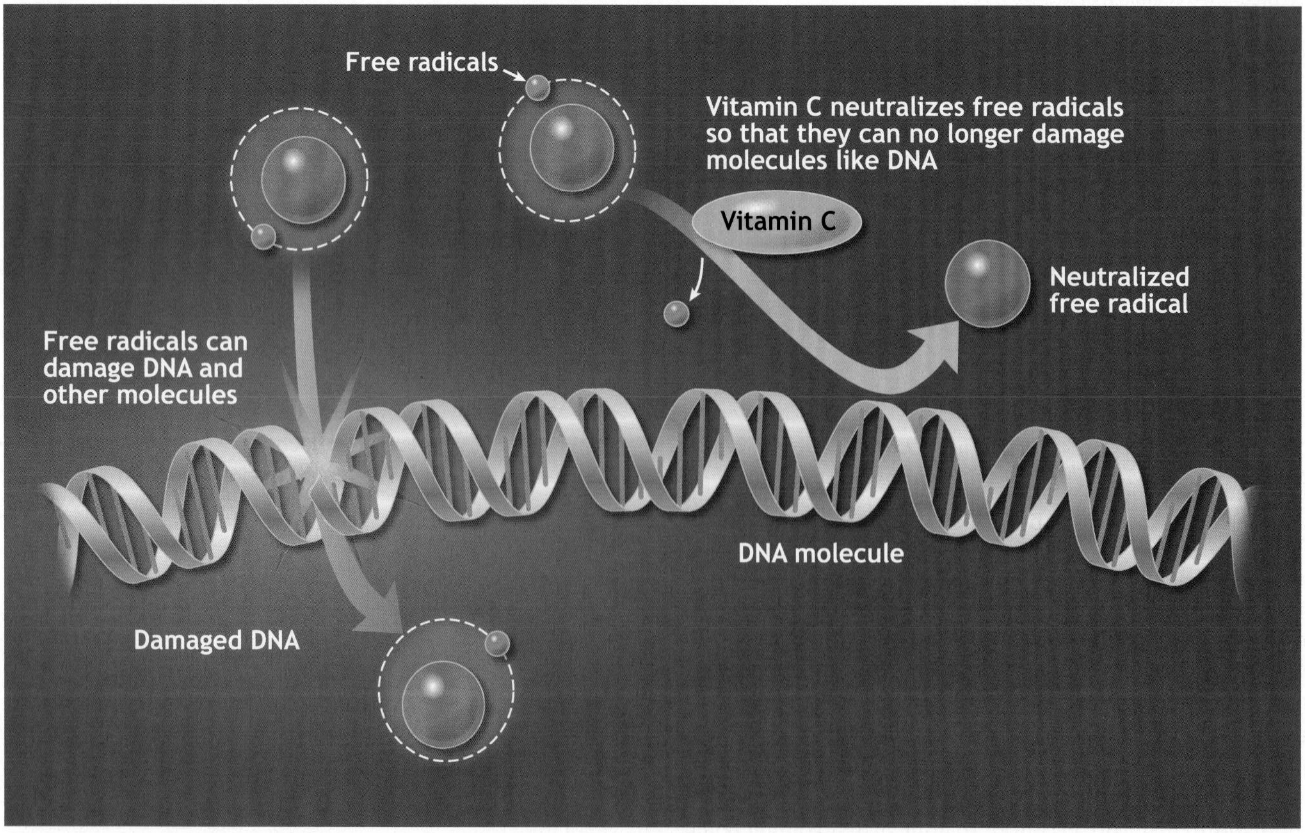

Free radicals

Vitamin C neutralizes free radicals so that they can no longer damage molecules like DNA

Vitamin C

Neutralized free radical

Free radicals can damage DNA and other molecules

Damaged DNA

DNA molecule

the chain reaction; they also blunt the damaging effects to cellular constituents of high serum homocysteine levels (see Chapter 31).[112] A diet with appropriate antioxidant vitamins and other chemoprotective agents (in the foods consumed) may reduce risk of cardiovascular disease, stroke, diabetes, osteoporosis, cataracts, premature aging, and diverse cancers, including breast, distal colon, prostate, pancreas, ovary, and endometrium.[43,69,111]

The **oxidative-modification hypothesis of atherosclerosis** maintains that the mild oxidation of LDL cholesterol—similar to butter turning rancid—contributes to the plaque-forming, artery-clogging process of atherosclerosis.[37,92,160] One model for heart disease protection proposes that antioxidant vitamins inhibit LDL cholesterol oxidation and its subsequent uptake into foam cells embedded in the arterial wall.

A multivitamin may prove beneficial if one's diet lacks the key nutrients vitamin B_{12}, vitamin D, or folic acid. *Nutritional guidelines now focus more on the consumption of a broad array of foods rather than on supplements containing isolated chemicals within these foods.* The current recommendations of nutrition and medical organizations increase the consumption of fruits, vegetables, and whole grains, and include lean meat or meat substitutes and low-fat dairy foods. Disease protection from a healthful diet links to the myriad accessory nutrients and substances within the nutrient-rich foods that include fruits, vegetables, and whole grains, as well as lean meat or meat substitutes and low-fat dairy foods.[67]

The National Cancer Institute (www.cancer.gov) encourages consumption of five or more servings (nine recommended for men) of fruits and vegetables daily, whereas the USDA's *Dietary Guidelines* recommend two to four servings of fruits and three to five servings of vegetables daily.

Obtain Vitamins From Food, Not Supplements

After a placebo-controlled 5-year study of nutritional supplementation, incident cancer was validated in 7.0% of the sample (145 events in men and 29 in women), and death from cancer occurred in 2.3% of the sample. No association emerged between cancer outcomes and supplementation with B vitamins and/or omega-3 fatty acids. A statistically significant interaction of treatment by sex occurred, with no effect of treatment on cancer risk among men and increased cancer risk among women for omega-3 fatty acid supplementation. Such findings provide another example of the wisdom of obtaining nutrients from whole foods and not from the isolated active substances in supplement form that may confer no benefit and may potentiate adverse effects.

Source: Andreeva VA, et al. B vitamin and/or omega-3 fatty acid supplementation and cancer: Ancillary findings from the supplementation with folate, vitamins B6 and B12, and/or omega-3 fatty acids (SU. FOL.OM3) randomized trial. *Arch Intern Med* 2012;172:540.

Vitamin-Rich Food Sources

The food sources below not only provide a rich source for specific vitamins but also supply them in a nutrient-rich package of accessory nutrients with potential health-promoting benefits.

- **Vitamin A** (carotenoids): organ meats, carrots, cantaloupe, sweet potatoes, pumpkin, apricots, spinach, milk, collards, eggs
- **Vitamin C**: guava, citrus fruits and juices, red, yellow, and green peppers, papaya, kiwi, broccoli, strawberries, tomatoes, sweet and white potatoes, kale, mango, cantaloupe
- **Vitamin D**: salmon, tuna, sardines, mackerel, oysters, cod liver oil, egg yolks, fortified milk, fortified orange juice, fortified breakfast cereal
- **Vitamin E**: vegetable oils, nuts, seeds, spinach, kiwi, wheat germ
- **Vitamin K**: spinach, kale, collards, Swiss chard, broccoli, romaine lettuce
- **Vitamin B_1** (thiamin): sunflower seeds, enriched bread, cereal, pasta, whole grains, lean meats, fish, beans, green peas, corn, soybeans
- **Vitamin B_2** (riboflavin): lean meats, eggs, legumes, nuts, green leafy vegetables, dairy products, enriched bread
- **Vitamin B_3** (niacin): dairy products, calf's liver, poultry, fish, lean meat, nuts, eggs, fortified bread and cereal
- **Pantothenic acid**: calf's liver, mushrooms, sunflower seeds, corn, eggs, fish, milk, milk products, whole-grain cereal, beans
- **Biotin**: eggs, fish, milk, liver and kidney, milk products, soybeans, nuts, Swiss chard, whole-grain cereal, beans
- **Vitamin B_6**: beans, bananas, nuts, eggs, meat, poultry, fish, potato, fortified bread and ready-to-eat cereals
- **Vitamin B_{12}**: liver, meat, eggs, poultry, fish (trout and salmon), shellfish, milk, milk products, fortified breakfast cereal
- **Folate**: (folic acid): beef liver, green leafy vegetables, avocado, green peas, enriched bread, fortified breakfast cereals

PHYSICAL ACTIVITY, FREE RADICALS, AND ANTIOXIDANTS

The benefits of physical activity are well documented, but the possibility for negative effects remains controversial. Potentially negative effects occur because an elevated aerobic exercise metabolism increases reactive oxygen and nitrogen free-radical production.[115,120,171] At relatively low cellular levels, free radicals may negatively influence metabolism through signaling mechanisms that maintain cellular balance.[89] Increased free radicals may overwhelm the body's natural defenses and pose a health risk from increased oxidative stress. Free radicals also can contribute to muscle injury and soreness from eccentric muscle actions and unaccustomed physical activity (see Chapter 22). Muscle damage of this nature releases muscle enzymes and initiates inflammatory cell infiltration into the damaged tissue.

An opposing position maintains that free-radical production increases during physical activity, yet the body's normal antioxidant defenses remain adequate or concomitantly improve. Improvement occurs as the natural enzymatic defenses (superoxide dismutase and glutathione peroxidase) "up-regulate" through exercise training adaptations.[125,145,173] *Research supports this latter position because the beneficial effects of regular physical activity decrease the incidence of heart disease and various cancers whose occurrences relate to oxidative stress.* Regular physical training also protects against myocardial injury from lipid peroxidation induced by short-term tissue ischemia followed by reperfusion.[35,60,158]

Increased Metabolism in Exercise and Free-Radical Production

Exercise produces reactive oxygen in at least two ways:

1. By an electron leak in the mitochondria, probably at the cytochrome level, to produce superoxide radicals.
2. During alterations in blood flow and oxygen supply—underperfusion during intense exercise followed by substantial reperfusion in recovery—that trigger excessive free-radical generation. The reintroduction of molecular oxygen in recovery also produces reactive oxygen species that magnify oxidative stress. Some argue that the potential for free-radical damage increases during trauma or stress, from muscle damage, and from environmental pollutants (e.g., smog).

The risk of oxidative stress increases with intense physical activity.[2,103,127] Exhaustive endurance exercise by untrained persons produces oxidative damage in the active muscles. Intense resistance exercise also increases free-radical production, indirectly measured by malondialdehyde, a lipid peroxidation byproduct.[102] **FIGURE 2.3** illustrates how regular aerobic physical activity affects oxidative response, the potential for tissue damage, and protective adaptive responses.

Important Questions

Two questions arise about the potential for increased oxidative stress with exercise:

1. Are physically active individuals more prone to free-radical damage?
2. Are protective agents with antioxidant properties required in increased quantities in the diets of physically active people?

In answer to the first question, the natural antioxidant defenses in well-nourished humans respond adequately to increased physical activity.[174] A single bout of submaximal exercise increases oxidant production, yet antioxidant defenses cope effectively in healthy individuals and trained heart transplant recipients.[75,172] Even with multiple bouts performed on consecutive days, the various indices of oxidative stress show no impairment of the body's antioxidant system.

The answer to the second question remains equivocal.[172] Some evidence indicates that consuming exogenous antioxidant compounds either slows activity-induced free-radical formation or augments the body's natural defense system.[35,74] If antioxidant supplementation proves beneficial, vitamin E

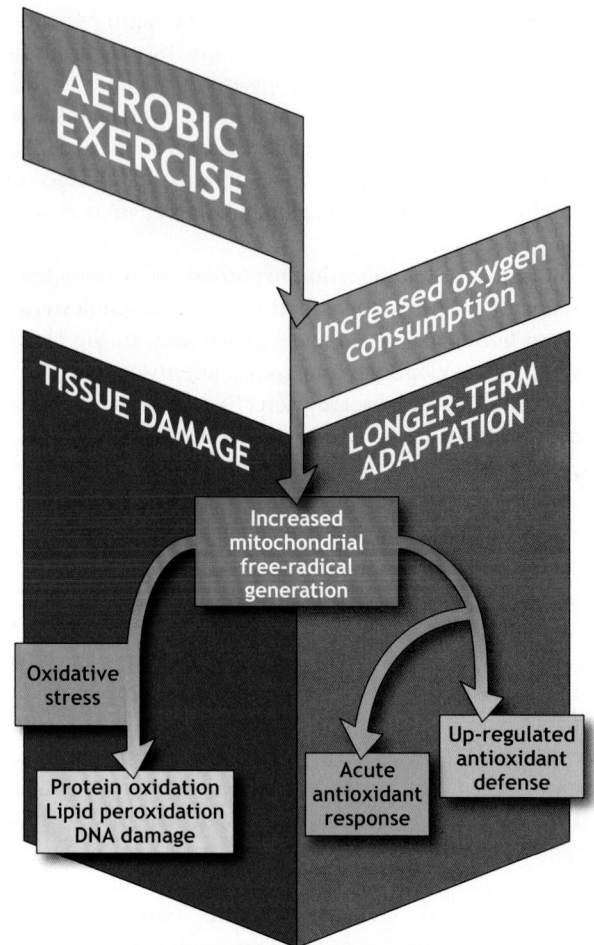

FIGURE 2.3 • Cascade of events and adaptations produced by regular aerobic exercise that lessen the likelihood of tissue damage from intense physical activity.

could be the most important antioxidant related to physical activity and physical training.[27,71]

In one study, vitamin E–deficient animals began training with plasma membrane function compromised from oxidative damage; they reached exhaustion earlier than animals with recommended vitamin E levels. In animals fed a normal diet, vitamin E supplements diminished oxidative damage to skeletal muscle fibers and myocardial tissue caused by exercise training.[55] Humans fed a daily antioxidant vitamin mixture of β-carotene, vitamin C, and vitamin E had lower serum and breath markers of lipid peroxidation at rest and following exercise than subjects not receiving supplements. Five months of vitamin E supplementation in racing cyclists reduced markers of oxidative stress induced by extreme endurance exercise. In another experiment using whole-body resistance training, 2 wk of supplementation with 120 IU of vitamin E daily decreased free-radical interaction with cellular membranes and blunted muscle tissue disruption caused by a single bout of intense exercise.[102] In contrast, antioxidant supplementation with vitamins C and E to individuals with no previous deficiencies in these vitamins had no effect on physical adaptations to strenuous endurance training.[23,56,180] Thirty days of vitamin E supplementation (1200 IU · d⁻¹) produced a 2.8-fold increase in serum vitamin E concentration without affecting contraction-induced indices of muscle damage (including postexercise force decrement) or inflammation caused by eccentric muscle actions.[14] Similarly, a 4-wk daily vitamin E supplement of 1000 IU produced no effect on biochemical or ultrastructural indices of muscle damage in experienced runners after a half marathon.[33] Differences in exercise severity and oxidative stress could account for discrepancies in research findings.

Recommended vitamin E supplementation ranges between 100 and 400 IU per day, but is not without risk. Vitamin E supplementation has produced internal bleeding by inhibiting vitamin K metabolism, particularly in persons taking anticoagulant medication. It also increased risk of prostate cancer among healthy men.[82]

DOES VITAMIN SUPPLEMENTATION PROVIDE A COMPETITIVE EDGE?

FIGURE 2.4 illustrates the progressive increase in money spent on dietary supplements in the United States between 1990 and 2010, with the growth rate exceeding 10% per year. Current estimates indicate that 40% of American adults take a daily vitamin/mineral supplement. More than 50% of competitive athletes in some sports consume supplements on a regular basis, either to ensure adequate micronutrient intake or to achieve an excess with the hope of enhancing exercise/sports performance, training responsiveness, and recovery.[26,42,80] Among elite Canadian athletes in predominantly "power"-based sports, 87% declared having taken three or more dietary supplements within the previous 6 months. Most of this supplementation was in the form of sports drinks, multivitamin and mineral preparations, carbohydrate sports bars, protein powder, and meal-replacement products.[97] When vitamin–mineral deficiencies appear in physically active people, they often occur among these three groups:

1. Vegetarians or groups with low energy intake such as dancers, gymnasts, and weight-class sport athletes who strive to maintain or reduce body weight.
2. Individuals who eliminate one or more food groups from their diet.
3. Individuals who consume large amounts of processed foods and simple sugars with low micronutrient density (e.g., endurance athletes).

Vitamins synthesized in the laboratory are no less effective for bodily functions than vitamins from food sources. When deficiencies exist, vitamin supplements reverse deficiency symptoms. When vitamin intake achieves recommended levels, supplements do not improve exercise performance. *More than 55 years of research on healthy persons with nutritionally adequate diets does not provide evidence that consuming vitamin (and mineral) supplements improves exercise performance, the hormonal and metabolic responses to exercise, or ability to train arduously and recover from such training.*[52,164,170,177]

 INTEGRATIVE QUESTION

Respond to an athlete who asks, "Is there anything wrong with taking megadoses of vitamin and mineral supplements to ensure I'm getting an adequate intake on a daily basis?"

Protection Against Upper Respiratory Tract Infection. Moderate physical activity and exercise training heightens immune function, whereas prolonged periods of intense endurance exercise or a strenuous training session transiently suppress the body's first line of defense against infectious agents.[118,178] An increased risk of upper respiratory tract infection (URTI) occurs within 1 or 2 wk of the exercise stress. Additional vitamin C and E and perhaps carbohydrate ingestion before, during, and following an intense training session may boost the normal immune mechanisms for combating infection.[73,113,117,121] Chapter 20 discusses more fully the relationship between physical activity at various intensity levels and immune function.

 A Healthful Way to Reduce Cold Risk

For overweight, sedentary, postmenopausal women who participated in a program of moderate-intensity exercise 5 days a week for 12 mo, the risk of colds decreased by more than three-fold compared to a control group of women who attended once-weekly stretching sessions.

Source: Chubak J, et al. Moderate-intensity exercise reduces incidence of colds among postmenopausal women. *Am J Med* 2006;119:937.

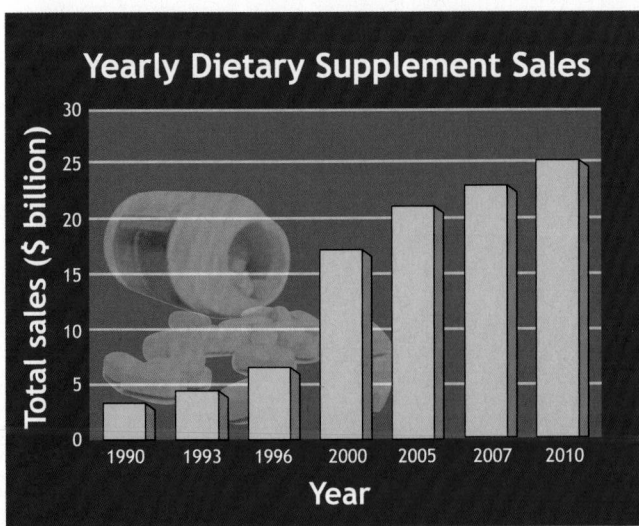

FIGURE 2.4 • Growth of an industry. Dietary supplement sales have increased tremendously as indicated by the supplement sales figures from 1990 to 2010. In 2006, estimates indicate that over one-half of the United States population used a dietary supplement. (Adapted with permission from McArdle WD, Katch FI, Katch VL. *Sports and Exercise Nutrition.* 4th Ed. Philadelphia: Wolters Kluwer Health, 2013.)

Vitamins and Exercise Performance

FIGURE 2.5 illustrates that B-complex and C vitamins play key roles as coenzymes to regulate energy-yielding reactions during carbohydrate, fat, and protein catabolism. They also contribute to hemoglobin synthesis and red blood cell production. The belief that "if a little is good, more must be better" has led many coaches, athletes, fitness enthusiasts, and even a prominent two-time Nobel Prize winner (http://www.quackwatch.com/01QuackeryRelatedTopics/pauling.html) to advocate using vitamin supplements above recommended levels. Nonetheless, the facts do not support such advice for individuals who consume an adequate diet.

Supplementing with vitamin B_6, an essential cofactor in glycogen and amino acid metabolism, did not benefit the metabolic mixture metabolized by women during intense aerobic

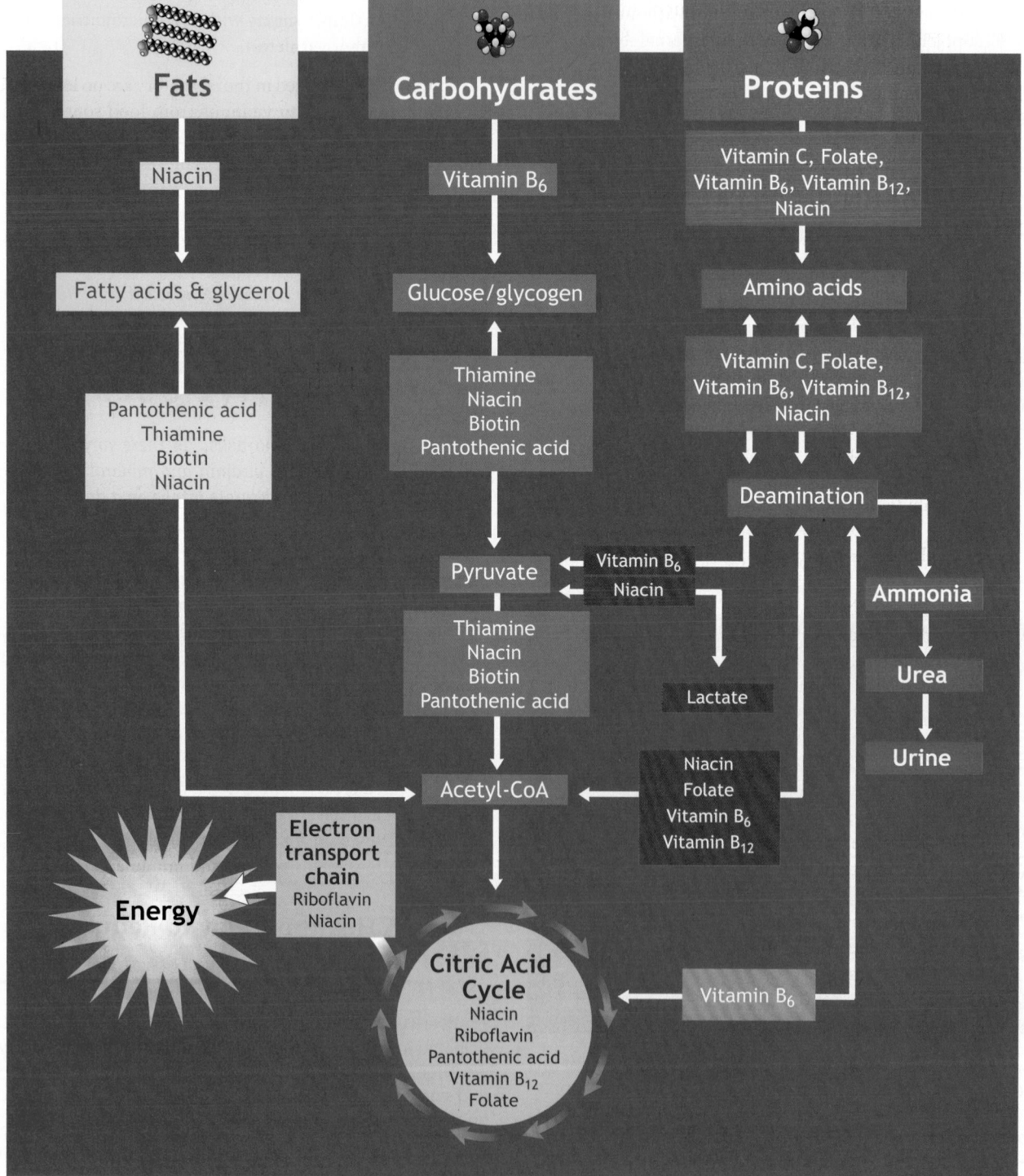

FIGURE 2.5 • General schema for the role of water-soluble vitamins in carbohydrate, fat, and protein metabolism. (Reprinted with permission from McArdle WD, Katch FI, Katch VL. *Sports and Exercise Nutrition*. 4th Ed. Philadelphia: Wolters Kluwer Health, 2013.)

activity. In general, athletes' status for this vitamin equals reference standards for the population[100] and does not decrease with strenuous exercise to a level warranting supplementation.[135] For endurance-trained men, 9 days of vitamin B$_6$ supplementation (20 mg per day) provided no ergogenic effect on cycling to exhaustion performed at 70% of aerobic capacity.[175]

Chronic high-potency, multivitamin–mineral supplementation for well-nourished, healthy individuals does not augment aerobic fitness, muscular strength, neuromuscular performance after prolonged running, and general athletic performance.[52,147] In addition to a lack of effectiveness for supplements of the B-complex group, no exercise benefits exist for excess vitamins C and E on stamina, circulatory function, or energy metabolism. Short-term daily supplementation with vitamin E (400 IU) produced no effect on normal neuroendocrine and metabolic responses to strenuous exercise or performance time to exhaustion.[148] Vitamin C status, assessed by serum concentrations and urinary ascorbate levels, in trained athletes does not differ from untrained individuals despite large differences in daily physical activity level.[138] Other investigators report similar findings for other vitamins.[48,136] Active persons typically increase daily energy intake to match their increased energy requirement; thus, a proportionate increase occurs in micronutrient intake, often in amounts that exceed recommended levels.

Summary

1. Vitamins serve crucial functions in almost all bodily processes. These organic compounds neither supply energy nor contribute to body mass.
2. With the exception of vitamin D, vitamins are obtained from food or dietary supplementation.
3. Plants synthesize vitamins; animals also produce them from precursor substances known as provitamins.
4. The 13 known vitamins are classified as either water soluble or fat soluble. The fat-soluble vitamins include A, D, E, and K; vitamin C and the B-complex vitamins constitute the water-soluble vitamins.
5. Excess fat-soluble vitamins accumulate in body tissues; when taken in excess, levels can increase to toxic concentrations. Excess water-soluble vitamins remain nontoxic and are excreted in the urine.
6. Vitamins regulate metabolism, facilitate energy release, and play key functions in bone and tissue synthesis.
7. Vitamins A, C, E, and the provitamin β-carotene serve important protective functions as antioxidants. An appropriate intake of these micronutrients reduces the potential for free-radical damage (oxidative stress) and may offer protection against heart disease and some types of cancer.
8. The Dietary Reference Intakes (DRIs) differ from their predecessor RDAs by focusing more on promoting health maintenance and risk reduction for nutrient-dependent diseases rather than the traditional criterion of preventing deficiency diseases.
9. The DRIs serve as an umbrella term that encompasses the RDAs, Estimated Average Requirements, Adequate Intakes, and Tolerable Upper Intake Levels for nutrient recommendations in planning and assessing diets for healthy persons.

10. DRI values include recommendations that apply to gender and life stages of growth and development based on age and during pregnancy and lactation.
11. Physical activity elevates metabolism and increases the production of potentially harmful free radicals. A daily diet that contains foods rich in antioxidant vitamins and minerals lessens oxidative stress.
12. The body's natural antioxidant defenses up-regulate in response to increased physical activity in well-nourished individuals.
13. Vitamin supplementation above recommended values does not improve exercise performance or the potential for intense physical training.

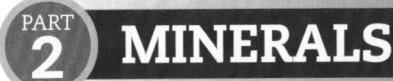

PART 2 · MINERALS

THE NATURE OF MINERALS

Approximately 4% of the body's mass consists of 22 mostly metallic elements, collectively called **minerals**. Minerals serve as constituents of enzymes, hormones, and vitamins; they combine with other chemicals (e.g., calcium phosphate in bone, iron in the heme of hemoglobin) or exist singularly (e.g., free calcium and sodium in body fluids).

The minerals essential to life include seven **major minerals** (required in amounts >100 mg daily) and 14 minor or **trace minerals** (required in amounts <100 mg daily). Trace minerals account for less than 15 g or 0.02% of the total body mass. Excess mineral intake serves no useful physiologic purpose but can produce toxic effects. DRIs have been established for many minerals; a diet that supplies these requirements ensures an adequate intake of the remaining minerals.

Most minerals, major or trace, occur freely in nature—mainly in the waters of rivers, lakes, and oceans; in topsoil; and beneath the earth's surface. Minerals exist in the root systems of plants and the body structure of animals that consume plants and water containing minerals. **TABLES 2.4 AND 2.5** present the RDA, AI, and UL values for the minerals, and **TABLE 2.6** lists the major bodily functions, dietary sources, and symptoms of deficiency or excess for the minerals.

ROLE OF MINERALS IN THE BODY

Minerals serve three broad functions in the body:

1. Provide *structure* in forming bones and teeth.
2. Help to maintain normal bodily *functions* (e.g., heart rhythm, muscle contractility, neural conductivity, acid-base balance).
3. *Regulate* metabolism by becoming constituents of enzymes and hormones that modulate cellular activity.

FIGURE 2.6 lists the participating minerals in catabolic and anabolic cellular processes. Minerals activate reactions that release energy during carbohydrate, fat, and protein catabolism. They play important roles in the biosynthesis of nutrients—glycogen

TABLE 2.4   Dietary Reference Intakes (DRIs): Recommended Mineral Intakes

Life-Stage Group	Calcium (mg/d)	Chromium (µg/d)	Copper (µg/d)	Fluoride (mg/d)	Iodine (µg/d)	Iron (mg/d)	Magnesium (mg/d)	Manganese (mg/d)	Molybdenum (µg/d)	Phosphorus (mg/d)	Selenium (µg/d)	Zinc (mg/d)
Infants												
0–6 mo	210*	0.2*	200*	0.01*	110*	0.27*	30*	0.003*	2*	100*	15*	2*
7–12 mo	270*	5.5*	220*	0.5*	130*	11*	75*	0.6*	3*	275*	20*	3
Children												
1–3 y	500*	11*	340	0.7*	90	7	80	1.2*	17	460	20	3
4–8 y	800*	15*	440	1*	90	10	130	1.5*	22	500	30	5
Males												
9–13 y	1300	25*	700	2*	120	8	240	1.9*	34	1250	40	8
14–18 y	1300*	35*	890	3*	150	11	410	2.2*	43	1250	55	11
19–30 y	1000*	35*	900	4*	150	8	400	2.3*	45	700	55	11
31–50 y	1000*	35*	900	4*	150	8	420	2.3*	45	700	55	11
51–70 y	1200*	30*	900	4*	150	8	420	2.3*	45	700	55	11
>70 y	1200*	30*	900	4*	150	8	420	2.3*	45	700	55	11
Females												
9–13 y	1300*	21*	700	2*	150	8	240	1.6*	34	1250	40	8
14–18 y	1300*	24*	890	3*	150	15	360	1.6*	43	1250	55	9
19–30 y	1000*	25*	900	3*	150	18	310	1.8*	45	700	55	8
31–50 y	1000*	25*	900	3*	150	18	320	1.8*	45	700	55	8
51–70 y	1200*	20*	900	3*	150	8	320	1.8*	45	700	55	8
>70 y	1200*	20*	900	3*	150	8	320	1.8*	45	700	55	8
Pregnancy												
≤18 y	1300*	29*	1000	3*	220	27	400	2.0*	50	1250	60	13
19–30 y	1000*	30*	1000	3*	220	27	350	2.0*	50	700	60	11
31–50 y	1000*	30*	1000	3*	220	27	360	2.0*	50	700	60	11
Lactation												
≤18 y	1300*	44*	1300	3*	290	10	360	2.6*	50	1250	70	14
19–30 y	1000*	45*	1300	3*	290	9	310	2.6*	50	700	70	12
31–50 y	1000*	45*	1300	3*	290	9	320	2.6*	50	700	70	12

Table presents Recommended Dietary Allowances (RDAs) in **bold type** and Adequate Intakes (AIs) in ordinary type followed by an asterisk (*). RDAs and AIs may both be used as goals for individual intake. RDAs are set to meet the needs of almost all (97–98%) individuals in a group. For healthy breastfed infants, the AI is the mean intake. The AI for other life-stage and gender groups is believed to cover the needs of all individuals in the group, but lack of data or uncertainty in the data prevent being able to specify with confidence the percentage of individuals covered by this intake.

Sources: Dietary Reference Intakes for Calcium, Phosphorous, Magnesium. Vitamin D, and Fluoride (1997) ; Dietary Reference Intakes for Thiamin, Riboflavin, Niacin, Vitamin B6, Folate, Vitamin B5, Pantothenic Acid, Biotin, and Choline (1998) ; Dietary Reference Intakes for Vitamin C, Vitamin E, Selenium, and Carotenoids (2000); and Dietary Reference Intakes for Vitamin A, Vitamin K, Arsenic, Boron, Chromium, Copper, Iodine, Iron, Manganese, Molybdenum, Nickel, Silicon, Vanadium, and Zinc (2001).

These reports may be accessed via www.nap.edu/catalog/dri. © National Academy of Sciences. Reprinted with permission.

TABLE 2.5 Dietary Reference Intakes (DRIs): Tolerable Upper Intake Levels (ULs[a])

Life-Stage Group	Arsenic[b] (mg/d)	Boron (mg/d)	Calcium (mg/d)	Chromium (mg/d)	Copper (µg/d)	Fluoride (mg/d)	Iodine (µg/d)	Iron (mg/d)	Magnesium (mg/d)[c]	Manganese (mg/d)	Molybdenum (µg/d)	Nickel (mg/d)	Phosphorus (g/d)	Selenium (µg/d)	Silicon[d]	Vanadium (mg/d)[e]	Zinc (mg/d)
Infants																	
0–6 mo	ND[f]	ND	ND	ND	ND	0.7	ND	40	ND	ND	ND	ND	ND	45	ND	ND	4
7–12 mo	ND	ND	ND	ND	ND	0.9	ND	40	ND	ND	ND	ND	ND	60	ND	ND	5
Children																	
1–3 y	ND	3	2.5	ND	1000	1.0	200	40	65	2	300	0.2	3	90	ND	ND	7
4–8 y	ND	6	2.5	ND	3000	2.2	300	40	110	3	600	0.3	3	150	ND	ND	12
Males, females																	
9–13 y	ND	11	2.5	ND	5000	10	600	40	350	6	1100	0.6	4	280	ND	ND	23
14–18 y	ND	17	2.5	ND	800	10	900	45	350	9	1700	1.0	4	400	ND	ND	34
19–70 y	ND	20	2.5	ND	10,000	10	1100	45	350	11	2000	1.0	4	400	ND	1.8	40
>70 y	ND	20	2.5	ND	10,000	10	1100	45	350	11	2000	1.0	3	400	ND	1.8	40
Pregnancy																	
≤18 y	ND	17	2.5	ND	8000	10	900	45	350	9	1700	1.0	3.5	400	ND	ND	34
19–50 y	ND	20	2.5	ND	10,000	10	1100	45	350	11	2000	1.0	3.5	400	ND	ND	40
Lactation																	
≤18 y	ND	17	2.5	ND	8,000	10	900	45	350	9	1700	1.0	4	400	ND	ND	34
19–50 y	ND	20	2.5	ND	10,000	10	1100	45	350	11	2000	1.0	4	400	ND	ND	40

[a]UL = The maximum level of daily nutrient intake that is likely to pose no risk of adverse effects. Unless otherwise specified, the UL represents total intake from food, water, and supplements. Due to lack of suitable data, ULs could not be established for arsenic, chromium, and silicon. In the absence of ULs, extra caution may be warranted in consuming levels above recommended intakes.

[b]Although the UL was not determined for arsenic, there is no justification for adding arsenic to food or supplements.

[c]The ULs for magnesium represent intake from a pharmacologic agent only and do not include intake from food and water.

[d]Although silicon has not been shown to cause adverse effects in humans, there is no justification for adding silicon to supplements.

[e]Although vanadium in food has not been shown to cause adverse effects in humans, there is no justification for adding vanadium to food and vanadium supplements should be used with caution. The UL is based on adverse effects in laboratory animals and this data could be used to set a UL for adults but not children and adolescents.

[f]ND = not determinable due to lack of data of adverse effects in this age group and concern with regard to lack of ability to handle excess amounts. Source of intake should be from food only to prevent high levels of intake.

Sources: Dietary Reference Intakes for Calcium, Phosphorous, Magnesium, Vitamin D, and Fluoride (1997); Dietary Reference Intakes for Thiamin, Riboflavin, Niacin, Vitamin B₆, Folate, Vitamin B₁₂, Pantothenic Acid, Biotin, and Choline (1998); Dietary Reference Intakes for Vitamin C, Vitamin E, Selenium, and Carotenoids (2000); and Dietary Reference Intakes for Vitamin A, Vitamin K, Arsenic, Boron, Chromium, Copper, Iodine, Iron, Manganese, Molybdenum, Nickel, Silicon, Vanadium, and Zinc (2001)

These reports may be accessed via www.nap.edu/catalog/dri. © National Academy of Sciences. Reprinted with permission.

TABLE 2.6	**The Important Major and Trace Minerals for Healthy Adults (Age 19–50 Years) and Their Food Sources, Functions, and the Effects of Deficiencies and Excesses**			
Mineral	**Dietary Sources**	**Major Bodily Functions**	**Deficiency**	**Excess**
Major				
Calcium	Milk, cheese, dark green vegetables, dried legumes	Bone and tooth formation, blood clotting, nerve transmission	Stunted growth, rickets, osteoporosis, convulsions	Not reported in humans
Phosphorus	Milk, cheese, yogurt, meat, poultry, grains, fish	Bone and tooth formation, acid-base balance, helps prevent loss of calcium from bone	Weakness, demineralization	Erosion of jaw (phossy jaw)
Potassium	Leafy vegetables, cantaloupe, lima beans, potatoes, bananas, milk, meats, coffee, tea	Fluid balance, nerve transmission, acid-base balance	Muscle cramps, irregular cardiac rhythm, mental confusion, loss of appetite; can be life-threatening	None if kidneys function normally; poor kidney function causes potassium buildup and cardiac arrhythmias
Sulfur	Obtained as part of dietary protein; present in food preservatives	Acid-base balance, liver function	Unlikely to occur with adequate dietary intake	Unknown
Sodium	Common salt	Acid-base balance, body water balance, nerve function	Muscle cramps, mental apathy, reduced appetite	Contributes to high blood pressure
Chlorine (chloride)	Chloride part of salt-containing food; some vegetables and fruits	Important part of extracellular fluids	Unlikely to occur with adequate dietary intake	Contributes to high blood pressure
Magnesium	Whole grains, green leafy vegetables	Activates enzymes involved in protein synthesis	Growth failure, behavioral disturbances	Diarrhea
Trace				
Iron	Eggs, lean meats, legumes, whole grains, green leafy vegetables	Constituent of hemoglobin and enzymes involved in energy metabolism	Iron-deficiency anemia (weakness, reduced resistance to infection)	Siderosis; cirrhosis of liver
Fluoride	Drinking water, tea, seafood	May be important in maintenance of bone structure	Higher frequency of tooth decay	Mottling of teeth, increased bone density
Zinc	Widely distributed in foods	Constituent of enzymes involved in digestion	Growth failure, small sex glands	Fever, nausea, vomiting, diarrhea
Copper	Meats, drinking water	Constituent of enzymes associated with iron metabolism	Anemia, bone changes (rare)	Rare metabolic condition (Wilson's disease)
Selenium	Seafood, meats, grains	Functions in close association with vitamin E	Anemia (rare)	Gastrointestinal disorders, lung irritations
Iodine (iodide)	Marine fish and shellfish, dairy products, vegetables, iodized salt	Constituent of thyroid hormones	Goiter (enlarged thyroid)	High intake depresses thyroid activity
Chromium	Legumes, cereals, organ meats, fats, vegetable oils, meats, whole grains	Constituent of some enzymes; involved in glucose and energy metabolism	Not reported in humans; impaired ability to metabolize glucose	Inhibition of enzymes Occupational exposures: skin and kidney damage

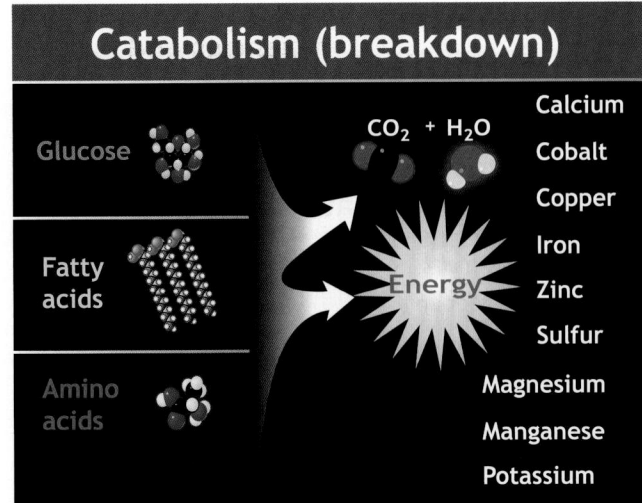

Catabolism (breakdown)

Glucose
Fatty acids
Amino acids

$CO_2 + H_2O$

Energy

Calcium
Cobalt
Copper
Iron
Zinc
Sulfur
Magnesium
Manganese
Potassium

Anabolism (buildup)

Glucose → Glycogen
Fatty acids → Fats
Amino acids → Proteins

Calcium
Chlorine
Magnesium
Manganese
Potassium

FIGURE 2.6 • Minerals that function in macronutrient catabolism and anabolism. (Reprinted with permission from McArdle WD, Katch FI, Katch VL. *Sports and Exercise Nutrition*. 4th Ed. Philadelphia: Wolters Kluwer Health, 2013.)

from glucose, triacylglycerols from fatty acids and glycerol, and proteins from amino acids. A lack of one or more essential minerals can disrupt the fine balance between catabolism and anabolism. Minerals also form important constituents of hormones. Inadequate thyroxine production from iodine insufficiency, for example, slows the body's resting metabolism. In extreme cases, this could predispose a person to develop obesity. Synthesis of insulin, the hormone that facilitates cellular glucose uptake, requires zinc (as do approximately 100 enzymes), whereas chlorine forms the key digestive acid hydrochloric acid.

The following sections describe specific functions of important minerals related to physical activity.

CALCIUM

Calcium, the body's most abundant mineral, combines with phosphorus to form bones and teeth. These two minerals represent about 75% of the body's total mineral content, or about 2.5% of body mass. In its ionized form (about 1% of 1200 g of endogenous calcium), calcium functions in muscle stimulation, blood clotting, nerve impulse transmission, activation of

several enzymes, synthesis of calcitriol (active form of vitamin D), and transport of fluids across cell membranes. It also may lessen symptoms of premenstrual syndrome, reduce colon cancer risk, and optimize blood pressure regulation.[41,101]

 See the animation "Calcium in Muscles" on **http://thePoint.lww.com/mkk8e** for a demonstration of this process.

Osteoporosis: Calcium, Estrogen, and Exercise

Bone, a dynamic tissue matrix of collagen and minerals, exists in a continual state of flux called **remodeling**. Most of the adult skeleton is replaced about every 10 years. Bone-destroying cells called *osteoclasts* (under the influence of parathyroid hormone) cause the breakdown or resorption of bone by enzyme action. In contrast, bone-forming *osteoblast* cells induce bone synthesis. Calcium availability affects the dynamics of bone remodeling. The two broad categories of bone include:

1. **Cortical bone:** dense, hard outer layer of bone such as the shafts of the long bones of the arms and legs
2. **Trabecular bone:** spongy, less dense, and relatively weaker bone, most prevalent in the vertebrae and ball of the femur

 See the animation "Bone Growth" on **http://thePoint.lww.com/mkk8e** for a demonstration of this process.

Calcium from food or derived from bone resorption maintains plasma calcium levels. Age and gender determine a person's calcium needs. As a general guideline from the Institute of Medicine (www.iom.edu), adolescents and young adults require 1300 mg of calcium daily or the calcium in five 8-oz glasses of milk (1000 mg for adults ages 19 to 50 and 1200 mg for those older than 50). Unfortunately, calcium remains one of the most frequent nutrients lacking in the diet of both sedentary and physically active individuals, particularly adolescent girls. For a typical adult, daily calcium intake only ranges between 500 and 700 mg. *Among athletes, female dancers, gymnasts, and endurance competitors are most prone to calcium dietary insufficiency.*[16,108]

Inadequate calcium intake or low levels of calcium-regulating hormones cause withdrawal of calcium "reserves" in bone to restore any deficit. Prolonging this restorative imbalance promotes one of two conditions:

1. **Osteopenia**—from the Greek words *osteo*, meaning "bone," and *penia*, meaning "poverty"—a midway condition where bones weaken with increased fracture risk.
2. **Osteoporosis**, literally meaning "porous bones," with bone density more than 2.5 standard deviations below normal for gender. Osteoporosis develops progressively as bone loses its calcium mass or bone mineral content and its calcium concentration or bone mineral density. This deterioration causes bone to progressively become more porous and brittle (**FIG. 2.7**). Eventually, the stresses of normal living cause bone to break, with compression fractures of the spine occurring most frequently (http://www.nof.org).

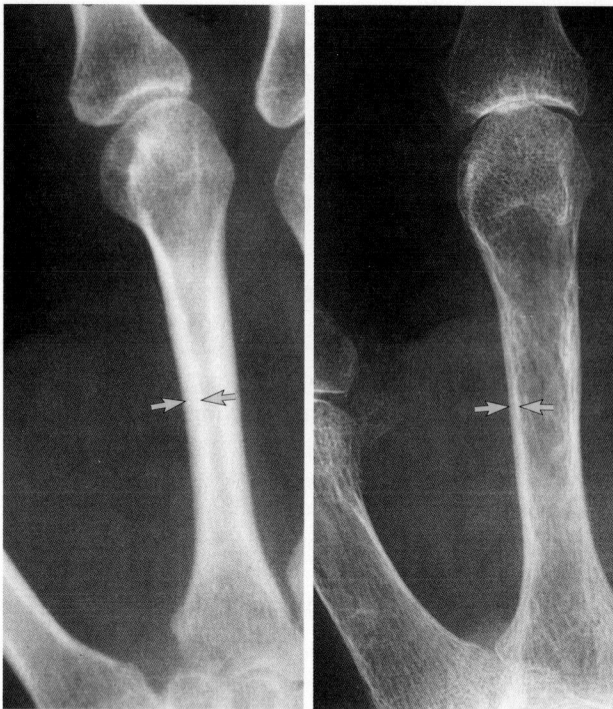

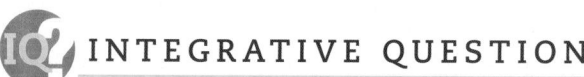

FIGURE 2.7 • Radiograph of mid-second metacarpal of person with normal mineralization (*left*) and of patient with severe osteoporosis (*right*). Under normal conditions, cortical width (*arrows*) is more than one-third of the total width of the metacarpal, whereas osteoporosis produces extreme cortical narrowing. Note the intracortical tunneling that occurs in more aggressive forms of osteoporosis. (Reprinted with permission from Brant W, Helms C. *Fundamentals of Diagnostic Radiology*. 3rd Ed. Baltimore: Lippincott Williams & Wilkins, 2006.)

INTEGRATIVE QUESTION

Discuss the role played by physical activity and calcium intake on bone health.

A Progressive Disease

Between 60 and 80% of an individual's susceptibility to osteoporosis links to genetic factors, while 20 to 40% remains lifestyle related. *The early teens serve as the prime years to maximize bone mass.*[15,107] Regular physical activity also enables females to gain bone mass throughout the third decade of life. Osteoporosis for many women begins early in life because the typical teenager consumes suboptimal calcium to support growing bones. This creates an irreversible deficit that cannot be fully eliminated after achieving skeletal maturity. A genetic predisposition can worsen calcium imbalance into adulthood.[53,94,169] Adequate intake of calcium, preferably from food, and vitamin D (600 international units [IU] a day for most adults and at least 800 IU daily after age 70), helps to maintain normal blood levels of calcium and bone mineralization.[18,88,163,176]

One of two women and one of eight men over age 50 can expect an osteoporosis-related fracture in their lifetime. Increased susceptibility to osteoporosis among older women

Bone Health Diagnostic Criteria Based on Variation (Standard Deviation [SD]) of Observed Bone Density Values Compared to Values for Sex-Matched Young Adult Population

Normal	<1.0 SD below mean
Osteopenia	1.0 to 2.5 SD below mean
Osteoporosis	>2.5 SD below mean
Severe osteoporosis	>2.5 SD below mean plus one or more fragility fractures

coincides with menopause and marked decrease in the secretion of estradiol, the most potent naturally occurring human estrogen. Most men normally produce some estrogen into old age—a major reason why they exhibit relatively lower osteoporosis prevalence. A portion of circulating testosterone converts to estradiol, which also promotes positive calcium balance.

Prevention of Bone Loss Through Diet

FIGURE 2.8A illustrates that a complex interaction among factors rather than the separate influence of each contributes to variations in bone mass.[98,153] That portion of bone mass variation attributable to diet may reflect how diet interacts with genetic factors, physical activity patterns, body weight, and drug or medication use (e.g., estrogen therapy). *Adequate calcium intake throughout life remains the prime defense against bone loss with age.*[15,76] For example, calcium supplementation in postmenarchal girls with suboptimal calcium intake enhanced bone mineral acquisition.[140] Adolescent girls should consume 1500 mg of calcium daily. Increasing daily calcium intake for middle-aged

Fifteen Risk Factors for Osteoporosis

1. Advancing age
2. History of fracture as an adult, regardless of cause
3. History of fracture in a parent or sibling
4. Cigarette smoking
5. Slight build or tendency toward underweight
6. White or Asian female
7. Sedentary lifestyle
8. Early menopause
9. Eating disorder
10. High protein intake (particularly animal protein)
11. Excess sodium intake
12. Alcohol abuse
13. Calcium-deficient diet before and after menopause
14. High caffeine intake (equivocal)
15. Vitamin D deficiency, either through inadequate exposure to sunlight or dietary insufficiency (prevalent in about 40% of adults)

National Academy of Sciences Recommended Daily Calcium Intake

Age	Amount (mg)
Birth to 6 mo	200 mg
Infants 7–12 mo	260 mg
Children 1–3 y	700 mg
Children 4–8 y	1000 mg
Children 9–13 y	1300 mg
Teens 14–18 y	1300 mg
Adults 19–50 y	1000 mg
Adult men 51–70 y	1000 mg
Adult women 51–70 y	1200 mg
Adults 71 y and older	1200 mg
Pregnant and breastfeeding teens	1300 mg
Pregnant and breastfeeding adults	1000 mg

women, particularly estrogen-deprived women following menopause, from 1200 to 1500 mg improves the body's calcium balance.[63,128] Adequate calcium intake and the addition of animal protein to the diet may reduce hip fracture risk.

Estrogen's Role in Bone Health

- Increases intestinal calcium absorption
- Reduces urinary calcium excretion
- Inhibits bone resorption
- Decreases bone turnover

Good dietary calcium sources include milk and milk products, sardines and canned salmon, kidney beans, and dark green leafy vegetables. Eight ounces of milk or 6 ounces of yogurt contains 300 mg of calcium, and one cup of spinach contains 270 mg. Americans spend more than $1 billion a year on calcium supplements hoping to stave off osteoporosis. Nearly 45% of American women, mostly older women, use dietary supplements containing calcium. Calcium supplements, best absorbed on an empty stomach, can correct dietary deficiencies regardless of whether the extra calcium comes from fortified foods or commercial supplements. Calcium citrate causes less stomach upset than other supplement forms; it also enhances iron absorption better than calcium gluconate, calcium carbonate, or other commercial products. Adequate availability of vitamin D facilitates calcium uptake. Calcium supplements should be taken in moderation as some research has linked excessive intake in supplement form (not food)

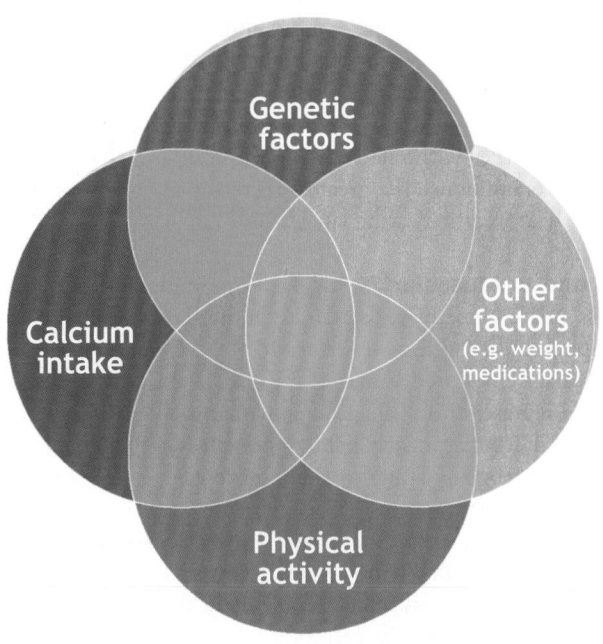

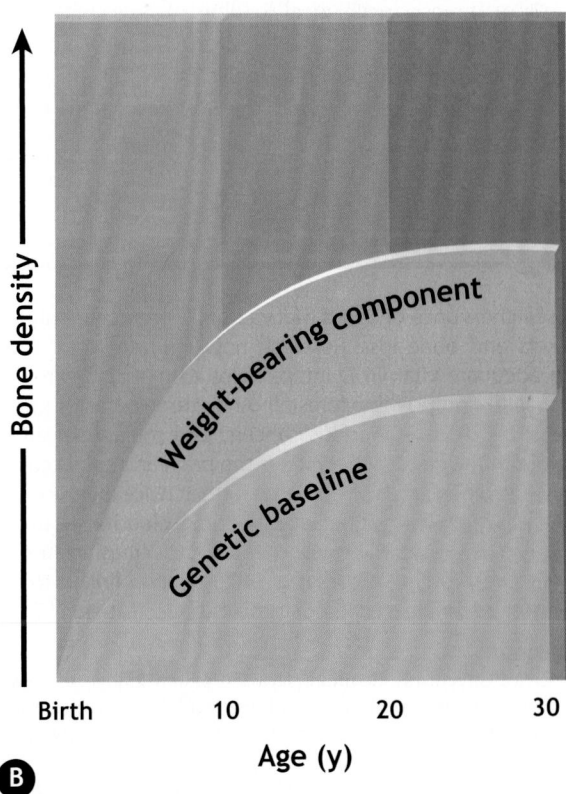

FIGURE 2.8 • (A) Variation in bone mass within the population is likely a function of how the different factors that affect bone mass interact with each other. (Adapted with permission from Specker BL. Should there be dietary guidelines for calcium intake? *Am J Clin Nutr* 2000;71:663.) **(B)** Weight-bearing exercise augments skeleton mass during growth above the genetic baseline. The degree of augmentation depends largely on the amount of mechanical loading on a particular bone. (Adapted with permission from Turner CH. Site-specific effects of exercise: Importance of interstitial fluid pressure. *Bone* 1999;24:161.)

with increased risk of heart attack and kidney stones. Excessive meat, salt, coffee, and alcohol consumption inhibits absorption. Individuals who live and train primarily indoors in northern latitudes should supplement with 200 IU of vitamin D daily.[7] Bone matrix formation also depends on vitamin K, prevalent in leafy green and cruciferous vegetables. The RDA for vitamin K is 90 mg for women and 120 mg for men.

Physical Activity Benefits. Mechanical loading through regular exercise slows the rate of skeletal aging. Regardless of age or gender, children and adults who maintain an active lifestyle have greater bone mass, size, and structure than their sedentary counterparts.[4,5,62,83,90,159] Benefits of regular physical activity on bone mass accretion, and perhaps bone shape and size, occur primarily during childhood and adolescence when peak bone mass increases to the greatest extent (**Fig. 2.8B**); the benefits may persist well beyond activity cessation.[6,59,105,114] These benefits often accrue into the seventh and eighth decades of life.[17,84,151] The decline in vigorous physical activity with a sedentary lifestyle with aging closely parallels age-related bone mass loss. In this regard, regular moderate physical activity coincides with higher values for cortical bone measures[144] and a substantially lower risk of hip fracture in postmenopausal women.[45,141]

The osteogenic effect of physical activity proves most effective during the growth periods of childhood and adolescence and may reduce fracture risk later in life.[15,72,78] Short bouts of intense mechanical loading of bone with dynamic exercise three to five times a week provide a potent stimulus to maintain or increase bone mass. **Figure 2.9** illustrates the beneficial effects of resistance training and circuit-resistance

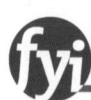

A More Important Role for Vitamin D

Researchers once believed that vitamin D protected only against rickets and bone loss. Research now indicates that maintaining adequate vitamin D intake helps to maintain cardiovascular health and possibly forestall other chronic health problems, including diabetes, various cancers, and multiple sclerosis, an autoimmune disease that affects the brain and spinal cord. Men with low blood levels of vitamin D were at twice the risk of a heart attack as those with higher levels. Optimal blood levels of vitamin D (20 ng · mL⁻¹) were also associated with decreasing amounts of C-reactive protein, a marker of inflammation linked to arterial stiffness and increased risk of cardiac abnormalities.

Sources:

Amer M, Qayyum R. Relation between serum 25-hydroxyvitamin D and C-reactive protein in asymptomatic adults (from the continuous National Health and Nutrition Examination Survey 2001 to 2006). *Am J Cardiol* 2012;109:226.

Giovannucci E, et al. 25-hydroxyvitamin D and risk of myocardial infarction in men: a prospective study. *Arch Intern Med* 2008;168:1174.

Salzer J, et al. Vitamin D as a protective factor in multiple sclerosis. *Neurology* 2012;79:2140.

Wilson C. Epidemiology: ethnicity, vitamin D, and CHD. *Nat Rev Cardiol* 2013;10:490.

Obtain Calcium From Food, Not Supplements

A recent report suggests that consuming calcium in supplement form may raise the risk of heart attack. Researchers from the University of Auckland in New Zealand reviewed 11 studies of nearly 12,000 people who consumed calcium supplements without also taking vitamin D. Of the 6166 individuals who consumed calcium supplements, a 30% greater incidence of myocardial infarction occurred compared to the 5805 individuals in the placebo group. These findings were consistent across trials and independent of age, sex, and supplement type.

Some researchers contend that the benefits of calcium supplements in reducing bone fracture risk and bone loss in older men and women with low calcium in their diets outweigh any potential heart attack risk. Ultimately, the potential risks of supplemental calcium must be weighed against the benefits of the supplements to prevent osteoporosis. Until this benefit-to-risk ratio debate settles, it seems prudent to advise people consuming calcium supplements to seek advice from their doctors, eat more calcium-rich foods, exercise, quit smoking, and maintain a healthy body weight to counter heart disease and reduce the risk of osteoporosis.

Source: Reid I, et al. Cardiovascular effects of calcium supplements. *Nutrients* 2013;5:2522

training or weight-bearing walking, running, dancing, rope skipping, or gymnastics. These modes of physical activity generate a considerable impact load and/or intermittent force against the long bones of the body.[39,91] Men and women in strength and power activities have as much or more bone mass than endurance athletes.[132] Volleyball, basketball, and gymnastic activities with relatively high impact and strain on the skeletal mass induce the greatest increases in bone mass, particularly at weight-bearing sites.[9,30,99,149]

Related to Muscular Strength. Bone mineral density and mass relate directly to measures of muscular strength and regional and total lean tissue mass.[32,49,124] Lumbar spine and proximal femur bone masses of elite teenage weightlifters exceed representative values for fully mature bone of reference adults.[29] Eccentric muscle training provides a more potent site-specific osteogenic stimulus than concentric muscle training because greater forces usually occur with eccentric loading.[61] Prior physical activity and sport experiences offer residual effects on an adult's bone mineral density. Exercise-induced increases in bone mass achieved during the teenage and young-adult years persist despite cessation of active competition.[81,83]

Site-Specific Effects. Muscle forces acting on specific bones during physical activity, particularly intermittent compression and tension mechanical loading, modify bone metabolism at the point of stress.[13,70,79] For example, the lower limb bones of older cross-country runners have greater bone mineral content than less-active counterparts. The throwing arm of baseball players also shows greater bone thickness than their less-used, nondominant arm. Likewise, the bone mineral content of

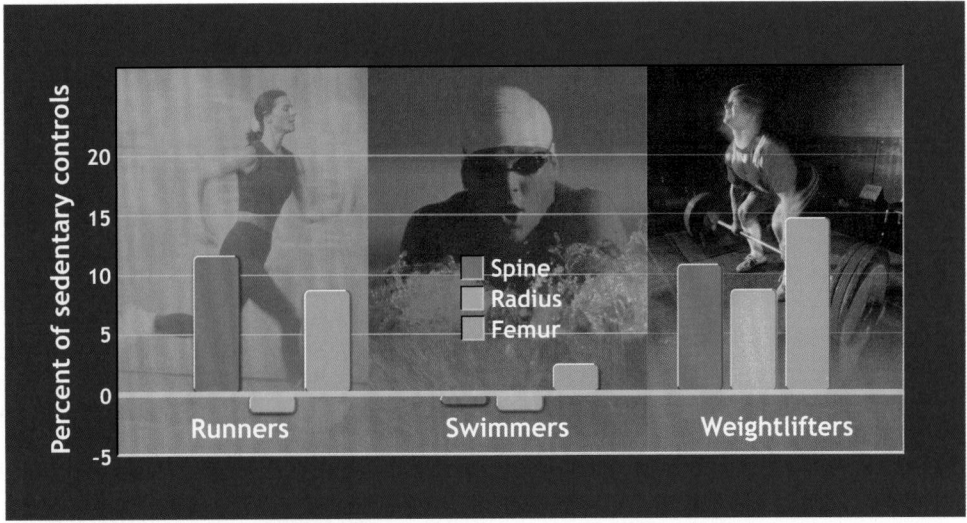

FIGURE 2.9 • Bone mineral density expressed as a percentage of sedentary control values at three skeletal sites for runners, swimmers, and weightlifters. (Adapted with permission from Drinkwater BL. Physical activity, fitness, and osteoporosis. In: Bouchard C, et al., eds. *Physical Activity, Fitness, and Health.* Champaign, IL: Human Kinetics, 1994.)

the humeral shaft and proximal humerus of the playing arm of tennis players averages 20 to 25% more than their non-dominant arm; side-to-side difference in the arms of nonplayers generally averages only 5%.[83] For females, this positive response to specific sports training occurs most noticeably in players who begin training before menarche.[77]

 INTEGRATIVE QUESTION

Why does resistance training for the body's major muscle groups offer unique benefits to bone mass compared with a typical weight-bearing program of brisk walking?

Mechanism for Bone Matrix Increase. Prevailing theory considers that dynamic loading creates hydrostatic pressure gradients within a bone's fluid-filled matrix. Fluid movement within this matrix in response to pressure changes from

 Six Principles to Promote Bone Health with Physical Activity

1. **Specificity:** Physical activity provides a local osteogenic effect.
2. **Overload:** Progressively increasing exercise intensity promotes continued bone deposition.
3. **Initial values:** Individuals with the smallest total bone mass show the greatest potential for bone deposition.
4. **Diminishing returns:** As one approaches the biologic ceiling for bone density, further density gains require greater effort.
5. **More not necessarily better:** Bone cells become desensitized in response to prolonged mechanical-loading sessions.
6. **Reversibility:** Discontinuing exercise overload reverses the positive osteogenic effects gained through increased levels of physical activity.

dynamic activity generates fluid shear stress on bone cells. This initiates a cascade of cellular events to ultimately stimulate the production of bone matrix protein.[168] Mechanosensitivity of bone and its subsequent buildup of calcium depends on two factors:

1. Magnitude of the applied force or strain magnitude
2. Frequency or number of cycles of application

Owing to the transient sensitivity of bone cells to mechanical stimuli, shorter, more frequent periods of high-frequency force (mechanical strain) with rest periods interspersed facilitate bone mass accretion.[58,87,133] As applied force and strain increase, the number of cycles required to initiate bone formation decrease.[31] Chemicals produced in bone itself also contribute to bone formation. Alterations in bone's geometric configuration to long-term exercise training enhance its mechanical properties.[11] **FIGURE 2.10** illustrates the anatomic structure and cross-sectional view of a typical long bone and depicts the dynamics of bone growth and remodeling.

THE FEMALE ATHLETE TRIAD: AN UNEXPECTED PROBLEM FOR WOMEN WHO TRAIN INTENSELY

A paradox exists between physical activity and bone dynamics for athletic premenopausal women, particularly in young athletes who have yet to attain peak bone mass. Women who train intensely and emphasize weight loss often engage in disordered eating behaviors that link to menstrual irregularities, primarily **amenorrhea** or cessation of menstrual flow. Disordered eating behaviors eventually lead to the **female athlete triad** (**FIG. 2.11**): energy drain, amenorrhea, and osteoporosis.[28,86,95,123,150]

The term *female triad* more accurately describes the syndrome of disorders because it afflicts physically active women in the general population who do not fit the typical profile of the competitive athlete.

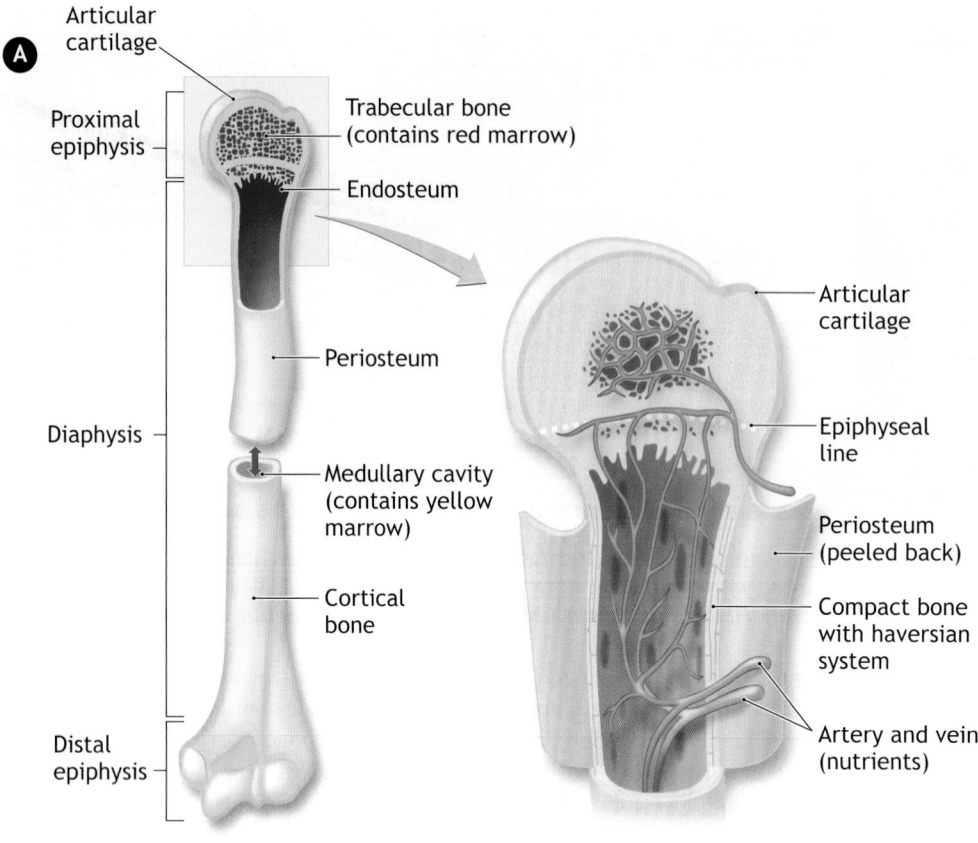

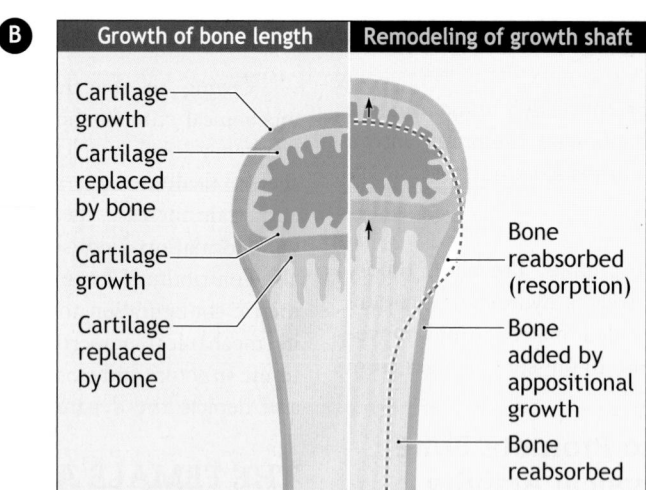

FIGURE 2.10 • Anatomic structure **(A)** and longitudinal view of a typical long bone, and **(B)** bone dynamics during growth and continual remodeling. (Reprinted with permission from McArdle WD, Katch FI, Katch VL. *Sports and Exercise Nutrition*. 4th Ed. Philadelphia: Wolters Kluwer Health, 2013.)

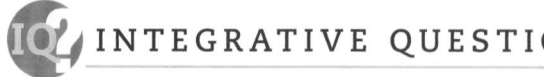 INTEGRATIVE QUESTION

Young girls and women who engage in sports likely suffer from at least one of the disorders of the female triad. Discuss factors related to this syndrome and how a coach might guard against their occurrence.

Many young women who play sports likely suffer from at least one of the triad's disorders, particularly disordered eating behaviors and accompanying energy deficit. This malady afflicts 15 to 60% of female athletes, particularly those involved in leanness-related sports.[116,166] **FIGURE 2.12** illustrates the contributing factors to exercise-related amenorrhea, considered the "red flag," or most recognizable symptom for the triad's presence. The prevalence of amenorrhea among athletes in body weight–emphasized sports—distance running, gymnastics, ballet, cheerleading, figure skating, and body building—probably ranges between 25 and 65%; no more than 5% of the general population of females of menstruating age experience this condition.

 INTEGRATIVE QUESTION

Advise a group of high school females about strategies to achieve weight loss to compete successfully and healthfully in competitive gymnastics.

Bone density relates closely to menstrual regularity and total number of menstrual cycles. Premature cessation of menstruation removes estrogen's protective effect on bone, making these young women more vulnerable to calcium loss with concomitant decrease in bone mass. The most severe menstrual disorders produce the greatest negative effect on bone mass.[24,165] Lowered bone density from extended amenorrhea often occurs at multiple sites, including bone areas regularly subjected to increased force and impact loading during exercise.[129] Concurrently, the problem worsens in individuals who undergo an energy deficit accompanied by low protein, lipid, and energy intakes.[181] In such cases, a poor diet also provides inadequate calcium intake.

Persistent amenorrhea that begins at an early age diminishes the benefits of regular physical activity on bone mass; it also increases the risk of musculoskeletal injuries, particularly repeated stress fractures, during exercise participation.[110] A 5% loss in bone mass increases the risk of stress fractures by nearly 40%. Reestablishing normal menses causes some regain in bone mass but not to levels achieved with normal menstruation. Bone mass often remains permanently at suboptimal levels throughout adult life—leaving the women at increased risk for osteoporosis and stress fractures, even years following competitive athletic participation.[38,104] Successful nonpharmacologic treatment of athletic amenorrhea uses a four-phase behavioral approach plus diet and training interventions:

1. Reduce training level by 10 to 20%
2. Gradually increase total energy intake
3. Increase body weight by 2 to 3%
4. Maintain calcium intake at 1500 mg daily

PHOSPHORUS

Phosphorus combines with calcium to form hydroxyapatite and calcium phosphate—compounds that confer rigidity to bones and teeth. Phosphorus also serves as an essential component of the intracellular mediator cyclic adenosine monophosphate (cAMP) and the intramuscular high-energy compounds adenosine triphosphate (ATP) and phosphocreatine (PCr). Phosphorus combines with lipids to form phospholipid compounds, integral components of the cells' bilayer plasma membrane. The phosphorous-containing phosphatase enzymes regulate cellular metabolism; phosphorus also buffers acid end products

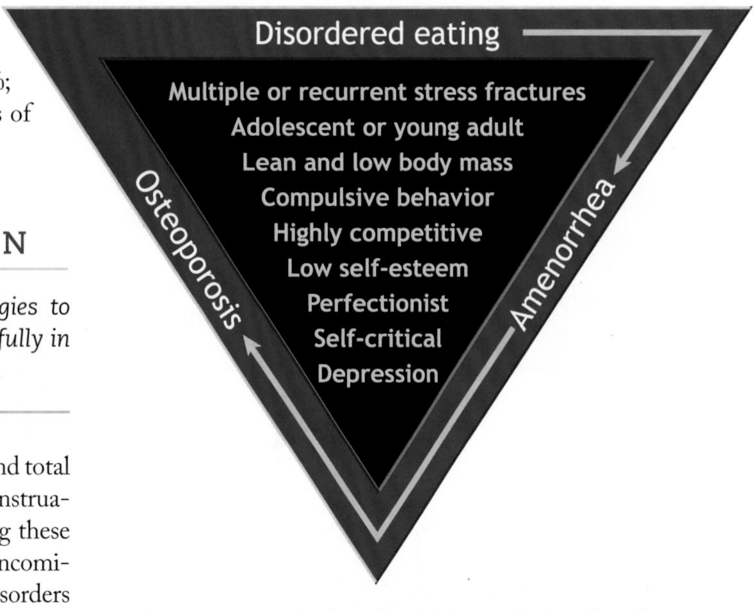

FIGURE 2.11 • The female athlete triad: disordered eating, amenorrhea, and osteoporosis. (Adapted with permission from American College of Sports Medicine Position Stand. The female athlete triad. *Med Sci Sports Exerc* 2007;39:1867.)

of energy metabolism. Chapter 23 discusses the usefulness of buffering agents for augmenting intense exercise performance. Athletes usually consume adequate phosphorus, with the possible exception of the low-energy diets of many female dancers and gymnasts.[16,108] Rich dietary sources of phosphorus include meat, fish, poultry, milk products, and cereals.

MAGNESIUM

Only about 1% of the body's 20 to 30 g of magnesium is found in blood, with about one-half of the stores present inside the cells of tissues and organs and the remainder combined with calcium and phosphorus in bone. About 400 enzymes that regulate metabolic processes contain magnesium. Magnesium plays an important role in glucose metabolism by facilitating muscle and liver glycogen formation from bloodborne glucose. It also participates as a cofactor in glucose, fatty acid, and amino acid breakdown during energy metabolism. Magnesium affects lipid and protein synthesis and contributes to optimal neuromuscular functioning. It acts as an electrolyte and, along with potassium and sodium, helps to maintain blood pressure.

By regulating DNA and ribonucleic acid (RNA) synthesis and structure, magnesium affects cell growth, reproduction, and plasma membrane integrity. Because of its role as a Ca^{+2} channel blocker, inadequate magnesium could precipitate hypertension and cardiac arrhythmias. Sweating produces only small losses of magnesium. Conflicting data exist concerning the possible effects of magnesium supplements on exercise performance and training response.[20,46,167]

The magnesium intake of athletes generally attains recommended levels, but female dancers and gymnasts have relatively low intakes.[16,108] Green leafy vegetables, legumes, nuts, bananas, mushrooms, and whole grains provide rich magnesium sources.

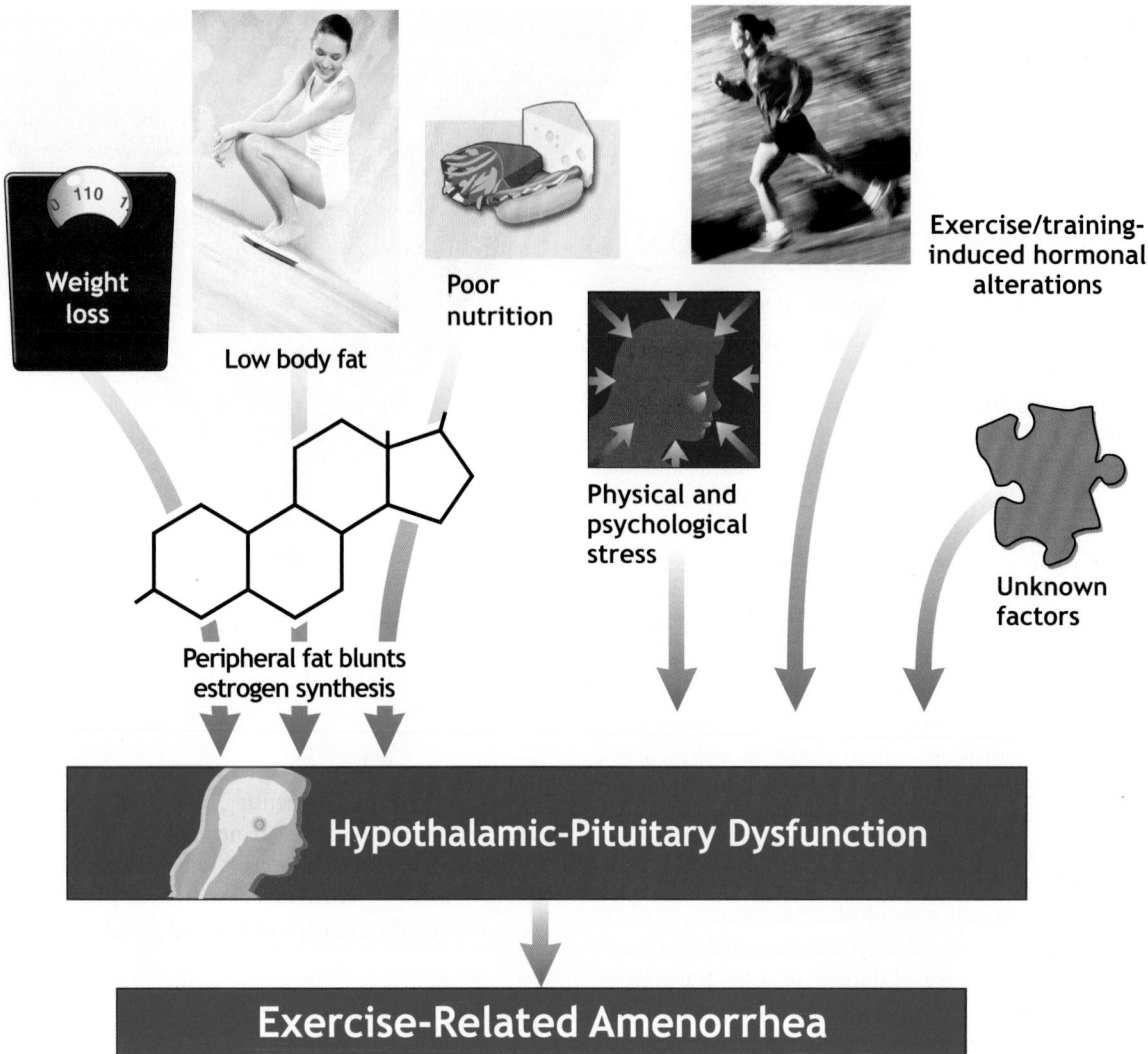

FIGURE 2.12 • Contributing factors to the development of exercise-related amenorrhea.

IRON

The body normally contains between 2.5 and 4.0 g (about 1/6 oz) of this trace mineral. Seventy to 80% of iron exists in functionally active compounds, predominantly combined with **hemoglobin** in red blood cells (85% of functional iron). This iron–protein compound increases the blood's oxygen-carrying capacity 65-fold. Iron serves other important exercise-related functions, as a structural component of **myoglobin** (12% of functional iron), a compound similar to hemoglobin that aids in oxygen storage and transport within the muscle cell. Small amounts of iron also exist in **cytochromes** that facilitate cellular energy transfer. About 20% of the body's iron does not combine in functionally active compounds and exists as **hemosiderin** and **ferritin** stored in the liver, spleen, and bone marrow. These stores replenish iron lost from the functional compounds and provide the iron reserve during periods of insufficient dietary iron intake. An iron-binding plasma glycoprotein, transferrin, transports iron from ingested food and damaged red blood cells to tissues in need, particularly the liver, spleen, bone marrow, and skeletal muscles. *Plasma levels of transferrin reflect the adequacy of the current iron intake.*

Physically active individuals should consume normal amounts of iron-rich foods in their diet. Persons with inadequate iron intake or with limited rates of iron absorption or high rates of iron loss often develop a reduced concentration of hemoglobin in red blood cells, commonly called iron-deficiency anemia, that produces general sluggishness, loss of appetite, pale skin, sore tongue, brittle nails, susceptibility to infection, difficulty keeping warm, frontal headaches, dizziness, and reduced capacity to sustain even mild physical activity. "Iron therapy" normalizes the blood's hemoglobin content and exercise capacity. TABLE 2.7 gives recommendations for iron intake for children and adults.

Females: A Population at Risk

According to the Centers for Disease Control and Prevention (CDC; www.cdc.gov), iron deficiency represents the most common nutritional deficiency and leading cause of anemia in the United States. Insufficient iron intake frequently occurs

TABLE 2.7	Recommended Dietary Allowances for Iron	
	Age (y)	**Iron (mg)**
Children	1–10	10
Males	11–18	12
	19+	10
Females	11–50	15
	51+	10
	Pregnant	30[a]
	Lactating	15[a]

Food and Nutrition Board, National Academy of Sciences–National Research Council, Washington, DC; www.iom.edu/CMS/3788.aspx
[a]Generally, this increased requirement cannot be met by ordinary diets; therefore, the use of 30–60 mg of supplemental iron is recommended.

among young children, teenagers, and females of childbearing age, including many physically active women. In the United States, between 10 and 13% of premenopausal women suffer from low iron intake and between 3 and 5% are anemic by conventional diagnostic criteria. Older women are not immune from this disorder; 6 to 9% of women age 50 and older suffer from iron deficiency. In addition, pregnancy can trigger a moderate iron-deficiency anemia from the increased iron demand placed on the mother by the fetus.

Iron loss ranges between 15 and 30 mg from the 30 to 60 mL of blood generally lost during a menstrual cycle. This loss requires an additional 5 mg of dietary iron daily for premenopausal females and increases the average monthly dietary iron requirement by 150 mg for synthesizing red blood cells lost during menstruation. In the United States, 30 to 50% of women experience dietary iron insufficiency from menstrual blood loss and limited dietary iron intake. The typical iron intake averages 6 mg of iron per 1000 calories of food consumed, with heme iron providing about 15% of the total iron.

Exercise-Induced Anemia: Fact or Fiction?

Interest in endurance sports, with increased participation by women, has focused research on the influence of intense training on the body's iron status. The term **sports anemia** describes reduced hemoglobin levels approaching clinical anemia ($12 \, \text{g} \cdot \text{dL}^{-1}$ of blood for women and $14 \, \text{g} \cdot \text{dL}^{-1}$ for men) attributable to physical training. *Strenuous* training may create an added demand for iron that often exceeds its intake. This would tax iron reserves and eventually lead to depressed hemoglobin synthesis and/or reduction in iron-containing compounds within the cell's energy transfer system. Individuals susceptible to an "iron drain" could experience reduced exercise capacity because of iron's crucial role in oxygen transport and use.

Intense physical training theoretically creates an augmented iron demand from three sources:

1. Small loss of iron in sweat
2. Loss of hemoglobin in urine from red blood cell destruction with increased temperature, spleen activity, and

circulation rates and from jarring of the kidneys and mechanical trauma from feet pounding on the running surface, known as foot-strike hemolysis
3. Gastrointestinal bleeding with distance running unrelated to age, gender, or performance time

Real Anemia or Pseudoanemia?

Apparent suboptimal hemoglobin concentrations and hematocrits occur more frequently among endurance athletes, supporting the possibility of an exercise-induced anemia. However, reduced hemoglobin concentration remains transient, occurring in the early phase of training and then returning toward pretraining values. **FIGURE 2.13** illustrates the general response for hematologic variables for high school female cross-country runners during a competitive season. The decrease in hemoglobin concentration generally parallels the disproportionately large expansion in plasma volume with endurance and resistance training (see Fig. 13.5 in Chapter 13).[36,54,143] Several days of training increase plasma volume by 20%, while total red blood cell volume remains unchanged. Consequently, *total* hemoglobin, an important factor in endurance performance, remains the same or increases slightly with training, while hemoglobin *concentration* decreases in the expanding plasma volume. Despite this hemoglobin dilution, aerobic capacity and exercise performance improve with training.

Mechanical destruction of red blood cells occurs with vigorous physical activity, along with some iron loss in sweat. No evidence indicates that these factors strain an athlete's iron reserves and precipitate clinical anemia if iron intake remains at recommended levels. Applying stringent criteria for both anemia and insufficiency of iron reserves makes sports anemia much less prevalent than generally believed. For male collegiate runners and swimmers, no indications of the early stages of anemia occurred despite large changes in training volume and intensity during the competitive season.[122] For female athletes, the prevalence of iron-deficiency anemia did *not* differ in comparisons among specific athletic groups or with nonathletic controls.[130]

Should Athletes Take an Iron Supplement?

Any increase in iron loss with training, when coupled with poor dietary habits in adolescent and premenopausal women, strains an already limited iron reserve. This does not mean that all individuals in training should supplement with iron or that dietary iron insufficiency or iron loss caused by physical activity produces sports anemia. It does suggest the importance of monitoring an athlete's iron status by periodic evaluation of hematologic characteristics and iron reserves, particularly those who consume iron supplements. Measuring serum ferritin concentration provides useful information about iron reserves. Values below $20 \, \text{mg} \cdot \text{L}^{-1}$ for females and $30 \, \text{mg} \cdot \text{L}^{-1}$ for males indicate depleted reserves.

For healthy individuals whose diets contain the recommended iron intake, excess iron either through diet or supplementation does *not* increase hemoglobin, hematocrit, or other measures of iron status or exercise performance. Potential harm exists from overconsumption or overabsorption of iron, particularly with the widespread use of vitamin C supplements, which facilitate iron absorption.[47] Iron supplements should not be used indiscriminately. Excessive iron, particularly heme iron, can accumulate to toxic levels and contribute to diabetes, liver disease, and heart and joint damage; it may even promote the growth of latent cancers (e.g., colon and prostate) and infectious organisms and create free radicals, which can damage cell membranes, vital proteins, and DNA.

Importance of Iron Source

The small intestine absorbs about 10 to 15% of the total ingested iron, depending on three factors:

1. Iron status
2. Form of iron ingested
3. Meal composition

For example, the small intestine usually absorbs 2 to 5% of iron from plants (trivalent ferric or **nonheme** elemental iron), whereas iron absorption from animal sources (divalent ferrous or **heme**) increases to 10 to 35%. The presence of heme iron, which represents between 35 and 55% of iron in animal sources, also increases iron absorption from nonheme sources.

 Factors Affecting Iron Absorption

Increase Iron Absorption
- Acid in the stomach
- Iron in heme form
- High body demand for red blood cells (blood loss, high-altitude exposure, physical training, pregnancy)
- Low iron stores in body
- Presence of mean protein factor (MPF)
- Presence of vitamin C in small intestine

Decrease Iron Absorption
- Phytic acid (in dietary fiber)
- Oxalic acid
- Polyphenols (in tea and coffee)
- High iron stores in body
- Excess of other minerals (Zn, Mg, Ca), particularly when taken as supplements
- Reduction in stomach acid
- Antacids

The low bioavailability of nonheme iron places women on vegetarian-type diets at risk for developing iron insufficiency. These individuals require almost twice the iron as meat eaters (14 mg per day for men and postmenopausal women and 32 mg a day for premenopausal women). Female vegetarian runners have a poorer iron status than counterparts who consume the same quantity of iron from predominantly animal sources.[152] Including foods rich in vitamin C (ascorbic acid) in the diet upgrades dietary iron bioavailability. Ascorbic acid prevents oxidation of ferrous iron to the ferric form, thus increasing nonheme iron's solubility for absorption at the alkaline pH of the small intestine. The ascorbic acid in one glass of orange juice stimulates a threefold increase in nonheme iron absorption from a typical breakfast meal.[142] Heme sources of iron include beef, beef liver, pork, tuna, and clams; oatmeal, dried figs, spinach, beans, and lentils are good nonheme sources. Fiber-rich foods, coffee, and tea contain compounds that interfere with the intestinal absorption of iron (and zinc).

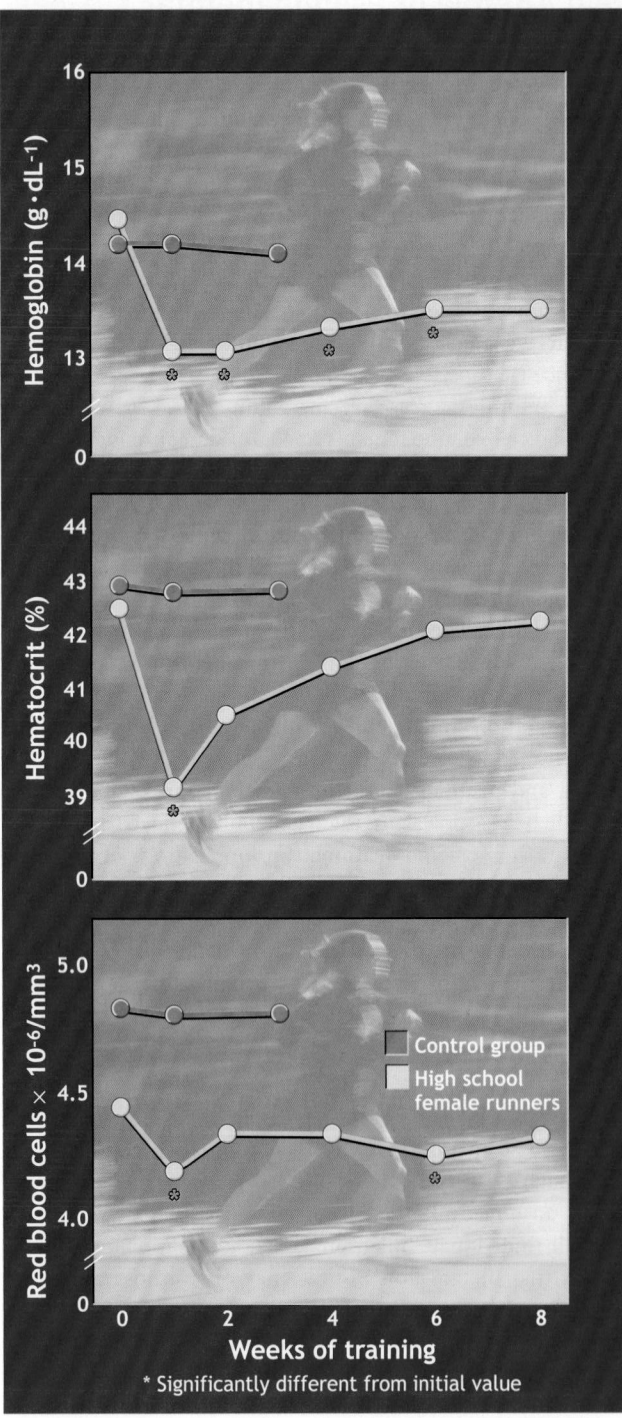

FIGURE 2.13 • Hemoglobin, red blood cell count, and hematocrit in female high school cross-country runners and a comparison group during the competitive season. (Adapted with permission from Puhl JL, et al. Erythrocyte changes during training in high school women cross-country runners. *Res Q Exerc Sport* 1981;52:484.)

Functional Anemia

A relatively high prevalence of nonanemic iron depletion exists among athletes in diverse sports as well as in recreationally active women and men.[34,40,57,146] Low values for hemoglobin within the "normal" range often reflect **functional anemia** or **marginal iron deficiency**. Depleted iron stores and reduced iron-dependent protein production (e.g., oxidative enzymes) with a relatively normal hemoglobin concentration characterize this condition. Ergogenic effects of iron supplementation on aerobic exercise performance and training responsiveness occur for these iron-deficient athletes.[21,22] Physically active but untrained women classified as iron depleted (serum ferritin <16 mg · L^{-1}) but not anemic (Hb >12 g · dL^{-1}) received either iron therapy (50 mg ferrous sulfate) or a placebo twice daily for 2 wk.[65] All subjects then completed 4 wk of aerobic training. The iron-supplemented group increased serum ferritin levels with only a small (nonsignificant) increase in hemoglobin concentration. The improvement in 15-km endurance cycling time in the supplemented group was twice that of women who consumed the placebo (3.4 vs. 1.6 min faster). Women with low serum ferritin levels but with hemoglobin concentrations above 12 g · dL^{-1}, although not clinically anemic, might still be functionally anemic and thus benefit from iron supplementation to augment exercise performance. Similarly, iron-depleted but nonanemic women received either a placebo or 20 mg of elemental iron as ferrous sulfate twice daily for 6 wk. **Figure 2.14** shows that the iron supplement attenuated the rate of decrease in maximal force measured sequentially during 8 min of dynamic knee-extension movements.

Current recommendations support iron supplementation for nonanemic physically active women with low serum ferritin levels. Supplementation in this case exerts little effect on hemoglobin concentration and red blood cell volume. Any improved exercise capacity likely occurs from increased muscle oxidative capacity, not the blood's increased oxygen transport capacity.

SODIUM, POTASSIUM, AND CHLORINE

Sodium, potassium, and chlorine, collectively termed *electrolytes*, remain dissolved in the body fluids as electrically charged particles, or ions. Sodium and chlorine represent the chief minerals contained in blood plasma and extracellular fluid. Electrolytes modulate fluid exchange within the body's

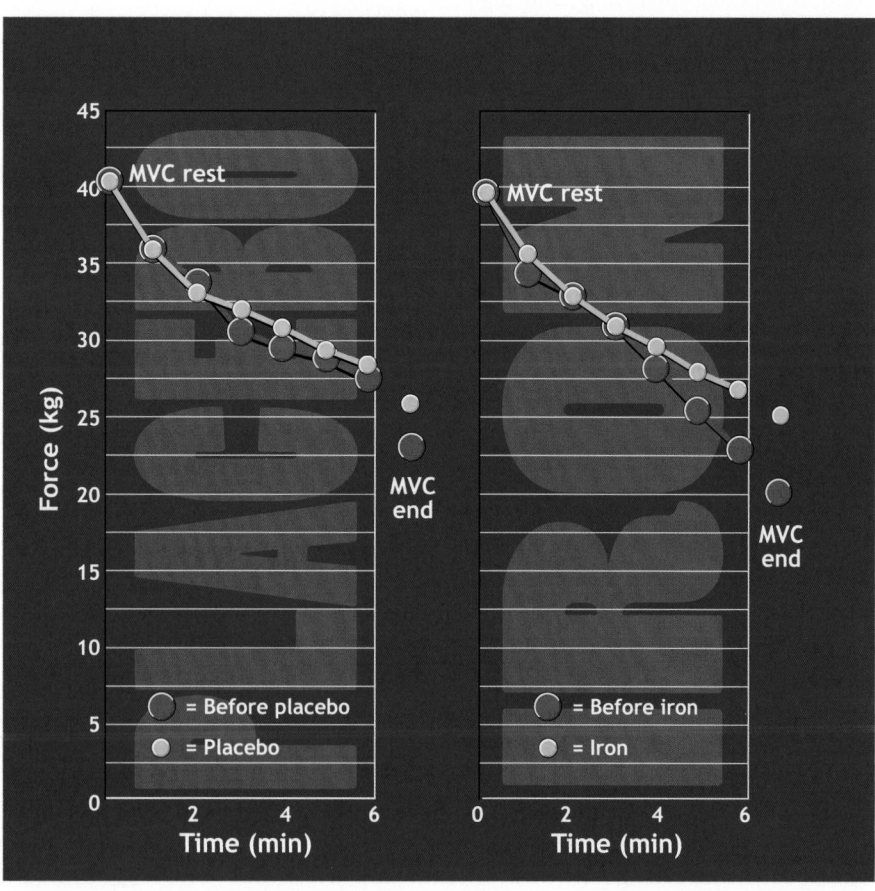

FIGURE 2.14 • Maximal voluntary static contractions (MVCs) over the first 6 min of a progressive fatigue test of dynamic knee extensions before (●) and after (◐) supplementation with either a placebo or iron. MVC$_{end}$ represents the last MVC of the protocol and occurred at different times (average < 8 min) for each subject. (Reprinted with permission from Brutsaert TD, et al. Iron supplementation improves progressive fatigue resistance during dynamic knee extensor exercise in iron-depleted, nonanemic women. *Am J Clin Nutr* 2003;77:441, as adapted in McArdle WD, Katch FI, Katch VL. *Sports and Exercise Nutrition.* 4th Ed. Philadelphia: Wolters Kluwer Health, 2013.)

TABLE 2.8 Electrolyte Concentrations in Blood Serum and Sweat, and Carbohydrate and Electrolyte Concentrations of Some Popular Beverages

Substance	Na⁺ (mEq·L⁻¹)ᵃ	K⁺ (mEq·L⁻¹)	Ca⁺⁺ (mEq·L⁻¹)	Mg⁺⁺ (mEq·L⁻¹)	Cl⁻ (mEq·L⁻¹)	Osmolality (mOsm·L⁻¹)ᵇ	CHO (g·L⁻¹)ᶜ
Blood serum	140	4.5	2.5	1.5–2.1	110	300	—
Sweat	60–80	4.5	1.5	3.3	40–90	170–220	—
Coca Cola	3.0	—	—	—	1.0	650	107
Gatorade	23.0	3.0	—	—	14.0	280	62
Fruit juice, typical	0.5	58.0	—	—	—	690	118
Pepsi Cola	1.7	Trace	—	—	Trace	568	81
Water	Trace	Trace	—	—	Trace	10–20	—

ᵃMilliequivalents per liter.
ᵇMilliosmoles per liter.
ᶜGrams per liter.

fluid compartments, promoting a constant, well-regulated exchange of nutrients and waste products between the cell and its external fluid environment. Potassium is the chief intracellular mineral. Even moderately low potassium levels (*Adequate Intake* for adults is 4.7 g daily, which represents roughly half of the average American intake) can negatively contribute to salt sensitivity, arterial stiffness, myocardial thickening, and high blood pressure. Bananas, apricots, sweet potatoes, fish, citrus fruits and nuts are good potassium food sources.

TABLE 2.8 lists normal values for serum and sweat electrolyte concentrations and the electrolyte and carbohydrate concentrations of common beverages.

Optimal Sodium Intake

The hormone **aldosterone** conserves sodium in the kidneys under conditions of low-to-moderate dietary sodium intake. In contrast, high dietary sodium blunts aldosterone release, with excess sodium voided in the urine. This maintains sodium balance throughout a wide range of intakes. Some individuals cannot adequately regulate excessive sodium intake. For these **"salt-sensitive"** individuals, abnormal sodium accumulation in bodily fluids increases fluid volume and elevates blood pressure to levels that pose a health risk.

Sodium intake in the United States regularly exceeds the recommended daily level for adults of 2300 mg, or the amount of one generous teaspoon of table salt (NaCl; sodium makes up about 40% of salt). The typical Western diet contains nearly 4000 mg of sodium (8 to 12 g of salt) each day, with three-quarters from processed food and restaurant meals. This represents 8 times the 500-mg minimum daily sodium requirement. Common sodium-rich dietary sources include monosodium glutamate (MSG), soy sauce, condiments, canned foods, baking soda, and baking powder. Estimates indicate that cutting salt intake by 3 g a day could reduce the national yearly number of heart disease cases by between 60,000 and 120,000 and strokes by 32,000 and 66,000, values on a par with disease reductions observed for declining tobacco use, obesity, and cholesterol levels.

Sodium-Induced Hypertension

One first line of defense in treating high blood pressure eliminates excess sodium from the diet. Reducing sodium intake can lower blood pressure via reduced plasma volume depending on the person's responsiveness to NaCl intake.[85] For "salt-sensitive" individuals, reducing dietary sodium to the low end of the recommended range and upgrading the quality of the diet (reducing intake of canned and packaged goods; increasing intake of fresh fruits and vegetables) reduces blood pressure in both normal-weight and obese hypertensives (see "In a Practical Sense").[1,157,179] Lowering salt intake reduces the risk of cardiovascular disease and stroke. A 5-g reduction in daily salt intake (about half of the 10-g daily intake in the American diet) related to a 23% lower risk of strokes and 17% lower risk of cardiovascular disease.[162] If dietary constraints prove ineffective in lowering blood pressure, diuretic drugs that induce water loss often become the next line of defense. Unfortunately, diuretics also produce losses in other minerals, particularly potassium. A potassium-rich diet (e.g., one that includes potatoes, bananas, oranges, tomatoes, and meat) should supplement diuretic use.

MINERALS AND EXERCISE PERFORMANCE

Consuming mineral supplements above recommended levels on a long- or short-term basis does not benefit exercise performance or enhance training responsiveness.

Mineral Loss in Sweat

Excessive water and electrolyte loss impairs heat tolerance and physical performance. It also leads to severe dysfunction that culminates in heat cramps, heat exhaustion, or heat stroke. The yearly toll of heat-related deaths during spring and summer football practice provides a tragic illustration of the importance of fluid and electrolyte replacement. An athlete may lose up to 5 kg of water from sweating during practice or an athletic event. This corresponds to about 8.0 g of salt depletion

IN A PRACTICAL SENSE

Lowering High Blood Pressure with Dietary Intervention: The DASH Diet

Consumer groups and the American Medical Association urge reducing salt intake to combat high blood pressure, a malady prevalent in about 40% of the U.S. population. Adults now consume about 4000 mg of sodium daily, almost double the recommended 2300 mg or 1 ts of table salt. Much excess salt consumption comes from restaurant and processed foods, similar to nearly all foods in the typical American diet.

About 75 million Americans have hypertension, a condition that if left untreated increases the risk of stroke, heart attack, arterial wall stiffness, and kidney disease. Only 50% of hypertensives seek treatment and only half of these individuals achieve long-term success. One reason for the lack of compliance concerns possible side effects of readily available antihypertensive medication. For example, fatigue and impotence often discourage patients from maintaining the medication

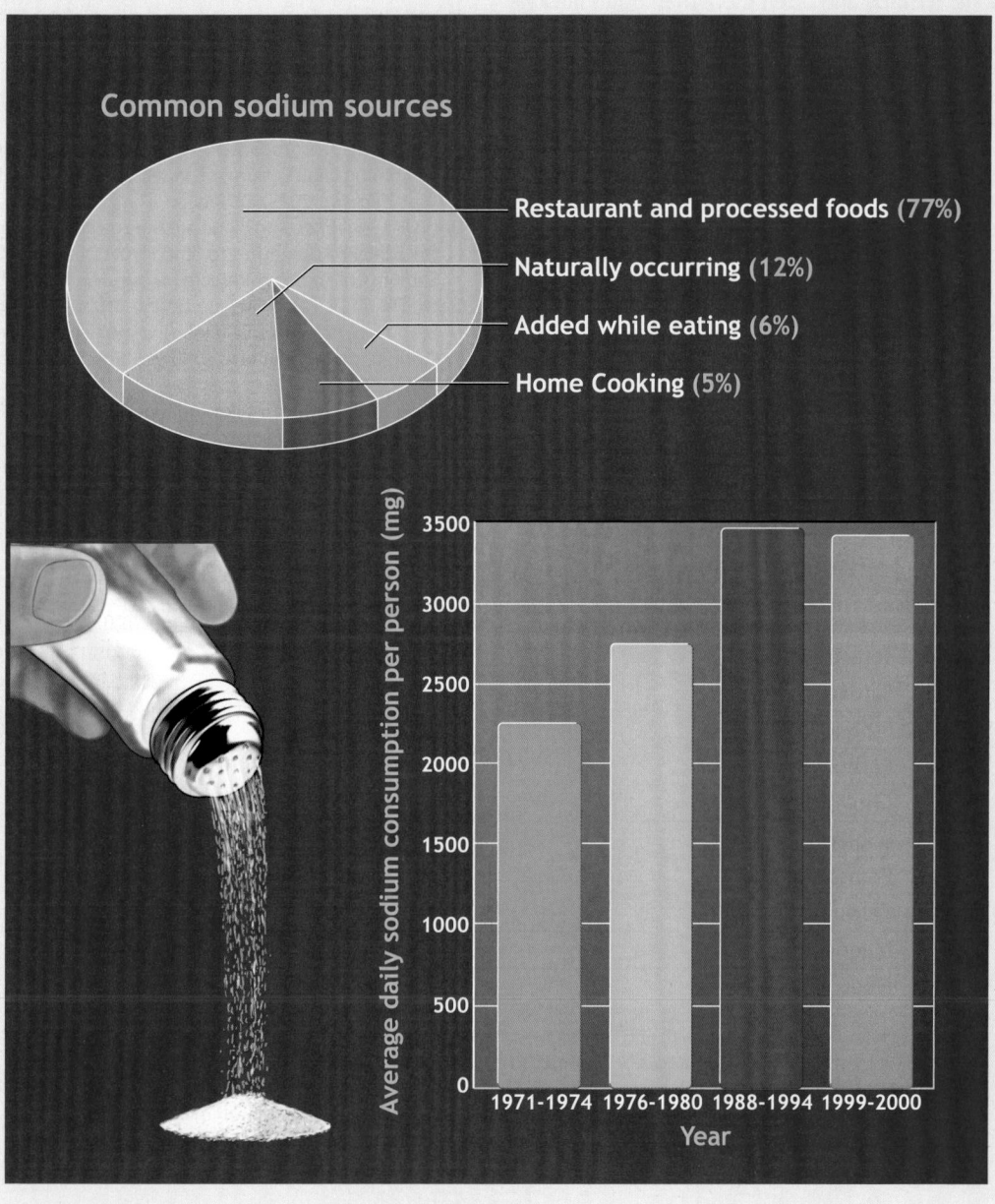

Common sodium sources

Restaurant and processed foods (77%)

Naturally occurring (12%)

Added while eating (6%)

Home Cooking (5%)

Average daily sodium consumption per person (mg)

1971–1974 1976–1980 1988–1994 1999–2000

Year

IN A PRACTICAL SENSE *(continued)*

schedule to treat hypertension. Particularly disturbing is children between ages 8 and 18 now consume on average about 3400 mg of sodium daily (range 1300 to 8100 mg), well above current guidelines. An association between sodium intake and high blood pressure existed among all children, with the response magnified among overweight and obese children.

THE DASH APPROACH

Research using **DASH (Dietary Approaches to Stop Hypertension;** www.nhlbi.nih.gov/health/public/heart/hbp/dash/new_dash.pdf) shows that this diet lowers blood pressure in some individuals to the same extent as pharmacologic therapy and often more than other lifestyle changes. Two months of the diet reduced systolic pressure by an average of 11.4 mm Hg; diastolic pressure decreased by 5.5 mm Hg. Every 2-mm Hg reduction in systolic pressure lowers heart disease risk by 5% and stroke risk by 8%. Further good news emerges from research that indicates that the standard DASH diet combined with a daily dietary salt intake of 1500 mg produced even greater blood pressure reductions than those achieved with the DASH diet only.

Table 1 shows the daily nutrient goals of the DASH diet. A 24-year follow-up of women whose diets most closely resembled the DASH plan showed they were 24% less likely to develop heart disease and 18% less likely to have a stroke. Further good news emerges from the latest research from the DASH group indicating that the standard DASH diet combined with a daily salt intake of 1150 mg—called

the DASH-Sodium diet—produced greater blood pressure reductions than achieved with the DASH diet only.

SAMPLE DASH DIET

Table 2 shows a sample DASH diet consisting of approximately 2100 kcal. This level of energy intake provides a stable body weight for a typical 70-kg person. More physically active and heavier individuals should boost portion size or the number of individual items to maintain weight. Individuals desiring to lose weight or who are lighter and/or sedentary should adjust intake in accordance with daily energy requirements.

Sources:
Bray GA, et al. A further subgroup analysis of the effect of the DASH diet and three sodium levels on blood pressure: results of the DASH-Sodium Trial. *Am J Cardiol* 2004;94:222.
Fung TT, et al. Adherence to a DASH-style diet and risk of coronary heart disease and stroke in women. *Arch Intern Med* 2008;168:713.
Miller PE, et al. Comparison of 4 established DASH diet indexes: examining associations of index scores and colorectal cancer. *Am J Clin Nutr* 2013;98:794.
Sacks FM, et al. Effects on blood pressure of reduced dietary sodium and the Dietary Approaches to Stop Hypertension (DASH) diet. DASH-Sodium Collaborative Research Group. *N Engl J Med* 2001;344:3.
Sacks FM, et al. Rationale and design of the Dietary Approaches to Stop Hypertension trial (DASH): a multicenter controlled feeding study of dietary patterns to lower blood pressure. *Ann Epidemiol* 1995;108:118.
Yang Q, et al. Sodium intake and blood pressure among US children and adolescents. *Pediatrics* 2012;130:611.

TABLE 1 — **Daily Nutrient Goals Used in the DASH Studies (for a 2100-Calorie Eating Plan)**

Total fat	27% of calories
Saturated fat	6% of calories
Protein	18% of calories
Carbohydrate	55% of calories
Cholesterol	150 mg
Sodium	2300 mg[a]
Potassium	4700 mg
Calcium	1250 mg
Magnesium	500 mg
Fiber	30 g

From US Department of Health and Human Services, National Institutes of Health, National Heart, Lung, and Blood Institute. *Your Guide to Lowering Your Blood Pressure with DASH.* 2006. Available at www.nhlbi.nih.gov/health/public/heart/hbp/dash/new_dash.pdf.

[a]1500 mg of sodium was a lower goal tested and found to be even better for lowering blood pressure. It was particularly effective for middle-aged and older individuals, African Americans, and those who already had high blood pressure.

IN A PRACTICAL SENSE *(continued)*

TABLE 2 — Sample DASH Diet (2100 kcal)

2300 mg sodium menu	Sodium (mg)	Substitution to reduce sodium to 1500 mg	Sodium (mg)
Breakfast			
¾ cup bran flakes cereal:	220	¾ cup shredded wheat cereal	1
1 medium banana	1		
1 cup low-fat milk	107		
1 slice whole wheat bread	149		
1 ts soft (tub) margarine	26	1 ts unsalted soft (tub) margarine	0
1 cup orange juice	5		
Lunch			
¾ cup chicken salad:	179	Remove salt from the recipe	120
2 slices whole wheat bread	299		
1 tbsp Dijon mustard	373	1 tbsp regular mustard	175
Salad and fruit:			
½ cup fresh cucumber slices	1		
½ cup tomato wedges	5		
1 tbsp sunflower seeds	0		
1 ts Italian dressing, low calorie	43		
½ cup fruit cocktail, juice pack	5		
Dinner			
3 oz beef, eye of the round:	35		
2 tbsp beef gravy, fat-free	165		
1 cup green beans, sauteed with:	12		
½ ts canola oil	0		
1 small baked potato:	14		
1 tbsp sour cream, fat-free	21		
1 tbsp grated natural cheddar cheese, reduced fat	67	1 tbsp natural cheddar cheese, reduced fat, low sodium	1
1 tbsp chopped scallions	1		
1 small whole wheat roll	148		
1 ts soft (tub) margarine	26	1 ts unsalted soft (tub) margarine	0
1 small apple	1		
1 cup low-fat milk	107		
Snacks			
⅓ cup almonds, unsalted	0		
¼ cup raisins	4		
½ cup fruit yogurt, fat-free, no sugar added	86		
Totals	2101		1507

From US Department of Health and Human Services, National Institutes of Health, National Heart, Lung, and Blood Institute. *Your Guide to Lowering Your Blood Pressure with DASH.* Available at: **http://www.nhlbi.nih.gov/health/public/heart/hbp/dash/new_dash.pdf.**

because each kg (1 L) of sweat contains about 1.5 g of salt. Despite this potential for mineral loss, replacement of water lost through sweating becomes a crucial and immediate need.

Defense Against Mineral Loss

Sweat loss during vigorous physical activity triggers a rapid, coordinated release of the hormones vasopressin and aldosterone and the enzyme renin, which reduce sodium and water loss through the kidneys. An increase in sodium conservation occurs even under extreme conditions (e.g., running a marathon in warm, humid weather when sweat output can equal 2 L per hour). Adding salt to the fluid or food ingested usually replenishes electrolytes lost in sweat, while facilitating rehydration. Salt supplements may be beneficial in prolonged activity in the heat when fluid loss exceeds 4 or 5 kg. This can be achieved by drinking a 0.1 to 0.2% salt solution (adding 0.3 ts of table salt per liter of water).[3] Although a mild potassium deficiency can occur with intense exercise training during heat stress, maintaining an adequate diet usually ensures optimum potassium levels. An 8-oz glass of orange or tomato juice replaces almost all of the calcium, potassium, and magnesium lost in 3 L (3 kg) of sweat.

Trace Minerals and Physical Activity

Strenuous physical activity may increase excretion of the following four trace elements:

1. *Chromium:* required for carbohydrate and lipid catabolism and proper insulin function and protein synthesis
2. *Copper:* required for red blood cell formation; influences gene expression and serves as a cofactor or prosthetic group for several enzymes
3. *Manganese:* component of superoxide dismutase in the body's antioxidant defense system
4. *Zinc:* component of lactate dehydrogenase, carbonic anhydrase, superoxide dismutase, and enzymes related to energy metabolism, cell growth and differentiation, and tissue repair

Urinary losses of zinc and chromium were 1.5- to 2.0-fold higher after a 6-mile run compared to a rest day.[8] Sweat loss of copper and zinc also can attain relatively high levels. Documentation of trace mineral losses with exercise does not necessarily mean athletes should supplement with these micronutrients. For example, short-term zinc supplementation (25 mg·d^{-1}) did not benefit metabolic and endocrine responses or endurance performance during intense exercise by eumenorrheic women.[148] Collegiate football players who supplemented with 200 mg of chromium (as chromium picolinate) daily for 9 wk experienced no beneficial changes in body composition and muscular strength during intense weightlifting compared with a control group that received a placebo.[25] Power and endurance athletes had higher plasma levels of copper and zinc than nontraining controls.[134]

Men and women who train intensely with large sweat production and with marginal nutrition (e.g., wrestlers, endurance runners, ballet dancers, and female gymnasts) should monitor trace mineral intake to prevent an overt deficiency. An excessive intake of one mineral may cause a deficiency in the other because iron, zinc, and copper interact with each other and compete for the same carrier during intestinal absorption. For well-nourished athletes, trace mineral supplementation does not enhance exercise performance or overall health.

Summary

1. Approximately 4% of body mass consists of 22 minerals distributed in all body tissues and fluids.
2. Minerals occur freely in nature in the waters of rivers, lakes, and oceans and in the soil. The root system of plants absorbs minerals, which eventually incorporate into the tissues of animals that consume plants.
3. Minerals function primarily in metabolism as important constituents of enzymes. Minerals provide structure to bones and teeth and serve in synthesizing the biologic macronutrients—glycogen, fat, and protein.

4. A balanced diet generally provides adequate mineral intake, except in some geographic locations that lack particular minerals in the soil (e.g., lack of iodine in the upper Midwest and Great Lakes regions).
5. Osteoporosis has reached epidemic proportions among older individuals, particularly women. Adequate calcium intake and regular weight-bearing physical activities and/or resistance training provide an effective way to stress the skeleton and defend against bone loss at any age.
6. Women who train intensely often do not match energy intake to energy output. This reduces body weight and body fat to a point that adversely affects menstruation, which contributes to bone loss at an early age. Restoration of normal menstruation does not fully restore bone mass.
7. About 40% of American women of childbearing age suffer from dietary iron insufficiency. This could lead to iron-deficiency anemia, which negatively impacts aerobic exercise performance and ability to train intensely.
8. For women on vegetarian-type diets, the relatively low bioavailability of nonheme iron increases their risk for developing iron insufficiency. Vitamin C in foods or supplements increases intestinal absorption of nonheme iron.
9. Regular physical activity probably does not drain the body's iron reserves. If it does, females, who have the greatest iron requirement and lowest iron intake, increase their risk for anemia.
10. Periodic assessment of the body's iron status should evaluate hematologic characteristics and iron reserves.
11. Excessive sweating during physical activity produces a considerable loss of body water and certain minerals, which should be replaced during and following physical activity. Sweat loss during exercise usually does not increase the mineral requirement above recommended values.

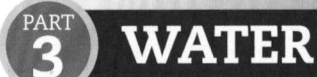

PART 3 **WATER**

THE BODY'S WATER CONTENT

Water makes up from 40 to 70% of body mass, depending on age, gender, and body composition (i.e., differences in lean vs. fat tissue). Water constitutes 65 to 75% of the weight of muscle and about 10% of the weight of fat. Body fat has a relatively low water content, so individuals with more total fat have a smaller overall percentage of their body weight as water.

FIGURE 2.15 depicts the fluid compartments of the body, normal daily body water variation, and specific terminology to describe the various states of human hydration. The body contains two fluid "compartments." One compartment, **intracellular**, refers to fluid inside the cells, whereas **extracellular** includes fluids that flow within the microscopic spaces between cells (**interstitial fluid**) as well as lymph, saliva, fluid in the eyes, fluid secreted by glands and the digestive tract,

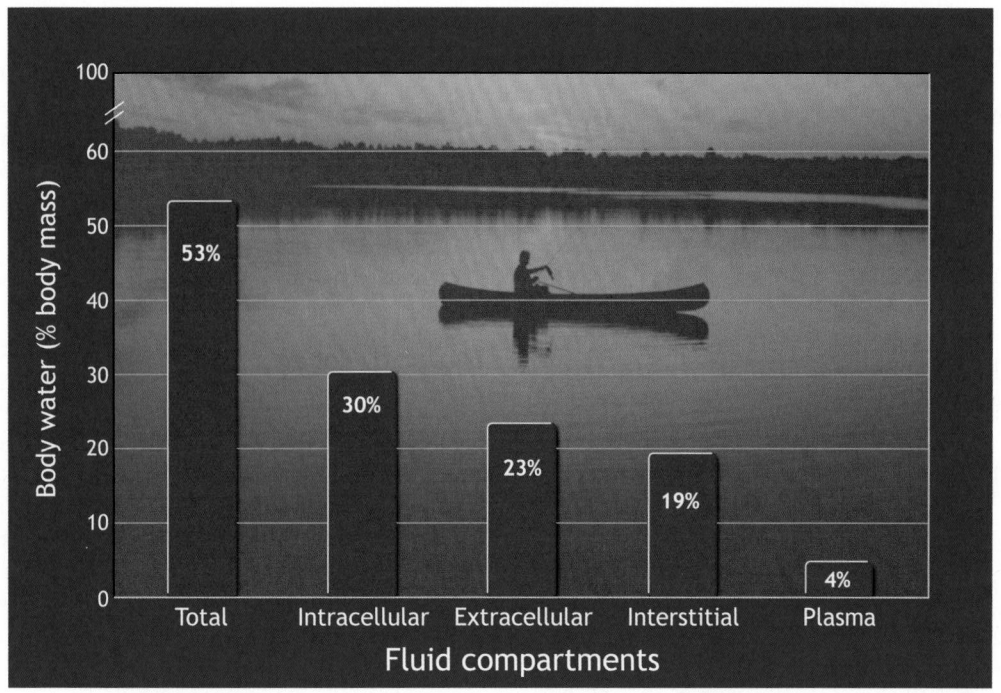

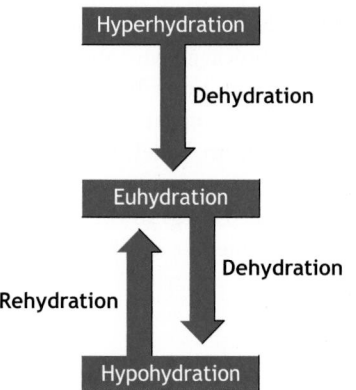

Daily euhydration variability of total body water
Temperature climate: ±0.165 L (±0.2% body mass)
Heat/exercise conditions: ±0.382 L (±0.5% body mass)

Daily plasma volume variability
All conditions: ±0.027 L (±0.6% blood volume)

Hydration terminology
Euhydration: normal daily water variation
Hyperhydration: new steady-state of increased water content
Hypohydration: new steady-state of decreased water content
Dehydration: process of losing water either from the hyperhydrated state to euhydration, or from euhydration downward to hypohydration
Rehydration: process of gaining water from a hypohydrated state toward euhydration

FIGURE 2.15 • Fluid compartments, average volumes and variability, and hydration terminology. Volumes represent an 80-kg man. Approximately 55% of the body mass consists of water in striated muscle, skeleton, and adipose tissue. For a man and woman of similar body mass, the woman contains less total water because of her larger ratio of adipose tissue (low water content) to lean body mass (striated muscle and skeleton). (Adapted with permission from Greenleaf JE. Problem: thirst, drinking behavior, and involuntary dehydration. *Med Sci Sports Exerc* 1992;24:645.)

fluid that bathes the spinal cord nerves, and fluid excreted from the skin and kidneys. Blood plasma accounts for nearly 20% of the extracellular fluid (3 to 4 L). *Extracellular fluid provides most of the fluid lost through sweating, predominantly from blood plasma.* Of the total body water, an average of 62% (26 L of the body's 42 L of water for an average 80-kg man) represents intracellular water, with 38% from extracellular sources. These volumes reflect averages from a dynamic exchange of fluid between compartments, particularly in physically active men and women. Moderate-to-intense physical training often increases the percentage of water distributed within the intracellular compartment because muscle mass typically increases, with its accompanying large water content. In contrast, an acute bout of exercise temporarily shifts fluid from plasma to interstitial and intracellular spaces from the increased hydrostatic (fluid) pressure within the circulatory system.

Functions of Body Water

Water is a ubiquitous, remarkable nutrient. Without water, death occurs within days. Water serves as the body's transport and reactive medium; diffusion of gases always takes place across water-moistened surfaces. Nutrients and gases travel in aqueous solution; waste products leave the body through the water in urine and feces. Water, in conjunction with proteins, lubricates joints and cushions a variety of "moving" organs such as the heart, lungs, intestines, and eyes. Water is noncompressible so it gives structure and form to the body through the turgor it provides for body tissues. Water has tremendous heat-stabilizing qualities because it absorbs considerable heat with only small changes in temperature. This latter quality, combined with water's high vaporization point, maintains a relatively stable body temperature during environmental heat stress and the increased internal heat load generated by physical activity.

WATER BALANCE: INTAKE VERSUS OUTPUT

The body's water content remains relatively stable over days, weeks, months, and even years. **Figure 2.16** displays the sources of water intake and output.

 See the animation "Water Balance" on **http:// thePoint.lww.com/mkk8e** for a demonstration of this process.

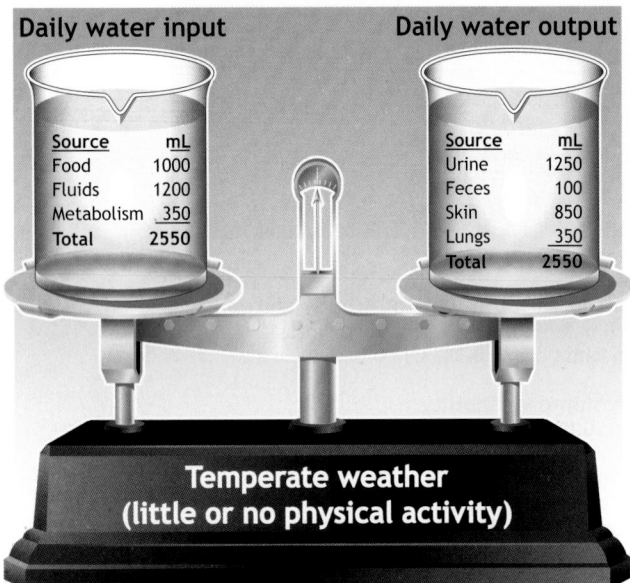

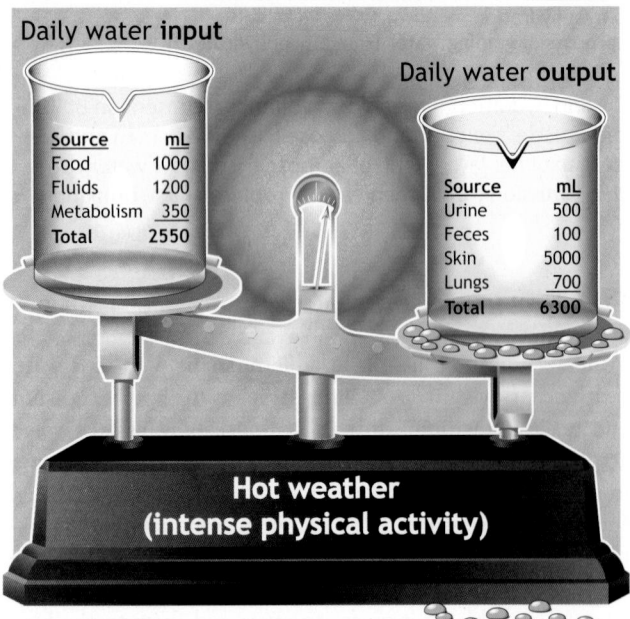

FIGURE 2.16 • Water balance in the body. **Top.** Little or no exercise with thermoneutral ambient temperature and humidity. **Bottom.** Moderate-to-intense exercise in a hot, humid environment.

Water Intake

A sedentary adult in a thermoneutral environment requires about 2.5 L of water daily. For an active person in a warm, humid environment, the water requirement often increases to between 5 and 10 L daily. Three sources provide this water:

1. Foods
2. Liquids
3. Metabolism

Water in Foods

Water from foods typically accounts for 20% of the recommended total fluid intake. Fruits and vegetables contain considerable water; in contrast, butter, oils, dried meats, and chocolate, cookies, and cakes have relatively low water content. The following foods exceed 90% of their weight as water—lettuce, raw strawberries, cucumbers, watercress, Swiss chard, boiled squash, green peppers, bean sprouts, boiled collards, watermelon and cantaloupe, canned pumpkin, celery, and raw peaches.

Water from Liquids

The average individual normally consumes 1200 mL, or 41 oz, of water daily. Physical activity and thermal stress increase fluid needs by five or six times this amount. At the extreme, an individual lost 13.6 kg of water weight during a 2-d, 17-hr, 55-mile run across Death Valley, California.[131] With proper fluid ingestion, including salt supplements, body weight loss amounted to only 1.4 kg. In this example, fluid loss and replenishment represented nearly 4 gallons of liquid!

Metabolic Water

The breakdown of macronutrient molecules in energy metabolism forms carbon dioxide and water. This metabolic water provides about 14% of the daily water requirement of a sedentary person. Glucose catabolism liberates 55 g of metabolic water. A larger amount of water also forms from protein (100 g) and fat (107 g) catabolism. Additionally, each gram of glycogen joins with 2.7 g of water as its glucose units link together; glycogen liberates this bound water during its breakdown for energy.

Water Output

Water loss from the body occurs in four ways:

1. In urine
2. Through skin
3. As water vapor in expired air
4. In feces

Water Loss in Urine

Under normal conditions, the kidneys reabsorb about 99% of the 140 to 160 L of renal filtrate formed each day. Consequently, the volume of urine excreted daily by the kidneys ranges from 1000 to 1500 mL, or about 1.5 quarts. Elimination of 1 g of solute by the kidneys requires about 15 mL of water. A portion of water in urine thus becomes "obligated" to rid the body of metabolic byproducts such as urea, an end product of protein breakdown. Large quantities of protein used for energy (as occurs with a high-protein diet where intake exceeds 2.0 g per kilogram body mass) may accelerate dehydration during exercise.

 See the animation "Renal Function" on http://thePoint.lww.com/mkk8e for a demonstration of this process.

Water Loss Through the Skin

On a daily basis, perhaps 350 mL of water continually seeps from the deeper tissues through the skin to the body's surface as insensible perspiration. Water loss also occurs through the skin in the form of sweat produced by specialized sweat glands beneath the skin. Evaporation of sweat provides the refrigeration mechanism to cool the body. The body produces 500 to 700 mL of sweat each day under normal thermal and physical activity conditions. This by no means reflects sweating capacity because a well-acclimatized person produces up to 12 L of sweat (at a rate of 1 L per hour) during prolonged, intense exercise in a hot environment.

Water Loss as Vapor

Insensible water loss through small water droplets in exhaled air amounts to between 250 and 350 mL a day from the complete moistening of inspired air as it traverses the pulmonary airways. Physical activity affects this source of water loss.[106] For physically active persons, the respiratory passages release 2 to 5 mL of water each minute during strenuous exercise, depending on climatic conditions. Ventilatory water loss is least in hot, humid weather and greatest in cold temperatures (inspired air contains little moisture) and at high altitudes. At high altitudes, inspired air volumes, requiring humidification, are considerably larger than at sea level.

Water Loss in Feces

Intestinal elimination produces between 100 and 200 mL of water loss as water constitutes approximately 70% of fecal matter. With diarrhea or vomiting, water loss increases up to 5000 mL, a potentially dangerous situation that can create fluid and electrolyte imbalance.

WATER REQUIREMENT IN PHYSICAL ACTIVITY

The loss of body water represents the most serious consequence of profuse sweating. Three factors determine the amount of water lost through sweating:

1. Physical activity intensity
2. Environmental temperature
3. Relative humidity

Sweating also occurs during physical activities in a water environment (e.g., vigorous swimming and water polo).

Relative humidity, the water content of the ambient air, affects efficiency of sweating in temperature regulation. Ambient air completely saturates with water vapor at 100% relative humidity. This blocks any evaporation of fluid from the skin's surface to the air, minimizing this important avenue for body cooling. Under high humidity, sweat beads on the skin and eventually rolls off without providing a cooling effect. On a dry day, air can hold considerable moisture, and fluid evaporates rapidly from the skin. Under these latter conditions, the sweat mechanism functions at optimal efficiency and body temperature remains regulated within a narrow range. Importantly, fluid loss from the vascular compartment when sweating strains circulatory function, which ultimately impairs exercise capacity and thermoregulation. *Monitoring changes in body weight (assessed following urination) conveniently assesses fluid loss during physical activity and/or heat stress. Each 0.45 kg (1 lb) of body weight loss corresponds to 450 mL (15 oz) of dehydration.*

Hyponatremia

The exercise physiology literature consistently confirms the need to consume fluid before, during, and after physical activity. In many instances, the recommended beverage remains plain, hypotonic water. Nevertheless, excessive water intake under certain exercise conditions can be counterproductive and produce the potentially serious medical complication of hyponatremia, or "water intoxication," first described in the medical literature among athletes in 1985 (FIG. 2.17).

A sustained low plasma sodium concentration creates an osmotic imbalance across the blood–brain barrier, allowing for rapid water influx into the brain. The resulting swelling of brain tissue produces a cascade of symptoms that range from mild (headache, confusion, malaise, nausea, and cramping) to severe (seizures, coma, pulmonary edema, cardiac arrest, and death).[10,51,139]

In general, mild hyponatremia exists when serum sodium concentration falls below 135 mEq · L⁻¹; serum sodium below 125 mEq · L⁻¹ triggers severe symptoms. The most conducive conditions for hyponatremia include water overload during ultramarathon-type, continuous activity lasting 6 to 8 hr, yet it can occur with activity of only 4 hr such as in standard marathons.[12,64,66,109]

 Five Predisposing Factors to Hyponatremia

1. Prolonged, high-intensity exercise in hot weather
2. Augmented sodium loss associated with sweat production containing high sodium concentration, often occurring in poorly conditioned individuals
3. Beginning physical activity in a sodium-depleted state because of "salt-free" or "low-sodium" diet
4. Use of diuretic medication for hypertension
5. Frequent intake of large quantities of sodium-free fluid during prolonged exercise

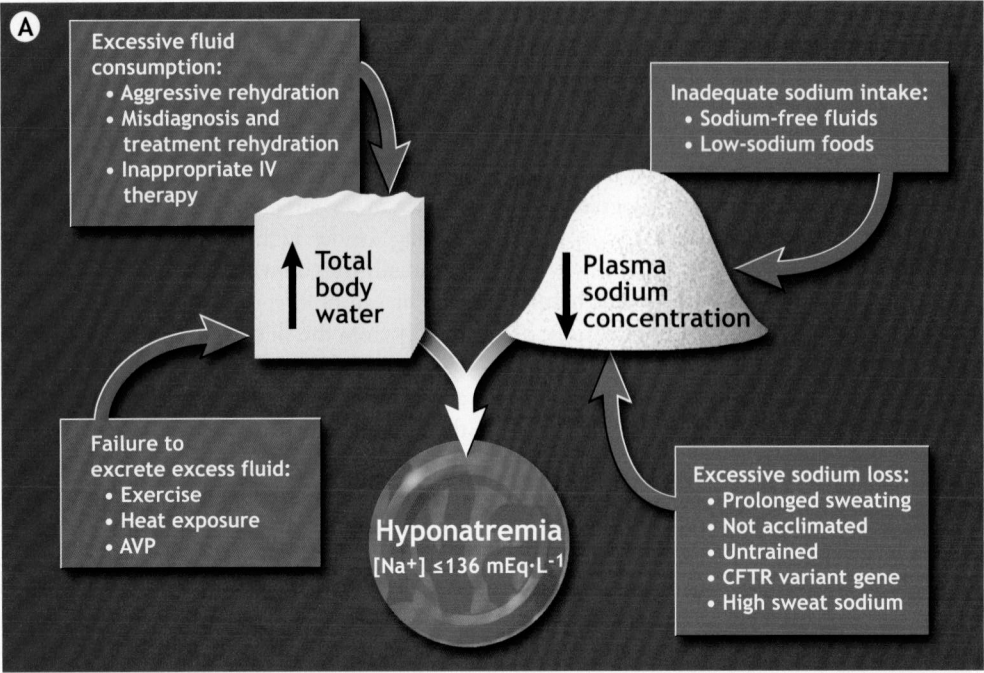

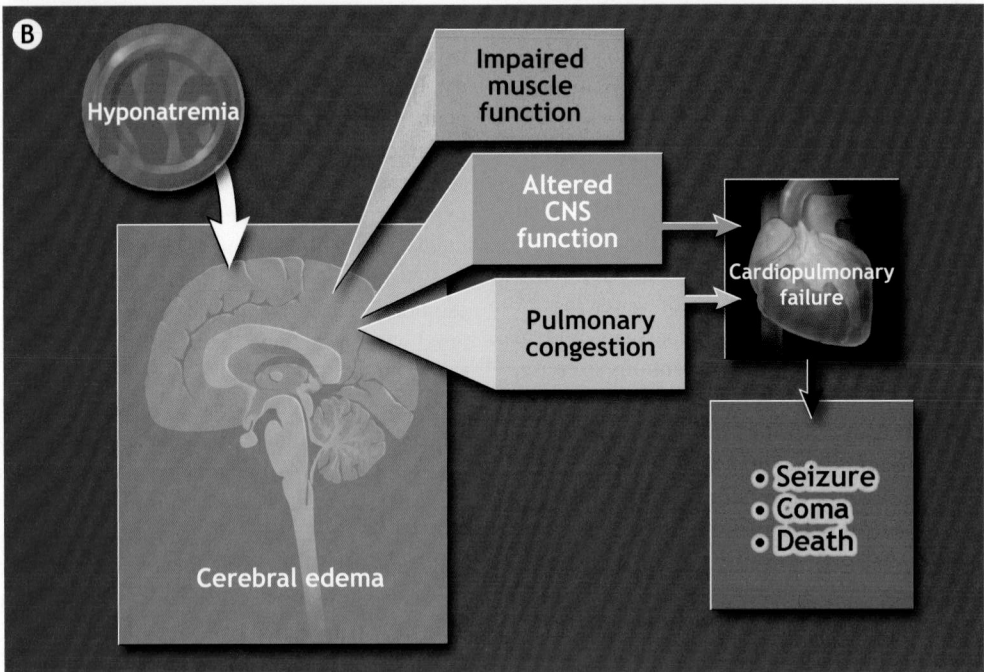

FIGURE 2.17 • **(A)** Factors that contribute to the development of hyponatremia. AVP, arginine vasopressin; CFTR, cystic fibrosis transmembrane regulatory gene. **(B)** Physiologic consequences of hyponatremia. CNS, central nervous system. (Adapted with permission from Montain SJ, et al. Hyponatremia associated with exercise: risk factors and pathogenesis. *Exerc Sport Sci Rev* 2001;29:113.)

Mild-to-severe hyponatremia has been reported with increasing frequency in ultraendurance athletes who compete in hot weather.[156] Nearly 30% of the athletes competing in the 1984 Ironman Triathlon had symptoms of hyponatremia, most frequently observed late in the race or in recovery. In a large study of more than 18,000 ultraendurance athletes including triathletes, approximately 9% of collapsed athletes during or following competition exhibited symptoms of hyponatremia.[119] The athletes, on average, drank fluids with low sodium chloride content (<6.8 mmol · L⁻¹). The runner with the most severe hyponatremia, with a serum Na level of 112 mEq · L⁻¹, excreted more than 7.5 L of dilute urine during the first 17 hr of hospitalization.

INTEGRATIVE QUESTION

In what way would knowledge about hyponatremia modify your recommendations concerning fluid intake prior to, during, and in recovery from long-duration physical activity?

Medical personnel monitored participants in the 1996 New Zealand Ironman Triathlon for changes in body mass and blood sodium concentration.[154] For athletes with clinical evidence of fluid or electrolyte disturbance, body mass declined 2.5 kg versus a decline of 2.9 kg in athletes not requiring medical care. Hyponatremia accounted for 9% of medical abnormalities. One athlete with hyponatremia (serum Na = 130 mEq·L^{-1}) drank 16 L of fluid during the race and gained 2.5 kg of body mass—consistent with the hypothesis that fluid overload causes hyponatremia. In an ultradistance multisport triathlon (kayak 67 km, cycle 148 km, run 23.8 km), the average competitors' body mass declined 2.5 kg, an amount equal to 3% of initial body mass.[155] None of the athletes gained weight, and six weighed the same pre- versus postrace; the one athlete who became hyponatremic (serum Na = 134 mEq·L^{-1}) maintained weight and did not seek medical attention. Serum sodium concentration at the end of the race for the 47 athletes averaged 139.3 mEq·L^{-1}.

Acclimatization level affects sodium loss. For example, sodium concentration in sweat ranges from 5 to 30 mmol·L^{-1} (115 to 690 mg·L^{-1}) in individuals fully acclimatized to the heat to 40 to 100 mmol·L^{-1} (920 to 2300 mg·L^{-1}) in the unacclimatized. In addition, some individuals produce highly concentrated sweat regardless of their degree of acclimatization. *Development of hyponatremia involves extreme sodium loss through prolonged sweating, coupled with dilution of existing extracellular sodium (reduced osmolality) from consuming fluids with low or no sodium* (Fig. 2.17A). A reduced extracellular solute concentration moves water into the cells (Fig. 2.17B). Water movement of sufficient magnitude congests the lungs, swells brain tissue, and adversely affects central nervous system function.

Several hours of physical activity in hot, humid weather often produces a sweating rate of more than 1 L per hour, with sweat sodium concentrations ranging from 20 to 100 mEq·L^{-1}. Frequently ingesting large volumes of plain water draws sodium from the extracellular fluid compartment into the unabsorbed intestinal water, further diluting serum sodium concentration. Physical activity magnifies the problem because urine production declines from reduced renal blood flow, which impedes ability to excrete excess water. Competitive athletes, recreational participants, and occupational workers should be aware of the dangers of excessive hydration and that fluid intake should not exceed fluid loss. The following six steps can reduce overhydration and hyponatremia risk in prolonged exercise:

1. Drink 400 to 600 mL (14 to 22 oz) of fluid 2 to 3 hr before exercise.
2. Drink 150 to 300 mL (5 to 10 oz) of fluid about 30 min before exercise.
3. Drink no more than 1000 mL·hr^{-1} (33 oz) of plain water spread over 15-min intervals during or after exercise.
4. Add a small amount of sodium (approximately ¼ to ½ ts of salt per 32 oz) to the ingested fluid.
5. Do not restrict salt in the diet.
6. Include some glucose in the rehydration drink (5 to 8% solution) to facilitate intestinal water uptake via the glucose–sodium transport mechanism.

Summary

1. Water makes up 40 to 70% of the total body mass. Muscle contains 70% water by weight; fat contains 10% water by weight.
2. Of the total body water, about 62% occurs intracellularly (inside the cells) and 38% extracellularly in plasma, lymph, and other fluids.
3. The typical average daily water intake of 2.5 L comes from liquid (1.2 L), food (1.0 L), and metabolic water produced during energy-yielding reactions (0.35 L).
4. Water loss from the body each day in an inactive person occurs from urine (1 to 1.5 L); skin, as insensible perspiration and sweat (0.85 L); water vapor in expired air (0.35 L); and feces (0.10 L).
5. Food and oxygen are always supplied in aqueous solution, and waste products exit via a watery medium.
6. Water also helps to provide structure and form to the body and plays a vital role in temperature regulation.
7. Physical activity and exercise training in hot weather increase the body's water requirement. Extreme conditions increase fluid needs five or six times above normal requirements.
8. Excessive sweating combined with consuming large volumes of plain water during prolonged physical activity set the "perfect storm" for hyponatremia or water intoxication. This dangerous condition relates to a significant decrease in serum sodium concentration.

the**Point** References are available online at **http://thepoint.lww.com/mkk8e.**

CHAPTER 3

Optimal Nutrition for Physical Activity

ANCILLARIES ◉ at-a-Glance

Visit http://thePoint.lww.com/mkk8e to access the following resources.

- References: Chapter 3
- Interactive Question Bank
- Animation: Digestion of Carbohydrate
- Animation: Fat Mobilization and Use
- Animation: Glycogen Synthesis
- Focus on Research: Potential Effect of Diet on Health Status

An optimal diet supplies required nutrients in adequate amounts for tissue maintenance, repair, and growth without excess energy intake. Less than optimal fluid, nutrient, and energy intakes profoundly affect these five factors:

1. Thermoregulatory function
2. Substrate availability
3. Capacity for physical activity
4. Recovery from physical activity
5. Training responsiveness

Dietary recommendations for physically active individuals must account for the energy requirements of a particular activity or sport and its training demands, including individual dietary preferences. No "one" food or diet exists for optimal health and exercise performance; careful planning and evaluation of food intake must follow sound nutritional guidelines. The physically active person must obtain sufficient energy and macronutrients to replenish liver and muscle glycogen, provide amino acid building blocks for tissue growth and repair, and maintain adequate lipid intake to provide essential fatty acids and fat-soluble vitamins.

In general, individuals who regularly engage in physical activity to keep fit do not require additional nutrients beyond those from a nutritionally well-balanced diet.[83]

NUTRIENT INTAKE AMONG THE PHYSICALLY ACTIVE

Inconsistencies exist among studies that relate diet quality to physical activity level or physical fitness. Part of the discrepancy relates to relatively crude and imprecise self-reported measures of physical activity, unreliable dietary assessments, and/or small sample size.[38,47,66,70] **TABLE 3.1** contrasts the nutrient and energy intakes with dietary recommendations of a large population-based cohort of about 7000 men and 2500 women classified as low, moderate, and high for cardiorespiratory fitness. The four most significant findings indicate the following:

1. Increasing physical fitness levels associated with a progressively lower body mass index
2. Remarkably small differences in energy intake related to physical fitness classification for women ($\leq$94 kcal daily)

TABLE 3.1 Average Values for Nutrient Intake Based on 3-Day Diet Records by Levels of Cardiorespiratory Fitness in 7059 Men and 2453 Women

Variable	Low Fitness ($n = 786$)	Moderate Fitness ($n = 2457$)	High Fitness ($n = 4716$)
Demographic and health data			
Age (y)	47.3 ± 11.1[a,b]	47.3 ± 10.3[c]	48.1 ± 10.5
Apparently healthy (%)	51.5[a,b]	69.1[c]	77.0
Current smokers (%)	23.4[a,b]	15.8[c]	7.8
BMI (kg · m^{-2})	30.7 ± 5.5[a,b]	27.4 ± 3.7[c]	25.1 ± 2.7
Nutrient data			
Energy (kcal)	2378.6 ± 718.6[a]	2296.9 ± 661.9[c]	2348.1 ± 664.3
kcal · kg^{-1} · d^{-1}	25.0 ± 8.1[a]	26.7 ± 8.4[c]	29.7 ± 9.2
Carbohydrate (% kcal)	43.2 ± 9.4[b]	44.6 ± 9.1[c]	48.1 ± 9.7
Protein (% kcal)	18.6 ± 3.8	18.5 ± 3.8	18.1 ± 3.8
Total fat (% kcal)	36.7 ± 7.2[b]	35.4 ± 7.1[c]	32.6 ± 7.5
SFA (% kcal)	11.8 ± 3.2[b]	11.3 ± 3.2[c]	10.0 ± 3.2
MUFA (% kcal)	14.5 ± 3.2[a,b]	13.8 ± 3.1[c]	12.6 ± 3.3
PUFA (% kcal)	7.4 ± 2.2[a,b]	7.5 ± 2.2	7.4 ± 2.3
Cholesterol (mg)	349.5 ± 173.2[b]	314.5 ± 147.5[c]	277.8 ± 138.5
Fiber (g)	21.0 ± 9.5[b]	22.0 ± 9.7[c]	26.2 ± 11.9
Calcium (mg)	849.1 ± 371.8[a,b]	860.2 ± 360.2[c]	924.4 ± 386.8
Sodium (mg)	4317.4 ± 1365.7	4143.0 ± 1202.3	4133.2 ± 1189.4
Folate (mcg)	336.4 ± 165.2[b]	359.5 ± 197.0[c]	428.0 ± 272.0
Vitamin B$_6$ (mg)	2.4 ± 0.9[b]	2.4 ± 0.9[c]	2.8 ± 1.1
Vitamin B$_{12}$ (mcg)	6.6 ± 5.5[a]	6.8 ± 6.0	6.6 ± 5.8
Vitamin A (RE)	1372.7 ± 1007.3[a,b]	1530.5 ± 1170.4[c]	1766.3 ± 1476.0
Vitamin C (mg)	117.3 ± 80.4[b]	129.2 ± 108.9[c]	166.0 ± 173.2
Vitamin E (AE)	11.5 ± 9.1[b]	12.1 ± 8.6[c]	13.7 ± 11.4

From Brodney S, et al. Nutrient intake of physically fit and unfit men and women. *Med Sci Sports Exerc* 2001;33:459.

BMI, body mass index; SFA, saturated fatty acid; PUFA, polyunsaturated fatty acid; MUFA, monounsaturated fatty acid; RE, retinol equivalents; AE, α-tocopherol units.

[a]Significant difference between low and moderate fit, $p < .05$.
[b]Significant difference between low and high fit, $p < .05$.
[c]Significant difference between moderate and high fit, $p < .05$.

and men (≤82 kcal daily); the moderate fitness group for both sexes consumed the fewest calories

3. A progressively higher dietary fiber intake and lower cholesterol intake occurred across fitness categories

4. Men and women with higher fitness levels consumed diets more closely linked to dietary recommendations for dietary fiber, percentage energy from total fat, percentage energy from saturated fat, and dietary cholesterol

 INTEGRATIVE QUESTION

In what ways might nutritional and energy intake goals for sports training differ from the requirements for actual competition?

Recommended Nutrient Intake

Figure 3.1 illustrates the recommended intakes for protein, lipid, and carbohydrate and the food sources for these macronutrients for a resting daily energy requirement of about 1200 kcal. A total daily energy requirement of about 2000 kcal for women and 3000 kcal for men represents the average values for typical young adults. *After meeting basic nutrient requirements as recommended in Figure 3.1, a variety of food*

sources with emphasis on unrefined complex carbohydrates should supply the extra energy demands for a variety of physical activities during a typical day.

Protein

As emphasized in Chapter 1, 0.83 g per kilogram of body mass represents the Recommended Dietary Allowance (RDA) for protein intake. A person weighing 77 kg (170 lb) requires about 64 g (2.2 oz) of protein daily. This protein recommendation remains adequate for most physically active individuals. The protein intake of the typical U.S. diet considerably exceeds the RDA for protein. For athletes who train intensely, a protein intake between 1.2 and 1.8 g per kilogram body mass should meet any added protein-related nutrient demands. This does not necessarily require protein supplementation because an athlete's diet typically exceeds the protein RDA by two to four times.

 INTEGRATIVE QUESTION

In what situations might a protein intake representing twice the RDA still prove inadequate for an individual involved in intense physical training?

Lipid

Precise standards for optimal lipid intake have not been established and vary with type of lipid consumed. The amount of dietary lipid differs widely depending on personal taste, economic status, geographic influences, and availability of lipid-rich foods. To promote good health, lipid intake should not exceed 30 to 35% of the diet's energy content. Of this, at least 70% should be unsaturated fatty acids. For a Mediterranean-type diet (refer to "The Essentials of Good Nutrition," later in this chapter), rich in mono- and polyunsaturated fatty acids, a somewhat higher total fat percentage of 35 to 40% remains reasonable.

The American Heart Association (www.heart.org) makes the following three recommendations concerning dietary lipid consumption:

1. Consume a diet with 25 to 35% of calories from fat, primarily unsaturated fatty acids of the polyunsaturated variety.
2. Limit saturated fat intake to less than 7% of total calories consumed.
3. Limit *trans* fat intake to less than 1% of total calories consumed.

As an example of these recommendations, a sedentary middle-aged woman with a 1600 kcal daily requirement should consume less than 12.4 g of saturated fat, less than 1.8 g of *trans* fat, and between 44 and 62 g of total fat daily. Most of the fat should come from heart-healthy mono- and

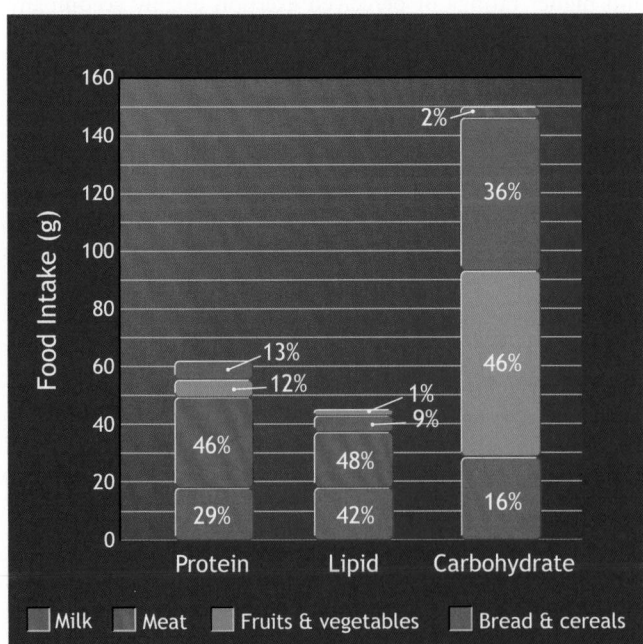

FIGURE 3.1 • General recommendations for carbohydrate, lipid, and protein components and the general categories of food sources in a balanced diet to meet resting daily energy requirement of about 1200 kcal. Values within bars represent percentage of that group's contribution to the specific macronutrient intake.

polyunsaturated fats (e.g., liquid vegetable oils, fatty fish, nuts, and seeds). Replacing "bad fats" with "good fats" in the diet requires keeping caloric intake in check and not substituting foods high in refined carbohydrates for foods high in fat.

High-Fat Versus Low-Fat Diets for Exercise Training and Performance

High-Fat Diets. Debate centers on the wisdom of maintaining a higher-than-average-fat diet during training or prior to endurance competition.[94,109,119] Adaptations to this type of diet have consistently shown a shift in substrate use toward higher fat oxidation during rest and exercise.[9,53,111] Proponents of high-fat diets argue that increasing daily dietary fat intake stimulates fat burning and augments capacity to mobilize and catabolize fat during intense aerobic physical activity. Any fat-burning enhancement could theoretically conserve glycogen reserves and/or contribute to improved endurance capacity under conditions of low glycogen reserves.

 See the animation "Fat Mobilization and Use" on http://thePoint.lww.com/mkk8e for a demonstration of this process.

To investigate possible benefits, endurance capacity was compared in two groups of 10 young men matched for aerobic capacity and fed either a high-carbohydrate diet (65% kcal from carbohydrate) or a high-fat diet (62% kcal from lipid) for 7 weeks. Each group trained for 60 to 70 min at 50 to 85% of aerobic capacity, 3 days a week during weeks 1 through 3 and 4 days a week during weeks 4 through 7. Following 7 weeks of training, the group consuming the high-fat diet switched to the high-carbohydrate diet. **FIGURE 3.2** displays the performance of both groups. The results for endurance were clear—the group consuming the high-carbohydrate diet performed considerably longer after training for 7 weeks than the group consuming the high-fat diet (102.4 min vs. 65.2 min). When the high-fat diet group switched to the high-carbohydrate diet during week 8 of the experiment, only a small improvement in endurance of 11.5 min occurred. Consequently, total overall improvement in endurance over the 8-week period reached 115% for the high-fat diet group, while endurance for the group receiving the high-carbohydrate diet improved by 194%! The upper portion of the graph shows the percentage contribution of macronutrients with the high-carbohydrate and high-fat diets. The authors concluded that the high-fat diet produced *suboptimal* adaptations in endurance performance, which did not become fully remedied by switching to a high-carbohydrate diet. Subsequent research from the same laboratory failed to demonstrate any endurance-enhancing effect of a high-fat diet containing only moderate carbohydrate (15% total calories) in rats, regardless of their current training status. For sedentary humans, maintaining a low- or high-dietary fat intake for 4 weeks produced no differences in maximal or submaximal aerobic performance.[80]

A high-fat diet may stimulate adaptive responses that augment fat use, but reliable research has yet to demonstrate consistent physical activity or training benefits from consistently consuming a high-fat diet. Compromised training capacity and symptoms of lethargy, increased fatigue, and higher ratings of perceived exertion usually accompany exercise when subsisting on a high-fat diet.[95,111] One must carefully consider recommending a high-fat diet from the

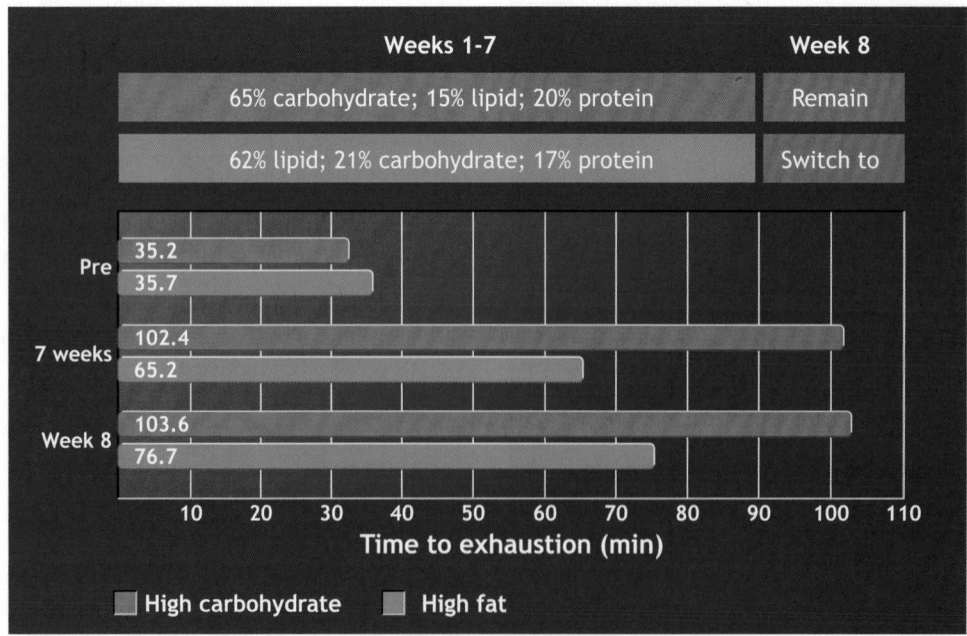

FIGURE 3.2 • Effects of a high-carbohydrate (CHO) versus a high-fat diet on endurance performance. The group consuming the high-fat diet for 7 weeks switched to the high-CHO diet during week 8. The endurance test consisted of pedaling a bicycle ergometer at the desired rate. (Adapted with permission from Helge JW, et al. Interaction of training and diet on metabolism and endurance during exercise in man. *J Physiol* 1996;492:293.)

standpoint of potential detrimental health risks. This concern may prove unwarranted for athletes with high daily levels of energy expenditure. Increasing the percentage of total lipid calories in the diet to 50% for physically active individuals who maintain a stable body weight and body composition does not compromise selected heart disease risk factors, including plasma lipoprotein profiles.[9,63] Considered in total, available research does *not* support the popular notion that reducing carbohydrate while increasing fat intake above a 30% level produces a more optimal metabolic "zone" for endurance performance.[87,99]

Low-Fat Diets. Restricting dietary fat below recommended levels also can impair exercise performance.[42,108] A diet of 20% lipid produced poorer endurance performance scores than a diet of identical caloric value containing about 40% lipid.[76] A low-fat diet also blunts the normal rise in plasma testosterone following an acute bout of resistance exercise, which may blunt the effects of such training.[112] Consuming low-fat diets during strenuous training also creates difficulty in increasing carbohydrate and protein intake enough to furnish "substitute" energy to maintain body weight and muscle mass.

Carbohydrate

No hazard to health exists when subsisting chiefly on a variety of fiber-rich whole food plant-based diet, with adequate intake of essential amino acids, fatty acids, minerals, and vitamins. The negative end of the nutrition continuum includes low-calorie "semistarvation" diets and other potentially harmful high-fat, low-carbohydrate diets, "liquid-protein" diets, single-food-centered diets, or time-centered diets that restrict food intake to certain times of the day (i.e., only consume foods within a continuous 8-hr period on any given day). Such extremes threaten good health, physical performance, and attainment of optimum body composition. *A low-carbohydrate diet rapidly compromises glycogen reserves for vigorous physical activity or regular training.* Excluding sufficient carbohydrate energy from the diet causes an individual to train in a state of relative glycogen depletion; this may eventually deplete muscle protein and produce "staleness" that hinders exercise performance.[12,48,68]

 See the animation "Digestion of Carbohydrate" on http://thePoint.lww.com/mkk8e for a demonstration of this process.

 ## Glycogen: An Important Fuel for Physical Activity

Muscle glycogen serves as the prime energy contributor during physical activity in the absence of an adequate oxygen supply to active muscles. In addition to this anaerobic energy role, muscle glycogen and blood glucose provide substantial energy during intense aerobic exercise.

 See the animation "Glycogen Synthesis" on http://thePoint.lww.com/mkk8e for a demonstration of this process.

Considering the body's limited glycogen reserves, the diet of physically active individuals should contain at least 55 to 60% of calories as carbohydrates, predominantly from fiber-rich, unprocessed grains, fruits, and vegetables. For many competitive athletes, the importance of maintaining a relatively high daily carbohydrate intake relates more to the considerable energy demands of training than to the short-term demands of competition.

Carbohydrate Needs in Intense Training. Athletes training for endurance running, ocean swimming, cross-country skiing, or cycling frequently experience a state of chronic fatigue when successive days of hard training become progressively more difficult. This condition of staleness often relates to the gradual depletion of the body's glycogen reserves, even if the diet contains the typical percentage of carbohydrate. **FIGURE 3.3** illustrates that three successive days of running 16.1 km or 10 miles nearly depletes glycogen in the thigh muscle. This occurred even though the runners' diet contained 40 to 60% carbohydrates. By the third day, the quantity of glycogen used during the run averaged considerably below that on the first day. Presumably, the body's fat reserves supplied the predominant energy for exercise on day 3. Unmistakably, a person who performs excessive strenuous exercise on a regular basis must adjust daily carbohydrate intake upward to permit optimal glycogen resynthesis to maintain high-quality training. The need for optimal replenishment of depleted glycogen reserves provides nutritional justification to gradually reduce or taper exercise intensity several days prior to competition.[101]

Carbohydrate intake recommendations for physically active individuals assume that daily energy intake balances daily energy expenditure. If it does not, even consuming a relatively large *percentage* of carbohydrate calories will not adequately replenish this important energy macronutrient. General recommendations for carbohydrate intake range between 6 and 10 g per kilogram of body mass daily. This amount varies with an individual's daily energy expenditure and type of physical activity performed. *Individuals who undergo intense endurance training should consume 10 g of carbohydrate per kilogram of body mass each day to induce protein-sparing and preserve glycogen reserves.* The daily carbohydrate intake for a small 46-kg (100-lb) athlete who expends about 2800 kcal per day should average 450 g or 1800 kcal. A 68-kg (150-lb) athlete should consume 675 g of carbohydrate (2700 kcal) daily to sustain an energy requirement averaging 4200 kcal. In both examples, carbohydrates exceed the minimum recommendation of 55 to 60% of total energy intake to represent 65%. This relatively high level of carbohydrate intake better maintains physical performance and mood state over the course of training.[1]

 ## INTEGRATIVE QUESTION

From a nutritional perspective, how can a reduced total volume of daily training (taper) improve training responsiveness and competitive performance?

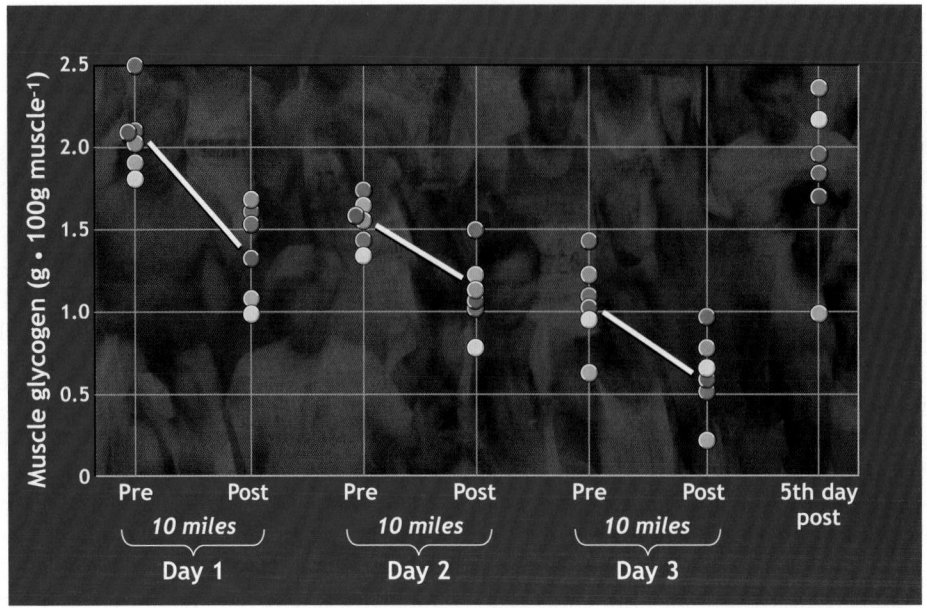

FIGURE 3.3 • Changes in muscle glycogen concentration (mean response) for six male subjects before and after each 10-mile (16.1-km) run performed on 3 successive days. Muscle glycogen measured 5 days after the last run is referred to as "5th day post." (Adapted with permission from Costill DL, et al. Muscle glycogen utilization during prolonged exercise on successive days. *J Appl Physiol* 1971;31:834.)

IN A PRACTICAL SENSE

Nutrition to Prevent Chronic Athletic Fatigue

Endurance runners, swimmers, cross-country skiers, and cyclists frequently experience chronic fatigue as successive days of hard training become progressively more difficult. Normal exercise performance deteriorates because the individual experiences increasing difficulty recovering from each workout session. The overtraining syndrome described in Chapter 21 relates to frequent infections, general malaise, and loss of interest in sustaining high-level training. Injuries occur more frequently in the overtrained, stale state.

DEPLETED CARBOHYDRATE PLAYS A ROLE

Gradually depleting carbohydrate reserves with repeated strenuous training most likely contributes to the overtraining syndrome. At least 1 to 2 days of rest or lighter physical activity combined with a high carbohydrate intake is required to reestablish pre-exercise muscle glycogen levels after exhaustive training or competition. Intense exercise performed regularly requires an upward adjustment of daily carbohydrate intake to optimize glycogen resynthesis and high-quality training. The guidelines below provide nutritional recommendations to reduce the likelihood of athletic fatigue or staleness.

Four Practical Nutritional Guidelines to Prevent Chronic Fatigue

1. Consume easily digested, high-carbohydrate drinks or solid foods 1 to 4 hr before training or competition. Consume about 1 g carbohydrate per kilogram of body mass 1 hr before exercise and up to 5 g carbohydrate per kilogram of body mass if the feeding occurs 4 hr prior to exercise. For example, a 70-kg swimmer would drink 350 mL (12 oz) of a 20% carbohydrate beverage 1 hr before exercise or eat 14 "energy bars," each containing 25 g carbohydrate, spread over the 4-hr period before exercise.

2. Consume a readily digested, high-carbohydrate liquid or solid food containing 0.35 to 1.5 g carbohydrate · kg body mass^{-1} · hr^{-1} immediately after exercise and for the first 4 hr after exercise. A 70-kg swimmer could drink 100 to 450 mL (3.6 to 16 oz) of a 25% carbohydrate beverage or one to four energy bars, each containing 25 g of carbohydrate immediately after exercise and every hour thereafter for 4 hr.

3. Consume a 15 to 25% carbohydrate drink or a solid, high-carbohydrate supplement with each meal. For example, reduce consumption of normal foods by 250 kcal and consume a high-carbohydrate beverage or solid food containing 250 kcal of carbohydrate with each meal.

4. Stabilize body weight during all phases of exercise training by matching energy consumption to training's energy demands. This also helps to maintain body glycogen reserves.

Source: Sherman WJ, Maglischo EW. Minimizing chronic athletic fatigue among swimmers: special emphasis on nutrition. *Sports Science Exchange* 1991;4(35).

THE ESSENTIALS OF GOOD NUTRITION

In the typical American diet, energy-dense but nutrient-poor foods frequently substitute for more nutrient-rich foods. Such a food intake pattern increases the risk for obesity, marginal micronutrient intakes, low high-density lipoprotein (HDL) and high low-density lipoprotein (LDL) cholesterol, and elevated homocysteine levels.

MYPLATE: THE HEALTHY EATING GUIDE

On June 2, 2011, the US Department of Agriculture unveiled **MyPlate**, a new icon with nutritional guidelines for healthy eating. MyPlate provides a stylized and colorful color-coded dinner plate to replace the 2005 MyPyramid. Supporters of the new icon claim it has greater practicality and intuitiveness than its MyPyramid predecessor; many nutritionists and healthcare professionals claimed MyPyramid was confusing and difficult to understand. The MyPlate strategy, emphasizing more plant-based eating habits from a variety of vegetables from all five subgroups, attempts to help Americans become healthier in their battle against the obesity crisis. The new guide, illustrated in FIGURE 3.4A, has different-sized plate portions to symbolize the recommended food groups and builds on the messages of the government's revised 2010 *Dietary Guidelines for Americans*.[55,60] Fruits and vegetables occupy one-half the plate, with vegetables predominating. Grains (particularly whole grains) and proteins

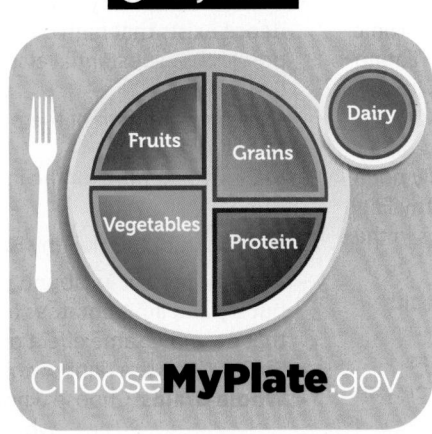

A My Plate

Fruits
- 2 cups a day.
- What counts as a cup?
  One cup or raw or cooked fruit or 100% fruit juice; a half-cup dried fruit.

Vegetables
- 2 ¹/₂ cups a day.
- What counts as a cup?
  One cup of raw or cooked vegetables or vegetable juice; two cups of leafy salad greens.

Dairy
- 3 cups a day.
- What counts as a cup?
  One cup of milk, yogurt, or fortified soy milk; 1-¹/₂ ounces natural or two ounces processed cheese.

Grains
- 6 ounces a day.
- What counts as an ounce?
  Once slide of bread; a half-cup of cooked rice, cereal, or poasta; one ounce of ready-to-eat cereal.

Protein foods
- 5 ¹/₂ ounces a day.
- What counts as an ounce?
  One ounce of lean meat, poultry, or fish; one egg; a tablespoon of peanut butter; a half-ounce of nuts or seeds; a quarter-cup of beans or peas.

ChooseMyPlate.gov

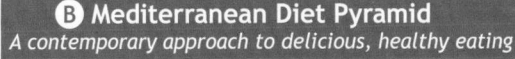

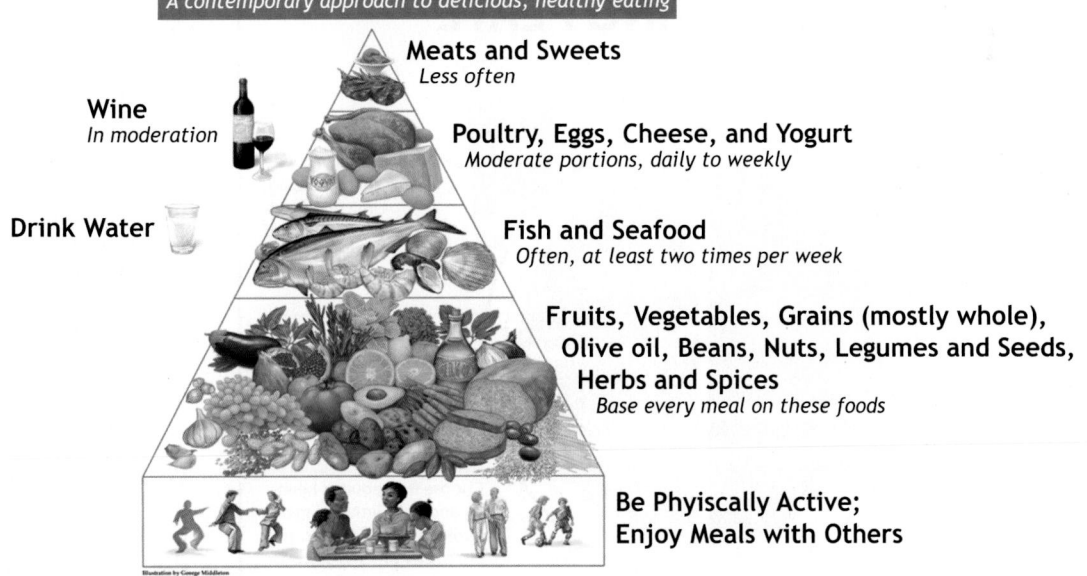

B Mediterranean Diet Pyramid
A contemporary approach to delicious, healthy eating

Meats and Sweets
Less often

Wine
In moderation

Poultry, Eggs, Cheese, and Yogurt
Moderate portions, daily to weekly

Drink Water

Fish and Seafood
Often, at least two times per week

Fruits, Vegetables, Grains (mostly whole), Olive oil, Beans, Nuts, Legumes and Seeds, Herbs and Spices
Base every meal on these foods

Be Phyiscally Active; Enjoy Meals with Others

© 2009 Oldways Preservation and Exchange Trust • www.oldwayspt.org

FIGURE 3.4 • **(A)** MyPlate: The new healthy eating guide. **(B)** Mediterrainian Diet Pyramid application to individuals whose diet consists largely of foods from the plant kingdom, or fruits, nuts, vegetables, and all manner of grains, and protein derived from fish, beans, and chicken, with dietary fat composed mostly of monounsaturated fatty acids and with mild alcohol consumption. (A, Courtesy USDA Center for Nutrition Policy and Promotion; B, reprinted with permission from Oldways Preservation & Exchange Trust, **www.oldwayspt.org**).

make up the other half, with grains taking up a majority of that half. MyPlate eliminates MyPyramid's references to sugars, fats, or oils. The protein category includes meat, poultry, seafood, eggs, and vegetarian options such as beans and peas, nuts and seeds, and tofu. A smaller blue circle adjoining the plate icon indicates dairy products (a glass of skim or reduced-fat milk, cheese, or yogurt). Daily caloric intake, portion size, fat intake, and energy expenditure are not represented. Similar to the new *Guidelines*, MyPlate stresses balanced portions among the different food categories. The Web site **www.ChooseMyPlate.gov** provides detailed advice about the *Guidelines*.

 ## Healthy Eating Plate: A Viable Alternative to MyPlate

Shortly following the U.S. government's release of MyPlate, nutrition experts at Harvard School of Public Health (HSPH) in conjunction with colleagues at Harvard Health Publications unveiled the *Healthy Eating Plate*, a visual guide as a blueprint for eating a healthy meal. The Healthy Eating Plate is based on the latest and best scientific evidence that shows that a plant-based diet rich in vegetables, whole grains, healthy fats, and healthy proteins lowers the risk of weight gain and chronic diseases. And like its MyPlate counterpart, the Healthy Eating Plate is simple and easy to understand—and addresses important deficiencies in the MyPlate's details.

Critics argue that MyPlate mixes science with the influence of powerful agricultural interests, which is generally not a recipe good for consumer health. Comparing the Healthy Eating Plate to the USDA's MyPlate shows the shortcomings in the government's guide. Criticisms of MyPlate include:

- Gives no indication that whole grains are better for health than refined grains
- The protein section offers no indication that some high-protein foods—fish, poultry, beans, nuts—are healthier than red meats and processed meats that often link to various chronic diseases
- It is silent on beneficial fats as part of a healthy diet
- Makes no differentiation between potatoes and other high glycemic vegetables that act like sugar in the body and their lower glycemic counterparts
- Recommends dairy at every meal, even though little evidence exists that high dairy intake protects against osteoporosis but substantial evidence exists that high intake can be harmful
- Makes no mention of the potential negative effect of sugary drinks
- Makes no mention of the importance of regular physical activity

The sections of the Healthy Eating Plate include:

- **Vegetables**: Eat an abundant variety, the more the better, but try and limit potatoes and other high glycemic starches that have the same effect on blood sugar as sweets.
- **Fruits**: Choose a rainbow of fruits every day.
- **Whole Grains**: Choose whole grains, such as oatmeal, whole wheat bread, and brown rice instead of refined grains, such as white bread and white rice that act like sugar in the body.
- **Healthy Proteins**: Choose fish, poultry, beans, or nuts; limit consumption of red meat and avoid processed meats since these have been shown to increase risk of heart disease, type 2 diabetes, colon cancer, and weight gain.
- **Healthy Oils**: Use olive, canola, and other plant oils in cooking, on salads, and at the table, since these healthy fats reduce harmful cholesterol and are good for the heart. Limit butter and avoid *trans* fat.
- **Water**: Drink water, tea, or coffee (with little or no sugar). Limit milk and dairy (1–2 servings per day) and juice (1 small glass a day) and avoid sugary drinks.
- **Stay Active**: Increased physical activity should be part of everyone's healthy eating program

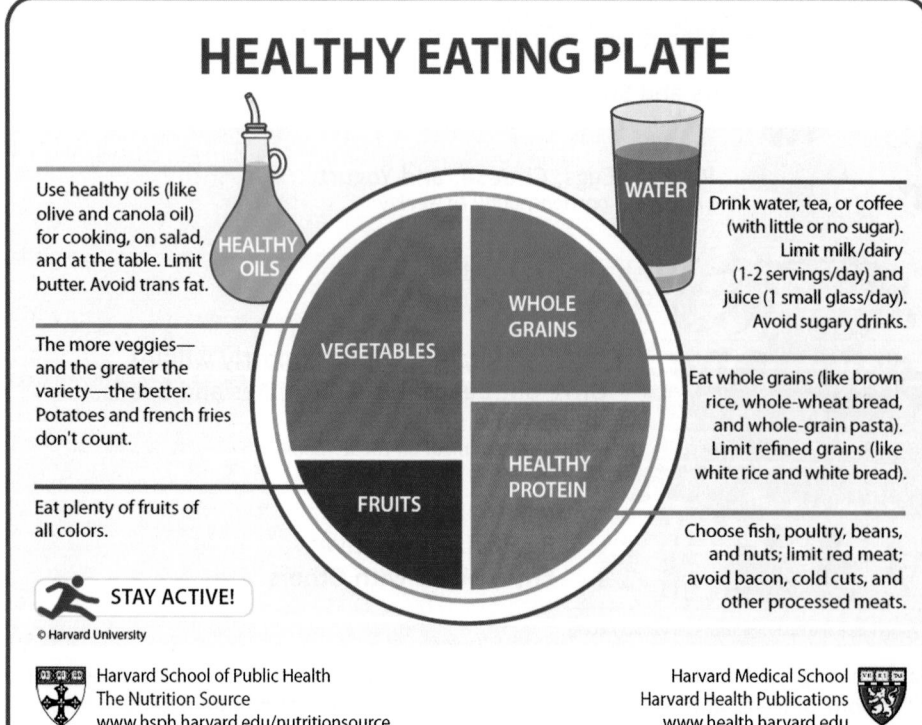

Goals and Guidelines for Healthful Eating

Population Goals	Major Guidelines
Overall healthy eating pattern	• Consume a varied diet that includes food from each of the major food groups, with an emphasis on fruits, vegetables, whole grains, low-fat or nonfat dairy products, fish, legumes, poultry, and lean meats. • Monitor portion size and number to ensure adequate, not excess, intake.
Approximate body weight 　BMI ≤25[a]	• Match energy intact to energy needs. • When weight loss is desirable, make appropriate changes to energy intake and expenditure (physical activity). • Limit foods with a high sugar content and those with a high caloric density.
Desirable cholesterol profile	• Limit food high in saturated fat, trans fat, and cholesterol. • Substitute unsaturated fat from vegetables, fish, legumes, and nuts.
Desirable blood pressure 　Systolic <140 mm Hg 　Diastolic <90 mm Hg	• Maintain a healthy body weight. • Consume a varied diet with an emphasis on vegetables, fruits, and low-fat or nonfat dairy products. • Limit sodium intake. • Limit alcohol intake.

Adapted from Krauss RM, et al. AHA dietary guidelines revision 2000: a statement for healthcare professionals from the Nutrition Committee of the American Heart Association. *Circulation* 2000;102:2284.
[a]BMI, body mass index (k·m^{-2}).

The latest 2010 *Dietary Guidelines for Americans* formulated for the general population also provide a sound framework for meal planning for physically active individuals. *The principle message advises consuming a varied but balanced diet.* To maintain a healthful body weight, attention must focus on portion size, number of calories, and increase in daily physical activity. A major point is to consume a reduced-sodium diet rich in fruits and vegetables, cereals and whole grains, nonfat and low-fat dairy products, legumes, nuts, fish, poultry, and lean meats with a concomitant reduction in calories from solid fats, added sugars, and refined grains.[4,16,21] According to the *Guidelines*, Americans consume far too many calories with too much solid fat, added sugars, refined grains, and sodium. They also consume too little potassium, dietary fiber, calcium, vitamin D, unsaturated fatty acids from oils, nuts, and seafood, and other important nutrients found mostly in vegetables, fruits, whole grains, and low-fat milk and milk products.

FIGURE 3.4B presents a dietary pyramid that applies to individuals whose diet consists largely of fruits, nuts, vegetables, fish, beans, and all manner of grains, with dietary fat composed mostly of monounsaturated fatty acids with mild ethanol consumption.

A Mediterranean-style diet protects individuals at high risk of death from heart disease, stroke, and metabolic syndrome, presumably from its association with increased total antioxidant capacity and low LDL-cholesterol levels.[26,31,78] Its high content of monounsaturated fatty acids (generally olive oil with its associated phytochemicals[93]) helps delay age-related memory loss, cancer, and overall mortality rate in healthy, elderly people.[29,62,90,103] The dietary focus of MyPlate and the two pyramids also reduces risk for ischemic stroke[54,55] and enhances the benefits of cholesterol-lowering drugs; it also associates with

less damage to small blood vessels in the brain.[30,57] The biggest impact of diet on cancer probably lies in its effect on minimizing overweight and obesity, risk factors for several forms of cancer.

 INTEGRATIVE QUESTION

How would you advise a high school soccer team with individuals from diverse ethnic backgrounds with unique food intake patterns about sound nutrition?

PHYSICAL ACTIVITY AND FOOD INTAKE

Balancing energy intake with energy expenditure represents a primary goal for the physically active individual of normal body weight. Energy balance optimizes physical performance and helps to maintain lean body mass, training responsiveness, and immune and reproductive function. The level of physical activity represents the most important factor that impacts daily energy expenditure.

FIGURE 3.5 illustrates that average energy intakes for males and females in the United States peak between ages 16 and 29 years and then decline for succeeding age groups. A similar pattern occurs for both males and females, with males reporting higher daily energy intakes than females at all ages. Between ages 20 and 29 years, women consume on average 35% fewer kcal than men on a daily basis (3025 kcal vs. 1957 kcal). Thereafter, the gender difference in energy intake becomes smaller; at age 70 years, women consume about 25% fewer kcal than men.

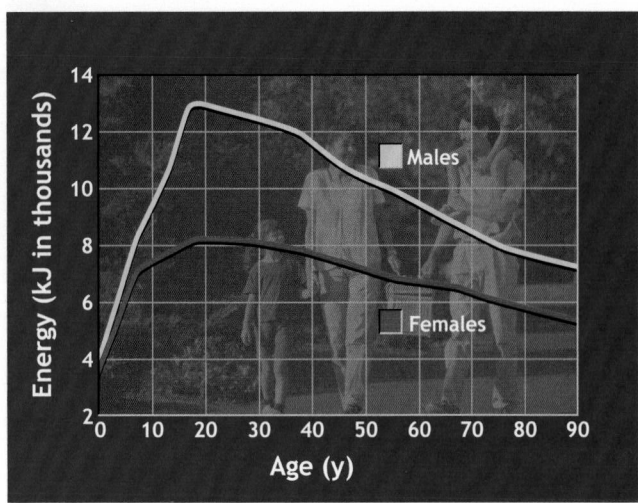

FIGURE 3.5 • Average daily energy intake for males and females by age in the U.S. population during the years 1988 to 1990. Multiply by 0.239 to convert kJ to kcal. (Adapted with permission from Briefel RR, et al. Total energy intake of the U.S. population: the third National Health and Nutrition Examination Survey, 1988–1991. *Am J Clin Nutr* 1995;62(suppl):1072S.)

Physical Activity Makes a Difference

Individuals who engage regularly in moderate-to-intense physical activity eventually increase daily energy intake to match higher energy expenditure levels. Lumber workers, who expend approximately 4500 kcal daily, unconsciously adjust energy intake to closely balance energy output. Consequently, body mass remains stable despite a relatively large food intake. The daily food intake of athletes in the 1936 Olympics supposedly averaged more than 7000 kcal, or roughly three times the average daily intake. These oft-quoted energy values justify what many believe to be an enormous food requirement of athletes in training. However, these figures probably depict inflated estimates because objective dietary data to support these claims do not exist. Distance runners who train upward of 100 miles weekly (6-min mile pace at 15 kcal per min) probably do not expend more than 800 to 1300 "extra" kcal each day above their normal energy requirements to balance the increased energy expenditure. FIGURE 3.6 presents energy intake data from a large sample of elite male and female endurance, strength, and team sport athletes in the Netherlands. Daily energy intake for males ranged between 2900 and 5900 kcal; female competitors consumed between 1600 and 3200 kcal. Daily energy intake generally did not exceed 4000 kcal for men and 3000 kcal for women (except for the large energy intakes of athletes at extremes of performance and training). For male and female recruits of the U.S. Marine Corps, daily energy expenditures averaged 6142 kcal for men and 4732 kcal for women during a 54-hr training exercise.[17]

To complement these observations, daily energy expenditure of elite female swimmers increased to 5593 kcal during high-volume training.[102] This value represents the highest

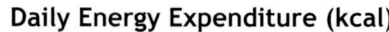

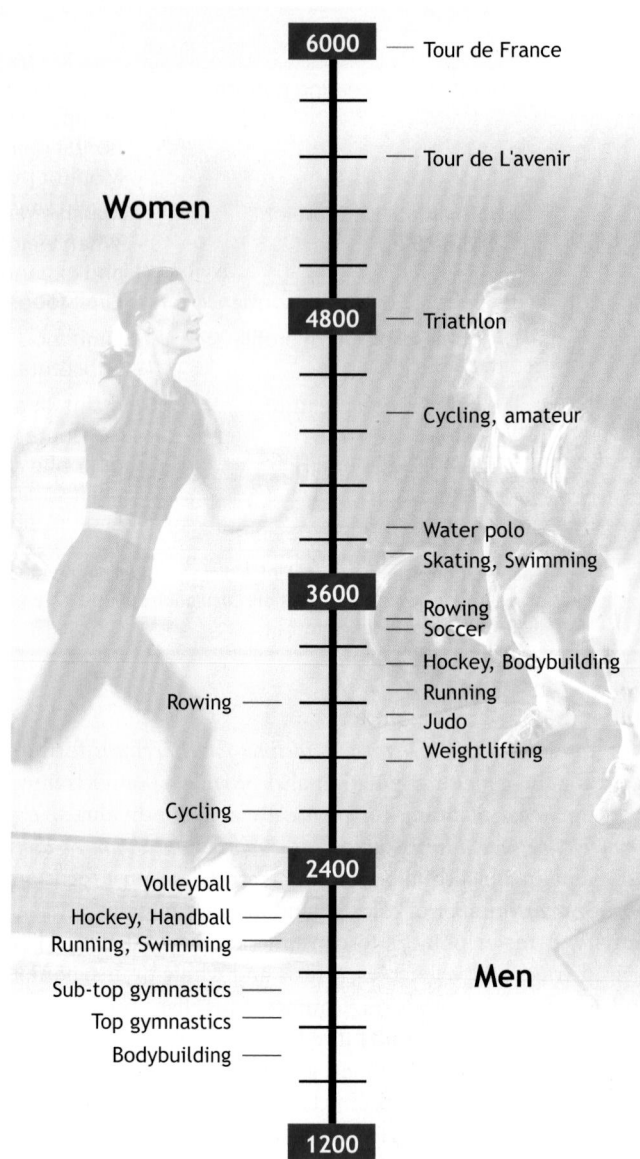

FIGURE 3.6 • Daily energy intake (kcal) of elite male and female endurance, strength, and team sport athletes. (Adapted with permission from van Erp-Baart AMJ, et al. Nationwide survey on nutritional habits in elite athletes. *Int J Sports Med* 1989;10:53.)

level of sustained daily energy expenditure reported for female athletes, yet energy intake did not increase to match training demands. It averaged only 3136 kcal, implying a negative energy balance of 43%. A negative energy balance in the transition from moderate to intense training can ultimately compromise an athlete's full potential to train and compete.

Tour de France and Other Endurance Activities

FIGURE 3.7 outlines the variation in daily energy expenditure for a male competitor during the Tour de France professional cycling race. In this grueling sporting event, energy expenditure averaged 6500 kcal daily for nearly 3 weeks. Large variation occurred depending on activity level for a particular day; the daily energy expenditure decreased to about 3000 kcal on a "rest" day and increased to 9000 kcal when cycling over a mountain pass. By combining liquid nutrition with normal meals, this cyclist nearly matched daily energy expenditure with energy intake. Unfortunately, the recent doping scandal involving the U.S. cycling team (the U.S. Anti-Doping Agency and International Cycling Union rescinded seven-time winner Lance Armstrong's consecutive first place finishes for blatant, serial use of illegal performance-enhancing drugs [http://cyclinginvestigation.usada.org], use that he later publicly admitted to [www.abc.com]) suggests that studies of such high levels of caloric expenditure could be "contaminated" by the undue influence of drugs.

Other sport and training activities also require extreme energy output and correspondingly high energy intake, sometimes in excess of 1000 kcal an hour in elite marathoners. Daily energy requirements of world-class cross-country skiers during 1 week of intense training averaged 3740 to 4860 kcal for women and 6120 to 8570 kcal for men.[89] The values for women agree with the average 3957 kcal daily energy expenditure over a 14-day training period reported for seven elite lightweight female rowers.[45] In another study,

the doubly labeled water technique (see Chapter 8) evaluated the energy balance for two men who pulled sledges with starting weights of 222 kg (10 hr · d^{-1} for 95 days) for 2300 km across Antarctica.[97] During a 10-day period, one man averaged a daily energy expenditure of 10,654 kcal, while his counterpart averaged an extraordinary output of 11,634 kcal. These values approach the 13,975-kcal theoretical daily energy expenditure ceiling attained by ultra long-distance runners.[18]

Ultra-Endurance Running Competition

Ultra-endurance events are increasingly popular, with significant physiologic challenges that potentially produce relatively large energy deficits during competitions. Deficits have been reported among ultraendurance cyclists in a 16-hr, 384-km cycle race.[7] For these athletes, mean energy intake averaged 18.7 MJ (4469 kcal) compared with an estimated energy requirement for the race of 25.5 MJ (6095 kcal). Of functional significance was the negative relationship between energy intake and time to complete the race, which suggests that reducing the energy deficit may be advantageous to race performance. Energy balance also was studied during a 1000-km (approximately 600-mile) race from Sidney to Melbourne, Australia. Greek ultramarathon champion Yiannis Kouros

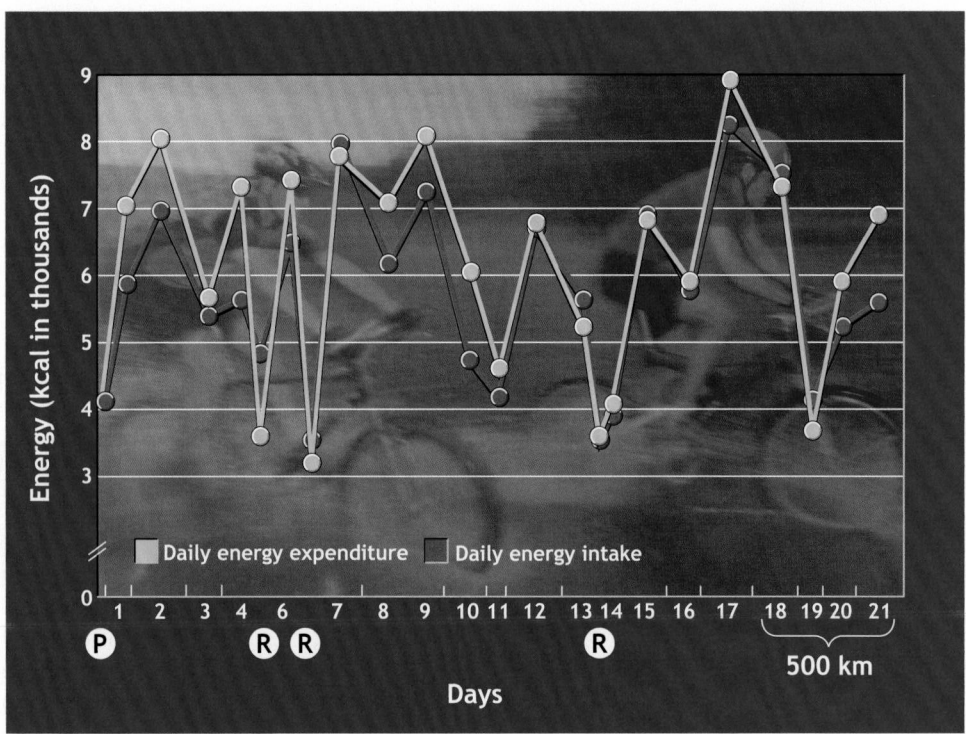

FIGURE 3.7 • Daily energy expenditure (*yellow circles*) and energy intake (*red circles*) for a cyclist during the Tour de France competition. For 3 weeks in July, nearly 200 cyclists ride over and around the perimeter of France, covering 2405 miles, more than 100 miles daily (only 1 day of rest), at an average speed of 24.4 mph. Note the extremely high energy expenditure values and ability to achieve energy balance with liquid nutrition plus normal meals. P, stage; R, rest day. (Adapted with permission from Saris WHM, et al. Adequacy of vitamin supply under maximal sustained workloads; the Tour de France. In: Walter P, et al., eds. *Elevated Dosages of Vitamins*. Toronto: Huber, 1989.)

TABLE 3.2 Race Conditions, Distance Covered, Average Daily Speed, Rest and Sleep Patterns, and Nutrient Balance During an Elite Ultraendurance Performance Race[a]

Course topography	SYDNEY		CANBERRA				MELBOURNE
Distance (km)	0 100 200	300 400	500 600	700 800 900	960		

Road conditions	← Continuous uphill →	← Level ground →	← Continuous hills →	← Plateau uphill course →	← Flat terrain →

Weather	Temperature 26°C Humidity 60% Spring weather	30°C + Summer weather	Gradual temp. drop (8–10°C) Drizzle + opposing winds Autumn weather	Rain	Winter conditions

Accumulated distance covered		270 km	463 km	615 km	780 km 915 km
days (d)	← d1 →	← d2 →	← d3 →	← d4 →	← d5 →

Average daily speed km · h^{-1} (m · s^{-1})	11.74 (3.26)	8.3 (2.31)	8.07 (2.24)	8.9 (2.47)	6.21 (1.72)

Rest (min)	60	30 15 75 10 10	60 10 10 10	10 15 10
		30 15 10 10		15 90 10 90

Sleep (min)		30	20 60	30 20 120

Adapted from Ronioyannis GP, et al. Energy balance in ultramarathon running. *Am J Clin Nutr* 1989;49:976.
[a]The runner Kouros weighed 65 kg, stature 171 cm, percentage body fat 8%, and $\dot{V}O_{2max}$ 62.5 mL · kg^{-1} · min^{-1}.

completed the race in 5 d, 5 hr, and 7 min, finishing 24 hr and 40 min ahead of the next competitor. TABLE 3.2 provides relevant features of race conditions, distance covered, average daily speed, and rest and sleep patterns. Kouros did not sleep during the first 2 days of competition. He covered 463 km (287.8 miles) at an average speed of 11.4 km · hr^{-1} (8.5 min · mile^{-1}) during day 1 and 8.3 km · hr^{-1} (11.6 min · mile^{-1}) on day 2. During the remaining days, he took frequent rest periods including periodic breaks for short "naps." Weather ranged from spring to winter conditions (86 to 46.4° F [30 to 8°C]) and terrain varied. TABLE 3.3 lists the pertinent details of food and water intake.

The near equivalence between Kouros's estimated total energy intake (55,970 kcal) and energy expenditure (59,079 kcal) represents a remarkable aspect of energy balance homeostasis to extremes of physical activity. Of the total energy intake, carbohydrates represented 95.3%, lipids 3%, with the remaining 1.7% from proteins. Protein intake from food averaged considerably below recommended levels, but Kouros did take protein supplements in tablet form. The

TABLE 3.3 Daily and Total Energy Balance, Nutrient Distributions in Food, and Water Intake During an Elite Ultraendurance Performance Race[a]

Race Day	Distance Covered (km)	Estimated Energy Expenditure (kcal)	Estimated Energy Intake (kcal)	Carbohydrates (g)	Carbohydrates (%)	Lipids (kcal)	Lipids (g)	Lipids (%)	Proteins (kcal)	Proteins (g)	Proteins (%)	(kcal)	H$_2$O (l)
1	270	15,367	13,770	3375	98.0	13,502	20	1.3	180	22	0.7	88	22.0
2	193	10,741	8600	1981	92.2	7923	53	5.6	477	50	2.3	200	19.2
3	152	8919	12,700	3074	96.8	12,297	27	1.9	243	40	1.3	160	22.7
4	165	9780	7800	1758	90.1	7032	56	6.5	504	66	3.4	264	14.3
5	135	7736	12,500	3014	96.4	12,058	30	2.2	270	43	1.4	172	18.3
5 hr	45	2536	550	138	100.0	550	—	—	—	—	—	—	3.2
Total	960	55,079	55,970	13,340		53,362	186		1674	221		734	99.7

Adapted from Rontoyannis GP, et al. Energy balance in ultramarathon running. *Am J Clin Nutr* 1989;49:976.
[a]The runner Kouros weighed 65 kg, stature 171 cm, percentage body fat 8%, and $\dot{V}O_{2max}$ 62.5 mL · kg^{-1} · min^{-1}.

unusually large daily energy intake, which ranged from 8600 to 13,770 kcal, came from Greek sweets (baklava, cookies, and doughnuts), some chocolate, dried fruit and nuts, various fruit juices, and fresh fruits. Every 30 min after the first 6 hr of running, Kouros replaced sweets and fruit with a small biscuit soaked in honey or jam. He consumed a small amount of roasted chicken on day 4 and drank coffee every morning. He took a 500-mg vitamin C supplement every 12 hr and a protein tablet twice daily.

Kouros's exceptional achievement exemplifies a highly conditioned athlete's exquisite regulatory control for energy balance during this demanding exercise. He performed at a pace that required an energy metabolism averaging 49% of aerobic capacity during the first 2 days of competition and 38% for days 3 through 5. He also finished the competition without muscular injuries or thermoregulatory problems, and his body mass remained unchanged; reported difficulties included a severe bout of constipation during the run and frequent urination that persisted for several days postrace.

Another case study of a 37-year-old male ultramarathoner further demonstrates the tremendous capacity for prolonged, high daily energy expenditure. The doubly labeled water technique evaluated energy expenditure during a 2-week period of a 14,500-km run around Australia in 6.5 months (average 70 to 90 km·d⁻¹; 43 to 56 miles·d⁻¹) with no days for rest.[44] Daily energy expenditure over the measurement period averaged 6321 kcal; daily water turnover equaled 6.1 L. The athlete ran about the same distance each day over the study period as in the entire race period. As such, these data likely represent energy dynamics for the entire run.

Extreme Ultra-Endurance Sports

The Iditasport ultramarathon consists of a choice of one race event from among the following options: run 120 km, snowshoe 120 km, bicycle 259 km, cross-country ski 250 km, or snowshoe, ski, and bicycle 250 km. Begun in 1983 as a single-event (Iditaski), a parallel competition emerged in 1987 consisting of long-distance cycling (Iditabike). In 1991, the two races merged along with foot, snowshoe, and triathlon events. The triathlon was discontinued in 1997, and the lengths of all other races changed to 160 km. The competition begins in late February, and the athletes traverse varied terrain, mostly in the wilderness over frozen rivers and lakes; wooded, rolling hills; and packed snow trails. On any given day, racers can experience extremes in weather conditions that range from calm, "balmy" 30°F (−1.1°C) to "harsh" −40°F (−40°C) with blizzard conditions. During the 48-hr time limit for the event, racers carry a minimum of 15 pounds of survival gear; this includes a sleeping bag rated to −20°F (−28.8°C), insulated sleeping pad, bivy sack or tent, stove and 8 ounces of fuel with fire starter (matches or lighter), pot to melt snow, insulated water containers to carry 2 quarts of water, headlamp or flashlight, and a minimum of 1 day's supply of emergency food. The supplies, weighing from 15 to 30 pounds, are carried in a backpack or pulled by sled.

Researchers estimated the total energy and macronutrient requirements for 13 males and 1 female in the 1995 race with 49 entrants (**Fig. 3.8**). The bikers consumed the most total calories (8458 kcal), 74.1% as carbohydrate, 9.4% as protein, and 16.5% as fat. A comparison study between 1997–1998 Iditasport athletes and their 1995 counterparts showed only small differences in energy and nutrient contents except for higher intakes of carbohydrate (78.5%) and less fat (14.5%) and protein (7.3%) for skiers. The authors concluded that even though the length of the events differed in 1994–1996 and 1997–1998, few differences existed in the energy content and macronutrient percentages of the diets among the four categories of competitors from the two time periods.

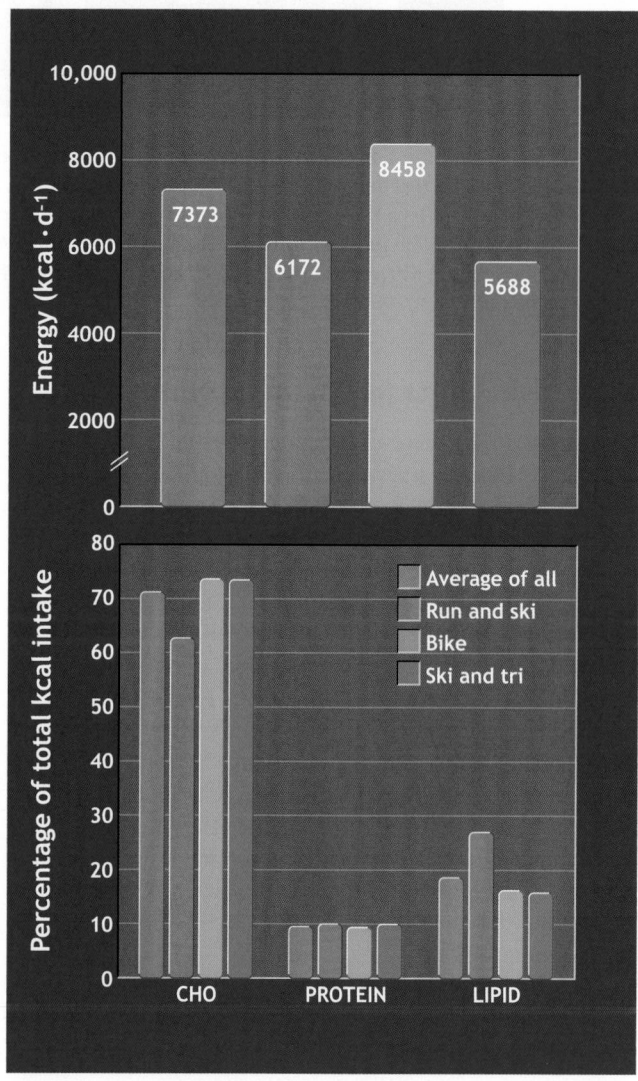

FIGURE 3.8 • Energy and macronutrient content of the diets of Iditasport competitors. Multiply kcal value by 4.182 to convert to kJ. (Data for 1995 from Case D, et al. Dietary intakes of participants in the Iditasport ultra-marathon. *Alaska Med* 1995;37:20. Data reported in the text for 1997–1998 from Stuempfle K, et al. Dietary factors of participants in the 1994–1998 Iditasport ultramarathon. *Med Sci Sports Exerc* 1999;31:S80.)

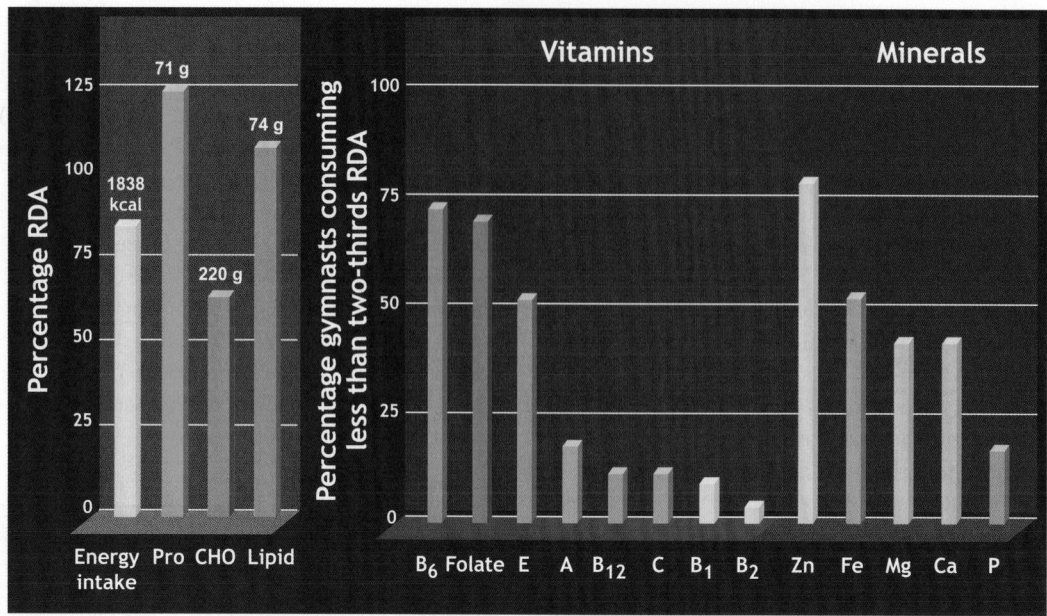

FIGURE 3.9 • Average daily nutrient intake for 97 adolescent female gymnasts (11 to 14 y) related to recommended values. The RDA on the *y* axis (*left*) reflects only protein, while energy, CHO, and lipid reflect "recommended" values. Percentage of gymnasts consuming less than two thirds of the RDA for micronutrients (*right*). Mean age, 13.1 years; mean stature, 152.4 cm (60 in.); mean body mass, 43.1 kg (94.8 lb). (Reprinted with permission from McArdle WD, Katch FI, Katch VL. *Sports and Exercise Nutrition*. 4th Ed. Philadelphia: Wolters Kluwer Health, 2013, as adapted with permission from Loosli AR, Benson J. Nutritional intake in adolescent athletes. *Ped Clin N Am* 1990;37(5):1143–1152.)

High-Risk Sports for Marginal Nutrition

Gymnasts, ballet dancers, ice dancers, and weight-class athletes in boxing, wrestling, rowing, and judo engage in arduous training. Owing to the nature of their sport, these athletes continually strive to maintain a lean, light body mass dictated by either esthetic or weight-class considerations. Energy intake often intentionally falls short of energy expenditure, and a relative state of malnutrition develops. Nutritional supplementation for these athletes may prove beneficial as suggested by the data in FIGURE 3.9 for daily nutrient intake (% of RDA) of 97 competitive female gymnasts aged 11 to 14 years. Twenty-three percent of the girls consumed less than 1500 kcal daily, and more than 40% consumed less than two thirds of the RDA for vitamins E and folic acid and the minerals iron, magnesium, calcium, and zinc. Clearly, many of these adolescent gymnasts needed to upgrade the nutritional quality of their diets or consider supplementation.

Eat More and Weigh Less

Physically active individuals generally consume more calories per kilogram of body mass than sedentary counterparts. The extra energy for physical activity accounts for the larger caloric intake. Paradoxically, the most active men and women, who eat more on a daily basis, weigh less than those who exercise at a lower total caloric expenditure. Regular physical activity allows a person to "eat more yet weigh less" while maintaining a lower percentage of body fat despite the age-related tendency toward weight gain in middle age.[10] *Physically active persons maintain a lighter and leaner body and a healthier heart disease risk profile, despite increased intake of food.* Chapter 30 discusses the important role of regular physical activity for weight control in more detail.

PRECOMPETITION MEAL

Athletes often compete in the morning following an overnight fast. As pointed out in Chapter 1, considerable depletion occurs in the body's carbohydrate reserves over an 8- to 12-hr period without eating, even if the person previously follows appropriate dietary recommendations. Consequently, precompetition nutrition takes on considerable importance. *The precompetition meal should provide adequate carbohydrate energy and ensure optimal hydration.* Fasting before competition or training makes no sense physiologically because it rapidly depletes liver and muscle glycogen, which impairs exercise performance. If a person trains or competes in the afternoon, breakfast becomes the important meal to optimize glycogen reserves. For late-afternoon training or competition, lunch becomes the important source for topping off glycogen stores. Consider the following three factors when individualizing the precompetition meal plan:

1. Athlete's food preference
2. "Psychological set" of competition
3. Digestibility of foods

As a general rule, on competition day exclude foods high in lipid and protein because they digest slowly and remain in the digestive tract longer than foods containing similar energy content as carbohydrate. Precompetition meal timing also deserves consideration. The increased stress and tension that accompany competition reduce blood flow to the digestive tract to produce depressed intestinal absorption. *A carbohydrate-rich, precompetition meal requires 1 to 4 hr to digest, absorb, and replenish muscle and liver glycogen (high glycemic carbohydrates digest and absorb more rapidly).*

Making a Choice—Protein or Carbohydrate?

The following five reasons justify modifying or even abolishing the high-protein precompetition meal in favor of one high in carbohydrates:

1. Dietary carbohydrates replenish liver and muscle glycogen depletion from the overnight fast.
2. Carbohydrate digestion and absorption occur more rapidly than either protein or lipid; this allows carbohydrate to provide energy faster and reduce the feeling of fullness after a meal.
3. A high-protein meal elevates resting metabolism more than a high-carbohydrate meal because of protein's greater energy requirements for digestion, absorption, and assimilation. This additional thermic effect could strain the body's heat-dissipating mechanisms and impair exercise performance in hot weather.
4. Protein catabolism for energy facilitates dehydration during exercise because the byproducts of amino acid breakdown require water for urinary excretion. The excretion of one gram of urea coincides with the elimination of about 50 mL of water.
5. Carbohydrate, not protein, represents the main energy nutrient for short-term anaerobic activity and intense aerobic exercise.

The ideal precompetition meal maximizes muscle and liver glycogen storage and provides glucose for intestinal absorption during physical activity. The meal should accomplish the following three goals:

1. Contain 150 to 300 g of carbohydrate (3 to 5 g per kilogram of body mass in either solid or liquid form)
2. Be consumed 1 to 4 hr before exercising for complete digestion and absorption and to optimize glycogen stores
3. Contain relatively little fat and fiber to facilitate gastric emptying and minimize gastrointestinal distress

The benefits of proper precompetition feeding occur only if the athlete maintains a nutritionally sound diet throughout training. Pre-exercise feedings cannot correct existing nutritional deficiencies or inadequate nutrient intake during the weeks before competition. Chapter 23 discusses how endurance athletes can augment precompetition glycogen storage in conjunction with specific exercise/diet modifications using "carbohydrate-loading" techniques.

INTEGRATIVE QUESTION

Outline how to eat well to establish a physically active and healthy lifestyle.

Liquid and Prepackaged Bars, Powders, and Meals

Commercially prepared nutrition bars, powders, and liquid meals offer an alternative approach to precompetition feeding or supplemental feedings during periods of competition. Nutrient supplements also effectively enhance energy and nutrient intake in exercise training, particularly when energy output exceeds energy intake from lack of interest or mismanagement of feedings.

Liquid Meals

Liquid meals provide high-carbohydrate content but contain enough lipid and protein to contribute to satiety. A liquid meal digests rapidly, leaving essentially no residue in the intestinal tract. Liquid meals prove particularly effective during daylong swimming and track meets or during tennis, soccer, softball, and basketball tournaments. In these outings, the person usually has little time for or interest in eating. Liquid meals offer a practical approach to supplementing caloric intake during the high-energy output phase of training. Athletes also can use liquid nutrition strategies to help maintain body weight and as a ready source of calories to gain weight.

Nutrition Bars

Nutrition bars (also called "energy bars," "protein bars," and "diet bars") contain a relatively high protein content that ranges between 10 and 30 g per bar. The typical 60-g bar contains 25 g (100 kcal) of carbohydrate with equal amounts of starch and sugar, 15 g (60 kcal) of protein, and 5 g (45 kcal) of lipid (3 g or 27 kcal of saturated fat), with the remaining weight as water. This represents about 49% of the average bar's total 205 calories from carbohydrates, 29% from protein, and 22% from lipid. The bars often include vitamins and minerals at 30 to 50% of recommended daily values; some contain dietary supplements such as β-hydroxy-β-methylbutyrate (HMB) and are labeled as dietary supplements rather than foods.

Nutrient Composition of Nutrition Bars Varies with Purpose

The currently popular "energy bars" contain a greater proportion of carbohydrates, whereas "diet" or "weight loss" bars are lower in carbohydrate content and higher in protein. "Meal replacement bars" have the largest energy content (240 to 310 kcal), with proportionally more of the three macronutrients. "Protein bars" simply contain a larger amount of protein.

Nutrition bars provide a relatively easy way to obtain important nutrients, but they should not totally substitute for normal food intake because they lack the broad array of plant fibers and phytochemicals found in food, and typically contain a relatively high level of saturated fatty acids. As an added warning, these bars, generally sold as dietary supplements, have no independent assessment by the Food and Drug Administration (FDA) through the Dietary Supplement Health and Education Act of 1994 (**www.health.gov/dietsupp/ch1.htm**). Shamefully, no other federal or state agency exists to validate the labeling claims for nutrient content and composition.

Nutrition Powders and Drinks

Nutrition powders and drinks have a high protein content, typically 10 to 50 g per serving. They also contain added vitamins, minerals, and other dietary supplement ingredients. The powders come in canisters or packets that mix with water or in liquid forms premixed in cans. These products often serve as an alternative to nutrition bars; they are marketed as meal replacements, diet aids, energy boosters, or concentrated protein sources.

The nutrient composition of powders and drinks varies considerably from nutrition bars. Most nutrition bars contain at least 15 g of carbohydrates to provide texture and taste, whereas powders and drinks do not. This accounts for the relatively high protein content of powders and drinks. Nutrition powders and drinks generally contain fewer calories per serving than do bars, but this can vary for a powder depending on the liquid used for mixing.

The recommended serving of a powder averages about 45 g (about 1.5 oz), the same amount as a nutrition bar minus its water content, but with wide variation in this recommendation. A typical serving of a high-protein powder mix contains about 10 g of carbohydrate (two thirds as sugar), 30 g of protein, and 2 g of lipid. This amounts to 178 kcal, or 23% of calories from carbohydrate, 67% from protein, and 10% from lipid. When mixed in water, these powdered nutrient supplements exceed the recommended protein intake percentage and fall below recommended lipid and carbohydrate percentages. A drink typically contains slightly more carbohydrate and less protein than does a powder. As with nutrition bars, the FDA and other federal or state agencies make no independent assessment of the validity of labeling claims for macronutrient content and composition.

CARBOHYDRATE FEEDINGS PRIOR TO, DURING, AND IN RECOVERY FROM PHYSICAL ACTIVITY

Intense aerobic activity for 1 hr decreases liver glycogen by about 55%, whereas a 2-hr strenuous workout almost depletes the glycogen content of the liver and active muscle fibers. Even supermaximal, repetitive 1- to 5-min bouts of activities interspersed with brief rest intervals—as in soccer, ice hockey, field hockey, European handball, and tennis—dramatically lower liver and muscle glycogen. The vulnerability of the body's glycogen stores during strenuous exercise has focused research on the potential benefits of carbohydrate feedings immediately before and during exercise. Fruitful areas of research also include different strategies to optimize glycogen replenishment in the postexercise recovery period.

Prior to Physical Activity

Confusion exists regarding the potential endurance benefits of pre-exercise ingestion of simple sugars. Some researchers argue that consuming rapidly absorbed high-glycemic carbohydrates within 1 hr before exercising accelerates glycogen depletion. This negatively affects endurance performance by two mechanisms:

1. A rapid rise in blood sugar triggers an overshoot in insulin release. An excess of insulin causes a relative hypoglycemia (also called **rebound hypoglycemia**, or reactive hypoglycemia). Significant blood sugar reduction impairs central nervous system function during physical activity.
2. A large insulin release facilitates the movement of glucose into muscle, which disproportionately increases glycogen catabolism in physical activity. At the same

Large Spike in Emergency Room Visits Linked to Energy Drinks

So-called energy drinks (e.g., 5-hr Energy, Red Bull Energy Drink, EnergyFizz, Red Rain Energy Shot, Full Throttle) are beverages, marketed as providing mental or physical stimulation, that contain stimulant drugs, chiefly caffeine (usually between 70 and 200 mg per container). Many also contain sugar or other sweeteners, herbal extracts, diverse vitamins and minerals, and amino acids (usually taurine that supports neurological development and helps to regulate the level of water and mineral salts in the blood). Energy drinks may or may not be carbonated.

These drinks have become a "rising health problem" according to a survey of U.S. hospitals by the federal Substance Abuse and Mental Health Services Administration (**www.samhsa.gov**), with the number of emergency-room visits linked to energy drink consumption doubling in 4 years—from 10,000 in 2007 to more than 20,000 in 2013. Of those visits in 2013, about 42% had mixed an energy drink with another stimulant such as Adderal or Ritalin or with alcohol. Fifty-eight percent of the individuals had consumed just the drink. Symptoms and adverse effects include rapid heart rate and breathing rate, increased blood pressure, panic attack symptoms, and cardiac rhythm irregularities.

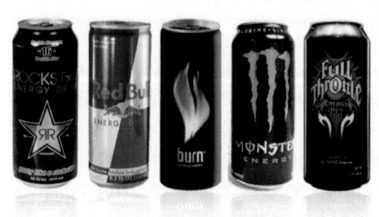

time, high insulin levels *inhibit* lipolysis, which reduces fatty acid mobilization from adipose tissue. Augmented carbohydrate breakdown and depressed fat mobilization contribute to premature glycogen depletion and early fatigue.

Research in the late 1970s showed that drinking a highly concentrated sugar solution before exercise precipitated early fatigue in endurance activities. When young men and women consumed a 300-mL solution containing 75 g of glucose 30 min before cycling, endurance declined by 19% compared to similar trials preceded by 300 mL of plain water or a liquid meal of protein, lipid, and carbohydrate.[28] Paradoxically, the concentrated sugar drink depleted muscle glycogen reserves prematurely compared with drinking plain water. The researchers hypothesized that the dramatic rise in blood sugar within 5 to 10 min after consuming the concentrated pre-event sugar drink caused the pancreas to oversecrete insulin (accentuated hyperinsulinemia). This, in turn, triggered rebound hypoglycemia as glucose moved rapidly into muscle.[40,117] Concomitantly, insulin inhibited mobilization and use of fat for energy, referred to as lipolysis suppression.[91] Consequently, intramuscular glycogen catabolized to a much greater extent, causing early glycogen depletion and fatigue compared with control conditions. Subsequent research has *not* corroborated these negative effects of concentrated pre-exercise sugar feedings on endurance.[3,27,91] The discrepancy in research findings has no clear explanation. One way to eliminate any potential for negative effects of pre-exercise simple sugars is to ingest them at least 60 min before activity.[36] This provides sufficient time to reestablish hormonal balance before exercise begins.

Debate Concerning Fructose

The small intestine absorbs fructose more slowly than either glucose or sucrose, causing a minimal insulin response with essentially no decline in blood glucose. The theoretical rationale for fructose use appears plausible, but its exercise benefits remain inconclusive. From a practical standpoint, gastrointestinal distress (vomiting and diarrhea) often accompanies high-fructose beverage consumption, which itself negatively affects exercise performance. After absorption, the liver must first convert the fructose to glucose; this further limits the rapidity of fructose availability as an energy source.

During Physical Activity

Physical and mental performance improves with carbohydrate supplementation *during* physical activity.[1,13,48,106,115] Adding protein to the carbohydrate-containing beverage (4:1 ratio of carbohydrate to protein) may delay fatigue and reduce muscle damage compared with supplementation during the activity with carbohydrate only.[51,86] When a person consumes carbohydrates during endurance activities, the carbohydrate form exerts little negative effect on hormonal response, metabolism, or endurance performance. The reason is straightforward:

Increased levels of sympathetic nervous system hormones (catecholamines) released during physical activity inhibit insulin release. Concurrently, exercise increases muscles' absorption of glucose, so any exogenous glucose moves into the cells with a lower insulin requirement.

Ingested carbohydrate provides a readily available energy nutrient for active muscles during intense exercise. Consuming about 60 g of liquid or solid carbohydrates each hour during exercise benefits high-intensity, long-duration (≥1 hr) aerobic activity and repetitive short bouts of near-maximal effort.[15,53,71] The beneficial effect reflect improved muscle function, possibly as a consequence of the protection of muscle membrane excitability. Supplemental carbohydrate during protracted intermittent exercise to fatigue also facilitates skill performance such as improved stroke quality during the final stages of prolonged tennis play. Supplementation also blunts the depression of neuromuscular functions associated with prolonged exercise, possibly as a consequence of protecting muscle membrane excitability.[96] Ingestion of multiple transportable carbohydrates may further enhance endurance performance.[24] Ingesting glucose plus fructose improved timed-trial cycling performance by 8% compared with glucose-only feedings. Combined glucose, fructose, and sucrose mixtures ingested at a high rate (about 1.8 to 2.4 $g \cdot min^{-1}$) produced 20 to 55% higher exogenous carbohydrate oxidation rates, peaking as high as 1.7 $g \cdot min^{-1}$ with reduced oxidation of endogenous carbohydrate, compared with ingestion of an isocaloric amount of glucose.[52,84]

Exogenous carbohydrate intake during intense physical activity provides the following three benefits:

1. Spares muscle glycogen, particularly in the highly active type I, slow-twitch muscle fibers, because the ingested glucose powers physical activity.[104,105]
2. Maintains a more optimal blood glucose level. This lowers the rating of perceived exertion; elevates plasma insulin; lowers cortisol and growth hormone levels; prevents headache, lightheadedness, and nausea; and attenuates other symptoms of central nervous system distress and diminished muscular performance.[11,73,74]
3. Blood glucose maintenance supplies muscles with glucose when glycogen reserves deplete in the later stages of prolonged exercise.[20,39]

Carbohydrate feedings during physical activity at 60 to 80% of aerobic capacity postpone fatigue by 15 to 30 min.[23] This effect contributes to enhanced performance in endurance competition because well-nourished athletes without supplementation usually fatigue within 2 hr. A single concentrated carbohydrate feeding about 30 min before anticipated fatigue (about 2 hr into the activity) proves as effective as periodic carbohydrate ingestion throughout exercise. The single concentrated feeding restores the blood glucose level (**FIG. 3.10**), which delays fatigue by increasing carbohydrate availability to active muscles.

The greatest benefits from carbohydrate feeding emerge during prolonged exercise at about 75% of aerobic capacity.[20] Fat provides the primary energy fuel in light-to-moderate exercise

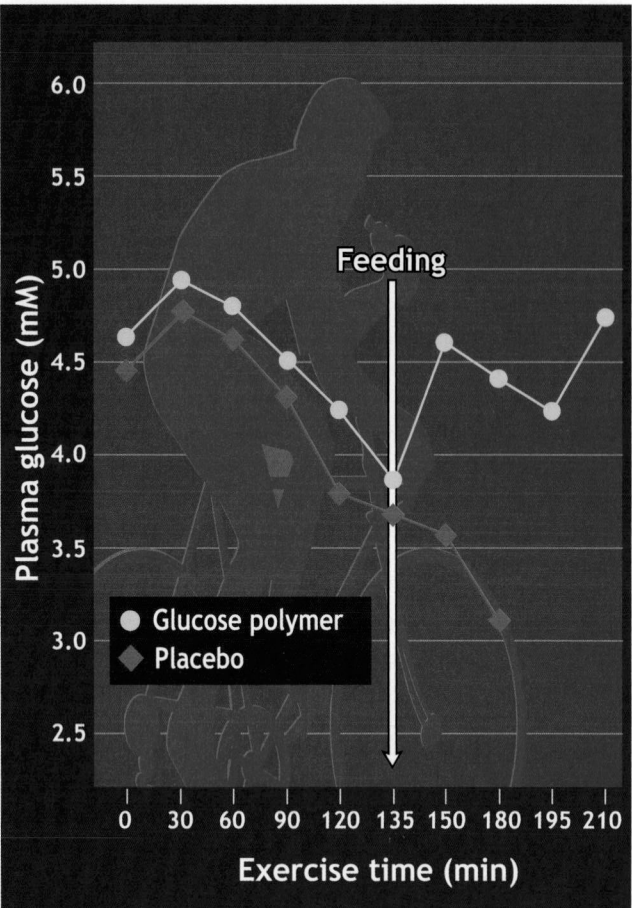

FIGURE 3.10 • Average plasma glucose concentration during prolonged intense aerobic exercise when subjects consumed a placebo or glucose polymer (3 g per kilogram of body mass in a 50% solution). (Adapted with permission from Coggan AR, Coyle EF. Metabolism and performance following carbohydrate ingestion late in exercise. *Med Sci Sports Exerc* 1989;21:59.)

below 50% of maximum; at this intensity, glycogen reserves do not decrease to a level that limits endurance.[2] Repeated feedings of carbohydrate in solid form (43 g sucrose with 400 mL water) at the beginning and at 1, 2, and 3 hr into the activity maintain blood glucose and slow glycogen depletion during 4 hr of cycling. Glycogen conservation not only extends endurance but also enhances sprint performance to exhaustion at the end of exercise.[82,92,98] *These findings demonstrate that carbohydrate feeding during prolonged, intense physical activity either conserves muscle glycogen for later use or maintains blood glucose for use as exercise progresses and muscle glycogen depletes, or both.*

The end result produced two effects:

1. Improved endurance at a high steady pace or during intense intermittent physical activity
2. Augmented sprint capacity toward the end of prolonged physical efforts

In a marathon run, a sustained high-energy output and final sprint to the finish contribute greatly to a winning performance.

Replenishing Glycogen Reserves: Refueling for the Next Bout of Intense Training or Competition

All carbohydrates and carbohydrate-containing foods do not digest and absorb at similar rates. Plant starch composed primarily of amylose is a resistant carbohydrate because of its relatively slow hydrolysis rate. Conversely, starch with a relatively high amylopectin content digests more rapidly. The **glycemic index** provides a relative measure of the increase in blood glucose concentration in the 2 hr after ingestion of a food containing 50 g of carbohydrate compared with a "standard" for carbohydrate (usually white bread or glucose) with an assigned value of 100. Ingesting 50 g of a food with a glycemic index of 45 raises blood glucose concentrations to levels that reach 45% of the value for 50 g of glucose. The glycemic index reflects the appearance of glucose in the systemic circulation (**Fig. 3.11**) and its uptake by peripheral tissues, which is influenced by the properties of the carbohydrate-containing food. For example, the food's amylose-to-amylopectin ratio and its fiber and fat content influence intestinal glucose absorption; in contrast, the food's protein content may augment insulin release to facilitate tissue glucose uptake. **Figure 3.12** presents a sample from the broad array of foods classified by their glycemic index. This sampling includes high- and low-glycemic index meals of similar calorie and macronutrient composition (see top inset tables).

Do not view the glycemic index as an unwavering standard because variability exists among individuals in their response to consuming a specific carbohydrate-containing food. Also, a high-glycemic index rating does not necessarily indicate poor nutritional quality.[77,116] For example, carrots, brown rice, and corn all have relatively high-glycemic index values yet contain rich quantities of health-protective micronutrients, phytochemicals, and dietary fibers. *A food with a moderate- to high-glycemic index rating offers more benefit for rapid replenishment of carbohydrate following prolonged physical activity than one rated low,[22,113] even if the replenishment meal contains a small amount of lipid and protein.*[14] Interestingly, the consumption of fat-free milk after an endurance activity replenishes carbohydrate as effectively as a non-nitrogenous carbohydrate control beverage, with the additional benefits of providing postexercise nutrition to support skeletal muscle and whole-body protein recovery.[67]

Optimal glycogen replenishment benefits individuals involved in regular intense training, tournament competition with qualifying rounds, or events scheduled with only 1 or 2 days for recuperation. An intense bout of resistance training also reduces muscle glycogen reserves. For athletes, acute weight loss by energy restriction without dehydration impairs anaerobic capacity.[81] Even without full glycogen replenishment, some restoration in recovery provides beneficial effects in the next workout bout. For example, consuming carbohydrate in the 4-hr recovery from a glycogen-depleting activity bout improves capacity in the subsequent bout compared with performance without carbohydrate in the 4-hr recovery.

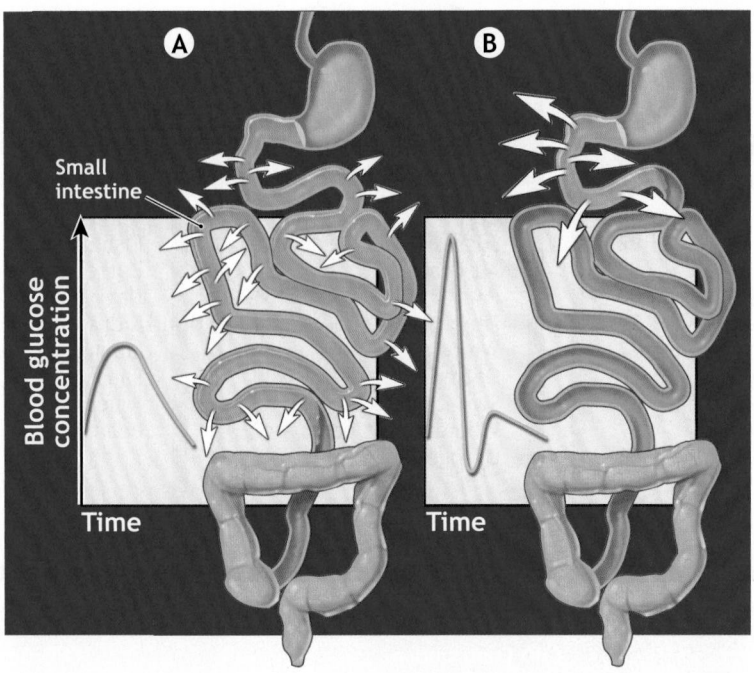

FIGURE 3.11 • General response of intestinal glucose absorption following feeding of foods with either **(A)** low or **(B)** high glycemic index. *Arrows* indicate absorption of glucose from the areas of the small intestine.

INTEGRATIVE QUESTION

Explain why foods with different glycemic index values dictate the nutritional recommendations for immediate pre-exercise versus immediate postexercise feedings.

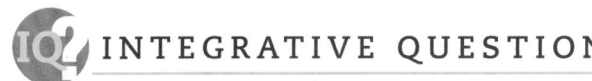

Glycogen depletion of previously exercised muscle augments the resynthesis of glycogen during recovery.[118] In addition, endurance-trained individuals restore more muscle glycogen than untrained counterparts.[43] Consuming foods after exercising facilitates glucose transport into muscle cells for three reasons:

1. Enhanced hormonal milieu, particularly higher insulin and lower catecholamine levels
2. Increased tissue sensitivity to insulin and intracellular glucose transporter proteins (e.g., GLUT 1 and GLUT 4, members of a family of facilitative monosaccharide transporters that mediate much of glucose transport activity; see Chapter 20)
3. Increased activity of a specific form of the glycogen-storing enzyme glycogen synthase

Practical Recommendations

Consuming carbohydrate-rich, high-glycemic foods immediately following intense training or competition speeds glycogen replenishment. Cereal is as good as commercially available sports drinks in initiating postexercise muscle recovery.[58] In one strategy, the individual consumes about 50 to 75 g (2 to 3 oz)

of high- to moderate-glycemic carbohydrates every 2 hr until achieving 500 to 700 g (7 to 10 g per kilogram of body mass) or until eating a large, high-carbohydrate meal. If immediately ingesting carbohydrate after exercise proves impractical, an alternative strategy entails eating meals that contain 2.5 g of high-glycemic carbohydrate per kilogram of body mass at 2, 4, 6, 8, and 22 hr postexercise. This replenishes glycogen to levels similar to those with the same protocol begun immediately postexercise.[75] Legumes and milk products have a slow rate of digestion and/or intestinal absorption and should be avoided in a glycogen replenishment strategy. Recent research reported that carbohydrate blends including fructose and galactose significantly improved postexercise liver glycogen resynthesis. Specifically, ingesting about 70 g · hr^{-1} of maltodextrin + fructose (2:1) or maltodextrin + galactose (2:1) during a 6.5-hr recovery period produced a twofold increase in the rates of liver glycogen replenishment compared with a maltodextrin + glucose control.[25] Glycogen resynthesis occurs more rapidly if the person remains inactive during the recovery period.[19]

Glycogen Replenishment Takes Time

Optimal carbohydrate intake replenishes glycogen stores at about 5 to 7% per hour. Even under the best of circumstances, it takes at least 20 hr to reestablish glycogen stores following glycogen-depleting exercise. Postexercise consumption of high-glycemic carbohydrates may speed recovery by facilitating removal of free ammonia that forms at an increased rate during strenuous exercise. Consuming glucose enhances glutamine and alanine synthesis in skeletal muscle; these compounds provide the primary vehicle to transport ammonia out of muscle tissue.[35]

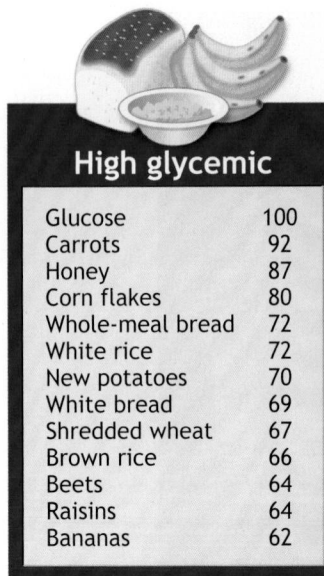
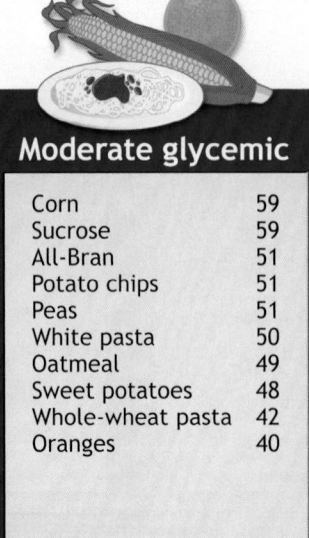

High glycemic

Glucose	100
Carrots	92
Honey	87
Corn flakes	80
Whole-meal bread	72
White rice	72
New potatoes	70
White bread	69
Shredded wheat	67
Brown rice	66
Beets	64
Raisins	64
Bananas	62

Moderate glycemic

Corn	59
Sucrose	59
All-Bran	51
Potato chips	51
Peas	51
White pasta	50
Oatmeal	49
Sweet potatoes	48
Whole-wheat pasta	42
Oranges	40

Low glycemic

Apples	39
Fish sticks	38
Butter beans	36
Navy beans	31
Kidney beans	29
Lentils	29
Sausage	28
Fructose	20
Peanuts	13

	High GI Diet			Low GI Diet		
		CHO (g)	Contribution to Total GI		CHO (g)	Contribution to Total GI
Breakfast				**Breakfast**		
	30 g corn flakes	25	9.9	30 g All-Bran	24	4.7
	1 banana	30	7.8	1 diced peach	8	1.1
	1 slice whole-meal bread	12	3.8	1 slice grain bread	14	2.2
	1 tsp margarine			1 tsp margarine		
				1 tsp jelly		
Snack				**Snack**		
	1 crumpet	20	6.4	1 slice grain fruit loaf	20	4.1
	1 tsp margarine			1 tsp margarine		
Lunch				**Lunch**		
	2 slices whole-meal bread	23.5	7.6	2 slices grain bread	28	4.5
	2 tsp margarine			2 tsp margarine		
	25 g cheese			25 g cheese		
	1 cup diced cantaloupe	8	10.4	1 apple	20	3.6
Snack				**Snack**		
	4 plain sweet biscuits	28	10.4	200 g low-fat fruit yogurt	26	4.1
Dinner				**Dinner**		
	120 g lean steak			120 g lean minced beef		
	1 cup of mashed potatoes	32	12.1	1 cup boiled pasta	34	6.4
	1/2 cup of carrots	4	1.7	1 cup of tomato and onion sauce	8	2.5
	1/2 cup of green beans	2	0.6	Green salad with vinaigrette	1	0.6
	50 g broccoli					
Snack				**Snack**		
	290 g watermelon	15	5.1	1 orange	10	2.1
	1 cup of reduced-fat milk throughout day	14	1.9	1 cup of reduced-fat milk throughout day	14	1.9
Total		212	69.8	**Total**	212	39.0

For each diet, the carbohydrate choices are maximized for differences between the two diets.

FIGURE 3.12 • Categorization for glycemic index (GI) of common food sources of carbohydrates. The inset table presents high- and low-glycemic index diets that contain the same amounts of energy and macronutrients and derive 50% of energy from carbohydrate (CHO) and 30% of energy from lipid. (From Brand-Miller J, Foster-Powell K. Diets with a low glycemic index: from theory to practice. *Nutr Today* 1999;34:64.)

Does the Coingestion of Caffeine and Protein with Carbohydrate Facilitate Postexercise Muscle Glycogen Synthesis? The Carbohydrate Amount May Be Crucial

Both protein and protein–caffeine coingestion with carbohydrate have been suggested as an effective strategy to facilitate the replenishment of muscle glycogen in recovery.[6,50] One proposed mechanism for the beneficial effects of postexercise amino acid and/or protein coingestion with carbohydrate is its stimulatory effect on insulin release and insulin's stimulatory effect on both glucose uptake and glycogen synthase activity in skeletal muscle. However, competing research results have demonstrated no benefit of protein coingestion on postexercise muscle glycogen synthesis with more than $1.0 \text{ g} \cdot \text{kg}^{-1} \cdot \text{hr}^{-1}$ of carbohydrate administered.[46,107] Recent research adds further support to these latter findings in that no additional benefit of coingestion of protein or caffeine was observed for accelerating postexercise muscle glycogen synthesis when ample amounts of carbohydrate ($1.2 \text{ g} \cdot \text{kg}^{-1} \cdot \text{hr}^{-1}$) were ingested.[5]

Cellular Uptake of Glucose

Normal blood glucose concentration, called **euglycemia**, approximates 5 mM, equivalent to 90 mg of glucose per dL (100 mL) of blood. Following a meal, blood glucose can rise above the hyperglycemic level to about 9 mM ($162 \text{ mg} \cdot \text{dL}^{-1}$). A decrease in blood glucose concentration well below normal to 2.5 mM ($<45 \text{ mg} \cdot \text{dL}^{-1}$) classifies as hypoglycemia and can occur during starvation or extremes of prolonged physical activity.

Glucose entry into red blood cells, brain cells, and kidney and liver cells depends on the maintenance of a positive concentration gradient of glucose across the cell membrane, termed *unregulated glucose transport*. In contrast, skeletal and heart muscle and adipose tissue require glucose transport via regulated uptake with insulin and GLUT 4, the predominant intracellular glucose transporter protein as regulating compounds.[69] Active skeletal muscle increases glucose uptake from the blood, independent of insulin's effect. This effect persists into the early postexercise period and helps to replenish glycogen stores. Maintaining adequate blood glucose levels during physical activity and in recovery decreases possible negative effects from a low blood glucose concentration.

The Glycemic Index and Pre-exercise Feedings

The ideal meal immediately before physical activity should provide a source of carbohydrate to sustain blood glucose and muscle metabolism while minimizing any increase in insulin release caused by the meal. Maintaining a relatively normal plasma insulin level should theoretically accomplish three ends:

1. Preserve blood glucose availability
2. Optimize fat mobilization and catabolism
3. Spare liver and muscle glycogen reserves

Coaches, trainers, and athletes should use the glycemic index to formulate the immediate pre-exercise feeding.[27,114] Consuming simple sugars (concentrated high-glycemic carbohydrates) immediately before physical activity could cause blood sugar to rise rapidly (**glycemic response**), triggering an excessive insulin release (**insulinemic response**). In contrast, consuming low-glycemic, carbohydrate-rich foods (starch with high amylose content or moderate-glycemic carbohydrate with high dietary fiber content) in the immediate 45- to 60-min pre-exercise period allows a slower rate of glucose absorption and reduces a potential rebound glycemic response. This strategy eliminates the insulin surge, while a steady supply of "slow-release" glucose remains available from the digestive tract throughout exercise. This effect should prove beneficial during prolonged, intense physical activity such as ocean swimming, where it often becomes impractical to consume carbohydrate during the activity. For trained cyclists who performed intense aerobic exercise, a pre-exercise low-glycemic meal of lentils extended endurance compared with feedings of glucose or a high-glycemic meal of potatoes of equivalent carbohydrate content.[100] A moderate-glycemic index breakfast cereal with added dietary fiber eaten 45 min before moderately intense physical activity increased time to fatigue by 16% over control conditions or a high-glycemic meal without fiber.[59]

Maintaining relatively high plasma glucose levels during prolonged physical activity following a pre-exercise meal of low-glycemic carbohydrate also enhances subsequent performance at maximal effort (**Fig. 3.13**). Ten trained cyclists consumed either a low-glycemic or high-glycemic meal 30 min before bicycling for 2 hr at 70% $\dot{V}O_{2max}$ followed by bicycling to exhaustion at 100% $\dot{V}O_{2max}$. The low-glycemic meal produced lower plasma insulin levels after 20 min of exercise. After 2 hr, carbohydrate oxidation and plasma glucose levels remained higher, with ratings of perceived exertion lower than under the high-glycemic conditions. Thereafter, time to exhaustion exercising at $\dot{V}O_{2max}$ averaged 59% longer than the high-glycemic maximal effort. Some research does not support the wisdom of pre-exercise low-glycemic feedings to enhance endurance performance.[37,38,113] Further study of the topic seems warranted.

INTEGRATIVE QUESTION

Advise an endurance athlete whose pre-event nutrition consists of a fast-food hamburger and high-protein shake consumed 1 hr before competition.

GLUCOSE FEEDINGS, ELECTROLYTES, AND WATER UPTAKE

As discussed in Chapter 25, ingesting fluid before and during exercise minimizes the detrimental effects of dehydration on cardiovascular dynamics, temperature regulation, and exercise performance. Adding carbohydrate to an **oral rehydration solution** also provides additional glucose energy. Determining the optimal fluid/carbohydrate mixture and volume becomes

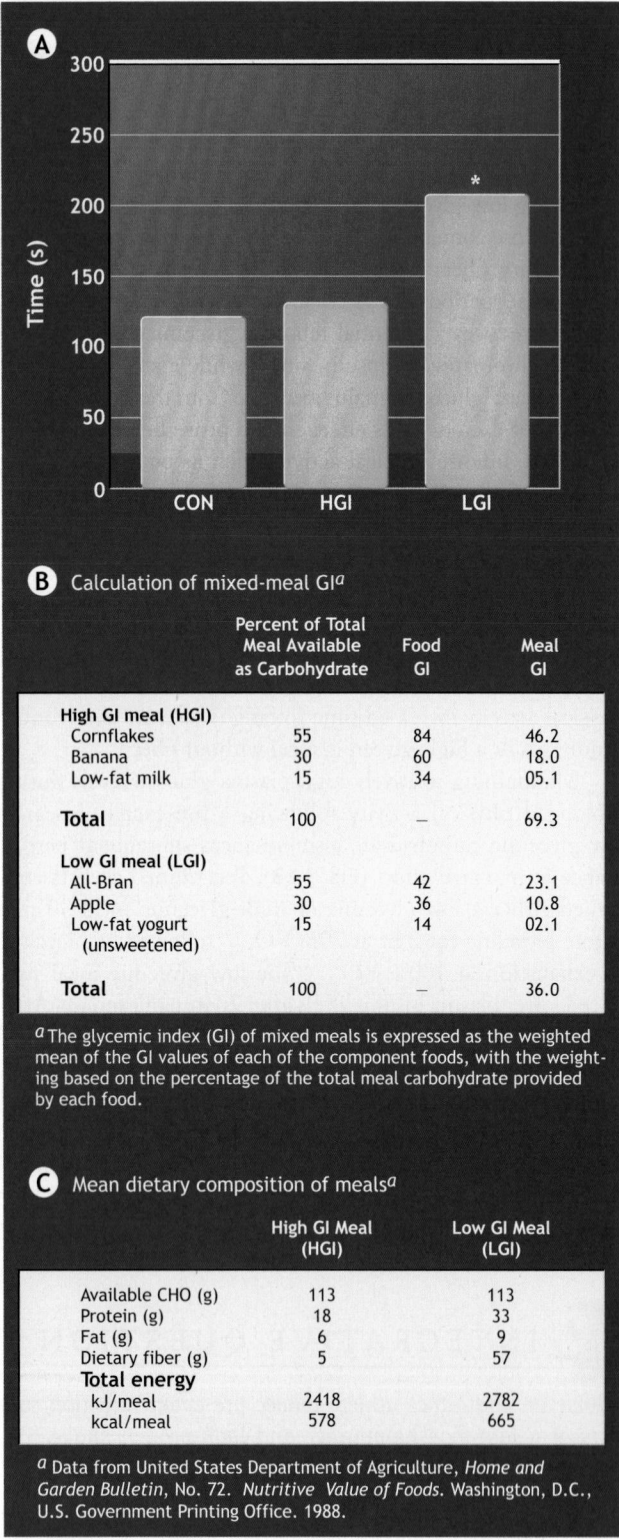

(A)

(B) Calculation of mixed-meal GI[a]

	Percent of Total Meal Available as Carbohydrate	Food GI	Meal GI
High GI meal (HGI)			
Cornflakes	55	84	46.2
Banana	30	60	18.0
Low-fat milk	15	34	05.1
Total	100	—	69.3
Low GI meal (LGI)			
All-Bran	55	42	23.1
Apple	30	36	10.8
Low-fat yogurt (unsweetened)	15	14	02.1
Total	100	—	36.0

[a] The glycemic index (GI) of mixed meals is expressed as the weighted mean of the GI values of each of the component foods, with the weighting based on the percentage of the total meal carbohydrate provided by each food.

(C) Mean dietary composition of meals[a]

	High GI Meal (HGI)	Low GI Meal (LGI)
Available CHO (g)	113	113
Protein (g)	18	33
Fat (g)	6	9
Dietary fiber (g)	5	57
Total energy		
kJ/meal	2418	2782
kcal/meal	578	665

[a] Data from United States Department of Agriculture, *Home and Garden Bulletin*, No. 72. *Nutritive Value of Foods*. Washington, D.C., U.S. Government Printing Office. 1988.

FIGURE 3.13 • (A) All-out cycling time to exhaustion (after 2 hr high-intensity exercise) for control (CON), moderately high-glycemic index (HGI) meal, and low-glycemic index (LGI) meal trials. Values represent the average cycling times for 10 trained cyclists. *Indicates LGI significantly longer than HGI and CON. Inset boxes indicate **(B)** calculation of mixed-meal glycemic index and **(C)** average dietary composition of the meals. (From DeMarco HM, et al. Pre-exercise carbohydrate meals: application of glycemic index. *Med Sci Sports Exerc* 1999;31:164.)

important to minimize fatigue and prevent dehydration. Concern centers on the dual observations that a large fluid volume intake impairs carbohydrate uptake, whereas a concentrated sugar solution impairs fluid replenishment.

Important Considerations

The rate the stomach empties affects fluid and nutrient absorption by the small intestine. **FIGURE 3.14** illustrates the major factors that influence gastric emptying. Little negative effect of exercise on gastric emptying occurs up to an intensity of about 75% of maximum, after which the emptying rate slows.[65] *A major factor to speed gastric emptying (and compensate for any inhibitory effects of the beverage's carbohydrate content) involves maintaining a high fluid volume in the stomach.* Consuming 400 to 600 mL of fluid immediately before physical activity optimizes the beneficial effect of increased stomach volume on fluid and nutrient passage into the intestine. Then, regularly drinking 150 to 250 mL of fluid at 15-min intervals throughout exercise continually replenishes fluid passed into the intestine.[61,64,72] This protocol produces a fluid delivery rate of about 1 L per hour, a volume sufficient to meet the fluid needs of most endurance athletes. Moderate hypohydration of up to 4% body mass does not impair the gastric emptying rate.[85] Fluid temperature does not exert a major effect during exercise, but highly carbonated beverages retard gastric emptying.[79] Beverages containing alcohol or caffeine induce a diuretic effect, with alcohol most pronounced, that facilitates water loss from the kidneys, making such beverages inappropriate for fluid replacement.

Particles in Solution

Gastric emptying slows when ingested fluids contain a high concentration of particles in solution (**osmolality**) or possess high caloric content.[8,85,110] The negative effect of concentrated sugar solutions on gastric emptying diminishes (and plasma volume remains unaltered) when the drink contains a short-chain glucose polymer (**maltodextrin**) rather than simple sugars. Short-chain polymers (3 to 20 glucose units) derived from cornstarch breakdown reduce the number of particles in solution. Fewer particles facilitate water movement from the stomach for intestinal absorption. Adding small amounts of glucose and sodium (glucose the more important factor) to oral rehydration solutions exert little negative effect on gastric emptying.[32,41] Glucose plus sodium facilitates fluid uptake by the intestinal lumen because of the rapid, active cotransport of glucose–sodium across the intestinal mucosa. Absorption of these particles stimulates water's passive uptake by osmotic action.[33,64] Extra glucose uptake also helps to preserve blood glucose. The additional glucose then spares muscle and liver glycogen and/or maintains blood glucose should glycogen reserves decrease as prolonged exercise continues.

Adding sodium to a fluid aids in maintaining plasma sodium concentrations. Extra sodium benefits ultraendurance athletes at risk for hyponatremia because of a large sweat–sodium loss coupled with the intake of copious amounts of plain water (see Chapter 2). Maintaining plasma osmolality by adding sodium to the rehydration beverage also reduces urine output and sustains

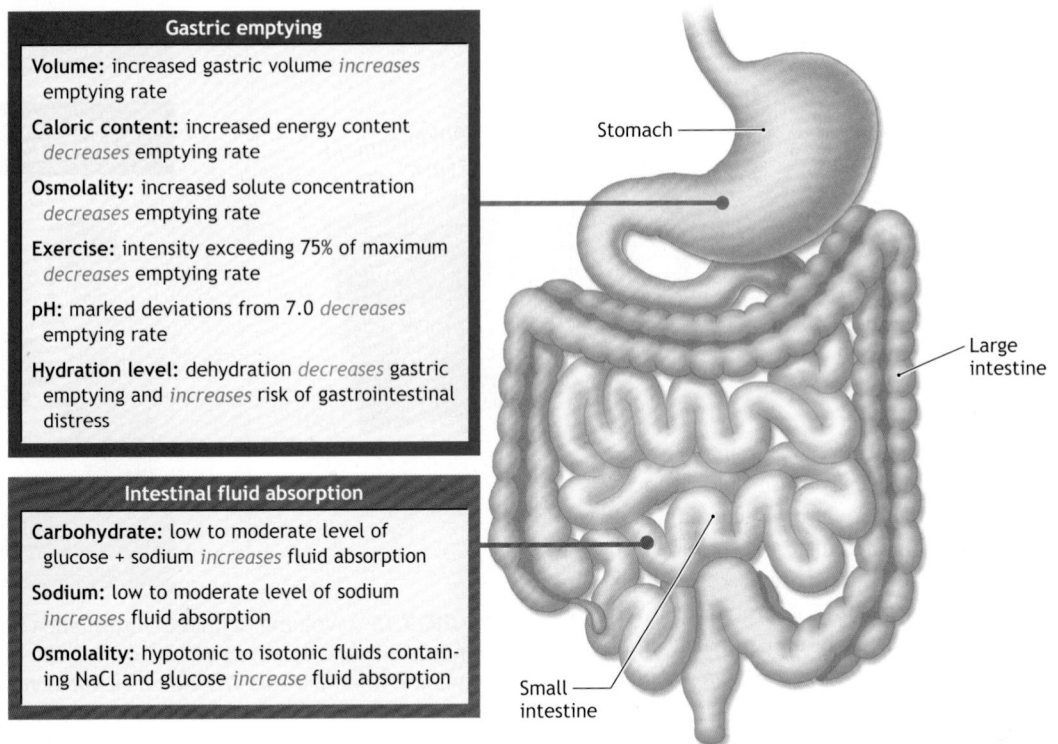

Gastric emptying

Volume: increased gastric volume *increases* emptying rate

Caloric content: increased energy content *decreases* emptying rate

Osmolality: increased solute concentration *decreases* emptying rate

Exercise: intensity exceeding 75% of maximum *decreases* emptying rate

pH: marked deviations from 7.0 *decreases* emptying rate

Hydration level: dehydration *decreases* gastric emptying and *increases* risk of gastrointestinal distress

Intestinal fluid absorption

Carbohydrate: low to moderate level of glucose + sodium *increases* fluid absorption

Sodium: low to moderate level of sodium *increases* fluid absorption

Osmolality: hypotonic to isotonic fluids containing NaCl and glucose *increase* fluid absorption

Stomach

Large intestine

Small intestine

FIGURE 3.14 • Major factors that affect gastric emptying (stomach) and fluid absorption (small intestine).

the sodium-dependent osmotic drive to drink (see Chapter 25). A normal plasma and extracellular fluid osmolality promotes continued fluid intake and fluid retention during recovery.

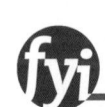

Three Recommendations for Fluid and Carbohydrate Replenishment During Exercise

1. Monitor dehydration rate from changes in body weight; require urination before postexercise body weight measurement for precise determination of the body's total fluid loss. Each pound of weight loss corresponds to 450 mL (15 oz) of dehydration.
2. Drink fluids at the same rate as their estimated depletion (or at least drink at a rate close to 80% of sweating rate) during prolonged exercise that increases cardiovascular stress, metabolic heat load, and dehydration.
3. Achieve carbohydrate (30 to 60 g · hr⁻¹) and fluid requirements by drinking a 4 to 8% carbohydrate beverage each hour (625 to 1250 mL; average 250 mL every 15 min).

Recommended Oral Rehydration Beverage

A 5 to 8% carbohydrate–electrolyte beverage consumed during exercise in the heat contributes to temperature regulation and fluid balance as effectively as plain water. As an added bonus, the drink provides intestinal energy delivery of approximately 5.0 kcal · min⁻¹; this helps to maintain glucose metabolism and glycogen reserves in prolonged exercise.[37,88] Consuming this solution in recovery from prolonged physical activity in a warm environment also improves endurance capacity for subsequent physical activity. To determine a drink's percentage carbohydrate, divide the carbohydrate content (g) by the fluid volume (mL) and multiply by 100. For example, 80 g of carbohydrate in 1 L (1000 mL) of water represents an 8% solution. Effective fluid absorption during prolonged physical activity occurs over a wide range of osmolalities. For example, total fluid absorption of carbohydrate–electrolyte beverages with osmolalities of 197 (hypotonic), 295 (isotonic), and 414 (hypertonic) mOsm per liter of H_2O did not differ from the absorption rate of a plain water placebo.[34]

Conventional Fluid Replacement Beverage Versus Carbohydrate/ Protein Powders and Drinks: Understanding the Difference

Do not confuse the conventional fluid replacement beverage designed as hydrating agents and as a means to replenish electrolytes and carbohydrates with more-concentrated carbohydrate/protein powders and drinks designed to provide significant carbohydrate and protein without concern for rapid fluid replenishment. The powders and drinks are good carbohydrate sources during recovery from intense training or competition but do not optimize fluid replenishment.

Environmental and physical activity conditions interact to influence the rehydration solution's optimal composition. Fluid replenishment becomes crucial to health and safety when intense aerobic effort performed under high thermal stress lasts 30 to 60 min. Under such conditions, the individual should consume a more dilute carbohydrate–electrolyte solution (5% carbohydrate). In cooler weather, when dehydration does not pose a problem, a more-concentrated 15% carbohydrate beverage would suffice. Little difference exists among liquid glucose, sucrose, or starch as the ingested carbohydrate fuel source during physical activity. Fructose is undesirable because of its potential to cause gastrointestinal distress. Furthermore, fructose absorption by the gut does not involve the active cotransport process required for glucose–sodium. This makes fructose absorption relatively slow and promotes less fluid uptake than an equivalent amount of glucose. *The optimal carbohydrate replacement rate during intense aerobic exercise ranges from 30 to 60 g (about 1 to 2 oz) per hour.*

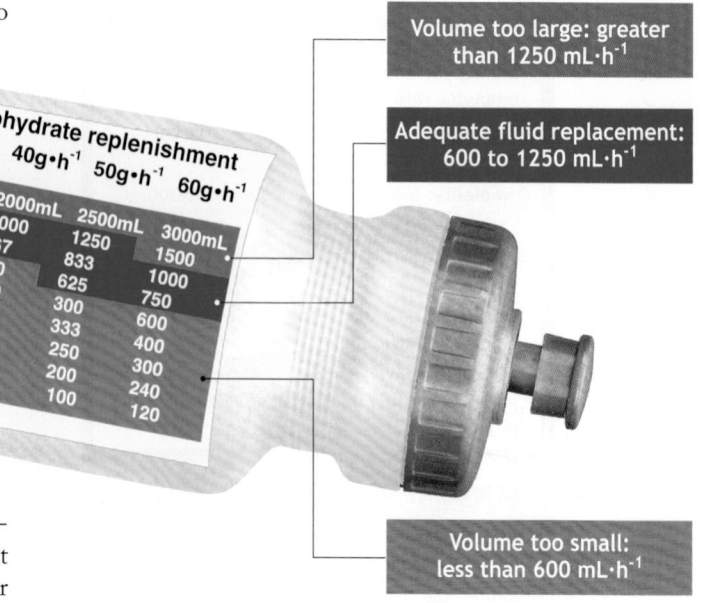

FIGURE 3.15 • Volume of fluid to ingest each hour to obtain the noted amount of carbohydrate ($g \cdot hr^{-1}$). (Reprinted with permission from McArdle WD, Katch FI, Katch VL. *Sports and Exercise Nutrition.* 4th Ed. Philadelphia: Wolters Kluwer Health, 2013, as adapted with permission from Coyle EF, Montain SJ. Benefits of fluid replacement with carbohydrate during exercise. *Med Sci Sports Exerc* 1992;24:S324.)

Five Qualities of the Ideal Oral Rehydration Beverage

fyi

1. Tastes good
2. Absorbs rapidly
3. Causes little or no gastrointestinal distress
4. Maintains extracellular fluid volume and osmolality
5. Offers the potential to enhance physical performance

FIGURE 3.15 presents a general guideline for fluid intake each hour during exercise for a given amount of carbohydrate replenishment. A tradeoff exists between how much carbohydrate to consume versus gastric emptying. The stomach still empties up to 1700 mL of water each hour, even when drinking an 8% carbohydrate solution. Approximately 1000 mL (about 1 qt) of fluid consumed each hour probably represents the optimal volume to offset dehydration as larger fluid volumes often produce gastrointestinal discomfort.

Summary

1. A balanced diet with as few as 1200 kcal provides the vitamin, mineral, and protein requirements of athletes and other individuals who train regularly.
2. The recommended protein intake of 0.83 g per kilogram of body mass represents a liberal requirement believed adequate for nearly all persons regardless of physical activity level.
3. A protein intake between 1.2 and 1.8 g per kilogram of body mass should adequately meet the possibility of added protein needed during intense exercise training.

Athletes generally consume two to four times the protein RDA because their greater caloric intake usually provides proportionately more protein.
4. No precise recommendations exist for daily lipid and carbohydrate intake. Prudent advice recommends no more than 30% of daily calories from lipids; of this amount, most should be unsaturated fatty acids. For physically active persons, unrefined polysaccharides should provide 60% or more of the daily calories (400 to 600 g on a daily basis).
5. A high-fat diet stimulates adaptive responses that augment fat catabolism. Consistent exercise or training benefits have not been demonstrated from this dietary modification.
6. Successive days of hard training gradually deplete the body's liver and muscle glycogen reserves and could lead to training staleness (making continued training more difficult).
7. ChooseMyPlate.gov provides recommendations for healthful nutrition for both sedentary and physically active individuals. It emphasizes fruits, grains, and vegetables and deemphasizes foods high in animal protein, lipids, and dairy products.
8. Intensity of daily physical activity largely determines energy intake requirements. The daily caloric needs of athletes in strenuous sports do not consistently exceed 4000 kcal.
9. The precompetition meal should include foods high in carbohydrates and relatively low in lipids and proteins. Three hours provides sufficient time to digest and absorb the precompetition meal.

10. Commercially prepared liquid meals offer well-balanced nutritive value, contribute to fluid need, absorb rapidly, and leave little residue in the digestive tract.

11. Carbohydrate-containing rehydration solutions consumed during physical activity enhance intense endurance performance by maintaining blood glucose concentration.

12. Glucose supplied via the blood can spare existing glycogen in active muscles during exercise and/or serve as reserve blood glucose for later use should muscle glycogen become depleted.

13. The glycemic index provides a relative measure of blood glucose increase after consuming a specific carbohydrate food. For rapid carbohydrate replenishment after exercise, individuals should consume 50 to 75 g of moderate- to high-glycemic index, carbohydrate-containing foods each hour.

14. Glycogen stores replenish at a rate of about 5 to 7% per hour with optimal carbohydrate intake. It takes about 20 hr for full liver and muscle glycogen replenishment following a glycogen-depleting physical activity bout.

15. Foods with a low glycemic index digest and absorb at a relatively slow rate to provide a steady supply of slow-release glucose during prolonged physical activity.

16. Consuming 400 to 600 mL of fluid immediately before exercise followed by regular fluid ingestion during exercise (250 mL every 15 min) optimizes gastric emptying by maintaining a relatively large fluid volume in the stomach.

17. The ideal oral rehydration solution to maintain fluid balance during physical activity and heat stress contains between 5 and 8% carbohydrates.

18. Adding a moderate amount of sodium to fluid stabilizes plasma sodium concentrations to minimize hyponatremia risk. Added sodium in the rehydration beverage also reduces urine production and sustains the sodium-dependent osmotic drive to drink.

thePoint References are available online at http://thepoint.lww.com/mkk8e.

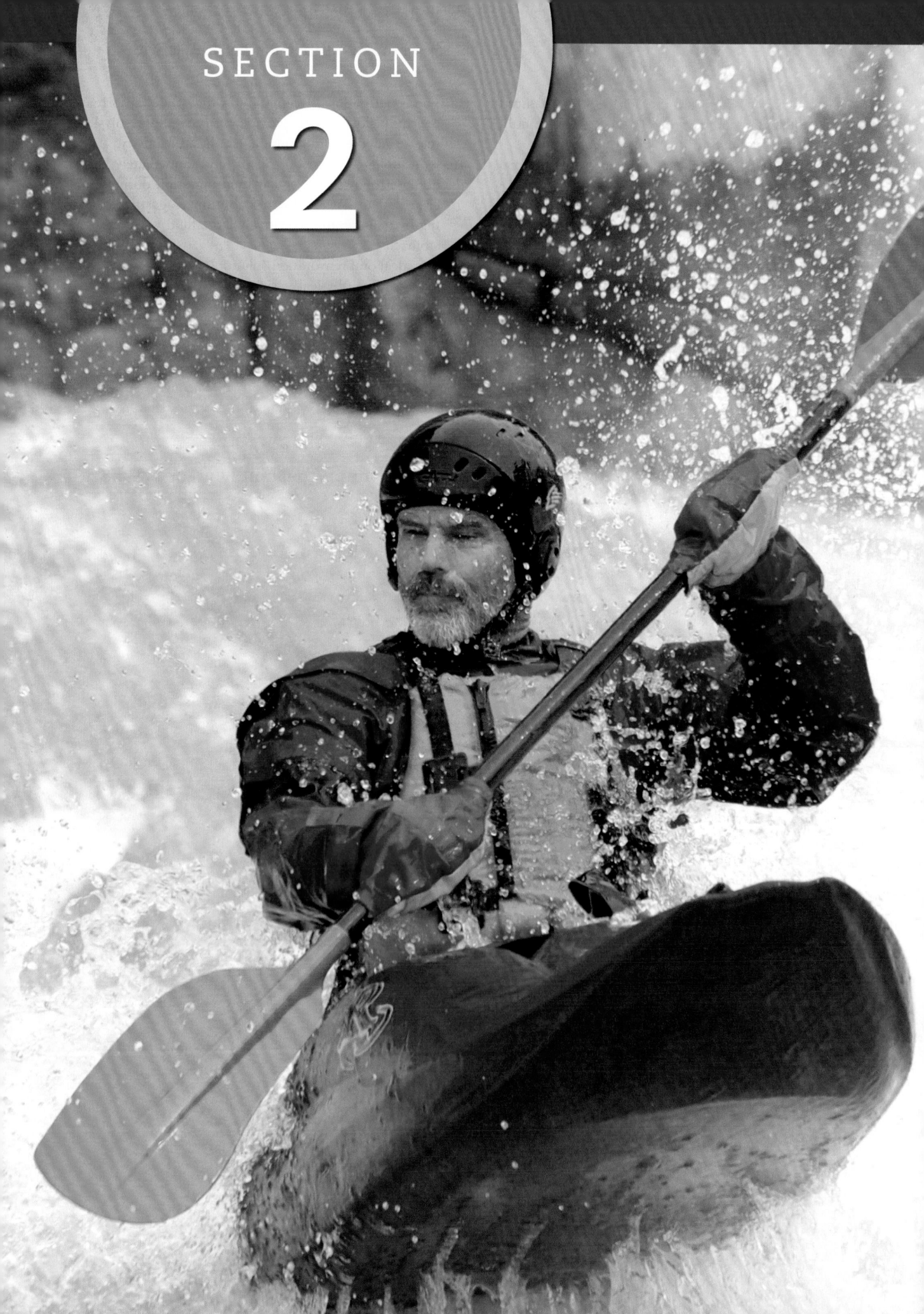

Energy for Physical Activity

Biochemical reactions that do not consume oxygen still generate considerable energy for short durations. This cellular strategy for rapid energy generation remains crucial in maintaining performance in sprint activities and other bursts of all-out physical activity. In comparison, longer-duration, less-intense activity relies on energy extraction from food through reactions that require oxygen. For greatest effectiveness, training the various physiologic systems requires an understanding of three important factors:

1. **How the body generates energy to sustain physical activity**

2. **Sources that provide energy**

3. **Energy requirements of diverse physical activities**

This section presents a broad overview of how cells extract chemical energy bound within food molecules and use it to power all forms of biologic work. We emphasize the importance of the food nutrients and processes of energy transfer to sustain physiologic function during light, moderate, and strenuous physical activity.

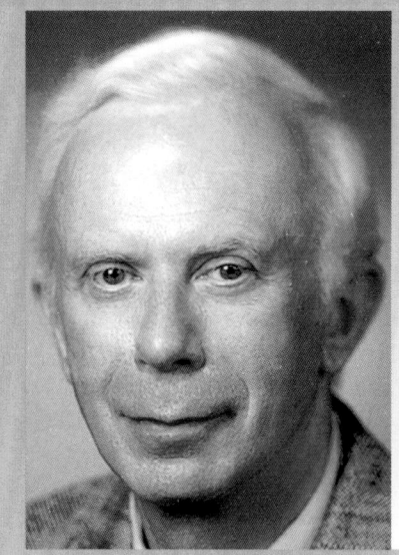

INTERVIEW WITH
Dr. John O. Holloszy

Education: BS (Oregon State College, Salem, OR); MD (Washington University School of Medicine, St. Louis, MO); postgraduate training (NIH Special Research Fellow, Department of Biological Chemistry, Washington University School of Medicine, St. Louis, MO)

Current Affiliation: Professor of Internal Medicine; Chief, Division of Geriatrics and Gerontology; and Director, Section of Applied Physiology, Washington University School of Medicine, St. Louis, MO

Honors, Awards, and ACSM Honor Award Statement of Contributions: See Appendix C, available online at http://thepoint.lww.com/mkk8e

Research Focus: The biological adaptations to exercise

Memorable Publication: Holloszy JO. Biochemical adaptations in muscle. *J Biol Chem* 1967;242:2278.

What first inspired you to enter the exercise science field? What made you decide to pursue your advanced degree and/or line of research?

➤ After completing medical school and 4 years of training in internal medicine and endocrinology and metabolism, I worked for 2 years as a Lieutenant Commander in the U.S. Public Health Service. Because of my interest in the prevention of coronary heart disease through diet and exercise, I was stationed at the Physical Fitness Research Laboratory at the University of Illinois.

At the time, Dr. Tom Cureton, Director of the Laboratory and pioneer in the area of endurance exercise training, conducted a year-round, daily exercise program, staffed by his graduate students, for university faculty and other individuals in the community. Most of the participants were middle-aged men, and I was tasked with obtaining information on the physiological and metabolic effects induced by the exercise program. With the help of some of Dr. Cureton's students and junior faculty, particularly James S. Skinner, who used this research for his doctoral dissertation, I conducted a series of studies on the effect of a 6-month exercise program on body composition, blood lipids, and cardiovascular function.

This was my first experience with the effects of endurance training. I became fascinated with the remarkable improvements in endurance and exercise capacity that developed rapidly in response to training. I was also impressed by the decrease in body fat, reduction in serum triglycerides, and improvement in cardiovascular function. I had become convinced by the epidemiological evidence that obesity, ischemic heart disease, and type 2 diabetes were largely diseases of exercise deficiency. But, at the time, there was little research being done on the effects of exercise and research on the biological effects of exercise was a low priority, generally viewed as unimportant and not prestigious. Therefore, because I had become

extremely interested in the biological mechanisms responsible for the adaptive responses to exercise at the cellular level, and because I thought that exercise deficiency had become the country's number one health problem, I decided to devote my career to research on the effects of exercise. My goals were to (1) elucidate the biological mechanisms underlying the improvements in performance and metabolism induced by exercise training; (2) evaluate the roles of exercise in the maintenance of health, treatment of disease, and prevention of loss of independence with advancing age; and, in the process, (3) bring research on the biology of exercise into the scientific mainstream.

Who were the most influential people in your career, and why?

➤ The only person who had a major influence on my career was Dr. Hiro Narahara, my mentor during my 2 years of postdoctoral research training in biochemistry. Like many physicians who come to basic research relatively late in their careers, I tended to be sloppy in laboratory work. Hiro forced me to become careful and accurate in my technical work, although, because of a lack of natural aptitude, I never did become a skilled bench researcher. My other mentors generally tried to dissuade me from devoting my research career to the biology of exercise because they thought that I would ruin my academic career by working in what was at the time a low-prestige area of science.

What has been the most interesting/enjoyable aspect of your involvement in science? What was the least interesting/enjoyable aspect?

➤ The most interesting and enjoyable aspects of my involvement in science have been the excitement and intellectual stimulation that comes from making new discoveries.

What is your most meaningful contribution to the field of exercise science, and why is it so important?

➤ Although it is difficult to single out, the most meaningful contribution that I have made to exercise science—the one that has probably had the greatest impact—is the discovery that endurance training induces an increase in muscle mitochondria. The importance of this finding is that it plays a major role in explaining how endurance training improves endurance and alters the metabolic response to exercise.

What advice would you give to students who express an interest in pursuing a career in exercise science research?

➤ A career in research in any area of biology can be extremely exciting and rewarding. This is particularly true of exercise science, a field in which there are still so many interesting, unanswered questions. However, biological research is extremely competitive in terms of coming up with novel, important ideas, obtaining research funding, keeping current with new methodology, and getting papers published. I would, therefore, strongly discourage students from pursuing a research career if they are not (1) highly intelligent, able to think independently and originally, with the ability to identify important problems and devise approaches for solving them; (2) highly motivated; (3) persevering and not easily discouraged; and (4) able to write well. There is probably nothing more discouraging than having to struggle for support and advancement, yet to be unsuccessful in one's chosen profession, but the chance for both is extremely high in biological research. A sensible approach for individuals who have an interest in exercise science but are not sure that they can succeed in a research career is to get a professional degree (MD, DO, PT, RN, RD, etc.), preferably along with a PhD. This way, one can remain associated with the research area and yet still be assured of making a good living.

What interests have you pursued outside of your professional career?

➤ My interests unrelated to my professional career include literature, particularly historical novels; opera; and gourmet food.

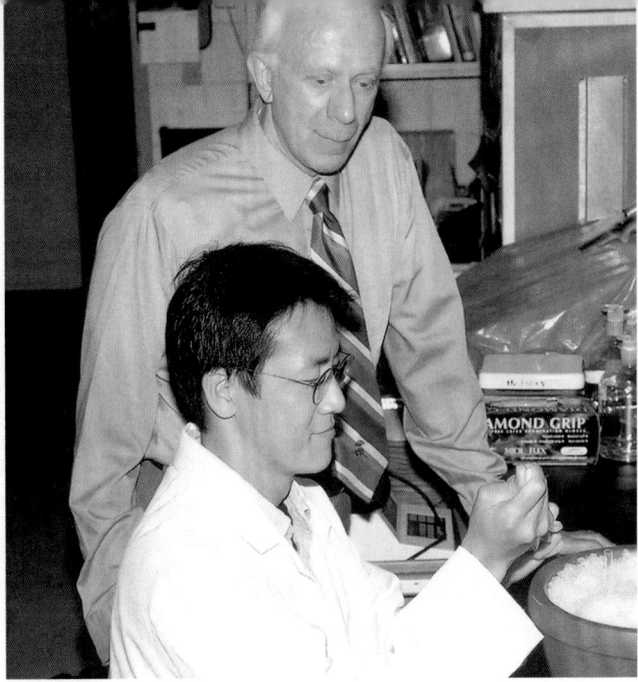

Where do you see the exercise science field (particularly your area of greatest interest) heading in the next 20 years?

➤ The most discouraging aspect of working in the field of exercise science is that, despite the now rather general perception that exercise is necessary for maintenance of health and functional capacity, the majority of people in North America are sedentary. Therefore, it seems likely to me that the major emphasis during the next 20 years will be (1) from a practical aspect, trying to get people to exercise, and (2) from a basic research perspective, trying to find pharmacological and other approaches that induce some of the same health benefits as exercise.

You have the opportunity to give a "last lecture." Describe its primary focus.

➤ The adaptive response of muscle mitochondria to endurance exercise.

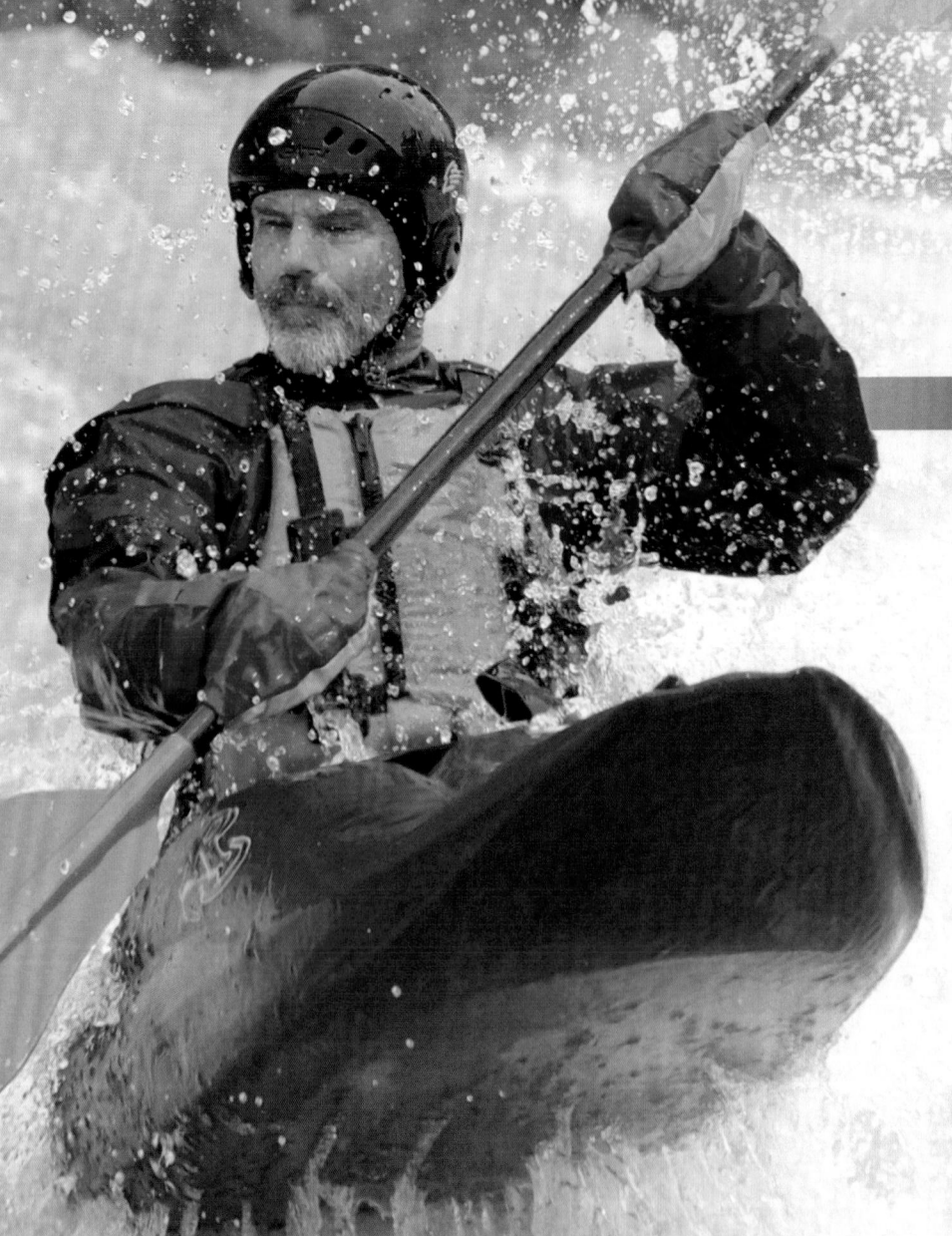

Energy Value of Food

CHAPTER OBJECTIVES

- Describe the laboratory method to directly determine the energy content of the macronutrients

- Discuss three factors that influence the difference between a food's gross energy value and its net physiologic energy value

- Define heat of combustion, digestive efficiency, and Atwater general factors

- Compute the energy content of a sample breakfast (8 oz orange juice, 2 soft-boiled eggs, 2 pieces whole-wheat toast, 1 pat butter, 1 tsp strawberry jam, ½ medium grapefruit) from its macronutrient composition

ANCILLARIES ◉ at-a-Glance

Visit http://thePoint.lww.com/mkk8e to access the following resources.

- Suggested Readings: Chapter 4
- Interactive Question Bank
- Appendix D: The Metric System and Conversion Constants in Exercise Physiology
- Appendix E: Nutritive Values for Common Foods, Alcoholic and Nonalcoholic Beverages, and Specialty and Fast-Food Items
- Animation: General Digestion
- Animation: Hydrolysis
- Focus on Research: Obesity-Related Thermogenic Response

MEASUREMENT OF FOOD ENERGY

The Calorie as a Measurement Unit

For food energy, 1 calorie or, more precisely, a **kilogram calorie** (abbreviated **kcal**), expresses the quantity of heat needed to raise the temperature of 1 kg or 1 L of water 33.8°F (1°C), specifically from 58.1 to 59.9°F (14.5 to 15.5°C). For example, if a particular food contains 400 kcal, then releasing the potential energy trapped within this food's chemical structure increases the temperature of 400 L of water 33.8°F (1°C). Different foods contain different amounts of potential energy. One-half cup of peanut butter with a caloric value of 759 kcal contains the equivalent heat energy to increase the temperature 33.8°F (1°C) of 759 L of water. The British thermal unit, BTU, represents a corresponding unit of heat using Fahrenheit degrees. One BTU represents the quantity of heat required to raise the temperature of 1 lb (weight) of water 1°F (−17.2°C) from 63 to 64°F (17.2 to 17.7°C).

Electrical, mechanical, and heat energy basically reflect the same state and can be changed from one form into another. Using the terminology of the Système International d'Unités (International System of Units or **SI units**), this energy is measured in units of **joules (J)**, named after English physicist James Prescott Joule (1818–1889) whose work formed the basis of the first law of thermodynamics—the law of conservation of energy. One J represents the work done or energy expended when one Newton (N) of force acts through a distance of 1 m along the direction of force; in other words, 1 J = 1 Newton-meter (Nm). The J, or more properly in nutritional science the **kilojoule (kJ**; equals 1000 J), represents the standard SI unit to express food energy. To convert kcal to kJ, multiply the kcal value by 4.184.

The kJ value for one-half cup of peanut butter, for example, equals 759 kcal × 4.184 or 3176 kJ. The **megajoule (MJ)** equals 1000 kJ; its use avoids unmanageably large numbers. The following conversions apply: 1000 cal = 1 kcal × 4184 J or 0.004184 kJ; 1 BTU = 778 foot-pounds (ft-lb) = 252 cal = 1055 J. Appendix D lists metric system transpositions and conversion constants commonly used in exercise physiology. Information on the history of the creation of the SI in the 1790s during the French Revolution can be found online at **http://physics.nist.gov/cuu/Units/history.html**; the system began with just the meter and kilogram as standards but now undergoes continuous updates and refinements

thePoint   Appendix D, available online at **http://thepoint. lww.com/mkk8e,** shows the relationship between metric units and U.S. units, including common expressions of work, energy, and power.

Gross Energy Value of Foods

Food and nutrition laboratories use bomb calorimeters similar to the one illustrated in **FIGURE 4.1** to measure the total or **gross energy value** of various food macronutrients. A bomb calorimeter (derived from the Latin *calor* = heat, and the Greek *metry* = measure) operates on the principle of **direct calorimetry** by measuring the heat liberated as the food completely burns. To accomplish this, oxygen under high pressure is forced into the sealed chamber containing the food. An electrical current moving through the fuse at the tip ignites the food–oxygen mixture. As the food burns, a water jacket surrounding the bomb absorbs the heat energy liberated. The calorimeter remains fully insulated from the ambient environment so the increase in water temperature directly reflects the heat released during a food's oxidation or burning.

Heat of combustion refers to the heat liberated by oxidizing a specific food; it represents the food's total energy

Clear Distinction Between Temperature and Heat

Distinct differences exist between temperature and heat. **Temperature** reflects a relative, quantitative measure of an object's hotness or coldness measured on a scale, usually with a numerical value. In essence, temperature relates to the average kinetic energy of a substance's molecules, but it is not energy. **Heat** describes thermal energy and its *transfer* or *exchange* from one object or system to another. Heat, measured in energy units, reflects the energy within a substance. Adding heat to a substance adds energy to the substance. To a molecular biologist, physicist, or chemist, the added heat (or energy) reflects an increase in the kinetic energy of the substance's molecules. If that energy changes the state of the substance (e.g., a melting ice cube as it enters the water phase), then the added energy breaks the ice molecule's bonds instead of changing its kinetic energy. In essence, when a substance gains heat, energy transfers to the substance.

Calories, Calories, or Kilocalories?

- The small calorie or gram calorie (symbol: cal or c) is the amount of energy needed to raise the temperature of one gram of water by one degree Celsius.
- The large calorie, kilogram calorie, dietary calorie, nutritionist's calorie, or food calorie (symbol: Cal or kcal) is the amount of energy needed to raise the temperature of one kilogram of water by one degree Celsius. The large calorie thus equals 1000 small calories or one kilocalorie (kcal).

In spite of its nonofficial status, the large calorie (kcal) is widely used as a unit of food energy in the United States, United Kingdom, and some other Western countries. The small calorie, often used in chemistry as the method of measurement, is fairly straightforward to quantify the relatively small amount of energy released in most chemical reactions.

Conversion Between Calories and Joules

An energy equivalency exists between 1 kcal of heat and 4.184 J of work. Energy and work unit conversion calculators on the Internet (**http://www.convert-me.com/en/convert/energy/**) easily perform the calculations among joules (J), kilojoules (kJ), and megajoules (MJ). For example, 10,000 J = 10 kJ = 0.01 MJ. Further interconversions include 73,760 ft-lb, 94.78 BTUs, and 23.88 kcal.

In terms of everyday life, one J = the energy *required* to lift a small apple with a mass of about 102 g 1 m off a table, and conversely the energy *released* when that same apple falls 1 m to the table. In human terms, one J = the energy released in 1 s as heat by an average-size person at rest. In engineering terms, one nanojoule (nJ) = one billionth of one J, and a microjoule (μJ) = one millionth of one J.

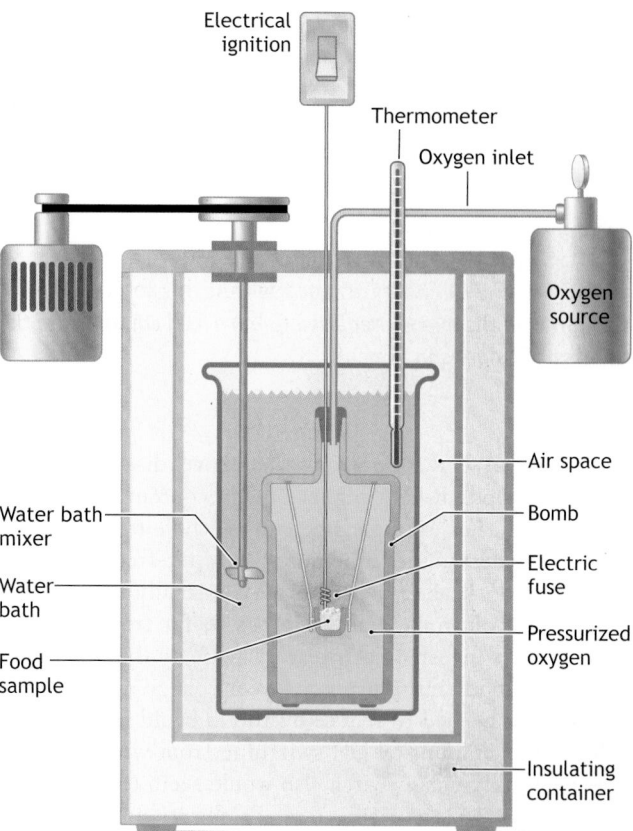

FIGURE 4.1 • A bomb calorimeter directly measures the energy value of food. **www.chem.hope.edu/~polik/Chem345-2000/bombcalorimetry.htm** provides calibration methods for bomb calorimetry, including explanations for different types of calorimeters and their methodology.

value. For example, a teaspoon of margarine releases 100 kcal of heat energy when burned completely in a bomb calorimeter. This equals the energy required to raise 1.0 kg or 2.2 lb of ice water to the boiling point. The oxidation pathways of an intact organism and the bomb calorimeter differ, yet the quantity of energy liberated remains the same in the food's complete breakdown.

Heat of Combustion: Lipids

The heat of combustion for lipid varies with the structural composition of the triacylglycerol molecule's fatty acids. One g of either beef or pork fat yields 9.50 kcal, whereas oxidizing 1 g of butterfat liberates 9.27 kcal. The average caloric value for 1 g of lipid in meat, fish, and eggs equals 9.50 kcal. In dairy products, the calorific equivalent amounts to 9.25 kcal per gram and in vegetables and fruits 9.30 kcal. *The average heat of combustion for lipid equals 9.4 kcal per gram.*

Heat of Combustion: Carbohydrates

Carbohydrate's heat of combustion varies depending on the arrangement of atoms in the particular carbohydrate molecule. The heat of combustion for glucose equals 3.74 kcal per gram, whereas glycogen (4.19 kcal) and starch (4.20 kcal) yield larger values. *The heat of combustion for 1 g of carbohydrate generally represents 4.2 kcal.*

Heat of Combustion: Proteins

Two factors affect energy release during combustion of a food's protein component:

1. The type of protein in the food
2. The relative nitrogen content of the protein

Common proteins in eggs, meat, corn, and beans (jack, lima, navy, soy) contain approximately 16% nitrogen and have corresponding heats of combustion that average 5.75 kcal per gram. Proteins in other foods have higher nitrogen content (e.g., most nuts and seeds [18.9%] and whole-kernel wheat, rye, millets, and barley [17.2%]). Whole milk (15.7%) and bran (15.8%) contain a slightly lower nitrogen percentage. *The heat of combustion for protein averages 5.65 kcal per gram.*

Comparing the Energy Value of Macronutrients

The average heats of combustion for the three macronutrients (carbohydrate, **4.2 kcal·g⁻¹**; lipid, **9.4 kcal·g⁻¹**; protein, **5.65 kcal·g⁻¹**) demonstrate that the complete oxidation of lipid in the bomb calorimeter liberates about 65% more energy per gram than protein oxidation and 120% more energy than carbohydrate oxidation. In Chapter 1, we showed that lipid molecules contain more hydrogen atoms than either carbohydrate or protein molecules. The common fatty acid palmitic acid, for example, has the structural formula $C_{16}H_{32}O_2$. The ratio of hydrogen atoms to oxygen atoms in fatty acids always exceeds the 2:1 ratio in carbohydrates. Simply stated, lipid molecules have more hydrogen atoms available for cleavage and subsequent oxidation for energy than carbohydrates and proteins.

 INTEGRATIVE QUESTION

Explain how the oxygen required to burn food can indicate the number of calories in a meal.

One can conclude from the above discussion that lipid-rich foods have a higher energy content than foods with less fat. For example, one cup of whole milk contains 160 kcal, whereas the same quantity of fat-free milk contains only 86 kcal. If a person who normally consumes 1 quart of whole milk daily switches to fat-free milk, the total calories ingested each year decrease by the equivalent of 25 lb of body fat. During a 4-year college experience, a person who needed to reduce by 100 lb could theoretically achieve this amount by just switching from whole milk to fat-free milk! Such a switch also would seem to be a viable strategy to stem the rising rates of obesity among young children and teens. Drinking fat-free rather than whole milk also reduces the intake of saturated fatty acids (0.4 vs. 5.1 g; 863%) and cholesterol (0.3 vs. 33 mg; 910%). In the 1960s and 1970s, parents who wished to reduce their child's intake of whole milk because of the milk's relatively high fat content (and relatively high cost) often switched to much cheaper powdered fat-free milk mixed with cold water to reduce the child's fat intake. The bottom line—small differences in energy intake (particularly lipid-rich foods) add up over time to potentiate large differences in energy balance.

Net Energy Value of Foods

Differences exist in the energy value of foods when the heat of combustion, known as the gross energy value determined by direct calorimetry, contrasts with the **net energy** available to the body. This pertains particularly to protein because the body cannot oxidize the nitrogen component of this nutrient. In the body, nitrogen atoms combine with hydrogen to form urea (NH_2CONH_2), which the kidneys excrete in the urine. Elimination of hydrogen in this manner represents a loss of approximately 19% of protein's potential energy. This hydrogen loss reduces protein's heat of combustion to approximately 4.6 kcal per gram instead of 5.65 kcal per gram released during oxidation in the bomb calorimeter. In contrast, the physiologic fuel values of carbohydrates and lipids, which contain no nitrogen, are identical to their heats of combustion in the bomb calorimeter.

Coefficient of Digestibility

The efficiency of digestive processes influences the ultimate energy yield from the food macronutrients. Numerically defined as the **coefficient of digestibility**, digestive efficiency indicates the percentage of ingested food digested and absorbed to meet metabolic needs. The feces contain the food residue that remains unabsorbed in the intestinal tract. Dietary fiber reduces the coefficient of digestibility; a high-fiber meal has less total energy absorbed than a fiber-free meal of equivalent energy content. This variance occurs because fiber moves food through the intestine more rapidly, reducing the food's absorption time.

TABLE **4.1** shows different digestibility coefficients, heats of combustion, and net energy values for nutrients from the various food groups. *The relative percentage of macronutrients digested and absorbed averages 97% for carbohydrate, 95% for lipid, and 92% for protein.* Considerable variability exists in efficiency percentages for any food within a particular category. Proteins in particular have digestive efficiencies ranging from a low of about 78% for protein in legumes to a high of 97% for protein from animal sources. Some advocates promote vegetables in weight-loss diets because of plant protein's relatively low coefficient of digestibility.

From the data in Table 4.1, one can round the average net energy values to whole numbers, referred to as **Atwater general factors**. Named for Wilbur Olin Atwater (1844–1907; pictured at left), the 19th-century chemist who pioneered the first, exacting human nutrition and energy balance studies at Wesleyan College, indicate the net metabolizable energy available to the body from ingested foods. The Atwater general factors provide a reasonable estimate of the energy content of the daily diet (see "In a Practical Sense," later in this chapter). For alcohol, 7 kcal (29.4 kJ) represents each g (mL) of pure 200-proof alcohol ingested. In terms of potential energy available to the body, alcohol's efficiency of use equals that of other carbohydrates.

 See the animation "General Digestion" on **http://thePoint.lww.com/mkk8e** for a demonstration of this process.

fyi Atwater General Factors

- Dietary carbohydrate: **4** kcal per gram
- Dietary protein: **4** kcal per gram
- Dietary lipid: **9** kcal per gram

A Calorie is a Calorie is a Calorie: Maybe, Maybe Not!

Based on conventional wisdom and research evidence, a gram of fat contains 9 kcal of energy while 4 kcal is ascribed to an equivalent weight of carbohydrate and protein. These values represent the classic Atwater factors developed over 105 years ago and currently used to estimate the average energy content computed from the proportions of the three. These computations assume that a given food digests and absorbs equally with little or no variation within the food's category. This simply is not the case. Because the cell walls of some plants are more difficult to break down than others, considerable variation exists in the useful energy available to the body. In addition, cooking generally disrupts the integrity of the cell wall to increase accessibility to the food's energy nutrients compared to the identical food in the raw state where some calories pass unavailable from the body. Some nuts (e.g., walnuts, hazelnuts, almonds, Brazil nuts) resist complete digestion so they too release fewer calories than "expected" computed from their actual macronutrient content. Diverse proteins demonstrate a broad range in variability in net energy available to the body owing to their specific requirements for complete digestion, absorption, and assimilation. Food processing also makes the energy in food more readily available than food in the unprocessed state. The standard Atwater model for computing a food's energy content appears relatively effective; the next time you assess the energy value of your diet, remember that the caloric values in food tables represent *averages*—averages that often fail to account for fluctuations related to the type, form, preparation (raw and whole, raw and pounded, cooked and whole, cooked and pounded), or whether the food is processed or consumed in a more natural unprocessed form. This also does not consider individual differences in digestive efficiency among individuals.

TABLE 4.1 Factors for Digestibility, Heats of Combustion, and Net Physiologic Energy Values[a] of Protein, Lipid, and Carbohydrate

Food Group	Digestibility (%)	Heat of Combustion (kcal · g⁻¹)	Net Energy (kcal · g⁻¹)
Protein			
Animal food	97	5.65	4.27
Meats, fish	97	5.65	4.27
Eggs	97	5.75	4.37
Dairy products	97	5.65	4.27
Vegetable food	85	5.65	3.74
Cereals	85	5.80	3.87
Legumes	78	5.70	3.47
Vegetables	83	5.00	3.11
Fruits	85	5.20	3.36
Average protein	*92*	*5.65*	*4.05*
Lipid			
Meat and eggs	95	9.50	9.03
Dairy products	95	9.25	8.79
Animal food	95	9.40	8.93
Vegetable food	90	9.30	8.37
Average lipid	*95*	*9.40*	*8.93*
Carbohydrate			
Animal food	98	3.90	3.82
Cereals	98	4.20	4.11
Legumes	97	4.20	4.07
Vegetables	95	4.20	3.99
Fruits	90	4.00	3.60
Sugars	98	3.95	3.87
Vegetable food	97	4.15	4.03
Average carbohydrate	*97*	*4.15*	*4.03*

From Merrill AL, Watt BK. Energy values of foods: basis and derivation. *Agricultural Handbook no. 74.* Washington, DC: USDA, 1973.
[a]Net physiologic energy values are computed as the coefficient of digestibility times the heat of combustion adjusted for energy loss in urine.

The Atwater 4-9-4 kcal rule generally proves useful to estimate the intake of food energy. Limitations do exist, particularly when consuming foods that include carbohydrate-bulking agents. For example, polysaccharides obtained from industrial gums, modified starches, and plant cell walls, which contain combinations of cellulose, hemicellulose, and a small amount of lignin, serve as common bulking agents in most prepared foods. These agents may be totally digestible, partially digestible, or indigestible, depending on their chemical structure. They pass through the intestinal tract with little breakdown because without naturally occurring enzymes, no hydrolysis

occurs; hence, they are of no energy value to the body. Determining digestibility coefficients by the use of bomb calorimetry also plays an essential role in animal husbandry research related to the care and feeding of livestock (**http://faculty.ksu. edu.sa/Hmetwally/Documents/Note%20in%20dig-energy-ff.pdf**), particularly as a measure of the animal' overall health (**http://ars.usda.gov/sp2UserFiles/Place/36553000/pdf's/02_ NIRSC_Mertens_Measuring%20Dig.pdf**).

 See the animation "Hydrolysis" on **http://thePoint. lww.com/mkk8e** for a demonstration of this process.

IN A PRACTICAL SENSE

Determining a Food's Macronutrient Composition and Energy Contribution

Food labels must indicate a food's macronutrient content (g) and total calories (kcal). Knowing the energy value per gram for carbohydrate, lipid, and protein in a food allows the ready computation of the percentage kcal derived from each macronutrient. The net energy value, referred to as Atwater general factors, equals 4 kcal for carbohydrate, 9 kcal for lipid, and 4 kcal for protein.

CALCULATIONS

The table shows the macronutrient composition for one large serving of McDonald's French fries (weight, 122.3 g [4.3 oz]). [*Note:* At their "Full Menu Explorer" (**http://www.mcdonalds. com/us/en/full_menu_explorer.html**), McDonald's provides the nutritional composition for each of the macronutrients for one serving along with the total kcal value for burgers and sandwiches, chicken and fish, breakfasts, salads, snacks and sides, beverages, and desserts and shakes.]

1. Calculate kcal of each macronutrient (column 4).

   Multiply the weight of each nutrient (column 2) by the appropriate Atwater general factor (column 3).

2. Calculate percentage weight of each nutrient (column 5).

   Divide the weight of each macronutrient (column 2) by the food's total weight.

3. Calculate percentage kcal for each macronutrient (column 6).

   Divide kcal value of each macronutrient (column 4) by the food's total kcal value.

LEARN TO READ FOOD LABELS

Computing the percentage weight and kcal of each macronutrient in a food promotes wise decisions in choosing foods. Manufacturers must state the absolute and percentage weights for each macronutrient, but computing their absolute and percentage energy contributions completes the more important picture. In the example for French fries, lipid represents only 17% of the food's total weight. The percentage of total calories from lipid increases to 48.3%, or about 195 kcal of this food's 402 kcal energy content. This information becomes crucial for those interested in maintaining a low-fat diet.

Similar computations can be used to estimate the caloric value of any food serving. Of course, increasing or decreasing portion sizes, adding lipid-rich sauces or creams, or using fruits or calorie-free substitutes affects the caloric content accordingly.

Macronutrient Energy Content and Percentage Composition of McDonald's French Fries, Large (Total Weight, 122.3 g [4.3 oz])

(1) Nutrient	(2) Weight (g)	(3) Atwater General Factor	(4) kcal	(5) % of Weight	(6) % of kcal
Protein	6	4 kcal·g^{-1}	24	4.9	6.0
Carbohydrate	45.9	4 kcal·g^{-1}	183.6	37.5	45.7
Lipid	21.6	9 kcal·g^{-1}	194.4	17.7	48.3
Ash	3.2		0	2.6	0
Water	45.6		0	37.3	0
Total	**122.3**		**402**	**100**	**100**

Use of Tabled Values

Computing the kcal content of foods requires considerable time and labor. Various governmental agencies in the United States and elsewhere have assessed nutritive values for thousands of foods. The most comprehensive data bank resources include the United States Nutrient Data Bank (USNDB; http://ndb.nal.usda.gov) maintained by the US Department of Agriculture's Consumer Nutrition Center and a computerized data bank maintained by the Bureau of Nutritional Sciences of Health and Welfare Canada.

thePoint Appendix E, available online at **http://thepoint. lww.com/mkk8e**, presents energy and nutritive values for common foods and lists resources for finding values of specialty and fast-food items.

A review of Appendix E indicates that large differences exist among the energy values of various foods. Consuming an equal number of calories from different foods often requires a tremendous intake of a particular food or a relatively little intake of another. For example, to consume 100 kcal from each of six common foods—carrots, celery, green peppers, grapefruit, medium-sized eggs, and mayonnaise—one must eat 5 carrots, 20 stalks of celery, 6.5 green peppers, 1 large grapefruit, or 1¼ eggs, but only 1 tablespoon of mayonnaise. Consequently, a typical sedentary adult female who expends 2100 kcal each day must consume about 420 celery stalks, 105 carrots, 136 green peppers, or 26 eggs, yet only 1½ cup of mayonnaise or 8 oz of salad oil to meet daily energy needs. These examples illustrate that foods high in lipid contain considerably more calories than foods low in lipid and correspondingly higher in water content.

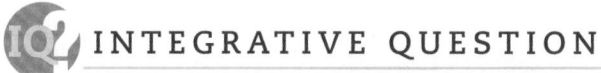

INTEGRATIVE QUESTION

What factors account for a discrepancy between computations of the energy value of daily food intake using the Atwater general factors and direct measurement by bomb calorimetry?

Also note that a calorie reflects food energy regardless of the food source. *From an energy standpoint, 100 calories from mayonnaise equals the same 100 calories in 20 celery stalks.* The more a person eats of any food, the more calories consumed. A small amount of fatty food represents a considerable number of calories; thus, the term *fattening* often describes these foods. An individual's caloric intake equals the sum of *all* energy consumed from either small or large quantities of foods. Celery would become a fattening food if consumed in excess!

Summary

1. A calorie or kilocalorie (kcal) represents a measure of heat that expresses a food's energy value.
2. Burning food in the bomb calorimeter permits direct quantification of the food's energy content.
3. A clear distinction exists between temperature and heat. Temperature reflects a relative, quantitative measure or number of an object's hotness or coldness measured on a scale. Heat describes thermal energy and its transfer or exchange from one object or system to another.
4. The heat of combustion quantifies the amount of heat liberated in the complete oxidation of a food. Average gross energy values equal 4.2 kcal per gram for carbohydrate, 9.4 kcal per gram for lipid, and 5.65 kcal per gram for protein.
5. The coefficient of digestibility represents the proportion of food consumed actually digested and absorbed.
6. Coefficients of digestibility average 97% for carbohydrates, 95% for lipids, and 92% for proteins. The net energy values equal 4 kcal per gram of carbohydrate, 9 kcal per gram of lipid, and 4 kcal per gram of protein. These Atwater general factors provide an accurate estimate of the net energy value of typical foods a person consumes.
7. The Atwater calorific values allow one to compute the energy (caloric) content of any meal from the carbohydrate, lipid, and protein compositions of the food.
8. Calories represent heat energy regardless of the food source (e.g., 500 kcal of peppermint ice cream = 500 kcal of raw carrots = 500 kcal pepperoni pizza = 500 kcal pistachio nuts).

thePoint Suggested readings are available online at **http://thepoint.lww.com/mkk8e.**

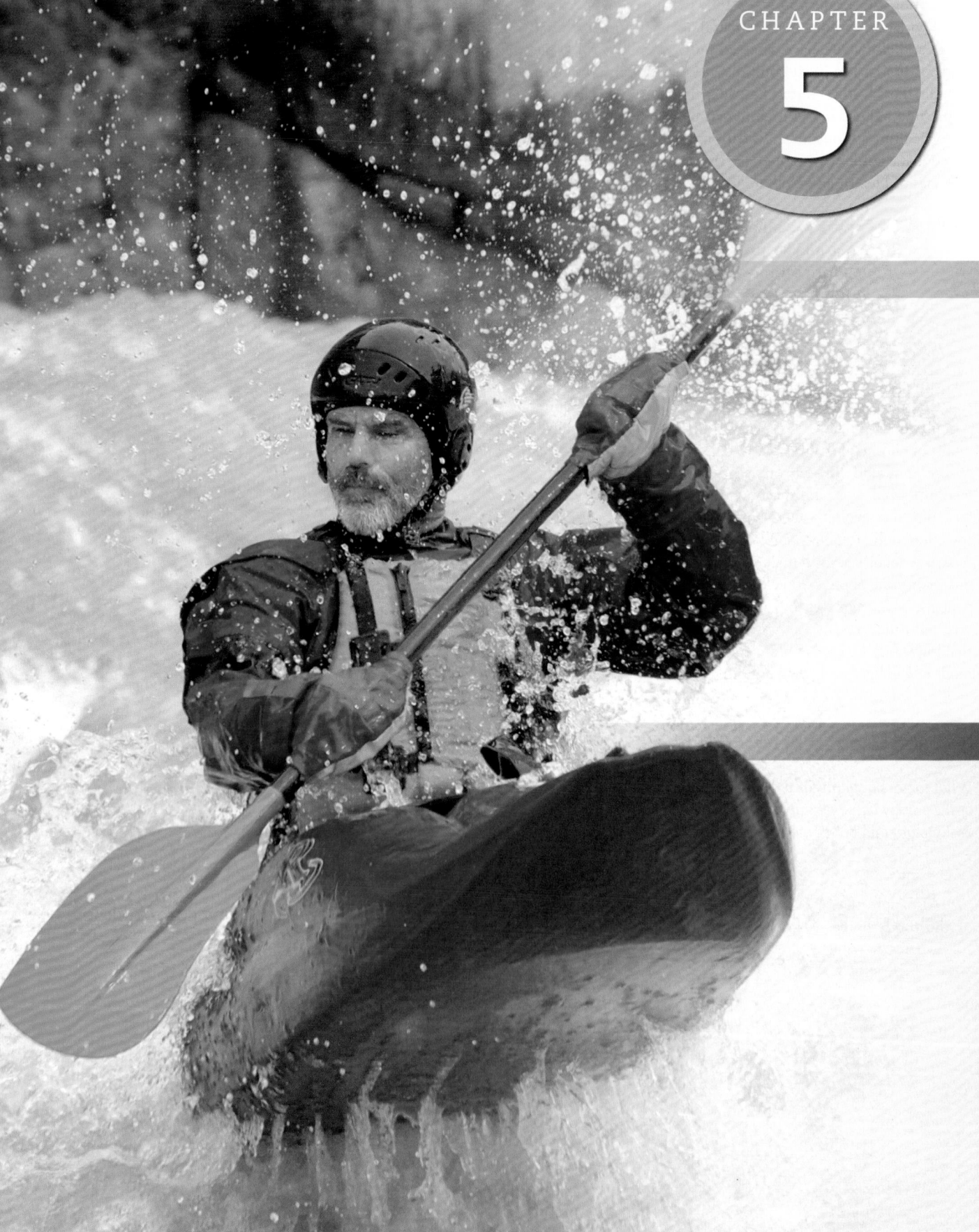

Introduction to Energy Transfer

CHAPTER OBJECTIVES

- Describe the first law of thermodynamics related to energy balance and work within biologic systems
- Define potential energy and kinetic energy and give examples of each
- Discuss the role of free energy in biologic work
- Give examples of exergonic and endergonic chemical reactions within the body and indicate their importance
- State the second law of thermodynamics and give a practical application of this law
- Discuss the role of coupled reactions in biologic processes
- Differentiate between photosynthesis and respiration and give the biologic significance of each
- Identify and give examples of the three forms of biologic work
- Describe how enzymes and coenzymes affect energy metabolism
- Differentiate between hydrolysis and condensation and explain their importance in physiologic function
- Discuss the role of redox chemical reactions in energy metabolism

ANCILLARIES 👁 at-a-Glance

Visit http://thePoint.lww.com/mkk8e to access the following resources.

- Suggested Readings: Chapter 5
- Interactive Question Bank
- Animation: Condensation
- Animation: Hydrolysis
- Focus on Research: Valid Determination of Oxygen Consumption

The capacity to extract energy from the food macronutrients and continually transfer it at a high rate to the contractile elements of skeletal muscle determines one's capacity for swimming, running, or skiing long distances. Likewise, specific energy-transferring capacities that demand all-out, "explosive" power output for brief durations determine success in weight-lifting, sprinting, jumping, and football line play. Muscular activity represents the main frame of reference in this text, yet al/ forms of biologic work require power generated from the direct transfer of chemical energy. *The breakdown of ingested food nutrients provides the energy source for synthesizing the chemical fuel that powers all forms of biologic work.*

The sections that follow introduce general concepts about bioenergetics that form the basis for understanding energy metabolism during all forms of physical activity.

ENERGY—THE CAPACITY FOR WORK

Unlike the physical properties of matter, one cannot define *energy* in concrete terms of size, shape, or mass. Rather, the term *energy* reflects a dynamic state related to change; thus, energy emerges only when change occurs. Within this context, energy relates to the performance of work—as work increases so also does energy transfer and thus change. From a mechanical perspective, work refers to the product of a given force acting through a given distance. In the body, cells more commonly accomplish chemical and electrical work than mechanical work. Because energy can be exchanged and converted from one form to another, we can express biologic work in mechanical units.

Bioenergetics refers to the flow and exchange of energy within a living system. The **first law of thermodynamics** describes a principle related to biologic work. Its basic tenet states that energy cannot be created or destroyed but transforms from one form to another without being depleted. In essence, this law describes the important **conservation of energy principle** that applies to both living and nonliving systems. In the body, chemical energy within the bonds of macronutrients does not immediately dissipate as heat during energy metabolism; instead, a large portion remains as chemical energy, which the musculoskeletal system changes into mechanical energy and ultimately to heat energy. *The first law of thermodynamics requires that the body does not produce, consume, or use up energy; instead, it transforms it from one state into another as physiologic systems undergo continual change.*

 INTEGRATIVE QUESTION

Based on the first law of thermodynamics, why is it imprecise to refer to energy "production" in the body?

Potential and Kinetic Energy

The total energy of a system includes potential energy and kinetic energy. **FIGURE 5.1** shows potential energy as energy of position,

similar to water flowing over the top of a dam. In the example of flowing water, energy change is proportional to the water's vertical drop—the greater the vertical drop, the greater the potential energy at the top. A waterwheel inserted into the flow of the falling water can harness some of the energy to produce useful work. For a falling boulder from the top, *all* potential energy transforms to kinetic energy and dissipates as unusable heat.

Other examples of potential energy include bound energy within the internal structure of a battery, a stick of dynamite, and a macronutrient before releasing its stored energy in metabolism. *The release of potential energy transforms into kinetic energy of motion.* In some cases, bound energy in one substance directly transfers to other substances to increase this substance's potential energy. Energy transfers of this type provide the necessary energy for the body's chemical work of **biosynthesis**. In this process, specific building-block atoms of carbon, hydrogen, oxygen, and nitrogen become activated and join other atoms and molecules to synthesize important biologic compounds and tissues. Some newly created compounds provide structure; examples include bone or the bilayer lipid-containing plasma membrane that encloses each cell. The synthesized compounds adenosine triphosphate (ATP) and phosphocreatine (PCr) contribute to the cell's energy requirements.

Energy-Releasing and Energy-Conserving Processes

The term **exergonic** describes any physical or chemical process that releases (frees) energy to its surroundings. Such reactions represent "downhill" processes because of a decline in free energy—"useful" energy for biologic work that encompasses all of the cell's energy-requiring, life-sustaining processes. Within a cell, where pressure and volume remain relatively

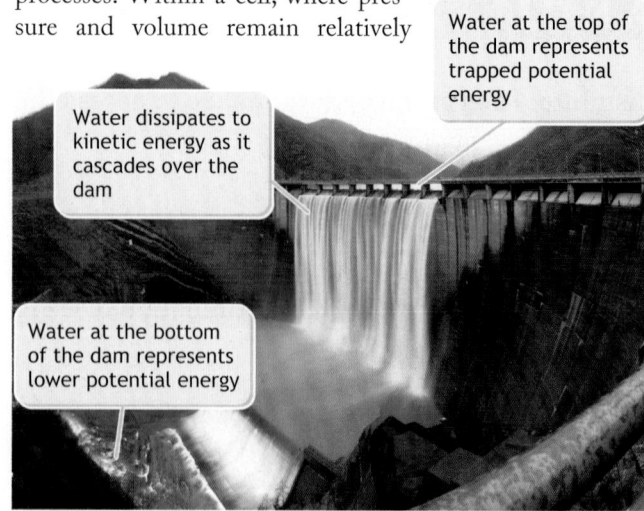

FIGURE 5.1 • High-grade potential energy capable of performing work degrades to a useless form of kinetic energy. In the example of falling water over a dam, the water at the crest, before it cascades to the next level, represents potential energy. All of this potential energy dissipates to kinetic energy (heat) as the water crashes to the surface below.

stable, free energy determines the potential energy within a molecule's chemical bonds. Free energy is described quantitatively as

$$G = H - TS$$

where G = free energy (denoted by the symbol G to honor American scientist Josiah Willard Gibbs [1839–1903] whose theoretical research provided the foundation of biochemical thermodynamics), H = enthalpy (thermodynamic measure of the thermal energy change in a reaction), S = randomness due to energy unavailability, and T = (temperature °C + 273).

Endergonic chemical reactions store or absorb energy; these reactions represent "uphill" processes and proceed with an increase in free energy for biologic work. Exergonic processes sometimes link or *couple* with endergonic reactions to transfer some energy to the endergonic process. In the body, coupled reactions conserve in usable form a large portion of the chemical energy stored within the macronutrients.

FIGURE 5.2 illustrates the flow of energy in endergonic and exergonic chemical reactions. Changes in free energy occur when the bonds in the reactant molecules form new product molecules with different bonding. In the endergonic reaction, energy is supplied to the product. In exergonic reactions, energy release occurs as the reactant "flows downhill." The equation that expresses these changes, under conditions of constant temperature, pressure, and volume, takes the following form:

$$\Delta G = \Delta H - T\Delta S$$

The symbol Δ (delta) designates change. The change in free energy represents a keystone of chemical reactions. In exergonic reactions, ΔG is negative; the products contain *less* free energy than the reactants, with the energy differential released as heat. For example, the union of hydrogen and

oxygen to form water releases 68 kcal per mole (molecular weight of a substance in grams) of free energy in the following reaction:

$$H_2 + O \rightarrow H_2O - \Delta G \ \ 68 \ kcal \cdot mole^{-1}$$

In the reverse endergonic reaction, ΔG remains positive because the product contains *more* free energy than the reactants. The release of 68 kcal of energy per mole of water causes the chemical bonds of the water molecule to split apart, freeing the original hydrogen and oxygen atoms. This "uphill" process of energy transfer allows the hydrogen and oxygen atoms with their original energy content to satisfy the principle of the first law of thermodynamics—*the conservation of energy.*

$$H_2 + O \leftarrow H_2O + \Delta G \ \ 68 \ kcal \cdot mole^{-1}$$

Energy transfer in cells follows the same principles as those in the waterfall example of Figure 5.1. Carbohydrate, lipid, and protein macronutrients possess considerable potential energy within their chemical bonds. The formation of product substances progressively reduces the nutrient molecule's original potential energy with a corresponding increase in kinetic energy. Enzyme-regulated transfer systems harness or conserve a portion of this chemical energy in new compounds for biologic work. In essence, living cells serve as transducers with the capacity to extract and use chemical energy stored within a compound's atomic structure. Conversely, and equally important, cells also bond atoms and molecules together to raise them to a higher level of potential energy.

The transfer of potential energy in any spontaneous process always proceeds in a direction that *decreases* the capacity to perform work. The tendency of potential energy to degrade to kinetic energy of motion with a lower capacity for work (i.e., increased **entropy**) reflects the **second law of thermodynamics**. A flashlight battery provides a good illustration—the

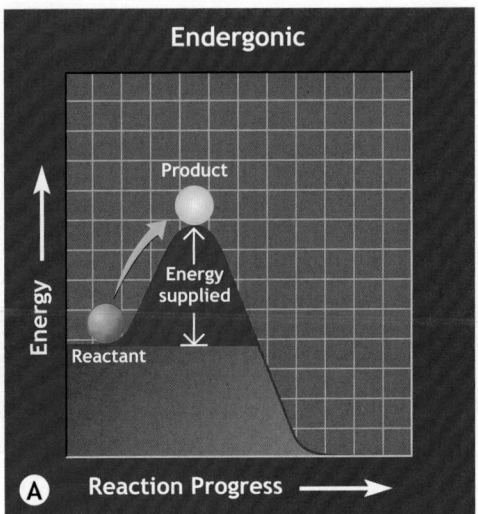

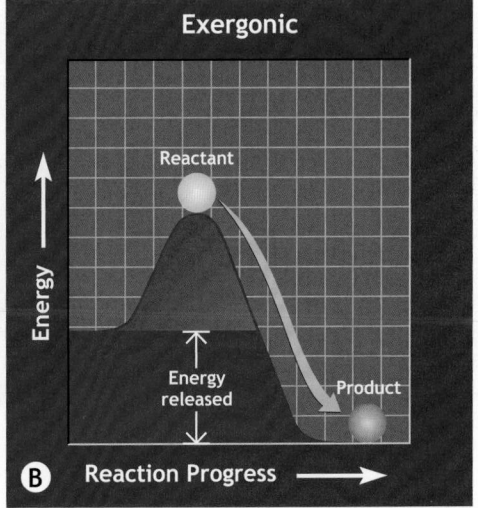

FIGURE 5.2 • Energy flow in chemical reactions. **(A)** Energy supply prepares an endergonic reaction to proceed because the reaction's product contains more energy than the reactant. **(B)** Exergonic reaction releases energy, resulting in less energy in the product than in the reactant.

electrochemical energy stored within its cells slowly dissipates, even if the battery remains unused. Energy from sunlight provides another illustration—it continually degrades to heat energy when light strikes an object and the surface it interacts with absorbs it. Food and other chemicals represent excellent stores of potential energy. This energy continually decreases as the compounds decompose through normal oxidative processes. Energy, like water, always runs downhill, so potential energy decreases. *Ultimately, all of the potential energy in a biological system degrades to the unusable form of kinetic or heat energy.*

INTERCONVERSIONS OF ENERGY

The total energy in a closed system remains constant, so a decrease in one form of energy matches an equivalent increase in another form. During energy conversions, a loss of potential energy from one source produces a temporary increase in the potential energy of another source. In this way, nature harnesses vast quantities of potential energy for useful purposes. Even in these favorable conditions, the net flow of energy in the biologic world moves toward entropy, ultimately producing a net loss of potential energy. Entropy reflects the continual process of energy change. All chemical and physical processes proceed in a direction where total randomness or disorder *increases* and the energy available for work *decreases*. In coupled reactions during biosynthesis, one part of a system may show a decrease in entropy while another part shows an increase. *No way exists to circumvent the second law—the entire system always shows a net increase in entropy.*

Forms of Energy

FIGURE 5.3 shows energy categorized into one of its six forms: chemical, mechanical, heat, light, electrical, and nuclear.

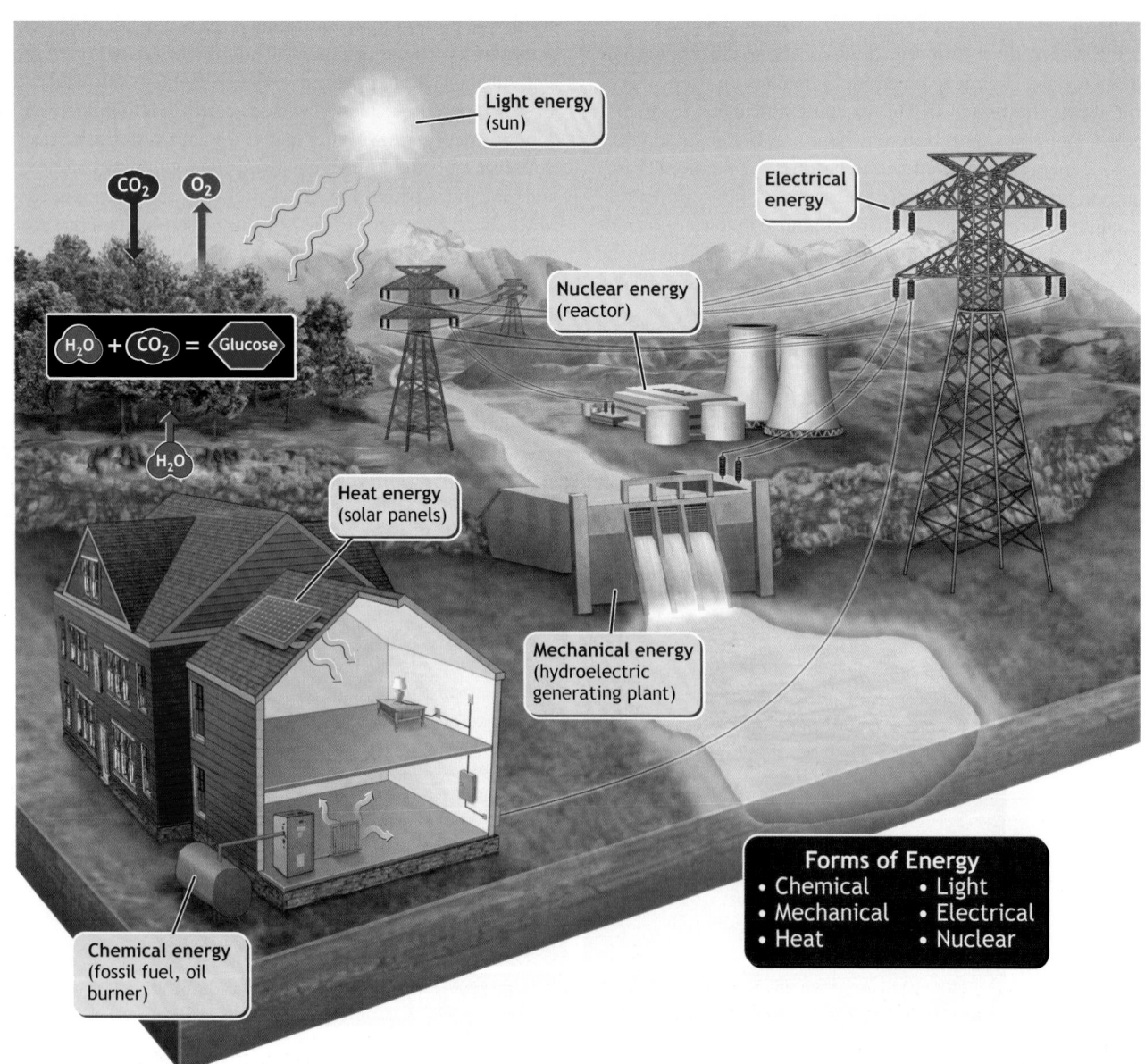

FIGURE 5.3 • Interconversions among six forms of energy.

Examples of Energy Conversions

The conversion of energy from one form to another occurs readily in the inanimate and animate worlds. **Photosynthesis** and **respiration** represent the most fundamental examples of energy conversion in living cells.

Photosynthesis. In the sun, nuclear fusion releases part of the potential energy stored in the nucleus of the hydrogen atom. This energy, in the form of gamma radiation, then converts to radiant energy.

FIGURE 5.4 depicts the dynamics of photosynthesis, an endergonic process powered by energy from sunlight. The pigment chlorophyll, contained in large chloroplast organelles within a leaf's cells, absorbs radiant (solar) energy to synthesize glucose from carbon dioxide and water, while oxygen flows to the environment. Plants also convert carbohydrates to lipids and proteins for storage as a future reserve for energy and to sustain growth. Animals then ingest plant nutrients to serve their own energy and growth needs. *In essence, solar energy coupled with photosynthesis provides animals with food and oxygen.*

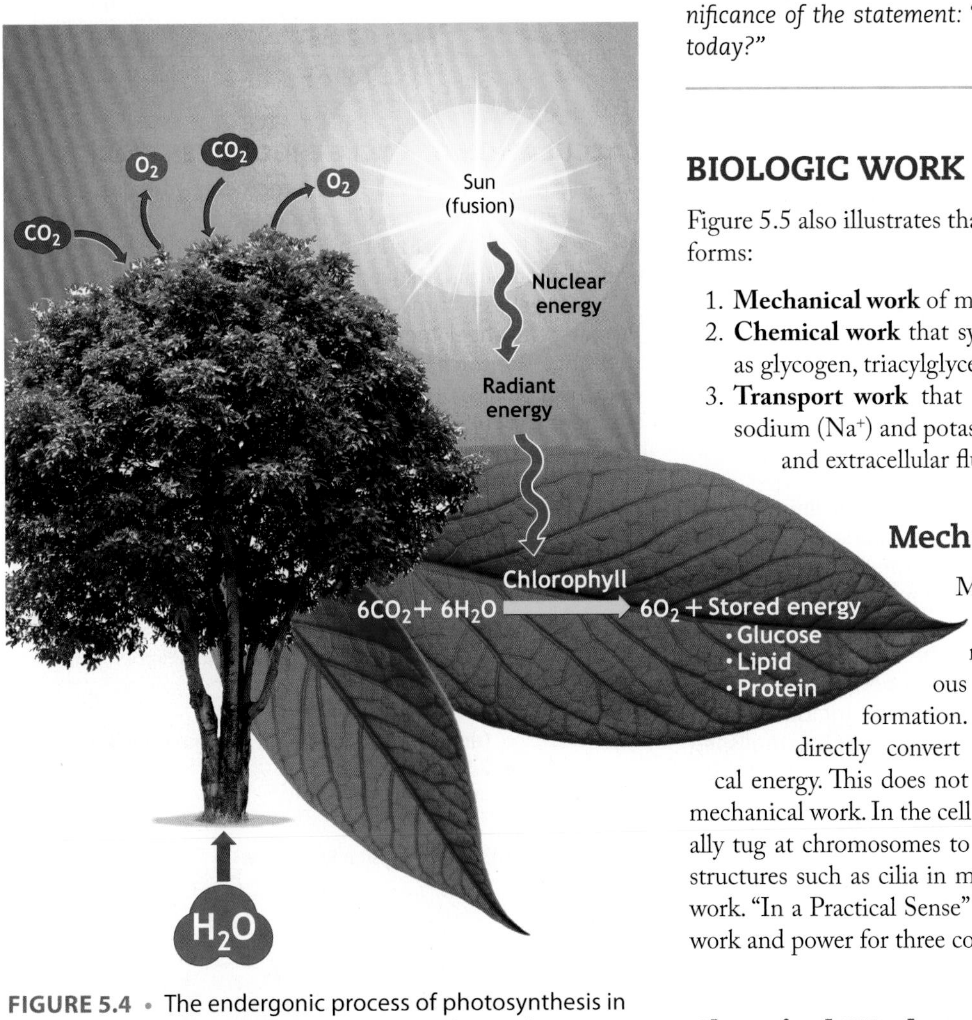

Respiration. FIGURE 5.5 illustrates the exergonic reactions of respiration (reverse of photosynthesis) as the plant's stored energy in the form of ATP transfers for mechanical work, chemical work, and transport work. With oxygen, the cells extract the chemical energy stored in the carbohydrate, lipid, and protein molecules. For the glucose molecule, respiration releases 689 kcal per mole (180 g) oxidized. *A portion of the energy released during cellular respiration is conserved in other chemical compounds for use in energy-requiring processes; the remaining energy flows to the environment as heat.*

INTEGRATIVE QUESTION

From the perspective of human bioenergetics, discuss the significance of the statement: "Have you thanked a green plant today?"

BIOLOGIC WORK IN HUMANS

Figure 5.5 also illustrates that biologic work takes one of three forms:

1. **Mechanical work** of muscle action
2. **Chemical work** that synthesizes cellular molecules such as glycogen, triacylglycerol, and protein
3. **Transport work** that concentrates substances such as sodium (Na^+) and potassium (K^+) ions in the intracellular and extracellular fluids

Mechanical Work

Mechanical work generated by muscle action and subsequent movement provides the most obvious physical example of energy transformation. A muscle fiber's protein filaments directly convert chemical energy into mechanical energy. This does not represent the body's only form of mechanical work. In the cell nucleus, contractile elements literally tug at chromosomes to facilitate cell division. Specialized structures such as cilia in many cells also perform mechanical work. "In a Practical Sense" shows the method for quantifying work and power for three common exercise forms.

Chemical Work

All cells perform chemical work for maintenance and growth. Continuous synthesis of cellular components takes place as other components degrade. Muscle tissue hypertrophy that

FIGURE 5.4 • The endergonic process of photosynthesis in plants, algae, and some bacteria serves as the mechanism to synthesize carbohydrates, lipids, and proteins. In this example, a glucose molecule forms when carbon dioxide binds with water with a positive free energy (useful energy) change (+ΔG).

O_2 CO_2 O_2 Sun (fusion)

CO_2

Nuclear energy

Radiant energy

Chlorophyll

$6CO_2 + 6H_2O \longrightarrow 6O_2 +$ Stored energy
• Glucose
• Lipid
• Protein

H_2O

IN A PRACTICAL SENSE

Measurement of Work on a Treadmill, Cycle Ergometer, and Step Bench

An ergometer is an exercise apparatus that quantifies and standardizes physical activity in terms of work and/or power output. The most common ergometers include treadmills, cycle and arm-crank ergometers, stair steppers, and rowers.

Work (W) represents application of force (F) through a distance (D):

$$W = F \times D$$

For example, for a body mass of 70 kg and vertical jump score of 0.5 m, work accomplished equals 35 kilogram-meters (70 kg × 0.5 m). The most common units of measurement to express work include kilogram-meters (kg-m), foot-pounds (ft-lb), joules (J), Newton-meters (Nm), and kilocalories (kcal).

Power (P) represents W performed per unit time (T):

$$P = F \times D \div T$$

CALCULATION OF TREADMILL WORK

Consider the treadmill as a moving conveyor belt with variable angle of incline and speed. Work performed on a treadmill equals the product of the weight (mass) of the person (F) and the vertical distance (*vert dist*) the person achieves walking or running up the incline. *Vert dist* equals the sine of the treadmill angle (theta, or θ) multiplied by the distance traveled (D) along the incline (treadmill speed × time):

$$W = body\ mass\ (force) \times vertical\ distance$$

Example

For an angle θ of 8° (measured with an inclinometer or determined by knowing the percent grade of the treadmill), the sine of angle θ equals 0.1392 (see table). The *vert dist* represents treadmill speed multiplied by exercise duration multiplied by sine θ. For example, *vert dist* on the incline while walking at 5000 m·hr⁻¹ for 1 hr equals 696 m (5000 × 0.1392). If a person with a body mass of 50 kg walked on a treadmill at an incline of 8° (grade approximately 14%) for 60 min at 5000 m·hr⁻¹, work accomplished computes as:

$$W = F \times \textbf{vert dist (sine θ} \times D)$$
$$= 50\ kg \times (0.1392 \times 5000\ m)$$
$$= 34,800\ kg\text{-}m$$

The value for power equals 34,800 kg-m ÷ 60 min, or 580 kg-m·min⁻¹.

Angle (°)	Sine (θ)	Grade (%)
1	0.0175	1.75
2	0.0349	3.49
3	0.0523	5.23
4	0.0698	6.98
5	0.0872	8.72
6	0.1045	10.51
7	0.1219	12.28
8	0.1392	14.05
9	0.1564	15.84
10	0.1736	17.63
15	0.2588	26.80
20	0.3420	36.40

CALCULATION OF CYCLE ERGOMETER WORK

The mechanically braked cycle ergometer contains a flywheel with a belt around it connected by a small spring at one end and an adjustable tension lever at the other end. A pendulum balance indicates the resistance against the flywheel as it turns. Increasing the tension on the belt increases flywheel friction, which increases resistance to pedaling. The force (flywheel friction) represents braking load in kg or kilopounds (kp = force acting on 1-kg mass at the normal acceleration of gravity). The distance traveled equals the number of pedal revolutions multiplied by the flywheel circumference.

Example

A person pedaling a bicycle ergometer with a 6-m flywheel circumference at 60 rpm for 1 min covers a distance (D) of 360 m each minute (6 m × 60). If the frictional resistance on the flywheel equals 2.5 kg, total work computes as:

$$W = F \times D$$
$$= frictional\ resistance \times distance\ traveled$$
$$= 2.5\ kg \times 360\ m$$
$$= 900\ kg\text{-}m$$

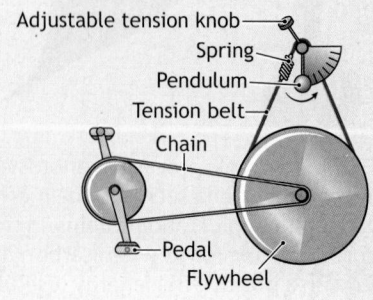

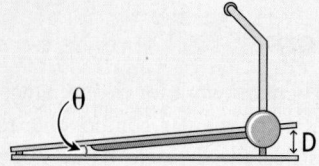

IN A PRACTICAL SENSE *(continued)*

Power generated by the effort equals 900 kg-m in 1 min or 900 kg-m · min⁻¹ (900 kg-m ÷ min).

CALCULATION OF WORK DURING BENCH STEPPING

Only the vertical (positive) work can be calculated in bench stepping. Distance (*D*) computes as bench height times the number of steps taken; force (*F*) equals the person's body mass (kg).

Example

If a 70-kg person steps on a bench 0.375-m high at a rate of 30 steps per minute for 10 min, total work computes as:

$$W = F \times D$$
$$= \text{body mass, kg} \times (\text{vertical distance [m]} \times \text{steps per min} \times 10 \text{ min})$$
$$= 70 \text{ kg} \times (0.375 \text{ m} \times 30 \times 10)$$
$$= 7875 \text{ kg-m}$$

Power generated during stepping equals 787 kg-m · min⁻¹ (7875 kg-m ÷ 10 min).

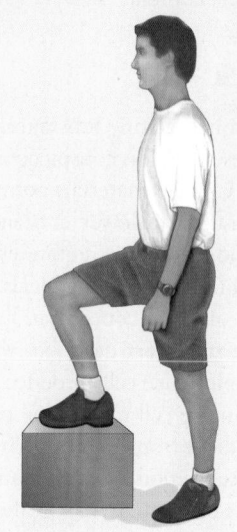

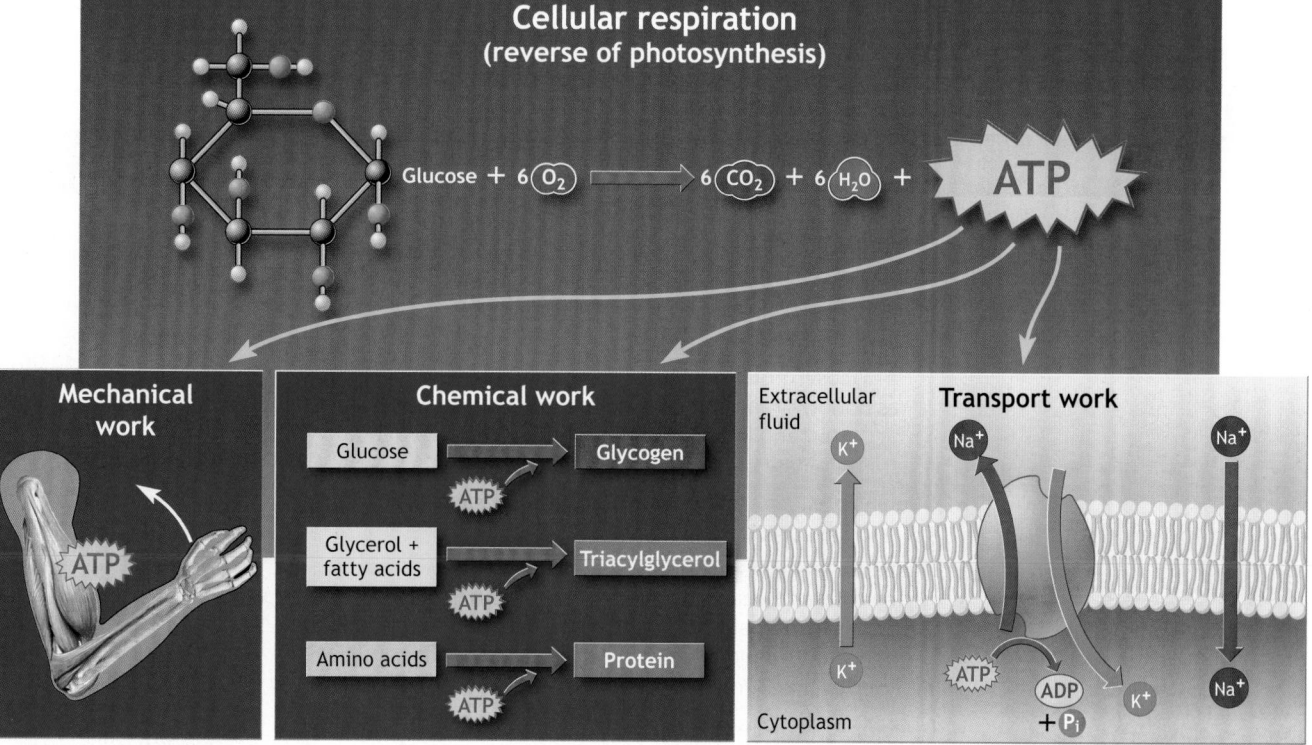

FIGURE 5.5 • The exergonic process of cellular respiration. Exergonic reactions, such as the burning of gasoline or the oxidation of glucose, release potential energy. This produces a negative standard free energy change (i.e., reduction in total energy available for work, or $-\Delta G$). In this illustration, cellular respiration harvests the potential energy in food to form ATP. Subsequently, the energy in ATP powers all forms of biologic work.

occurs in response to chronic overload in resistance training vividly illustrates chemical work as individual fibers increase their protein contractile content.

Transport Work

The biologic work of concentrating substances in the body's trillions of cells progresses much less conspicuously than mechanical or chemical work. Cellular materials normally flow from an area of high concentration to lower concentration. This passive process of **diffusion** does not require energy. Under normal physiologic conditions, some chemicals require transport "uphill" from an area of lower concentration to one of higher concentration. **Active transport** describes this energy-requiring process. For example, when cells produce ATP in the mitochondria, organelles in the cell membrane pump the ATP up the concentration gradient from an area of lower concentration to one of higher concentration. Secretion and reabsorption in the kidney tubules rely on active transport mechanisms, as does neural tissue to establish the proper electrochemical gradients about its plasma membranes. These "quiet" forms of biologic work require a continual expenditure of stored chemical energy.

ENZYMES AND COENZYMES ALTER THE RATE OF ENERGY RELEASE

The upper limits of exercise intensity ultimately depend on the rate that cells extract, conserve, and transfer chemical energy from food nutrients to the skeletal muscle's contractile filaments. *The sustained pace of a marathon runner at close to 90% of aerobic capacity, or the sprinter's rapid speed in all-out running, directly reflects the body's capacity to transfer chemical energy into mechanical work.*

Enzymes as Biologic Catalysts

Enzymes, highly specific and large protein catalysts, accelerate the forward and reverse rates of chemical reactions without themselves being consumed or changed during the reaction. Enzymes only govern reactions that normally take place, but at a much slower rate. In a way, enzymes reduce required **activation energy**—the energy input to initiate a reaction—so the reaction's rate changes. Enzyme action takes place without altering equilibrium constants and total energy released (free energy change or ΔG) in the reaction.

Enzymes possess the unique property of not being readily altered by the reactions they affect. Consequently, enzyme turnover in the body remains slow, and specific enzymes are continually reused. A typical mitochondrion may contain up to 10 billion enzyme molecules, each carrying out millions of operations within a brief time. During all-out physical activity, enzyme activity increases as energy demands rise about 100 times the resting levels. A single cell can contain thousands of different enzymes, each with a specific function that catalyzes a distinct cellular reaction. For example, glucose breakdown to carbon dioxide and water requires 19 different

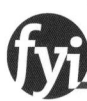 **Six Classifications of Enzymes**

Name	Action	Example
Oxidoreductases	Catalyze oxidation-reduction reactions where the substrate oxidized is regarded as hydrogen or electron donor; includes dehydrogenases, oxidases, oxygenases, reductases, peroxidases, and hydroxylases.	Lactate dehydrogenase
Transferases	Catalyze the transfer of a group (e.g., the methyl group or a glycosyl group) from one compound (generally regarded as donor) to another compound (generally regarded as acceptor) and include kinases, transcarboxylases, and transaminases.	Hexokinase
Hydrolases	Catalyze reactions that add water; include esterases, phosphatases, and peptidases.	Lipase
Lyases	Catalyze reactions that cleave C–C, C–O, C–N, and other bonds by different means than by hydrolysis or oxidation. They differ from other enzymes in that two substrates are involved in one reaction direction, but only one in the other direction. Include synthases, deaminases, and decarboxylases.	Carbonic anhydrase
Isomerases	Catalyze reactions that rearrange molecular structure; include isomerases and epimerases. These enzymes catalyze changes within one molecule.	Phosphoglycerate mutase
Ligases	Catalyze bond formation between two substrate molecules with concomitant hydrolysis of the diphosphate bond in ATP or a similar triphosphate.	Pyruvate carboxylase

chemical reactions, each catalyzed by its own specific enzyme. Many enzymes operate outside the cell—in the bloodstream, digestive mixture, or intestinal fluids.

Enzymes Alter Reaction Rates

Enzymes do not all operate at the same rate; some operate slowly, others more rapidly. Consider the enzyme carbonic anhydrase, which catalyzes the hydration of carbon dioxide to form carbonic acid. Its maximum **turnover number**—number of moles of substrate that react to form product per mole of enzyme per unit time—is 800,000. In contrast, the turnover number is only two for tryptophan synthetase, which catalyzes the final step in tryptophan synthesis. Enzymes also act along small regions of substrate, each time working at a different rate than previously. Some enzymes delay initiating their work. The precursor digestive enzyme trypsinogen, manufactured by the pancreas in its inactive form, serves as a good example. Trypsinogen enters the small intestine where enzyme action activates it and changes its molecular configuration so it now becomes the active enzyme trypsin. This "changed" enzyme digests complex proteins into simple amino acids. **Proteolytic action** describes this catabolic process. Without the delay in activity, trypsinogen would literally digest the pancreatic tissue that produced it.

FIGURE 5.6 shows that pH and temperature dramatically alter enzyme activity to change reaction rates. For some enzymes, peak activity requires high acidity, whereas others function optimally on the alkaline side of neutrality. Note that the two enzymes pepsin and trypsin (Fig. 5.6B) exhibit different pH profiles that modify their activity rates and determine optimal function. Pepsin operates optimally at a pH between 2.4 and 2.6, whereas trypsin's optimum range approximates that of saliva and milk (6.2 to 6.6). This pH effect on enzyme dynamics takes place because changing a fluid's hydrogen ion concentration alters the balance between positively and negatively charged molecular complexes in the enzyme's amino acids. Increases in temperature generally accelerate enzyme

reactivity. As temperature rises above 104 to 122°F (40 to 50°C), the protein enzymes permanently change the nature of their natural qualities (denature) and their activity ceases.

Enzyme Mode of Action

The unique characteristic of an enzyme's three-dimensional globular protein structure defines the interaction with its specific substrate. FIGURE 5.7 illustrates how interaction works similar to a key fitting a lock. The enzyme "turns on" when its **active site**, usually a groove, cleft, or cavity on the protein's surface, joins in a "perfect fit" with the substrate's active site. Upon forming an **enzyme–substrate complex**, the splitting of chemical bonds forms a new product with new bonds. This immediately frees the enzyme to act on additional substrate. A more contemporary hypothesis considers the lock and key more of an "induced fit" because of the required conformational characteristics of enzymes. The example depicts the interaction sequence of the enzyme maltase as it disassembles or hydrolyzes maltose into its component two glucose building blocks:

Step 1: The active site of the enzyme and substrate line up to achieve a perfect fit and form an enzyme–substrate complex.
Step 2: The enzyme catalyzes or greatly speeds up the chemical reaction with the substrate. Note that the hydrolysis reaction adds a water molecule.
Step 3: An end product forms (two glucose molecules) to release the enzyme to act on another substrate.

German chemist and 1902 Nobel laureate Emil Fischer (1852–1919) first proposed the "**lock-and-key mechanism**" to describe the enzyme–substrate interaction (http://www.nobelprize.org/nobel_prizes/chemistry/laureates/1902/fischer-bio.html). This process ensures that the correct enzyme "mates" with its specific substrate to perform a particular function. Once the enzyme and substrate join, a *conformational change* in enzyme shape takes place as it molds to the substrate. Even if an enzyme links with a substrate, unless the specific conformational change

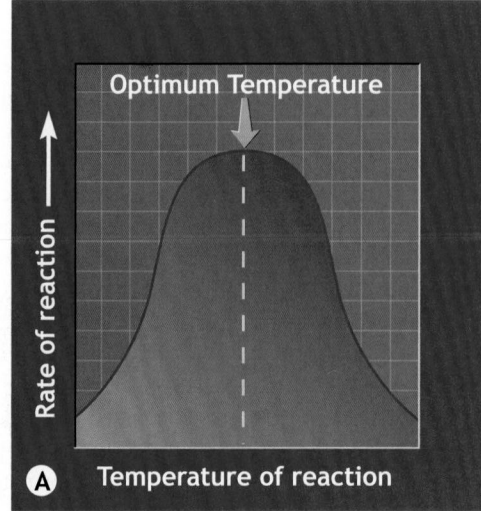
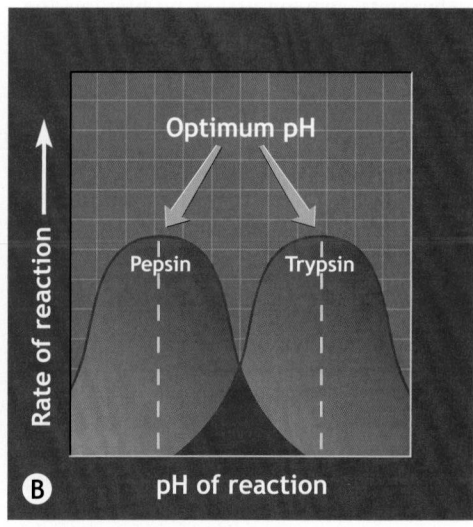

FIGURE 5.6 • Effects of **(A)** temperature and **(B)** pH on the enzyme action turnover rate.

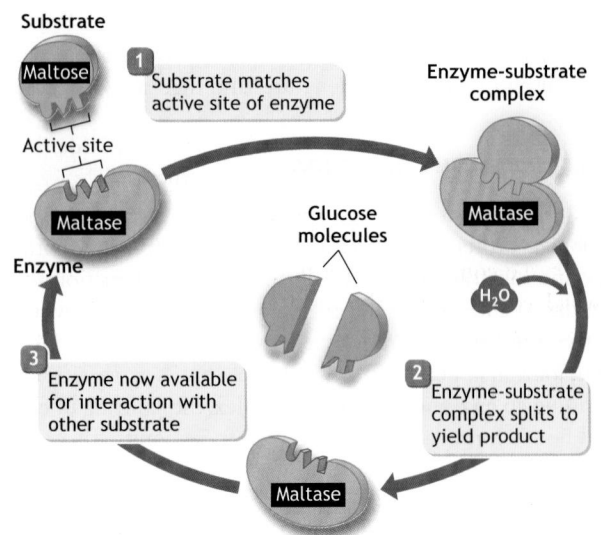

FIGURE 5.7 • Sequence of steps in the "lock-and-key mechanism" of an enzyme with its substrate. The example shows how two monosaccharide glucose molecules form when maltase interacts with its disaccharide substrate maltose.

occurs in the enzyme's shape, it will not interact chemically with the substrate.

The lock-and-key mechanism serves a protective function so only the correct enzyme activates a given substrate. Consider the enzyme hexokinase, which accelerates a chemical reaction by linking with a glucose molecule. When this occurs, a phosphate molecule transfers from ATP to a specific binding site on one of glucose's carbon atoms. Once the two binding sites join to form a glucose–hexokinase complex, the substrate begins its stepwise degradation, controlled by other specific enzymes, to form less complex molecules during energy metabolism.

Coenzymes

Some enzymes remain totally dormant unless activated by additional substances called **coenzymes**. These nonprotein organic substances facilitate enzyme action by binding the substrate with a specific enzyme. Coenzymes then regenerate to assist in further similar reactions. The metallic ions iron and zinc play coenzyme roles, as do the B vitamins or their derivatives. Oxidation–reduction reactions use the B vitamins riboflavin and niacin, while other vitamins serve as transfer agents for groups of compounds in different metabolic processes (see Table 2.1).

 **Vitamins Serve as Coenzymes But Do Not Provide Energy**

Some advertisements for vitamins imply that taking vitamin supplements provides immediate usable energy for exercise. This simply does not occur. Vitamins often serve as coenzymes to "make reactions go," but they contain no chemical energy for biologic work.

A coenzyme requires less specificity in its action than an enzyme because the coenzyme affects a number of different reactions. It acts either as a "cobinder" or as a temporary carrier of intermediary products in the reaction. For example, the coenzyme **nicotinamide adenine dinucleotide** (**NAD⁺**) forms NADH in transporting hydrogen atoms and electrons released from food fragments during energy metabolism. The electrons then pass to other special transporter molecules in another series of chemical reactions that ultimately deliver the electrons to oxygen.

Enzyme Inhibition

Many substances inhibit enzyme activity to slow a reaction rate. **Competitive inhibitors** closely resemble the structure of the normal substrate for an enzyme. They bind to the enzyme's active site but the enzyme cannot change them. The inhibitor repetitively occupies the active site and blunts the enzyme's interaction with its substrate. **Noncompetitive inhibitors** do not resemble the enzyme's substrate and do not bind to its active site. Instead, they bind to the enzyme at a site other than the active site. This changes the enzyme's structure and ability to catalyze the reaction because of the presence of the bound inhibitor. Some drugs used in the treatment of cancer, depression, and acquired immunodeficiency syndrome act as noncompetitive enzyme inhibitors (as do some poisons, pesticides, antibiotics, and painkillers).

HYDROLYSIS AND CONDENSATION: THE BASIS FOR DIGESTION AND SYNTHESIS

In general, hydrolysis reactions digest or degrade complex molecules into simpler subunits; condensation reactions build larger molecules by bonding their subunits.

Hydrolysis Reactions

Hydrolysis catabolizes carbohydrates, lipids, and proteins into simpler forms that the body absorbs and assimilates. This basic decomposition process splits chemical bonds by adding H^+ and OH^- (constituents of water) to the reaction byproducts. Examples of hydrolytic reactions include digestion of starches and disaccharides to monosaccharides, proteins to amino acids, and lipids to their glycerol and fatty acid constituents. Specific enzymes catalyze each step of the breakdown process. For disaccharides, the enzymes are lactase (lactose), sucrase (sucrose), and maltase (maltose). The lipid enzymes called lipases degrade the triacylglycerol molecule by adding water. This cleaves the fatty acids from their glycerol backbone. During protein digestion, protease enzymes accelerate amino acid release when the addition of water splits the peptide linkages. The following represents the general form for all hydrolysis reactions:

$$AB + HOH \rightarrow A\text{-}H + B\text{-}OH$$

Water added to the substance AB causes the chemical bond that joins AB to decompose and produce the breakdown products A-H (H refers to a hydrogen atom from water) and B-OH (OH refers to the hydroxyl group from water). FIGURE 5.8A illustrates the hydrolysis reaction for the disaccharide sucrose to its end-product molecules, glucose and fructose. The figure also shows the hydrolysis of a dipeptide (a protein) into its two constituent amino acid units. Intestinal absorption occurs following hydrolysis of the carbohydrate, lipid, and protein macronutrients.

 See the animation "Hydrolysis" on **http://thePoint. lww.com/mkk8e** for a demonstration of this process.

Condensation Reactions

The reactions of hydrolysis can reverse direction as the compound AB synthesizes from A-H and B-OH. A water molecule also forms in this building process of **condensation** (also termed *dehydration synthesis*). The structural components of the nutrients bind together in condensation reactions to form more complex molecules and compounds. FIGURE 5.8B shows the condensation reactions for maltose synthesis from two glucose units and the synthesis of a more complex protein from two amino acid units. During protein synthesis, a hydroxyl removed from one amino acid and a hydrogen removed from the other amino acid join to create a water molecule. The term

Ⓐ Hydrolysis

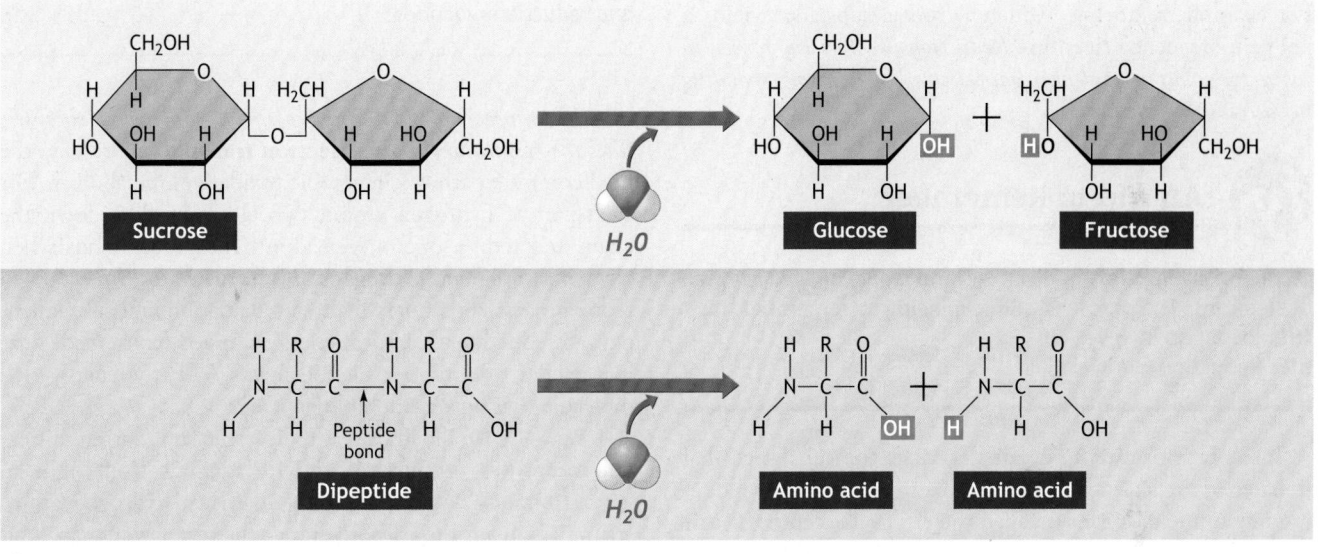

Ⓑ Condensation

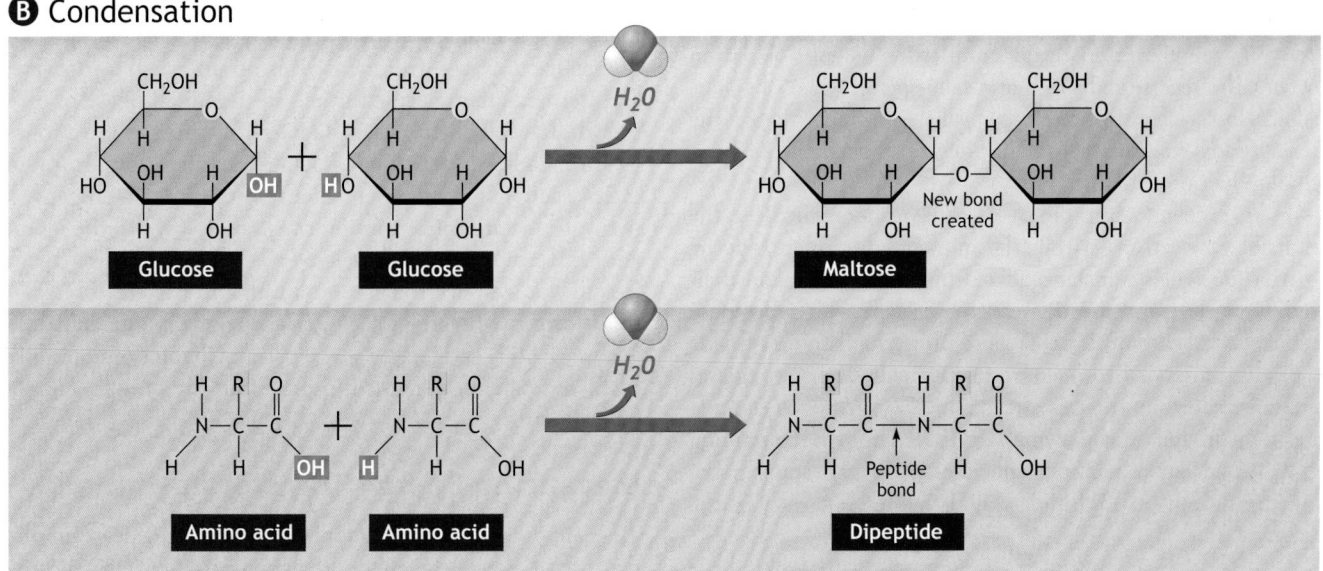

FIGURE 5.8 • **(A)** Hydrolysis of the disaccharide sucrose to the end-product molecules glucose and fructose and the hydrolysis of a dipeptide (protein) into two amino acid constituents. **(B)** A condensation chemical reaction for synthesizing maltose from two glucose units and creation of a protein dipeptide from two amino acid subunits. Note that the reactions in **B** illustrate the reverse of the hydrolysis reaction for the dipeptide. The symbol R represents the remainder of the molecule.

peptide bond describes the new bond that forms for the protein. Water also forms in the synthesis of more complex carbohydrates from simple sugars; for lipids, water forms when glycerol and fatty acid components combine to form a triacylglycerol molecule.

 See the animation "Condensation" on **http://the Point.lww.com/mkk8e** for a demonstration of this process.

Oxidation and Reduction Reactions

Literally thousands of simultaneous chemical reactions occur in the body involving the transfer of electrons from one substance to another. *Oxidation reactions transfer oxygen atoms, hydrogen atoms, or electrons.* A loss of electrons always occurs in oxidation reactions, with a corresponding net gain in valence. For example, removing hydrogen from a substance yields a net gain of valence electrons. *Reduction involves any process in which the atoms in an element gain electrons, with a corresponding net decrease in valence.*

 An Aid to Remember

Oxidation involves loss of electrons and *reduction involves gain* of electrons . The phrase OIL RIG can help you remember this:
OIL: Oxidation Involves Loss
RIG: Reduction Involves Gain

The term **reducing agent** describes the substance that donates or loses electrons as it oxidizes. The substance reducing or gaining electrons is called the electron acceptor or **oxidizing agent**. Electron transfer requires both oxidizing and reducing agents, and the process of oxidation and reduction reactions are characteristically **coupled**. Whenever oxidation occurs, the reverse reduction also takes place; when one substance loses electrons, the other substance gains them. The term **redox reaction** commonly describes a coupled oxidation–reduction reaction.

An excellent example of a redox reaction involves the transfer of electrons within the mitochondria. Here, special carrier molecules transfer oxidized hydrogen atoms and their removed electrons for delivery to oxygen, which becomes reduced. The carbohydrate, fat, and protein substrates provide a ready source of hydrogen atoms. Dehydrogenase (oxidase) enzymes speed up the redox reactions. Two hydrogen-accepting dehydrogenase coenzymes are the vitamin B–containing NAD^+ and flavin adenine dinucleotide (FAD). Transferring electrons from NADH and $FADH_2$ harnesses energy in the form of ATP.

Energy release in glucose oxidation occurs when electrons reposition or shift as they move closer to oxygen atoms—their final destination. The close-up illustration of a mitochondrion in **FIGURE 5.9** shows the different chemical events that occur on the outer and inner mitochondrial membranes and matrix. The inset table summarizes the mitochondrion's various chemical reactions related to its structures in the outer membrane (4 reactions), inner membrane (5 reactions), and matrix (8 reactions). Most of the energy-generating "action," including the redox reactions, takes place within the mitochondrial matrix. The inner membrane is rich in protein (70%) and lipid (30%), two key macromolecules whose configurations encourage transfer of chemicals through membranes.

 INTEGRATIVE QUESTION

What biologic benefit comes from the coupling of oxidation and reduction reactions?

*The transport of electrons by specific carrier molecules constitutes the **respiratory chain**.* **Electron transport** represents the final common pathway in aerobic (oxidative) metabolism. For each pair of hydrogen atoms, two electrons flow down the chain and reduce one oxygen atom. The process ends when oxygen accepts two hydrogens and forms water. This coupled redox process constitutes hydrogen oxidation and subsequent oxygen reduction. Chemical energy trapped (conserved) during cellular oxidation–reduction forms ATP, the energy-rich molecule that powers all biologic work.

FIGURE 5.10 illustrates a redox reaction during different intensities of physical activity ranging from light to very strenuous. With increasing intensity, hydrogen atoms strip away from the carbohydrate substrate faster than their oxidation along the respiratory chain. To continue energy metabolism, a substance other than oxygen must "accept" the nonoxidized excess hydrogens. This occurs when a pyruvate, an intermediate molecule formed in the initial phase of carbohydrate catabolism, accepts a pair of hydrogens (electrons) to form ionized lactic acid (lactate) in the body. As more intense activity produces a greater flow of excess hydrogens to pyruvate, lactate concentration rises rapidly within the blood and active muscle. During recovery, the excess hydrogens in lactate oxidize (electrons are removed and passed to NAD^+) to re-form a pyruvate molecule. The enzyme lactate dehydrogenase (LDH) accelerates this reversal. Chapter 6 more fully discusses oxidation–reduction reactions in human energy metabolism.

Measuring Energy Transfer in Humans

The gain or loss of heat in a biologic system provides a simplified way to assess the energy dynamics of any chemical process. In food catabolism within the body, a human calorimeter

Cell

Mitochondrion

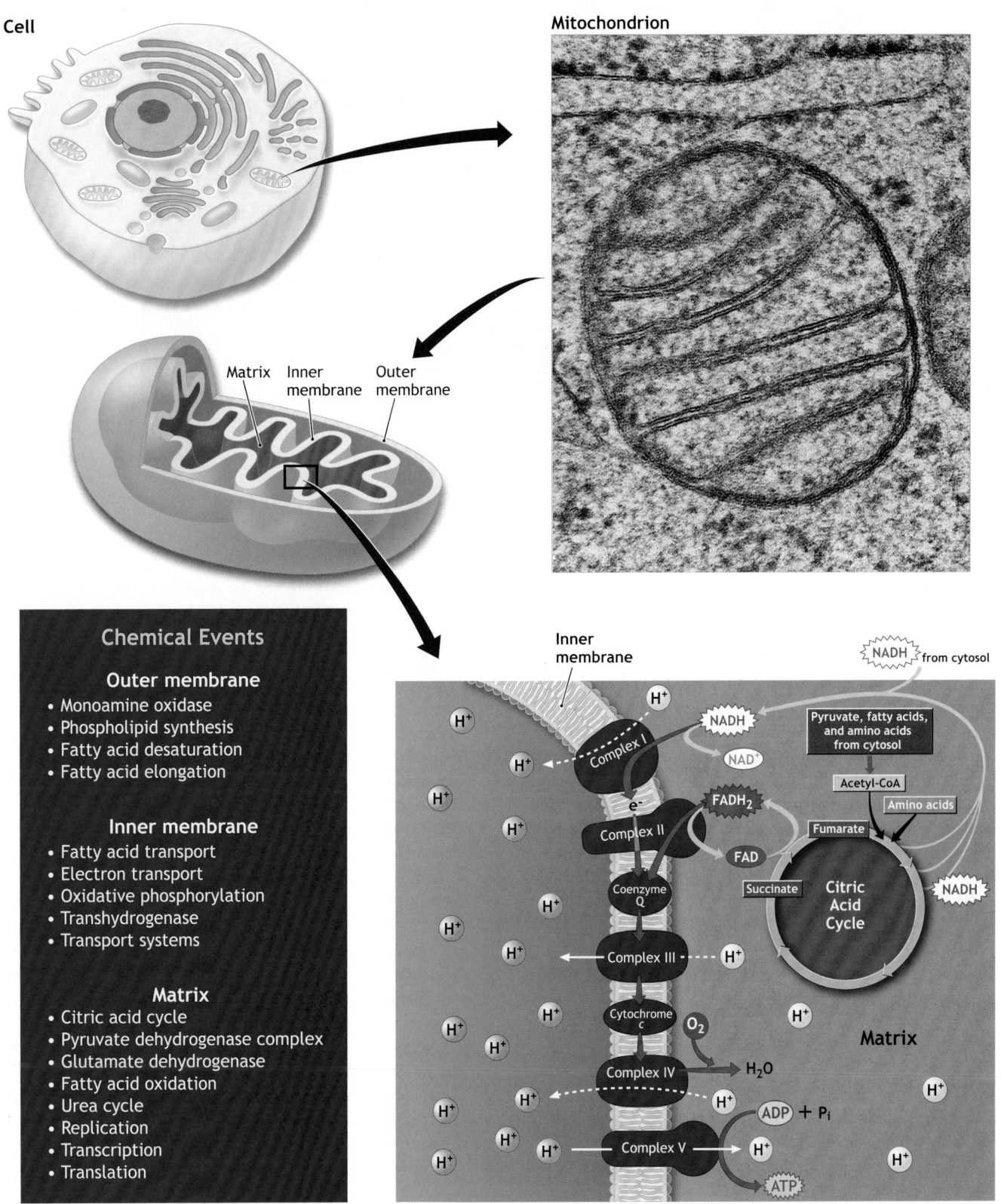

Matrix   Inner membrane   Outer membrane

Chemical Events

Outer membrane
- Monoamine oxidase
- Phospholipid synthesis
- Fatty acid desaturation
- Fatty acid elongation

Inner membrane
- Fatty acid transport
- Electron transport
- Oxidative phosphorylation
- Transhydrogenase
- Transport systems

Matrix
- Citric acid cycle
- Pyruvate dehydrogenase complex
- Glutamate dehydrogenase
- Fatty acid oxidation
- Urea cycle
- Replication
- Transcription
- Translation

Inner membrane

NADH from cytosol

Complex I   NADH   NAD$^+$

Pyruvate, fatty acids, and amino acids from cytosol

Acetyl-CoA   Amino acids

e$^-$

Complex II   FADH$_2$ FAD   Fumarate

Coenzyme Q   Succinate   **Citric Acid Cycle**   NADH

Complex III   H$^+$

Cytochrome c O$_2$ **Matrix**

Complex IV   H$_2$O

ADP + P$_i$

Complex V   H$^+$

ATP

FIGURE 5.9 • The mitochondrion, its intramitochondrial structures, and primary chemical reactions. The inset table summarizes the different chemical events in relation to mitochondrial structures.

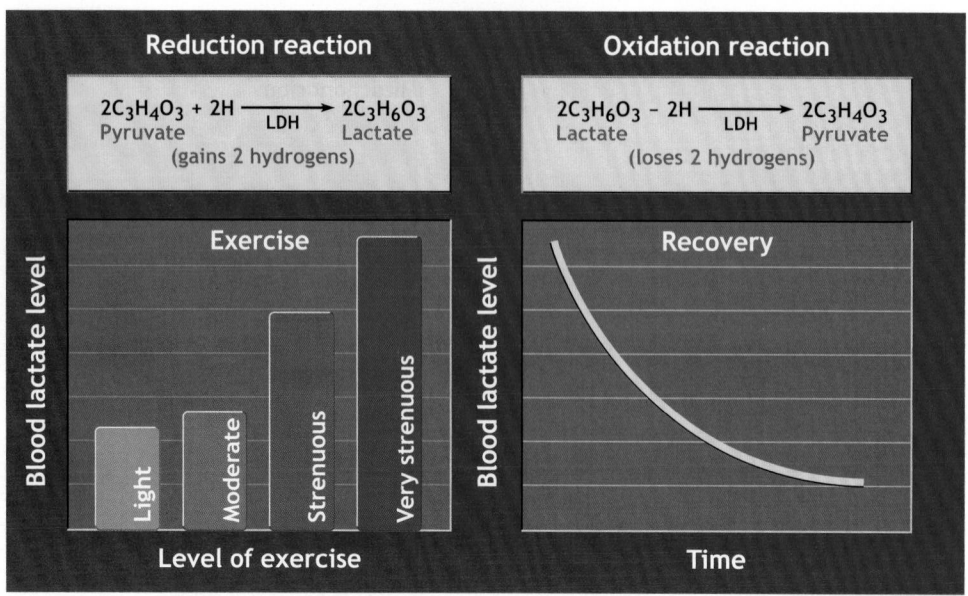

FIGURE 5.10 • Example of a redox (oxidation–reduction) reaction. During progressively more strenuous exercise when oxygen supply (or use) becomes inadequate, some pyruvate formed in energy metabolism gains two hydrogens (two electrons) and becomes reduced to a new compound, lactate. In recovery, when oxygen supply (or use) becomes adequate, lactate loses two hydrogens (two electrons) and oxidizes back to pyruvate. This example shows how a redox reaction continues energy metabolism, despite limited oxygen availability (or use) in relation to exercise energy demands.

(see Fig. 8.1 in Chapter 8), similar to the bomb calorimeter described in Chapter 4 (see Fig. 4.1), measures the energy change directly as heat (kcal) released from the chemical reactions.

The complete combustion of food takes place at the expense of molecular oxygen, so the heat generated in these exergonic reactions can be inferred readily from oxygen consumption measurements. Oxygen consumption measurement forms the basis of indirect calorimetry to determine the energy expended by humans during rest and diverse physical activities. Chapter 8 discusses how direct and indirect calorimetry determine heat production or energy metabolism in humans.

 INTEGRATIVE QUESTION

Discuss the implications of the second law of thermodynamics for measuring energy expenditure.

Summary

1. *Energy*, defined as the ability to perform work, emerges only when a change takes place.
2. Energy exists in either potential or kinetic form. *Potential energy* refers to energy associated with a substance's structure or position; *kinetic energy* refers to energy of motion. Potential energy can be measured when it transforms into kinetic energy.
3. The six forms of energy are chemical, mechanical, heat, light, electrical, and nuclear. Each energy form can convert or transform to another form.
4. Exergonic energy reactions release energy to the surroundings. Endergonic energy reactions store, conserve, or increase free energy. All potential energy ultimately degrades into kinetic or heat energy.
5. Living organisms temporarily conserve a portion of potential energy within the structure of new compounds, some of which power biologic work.
6. Entropy describes the tendency of potential energy to degrade to kinetic energy with a lower capacity for work.
7. Plants transfer the energy of sunlight to the potential energy bound within carbohydrates, lipids, and proteins through the endergonic process of photosynthesis.
8. Respiration, an exergonic process, releases stored energy in plants for coupling to other chemical compounds for biologic work.
9. Energy transfer in humans supports three forms of biologic work: chemical (biosynthesis of cellular molecules), mechanical (muscle contraction), or transport (transfer of substances among cells).
10. Enzymes represent highly specific protein catalysts that accelerate chemical reaction rates without being consumed or changed in the reaction.
11. Coenzymes consist of nonprotein organic substances that facilitate enzyme action by binding a substrate to its specific enzyme.

12. Hydrolysis (catabolism) of complex organic molecules performs critical functions in macronutrient digestion and energy metabolism. Condensation (anabolism) reactions synthesize complex biomolecules for tissue maintenance and growth.

13. The linking or coupling of oxidation–reduction (redox) reactions enables oxidation (substance loses electrons) to coincide with the reverse reaction of reduction (substance gains electrons).

14. Redox reactions provide the basis for the body's energy-transfer processes.

15. The transport of electrons by specific carrier molecules constitutes the respiratory chain. Electron transport represents the final common pathway in aerobic metabolism.

thePoint Suggested readings are available online at
http://thepoint.lww.com/mkk8e.

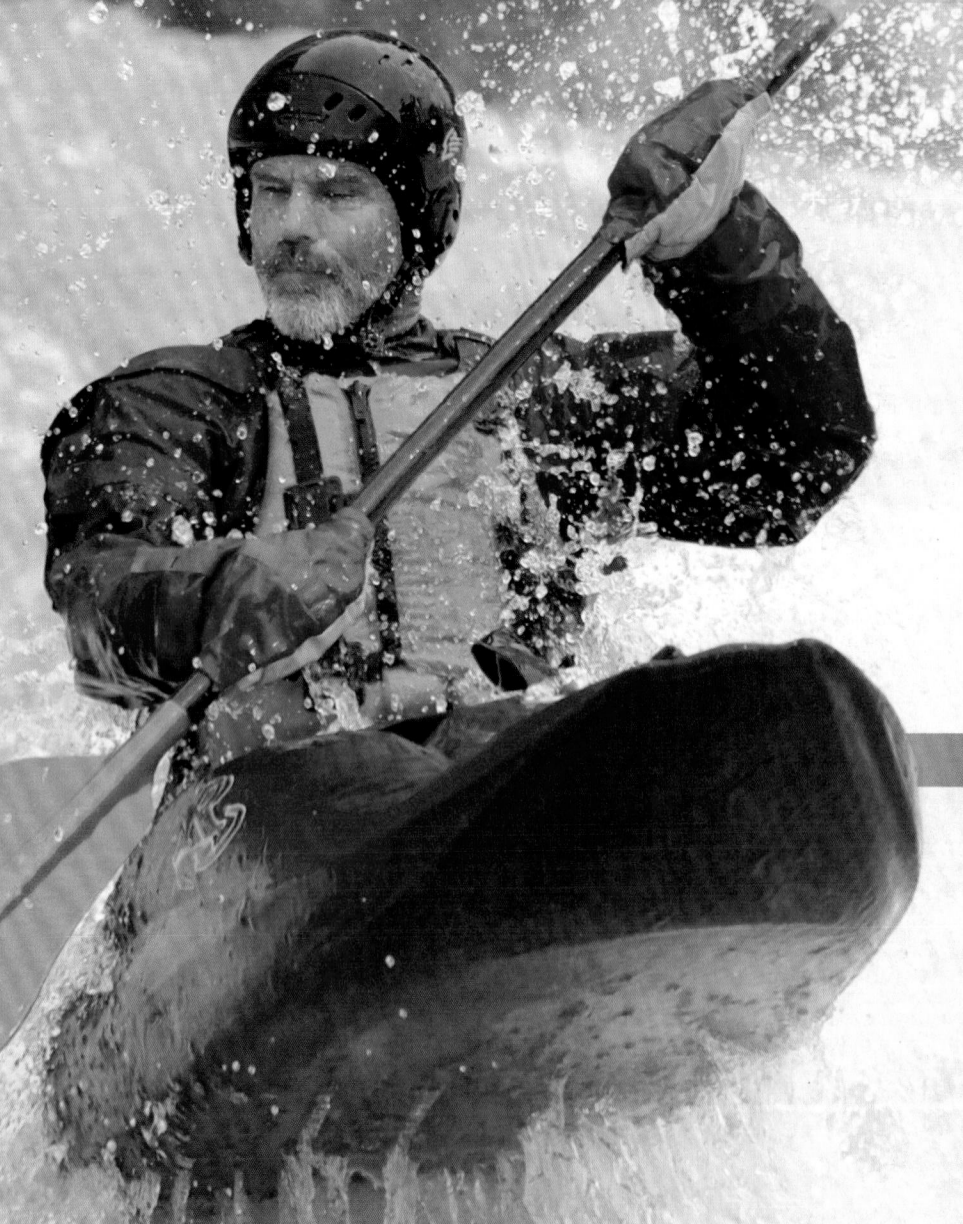

Energy Transfer in the Body

Humans require a continual supply of chemical energy to maintain numerous complex physiologic functions. Energy derived from food oxidation does not release suddenly at some kindling temperature, as occurs when organic materials combust and release heat. The body, unlike a mechanical engine, cannot use heat energy. If the body required only heat energy, body fluids would boil and tissues would burst into flames.

Instead, human energy dynamics involve transferring energy via chemical bonds. Potential energy within carbohydrate, fat, and protein bonds releases stepwise in small quantities with the splitting of chemical bonds. A portion of this energy is conserved when new bonds form during enzymatically controlled reactions in the cool, watery medium of the cell. Energy lost by one molecule transfers to the chemical structure of other molecules without appearing as heat. This provides for a high efficiency of energy transformations.

Biologic work occurs when compounds low in potential energy become "juiced up" from energy transfer via high-energy phosphate bonds. In a sense, the cells receive as much energy as they require. The story of how the body maintains its continuous energy supply begins with ATP, the special carrier molecule of free energy.

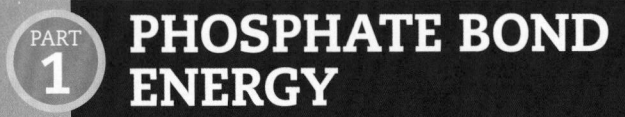

PART 1 — PHOSPHATE BOND ENERGY

ADENOSINE TRIPHOSPHATE: THE ENERGY CURRENCY

Energy in food does not transfer directly to cells for biologic work. Rather, energy from macronutrient oxidation is harvested and funneled through the energy-rich compound **adenosine triphosphate (ATP)**. The potential energy within this nucleotide molecule powers all of the cell's energy-requiring processes. In essence, the energy donor–energy receiver role of ATP represents the cells' two major energy-transforming activities:

1. Extract potential energy from food and conserve it within the bonds of ATP
2. Extract and transfer the chemical energy in ATP to power biologic work

ATP serves as the ideal energy-transfer agent. It "traps" within its phosphate bonds a large portion of the original food molecule's potential energy. ATP also readily transfers this trapped energy to other compounds to raise them to a higher activation level. The cell contains other high-energy compounds (e.g., phosphoenolpyruvate; 1,3-diphosphoglycerate; phosphocreatine), but ATP remains the most important. **Figure 6.1** shows how ATP forms from a molecule of adenine and ribose (called adenosine) linked to three phosphates

(triphosphate), each consisting of phosphorus and oxygen atoms. The bonds that link the two outermost phosphates (symbolized by) represent high-energy bonds because they release useful energy during hydrolysis. The released energy powers body functions including glandular secretion, digestion, tissue synthesis, circulatory function, muscle action, and nerve transmission. In muscle, the energy stimulates specific sites on the contractile elements to activate the molecular motors that power muscle fibers to shorten. A new compound, **adenosine diphosphate (ADP)**, forms when ATP joins with water, catalyzed by the enzyme **adenosine triphosphatase (ATPase).**

See the animation "ATPase" on **http://thePoint.lww.com/mkk8e** for a demonstration of this process.

This reaction cleaves ATP's outermost phosphate bond to release an inorganic phosphate ion and approximately 7.3 kcal of free energy, or $-\Delta G$ (i.e., energy available for work) per mole of ATP hydrolyzed to ADP. The symbol ΔG refers to the standard free energy change measured under laboratory conditions (77°F [25°C]; 1 atmosphere pressure; concentrations maintained at 1 molal at pH = 7.0). Standard laboratory conditions are seldom achieved in the body, yet this expression of free energy change makes comparisons possible under different conditions. In the intracellular environment, the value may actually approach 10 kcal·mol^{-1}.

$$ATP + H_2O \xrightarrow{ATPase} ADP + P_i - \Delta G\ 7.3\ kcal \cdot mol^{-1}$$

The free energy liberated in ATP hydrolysis reflects the energy difference between reactant and end product. This reaction generates considerable free energy, making ATP a **high-energy phosphate** compound. Infrequently, additional energy releases when another phosphate splits from ADP. In some reactions of biosynthesis, ATP donates its two terminal phosphates simultaneously to construct new cellular material. The remaining molecule, adenosine monophosphate (AMP), has a single phosphate group.

The energy liberated during ATP breakdown directly transfers to other energy-requiring molecules. *Energy from ATP hydrolysis powers all forms of biologic work; thus, ATP constitutes the cell's "energy currency."*

Figure 6.2 illustrates ATP's role as energy currency for the biologic work of macronutrient synthesis in anabolic (endergonic) processes and its subsequent reconstruction from ADP and a phosphate ion (P_i) via oxidation of stored macronutrients via catabolic or exergonic processes.

ATP splits almost instantly without the need for molecular oxygen. This capability to hydrolyze ATP without oxygen (anaerobically) generates rapid energy transfer. Bodily movements requiring this type of "rapid" energy include sprinting 10 s to catch a bus, lifting an object, swinging a golf club, spiking a volleyball, or performing a pull-up or push-up. In each case, energy metabolism proceeds uninterrupted because the energy required for the activity derives almost exclusively from intramuscular ATP hydrolysis.

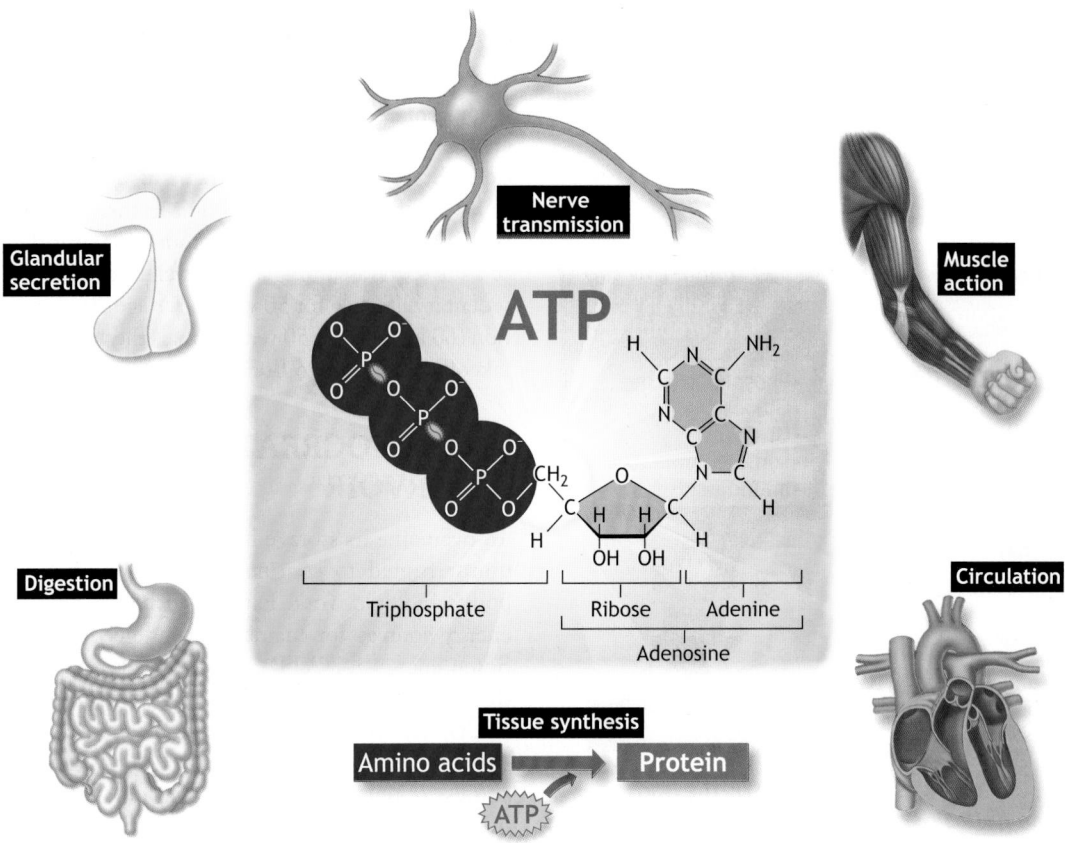

FIGURE 6.1 • Structure of ATP, the energy currency that powers all forms of biologic work. The symbol ⬤ represents high-energy bonds.

The body always attempts to maintain a continuous ATP supply through different metabolic pathways; some are located in the cell's cytosol, whereas others operate within the mitochondria (**FIG. 6.3**). For example, the cytosol contains the pathways for ATP production from the anaerobic breakdown of PCr, glucose, glycerol, and the carbon skeletons of some deaminated amino acids. Within the mitochondria, reactive processes harness cellular energy to generate ATP aerobically (see "Cellular Oxidation," later in this chapter)—the citric acid cycle and respiratory chain—from the catabolism of fatty acids, pyruvate, and some amino acids.

ATP: A Limited Currency

Cells contain a small quantity of ATP and must therefore continually resynthesize it at its rate of use. Only under extreme conditions of physical activity do ATP levels in skeletal muscle decrease. A limited ATP supply provides a biologically useful

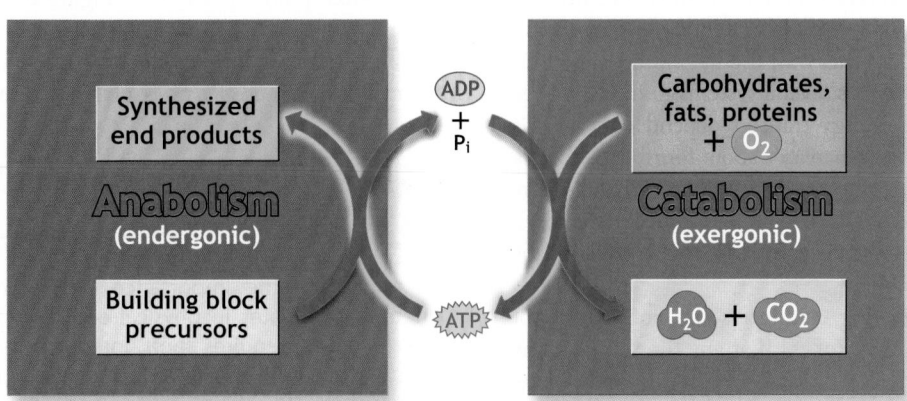

FIGURE 6.2 • Catabolism–anabolism interactions. Continual recycling of ATP for biologic work of macronutrient synthesis (anabolic or endergonic processes) and its subsequent reconstruction from ADP and a phosphate ion (P_i) via oxidation of the stored macronutrients (catabolic or exergonic processes).

Cell

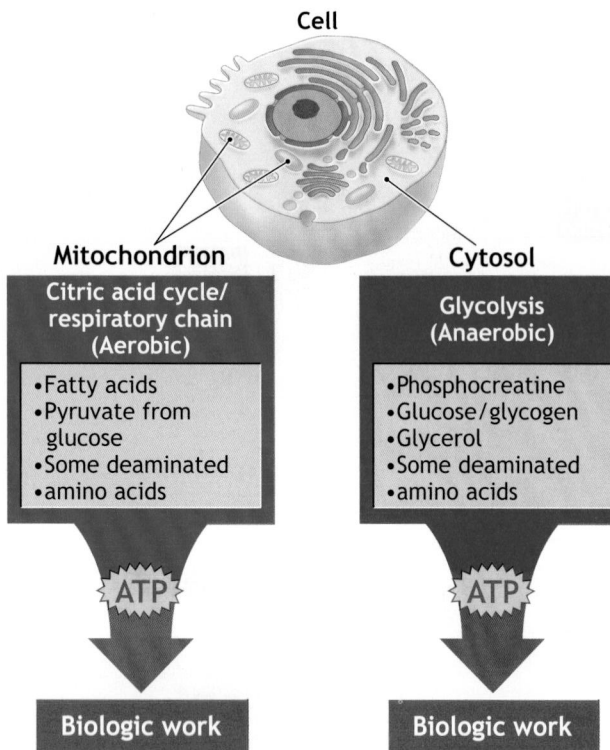

Mitochondrion

Citric acid cycle/ respiratory chain (Aerobic)
• Fatty acids • Pyruvate from glucose • Some deaminated • amino acids

Cytosol

Glycolysis (Anaerobic)
• Phosphocreatine • Glucose/glycogen • Glycerol • Some deaminated • amino acids

Biologic work   **Biologic work**

FIGURE 6.3 • Diverse ways to produce ATP. The body maintains a continuous ATP supply through different metabolic pathways: Some are located in the cell's cytosol, whereas others operate within the mitochondria. Reactions that harness cellular energy to generate ATP aerobically—the citric acid cycle and respiratory chain (including β-oxidation)—reside within the mitochondria. (Adapted with permission from McArdle WD, Katch FI, Katch VL. *Sports and Exercise Nutrition.* 4th Ed. Philadelphia: Wolters Kluwer Health, 2013.)

mechanism to regulate energy metabolism. By maintaining a small amount of ATP, the relative ATP concentration (and corresponding ADP, P_i, and AMP concentrations) changes rapidly in response to only a minimal ATP decrease. Any increase in energy requirement immediately disrupts the balance between ATP and ADP and P_i. The imbalance stimulates the breakdown of other stored energy-containing compounds to resynthesize ATP. In this way, the beginning of muscular movement rapidly activates several systems to increase energy transfer. Increases in energy transfer depend on movement intensity. Energy transfer increases about fourfold in the transition from sitting in a chair to slow walking. Changing from a slow walk to an all-out sprint almost immediately accelerates the rate of energy transfer within active muscles about 120-fold!

Under normal resting conditions the body stores only 80 to 100 g (about 3.0 oz) of ATP at any time. This quantity makes available each second approximately 2.4 mmol of ATP per kilogram wet muscle weight, or about 1.44×10^{10} molecules of ATP. This represents enough intramuscular stored energy to power several seconds of explosive, all-out physical activity.

ATP alone does not represent a significant energy reserve. This provides an advantage because of the relatively heavy weight of the ATP molecule. A sedentary person resynthesizes an amount of ATP each day equal to about 75% of body mass. For endurance athletes who generate 20 times their resting energy expenditure throughout a 2.5-hr marathon race, this amounts to 80 kg of ATP resynthesis during the run. To appreciate the tremendous quantity of ATP production over the adult portion of a life span (assuming a body weight of 80 kg and a relatively sedentary lifestyle for 50 years after age 20), total ATP production (60 kg daily for 50 years) equals the approximate maximum takeoff weight of two Boeing 787 Dreamliner aircraft.

PHOSPHOCREATINE: THE ENERGY RESERVOIR

To overcome its storage limitation, ATP resynthesis proceeds uninterrupted to continuously supply energy for all of the body's biologic work. Fat and glycogen represent the major energy sources for maintaining as-needed ATP resynthesis. Some energy for ATP resynthesis also comes directly from the anaerobic splitting of a phosphate from **phosphocreatine** (**PCr**), another intracellular high-energy phosphate compound. **FIGURE 6.4** schematically illustrates the reversible release and use of phosphate-bond energy in ATP and PCr. The term **high-energy phosphates** describes these compounds.

Specificity of Training the Immediate Energy System

Physical training increases the muscles' quantity of high-energy phosphates. The most effective training uses repeat 6- to 10-s intervals of maximal movement in the specific activity requiring improved sprint-power capacity.

The PCr and ATP molecules share a similar characteristic; a large amount of free energy releases when the bond cleaves between the PCr's creatine and phosphate molecules. The double-pointing arrow in Figure 6.4 indicates a reversible reaction. In other words, phosphate (P) and creatine (Cr) rejoin to form PCr. This also applies to ATP: ADP plus P reforms ATP. Because PCr has a larger free energy of hydrolysis

The Fuel for Explosive, Short-Term Exercise

To appreciate the importance of the intramuscular high-energy phosphates in physical activity, consider activities in which success requires short, intense bursts of energy. These include football, tennis, track and field, golf, volleyball, field hockey, baseball, weightlifting, and wood chopping that often require bursts of maximal effort for only up to 8 s.

than ATP, its hydrolysis catalyzed by the enzyme **creatine kinase** (4 to 6% on the outer mitochondrial membrane, 3 to 5% in the sarcomere, and 90% in the cytosol) drives ADP phosphorylation to ATP. Cells store approximately four to six times more PCr than ATP.

Transient increases in ADP within the muscle's contractile unit during exercise shift the creatine kinase reaction toward PCr hydrolysis and ATP production (the upper reaction in Fig. 6.4); the reaction does not require oxygen and reaches a maximum energy yield in about 10 s.[39] Thus, PCr serves as a "reservoir" of high-energy phosphate bonds. The rapidity of ADP phosphorylation considerably exceeds energy transfer from stored muscle glycogen because of the high activity rate of creatine kinase.[18] If maximal effort continues beyond 10 s, energy for continual ATP resynthesis must originate from less-rapid catabolism of the stored macronutrients. Chapter 23 discusses the potential for exogenous creatine supplementation to enhance short-term, explosive exercise performance.

The **adenylate kinase reaction** represents another single-enzyme–mediated reaction for ATP regeneration. The reaction uses two ADP molecules to produce one molecule of ATP and AMP as follows:

$$2 \text{ ADP} \xleftrightarrow{\text{ adenylate kinase }} \text{ATP} + \text{AMP}$$

The adenylate kinase and creatine kinase (lower reaction in Fig. 6.4) reactions not only augment the muscle's ability to rapidly increase energy output (ATP availability), but also produce the molecular byproducts AMP, P_i, and ADP that activate the initial stages of glycogen and glucose catabolism and the cellular oxidation (respiration) pathways of the mitochondrion.

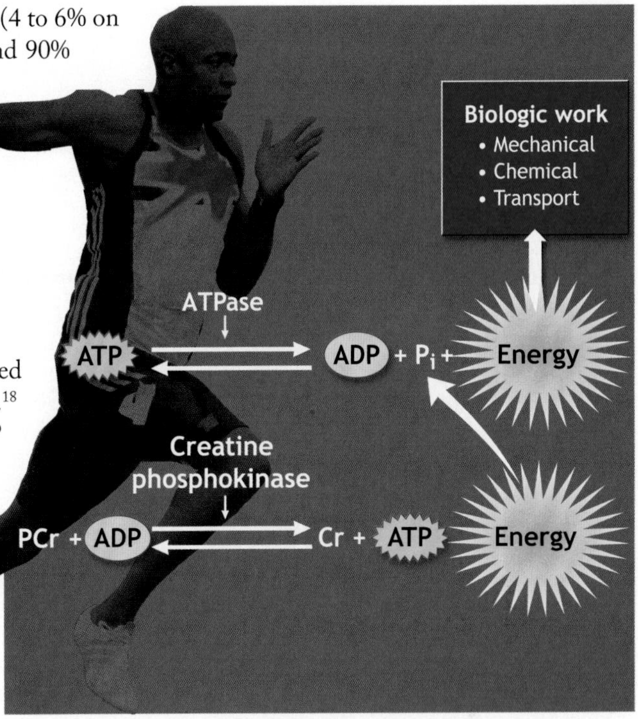

CELLULAR OXIDATION

Most energy for phosphorylation derives from the oxidation ("biologic burning") of dietary carbohydrate, lipid, and protein macronutrients. Recall from Chapter 5 that a molecule becomes reduced when it accepts electrons from an electron donor. In turn, the molecule that gives up the electron becomes oxidized. *Oxidation reactions (those that donate electrons) and reduction reactions (those that accept electrons) remain coupled and constitute the biochemical mechanism that underlies energy metabolism.* This process continually provides hydrogen atoms from the catabolism of stored macronutrients. The mitochondria, the cell's "energy factories," contain carrier molecules that remove electrons from hydrogen (oxidation) and eventually pass them to oxygen (reduction). ATP synthesis occurs during oxidation–reduction (redox) reactions.

Electron Transport

FIGURE **6.5** illustrates the general schema for hydrogen oxidation and accompanying electron transport to oxygen.

FIGURE 6.4 • ATP and PCr provide anaerobic sources of phosphate-bond energy. The energy liberated from the hydrolysis (splitting) of PCr rebonds ADP and P_i to form ATP. (Adapted with permission from McArdle WD, Katch FI, Katch VL. *Sports and Exercise Nutrition.* 4th Ed. Philadelphia: Wolters Kluwer Health, 2013.)

See the animation "Electron Transfer Chain" on http://thePoint.lww.com/mkk8e for a demonstration of this process.

During cellular oxidation, hydrogen atoms are not merely turned loose in intracellular fluids. Rather, substrate-specific **dehydrogenase enzymes** catalyze hydrogen's release from the nutrient substrate. The coenzyme component of the dehydrogenase (usually the niacin-containing **nicotinamide adenine dinucleotide [NAD⁺]**) accepts pairs of electrons (energy) from hydrogen. Although the substrate oxidizes and gives up hydrogens (electrons), NAD⁺ gains hydrogen and two electrons and reduces to NADH; the other hydrogen appears as H⁺ in the cell fluid. The riboflavin-containing coenzyme **flavin adenine dinucleotide (FAD)** serves as another electron acceptor to oxidize food fragments. Like NAD⁺, FAD catalyzes dehydrogenation and accepts electron pairs. Unlike NAD⁺, FAD becomes FADH₂ by accepting both hydrogens. *NADH and FADH₂ provide energy-rich molecules because they carry electrons with high energy-transfer potential.*

The **cytochromes**, a series of iron-protein electron carriers dispersed on the inner membranes of the mitochondrion, then pass in "bucket brigade" fashion pairs of electrons carried by NADH and FADH₂. The iron portion of each

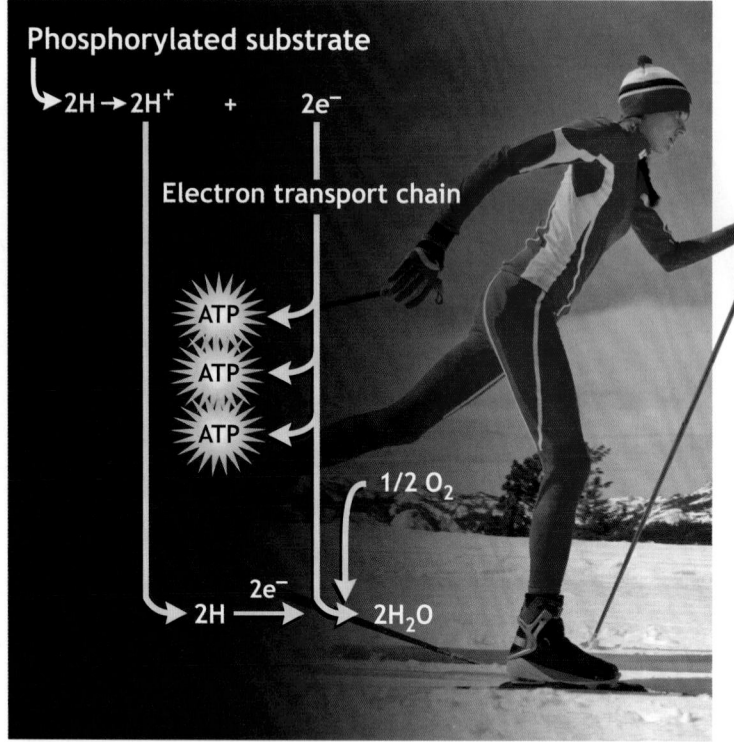

Phosphorylated substrate

Electron transport chain

FIGURE 6.5 • General scheme for oxidizing (removing electrons) hydrogen and the accompanying electron transport. In this process, oxygen is reduced (gain of electrons) and water forms. The liberated energy powers the synthesis of ATP from ADP.

cytochrome exists in either its oxidized (ferric or Fe^{3+}) or reduced (ferrous, or Fe^{2+}) ionic state. By accepting an electron, the ferric portion of a specific cytochrome reduces to its ferrous form. In turn, ferrous iron donates its electron to the next cytochrome and so on down the line. By shuttling between these two iron forms, the cytochromes transfer electrons to ultimately reduce oxygen to form water. NAD^+ and FAD then recycle for subsequent electron transfer. The NADH generated during glycolysis (see section "Glycolysis Generates Energy from Glucose") converts back to NAD via "shuttling" of the hydrogens from NADH across the mitochondrial membrane.

Electron transport by specific carrier molecules constitutes the **respiratory** (or cytochrome) **chain**, the final common pathway where electrons extracted from hydrogen pass to oxygen. For each pair of hydrogen atoms, two electrons flow down the chain and reduce one atom of oxygen to form one water molecule. During the passage of electrons down the five-cytochrome chain, enough energy releases to rephosphorylate ADP to ATP at three of the sites. At the last cytochrome site, cytochrome oxidase (cytochrome aa_3, with strong affinity for oxygen), discharges its electron directly to oxygen. **FIGURE 6.6B** shows the route for hydrogen oxidation, electron transport, and energy transfer in the respiratory chain that releases free

energy in relatively small amounts. In several of the electron transfers, the formation of high-energy phosphate bonds conserves energy. Each electron acceptor in the respiratory chain has a progressively greater affinity for electrons. In biochemical terms, this affinity for electrons represents a substance's **reduction potential**. Oxygen, the last electron receiver in the transport chain, possesses the largest reduction potential. Mitochondrial oxygen ultimately drives the respiratory chain and other catabolic reactions that require continual availability of NAD^+ and FAD.

Oxidative Phosphorylation

Oxidative phosphorylation synthesizes ATP by transferring electrons from NADH and FADH$_2$ to oxygen. **FIGURE 6.7** illustrates how the energy generated in the reactions of electron transport pumps protons across the inner mitochondrial membrane into the intermembrane space. The electrochemical gradient generated by this reverse flow of protons across the inner membrane (see arrow pointing into the intermembrane space) represents stored potential energy and provides the coupling mechanism that binds ADP and a phosphate ion to synthesize ATP. The mitochondrion's inner membrane remains impermeable to ATP, so the protein complex ATP/ADP translocase exports the newly synthesized ATP molecule. In turn, ADP and P_i move into the mitochondrion for subsequent synthesis to ATP. Biochemists refer to this union as **chemiosmotic coupling**, the cell's primary endergonic means to extract and trap chemical energy in the high-energy phosphates. *More than 90% of ATP synthesis takes place in the respiratory chain by oxidative reactions coupled with phosphorylation.*

In a way, oxidative phosphorylation can be likened to a waterfall divided into several separate cascades by intervention of turbines at different heights. **FIGURE 6.6A** depicts the turbines that harness the energy of falling water; similarly, electrochemical energy generated during electron transport becomes harnessed and transferred (coupled) to ADP. Energy transfer from NADH to ADP to re-form ATP happens at three distinct coupling sites during electron transport (Fig. 6.6B). Oxidation of hydrogen and subsequent phosphorylation occurs as follows:

$$NADH + H^+ + 3\,ADP + 3\,P_i + 1/2\,O_2 \rightarrow NAD^+ + H_2O + 3\,ATP$$

The ratio of phosphate bonds formed to oxygen atoms consumed (P/O ratio) reflects quantitatively the coupling of ATP production to electron transport. In the preceding equation, note that the P/O ratio equals 3 for each NADH plus H^+ oxidized. However, if $FADH_2$ originally donates hydrogen, only two ATP molecules form for each hydrogen pair oxidized (P/O ratio = 2). This occurs because

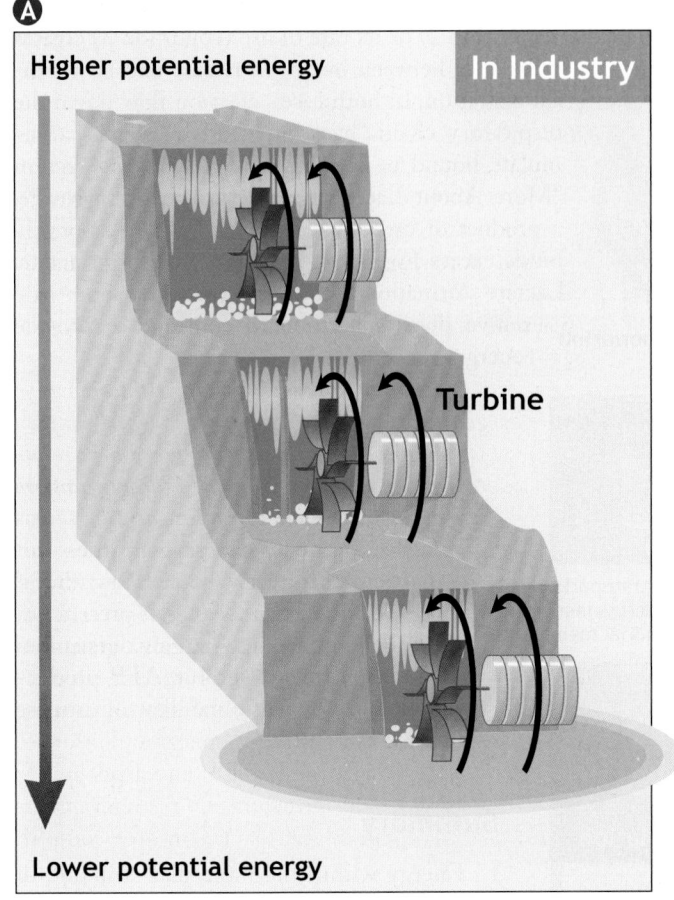

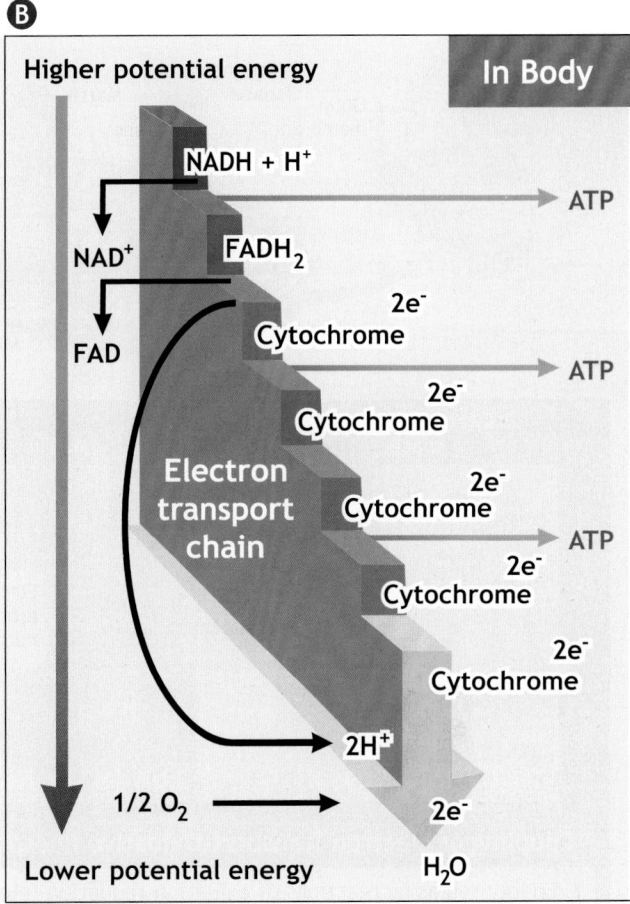

FIGURE 6.6 • Examples of harnessing potential energy. **(A)** In industry, energy from falling water becomes harnessed to turn the waterwheel, which in turn performs mechanical work. **(B)** In the body, the electron transport chain removes electrons from hydrogens for ultimate delivery to oxygen. In oxidation–reduction, much of the chemical energy stored within the hydrogen atom does not dissipate to kinetic energy, but instead is conserved within ATP. (Reprinted with permission from McArdle WD, Katch FI, Katch VL. *Sports and Exercise Nutrition*. 4th Ed. Philadelphia: Wolters Kluwer Health, 2013.)

$FADH_2$ enters the respiratory chain at a lower energy level at a point beyond the site of the first ATP synthesis (Fig. 6.6B).

Biochemists have recently adjusted their accounting transpositions regarding conservation of energy in the resynthesis of an ATP molecule in aerobic pathways. Energy provided by oxidation of NADH and $FADH_2$ resynthesizes ADP to ATP. Additional energy (H^+) is also required to shuttle the NADH from the cell's cytoplasm across the mitochondrial membrane to deliver H^+ to electron transport. This added energy exchange of NADH shuttling across the mitochondrial membrane reduces the net ATP yield for glucose metabolism and changes the overall efficiency of ATP production (see the section "Efficiency of Electron Transport–Oxidative Phosphorylation"). The oxidation of one NADH molecule produces on average only 2.5 ATP molecules. This decimal value for ATP does not indicate formation of one-half of an ATP molecule but rather indicates the average number of ATP produced per

NADH oxidation with the energy for mitochondrial transport subtracted. When $FADH_2$ donates hydrogen, then on average only 1.5 molecules of ATP form for each hydrogen pair oxidized.

Efficiency of Electron Transport–Oxidative Phosphorylation

Each mole of ATP formed from ADP conserves approximately 7 kcal of energy. Because 2.5 moles of ATP regenerate from the total of 52 kcal of energy released to oxidize 1 mole (1-g molecular weight) of NADH, about 18 kcal (7 kcal · mol^{-1} × 2.8) is conserved as chemical energy. This represents a relative efficiency of 34% for harnessing chemical energy via electron transport oxidative phosphorylation (18 kcal ÷ 52 kcal × 100). Considering that a steam engine transforms its fuel into useful energy at only about 30% efficiency, the value of 34% or above for the human body represents a relatively high efficiency rate.

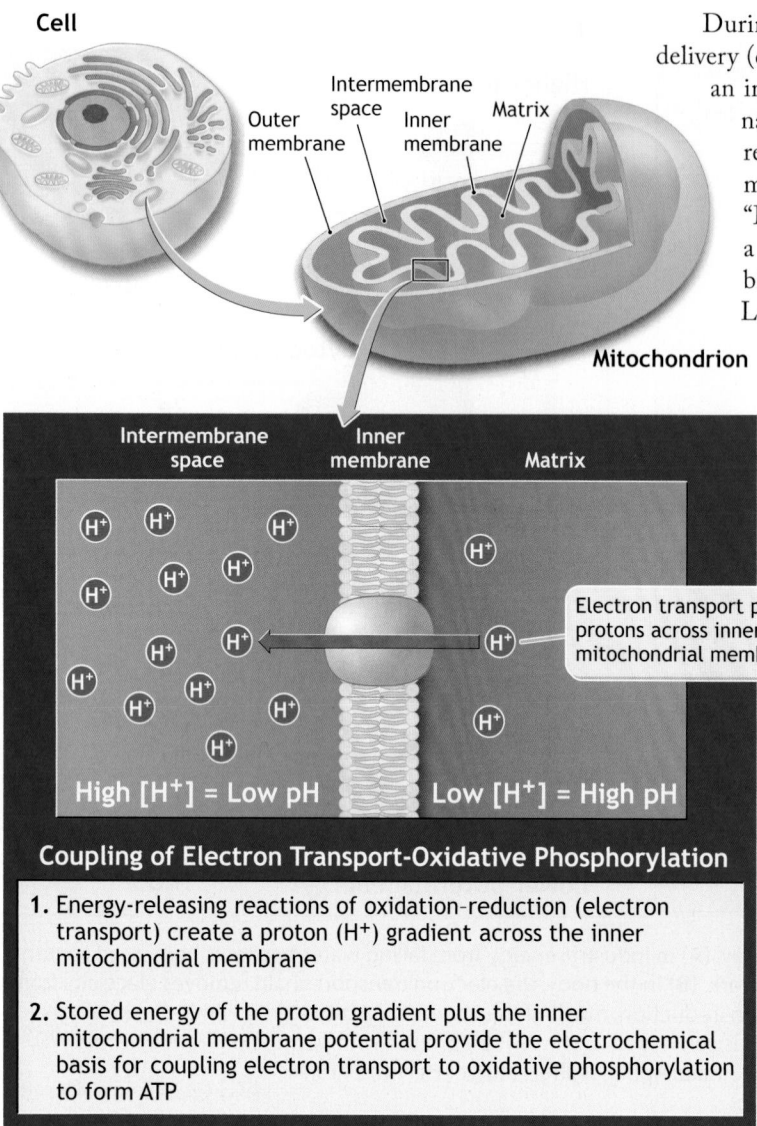

During strenuous physical activity, inadequacy in oxygen delivery (condition 2) or its rate of use (condition 3) creates an imbalance between hydrogen release and its terminal oxidation. In both cases, electron flow down the respiratory chain "backs up" and hydrogens accumulate bound to NAD^+ and FAD. In the section "More About Lactate," we describe how pyruvate, a product of carbohydrate breakdown, temporarily binds excess hydrogens (electrons) to form lactate. Lactate formation allows electron transport–oxidative phosphorylation to continue to provide energy as needed.

Aerobic metabolism refers to energy-generating catabolic reactions where oxygen serves as the final electron acceptor in the respiratory chain to combine with hydrogen to form water. In one sense, the term *aerobic* seems misleading because oxygen does not participate directly in ATP synthesis. On the other hand, oxygen's presence at the "end of the line" largely determines the capacity for aerobic ATP production and the sustainability of intense endurance exercise.

FIGURE 6.7 • The mitochondrion: the site for aerobic energy metabolism. Electron transport creates a proton (H^+) gradient across the inner mitochondrial membrane. This produces a net flow of protons to provide the coupling mechanism to drive ATP resynthesis.

OXYGEN'S ROLE IN ENERGY METABOLISM

Three prerequisites exist for the continual resynthesis of ATP during coupled oxidative phosphorylation. Satisfying the following three conditions causes hydrogen and electrons to shuttle uninterrupted down the respiratory chain to oxygen during energy metabolism:

1. Tissue availability of the reducing agent NADH (or $FADH_2$)
2. Presence of the oxidizing agent oxygen in the tissues
3. Sufficient concentration of enzymes and mitochondria to ensure that energy transfer reactions proceed at their appropriate rate

Summary

1. Energy within the molecular structure of carbohydrate, fat, and protein does not suddenly release in the body at some kindling temperature. Rather, energy releases slowly in small amounts during complex, enzymatically controlled reactions to promote more efficient energy transfer and conservation.

2. About 40% of the potential energy in food nutrients transfers to the high-energy compound ATP.

3. Splitting the terminal phosphate bond from ATP liberates free energy to power all forms of biologic work. This makes ATP the body's energy currency despite its limited quantity of only about 3.0 oz.

4. PCr interacts with ADP to form ATP; this nonaerobic, high-energy reservoir replenishes ATP almost instantaneously.

5. Phosphorylation refers to energy transfer via phosphate bonds as ADP with creatine continually recycle into ATP and PCr.

6. Cellular oxidation occurs on the inner lining of the mitochondrial membranes; it involves transferring electrons from NADH and $FADH_2$ to oxygen.

7. Electron transport–oxidative phosphorylation produces coupled transfer of chemical energy to form ATP from ADP plus phosphate ion.

8. During aerobic ATP resynthesis, oxygen serves as the final electron acceptor in the respiratory chain to combine with hydrogen to form water.

PART 2 ENERGY RELEASE FROM MACRONUTRIENTS

Energy release in macronutrient catabolism serves one crucial purpose: to phosphorylate ADP to reform the energy-rich compound ATP. FIGURE 6.8 outlines three broad stages that ultimately lead to the release and conservation of energy by the cell for biologic work:

1. *Stage 1* involves the digestion, absorption, and assimilation of large food macromolecules into smaller subunits for use in cellular metabolism.

2. *Stage 2* degrades amino acid, glucose, and fatty acid and glycerol units within the cytosol into acetyl-coenzyme A (formed within the mitochondrion), with limited ATP and NADH production.

3. *Stage 3* within the mitochondrion, acetyl-coenzyme A degrades to CO_2 and H_2O with considerable ATP production.

The specific pathways of degradation differ depending on the nutrient substrate catabolized. In the sections that follow, we show how ATP resynthesis occurs from extraction of the potential energy in carbohydrate, fat, and protein macronutrients.

FIGURE 6.9 outlines the six fuel sources that supply substrate for ATP formation.

1. Triacylglycerol and glycogen molecules stored within muscle cells
2. Blood glucose (derived from liver glycogen)
3. Free fatty acids (derived from triacylglycerols in liver and adipocytes)
4. Intramuscular- and liver-derived carbon skeletons of amino acids
5. Anaerobic reactions in the cytosol in the initial phase of glucose or glycogen breakdown (small amount of ATP)
6. Phosphorylation of ADP by PCr under enzymatic control by creatine kinase and adenylate kinase

ENERGY RELEASE FROM CARBOHYDRATE

Carbohydrate's primary function supplies energy for cellular work. Our discussion of macronutrient energy metabolism begins with carbohydrate for five reasons:

1. Carbohydrate provides the only macronutrient substrate whose stored energy generates ATP without oxygen (anaerobically). This takes on importance in activities requiring rapid energy release above levels supplied by aerobic metabolism. In such a case, intramuscular glycogen supplies most of the energy for ATP resynthesis.

2. During light and moderate physical activity, carbohydrate supplies about one-third of the body's energy requirements.

3. Processing a large quantity of fat for energy requires minimal carbohydrate catabolism.

4. Aerobic breakdown of carbohydrate for energy occurs more rapidly than energy generation from fatty acid breakdown. Thus, depleting glycogen reserves considerably reduces exercise power output. In prolonged aerobic exercise such as marathon running, athletes often experience nutrient-related fatigue—a state associated with muscle and liver glycogen depletion (see Chapters 3 and 23).

5. The central nervous system requires an uninterrupted supply of carbohydrate to function properly. The brain normally uses blood glucose almost exclusively as its fuel. In poorly regulated diabetes, during starvation, or with prolonged low carbohydrate intake, the brain adapts after about 8 days and metabolizes large amounts of fat (as ketones) for an alternative fuel.

The complete breakdown of one mole of glucose to carbon dioxide and water yields a maximum of 686 kcal of chemical free energy available for work.

$$C_6H_{12}O_6 + 6\,O_2 \rightarrow 6\,CO_2 + 6\,H_2O - \Delta G\ 686\ \text{kcal} \cdot \text{mol}^{-1}$$

Complete glucose breakdown conserves only some of the released energy as ATP. Recall that the synthesis of 1 mole of ATP from ADP and a phosphate ion requires 7.3 kcal of energy. Coupling all of the energy from glucose oxidation to phosphorylation could theoretically form 94 moles of ATP per mole of glucose (686 kcal ÷ 7.3 kcal · mol⁻¹ = 94 mol). In the muscle, phosphate bond formation conserves only 34%, or 233 kcal, of energy, with the remainder dissipated as heat (see "Efficiency of Electron Transport-Oxidative Phosphorylation"). As such, glucose breakdown regenerates 32 moles of ATP (233 kcal ÷ 7.3 kcal · mol⁻¹ = 32 mol) with an accompanying free energy gain of 233 kcal.

Anaerobic Versus Aerobic Glycolysis

Two forms of carbohydrate breakdown occur in a series of fermentation reactions collectively termed **glycolysis** ("the dissolution of sugar"), or the Embden–Meyerhof pathway, named for its two German chemist discoverers (Otto Meyerhof [1884–1951]; 1922 Nobel Prize in Physiology or Medicine; http://www.nobelprize.org/nobel_prizes/medicine/laureates/1922/meyerhof-bio.html and Gustav Embden [1874–1933]). In one form, lactate, formed from pyruvate, becomes the end product. In the other form, pyruvate remains the end product. With pyruvate as the end substrate, carbohydrate catabolism proceeds and couples to further break down in the citric acid cycle with subsequent electron transport production of ATP. Carbohydrate breakdown of this form (sometimes

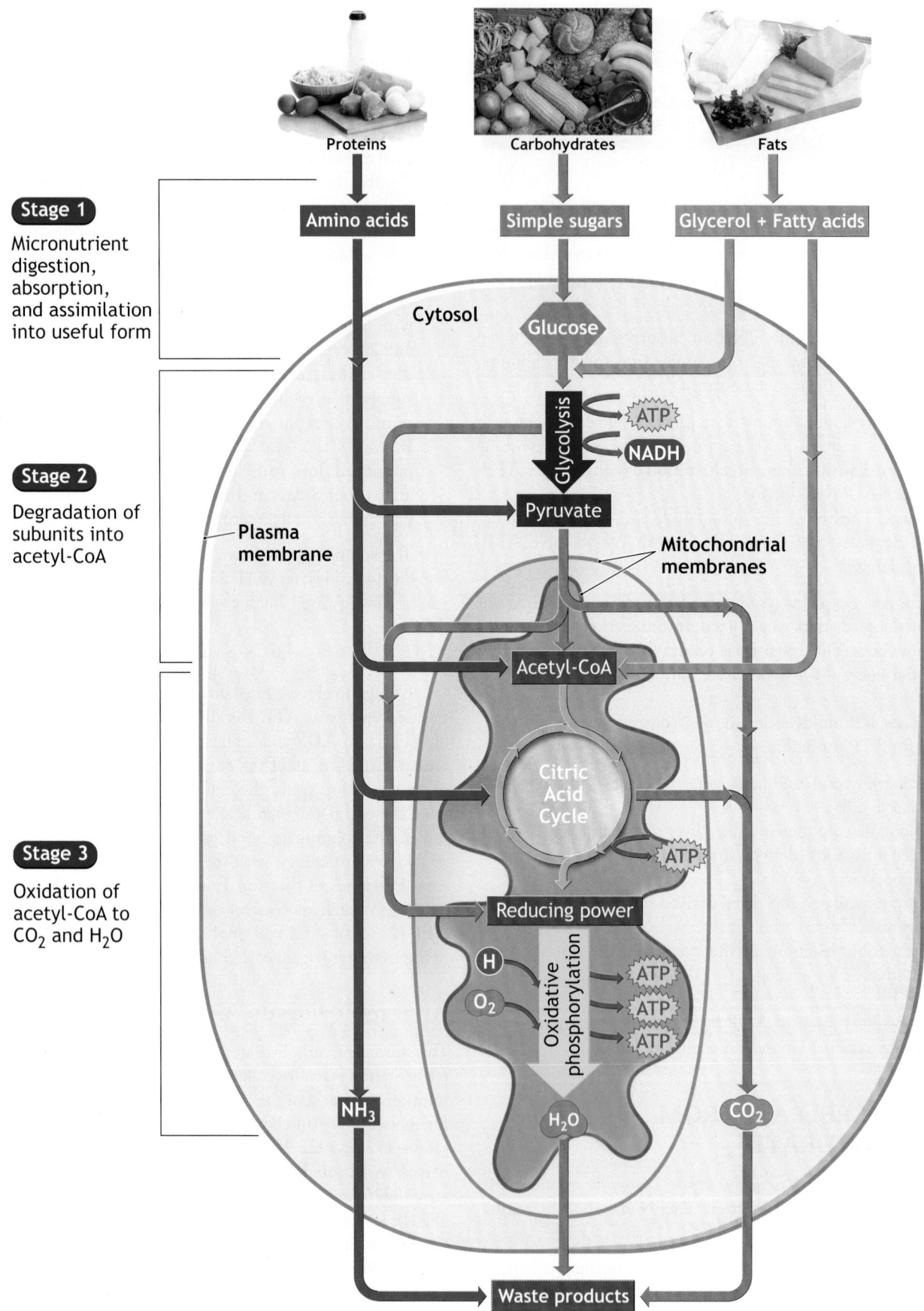

FIGURE 6.8 • Three broad stages for macronutrient use in energy metabolism.

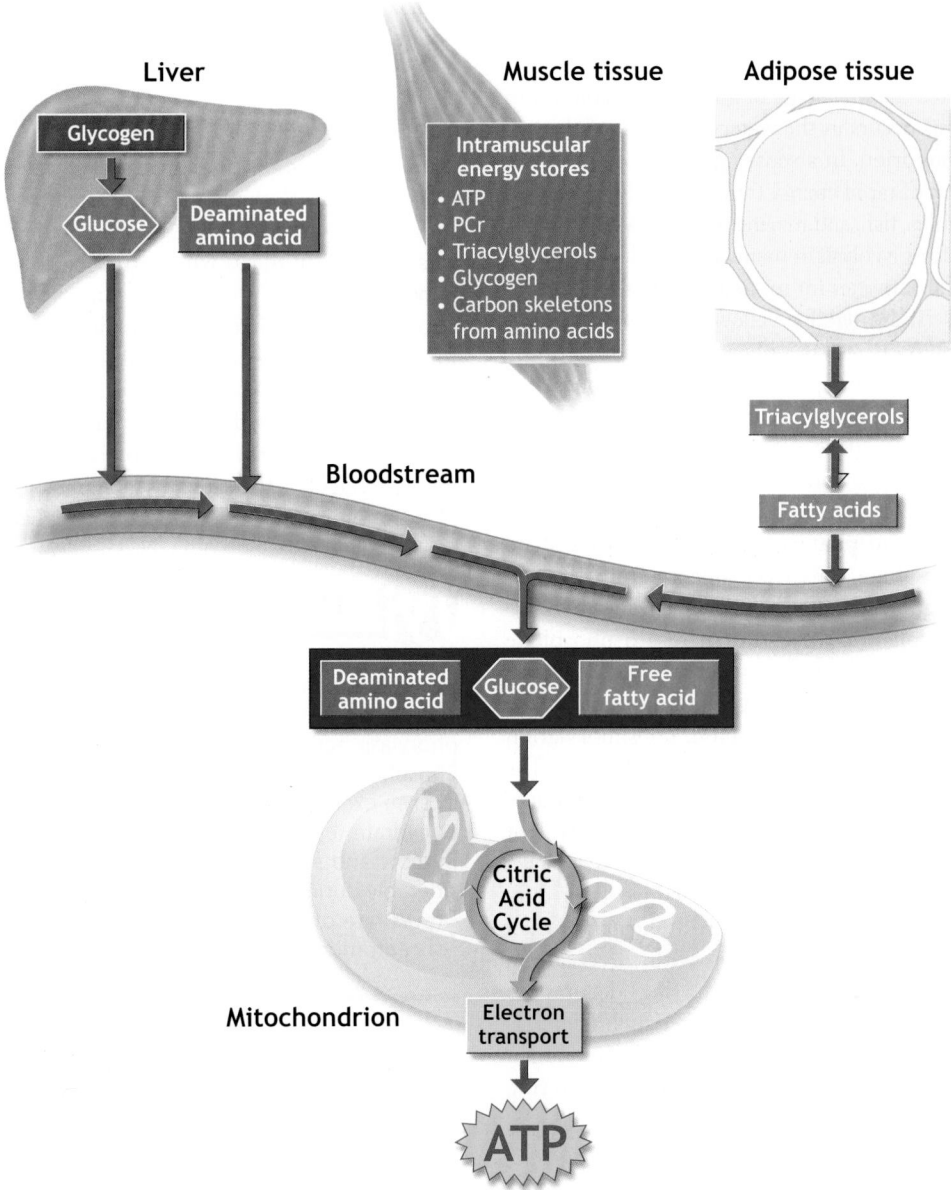

FIGURE 6.9 • Fuel sources that supply substrate to regenerate ATP. The liver provides a rich source of amino acids and glucose, while adipocytes generate large quantities of energy-rich fatty acid molecules. After their release, the bloodstream delivers these compounds to the muscle cell. Most of the cells' energy production takes place within the mitochondria. Mitochondrial proteins carry out their roles in oxidative phosphorylation on the inner membranous walls of this architecturally elegant complex. The intramuscular energy sources consist of the high-energy phosphates ATP and PCr and triacylglycerols, glycogen, and amino acids.

termed *aerobic* [with oxygen] *glycolysis*) is a relatively *slow* process resulting in substantial ATP formation. In contrast, glycolysis that results in lactate formation (referred to as *anaerobic* [without oxygen] *glycolysis*) represents rapid but limited ATP production. The net formation of either lactate or pyruvate depends more on the relative glycolytic and mitochondrial activities than on the presence of molecular oxygen. The relative demand for rapid or slow ATP production determines the form of glycolysis. The glycolytic process itself, from beginning substrate (glucose) to end substrate (lactate or pyruvate), does

not involve oxygen. We agree with other exercise physiology textbook authors that *rapid* (anaerobic) and *slow* (aerobic) glycolysis are the appropriate terms to describe glycolysis.

Glucose degradation occurs in two stages. In stage one, glucose breaks down rapidly into two molecules of pyruvate. Energy transfer for phosphorylation occurs without oxygen (anaerobic). In stage two, pyruvate degrades further to carbon dioxide and water. Energy transfers from these reactions require electron transport and accompanying oxidative phosphorylation (aerobic).

Anaerobic Energy Release From Glucose: Rapid Glycolysis

FIGURE 6.10 illustrates the first stage of glucose degradation in glycolysis. Glycolysis occurs in the watery medium of the cell outside the mitochondrion. In a sense, glycolysis represents a more primitive form of rapid energy transfer highly developed in amphibians, reptiles, fish, and marine mammals. In humans, the cells' capacity for glycolysis remains crucial during maximum-effort physical activities for up to about 90 s.

In reaction 1 (indicated by yellow number 1 on left within black circle), ATP acts as a phosphate donor to phosphorylate glucose to glucose 6-phosphate. In most tissues, this "traps" the glucose molecule in the cell. In the presence of the enzyme *glycogen synthase*, glucose links, or polymerizes, with other glucose molecules to form a large glycogen molecule (see Fig. 1.3 in Chapter 1). The liver and kidney cells, however, contains the enzyme **phosphatase** that splits the phosphate from glucose 6-phosphate. This frees glucose from the cell for transport throughout the body. During energy metabolism, glucose 6-phosphate changes to fructose 6-phosphate (reaction 2). At this stage, energy is not yet released, yet some energy incorporates into the original glucose molecule at the expense of one ATP molecule. In a sense, phosphorylation "primes the pump" for continued energy metabolism. The fructose 6-phosphate molecule gains an additional phosphate and changes to fructose 1,6-diphosphate under control of **phosphofructokinase** (**PFK**; reaction 3). The activity level of this enzyme probably limits the rate of glycolysis during maximum-effort activity. Fructose 1,6-diphosphate then splits into two phosphorylated molecules with three carbon chains (*3-phosphoglycerasdehyde*); these further decompose to *pyruvate* in five successive reactions. Fast-twitch (type II) muscle fibers (see Chapter 7) contain relatively large quantities of PFK; this makes them ideally suited for generating anaerobic energy via glycolysis.

Metabolism of Glucose to Glycogen and Glycogen to Glucose

The cytoplasm of liver and muscle cells contains glycogen granules and the enzymes for glycogen synthesis (**glycogenesis**) and glycogen breakdown (**glycogenolysis**). Under normal conditions following a meal, glucose does not accumulate in the blood. Rather, surplus glucose either enters the pathways of energy metabolism, stores as glycogen, or converts to fat. In high cellular activity, available glucose oxidizes via the glycolytic pathway, citric acid cycle, and respiratory chain to form ATP. In contrast, low cellular activity and/or depleted glycogen reserves inactivate key glycolytic enzymes. This causes surplus glucose to form glycogen.

Glycogenolysis describes the cleavage of glucose from the glycogen molecule. The glucose residue then reacts with a phosphate ion to produce glucose 6-phosphate, bypassing step 1 of the glycolytic pathway. When glycogen provides a glucose molecule for glycolysis, a net gain of three ATPs occurs rather than two ATPs during glucose breakdown.

Regulation of Glycogen Metabolism

In the liver, **glycogen phosphorylase** enzymes become inactive following a meal, while **glycogen synthase** activity increases to facilitate storage of the glucose obtained from food. Conversely, between meals when glycogen reserves decrease, liver phosphorylase becomes active (concurrent depression of glycogen synthase activity) to maintain stability in blood glucose for use by body tissues. Skeletal muscle at rest shows higher synthase activity, whereas physical activity increases phosphorylase activity with a concomitant blunting of the synthase enzyme. **Epinephrine**, a sympathetic nervous system hormone, accelerates the rate at which phosphorylase cleaves one glucose component at a time from the glycogen molecule.[7,9]

 The Glycogenolysis Cascade

Epinephrine's action has been termed the *glycogenolysis cascade* because this hormone affects progressively greater phosphorylase activation to ensure rapid glycogen mobilization. Phosphorylase activity remains at the highest level during intense exercise when sympathetic activity increases and carbohydrate represents the optimum energy fuel. Sympathetic outflow and subsequent glycogen catabolism decrease considerably during low-to-moderate intensity exercise when the slower rate of fatty acid oxidation adequately maintains ATP concentrations in active muscle.

Substrate-Level Phosphorylation in Glycolysis

Most energy generated in glycolysis does not result in ATP resynthesis but instead dissipates as heat. Note that in reactions 7 and 10 in Figure 6.10, the energy released from glucose intermediates stimulates direct transfer of phosphate groups to four ADP molecules, generating four ATP molecules. *Because two molecules of ATP contribute to the initial phosphorylation of the glucose molecule, glycolysis generates a net gain of two ATP molecules. This represents an endergonic conservation of 14.6 kcal·mol^{-1}, all without involvement of molecular oxygen.* Instead, the energy transferred from substrate to ADP by phosphorylation in rapid glycolysis occurs via phosphate bonds in the anaerobic reactions, often called **substrate-level phosphorylation**. Energy conservation during this form of glycolysis operates at an efficiency of about 30%.

Rapid glycolysis generates only about 5% of the total ATP during the glucose molecule's complete degradation to energy. Examples of activities that rely heavily on ATP generated by rapid glycolysis include sprinting at the end of a mile run, swimming all-out from start to finish in a 50- or a 100-m swim, routines on gymnastics apparatus, and sprint-running up to 200 m.

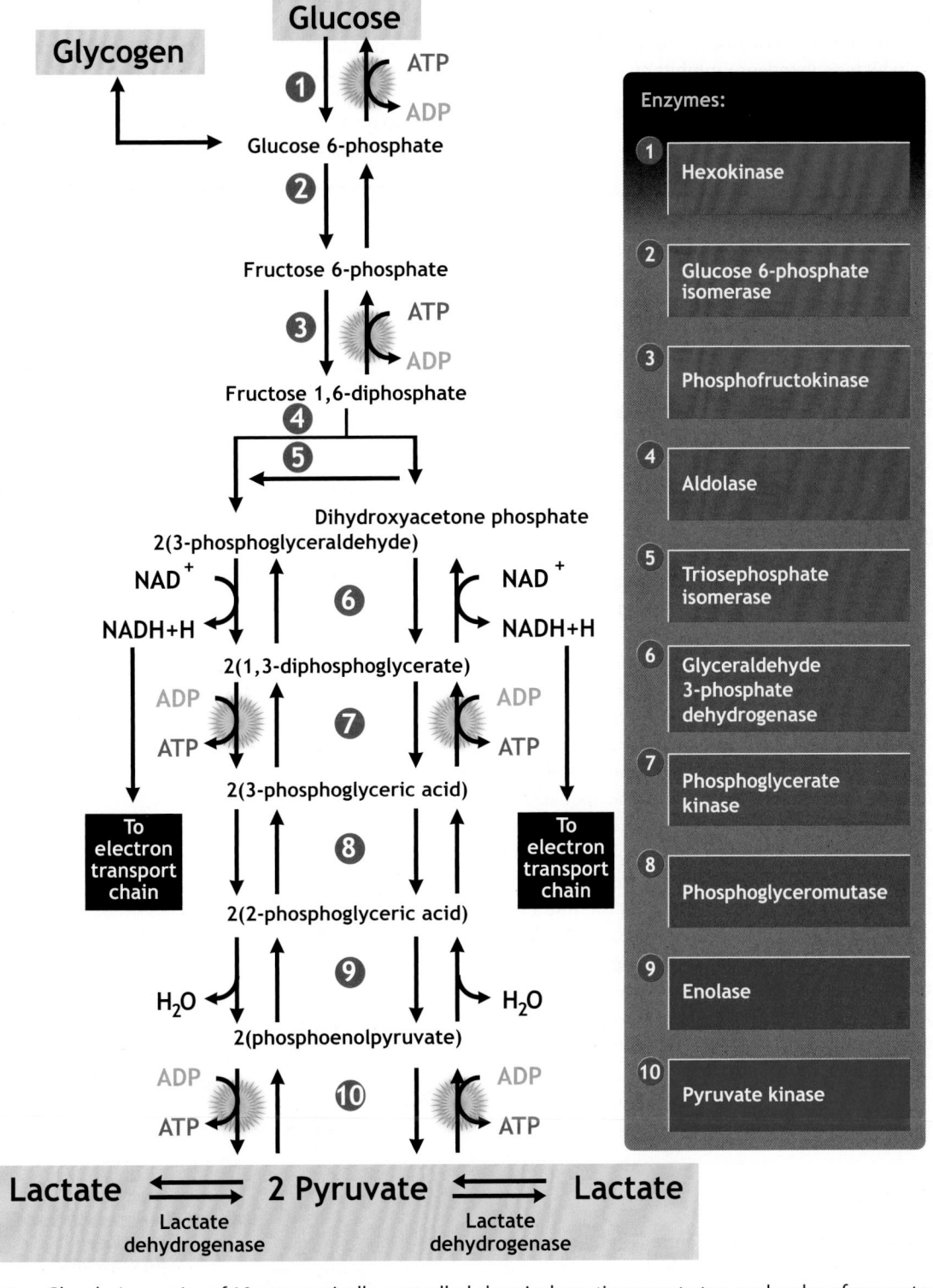

FIGURE 6.10 • Glycolysis: a series of 10 enzymatically controlled chemical reactions create two molecules of pyruvate from the anaerobic breakdown of glucose. Lactate forms when NADH oxidation does not keep pace with its formation in glycolysis. Enzymes colored yellow/purple play a key regulatory role in these metabolic reactions. (Adapted with permission from McArdle WD, Katch FI, Katch VL. *Sports and Exercise Nutrition*. 4th Ed. Philadelphia: Wolters Kluwer Health, 2013.)

Regulation of Glycolysis

Three factors regulate glycolysis:

1. Concentrations of the four key glycolytic enzymes: hexo-kinase, phosphorylase, phosphofructokinase, and pyruvate kinase
2. Levels of the substrate fructose 1,6-disphosphate
3. Oxygen, which in abundance inhibits glycolysis

In addition, glucose delivery to cells influences its subsequent use in energy metabolism.

Glucose locates in the surrounding extracellular fluid for transport across the cell's plasma membrane. A family of five proteins, collectively termed *facilitative glucose transporters*, mediates this process of **facilitative diffusion**. Muscle fibers and adipocytes contain an insulin-dependent transporter known as Glu T4, or **GLUT 4**. In response to both insulin and physical activity (independent of insulin), this transporter migrates from vesicles within the cell to the plasma membrane.[33] Its action facilitates glucose transport into the sarcoplasm, where it subsequently catabolizes to form ATP. Another glucose transporter, GLUT 1, accounts for basal levels of glucose transport into muscle.

Hydrogen Release in Glycolysis

Glycolytic reactions strip two pairs of hydrogen atoms from the glucose substrate and pass their electrons to NAD^+ to form NADH (Fig. 6.10, reaction 6). Normally, if the respiratory chain processed these electrons directly, 2.5 ATP molecules would form for each NADH molecule oxidized (P/O ratio = 2.5). Within heart, kidney, and liver cells, extramitochondrial hydrogen (NADH) appears as NADH in the mitochondrion (via a mechanism termed the **malate–aspartate shuttle**). This produces 2.5 ATP molecules from the oxidation of each NADH molecule. The mitochondria in skeletal muscle and brain cells remain impermeable to cytoplasmic NADH formed during glycolysis. Consequently, electrons from extramitochondrial NADH shuttle indirectly into the mitochondria. This route terminates when electrons pass to FAD to form $FADH_2$ (via a mechanism termed the **glycerol–phosphate shuttle**) at a point below the first formation of ATP. *Thus, 1.5 rather than three ATP molecules form when the respiratory chain oxidizes cytoplasmic NADH (P/O ratio = 1.5).* From two molecules of NADH formed in glycolysis, four molecules of ATP generate aerobically by subsequent coupled electron transport–oxidative phosphorylation in skeletal muscle.

More About Lactate

Sufficient oxygen bathes the cells during light-to-moderate levels of energy metabolism. The hydrogens (electrons) stripped from the substrate and carried by NADH oxidize within the mitochondria to form water when they join with oxygen. In a biochemical sense, a "steady state," or more precisely a "steady rate," exists because hydrogen oxidizes at about the same rate it becomes available.

 Lactic Acid Versus Lactate

Lactic acid ($C_3H_6O_3$), also known as "milk acid," and **lactate** should not be confused as they are different substances. Lactic acid is an acid formed during anaerobic glycolysis that in the body quickly dissociates to release a hydrogen ion (H^+). The remaining compound binds with a positively charged sodium or potassium ion to form the acid salt called lactate. Under physiological conditions, the majority of lactic acid dissociates and presents as lactate.

In strenuous physical activity, when energy demands exceed either oxygen supply or its rate of use, the respiratory chain cannot process all of the hydrogen joined to NADH. Continued release of anaerobic energy in glycolysis depends on NAD^+ availability to oxidize 3-phosphoglyceraldehyde (see reaction 6, Fig. 6.10); otherwise, the rapid rate of glycolysis "grinds to a halt." During rapid **anaerobic glycolysis**, NAD^+ "frees up" or regenerates when pairs of "excess" nonoxidized hydrogens combine with pyruvate to form lactate. Lactate formation requires one additional step (catalyzed by **lactate dehydrogenase**) in a reversible reaction. as shown in **Figure 6.11**.

During rest and moderate physical activity, some lactate continually forms in two ways:

1. Energy metabolism of red blood cells (they contain no mitochondria)
2. Limitations posed by enzyme activity in muscle fibers with high glycolytic capacity

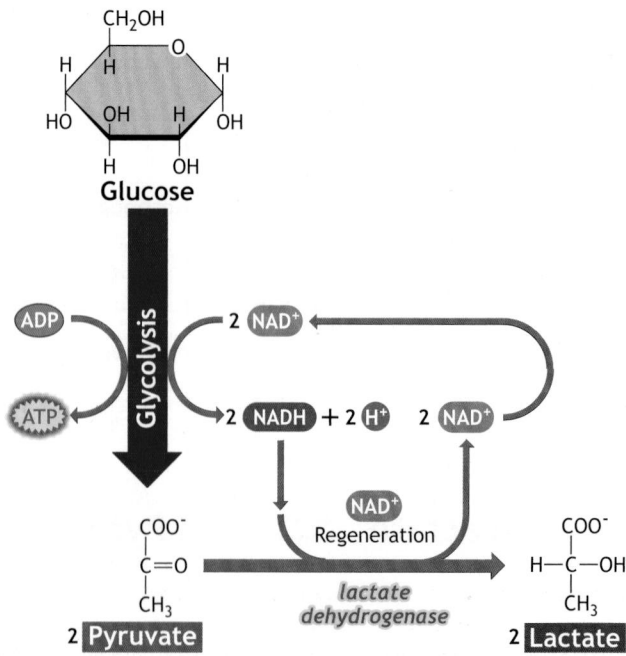

FIGURE 6.11 • Under physiologic conditions within muscle, lactate forms when hydrogens from NADH combine temporarily with pyruvate. This frees up NAD to accept additional hydrogens generated in glycolysis.

Any lactate that forms in this manner readily oxidizes for energy in neighboring muscle fibers with high oxidative capacity or in more distant tissues such as the heart and ventilatory muscles. Lactate also serves as an indirect precursor of liver glycogen. Consequently, lactate does not *accumulate* because its removal rate equals its rate of production. Endurance athletes show an enhanced ability for lactate clearance (or turnover) during exercise.[22]

As previously discussed, a direct pathway exists for liver glycogen synthesis from dietary carbohydrate. Liver glycogen synthesis also occurs indirectly from the conversion of the 3-carbon precursor lactate to glucose. Other tissues (e.g., erythrocytes and adipocytes) also contain glycolytic enzymes, but skeletal muscle possesses the largest quantity. Thus, much of the lactate-to-glucose conversion likely occurs in this tissue. This indirect pathway, from lactate to liver glycogen synthesis (particularly after eating), is known as the "**glucose paradox**." Later in this chapter, we discuss the glucose paradox as part of the lactate shuttle to explain formation, distribution, and utilization of lactate in carbohydrate metabolism.

The temporary storage of hydrogen with pyruvate represents a unique aspect of energy metabolism because it provides a ready "collector" for temporary storage of the end product of rapid glycolysis. Once lactate forms in muscle it takes two different routes:

1. It diffuses into the interstitial space and blood for buffering and removal from the site of energy metabolism
2. It provides gluconeogenic substrate for glycogen synthesis

In this way, rapid glycolysis continues to supply anaerobic energy for ATP resynthesis. This avenue for extra energy remains temporary, however, when blood and muscle lactate levels increase and ATP formation fails to keep pace with its rate of use. The end result—fatigue—soon sets in and exercise performance diminishes. Increased intracellular acidity under anaerobic conditions mediates fatigue by inactivating various enzymes in energy transfer, thus impairing the muscle's contractile properties.[2,6,17,23]

Lactate: A Valuable "Waste Product." Lactate should not be viewed as a metabolic waste product—a common belief termed *the mythology of lactic acid*. To the contrary, it provides a valuable source of chemical energy that accumulates with intense physical activity.[12,13] When sufficient oxygen becomes available during recovery, or when pace slows, NAD^+ scavenges hydrogens attached to lactate to form ATP via oxidation. The carbon skeletons of the pyruvate molecules re-formed from lactate during activity (one pyruvate molecule + 2 hydrogens form a molecule of lactate) become either oxidized for energy or synthesized to glucose (gluconeogenesis) in muscle itself or in the **Cori cycle** (Fig. 6.12). The Cori cycle removes lactate released from active muscles and uses it to replenish glycogen reserves depleted from intense physical activity.[37]

In intense physical activity (>80% aerobic capacity) with elevated carbohydrate catabolism, the glycogen within inactive tissues supplies the needs of active muscle. Active glycogen turnover through the **exchangeable lactate pool** progresses because inactive tissues release lactate into the circulation. The

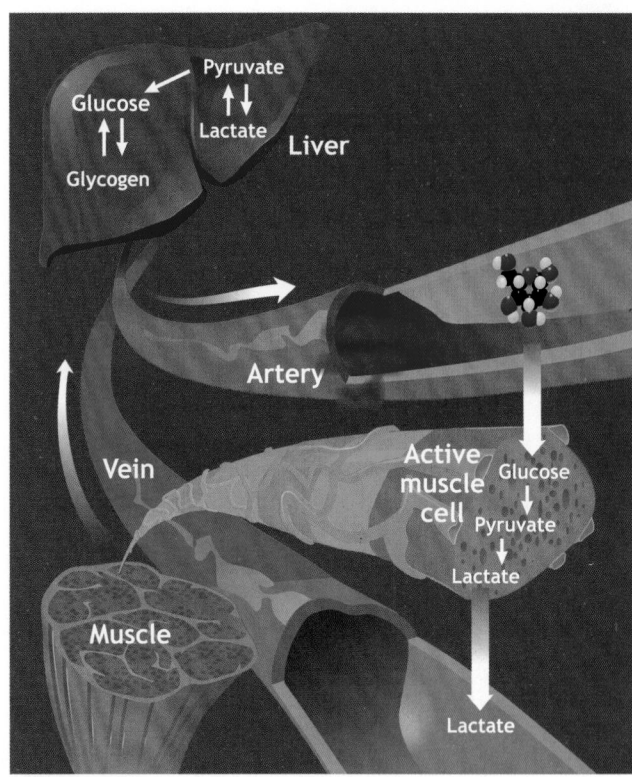

FIGURE 6.12 • The biochemical reactions of the Cori cycle in the liver synthesize glucose from the lactate released from active muscles. This gluconeogenic process helps to maintain carbohydrate reserves. (Adapted with permission from McArdle WD, Katch FI, Katch VL. *Sports and Exercise Nutrition.* 4th Ed. Philadelphia: Wolters Kluwer Health, 2013.)

lactate provides a precursor to synthesize carbohydrate (via the Cori cycle in liver and kidneys) to support blood glucose levels and concomitant exercise energy requirements.[3,22]

Lactate Shuttle: Blood Lactate as an Energy Source. Isotope tracer studies show that lactate produced in fast-twitch muscle fibers (and other tissues) circulates to other fast-twitch or slow-twitch fibers for conversion to pyruvate. Pyruvate, in turn, converts to acetyl-CoA and enters into the citric acid cycle (see the next section) for aerobic energy metabolism. This process of **lactate shuttling** among cells enables glycogenolysis in one cell to supply other cells with fuel for oxidation. *This makes muscle not only a major site of lactate production, but also a primary tissue for lactate removal via oxidation.*[4,13,15]

Aerobic (Slow) Glycolysis: The Citric Acid Cycle

The anaerobic reactions of glycolysis release only about 5% of the energy within the original glucose molecule. Extraction of the remaining energy continues when pyruvate irreversibly converts to **acetyl-CoA**, a form of acetic acid. Acetyl-CoA enters the **citric acid cycle** (also termed Krebs cycle for its discoverer, 1953 Nobel Prize–winning chemist Sir Hans Adolf Krebs, or tricarboxylic acid cycle; http://www.nobelprize.org/nobel_prizes/medicine/laureates/1953/press.html), the second stage of carbohydrate breakdown. As shown schematically in FIGURE 6.13, the citric acid cycle degrades the acetyl-CoA substrate to carbon dioxide and hydrogen atoms within the mitochondria. The reduced coenzyme carrier molecules transfer hydrogen to the electron transport chain. ATP forms when hydrogen atoms oxidize during electron transport–oxidative phosphorylation.

 See the animation "Tricarboxylic Acid Cycle" on http://thePoint.lww.com/mkk8e for a demonstration of this process.

FIGURE 6.14 shows pyruvate preparing to enter the 10-step enzymatically-controlled citric acid cycle by joining with coenzyme A (A for acetic acid) to form the 2-carbon compound acetyl-CoA. The two released hydrogens transfer their electrons to NAD^+ to form one molecule of carbon dioxide as follows:

$$Pyruvate + NAD^+ + CoA \rightarrow Acetyl\text{-}CoA + CO_2 + NADH^+ + H^+$$

 ### Free Radicals Form During Aerobic Metabolism

Passage of electrons along the electron transport chain sometimes forms free radicals, which are atoms, molecules, or ions with an unpaired electron in their outer shell, making them highly reactive. These reactive free radicals bind quickly to other molecules and promote potential damage to the combining molecule. Free radical formation in muscle, for example, might contribute to muscle fatigue or soreness or a possible reduction in metabolic potential.

The acetyl portion of acetyl-CoA joins with **oxaloacetate** to form **citrate** (the same 6-carbon citric acid compound found in citrus fruits), which then proceeds through the citric acid cycle. This cycle continues to operate because it retains the original oxaloacetate molecule to join with a new acetyl fragment that enters the cycle.

Each acetyl-CoA molecule entering the citric acid cycle releases two carbon dioxide molecules and four pairs

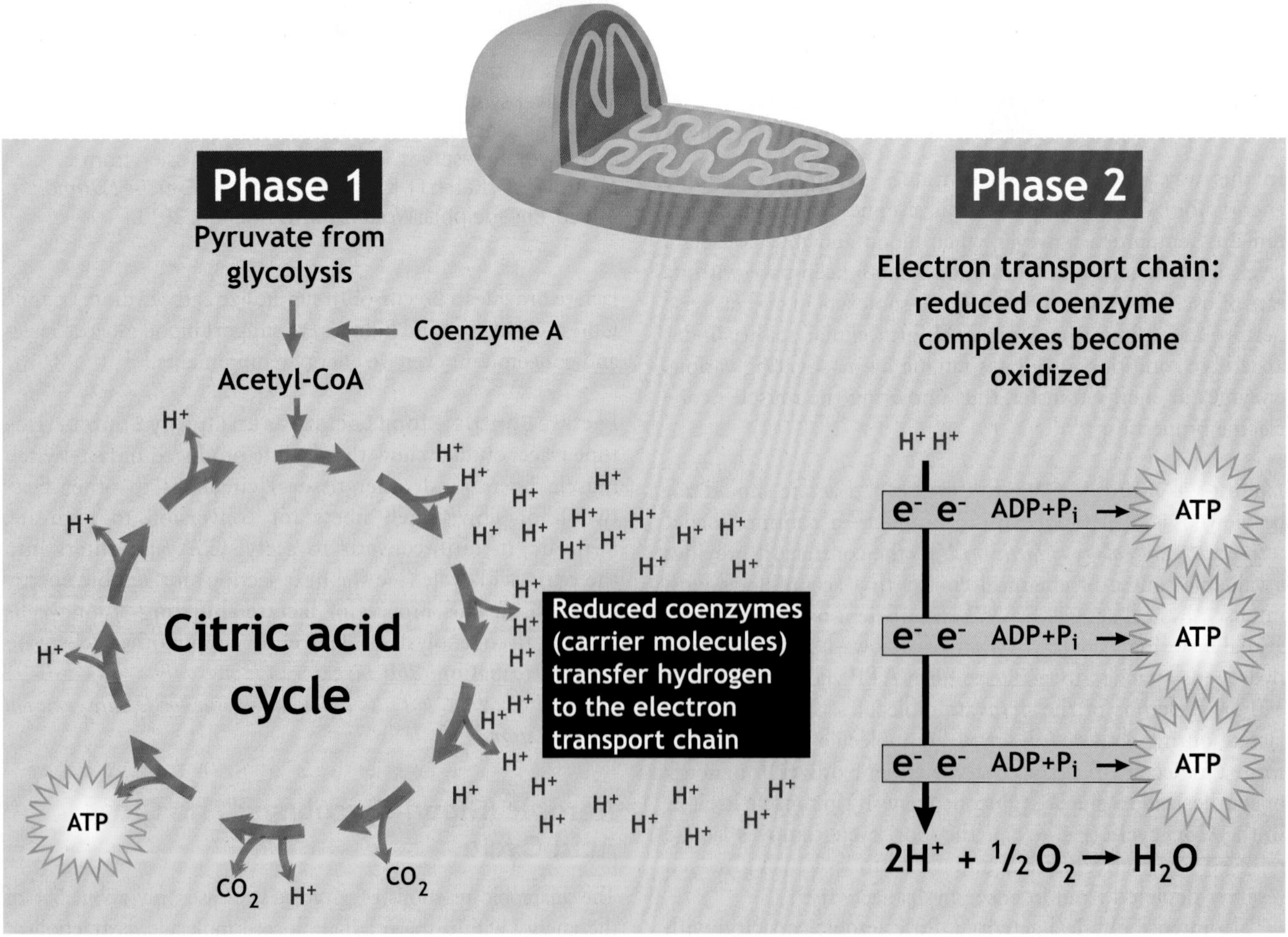

FIGURE 6.13 • Aerobic energy metabolism. Phase 1. In the mitochondria, the citric acid cycle generates hydrogen atoms during acetyl-CoA breakdown. Phase 2. Significant quantities of ATP regenerate when these hydrogens oxidize via the aerobic process of electron transport–oxidative phosphorylation (electron transport chain). (Adapted with permission from McArdle WD, Katch FI, Katch VL. *Sports and Exercise Nutrition*. 4th Ed. Philadelphia: Wolters Kluwer Health, 2013.)

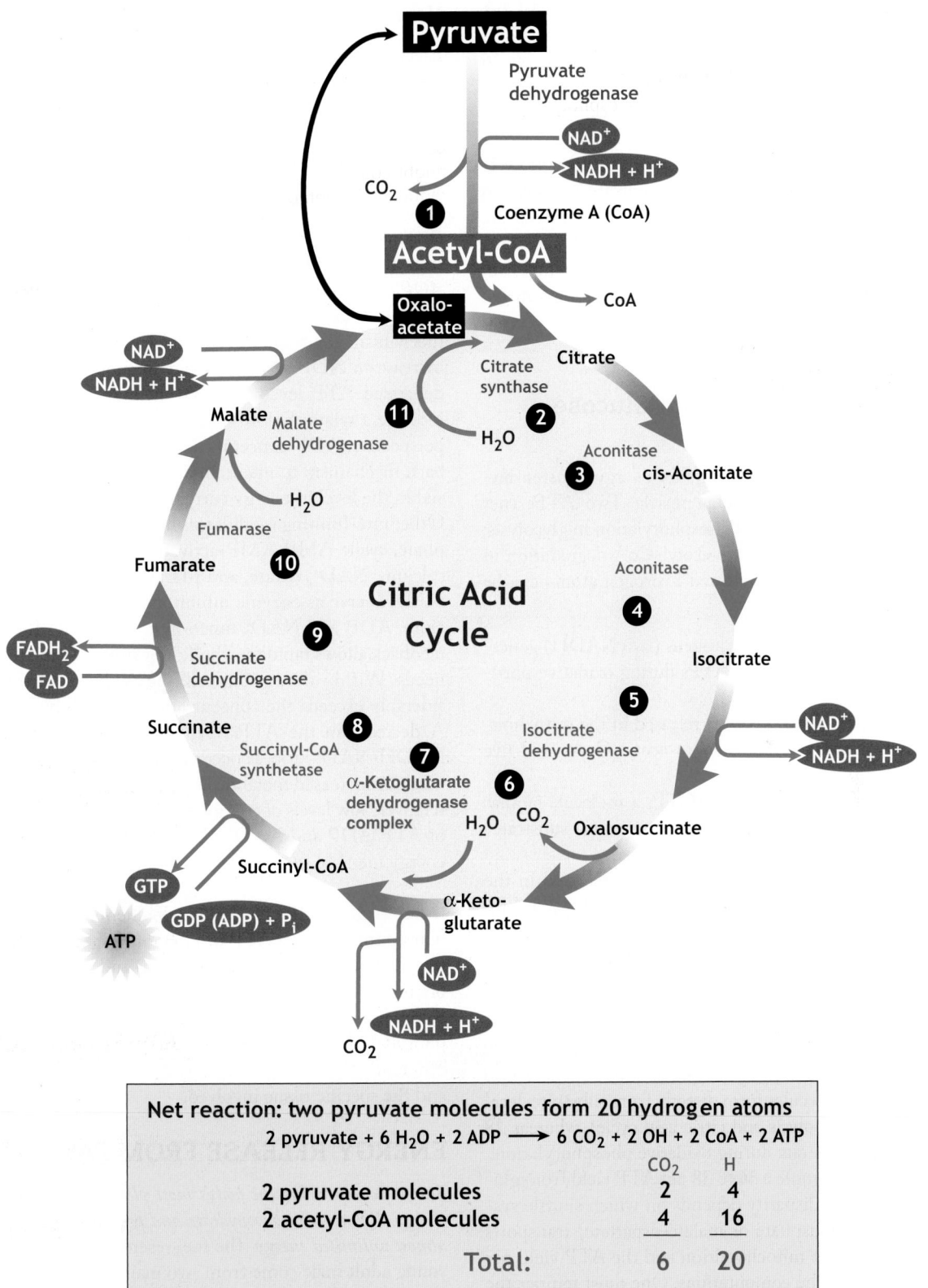

Net reaction: two pyruvate molecules form 20 hydrogen atoms

2 pyruvate + 6 H_2O + 2 ADP ⟶ 6 CO_2 + 2 OH + 2 CoA + 2 ATP

	CO_2	H
2 pyruvate molecules	2	4
2 acetyl-CoA molecules	4	16
Total:	6	20

FIGURE 6.14 • Flow sheet for the release of hydrogen and carbon dioxide in the mitochondrion during the breakdown of one pyruvate molecule. All values are doubled when computing the net gain of hydrogen and carbon dioxide because two molecules of pyruvate form from one glucose molecule in glycolysis. Enzymes colored purple are key regulatory enzymes. (Reprinted with permission from McArdle WD, Katch FI, Katch VL. *Sports and Exercise Nutrition*. 4th Ed. Philadelphia: Wolters Kluwer Health, 2013.)

of hydrogen atoms. One molecule of ATP also regenerates directly by substrate-level phosphorylation from citric acid cycle reactions (reactions 7–8, Fig. 6.14). As summarized at the bottom of Figure. 6.14, the formation of two acetyl-CoA molecules from two pyruvate molecules created in glycolysis releases four hydrogens, while the citric acid cycle releases 16 hydrogens for a total of 20 hydrogens. *The primary function of the citric acid cycle generates electrons (H^+) for passage in the respiratory chain to NAD^+ and FAD.*

Oxygen does not participate directly in citric acid cycle reactions. The chemical energy within pyruvate transfers to ADP through electron transport–oxidative phosphorylation. With adequate oxygen, including enzymes and substrate, NAD^+ and FAD regenerate, and citric acid cycle metabolism proceeds unimpeded. *Citric acid cycle, electron transport, and oxidative phosphorylation represent the three components of aerobic metabolism.*

Total Energy Transfer From Glucose Catabolism

Figure **6.15** summarizes the pathways for energy transfer during glucose catabolism in skeletal muscle. Two ATPs (net gain) form from substrate-level phosphorylation in glycolysis; similarly, two ATPs emerge from acetyl-CoA degradation in the citric acid cycle. The 24 released hydrogen atoms can be accounted for as follows:

1. Four extramitochondrial hydrogens (two NADH) generated in glycolysis yield five ATPs during oxidative phosphorylation.
2. Four hydrogens (two NADH) released in the mitochondrion when pyruvate degrades to acetyl-CoA yield five ATPs.
3. Two guanosine triphosphates (GTP; a molecule similar to ATP) produced in the citric acid cycle via substrate-level phosphorylation.
4. Twelve of the 16 hydrogens (6 NADH) released in the citric acid cycle, to yield 15 ATPs (6 NADH × 2.5 ATP per NADH = 15 ATP).
5. Four hydrogens joined to FAD (two $FADH_2$) in the citric acid cycle to yield three ATPs.

The complete breakdown of glucose yields a total of 34 ATPs. *Because two ATPs initially phosphorylate glucose, 32 ATP molecules equal the net ATP yield from glucose catabolism in skeletal muscle.* Four ATP molecules form directly from substrate-level phosphorylation (glycolysis and citric acid cycle), whereas 28 ATP molecules regenerate during oxidative phosphorylation.

Some textbooks quote a 36 to 38 net ATP yield from glucose catabolism. The disparity depends on which shuttle system (the glycerol–phosphate or malate–aspartate) transports $NADH + H^+$ into the mitochondrion and the ATP yield per H oxidation used in the computations. One must temper the theoretical values for ATP yield in energy metabolism in light of biochemical information that suggests they overestimate because only 30 to 32 ATP actually enter the cell's cytoplasm. The differentiation between theoretical versus actual ATP yield may result from the added energy cost to transport ATP out of the mitochondria.[10]

What Regulates Energy Metabolism?

Electron transport and subsequent energy release normally tightly couple to ADP phosphorylation. Without ADP availability for phosphorylation to ATP, electrons generally do not shuttle down the respiratory chain to oxygen. *Metabolites that either inhibit or activate enzymes at key control points in the oxidative pathways modulate regulatory control of glycolysis and the citric acid cycle.*[14,16,28,31] Each pathway contains at least one enzyme considered rate limiting because the enzyme controls the overall speed of that pathway's reactions. *Cellular ADP concentration exerts the greatest effect on the rate-limiting enzymes that control macronutrient energy metabolism.* This mechanism for respiratory control makes sense because any increase in ADP signals a need to supply energy to restore depressed ATP levels. Conversely, high cellular ATP levels indicate a relatively low energy requirement. From a broader perspective, ADP concentrations function as a cellular feedback mechanism to maintain a relative constancy (homeostasis) in the level of energy currency required for biologic work. Other rate-limiting modulators include cellular levels of phosphate, cyclic AMP, AMP-activated protein kinase (AMPK), calcium, NAD^+, citrate, and pH. More specifically, ATP and NADH serve as enzyme inhibitors, whereas intracellular calcium, ADP, and NAD^+ function as activators. This chemical feedback allows rapid metabolic adjustment to the cells' energy needs. Within the resting cell, the ATP concentration considerably exceeds the concentration of ADP by about 500:1. A decrease in the ATP/ADP ratio and intramitochondrial $NADH/NAD^+$ ratio, as occurs when exercise begins, signals a need for increased metabolism of stored nutrients. In contrast, relatively low levels of energy metabolism maintain high ratios of ATP/ADP and $NADH/NAD^+$, which depress the rate of energy metabolism.[1]

Independent Effects. No single chemical regulator dominates mitochondrial ATP production. In vitro (artificial environment outside the living organism) and in vivo (in the living organism) experiments show that changes in each of these compounds independently alter the rate of oxidative phosphorylation. All exert regulatory effects, each contributing differently depending on energy demands, cellular conditions, and the specific tissue involved.

ENERGY RELEASE FROM FAT

Stored fat represents the body's most plentiful source of potential energy. Relative to carbohydrate and protein, stored fat provides almost unlimited energy. The fuel reserves from fat in a typical young adult male come from two main sources:

1. Between 60,000 and 100,000 kcal (enough energy to power about 25 to 40 marathon runs) from triacylglycerol in fat cells (adipocytes) distributed throughout the body (see Chapter 28)

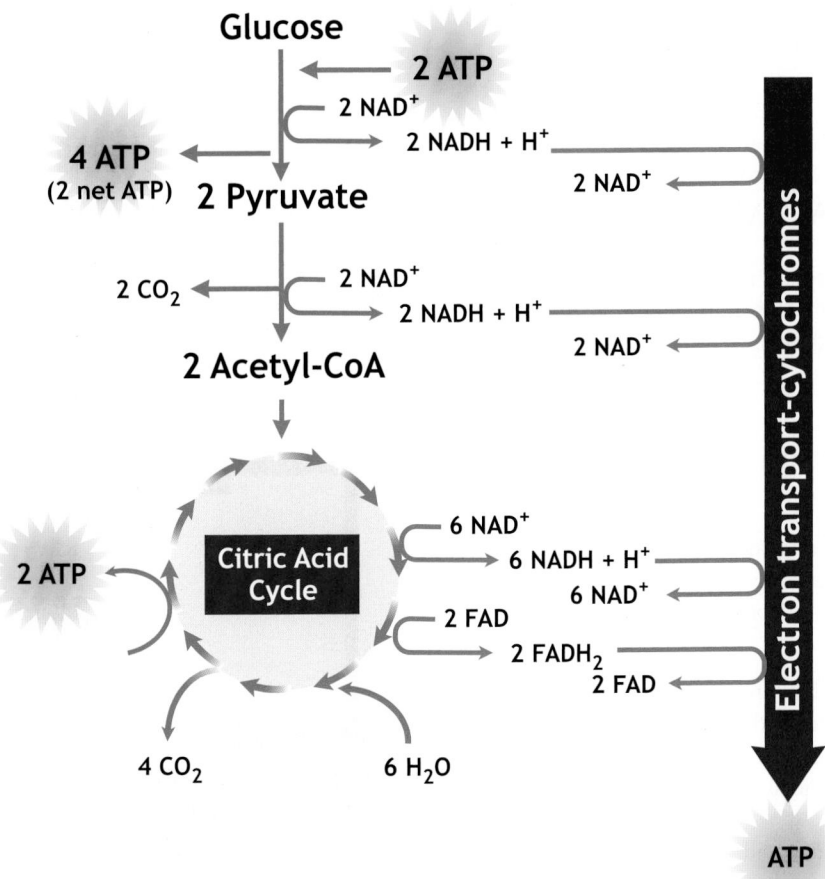

FIGURE 6.15 • A net yield of 32 ATPs from energy transfer during the complete oxidation of one glucose molecule in glycolysis, citric acid cycle, and electron transport. (Adapted with permission from McArdle WD, Katch FI, Katch VL. *Sports and Exercise Nutrition*. 4th Ed. Philadelphia: Wolters Kluwer Health, 2013.)

2. About 3000 kcal from intramuscular triacylglycerol (12 mmol · kg muscle^{-1})

In contrast, carbohydrate energy reserves generally amount to less than 2000 kcal.

Three specific energy sources for fat catabolism include:

1. Triacylglycerols stored directly within the muscle fiber in close proximity to the mitochondria (more in slow-twitch than in fast-twitch muscle fibers)

2. Circulating triacylglycerols in lipoprotein complexes that become hydrolyzed on the surface of a tissue's capillary endothelium

3. Circulating free fatty acids mobilized from triacylglycerols in adipose tissue

Prior to energy release from fat, hydrolysis (**lipolysis**) in the cell's cytosol splits the triacylglycerol molecule into a glycerol molecule and three water-insoluble fatty acid molecules. **Hormone-sensitive lipase** (activated by cyclic AMP;

see section on "Hormonal Effects" and Chapter 20) catalyzes triacylglycerol breakdown as follows:

$$\text{Triacylglycerol} + 3\,H_2O \xrightarrow{\text{lipase}} \text{Glycerol} + 3\,\text{Fatty acids}$$

INTEGRATIVE QUESTION

Discuss the claim that regular low-intensity physical activity stimulates greater body fat loss than high-intensity activity of equal total caloric expenditure.

Adipocytes: The Site of Fat Storage and Mobilization

FIGURE 6.16 outlines the dynamics of fatty acid mobilization (lipolysis) in adipose tissue and delivery to skeletal muscle. Lipid mobilization and catabolism involves seven discrete processes:

1. Breakdown of triacylglycerol to free fatty acids
2. Transport of free fatty acids in the blood
3. Uptake of free fatty acids from blood to muscle
4. Preparation of fatty acids for catabolism (energy activation)
5. Entry of activated fatty acid into muscle mitochondria
6. Breakdown of fatty acid to acetyl-CoA via β-oxidation and the production of NADH and $FADH_2$
7. Coupled oxidation in citric acid cycle and electron transport chain

All cells store some fat, but adipose tissue serves as the major supplier of fatty acid molecules. Adipocytes specialize in synthesizing and storing triacylglycerols. Triacylglycerol fat droplets occupy up to 95% of adipocyte cell volume. Once hormone-sensitive lipase stimulates fatty acids to diffuse from the adipocyte into the circulation, nearly all of them bind to plasma albumin for transport to active tissues as **free fatty acids (FFAs)**.[8,34] Hence, FFAs are not truly "free" entities. At the muscle site, the albumin–FFA complex releases FFAs for transport by diffusion and/or a protein-mediated carrier system across the plasma membrane. Once inside the muscle fiber, FFAs accomplish two tasks:

1. Re-esterify to form triacylglycerols
2. Bind with intramuscular proteins and enter the mitochondria for energy metabolism by action of **carnitine acyltransferase** located on the inner mitochondrial membrane

Carnitine acyltransferase catalyzes the transfer of an acyl group to carnitine to form acylcarnitine, a compound that readily crosses the mitochondrial membrane. Medium- and short-chain fatty acids do not depend on this enzyme-mediated transport. Instead, these fatty acids diffuse freely into the mitochondria.

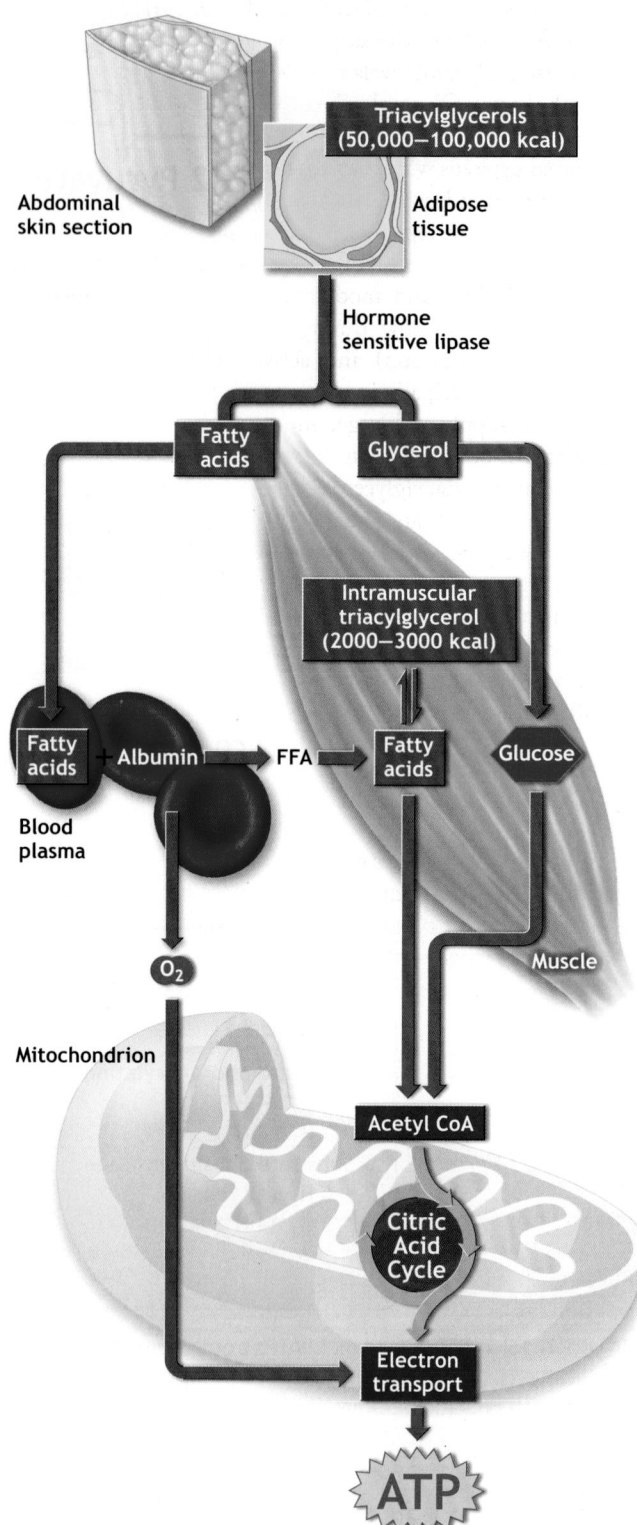

FIGURE 6.16 • Dynamics of fat mobilization and fat use. Hormone-sensitive lipase stimulates triacylglycerol breakdown into its glycerol and fatty acid components. The blood transports free fatty acids (FFAs) released from adipocytes and bound to plasma albumin. Energy is released when triacylglycerols stored within the muscle fiber also degrade to glycerol and fatty acids.

The water-soluble glycerol molecule formed during lipolysis diffuses from the adipocyte into the circulation. This allows plasma glycerol levels to reflect the level of triacylglycerol catabolism.[32] Glycerol, when delivered to the liver, serves as a precursor for glucose synthesis. The relatively slow rate of this process explains why supplementing with exogenous glycerol (consumed in liquid form) contributes little as an energy substrate or glucose replenisher during exercise.[27]

Adipose tissue release of FFAs and their subsequent use for energy in light and moderate physical activity increase directly with blood flow through adipose tissue (threefold increase not uncommon) and active muscle. FFA catabolism increases principally in slow-twitch muscle fibers whose ample blood supply and large, numerous mitochondria make them ideal for fat breakdown.

Circulating triacylglycerols carried in lipoprotein complexes also provide an energy source. **Lipoprotein lipase (LPL)**, an enzyme synthesized within the cell and localized on the surface of its surrounding capillaries, catalyzes the hydrolysis of these triacylglycerols. LPL also facilitates a cell's uptake of fatty acids for energy metabolism or for resynthesis (called *reesterfication*) of triacylglycerols stored within muscle and adipose tissues.[34]

 INTEGRATIVE QUESTION

If an average person stores enough energy as body fat to power a 750-mile run, why do athletes often experience impaired performance toward the end of a 26.2-mile marathon performed under intense, steady-rate aerobic metabolism?

Hormonal Effects

Epinephrine, norepinephrine, glucagon, and growth hormone augment lipase activation and subsequent lipolysis and FFA mobilization from adipose tissue. Plasma concentrations of these lipogenic hormones increase during exercise to continually supply active muscles with energy-rich substrate. An intracellular mediator, **adenosine 3′,5′-cyclic monophosphate (cyclic AMP)**, activates hormone-sensitive lipase and thus regulates fat breakdown. Various lipid-mobilizing hormones, which themselves do not enter the cell, activate cyclic AMP.[35] Circulating lactate, ketones, and particularly insulin inhibit cyclic AMP activation.[8] Physical training–induced increases in the activity level of skeletal muscle and adipose tissue lipases, including biochemical and vascular adaptations in the muscles themselves, enhance fat use for energy during moderate activity.[19,20,21,24] Paradoxically, excess body fat decreases the availability of fatty acids during physical activity.[25] Chapter 20 presents a more detailed evaluation of hormone regulation in exercise and training.

The availability of fatty acid molecules regulates fat breakdown or synthesis. After a meal, when energy metabolism remains relatively low, digestive processes increase FFA and triacylglycerol delivery to cells; this in turn stimulates triacylglycerol synthesis. In contrast, moderate physical activity increases fatty acid use for energy, which reduces their cellular concentration. The decrease in intracellular FFAs stimulates triacylglycerol breakdown into glycerol and fatty acid components. Concurrently, hormonal release triggered by movement stimulates adipose tissue lipolysis to further augment FFA delivery to active muscle.

Catabolism of Glycerol and Fatty Acids

Figure 6.17 summarizes the pathways for degrading the glycerol and fatty acid fragments of the triacylglycerol molecule.

Glycerol

The anaerobic reactions of glycolysis accept glycerol as 3-phosphoglyceraldehyde. This molecule then degrades to pyruvate to form ATP by substrate-level phosphorylation. Hydrogen atoms pass to NAD⁺, and the citric acid cycle oxidizes pyruvate. *The complete breakdown of a single glycerol molecule synthesizes 19 ATP molecules.* Glycerol also provides carbon skeletons for glucose synthesis (see "In a Practical Sense"). The gluconeogenic role of glycerol becomes important when glycogen reserves deplete from either dietary restriction of carbohydrates, long-term physical activity, or intense training.

 INTEGRATIVE QUESTION

If elite marathoners run at an exercise intensity that does not cause appreciable accumulation of blood lactate, why do some athletes appear disoriented and fatigued and forced to slow down toward the end of a 26.2-mile competition?

Fatty Acids

Fatty acid molecules transform into acetyl-CoA in the mitochondria during **beta (β)-oxidation**. This involves successive splitting of 2-carbon acyl fragments from the long chain of the fatty acid. ATP phosphorylates the reactions, water is added, hydrogens pass to NAD⁺ and FAD, and the acyl fragment joins with coenzyme A to form acetyl-CoA. β-oxidation provides the same acetyl unit as that generated from glucose catabolism. β-oxidation continues until the entire fatty acid molecule degrades to acetyl-CoA for direct entry into the citric acid cycle. The hydrogens released during fatty acid catabolism oxidize through the respiratory chain. *Note that fatty acid breakdown relates directly to oxygen consumption. Oxygen* must join with hydrogen for β-oxidation to proceed. Under anaerobic conditions, hydrogen remains with NAD⁺ and FAD, thus halting fat catabolism.

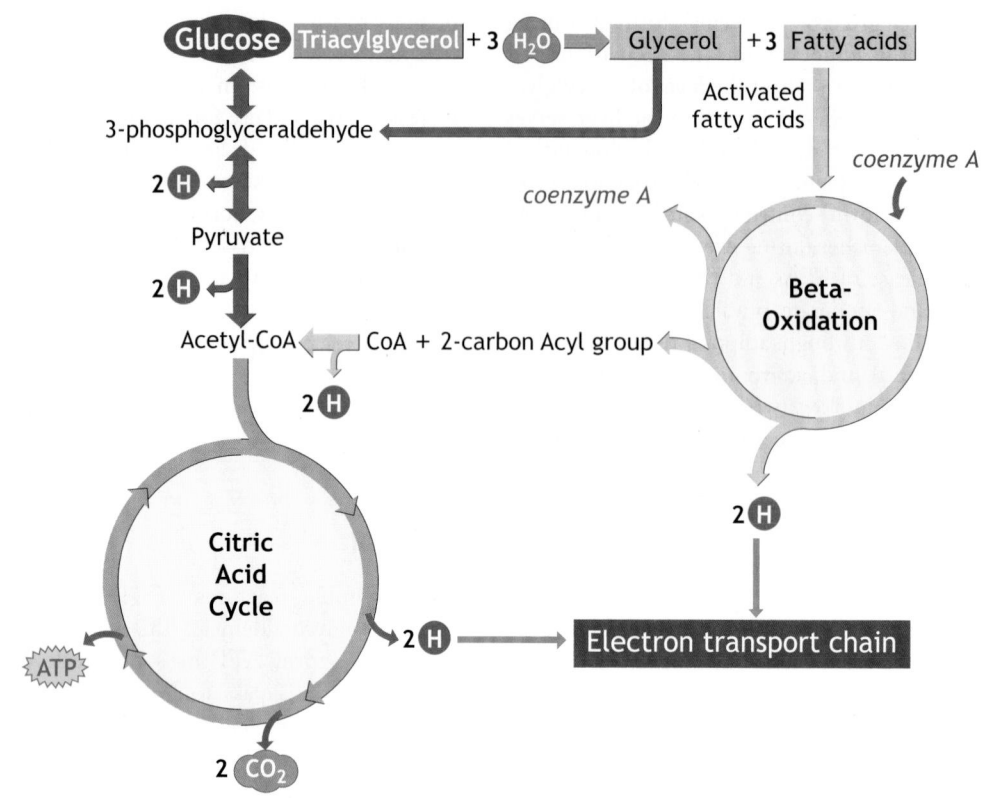

Source	Pathway	ATP yield per molecule neutral fat
1 molecule glycerol	Glycolysis + Citric acid cycle	19
3 molecules of 18-carbon fatty acid	ß-oxidation + Citric acid cycle	441
		TOTAL: 460

FIGURE 6.17 • General schema for the breakdown of the glycerol and fatty acid components of a triacylglycerol molecule. Glycerol enters the energy pathways during glycolysis. Fatty acids prepare to enter the citric acid cycle through β-oxidation. The electron transport chain accepts hydrogens released during glycolysis, β-oxidation, and citric acid cycle metabolism.

Total Energy Transfer From Fat Catabolism

The breakdown of a fatty acid molecule progresses in three stages as follows:

1. β-oxidation produces NADH and $FADH_2$ by cleaving the fatty acid molecule into 2-carbon acyl fragments.
2. Citric acid cycle degrades acetyl-CoA into carbon dioxide and hydrogen atoms.
3. Hydrogen atoms oxidize via electron transport–oxidative phosphorylation.

For each 18-carbon fatty acid molecule, 147 molecules of ADP phosphorylate to ATP during β-oxidation and citric acid cycle metabolism. Each triacylglycerol molecule contains three fatty acid molecules to form 441 ATP molecules from the fatty acid components (3×147 ATP). Also, 19 ATP molecules form during glycerol breakdown to generate 460 molecules of ATP for each triacylglycerol molecule catabolized. This represents a considerable energy yield compared to the net 32 ATPs formed when a skeletal muscle catabolizes a glucose molecule. The efficiency of energy conservation for fatty acid oxidation amounts to about 40%, a value slightly higher than glucose oxidation.

Intracellular and extracellular lipid molecules usually supply between 30 and 80% of the energy for biologic work, depending on a person's nutritional status, level of training, and the intensity and duration of physical activity.[38] Fat becomes the *primary* energy fuel for exercise and recovery when intense, long-duration exercise depletes glycogen.[21] Furthermore, enzymatic adaptations occur with prolonged exposure to a high-fat, low-carbohydrate diet because this dietary regimen enhances capacity for fat oxidation during physical activity.[26]

IN A PRACTICAL SENSE

Potential for Glucose Synthesis from Triacylglycerol Components

Circulating glucose provides vital fuel for brain and red blood cell functions. Maintaining blood glucose homeostasis remains a challenge in prolonged starvation or intense endurance activity because muscle and liver glycogen reserves deplete rapidly. When this occurs, the central nervous system eventually metabolizes ketone bodies as an energy fuel. The ketones consist of three water-soluble dissolved compounds—acetone, acetoacetic acid, and β-hydroxybutyric acid—produced when fatty acids break down for energy in the liver. Concurrently, muscle protein (amino acids) degrades to gluconeogenic constituents to sustain plasma glucose levels. Excessive muscle protein catabolism eventually produces a muscle-wasting effect. Reliance on protein catabolism, coincident with depleted glycogen, continues because fatty acids from triacylglycerol hydrolysis in muscle and adipose tissue fail to provide gluconeogenic substrates.

NO GLUCOSE SYNTHESIS FROM FATTY ACIDS

The accompanying figure illustrates why humans cannot convert fatty acids (palmitate in example) from triacylglycerol breakdown to glucose. Fatty acid oxidation within the mitochondria produces acetyl-CoA. Because the *pyruvate dehydrogenase* and *pyruvate kinase* reactions proceed irreversibly, acetyl-CoA cannot simply form pyruvate by carboxylation and synthesize glucose by reversing glycolysis. Instead, the 2-carbon acetyl group formed from acetyl-CoA degrades further when it enters the citric acid cycle. In humans, fatty acid hydrolysis produces no net synthesis of glucose.

LIMITED GLUCOSE FROM TRIACYLGLYCEROL-DERIVED GLYCEROL

The figure also shows that triacylglycerol hydrolysis via hormone-sensitive lipase (HSL) produces a single 3-carbon glycerol molecule. Unlike fatty acids, the liver can use glycerol for glucose synthesis. After delivery of glycerol in the blood to the liver, glycerol kinase phosphorylates it to glycerol 3-phosphate. Further reduction produces dihydroxyacetone phosphate, a substance that provides the carbon skeleton for continued glucose synthesis.

There is a clear "practical application" to sports and exercise nutrition from an understanding of the limited metabolic pathways available for glucose synthesis from the body's triacylglycerol energy depots. Replenishment and maintenance of liver and muscle glycogen reserves depend on exogenous carbohydrate intake. The physically active person must make a concerted effort to regularly consume nutritious, low-to-moderate glycemic sources of this macronutrient.

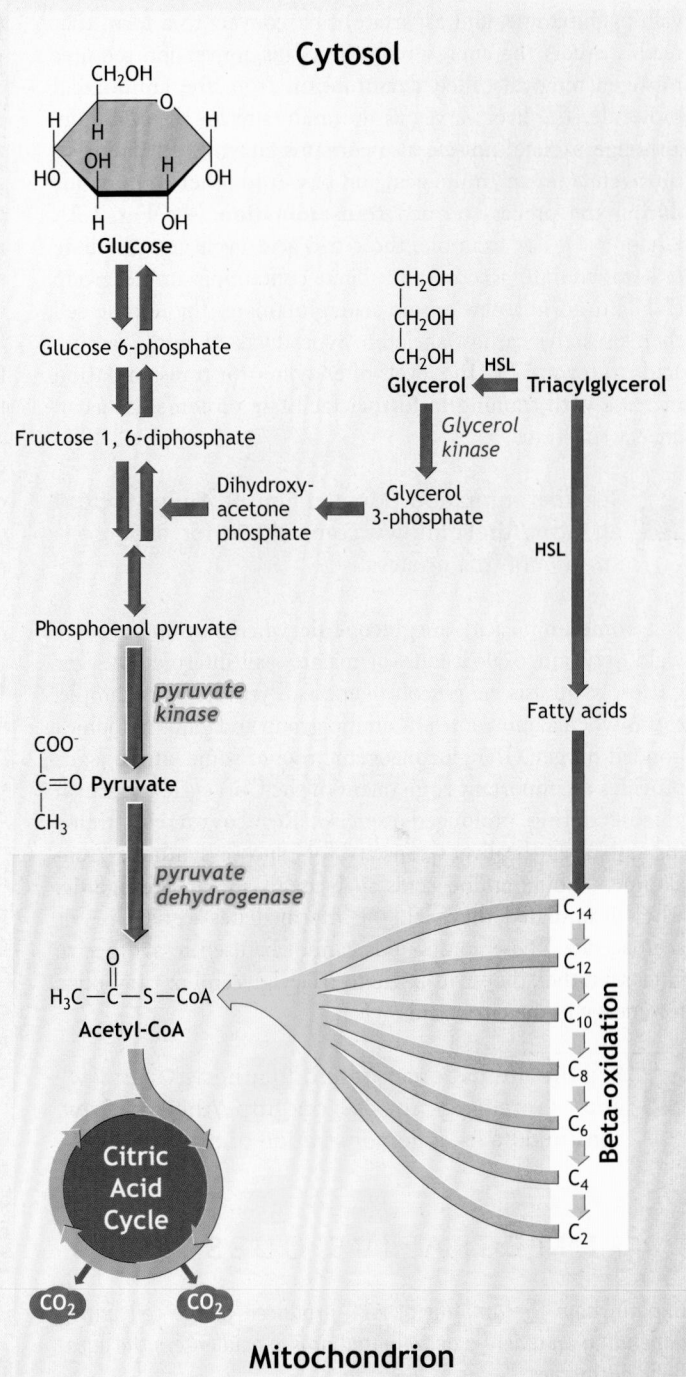

ENERGY RELEASE FROM PROTEIN

Chapter 1 emphasized that protein plays a contributory role as an energy substrate during endurance activities and intense training. When used for energy, the amino acids (primarily the branched-chain amino acids leucine, isoleucine, valine, glutamine, and aspartate) first convert to a form that readily enters the energy pathways. This conversion requires nitrogen removal called **deamination** from the amino acid molecule. The liver serves as the main site for deamination, although skeletal muscle also contains enzymes that remove nitrogen from an amino acid and pass it to other compounds during the process termed **transamination** (see Fig. 1.21, Chapter 1). For example, the citric acid cycle intermediate α-ketoglutarate accepts a nitrogen-containing amine group (NH_2) to form a new amino acid, glutamate. The muscle cell then uses the carbon-skeleton byproducts of donor amino acids to form ATP. The levels of enzymes for transamination increase with training to further facilitate protein's use as an energy substrate.

 See the animation "Metabolism of Amino Acids" on http://thePoint.lww.com/mkk8e for a demonstration of this process.

Some amino acids are **glucogenic**; when deaminated, they yield pyruvate, oxaloacetate, or malate—all intermediates for glucose synthesis via gluconeogenesis. Pyruvate, for example, forms when alanine loses its amino group and gains a double-bonded oxygen. The gluconeogenic role of some amino acids provides an important component of the Cori cycle to furnish glucose during prolonged exercise. Regular exercise training enhances the liver's capacity for glucose synthesis from alanine.[37] Some amino acids such as glycine are **ketogenic**; when deaminated, they yield the intermediates acetyl-CoA or acetoacetate. These compounds cannot be used to synthesize glucose; rather, they synthesize to triacylglycerol or catabolize for energy in the citric acid cycle.

 See the animations "Protein Synthesis Overview" and "Protein Synthesis" on http://thePoint.lww.com/mkk8e for a demonstration of this process.

 INTEGRATIVE QUESTION

Explain how the amount of ATP produced in the cell varies depending on where a deaminated amino acid enters the catabolic pathways.

Protein Breakdown Facilitates Water Loss

When protein provides energy, the body must eliminate the nitrogen-containing amine group and other solutes produced from protein breakdown. These waste products leave the body dissolved in "obligatory" fluid (urine). For this reason, excessive protein catabolism increases the body's water needs.

THE METABOLIC MILL: INTERRELATIONSHIPS AMONG CARBOHYDRATE, FAT, AND PROTEIN METABOLISM

The "metabolic mill" illustrated in FIGURE 6.18 depicts the citric acid cycle as the vital link between macronutrient (carbohydrate, fat, protein) energy and chemical energy in ATP. The citric acid cycle also serves as a metabolic hub to provide intermediates that cross the mitochondrial membrane into the cytosol to synthesize bionutrients for maintenance and growth. For example, excess carbohydrates provide the glycerol and acetyl fragments to synthesize triacylglycerol, which can contribute to increased body fatness. Acetyl-CoA functions as the starting point for synthesizing cholesterol and many hormones. Fatty acids *cannot* contribute to glucose synthesis because the conversion of pyruvate to acetyl-CoA does not reverse (notice the one-way arrow in Fig. 6.17). Many of the carbon compounds generated in citric acid cycle reactions also provide the organic starting points to synthesize nonessential amino acids.

Glucose Conversion to Fat

Lipogenesis describes the formation of fat, mostly in the cytoplasm of liver cells. It occurs when ingested glucose or protein not used to sustain energy metabolism converts into stored triacylglycerol. For example, when muscle and liver glycogen stores fill (as after a large carbohydrate meal), pancreatic release of insulin causes a 30-fold increase in glucose transport into adipocytes. Insulin initiates the translocation of a latent pool of GLUT 4 transporters from the adipocyte cytosol to the plasma membrane. GLUT 4 facilitates glucose transport into the cytosol for synthesis to triacylglycerols and subsequent storage within the adipocyte. This lipogenic process requires ATP energy working in concert with the B vitamins biotin, niacin, and pantothenic acid.

Lipogenesis begins with carbons from glucose and the carbon skeletons from amino acid molecules that metabolize to acetyl-CoA (see the section "Energy Release From Protein") Liver cells bond the acetate parts of the acetyl-CoA molecules in a series of steps to form the 16-carbon saturated fatty acid palmitic acid. This molecule then lengthens to an

 Excess Dietary Protein Accumulates as Fat

Athletes and others who believe that taking protein supplements builds muscle should take pause. Extra protein consumed above the body's requirement (easily achieved with a well-balanced "normal" diet) ends up either catabolized for energy or converted to body fat! This excess does *not* contribute to the synthesis of muscle tissue.

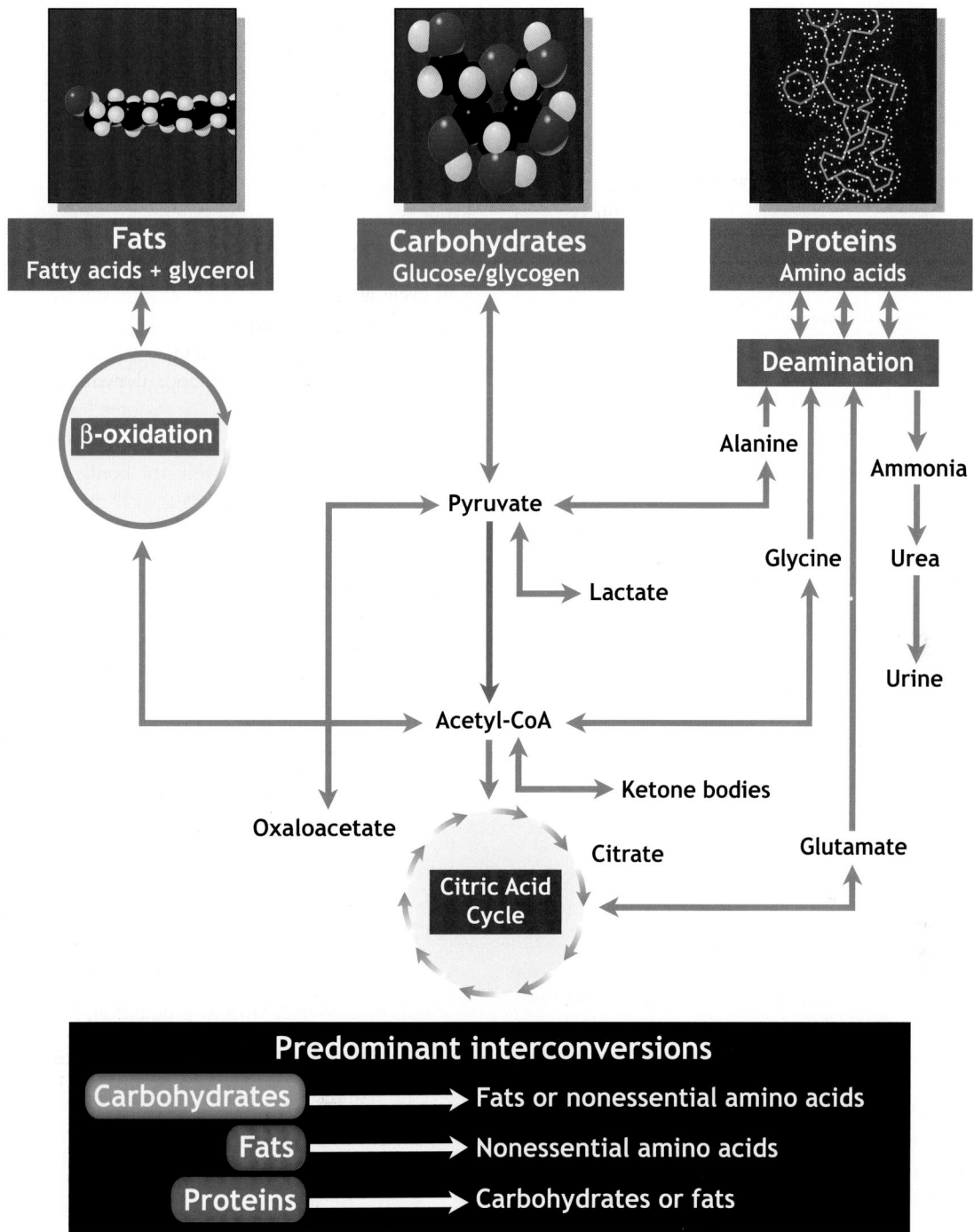

FIGURE 6.18 • The "metabolic mill" allows important interconversions for catabolism and anabolism among carbohydrates, fats, and proteins. (Adapted with permission from McArdle WD, Katch FI, Katch VL. *Sports and Exercise Nutrition*. 4th Ed. Philadelphia: Wolters Kluwer Health, 2013.)

18- or 20-carbon chain fatty acid in either the cytosol or the mitochondria. Three fatty acid molecules ultimately join (esterify) with one glycerol molecule (produced during glycolysis) to yield one triacylglycerol molecule. Triacylglycerol releases into the circulation as a very low-density lipoprotein (VLDL); cells can use VLDL for ATP production or store it in adipocytes along with other fats from dietary sources.

Protein Conversion to Fat

Surplus dietary protein (similar to carbohydrate) readily converts to fat. After protein's digestion, the circulation transports the amino acids absorbed by the small intestine to the liver. Figure 6.18 illustrates that the carbon skeletons from these amino acids after deamination convert to pyruvate. This six-carbon molecule then enters the mitochondrion for conversion to acetyl-CoA for one of two purposes:

1. Catabolism in the citric acid cycle
2. Fatty acid synthesis

Fats Burn in a Carbohydrate Flame

In metabolically active tissues, fatty acid breakdown depends somewhat on continual background levels of carbohydrate catabolism. Recall that acetyl-CoA enters the citric acid cycle by combining with oxaloacetate to form citrate. Oxaloacetate then regenerates from pyruvate during carbohydrate breakdown. This conversion occurs under enzymatic control of pyruvate carboxylase, which adds a carboxyl group to the pyruvate molecule. The degradation of fatty acids in the citric acid cycle continues only if sufficient oxaloacetate and other intermediates from carbohydrate breakdown combine with the acetyl-CoA formed during β-oxidation. These intermediates are continually lost or removed from the cycle and need to be replenished. Pyruvate formed during glucose catabolism plays an important role in maintaining a proper level of oxaloacetate (Figs. 6.14 and 6.18). Low pyruvate levels (as occurs with inadequate carbohydrate breakdown) reduce levels of the citric acid cycle intermediates (oxaloacetate and malate). Fats require such intermediates generated during carbohydrate breakdown for their continual catabolism for energy in the metabolic mill.[5,11,30,36,40] In the sense that carbohydrate acts as a metabolic primer, we can state that "fats burn in a carbohydrate flame."

A Slower Rate of Energy Release From Fat

A rate limit exists for fatty acid use by active muscle.[41] *The power generated solely by fat breakdown represents only about one-half that achieved with carbohydrate as the chief aerobic energy source.* Thus, depleting muscle glycogen must decrease a muscle's maximum aerobic power output. Just as the hypoglycemic condition coincides with a "central" or neural fatigue, muscle glycogen depletion probably causes "peripheral" or local muscle fatigue during exercise.[29]

Gluconeogenesis provides a metabolic option to synthesize glucose from noncarbohydrate sources. This process does not replenish or even maintain glycogen stores without adequate carbohydrate consumption. Appreciably reducing carbohydrate availability seriously limits energy transfer capacity. Glycogen depletion can occur under the following five conditions:

1. Prolonged physical activity (e.g., marathon running)
2. Consecutive days of intense training
3. Inadequate energy intake (routinely skipping meals)
4. Dietary elimination of carbohydrates (as advocated with high-fat, low-carbohydrate "ketogenic diets")
5. Diabetes, which impairs cellular glucose uptake

Depletion of glycogen depresses aerobic exercise intensity, even if large amounts of fatty acid substrate still circulate to muscle. With extreme carbohydrate depletion, the acetate fragments acetoacetate and α-hydroxybutyrate produced in β-oxidation accumulate in extracellular fluids because they cannot enter the citric acid cycle. The liver then converts these compounds to ketone bodies, some of which pass in the urine. If ketosis persists, the acid quality of the body fluids can increase to potentially toxic levels.

Summary

1. Food macronutrients provide the major sources of potential energy to form ATP (when ADP and a phosphate ion rejoin).
2. The complete breakdown of 1 mole of glucose liberates 689 kcal of energy. Of this, the bonds within ATP conserve about 224 kcal (34%), with the remaining energy dissipated as heat.
3. During glycolytic reactions in the cell's cytosol, a net of two ATP molecules forms during anaerobic substrate-level phosphorylation.
4. Pyruvate converts to acetyl-CoA during the second stage of carbohydrate breakdown within the mitochondrion. Acetyl-CoA then progresses through the citric acid cycle.
5. The respiratory chain oxidizes the hydrogen atoms released during glucose breakdown; a portion of the released energy couples with ADP phosphorylation.
6. Complete oxidation of a glucose molecule in skeletal muscle yields a total (net gain) of 32 ATP molecules.
7. Oxidation of hydrogen atoms at their rate of formation establishes a biochemical steady state or "steady rate" of aerobic metabolism.
8. During intense physical activity when hydrogen oxidation fails to keep pace with its production, pyruvate temporarily binds hydrogen to form lactate. This allows progression of anaerobic glycolysis for an additional duration.
9. Compounds that either inhibit or activate enzymes at key control points in the oxidative pathways modulate regulatory control of glycolysis and the citric acid cycle.
10. Cellular ADP concentration exerts the greatest effect on the rate-limiting enzymes that control energy metabolism.
11. The complete oxidation of a triacylglycerol molecule yields about 460 ATP molecules. Fatty acid catabolism requires oxygen; the term *aerobic* describes such reactions.
12. Protein serves as a potentially important energy substrate. After nitrogen removal from the amino acid molecule during deamination, the remaining carbon skeleton enters metabolic pathways to produce ATP aerobically.
13. Numerous interconversions take place among the food nutrients. Fatty acids represent a noteworthy exception because they cannot produce glucose.

14. Fats require intermediates generated in carbohydrate breakdown for their continual catabolism for energy in the metabolic mill. To this extent, "fats burn in a carbohydrate flame."

15. The power generated solely by fat breakdown represents only about half of that achieved with carbohydrate as the chief aerobic energy source. Thus, muscle glycogen depletion considerably decreases a muscle's maximum aerobic power output.

thePoint References and Suggested Readings are available online at http://thepoint.lww.com/mkk8e.

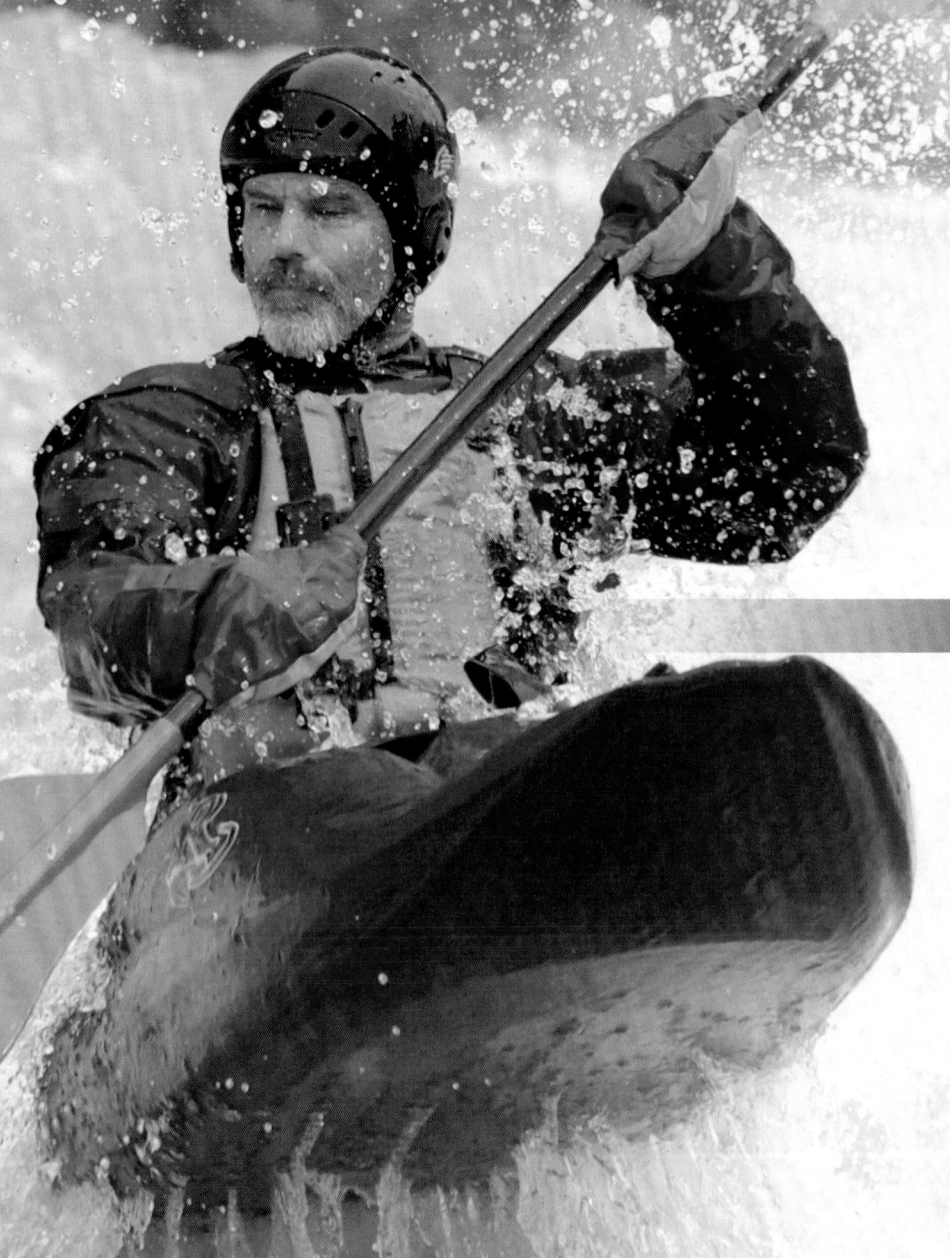

Energy Transfer During Physical Activity

CHAPTER OBJECTIVES

- Identify the three energy systems and outline the relative contribution of each for intensity and duration of physical activity; relate your discussion to specific sport activities

- Discuss the blood lactate threshold and indicate differences between sedentary and endurance-trained individuals

- Outline the time course for oxygen consumption during 10 min of moderate-intensity physical activity

- Draw a figure to illustrate oxygen consumption during progressive increments in exercise intensity up to maximum

- Differentiate between type I and type II muscle fibers

- Discuss differences in recovery oxygen consumption patterns from moderate and exhaustive physical activity. What factors account for the excess postexercise oxygen consumption (EPOC) from each form of activity?

- Outline optimal recovery procedures from steady-rate and non–steady-rate exercise

- Discuss the rationale for intermittent exercise applied to interval training

ANCILLARIES at-a-Glance

Visit http://thepoint.lww.com/mkk8e to access the following resources.

- References: Chapter 7
- Interactive Question Bank
- Focus on Research: A Challenge to Conventional Wisdom

Physical activity provides the greatest demand for energy transfer. In sprint running and swimming, for example, energy output from the active muscles exceeds their resting value by 120 times or more. During less intense but sustained marathon running, whole-body energy requirement increases 20 times or more above resting levels. The relative contribution of the body's energy transfer systems differs markedly depending on intensity and duration of physical activity and the participant's current fitness status.

IMMEDIATE ENERGY: THE ATP–PCR SYSTEM

Intense physical activity of short duration requires immediate energy, as in a 100-m dash, 25-m swim, or lifting a heavy weight. This energy comes almost exclusively from the intramuscular high-energy phosphate or phosphagen sources: adenosine triphosphate (ATP) and phosphocreatine (PCr). Each kilogram of skeletal muscle contains 3 to 8 mmol of ATP and four to five times more PCr. For a 70-kg person with a muscle mass of 30 kg, this represents between 570 and 690 mmol of high-energy phosphates. Assuming that 20 kg of muscle becomes active during "big-muscle" activity, sufficient stored phosphagen energy can power brisk walking for 1 min, running at a marathon pace for 20 to 30 s, or sprint-running for 5 to 8 s. The quantity of these high-energy compounds probably becomes fully depleted within 20 to 30 s of all-out exercise.[8,19] The maximum rate of energy transfer from the high-energy phosphates exceeds by four to eight times the maximal energy transfer from aerobic metabolism. In a world and Olympic record 100-m sprint by Usain Bolt of Jamaica (world record 9.58 s [10.44 m·s⁻¹], August 16, 2009; Olympic record 9.63 s; [10.38 m·s⁻¹], August 5, 2012), the runner cannot maintain maximum speed throughout the run. Toward the end of the race, the runner begins to slow; often, the winner is the one who slows down least.

SHORT-TERM GLYCOLYTIC (LACTATE-FORMING) ENERGY SYSTEM

Resynthesis of the high-energy phosphates proceeds at a rapid rate for intense, short-duration physical activity. The energy to phosphorylate ADP during such movements comes mainly from stored muscle glycogen breakdown via rapid anaerobic glycolysis with resulting lactate formation. Recall that this process allows ATP to form rapidly without oxygen. Rapid anaerobic glycolysis for ATP resynthesis can be considered reserve fuel. It comes into play when a person accelerates at the start of movement or during the last few hundred yards of a mile run, or performs all-out from start to finish during a 440-m run or 100-m swim. *Rapid and considerable accumulations of blood lactate occur during large muscle, maximal movements of between 60 and 180 seconds' duration.* Decreasing intensity to extend the movement period correspondingly decreases the rate of lactate accumulation and the final blood lactate level.

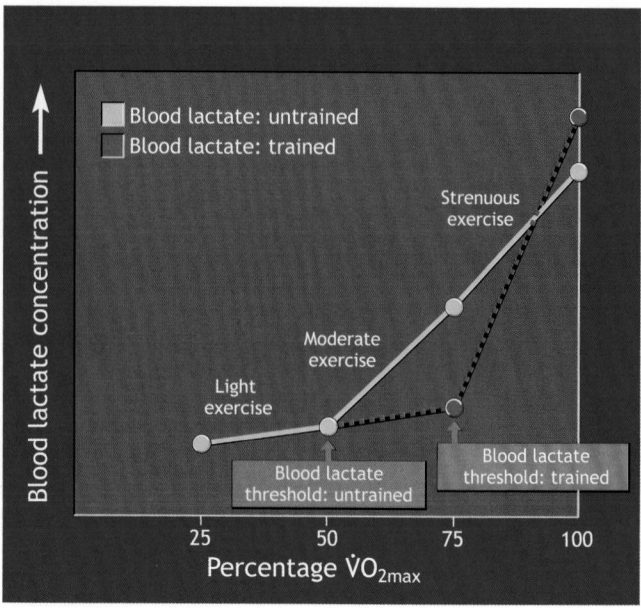

FIGURE 7.1 • Blood lactate concentration for trained and untrained subjects at different levels of physical activity expressed as a percentage of maximal oxygen consumption ($\dot{V}O_{2max}$).

Lactate Accumulation

Blood lactate does not accumulate at all levels of physical activity. FIGURE 7.1 illustrates for endurance athletes and untrained subjects the general relationship between oxygen consumption, expressed as a percentage of maximum, and blood lactate during light, moderate, and strenuous activity. During light and moderate activity (<50% aerobic capacity), blood lactate formation equals lactate disappearance and oxygen-consuming reactions adequately meet the energy demands. In biochemical terms, energy generated from hydrogen oxidation provides the predominant ATP "fuel" for muscular activity. Any lactate formed in one part of a working muscle becomes oxidized by muscle fibers with high oxidative capacity in the same muscle or less active nearby muscles such as the heart and other tisues.[11,32] When lactate oxidation equals its production, blood lactate level remains stable even though increases may occur in movement intensity and oxygen consumption.

For healthy, untrained persons, blood lactate begins to accumulate and rise in an exponential manner at about 50 to 55% of the maximal capacity for aerobic metabolism. The traditional explanation for blood lactate accumulation in physical activity assumes a relative tissue hypoxia. When glycolytic metabolism predominates, nicotinamide adenine dinucleotide (NADH) production exceeds the cell's capacity for shuttling its hydrogens (electrons) down the respiratory chain because of insufficient oxygen supply or oxygen use at the tissue level, or even stimulated by the hormones epinephrine and norepinephrine independent of tissue hypoxia. The imbalance in hydrogen release and subsequent oxidation (more precisely, the cytoplasmic NAD⁺/NADH ratio) causes pyruvate to accept the excess hydrogens (i.e., two hydrogen ions attach to the pyruvate molecule). The original pyruvate with two additional hydrogens forms a new molecule—lactic acid (changed to lactate in the body), which begins to accumulate.[33]

Radioactive tracer studies that label the carbon in the glucose molecule spawned a hypothesis to explain lactate buildup in muscle and its subsequent appearance in blood.[10] The research revealed that while lactate continuously forms in muscle during rest and moderate physical activity, about 70% of the lactate oxidizes, 20% converts to glucose in muscle and liver, and 10% synthesizes to amino acids. No *net* lactate accumulation results (i.e., blood lactate concentration remains stable). *Blood lactate accumulates only when its disappearance by oxidation or substrate conversion does not match its production.*

Aerobic training adaptations allow high rates of lactate turnover at a given movement intensity; lactate begins to accumulate at higher intensity levels than in the untrained state.[44] Another explanation for lactate buildup during physical activity includes the tendency for the enzyme lactate dehydrogenase (LDH) in fast-twitch muscle fibers to favor the conversion of pyruvate to lactate. In contrast, the LDH level in slow-twitch fibers favors lactate-to-pyruvate conversion. Recruitment of fast-twitch fibers with increasing exercise intensity therefore favors lactate formation, independent of tissue oxygenation.

Lactate production and accumulation accelerate as exercise intensity increases. In such cases, the muscle cells can neither meet the additional energy demands aerobically nor oxidize lactate at its rate of formation. A similar pattern exists for untrained subjects and endurance athletes, except the threshold for lactate buildup, termed the **blood lactate threshold**, occurs at a *higher percentage* of the athlete's aerobic capacity.[21,51,52] Trained endurance athletes perform steady-rate aerobic exercise at intensities between 80 and 90% of maximum capacity for aerobic metabolism.[48] This favorable aerobic response most likely relates to three factors[11,14,20,35]:

1. Athletes' specific genetic endowment (e.g., muscle fiber type, muscle blood flow responsiveness)
2. Specific local training adaptations that favor less lactate production
3. More rapid rate of lactate removal via greater lactate turnover and/or conversion at any intensity of physical activity

Endurance training increases capillary density and the size and number of mitochondria, including the concentration of enzymes and transfer agents in aerobic metabolism,[30,45] a response that remains unimpaired with aging.[15] Such training adaptations enhance cellular capacity to generate ATP aerobically through glucose and fatty acid catabolism. Maintaining a low lactate level also conserves glycogen reserves to inhibit the processes of muscular fatigue and extend the duration of intense aerobic effort.[49] Chapter 14 further develops the concept of the blood lactate threshold, its measurement, and its relation to endurance performance. In Chapter 21, we discuss how training impacts blood lactate threshold adaptations.

Lactate-Producing Capacity

Producing high blood lactate levels during maximal physical activity increases with specific sprint-power anaerobic training and decreases when training stops. Sprint-power athletes often achieve 20 to 30% higher blood lactate levels than untrained counterparts during maximal short-duration exercise. One or more of the following three mechanisms explains this response:

1. Improved motivation that accompanies training
2. Increased intramuscular glycogen stores that accompany training may allow a greater contribution of energy via anaerobic glycolysis
3. Training-induced increase in glycolytic-related enzymes, particularly phosphofructokinase. The 20% increase in glycolytic enzymes falls well below the two- to threefold increase in aerobic enzymes with endurance training

LONG-TERM ENERGY: THE AEROBIC SYSTEM

As discussed previously, glycolytic reactions produce relatively few ATP. Consequently, aerobic metabolism provides nearly all of the energy transfer when intense physical activity continues beyond several minutes.

Oxygen Consumption During Exercise

FIGURE 7.2 illustrates oxygen consumption—also referred to as *pulmonary oxygen uptake* because oxygen measurements occur at the lung and not the active muscles—during each minute of a slow 10-min run. Oxygen consumption rises exponentially during the first minutes of physical activity, called the *fast component* of exercise oxygen consumption, to attain a plateau between the third and fourth minutes. It then remains relatively stable

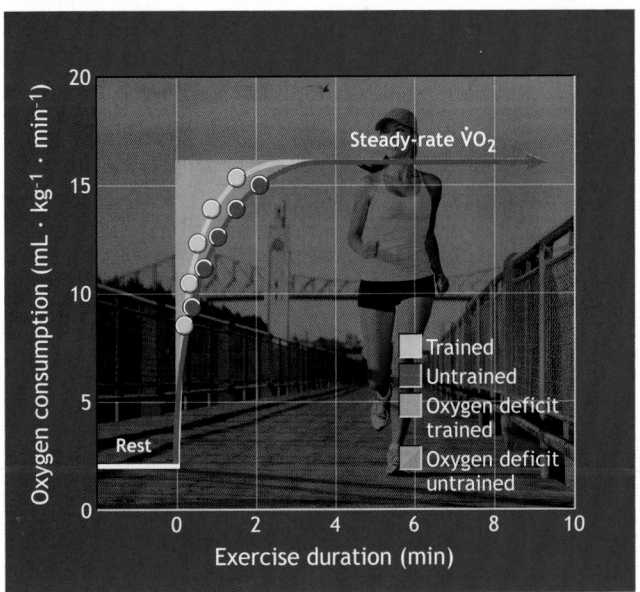

FIGURE 7.2 • Time course for oxygen consumption during a continuous jog at a relatively slow pace by an endurance-trained and an untrained individual. The orange and purple regions indicate the oxygen deficit—the quantity of oxygen that would have been consumed had oxygen consumption reached steady rate immediately.

for the duration of effort. *Steady state* or *steady rate* generally describes the flat portion or plateau of the oxygen consumption curve. Steady rate reflects a balance between energy required by the working muscles and ATP production in aerobic metabolism. Within the steady-rate region, coupled redox reactions supply the energy for physical activity; any lactate produced either oxidizes or reconverts to glucose. *No appreciable blood lactate accumulates under steady-rate, aerobic metabolic conditions.*

 ## Lactic Acid, Lactate, and pH

Hydrogen ions (H^+) that dissociate from lactic acid present a primary problem to the body's homeostatic mechanisms. At normal pH levels, lactic acid almost immediately and completely dissociates to H^+ and lactate (La^-). Few disruptions exist if the amount of free H^+ does not exceed the body's ability to buffer them and maintain pH at a relatively stable level. The pH decreases when excessive lactic acid exceeds the body's immediate buffering capacity. Discomfort occurs as the blood becomes more acidic, impairing exercise performance.

Once a steady rate of aerobic metabolism occurs, physical activity theoretically could progress indefinitely if the individual possessed the "will" to continue. This assumes that steady-rate aerobic metabolism singularly determines the capacity to sustain steady-rate exercise. Fluid loss and electrolyte depletion during activity often pose limiting factors, especially in hot weather. Maintaining adequate reserves of both liver glycogen for central nervous system function and muscle glycogen to power exercise takes on added importance at high intensities of prolonged aerobic effort. Glycogen depletion dramatically reduces exercise capacity.

Individuals possess many steady-rate levels during physical activity. For some, the spectrum ranges from sitting and working at the computer to mowing the lawn continuously for 45 min. An elite endurance runner can maintain a steady rate of aerobic metabolism throughout a 26.2-mile marathon, averaging slightly less than 5 min a mile, or during a 658-mile ultramarathon, averaging 118 miles a day slightly over 5 d and 5 hr! Two factors help explain these exceptional endurance accomplishments:

1. High capacity of the central circulation to *deliver* oxygen to active muscles
2. High capacity of the active muscles to *use* available oxygen

Oxygen Deficit

At activity onset, the oxygen consumption curve in Figure 7.2 does not increase instantaneously to steady rate. In the initial, transitional stage of constant-load effort, oxygen consumption remains below a steady-rate level even though the exercise-energy requirement remains unchanged throughout exercise. A lag in oxygen consumption early in exercise should not be surprising because energy for muscle action comes directly from the immediate anaerobic breakdown of ATP. Even with experimentally increased oxygen availability and increased oxygen diffusion gradients at the tissue level, the initial increase in

exercise oxygen consumption is always lower than the steady-rate oxygen consumption.[24,25] Owing to the interaction of intrinsic inertia in cellular metabolic signals and enzyme activation and relative sluggishness of oxygen delivery to the mitochondria, the hydrogens produced in energy metabolism do not immediately oxidize and combine with oxygen.[40,46] Oxygen consumption increases rapidly in subsequent energy transfer reactions under three conditions: when oxygen combines with the hydrogens liberated in (1) glycolysis, (2) β-oxidation of fatty acids, or (3) citric acid cycle reactions. After several minutes of submaximal physical activity, hydrogen production and subsequent oxidation and ATP production become proportional to the exercise-energy requirement. At this stage, oxygen consumption attains a balance indicating a relative steady rate between energy requirement and aerobic energy transfer.

The **oxygen deficit** *quantitatively expresses the difference between the total oxygen consumption during activity and the total that would be consumed had steady-rate oxygen consumption been achieved at the onset.* This oxygen deficit represents the immediate anaerobic energy transfer from the hydrolysis of intramuscular high-energy phosphates and rapid glycolysis until steady-rate energy transfer matches the energy requirements.

FIGURE 7.3 depicts the relationship between the contribution of energy from the ATP–PCr and lactate energy systems

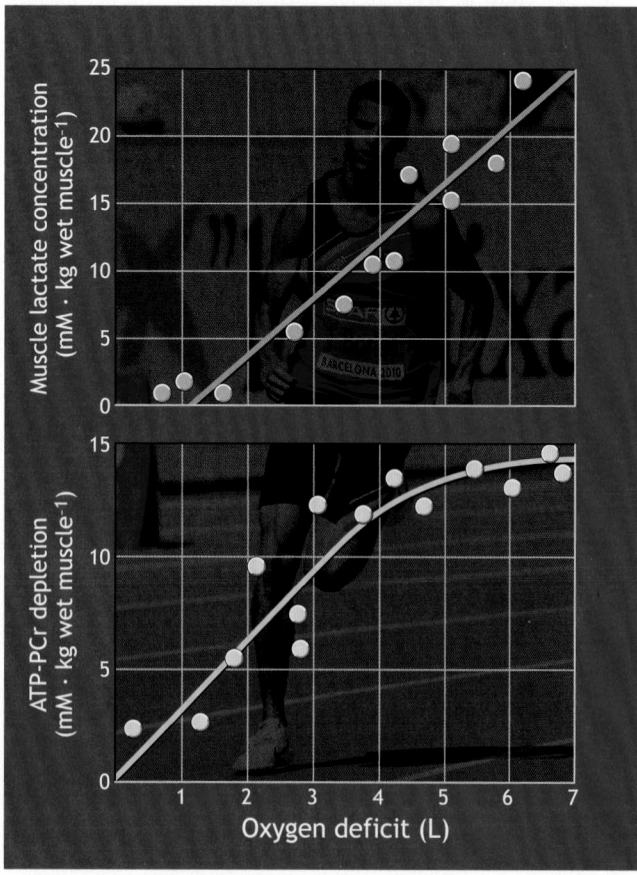

FIGURE 7.3 • Muscle ATP and PCr depletion and muscle lactate concentration plotted versus oxygen deficit. (Adapted with permission from Karlsson J. Muscle ATP, PCr and lactate in submaximal and maximal exercise. In: Pernow B, Saltin B, eds. *Muscle Metabolism During Exercise.* New York: Plenum Press, 1971.)

and the size of the oxygen deficit. High-energy phosphates substantially deplete during physical activity that generates about a 3- to 4-L oxygen deficit. Consequently, further activity progresses only with ATP resynthesis via either anaerobic glycolysis or the aerobic breakdown of macronutrients. Interestingly, lactate begins to increase in active muscle well before the high-energy phosphates reach their lowest levels. This indicates that rapid glycolysis also contributes anaerobic energy in the initial stages of vigorous physical activity, well before full use of the high-energy phosphates. *Energy for physical activity does not simply occur from activating a series of energy systems that "switch on" and "switch off," but rather from smooth blending with considerable overlap of one mode of energy transfer to another.*[26,43]

Oxygen Deficit in the Trained and Untrained

Oxygen consumption kinetics at the onset of activity do not differ between children and adults.[27] The endurance-trained person achieves steady rate more rapidly, with a smaller oxygen deficit than sprint-power athletes, cardiac patients, older adults, or untrained individuals.[7,16,31,34] Consequently, a faster aerobic kinetic response allows the trained person to consume a greater total amount of oxygen to steady-rate exercise and makes the anaerobic component of energy transfer proportionately smaller. The following three aerobic training adaptations facilitate the rate of aerobic metabolism when exercise begins:

1. More rapid increase in muscle bioenergetics
2. Increase in overall cardiac output
3. Disproportionately large regional blood flow to active muscle complemented by cellular adaptations

These adaptations increase capacity to generate ATP aerobically (see Chapter 21).

 INTEGRATIVE QUESTION

How would you answer the question: At what level of physical activity does the body switch to anaerobic energy metabolism?

Maximal Oxygen Consumption

Figure 7.4 depicts oxygen consumption during a series of constant-speed runs up six progressively steeper "hills." Hills are simulated in the laboratory by increasing treadmill elevation, step bench height and/or stepping rate, increasing resistance to pedaling at a constant rate on a bicycle ergometer, and increasing rate of water flow toward the swimmer in a swim flume. Each successive "hill" requires a greater energy output that places additional demand on the capacity for aerobic ATP resynthesis. During the first several hills, oxygen consumption increases rapidly, with each new steady-rate value in direct proportion to exercise intensity. The runner maintains speed up the two last hills, but oxygen consumption fails to increase as rapidly or to the same extent as in the previous hills. No increase in oxygen consumption occurs during the run up the last hill. *The region in yellow at the top right of the figure where oxygen consumption plateaus or increases only slightly with additional increases in exercise intensity represents the* **maximal oxygen consumption**—*also called* **maximal oxygen uptake**,

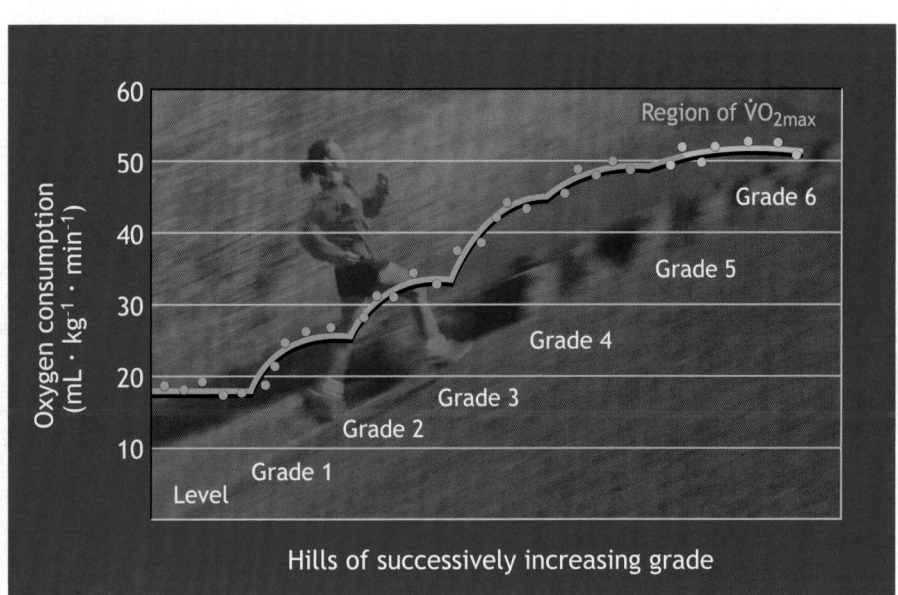

FIGURE 7.4 • Attainment of maximal oxygen consumption ($\dot{V}O_{2max}$) while running up hills of progressively increasing slope. $\dot{V}O_{2max}$ occurs in the region (designated by *yellow* data points along the *yellow* part of the curve and not a single point) where further increases in exercise intensity produce a less-than-expected increase (or no increase) in oxygen consumption. Dots represent measured values of oxygen consumption while traversing the hills.

maximal aerobic power, aerobic capacity, or simply $\dot{V}O_{2max}$. Energy transfer via anaerobic glycolysis allows performance of more-intense physical activity with resulting lactate accumulation. Under these conditions, the runner soon becomes exhausted and fails to continue.

The $\dot{V}O_{2max}$ provides a quantitative measure of a person's capacity for aerobic ATP resynthesis. This makes the $\dot{V}O_{2max}$ an important indicator of how well a person can maintain intense activity for longer than 4 or 5 min. Attainment of a high $\dot{V}O_{2max}$ has important physiologic meanings in addition to its role in sustaining energy metabolism in exercise. A high $\dot{V}O_{2max}$ requires the integrated and high-level response of diverse physiologic support systems (pulmonary ventilation, hemoglobin concentration, blood volume and cardiac output, peripheral blood flow, and cellular metabolic capacity), illustrated in FIGURE 7.5. In subsequent chapters, we discuss various aspects of $\dot{V}O_{2max}$, including its physiologic significance, measurement, and role in determining physical performance and improved cardiovascular health.

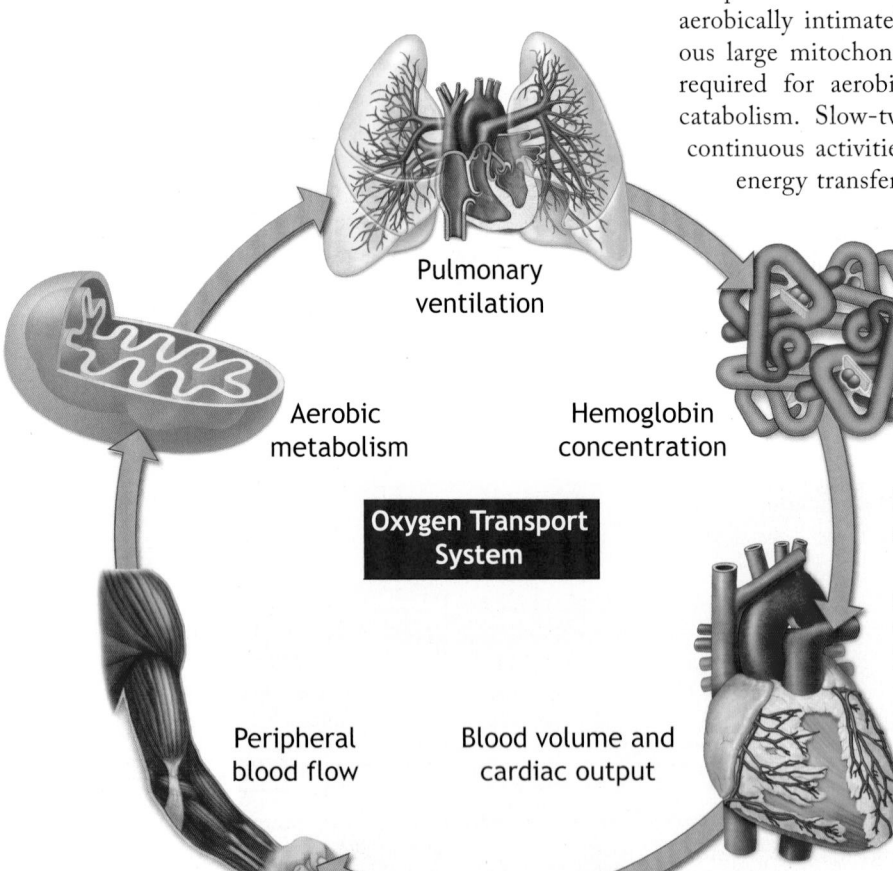

FIGURE 7.5 • The oxygen transport system. The physiologic significance of $\dot{V}O_{2max}$ depends on the functional capacity and integration of systems required for oxygen supply, transport, delivery, and use. (Lung and heart images adapted with permission from Moore KL, Dalley AF, Agur AMR. *Clinically Oriented Anatomy*, 7th ed., as used with permission from Agur AMR, Dalley AF. *Grant's Atlas of Anatomy*. 13th Ed. Baltimore: Wolters Kluwer Health, 2013.)

Fast- and Slow-Twitch Muscle Fibers Generate ATP Differently

Two distinct types of muscle fibers exist in humans, with each generating ATP differently. **Fast-twitch (FT)** or **type II** fibers have two primary subdivisions, type IIa and type IIx. Each fiber type possesses rapid contraction speed and high capacity for anaerobic ATP production via glycolysis. The subdivision type IIa fiber also possesses somewhat high aerobic capacity. Type II fibers become active during change-of-pace and stop-and-go activities such as basketball, field hockey, lacrosse, soccer, and ice hockey. They also increase force output when running or cycling up hills while maintaining a constant speed or during all-out effort that requires rapid, powerful movements that depend almost exclusively on energy from anaerobic metabolism.

The second fiber type, the **slow-twitch (ST)** or **type I** muscle fiber, generates energy primarily through aerobic pathways. This fiber possesses a slower contraction speed compared with fast-twitch fibers. Capacity to generate ATP aerobically intimately relates to the type I fiber's numerous large mitochondria including high levels of enzymes required for aerobic metabolism, particularly fatty acid catabolism. Slow-twitch muscle fibers primarily sustain continuous activities that require a steady rate of aerobic energy transfer. Fatigue in prolonged running associates with glycogen depletion in the leg muscles' type I and type IIa muscle fibers.[2,22] This selective glycogen depletion pattern also occurs in the arms of wheelchair-dependent athletes during extended exercise durations.[42] More than likely, the predominance of slow-twitch muscle fibers contributes to high blood lactate thresholds observed among elite endurance athletes.

Athletes who excel in different sporting events such as high-power versus endurance activities usually have a large percentage of the specific muscle fiber type that supports the sport's energy demands. For example, FIGURE 7.6 illustrates the muscle-fiber composition of two athletes in sports that rely on distinctly different energy transfer systems favored by specific muscle fiber type predominance. For the 50-m sprint swim champion (*left panel*), type II fibers represent nearly 80% of the total muscle fibers, whereas the endurance cyclist possesses 80% type I fibers. From a practical perspective, most sports require relatively slow, sustained muscle actions interspersed with short bursts of powerful effort (e.g., basketball, soccer, lacrosse, field hockey). Not surprisingly, these activities require an equal percentage and activation of *both* muscle fiber types.

IN A PRACTICAL SENSE

Interpreting $\dot{V}O_{2MAX}$—Establishing Cardiovascular Fitness Categories

Cardiovascular fitness reflects the maximal amount of oxygen consumed during each minute of near-maximal exercise. Values for maximal oxygen consumption, or $\dot{V}O_{2max}$, generally are expressed in milliliters of oxygen per kilogram of body mass per minute $(mL \cdot kg^{-1} \cdot min^{-1})$. Individual values can range from about 10 $mL \cdot kg^{-1} \cdot min^{-1}$ in cardiac patients to 80 or 90 $mL \cdot kg^{-1} \cdot min^{-1}$ in world-class runners and cross-country skiers. Men and women distance runners, swimmers, cyclists, and cross-country skiers generally attain $\dot{V}O_{2max}$ values nearly double those of sedentary persons (see Fig. 11.7 in Chapter 11).

Researchers have measured the $\dot{V}O_{2max}$ of thousands of individuals of different ages. The average values and respective ranges for men and women of different ages establish category values to classify individuals for cardiovascular fitness. The table presents a five-part classification based on data from the literature for nonathletes.

Cardiovascular Fitness Classifications

Gender	Age	Poor	Fair	Average	Good	Excellent
Men	≤29	≤24.9	25–33.9	34–43.9	44–52.9	≥53
	30–39	≤22.9	23–30.9	31–41.9	42–49.9	≥50
	40–49	≤19.9	20–26.9	27–38.9	39–44.9	≥45
	50–59	≤17.9	18–24.9	25–37.9	38–42.9	≥43
	60–69	≤15.9	16–22.9	23–35.9	36–40.9	≥41
Women	≤29	≤23.9	24–30.9	31–38.9	39–48.9	≥49
	30–39	≤19.9	20–27.9	28–36.9	37–44.9	≥45
	40–49	≤16.9	17–24.9	25–34.9	35–41.9	≥42
	50–59	≤14.9	15–21.9	22–33.9	34–39.9	≥40
	60–69	≤12.9	13–20.9	21–32.9	33–36.9	≥37

The preceding discussion suggests that a muscle's predominant fiber type contributes to success in certain sports or physical activities. Chapter 18 explores this idea more fully, including other considerations concerning metabolic, contractile, and fatigue characteristics of each fiber type, the various subdivisions, proposed classification system, and effects of exercise training.

ENERGY SPECTRUM OF PHYSICAL ACTIVITY

FIGURE 7.7 illustrates the relative contribution of anaerobic and aerobic energy sources related to maximal exercise time. **TABLE 7.1** also shows the relative contributions of the major energy fuels during various running competitions. These data, based on laboratory experiments that involve all-out running, readily transpose to other activities by drawing the appropriate time relationships. For example, a 100-m sprint run corresponds to any all-out physical activity for about 10 s, while an 800-m run and 200-m swim last approximately 2 min. All-out 1-min activity includes the 400-m run, the 100-m swim, and repeated full-court presses during basketball.

The allocation of energy for physical activity from each energy transfer form progresses along a continuum. At one extreme, the intramuscular high-energy phosphates supply almost all of the exercise energy needs. The ATP–PCr and lactic acid systems supply about half the energy for intense activity lasting 2 min, with the remainder supplied by aerobic reactions. To excel under these exercise conditions requires a well-developed anaerobic and aerobic metabolic capacity. Intense physical activity of intermediate duration performed for 5 to 10 min (e.g., middle-distance running and swimming, or basketball) places greater demand on aerobic energy transfer. Long-duration marathon running, distance swimming, cycling, recreational jogging, and trekking require a constant aerobic energy supply with little reliance on energy transfer from anaerobic sources.

An understanding of the energy demands of diverse physical activities helps to explain why a world-record holder in the 1-mile run does not necessarily excel in distance running. Conversely, premier marathon runners rarely run 1 mile in less than 4 min, yet can complete a 26.2-mile marathon at a 5-min-per-mile pace. *The appropriate approach to physical training analyzes an activity for its specific energy components and then formulates training strategies to ensure*

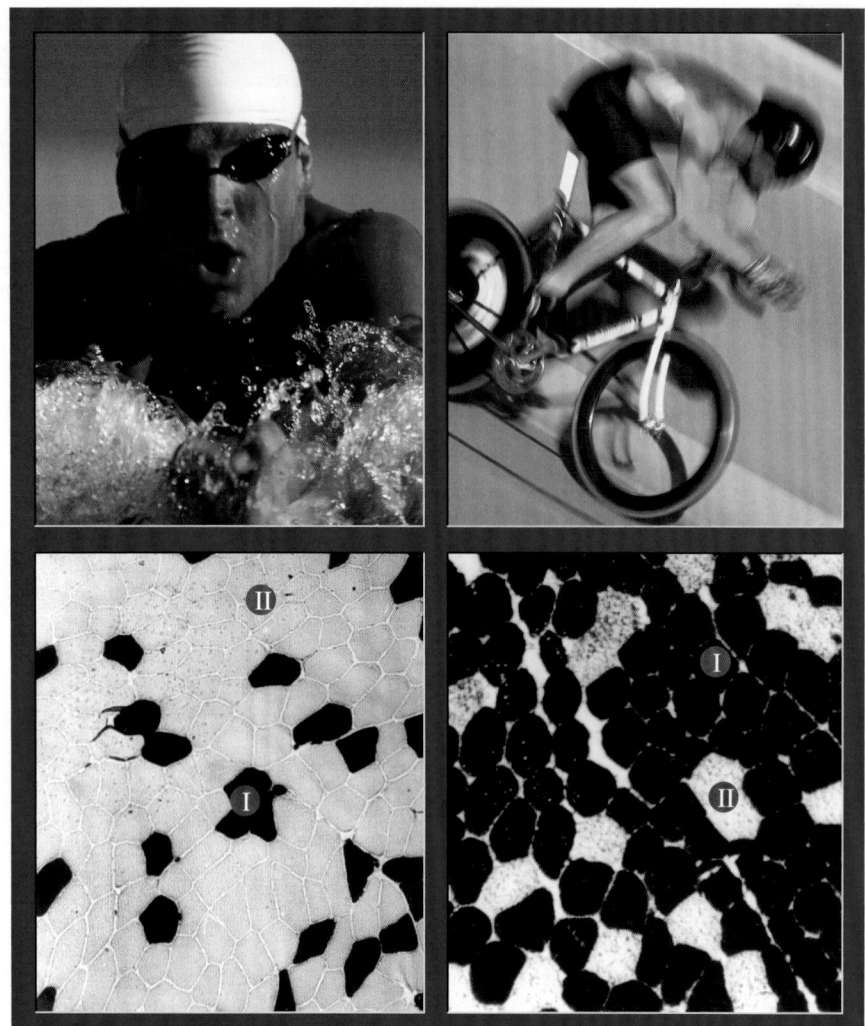

FIGURE 7.6 • Differences in muscle-fiber type composition between a sprint swimmer and endurance cyclist. The type I and type II muscle fibers were sampled from the *vastus lateralis* muscle and stained for myofibrillar ATPase after incubation at pH 4.3. Type I fibers stain dark, while type II fibers remain unstained. (Photos and photomicrographs courtesy of Dr. R. Billeter, School of Life Sciences, University of Nottingham, Great Britain.)

optimal adaptations in physiologic and metabolic function. Improved capacity for energy transfer usually translates into improved performance.

 INTEGRATIVE QUESTION

If athletes generally perform marathon running under intense but steady-rate aerobic conditions, explain why some have reduced capacity to sprint to the finish at race end.

OXYGEN CONSUMPTION DURING RECOVERY

Following physical activity, bodily processes do not immediately return to resting levels. After relatively light, short-duration physical effort, recovery proceeds rapidly and unnoticed. In contrast, more strenuous running for one-half mile or swimming 200 yards as fast as possible requires considerable time for resting metabolism to return to pre-activity levels. How rapidly an individual responds in recovery from light, moderate, and strenuous physical activity depends on specific metabolic and physiologic processes during and in recovery from each type of effort.

FIGURE **7.8** illustrates oxygen consumption during activity and recovery from different movement intensities. Light activity (**A**), with rapid attainment of steady-rate oxygen consumption, produces a small oxygen deficit. The magnitude of recovery oxygen consumption, coincidently, approximates the size of the oxygen deficit at the beginning of exercise. Recovery proceeds rapidly. Oxygen consumption follows a logarithmic curve, decreasing by about 50% over each subsequent 30-s period until reaching the pre-exercise level.

Oxygen consumption, usually expressed as $mL \cdot min^{-1}$, $L \cdot min^{-1}$, or $mL \cdot kg^{-1} \cdot min^{-1}$ during steady-rate and non–steady-rate activity and recovery, plots as a logarithmic function related to time.[6,50] The function increases in activity or decreases

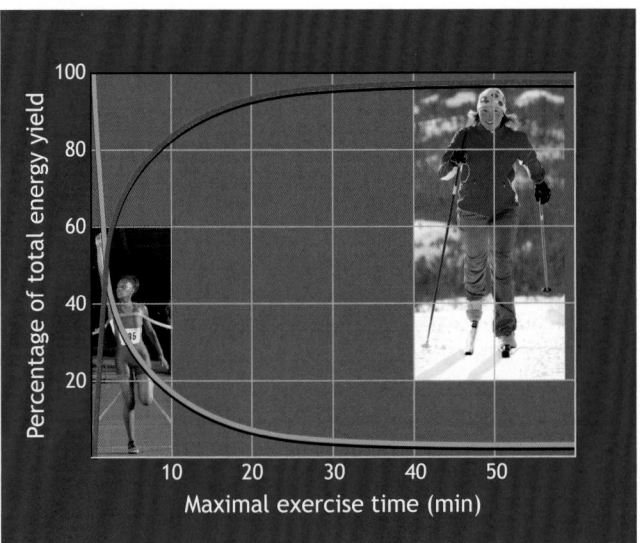

Duration of maximal exercise

	Seconds			Minutes					
	10	30	60	2	4	10	30	60	120
Percentage anaerobic	90	80	70	50	35	15	5	2	1
Percentage aerobic	10	20	30	50	65	85	95	98	99

FIGURE 7.7 • Relative contribution of aerobic and anaerobic energy metabolism during maximal physical effort of various durations. Note that 2 min of maximal effort requires about 50% of the energy from combined aerobic and anaerobic processes. A world-class 4-min-mile pace derives approximately 65% of its energy from aerobic metabolism, with the remainder generated from anaerobic processes. A 2.5-hr marathon, in contrast, generates almost all of its energy from aerobic processes. (Adapted with permission from Åstrand PO, Rodahl K. *Textbook of Work Physiology*. New York: McGraw-Hill, 1977.)

in recovery by a constant fraction for each unit of time as oxygen consumption approaches an asymptote or level value. Consider the example of recovery from 10 min of steady-rate physical activity at an oxygen consumption of 2000 mL · min⁻¹. If recovery oxygen consumption decreased by half over 30 s, then oxygen consumption would equal 1000 mL · min⁻¹ at 30-s recovery and 500 mL · min⁻¹ at 60 s, with the resting value of 250 mL · min⁻¹ achieved in about 90 s.

Moderate-to-intense aerobic activity (Fig. 7.8B) requires a longer time to achieve steady-rate oxygen consumption and creates a larger oxygen deficit than less-intense effort. Consequently, it takes longer for the recovery oxygen consumption to return to pre-activity levels. The oxygen consumption recovery curve demonstrates an initial rapid decline, similar to recovery from light activity, followed by a more gradual decline to baseline resting levels. In Figure 7.8A and B, the oxygen deficit and recovery oxygen consumption compute by using the steady-rate oxygen consumption to represent the oxygen or energy requirement of physical activity. Figure 7.8C shows that all-out, exhaustive physical effort does not produce steady-rate oxygen consumption. Such effort demands a larger energy requirement than aerobic processes can supply. Consequently, anaerobic energy transfer increases and blood lactate accumulates, with considerable time required to achieve complete recovery. Failure to achieve steady-rate oxygen consumption makes it unfeasible to accurately quantify the true oxygen deficit.

Each of the curves in Figure 7.8 shows that oxygen consumption during recovery always exceeds the resting value, independent of exercise intensity. The excess oxygen consumption has classically been termed **oxygen debt** or **recovery oxygen consumption**, with the newer preferred term the **excess postexercise oxygen consumption** or **EPOC** (indicated by the *dark blue* shaded area under each recovery curve). EPOC computes as the total oxygen consumed in recovery minus the total oxygen theoretically consumed at rest during

TABLE 7.1 — **Estimate of the Percent Contribution of Different Fuels to ATP Generation in Various Running Events (Assumes 70-kg Male)**

	Percent Contribution to ATP Generation				
		Glycogen		Blood Glucose	Triacylglycerol
Event	**Phosphocreatine**	**Anaerobic**	**Aerobic**	**(Liver Glycogen)**	**(Fatty Acids)**
100 m	50	50	—	—	—
200 m	25	65	10	—	—
400 m	12.5	62.5	25	—	—
800 m	6	50	44	—	—
1500 m	a	25	75	—	—
5000 m	a	12.5	87.5	—	—
10,000 m	a	3	97	—	—
Marathon	—	—	75	5	20
Ultramarathon (80 km)	—	—	35	5	60
24-h race	—	—	10	2	88
Soccer game	10	70	20	—	—

From Newsholme EA, et al. Physical and mental fatigue: metabolic mechanisms and importance of plasma amino acids. *Br Med Bull* 1992;48:477.
ᵃIn such events phosphocreatine is used for the first few seconds and, if it has been resynthesized during the race, in the sprint to the finish.

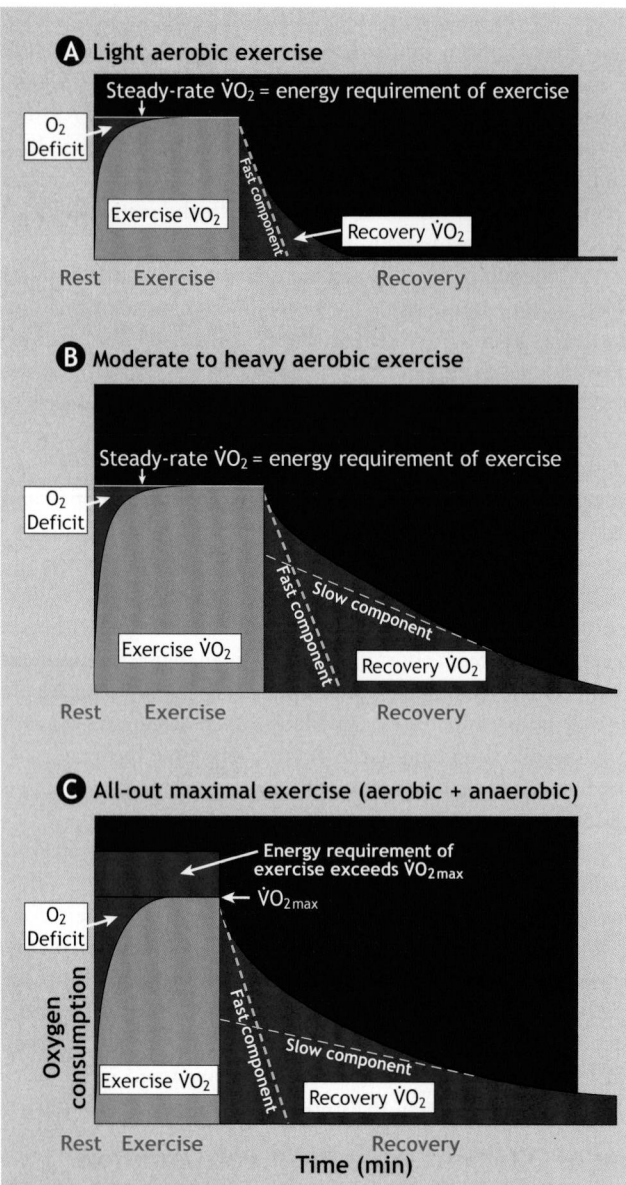

FIGURE 7.8 • Oxygen consumption during physical activity and in recovery from **(A)** light steady-rate effort, **(B)** moderate-to-intense steady-rate effort, and **(C)** exhaustive effort that does not produce a steady rate of aerobic metabolism. Note that in exhaustive effort, the exercise oxygen requirement exceeds the actual exercise oxygen consumption. (Adapted with permission from Katch VL, McArdle WD, Katch FI. *Essentials of Exercise Physiology*. 4th Ed. Philadelphia: Wolters Kluwer Health, 2011.)

during activity and recovery. As we discuss later in the section on Contemporary Concepts, this assumption may not be entirely correct, particularly following strenuous physical activity.

The curves in Figure 7.8 illustrate two important characteristics of recovery oxygen consumption:

1. With mild aerobic activity of relatively short duration and little disruption in body temperature and hormonal milieu, about half of the total recovery oxygen consumption occurs within 30 s, and complete recovery within 2 to 4 min. The decline in oxygen consumption follows a single-component exponential curve termed the **fast component** of recovery oxygen consumption.

2. Recovery from strenuous activity presents a different picture, presumably because three factors—blood lactate, body temperature, and thermogenic hormone levels—increase substantially. In addition to the fast component of the recovery phase, a second phase of recovery exists: the **slow component**. Depending on the intensity and duration of the previous physical activity, the slow component can take up to 24 hr to return to pre-exercise oxygen consumption.[5,23,43] Even with shorter, intermittent bouts of "supermaximal" effort (e.g., three 2-min bouts at 108% $\dot{V}O_{2max}$ interspersed with 3-min rest intervals), recovery oxygen consumption remains elevated for 1 hr or longer.[4]

Trained subjects have a faster rate of recovery oxygen consumption when exercising at either the same absolute or relative intensities compared to untrained counterparts.[42] More than likely, training adaptations that facilitate the rapid achievement of steady-rate oxygen consumption also facilitate a rapid recovery process.

Metabolic Dynamics of Recovery Oxygen Consumption

A precise biochemical explanation for the recovery oxygen consumption, particularly the role of lactate, remains elusive because no comprehensive explanation exists about the interaction of specific contributory factors.

Early Theories About Postexercise Oxygen Consumption (the So-Called "Oxygen Debt")

In 1922, Nobel laureate Archibald Vivian Hill 🖼 (http://www.nobelprize.org/nobel_prizes/medicine/laureates/1922/hill-bio.html) and colleagues first coined the term *oxygen debt*. These pioneer scientists discussed energy metabolism during physical activity and recovery in financial–accounting terms.[28] The body's carbohydrate stores were likened to energy "credits." Expending stored credits during physical activity incurred an energy "debt." The greater energy "deficit" or use of available stored energy credits, the larger the energy debt. Hill believed that the recovery oxygen consumption represented the cost of repaying this debt—hence the term *oxygen debt*.

the recovery period. For example, if a total of 5.5 L of oxygen were consumed in recovery until attaining the resting value of 0.310 L · min⁻¹, and recovery required 10 min, the recovery oxygen consumption would equal 5.5 L minus 3.1 L (0.310 L × 10 min) or 2.4 L. This indicates that the preceding exercise caused physiologic alterations during activity *and* during recovery that required an additional 2.4 L of oxygen before it returned to pre-exercise rest. These calculations assume that resting oxygen consumption remains unaltered

Lactate accumulation from the anaerobic component of physical activity represented the use of glycogen, the stored energy credit. The ensuing oxygen debt served two purposes:

1. Reestablish the original glycogen stores or credits by synthesizing approximately 80% of the lactate back to glycogen in the liver via the Cori cycle.
2. Catabolize the remaining lactate through the pyruvate–citric acid cycle pathway, with the new ATP presumably powering glycogen resynthesis from lactate.

This early explanation of the dynamics of recovery oxygen consumption was subsequently termed the "*lactic acid theory of oxygen debt.*"

In 1933, following the work of Hill, researchers at the Harvard Fatigue Laboratory (**http://hper.usu.edu/files/uploads/Courses/Fall%202010/PEP/PEP-2000-Harvard-Fatigue-Lab.pdf**) deduced that the initial phase of recovery oxygen consumption terminated before blood lactate could decline.[36] They showed that a physically active individual could incur an oxygen debt of almost 3 L without any appreciable blood lactate accumulation. To resolve these findings, they proposed two phases of oxygen debt:

1. **Alactic** or **alactacid oxygen debt** (meaning without lactate buildup).
2. **Lactic acid** or **lactacid oxygen debt** associated with elevated blood lactate levels.

The researchers speculated that these two explanations occurred because the early chemical methodology did not allow them to measure ATP and PCr replenishment or the relationship between blood lactate and glucose and glycogen levels.

Contemporary Concepts

The elevated aerobic metabolism in recovery restores the body to its pre-exercise condition. In short-duration, light-to-moderate activity, recovery oxygen consumption generally replenishes the high-energy phosphates depleted by the activity. Recovery from activity typically proceeds rapidly within several minutes. In longer-duration intense aerobic exercise of 60 min or more, recovery oxygen consumption remains elevated considerably longer.[9] **Figure 7.9** illustrates the effect of exercise duration on the magnitude of recovery oxygen consumption.[40] Eight trained women walked at 70% of $\dot{V}O_{2max}$ for 20, 40, or 60 min. Recovery oxygen consumption totaled 8.6 L for the 20-min workout period and 9.8 L for the 40-min session. The amount of oxygen consumed during the 60-min workout nearly doubled to 15.2 L. The increase in recovery oxygen consumption in each bout of steady-rate walking failed to relate to lactate accumulation. Rather, disequilibrium in other physiologic functions elevate the recovery metabolism.

In exhaustive physical effort with its large anaerobic component and lactate accumulation, a small portion of EPOC resynthesizes lactate to glycogen. There is some suggestion that this gluconeogenic mechanism also progresses during exercise, particularly in trained individuals.[17,35] A significant component of EPOC relates to physiologic processes that take place during

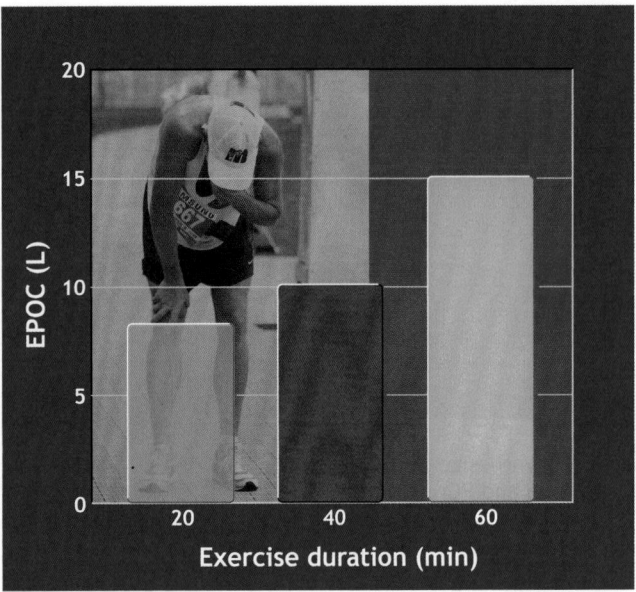

FIGURE 7.9 • Total excess postexercise oxygen consumption (EPOC) during a 3-hr recovery from 20, 40, and 60 min of treadmill walking at 70% $\dot{V}O_{2max}$. EPOC for the 60-min walk significantly exceeded the 20- or 40-min walks. (Adapted with permission from Quinn TJ, et al. Postexercise oxygen consumption in trained females: effect of exercise duration. *Med Sci Sports Exerc* 1994;26:908.)

recovery, in addition to metabolic events during physical activity. Such factors likely account for the considerably larger oxygen debt than oxygen deficit in prolonged aerobic exercise and exhaustive anaerobic exercise. Body temperature, for example, rises about 5.4°F (3°C) during a long bout of intense aerobic activity and can remain elevated for several hours in recovery. Elevated body temperature directly stimulates metabolism to increase recovery oxygen consumption.

Other factors also affect EPOC. Up to 10% of the recovery oxygen consumption reloads the blood returning to the lungs from the previously active muscles. An additional 2 to 5% restores oxygen dissolved in bodily fluids and bound to myoglobin within muscle. Ventilation volumes in recovery from intense physical activity remain 8 to 10 times above the resting requirement, a cost that can equal 10% of EPOC. The heart also works harder and requires a greater oxygen supply during recovery. Tissue repair and redistribution of calcium, potassium, and sodium ions within muscle and other body compartments also require additional energy. The residual effects of the thermogenic hormones epinephrine, norepinephrine, and thyroxine, including the glucocorticoids released in physical activity, elevate metabolism in recovery. *In essence, all of the physiologic systems activated in physical activity increase their own particular need for oxygen during recovery (see yellow text boxes in* **Fig. 7.10***).* Two factors impact recovery oxygen consumption:

1. Level of anaerobic metabolism *during* physical activity
2. Respiratory, circulatory, hormonal, ionic, and thermal adjustments that elevate metabolism *during* recovery

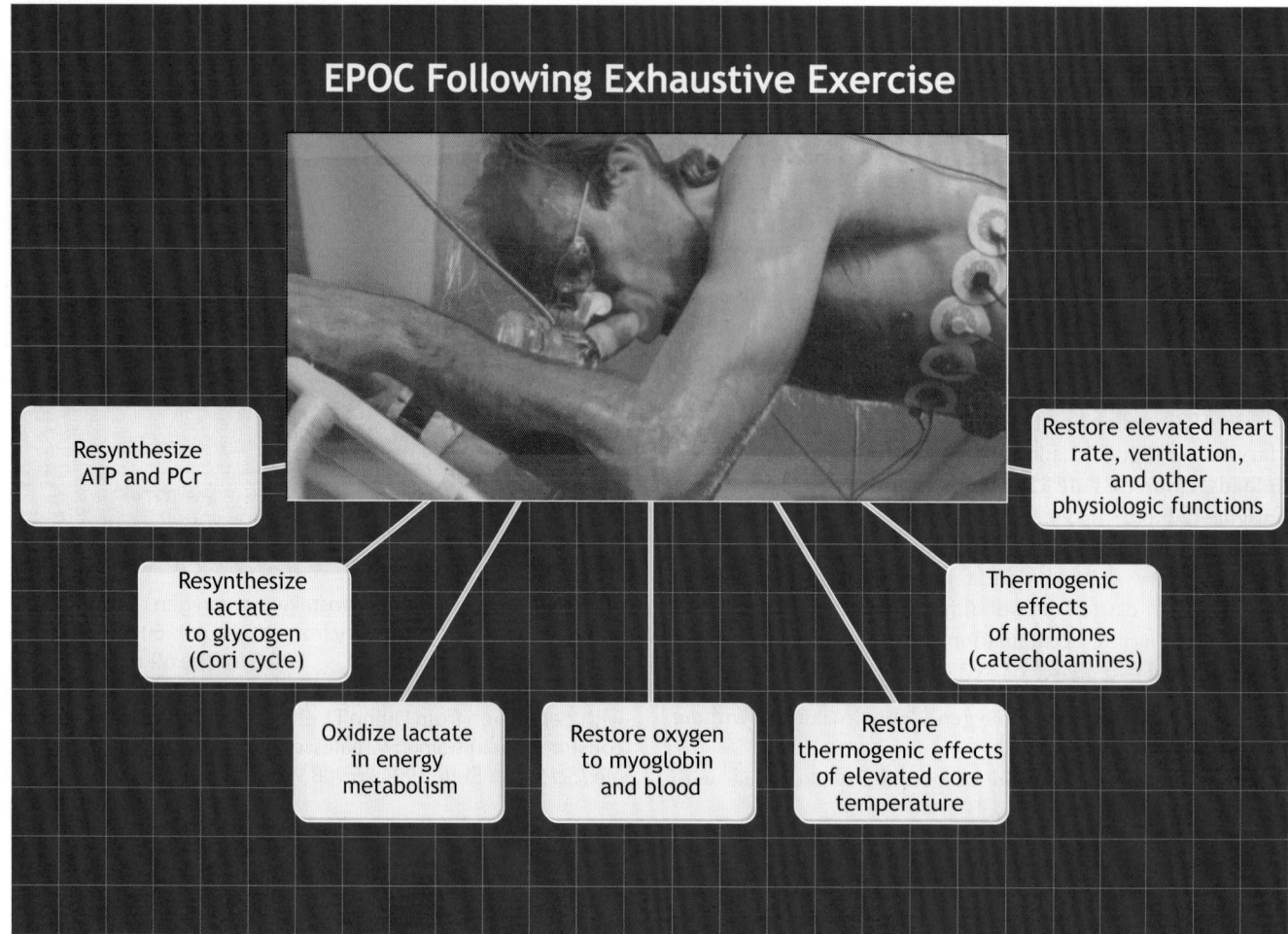

FIGURE 7.10 • Factors that contribute to the EPOC following exhaustive physical activity.

Implications of EPOC for Exercise and Recovery

Understanding the dynamics of EPOC provides a basis for structuring activity intervals and optimizing recovery. No appreciable lactate accumulates either with steady-rate aerobic activity or with brief 5- to 10-s bouts of all-out effort powered by the intramuscular high-energy phosphates. Consequently, recovery progresses rapidly and activity can begin again with only a short rest period, with passive recovery most desirable.[18] In contrast, prolonged durations of anaerobic effort for longer than 2 min produce considerable lactate buildup in active muscles and blood, with disruption in various physiologic systems. As such, recovery oxygen consumption often requires considerable time to return to pre-activity baseline levels. Prolonged recovery between exercise intervals would impair performance in basketball, hockey, soccer, tennis, and badminton. An athlete pushed to a high level of anaerobic metabolism may not fully recover during brief time-out periods or intermittent intervals of less intense physical activity.

Procedures for speeding recovery from physical activity generally are either active or passive. In **active recovery**, often termed "cooling down" or "tapering off," the individual performs submaximal effort with large muscle groups, believing that continued physical activity in some way prevents muscle cramps and stiffness and facilitates lactate removal and overall recovery. With **passive recovery**, the person usually lies down, presuming that total inactivity reduces the resting energy requirements and thus "frees" oxygen to fuel the recovery process. Modifications of passive recovery have included massage, cold showers, specific body positions, and consuming cold liquids.

Optimal Recovery from Steady-Rate Physical Activity

For most individuals, little lactate accumulates during steady-rate physical activity below 55 to 60% $\dot{V}O_{2max}$. Recovery entails resynthesis of high-energy phosphates and replenishment of oxygen in the blood, bodily fluids, and muscle myoglobin, with a small energy cost to sustain elevated circulation and ventilation. Passive procedures facilitate recovery because any additional activity under these circumstances only elevates total metabolism and delays recovery.

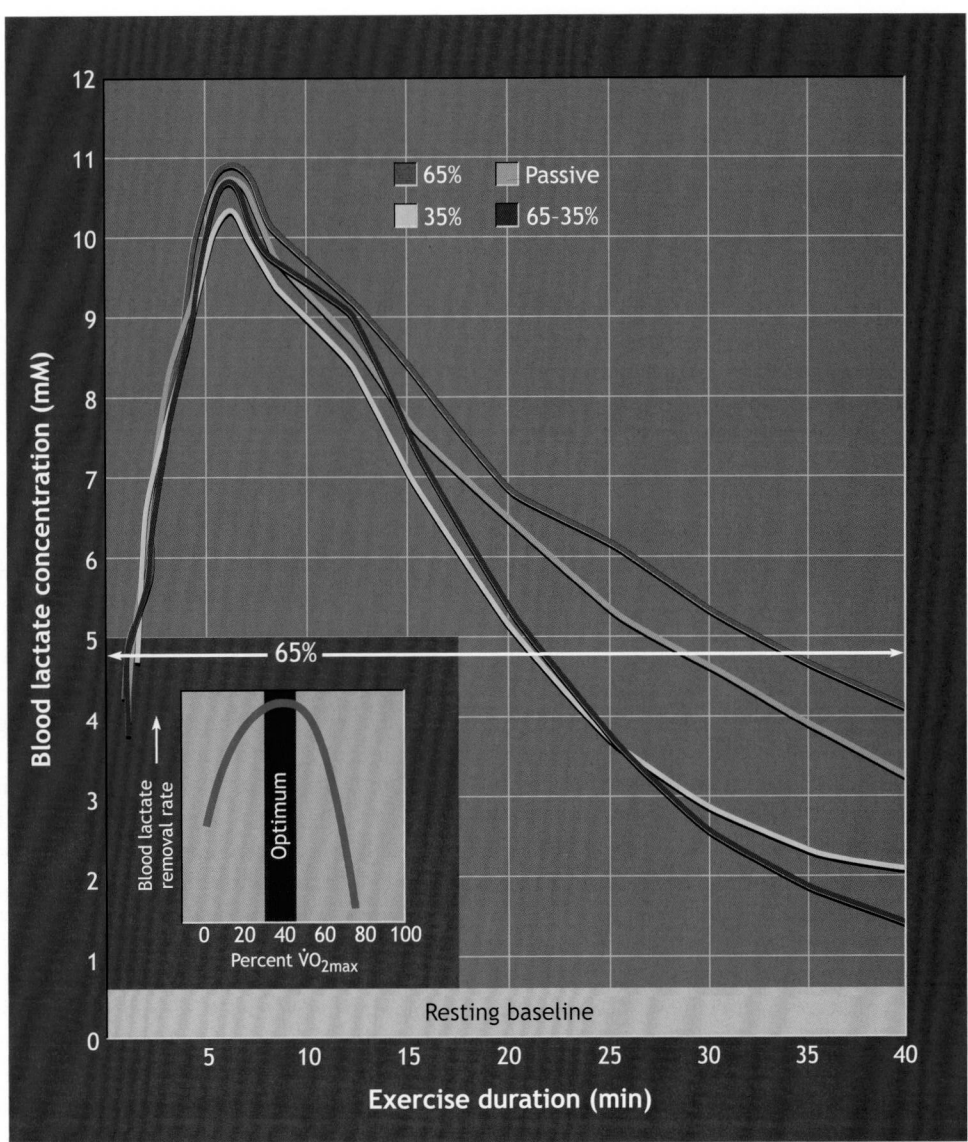

FIGURE 7.11 • Blood lactate concentration following maximal exercise using passive recovery and active recoveries at 35%, 65%, and a combination 35 and 65% $\dot{V}O_{2max}$. The horizontal *white line* indicates the blood lactate level produced by exercise at 65% $\dot{V}O_{2max}$ without previous exercise. The bottom *inset curve* depicts the generalized relationship between exercise intensity and rate of lactate removal. (Adapted with permission from Dodd S, et al. Blood lactate disappearance at various intensities of recovery exercise. *J Appl Physiol: Respir Environ Exerc Physiol* 1984;57:1462.)

Optimal Recovery from Non-Steady-Rate Physical Activity

Blood lactate accumulates when physical activity intensity exceeds the maximum steady-rate level and lactate formation in muscle exceeds its removal rate. With increasing intensity, blood lactate levels rise sharply and the exerciser soon becomes exhausted. Although the precise mechanisms for exhaustion during anaerobic activity remain unclear, blood lactate levels provide an objective indication of the relative strenuousness of exercise; they also reflect the adequacy of recovery. Because lactate anions induce a fatiguing effect on skeletal muscle (independent of associated reductions in pH),[29] any procedure that accelerates lactate removal probably augments any subsequent physical performance.[1]

Performing aerobic physical activity in recovery accelerates blood lactate removal.[13,2139,41,47] The optimal level of recovery activity ranges between 30 and 45% $\dot{V}O_{2max}$ for cycling and 55 to 60% $\dot{V}O_{2max}$ when the recovery involves running.[38] This difference between activity modes reflects more localized muscle involvement in bicycling that lowers the threshold for blood lactate accumulation.

FIGURE 7.11 illustrates blood lactate recovery patterns for trained men who performed 6 min of supermaximal exercise on a bicycle ergometer. Active recovery involved 40 min of continuous cycling at either 35 or 65% $\dot{V}O_{2max}$. A combination of 65% $\dot{V}O_{2max}$ (7 min) followed by 35% $\dot{V}O_{2max}$ (33 min) evaluated whether a higher-intensity exercise interval early in recovery would expedite lactate removal. The results indicated that moderate aerobic activity (35%

	Classic Study Results with Intermittent Physical Activity		
TABLE 7.2			
Exercise–Rest Periods	**Total Distance Run (yards)**	**Average Oxygen Consumption ($L \cdot min^{-1}$)**	**Blood Lactate Level ($mg \cdot dL$ $Blood^{-1}$)**
4-min continuous	1422	5.6	150
10-s exercise 5-s rest	7294	5.1	44
10-s exercise 10-s rest	5468	4.4	20
15-s exercise 30-s rest	3642	3.6	16

From data of Christenson EH, et al. Intermittent and continuous running. *Acta Physiol Scand* 1960;60:269.

$\dot{V}O_{2max}$, *yellow curve*) performed in recovery better facilitates lactate removal compared with a passive recovery procedure (*aqua curve*). Combining higher-intensity followed by lower-intensity activity (*purple curve*) provided no greater benefit than a single exercise level at moderate intensity. Performing recovery physical activity above the lactate threshold (65% $\dot{V}O_{2max}$, *red curve*) offers no advantage and may even prolong recovery by initiating lactate formation and accumulation. The inset graph illustrates that optimal recovery intensity probably ranges between 30 and 40% $\dot{V}O_{2max}$.

The facilitated lactate removal with active recovery likely results from increased blood perfusion through the "lactate-using" liver, heart, and inspiratory muscles. These structures serve as net consumers of lactate during recovery from intense physical activity.[3,12] Increased blood flow through the muscles in active recovery also enhances lactate removal because citric acid cycle metabolism readily oxidizes lactate from muscle tissue.

Intermittent (Interval) Physical Activity

One approach to performing physical activity that normally produces exhaustion within several minutes if performed continuously requires exercising *intermittently* with preestablished spacing of activity and rest intervals. The physical conditioning strategy of **interval training** characterizes this approach. This training regimen applies different work-to-rest intervals with supermaximal effort to overload the energy transfer systems. For example, with all-out movement of up to 8 seconds' duration, the intramuscular high-energy phosphates provide most of the energy with only minimal reliance on the glycolytic pathway. This produces rapid recovery in the alactic or fast component of postexercise oxygen uptake, enabling a subsequent bout of intense activity to begin following a brief recovery.

TABLE 7.2 summarizes the results of a classic series of experiments that combined exercise and rest intervals. On one day, the subject ran at a speed that would normally exhaust him within 5 min. The continuous run covered about 0.8 mile, and the runner attained a $\dot{V}O_{2max}$ of 5.6 $L \cdot min^{-1}$. A high blood lactate level owing to substantial anaerobic metabolism verified a relative state of exhaustion (last column in the table).

On another day, he ran at the same fast speed but intermittently, with periods of 10 s of running and 5 s of recovery. During 30 min of intermittent running, the time running amounted to 20 min and the distance covered equaled 4 miles, compared with less than 5 min and 0.8 miles with a continuous run! The effectiveness of the intermittent activity protocol becomes even more impressive considering that blood lactate remained low, even though oxygen consumption averaged 5.1 $L \cdot min^{-1}$ (91% $\dot{V}O_{2max}$) during the 30-min period. A relative balance existed between the energy requirements of physical activity and aerobic energy transfer within the muscles throughout the exercise and rest intervals.

Manipulating the duration of physical activity and rest intervals can effectively overload a specific energy-transfer system. When the rest interval increased from 5 to 10 s, oxygen consumption averaged 4.4 $L \cdot min^{-1}$; 15-s work and 30-s recovery intervals produced only a 3.6 L oxygen consumption. For each 30-min bout of intermittent running, the runner achieved a longer distance and substantially lower blood lactate level than when running continuously at the same intensity. Chapter 21 focuses on the specific application of the principles of intermittent physical activity for aerobic and anaerobic training and sports performance.

Summary

1. Intensity and duration of physical effort impact the relative contribution of the pathways for ATP production.
2. The intramuscular stores of ATP and PCr (immediate energy system) provide the energy for short-duration, intense physical activity (100-m dash, repetitive lifting of heavy weights).
3. For less intense activity of longer duration (1 to 2 min), the anaerobic reactions of glycolysis (short-term, lactate-forming energy system) generate most of the energy.
4. The aerobic system (long-term energy system) predominates as physical activity progresses beyond several minutes.
5. Humans possess two distinct muscle fiber types, each with unique metabolic and contractile properties: low glycolytic–high oxidative, slow-twitch fibers (type I) and

low oxidative–high glycolytic, fast-twitch fibers (type II). Intermediate fibers of the fast-twitch type also exist with overlapping metabolic characteristics.

6. Understanding the energy spectrum of physical activity allows individuals to train for specific improvement in each of the body's energy transfer systems.

7. A steady rate of oxygen consumption represents a balance between the energy requirements of the active muscles and aerobic ATP resynthesis.

8. Oxygen deficit defines the difference between the oxygen requirement of physical activity and the oxygen consumed during physical activity.

9. Maximum oxygen consumption ($\dot{V}O_{2max}$) quantitatively defines a person's maximum capacity to resynthesize ATP aerobically. The $\dot{V}O_{2max}$ serves as an important indicator of physiologic functional capacity to sustain intense aerobic activity.

10. Oxygen consumption remains elevated above the resting level following physical activity. Recovery oxygen consumption reflects the metabolic demands of exercise and the exercise-induced physiologic imbalances in recovery.

11. Moderate physical activity following intense physical activity (referred to as active recovery) facilitates recovery compared with passive procedures.

12. Proper spacing of the work-to-rest intervals provides a way to augment physical activity at an intensity that would normally prove fatiguing if performed continuously.

thePoint References are available online at http://thepoint.lww.com/mkk8e.

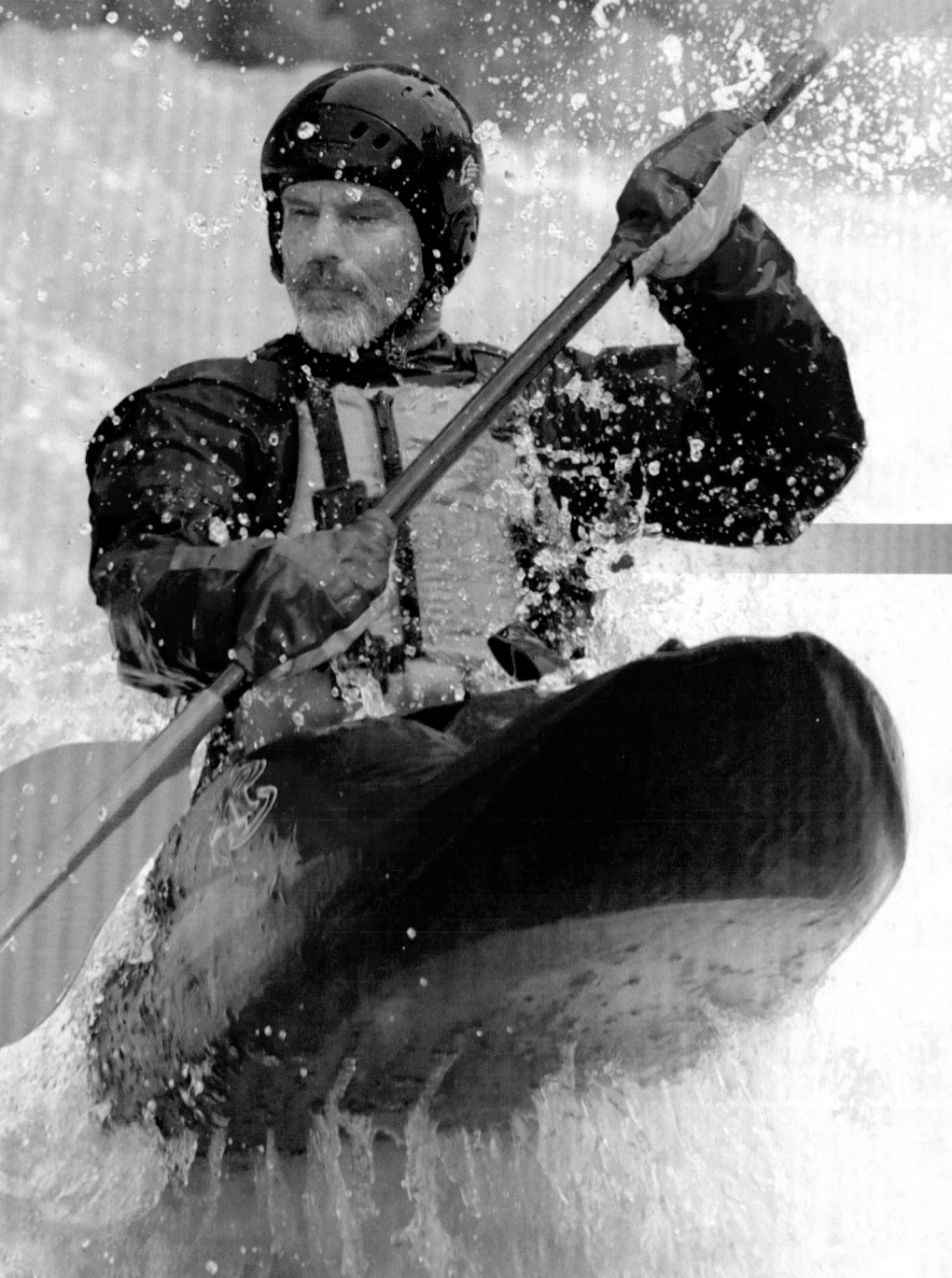

Measurement of Human Energy Expenditure

CHAPTER OBJECTIVES

- Define direct calorimetry, indirect calorimetry, closed-circuit spirometry, and open-circuit spirometry

- Diagram the closed-circuit spirometry system for oxygen consumption determinations

- Describe portable spirometry, bag technique, and computerized instrumentation systems of open-circuit spirometry

- Outline the basics of the micro-Scholander and Haldane techniques to chemically analyze expired air samples

- Discuss how the doubly labeled water technique estimates human energy expenditure and give advantages and limitations of the method

- Define respiratory quotient (RQ), and discuss its use to quantify energy release in metabolism and the composition of the food mixture metabolized during rest and steady-rate physical activity

- Discuss the difference between RQ and respiratory exchange ratio (RER) and factors that affect each

ANCILLARIES at-a-Glance

Visit http://thepoint.lww.com/mkk8e to access the following resources.

- References: Chapter 8
- Interactive Question Bank
- Appendix F: Energy Expenditure in Household, Occupational, Recreational, and Sports Activities
- Appendix G: Standardizing Gas Volumes: Environmental Factors
- Focus on Research: Respiratory Gas Exchange Implies Metabolic Mixture

MEASURING THE BODY'S HEAT PRODUCTION

All metabolic processes within the body ultimately result in heat production. Thus, the rate of heat production by cells, tissues, and even the whole body operationally defines the rate of energy metabolism. The calorie represents the basic unit of heat measurement, and the term *calorimetry* defines the measurement of heat transfer. **FIGURE 8.1** illustrates two different approaches, *direct calorimetry* and *indirect calorimetry*, to accurately quantify human energy (heat) transfer.

Direct Calorimetry

The early experiments of French chemist Antoine Lavoisier (1743–1794) and his contemporaries (**http://scienceworld. wolfram.com/biography/Lavoisier.html**) in the 1770s provided the impetus to directly measure energy expenditure during rest and physical activity. The idea, similar to that used in the bomb calorimeter described in Chapter 4 to determine food energy, provides a convenient though elaborate methodology to measure heat production in humans.

In the 1890s at Wesleyan University, professors Wilber Olin Atwater (a chemist; 1844–1907; see, for example, **http:// jn.nutrition.org/content/124/9_Suppl/1707S.full.pdf**) and Edward Bennett Rosa (a physicist; 1861–1921; see, for example, **http://www.nasonline.org/publications/biographical-memoirs/memoir-pdfs/rosa-e-b.pdf**) used the first human calorimeter of major scientific importance.[1,30] Their pioneering

and elegant calorimetric experiments relating energy input (food consumption) to energy expenditure verified the law of the conservation of energy and established the validity of indirect calorimetry. The calorimeter, diagramed schematically in **FIGURE 8.2**, consisted of a chamber where a subject could live, eat, sleep, and exercise on a bicycle ergometer. The experiments lasted from several hours to 13 days, and some involved cycling performed for up to 16 hr with total energy expenditure exceeding 10,000 kcal! A staff of 16, working in teams for 8- to 12-hr shifts, operated the airtight, thermally insulated calorimeter. A known volume of water at a specified temperature that circulated through a series of coils at the top of the chamber absorbed the heat produced and radiated by the subject. Insulation surrounded the entire chamber so that any change in water temperature, measured in units of 0.01°C with a microscope mounted alongside a thermometer, reflected the subject's energy metabolism. For adequate ventilation, exhaled air continually passed from the room through chemicals that removed moisture and absorbed carbon dioxide. Oxygen was added to the air recirculated through the chamber.

Since publication of the seminal papers by Atwater and Rosa, other calorimetric methods have emerged for inferring energy expenditure from metabolic gas exchange for extended periods in respiration chambers, and by metabolic and thermal balance with water flow and airflow calorimeters.[5,8,13,19–21] The modern space suit worn by astronauts during extravehicular activities, for example, represents a "suit calorimeter" designed to maintain respiratory gas exchange, thermal balance, and protection from a potentially hostile ambient environment. These suits have application for performing extended work outside an orbiting space vehicle (the current International Space Station), and will play an even more crucial role when establishing a manned Mars outpost within the next two decades.[23]

Over the years, various other heat-measuring devices have been developed, each based on a different principle of operation.

1. In an **airflow calorimeter**, temperature change in air that flows through an insulated space, multiplied by the air's mass and specific heat, including calculations for evaporative heat loss, determines heat production.
2. A **water flow calorimeter** operates similarly, except that a change in temperature occurs in water flowing through coils that make up part of an environmentally self-contained body suit worn by astronauts.
3. **Gradient layer calorimetry** measures body heat that flows from the subject through a sheet of insulating materials with appropriate piping and cooler water flowing on the outside of the gradient.

Direct measurement of heat production in humans has considerable theoretical implications but limited practical applications. Accurate measurements of heat production in the calorimeter require considerable time and expense and formidable engineering expertise. Thus, calorimeters remain inapplicable for energy determinations for most sport, occupational, and recreational activities.

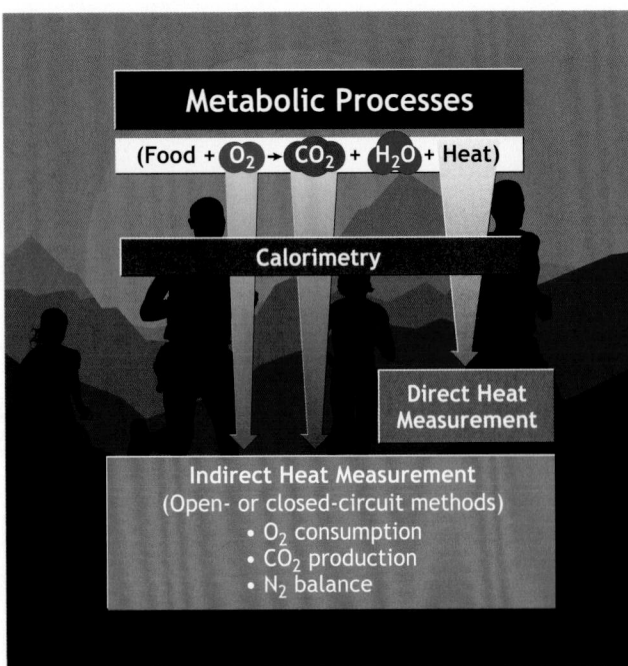

FIGURE 8.1 • Measurement of the body's rate of heat production gives a direct assessment of metabolic rate. Heat production (metabolic rate) can also be estimated indirectly by measuring the exchange of carbon dioxide and oxygen during the breakdown of food macronutrients and nitrogen excretion.

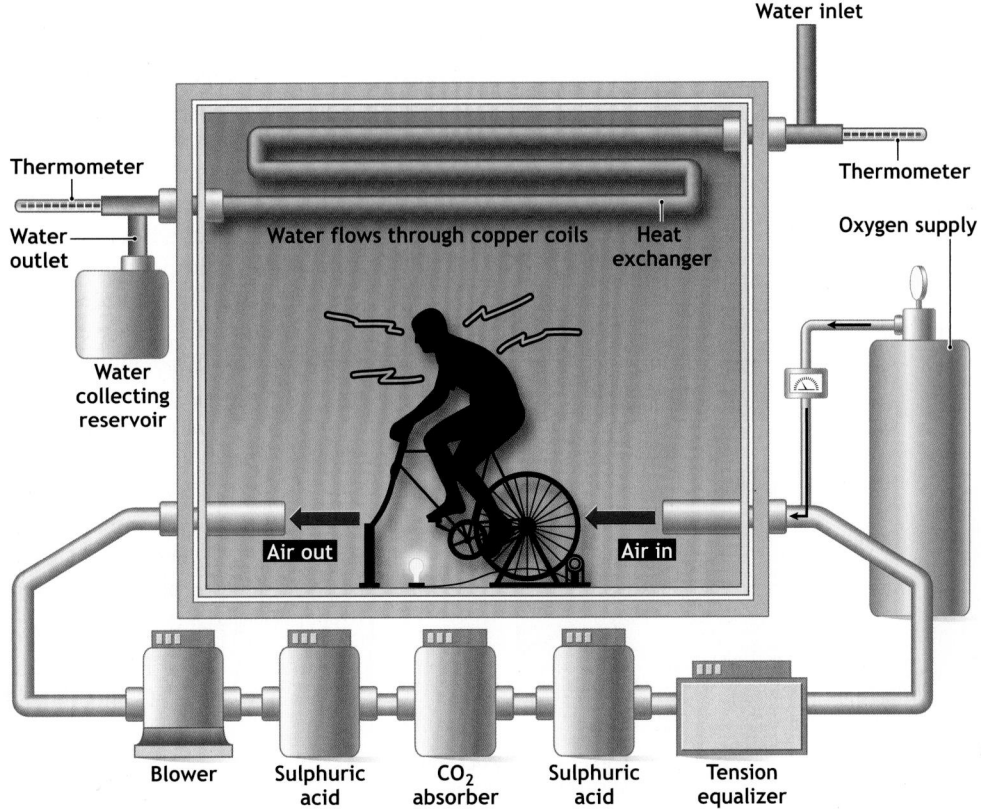

FIGURE 8.2 • A human calorimeter directly measures the body's rate of energy metabolism (heat production). In the Atwater-Rosa calorimeter, a thin sheet of copper lines the interior wall to which heat exchangers attach overhead and through which cold water passes. Water cooled to 35.6°F (2°C) moves at a high flow rate, absorbing the heat radiated from the subject during exercise. As the subject rests, warmer water flows at a slower rate. In the original bicycle ergometer shown in the schematic, the rear wheel contacts the shaft of a generator that powers a light bulb. In later versions of ergometers, copper composed part of the rear wheel. The wheel rotated through the field of an electromagnet to produce an electric current for determining power output.

Indirect Calorimetry

All energy-releasing reactions in humans ultimately depend on oxygen use. Measuring a person's oxygen consumption during physical activities provides researchers with an indirect yet highly accurate estimate of energy expenditure. Compared with direct calorimetry, indirect calorimetry remains simpler and less expensive.

Studies with bomb calorimetry show the release of approximately 4.82 kcal of energy when a mixed-diet blend of carbohydrate, lipid, and protein burns with 1 L of oxygen. Even with large variations in metabolic mixture, this **calorific value for oxygen** varies only slightly, generally within 2 to 4%. Thus, a rounded value of 5.0 kcal per liter of oxygen consumed provides an appropriate conversion factor to estimate energy expenditure under steady-rate conditions of aerobic metabolism. This energy–oxygen equivalent of 5.0 kcal per liter provides a suitable yardstick to express any aerobic physical activity in energy units (see Appendix F).

thePoint Appendix F, available online at **http://thepoint. lww.com/mkk8e**, provides energy expenditure in household, occupational, recreational, and sports activities.

Indirect calorimetry yields results comparable to direct measurement with the human calorimeter. **Closed-circuit spirometry** and **open-circuit spirometry** represent the two applications of indirect calorimetry.

 INTEGRATIVE QUESTION

What rationale underlies early experiments that quantified energy metabolism of small animals by measuring the rate that ice melted in a container that surrounded the animal?

Closed-Circuit Spirometry

FIGURE 8.3 illustrates the closed-circuit spirometric apparatus developed in the late 1800s and used in hospitals and research laboratories through the 1980s to estimate resting energy expenditure. The simplicity of this method to directly measure oxygen consumption has considerable theoretical importance but limited practical applications. The subject breathes 100% oxygen from a prefilled container or spirometer. The equipment is called "closed" because the subject

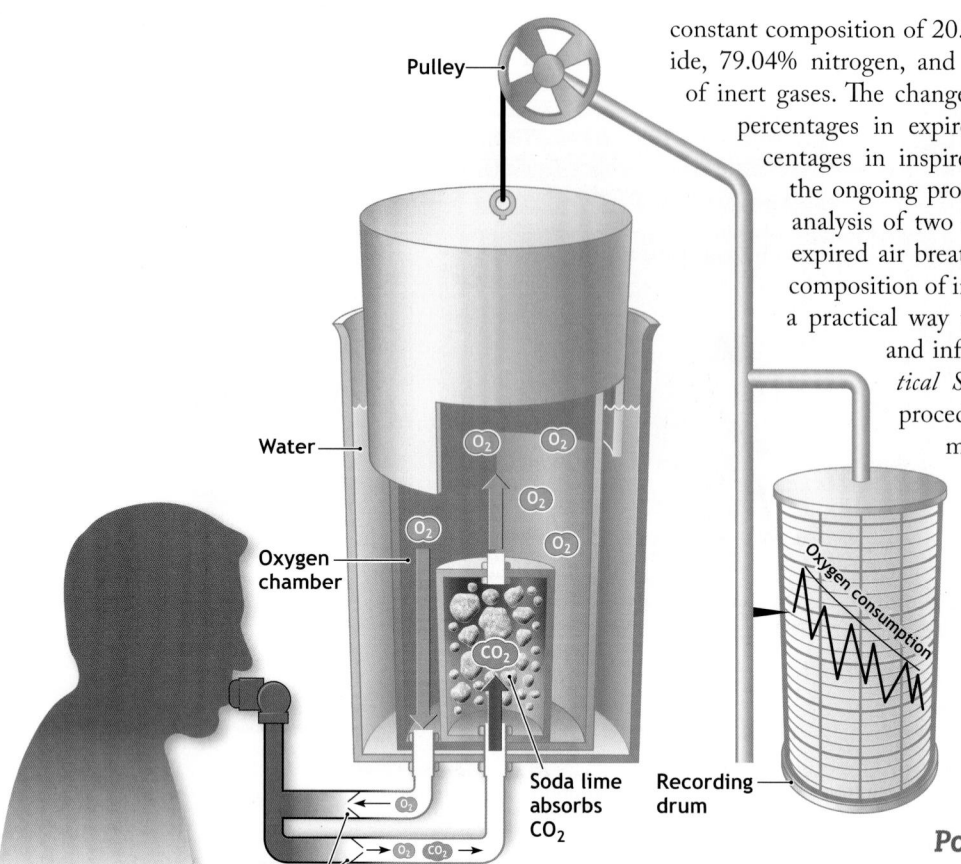

FIGURE 8.3 • The closed-circuit method uses a spirometer prefilled with 100% oxygen. As the subject rebreathes from the spirometer, soda lime removes the expired air's carbon dioxide. The difference between the initial and final volumes of oxygen in the calibrated spirometer indicates oxygen consumption during the measurement interval.

rebreathes only the gas from the spirometer. A canister of potassium hydroxide (soda lime) placed in the breathing circuit absorbs the exhaled carbon dioxide. A drum attached to the spirometer revolves at a known speed to record the oxygen removed (i.e., oxygen consumed) from changes in the system's total volume.

During physical activity, closed-circuit spirometry measurement becomes problematic. The subject must remain close to the bulky equipment, the circuit offers considerable resistance to accommodate large breathing volumes, and carbon dioxide removal lags behind its production rate during intense effort. For these reasons, open-circuit spirometry remains the most widely used laboratory procedure to measure oxygen consumption during human movement.

Open-Circuit Spirometry

The open-circuit method provides a simple way to measure oxygen consumption. A subject inhales ambient air with a

constant composition of 20.93% oxygen, 0.03% carbon dioxide, 79.04% nitrogen, and a small but negligible quantity of inert gases. The changes in oxygen and carbon dioxide percentages in expired air compared with the percentages in inspired ambient air indirectly reflect the ongoing process of energy metabolism. Thus, analysis of two factors—volume of inspired and expired air breathed during a specified time and composition of inspired and expired air—provides a practical way to measure oxygen consumption and infer energy expenditure. *In a Practical Sense* illustrates the step-by-step procedure for computing the important metabolic variables via open-circuit spirometry.

Three common indirect calorimetry procedures measure oxygen consumption during physical activity:

1. Portable spirometry
2. Bag technique
3. Computerized instrumentation

Portable Spirometry

Two German scientists at the Max Plank Institute for Nutritional Research in the early 1940s perfected a lightweight, portable system, first devised by German respiratory physiologist and pioneer of modern altitude physiology and aviation medicine Nathan Zuntz (1847–1920; www.ncbi.nlm.nih.gov/pubmed/7726784) at the turn of the century, to determine energy expenditure indirectly during physical activity.[15] The activities included war-related operations such as traveling over different terrain with full battle gear, operating transportation vehicles including tanks and aircraft, and performing physical tasks that soldiers encounter during combat operations. Carrying the portable spirometer allowed for considerable freedom of movement in physical activities as diverse as mountain climbing, downhill skiing, sailing, golf, and common household activities (Appendix F, http://thepoint.lww.com/mkk8e). Nevertheless, the equipment becomes cumbersome during vigorous activity, and the meter begins to underrecord airflow volume during intense activity with rapid breathing.[17]

thePoint Appendix F, available online at http://thepoint.lww.com/mkk8e, lists the calorie expenditure for different physical activities, including common household activities.

Over time, different portable systems have been designed, tested, and used in many applications. For the most part, portable systems now use the latest advances in miniaturized computer technology to produce acceptable results compared to more fixed, dedicated desktop systems or the traditional Douglas bag system described in the section on

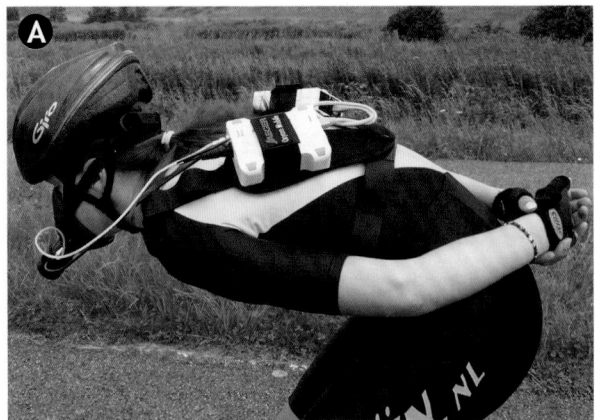

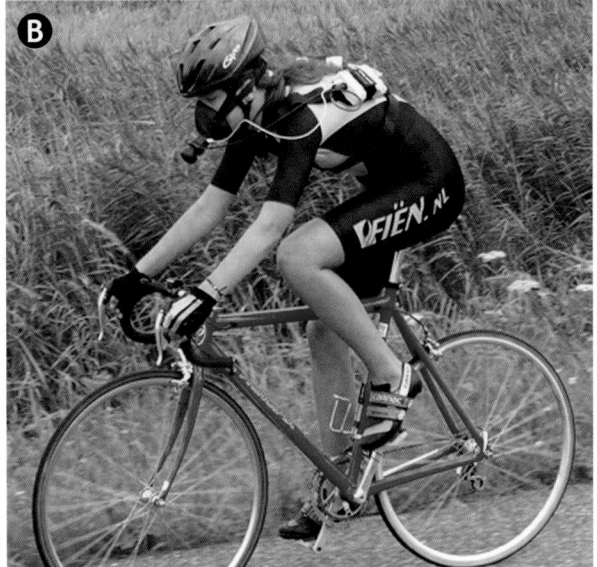

FIGURE 8.4 • Portable metabolic collection systems use the latest in miniature computer technology. Built-in oxygen and carbon dioxide analyzer cells coupled with a highly sensitive micro-flow meter measure oxygen uptake by the open-circuit method during different activities such as **(A)** in-line skating and **(B)** cycling. (Adapted with permission from McArdle WD, Katch FI, Katch VL. *Sports and Exercise Nutrition.* 4th Ed. Philadelphia: Wolters Kluwer Health, 2013.)

Bag Technique. **FIGURES 8.4A AND B** show applications of commerically available portable metabolic collection systems. The most current miniaturized systems include whole-body multisensor devices worn on the wrist or arm, or a collection system similar to a lightweight headset microphone. In these applications, an integrated computer performs the metabolic calculations based on electronic signals it receives from microdesigned instruments that measure oxygen and carbon dioxide in expired air, and respiratory flow dynamics and volumes. Microchips store the data for later analyses. More comprehensive advanced systems also include automated blood pressure, heart rate, and temperature monitors, with preset instructions to regulate speed, duration, and workload of a treadmill, bicycle ergometer, stepper, rower, swim flume, resistance device, or other exercise apparatus.

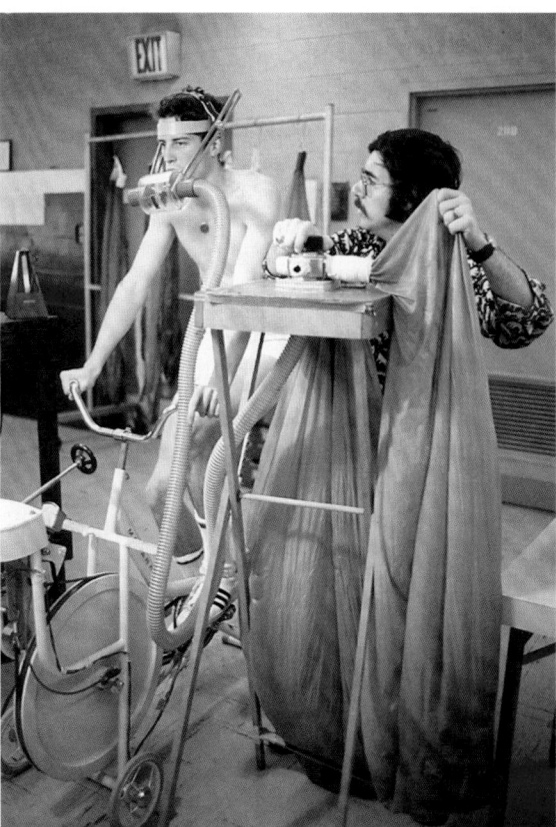

FIGURE 8.5 • Oxygen uptake measurement by open-circuit spirometry (bag technique) during stationary cycle ergometer exercise.

Bag Technique

FIGURE 8.5 depicts the classic bag technique. The subject rides a stationary bicycle ergometer wearing headgear attached to a two-way, high-velocity, low-resistance breathing valve. He breathes ambient air through one side of the valve and expels it through the other side. The expired air then passes into either large plastic or canvas Douglas bags (named for distinguished British respiratory physiologist Claude G. Douglas [1882–1963]) or rubber meteorological balloons or directly through a gas meter that continually measures expired air volume. The meter draws off an aliquot sample of expired air for analysis of O_2 and CO_2 composition with subsequent calculations of oxygen consumed and carbon dioxide produced.

Computerized Instrumentation

With advances in computer and microprocessor technology, the exercise scientist can rapidly measure metabolic and physiologic responses to exercise. A computer interfaces with at least three instruments: a system to continuously sample the subject's expired air volume, and oxygen and carbon dioxide analyzers to measure the expired gas mixture's composition. The computer performs metabolic calculations based on electronic signals it receives from the instruments. A printed or graphic display of the data appears throughout the

IN A PRACTICAL SENSE

Calculating Oxygen Consumption ($\dot{V}O_2$), Carbon Dioxide Production ($\dot{V}CO_2$), and the Respiratory Quotient (RQ) Using Open-Circuit Spirometry

Because the percentage composition of inspired air remains relatively constant ($CO_2 = 0.03\%$, $O_2 = 20.93\%$, $N_2 = 79.04\%$), determining a person's oxygen consumption requires measuring the amount and composition of the expired air. Expired air always contains more CO_2 (usually 2.5 to 5.0%), less O_2 (usually 15.0 to 18.5%), and more N_2 (usually 79.04 to 79.60%) than the air inspired.

NITROGEN EXCHANGE: THE HALDANE TRANSFORMATION

Nitrogen is inert in terms of energy metabolism; any change in its concentration in expired air reflects that the number of oxygen molecules removed from inspired air are not replaced by the same number of carbon dioxide molecules produced in metabolism. This results in the volume of expired air ($\dot{V}_{E,STPD}$) being unequal to the inspired volume ($\dot{V}_{I,STPD}$). For example, if the respiratory quotient is less than 1.00 (i.e., less CO_2 produced in relation to O_2 consumed), and 3 liters (L) of air are inspired, less than 3 L of air will be expired. In this case, the nitrogen concentration is higher in expired air than in inspired air. This is not because nitrogen has been produced; rather, nitrogen molecules now represent a larger percentage of $\dot{V}_E$ compared to $\dot{V}_I$. $\dot{V}_E$ differs from $\dot{V}_I$ in direct proportion to the change in nitrogen concentration between the inspired and expired air volumes. Thus, $\dot{V}_I$ can be determined from $\dot{V}_E$ using the ratio of nitrogen expired compared to the nitrogen inspired in an equation known as the *Haldane transformation*.

$$\dot{V}_{I,STPD} = \dot{V}_{E,STPD} \times \frac{\%N_2E}{\%N_2I} \qquad \textbf{Equation 1}$$

where $\%N_2I = 79.04$ and $\%N_2I$ = percent nitrogen in expired air computed from gas analysis as $[(100 - (\%O_{2E} + \%CO_{2E})]$.

CALCULATING $\dot{V}O_2$ USING EXPIRED AIR VOLUME

The following examples assume that all ventilation volumes are expressed as standard temperature, pressure, dry (STPD).

thePoint   Appendix G, available online at http://thepoint.lww.com/mkk8e, explains how to standardize gas volumes to reference conditions (STPD and BTPS).

The volume of O_2 in inspired air per minute ($\dot{V}O_{2I}$) can be determined as follows:

$$\dot{V}O_{2I} = \dot{V}_I \times \%O_{2I} \qquad \textbf{Equation 2}$$

Using the Haldane transformation and substituting equation (1) for $\dot{V}_I$,

$$\dot{V}O_{2I} = \dot{V}_E \times \frac{\%N_2E}{79.04} \times \%O_{2I} \qquad \textbf{Equation 3}$$

where $\%O_2 = 20.93\%$.

The amount or volume of oxygen in expired air ($\dot{V}O_{2E}$) computes as

$$\dot{V}O_{2E} = \dot{V}_E \times \%O_{2E} \qquad \textbf{Equation 4}$$

where $\%O_{2E}$ is the fractional concentration of oxygen in expired air determined by gas analysis (chemical or electronic methods).

The amount of O_2 removed from inspired air each minute ($\dot{V}O_2$) can then be computed as follows:

$$\dot{V}O_2 = \dot{V}_I \times \%O_{2I} - \dot{V}_E \times \%O_{2E} \qquad \textbf{Equation 5}$$

By substitution,

$$\dot{V}O_2 = \left\langle \left[\left(\dot{V}_E \times \frac{\%N_2E}{79.04\%} \right) \times 20.93\% \right] - \left(\dot{V}_E \times \%O_{2E} \right) \right\rangle$$

$$\textbf{Equation 6}$$

where $\dot{V}O_2$ = volume of oxygen consumed per minute, expressed in mL or L, and $\dot{V}_E$ = expired air volume consumed per minute, expressed in mL or L, and $\dot{V}_E$ = expired air volume per minute, expressed in mL or L, STPD. Equation 6 can be simplified to:

$$\dot{V}O_2 = \dot{V}_E \left[\left(\frac{\%N_2E}{79.04\%} \times 20.93\% \right) - \%O_{2E} \right] \qquad \textbf{Equation 7}$$

After dividing 20.93 by 79.04, the final form of the equation becomes:

$$\dot{V}O_2 = \dot{V}_E \left[(\%N_{2E} \times 0.265) - \%O_{2E} \right] \qquad \textbf{Equation 8}$$

Equation 8 is the equation of choice to calculate $\dot{V}O_2$ when ventilation expired (STPD) is determined.

True O_2

The value obtained within the brackets in equations 7 and 8 is referred to as the *True O_2* and represents the "oxygen extraction" or, more precisely, the percentage of oxygen consumed for any volume of air expired.

CALCULATING $\dot{V}O_2$ USING INSPIRED AIR VOLUME

In situations where only $\dot{V}_I$ is measured, the $\dot{V}_E$ can be calculated from the Haldane transformation as:

$$\dot{V}_E = \dot{V}_I \frac{\%N_{2I}}{\%N_{2E}} \qquad \textbf{Equation 9}$$

By substitution in equation (5), the computational equation becomes:

$$\dot{V}O_2 = \dot{V}_I \left[\%O_{2I} - \left(\frac{\%N_{2I}}{\%N_{2E}} \times \%O_{2E} \right) \right] \qquad \textbf{Equation 10}$$

CALCULATING CARBON DIOXIDE PRODUCTION ($\dot{V}CO_2$)

The carbon dioxide production per minute ($\dot{V}CO_2$) calculates as follows:

$$\dot{V}CO_2 = \dot{V}_E \left(\%CO_{2E} - \%CO_{2I} \right) \qquad \textbf{Equation 11}$$

where $\%CO_{2E}$ = percent carbon dioxide in expired air determined by gas analysis, and $\%CO_2$ = percent carbon dioxide in inspired air, which is essentially constant at 0.003%.

The final form of the equation becomes:

$$\dot{V}CO_{2E} = \dot{V}_E \left(\%CO_{2E} - 0.003\% \right) \qquad \textbf{Equation 12}$$

CALCULATING THE RESPIRATORY QUOTIENT (RQ)

The respiratory quotient (RQ) calculates in one of two ways:

$$RQ = \frac{\dot{V}CO_2}{\dot{V}O_2} \qquad \textbf{Equation 13}$$

or

$$RQ = \frac{\%CO_{2E} - 0.03\%}{"True"O_2}$$

Example

Compute $\dot{V}O_2$, $\dot{V}CO_2$, and RQ from the following data:

a. $\dot{V}_{E, STPD}$ = 60.0 L
b. $\%O_{2E}$ = 16.86 or (0.1686)
c. $\%CO_{2E}$ = 3.62 or (0.0362)

$$\dot{V}O_2 = \dot{V}_E \left[(\%N_{2E} \times 0.265) - \%O_{2E} \right] \qquad \textbf{Equation 8}$$

$\dot{V}O_2$ = 60.0 [(1.00 − (0.1686 + 0.0362)) × 0.265 − 0.1686]
$\dot{V}O_2$ = 60.0 [(0.7952 × 0.265) − 0.1686]
$\dot{V}O_2$ = 2.527 L·min⁻¹

$$\dot{V}CO_{2E} = \dot{V}_E \left(\%CO_{2E} - 0.003\% \right) \qquad \textbf{Equation 12}$$

$$\dot{V}CO_{2E} = 60.0 \left(0.0362 - 0.003\% \right)$$

$\dot{V}CO_{2E}$ = 1.992 L·min⁻¹

$$RQ = \frac{\dot{V}CO_2}{\dot{V}O_2} \qquad \textbf{Equation 13}$$

$$RQ = \frac{1.992}{2.527}$$

$$RQ = 0.79$$

---

measurement period. FIGURE 8.6 depicts a typical computerized system to assess and monitor metabolic and physiologic responses during physical activity. The flowchart in the figure illustrates the sequence of events, usually breath by breath, to compute ventilation volume and the amount of oxygen consumed and carbon dioxide produced during the measurement period. "In a Practical Sense" presents the computations of pulmonary and metabolic data using open-circuit spirometry.

Computerized systems offer advantages in ease of operation and speed of data analysis, but disadvantages also exist.[4,10,32] These include the high cost of equipment and delays from system breakdowns. *Regardless of the sophistication of a particular automated system, the output data still reflect the accuracy of the measuring devices.* The reliability and validity of measurement instruments require careful and frequent calibration that employs established reference or criterion standards.

Chemical Gas Analyzers for Calibration Purposes. Metabolic measurements require frequent calibration of equipment that assess the air volume breathed and measure the expired air volume's oxygen and carbon dioxide fractional concentrations. In this regard, most laboratories use criterion instruments for calibration purposes. FIGURE 8.7 illustrates two classic chemical procedures to analyze gas mixtures for oxygen, carbon dioxide, and nitrogen, and for subsequent calibration and/or validation of electronic analyzers. Before the conversion to electronic and computerized instrumentation, oxygen consumption determinations used either the Scholander or Haldane gas analysis methods. The Scholander technique, developed by Swedish physician and biologist Per Scholander (1905–1980; http://www.nasonline.org/publications/biographical-memoirs/memoir-pdfs/Scholander_Per.pdf), remained the method of choice through the 1980s to validate gas analysis procedures. The Haldane analyzer, also used in the early years of exercise physiology research, was devised by the British physiologist who invented the gas mask used in World War I, John Scott Haldane (1860–1936; http://navxdivingu.blogspot.com/2009/10/diving-history-john-scott-haldane.html). Both of these methods involved hundreds of time-consuming separate analyses for a single experiment, with frequent duplicate measurements to verify

INTEGRATIVE QUESTION

Discuss the common energy basis to equate food intake and physical activity.

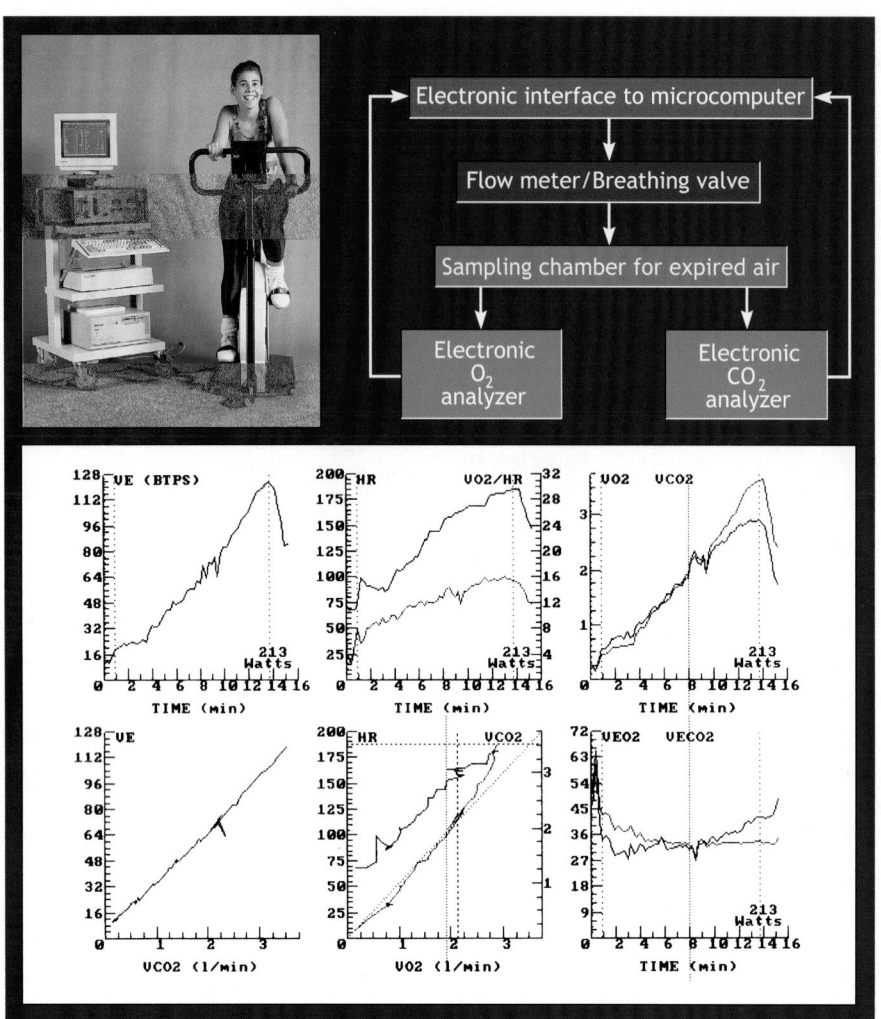

FIGURE 8.6 • Computer systems approach to collect, analyze, and monitor physiologic and metabolic data.

results. This partly explains why energy metabolism studies from the early exercise physiology literature often only relied on one or two subjects and took so long to complete. When performed properly with attention to detail, these chemical analyzers produced highly accurate and reliable data.

The **micro-Scholander technique** measures oxygen and carbon dioxide concentration in expired air to an accuracy of ± 0.015 mL per 100 mL of gas.[22] A skilled technician can perform one analysis of a 0.5-mL gas microsample in about 10 min. The **Haldane method** provides another technique for gas analysis.[11] It uses a larger air sample and requires between 10 and 15 min to complete one analysis.

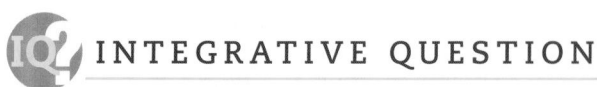 INTEGRATIVE QUESTION

Justify measuring only CO_2 production to estimate energy expenditure during steady-rate physical activity.

Direct Versus Indirect Calorimetry

Comparisons of energy metabolism with direct and indirect calorimetry provide convincing evidence for the validity of the indirect method. Research in the early part of the 19th century compared the two calorimetry methods over 40 days on three men who lived in a calorimeter similar to the one shown in Figure 8.2. Daily energy expenditure averaged 2723 kcal when measured directly by heat production and 2717 kcal when computed indirectly by closed-circuit oxygen consumption measures. Other experiments with animals and humans, using rest and light and moderate (steady-rate) physical activity, also show close agreement between direct and indirect methods; in most instances, the difference averages less than ±1%. In Atwater and Rosa's calorimetry experiments, methodological errors averaged only ±0.2%. This remarkable achievement, using mostly handmade instruments, resulted from the scientists' dedication to precise calibration methods long before the availability of electronic instrumentation.

DOUBLY LABELED WATER TECHNIQUE

The doubly labeled water technique provides an isotope-based method to safely estimate total (average) daily energy expenditure of groups of children and adults, in free-living

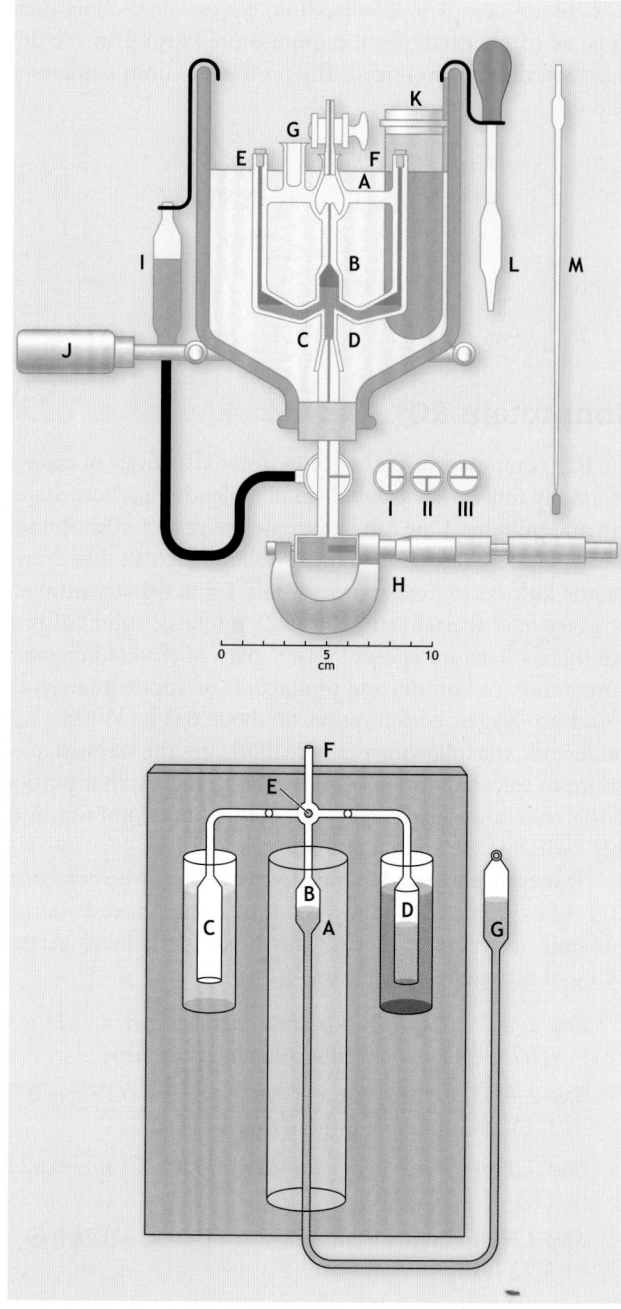

FIGURE 8.7 • General schematic for two common analytical procedures for gas analysis. **(Top)** Micro-Scholander gas analyzer. (A) Compensating chamber; (B) reaction chamber; (C) side arm for CO_2 absorber; (D) side arm for O_2 absorber; (E) and (F) solid vaccine bottle stoppers; (G) receptacle for stopcock; (H) micrometer burette; (I) leveling bulb containing mercury; (J) handle for tilting apparatus; (K) tube for storing the acid rinsing solution; (L) pipette for the rinsing acid; (M) transfer pipette. **(Bottom)** Haldane gas analyzer. (A) Water jacket surrounding the measuring burette; (B) calibrated measuring burette containing a gas sample for measurement; (C) vessel containing CO_2 absorber (potassium hydroxide); (D) vessel containing O_2 absorber (pyrogallate); (E) glass valve; (F) entry for gas sample; (G) mercury-leveling bulb. The gas introduced into the burette is exposed to the O_2 and CO_2 absorbers by alternately lowering and raising the mercury-leveling bulb. The O_2 and CO_2 gas volumes are determined by subtraction from the initial volume.

conditions without the normal constraints imposed by laboratory procedures.[7,24,25,27,33] Few studies routinely use this method, and subject number remains small because of the expense in using doubly labeled water and the need for sophisticated measurement equipment. Nevertheless, its measurement does serve as a criterion or standard to validate other methods that estimate total daily energy expenditure over prolonged periods.[3,6,9,17,23,28]

The subject consumes a quantity of water with a known concentration of the heavy, nonradioactive forms of the stable isotopes of hydrogen (^{2}H, or deuterium) and oxygen (^{18}O, or oxygen-18)—hence the term *doubly labeled water*. The isotopes distribute throughout bodily fluids. Labeled hydrogen leaves the body as water (^{2}H$_2$O) in sweat, urine, and pulmonary water vapor, while labeled oxygen leaves as both water (H$_2^{18}$O) and carbon dioxide (C^{18}O$_2$) produced during macro-nutrient oxidation in energy metabolism. Differences between elimination rates of the two isotopes (determined by an isotope ratio mass spectrometer) relative to the body's normal background levels estimate total CO_2 production during the measurement period. Oxygen consumption is easily estimated on the basis of CO_2 production and an assumed (or measured) respiratory quotient (see the next section) value of 0.85.

Under normal circumstances, analysis of urine or saliva before consuming the doubly labeled water serves as the control baseline values for ^{18}O and ^{2}H. Ingested isotopes require about 5 hr to distribute throughout the body water. The researchers then measure the enriched urine or saliva sample initially and then every day (or week) thereafter for the study's duration (usually up to 3 weeks). The progressive decrease in the sample concentrations of the two isotopes permits computation of the CO_2 production rate.[26] Accuracy of the doubly labeled water technique versus directly measured energy expenditure in controlled settings averages between 3 and 5%. This magnitude of error probably increases in field studies, particularly among physically active individuals.[31]

The doubly labeled water technique provides an ideal way to assess total energy expenditure of individuals over prolonged periods, including bed rest and extreme activities like climbing Mt. Everest, cycling the Tour de France, trekking across Antarctica, military activities, extravehicular activities in space, and endurance running and swimming.[2,12,18,29] Drawbacks to the method include the cost of enriched ^{18}O and expense incurred in spectrometric analysis of both isotopes.

RESPIRATORY QUOTIENT

Research in the early part of the 20th century discovered a way to evaluate the metabolic mixture metabolized during rest and steady-rate exercise from measures of pulmonary gas exchange.[16] Because of inherent chemical differences in carbohydrate, fat, and protein composition, they require different amounts of oxygen for complete oxidation of each molecule's carbon and hydrogen atoms to the carbon dioxide and water end products. Thus, carbon dioxide produced per unit of oxygen consumed varies with the type of substrate catabolized. The **respiratory quotient (RQ)** describes this ratio of metabolic gas exchange measured at the lungs as follows:

$$RQ = CO_2 \text{ produced} \div O_2 \text{ consumed}$$

The RQ provides a convenient guide to approximate the nutrient mixture catabolized for energy during rest and aerobic physical activity. Also, because the caloric equivalents for oxygen differ somewhat depending on the nutrient oxidized, *precise* determination of the body's heat production by indirect calorimetry requires measuring both RQ and oxygen consumption.

RQ for Carbohydrate

The complete oxidation of one glucose molecule requires six oxygen molecules and produces six molecules of carbon dioxide and water as follows:

$$C_6H_{12}O_6 + 6\,O_2 \rightarrow 6\,CO_2 + 6\,H_2O$$
$$RQ = 6\,CO_2 \div 6\,O_2$$
$$= 1.00$$

Gas exchange during glucose oxidation produces a number of CO_2 molecules equal to the number of O_2 molecules consumed; therefore, the RQ for carbohydrate equals 1.00.

RQ for Fat

The chemical composition of fats differs from carbohydrates because fats contain considerably more hydrogen and carbon atoms than oxygen atoms. Consequently, fat catabolism requires more oxygen in relation to carbon dioxide production. For example, palmitic acid, a typical fatty acid, oxidizes to carbon dioxide and water, producing 16 carbon dioxide molecules for every 23 oxygen molecules consumed. The following equation summarizes this exchange to compute the RQ:

$$C_{16}H_{32}O_2 + 23\,O_2 \rightarrow 16\,CO_2 + 16\,H_2O$$
$$RQ = 16\,CO_2 \div 23\,O_2$$
$$= 0.696$$

Generally, a value of 0.70 represents the RQ for fat, with values ranging between 0.69 and 0.73 depending on the oxidized fatty acid's carbon-chain length.

RQ for Protein

Proteins do not simply oxidize to carbon dioxide and water during energy metabolism in the body. Rather, the amino acid molecule is first deaminated in the liver. The body then excretes the nitrogen and sulfur fragments in the urine, sweat, and feces. The remaining keto acid fragment oxidizes to carbon dioxide and water to provide energy for biologic work.

To achieve complete combustion, these short-chain keto acids, as in fat catabolism, require more oxygen in relation to carbon dioxide produced. The protein albumin oxidizes as follows:

$$C_{72}H_{112}N_2O_{22}S + 77\,O_2 \rightarrow 63\,CO_2$$
$$+ 38\,H_2O + SO_3 + 9\,CO(NH_2)_2$$
$$RQ = 63\,CO_2 \div 77\,O_2$$
$$= 0.818$$

The general value 0.82 characterizes the RQ for protein.

Nonprotein RQ

The RQ computed from the compositional analysis of expired air usually reflects the catabolism of a blend of carbohydrates, fats, and proteins. One can determine the precise contribution of each of these nutrients to the metabolic mixture. For example, the kidneys excrete approximately 1 g of urinary nitrogen for every 5.57 (current value) to 6.25 g (classic value) of protein metabolized for energy.[14] Each gram of excreted nitrogen represents a carbon dioxide production of approximately 4.8 L and an oxygen consumption of about 6.0 L. Within this framework, the following example illustrates the stepwise procedure to calculate the **nonprotein RQ**; that is, that portion of the respiratory exchange attributed to the combustion of only carbohydrate and fat excluding protein.

This example considers data from a subject who consumes 4.0 L of oxygen and produces 3.4 L of carbon dioxide during a 15-min rest period. During this time, the kidneys excrete 0.13 g of nitrogen in the urine.

Step 1. 4.8 L CO_2 per g protein metabolized × 0.13 g = 0.62 L CO_2 produced in protein catabolism

Step 2. 6.0 L O_2 per g protein metabolized × 0.13 g = 0.78 L O_2 consumed in protein catabolism

Step 3. Nonprotein CO_2 produced = 3.4 L CO_2 − 0.62 L CO_2 = 2.78 L CO_2

Step 4. Nonprotein O_2 consumed = 4.0 L O_2 − 0.78 L O_2 = 3.22 L O_2

Step 5. Nonprotein RQ = 2.78 ÷ 3.22 = 0.86

TABLE 8.1 presents the thermal energy equivalents for oxygen consumption for different nonprotein RQ values and the percentage of fat and carbohydrate catabolized for energy. For the nonprotein RQ of 0.86 computed in the previous example, each liter of oxygen consumed liberates 4.875 kcal. Also, for this RQ, 54.1% of the nonprotein calories derive from carbohydrate, and 45.9% come from fat. The total 15-min heat production at rest attributable to fat and carbohydrate catabolism equals 15.70 kcal (4.875 kcal·L^{-1} × 3.22 L O_2); the energy from the breakdown of protein equals 3.51 kcal (4.5 kcal·L^{-1} × 0.78 L O_2). The total energy from the combustion of protein and nonprotein macronutrients during the 15-min period equals 19.21 kcal (15.70 kcal nonprotein + 3.51 kcal protein).

IN A PRACTICAL SENSE

The Weir Method to Calculate Energy Expenditure

In 1949, John Brash de Vere Weir (1908–1985), a senior lecturer in physiology from Glasgow University, presented a simple method to estimate caloric expenditure (kcal · min^{-1}) from measures of pulmonary ventilation and expired oxygen percentage, accurate to within ±1% of the traditional respiratory quotient (RQ) method.

BASIC EQUATION

Weir showed that the following formula could calculate energy expenditure if total energy production from protein breakdown equaled 12.5% (a reasonable percentage for most people under most conditions):

$$\text{kcal} \cdot \text{min}^{-1} = \dot{V}_{E(STPD)} \times (1.044 - 0.0499 \times \%O_{2E})$$

where $\dot{V}_{E(STPD)}$ represents expired minute ventilation (L · min^{-1}) corrected to STPD conditions, and $\%O_{2E}$ represents expired oxygen percentage. The value in parentheses (1.044 − 0.0499 × $\%O_{2E}$) represents the "Weir factor." The table displays Weir factors for different $\%O_{2E}$ values.

To use the table, locate the $\%O_{2E}$ and corresponding Weir factor. Compute energy expenditure in kcal · min^{-1} by multiplying the Weir factor by $\dot{V}_{E(STPD)}$.

EXAMPLE

A person runs on a treadmill and $\dot{V}_{E(STPD)} = 50$ L · min^{-1} and $\%O_{2E} = 16.0\%$. Compute energy expenditure by the de Weir method as follows:

$$\begin{aligned}
\text{kcal} \cdot \text{min}^{-1} &= \dot{V}_{E(STPD)} \times (1.044 - [0.0499 \times \%O_{2E}]) \\
&= 50 \times (1.044 - [0.0499 \times 16.0]) \\
&= 50 \times 0.2456 \\
&= 12.3
\end{aligned}$$

de Weir also derived the following equation to calculate kcal · min^{-1} from RQ and $\dot{V}O_2$ in L · min^{-1}:

$$\text{kcal} \cdot \text{min}^{-1} = ([1.1 \times RQ] + 3.9) \times \dot{V}O_2$$

Weir Factors

%O$_{2E}$	Weir Factor	%O$_{2E}$	Weir Factor
14.50	0.3205	17.00	0.1957
14.60	0.3155	17.10	0.1907
14.70	0.3105	17.20	0.1857
14.80	0.3055	17.30	0.1807
14.90	0.3005	17.40	0.1757
15.00	0.2955	17.50	0.1707
15.10	0.2905	17.60	0.1658
15.20	0.2855	17.70	0.1608
15.30	0.2805	17.80	0.1558
15.40	0.2755	17.90	0.1508
15.50	0.2705	18.00	0.1468
15.60	0.2656	18.10	0.1408
15.70	0.2606	18.20	0.1368
15.80	0.2556	18.30	0.1308
15.90	0.2506	18.40	0.1268
16.00	0.2456	18.50	0.1208
16.10	0.2406	18.60	0.1168
16.20	0.2366	18.70	0.1109
16.30	0.2306	18.80	0.1068
16.40	0.2256	18.90	0.1009
16.50	0.2206	19.00	0.0969
16.60	0.2157	19.10	0.0909
16.70	0.2107	19.20	0.0868
16.80	0.2057	19.30	0.0809
16.90	0.2007	19.40	0.0769

From Weir JB. New methods for calculating metabolic rates with special reference to protein metabolism. *J Physiol* 1949;109:1.
If %O$_{2E}$ does not appear in the table, compute individual Weir factors as 1.044 − 0.0499 × %O$_{2E}$.

Interestingly, if the thermal equivalent for a mixed diet (RQ = 0.82) had been used in the caloric transformation, or if RQ had been computed from total respiratory gas exchange and applied to Table 8.1 without considering the protein component, the estimated energy expenditure would be 19.3 kcal (4.825 kcal · L^{-1} × 4.0 L O$_2$; assuming a mixed diet). This corresponds to a difference of only 0.5% from the value obtained with the more elaborate and time-consuming method requiring urinary nitrogen analysis. *In most cases, the gross metabolic nonprotein RQ calculated from pulmonary gas exchange and applied to Table 8.1 without measures of urinary and other nitrogen sources introduces only minimal error because the contribution of protein to energy metabolism usually remains small.*

How Much Food Metabolizes for Energy?

The last two columns of Table 8.1 present conversions for the nonprotein RQ to grams of carbohydrate and fat metabolized per liter of oxygen consumed. For the subject with an RQ of 0.86, this represents approximately 0.62 g of carbohydrate

TABLE 8.1 Thermal Equivalents of Oxygen for the Nonprotein RQ, Including Percentage Kilocalories and Grams Derived from Carbohydrate and Fat

Nonprotein RQ	kcal Per LO_2	Percentage kcal Derived from		Grams per LO_2	
		Carbohydrate	Fat	Carbohydrate	Fat
0.707	4.686	0.0	100.0	0.000	0.496
0.71	4.690	1.1	98.9	0.012	0.491
0.72	4.702	4.8	95.2	0.051	0.476
0.73	4.714	8.4	91.6	0.090	0.460
0.74	4.727	12.0	88.0	0.130	0.444
0.75	4.739	15.6	84.4	0.170	0.428
0.76	4.750	19.2	80.8	0.211	0.412
0.77	4.764	22.8	77.2	0.250	0.396
0.78	4.776	26.3	73.7	0.290	0.380
0.79	4.788	29.9	70.1	0.330	0.363
0.80	4.801	33.4	66.6	0.371	0.347
0.81	4.813	36.9	63.1	0.413	0.330
0.82	4.825	40.3	59.7	0.454	0.313
0.83	4.838	43.8	56.2	0.496	0.297
0.84	4.850	47.2	52.8	0.537	0.280
0.85	4.862	50.7	49.3	0.579	0.263
0.86	4.875	54.1	45.9	0.621	0.247
0.87	4.887	57.5	42.5	0.663	0.230
0.88	4.899	60.8	39.2	0.705	0.213
0.89	4.911	64.2	35.8	0.749	0.195
0.90	4.924	67.5	32.5	0.791	0.178
0.91	4.936	70.8	29.2	0.834	0.160
0.92	4.948	74.1	25.9	0.877	0.143
0.93	4.961	77.4	22.6	0.921	0.125
0.94	4.973	80.7	19.3	0.964	0.108
0.95	4.985	84.0	16.0	1.008	0.090
0.96	4.998	87.2	12.8	1.052	0.072
0.97	5.010	90.4	9.6	1.097	0.054
0.98	5.022	93.6	6.4	1.142	0.036
0.99	5.035	96.8	3.2	1.186	0.018
1.00	5.047	100.0	0	1.231	0.000

From Zuntz N. Ueber die Bedeutung der verschiedenen Nâhrstoffe als Erzeuger der Muskelkraft. *Arch Gesamte Physiol* 1901;LXXXIII:557–571; *Pflugers Arch Physiol* 1901;83:557.

and 0.25 g of fat. For the 3.22 L of oxygen consumed during the 15-min rest period, this represents 2.0 g of carbohydrate (3.22 L O_2 × 0.62) and 0.80 g of fat (3.22 L O_2 × 0.25) metabolized for energy.

RQ for a Mixed Diet

The RQ seldom reflects the oxidation of pure carbohydrate or pure fat during activities ranging from complete bed rest to mild aerobic walking or slow jogging. Instead, catabolism of a mixture of these nutrients occurs with an RQ intermediate between 0.70 and 1.00. *For most purposes, assume an RQ of 0.82 (metabolism of a mixture of 40% carbohydrate and 60% fat) and apply the caloric equivalent of 4.825 kcal per liter of oxygen for energy transformations.* In using 4.825, the maximum error possible in estimating energy expenditure from steady-rate oxygen consumption averages about 4%. When requiring greater precision, compute the actual RQ and refer to Table 8.1 to obtain the exact caloric transformation and percentage contribution of carbohydrate and fat to the metabolic mixture.

INTEGRATIVE QUESTION

How have exercise physiologists determined that between 70 and 80% of the energy during the last phases of a marathon run comes from the combustion of fat?

RESPIRATORY EXCHANGE RATIO (RER)

The RQ assumes that the exchange of oxygen and carbon dioxide measured at the lungs reflects gas exchange from macronutrient catabolism in the cell. This assumption remains reasonable during rest and steady-rate conditions with little reliance on anaerobic metabolism. Several factors other than food combustion can spuriously alter the exchange of oxygen and carbon dioxide in the lungs. When this occurs, the ratio of gas exchange no longer reflects only the substrate mixture of energy metabolism. Respiratory physiologists refer to the ratio of carbon dioxide produced to oxygen consumed under such conditions as the **respiratory exchange ratio (RER)**. In this case, the pulmonary exchange of oxygen and carbon dioxide no longer reflects cellular oxidation of specific foods. One computes this exchange ratio in exactly the same manner as RQ.

For example, carbon dioxide elimination increases during hyperventilation because breathing increases to disproportionately higher levels compared with metabolic demands (see Chapter 14). Overbreathing decreases the blood's normal level of carbon dioxide because this nonmetabolic carbon dioxide "blows off" from the lungs in the expired air without a corresponding increase in oxygen consumption. This creates a rise in the respiratory exchange ratio (usually above 1.00) that does not reflect macronutrient oxidation.

Exhaustive activity presents another situation in which R rises above 1.00. Sodium bicarbonate in the blood buffers or neutralizes the lactate generated during anaerobic metabolism to maintain proper acid-base balance (see Chapter 14). Lactate buffering produces carbonic acid, a weaker acid as follows:

$$HLa + NaHCO_3 \rightarrow NaLa + H_2CO_3$$

In the pulmonary capillaries, carbonic acid degrades to its component carbon dioxide and water molecules. Carbon dioxide readily exits the lungs in the reaction:

$$H_2CO_3 \rightarrow H_2O + CO_2 \rightarrow Lungs$$

The RER increases above 1.00 because buffering adds "extra" nonmetabolic-created carbon dioxide to the expired air above the quantity normally released during energy metabolism. In rare instances, the exchange ratio exceeds 1.00 when a person gains body fat through excessive dietary carbohydrate intake. In this lipogenic situation, the conversion of carbohydrate to fat liberates oxygen as the excess calories accumulate in adipose tissue. The released oxygen then supplies energy metabolism; this reduces the lungs' uptake of atmospheric oxygen despite normal carbon dioxide production.

Relatively low RER values can also occur. Following exhaustive physical activity, the cells and bodily fluids retain carbon dioxide to replenish the sodium bicarbonate that buffered the accumulating lactate. This replenishment of alkaline reserve decreases the expired carbon dioxide level without affecting oxygen consumption and may cause a decrease in the respiratory exchange ratio to below 0.70.

Summary

1. Direct calorimetry and indirect calorimetry represent two methods to determine human energy expenditure.
2. Direct calorimetry measures heat production in an appropriately insulated calorimeter. Indirect calorimetry infers energy expenditure from oxygen consumption and carbon dioxide production, using either closed-circuit spirometry or open-circuit spirometry.
3. The doubly labeled water technique estimates energy expenditure in free-living conditions without the normal constraints imposed by laboratory procedures. It serves as a "gold standard" to validate other long-term energy expenditure estimates.
4. The complete oxidation of each macronutrient requires a different quantity of oxygen consumption for comparable carbon dioxide production. The ratio of carbon dioxide produced to oxygen consumed, the respiratory quotient (RQ), quantifies the macronutrient mixture catabolized for energy.
5. The RQ averages 1.00 for carbohydrate, 0.70 for fat, and 0.82 for protein.
6. For each RQ, a corresponding caloric value exists per liter of oxygen consumed. The RQ–kcal relationship can accurately determine energy expenditure during physical activity.
7. The respiratory exchange ratio (RER) reflects the pulmonary exchange of carbon dioxide and oxygen under differing physiologic and metabolic conditions; RER does not fully mirror the gas exchange of the macronutrient mixture catabolized.

thePoint References are available online at
http://thepoint.lww.com/mkk8e.

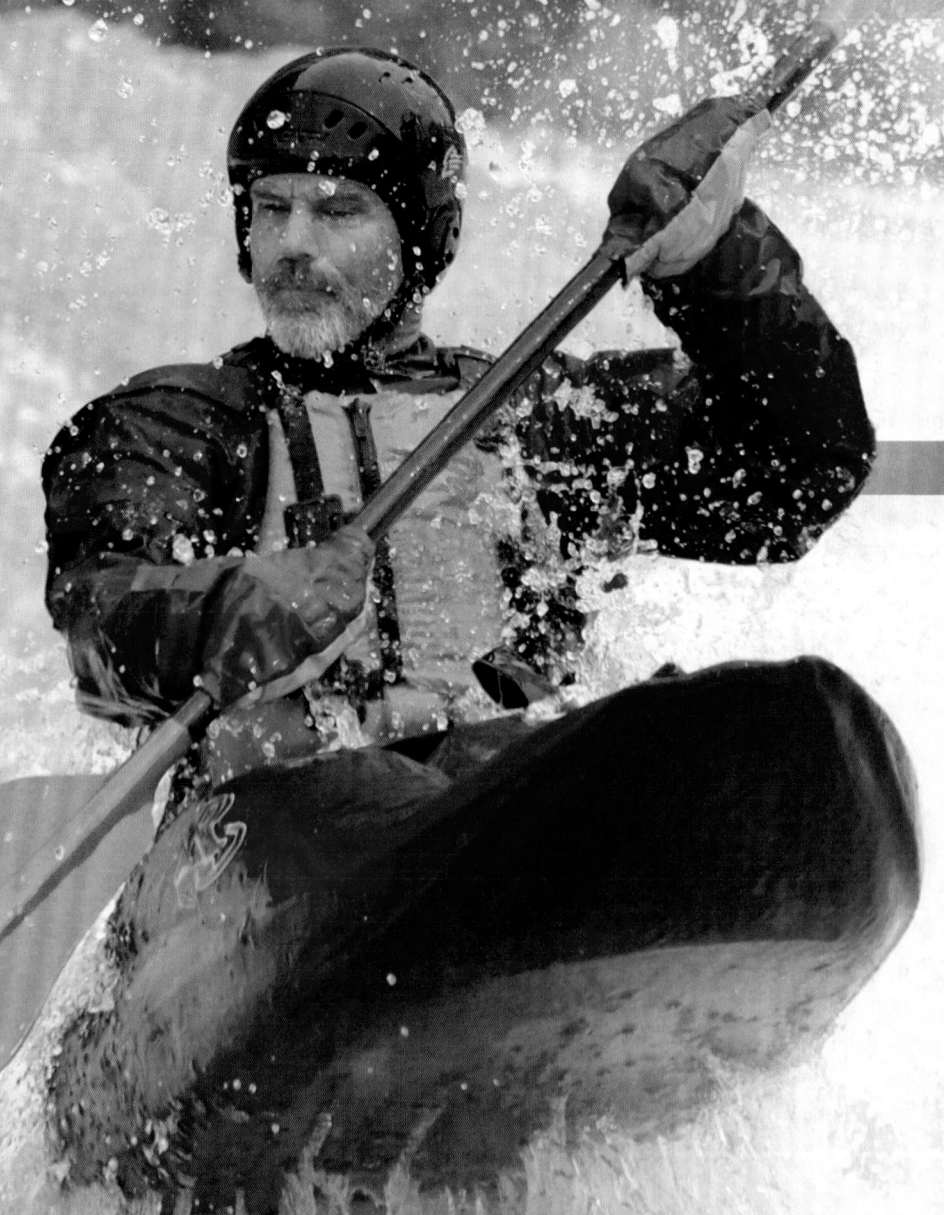

Human Energy Expenditure During Rest and Physical Activity

CHAPTER OBJECTIVES

- Define basal metabolic rate and list three factors that affect it

- Discuss three factors that affect total daily energy expenditure

- Outline two classification systems to rate the relative strenuousness of physical activity

- Explain the role of body weight in calculating the energy cost of diverse physical activities

- Present the rationale including advantages and limitations of heart rate to estimate energy expenditure of physical activities

ANCILLARIES ◉ at-a-Glance

Visit http://thepoint.lww.com/mkk8e to access the following resources.

- References: Chapter 9
- Interactive Question Bank
- Appendix F: Energy Expenditure in Household, Occupational, Recreational, and Sports Activities
- Focus on Research: Factors that Affect Recovery Oxygen Consumption

Metabolism involves all of the chemical reactions of the body's biomolecules that encompass synthesis or **anabolism** and breakdown or **catabolism**. FIGURE 9.1 illustrates the following three general factors that impact **total daily energy expenditure** (**TDEE**). Combined, these three components comprise the dietary energy requirements for nongrowing individuals.

1. Thermogenic effect of feeding
2. Thermic effect of physical activity
3. Resting metabolic rate

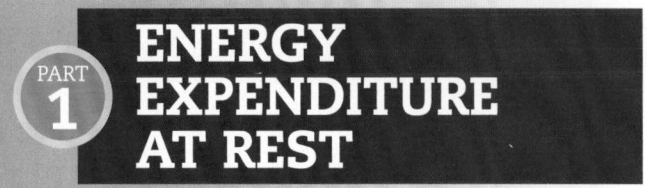

ENERGY EXPENDITURE AT REST

PART 1

BASAL AND RESTING METABOLIC RATE

Each individual requires a minimum level of energy to sustain vital functions in the waking state. This energy requirement—termed **basal metabolic rate** or simply **BMR** (also referred to as basal energy expenditure [BEE])—reflects the sum total of the body's many avenues for heat production. Measuring oxygen consumption under stringent laboratory conditions indirectly determines the BMR. For example, the person must remain in the postabsorptive (fasting) state without food consumed for the 12 to 18 previous hours to avoid increases in metabolism from digestion, absorption, and assimilation of ingested nutrients. To reduce other calorigenic influences, the person cannot perform any physical activity for a minimum of 2 hr prior to the assessment. In the laboratory, the person rests supine for about 30 min in a comfortable, thermoneutral environment before measuring oxygen consumption for a minimum of 10 min. Oxygen consumption values for BMR usually range between 160 and 290 mL·min⁻¹ (0.8 to 1.43 kcal·min⁻¹) depending on gender, age, overall body size (stature and body mass), and fat-free body mass (FFM).

Knowledge of BMR est-ablishes the energy baseline required to develop prudent weight control strategies through food restriction, regular physical activity, or their combination. Basal values measured under controlled laboratory conditions are only

slightly below values for **resting metabolic rate** (**RMR**) measured 3 to 4 hr after a light meal without prior physical activity. For this reason, the RMR often substitutes and is used interchangeably with BMR. Nevertheless, their differences need acknowledgment. For example, BMR is always slightly lower than RMR, depending on such factors as body size, amount of muscle mass, age, health/fitness status, hormonal status, and body temperature. When measured under standardized conditions, both BMR and RMR show high reproducibility and stability.[8]

Essentially, BMR and RMR refer to the sum of the metabolic processes of the active cell mass required to sustain normal regulatory balance and body functions during the basal or less stringent resting state. For the typical person, RMR accounts for about 60 to 75% of TDEE, whereas thermic effects from eating account for approximately 10%, and physical activity for the remaining 15 to 30%.

METABOLIC SIZE CONCEPT

Experiments in the late 1800s showed that resting energy expenditure varied in proportion to the body's surface area. A series of carefully conducted experiments determined energy metabolism of a dog and a man over a 24-hr period. The total heat generated by the larger man exceeded the energy metabolism of the dog by about 200%. Expressing heat production in relation to surface area reduced the metabolic difference between man and dog to only about 10%. This provided the basis for the common practice of expressing basal or resting metabolic rate (energy expenditure) by body surface area (in square meters) per hour (kcal·m⁻²·hr⁻¹). This expression acknowledges the fundamental relationship between heat production and body size that has become known as the "*surface area law.*"

Further research in the 1920s provided solid evidence that the surface area law did not apply universally to all temperature-regulating species or homeotherms. To more fully describe the relationship between metabolic heat production and body size, the concept of *metabolic size* related basal metabolism to body mass raised to the 0.75 power (body mass$^{0.75}$). BMR expressed relative to body mass$^{0.75}$ holds true for humans and a wide variety of mammals and birds that differ considerably in size and shape. FIGURE 9.2 illustrates the logarithmic plot of body mass (range: 0.01 to 10,000 kg) and metabolic rate expressed in watts (W), where 1 W = 0.01433 kcal·m⁻² (range: 0.1 to 1000 W). The best-fitting straight line

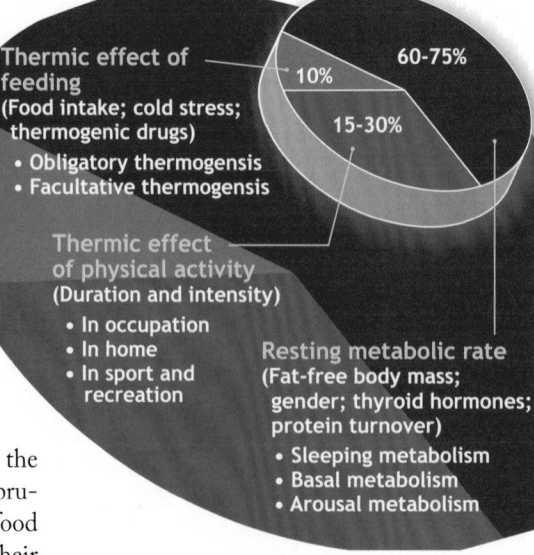

FIGURE 9.1 • Components of total daily energy expenditure (TDEE).

describing this relationship truly represents one of the more striking biologic concepts related to animal size and metabolic and physiologic functions. Such intrinsic relationships help evolutionary biologists understand physiologic function among different animal species, particularly thermoregulation in large mammals (referred to as *gigantothermy*), migration patterns, and an animal's ability to adapt to different ecosystems during their early biological development. Chapter 22 discusses the use of allometric scaling as a mathematical procedure to establish a scientifically defensible relationship between a body size variable (e.g., stature, body mass, FFM) and some other variable of interest such as muscular strength or aerobic capacity. This allometric "correction" permits statistically correct comparisons among individuals or groups that exhibit large differences in body size, and not simply a ratio determined by dividing one variable such as oxygen consumption by the another such as body mass.

Many subsequent studies have shown that indexing BMR or RMR to lean body mass (representing the non-adipose tissue component of the body) or the FFM (representing nonlipid mass) also accounts for gender differences in energy expenditure (see inset Fig. 9.3). For an individual or group of individuals of the same gender, body surface area provides as good an index of RMR as does FFM because of the strong within-gender association between body surface area and FFM.

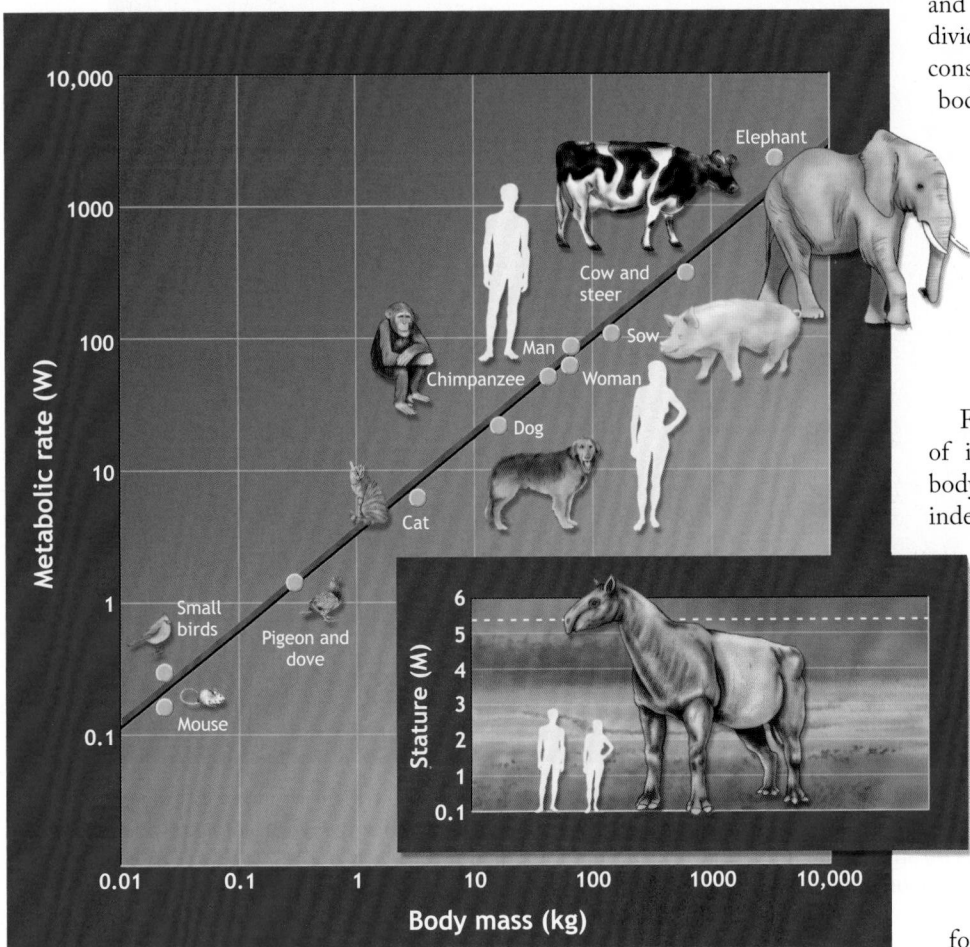

FIGURE 9.2 • Metabolic rate (in watts) from mouse to elephant. Logarithmic plot of body mass and metabolic rate for a variety of birds and mammals differing considerably in body size and shape. Numerous experiments have confirmed the "mouse-to-elephant curve" for metabolism using body mass to the 0.75 power, whereas metabolic rate relates to body surface area to the 0.67 power. The schematic inset figure compares the body size of the world's tallest male (2.89 m [9 ft 5¾ in]) and female (2.48 m [8 ft 1¾ in]) with the world's largest land mammal (*Baluchitherium*, predecessor of the rhinoceros), whose body mass approximated 30 tons at a stature of 5.26 m (17 ft 3 in). Comparisons between a microorganism (amoeba: mass, 0.1 mg) and a 100-ton blue whale (*Balaenoptera musculus*)—or the smallest Gabon dwarf shrew specimen, recently discovered in the Philippines, that weighed 1.4 g, one-tenth the size of a small mouse mammal or one-millionth the size of an elephant—illustrate the importance of appropriate scaling procedures when relating oxygen consumption, heart size, and blood volume to body mass.

METABOLIC RATES OF HUMANS: AGE AND GENDER COMPARISONS

FIGURE 9.3 presents BMR data for men and women over a wide range of age and body weight, expressed as $kcal \cdot m^{-2} \cdot hr^{-1}$. An individual's BMR or RMR estimated from the curves generally falls within ±10% of the value obtained during laboratory measurements. The inset figure illustrates the relatively strong association between FFM and daily RMR for men and women. Females exhibit an average 5 to 10% lower rate than males of the same age. This does not necessarily reflect true "gender differences" in metabolic rates of specific tissues. Rather, it results largely because women possess more body fat and less fat-free tissue than men of similar size (i.e., fat tissue has lower metabolic activity than muscle). Changes in body composition, either a decrease in FFM and/or increase in body fat during adulthood, help to explain the 2 to 3% per decade BMR reduction observed for adult men and women.[2,7,22] Some depression of the metabolic activity of lean tissue components also may progress with increasing age,[19] and contribute to an age-related increase in body fat.

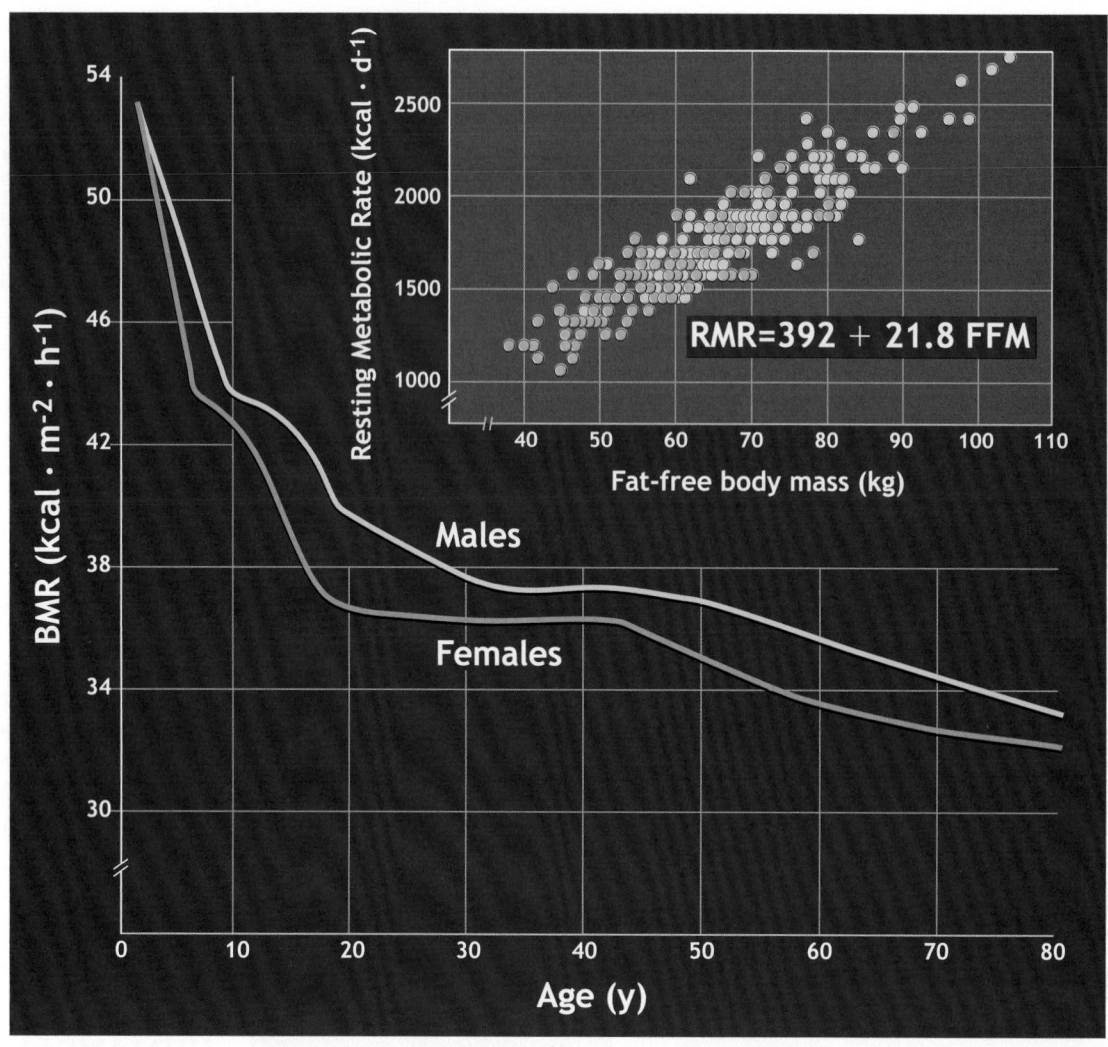

FIGURE 9.3 • Basal metabolic rate (BMR) as a function of age and gender. (Data from Altman PL, Dittmer D. *Metabolism*. Bethesda, MD: Federation of American Societies for Experimental Biology, 1968.) Inset graph shows the relatively strong relationship between fat-free body mass (FFM) and resting metabolic rate (RMR) for men and women. (Adapted with permission from Ravussin E, et al. Determination of 24-hour energy expenditure in man: Methods and results using a respiratory chamber. *J Clin Invest* 1986;78:1568.)

Effects of Regular Physical Activity

Similar BMR measures occur when comparing young and middle-aged endurance-trained men who showed no group difference for FFM.[16] Moreover, resting metabolism increased by 8% when 50- to 65-year-old men increased their FFM with resistance training.[23] An 8-week aerobic training program for older individuals produced a 10% increase in resting metabolism without a change in FFM.[20] This suggests that regular physical activity affects factors in addition to body composition to stimulate resting metabolism. *Regular endurance and resistance exercise offsets the decrease in resting metabolism that usually accompanies aging.* For athletes, an added bonus occurs in that maintaining FFM during weight reduction counters the potential negative effects of weight loss on exercise performance.

The curves in Figure 9.3 fairly accurately estimate a person's resting metabolic rate. For example, between ages 20 and 40

years, the BMR of men averages about 38 kcal per m² per hour, whereas for women the corresponding value equals 35 kcal per m² per hour. For greater precision, read the specific age-related value directly from the appropriate curve. To estimate total metabolic rate per hour, multiply the BMR value by the person's calculated surface area (see calculation method, next paragraph). This hourly total provides important information to estimate the daily energy baseline requirement for caloric intake.

Accurate measurement of the body's surface area poses a considerable challenge. Experiments in the early 1900s provided the data to formulate **FIGURE 9.4**. The studies clothed eight men and two women in tight whole-body underwear and applied melted paraffin and paper strips to prevent modification of the body surface. The treated cloth was then removed and cut into flat pieces to allow for precise measurements of body surface area (length × width). The close relationship between height (stature) and body weight (mass) and body surface area enabled derivation of

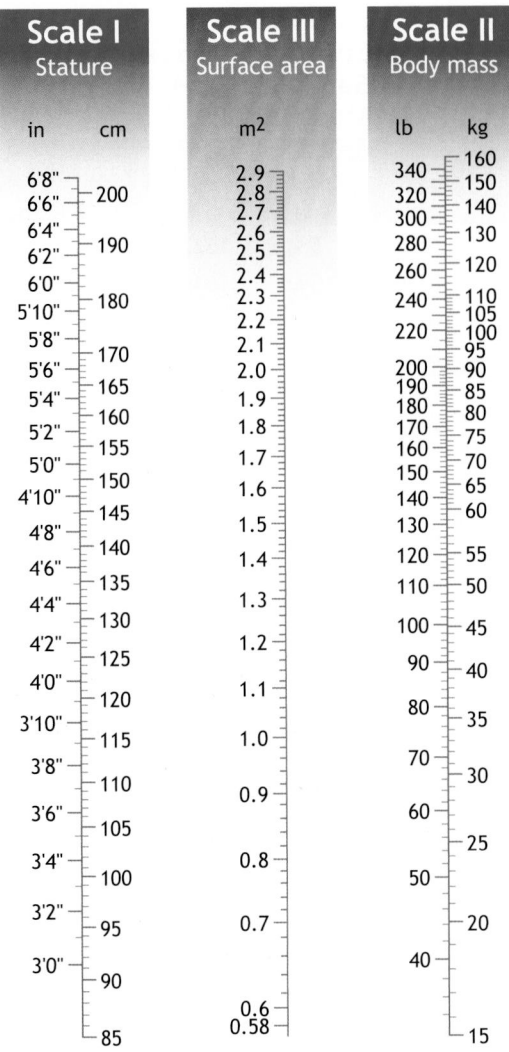

FIGURE 9.4 • Nomogram to estimate body surface area from stature and body mass. (From DuBois EF, *Basal Metabolism in Health and Disease*. Philadelphia: Lea & Febiger, 1936. Copyright 1920 by WM Boothby & RB Sandiford.)

the following empirical formula to predict body surface area (BSA):

$$BSA, m^2 = H^{0.725} \times W^{0.425} \times 71.84$$

where H = stature in cm and W = mass in kg. This formula yields results similar to the nomogram values in Figure 9.4.

To determine surface area from the nomogram, locate stature on scale I and body mass on scale II. Connect these two points with a straightedge; the intersection on scale III gives the surface area in square meters (m²). Repeat the procedure twice to verify the numbers. For example, if stature equals 185 cm and body mass equals 75 kg, surface area from scale III on the nomogram equals 1.98 m². Careful measurement should yield similar results.

"Normalcy" of BMR Values

Classical assessment of the normalcy of thyroid function compares a person's measured BMR with "standard metabolic rates" based on age and gender (TABLE 9.1 and Figure 9.3). Any value within ±10% of the standard represents a normal BMR. The following formula computes the deviation expressed as a percentage:

$$\Delta BMR = (\text{measured BMR} - \text{standard BMR}) \times 100$$
$$\div \text{ standard BMR}$$

For example, a BMR of 35 kcal·m²·hr⁻¹ for a 19-year-old male, determined by indirect calorimetry, falls 10.7% below the standard BMR.

$$\Delta BMR = (35 - 39.2) \times 100 \div 39.2$$
$$= -10.7\%$$

Estimating Resting Daily Energy Expenditure

To estimate a person's **resting daily energy expenditure** (RDEE), multiply the appropriate BMR value in Table 9.1 by the surface area computed from stature and mass. For a 50-year-old woman, for example, the estimated BMR equals 33.9 kcal per m² per hour. For a surface area of 1.40 m², the hourly energy expenditure equals 47.5 kcal per hour (33.9 kcal × 1.40 m²). On a daily basis, this amounts to a RDEE of 1140 kcal (47.5 kcal × 24).

TABLE 9.2 provides an estimate of RDEE from FFM estimated from several indirect procedures described in Chapter 28. The data in the table were computed from the following generalized equation, applicable to males and females over a wide range of body weights:

$$RDEE (kcal) = 370 + 21.6 (FFM, kg)$$

A male who weighs 90.9 kg at 21% body fat has an estimated FFM of 71.7 kg. Rounding to 72 kg translates to an RDEE of 1925 kcal or 8047 kJ (8.08 MJ).

Contribution of Diverse Tissues to Human Metabolism

TABLE 9.3 presents estimates of absolute and relative energy needs, expressed as oxygen consumption, of various organs and tissues of adults at rest. The brain and skeletal muscles consume about the same total quantity of oxygen even though the brain weighs only 1.6 kg (2.3% of body mass), while muscle constitutes almost 50% of the body mass. For children, brain metabolism represents nearly 50% of total resting energy expenditure. This similarity in metabolism does not transfer to maximal exercise because the energy generated by active muscle increases nearly 100 times; the total energy expended by the brain increases only marginally.

 INTEGRATIVE QUESTION

Discuss why middle-aged men and women should try to maintain or increase muscle mass for purposes of weight control.

TABLE 9.1	Standard Basal Metabolic Rates			
	kcal·m⁻²·hr⁻¹		kJ·m⁻²·hr⁻¹	
Age (y)	Men	Women	Men	Women
1	53.0	53.0	222	222
2	52.4	52.4	219	219
3	51.3	51.2	215	214
4	50.3	49.8	211	208
5	49.3	48.4	206	203
6	48.3	47.0	202	197
7	47.3	45.4	198	190
8	46.3	43.8	194	183
9	45.2	42.8	189	179
10	44.0	42.5	184	178
11	43.0	42.0	180	176
12	42.5	41.3	178	173
13	42.3	40.3	177	169
14	42.1	39.2	176	164
15	41.8	37.9	175	159
16	41.4	36.9	173	154
17	40.8	36.3	171	152
18	40.0	35.9	167	150
19	39.2	35.5	164	149
20	38.6	35.3	162	148
25	37.5	35.2	157	147
30	36.8	35.1	154	147
35	36.5	35.0	153	146
40	36.3	34.9	152	146
45	36.2	34.5	152	144
50	35.8	33.9	150	142
55	35.4	33.3	148	139
60	34.9	32.7	146	137
65	34.4	32.2	144	135
70	33.8	31.7	141	133
75 +	33.2	31.3	139	131

Adapted from Fleish A. Le metabolisme basal standard et sa determination aumoyen du "Metabocalculator." *Helv Med Acta* 1951;18:23.

TABLE 9.2	Estimation of Resting Daily Energy Expenditure (RDEE) Based on Fat-Free Body Mass (FFM)				
FFM (kg)	RDEE[a] (kcal)[b]	FFM (kg)	RDEE (kcal)	FFM (kg)	RDEE (kcal)
30	1018	58	1623	86	2228
31	1040	59	1644	87	2249
32	1061	60	1666	88	2271
33	1083	61	1688	89	2292
34	1104	62	1709	90	2314
35	1126	63	1731	91	2336
36	1148	64	1752	92	2357
37	1169	65	1774	93	2379
38	1191	66	1796	94	2400
39	1212	67	1817	95	2422
40	1234	68	1839	96	2444
41	1256	69	1860	97	2465
42	1277	70	1882	98	2487
43	1299	71	1904	99	2508
44	1320	72	1925	100	2530
45	1342	73	1947	101	2552
46	1364	74	1968	102	2573
47	1385	75	1990	103	2595
48	1407	76	2012	104	2616
49	1428	77	2033	105	2638
50	1450	78	2055	106	2660
51	1472	79	2076	107	2681
52	1493	80	2098	108	2703
53	1515	81	2120	109	2724
54	1536	82	2141	110	2746
55	1558	83	2163	111	2768
56	1580	84	2184	112	2789
57	1601	85	2206	113	2811

Data from Katch V. *Exercise Physiology Laboratory*. University of Michigan.
[a]Prediction equation for RDEE derived as the weighted mean constants from studies of large samples of males and females.
[b]To convert kcal to kJ, multiply by 4.18; to convert kcal to MJ, multiply by 0.0042.

FIVE FACTORS THAT AFFECT TOTAL DAILY ENERGY EXPENDITURE

Five important factors affect TDEE:

1. Physical activity
2. Diet-induced thermogenesis
3. Calorigenic effect of food on exercise metabolism
4. Climate
5. Pregnancy

Physical Activity

Under typical circumstances, physical activity accounts for between 15 and 30% of a person's TDEE. As we discuss and illustrate throughout this text, *physical activity exerts by far the most profound effect on human energy expenditure.* World-class athletes nearly double their TDEE with 3 or 4 hr of intense training. Most persons can sustain metabolic rates 10 times the resting value during continuous "big muscle" fast walking, running, uphill hiking, bicycling, and swimming.

IN A PRACTICAL SENSE

Estimating Resting Daily Energy Expenditure from Body Mass, Stature, and Age

Body mass, stature, and age contribute to individual differences in resting daily energy expenditure (RDEE), making it possible to accurately estimate RDEE using these variables. The method, validated in the early 1900s by Drs. Jay Arthur Harris and Francis G. Benedict (**http://www.ncbi.nlm.nih.gov/pmc/articles/PMC1091498/**), used closed-circuit spirometry to carefully measure oxygen uptake in individuals who varied widely in body size and age.

HARRIS-BENEDICT EQUATIONS FOR PREDICTING BMR

Women

RDEE, (kcal · 24 h^{-1}) = 655 + (9.6 × body mass, kg) + (1.85 × stature, cm) − (4.7 × age, y)

Men

RDEE, (kcal · 24 h^{-1}) = 66.0 + (13.7 × body mass, kg) + (5.0 × stature, cm) − (6.8 × age, y)

Example—Female

Data: Body mass = 62.7 kg; Stature = 172.5 cm; Age = 22.4 y

RDEE = 655 + (9.6 × body mass, kg) + (1.85 × stature, cm) − (4.7 × age, y)
RDEE = 655 + (9.6 × 62.7) + (1.85 × 172.5) − (4.7 × 22.4)
RDEE = 655 + 601.92 + 319.13 − 105.28
RDEE = 1471 kcal

Example—Male

Data: Body mass, 80 kg; Stature, 189.0 cm; Age, 30 y

RDEE = 66.0 + (13.7 × body mass, kg) + (5.0 × stature, cm) − (6.8 × age, y)
RDEE = 66.0 + (13.7 × 80, kg) + (5.0 × 189.0, cm) − (6.8 × 30.0, y)
RDEE = 66.0 + 1096 + 945 − 204
RDEE = 1903 kcal

Source: Harris JA, Benedict FG. *A Biometric Study of Basal Metabolism in Man.* Publ. No. 279. Washington, DC: Carnegie Institute, 1919.

Diet-Induced Thermogenesis

Food consumption generally increases energy metabolism. **Diet-induced thermogenesis** (**DIT**; sometimes referred to as **thermic effect of food** [**TEF**]) consists of two components. One component, **obligatory thermogenesis** (formerly called specific dynamic action [SDA]), results from energy required to digest, absorb, and assimilate food nutrients. The second component, **facultative thermogenesis**, relates to activation of the sympathetic nervous system and its stimulating influence on metabolic rate.

To our knowledge, the first experiment on DIT, performed by influential German nutritional physiologist Max Rubner (1854–1932; **http://www.mri.bund.de/en/de/max-rubner-institut/max-rubner.html**) in 1891, used indirect calorimetry. This classic research established the 24-hr energy expenditure of 742 kcal for a fasting dog.[13] Rubner then fed the dog 2 kg of meat that contained 1926 kcal. Food consumption increased the dog's daily energy expenditure to 1046 kcal. Rubner attributed the 41% increase of 304 kcal to the "chemical work of glands in metabolizing absorbed nutrients" or the "work of digestion." The increased metabolism represented 16% of the total energy ingested. Numerous subsequent experiments indicate that the meal's size and macronutrient composition, time elapsed since the previous meal, and nutritional and the subject's health status differentially affect the magnitude of DIT.

The thermic effect of food generally reaches maximum within 1 hr following a meal. Considerable variability exists among individuals; the magnitude of DIT usually varies between 10 and 30% of the ingested food energy, depending on the quantity and type of food consumed. A meal of pure protein, for example, elicits a thermic effect nearly 25% of the meal's total caloric value. This large thermic effect results largely from activation of digestive processes. It also includes extra energy required by the liver to assimilate and synthesize protein and/or to deaminate amino acids and convert them to glucose or triacylglycerols.

Overweight individuals often have a blunted thermic response to eating that contributes to excess body fat accumulation.[24,25] Interestingly, the magnitude of DIT also may be lower in endurance-trained individuals than in untrained

	Oxygen Consumption of Various Body Tissues at Rest for a 65-kg Man		
TABLE 9.3			
Organ	**Oxygen Consumption (mL · min^{-1})**		**Percentage of Resting Metabolism**
Liver	67		27
Brain	47		19
Heart	17		7
Kidneys	26		10
Skeletal muscle	45		18
Remainder	48		19
	250		100

IN A PRACTICAL SENSE

Predicting $\dot{V}O_{2max}$ During Pregnancy from Submaximum Exercise Heart Rate and Oxygen Consumption

Authorities recommend that a woman participate in regular physical activity during an uncomplicated pregnancy. Most agree that an individualized prescription should guide physical activity because of concern for fetal well-being. The prescription typically specifies intensity, duration, and frequency of activity. Intensity usually represents some percentage of the maximal oxygen consumption ($\%\dot{V}O_{2max}$) obtained from equations relating heart rate (HR) to $\%\dot{V}O_{2max}$. The direct determination of $\dot{V}O_{2max}$ requires that subjects perform near-exhaustive exercise, an unacceptable requirement for most pregnant women.

PREDICTING $\dot{V}O_{2MAX}$ FROM SUBMAXIMUM EXERCISE

Predicting $\dot{V}O_{2max}$ during pregnancy involves a three-stage, submaximum cycle ergometer testing. Oxygen consumption ($\dot{V}O_2$) and HR, measured toward the end of the final exercise stage, predict $\dot{V}O_{2max}$ via regression analyses.

SUBMAXIMUM CYCLE ERGOMETER TEST

Subject rests for 10 min and then performs a continuous three-stage, 6-min per stage, cycle ergometer test as follows:
Stage 1: 0 watts (W) (unloaded cycling)
Stage 2: 30 W (184 kg-m $\cdot$ min^{-1})
Stage 3: 60 W (367 kg-m $\cdot$ min^{-1})

PREDICTION EQUATIONS

Measure $\dot{V}O_2$ (L $\cdot$ min^{-1} and HR (b $\cdot$ min^{-1}) for each of the last 3 min of the final exercise stage. Use the average of the three HR values to predict $\%\dot{V}O_{2max}$ in the following equation:

$$\text{Predicted } \%\dot{V}O_{2max} = (0.634 \times HR\,[b \cdot min^{-1}]) - 30.79$$

Use the predicted $\dot{V}O_{2max}$ and the measured $\dot{V}O_2$ (L $\cdot$ min^{-1}) during the last exercise stage to predict $\dot{V}O_{2max}$ (L $\cdot$ min^{-1}) in the following equation:

$$\text{Predicted } \dot{V}O_{2max} = \dot{V}O_2 \div \text{predicted } \%\dot{V}O_{2max} \times 100$$

EXAMPLE

A woman 20 weeks' pregnant, weighing 70.4 kg, performs the three-stage cycle ergometer test. The average value for final-stage HR equals 155 b $\cdot$ min^{-1}; the average value for $\dot{V}O_2$ equals 1.80 L $\cdot$ min^{-1}.

$$
\begin{aligned}
\text{Predicted} &\,\%\dot{V}O_{2max} \\
&= (0.634 \times HR\,[b \cdot min^{-1}]) - 30.79 \\
&= (0.634 \times 155) - 30.79 \\
&= 67.5\%
\end{aligned}
$$

$$
\begin{aligned}
\text{Predicted} &\,\dot{V}O_{2max} \\
&= \dot{V}O_2 \div \text{predicted } \%\dot{V}O_{2max} \times 100 \\
&= 1.80 \div 67.5 \times 100 \\
&= 2.67\,L \cdot min^{-1}\,(2670\,mL \cdot min^{-1}) \\
&= 2670\,mL \cdot min^{-1} \div 70.4\,kg \\
&= 37.9\,mL \cdot kg^{-1} \cdot min^{-1}
\end{aligned}
$$

Source: Sady SP, et al. Prediction of $\dot{V}O_{2max}$ during cycle exercise in pregnant women. *J Appl Physiol* 1988;65:657.

---

counterparts.[11,21,27] Any "training effect" probably reflects a calorie-sparing adaptation to conserve energy and glycogen during periods of increased physical activity. Energy conservation in any form seems counterproductive to the potential of increased physical activity for weight control. For the physically active person, DIT represents only a small portion of TDEE compared with energy expenditure through regular physical activity.

Calorigenic Effect of Food on Exercise Metabolism

DIT has been compared in resting and exercising subjects after consuming meals of identical macronutrient composition and caloric content. In one study, six men performed moderate physical activity on a bicycle ergometer before breakfast on one day; then on separate days, they performed exercise for 30 min after a breakfast containing either 350,

1000, or 3000 kcal.[3] The results indicated that (1) breakfast increased resting metabolism by 10%, (2) variations in the caloric value of the meal exerted no influence on the thermic effect, and (3) performing physical activity following a meal of 1000 or 3000 kcal produced a larger energy expenditure than exercise without prior food. The calorigenic effect of food on energy metabolism during physical activity nearly doubled the food's thermic effect at rest. Apparently, physical activity augments DIT. This agrees with previous findings in which the thermic response to a 1000-kcal meal averaged 28% of the basal requirement at rest, yet increases to 56% of the basal requirement when subjects exercised following eating.[17] The DIT of carbohydrate and protein exceeded that for lipid. As with their response during rest, some obese men and women exhibit a depressed DIT when they exercise after eating. For most individuals, it seems reasonable to encourage moderate physical activity after a meal to potentially augment a diet-induced increase in caloric expenditure.

Climate

Environmental factors influence resting metabolic rate. The resting metabolism of people in a tropical climate averages 5 to 20% higher than for counterparts living in more temperate areas. Physical activity performed in hot weather also imposes a small additional metabolic load; it causes about 5% higher oxygen consumption compared to a thermoneutral environment, probably from the thermogenic effect of an elevated core temperature per se. This would include additional energy required for sweat gland activity and altered circulatory dynamics performing work in the heat.

Cold environments generally increase energy metabolism during rest and physical activity. The magnitude of the effect depends largely on the individual's body fat content and effectiveness of the clothing ensemble to retain heat. Metabolic rate increases up to fivefold at rest during extreme cold stress because shivering generates body heat to maintain a stable core temperature. Exercising in cold water serves as a good example of the effects of cold stress because of the difficulty in maintaining a stable core temperature in such a stressful thermal environment.[26]

Pregnancy

One area of interest concerns the degree that pregnancy affects the metabolic cost and physiologic strain imposed by physical activity.[4] One investigation studied 13 women from the sixth month of pregnancy to 6 weeks after the end of gestation.[9] Physiologic measures taken every 4 weeks included heart rate and oxygen consumption during bicycle and treadmill exercise. Heart rate and oxygen consumption during walking (weight-bearing exercise) increased progressively during the measurement period. Exercise heart rate and oxygen consumption remained unchanged during weight-supported bicycle riding at a constant intensity. The added energy cost to weight-bearing locomotion in walking, jogging, and stair climbing during pregnancy results *primarily* from the additional weight transported (and reduced economy of effort from encumbrance of fetal tissue) with a relatively small effect from the developing fetus per se. Chapter 21 more fully discusses the physiologic and metabolic impact of physical activity on both mother and fetus during pregnancy.

Summary

1. Total daily energy expenditure equals the sum of resting metabolism, thermogenic influences (e.g., thermic effect of food), and the energy generated in physical activity.
2. The BMR represents the minimum energy required to maintain vital functions in the waking state measured under controlled laboratory conditions. The BMR averages only slightly lower than the resting metabolic rate (RMR) and relates closely to body surface area (BSA).
3. RMR, as does BMR, decreases with age from variations in fat-free body mass (FFM). The RMR for men generally exceeds values for women of similar body size. One can accurately predict RMR from FFM in men and women who vary considerably in body size.
4. Different organs expend different amounts of energy during rest and physical activity. At rest, muscles generate about 20% of the body's total energy expenditure. During all-out effort, the energy expended by skeletal muscles can increase more than 100 times above its resting value to account for nearly 85% of the total energy expenditure.
5. Five major factors affect a person's metabolic rate: physical activity, diet-induced thermogenesis, calorigenic effect of food on exercise metabolism, climate, and pregnancy, with physical activity exerting the greatest effect.

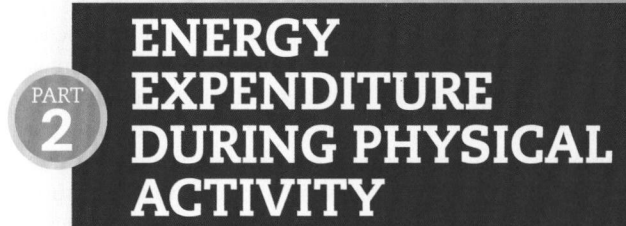

CLASSIFICATION OF PHYSICAL ACTIVITIES BY ENERGY EXPENDITURE

Most individuals have performed some type of physical work they would classify as "exceedingly difficult." This might include walking up a long flight of stairs, shoveling snow for 60 min, running a long block to catch a bus, digging a deep trench, skiing or snowshoeing through a blizzard, or hiking up steep terrain. *Intensity and duration represent two important factors that impact the relative strenuousness of a particular physical task.* It requires about the same net number of calories to complete a 26.2-mile marathon at various running speeds. One person might expend a considerable rate of energy expenditure running at maximum steady-rate pace (e.g., 80% $\dot{V}O_{2max}$) and complete the distance in a little more than 2 hr. Another runner of equal fitness might select a slower, more comfortable pace (e.g., 55% $\dot{V}O_{2max}$) and complete the run in 3 hr. In this example, the intensity of effort distinguishes the physical demands of the task. In another example, two persons of equal fitness may run at the same speed, but one person runs for twice as long as the other. In this case, exercise duration becomes the important consideration in classifying the strenuousness of the physical effort.

Several classification systems rate sustained physical activity for "strenuousness." One system recommends classification of work by the ratio of energy required for the task to the resting energy requirement.[1] This system uses the **physical activity ratio (PAR)**. **Light work** for men elicits an oxygen consumption (energy expenditure) up to three times the resting requirement. **Heavy work** encompasses physical activity requiring six to eight times resting metabolism, whereas **maximal work** includes any task that requires metabolism to increase nine times or more above rest. As a frame of reference, most industrial jobs and household tasks require less than three times resting energy expenditure. These work classifications rated in multiples of resting metabolism average slightly lower for women because of their generally lower aerobic capacity. Work classification based on the PAR model rates the strenuousness of occupational tasks at a somewhat lower level than typical classifications for general exercise. This occurs because occupational and industrial work usually extends for much longer durations than exercise training, often requiring the use of a smaller muscle mass performed under varying and stressful environmental conditions and physical constraints.

THE MET

TABLE **9.4** presents a five-level classification system based on the energy or kcal required by untrained men and women who perform different physical activities including a broad range of occupational tasks.[6] Fortuitously, a 5-kcal energy output equals approximately 1 L of oxygen consumed, thus enabling transposition of these calorie values into liters of oxygen consumed per minute ($L \cdot min^{-1}$) or milliliters of oxygen per kilogram of body mass per minute ($mL \cdot kg^{-1} \cdot min^{-1}$) or **METs**, the latter *defined as multiples of the resting metabolic rate.* One MET equals a resting oxygen consumption of about $250 \ mL \cdot min^{-1}$ for an average-sized man and $200 \ mL \cdot min^{-1}$ for an average-sized woman. Physical activity performed at 2 METs requires twice the resting metabolism, about $500 \ mL \cdot min^{-1}$ for a man, 3 METs equals three times rest, and so on. For a different but usually more accurate classification that considers variations in body size, one should express the MET as oxygen consumption per unit body mass: *1 MET equals $3.5 \ mL \cdot kg^{-1} \cdot min^{-1}$; 2 METs equals $7.0 \cdot mL \cdot kg^{-1} \cdot min^{-1}$, and so on.*

TABLE **9.5** presents a classification system for characterizing the intensity of leisure-time physical activity in absolute (METs) and relative (%$\dot{V}O_{2max}$) intensity by age categories. To account for the general aging effect on aerobic capacity, the categories for activity intensity in METs adjust lower as age increases.

DAILY RATES OF AVERAGE ENERGY EXPENDITURE

TABLE **9.6** presents averages for stature and body mass and daily energy expenditure for males and females living in the United States. The average man age 19 to 50 years expends 2900 kcal daily, whereas the female expends 2200 kcal. These individuals spend nearly 75% of the day in activities that require only light energy expenditure (e.g., sleeping/lying down, 8 hr; sitting, 6 hr; standing, 6 hr; walking, 2 hr; recreational activity, 2 hr). For most individuals, energy expenditure rarely rises substantially above the resting level, with walking the most common physical activity. The term *homo sedentarius* all too appropriately describes most of the world's population! This descriptor is compelling, as physical inactivity in highly mechanized societies has become a pandemic despite the admonitions of scientists, educators, and governmental agencies. The Centers for Disease Control and Prevention (**www.cdc.gov**) estimates that physical inactivity and poor eating habits in the United States account for about 300,000 deaths yearly, and probably more in 2013–2014. Such estimates are currently unavailable for other industrialized countries worldwide.

TABLE 9.4	Five-Level Classification of Physical Activity Based on Energy Expenditure			
	Energy Expenditure[a]			
Level	**kcal · min⁻¹**	**L · min⁻¹**	**mL · kg⁻¹ · min⁻¹**	**METs**
Men				
Light	2.0–4.9	0.40–0.99	6.1–15.2	1.6–3.9
Moderate	5.0–7.4	1.00–1.49	15.3–22.9	4.0–5.9
Heavy	7.5–9.9	1.50–1.99	23.0–30.6	6.0–7.9
Very heavy	10.0–12.4	2.00–2.49	30.7–38.3	8.0–9.9
Unduly heavy	≥12.5	≥2.50	≥38.4	≥10.0
Women				
Light	1.5–3.4	0.30–0.69	5.4–12.5	1.2–2.7
Moderate	3.5–5.4	0.70–1.09	12.6–19.8	2.8–4.3
Heavy	5.5–7.4	1.10–1.49	19.9–27.1	4.4–5.9
Very heavy	7.5–9.4	1.50–1.89	27.2–34.4	6.0–7.5
Unduly heavy	≥9.5	≥1.90	≥34.5	≥7.6

[a] $L \cdot min^{-1}$ based on 5 kcal per liter of oxygen; $mL \cdot kg^{-1} \cdot min^{-1}$ based on 65-kg man and 55-kg woman; one MET equals the average resting oxygen consumption ($250 \ mL \cdot min^{-1}$ for men, $200 \ mL \cdot min^{-1}$ for women).

| TABLE 9.5 | **Characterization of the Intensity of Leisure-Time Physical Activity Related to Age** |

		Absolute Intensity (METs)			
Categorization	Relative Intensity (%$\dot{V}O_{2max}$)	Young	Middle-Aged	Old	Very Old
Rest	<10	1.0	1.0	1.0	1.0
Light	<35	<4.5	<3.5	<2.5	<1.5
Fairly light	<50	<6.5	<5.0	<3.5	<2.0
Moderate	<70	<9.0	<7.0	<5.0	<2.8
Heavy	<70	>9.0	>7.0	>5.0	>2.8
Maximal	100	13.0	10.0	7.0	4.0

Adapted with permission from Bouchard C, et al. *Exercise, Fitness, and Health: A Consensus of Current Knowledge*. Champaign, IL: Human Kinetics, 1990.

| TABLE 9.6 | **Reference Heights, Weights, and Energy Expenditures of Children and Adults Living in the United States** |

		Height, Weight, and Body Mass Index		
Gender	Age	Median Body Mass Index[a]	Reference Height (cm [in])	Reference Weight[b] (kg [lb])
Male, female	2–6 mo	—	64 (25)	7 (16)
	7–11 mo	—	72 (28)	9 (20)
	1–3 y	—	91 (36)	13 (29)
	4–8 y	15.8	118 (46)	22 (48)
Male	9–13 y	18.5	147 (58)	40 (88)
	14–18 y	21.3	174 (68)	64 (142)
	19–30 y	24.4	176 (69)	76 (166)
Female	9–13 y	18.3	148 (58)	40 (88)
	14–18 y	21.3	163 (64)	57 (125)
	19–30 y	22.8	163 (64)	61 (133)

[a]In kg per m^2.
[b]Calculated from median body mass index and median heights for ages 4 to 8 years and older.
Adapted from *Dietary Reference Intakes: A Risk Assessment Model for Establishing Upper Intake Levels for Nutrients*. Food and Nutrition Board, Institute of Medicine. Washington, DC: National Academy Press, 1998.

Gender, Age, and Energy Expenditure		
	Age (y)	Energy Expenditure (kcal)
Males	15–18	3000
	19–24	2900
	25–50	2900
	51 +	2300
Females	15–18	2200
	19–24	2200
	25–50	2200
	50+	1900

Data from Food and Nutrition Board, National Research Council. *Recommended Dietary Allowances, Revised*. Washington, DC: National Academy of Sciences, 1989.

ENERGY COST OF HOUSEHOLD, INDUSTRIAL, AND RECREATIONAL ACTIVITIES

Appendix F lists examples of energy expenditures expressed by body mass (kcal·kg⁻¹) for common household activities, selected industrial tasks, and popular recreational and sports activities. These data highlight the large variation in energy expenditure for such diverse physical activities as lawn bowling and kite flying. The caloric values also represent averages, with values for an individual varying considerably depending on skill, pace, and fitness level.

thePoint | Appendix F, available online at http://thepoint. lww.com/mkk8e, provides examples of energy expenditure in household, occupational, recreational, and sports activities.

The values listed in the column for body mass represent the activity's caloric expenditure for 1 min. This equals the gross energy value (see Chapter 10) because it includes the energy expenditure of rest for a 1-min interval. To estimate the total expenditure of performing an activity, multiply the caloric value in the table by the number of minutes of participation. For example, if a 70-kg man spends 30 min vacuuming (carpet sweeping), his total energy expenditure for this household task equals 102 kcal (3.4 kcal × 30 min). The same individual expends approximately 690 kcal during a 50-min judo workout, but only 90 kcal while sitting quietly watching television for 2 hr. Golf (without a cart) requires about 6.0 kcal each minute, or 360 kcal·hr⁻¹. The same person expends almost twice this energy, or 708 kcal·hr⁻¹, while swimming backstroke. Viewed somewhat differently, 25 min of swimming backstroke requires about the same number of calories as playing golf for 1 hr. Increasing the pace of either the swim or the golf game proportionally increases the energy expenditure.

Influence of Body Mass

Increases in body mass raise the energy expended in many physical activities (see Appendix F), particularly in **weight-bearing physical activity** like walking and running. FIGURE 9.5 clearly illustrates that the energy cost of walking increases proportionately with body mass (i.e., a larger body mass requires greater energy expenditure). For persons with the same body mass, there are little practical variations in oxygen consumption; thus, body mass accurately predicts the energy expended during walking.

The influence of body mass on energy metabolism during weight-bearing activity occurs whether the person gains weight naturally as body fat or FFM, or as a short-term added load from sports equipment or a weighted vest worn on the torso.[5,28] With **weight-supported physical activity** (e.g., stationary cycling or elliptical exercise), the influence of body mass on energy cost decreases considerably. It averages only about 5% higher in stationary cycling among heavy people

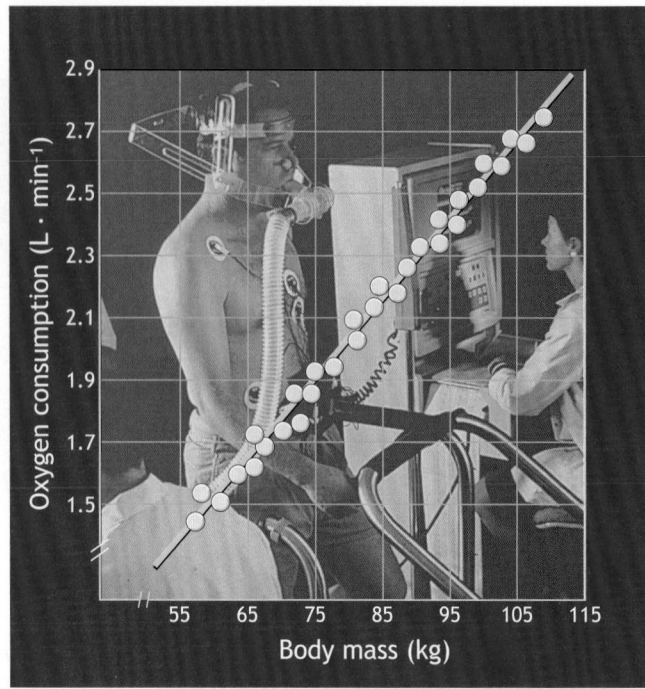

FIGURE 9.5 • Relationship between body mass and oxygen consumption measured during submaximal, brisk treadmill walking. (Adapted with permission from Laboratory of Applied Physiology, Queens College, NY.)

because of extra energy required to lift the heavier lower limbs.[10,12] This body weight effect during stationary cycling slightly lowers energy cost values for women compared with men. For overweight persons desiring to use physical activity for weight loss, this activity form generates a considerable caloric expenditure compared to weight-supported activity simply from the added cost of transporting a heavier body weight.

Appendix F also shows that the energy cost for cross-country running ranges between 8.2 kcal per minute for a 50-kg person and almost twice as much at 16.0 kcal for a person who weighs 98 kg. Expressing the energy requirement by body mass as kcal·kg⁻¹·min⁻¹ attempts to eliminate this variation. In this case, energy cost averages about 0.164 kcal·kg⁻¹·min⁻¹. Expressing energy cost per kilogram of body mass reduces differences between individuals regardless of age, race, gender, and body mass. Nevertheless, a heavier person still expends more *total* calories than a lighter person for an equivalent exercise period because the activity mainly requires the transport of body mass—and this requires proportionately more energy.

HEART RATE TO ESTIMATE ENERGY EXPENDITURE

For each person, heart rate and oxygen consumption relate linearly over a large range of exercise intensities to about 80% of maximum. From this intrinsic relationship, the heart rate provides an estimate of oxygen consumption and thus energy

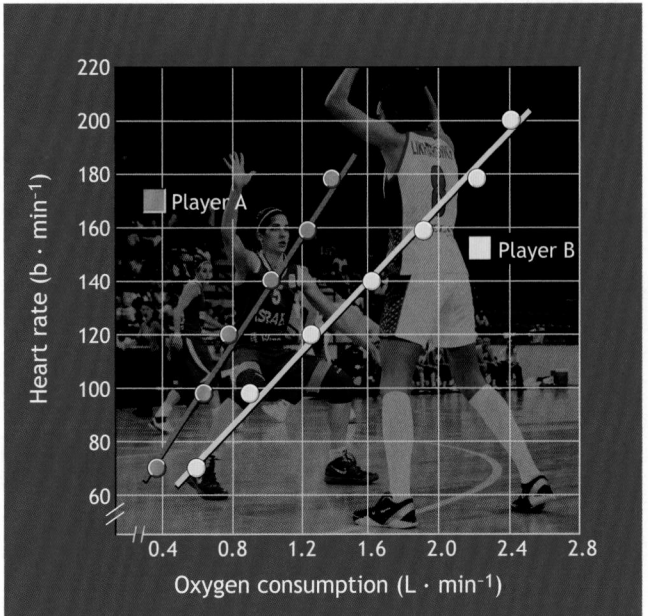

FIGURE 9.6 • Linear relationship between heart rate and oxygen consumption for two women collegiate basketball players of different aerobic fitness levels. Measurements made during a graded exercise test on a motor-driven treadmill. (Adapted with permission from Laboratory of Applied Physiology, Queens College, NY.)

expenditure during aerobic activity. This approach has proved useful when the oxygen consumption could not be measured during the desired activity.

FIGURE 9.6 presents data for two members of a women's basketball team during a laboratory treadmill running test. For each woman, heart rate increased linearly with oxygen consumption—a proportionate increase in heart rate (HR) accompanied each increase in oxygen consumption ($\dot{V}O_2$). Both HR–$\dot{V}O_2$ lines display linearity, but the same heart rate does not correspond to the same oxygen consumption for both women because the slopes or rate of change of the lines differ. Heart rate for subject B increases less than that for subject A for a given increase in oxygen consumption. Chapters 11, 17, and 21 discuss the significance of the difference in heart rate increase with physical activity and its relation to cardiovascular fitness. For the current discussion, exercise heart rate estimates exercise oxygen consumption with reasonable accuracy. For player A, a heart rate of 140 b·min⁻¹ corresponds to an oxygen consumption of 1.08 L·min⁻¹, whereas the same heart rate for player B corresponds to a 1.60 L·min⁻¹ oxygen consumption. Heart rates obtained by radiotelemetry during basketball competition were then applied to each player's HR–$\dot{V}O_2$ line to estimate energy expenditure under game conditions.[15]

Heart rate to estimate energy expenditure appears practical but has limited research applications because it has been validated for only a few general, large muscle activities. One major problem concerns the degree of similarity between the laboratory test to establish the HR–$\dot{V}O_2$ line and specific activities to which it applies. For example, factors other than oxygen consumption influence exercise heart rate response. These include environmental temperature, emotions, previous food intake, body position, muscle groups exercised, continuous or discontinuous (stop-and-go) activity, or whether muscles act statically or more dynamically. In aerobic dance, for example, heart rates while dancing at a specific oxygen consumption exceed heart rates at the same oxygen consumption during treadmill walking or running.[18] Consistently higher heart rates occur in upper-body physical activity; they also are higher when muscles act statically in straining-type movements than in dynamic movements at any submaximal oxygen consumption. Applying heart rate during upper-body or static-type activity to a HR–$\dot{V}O_2$ line developed during running or cycling overpredicts the measured oxygen consumption.[14]

INTEGRATIVE QUESTION

A high-tech computer company asks you to validate a wrist-mounted device to measure energy expenditure. The person exhales one breath onto the top of the instrument while moving. The device's electronic components and microprocessor analyze expired air to compute oxygen consumption and energy expenditure. Outline the steps to establish the instrument's validity.

Summary

1. Different classification systems rate the strenuousness of physical activities. These include ratings based on three factors: ratio of the energy cost of the task to the resting energy requirement, oxygen requirement in mL·kg⁻¹·min⁻¹, or multiples of resting metabolism as METs.
2. Total daily energy expenditure averages 2900 kcal for men and 2200 kcal for women ages 19 to 50 years.
3. Considerable variability among individuals exists for daily energy expenditure, with the largest variation determined by the intensity level of the physical activity.
4. Daily energy expenditure provides a framework to classify different occupations. Within any classification, energy expended during leisure-time recreational pursuits contributes considerable additional variability.
5. Heavier individuals expend more total energy in physical activity than lighter counterparts, particularly in weight-bearing walking, climbing, and running activities.
6. Heart rate offers only limited practical benefit to predict oxygen consumption and caloric expenditure for most physical activities.

thePoint References are available online at
http://thepoint.lww.com/mkk8e.

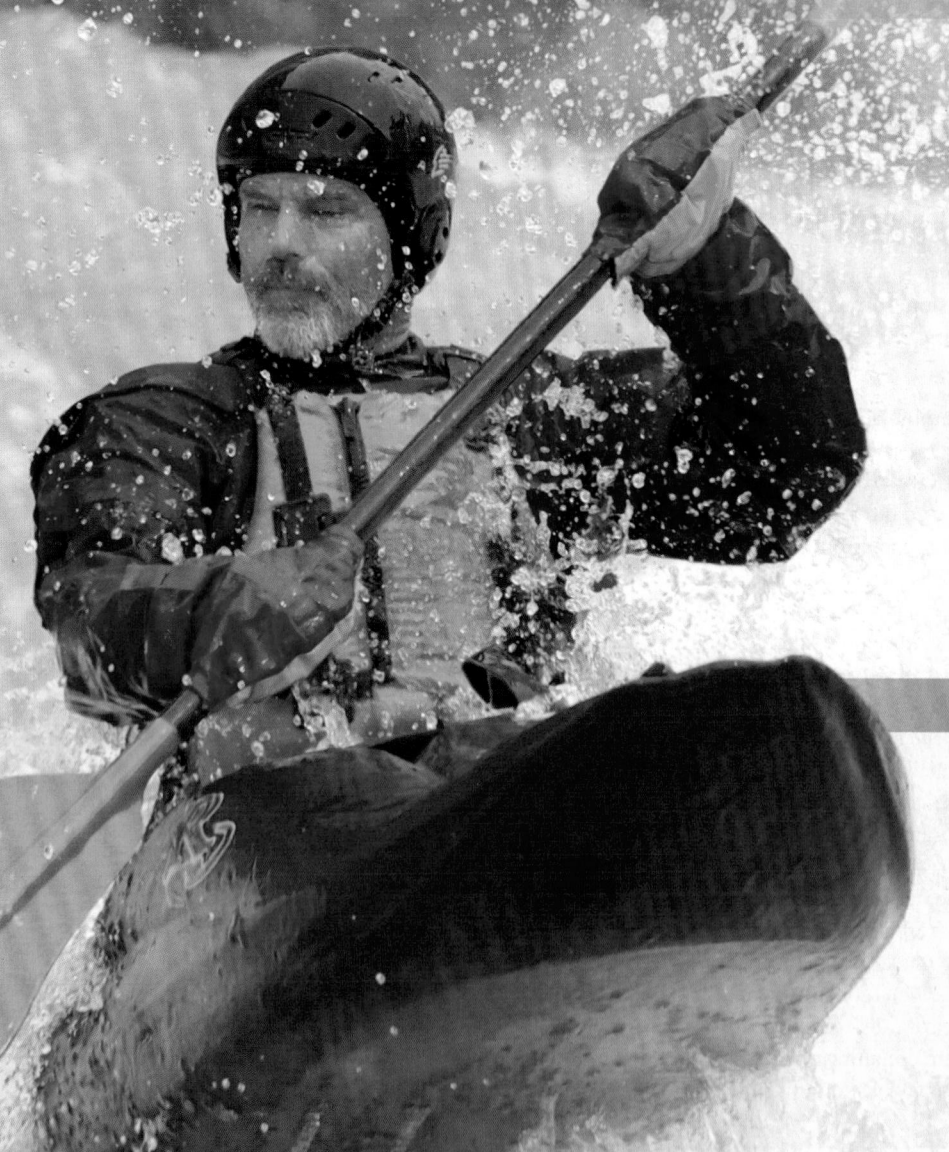

CHAPTER

10

Energy Expenditure During Walking, Jogging, Running, and Swimming

The following sections explore energy expenditure data for the popular activities of walking, running, and swimming. These modes of physical activity take on special significance for their important roles in weight control, physical conditioning, and health maintenance and rehabilitation.

GROSS VERSUS NET ENERGY EXPENDITURE

The following example illustrates the use of oxygen consumption to estimate energy expenditure during swimming. A 25-year-old man swimming for 40 min at a moderate, steady pace consumes oxygen at a rate of 2.0 L per minute for a total 80 L of oxygen consumed. To compute energy expenditure in kcal·min^{-1} from oxygen consumption, use the calorific transformation of 5.0 kcal per liter of oxygen consumed, assuming carbohydrate as the sole energy fuel (see Chapter 8). In this example, the swimmer expends about 400 kcal (80 L O$_2$ × 5 kcal) during the swim. This computation does not assess energy expenditure of the swim per se because the 400 kcal, called **gross energy expenditure**, also includes energy that would have been expended if the person only rested for 40 min. To obtain the **net energy expenditure** of *only* the 40-min swim, subtract resting metabolism from the gross energy expenditure of the activity.

Net energy expenditure = Gross energy expenditure
− Resting metabolism for the
equivalent time

Knowing the swimmer's body mass and stature (assume 65 kg; 1.74 cm) permits computation of his surface area of 1.78 m^2 from the nomogram in Figure 9.4 in Chapter 9. Multiplying this value by the average basal metabolic rate (BMR) for young men, 38 kcal·m^{-2}·hr^{-1} (Fig. 9.3 in Chapter 9), results in an estimated resting energy expenditure of 67.6 kcal per hour (1.78 m^2 × 38 kcal), equivalent to about 45 kcal for the 40-min swim. The net energy expended for the swim computes as gross energy expenditure (400 kcal) minus the 40-min resting value (45 kcal), for an estimated net energy expenditure of 355 kcal for swimming.

Figure 7.2 in Chapter 7 showed that oxygen consumption during constant-load light-to-moderate exercise increased rapidly during the first several minutes, then leveled off or achieved a steady-rate value and remained stable thereafter. Only one or two oxygen consumption measures under these conditions are required to estimate total energy expenditure. In contrast, tennis, soccer, lacrosse, field hockey, basketball, and other stop-and-go, moderately vigorous activities require more frequent oxygen consumption values to accurately estimate total energy expenditure. Strenuous physical activity, when energy requirements considerably exceed aerobic energy transfer, derives considerable energy anaerobically with accompanying blood lactate accumulation. These confounding factors preclude accurately estimating energy expenditure.

ECONOMY OF HUMAN MOVEMENT

Human **efficiency** of movement, often referred to as **mechanical efficiency**, considers the ratio between energy expenditure of movement (calculated from the rate of external work performed times the duration of the movement) and that fraction of energy expenditure that appears as external work, often called *energy output*. Efficiency of human movement equals the calculated amount of energy required to perform a particular task relative to the actual energy requirement of the work accomplished. **Movement economy**, in contrast, refers to the energy required, usually inferred from measurement of oxygen consumption, to maintain a constant movement velocity.

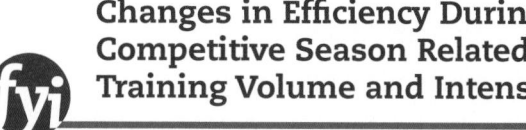

Changes in Efficiency During a Competitive Season Related to Training Volume and Intensity

Cyclists who spend the most time training at or above their lactate threshold (LT) increase gross efficiency cycling compared to preseason and post-season. The increase in gross efficiency averages a modest 1%, yet this can make a difference in winning or losing, and posting a rider's best times.

Source: Hopker J, et al. Changes in cycling efficiency during a competitive season. *Med Sci Sports Exer* 2009;41:912.

Economy of Movement

Assessing movement economy involves measuring the oxygen consumed during steady-rate exercise at a constant power output or velocity. During steady-rate exercise, oxygen consumption closely mirrors energy expenditure. At submaximal running, cycling, or swimming, an individual with greater movement economy consumes *less* oxygen (lower steady-rate $\dot{V}O_2$). African women who balance heavy loads on their heads have mastered a subtle adjustment in walking technique that allows them to carry up to 20% of their body weight with no increase in energy expenditure. Stated somewhat differently, they exhibit greater movement economy. Europeans, in contrast, exerted proportionately more effort (increased oxygen consumption and decreased movement economy) from the added weight on their heads.

Economy of movement takes on added importance during longer-duration activity where success largely depends on the individual's aerobic capacity and ability to maintain the lowest oxygen consumption at any given work rate. From age 21 to 28 years, six-time Grand Champion of the Tour de France Lance Armstrong improved 8% in movement economy, which translated to increased power production when cycling at a given oxygen uptake. The researchers speculated this occurred from changes in muscle myosin type stimulated from years of training intensely for 3 to 6 hr on most days.[20,21] Despite this remarkable change in power production and hypothesized change in muscle myosin type, one must wonder to what extent this athlete's confession in 2013 of using performance-enhancing drugs contributed to his success in the races and associated changes in the metabolic profile.

For children and adults, any training adjustment that improves economy of effort and reduces oxygen uptake usually improves performance.[23,40] **FIGURE 10.1** displays the strong association between running economy and endurance performance in elite athletes of comparable aerobic fitness. Clearly, athletes with greater running economies (i.e., lower oxygen consumption at a predetermined speed) achieve faster race times. Variations in running economy among this homogeneous group explained approximately 64% of the total variation in 10-km running performance.

Running Economy Improves With Age

Running economy improves steadily from ages 10 to 18 years. This partly explains the relatively poor performance of young children in distance running and their progressive improvements throughout adolescence. Improved endurance occurs even though aerobic capacity relative to body mass ($mL\ O_2 \cdot kg^{-1} \cdot min^{-1}$) remains constant during this time.

Even among trained runners, notable variation in economy emerges at submaximal running speeds.[58,61,79] In general, long-term programs of run training improve running economy, due partly to training-induced reductions in pulmonary ventilation during submaximal running.[13,32,84] It remains unclear whether the first 6 weeks of run training affect running mechanics or economy despite improvements in performance and physiologic function.[32,46] Short-term training emphasizing "proper" running technique that includes better sequencing of arm movements and body alignment does not enhance running economy.[42] In contrast, distance runners with an uneconomical stride-length pattern benefit from a short-term audiovisual feedback program that focuses on optimizing stride length,[60] including biofeedback and relaxation psychophysiologic interventions.[13] An 8-week program of heavy resistance training emphasizing half squats improved running economy in well-trained male and female distance runners.[83]

No single biomechanical factor accounts for individual differences in running economy, although muscle structural and compositional factors probably play a role.[45] Indirect evidence from studies of cyclists indicates that muscle

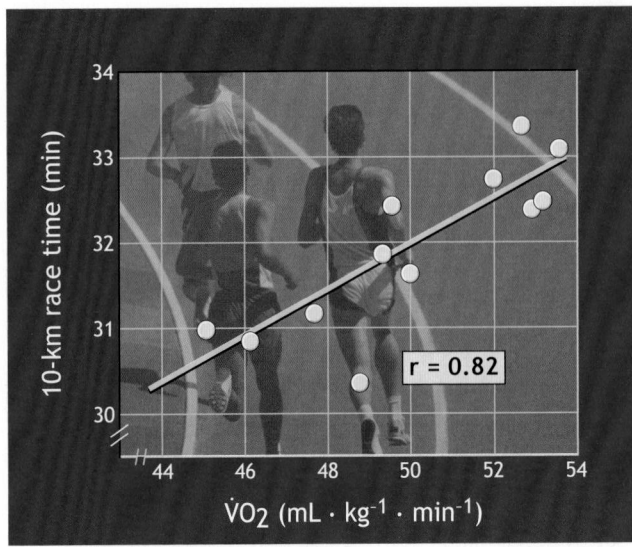

FIGURE 10.1 • Relationship between submaximal oxygen consumption running at 268 m · min⁻¹ and 10-km race time in elite male runners of comparable aerobic capacity. (Adapted with permission from Morgan DW, Craib M. Physiological aspects of running economy. *Med Sci Sports Exerc* 1992;24:456.)

fiber-type distribution in active muscles affects the economy of physical effort. During submaximal cycling, the economy of well-trained cyclists varies by ±15%.[23] Cyclists with greater economy possessed a larger percentage of slow-twitch (type I) muscle fibers in the vastus lateralis muscle. Aerobic, type I muscle fibers respond with greater mechanical efficiency than faster-contracting, highly anaerobic type II muscle fibers.[22]

Mechanical Efficiency

Mechanical efficiency reflects the percentage of total chemical energy expended that contributes to external work, with the remainder lost as heat.

Mechanical efficiency (%) = External work accomplished ÷ Energy expenditure × 100

External work accomplished (or energy output) equals force acting through a vertical distance (F × D), usually recorded as foot-pounds (ft-lb) or kilogram-meters (kg-m) and expressed in kcal units (1 kcal = 3087 ft-lb, or 426.4 kg-m in a perfect machine without loss in efficiency). External work is easily determined during cycle ergometry, or stair climbing or bench stepping—both require lifting the body mass a given distance (see "In A Practical Sense," Chapter 5). One cannot compute mechanical efficiency during horizontal walking or running because no external work is accomplished; reciprocal arm and leg movements negate each other without a net gain in vertical distance. If a person walks or runs up a grade, the work component can be estimated from body mass and vertical distance or lift achieved. Total oxygen consumed represents the denominator (energy expenditure) of the efficiency ratio. During steady-rate exercise, oxygen consumption converts to energy units—roughly 1.0 L O_2 = 5.0 kcal (see Table 8.1 in Chapter 8 for precise calorific transformations).

As an example, consider a 15-min ride on a stationary bicycle that generates 13,300 kg-m of work with net oxygen consumed to produce work totaling 25 L (RQ = 0.88).

Oxygen consumed converts to kcal as follows:

1. For RQ = 0.88, each liter of oxygen consumed generates an energy equivalent of 4.9 kcal (Table 8.1).
2. 25 L of oxygen consumption during the 15-min ride generates 122.5 kcal of energy (25 × 4.9 kcal).

The energy equivalent of 13,300 kg-m of external work equals 31.19 kcal (13,300 kg-m ÷ 426.4 kg-m per kcal).

Mechanical efficiency computes as follows:

$$\text{Mechanical efficiency} = 31.19 \text{ kcal} \div 122.5 \text{ kcal} \times 100$$
$$= 25.5\%$$

Like all machines, the human body's efficiency for mechanical work falls considerably below 100%. The energy required to overcome internal and external friction represents the largest factor to affect mechanical efficiency. This constitutes wasted energy because it does not contribute to work accomplished; consequently, work input (denominator in the equation) *always* exceeds work output (numerator in the equation).

On average, mechanical efficiency ranges between 20 and 25% for walking, running, and stationary cycling. Body size, gender, fitness level, and skill affect individual differences in efficiency. Efficiency falls below 20% for activities with substantial drag force that resists movement, as, for example, road cycling, cross-country skiing, ice skating, rowing, and swimming. Competitors in these sports focus attention on reducing drag by improving aerodynamics and/or hydrodynamics through alterations in clothing, equipment, and technique. For the elite athlete, small improvements in efficiency translate to increased likelihood of success.

Delta Efficiency

The calculation of **delta efficiency** provides an alternative approach to determine mechanical efficiency (not affected by body weight or changes in body weight):[5,68]

$$\text{Delta efficiency} = \Delta \text{ Work production} \div \Delta \text{ Energy expenditure} \times 100$$

where Δ work production equals the calculated difference in work output at two different activity levels, and Δ energy expenditure equals the difference in energy expenditure between the two activity levels.

For example, suppose an individual initially cycles at 100 W at a $\dot{V}O_2$ of 1.50 L·min^{-1} with an RQ of 0.89. Work intensity then increases to 200 W, with a corresponding $\dot{V}O_2$ of 2.88 L·min^{-1} and RQ of 0.95. Delta efficiency computes as

follows, where 1 W = 0.014 kcal·min^{-1}; RQ of 0.89 = 4.911 kcal·LO_2^{-1}; RQ of 0.95 = 4.985 kcal·LO_2^{-1}:

$$\text{Delta efficiency} = 200 \text{ W} - 100 \text{ W} \div 2.88 \text{ L·min}^{-1}$$
$$- 1.50 \text{ L·min}^{-1} \times 100$$
$$= (200 \times 0.014) - (100 \times 0.014)$$
$$\div (2.88 \times 4.985) - (1.50 \times 4.911)$$
$$\times 100$$
$$= 1.4 \text{ kcal·min}^{-1} \div 6.99 \text{ kcal·min}^{-1}$$
$$\times 100$$
$$= 0.2003 \times 100$$
$$= 20.0\%$$

ENERGY EXPENDITURE DURING WALKING

Walking represents the major daily physical activity for most persons. FIGURE 10.2 displays the combined research from five countries on energy expenditure of men walking at speeds from 1.5 to 9.5 km·hr^{-1} (0.9 to 5.9 mph). The relationship between walking speed and oxygen consumption remains approximately linear between 3.0 and 5.0 km·hr^{-1} (1.9 and 3.1 mph); as walking economy decreases at faster speeds, the relationship curves upward with a disproportionate increase in energy expenditure with increasing speed. This explains why, per unit distance traveled, faster, less-efficient walking speeds require more total calories expended per unit distance traveled.

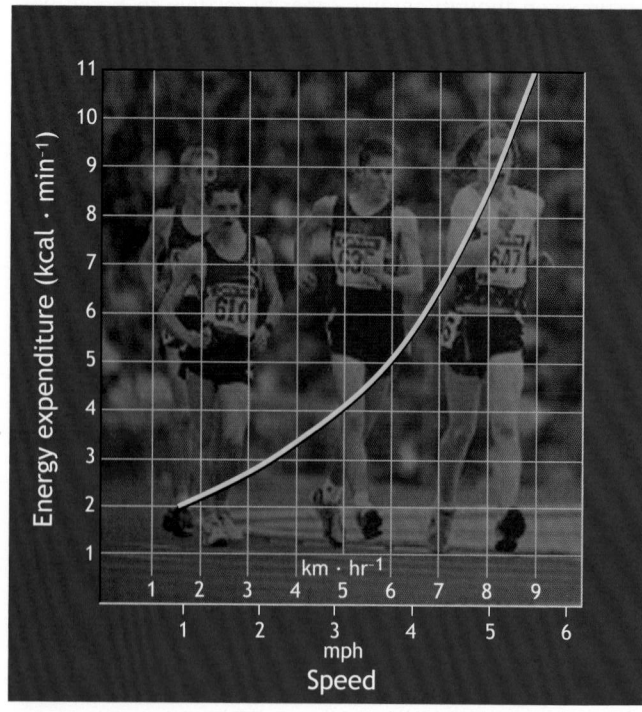

FIGURE 10.2 • Energy expenditure walking on a level surface at different speeds. The *yellow line* represents average values from various studies reported in the literature.

TABLE 10.1	Prediction of Energy Expenditure (kcal·min⁻¹) from Speed of Level Walking and Body Mass[a]						
Walking Speed		Body Mass						
mph	km·hr⁻¹	kg 36 lb 80	45 100	54 120	64 140	73 160	82 180	91 200
2.0	3.22	1.9	2.2	2.6	2.9	3.2	3.5	3.8
2.5	4.02	2.3	2.7	3.1	3.5	3.8	4.2	4.5
3.0	4.83	2.7	3.1	3.6	4.0	4.4	4.8	5.3
3.5	5.63	3.1	3.6	4.2	4.6	5.0	5.4	6.1
4.0	6.44	3.5	4.1	4.7	5.2	5.8	6.4	7.0

Data from Passmore R, Durnin JVGA. Human energy expenditure. *Physiol Rev* 1955;35:801.

[a]How to use the table: A 120-lb (54-kg) person who walks at 3.0 mph (4.83 km·hr⁻¹) expends 3.6 kcal·min⁻¹. This person expends 216 kcal in a 60-min walk (3.6 × 60).

Influence of Body Mass

With an equation based on the combined data in Figure 10.2 and additional studies,[1,30] one can accurately predict energy expenditure of horizontal walking at speeds between 3.2 and 6.4 km·hr⁻¹ (2.0 and 4.0 mph) for men and women who differ in body weight. These values, listed in TABLE 10.1, achieve accuracy to within ±15% of measured energy expenditure. On a daily basis, error estimates of energy expended in walking generally range from 50 to 100 kcal, assuming the person walks 2 hours daily. The predictions are less accurate when extrapolations are made for light (<36 kg) and heavy (>91 kg) individuals.

Terrain and Walking Surface

TABLE 10.2 summarizes the influence of terrain and different surfaces on energy expenditure of walking. Similar economies exist for level walking on a grass track or paved surface. In contrast, walking in sand requires almost twice the energy

TABLE 10.2	Effect of Different Terrain on the Energy Expenditure of Walking Between 5.2 and 5.6 km·hr⁻¹
Terrain	Correction Factor [a]
Paved road (similar to grass track)	0.0
Plowed field	1.5
Hard snow	1.6
Sand dune	1.8

First entry from Passmore R, Durnin JVGA. Human energy expenditure. *Physiol Rev* 1955;35:801. Last three entries from Givoni B, Goldman RF. Predicting metabolic energy cost. *J Appl Physiol* 1971;30:429.

[a]The correction factor is a multiple of the energy expenditure for walking on a paved road or grass track. For example, the energy expenditure of walking in a plowed field equals 1.5 times that of walking on a paved road. Divide by 1.61 to convert to mph.

expenditure compared to walking on a hard surface because of sand's hindering effects on the forward movement of the foot and the added force required by calf muscles to compensate for foot slippage. Walking in soft snow triples energy expenditure compared with similar walking on a treadmill.[82] A brisk walk or jog along a beach or in freshly fallen snow provides an excellent way to "burn" additional calories or improve physiologic fitness.[80]

Individuals generate essentially the same energy expenditure walking on a firm, level surface or walking on a treadmill at an equivalent speed and distance.[72] Such data confirm the belief that energy expenditure results from laboratory studies provide confidence in translating human energy expenditure data to "real-life" situations.

Downhill Walking

Walking downhill on a mountain hike or golf course provides welcome relief compared with uphill walking. Downhill walking or running represents a form of **negative work** as the body's center of mass moves in a downward vertical direction with each step cycle. At the same speed and elevation, it requires less energy to perform eccentric muscle actions (negative work) than the concentric actions of positive work.

FIGURE 10.3 illustrates the net oxygen consumption for both level and negative-grade walking at constant speeds of either 6.3 or 5.4 km·hr⁻¹. Compared with walking on level ground, progressive negative-grade walking decreases oxygen consumption down to a −9% grade for speeds of 5.4 km·hr⁻¹ and −12% for speeds of 6.3 km·hr⁻¹. Energy expenditure begins to increase at more severe negative grades. The additional energy expenditure to resist or "brake" the body from gravity's pull while trying to achieve a proper and safe walking rhythm increases the oxygen consumption for walking down steeper grades.

Footwear and Other Distal Leg Loads

It requires considerably more energy to carry weight on the feet or ankles than to carry the same weight on the torso.[12] A weight

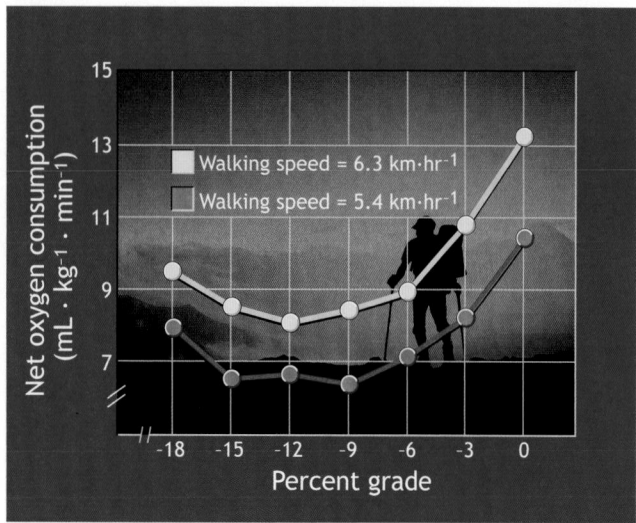

FIGURE 10.3 • Net oxygen consumption of level (0% grade) and downhill walking at grades between −3 and −18% and speeds between 5.4 and 6.3 km·hr⁻¹. Percent grade reflects the vertical distance moved downward per unit horizontal distance traversed. (Adapted with permission from Wanta DM, et al. Metabolic response to graded downhill walking. *Med Sci Sports Exerc* 1993;25:159.)

equal to 1.4% of body mass placed on the ankles increases energy expenditure of walking an average of 8%, or nearly six times more than with the same weight on the torso.[39] In a practical sense, wearing boots disproportionately increases the energy expenditure of walking and running compared with energy expenditure wearing lighter running shoes. Adding an additional 100 g to each shoe increases oxygen consumption during moderate running by 1%. Running barefoot offers no metabolic advantage over running in light-weight, cushioned shoes.[33] In the design of running shoes, hiking and climbing boots, and work boots for mining, forestry, fire-fighting, and the military, small changes in shoe weight produce meaningful changes in movement economy and hence total energy expenditure.[36] Minimally shod runners show greater running economy (2.4 to 3.3%) than traditionally shod runners, after accounting for the effects of shoe mass and stride frequency.[66] Greater elastic energy storage and release in the lower extremity during minimal-shoe running helps to explain this difference. The cushioning properties and longitudinal bending stiffness of shoes also affect walking and running economy. A more flexible and softer-soled running shoe reduced oxygen consumption with increased economy of running at a moderate speed by −2.4% compared with a similar shoe with a firmer cushioning system, even though the pair of softer-soled shoes weighed an additional 31 g.[34,64,77]

Walking

Ankle weights increase energy expenditure of walking to values usually observed for running.[54] The effect benefits individuals who use only walking as a low-impact training modality yet require greater energy expenditures than during normal walking. Handheld weights, walking poles that simulate arm action in cross-country skiing, power belts worn around the waist with resistance cords with handles for arm action, weighted vests, and swinging the arms in upper-body exercise increase walking's energy expenditure.[29,71,73,91]

Handheld weights and walking poles may disproportionately increase exercise systolic blood pressure, perhaps from the pressure-elevating effects of upper-body exercise (see Chapter 15, "Blood Pressure in Upper-Body Exercise") and increased intramuscular tension from gripping. An augmented blood pressure response contraindicates using handheld weights for individuals with existing hypertension or coronary heart disease.

Running

Considering the relatively small increase in energy expenditure with hand or ankle weights in running, it seems more practical to simply increase unweighted running speed or distance. This reduces injury potential from the added impact force imparted by the weights and eliminates any discomfort from carrying them. For individuals with orthopedic limitations, in-line skating offers a less-stressful alternative for an equivalent aerobic demand.[48,53]

 INTEGRATIVE QUESTION

Give recommendations for mode–specific aerobic physical activities for training individuals with osteoarthritis of the knees?

Competition Walking

For Olympic-caliber walkers, walking speed during competition averaged 13.0 km·hr⁻¹ (11.5 to 14.8 km·hr⁻¹ [7.1 to 9.2 mph]) over distances from 1.6 to 50 km. This represents a relatively fast speed; the world record for the 20-km walk (12.6-mile) for men of 1:16:43 (Sergey Morozov of Russia, 2008; women, Yelena Lashmanova of Russia, 2012:1:25:02) equals a speed of 15.74 km·hr⁻¹ (9.78 mph) and 16 km·hr⁻¹ (9.94 mph) for women! **FIGURE 10.4** illustrates that the break point in economy of locomotion between walking and running ranged between 8.0 and 9.0 km·hr⁻¹. These data, plus biomechanical evidence, indicate about the same crossover speed—when running becomes more economical than walking—for conventional and competitive styles of walking (**FIG. 10.5**). The preferred transition speed of 7.2 km·hr⁻¹ (4.5 mph) (nonrunners) and 7.4 km·hr⁻¹ (4.6 mph) (runners) is slower than the energetically optimal speed, and these speeds remain independent of training state or aerobic capacity.[75] In addition, treadmill walking at competition speeds produced only slightly lower oxygen consumptions for race-walkers than their highest oxygen consumptions during treadmill running. A linear relationship exists between oxygen consumption and walking

Speed, Pace Times, and Target Distance Conversions

The following table provides useful conversions for different speeds, pace, and distances.

MPH	km/hr	min/mi	min/km	3 mi	5 km	8 km	10 km	1/2 mar	Marathon
3.0	**4.8**	**0:20:00**	**0:12:26**	**1:00:00**	**1:02:08**	**1:39:25**	**2:04:16**	**4:22:13**	**8:44:26**
3.2	5.1	0:18:45	0:11:39	0:56:15	0:58:15	1:33:12	1:56:30	4:05:50	8:11:40
3.4	5.5	0:17:39	0:10:58	0:52:56	0:54:50	1:27:43	1:49:39	3:51:22	7:42:44
3.6	5.8	0:16:40	0:10:21	0:50:00	0:51:47	1:22:51	1:43:34	3:38:31	7:17:02
3.8	6.1	0:15:47	0:09:49	0:47:22	0:49:03	1:18:29	1:38:07	3:27:01	6:54:02
4.0	**6.4**	**0:15:00**	**0:09:19**	**0:45:00**	**0:46:36**	**1:14:34**	**1:33:12**	**3:16:40**	**6:33:20**
4.2	6.8	0:14:17	0:08:53	0:42:51	0:44:23	1:11:01	1:28:46	3:07:18	6:14:36
4.4	7.1	0:13:38	0:08:28	0:40:55	0:42:22	1:07:47	1:24:44	2:58:47	5:57:34
4.6	7.4	0:13:03	0:08:06	0:39:08	0:40:31	1:04:50	1:21:03	2:51:01	5:42:01
4.8	7.7	0:12:30	0:07:46	0:37:30	0:38:50	1:02:08	1:17:40	2:43:53	5:27:46
5.0	**8.0**	**0:12:00**	**0:07:27**	**0:36:00**	**0:37:17**	**0:59:39**	**1:14:34**	**2:37:20**	**5:14:40**
5.2	8.4	0:11:32	0:07:10	0:34:37	0:35:51	0:57:21	1:11:42	2:31:17	5:02:34
5.4	8.7	0:11:07	0:06:54	0:33:20	0:34:31	0:55:14	1:09:02	2:25:41	4:51:21
5.6	9.0	0:10:43	0:06:39	0:32:09	0:33:17	0:53:16	1:06:35	2:20:28	4:40:57
5.8	9.3	0:10:21	0:06:26	0:31:02	0:32:08	0:51:25	1:04:17	2:15:38	4:31:16
6.0	**9.7**	**0:10:00**	**0:06:13**	**0:30:00**	**0:31:04**	**0:49:43**	**1:02:08**	**2:11:07**	**4:22:13**
6.2	10.0	0:09:41	0:06:01	0:29:02	0:30:04	0:48:06	1:00:08	2:06:53	4:13:46
6.4	10.3	0:09:22	0:05:50	0:28:07	0:29:08	0:46:36	0:58:15	2:02:55	4:05:50
6.6	10.6	0:09:05	0:05:39	0:27:16	0:28:15	0:45:11	0:56:29	1:59:11	3:58:23
6.8	10.9	0:08:49	0:05:29	0:26:28	0:27:25	0:43:52	0:54:50	1:55:41	3:51:22
7.0	**11.3**	**0:08:34**	**0:05:20**	**0:25:43**	**0:26:38**	**0:42:36**	**0:53:16**	**1:52:23**	**3:44:46**
7.2	11.6	0:08:20	0:05:11	0:25:00	0:25:53	0:41:25	0:51:47	1:49:15	3:38:31
7.4	11.9	0:08:06	0:05:02	0:24:19	0:25:11	0:40:18	0:50:23	1:46:18	3:32:37
7.6	12.2	0:07:54	0:04:54	0:23:41	0:24:32	0:39:15	0:49:03	1:43:30	3:27:01
7.8	12.6	0:07:42	0:04:47	0:23:05	0:23:54	0:38:14	0:47:48	1:40:51	3:21:42
8.0	**12.9**	**0:07:30**	**0:04:40**	**0:22:30**	**0:23:18**	**0:37:17**	**0:46:36**	**1:38:20**	**3:16:40**
8.2	13.2	0:07:19	0:04:33	0:21:57	0:22:44	0:36:22	0:45:28	1:35:56	3:11:52
8.4	13.5	0:07:09	0:04:26	0:21:26	0:22:12	0:35:30	0:44:23	1:33:39	3:07:18
8.6	13.8	0:06:59	0:04:20	0:20:56	0:21:41	0:34:41	0:43:21	1:31:28	3:02:57
8.8	14.2	0:06:49	0:04:14	0:20:27	0:21:11	0:33:54	0:42:22	1:29:24	2:58:47
9.0	**14.5**	**0:06:40**	**0:04:09**	**0:20:00**	**0:20:43**	**0:33:08**	**0:41:25**	**1:27:24**	**2:54:49**
9.2	14.8	0:06:31	0:04:03	0:19:34	0:20:16	0:32:25	0:40:31	1:25:30	2:51:01
9.4	15.1	0:06:23	0:03:58	0:19:09	0:19:50	0:31:44	0:39:40	1:23:41	2:47:22
9.6	15.4	0:06:15	0:03:53	0:18:45	0:19:25	0:31:04	0:38:50	1:21:57	2:43:53
9.8	15.8	0:06:07	0:03:48	0:18:22	0:19:01	0:30:26	0:38:03	1:20:16	2:40:33
10.0	**16.1**	**0:06:00**	**0:03:44**	**0:18:00**	**0:18:38**	**0:29:50**	**0:37:17**	**1:18:40**	**2:37:20**
10.2	16.4	0:05:53	0:03:39	0:17:39	0:18:17	0:29:14	0:36:33	1:17:07	2:34:15
10.4	16.7	0:05:46	0:03:35	0:17:18	0:17:55	0:28:41	0:35:51	1:15:38	2:31:17
10.6	17.1	0:05:40	0:03:31	0:16:59	0:17:35	0:28:08	0:35:10	1:14:13	2:28:26
10.8	17.4	0:05:33	0:03:27	0:16:40	0:17:16	0:27:37	0:34:31	1:12:50	2:25:41
11.0	**17.7**	**0:05:27**	**0:03:23**	**0:16:22**	**0:16:57**	**0:27:07**	**0:33:54**	**1:11:31**	**2:23:02**
11.2	18.0	0:05:21	0:03:20	0:16:04	0:16:39	0:26:38	0:33:17	1:10:14	2:20:28
11.4	18.3	0:05:16	0:03:16	0:15:47	0:16:21	0:26:10	0:32:42	1:09:00	2:18:01
11.6	18.7	0:05:10	0:03:13	0:15:31	0:16:04	0:25:43	0:32:08	1:07:49	2:15:38
11.8	19.0	0:05:05	0:03:10	0:15:15	0:15:48	0:25:17	0:31:36	1:06:40	2:13:20
12.0	**19.3**	**0:05:00**	**0:03:06**	**0:15:00**	**0:15:32**	**0:24:51**	**0:31:04**	**1:05:33**	**2:11:07**

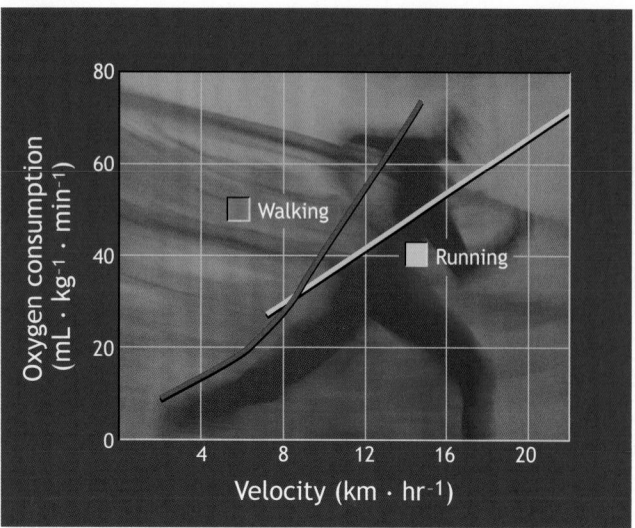

FIGURE 10.4 • Relationship between oxygen consumption and horizontal velocity for walking and running in competition walkers. (Adapted with permission from Menier DR, Pugh LGCE. The relation of oxygen intake and velocity of walking and running in competition walkers. *J Physiol* 1968;197:717.)

at speeds above 8 km·hr^{-1} (5.0 mph), but the slope of the line was *twice* as steep compared to running at the same speeds. The athletes walked at velocities of nearly 16 km·hr^{-1} (9.9 mph). *The economy of walking faster than 8 km·hr^{-1} equaled only one-half the economy for running at the same speeds.* Attainment of similar values for $\dot{V}O_{2max}$ during race-walking and running by elite competitors further supports the model for aerobic

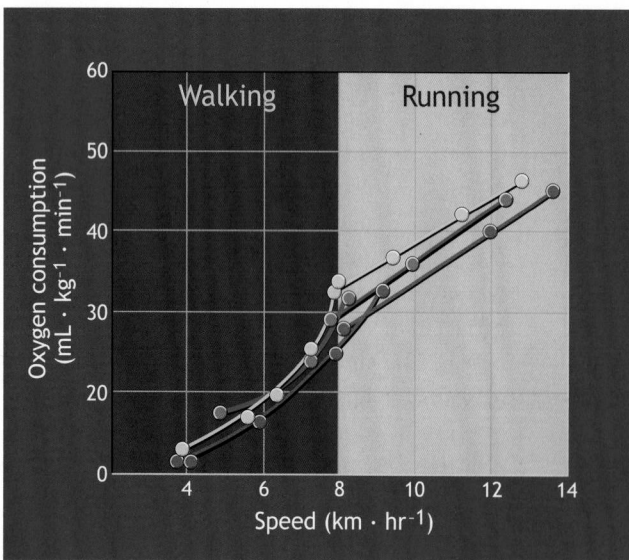

FIGURE 10.5 • Relationship between oxygen consumption and speed of horizontal walking and running in men and women. Different *colored lines* represent values from various research studies. (Adapted with permission from Falls HB, Humphrey LD. Energy cost of running and walking in young women. *Med Sci Sports* 1976;8:9.)

training specificity because $\dot{V}O_{2max}$ in untrained subjects during walking generally remains 5 to 15% below running values.[35,51]

Competition walkers achieve high yet uneconomical rates of movement unattainable during conventional walking, with a distinctive modified walking technique that constrains the athlete to certain movement patterns regardless of walking speed (http://www.youtube.com/watch?v=FMwSAPp_iIU). The athlete must maintain this gait despite progressive decreases in walking economy as exercise duration progresses and fatigue increases.[10,11] Among elite race-walkers, variations in walking economy contribute more to successful performance than in competitive running.[35]

ENERGY EXPENDITURE DURING RUNNING

Primary biomechanical factors that determine energy expenditure of running in relation to velocity among mammals include the magnitude and rate of muscular force generation to counteract gravity and to operate the springlike properties of the muscle-tendon system.[43] Energy expenditure for running has been quantified during performance of the actual activity and on a treadmill with precise control of speed and grade. The terms *jogging* and *running* reflect qualitative assessments related to speed and strenuousness. At identical submaximal speeds, an endurance athlete runs at a lower percentage of $\dot{V}O_{2max}$ than an untrained person, although both maintain nearly similar oxygen consumption rates while running. The demarcation between a jog and a run relates more to the participant's fitness level: *A jog for one person represents a run for another.*

Independent of fitness, it becomes more economical from an energy expenditure standpoint to discontinue walking and begin running at speeds above about 8 km·hr^{-1}. Figure 10.5 illustrates the relationship between oxygen consumption and horizontal walking and running for men and women at speeds between 4 and 14 km·hr^{-1}. For data depicted in green and yellow, the lines relating oxygen consumption and speed intersect at a running speed of 8.0 km·hr^{-1}; the breakpoint in locomotion economy for competition walkers shown in red occurs at about 8.7 km·hr^{-1}.

 ## Elite Runners Run More Economically

At a particular speed, elite endurance runners run at a lower oxygen uptake than less trained or less successful counterparts of similar age. This holds for 8- to 11-year-old cross-country runners and adult marathoners. Elite distance athletes as a group run with 5 to 10% greater economy than well-trained middle-distance runners.

IN A PRACTICAL SENSE

Predicting Energy Expenditure During Treadmill Walking and Running

An almost linear relationship exists between oxygen consumption (energy expenditure) and walking speeds between 3.0 and 5.0 km·hr⁻¹ (1.9 and 3.1 mph), and running at speeds faster than 8.0 km·hr⁻¹ (5 to 10 mph; see Fig. 10.5). Adding the resting oxygen consumption to the oxygen requirements of the horizontal and vertical components of the walk or run makes it possible to estimate total (gross) exercise oxygen consumption ($\dot{V}O_2$) and energy expenditure.

BASIC EQUATION

$\dot{V}O_2$ (mL·kg⁻¹·min⁻¹) = Resting component (1 MET [3.5 mL O_2·kg⁻¹·min⁻¹]) + Horizontal component (speed, [m·min⁻¹] × oxygen consumption of horizontal movement) + Vertical component (percentage grade × speed [m·min⁻¹] × oxygen consumption of vertical movement).

[To convert mph to m·min⁻¹, multiply by 26.82; to convert m·min⁻¹ to mph, multiply by 0.03728.]

Walking

Oxygen consumption of the horizontal component of movement equals 0.1 mL·kg⁻¹·min⁻¹, and 1.8 mL·kg⁻¹·min⁻¹ for the vertical component.

Running

Oxygen consumption of the horizontal component of movement equals 0.2 mL·kg⁻¹·min⁻¹, and 0.9 mL·kg⁻¹·min⁻¹ for the vertical component.

PREDICTING ENERGY EXPENDITURE OF TREADMILL WALKING

Problem

A 55-kg person walks on a treadmill at 2.8 mph (2.8 × 26.82 = 75 m·min⁻¹ up a 4% grade. Calculate (1) $\dot{V}O_2$ (mL·kg⁻¹·min⁻¹), (2) METs, and (3) energy expenditure (kcal·min⁻¹).

[Note: Express % grade as a decimal value (i.e., 4% grade = 0.04)]

Solution

1. $\dot{V}O_2$ (mL·kg⁻¹·min⁻¹) = Resting component + Horizontal component + Vertical component

   $\dot{V}O_2$ = Resting $\dot{V}O_2$ (mL·kg⁻¹·min⁻¹)

   + [speed (m·min⁻¹) × 0.1 mL·kg⁻¹·min⁻¹]

   + [% grade × speed (m·min⁻¹)

   × 1.8 mL·kg⁻¹·min⁻¹]

   = 3.5 + (75 × 0.1) + (0.04 × 75 × 1.8)

   = 3.5 + 7.5 + 5.4

   = 16.4 mL·kg⁻¹·min⁻¹

2. METs = $\dot{V}O_2$ (mL·kg⁻¹·min⁻¹)

   ÷ 3.5 mL·kg⁻¹·min⁻¹

   = 16.4 4 ÷ 3.5

   = 4.7

3. kcal·min⁻¹ = $\dot{V}O_2$ (mL·kg⁻¹·min⁻¹)

   × Body mass (kg) × 5.05 kcal·LO_2^{-1}

   = 16.4 mL·kg⁻¹·min⁻¹

   × 55 kg × 5.05 kcal·L⁻¹

   = 0.902 L·min⁻¹ × 5.05 kcal·L⁻¹

   = 4.6

PREDICTING ENERGY EXPENDITURE OF TREADMILL RUNNING

Problem

A 55-kg person runs on a treadmill at 5.4 mph (5.4 × 26.82 = 145 m·min⁻¹) up a 6% grade. Calculate (1) $\dot{V}O_2$ in mL·kg⁻¹·min⁻¹, (2) METs, and (3) energy expenditure (kcal·min⁻¹).

Solution

1. $\dot{V}O_2$ (mL·kg⁻¹·min⁻¹) = Resting component + Horizontal component + Vertical component

   $\dot{V}O_2$ = Resting $\dot{V}O_2$ (mL·kg⁻¹·min⁻¹)

   + [speed (m·min⁻¹)

   × 0.2 mL·kg⁻¹·min⁻¹]

   + [% grade × speed (m·min⁻¹)

   × 0.9 mL·kg⁻¹·min⁻¹]

   = 3.5 + (145 × 0.2) + (0.06 × 145 × 0.9)

   = 3.5 + 29.0 + 7.83

   = 40.33 mL·kg⁻¹·min⁻¹

2. METs = $\dot{V}O_2$ (mL·kg⁻¹·min⁻¹)

   × 3.5 mL·kg⁻¹·min⁻¹

   = 40.33 ÷ 3.5

   = 11.5

3. kcal·min⁻¹ = $\dot{V}O_2$ (mL·kg⁻¹·min⁻¹)

   × Body mass (kg)

   × 5.05 kcal·LO_2^{-1}

   = 40.33 mL·kg⁻¹·min⁻¹

   × 55 kg × 5.05 kcal·L⁻¹

   = 2.22 L·min⁻¹ × 5.05 kcal·L⁻¹

   = 11.2

Adapted with permission from *ACSM Guidelines for Exercise Testing and Prescription*. 9th Ed. Baltimore: Lippincott Williams & Wilkins, 2014.

Economy of Running Fast or Slow

The data for running in Figure 10.5 illustrate an important principle about running speed and energy expenditure. *The linear relationship between oxygen consumption and running speed indicates an equivalency in total energy requirement for running a given distance (in steady rate) that is about the same regardless of speed throughout a broad range of running speeds.* Simply stated, running a mile at 10 mph requires about twice the energy a minute as running a mile at 5 mph; at the faster speed, completing the mile requires 6 min, but running at the slower speed takes about twice as long or about 12 min. The *net* energy expenditure to traverse a mile remains about the same.[74] Equivalent energy expenditure per mile regardless of running speed occurs for horizontal running and for running at a specific grade that ranges from −45 to +15%.[24,49] *During horizontal running, the net energy expenditure per kilogram of body mass per kilometer traveled averages 1 kcal or 1 kcal $\cdot$ kg^{-1} $\cdot$ km^{-1}.* The net energy expenditure running 1 km for individuals who weigh 78 kg averages 78 kcal, independent of running speed. Expressed as oxygen consumption (5 kcal = 1 L O$_2$), this amounts to 15.6 L of oxygen consumed per kilometer (78 kcal $\cdot$ km^{-1} ÷ 5 kcal). Comparisons of net energy expenditure of locomotion per unit distance traveled for walking and running indicate greater energy expenditure when running a given distance.[6]

INTEGRATIVE QUESTION

An elite 140-lb female runner claims she consistently consumes 12,000 kcal daily simply to maintain body weight owing to the strenuousness of her training. Using examples of exercise energy expenditures, discuss the plausibility of this level of caloric intake.

Net Energy Expenditure Values

Table 10.3 presents values for *net energy expenditure* during running for 1 hr at various speeds—expressed in kilometers per hour, miles per hour, and the number of minutes required to complete 1 mile at a specific speed. Bolded values indicate net calories expended running 1 mile for a given body mass. Recall that energy requirement for each mile remains fairly constant regardless of running speed. *A person who weighs 62 kg requires approximately 2600 kcal (net) to run a 26.2-mile marathon regardless of whether the run takes just over 2 hr, 3 hr, or 4 hr!*

Table 10.3 also reveals that energy expenditure per mile increases proportionally with body mass. A 102-kg person who runs 5 miles each day at a comfortable pace expends 163 kcal for each mile run, or 815 kcal for 5 miles. The influence of body mass on an activity's energy expenditure supports

TABLE 10.3 — Net Energy Expenditure Per Hour of Horizontal Running Related to Velocity and Body Mass[a]

Body Mass (kg)	(lb)	km·hr⁻¹[b] mph min per mile kcal per mile	8 4.97 12:00	9 5.60 10:43	10 6.20 9:41	11 6.84 8:46	12 7.46 8:02	13 8.08 7:26	14 8.70 6:54	15 9.32 6:26	16 9.94 6:02
50	110	**80**	400	450	500	550	600	650	700	750	800
54	119	**86**	432	486	540	594	648	702	756	810	864
58	128	**93**	464	522	580	638	696	754	812	870	928
62	137	**99**	496	558	620	682	744	806	868	930	992
66	146	**106**	528	594	660	726	792	858	924	990	1056
70	154	**112**	560	630	700	770	840	910	980	1050	1120
74	163	**118**	592	666	740	814	888	962	1036	1110	1184
78	172	**125**	624	702	780	858	936	1014	1092	1170	1248
82	181	**131**	656	738	820	902	984	1066	1148	1230	1312
86	190	**138**	688	774	860	946	1032	1118	1204	1290	1376
90	199	**144**	720	810	900	990	1080	1170	1260	1350	1440
94	207	**150**	752	846	940	1034	1128	1222	1316	1410	1504
98	216	**157**	784	882	980	1078	1176	1274	1372	1470	1568
102	225	**163**	816	918	1020	1122	1224	1326	1428	1530	1632
106	234	**170**	848	954	1060	1166	1272	1378	1484	1590	1696

[a]Interpret the table as follows: For a 50-kg person, the net energy expenditure for running for 1 hr at 8 km $\cdot$ hr^{-1} or 4.97 mph equals 400 kcal; this speed represents a 12-min per mile pace. Thus, 5 miles would be run in 1 hr and 400 kcal would be expended. Increasing the pace to 12 km $\cdot$ hr^{-1} expends 600 kcal during the hour of running.

[b]Running speeds are expressed as kilometers per hour (km $\cdot$ hr^{-1}), miles per hour (mph), and minutes required to complete each mile (min per mile). The values in **boldface type** are *net* calories expended to run 1 mile for a given body mass, independent of running speed.

| TABLE 10.4 | Energy Requirements (METs) for Horizontal and Grade Walking and Running on a Solid Surface | | | | | | |

Horizontal and Grade Walking

% Grade	mph	1.7	2.0	2.5	3.0	3.4	3.75
	m · min⁻¹	45.6	53.7	67.0	80.5	91.2	100.5
0		2.3	2.5	2.9	3.3	3.6	3.9
2.5		2.9	3.2	3.8	4.3	4.8	5.2
5.0		3.5	3.9	4.6	5.4	5.9	6.5
7.5		4.1	4.6	5.5	6.4	7.1	7.8
10.0		4.6	5.3	6.3	7.4	8.3	9.1
12.5		5.2	6.0	7.2	8.5	9.5	10.4
15.0		5.8	6.6	8.1	9.5	10.6	11.7
17.5		6.4	7.3	8.9	10.5	11.8	12.9
20.0		7.0	8.0	9.8	11.6	13.0	14.2
22.5		7.6	8.7	10.6	12.6	14.2	15.5
25.0		8.2	9.4	11.5	13.6	15.3	16.8

Horizontal and Grade Jogging/Running

% Grade	mph	5	6	7	7.5	8	9	10
	m · min⁻¹	134	161	188	201	215	241	268
0		8.6	10.2	11.7	12.5	13.3	14.8	16.3
2.5		10.3	12.3	14.1	15.1	16.1	17.9	19.7
5.0		12.0	14.3	16.5	17.7	18.8		
7.5		13.9	16.4	18.9				
10.0		15.5	18.5					

Adapted with permission from *ACSM Guidelines for Exercise Testing and Prescription*. 9th Ed. Baltimore: Lippincott Williams & Wilkins, 2014.

the role of weight-bearing physical activity as an additional caloric stressor for overly fat persons who should increase daily energy expenditure for weight loss. Increasing or decreasing the speed within the broad range of steady-rate pacing simply alters the duration of the 5-mile run; it has little effect on the total energy or kcal expended.

TABLE 10.4 summarizes data from studies of energy expenditure using horizontal and grade walking and running on a firm surface. The energy requirement represents multiples of the resting metabolic rate or METs (1 MET = 3.5 mL $O_2 \cdot kg^{-1} \cdot min^{-1}$).

Stride Length, Stride Frequency, and Speed

Running

One can increase running speed in three ways:

1. Increase number of steps each minute (*stride frequency*)
2. Increase distance between steps (*stride length*)
3. Increase *both* length and frequency of strides

The third option may seem obvious, but several experiments have provided objective data concerning this alternative.

Research in 1944 evaluated the stride pattern for a Danish champion in 5- and 10-km running events.[8] At a running speed of 9.3 km · hr⁻¹, this athlete's stride frequency equaled 160 per minute, with a corresponding stride length of 97 cm. When running speed increased 91% to 17.8 km · hr⁻¹, stride frequency increased only 10%, to 176 per minute, whereas stride length increased 83%, to 168 cm. FIGURE 10.6A displays the interaction between stride frequency and stride length as running speed increases. Doubling speed from 10 to 20 km · hr⁻¹ increases stride length by 85%, whereas stride frequency increases only about 9%. Running at speeds above 23 km · hr⁻¹ occurs mainly by increasing stride frequency. *As a general rule, running speed increases mainly by lengthening stride: At faster speeds stride frequency becomes important.* Relying on increasing length of the "stroke" cycle, not frequency, to achieve rapid speeds in endurance performance also occurs among top-flight kayakers, rowers, cross-country skiers, and speed skaters.

Competition Walking

A competitive walker does not increase speed the same way as a runner. FIGURE 10.6B illustrates the stride length–stride frequency relationship for an Olympic 10-km medal

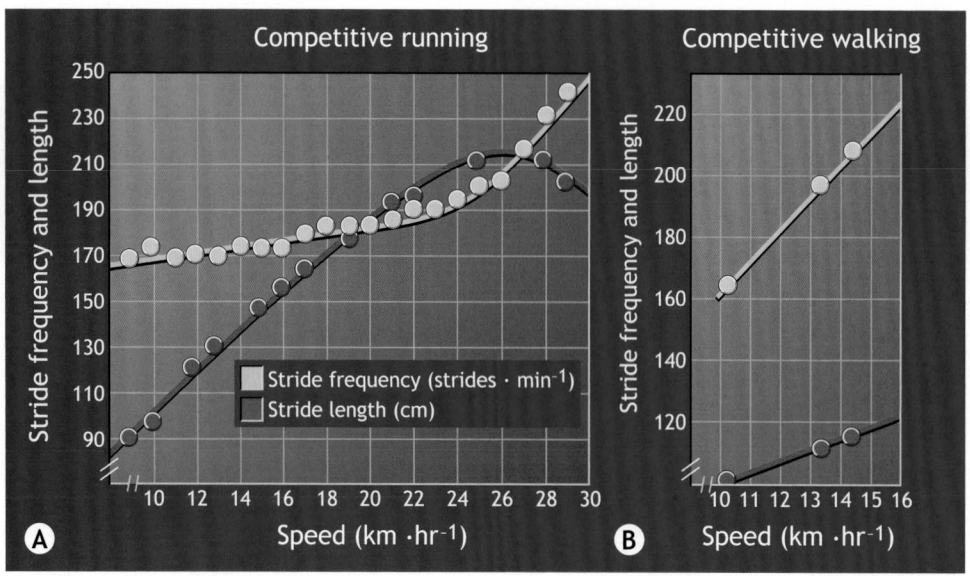

FIGURE 10.6 • **(A)** Stride frequency and stride length as a function of running speed. **(B)** Data for an Olympic walker during race-walking. (Adapted with permission from Hogberg P. Length of stride, stride frequency, flight period and maximum distance between the feet during running with different speeds. *Int Z Angew Physiol* 1952;14:431.)

winner who walked at speeds from 10 to 14.4 km·hr⁻¹. When walking speed increased within this range, stride frequency increased 27% and stride length increased 13%. Faster speeds produced an even greater increase in stride frequency. Unlike running, where the body essentially "glides" through the air, competitive race-walking requires that the back foot remain on the ground until the front foot makes contact. Thus, lengthening stride becomes difficult and ineffectual to increase speed. Involving trunk and arm musculature to move the leg forward rapidly requires additional energy expenditure; this explains the poorer economy for walking than running at speeds above 8 or 9 km·hr⁻¹ (see Fig. 10.4).

Optimum Stride Length

Each person runs at a constant speed with an optimum combination of stride length and stride frequency. This optimum depends largely on the person's mechanics or "style" of running, and cannot be determined from body measurements.[16] Nevertheless, energy expenditure increases more for overstriding than understriding. **FIGURE 10.7** relates oxygen consumption to different stride lengths altered by a subject running at the relatively fast speed of 14 km·hr⁻¹.

For this runner, a stride length of 135 cm produced the lowest oxygen consumption of 3.35 L·min⁻¹. When stride length decreased to 118 cm, oxygen consumption increased 8%;

 ## Edward Payson Weston: Walker Extraordinaire

Born in 1839, when life span averaged 40 years, Edward Payson Weston (1839–1929) in his prime would walk 50 to 100 miles a day. In 1861, he walked 453 miles from Boston to Washington, DC, in 10 days and 10 hours to attend Lincoln's inauguration on March 4. The new 16th president, Abraham Lincoln, gave Weston a congratulatory handshake, which inspired Weston to compete in many professional "pedestrian" competitions. These included 6-day ultramarathon races before huge crowds in New York City's Madison Square Garden and in London's Agricultural Hall. At age 71, Weston was the first to walk across America from Los Angeles to New York City, covering approximately 3600 miles in 88 days, averaging 41 miles daily. In his mid-80s, Weston still walked 25 miles a day. Other notable achievements included walking from Philadelphia to New York, a distance of over 100 miles, in less than 24 hours; at age 68, he repeated his Maine-to-Chicago walk of 1867, beating his prior time by over 24 hours. In 1909, Weston walked for 100 days, covering a distance of nearly 4000 miles from New York City to San Francisco following many routes not on the standard trail of that time.

Weston, a professional race walker and early American advocate of vigorous exercise, died in 1929 at age 90, 2 years after being struck by a New York City taxicab that caused him to lose the use of his legs.

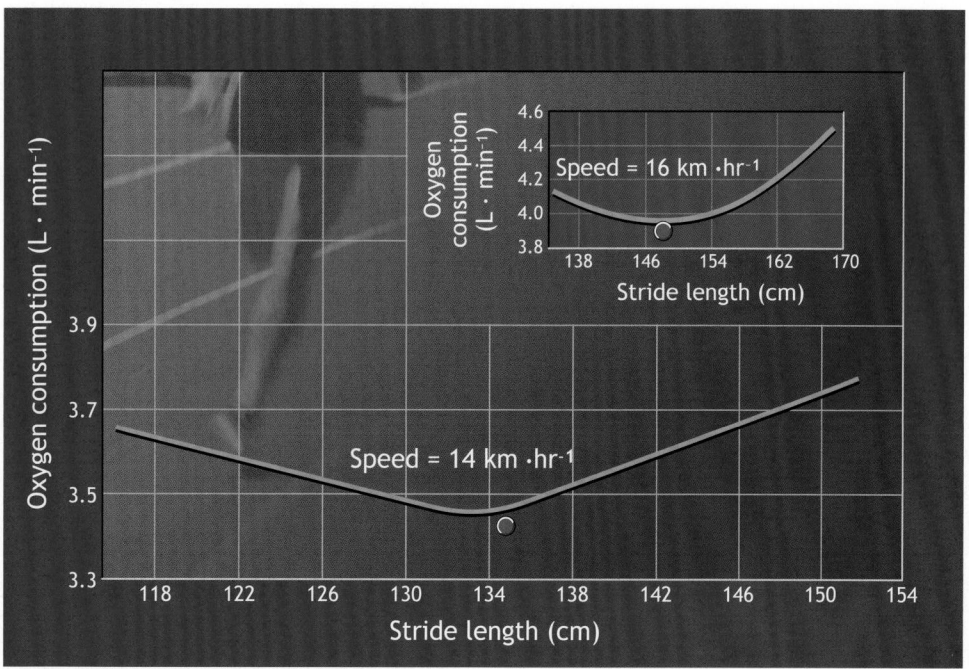

FIGURE 10.7 • Oxygen consumption while running at 14 km·hr^{-1} affected by different stride lengths. The inset graph plots oxygen consumption at a faster speed of 16 km·hr^{-1}. (Adapted with permission from Hogberg P. Length of stride, stride frequency, flight period and maximum distance between the feet during running with different speeds. *Int Z Angew Physiol* 1952;14:431.)

lengthening the distance between steps to 153 cm increased oxygen consumption by 12%. The inset graph shows a similar pattern for oxygen consumption when running speed increased to 16 km·hr^{-1} and stride lengths varied between 135 and 169 cm. Decreasing this runner's stride length from the optimum of 149 to 135 cm increased oxygen consumption by 4.1%; lengthening the stride to 169 cm increased aerobic energy expenditure nearly 13%. As one might expect, stride length selected by the subject (marked in the figure by the *solid red circle*) produced the most economical stride length (lowest $\dot{V}O_2$). Lengthening the stride above the optimum produced a larger increase in oxygen consumption than a shorter-than-optimum length. Urging a runner who shows signs of fatigue to "lengthen your stride" to maintain speed actually proves counterproductive in terms of economy of effort and subsequent performance.

Well-trained runners have "learned" through experience to run at the stride length they are accustomed to. In keeping with the concept that the body attempts to achieve a **level of minimum effort**, a self-selected stride length and frequency generally produce the most economical running performance. This reflects an individual's unique body size, inertia of limb segments, and anatomic development.[15,55,56] *No "best" style characterizes elite runners.* For the competitive runner, any minor improvement in running economy generally improves race performance.

Running Economy: Children and Adults, Trained and Untrained

Children are less economical runners than adults; they require 20 to 30% more oxygen per unit body mass to run at a given

speed.[2,42,63] Adult models to predict energy expenditure during weight-bearing locomotion fail to account for the increased and changing energy expenditures in children and adolescents.[37,62]

FIGURE 10.8 illustrates the relationship between walking and running speeds of 2 and 8 mph in male and female adolescent volunteers and (**A**) oxygen consumption and (**B**) energy expenditure. Despite higher oxygen consumption and energy expenditure values during walking and running for adolescents than adults (Fig. 10.5), the shape of the curves for both groups remains remarkably similar.

Differences exist in energy expenditure among children and adolescents in weight-bearing physical activities. This has been attributed to a larger ratio of surface area to body mass, greater stride frequencies, and shorter stride lengths, and to differences in anthropometric variables and mechanics that reduce movement economy.[31,76] Economy of movement in weight-bearing activity also improves in obese adolescents and adults following weight loss.[27,67] **FIGURE 10.9B** illustrates that running economy improves steadily during years 10 through 18. Poor running economy among young children partly explains their poorer performance in distance running compared with adults and their progressive performance improvement through adolescence, while aerobic capacity (mL O$_2$·kg^{-1}·min^{-1}; **FIG. 10.9A**) remains relatively unchanged throughout this period. Consequently, improvement in weight-bearing fitness tests as the 1-mile walk-run during the growth years does not necessarily imply concomitant improvement in $\dot{V}O_{2max}$.[23]

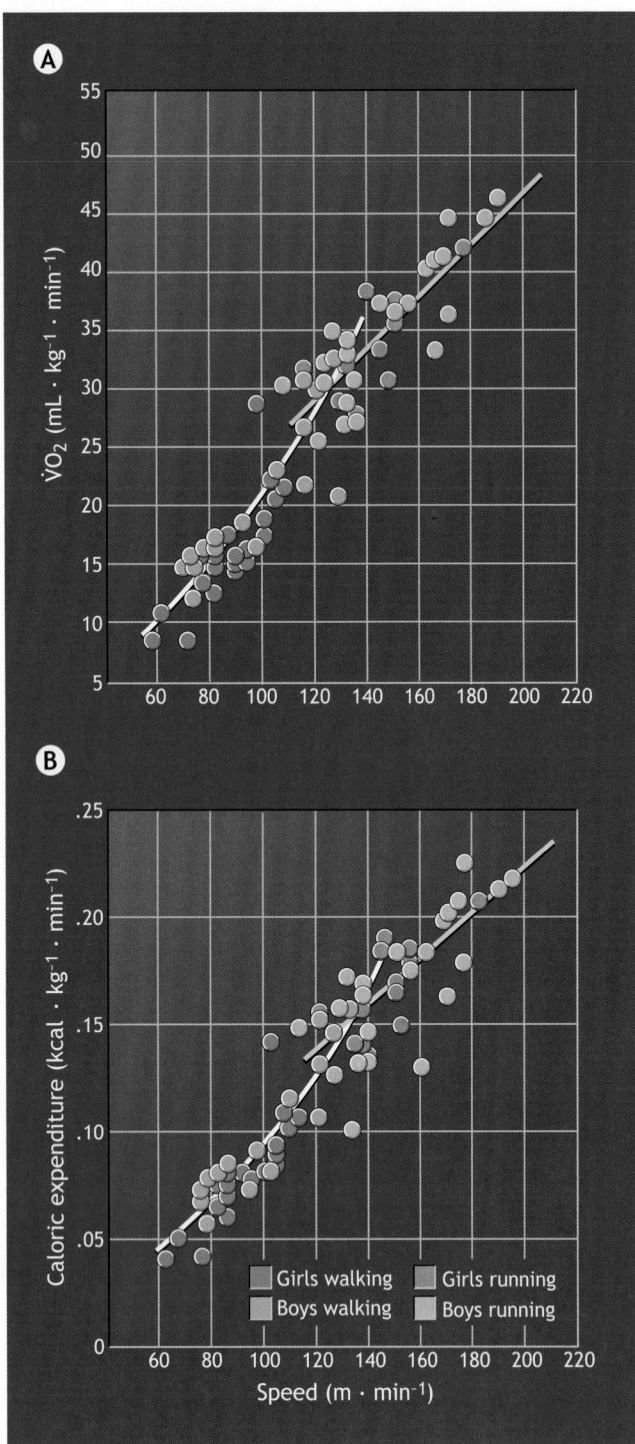

FIGURE 10.8 • Relationship between walking speed and running speed and oxygen consumption **(A)** and energy expenditure **(B)** in adolescent boys (N = 47) and girls (N = 35). The *white line* represents the curve of best fit for walking; the *orange line* represents the best-fit line for running. (Adapted with permission from Walker JL, et al. The energy cost of horizontal walking and running in adolescents. *Med Sci Sports Exerc* 1999;31:311.)

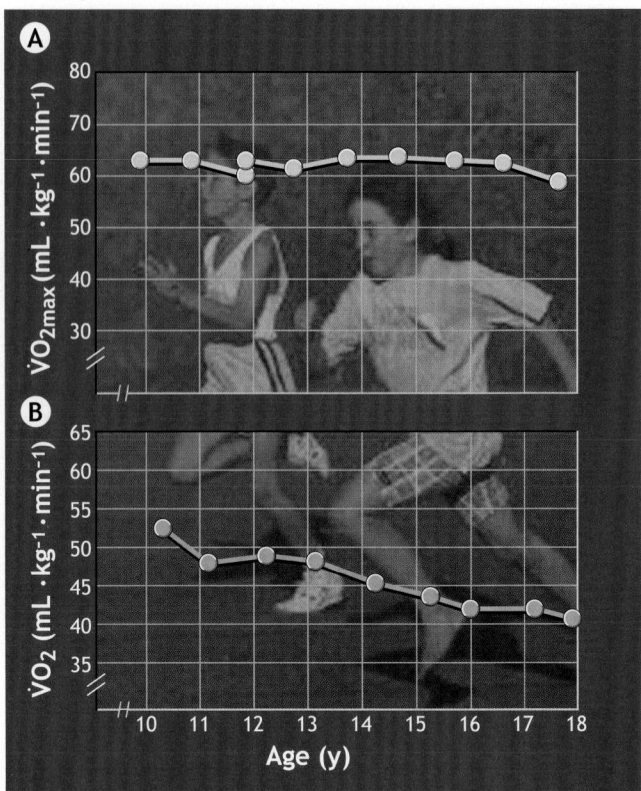

FIGURE 10.9 • Effects of age during childhood and adolescence on **(A)** aerobic capacity and **(B)** submaximal oxygen consumption during running at 202 m · min⁻¹. (Adapted with permission from Daniels J, et al. Differences and changes in $\dot{V}O_2$ among runners 10 to 18 years of age. *Med Sci Sports* 1978;10:200.)

 INTEGRATIVE QUESTION

Discuss the practical implications of knowing that children demonstrate lower economy for walking and running than adults.

Elite adolescent and adult endurance runners generally have lower oxygen consumption scores when running at a particular speed than less trained or less successful age-matched counterparts.[40,51] For trained runners, economy values and biomechanical characteristics during running remain fairly stable from day to day, even during intense running, with probably no difference between genders.[25,58,59]

Air Resistance

Anyone who has run into a headwind knows it requires greater effort or energy to maintain a given pace than running in calm air or with the wind at one's back. The effect of air resistance on energy expenditure of running varies with three factors:

1. Air density
2. Runner's projected surface area
3. Square of wind velocity

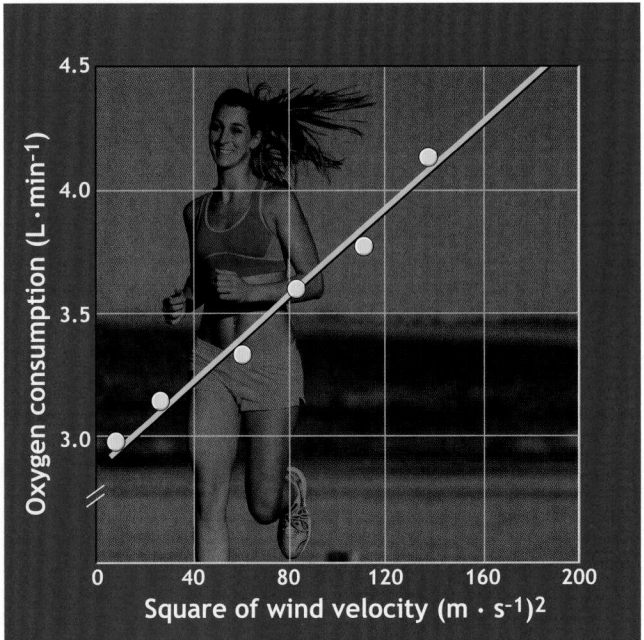

FIGURE 10.10 • Oxygen consumption as a function of the square of the wind velocity while running at 15.9 km · hr^{-1} against various headwinds. (Adapted with permission from Pugh LGCE. Oxygen intake and treadmill running with observations on the effect of air resistance. *J Physiol* 1970;207:823.)

Depending on speed, overcoming air resistance requires 3 to 9% of the total energy expenditure of running in calm air.[69] Running into a headwind creates an additional energy "expense." **Figure 10.10** shows that oxygen consumption while running at 15.9 km · hr^{-1} in calm conditions averaged 2.92 L · min^{-1}. This increased 5.5% to 3.09 L · min^{-1} against a 16-km · hr^{-1} headwind, and further to 4.1 L · min^{-1} when running against the strongest wind (66 km · hr^{-1}; 41 mph)—an additional 41% expenditure of energy to maintain running velocity.

Some have argued that running with a tailwind counterbalances the negative effects of running into a headwind. This does not occur, however, because the energy expenditure of cutting through a headwind exceeds the reduced oxygen consumption with an equivalent wind velocity at one's back.

Wind tunnel tests show that clothing modification or even trimming one's hair improves aerodynamics and reduces air resistance effects up to 6%. This magnitude of reduction translates into improved running performance, particularly for elite athletes. Wind velocity has less effect on energy expenditure at higher altitudes than at sea level because of the lower air density at higher elevations. Moderate altitude lowers oxygen consumption of competitive ice skating at a given speed compared with sea level.[3] An altitude effect also applies to the energy expenditure of running, cross-country skiing, and cycling.

Drafting: Beneficial Outcomes

The negative effect of air resistance and headwind on energy expenditure of running confirms the wisdom of running in an aerodynamically desirable position directly behind a competitor. This technique, called **drafting,** shelters the person taking advantage of it. Running 1 m behind another runner at a speed of 21.6 km · hr^{-1}, for example, decreases total energy expenditure by about 7%.[68] The beneficial effect of drafting on economy of effort also impacts cross-country skiing, short-track speed skating, and bicycling.[7,28,78] Bicycling at 40 km · hr^{-1} on a calm day requires about 90% of the total exercise power simply to overcome air resistance. At this speed, energy expenditure decreases 26 to 38% when a competitor closely follows another cyclist.[44]

For elite speed skaters, drafting within 1 meter of the leader during controlled-pace 4-min skating trials lowers exercise heart rate and blood lactate concentration.[78] A reduced level of physical stress with drafting should theoretically give the competitor an additional energy reserve for the crucial sprint to the finish. When triathletes draft during the cycling leg of a sprint-distance triathlon (0.75-km swim, 20-km bike, 5-km run), oxygen consumption, heart rate, and blood lactate concentrations remain lower than when the athletes cycle at the same speed without drafting.[38] These physiologic benefits translate into improved subsequent performance; maximal running speed after biking with drafting translates to faster running performance than without prior drafting.

More modern equipment also plays a role. For elite cyclists, helmets now weigh under 6 oz—less than a full can of soda. Helmet shape reduces drag by directing wind over the head and past the rider's back when leaning forward; adding dimples to the jersey reduces the drag, and microfiber polyester garments suck moisture away from the body to facilitate a cooler and drier ride. These economy-enhancing and thermal-optimizing modifications to equipment surely benefit world class–level performance.[20]

Treadmill Versus Track Running

The treadmill provides the primary exercise mode to evaluate the physiology of running. One might question the validity of this procedure for determining energy metabolism during running and relating it to competitive track performance. For example, does the energy required to run at a given treadmill speed equal that required to run on a track in calm weather? To answer this question, eight distance runners ran on a treadmill and track under calm air conditions at three submaximal speeds of 180 m · min^{-1}, 210 m · min^{-1}, and 260 m · min^{-1}. Graded running tests determined possible differences between treadmill and track running on maximal oxygen consumption. **Table 10.5** summarizes the results for one submaximal running speed and maximal exercise.

From a practical standpoint, no measurable differences emerged in the energy requirements of submaximal running up to 286 m · min^{-1} on the treadmill and track, either on level or up a grade, or between $\dot{V}O_{2max}$ in both activity modes. The possibility exists that at faster speeds achieved by elite endurance runners, the impact of air resistance on a calm day increases oxygen consumption in track running

TABLE 10.5	Comparison of Average Metabolic Responses During Treadmill and Track Running		
Measurement	**Treadmill**	**Track**	**Difference**
Submaximal Exercise			
Oxygen consumption, mL·kg⁻¹·min⁻¹	42.2	42.7	0.5
Respiratory exchange ratio	0.89	0.87	−0.02
Running speed, m·min⁻¹	213.7	216.8	3.1
Maximal Exercise			
Oxygen consumption, L·min⁻¹	4.40	4.44	0.04
mL·kg⁻¹·min⁻¹	66.9	66.3	−0.6
Ventilation, L·min⁻¹, BTPS	142.5	146.5	4.0
Respiratory exchange ratio	1.15	1.11	0.04

Adapted from McMiken DF, Daniels JT. Aerobic requirements and maximum aerobic power in treadmill and track running. *Med Sci Sports* 1976;8:14.

compared with "stationary" treadmill running at the same fast speed. This certainly occurs in activities requiring the athlete to move at high velocities in cycling and speed skating, where the retarding effects of air resistance become considerable.

Marathon Running

The current men's fastest marathon ever run is 2 hr:03 min:02 s (Geoffrey Mutai of Kenya, April 18, 2011, Boston Marathon). (Note: This run did not count as an official world record because the course did not meet international standards—too much downhill, too much tailwind; 5 months later, Kenyan Patrick Makau lowered the official world record to 2:03:38 in Berlin.) This average speed of 4 min:44 s per mile over the 26.2-mile course represents an extraordinary achievement in human running capacity. Not only does this blistering pace require a steady-rate oxygen consumption that exceeds the aerobic capacity of most male college students, it also demands that the marathoner sustain 80 to 90% of $\dot{V}O_{2max}$ for over 2 hr.

Researchers measured two distance runners during a marathon to assess minute-by-minute and total energy expenditure.[50] They determined oxygen consumption every 3 miles using open-circuit spirometry (see Chapter 8). Marathon times were 2 hr:36 min:34 s ($\dot{V}O_{2max}$ = 70.5 mL·kg⁻¹·min⁻¹) and 2 hr:39 min:28 s ($\dot{V}O_{2max}$ = 73.9 mL·kg⁻¹·min⁻¹). The first runner maintained an average speed of 16.2 km·hr⁻¹ that required an oxygen consumption equal to 80% of his $\dot{V}O_{2max}$. For the second runner, who averaged a slower speed of 16.0 km·hr⁻¹, the aerobic component averaged 78.3% of his maximum. For both men, the total energy required to run the marathon ranged between 2300 and 2400 kcal.

Exercise Economy and Muscle Fiber Type

Muscle fiber type affects economy of cycling effort. During submaximal cycling, the economies of trained cyclists varied up to 15%. Differences in muscle fiber types in the active muscles account for an important component of this variation. Cyclists

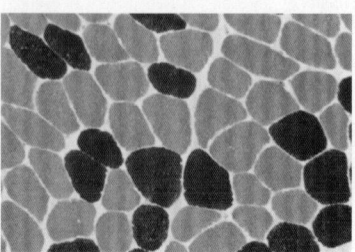

who exhibit the most economical cycling pattern possessed the greater percentage of slow-twitch (type I) muscle fibers in their legs. Type I fibers probably act with greater mechanical efficiency than faster-acting type II fibers.

SWIMMING

Swimming differs in several important aspects from walking or running. One obvious difference entails expenditure of energy to maintain buoyancy while simultaneously generating horizontal movement by using arms and legs, either in combination or separately. Other differences include requirements for overcoming **drag forces** that impede a swimmer's forward movement. The amount of drag depends on the fluid medium and the swimmer's size, shape, and velocity. These four factors contribute to a mechanical efficiency in front-crawl swimming that ranges between only 5 and 9.5%.[88] *A considerably lower mechanical efficiency makes the energy expenditure during swimming a given distance average about four times more than the energy expenditure running the same distance.*

Methods of Measurement

Subjects can hold their breath for short swims of 25 yards at different velocities. Oxygen consumption during a 20- to 40-min recovery provides an estimate of energy expenditure. For longer swims, including 12- to 14-hr endurance events, one can compute energy expenditure from oxygen consumption measured with open-circuit spirometry during portions of the swim. **FIGURE 10.11A AND B** shows the first attempts to measure oxygen uptake of a swimmer in 1919 by pioneering Swedish researcher-physicians Göran Liljestrand and Nils Stenström.[47] **FIGURE 10.11C** illustrates the oxygen uptake measurement conducted in a swimming pool where the researcher walks alongside the swimmer and carries portable gas-collection equipment.[41]

For another form of swimming test to estimate maximum capacity, the subject remains stationary while attached or tethered to a cable and pulley system by a belt worn around the waist. Periodic increases in the weight stack attached to the cable force the swimmer to exert greater effort to maintain a constant body position. Another form of measurement makes use of a flume or "swimming treadmill." Water circulates at velocities varying from a slow swimming speed to near-record pace for a freestyle sprint. Aerobic capacity measurements using tethered, free, or flume swimming produce

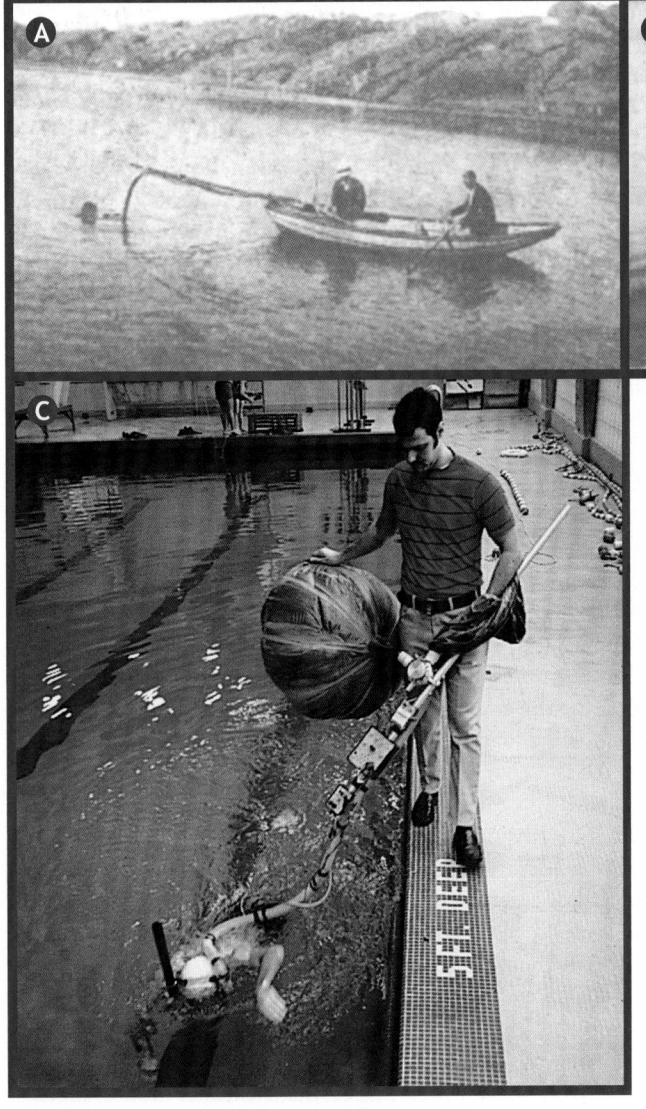

FIGURE 10.11 • (A, B) First recorded open-circuit spirometry measurements in 1919 of oxygen consumption during swimming. The swimmer used a snorkel-type mouthpiece connected to a flexible hose, and the investigators rowed alongside the swimmer. Expired air was collected in canisters and taken back to the laboratory for analysis. (Reprinted with permission from Liljestrand G, Stenström. Studien über die physiologie des schwimmens. *N Scan Arch Physiol* 1920;39:1.) **(C)** In this example of open-circuit spirometry, the investigator walks alongside the swimmer to collect expired air for later laboratory analyses for oxygen consumption.

essentially identical values.[9] Any of these modes of measurement objectively evaluate metabolic and physiologic dynamics and capacities during swimming.

Energy Expenditure and Drag

Total drag force encountered by a swimmer consists of three components:

1. **Wave drag**—caused by waves that build up in front of and form hollows behind the swimmer moving through the water. This component of drag does not significantly affect swimming at slow velocities, but its influence increases at faster swimming speeds.
2. **Skin friction drag**—produced as water slides over the skin surface. Even at fast swimming velocities, the quantitative contribution of skin friction drag to the total drag remains small. Research supports the common practice of swimmers "shaving down" to reduce skin friction drag and thereby decrease energy expenditure.[81]
3. **Viscous pressure drag**—caused by the pressure differential created in front of and behind the swimmer, which substantially counters propulsive efforts at slow velocities. Viscous pressure drag forms adjacent to the swimmer from separation of a thin sheet of water or boundary layer. Its effect decreases for highly skilled swimmers who master streamline stroke mechanics. The effect of such enhanced techniques reduce the separation region by moving it closer to the trailing edge of the water, akin to an oar slicing through water with the blade parallel rather than perpendicular to the water flow.

Ways to Reduce Drag Force Effects

Figure 10.12 depicts a curvilinear relationship between body drag and velocity when towing a swimmer through the water. As velocity increases above 0.8 m·s⁻¹, drag decreases by supporting the legs with a flotation device that places the body in a more hydrodynamically desirable horizontal position. Generally, drag force averages 2 to 2.5 times more during swimming than passive towing.[86]

Variations in swimsuit designs tend to reduce overall drag when compared to conventional suits, with positive effects noted for suits that cover the body from the shoulder to either the ankle or knee and for those that cover only the lower body.[17,57] Wet suits worn by triathletes during swimming reduce body drag by about 14%, thus lowering oxygen consumption at a given speed.[87,89] Improved swimming economy largely explains the faster swim times of triathletes who wear wet suits. As in running, cross-country skiing, and cycling, drafting in swimming by following up to 50 cm behind the toes of a lead swimmer reduces drag force, metabolic cost (by 11 to 38%), and physiologic demand,[4,19] and improves economy in a subsequent cycling session.[26] This effect enables an endurance triathlete or ocean racer to conserve energy and possibly improve performance toward the end of competition. Triathletes swimming 400 m swam the total distance 3% faster in a drafting position with lower blood lactate and stroke rate compared to swimming in the lead position.[18] Performance changes coincided with large reductions in passive drag

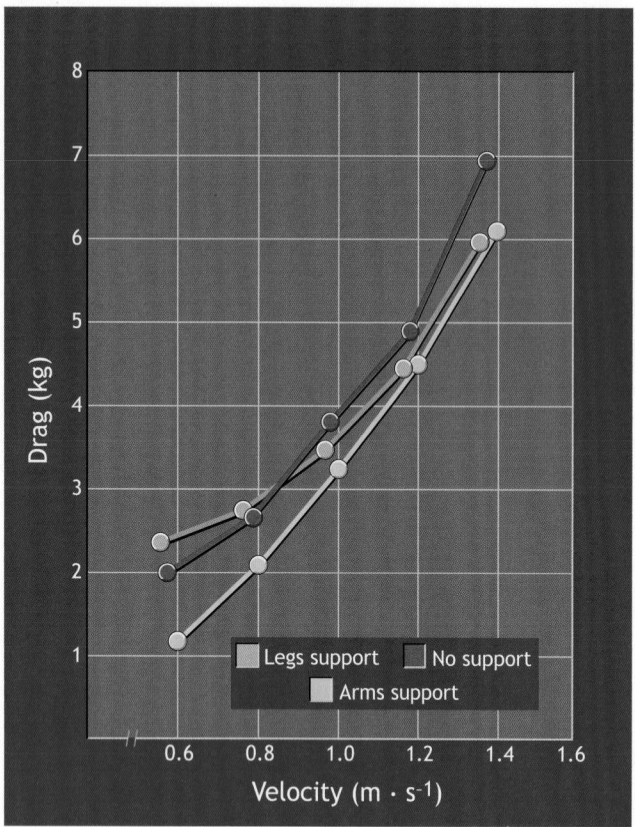

FIGURE 10.12 • Drag force in three different prone positions related to towing velocity. (Adapted with permission from Holmér I. Energy cost of arm stroke, leg kick, and the whole stroke in competitive swimming styles. *Eur J Appl Physiol* 1974;33:105.)

force in the drafting position; faster and leaner swimmers showed the greatest drag force reduction and performance improvement.

In the 2004 Athens Summer Olympic Games, swimmers for the first time wore neck-to-ankle body suits. Proponents maintain that the technology-driven approach to competitive swimming maximizes swimming economy by trapping air between the suit and the body and allows swimmers to achieve 3% faster times than times with standard swimsuits. These hi-tech suits were used up to 2009, when the International Swimming Federation (FINA; www.fina.org) banned them after the world championships. All world records using these suits were allowed up to 2010. Male and female swimmers who used these suits set 108 world records (30 in 2009).

Kayaking. The energy demands of kayaking largely reflect the resistance provided by the water to the craft's forward movement. Consequently, drafting or "wash riding" behind a competitor reduces the energy requirements of paddling between 18 and 32%.[65] The assist to forward movement provided by the wash generated by the lead boat improves kayaking economy. This effect decreases resistance and water pressure that impacts boat movement.

Energy Expenditure, Swimming Velocity, and Skill

Elite swimmers swim a particular stroke at a given velocity with greater economy than less trained or recreational swimmers. Highly skilled swimmers use more of the energy they generate per stroke to overcome drag forces. Consequently, they cover a greater distance per stroke than less skilled swimmers who in effect "waste" considerable energy in moving the water during the swim. FIGURE 10.13A compares the oxygen consumptions and velocities for breaststroke, back crawl, and front crawl at three levels of swimming ability. One subject, a recreational swimmer, did not participate in swim training; the trained subject, a top Swedish swimmer, swam on a daily basis; the elite swimmer was a European champion. Except during the breaststroke, the elite swimmer had a lower oxygen consumption at a given speed than trained and untrained swimmers. FIGURE 10.13B illustrates that the breaststroke required greater oxygen consumption for the trained swimmers at any speed, followed by the backstroke, with the front crawl being the least "expensive" of the three strokes. The marked accelerations and decelerations within each stroke cycle cause the energy expended for the butterfly and breaststroke to nearly double that for front and back crawl at the same speeds.[85] At comparable speeds sustained aerobically, the energy expenditure of surface swimming with fins was about 40% lower than swimming without them.[90]

Effects of Water Temperature

Relatively cold water places the swimmer under thermal stress. Swimming in colder water initiates different metabolic and cardiovascular adjustments than swimming in warmer water. These responses primarily maintain a stable core temperature by compensating for considerable heat loss from the body, particularly at water temperatures below 77°F (25°C). Body heat loss occurs most readily in lean swimmers who lack the benefits of the insulatory effects of subcutaneous fat.

FIGURE 10.14 illustrates oxygen consumption during breaststroke swimming at water temperatures of 64.4°F (18°C), 78.8°F (26°C), and 91.4°F (33°C). Regardless of swimming speed, cold water produced the highest oxygen consumptions. The body begins to shiver in cold water to regulate core temperature; this accounts for the higher energy expenditure when swimming in lower water temperatures. For individuals with an average body fat percentage , optimal water temperature for competitive swimming ranges between 82°F and 86°F (28°C and 30°C). Within this range, metabolic heat generated during this mode of exercise readily transfers to the water. Nevertheless, the heat flow gradient from the body is not large enough to stimulate shivering (which would

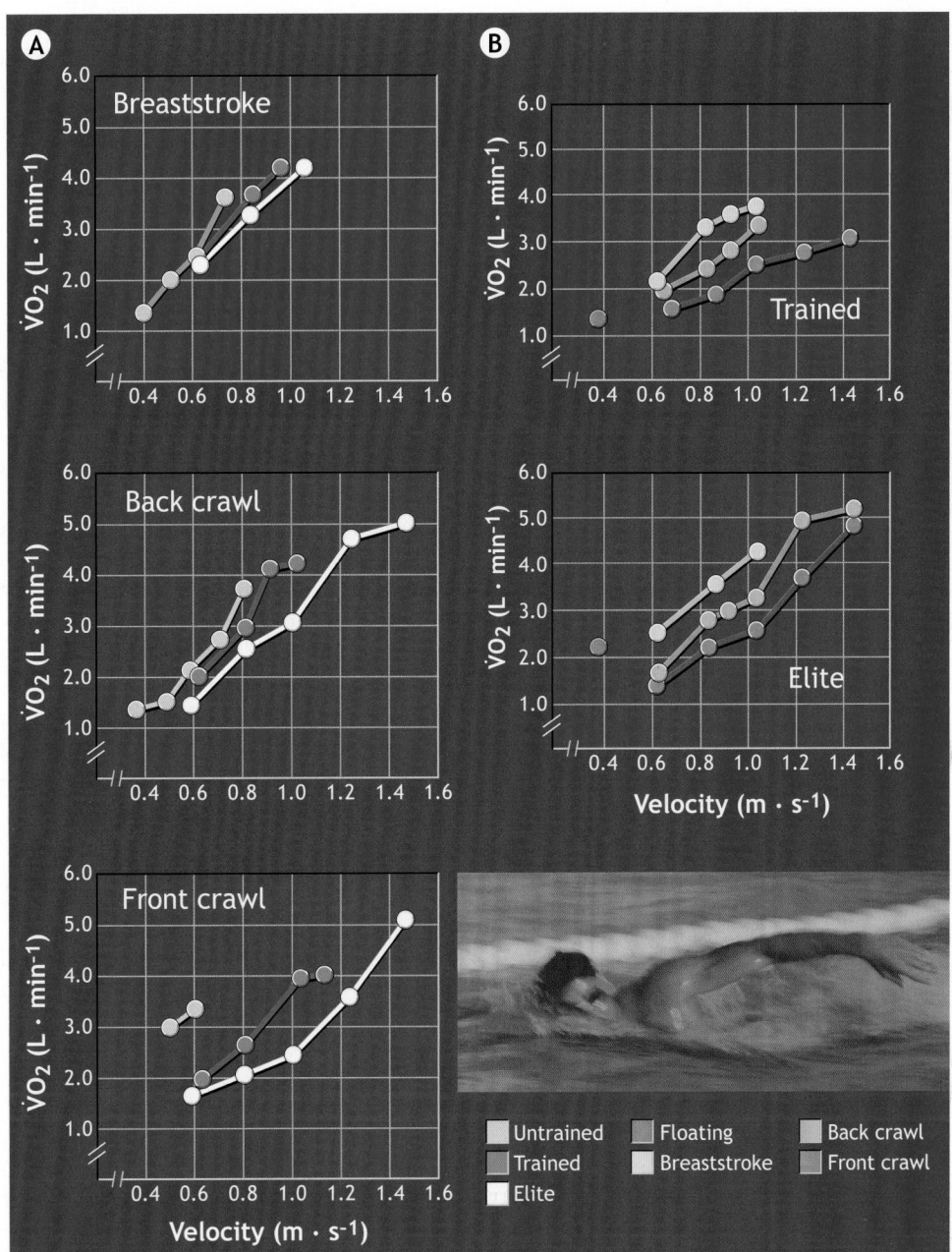

FIGURE 10.13 • **(A)** Oxygen consumption related to swimming velocity for the breaststroke, front crawl, and back crawl in subjects at three levels of skill ability. **(B)** Oxygen consumption for two trained swimmers during three competitive strokes. (Adapted with permission from Holmér I. Oxygen uptake during swimming in man. *J Appl Physiol* 1972;33:502.)

increase energy metabolism) or to reduce core temperature from cold stress.

Effects of Buoyancy: Men Versus Women

Women of all ages possess, on average, a higher body fat percentage than men. Fat readily floats and muscle and bone sink in water, allowing the average woman to gain a hydrodynamic lift and expends less energy to stay afloat than the average man. More than likely, gender differences in percentage body

fat and thus body buoyancy partially explain women's greater swimming economy. For example, women swim a given distance at about 30% lower total energy expenditure than men. Expressed another way, women achieve higher swimming velocities than men at the same energy expenditure.

Women also show a greater peripheral body fat distribution. This causes their legs and arms to float relatively high in water, making them more streamlined. In contrast, the leaner legs of men tend to swing down and float lower in the water.[14] Lowering the legs to a deeper position increases body drag and reduces swimming economy (see Fig. 10.12). Enhanced

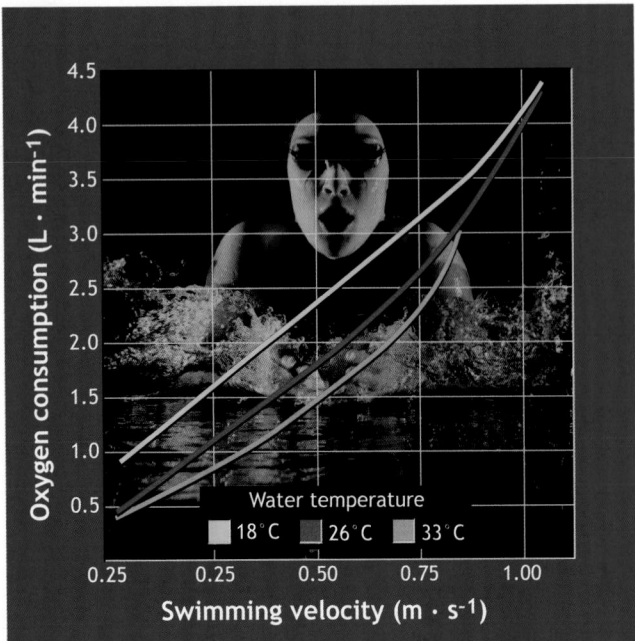

FIGURE 10.14 • Energy expenditure for the breaststroke at three water temperatures related to swimming velocity. (Adapted with permission from Nadel ER, et al. Energy exchanges of swimming man. *J Appl Physiol* 1974;36:465.)

flotation and the females' smaller body size, which also reduces drag, contribute to the gender difference in swimming economy.[85,86] The potential hydrodynamic benefits that women possess become evident during longer distance ocean swims because swimming economy and body insulation contribute to success. For example, the women's record for swimming the 21-mile English Channel from England to France equals

7 hr:25 min:15 s (Yvetta Hlavacova; Czech Republic, 2006). The men's record (Trent Grimsey; Australia, 2012) equals 6 hr:55 min, a difference of only 6.8% (**http://www.channelswimming.com/swim-list.htm**). In several instances, women swam faster than men. In fact, the first woman to successfully cross the Channel in 1926 swam 35% faster than the first male to complete the swim in 1875 (**TABLE 10.6**).

Endurance Swimmers

Distance swimming in ocean water poses a severe metabolic and physiologic challenge. A study of nine English Channel swimmers included measurements taken under race conditions in a saltwater pool at swimming speeds that ranged from 2.6 to 4.9 km·hr^{-1}.[70] During the race, competitors maintained a constant stroke rate and pace until the last few hours, when fatigue set in. From detailed observations of one male subject, the average speed of 2.85 km·hr^{-1} during a 12-hr swim required an average oxygen consumption of 1.7 L O$_2$·min^{-1}, or an equivalent energy expenditure of 8.5 kcal·min^{-1}. The gross caloric expenditure for the 12-hour swim was about 6120 kcal (8.5 kcal × 60 min × 12 hr). The net energy expenditure of swimming the English Channel, assuming a resting energy expenditure of 1.2 kcal·min^{-1} (0.260 L O$_2$·min^{-1}), exceeded 5200 kcal or approximately twice the number of calories expended running a marathon.

 INTEGRATIVE QUESTION

Discuss whether swim training improves swimming economy more than run training improves running economy.

| TABLE 10.6 | Comparisons of English Channel World Record Swimming Times Between Men and Women |

English Channel Records (Hr:Min): Male Versus Female			
Record	**Male**	**Female**	**% Difference (male:female)**
First attempt–one way	21:45 (1875)	14:39 (1926)	34.9
Fastest–one way	**07:17 (1994)**	**7:40 (1978)**	**−5.26**
Youngest–one way	11:54 (11 y, 11 mo; 1988)	15:28 (12 y, 11 mo; 1983)	−29.9
Oldest–one way	18:37 (67 y; 1987)	12:32 (57 y; 1999)	32.69
Fastest–two way	16:10 (1987)	17:14 (1991)	−6.6
Fastest–three way	28:21 (1987)	34:40 (1990)	−22.2

Adapted with permission from Katch VL, McArdle WD, Katch FI. *Essentials of Exercise Physiology.* 4th Ed. Philadelphia: Wolters Kluwer Health, 2011. Note that for two records (first attempt, oldest) females bettered the male record by more than 30%.

Summary

1. Total or gross energy expenditure includes the resting energy requirement; net energy expenditure represents the energy expenditure of the activity excluding the resting value.

2. Economy of movement refers to the oxygen consumed during steady-rate exercise.

3. Mechanical efficiency evaluates the relationship between work accomplished and energy expended doing the work.

4. Walking, running, and cycling produce mechanical efficiencies between 20 and 25%. Efficiencies decrease below 20% for activities with considerable resistance to movement (drag).

5. A linear relationship exists between walking speed and oxygen consumption at normal walking speeds. Walking on sand requires about twice the energy as walking on firm surfaces. A proportionately larger energy expenditure exists for heavier persons during weight-bearing physical activities.

6. Running becomes more economical than walking at speeds that exceed 8 km·hr^{-1}.

7. Handheld and ankle weights can increase the energy expenditure of walking to values similar to running.

8. The total caloric expenditure of running a given distance at steady-rate oxygen consumption remains about the same independent of running speed.

9. Net energy expenditure during horizontal running approximates 1 kcal·kg^{-1}·km^{-1}.

10. Shortening running stride and increasing stride frequency to maintain a constant running speed requires less energy than lengthening stride and reducing frequency.

11. An individual subconsciously "selects" the combination of stride length and frequency to favor optimal economy of movement, which represents a level of minimum effort.

12. Energy expended to overcome air resistance accounts for 3 to 9% of the energy expenditure of running in calm air. This percentage increases considerably when a runner maintains pace while running into a brisk headwind.

13. Children generally require more oxygen to transport their body mass while running than do adults. A relatively lower running economy accounts for the poorer endurance performance of children compared with adults of similar aerobic capacity.

14. Running a given distance or speed on a treadmill requires similar energy output as running on a track under identical environmental conditions.

15. A person expends about four times more energy to swim a given distance than to run the same distance because of greater energy to maintain buoyancy and overcome drag forces in swimming.

16. Elite swimmers expend fewer calories to swim a given stroke at any velocity than less skilled counterparts.

17. Significant gender differences exist in body drag, mechanical efficiency, and net oxygen consumption during swimming. Women swim a given distance at approximately 30% lower energy expenditure than men.

18. The net energy expenditure of swimming the English Channel exceeds 5200 kcal or approximately twice the calories expended running a marathon.

the**Point** References are available online at
http://thepoint.lww.com/mkk8e.

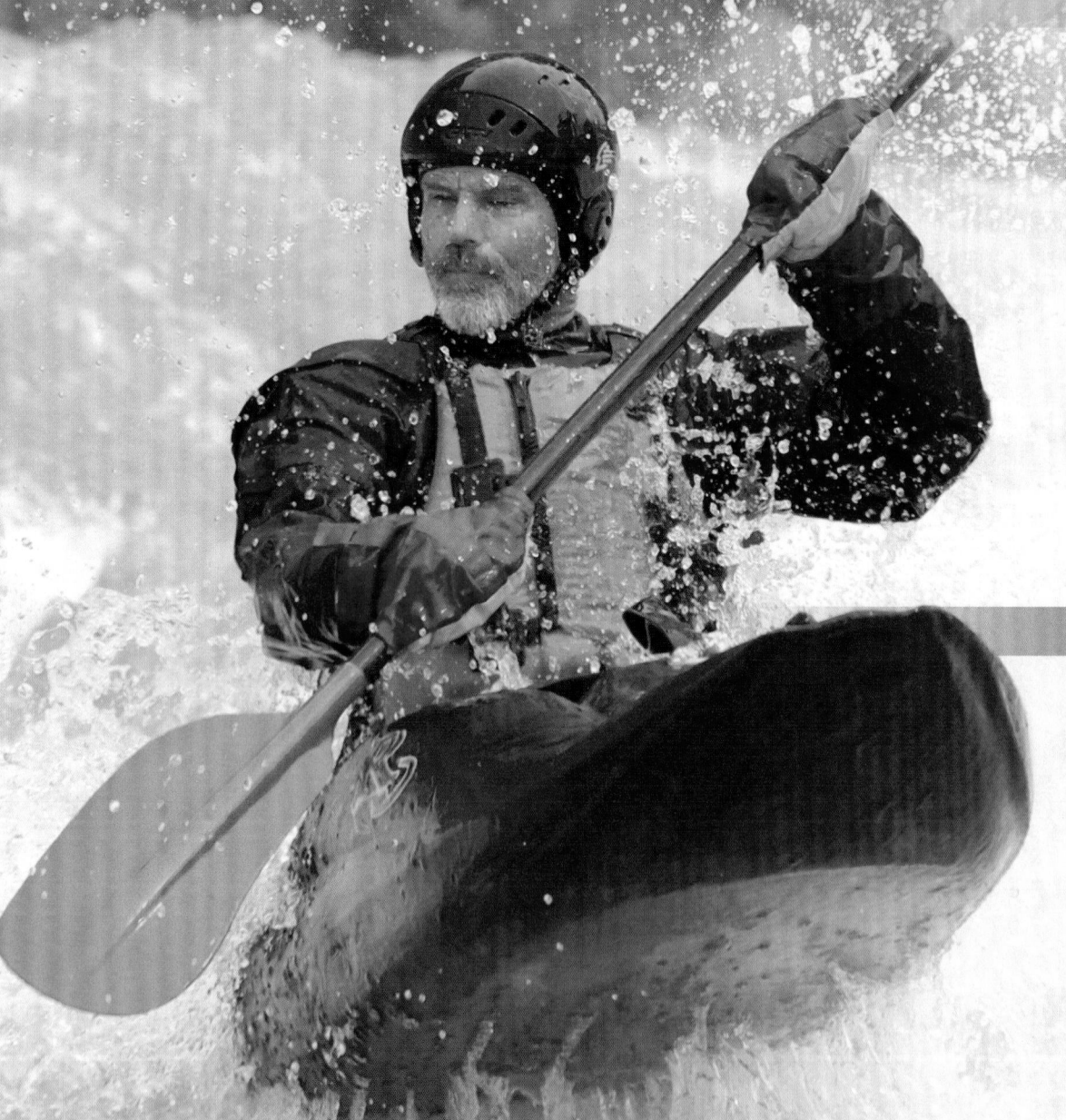

Individual Differences and Measurement of Energy Capacities

CHAPTER OBJECTIVES

- Explain specificity and generality as they apply to physical performance and physiologic functions

- Outline the anaerobic-to-aerobic exercise energy transfer continuum

- Describe two practical "field tests" to evaluate power output capacity of the immediate energy system

- Describe a common test to evaluate power output capacity of the short-term energy system

- Explain how motivation, buffering, and physical training influence the glycolytic energy pathway

- Define maximal oxygen consumption and its physiologic significance

- Differentiate between maximal oxygen consumption and peak oxygen consumption

- Define graded exercise test and list criteria that indicate attainment of a "true" $\dot{V}O_{2max}$ during graded exercise testing

- Outline three common treadmill protocols to assess $\dot{V}O_{2max}$

- Indicate the influence of each of the following six factors on $\dot{V}O_{2max}$: activity mode, heredity, state of training, gender, body composition, and age

- Describe a walking field test to predict $\dot{V}O_{2max}$

- List three assumptions to predict $\dot{V}O_{2max}$ from submaximal exercise heart rate

ANCILLARIES ● at-a-Glance

Visit http://thePoint.lww.com/mkk8e to access the following resources.

- References: Chapter 11
- Interactive Question Bank
- Focus on Research: An important Measure of Cardiorespiratory Functional Capacity

SPECIFICITY VERSUS GENERALITY OF METABOLIC CAPACITY AND EXERCISE PERFORMANCE

The body derives useful energy from different metabolic pathways, yet considerable variability exists among individuals in capacity for each form of energy transfer. The extent of individual variability underlies the concept of **individual differences** in metabolic capacity. A high $\dot{V}O_{2max}$ in running, for example, does not necessarily ensure a similarly high $\dot{V}O_{2max}$ when using the different muscle groups required in swimming and rowing. That some individuals with high aerobic power in one activity possess above-average aerobic power in other activities illustrates the **generality principle** of metabolic function.

The nonoverlapped areas in **FIGURE 11.1** represent **specificity** of metabolic function among the body's three energy systems, while the three overlapped portions represent generality. In the broadest sense, specificity indicates a low likelihood for an individual to excel in each of a particular sport's sprint, middle-distance, and long-distance competitions. In a more narrow definition of metabolic and physiologic specificity, most individuals do not possess an equally high energy-generating capacity for aerobic activities as different as running (lower-body) and swimming or arm-crank (upper-body) exercises.

Based on the **specificity concept**, training to achieve a high aerobic power ($\dot{V}O_{2max}$) contributes little to one's capacity to generate energy anaerobically, and vice versa. A high degree of specificity also exists for the effects of physical training on neuromuscular patterning and demands. *Terms such as "speed," "power," and "endurance" must be applied precisely within the context of the specific movement patterns and specific metabolic and physiologic requirements of the activity.*

This chapter evaluates the capacity of the three energy-transfer systems discussed in Chapters 6 and 7, with emphasis on individual differences, specificity, and appropriate measurement.

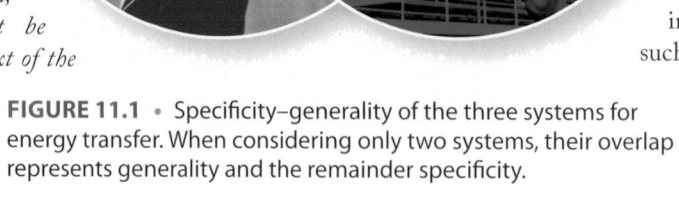

FIGURE 11.1 • Specificity–generality of the three systems for energy transfer. When considering only two systems, their overlap represents generality and the remainder specificity.

Long-term energy system

Immediate energy system

Short-term energy system

INTEGRATIVE QUESTION

Explain why it is important that a triathlete train in each of the sport's three events.

OVERVIEW OF ENERGY-TRANSFER CAPACITY DURING EXERCISE

The immediate and short-term energy systems predominantly power all-out movements for up to 2 min. Both systems operate anaerobically. A greater reliance on anaerobic energy exists for fast, short-duration movements or when increasing resistance to movement at a given speed.

FIGURE 11.2 illustrates the relative activation of anaerobic and aerobic energy-transfer systems for different durations of all-out effort. When movement begins at either fast or slow speed, intramuscular high-energy phosphates adenosine triphosphate (ATP) and phosphocreatine (PCr) provide immediate energy to power muscle action. Following the first few seconds of movement, glycolytic pathways generate an increasingly greater percentage of total energy required for continuous ATP resynthesis. Continued activity places progressively greater demands on the long-term aerobic system. All physical activities and sports lend themselves to classification on an immediate-to-glycolytic-to-aerobic continuum. Some activities rely predominantly on a single system of energy transfer, whereas most require activation of more than one energy system depending on intensity and duration. Performing at a higher intensity but shorter duration of effort requires a markedly increased demand on anaerobic energy transfer. The fact that specific metabolic requirements of intense physical activity vary with the duration of effort and because of the highly specific nature of one's metabolic capacity (nonoverlapped areas in Fig. 11.1) largely explain the great difficulty to excel in diverse sport performances such as sprint, middle-distance, endurance, and ultraendurance running events.

ANAEROBIC ENERGY TRANSFER: THE IMMEDIATE AND SHORT-TERM ENERGY SYSTEMS

Performance Tests to Evaluate the Immediate Energy System

Football, weightlifting, and other short-duration, maximal-effort activities that require rapid energy release rely nearly exclusively on energy from the intramuscular high-energy phosphates. Performance tests that maximally activate the

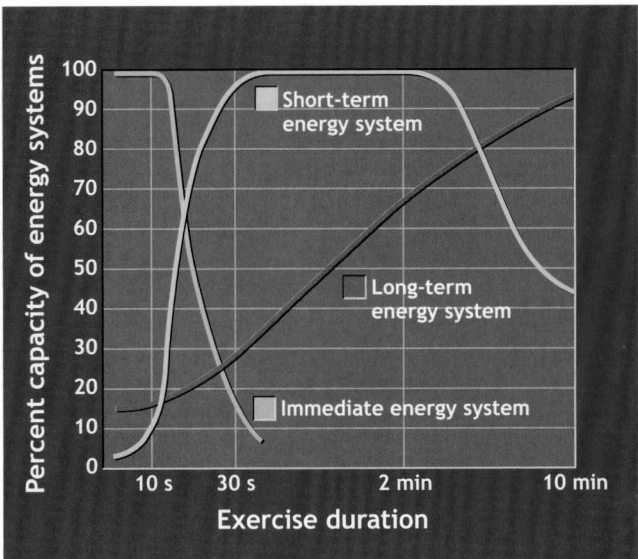

FIGURE 11.2 • Three systems of energy transfer and percentage use of their total capacity during all-out physical activity of different durations.

ATP–PCr energy system serve as practical field tests to evaluate the capacity for "immediate" energy transfer. Two assumptions underlie use of performance test scores to infer the power-generating capacity of the high-energy phosphates:

1. All ATP at maximal power output regenerates via ATP–PCr hydrolysis
2. Adequate ATP and PCr exist to support maximal effort for about 6 s duration.

The term *power test* generally describes these measures of brief, maximal capacity. Power in this context refers to the time-rate of accomplishing work; it computes as follows:

$$P = (FD) \div T$$

where F equals *force* generated, D equals *distance* the force moves, and T represents exercise *time* or duration. Power is expressed in watts: 1 watt equals 0.73756 ft-lb·s⁻¹, 0.01433 kcal·min⁻¹, 1.341 × 10⁻³ hp (or 0.0013 hp), or 6.12 kg-m·min⁻¹.

Stair-Sprinting Power Tests

Figure 11.3 illustrates a practical way to evaluate high-energy phosphate power output. This relatively simple performance test assesses power output by recording the time required to run up a staircase, three steps at a time, as fast as possible. External work accomplished consists of total vertical distance traversed up the stairs; the distance for six stairs usually equals 1.05 m. For example, the power output of a 65-kg woman who traverses six steps in 0.52 s computes as follows:

$$F = 65 \text{ kg}$$
$$D = 1.05 \text{ m}$$
$$T = 0.52 \text{ s}$$
$$\text{Power} = (65 \text{ kg} \times 1.05 \text{ m}) \div 0.52 \text{ s}$$
$$= 131.3 \text{ kg-m} \cdot \text{s}^{-1} \text{ (1287 watts)}$$

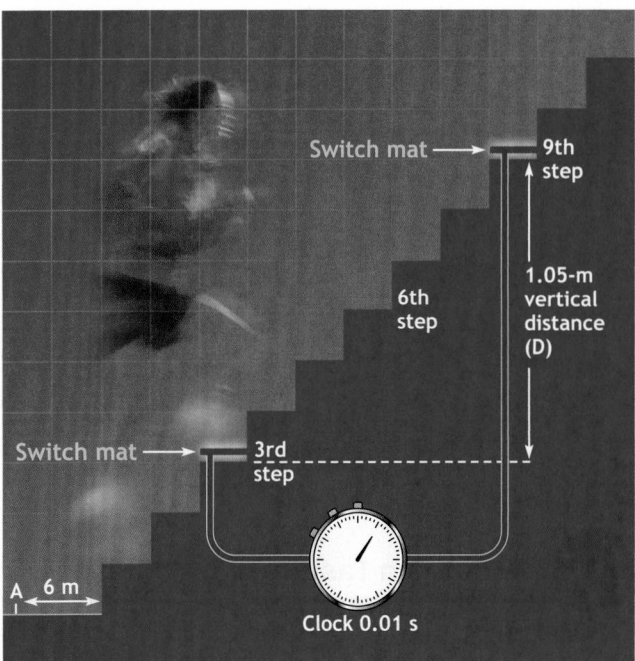

FIGURE 11.3 • Stair-sprinting power test. The subject begins at point A and runs as fast as possible up a flight of stairs, taking three steps at a time. Electric switch mats placed on the steps record the time needed to cover the distance between stairs 3 and 9 to the nearest 0.01 s. Power output equals the product of the subject's body mass (F) and vertical distance covered (D), divided by the time (T).

Based on the equation, body mass influences power calculations in stair-sprinting tests because a heavier person who achieves the same speed as a lighter counterpart would achieve a higher power score. This implies that the heavier person possesses a more highly developed immediate energy system. Unfortunately, no direct evidence justifies this conclusion; athletes, coaches, and trainers must use care interpreting differences in stair-sprinting power scores and inferring individual differences in ATP–PCr energy-transfer capacity among individuals who differ in body weight. *The test should be used with individuals of similar body mass or the same individuals before and after specific training designed to develop leg power output from the immediate energy system (assuming no change in body mass).*

 ## INTEGRATIVE QUESTION

Considering training specificity, describe how to test the power output capacity of the immediate energy system of volleyball players, swimmers, and soccer players.

Jumping-Power Tests

The popular vertical jump-and-reach test or a standing broad jump often appear in physical fitness test batteries as measures of immediate energy power output. The vertical jump score reflects the difference between a person's standing reach and maximum vertical jump-and-touch height. The broad jump score consists of the horizontal distance traversed in a leap from a semi-crouched position. Both tests purport to measure leg power, but they probably fail to achieve this goal. For example, jump tests generate power to propel the body from the crouched position only while the feet maintain contact with the surface. *This extremely brief period of muscle activation probably does not adequately evaluate a person's maximal ATP/PCr energy transfer capacity.* Also, we are aware of no data to show a relationship between jump-test scores and actual ATP–PCr levels or depletion patterns in the primary muscles activated during the jump.

What is a Fast Runner?

The world's fastest human, Jamaican sprinter Usain Bolt, reached a top speed of nearly 28 mph during his world record 100-m dash at the 2012 London Olympics. But this speed appears rather sluggish among other land animals. The cheetah captures gold every time by accelerating to a speed of 60 mph in just 3 s while reaching a top speed of 70 mph over distances of up to 1000 ft. The pronghorn antelope garners the silver medal in a sprint with a top speed of 60 mph over short distances, while averaging a speed of 40 mph for more than 30 min. At this speed, the pronghorn would complete the Boston Marathon in 40 min compared to the fastest human's time for the 26.2-mile run of 123 min.

Other Power Performance Tests

Figure 11.2 suggests that any all-out physical effort of 6 to 8 s probably reflects a person's capacity for immediate power performance from high-energy phosphates in the specific muscles activated. Other possible tests include sprint-running or cycling, brief shuttle runs, and localized movements produced by arm-cranking or leg movements.

Interrelationships Among Power Performance Tests

If the various power tests measure the same "general" metabolic capacity, then individuals who perform best on one test should rank correspondingly high on a second or third different test. Unfortunately, this does not usually occur to any great extent. Although some individuals who score well on one power performance test tend to score well on another test, a poor relationship generally exists.[87] **Table 11.1** shows the interrelationship (expressed statistically as a correlation coefficient) between several tests purported to measure immediate energy power output. The relationship ranges from poor

TABLE 11.1	Correlations Among Measures of Immediate Anaerobic Power Output	
Variable	Jump and Reach	Stair-Sprinting
40-yard dash	−0.48[a]	−0.88[a]
Jump and reach	—	−0.31[a]

From the Applied Physiology Laboratory, University of Michigan ($N = 31$ males).
[a]Negative correlations mean faster times (lower scores) associate with higher jumps or greater power outputs.

to good, depending on the test. The fairly strong relationship between stair-sprinting power test scores and 40-yard dash scores ($r = -0.88$) indicates that one can obtain almost the same information on short-term power performance through sprint running on a track as the more elaborate procedures required in the stair sprint.

Several factors explain relatively low relationships among the other power test scores. First, human exercise performance remains highly task specific. From a metabolic and performance perspective, this means that the best sprint runner does not necessarily rank as the best sprint swimmer, sprint cyclist, "stair sprinter," or "arm cranker." While it is true that identical metabolic reactions generate energy to power each performance, these reactions occur within the specific muscles activated by exercise. Each specific test also requires different neuromuscular and skill components that introduce variability and specificity into test scores.

Power tests offer an excellent means for self-testing and motivation. They also can serve as a means for training the immediate energy system. For example, football coaches use the 40-yard dash for power training and as a test to evaluate football speed. Forty-yard dash test scores may provide relevant information concerning "speed" in football, even though no data exist to quantify how a 40-yard sprint in a straight line relates to all of the complex skills and movements involved in game performance, let alone some general factor of overall football ability. A run test of shorter distances (up to 20 yards) and/or with multiple changes in direction and pacing would probably provide a more appropriate, task-specific performance to assess the likelihood of football success.

Tests to Evaluate the Immediate Energy System

Several physiologic and biochemical measures evaluate energy-generating capacity of the immediate energy system. These include the following:

1. Size of the intramuscular ATP–PCr pool
2. Depletion rates of ATP and PCr in all-out, short-duration activity.

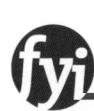

High-Intensity Interval Training (HIIT) Reduces Fat in Overweight Young Males

Forty-six overweight males (BMI = 48.4) participated in a 12-week high-intensity interval training (HIIT) program that included supervised 8-s sprints with 12-s recovery continuously throughout a 20-min session once daily for 12 weeks. Aerobic power improved by 15% for the training group compared to controls. Abdominal and trunk adiposity also were reduced in the training group by 0.1 kg and 1.5 kg, and a 17% reduction in visceral fat after 12 weeks of HIIT.

Source: Heydari M, et al. The effect of high-intensity intermittent exercise on body composition of overweight young males. *J Obes* 2012;2012:480467.

ATP and PCr depletion rates provide the most direct estimate and correlate highly with physical performance assessments of the immediate energy system. For example, one experiment determined muscle PCr depletion at different intervals of a 100-m sprint, using the muscle biopsy technique.[35] Compared with resting values (22 mmol·kg wet weight^{-1}), PCr decreased by 60% during the first 40 m (<6 s) and only another 20% for the remainder of the sprint. It remains nearly impossible with current technology to readily obtain precise biochemical data during all-out effort of brief duration. Researchers must rely on the "face validity" of the various specific performance measures as satisfactory markers to evaluate capacity for ATP–PCr energy transfer in physical activity.

Performance Test Evaluation of the Short-Term Energy System

Figure 11.2 shows that when all-out physical effort continues for longer than a few seconds, the short-term energy system (glycolysis) generates increasingly more of the energy for ATP resynthesis. This does not mean that aerobic metabolism is unimportant at this stage of activity or that oxygen-consuming reactions have not "switched on." To the contrary, the contribution of aerobic energy transfer increases early in physical activity.[83] During short-duration maximal effort, the energy requirement greatly exceeds energy generated by hydrogen oxidation in the respiratory chain. Consequently, glycolytic production of ATP predominates, with subsequent quantities of lactate accumulating in active muscle and ultimately in blood. *Blood lactate level provides the most common indicator of activation of the short-term glycolytic energy system.*

Unlike tests for maximal oxygen consumption, no specific criteria exist to indicate that a person has attained maximal glycolytic effort. More than likely, self-motivation and testing environment greatly influence performance on such tests.[104] Performance test scores show good reproducibility from day to day, particularly under standardized conditions.[4,51,63]

Performances that activate the short-term energy system require maximal effort for up to 3 min. All-out runs and stationary cycling have usually assessed anaerobic power, as have shuttle runs and repetitive weightlifting at a certain percentage of maximum capacity. The influence of age, gender, skill, motivation, and body size creates difficulty selecting a suitable criterion test or developing appropriate norms to evaluate anaerobic power. Above-normal intramuscular glycogen levels do not affect test performance or final level of blood lactate accumulation.[91] Based on the principle of exercise specificity, one should *not* use a test that requires maximal activation of the leg musculature to assess short-term anaerobic capacity for an upper-body activity such as rowing or swimming. *The performance test must closely resemble the activity that requires energy capacity assessment.* In most cases, the activity itself best serves as the performance test.

In 1973, the **Katch test** of all-out stationary cycling of short duration estimated the power of the anaerobic energy systems.[42] Subsequent extension of this work created a stationary bicycle test with frictional resistance against the flywheel preset at a high load (6 kg for men; 5 kg for women). Subjects turned as many revolutions as possible in 40 s, with pedal rate continuously recorded with a microswitch assembly. Peak cycling power during any portion of the test (properly reported in watts) represented the subject's anaerobic power, whereas total work accomplished indicated anaerobic capacity reported in joules. A later modification, the popular **Wingate test**, involves 30 s of supermaximal effort on either an arm-crank or leg-cycle ergometer.[4,106] Body mass determines resistance to pedaling (originally set to 0.075 kg per kg body mass but now can exceed 0.12 kg in athletes) with resistance applied within 3 s after overcoming the initial inertia and unloaded frictional resistance of the ergometer. **Peak power** represents the highest mechanical power generated during any 3- to 5-s period of the test; **relative power** represents peak power divided by body mass. **Anaerobic fatigue** represents the percentage decline in power output during the test and **anaerobic capacity** is the total work accomplished over the 30 s. **Rate of fatigue** corresponds to the decline in power relative to the peak value. The Katch and Wingate tests assume that peak power output reflects the energy-generating capacity of the high-energy phosphates, while average power reflects glycolytic capacity.

Confusion regarding use of the terms *power* and *capacity* emerges with use of these tests. Originally, the desire was to create measures of anaerobic performance, similar to

A Considerable Energy Output

During a marathon, elite athletes generate a steady-rate energy expenditure of about 25 kcal per minute for the duration of the run! Among elite rowers, a 5- to 7-min competition generates about 36 kcal per minute.

| TABLE 11.2 | Wingate Percentile Norms for Average Power and Peak Power for Physically Active Young Adult Men and Women | | | | | | | |

	Male		Female		Male		Female	
% Rank	Avg Power Watts	Avg Power Watts·kg BM⁻¹ᵃ	Avg Power Watts	Avg Power Watts·kg BM⁻¹ᵃ	Peak Power Watts	Peak Power Watts·kg BM⁻¹ᵃ	Peak Power Watts	Peak Power Watts·kg BM⁻¹ᵃ
90	662	8.24	470	7.31	822	10.89	560	9.02
80	618	8.01	419	6.95	777	10.39	527	8.83
70	600	7.91	410	6.77	757	10.20	505	8.53
60	577	7.59	391	6.59	721	9.80	480	8.14
50	565	7.44	381	6.39	689	9.22	449	7.65
40	548	7.14	367	6.15	671	8.92	432	6.96
30	530	7.00	353	6.03	656	8.53	399	6.86
20	496	6.59	336	5.71	618	8.24	376	6.57
10	471	5.98	306	5.25	570	7.06	353	5.98

Adapted with permission from Maud PJ, Schultz BB. Norms for the Wingate anaerobic test with comparisons in another similar test. *Res Q Exerc Sport* 1989;60:144.
ᵃW·kg BM⁻¹, watts per kilogram of body mass.

aerobic performance, as a power measurement. However, some authors incorrectly use the term *capacity* to infer total work (joules) but use power scores (joules · s⁻¹ = watts) to represent this entity. To represent anaerobic power in this context, the term *capacity* must be a power score (much like $\dot{V}O_{2max}$) and not a work score; thus, the correct expression is watts. The joule is used to compute total anaerobic work.

"In a Practical Sense" provides the procedures to determine anaerobic power and capacity using the Wingate cycle ergometer test. TABLE 11.2 presents normative standards for average and peak power outputs in young, physically active men and women during the Wingate cycling test. Performance scores, blood lactate concentrations, and peak heart rates show high test–retest reproducibility and moderate validity compared with other anaerobic capacity criteria.[66,101] Elite volleyball and ice hockey players have achieved some of the highest Wingate power scores.

FIGURE 11.4 A AND 11.4B present the relative contributions of each energy system during three cycle ergometer anaerobic power tests of different durations. The lower figure (**B**) gives estimated kilojoules of total energy; the upper figure presents the percentage contribution of each system to total work accomplished. Note the progressive change in the percentage contribution of each energy system as a function of increasing duration of effort.

Lower in Children. The reason for the poor performance of children compared with adolescents and young adults on the Wingate test remains unclear. Possible explanations include children's relatively lower intramuscular glycogen concentrations, poorer motivation, and their slower rate of glycogen hydrolysis during physical activity.

Gender Differences. Large gender differences exist in anaerobic power when comparing test scores on an absolute basis.[22,77] These observations, as with most physiologic and performance tests, seem readily explained by the clear gender differences in factors that affect absolute anaerobic power output—body mass, active muscle mass, and fat-free body mass (FFM). Expressing power output capacity relative to a component of body mass or composition should minimize or even eliminate the gender difference in anaerobic capacity. This adjustment should offer insight into whether gender effects truly exist in a muscle's capacity to generate energy anaerobically.

Gender differences in body composition, physique, muscular strength, or neuromuscular factors do *not* fully explain the

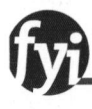

The Fastest Creatures in the Sky, On Land, and in Water

In the Sky
The *peregrine falcon* is not only considered the fastest creature in the sky, it can fly horizontally at speeds up to 55 mph and dive downward at over 280 mph.

On Land
The *cheetah* can reach speeds up to 75–80 mph (at its top speed it only has one foot touching the ground at a time); also, the cheetah can reach a speed of nearly 70 mph in a little over 3 s.

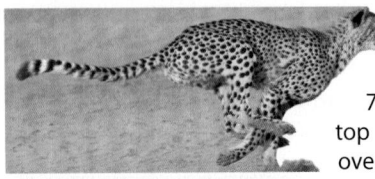

In the Sea
The Indo-Pacific *sailfish* measures about 7 ft in length; it reaches a top speed of about 68 mph over a brief time period.

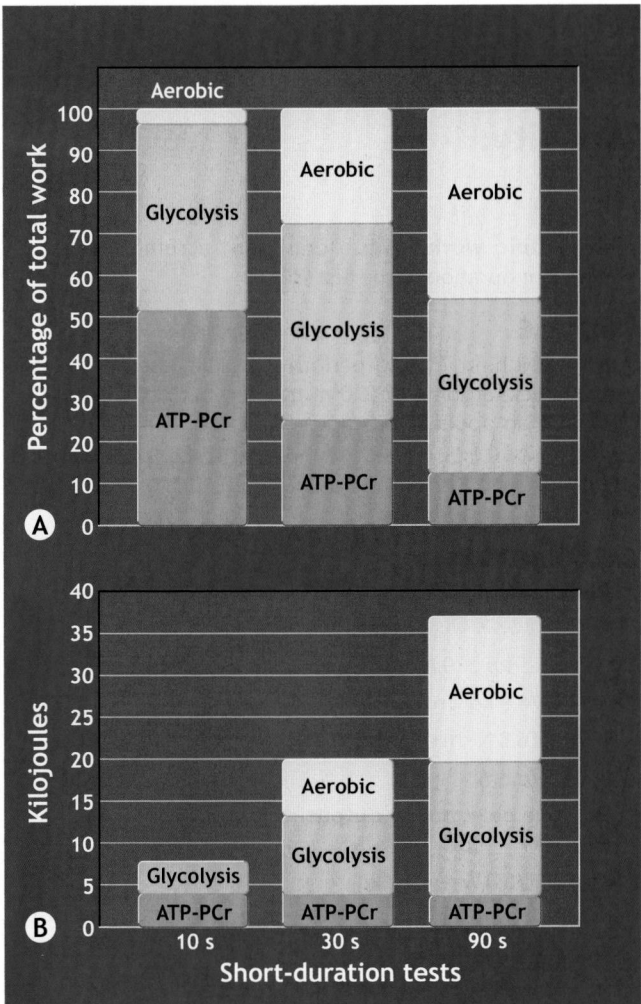

FIGURE 11.4 • Relative contribution of each energy system to total work accomplished in three short-duration exercise tests. **(A)** Percentage of total work output. **(B)** Total kilojoules of energy. Test results based on Katch test protocol (see section "Performance Test Evaluation of the Short-Term Energy System"). (Data from Applied Physiology Laboratory, University of Michigan, Ann Arbor, MI.)

lower anaerobic performance of women.[52,67] For a given fat-free leg volume, the peak oxygen deficit, considered by some a measure of anaerobic power[3,57] during supermaximal cycling, remained higher in men than in women.[102] These differences averaged about 20%, even when adjusting for the estimated difference in active muscle mass between genders. Similar gender differences in anaerobic performance exist for children and adolescents.[65,77] The gender effect among adolescents remains apparent for the lower body musculature even when considering differences in body composition.[67] Males' greater relative muscle area and metabolic capacity of the fast-twitch fiber type and larger catecholamine response to physical activity may help to explain their larger anaerobic performance.

Available evidence indicates an inherent biologic gender difference in glycolytic exercise power/capacity. Physical testing that focuses on this fitness component would inflate typically observed performance differences between men and women. Even adjusting the performance score to body size or body composition does not eliminate this difference. In occupational settings, the justifiable concern when using all-out anaerobic physical effort to predict job performance relates to the potential to exacerbate gender differences in performance scores and magnify any adverse impact on females. Female maximal anaerobic performance remains unaffected by variations in menstrual cycle phase.[30]

Marathon Records Difficult to Repeat

Only five men and eight women have been able to follow one marathon world record with another. James Peters set four marathon records between 1952 and 1954, while Abebe Bikila, Derek Clayton, Khalid Khannouchi, and most recently Haile Gebrselassie each set two world records back-to-back. On the women's side, Greta Weitz set four consecutive world records from 1978 to 1983 (the last stood only for one day!), while Chantal Langlace, Jacqueline Hansen, Christa Vahlensieck, Joyce Smith, Tegla Loroupe, and, most recently, Paula Radcliffe each broke the marathon record twice. Perhaps the most famous of all of the world records were the races of Abebe Bikila the barefoot Ethiopian, who set world records four years apart while winning Olympic Marathons in 1960 (Rome, barefoot) and 1964 (Tokyo, wearing shoes).

Maximally Accumulated Oxygen Deficit

Determination of the **maximally accumulated oxygen deficit (MAOD)** provides another indirect measure of anaerobic metabolic capacity.[57,58,80,99] MAOD determination relies on an extrapolation procedure using the linear exercise intensity–oxygen consumption relationship established from several levels of submaximal treadmill exercise. From these data, a regression line predicts the individual's supramaximal oxygen consumption, usually set at 125% of the subject's directly measured $\dot{V}O_{2max}$. MAOD calculates as the difference between the predicted supramaximal oxygen consumption from the exercise intensity–oxygen consumption relationship and oxygen consumption measured during a 2- to 3-min all-out treadmill run to fatigue. The measure correlates positively with Wingate test, sprint-running, and stair-climbing anaerobic performance test scores; it demonstrates independence from aerobic energy estimates, differentiates between aerobically and anaerobically trained individuals, and remains unchanged with high-intensity physical effort of varying durations.

Assessing the Short-Term Energy System

Blood Lactate Levels

Physiologists have traditionally interpreted the appearance of "excess" lactate in muscle and blood following exercise to indicate contributions of anaerobic metabolism to the activity's

IN A PRACTICAL SENSE

Determining Anaerobic Power and Capacity: The Wingate Cycle Ergometer Test

The Wingate cycle ergometer test represents the most popular test to assess anaerobic capacity. Developed at the Wingate Institute in Israel in the 1970s, its scores can reliably determine peak anaerobic power and anaerobic fatigue.

THE TEST

A mechanically braked bicycle ergometer serves as the testing device. After warming up (3 to 5 min), the subject begins pedaling as fast as possible, without resistance. Within 3 s, a fixed resistance is applied to the flywheel; the subject continues to pedal "all out" for 30 s. An electrical or mechanical counter continuously records flywheel revolutions in 5-s intervals. Total work during the 30 s computes in joules and power computes as joules $\cdot$ s^{-1}, or watts.

RESISTANCE

Flywheel resistance equals 0.075 kilogram per kg body mass. For a 70-kg person, the flywheel resistance would equal 5.25 kg (70 kg $\times$ 0.075). Resistance often increases to 0.10 kg per kilogram body mass or higher (up to 0.12 kg) when testing power- and sprint-type athletes. The Wingate test was originally designed using the Swedish Monarch cycle ergometer. The unit of resistance was the former standard Swedish unit of force called the *kilopond*. Measurement of the kilopond (kp) was a cleverly engineered system composed of a basket containing a weight representing the braking force applied to the flywheel, equal to the weight of the basket and its contents. The standard corresponded to the weight of a 1 kg mass; hence, 1 kp has come to represent 1 kg. The proper unit of force when using the Monarch bike should be kp-m $\cdot$ min^{-1}, not kg-m $\cdot$ min^{-1}. When Sweden joined the European Union, they switched to the SI unit of force, the Newton (N). [One kp corresponds to the force exerted by Earth's gravity (9.80665 m $\cdot$ s^{-2}) on 1 kilogram of mass; thus, one kilogram-force equals 9.80665 Newtons (N).]

TEST SCORES

1. **Peak power (PP) output**—The highest power output, observed during the first 5-s exercise interval, indicates the energy-generating capacity of the immediate energy system (intramuscular high-energy phosphates ATP and PCr). PP, expressed in watts (1 W = 6.12 kp-m $\cdot$ min^{-1}), computes as Force in Newtons (kp resistance $\times$ acceleration due to gravity) $\times$ Distance (number of revolutions $\times$ distance per revolution) $\div$ Time in minutes (5 s = 0.0833 min).

2. **Relative peak power (RPP) output**—Peak power output (W) relative to body mass: PP $\div$ Body mass (kg).

3. **Anaerobic fatigue (AF)**—Percentage decline in power output during the test; AF is thought to represent the total capacity to produce ATP via the immediate and short-term energy systems. AF computes as (Highest 5-s PP − Lowest 5-s PP) $\div$ Highest 5-s PP $\times$ 100.

4. **Anaerobic work (AW)**—Total work accomplished in watts for duration of the test (30 s).

EXAMPLE

A male weighing 73.3 kg performs the Wingate test on a Monark cycle ergometer (6.0 m traveled per pedal revolution) with an applied resistance (force) of 5.5 kp (73.3-kg body mass $\times$ 0.075 = 5.497, rounded to 5.5 kg); pedal revolutions for each 5-s interval equal 12, 10, 8, 7, 6, and 5 (48 total revolutions in 30 s).

CALCULATIONS

1. **Peak power output**

   PP = Force $\times$ Distance $\div$ Time

   $\quad$ = (5.5 kp $\times$ 9.8 m $\cdot$ s^{-2}) $\times$ (12 rev $\cdot$ 6 m/rev) $\div$ 5 s

   $\quad$ = 776.8 kg $\cdot$ m^2 $\cdot$ s^{-3}

   $\quad$ = 776.8 N $\cdot$ m $\cdot$ s^{-2}

   $\quad$ = 776.8 W

2. **Relative peak power output**

   RPP = PP $\div$ Body mass, kg

   $\quad$ = 776.8 W $\div$ 73.3 kg

   $\quad$ = 10.6 W $\cdot$ kg^{-1}

3. **Anaerobic fatigue**

   AF = (Highest PP − Lowest PP) $\div$ Highest PP $\times$ 100

   [Highest PP = Force $\times$ Distance $\div$ Time = 5.5 kp $\times$ 9.8 m $\cdot$ s^{-2})

   $\quad\quad$ $\times$ (12 rev $\times$ 6 m) $\div$ 0.0833 min

   $\quad\quad$ = 4753.9 kp-m $\cdot$ min^{-1}, or 776.8 W]

   [Lowest PP = Force $\times$ Distance $\div$ Time = (5.5 kp $\times$ 9.8 m $\cdot$ s^{-2})

   $\quad\quad$ $\times$ (5 rev $\times$ 6 m) $\div$ 0.0833 min

   $\quad\quad$ = 1980.8 kp-m $\cdot$ min^{-1}, or 323.7 W]

   $\quad$ AF = 776.8 W − 323.7 W $\div$ 776.8 W $\times$ 100

   $\quad$ = 58.3%

4. **Anaerobic work**

   AW = Force $\times$ Total Distance (in 30 s)

   $\quad$ = (5.5 kg $\times$ 9.8 m $\cdot$ s^{-2}) $\times$ [(12 rev + 10 rev + 8 rev + 7 rev + 6 rev + 5 rev) $\times$ 6 m]

   $\quad$ = 15,523 joules, or 15.5 kJ

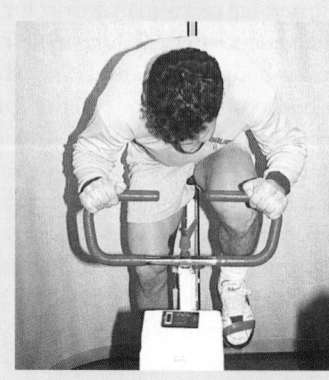

energy requirement. Measurements of muscle or venous blood lactate routinely verified steady-rate exercise or magnitude of glycolytic activity consequent to non–steady-rate exercise. This view now appears overly simplified in light of research showing lactate's role as a metabolic intermediate rather than a metabolic "dead end" whose only fate involves reconversion to pyruvate. Lactate serves as an important substrate in energy-storing *and* energy-generating pathways in different tissues. Lactate measured during or following physical activity does not necessarily reflect absolute levels of anaerobic energy transfer via glycolysis.[12,19,31,32] With increasing intensity, including near-maximal and supramaximal levels of effort, greater lactate production reflects increasing ATP resynthesis from anaerobic pathway.[84] Anaerobic glycolysis and PCr degradation provide about 70% of the total energy yield for 30 s of all-out physical effort, with aerobic pathways generating the remaining energy (see Fig. 11.4).

 INTEGRATIVE QUESTION

Explain why females score poorly when using absolute scores for "average power" and "peak power" on the Wingate leg-cycle ergometer test.

Glycogen Depletion

The pattern of glycogen depletion reveals the glycolytic contribution to physical activity because glycogen stored in specific muscles activated by the activity powers the short-term energy system. **FIGURE 11.5** illustrates the close connection between glycogen depletion rate in the quadriceps femoris muscle during cycling and exercise intensity.

During prolonged but relatively light activity ($31\% \dot{V}O_{2max}$), a considerable muscle glycogen reserve remains even after 180 min. Relatively large quantities of fatty acids provide fuel for exercise at this intensity, with only minimal reliance on stored glycogen. The two intense supermaximal workloads (120% and $150\% \dot{V}O_{2max}$) produced the most rapid and pronounced glycogen depletion. This outcome makes sense from a metabolic standpoint: Glycogen provides the most rapid phosphorylation of ATP of the three macronutrients, and glycogen serves as the only stored macronutrient that anaerobically resynthesizes ATP.

Changes in *total* muscle glycogen, like those illustrated in Figure 11.5, do not necessarily indicate precise amounts of glycogen catabolism in specific fibers within active muscle. Depending on intensity, glycogen depletion progresses selectively in either fast- or slow-twitch muscle fibers. Fast-twitch fibers provide most of the power requirements for all-out effort (e.g., repeated 1-min sprints on a bicycle ergometer at an intense load). The glycogen content of these fibers becomes almost totally depleted because of the activity's anaerobic nature. In contrast, during moderately intense but more prolonged aerobic activities, slow-twitch muscle fibers become glycogen depleted first. Specificity in glycogen

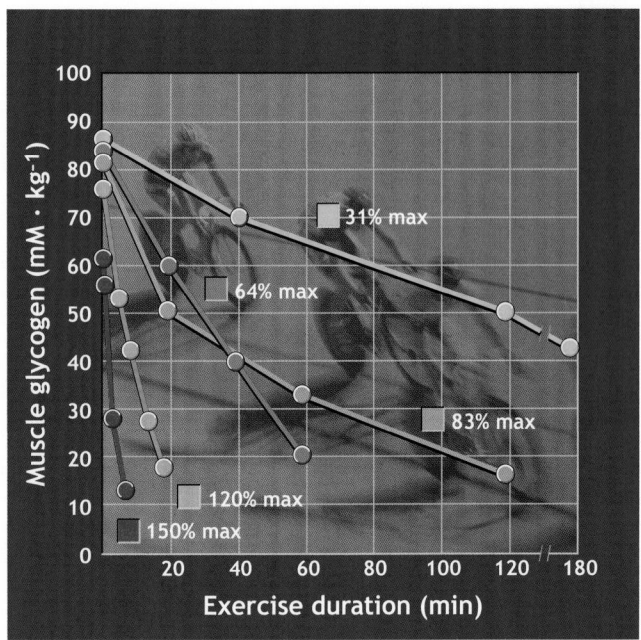

FIGURE 11.5 • Glycogen depletion from the vastus lateralis of the quadriceps femoris muscles during bicycle exercise of different intensities and durations. Exercise at 31% of $\dot{V}O_{2max}$ (the lightest workload) caused some depletion of muscle glycogen, but the most rapid depletion occurred during exercise between 83 and 150% of $\dot{V}O_{2max}$. (Adapted with permission from Gollnick PD. Selective glycogen depletion pattern in human muscle fibers after exercise of varying intensity and at varying pedaling rates. *J Physiol* 1974;241:45.)

use and depletion by specific fiber types makes it difficult to evaluate the anaerobic involvement of distinct fibers from changes in a muscle's total glycogen content before and after exercise.

Individual Differences in Short-Term Energy-Transfer Capacity

Three factors contribute to differences among individuals in capacity to generate short-term anaerobic energy:

1. Effects of previous training
2. Capacity to buffer acid metabolites
3. Motivation

Effects of Training

Many factors relate to differences in anaerobic metabolism between sprint-trained athletes and untrained subjects. Swedish researchers in a classic 1971 experiment determined that trained subjects always exhibit higher levels of muscle lactic acid, blood lactate, and more pronounced muscle glycogen depletion following short-term maximal bicycle ergometer exercise. Significant reductions occurred in the intramuscular high-energy phosphates with essentially no differences observed between groups.[38a]

Buffering of Acid Metabolites

Buffering capacity refers to how well different substances resist increases in free hydrogen ion concentration by binding free protons to prevent a decrease in pH. When anaerobic energy transfer predominates, lactate accumulates and muscle and blood acidity increase to negatively affect the intracellular environment and the contractile capacity of active muscles. Anaerobic training might enhance short-term energy capacity by improving the body's alkaline reserve for buffering. Such a training adaptation would theoretically enable greater lactate production through more effective buffering. This reasoning seems appealing, yet athletes have only a slightly larger alkaline reserve than sedentary counterparts. Additionally, no appreciable change in alkaline reserve occurs following intense physical training. *Exercise training most likely confers a buffering capability within the range expected for healthy untrained individuals.* Chapter 23 discusses the potential ergogenic effects of pre-exercise-induced alkalosis.

Motivation

Individuals with a higher "pain tolerance," "toughness," or ability to "push" beyond the discomforts of intense, fatiguing effort can accomplish more work anaerobically. This coincides with higher blood lactate concentrations and greater glycogen depletion. Motivational factors prove difficult to categorize or quantify yet undoubtedly play an integral role in achieving superior performance at most levels of competition.

AEROBIC ENERGY: THE LONG-TERM ENERGY SYSTEM

FIGURE 11.6 illustrates that male and female athletes who excel in endurance sports generally have a superior capacity for aerobic energy transfer. The maximal oxygen consumption of elite cross-country skiers, distance runners, swimmers, bicyclists, and skaters exceeds that of sedentary men and women by almost twofold. This does not mean that $\dot{V}O_{2max}$ provides the sole determinant of endurance performance. Other factors, principally those at the local tissue level, include improved capillary density, enzymes, mitochondrial size and number, and muscle fiber type. These intrinsic qualities strongly influence a muscle's capacity to sustain a high level of aerobic activity.[36] The $\dot{V}O_{2max}$ does provide important information about the capacity of the long-term energy system. This measure also conveys important physiologic meaning because attaining a high $\dot{V}O_{2max}$ requires integration of high levels of pulmonary, cardiovascular, and neuromuscular function (see Fig. 7.5). *This makes $\dot{V}O_{2max}$ a fundamental measure of physiologic functional capacity for physical activity.*

Physiologic Tests to Evaluate the Long-Term Aerobic Energy System Assessment of Maximal Oxygen Consumption

Over the past 75 years, considerable research effort has developed methodology to assess maximal aerobic power. Normative standards exist related to age, gender, state of training, and body size.

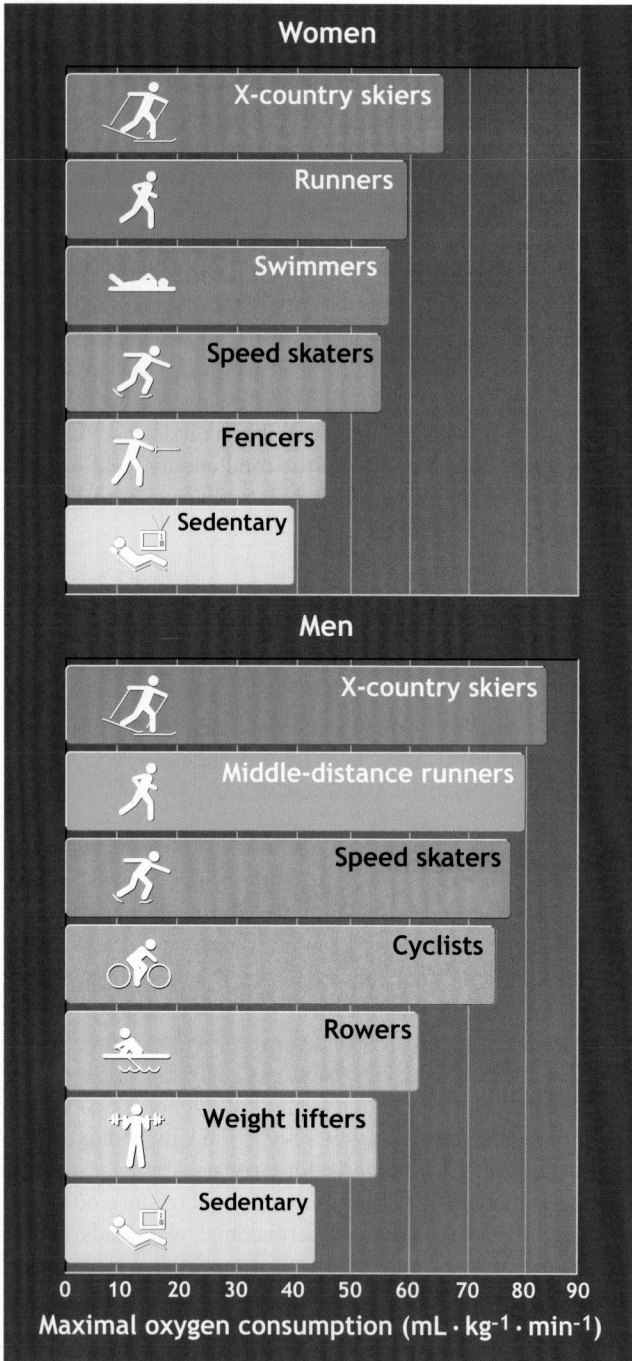

FIGURE 11.6 • Maximal oxygen consumption of male and female Olympic-caliber athletes in different sport categories compared with healthy sedentary subjects. (Adapted with permission from Saltin B, Åstrand PO. Maximal oxygen consumption in athletes. *J Appl Physiol* 1967;23:353.)

Criteria for Maximal Oxygen Consumption

The plot in FIGURE 11.7 relates oxygen consumption and exercise intensity during progressive increases in treadmill effort. The test terminated when the subject could not complete the

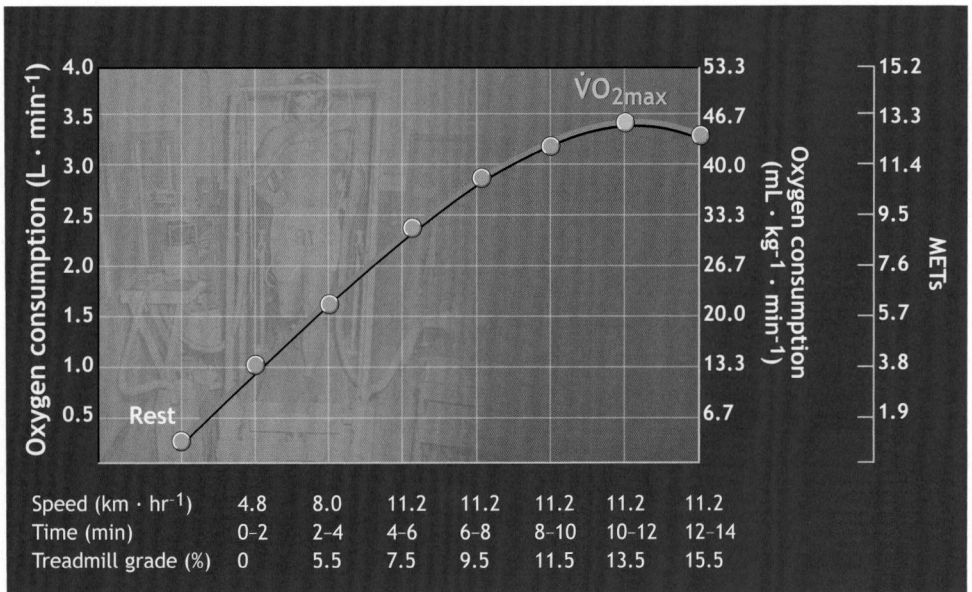

FIGURE 11.7 • Peaking-over in oxygen consumption with increasing treadmill exercise intensity. Each point represents the average oxygen consumption of 18 sedentary males. The region where oxygen consumption fails to increase the expected amount or even decreases slightly with increasing intensity represents the $\dot{V}O_{2max}$. (Data from the Applied Physiology Laboratory, University of Michigan, Ann Arbor, MI.)

full duration of a particular interval. The highest oxygen consumption (average of 18 subjects) occurred before subjects attained their maximum level of effort. *Demonstration of a leveling-off or peaking-over in oxygen consumption with increasing exercise intensity generally provides assurance that a person has reached maximum aerobic metabolism (i.e., achieved "true" $\dot{V}O_{2max}$).* Agreement on a precise standard for the criterion remains controversial.[21,37,82] Less stringent criteria, besides failure for oxygen consumption to increase in graded exercise, also establish attainment of $\dot{V}O_{2max}$. Oxygen consumption that fails to increase by the value expected on the basis of previous observations with the specific test protocol often serves as an appropriate criterion.[1,37,86]

Oxygen consumption at higher levels of effort does not readily plateau, particularly among children,[75] except in treadmill running. The term **peak oxygen consumption**, or $\dot{V}O_{2peak}$, applies when leveling-off does not occur or maximum performance appears limited by local muscular factors rather than central circulatory dynamics. *$\dot{V}O_{2peak}$ refers to the highest value of oxygen consumption measured during a graded exercise test.* The highest oxygen consumption value often occurs in the last minute of the activity. Secondary criteria that objectify $\dot{V}O_{2peak}$ include attainment of the age-predicted maximum heart rate or a respiratory exchange ratio (R) that exceeds 1.15. Some also argue that to accept an oxygen consumption value as near maximum, blood lactate should attain 70 or 80 mg per dL of blood (8 to 10 mmol) or above.[21]

Maximal Oxygen Consumption Tests

A variety of tests that activate the body's large muscle groups can determine $\dot{V}O_{2max}$, provided exercise intensity and duration maximize aerobic energy transfer. Usual activity modes include treadmill running or walking, bench stepping, and stationary cycling. In accord with exercise test and training specificity, other forms of testing employ free, tethered, and flume swimming[6,47]; swim-bench ergometry[29]; in-line skating[96]; roller skiing[76]; simulated arm–leg climbing[11]; rowing[15]; ice skating[24]; and arm-crank and wheelchair exercise.[79,90,92] Such performance tests remain substantially unaffected by a subject's strength, speed, body size, and skill, with the exception of specialized tests that measure aerobic capacity in sport-specific activities.

The $\dot{V}O_{2max}$ test may require a single, continuous 3- to 5-min supermaximal effort. The test usually consists of progressive increments in **graded exercise** (and effort) until the subject simply refuses to continue the activity. Some researchers term this end point "exhaustion." In reality, the person terminates the test—a decision often influenced by motivational factors that do not necessarily reflect true physiologic strain. Bringing the subject to the point of acceptable criteria for either $\dot{V}O_{2max}$ or $\dot{V}O_{2peak}$ often requires considerable urging and prodding.[95] Practical experience indicates that attaining a plateau in oxygen consumption during a graded exercise test in well-trained athletes requires a high level of anaerobic energy output. This poses some difficulty for untrained and elderly persons who normally do not perform strenuous physical activity with its associated discomforts and potential health concerns.

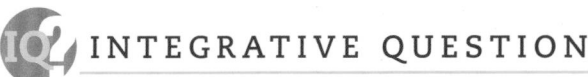 INTEGRATIVE QUESTION

Explain why $\dot{V}O_{2max}$ provides important insights about the functional capacities of different physiologic systems.

TABLE 11.3	Average $\dot{V}O_{2max}$ for 15 Male College Students During Continuous and Discontinuous Tests on the Treadmill and Bicycle Ergometer[a]					
Variable	**Bike, Discontinuous**	**Bike, Continuous**	**Treadmill, Discontinuous Run-Walk**	**Treadmill, Continuous Walk**	**Treadmill, Discontinuous Run**	**Treadmill, Continuous Run**
$\dot{V}O_{2max}$, mL·min^{-1}	3691 ± 453	3683 ± 448	4145 ± 401	3944 ± 395	4157 ± 445	4109 ± 424
$\dot{V}O_{2max}$, mL·kg^{-1}·min^{-1}	50.0 ± 6.9	49.9 ± 7.0	56.6 ± 7.3	53.7 ± 7.6	56.6 ± 7.6	55.5 ± 6.8

Adapted with permission from McArdle WD, et al. Comparison of continuous and discontinuous treadmill and bicycle tests for max $\dot{V}O_2$. *Med Sci Sports* 1973;5:156.
[a]Values are means ± standard deviations.

Test Comparisons

There are two popular maximal oxygen consumption test protocols:

1. *Continuous*—progressively increasing exercise increments without recovery or rest intervals
2. *Discontinuous*—progressively increasing exercise increments interspersed with recovery intervals

Both test protocols yield similar $\dot{V}O_{2max}$ values.[21] The data in **TABLE 11.3** reveal a systematic comparison of $\dot{V}O_{2max}$ scores measured using six common continuous and discontinuous treadmill and bicycle protocols. Only an 8-mL difference in $\dot{V}O_{2max}$ occurred between the continuous and discontinuous bicycle tests, but $\dot{V}O_{2max}$ during cycling averaged 6.4 to 11.2% below treadmill values. The largest difference among the three treadmill running tests equaled only 1.2%. In contrast, the walking test elicited $\dot{V}O_{2max}$ scores nearly 7% higher than values on the bicycle, but 5% lower than the three running tests.

Subjects commonly complained of intense local discomfort in the thigh muscles during intense activity, limiting their ability to continue, in both continuous and discontinuous bicycle tests. They experienced discomfort in the lower back and calf muscles during treadmill walking, notably at higher treadmill elevations. Running tests rarely produced local discomfort; subjects complained more of general fatigue usually categorized as feeling "winded." For ease of administration, the continuous treadmill run provides a practical test of aerobic capacity for most healthy individuals. The total time to administer the test should average between 8 and 10 min for moderately to highly trained individuals, compared with 65 min for the discontinuous running test. Subjects tolerate the continuous test well and prefer the shorter time.[105] Achievement of $\dot{V}O_{2max}$ also occurs with a continuous protocol that increases effort intensity progressively in 15-s intervals.[23] Total test time for either bicycle or treadmill exercise with this approach averages only about 5 min.

Common Treadmill Protocols. **FIGURE 11.8** summarizes six common treadmill protocols to assess aerobic capacity in normal individuals and cardiac patients. Manipulation of exercise duration and treadmill speed and grade share common features. The Bruce protocol (example **C**, which employs an increase in speed and/or grade every 3 min, is most popular for assessing cardiovascular parameters during physician-monitored stress tests (see Chapter 32, "Stress Test Protocols"). The Harbor treadmill test (example **F**), referred to as a *ramp test*, depicts a unique application. With this protocol, treadmill grade increases by a constant amount (between 1 and 4%) each minute for up to 10 min, depending on the person's capacity. This relatively quick procedure—well tolerated by both healthy subjects and cardiac patients—elicits a linear increase in oxygen consumption up to maximum.[13,18,70,98]

 INTEGRATIVE QUESTION

Discuss why training studies should objectively demonstrate attainment of true $\dot{V}O_{2max}$ in both pre- and posttest measures. How can this goal be verified?

Factors That Affect Maximal Oxygen Consumption

The six most important factors that influence the maximal oxygen consumption score include:

1. Mode of activity
2. Heredity
3. State of training
4. Gender
5. Body size and composition
6. Age

Mode of Activity

Variations in $\dot{V}O_{2max}$ with different forms of physical activity generally reflect variations in the quantity of muscle mass activated. Treadmill exercise usually produces the highest values among diverse activity modes. Bench stepping produces $\dot{V}O_{2max}$ *scores similar to treadmill values and higher than values on a cycle ergometer.*[39] *During arm-crank exercise, aerobic capacity averages only about 70% of the treadmill*

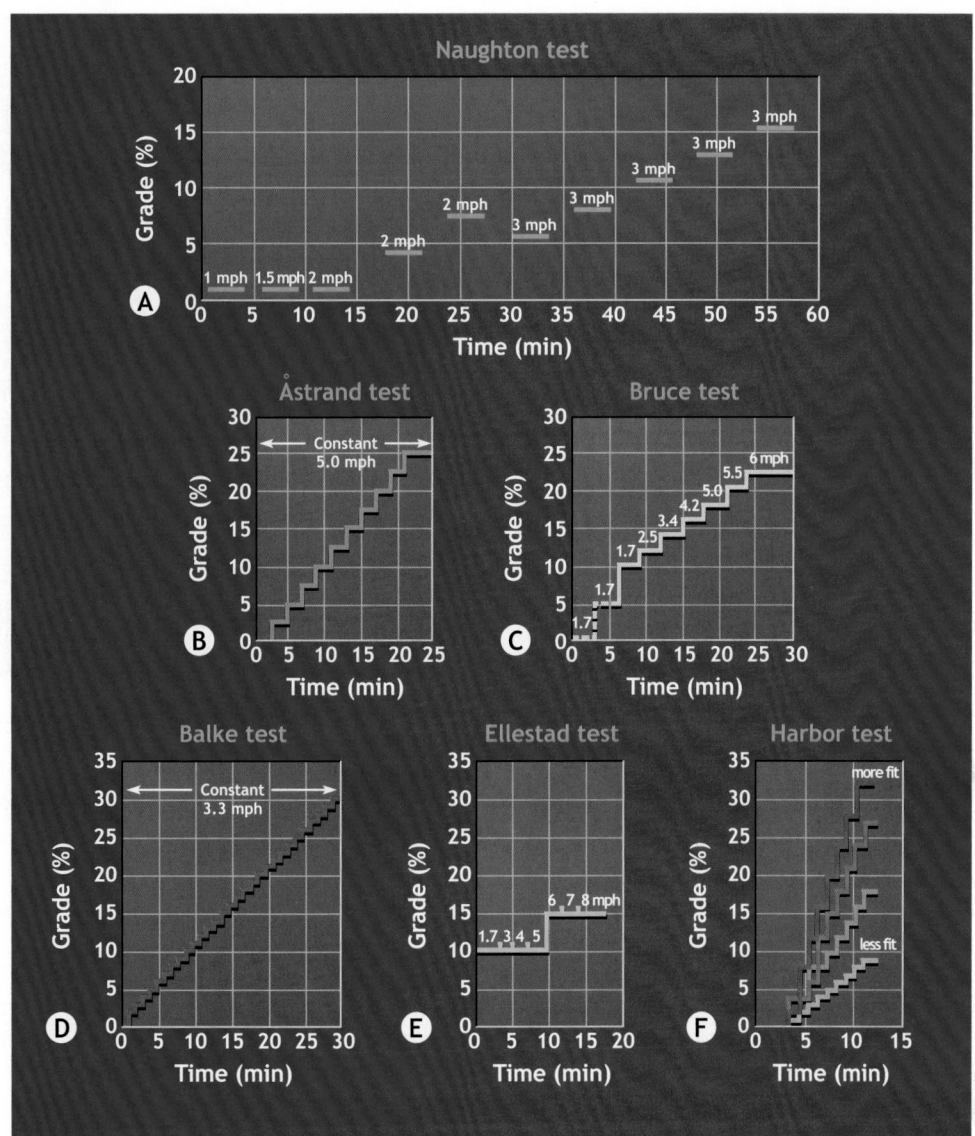

FIGURE 11.8 • Six commonly used treadmill protocols to assess $\dot{V}O_{2max}$. **(A)** Naughton protocol. Three-minute exercise periods of increasing intensity alternate with 3 min of rest. Exercise periods vary in % grade and speed. **(B)** Åstrand protocol. Constant speed at 5 mph. After 3 min at 0% grade, the grade increases 2½% every 2 min. **(C)** Bruce protocol. Grade and/or speed change every 3 min. Omit the 0% and 5% grades for healthy subjects. **(D)** Balke protocol. After 1 min at 0% grade and 1 min at 2% grade, the grade increases 1% per minute; speed is maintained at 3.3 mph. **(E)** Ellestad protocol. Initial grade of 10% and later grade of 15%, while speed increases every 2 or 3 min. **(F)** Harbor protocol. After 3 min of walking at a comfortable speed, the grade increases at a constant preselected amount each minute: 1%, 2%, 3%, or 4%, so that the subject achieves $\dot{V}O_{2max}$ in approximately 10 min. (Adapted with permission from Wasserman K, et al. *Principles of Exercise Testing and Interpretation*. 2nd Ed. Philadelphia: Lea & Febiger, 1994.)

score.[90] For skilled but untrained swimmers, the $\dot{V}O_{2max}$ during swimming usually equals about 80% of treadmill values.[47,55] A definite test specificity emerges for this activity form because trained collegiate swimmers achieve $\dot{V}O_{2max}$ values swimming only 11% below treadmill values.[53] Some elite swimmers equal or even exceed their treadmill scores during swimming tests.[47] Similarly, a distinct exercise specificity exists for competitive race-walkers who achieve similar $\dot{V}O_{2max}$ values during treadmill walking and treadmill running.[59] When competitive cyclists pedal at the rapid

frequencies of competition, they too achieve $\dot{V}O_{2max}$ values equivalent to treadmill $\dot{V}O_{2max}$ scores.[33,85]

Treadmill exercise proves highly desirable for determining $\dot{V}O_{2max}$ in healthy subjects in the laboratory. One can easily quantify and regulate effort intensity. Compared with other forms of activity, the treadmill allows subjects to more readily meet one or more of the criteria to attain $\dot{V}O_{2max}$ or $\dot{V}O_{2peak}$. In field experiments (outside the laboratory setting), bench stepping and cycle ergometry remain suitable alternatives.

Heredity

The interaction between inherited factors (DNA sequence variation; see Section 8, "A Look to the Future") and physical activity enhances our understanding of individual variations in training responsiveness, including anticipated health-related benefits from regular physical activity.[7,34,62,74] Frequent questions concern the relative contribution of natural endowment (genotype) to physiologic function, daily physical activity level, neuromuscular coordination, and physical performance (phenotype).[10,27,46,61,64,73,103] For example, to what extent does heredity determine the extremely high aerobic capacities of the endurance athletes in Figure 11.6. Do these exceptionally high levels of functional capacity simply reflect intensive training? How does familial aggregation affect skeletal muscle capillary density and enzyme activity and their response to training?

In general, most physical fitness characteristics demonstrate high heritability. Early research focused on 15 pairs of identical twins (monozygous; same heredity from a single fertilized ovum) and 15 pairs of fraternal twins (dizygous; like ordinary siblings, derived from two separate fertilized ovum) raised in the same city and with parents of similar socioeconomic backgrounds. Heredity alone accounted for up to 93% of observed differences in $\dot{V}O_{2max}$. The capacity of the short-term glycolytic energy system indicated a genetic determination of approximately 81%, while maximum heart rate showed approximately 86% genetic determination.[44] In larger groups of brothers, fraternal twins, and identical twins, a smaller effect of inherited factors occurred for aerobic capacity and endurance performance.[8,9] **Figure 11.9** presents data for $\dot{V}O_{2max}$ for identical twin and fraternal twin brothers. Lesser variation in aerobic capacity between brother pairs emerged for identical twins (yellow circles) with identical genetic constitutions. Chapters 21 and 33 discuss the potential contribution of genetic makeup to one's responsiveness to aerobic training.

Researchers estimate the genetic effect at about 20 to 30% for $\dot{V}O_{2max}$, 50% for maximum heart rate, and 70% for physical working capacity.[7,8,69] Combining the estimated effects of genetics and familial environment raises the upper limit of genetic determination to about 50% for $\dot{V}O_{2max}$ when adjusted for age, gender, and body mass and/or body composition.[9] Identical twins have similar muscle fiber type composition, whereas fiber type varies widely between fraternal twins and brothers.[45] Between 15 and 40% of the variation in muscular strength among individuals probably results from genetic factors.[68,89] Future research may determine a precise upper limit of genetic determination; at this time, we can assume that inherited factors contribute considerably to physiologic function, daily physical activity level, exercise performance, training responsiveness, and specific components of health-related physical fitness.[26,46,72,74,93]

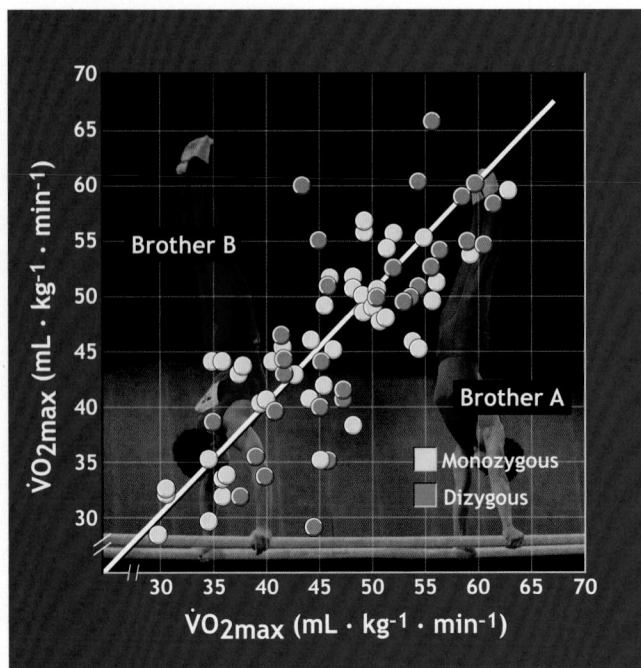

FIGURE 11.9 • Maximal oxygen consumptions ($\dot{V}O_{2max}$) for pairs of monozygotic (identical) and dizygotic (fraternal) twin brothers. (From Bouchard C, et al. Aerobic performance in brothers, dizygotic and monozygotic twins. *Med Sci Sports Exerc* 1986;18:639.)

State of Training

A person's state of aerobic training contributes substantially to their $\dot{V}O_{2max}$, which normally varies between 5 and 20% depending on a person's fitness at the time of testing. Chapter 21 discusses further the influence of training on aerobic capacity.

Gender

Women typically achieve $\dot{V}O_{2max}$ scores 15 to 30% below values of male counterparts.[81,94] Even among trained endurance athletes, the gender difference ranges between 15 and 20%.[5] These differences remain considerably larger for $\dot{V}O_{2max}$ expressed in absolute units (L·min⁻¹) rather than to body mass (mL·kg⁻¹·min⁻¹).[100] Among world-class cross-country skiers, for example, a 43% lower $\dot{V}O_{2max}$ absolute value for women (6.54 vs. 3.75 L·min⁻¹) becomes 15% lower when expressed relative to body mass (83.8 vs. 71.2 mL·kg⁻¹·min⁻¹).

Differences in body composition discussed in the next section and hemoglobin concentration usually explain the gender difference in $\dot{V}O_{2max}$. Untrained young adult women generally average about 25% body fat, whereas men average 15%. The average male generates more total aerobic energy simply because he possesses more muscle mass and has less fat than the average female. Trained athletes have lower percentages of fat than average individuals, yet trained women still possess more body fat than male counterparts. Perhaps because of higher testosterone levels, men also have a 10 to 14% greater hemoglobin concentration than women. This difference in the blood's oxygen-carrying capacity enables men to circulate more oxygen during physical activity. This advantage increases their aerobic capacities above those of women.

Factors other than lower body fat and higher hemoglobin concentrations may help to explain male–female aerobic capacity differences. For example, normal physical activity levels differ between the average male and average female. One could argue that social constraints reduce opportunities for females of all ages to participate in extracurricular athletic activities and recreational pursuits. Among prepubertal children, boys engage in more daily physical activity than girls of the same age. Despite these fitness-inhibiting factors, the aerobic capacities of physically active females generally exceed those of sedentary males. $\dot{V}O_{2max}$ of female cross-country skiers, for example, exceeds untrained males by 40%.[5] Even among "normal" populations, considerable variability exists within each gender, and the $\dot{V}O_{2max}$ scores for many women exceed average values for men.

Body Size and Composition

Variations in body mass explain nearly 70% of the differences in $\dot{V}O_{2max}$ scores among individuals. This limits interpretations of physical performance or absolute values for oxygen consumption when comparing individuals who differ in body size or composition. The effect of body size on aerobic capacity has led to the common practice of expressing oxygen consumption related to surface area, body mass, FFM, or limb volume. TABLE 11.4 reveals a 43% difference in $\dot{V}O_{2max}$ ($L \cdot min^{-1}$) for an untrained man and woman differing considerably in body size and composition. When expressed per unit of body mass as $mL \cdot kg^{-1} \cdot min^{-1}$, the $\dot{V}O_{2max}$ of the woman remains about 20% lower than for the man. Expressing aerobic capacity by FFM reduces between-subject difference even more (29%).

Adjusting for variation in muscle mass activated in physical activity provides additional information to explain interindividual variation in $\dot{V}O_{2max}$. For example, adjusting oxygen consumption values obtained during maximal arm-cranking for variations in estimated arm and shoulder size eliminates gender differences in $\dot{V}O_{2peak}$.[97] Expressing oxygen consumption per unit of appendicular skeletal muscle mass often negates the difference in $\dot{V}O_{2max}$ between men and women of similar training status.[14] The size of the contracting muscle mass activated in an activity largely accounts for gender differences in aerobic capacity.

Age

Age does not spare its effect on maximal oxygen consumption.[40,56,71] Available data provide insight into the possible effects of aging on physiologic function, although one can draw only limited inferences from cross-sectional studies of persons of different age groups. FIGURE 11.10 summarizes trends in aerobic capacity of children and adults.

Children. Figure 11.10A and 11.10B illustrates age trends in the absolute and relative aerobic capacities of boys and girls ages 6 to 16 years.

- **Absolute values:** $\dot{V}O_{2max}$ values in $L \cdot min^{-1}$ for boys and girls remain similar until about age 12; at age 14, $\dot{V}O_{2max}$ for boys averages 25% higher than that for girls, and by age 16 the difference exceeds 50%. The difference generally relates to the combined effect of a greater muscle mass in boys and their greater daily physical activity levels.
- **Relative values:** For boys, average aerobic capacity in $mL \cdot kg^{-1} \cdot min^{-1}$ remains level at about 52 $mL \cdot kg^{-1} \cdot min^{-1}$ from ages 6 to 16 (Fig. 11.10B); for girls, the line slopes downward with age, reaching about 40 $mL \cdot kg^{-1} \cdot min^{-1}$ at age 16, a value 32% below male counterparts. The greater accumulation of body fat in adolescent females partially accounts for the lower values; females must transport this extra fat that does not enhance the capacity for aerobic metabolism.

Adults. $\dot{V}O_{2max}$ declines steadily after age 25 at a rate of about 1% per year, so at age 55 it averages about 27% below values reported for 20-year-olds (Fig. 11.10C). $\dot{V}O_{2max}$ declines at an accelerated rate during aging.[25] For eight women nearly 80 years of age, $\dot{V}O_{2max}$ averaged 13.4 $mL \cdot kg^{-1} \cdot min^{-1}$, or about 3.7 METs.[26] Despite this apparent aging effect, strong evidence indicates that a person's habitual physical activity level exerts far greater influence on aerobic capacity than chronological age per se.[60] Refer to Chapter 31 for further discussion about age-related influences on physiologic function.

Prediction Test Evaluation of the Long-Term Aerobic Energy System

Direct $\dot{V}O_{2max}$ measurement requires an extensive laboratory, specialized equipment, and considerable subject physical

TABLE 11.4　Different Ways to Express Oxygen Consumption

Variable	Female	Male	Female vs. Male % Difference
$\dot{V}O_{2max}$, $L \cdot min^{-1}$	2.00	3.50	−43
$\dot{V}O_{2max}$, $mL \cdot kg^{-1} \cdot min^{-1}$	40.0	50.0	−20
$\dot{V}O_{2max}$, $mL \cdot kg\,FFM^{-1} \cdot min^{-1}$	53.3	58.8	−9
Body mass, kg	50	70	−29
Percentage body fat	25	15	+67
Fat-free body mass, kg	37.5	59.5	−37

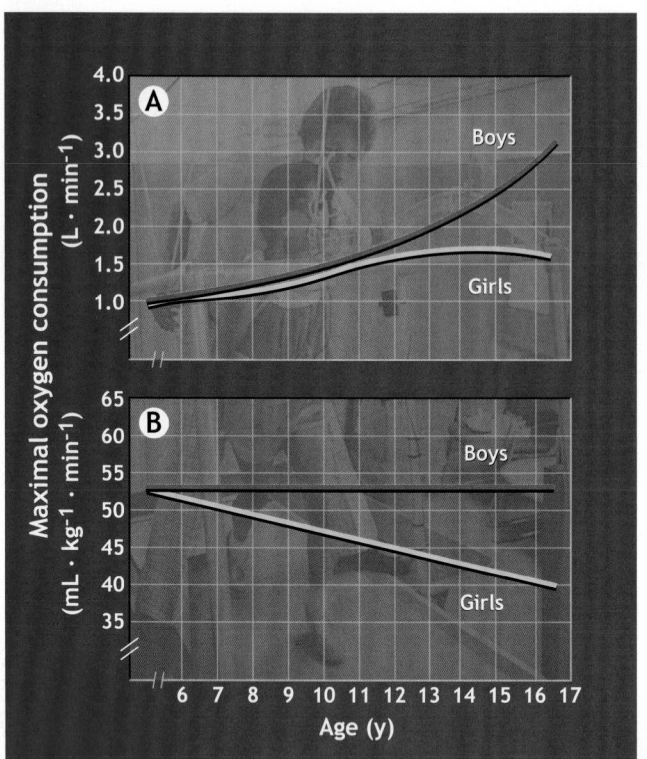

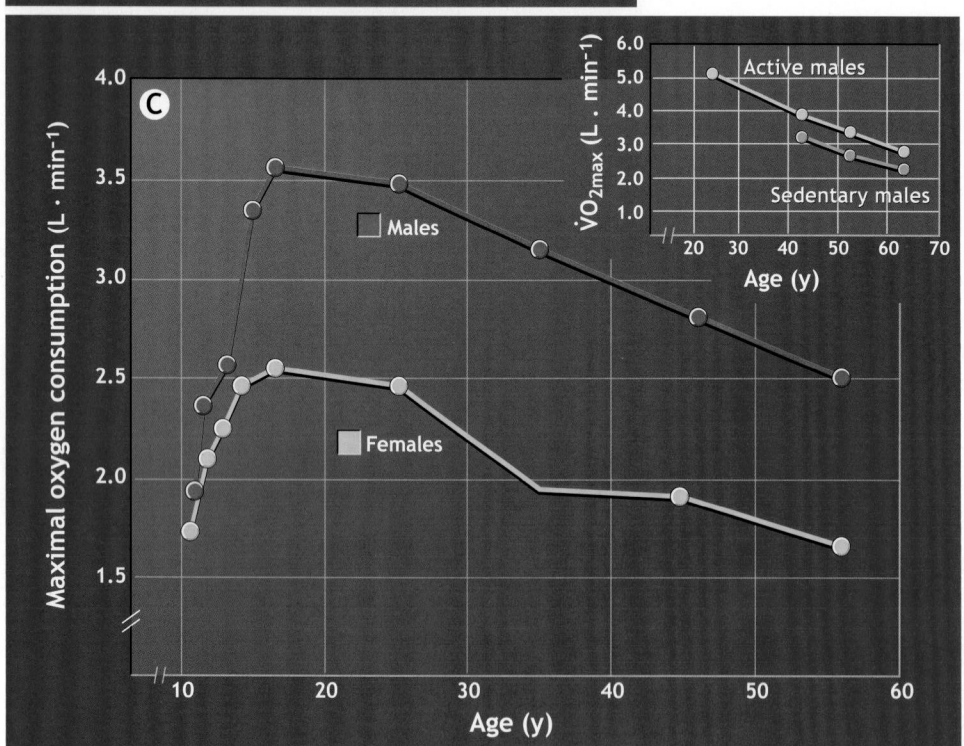

FIGURE 11.10 • Maximal oxygen consumption related to age in boys and girls **(A and B)** and men and women **(C)**. (**A and B** adapted with permission from Krahenbuhl GS, et al. Developmental aspects of maximal aerobic power in children. *Exerc Sport Sci Rev* 1985;13:503. Terjung RL, ed. *Vol. 13.* New York: Macmillan, 1985; **C** adapted with permission from Hermansen L. Individual differences. In: Larson LA, ed. *Fitness, Health, and Work Capacity: International Standards for Assessment.* New York: Macmillan, 1974. Inset graph in C redrawn from table data of Åstrand PO, Rodahl KR. *Textbook of Work Physiology.* New York: McGraw-Hill, 1970.)

effort and motivation. Consequently, laboratory tests remain impractical to assess large groups of untrained subjects. In addition, strenuous exertion could prove risky to adults who do not receive proper medical clearance and appropriate supervision. These considerations increase the importance of submaximal exercise testing to *predict* $\dot{V}O_{2max}$ from performance during walking and running or from heart rate during or immediately postexercise.

A Word of Caution About Predictions

All predictions contain error, referred to as the **standard error of estimate** (**SEE**). Errors of estimate are expressed in measurement units of the predicted variable (e.g., kg, mL, min, s) or as a percentage. For example, suppose the $\dot{V}O_{2max}$ (mL·kg^{-1}·min^{-1}) predicted from time on a walking test equals 55 mL·kg^{-1}·min^{-1}, with SEE 610 mL·kg^{-1}·min^{-1}. This means that the actual $\dot{V}O_{2max}$ probably (68% confidence) lies within ±10 mL·kg^{-1}·min^{-1}, or between 45 and 65 mL·kg^{-1}·min^{-1} of the predicted value. This represents a relatively large error (±18% of the absolute value).

Some predictions are associated with small errors (SEE ±5%) and others with larger errors. Obviously, a larger error translates to a less useful predicted score because the likely true score encompasses such a large range of possible values. Without knowing the magnitude of the SEE, one cannot judge the usefulness of a predicted score. With predictions, one must interpret the predicted score in light of the magnitude of the prediction error. With a relatively small prediction error, prediction of $\dot{V}O_{2max}$ proves useful in appropriate situations in which direct measurement is not possible.

Walking Tests

Walking tests can predict $\dot{V}O_{2max}$ with reasonable accuracy. The following equation predicts $\dot{V}O_{2max}$ in L·min^{-1} from walking speed, heart rate, body weight, age, and gender in men and women:[43]

$$\dot{V}O_{2max} = 6.9652 + (0.0091 \times Wt) - (0.0257 \times Age) + (0.5955 \times Gender) - (0.224 \times T1) - (0.0115 \times HR1{-}4)$$

where Wt is body weight in pounds; Age is in years; Gender is 0 for females, 1 for males; T1 is time for the 1-mile track walk, expressed as minutes and hundredths of a minute; and HR1–4 is heart rate in beats per minute measured immediately at the end of the last quarter-mile.

The following equation predicts $\dot{V}O_{2max}$ in $mL \cdot kg^{-1} \cdot min^{-1}$ using the same variables:

$$\dot{V}O_{2max} = 132.853 - (0.0769 \times Wt) - (0.3877 \times Age) \\ + (6.315 \times Gender) - (3.2649 \times T1) \\ - (0.1565 \times HR1\text{–}4)$$

The multiple correlation is $r = 0.92$ for predicting $\dot{V}O_{2max}$ from 1-mile walking performance for both equations with a SEE of ±0.335 $L \cdot min^{-1}$, or ±4.4 $mL \cdot kg^{-1} \cdot min^{-1}$. This means that about 68% of the people tested have an actual $\dot{V}O_{2max}$ within ±0.335 $L \cdot min^{-1}$ (±4.4 $mL \cdot kg^{-1} \cdot min^{-1}$) of the predicted value. The group studied ranged in age from 30 to 69 years; thus, the prediction method applies to a large segment of the adult population.

The following data for a 30-year-old female illustrate the prediction method:

$$Body\ weight = 155.5\ lb$$
$$T1 = 13.56\ min$$
$$HR1\text{–}4 = 145\ b \cdot min^{-1}$$

Substituting in the equation to predict $\dot{V}O_{2max}$ in $mL \cdot kg^{-1} \cdot min^{-1}$:

$$\dot{V}O_{2max} = 132.853 - (0.0769 \times 155.5) - (0.3877 \times 30.0) \\ + (6.315 \times 0) - (3.2649 \times 13.56) - (0.1565 \times 145)$$
$$\dot{V}O_{2max} = 132.853 - (11.96) - (11.63) + (0) \\ - (44.27) - (22.69)$$
$$\dot{V}O_{2max} = 42.3\ mL \cdot kg^{-1} \cdot min^{-1}$$

Endurance Runs

As with walking tests, runs of various durations or distances evaluate aerobic fitness. Test use reasonably assumes that a person's ability to maintain a high, steady-rate oxygen consumption largely determines the distance run over at least 5 min duration. This ability depends on the maximum capacity to generate energy aerobically (i.e., $\dot{V}O_{2max}$). This rationale provided the framework for a field performance test devised in 1959 to evaluate aerobic fitness of military personnel.[2] The test required subjects to run as far as possible in 15 min. A 1968 study by Cooper shortened run time to 12 min.[16]

In his original validation of the 12-min test, Cooper reported a strong association between $\dot{V}O_{2max}$ of Air Force personnel and distances run-walked in 12 min. The correlation coefficient was $r = 0.90$ between 12-min run-walk distance and $\dot{V}O_{2max}$ ($mL \cdot kg^{-1} \cdot min^{-1}$) in 47 men who varied considerably in age (17 to 54 years), body mass (52 to 123 kg), and $\dot{V}O_{2max}$ (31 to 59 $mL \cdot kg^{-1} \cdot min^{-1}$). Other researchers reported the same correlation for 9 ninth-grade boys.[20] Subsequent studies have failed to demonstrate as strong a connection between "Cooper 12-min run scores" and aerobic capacity. For example, one study measured 11- to 14-year-old boys and reported a correlation of $r = 0.65$.[48] For a group of 26 female athletes, the correlation between the run-walk scores and $\dot{V}O_{2max}$ was

$r = 0.70$,[49] and for 36 untrained college women, a similar correlation of $r = 0.67$ emerged.[41]

Importantly, a simple correlation between run-walk scores and $\dot{V}O_{2max}$ does not consider the interacting effects of age and body mass. These variables themselves relate to both run-walk times and $\dot{V}O_{2max}$ scores. When restricting these original data to the same age range as subjects in the preceding study of 36 untrained women, the computed correlation coefficient decreased dramatically from $r = 0.90$ to $r = 0.59$.

One must view $\dot{V}O_{2max}$ predictions based on running performance with caution. The need to establish a consistent level of motivation and effective pacing during running becomes critical with inexperienced subjects. Some individuals achieve an optimal pace throughout the run while some may run too fast early in the run and be forced to slow down or even stop before completing the test. Other individuals may begin too slowly and continue this way, so that their final performance scores reflect inappropriate pacing or lack of motivation rather than poor physiologic capacity. The $\dot{V}O_{2max}$ does not singularly determine endurance running performance. Body mass and fatness, running economy, and percentage of aerobic capacity sustained without blood lactate buildup also contribute to successful running. *Generally, the SEE of predicting $\dot{V}O_{2max}$ from run-walk performance averages about ±8 to $\pm10\%$ of the predicted value.*

Limitations for Use with Children

Maximum 1-mile run or walk times serve only limited use for $\dot{V}O_{2max}$ prediction in growing children because the age-related exercise performance improvements in youth relate poorly to changes in aerobic capacity.[17] The largest contributions to test score improvement in children as they grow older result from increased percentage of $\dot{V}O_{2max}$ sustained during the activity (i.e., increased blood lactate threshold) and improved running economy. Both factors contribute substantially to faster times independent of any improvement in $\dot{V}O_{2max}$.

Predictions Based on Heart Rate

Tests to predict $\dot{V}O_{2max}$ use exercise or postexercise heart rate during a standardized regimen of submaximal effort performed on either a bicycle ergometer, treadmill, or step test. These tests apply the essentially linear relationship between heart rate (HR) and oxygen consumption ($\dot{V}O_2$) during increasing intensities of light to relatively intense aerobic activity. The slope of the line to describe the HR–$\dot{V}O_2$ relationship (i.e., rate of heart rate increase) reflects the adequacy of the cardiovascular response and aerobic fitness capacity. The $\dot{V}O_{2max}$ is estimated by drawing a best-fit straight line through several submaximal points that relate heart rate and oxygen consumption (or exercise intensity); the **HR–$\dot{V}O_2$ line** is then extended to an assumed maximum heart rate for the subject's age.

FIGURE 11.11 illustrates the **extrapolation procedure** for an untrained and an endurance-trained college student. Four submaximal measures during graded exercise provided the data points to construct the HR–$\dot{V}O_2$ line. Each person's HR–$\dot{V}O_2$ line tends toward linearity, although the slope of the line often differs considerably. A person of relatively high

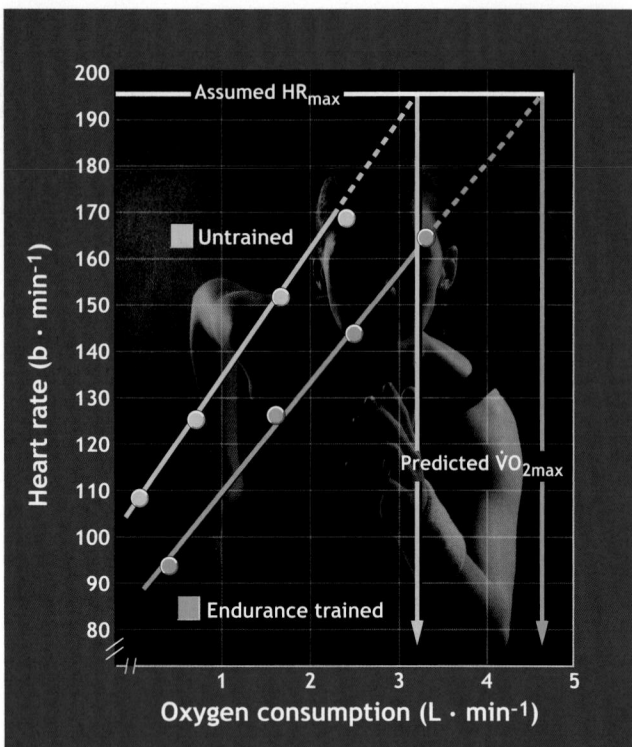

FIGURE 11.11 • Extrapolating the linear relationship between submaximal heart rate and oxygen consumption up to an assumed maximum heart rate during graded exercise by an untrained subject and an endurance-trained subject.

aerobic fitness performs more intense effort (i.e., achieves higher $\dot{V}O_2$) before reaching a heart rate of 140 or 160 b·min⁻¹ than a less-fit person. Heart rate increases linearly with exercise intensity ($\dot{V}O_2$), so the person with the smallest heart rate increase tends to achieve the highest exercise capacity and highest $\dot{V}O_{2max}$. Extrapolation of the HR–$\dot{V}O_2$ line to a heart rate of 195 b·min⁻¹—the assumed maximum heart rate for subjects of college age—predicted the $\dot{V}O_{2max}$ of the two subjects depicted in Figure 11.11.

The following four assumptions impact the accuracy of the $\dot{V}O_{2max}$ prediction from submaximal exercise heart rate:

1. *Linearity of heart rate–oxygen consumption or exercise intensity relationship.* This assumption generally holds, particularly during light to moderate physical activity. In some subjects, the HR–$\dot{V}O_2$ line curves or asymptotes at more intense workloads in a direction to indicate a larger than expected increase in oxygen consumption per unit increase in heart rate. Oxygen consumption increases more than predicted by linear extrapolation of the HR–$\dot{V}O_2$ line, thereby underestimating these subjects' $\dot{V}O_{2max}$.

2. *Similar maximum heart rates for all subjects.* One standard deviation from the average maximum heart rate for individuals of the same age equals ±10 b·min⁻¹. Extrapolating the HR–$\dot{V}O_2$ line of a young adult to 195 b·min⁻¹, for example, overestimates the $\dot{V}O_{2max}$ of a person whose actual maximum heart rate is 185 b·min⁻¹. The opposite

occurs for a subject with an actual maximum heart rate of 210 b·min⁻¹. Maximum heart rate also decreases with age. Failure to consider this age effect (i.e., extrapolating to an average heart rate of 195 b·min⁻¹ for 25-year-olds) consistently overestimates $\dot{V}O_{2max}$ in older subjects. Chapter 31 discusses the effect of age on maximum heart rate.

3. *Assumed constant economy and mechanical efficiency during activity.* Variations in exercise economy contribute to $\dot{V}O_{2max}$ prediction errors with tests that estimate submaximal oxygen consumption from the external workload (rather than measuring $\dot{V}O_2$ directly). More specifically, an underestimation of $\dot{V}O_{2max}$ occurs for a subject with poor exercise economy whose submaximal oxygen consumption increases more than assumed on the basis of estimates from exercise intensity. This occurs because of an elevated heart rate from the added oxygen cost of uneconomical movement. Variation in walking or cycling economy among individuals usually does not exceed 6%; for bench stepping, the variation can equal about 10%, a value unrelated to age, leg length, aerobic fitness, or percentage body fat.[88] Seemingly small modifications in test procedures profoundly affect exercise economy. Simply allowing individuals to support themselves with the treadmill handrails reduces the oxygen cost of physical activity by as much as 30%.[107]

4. *Day-to-day heart rate variation.* Under highly standardized conditions, the day-to-day variation in heart rate still averages about 5 b·min⁻¹ during submaximal exercise.

Within the framework of these limitations, $\dot{V}O_{2max}$ predicted from submaximal heart rate generally falls within 10 to 20% of the person's actual value. This accuracy level remains *unacceptable* for research purposes, yet the prediction tests can effectively screen and classify individuals for aerobic fitness in a gymnasium or health-club setting. The technique also has proved useful to estimate aerobic capacity during pregnancy (see "In a Practical Sense," Chapter 9).[78]

The Step Test

"Prediction equations" applied to step-test results can estimate $\dot{V}O_{2max}$ with reasonable accuracy.

In one of our laboratories, we devised a 3-min step test to evaluate the heart rate responses of thousands of college men and women.[54] The test used gymnasium bleachers (16¼ in. high) to test large numbers of students at the same time. Subjects performed each stepping cycle to a four-step cadence, "up-up-down-down." The women performed 22 complete step-ups per minute, regulated by a metronome set at 88 beats per minute. Males tended to be "fitter" for step-up exercise than females, so their cadence was 24 step-ups per minute, or 96 beats per minute on the metronome. The step test began after a brief demonstration and practice period. At the completion of stepping, students remained standing while pulse rate was measured for 15 s, 5 to 20 s into recovery. Recovery heart rate was converted to beats per minute (15-s HR × 4).

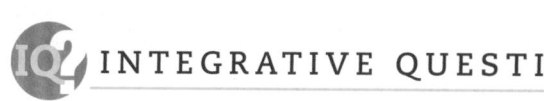

INTEGRATIVE QUESTION

Explain why $\dot{V}O_{2max}$ values do not always agree when measured directly in the laboratory and predicted with a 12-min run.

Based on the linear relationship between heart rate and oxygen consumption during submaximal effort, one would expect a person with a low step-test heart rate (i.e., farther from maximum) to experience less stress than someone of the same age who performed the identical exercise with a relatively high heart rate. In other words, a lower heart rate during a standard exercise corresponds to a higher $\dot{V}O_{2max}$. To determine validity of the step test to estimate aerobic capacity, we then measured the $\dot{V}O_{2max}$ for a group of untrained, young adult men and women who also performed the step test. FIGURE 11.12 illustrates the relationship between $\dot{V}O_{2max}$ and the women's step-test scores. The results clearly indicated that step-test heart rate provided useful information about $\dot{V}O_{2max}$. Subjects with a high recovery heart rate tended to have a lower $\dot{V}O_{2max}$, whereas a faster recovery (lower heart rate) related to a relatively high $\dot{V}O_{2max}$. The following equations predict $\dot{V}O_{2max}$ (mL·kg⁻¹·min⁻¹) from step-test pulse rate (ST$_{pulse}$) for similar groups of young adult men and women:

Men:

$$\dot{V}O_{2max} = 111.33 - (0.42 \times ST_{pulse} \text{ [b·min}^{-1}\text{]})$$

Women:

$$\dot{V}O_{2max} = 65.81 - (0.1847 - ST_{pulse} \text{ [b·min}^{-1}\text{]})$$

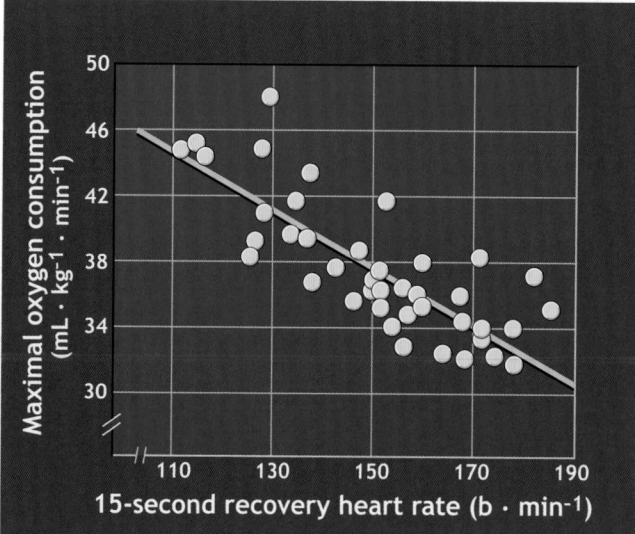

FIGURE 11.12 • Scattergram and line of "best fit" that relates step-test heart rate score and maximal oxygen consumption in untrained college women.

For example, an untrained college-age male with a step-test recovery pulse rate of 152 b·min⁻¹ has a predicted $\dot{V}O_{2max}$ of 47.5 mL·kg⁻¹·min⁻¹ (111.33 – [0.42 × 152]). For predictive accuracy, one can be 95% confident that the predicted $\dot{V}O_{2max}$ falls within ±16% of the person's true $\dot{V}O_{2max}$.

A Novel Approach to Predicting $\dot{V}O_{2max}$ from Nonexercise Data

A unique approach to $\dot{V}O_{2max}$ prediction for quick screening of large groups of individuals requires specific nonexercise data from a questionnaire[28,38] (see TABLE 11.5). The SEE for a predicted score from the method described below equals ±3.44 mL O_2·kg⁻¹·min⁻¹.

Data input to predict $\dot{V}O_{2max}$ from nonexercise data:

1. **Sex**—(female = 0; male = 1).
2. **Body mass index (BMI; kg·m⁻²)**—Self-reported body mass (kg) and stature (m) used to compute BMI as follows:

$$BMI = \text{Body mass (kg)} \div \text{Stature (m}^2\text{)}$$

3. **Physical activity rating (PA-R)**—A point value between 0 and 10 represents overall physical activity level for the previous 6 months (Table 11.5A).
4. **Perceived functional ability (PFA)**—Sum of the point values between 0 and 13 for questions about current level of perceived functional ability to maintain a continuous pace on an indoor track for 1 mile and perceived pace to cover a distance of 3 miles without becoming breathless or overly fatigued (Table 11.5B).

Equation

$$\dot{V}O_{2max} \text{ (mL·kg}^{-1}\text{·min}^{-1}\text{)} = 44.895 + (7.042 \times \text{Sex}) - (0.823 \times BMI) + (0.738 \times PFA) + (0.688 \times \text{PA-R})$$

Example

1. Sex, female
2. BMI = 22.66 (self-reported body mass = 136 lb [61.7 kg]; self-reported height = 5 feet 5 inches [1.65 m]); BMI = 61.7 ÷ (1.65 × 1.65) = 22.66
3. PA-R score = 5 (see Table 11.5)
4. PFA score = 15 (sum of 7 scored on first set of questions and 8 on second set; see Table 11.5B.)

Computation

$$
\begin{aligned}
\dot{V}O_{2max} &= 44.895 + (7.042 \times \text{Sex}) - (0.823 \times BMI) \\
&\quad + (0.738 \times PFA) + (0.688 \times \text{PA-R}) \\
&= 44.895 + (7.042 \times 0) - (0.823 \times 22.66) \\
&\quad + (0.738 \times 15) + (0.688 \times 5) \\
&= 44.895 - 18.65 + 11.07 + 3.77 \\
&= 41.1 \text{ mL·kg}^{-1}\text{·min}^{-1}
\end{aligned}
$$

| TABLE 11.5 | Input Information on Level of Physical Activity and Perceived Functional Capacity for Predicting $\dot{V}O_{2max}$ from Nonexercise Data |

A. Physical Activity Rating (PA-R)

Select the number that best describes your overall level of physical activity for the previous 6 months:

Points	Description
0	**Inactive:** avoid walking or exertion (e.g., always use elevator, drive when possible instead of walking)
1	**Light activity:** walk for pleasure, routinely use stairs, occasionally exercise sufficiently to cause heavy breathing or perspiration
2	**Moderate activity:** 10 to 60 min per week of moderate activity such as golf, horseback riding, calisthenics, table tennis, bowling, weightlifting, yard work, cleaning house, walking for exercise
3	**Moderate activity:** over 1 hr per week of moderate activity described above
4	**Vigorous activity:** run less than 1 mile per week or spend less than 30 min per week in comparable activity such as running or jogging, lap swimming, cycling, rowing, aerobics, skipping rope, running in place, or engaging in vigorous aerobic-type activity such as soccer, basketball, tennis, racquetball, or handball
5	**Vigorous activity:** run 1 mile to less than 5 miles per week or spend 30 min to less than 60 min per week in comparable physical activity as described above
6	**Vigorous activity:** run 5 miles to less than 10 miles per week or spend 1 hr to less than 3 hr per week in comparable physical activity as described above
7	**Vigorous activity:** run 10 miles to less than 15 miles per week or spend 3 hr to less than 6 hr per week in comparable physical activity as described above
8	**Vigorous activity:** run 15 miles to less than 20 miles per week or spend 6 hr to less than 7 hr per week in comparable physical activity as described above
9	**Vigorous activity:** run 20 to 25 miles per week or spend 7 to 8 hr per week in comparable physical activity as described above
10	**Vigorous activity:** run over 25 miles per week or spend over 8 hr per week in comparable physical activity as described above

B. Perceived Functional Ability (PFA) Questions

Suppose you exercise continuously on an indoor track for 1 mile. Which exercise pace is right for you—not too easy or not too hard? Circle the appropriate number from 1 to 13.

Points	Description
1	Walking at a slow pace (18-min per mile or more)
2	
3	Walking at a medium pace (16-min per mile)
4	
5	Walking at a fast pace (14-min per mile)
6	
7	Jogging at a slow pace (12-min per mile)
8	
9	Jogging at a medium pace (10-min per mile)
10	
11	Jogging at a fast pace (8-min per mile)
12	
13	Running at a fast pace (7-min per mile or less)

TABLE 11.5	**Input Information on Level of Physical Activity and Perceived Functional Capacity for Predicting $\dot{V}O_{2max}$ from Nonexercise Data** *(Continued)*

How fast could you cover a distance of 3 miles and NOT become breathless or overly fatigued? Be realistic. Circle the appropriate number from 1 to 13.

Points	Description
1	I could walk the entire distance at a slow pace (18-min per mile or more)
2	
3	I could walk the entire distance at a medium pace (16-min per mile)
4	
5	I could walk the entire distance at a fast pace (14-min per mile)
6	
7	I could jog the entire distance at a slow pace (12-min per mile)
8	
9	I could jog the entire distance at a medium pace (10-min per mile)
10	
11	I could jog the entire distance at a fast pace (8-min per mile)
12	
13	I could run the entire distance at a fast pace (7-min per mile or less)

Adapted with permission from George JD, et al. Non-exercise $\dot{V}O_{2max}$ estimation for physically active college students. *Med Sci Sports Exerc* 1997;29:415.

Summary

1. The concepts of individual differences and exercise specificity provide an important underlying framework to understand anaerobic and aerobic power capacities.
2. Precise contributions of anaerobic and aerobic energy transfer depend largely on the intensity and duration of effort.
3. During strength and power-sprint activities, energy transfer primarily involves the immediate and short-term (anaerobic) energy systems. The long-term (aerobic) energy system becomes progressively more active during activity lasting longer than 2 min.
4. Appropriate physiologic measurements and performance tests evaluate the capacity of each energy-transfer system. These tests evaluate energy-transfer capacity at a particular point in time or show changes consequent to a specific training program.
5. The stair-sprinting test commonly measures the power capacity of the intramuscular high-energy phosphates ATP and PCr.
6. The 30-s, all-out Wingate test evaluates peak power and average power output capacity from the glycolytic pathway. Interpretations of test results must consider body size and the exercise specificity principle.
7. The maximal accumulated oxygen deficit (MAOD) correlates positively with other anaerobic performance tests; it demonstrates independence from aerobic energy sources and differentiates between aerobically and anaerobically trained individuals.

8. Training status, acid-base regulation, and motivation contribute to individual differences in the capacities of the immediate and short-term anaerobic energy systems.
9. Maximal oxygen consumption ($\dot{V}O_{2max}$) provides important, reproducible information about the power capacity of the long-term energy system, including the functional capacity of the physiologic support systems.
10. Heredity, state and type of training, age, gender, and body composition contribute uniquely to an individual's $\dot{V}O_{2max}$.
11. Expressing aerobic capacity by a ratio of body size or composition (e.g., $mL \cdot kg^{-1} \cdot min^{-1}$ or $mL \cdot kg\ FFM^{-1} \cdot min^{-1}$) reduces gender difference in $\dot{V}O_{2max}$.
12. Tests to predict $\dot{V}O_{2max}$ from submaximal physiologic and performance data often prove useful for fitness classification purposes.
13. Tests to predict $\dot{V}O_{2max}$ from submaximal physiologic and performance data rely on the validity of four assumptions: linearity of the HR–$\dot{V}O_2$ relationship, constancy in maximum heart rate, relatively constant exercise economy, and minimal day-to-day variation in exercise heart rate.
14. Field methods provide useful information about cardiovascular-aerobic function in the absence of more valid laboratory methods.
15. Nonexercise data predict $\dot{V}O_{2max}$ accurately for screening and classification purposes.

thePoint References are available online at
http://thepoint.lww.com/mkk8e.

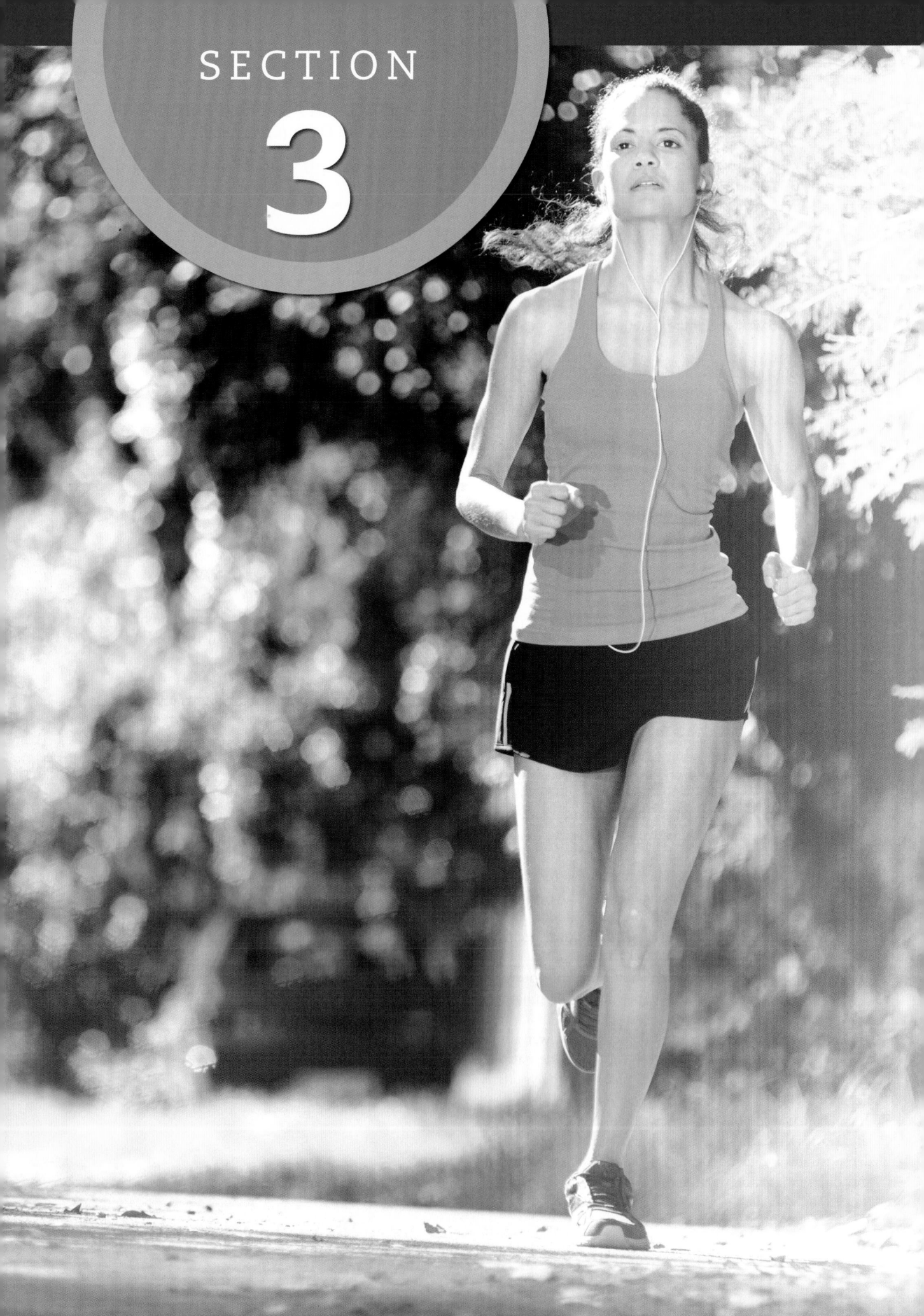

Aerobic Systems of Energy Delivery and Utilization

OVERVIEW

Many sports, recreational, and occupational activities require a moderately intense and sustained energy release. The aerobic breakdown of carbohydrates, fats, and proteins provides energy for such activities by phosphorylating adenosine diphosphate (ADP) to adenosine triphosphate (ATP). Two factors influence how well individuals sustain a high level of steady-rate (aerobic) physical activity with minimal fatigue:

1. **Capacity and integration of physiologic systems for oxygen delivery**
2. **Capacity of specific muscle fibers activated in physical activity to generate ATP aerobically**

Individual differences in aerobic capacity depend on the combined influence of ventilatory, circulatory, muscular, and endocrine systems described in this section. Knowledge about the energy requirements and corresponding physiologic adjustments to physical activity provides a solid basis to formulate an effective training program and evaluate its results.

INTERVIEW WITH
Dr. Loring B. Rowell

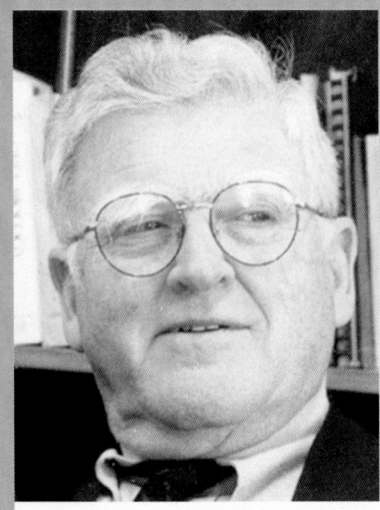

Education: BS (Springfield College, Springfield, MA); PhD (Physiology, University of Minnesota, MN); postgraduate training (Senior Fellow, Department of Physiology and Biophysics, and of Medicine in Cardiology, University of Washington School of Medicine, St. Louis, MO)

Current Affiliation: Professor Emeritus, University of Washington

Honors, Awards, and ACSM Honor Award Statement of Contributions: See Appendix C, available online at http://thepoint.lww.com/mkk8e.

Research Focus: Human cardiovascular system control and adjustments to exercise

Memorable Publication: Rowell LB. Neural control of muscle blood flow: Importance during dynamic exercise. *Clin Exp Pharm Physiol* 1997;24:117.

What first inspired you to enter the exercise science field? What made you decide to pursue your advanced degree and/or line of research?

➤ Dr. Peter V. Karpovich at Springfield College (MA) provided my first exposure to the science of physiology. His precise and demanding teaching provided the motivation to seek an advanced degree in physiology and to do research in that field.

What influence did your undergraduate education have on your final career choice?

➤ Again, the undergraduate teaching of Dr. Karpovich, my experience working in his laboratory, and his urging and support paved the way. His influence led me to the Department of Physiology at the University of Minnesota Medical School and the laboratories of Ancel Keys, Henry L. Taylor, and Francisco Grande and colleagues.

Who were the most influential people in your career, and why?

➤ First, Drs. Henry L. Taylor and Francisco Grande guided my graduate education and taught me how to do research. They became lifelong models for an approach to research and scholarship that I admire greatly. Second, my scientific colleagues, students, and fellows have all provided me with constant stimulation and education, and have enriched my career.

What has been the most interesting/enjoyable aspect of your involvement in science? What was the least interesting/enjoyable aspect?

➤ Regarding the most interesting and enjoyable aspects: First are the wonderful colleagues from all over the world who became lifelong friends and enormous positive influences on my life. Second was the research, the excitement of developing methods to answer a scientific question, getting an answer, having it accepted by peers, and seeing it published. The least enjoyable aspects were not having our answers accepted by our peers and any breakdown or failure of our developed methods.

What is your most meaningful contribution to the field of exercise science, and why is it so important?

➤ Time and history must judge. I think it is the collection of experiments (1964–1974) in which we quantified the reductions in regional organ blood flow, which were closely related to exercise intensity expressed as percent of $\dot{V}O_{2max}$ and heart rate. They revealed the quantitative significance of this regional vasoconstriction to blood pressure regulation and to the redistribution of oxygen from resting organs to active muscle. And they showed how this regional vasoconstriction determines the volume of blood available to fill the heart (and thus stroke volume) in exercising humans and how this crucial adjustment is upset by skin vasodilation during heat stress.

What advice would you give to students who express an interest in pursuing a career in exercise science research?

➤ My advice is based on physiology because that is what I do. I am a cardiovascular physiologist who has used exercise as a powerful precision tool to understand how the cardiovascular system works. Acquisition of a strong background in general physics, mathematics, and chemistry (inorganic, analytical, organic, and especially basic physical chemistry) is essential. In as much as the physiology of exercise is actually the total physiology of a nonresting, nonsupine individual, all areas of physiology are essential because there is no physiological function, regulation, or control that is not vital (i.e., exercise physiology = physiology in toto). Thus, the broader and deeper the training in physiology, the more likely the research will yield basic new information. To quote Sir Joseph Barcroft (1934), "The condition of exercise is not a mere variant of the condition of rest, it is the essence of the machine."

What interests have you pursued outside your professional career?

➤ Competitive and recreational alpine skiing, plus coaching and instruction; alpinism (glacier and rock climbing); road and mountain bicycling; tennis; landscape painting (oil); and historical literature.

Where do you see the exercise science field (particularly your area of greatest interest) heading in the next 20 years?

➤ This field may play a more vital role in the biological sciences than we had once imagined. If the basic life scientists rush to apply their expertise to provide functional meaning to the genetic code, as is expected, who will be left to teach basic human biology and physiology? Who will explore the functional consequences of aging, for example? Who will discover what controls breathing and circulation during exercise? Who will do the systematic, integrative science that reveals how whole organ systems and organisms actually work? These questions are not likely to be answered by reductionists (e.g., molecular biologists) working upward from molecules to cells to systems—this is in the wrong direction!

You have the opportunity to give a "last lecture." Describe its primary focus.

➤ Its primary focus would be on the question, "What reflexes govern cardiovascular function in exercise?" This century-old, unanswered question concerns what is being controlled (and how), and what signals or errors are being sensed (and how) and corrected (and how) by the autonomic nervous system. The lecture would present the currently dominant ideas and would argue which ones do not seem feasible (and why) and

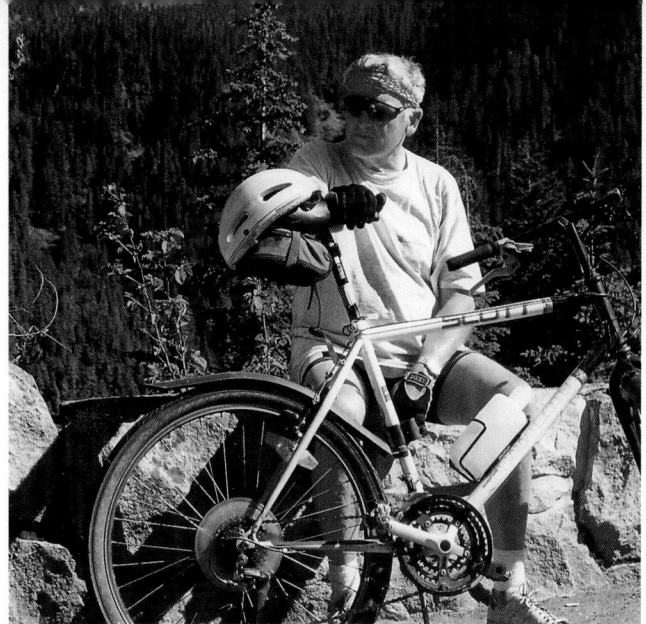

which ones seem feasible based on current knowledge. It would ask where we turn next. And, finally, it would warn us of the great danger of ignoring history—a danger now encouraged by exclusion of all literature published before 1970 from the computer indexing services.

CHAPTER

12

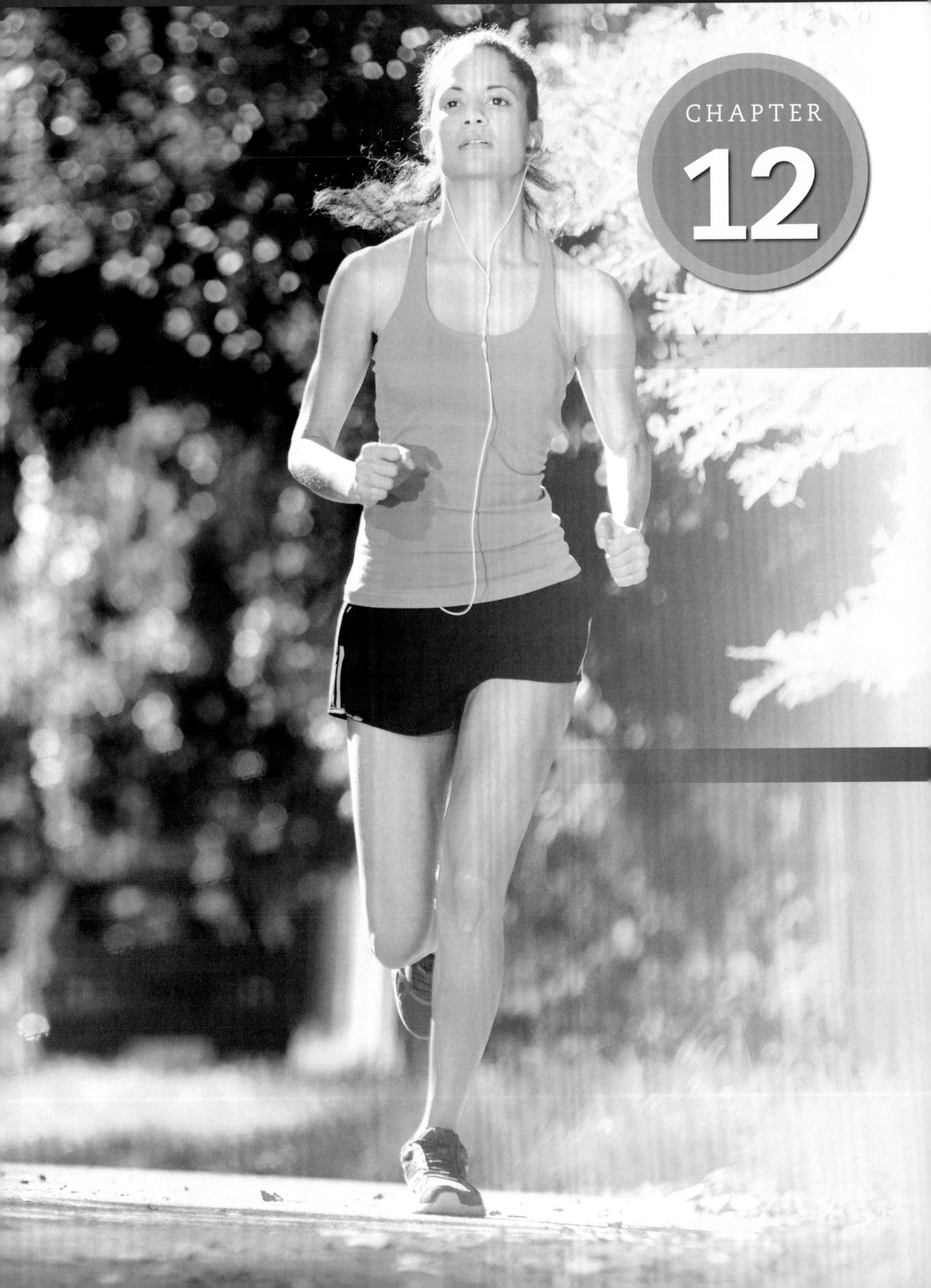

Pulmonary Structure and Function

- Diagram the ventilatory system—label the glottis, trachea, bronchi, bronchioles, and alveoli

- Describe the ventilatory system's conducting zone and the transitional and respiratory zones

- Discuss the mechanical and muscular aspects of inspiration and expiration during rest and physical activity

- Define and quantify static and dynamic lung function measures and their relation to physical performance

- Define minute ventilation, alveolar ventilation, ventilation–perfusion ratio, and anatomic and physiologic dead space

- Discuss the contributions of breathing rate and tidal volume to minute ventilation and alveolar minute ventilation at rest and during physical activity

- Discuss factors that account for variations in ventilation–perfusion ratio among healthy individuals and those with pulmonary limitations, and why this ratio varies within different lung areas

- Explain the four phases of the Valsalva and discuss the physiologic consequences of this maneuver

- Describe the effects of cold-weather exercise on the respiratory tract

Visit http://thePoint.lww.com/mkk8e to access the following resources.

- References: Chapter 12
- Interactive Question Bank
- Animation: Accessory Muscles of Respiration
- Animation: Asthma
- Animation: Perform a Pulmonary Function Test
- Animation: Pulmonary Ventilation
- Animation: The Respiratory System
- Focus on Research: Physiological Control of Pulmonary Ventilation

SURFACE AREA AND GAS EXCHANGE

If oxygen supply to muscle depended only on diffusion through the skin surface, one could not sustain the basal oxygen requirement of 0.2 to 0.4 L per min, let alone the 4- to 5-L per minute oxygen consumption and carbon dioxide elimination required to run a world-class, 5-min per mile marathon pace. The body's relatively compact and remarkably efficient **ventilatory system** meets the requirements for gas exchange. This system, depicted in FIGURE 12.1, regulates the gaseous state of the body's "external" pulmonary environment to effectively aerate body fluids.

ANATOMY OF VENTILATION

Pulmonary ventilation describes the process of moving and exchanging ambient air with air in the lungs. Air entering the nose and mouth flows into the conductive portions of the ventilatory system where it adjusts to body temperature and is filtered and almost completely humidified as it travels through the **trachea**. The inspired air then passes into two **bronchi**, the large first generation of airways

that serve as primary conduits into each of the lungs. The bronchi further subdivide into numerous **bronchioles** that conduct inspired air through a winding, narrow route until it eventually mixes with existing air in the alveolar ducts. Microscopic alveoli, hollow terminal cavities that are spherical outcroppings of the respiratory bronchioles, completely envelop these ducts.

Pulmonary Respiration Versus Cellular Respiration: A Conflict in Terms?

Physiologists apply the term *respiration* within two different contexts, yet both forms are inexorably linked. In one sense, *cellular respiration* defines metabolic processes that occur within the cell that generate energy via oxygen utilization and carbon dioxide production. Within the second context, *pulmonary respiration* defines lung ventilation with a resulting uptake of oxygen and elimination of carbon dioxide to maintain blood–gas homeostasis.

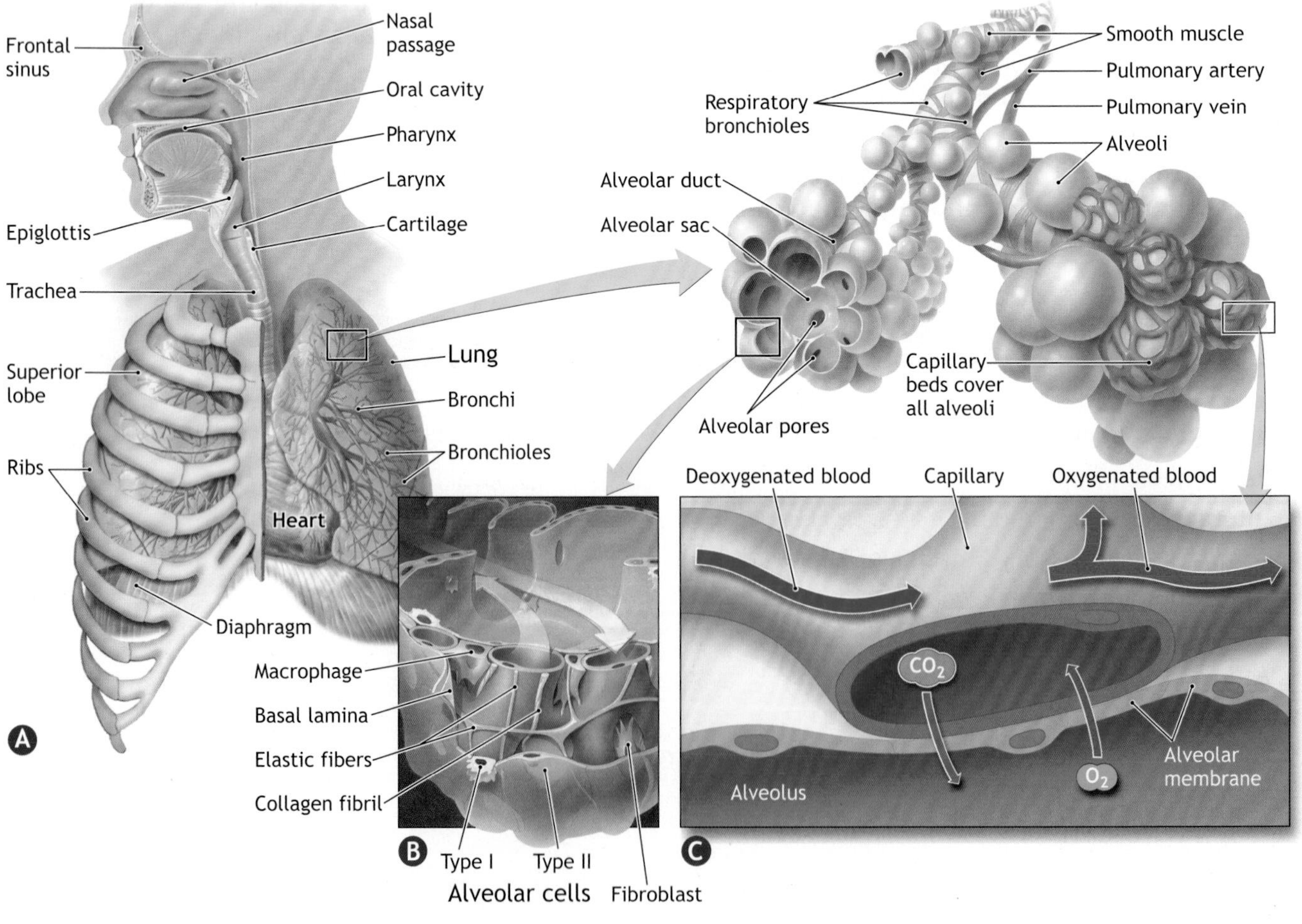

FIGURE 12.1 • **(A)** Major pulmonary structures within the thoracic cavity including the terminal branches of the respiratory tree. **(B)** Section of lung tissue showing individual alveolus including type I cells that form the structure of the alveolar wall, type II cells that secrete pulmonary surfactant, and macrophages that destroy foreign substances including bacteria. **(C)** Gas exchange function in alveolus.

The Lungs

The lungs provide the **gas exchange surface** that separates blood from the surrounding alveolar gaseous environment. Oxygen transfers from alveolar air into alveolar capillary blood; simultaneously, the blood's carbon dioxide moves into the alveolar chambers where it subsequently flows into ambient air. The lungs of an average-sized adult weigh approximately 2.3 kg, and the volume varies between 4 and 6 L, about the volume of air in a basketball. The lungs consist of about 10% solid tissue, with the remainder filled by air and blood. If spread out, lung tissue would cover an area of 50 to 100 m², an area 20 to 50 times larger than the body's external surface or about half of a tennis court (**Fig. 12.2**).

The highly vascularized, moist lung surface consisting of 1500 miles of airways and 600 miles of capillaries fits within the chest cavity. The lung membranes fold over onto themselves to provide a considerable interface to aerate blood. At rest, a single red blood cell remains in a pulmonary capillary for only about 0.5 to 1.0 s as it traverses past two to three individual alveoli. During any 1 s of maximal effort, no more than 1 pint of blood flows within the delicate mesh network of lung tissue blood vessels.

The Alveoli

The lungs contain more than 600 million **alveoli**, the final branching of the respiratory tree. These elastic, thin-walled membranous sacs approximately 0.3 mm in diameter composed of simple squamous epithelial cells provide the vital surface for gas exchange between lung tissue and blood. Alveolar tissue receives the largest blood supply of any of the body's organs. Millions of short, thin-walled capillaries and alveoli lie side by side; air moves along one side and blood along the other. Gases diffuse across the extremely thin barrier of alveolar and capillary cells (~0.3 μm); the diffusion distance remains relatively constant throughout varying levels of physical activity. The integrity of the thin pulmonary blood-gas barrier remains constant during sustained effort. The surface remains as thin as possible without compromising structural integrity to facilitate rapid exchange of respiratory gases. In elite endurance athletes, alveolar mechanical stress from large ventilation and accompanying pulmonary blood flow in near-maximal exercise can impair the blood–gas barrier's permeability. For these individuals, an increased permeability is reflected by elevated concentrations of red blood cells, total protein, and leukotriene B_4 (a potent chemotactic agent that initiates, coordinates, and amplifies the inflammatory response) in bronchoalveolar lavage fluid with maximal exertion.[22,23,46]

Small **pores of Kohn** within each alveolus evenly disperse surfactant (see the section titled "Surfactant"

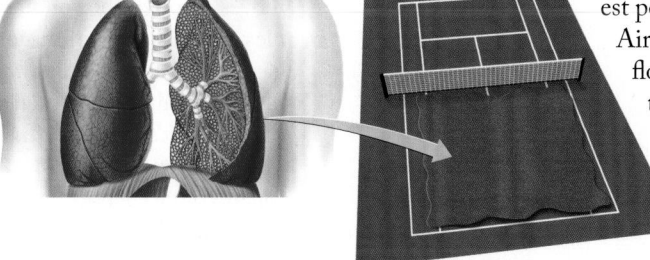

FIGURE 12.2 • The lungs provide an exceptionally large surface for gas exchange.

below) over the respiratory membranes to reduce surface tension for easier alveolar inflation. The pores also provide for gas interchange between adjacent alveoli. Mixing in this manner sustains the indirect ventilation of alveoli damaged or blocked from lung disease (see Chapter 32).

Each minute at rest, approximately 250 mL of oxygen leaves the alveoli and enters the blood, and 200 mL of carbon dioxide diffuses in the opposite direction. When endurance athletes perform intensely, nearly 25 times this quantity of oxygen and carbon dioxide transfers across the alveolar–capillary membrane. In healthy individuals, pulmonary ventilation during rest and physical activity primarily maintains a constant and favorable oxygen and carbon dioxide concentration in the alveolar chambers to ensure complete gaseous exchange before the blood leaves the lungs for transport throughout the body.

 See the animation "The Respiratory System" on http://thePoint.lww.com/mkk8e for a demonstration of this process.

MECHANICS OF VENTILATION

Figure 12.3 illustrates the physical principle that underlies breathing dynamics. Note the two lung-shaped balloons suspended in a jar with its glass bottom replaced by a thin rubber membrane. Pulling the membrane down increases jar volume. This reduces air pressure within the jar compared with ambient air outside the jar. This imbalance causes air to rush in to inflate the balloons. Conversely, as the elastic membrane recoils, pressure within the jar temporarily increases and air rushes out. Increasing the depth and rate of descent and ascent of the rubber membrane exchanges a considerable air volume within the balloons in a given time.

Figure 12.4 illustrates the ventilatory system subdivided into two parts:

1. **Conducting zones** (zones 1–16 *shown in blue at the right*) that includes the trachea and terminal bronchioles
2. **Transitional** and **respiratory zones** (zones 17–23 *shown in brown at the right*) that comprise bronchioles, alveolar ducts, and alveoli.

The structures of the conducting zone contain no alveoli, so the term *anatomic dead space* describes this area. The respiratory zone represents the site of gas exchange. It occupies about 2.5 to 3.0 L and constitutes the largest portion of the total lung volume. Air moving into the lungs literally flows down the trachea to the terminal bronchi, much like water flowing through a hose. As air reaches the smaller air passages in the transitional zone, the tremendous increase in surface area slows airflow into the alveoli.

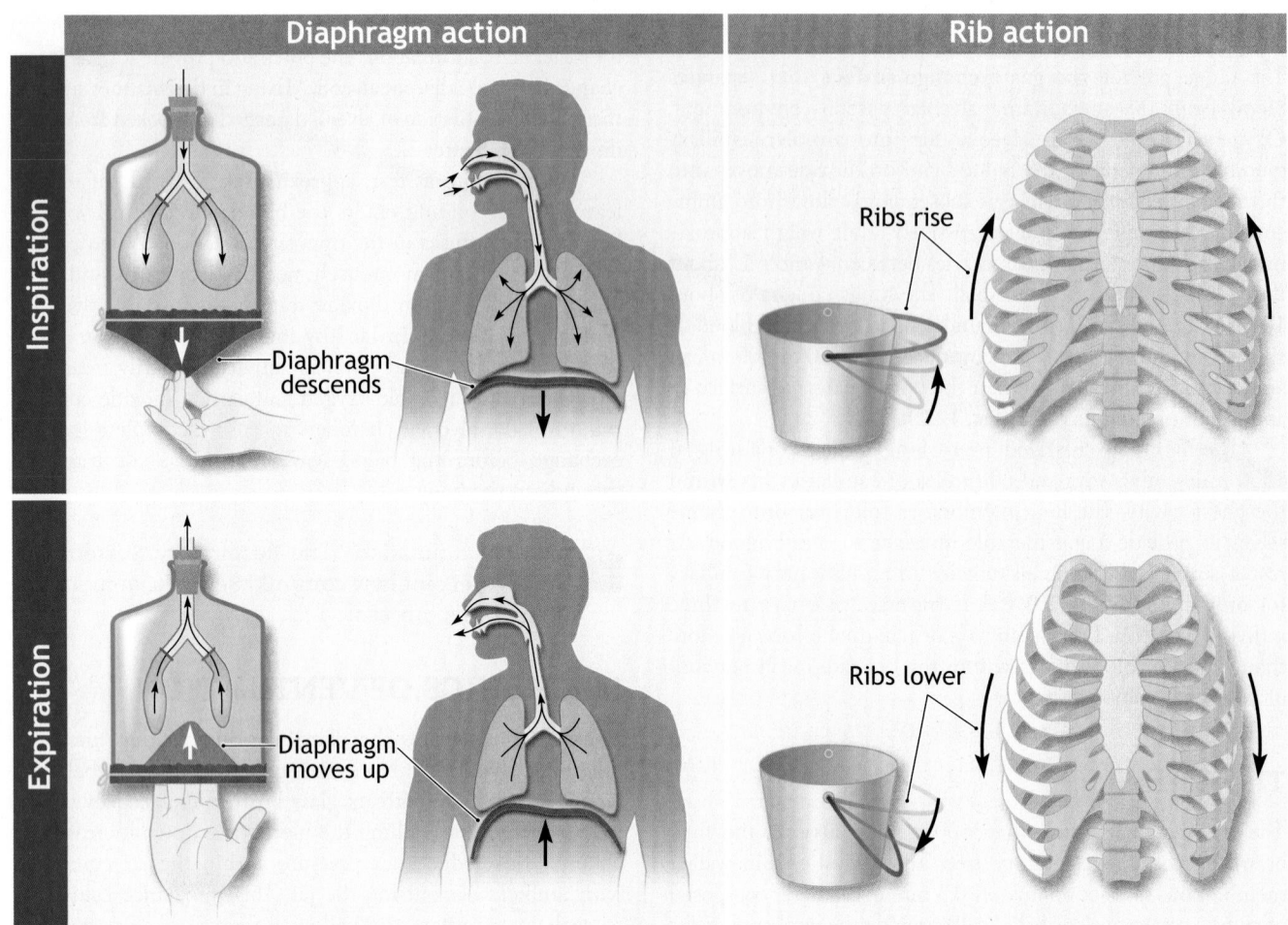

FIGURE 12.3 • Mechanics of breathing. During *inspiration*, the chest cavity increases in size because the ribs raise and the diaphragm descends, causing air to flow into the lungs. Inhalation increases in the anterior–posterior (A–P) and vertical diameters of the rib cage. Approximately 70% of lung expansion results from A–P enlargement and 30% from diaphragmatic descent. In addition to diaphragmatic action, the external intercostal muscles become active and the internal intercostal muscles relax during inhalation. During *expiration*, the ribs swing down and the diaphragm returns to a relaxed position. This reduces thoracic cavity volume and air rushes out. The movement of the jar's rubber bottom causes air to enter and exit the two balloons, simulating the action of the diaphragm. The movement of the bucket handle simulates rib action. The diaphragm, external intercostals, sternocleidomastoids, scapular elevators, anterior serrati scleni, and spinal erector muscles compose the inspiratory muscles that elevate and enlarge the thorax; muscles of expiration (rectus abdominis, internal intercostals, posterior inferior serrati muscles) depress the thorax and reduce its size.

The ventilatory conducting zone functions also include the following:

1. Air transport
2. Humidification
3. Warming
4. Particle filtration
5. Vocalization
6. Immunoglobulin secretion

The four respiratory zone functions encompass:

1. Surfactant production (in the alveolar endothelium)
2. Molecule activation and inactivation (in the capillary endothelium)
3. Blood clotting regulation
4. Endocrine function

FIGURE **12.5** depicts the relationship between airway generation (forward velocity) and total cross-sectional area of the conducting passages of various lung segments. Airway cross section increases considerably and velocity slows as air moves through the conducting zone to the terminal bronchioles. At this stage, diffusion provides the primary means for gas movement and distribution. In the alveoli, gas pressures rapidly equilibrate on each side of the alveolar–capillary membrane. **Fick's law of diffusion** (derived in 1845 by German physiologist Adolf Gaston Eugen Fick [1852–1937], inventor of contact lenses and first to devise a technique to measure cardiac output [see Chapter 17]) governs gas diffusion across a fluid membrane. This two-part law states that a gas diffuses through a sheet of tissue at a rate (1) directly proportional to the tissue area, a diffusion constant, and the pressure

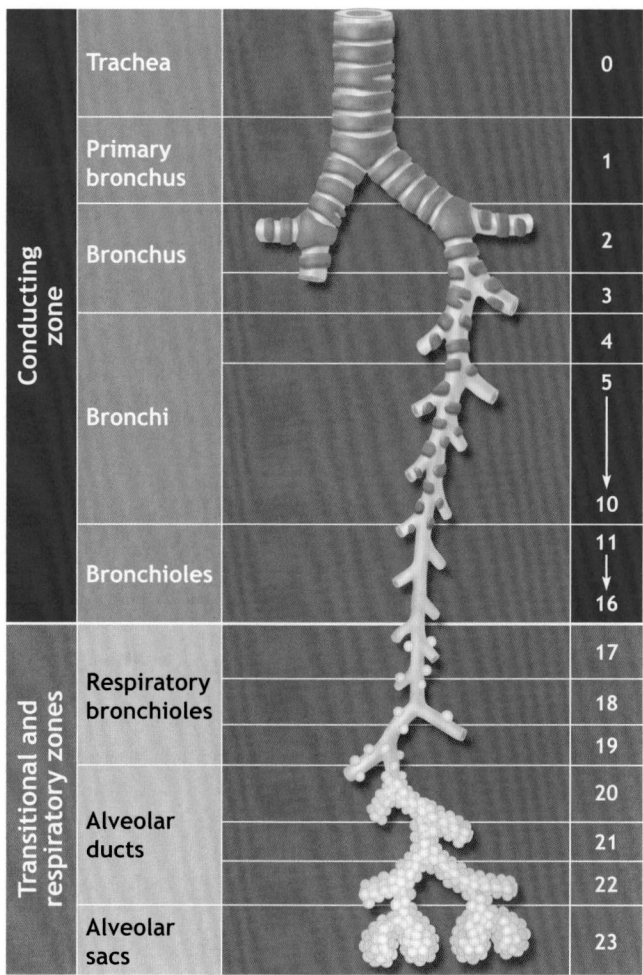

Conducting zone	Trachea	0
	Primary bronchus	1
	Bronchus	2
		3
		4
	Bronchi	5 ↓ 10
	Bronchioles	11 ↓ 16
Transitional and respiratory zones		17
	Respiratory bronchioles	18
		19
		20
	Alveolar ducts	21
		22
	Alveolar sacs	23

FIGURE 12.4 • Separation of human lung tissue into a series of discrete *conduction zones* (zones 1 through 16) and *transitional* and *respiratory* zones (zones 17 through 23).

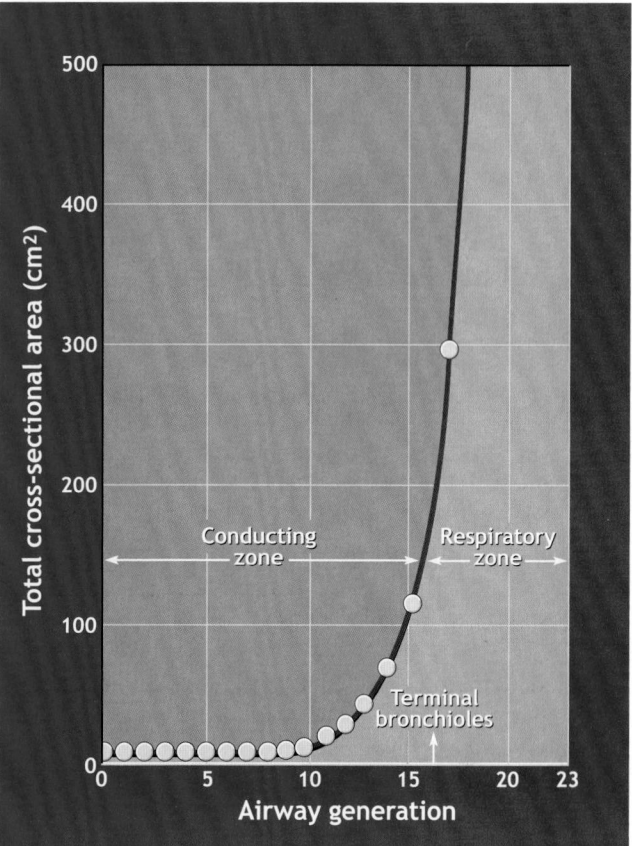

FIGURE 12.5 • Airflow in the lungs in relation to the total cross-sectional tissue area. Forward airflow velocity during inspiration decreases considerably because of the large increase in tissue cross-sectional area beginning in the region of the terminal bronchioles. (Adapted with permission from West JB. *Respiratory Physiology—The Essentials*. 8th Ed. Baltimore: Lippincott Williams & Wilkins, 2008.)

differential of the gas on each side of the membrane and (2) inversely proportional to tissue thickness. The diffusion constant (D) relates directly to gas solubility (S) and inversely to the square root of the gas molecular weight (MW). On a per-molecule basis, carbon dioxide (MW = 44) diffuses about 20 times faster through thin membranous tissues than oxygen (MW = 32) because of carbon dioxide's higher solubility despite the relatively similar MWs of the two gases.

The lungs do not merely remain suspended in the chest cavity as the balloons do in Figure 12.3. Instead, the pressure differential between the air in the lungs and the lung–chest wall interface causes them to adhere to the chest wall and literally follow its every movement. Any change in thoracic cavity volume correspondingly alters lung volume.

Inspiration

The **diaphragm**, a large, dome-shaped sheet of striated musculofibrous tissue, serves the same purpose as the jar's lower rubber membrane depicted in Figure 12.3. This primary ventilatory muscle—whose mitochondrial volume density, oxidative capacity of muscle fibers, and aerobic capacity exceed by up to fourfold that

of most other skeletal muscles[33]—creates an airtight separation between the abdominal and thoracic cavities. The diaphragm contains a series of openings through which the esophagus, blood vessels, and nerves pass. This separating membrane possesses high oxidative potential and the greatest capacity of all the respiratory muscles for shortening and volume displacement.[13,34]

During **inspiration**, the diaphragm muscle contracts, flattens, and moves downward toward the abdominal cavity by as much as 10 cm. Elongation and enlargement of the chest cavity expands the air in the lungs, causing its **intrapulmonic pressure** to decrease to slightly below atmospheric pressure. The lungs inflate as the nose and mouth literally suck air inward. The degree of filling depends on the magnitude of inspiratory movements. Maximal activation of the inspiratory muscles of healthy individuals produces pressures that range between 80 and 140 mm Hg. Inspiration ends when thoracic cavity expansion ceases. This causes equality between intrapulmonic pressure and ambient atmospheric pressure.

During physical activity, the highly efficient movements of the diaphragm, rib cage (ribs and sternum), and abdominal muscles synchronize to contribute to inspiration and expiration.[2,25] During inspiration, the **scaleni** and **external intercostal** muscles between the ribs contract, causing the ribs to rotate and lift up and away from the body. This action corresponds to the movement of the handle lifted up and away from the side of the bucket (see Fig. 12.3, *upper right*). Inspiratory action increases during activity when the diaphragm descends, the ribs swing upward, and the sternum thrusts outward to increase the lateral and anterior–posterior diameter of the thorax.

Body Position Facilitates Breathing

Athletes often bend forward from the waist to facilitate breathing following sustained physical effort. This body position serves two purposes: (1) promotes blood flow to the heart and (2) minimizes the antagonistic effects of gravity on the usual upward direction of inspiratory movements.

Expiration

Expiration during rest and light physical activity represents a passive process of air movement out of the lungs and results from two factors: (1) natural recoil of the stretched lung tissue and (2) relaxation of the inspiratory muscles. The sternum and ribs swing down and the diaphragm rises toward the thoracic cavity. These movements decrease chest cavity volume and compress alveolar gas so air moves from the respiratory tract to the atmosphere. Expiration ends when the compressive force of expiratory muscles ceases and intrapulmonic pressure decreases to atmospheric pressure. During strenuous activity, **internal intercostal** and **abdominal muscles** act powerfully on the ribs and abdominal cavity to reduce thoracic dimensions.[14] This makes exhalation rapid and more extensive.

No major differences exist in ventilatory mechanics between men and women of different ages. At rest in the supine position, most persons breathe diaphragmatically ("abdominal breathers"), whereas in the upright position rib and sternum actions become more apparent. Rib cage movement dictates the rapid alterations in thoracic volume in strenuous exertion. Distinct biochemical differences among muscles that compose the respiratory pump provide the evidence that the rib musculature acts more rapidly than the diaphragm and abdominal muscles.[35] The position of the head and back naturally adopted by distance runners—forward lean from the waist, neck flexed, and head extended forward with mandible parallel to the ground—favors pulmonary ventilation during intense activity.

Surfactant

Pressures vary continually within the alveolar and pleural spaces throughout the ventilatory cycle. Resistance to normal expansion of the lung cavity and alveoli progressively increases during inspiration from the effect of **surface tension**, primarily in the alveoli. Surface tension relates to a resisting force created at the surface of a liquid in contact with a gas, structure, or another liquid. In the alveoli, surface tension results from the attractive forces between the liquid molecules that

line these structures. The tension or force created causes the liquid to assume a shape that presents the smallest surface area to the surrounding medium. The greater the surface tension surrounding a spherical object such as an alveolus, the greater the force required to overcome pressure within the sphere and cause it to enlarge or inflate. **Surfactant** (a contraction of "surface active agent," or literally a wetting agent) consists of a lipoprotein mixture of phospholipids, proteins, and calcium ions produced by alveolar epithelial cells. The main component of surfactant, the phospholipid dipalmitoylphosphatidylcholine, reduces surface tension. It mixes with the fluid that encircles the alveolar chambers. Its action interrupts the surrounding water layer, reducing the alveolar membrane's surface tension to increase overall lung compliance. This effect reduces the energy required for alveolar inflation and deflation.[48] In the absence of surfactant, small alveoli have a tendency to collapse (called *atelextasis*) due to high collapsing pressures, which makes it more difficult for them to remain open. The opposite effect occurs in larger alveoli with larger radii and thus low collapsing pressure.

LUNG VOLUMES AND CAPACITIES

FIGURE 12.6 illustrates various lung volume measurements and average values for men and women that affect the ability to increase breathing depth. To obtain these measurements, the subject rebreathes through a water-sealed, volume-displacement recording spirometer, similar to the one described in Chapter 8 (Fig. 8.3), for measuring oxygen consumption by the closed-circuit method. As with many anatomic and physiologic measures, lung volumes vary with age, gender, and body size and composition, but particularly with stature. Common practice evaluates lung volumes by comparing them to established standards that consider these factors.

 See the animation "Perform a Pulmonary Function Test" on **http://thePoint.lww.com/mkk8e** for a demonstration of this process.

Static Lung Volumes

The spirometer bell falls and rises during inhalation and exhalation to provide a record of ventilatory volume and breathing rate. **Tidal volume** (**TV**) describes air volume moved during either the inspiratory or expiratory phase of each breathing cycle (first portion of the record). Under resting conditions, TV usually ranges between 0.4 and 1.0 L of air per breath.

After recording several trials of TV, the subject inspires as deeply as possible following a normal inspiration. The additional 2.5- to 3.5-L volume above inspired tidal air represents the reserve ability for inhalation, referred to as the **inspiratory reserve volume (IRV)**. Following IRV measurement, the subject reestablishes the normal breathing pattern. After a normal exhalation, the subject continues to exhale and forces as much air as possible from the lungs. This additional volume represents **expiratory reserve volume** (**ERV**), which ranges between 1.0 and 1.5 L for an average-sized man. During physical activity, encroachment on IRV and ERV, particularly IRV, considerably increases TV.

The total volume of air voluntarily moved in one breath, from full inspiration to maximum expiration, represents the vital capacity (VC), or more precisely, **forced vital capacity (FVC)**. FVC includes TV plus IRV and ERV. FVC usually ranges between 4 and 5 L in healthy young men and between 3 and 4 L in healthy young women. Values of 6 to 7 L are not uncommon for tall individuals, and unusually large FVC values have been published for a professional football player (7.6 L) and an Olympic gold medalist in cross-country skiing (8.1 L).[3,47] These athletes' large lung volumes generally reflect genetic influences and body size characteristics because exercise training does not appreciably change static lung volumes.

Residual Lung Volume

The **residual lung volume (RLV)** represents the air volume remaining in the lungs after exhaling as deeply and forcibly as possible. This volume averages between 0.8 and 1.2 L for college-age, healthy women and between 0.9 and 1.4 L for college-age, healthy men. RLV for apparently healthy professional football players ranges between 0.96 and 2.46 L.[45] RLV increases with age, whereas IRV and ERV decrease proportionally. A decline in lung tissue elasticity components with aging probably decreases breathing reserve and concomitantly increases residual lung volume. Alterations in pulmonary function may not entirely reflect an aging phenomenon because regular aerobic training diminishes the typical age-related decline in static and dynamic lung functions.[16] The RLV allows an uninterrupted exchange of gas between the blood and alveoli to prevent fluctuations in blood gases during phases of the breathing cycle including deep breathing. RLV plus FVC constitutes **total lung capacity (TLC)**.

Effects of Previous Physical Activity. The RLV temporarily increases from an acute bout of either short-term or prolonged activity. In one study, RLV increased during recovery from a maximal treadmill test by 21% after 5 min, 17% after 15 min, and 12% after 30 min.[5] RLV generally reverts to its original value within 24 hr. Two possible factors that increase RLV with physical activity are:

1. Closure of small peripheral airways
2. Increase in thoracic blood volume

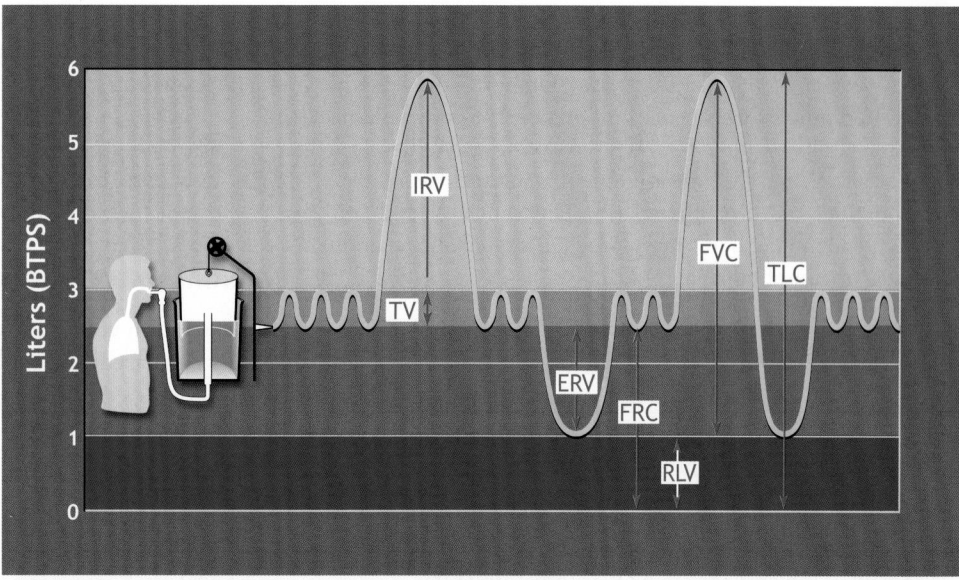

Lung volume/capacity	Definition	Average values (mL)	
		Men	Women
Tidal Volume (TV)	Volume inspired or expired per breath	600	500
Inspiratory Reserve Volume (IRV)	Maximum inspiration at end of tidal inspiration	3000	1900
Expiratory Reserve Volume (ERV)	Maximum expiration at end of tidal expiration	1200	800
Total Lung Capacity (TLC)	Volume in lungs after maximum inspiration	6000	4200
Residual Lung Volume (RLV)	Volume in lungs after maximum expiration	1200	1000
Forced Vital Capacity (FVC)	Maximum volume expired after maximum inspiration	4800	3200
Inspiratory Capacity (IC)	Maximum volume inspired following tidal expiration	3600	2400
Functional Residual Capacity (FRC)	Volume in lungs after tidal expiration	2400	1800

Equation to predict RLV in normal-weight and overweight men and women*

Normal-weight men and women	R	SEE
RLV = 0.0275 AGE + 0.0189 HT − 2.6139	0.70	0.405

Overweight men and women	R	SEE
RLV = 0.0277 AGE + 0.0048 WT + 0.0138 HT − 2.3967	0.65	0.404

R, multiple correlation coefficient; Age (y); HT, height (cm); WT, weight (kg); SEE, standard error of estimate.
*From Miller WC, et al. Derivation of prediction equations for RV in overweight men and women. Med Sci Sports Exerc 1998;30:322.

FIGURE 12.6 • Static measurements of lung volumes.

The added blood volume does not alter the lungs' mechanical properties, but it does displace air, thus preventing complete exhalation (reduced FVC).[8] Any temporary increase in RLV would affect subsequent computations of body volume by hydrostatic weighing for body composition studies (see Chapter 28). When RLV measurement is impractical, prediction equations based on the relation between RLV and age, stature, gender, and body mass provide reasonably accurate estimates (see inset table, Fig. 12.6).

Dynamic Lung Volumes

Adequacy of pulmonary ventilation depends on how well an individual sustains high airflow levels rather than on air movement in a single breath. Dynamic ventilation depends on two factors:

1. Maximum "stroke volume" of the lungs (FVC)
2. Speed of moving a volume of air (breathing rate)

In turn, airflow velocity depends on the resistance of the respiratory passages to the smooth flow of air and the "stiffness" imposed by the mechanical properties of the chest and lung tissue to a change in shape during breathing, termed *lung compliance*. Patients with lung disease rarely experience symptoms of distress until a large part of their ventilatory capacity decreases. Individuals with mild airway obstruction successfully engage in competitive distance running.[29]

FEV-to-FVC Ratio

Some individuals with severe lung disease achieve near-normal FVC values if measured with no time limit for this maneuver. For this reason, clinicians prefer a "dynamic" measurement of lung function such as **forced expiratory volume** (**FEV**), usually measured over 1 s (**FEV$_{1.0}$**). FEV$_{1.0}$ divided by FVC (**FEV$_{1.0}$ ÷ FVC**) indicates pulmonary airflow capacity. It reflects pulmonary expiratory power and overall resistance to air movement upstream in the lungs. Healthy individuals normally expel about 85% of the vital capacity in 1 s. Severe obstructive lung disease (emphysema or bronchial asthma)—with accompanying reduced airway caliber and loss of elastic recoil of lung tissue— considerably reduces FEV$_{1.0}$/FVC, often to values less than 40% of the vital capacity.[28,42] The demarcation point for airway obstruction during dynamic spirometry represents an FEV$_{1.0}$/FVC of 70% or less. FIGURE 12.7 presents pulmonary function test results for FEV$_{1.0}$ and FVC in individuals with normal lung function (*left*) and those with obstructive (*middle*) and restrictive (*right*) lung diseases. Clinicians also compute other values from portions of the curve generated in the forced spirometry maneuver (e.g., mid-50%

of the expiratory curve or instantaneous flows at 25, 50, or 75% FVC) to assess airflow dynamics in the small airways of the pulmonary tract.[44]

 See the animation "Asthma" on **http://thePoint. lww.com/mkk8e** for a demonstration of the effects of asthma on the pulmonary system.

Maximum Voluntary Ventilation

The **maximum voluntary ventilation** (**MVV**) evaluates ventilatory capacity with rapid and deep breathing for 15 s. The 15-s volume, extrapolated to the volume if the subject continued for 1 min, represents MVV and typically ranges between 35 and 40 times the FEV$_{1.0}$.[45] MVV also averages 25% higher than the ventilation during maximal exercise because exercise does not maximally stress how a healthy person breathes. For healthy, college-age men, MVV ranges between 140 and 180 L·min^{-1}; values for women range between 80 and 120 L·min^{-1}. MVV in male members of the United States Nordic Ski Team averaged 192 L·min^{-1}; the individual high was 239 L·min^{-1}.[17] Conversely, patients with obstructive lung disease achieve only about 40% of the MVV considered normal for their age and body size.

 INTEGRATIVE QUESTION

How does regular resistance and aerobic training affect the typical aging decline in measures of lung function?

Physical Activity Implications of Gender Differences in Static and Dynamic Lung Function Measures

Adult women consistently have a reduced lung size and smaller static and dynamic lung function measures, reduced airway diameters, and a smaller diffusion surface than men even after

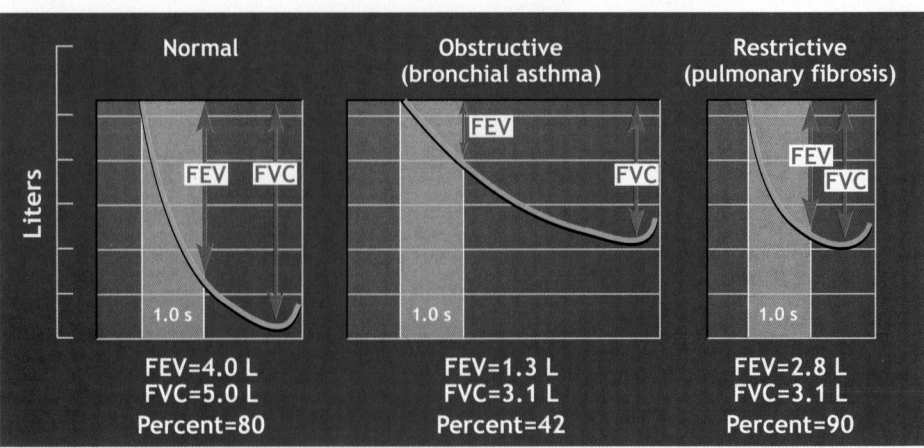

FIGURE 12.7 • Examples of spirometric tracings during standard pulmonary function tests for FEV$_{1.0}$ and FVC in individuals with normal dynamic lung function and in patients with either obstructive or restrictive lung disease.

Ventilatory Muscles Respond to Training

Specific training of the ventilatory muscles improves their strength and endurance and increases both inspiratory muscle function and MVV.[1,37,42] Ventilatory training in patients with chronic pulmonary disease enhances exercise capacity and reduces physiologic strain.[9,39] Progressive desensitization to the feeling of breathlessness and greater self-control of respiratory symptoms represent important benefits of ventilatory muscle training and regular physical activity for patients with chronic obstructive lung disease.

accounting for differences in stature. This disparity produces expiratory flow limitations, greater respiratory muscle work, and relatively greater use of ventilatory reserve compared with men during maximal physical effort. This is particularly true for highly trained women compared to trained men and less-fit women.[31] A relatively smaller lung volume plus a high expiratory flow rate requirement in trained women during intense activity places considerable demand on the maximum flow–volume envelope of the airways (i.e., mechanical constraints of TV and pulmonary minute ventilation). This adversely affects how highly fit women maintain alveolar-to-arterial oxygen exchange, which could compromise arterial oxygen saturation and aerobic capacity to a greater degree than observed for men.[19,20]

LUNG FUNCTION, AEROBIC FITNESS, AND PHYSICAL PERFORMANCE

Unlike the other components of the aerobic system, regular endurance activity does not stimulate large increases in the functional capacity of the pulmonary system. Dynamic lung function tests indicate the severity of obstructive and restrictive lung diseases, yet generally provide little information about aerobic fitness or performance when values fall within the normal range. For example, no difference emerges when comparing the average FVC of prepubescent and Olympic wrestlers, middle-distance athletes, and untrained, healthy subjects.[36,38] Professional football players averaged only 94% of their predicted FVC; the defensive backs achieved only 83% of predicted "normal" values for body size (see "In a Practical Sense"). Somewhat surprisingly, similar values emerged for static and dynamic lung function of accomplished marathon runners and other endurance-trained athletes compared with untrained controls of similar body size.[16,30]

Swimming and scuba diving stimulate development of larger than normal static lung volumes. These sports strengthen the inspiratory muscles, which must work against the additional resistance of the mass of water that compresses the thorax. Enhanced ventilatory muscle strength and power explain the relatively large FVC of scuba divers and competitive swimmers.[6,10,11]

Little relationship exists among different lung volumes and capacities and various track performances. This includes distance running for a large group of teenage boys and girls,

even after adjusting for differences in body size.[12] For marathon runners versus sedentary subjects of similar body size, no difference existed for lung function values (TABLE 12.1).[24,29] For healthy, untrained individuals, no relationship exists between maximal oxygen consumption and FVC or MVV (adjusted for body size). Fatigue from strenuous physical activity frequently relates to feeling "out of breath," or "winded," yet normal capacity for pulmonary ventilation for most individuals does not limit maximal aerobic performance. The larger than normal lung volumes and breathing capacities of some athletes probably reflect genetic endowment. Specific muscular training can increase pulmonary function by strengthening the respiratory muscles.

PULMONARY VENTILATION

One can view pulmonary ventilation from two perspectives: (1) volume of air moved into or out of the total respiratory tract each minute and (2) air volume that ventilates only the alveolar chambers each minute.

 See the animation "Pulmonary Ventilation" on **http://thePoint.lww.com/mkk8e** for a demonstration of this process.

Minute Ventilation

The normal breathing rate during quiet breathing at rest in a thermoneutral environment averages 12 breaths per minute and TV averages 0.5 L of air per breath. Consequently, the volume of air breathed each minute, referred to as **minute ventilation,** equals 6 L.

$$\text{Minute ventilation } (\dot{V}_E) = \text{Breathing rate} \times \text{Tidal volume}$$
$$= 12 \times 0.5 \text{ L}$$
$$= 6 \text{ L} \cdot \text{min}^{-1}$$

An increase in either the rate or depth of breathing or both increases minute ventilation. During strenuous physical activity, healthy young adults readily increase their breathing rate to 35 to 45 breaths per minute. Some elite endurance athletes breathe as rapidly as 60 to 70 times each minute during maximal effort. TVs of 2.0 L and higher commonly occur in most adults during physical activity. Such increases in breathing rate and TV increase minute ventilation to 100 L or more (about 17 to 20 times the resting value). In male endurance athletes, ventilation may increase to 160 L · min⁻¹ during maximal effort. Minute ventilation volumes of 200 L, with a high volume of 208 L in a professional football player, have been observed during maximal bicycle exercise.[47] *Even with such large minute ventilations, TVs for trained and untrained individuals rarely exceed 60% of vital capacity.*

Alveolar Ventilation

A portion of the air in each breath does not enter the alveoli and participate in gaseous exchange with the blood. The term *anatomic dead space* describes this air that fills the upper airway structures (mouth, nasal passages, nasopharynx, larynx,

IN A PRACTICAL SENSE

Predicting Pulmonary Function Variables in Men and Women

Pulmonary function variables do not directly relate to measures of physical fitness in healthy individuals. Instead, their measurement often forms part of a standard medical/health/fitness examination, particularly for individuals at risk for limited pulmonary function (e.g., chronic cigarette smokers, asthmatics). Measurement of pulmonary dimensions and lung functions with a water-filled spirometer (see Fig. 12.6) or electronic spirometer provides the framework for discussions of pulmonary dynamics during rest and physical activity. Proper evaluation of measured values for pulmonary function requires comparison to "expected" values (norms) from the clinical literature.

EQUATIONS

Pulmonary function scores associate closely with stature (ST) and age (A), enabling these two variables to predict the expected average (normal) lung function value for an individual.

Data

Woman: A, 22 y; ST, 165.1 cm (65 in)
Man: A, 22 y; ST, 182.9 cm (72 in)

EXAMPLES

Woman

1. *Forced vital capacity (FVC)*
   FVC (L) = $(0.0414 \times ST\,[cm]) - (0.0232 \times A\,[y]) - 2.20$
   = 6.835 − 0.5104 − 2.20
   = 4.12 L

2. *Forced expiratory volume in 1 s (FEV$_{1.0}$)*
   FEV$_{1.0}$ (L) = $(0.0268 \times ST\,[cm]) - (0.0251 \times A\,[y]) - 0.38$
   = 4.425 − 0.5522 − 0.38
   = 3.49 L

3. *Percentage forced vital capacity in 1 s (FEV$_{1.0}$/FVC):*
   FEV$_{1.0}$/FVC(%) = $(-0.2145 \times ST\,[cm]) - (0.1523 \times A\,[y]) + 124.5$
   = −35.41 − 3.35 + 124.5
   = 85.7%

4. *Maximum voluntary ventilation (MVV)*
   MVV (L·min^{-1}) = $40 \times$ FEV$_{1.0}$
   = 40 × 3.49 (from #2)
   = 139.6 L·min^{-1}

Man

1. *Forced vital capacity (FVC)*
   FVC (L) = $(0.0774 \times ST\,[cm] - (0.0212 \times A\,[y]) - 7.75)$
   = 14.156 − 0.4664 − 7.75
   = 5.49 L

2. *Forced expiratory volume in 1 s (FEV$_{1.0}$)*
   FEV$_{1.0}$ (L) = $(0.0566 \times ST\,[cm]) - (0.0233 \times A\,[y]) - 0.491$
   = 10.35 − 0.5126 − 4.91
   = 4.93 L

3. *Percentage forced vital capacity in 1 s (FEV$_{1.0}$/FVC)*
   FEV$_{1.0}$/FVC (%) = $(-0.1314 \times ST\,[cm]) - (0.1490 \times A\,[y]) + 110.2$
   = −24.03 − 3.35 + 110.2
   = 82.8%

4. *Maximum voluntary ventilation (MVV)*
   MVV (L·min^{-1}) = $40 \times$ FEV$_{1.0}$
   = 40 × 4.93 L (from #2)
   = 197.2 L·min^{-1}

Equations to Predict Pulmonary Function Variables by Age and Gender

Variable	Men <25Y	Men >25 Y	Female <25 Y	Female >25 Y
Forced vital capacity (FVC): Maximum volume expired following a maximum inspiration	FVC (L) = $(0.0774 \times ST) - (0.0212 \times A) - 7.75$	FVC (L) = $(0.065 \times ST) + (0.029 \times A) - 5.459$	FVC (L) = $(0.0414 \times ST) - (0.0232 \times A) - 2.20$	FVC (L) = $(0.037 \times ST) + (0.092 \times A) - 3.469$
Forced expiratory volume in 1 s (FEV$_{1.0}$): Volume forcibly expired in 1 s following a maximum inspiration	FEV$_{1.0}$(L) = $(0.0566 \times ST) - 0.0233 \times A) - 0.491$	FEV$_{1.0}$(L) = $(0.052 \times ST) + (0.027 \times A) - 4.203$	FEV$_{1.0}$(L) = $(0.0268 \times ST) - (0.0251 \times A) - 0.38$	FEV$_{1.0}$(L) = $(0.027 \times ST) - (0.021 \times A) - 0.794$
FEV$_{1.0}$/FVC: Percentage of forced vital capacity expired in 1 s	FEV$_{1.0}$/FVC (%) = $(-0.1314 \times ST) - (0.1490 \times A) + 110.2$	FEV$_{1.0}$/FVC (%) = $103.64 - (0.87 \times ST) - (0.14 \times A)$	FEV$_{1.0}$/FVC (%) = $(-0.2145 \times ST) - (0.1523 \times A) + 124.5$	FEV$_{1.0}$/FVC (%) = $107.38 - (0.111 \times ST) - (0.109 \times A)$
Maximum voluntary ventilation (MW): Maximum amount of air forcibly breathed in 1 min	MMV ((L·min^{-1}) = $40 \times$ FEV$_{1.0}$	MMV (L·min^{-1}) = $(1.15 \times H) - (1.27 \times A) + 14$	MMV (L·min^{-1}) = $40 \times$ FEV	MMV (L·min^{-1}) = $(0.55 \times ST) - (0.72 \times A) + 50$

ST, stature (height) in centimeters; A, age in years.

Comroe JH, et al. *The Lung*. Chicago: Year Book Medical Publishers, 1962.
Miller A. *Pulmonary Function Tests in Clinical and Occupational Disease*. Philadelphia: Grune & Stratton, 1986.
Taylor AE, et al. *Clinical Respiratory Physiology*. Philadelphia: WB Saunders, 1989.
Wasserman K, et al. *Principles of Exercise Testing and Interpretation*. Baltimore: Lippincott Williams & Wilkins, 2004.

TABLE 12.1 — Anthropometric Data, Pulmonary Function, and Resting Minute Ventilation in 20 Marathon Runners and Healthy Controls

Measure	Runners	Controls	Difference[a]
Anthropometric			
Age, y	27.8	27.4	0.4
Stature, cm	175.8	176.7	0.9
Surface area, m^2	1.82	1.89	0.07
Pulmonary Function			
FVC, L	5.13	5.34	0.21
TLC, L	6.91	7.13	0.22
FEV$_{1.0}$, L	4.32	4.47	0.15
FEV$_{1.0}$ / FVC, %	84.3	83.8	0.5
MVV, L · min^{-1}	179.8	176.0	3.8
Resting Ventilation			
$\dot{V}_e$, L · min^{-1}	11.9	11.9	0.9
Breathing rate, breaths · min^{-1}	10.9	11.1	0.2
Tidal volume, L	1.16	1.06	0.10

Adapted with permission from Mahler DA, et al. Ventilatory responses at rest and during exercise in marathon runners. *J Appl Physiol* 1982;52:388.
[a]All differences not statistically significant.

fyi Typical Values for Pulmonary Ventilation During Rest and Moderate and Intense Physical Activity

Condition	Breathing Rate (Breaths · min^{-1})	Tidal Volume (L · min^{-1})	Pulmonary Ventilation (L · Breath^{-1})
Rest	12	0.5	6
Moderate exercise	30	2.5	75
Intense exercise	50	3.0	150

reaching the alveoli and participating in gas exchange—prevents drastic changes in alveolar air composition to ensure consistency in arterial blood gases throughout the breathing cycle.

TABLE 12.2 indicates that minute ventilation does not always reflect alveolar ventilation. The first example of shallow breathing shows that one can reduce TV to 150 mL, yet still maintain a 6-L minute ventilation by increasing breathing rate to 40 breaths per minute. The same 6-L minute volume results from decreasing breathing rate to 12 breaths per minute and increasing TV to 500 mL. In contrast, doubling TV and halving the breathing rate, as in the example of deep breathing, also produces a 6-L minute ventilation. Each of these ventilatory adjustments drastically affects alveolar ventilation. In the example of shallow breathing, dead-space air represents the only air volume moved without any alveolar ventilation. In the other examples, deeper breathing causes a larger portion of each breath to enter into and mix with alveolar air. Alveolar ventilation determines the gaseous concentrations at the alveolar-capillary membrane.

Dead Space Versus Tidal Volume

The preceding examples of alveolar ventilation represent oversimplifications because they assumed a constant dead space despite changes in TV. Actually, anatomic dead space

trachea, and other nondiffusible conducting portions of the respiratory tract). The anatomic dead space generally ranges between 150 and 200 mL (about 30% of the resting TV) in healthy individuals. The composition of dead-space air remains almost identical to ambient air except for its full saturation with water vapor.

The dead-space volume permits about 350 mL of the 500 mL of inspired TV at rest to enter into and mix with existing alveolar air. This does not mean that only 350 mL of air enters and leaves the alveoli with each breath. Instead, if TV equals 500 mL, then 500 mL of air enters the alveoli, but only 350 mL of this is fresh air. This represents about one-seventh of total alveolar air. Such relatively small and seemingly inefficient **alveolar ventilation**—that portion of inspired air

TABLE 12.2 — Relationships Among Tidal Volume, Breathing Rate, and Both Total and Alveolar Minute Ventilation

Condition	Tidal Volume (mL)	× Breathing Rate (Breaths · min^{-1})	= Total Minute Ventilation (mL · min^{-1})	− Dead Space Minute Ventilation (mL · min^{-1})	= Alveolar Minute Ventilation (mL · min^{-1})
Shallow breathing	150	40	6000	(150 mL × 40)	0
Normal breathing	500	12	6000	(150 mL × 12)	4200
Deep breathing	1000	6	6000	(150 mL × 6)	5100

increases as TV becomes larger; it often doubles during deep breathing from some stretching of the respiratory passages with a fuller inspiration. Importantly, any increase in dead space still represents proportionately less volume than the accompanying increase in TV. *Consequently, deeper breathing provides more effective alveolar ventilation than similar minute ventilation achieved through increased breathing rate.*

Ventilation–Perfusion Ratio

Adequate gas exchange between alveoli and blood requires effective matching of alveolar ventilation to the blood perfusing the pulmonary capillaries. Approximately 4.2 L of air normally ventilates the alveoli each minute at rest, and an average of 5.0 L of blood flows through the pulmonary capillaries. In this case, the ratio of alveolar ventilation to pulmonary blood flow, termed the **ventilation–perfusion ratio**, equals 0.84 (4.2 ÷ 5.0). This ratio means that alveolar ventilation of 0.84 L matches each liter of pulmonary blood flow. In light activity, the ventilation–perfusion ratio remains approximately 0.8. In contrast, intense physical activity produces a disproportionate increase in alveolar ventilation. In healthy individuals, the ventilation–perfusion ratio may exceed 5.0; in most instances, this response ensures adequate aeration of venous blood. The mismatching of alveolar ventilation to perfusion (blood flow) accounts for many of the gas exchange problems occurring in pulmonary disease and possibly during intense activity among highly trained endurance athletes. The ventilation–perfusion ratio varies depending on the region (zone) of the lung because of gravitational effects and because the base (lower region) of the lung positions below the heart and its apex (upper region) lies above the heart (see FYI, "Bronchopulmonary Segments").[4]

the ratio at the apex of the lung exceeds 1.0 (indicative of underperfusion or overventilation). In essence, abnormally large ventilation–perfusion ratios waste a large amount of pulmonary ventilation in overventilating alveoli that cannot use the oxygen while at the same time providing inadequate oxygen for alveoli in need. Despite these regional variations in ventilation in relation to blood flow, ventilation–perfusion ratios that exceed 0.50 are sufficient to meet gas exchange demands at rest.

Physiologic Dead Space

Sometimes the alveoli may not function adequately in gas exchange because of two factors:

1. Underperfusion of blood
2. Inadequate ventilation relative to alveolar surface

The term *physiologic dead space* describes the portion of the alveolar volume with a ventilation–perfusion ratio that approaches zero. FIGURE 12.8 shows the negligible physiologic dead space (*yellow horizontal bar*) in the healthy lung. In certain pathologic situations, physiologic dead space increases to 50% of the TV, as with inadequate perfusion from hemorrhage or blockage of the pulmonary circulation by an embolism or inadequate ventilation in emphysema, asthma, and pulmonary fibrosis. An increased physiologic dead space from decreased functional alveolar surface in emphysema produces extreme ventilation even at low intensities of physical activity. Many patients cannot achieve maximal circulatory capacity because of ventilatory muscle fatigue from excessive breathing. Adequate gas exchange becomes impossible when the dead space of the lung exceeds 60% of total lung volume.

Breathing Rate Versus Tidal Volume

Increasing the rate and depth of breathing increases alveolar ventilation in physical activity. In moderate activity, well-trained athletes maintain alveolar ventilation by increasing TV with only a small increase in breathing rate.[15] As breathing

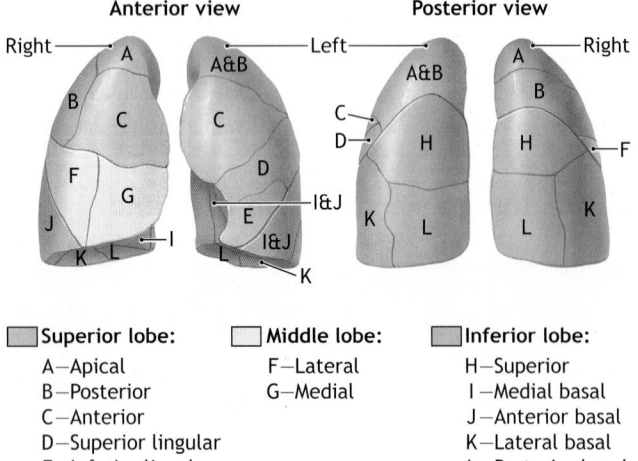

Bronchopulmonary Segments

Anterior view   **Posterior view**

Superior lobe:
A–Apical
B–Posterior
C–Anterior
D–Superior lingular
E–Inferior lingular

Middle lobe:
F–Lateral
G–Medial

Inferior lobe:
H–Superior
I–Medial basal
J–Anterior basal
K–Lateral basal
L–Posterior basal

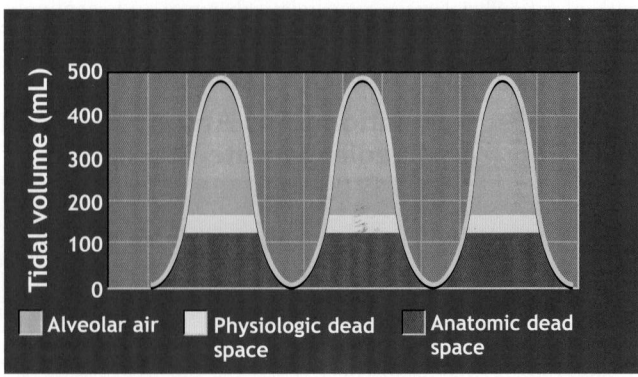

FIGURE 12.8 • Distribution of tidal volume (TV) in a healthy subject at rest. TV includes about 350 mL of ambient air that mixes with alveolar air, 150 mL of ambient air that remains in the larger air passages (anatomic dead space), and a small portion of air distributed to either poorly ventilated or poorly perfused alveoli (physiologic dead space).

The volume of blood flowing through the lung is greatest at the base (indicative of overperfusion or underventilation) and least at its apex. This results in a ratio less than 1.0 whereas

becomes deeper during activity, alveolar ventilation increases from 70% of the total minute ventilation at rest to more than 85% of the exercise ventilation. FIGURE 12.9 shows that encroachment on the IRV, with a smaller decrease in the end-expiratory level, increases exercise TV. With more intense activity, the increase in TV plateaus at approximately 60% of vital capacity; minute ventilation increases further through nonconscious increases in breathing rate. Each person develops a "style" of breathing where breathing rate and TV blend to provide efficient alveolar ventilation. Conscious manipulation of breathing usually disturbs the exquisitely regulated physiologic adjustments to physical activity. Attempts to modify breathing during running or other general physical activities offer no benefit to exercise performance. During rest and all levels of exertion, a healthy person should breathe in the manner that seems most natural.

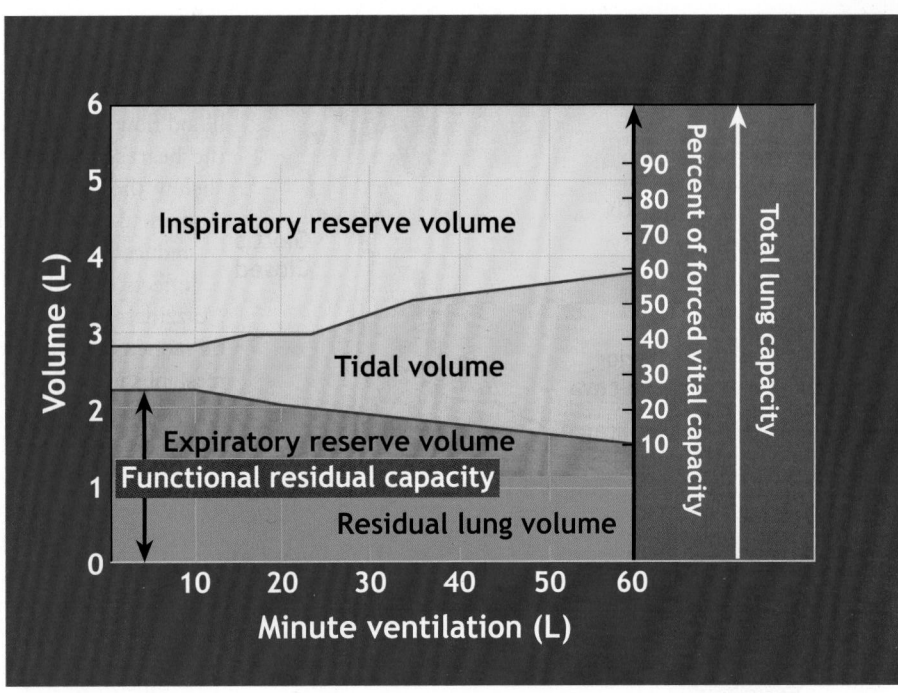

FIGURE 12.9 • Tidal volume and subdivisions of pulmonary air during rest and exercise.

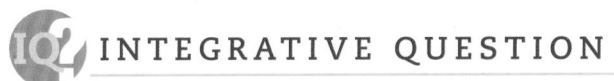

INTEGRATIVE QUESTION

How can a person accelerate breathing rate at rest without disrupting normal alveolar ventilation?

VARIATIONS FROM NORMAL BREATHING PATTERNS

Breathing patterns during physical activity generally progress in an effective and highly economical manner, yet some pulmonary responses can adversely affect performance and/or physiologic balance.

Hyperventilation

Hyperventilation refers to an increase in pulmonary ventilation that exceeds the oxygen consumption and carbon dioxide elimination needs of metabolism. This "overbreathing" quickly lowers normal alveolar carbon dioxide concentration and causes excess carbon dioxide to leave bodily fluids via the expired air. An accompanying decrease in hydrogen ion concentration [H+] increases plasma pH. Several seconds of hyperventilation generally produce light-headedness; prolonged hyperventilation leads to unconsciousness from excessive carbon dioxide unloading.

Dyspnea

Dyspnea refers to an inordinate shortness of breath or subjective distress in breathing. The sense of breathing incapacity during physical activity, particularly in novice exercisers, usually accompanies elevated arterial carbon dioxide and [H+]. Both conditions excite the inspiratory center to increase breathing rate and depth. Failure to adequately regulate arterial carbon dioxide and [H+] most likely relates to low aerobic fitness levels and a poorly conditioned ventilatory musculature.

Valsalva Maneuver

The expiratory muscles, besides their normal role in pulmonary ventilation, provide for the ventilatory maneuvers of coughing and sneezing. They also contribute to stabilizing the abdominal and chest cavities during heavy lifting. In quiet breathing, intrapulmonic pressure decreases only about 3 mm Hg during inspiration and rises a similar amount above atmospheric pressure in exhalation (FIG. 12.10A). Closing the **glottis** (narrowest part of the larynx through which air passes into the trachea) following a full inspiration while maximally activating the expiratory muscles creates compressive forces that increase **intrathoracic pressure** more than 150 mm Hg above atmospheric pressure (FIG. 12.10B). Pressures increase to higher levels within the abdominal cavity during a maximal exhalation against a closed glottis.[18] Forced exhalation against a closed glottis, termed the *Valsalva maneuver*, occurs commonly in weightlifting and other activities that require a rapid, maximum application of force of short duration. The Valsalva stabilizes the abdominal and thoracic cavities to enhance muscle action.

Physiologic Consequences of Performing the Valsalva Maneuver

A prolonged Valsalva maneuver produces an acute drop in blood pressure. Increased intrathoracic pressure during a Valsalva

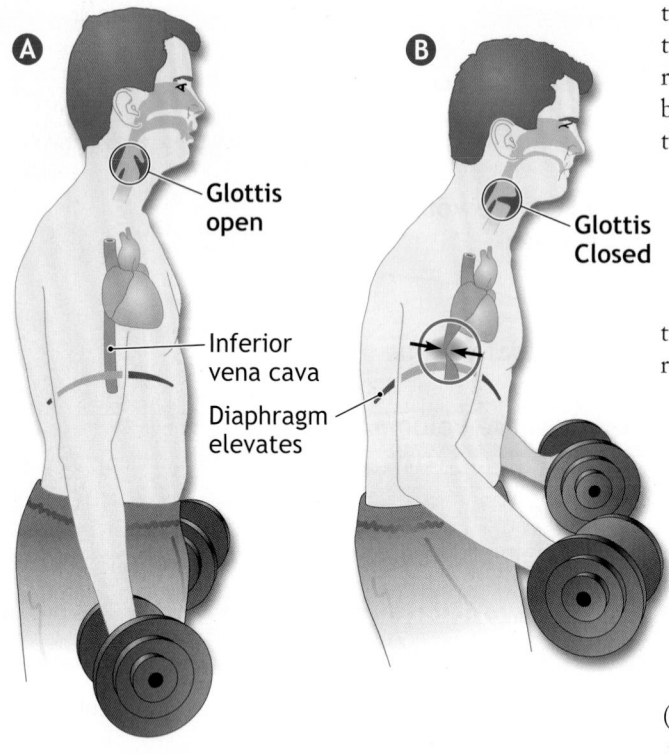

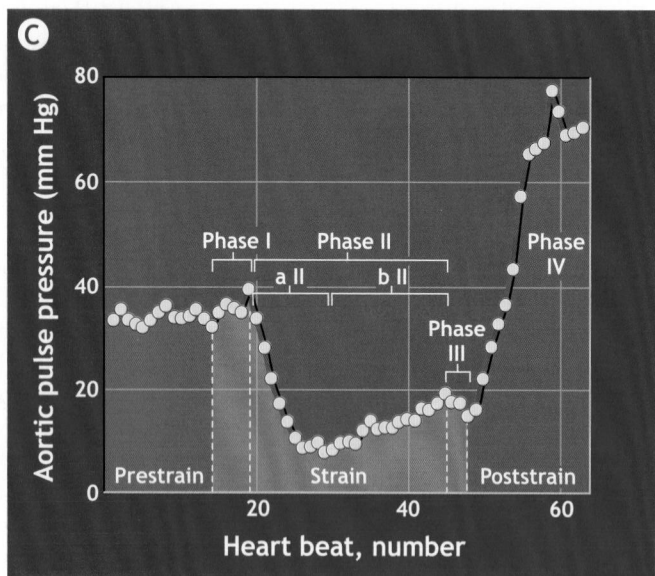

transmits through the thin walls of the veins that pass through the thoracic region. Because venous blood remains under relatively low pressure, thoracic veins collapse, which reduces blood flow to the heart. Reduced venous return sharply lowers the heart's stroke volume, triggering a fall in blood pressure below the resting level.[7,26] Performing a prolonged Valsalva maneuver during static, straining-type exercise dramatically reduces venous return and arterial blood pressure. These effects diminish the brain's blood supply, often producing dizziness, "spots before the eyes," or fainting. Once the glottis reopens and intrathoracic pressure normalizes, blood flow reestablishes with an "overshoot" in arterial blood pressure.[41,43]

FIGURE 12.10C illustrates four phases of the typical blood pressure response (heartbeat by heartbeat) during the Valsalva maneuver in a healthy subject. Aortic pulse pressure increases slightly as the Valsalva begins (phase I), probably from the mechanical effect of elevated intrathoracic pressure that expels blood from the left ventricle into the aorta. A biphasic response occurs within six heartbeats of Valsalva onset. This consists of a large reduction in aortic pulse pressure (phase IIa) followed by a relatively small gradual rise (phase IIb) and secondary decrease (phase III) during the continued Valsalva strain. When the maneuver ceases (release of strain), blood pressure rises rapidly and overshoots the resting value (phase IV).

A Common Misconception. The Valsalva maneuver does not cause the large increases in blood pressure during heavy resistance exercises. Recall from the preceding figure that a prolonged Valsalva dramatically reduces blood pressure. Confusion arises because a Valsalva maneuver of insufficient duration to lower blood pressure usually accompanies straining muscular efforts common during isometric and dynamic resistance exercise. These activities, with or without Valsalva, greatly increase resistance to blood flow in active muscle with a resulting rise in systolic blood pressure.[21] For example, intramuscular fluid pressure increases linearly with all levels of isometric force to the maximum.[40] Increased peripheral vascular resistance increases the arterial blood pressure and workload of the heart throughout exercise. These responses pose a potential danger to individuals with cardiovascular disease; they form the basis for advising cardiac patients to refrain from heavy resistance training. In contrast, performing rhythmic muscular activity, including moderate weightlifting, promotes a steadier blood flow and only modest increase in blood pressure and work of the heart. Chapter 15 more fully discusses the blood pressure response to different activity modes.

FIGURE 12.10 • The Valsalva maneuver reduces the return of blood to the heart because increased intrathoracic pressure collapses the inferior vena cava that passes through the chest cavity. **(A)** Normal breathing. **(B)** Straining exercise with accompanying Valsalva maneuver. **(C)** Typical normal response of aortic pulse pressure with a Valsalva maneuver during calibrated muscle strain. The figure illustrates 63 consecutive heartbeats (○). High-fidelity aortic pressure recordings were obtained at the aortic root level. Pulse pressure represents systolic pressure minus diastolic pressure. (Data from Hébert J-L, et al. Pulse pressure response to the strain of the Valsalva maneuver in humans with preserved systolic function. *J Appl Physiol* 1998;85:817.)

 INTEGRATIVE QUESTION

After completing a maximum-lift standing press, a person exclaims, "I feel slightly dizzy and see spots before my eyes." Provide a plausible physiologic explanation.

THE RESPIRATORY TRACT DURING COLD-WEATHER PHYSICAL ACTIVITY

Cold ambient air normally does not damage the respiratory passages. Even in extreme cold weather, the incoming air generally warms to 79.7 to 89.9°F (26.5 to 32.2°C) by the time it reaches the bronchi. Nonetheless, values as low as 68°F (20°C) can occur in the bronchi when breathing large volumes of cold, dry air.[32] Airway warming of inspired air greatly increases the air's capacity to hold moisture, which produces considerable water loss from the respiratory passages. In cold weather, the respiratory tract loses considerable water and heat, most notably during strenuous exercise with large ventilatory volumes. Fluid loss from the airways often contributes to overall dehydration, dry mouth, burning sensation in the throat, and generalized irritation of the respiratory passages. Wearing a scarf or cellulose mask-type "balaclava" that covers the nose and mouth traps the water in exhaled air and subsequently warms and moistens the next incoming breath of air. This effect reduces the symptoms of respiratory discomfort.

Postexercise Coughing

Physical activity in cold weather can dry the throat and trigger coughing during the recovery period. The response becomes prevalent following exercise in cold weather when the respiratory tract loses considerable water. Postexercise coughing relates directly to the overall respiratory water loss (not respiratory heat loss) associated with the large ventilatory volumes breathed during exercise.

Summary

1. The lungs provide a large surface between the body's internal fluid environment and the gaseous external environment. During any 1 s of physical activity, no more than 1 pint of blood flows in the pulmonary capillaries.
2. Normal regulation of pulmonary ventilation maintains a favorable concentration of alveolar oxygen and carbon dioxide to ensure adequate aeration of blood flowing through the lungs.
3. Fick's law of diffusion governs gas movement across a fluid membrane. This law states that a gas diffuses through a sheet of tissue at a rate directly proportional to the tissue area, a diffusion constant, and the pressure differential of the gas on each side of the membrane and inversely proportional to tissue thickness.
4. Surfactant consists of a lipoprotein mixture secreted within lung tissue that reduces surface tension between the alveolar membrane and surrounding tissues. Its action reduces the alveolar membrane's surface tension to increase overall lung compliance. This effect reduces the energy required for alveolar inflation and deflation.
5. Pulmonary airflow depends on small pressure differentials between ambient air and air within the lungs. Muscle actions that alter thoracic cavity dimensions produce these pressure differences.
6. Lung volumes vary with age, gender, and body size (particularly stature) and should only be evaluated with established norms based on these factors.
7. The residual lung volume represents air remaining in the lungs following maximal exhalation. This air volume allows uninterrupted exchange of gas during all phases of the breathing cycle.
8. Forced expiratory volume and maximum voluntary ventilation dynamically measure the ability to sustain a high airflow level. These lung function measures serve as excellent screening tests to detect lung disease.
9. Measures of static and dynamic lung function within the normal range poorly predict aerobic fitness and exercise performance.
10. Breathing rate and tidal volume (TV) determine pulmonary minute ventilation. Minute ventilation averages $6 \text{ L} \cdot \text{min}^{-1}$ at rest and can increase to $200 \text{ L} \cdot \text{min}^{-1}$ during maximal effort.
11. Alveolar ventilation reflects the portion of minute ventilation that enters the alveoli for gaseous exchange with the blood.
12. The ventilation–perfusion ratio reflects the association between alveolar minute ventilation and pulmonary blood flow.
13. At rest, alveolar ventilation of 0.8 L matches each L of pulmonary blood flow. During intense physical activity, alveolar ventilation increases disproportionately to increase the ventilation–perfusion ratio to 5.0.
14. TV increases during physical activity by encroachment into inspiratory and expiratory reserve volumes. During intense exercise, TV plateaus at approximately 60% of the vital capacity; minute ventilation increases further through increases in breathing rate.
15. A healthy person should breathe in a manner that seems most natural during rest, physical activity, and recovery.
16. Hyperventilation refers to increased pulmonary ventilation that exceeds gas exchange needs of metabolism. This "overbreathing" quickly lowers normal alveolar carbon dioxide concentration, causing excess carbon dioxide to leave body fluids via expired air.
17. A Valsalva maneuver describes a forced exhalation against a closed glottis. This action causes large pressure increases within the chest and abdominal cavities that compress the thoracic veins, thereby reducing venous return to the heart. This ultimately reduces arterial blood pressure.
18. The straining muscular effort that typically accompanies the Valsalva temporarily elevates blood pressure and adds to the heart's workload. Individuals with heart and vascular disease should refrain from heavy weightlifting and isometric muscle actions.
19. Breathing cold ambient air normally does not damage the respiratory passages.

thePoint   References are available online at
http://thepoint.lww.com/mkk8e.

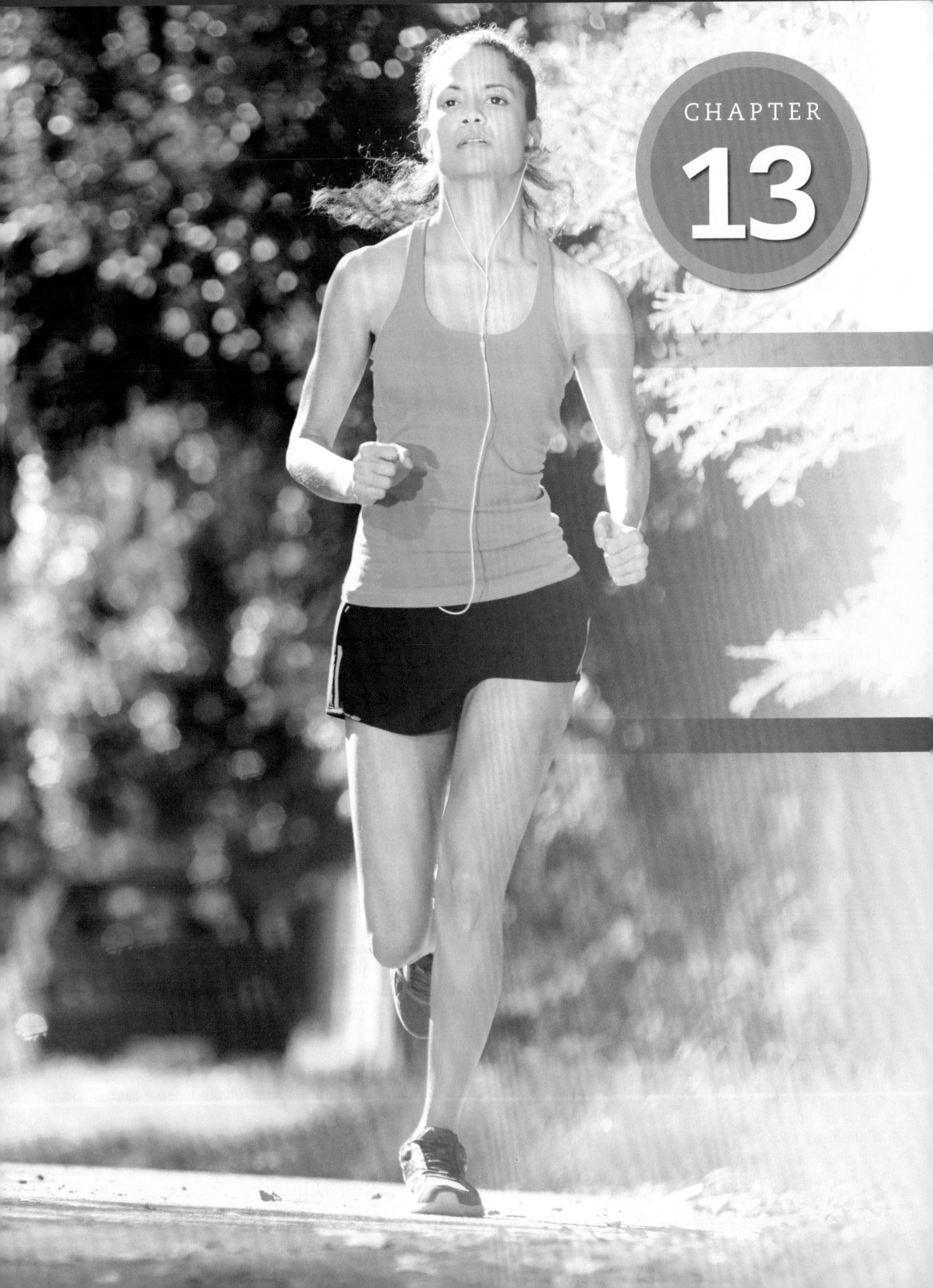

Gas Exchange and Transport

CHAPTER OBJECTIVES

- List the partial pressures of respired gases during rest and maximal physical activity in the alveoli, arterial blood, active muscles, and mixed-venous blood

- Explain the impact of Henry's law on pulmonary gas exchange

- Discuss the role partial pressure plays in the loading and unloading of metabolic gases in the lungs and tissues

- Quantify oxygen transport in arterial plasma and combined with hemoglobin under sea-level, ambient conditions

- Discuss the physiologic advantages of oxyhemoglobin's S-shaped dissociation curve

- Describe myoglobin's role in oxygen delivery to the tissues during physical exertion

- Describe factors that produce the "Bohr effect" and outline its major benefit in physical activity

- Explain the role of myoglobin during intense physical activity

- List and quantify three ways for carbon dioxide transport in blood

ANCILLARIES 👁 *at-a-Glance*

Visit http://thePoint.lww.com/mkk8e to access the following resources.

- References: Chapter 13
- Interactive Question Bank
- Animation: Gas Exchange in Alveoli
- Animation: Oxygen Transport
- Focus on Research: Muscle: A Remarkably Adaptable Tissue

The body's supply of oxygen in ambient air depends on two factors: (1) concentration and (2) pressure. Ambient air remains relatively constant in composition at 20.93% oxygen, 79.04% nitrogen, including small quantities of other inert gases that behave physiologically like nitrogen, 0.03% carbon dioxide, and usually small quantities of water vapor. The gas molecules move at relatively high speeds and exert a pressure against any contacted surface. At sea level, the pressure of air molecules raises a column of mercury in a barometer to a height of 760 mm (29.9 in.), or 1 torr. The **torr**—named for Italian physicist and mathematician Evangelista Torricelli (1608–1647; see, for example, http://inventors.about.com/od/gstartinventors/a/Galileo_Galilei.htm) who invented the barometer in 1644—is not an SI unit but an expression of gas pressure. *One torr equals the pressure necessary to raise a 1-mm column of mercury 1 mm high at 0°C against the standard acceleration of gravity at 45° north latitude (980.6 cm·s⁻²). One standard atmosphere equals 760 torr.* The barometric reading varies with changing weather conditions and becomes lower with increasing altitude (see Chapter 24).

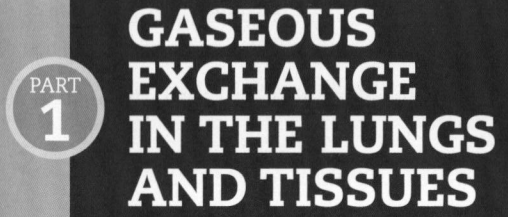

PART 1 — GASEOUS EXCHANGE IN THE LUNGS AND TISSUES

CONCENTRATIONS AND PARTIAL PRESSURES OF RESPIRED GASES

The molecules of each specific gas in a mixture of gases exert their individual **partial pressure**. The mixture's total pressure equals the sum of the partial pressures of the individual gases in the mixture. This association, known as **Dalton's law**, was named to honor the British chemist and physicist John Dalton (1766–1844; www.famousscientists.org/john-dalton), who also developed the atomic theory of matter. Partial pressure computes as follows:

Partial pressure = Percentage concentration of specific gas
× Total pressure of gas mixture

Ambient Air

TABLE 13.1 lists the volumes, percentages, and partial pressures of the gases in dry ambient air at sea level. The partial pressure of oxygen equals 20.93% of the total 760 mm Hg pressure exerted by air or 159 mm Hg (20.93 ÷ 100 × 760 mm Hg). Carbon dioxide exerts a pressure of only 0.23 mm Hg (0.03 ÷ 100 × 760 mm Hg), whereas the molecules of nitrogen exert a pressure that raises the mercury in a manometer about 600 mm (79.04 ÷ 100 × 760 mm Hg). A *P* placed in front of the gas symbol denotes partial pressure. The

Mercury Instead of Water

During the last 3 months of his life, Galileo (1564–1642; see, for example, http://inventors.about.com/od/gstartinventors/a/Galileo_Galilei.htm) suggested to Torricelli that he include mercury in his ongoing vacuum experiments. Two years later, Torricelli filled a 4-foot-long glass tube with mercury (13.6 times heavier than water, reducing dramatically the need for an extremely long water-filled tube that was taller than his house), and inverted the tube into a dish to create a sustained vacuum. He observed that the mercury did not flow, leaving the air above the mercury undisturbed in a vacuum. Thus, Torricelli became the first scientist to discover the basic principle of a barometer—that changes in atmospheric pressure could be measured by changes in the height of mercury in a tube. He also deduced that day-to-day changes in atmospheric pressure (i.e., cloudy, rainy, stormy) affected atmospheric pressure, in effect paving the way for modern weather forecasting. Vice Admiral Robert Fitzroy (1805–1865), captain of Charles Darwin's exploration ship the *HMS Beagle*, is credited with beginning the first published daily weather forecasting in London in 1860 that detailed the rise and fall of air pressure.

partial pressures at sea level for the principal components of ambient air average as follows: oxygen (Po_2) = 159 mm Hg, carbon dioxide (Pco_2) = 0.2 mm Hg, and nitrogen (P_{N_2}) = 600 mm Hg.

Tracheal Air

Air completely saturates with water vapor as it enters the nasal cavities and mouth and passes down the respiratory tract. The vapor dilutes the inspired air mixture somewhat. At a body temperature of 98.6°F (37°C), for example, the pressure of water molecules in humidified air equals 47 mm Hg; this leaves

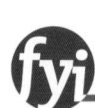

Common Symbols for Gas Pressure in Respiratory Physiology

- P_Ao_2: Partial pressure of oxygen in alveolar chambers
- Pao_2: Partial pressure of oxygen in arterial blood
- $Sao_2\%$: Percent saturation of arterial blood with oxygen
- Pvo_2: Partial pressure of oxygen in venous blood
- P_Aco_2: Partial pressure of carbon dioxide in alveolar chambers
- $Paco_2$: Partial pressure of carbon dioxide in arterial blood
- $Pvco_2$: Partial pressure of carbon dioxide in venous blood
- $Svo_2\%$: Percent saturation of venous blood with oxygen
- **a-vO₂ diff**: Arteriovenous oxygen difference; difference between oxygen carried in arterial blood and carried in venous blood
- **a-v̄O₂ diff**: Arterial–mixed-venous oxygen difference; difference between oxygen carried in arterial blood and carried in mixed-venous blood
- **v̄**: Mixed-venous blood

TABLE 13.1 — Partial Pressure and Volume of Gases in Dry Ambient Air at Sea Level

Gas	Percentage	Partial Pressure[a] (mm Hg)	Gas Volume (mL · L^{-1})
Oxygen	20.93	159	209.3
Carbon dioxide	0.03	0.2	0.4
Nitrogen	79.04[b]	600	790.3

[a]At 760 mm Hg ambient air pressure.
[b]Includes 0.93% argon and other trace rare gases.

713 mm Hg (760 − 47 mm Hg) as the total pressure exerted by the inspired dry air molecules. Consequently, the effective P_{O_2} in **tracheal air** decreases by about 10 mm Hg from its ambient value of 159 mm Hg to 149 mm Hg [0.2093 × (760 − 47 mm Hg)]. Carbon dioxide's negligible contribution to inspired air means that humidification exerts little effect on inspired P_{CO_2}.

Alveolar Air

Alveolar air composition differs considerably from the incoming breath of moist ambient air because carbon dioxide continually enters the alveoli from the blood; in contrast, oxygen flows from the lungs into the blood for transport throughout the body. TABLE 13.2 shows that alveolar air contains on average 14.5% oxygen, 5.5% carbon dioxide, and 80.0% nitrogen. After subtracting the vapor pressure from moist alveolar gas, the average alveolar P_{O_2} becomes 103 mm Hg [0.145 × (760 − 47 mm Hg)] and 39 mm Hg [0.055 × (760 − 47 mm Hg)] for P_{CO_2}. *These values represent average pressures exerted by oxygen and carbon dioxide molecules against*

TABLE 13.2 — Partial Pressure and Volume of Dry Alveolar Gases at Sea Level (98.6°F [37°C])

Gas	Percentage	Partial Pressure[a] (mm Hg)	Gas Volume (mL · L^{-1})
Oxygen	14.5	103	145
Carbon dioxide	5.5	39	55
Nitrogen[b]	80.0	571	800
Water vapor		47	

[a]At 760 − 47 mm Hg alveolar gas pressure.
[b]Nitrogen occupies a slightly greater percentage of alveolar air than ambient air because energy metabolism generally produces less carbon dioxide than oxygen consumed (i.e., the respiratory quotient [RQ = $\dot{V}_{CO_2} \div \dot{V}_{O_2}$] equals less than 1.00). The nitrogen percentage increases because of this exchange imbalance.

the alveolar side of the alveolar–capillary membrane. They do not remain physiologic constants; rather, they vary somewhat with the ventilatory cycle phase and the adequacy of ventilation in various lung regions. Recall that a relatively large volume of air remains in the lungs after each normal exhalation. This functional residual capacity (FRC) serves as a damper, so each incoming breath exerts only a small effect on alveolar air composition. This explains why the partial pressures of alveolar gases remain relatively stable.

GAS MOVEMENT IN AIR AND FLUIDS

In accordance with **Henry's law** (named for English chemist and physician William Henry [1774–1836]), the mass of a gas that dissolves in a fluid at a given temperature varies directly with the pressure of the gas over the liquid (provided no chemical reaction takes place between the gas and liquid). Two factors govern the rate of gas diffusion into a fluid:

1. The **pressure differential** between the gas above the fluid and the gas dissolved in the fluid
2. The **solubility** of the gas in the fluid

Pressure Differential

FIGURE 13.1 illustrates the concept of pressure differential. In this example, oxygen molecules continually bombard the water surface in three chambers. The pure water in chamber A contains no oxygen (P = 0 mm Hg), and a large number of oxygen molecules enter the water and dissolve in it. Dissolved gas molecules also move randomly, allowing for the exit of some oxygen molecules. In chamber B, oxygen still shows a *net* movement into the fluid from the gaseous state. Eventually, the number of molecules entering and leaving the fluid equalizes, as in chamber C. In this latter case, the gas pressures equilibrate without net oxygen diffusion into or out of the water. Conversely, if the pressure of dissolved oxygen molecules exceeds the pressure of the free gas in air, oxygen leaves the fluid until it attains a new pressure equilibrium. *In humans, the pressure difference between alveolar and pulmonary blood gases creates the driving force for gas diffusion across the pulmonary membrane.*

Solubility—The Dissolving Power of a Gas

For two different gases at identical pressure differentials, the solubility of each gas determines the number of molecules that move into or out of a fluid. Gas solubility is expressed as milliliters of a gas per 100 mL (dL) of a fluid. Oxygen, carbon dioxide, and nitrogen have different solubility coefficients in whole blood. Carbon dioxide dissolves most readily with a solubility coefficient of 57.03 mL of carbon dioxide per dL of fluid at 760 mm Hg and 98.6°F (37°C). Oxygen, with a solubility coefficient of 2.26 mL, remains relatively insoluble. Nitrogen is least soluble with a coefficient of 1.30 mL.

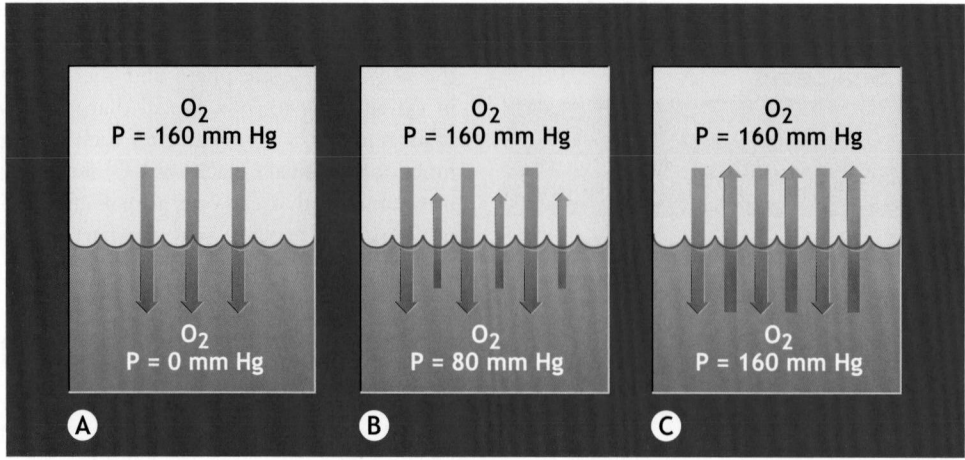

FIGURE 13.1 • Solution containing oxygen in water. **(A)** When oxygen first comes in contact with pure water. **(B)** Dissolved oxygen halfway to equilibrium with gaseous oxygen. **(C)** Equilibrium between oxygen in air and in water.

The amount of gas dissolved in a fluid computes as follows:

Quantity of gas (mL · dL^{-1}) = Solubility coefficient × (Gas partial pressure ÷ Total barometric pressure)

For example, the amount of oxygen dissolved in 1 dL of arterial whole blood (P_{O_2} = 100 mm Hg) at sea level (760 mm Hg) computes as:

$$\text{Quantity of gas} = 2.26 \times (100 \div 760)$$
$$= 0.3 \text{ mL} \cdot \text{dL}^{-1}$$

For each unit of pressure that favors diffusion, approximately 25 times more carbon dioxide than oxygen moves into (or out of) a fluid. Viewed another way, equal quantities of oxygen and carbon dioxide enter or leave a fluid under considerably different pressure gradients for each gas—precisely what occurs in the body.

At rest, dissolved oxygen contributes about 4% of the total oxygen consumed by the body each minute; in maximal physical activity, it provides less than 2% of the total requirement. Even increasing arterial P_{O_2} by breathing 100% oxygen (ambient P_{O_2} = 760 mm Hg), dissolved oxygen (1.5 to 2.0 mL · dL blood^{-1}) still supplies only 40% of the total oxygen for rest and about 10% during maximal exertion. The physiologic significance of dissolved oxygen and carbon dioxide comes not from its role as a transport vehicle, but in determining the partial pressures of these gases. Partial pressure plays a central role in loading and unloading oxygen and carbon dioxide in the lungs and tissues.

GAS EXCHANGE IN THE LUNGS AND TISSUES

Exchange of gases between the lungs and blood and gas movement at the tissue level progress passively by diffusion, depending on their pressure gradients. **FIGURE 13.2** illustrates pressure gradients that favor gas transfer in different regions of the body at rest.

 See the animation "Oxygen Transport" on **http://thePoint.lww.com/mkk8e** for a demonstration of this concept.

Gas Exchange in the Lungs

Figure 13.2A shows that at rest, the 100-mm Hg pressure of oxygen molecules in the alveoli exceeds by about 60 mm Hg the 40-mm Hg oxygen pressure in blood that enters the pulmonary capillaries. Consequently, oxygen travels from higher to lower pressure as it dissolves and diffuses through the alveolar membranes into the blood. In contrast, carbon dioxide exists under slightly greater pressure in returning venous blood than in the alveoli; this causes net diffusion of carbon dioxide from the blood into the lungs. Despite the relatively small pressure gradient of 6 mm Hg for carbon dioxide diffusion (compared with the 60-mm Hg diffusion gradient for oxygen), carbon dioxide transfer occurs rapidly because of its high solubility in plasma. Nitrogen, neither used nor produced

 ## Approximate Solubility Coefficients of Gases in Physiologic Fluids

Gas	Water	Plasma	Blood	Quantity Dissolved (per dL Blood)
Oxygen	2.39	2.14	2.26	0.3 mL
Carbon dioxide	56.7	51.5	57.03	3.0 mL
Nitrogen	1.23	1.18	1.30	0.8 mL

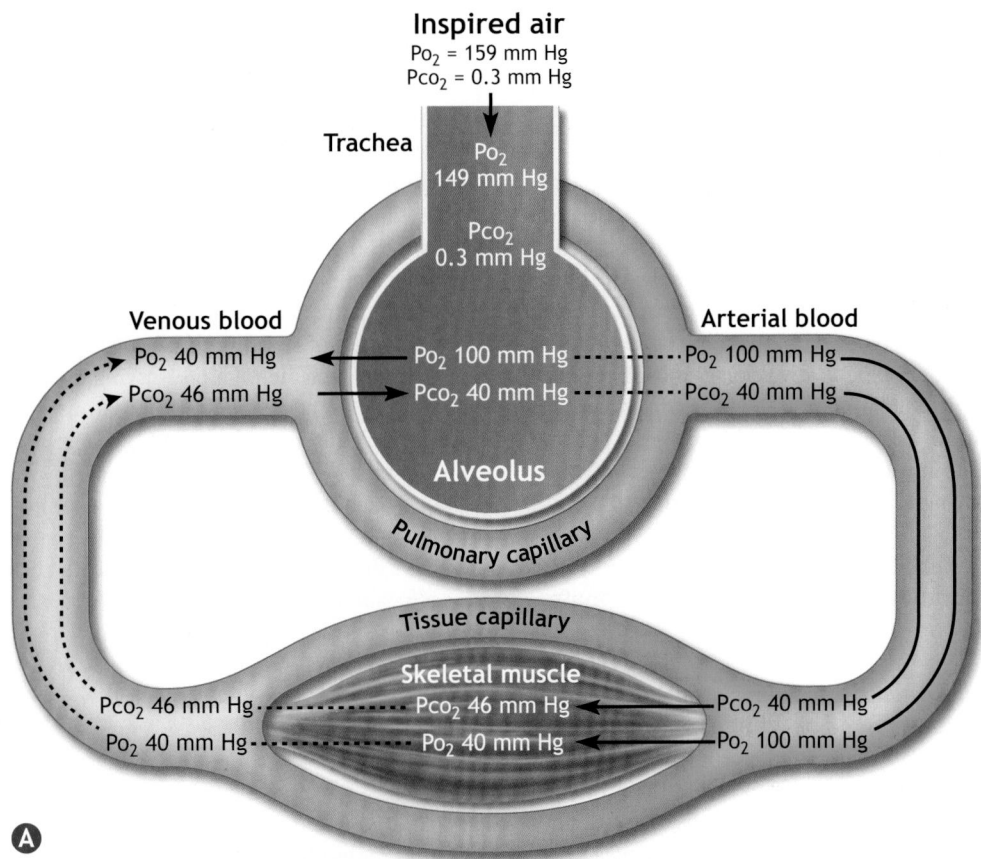

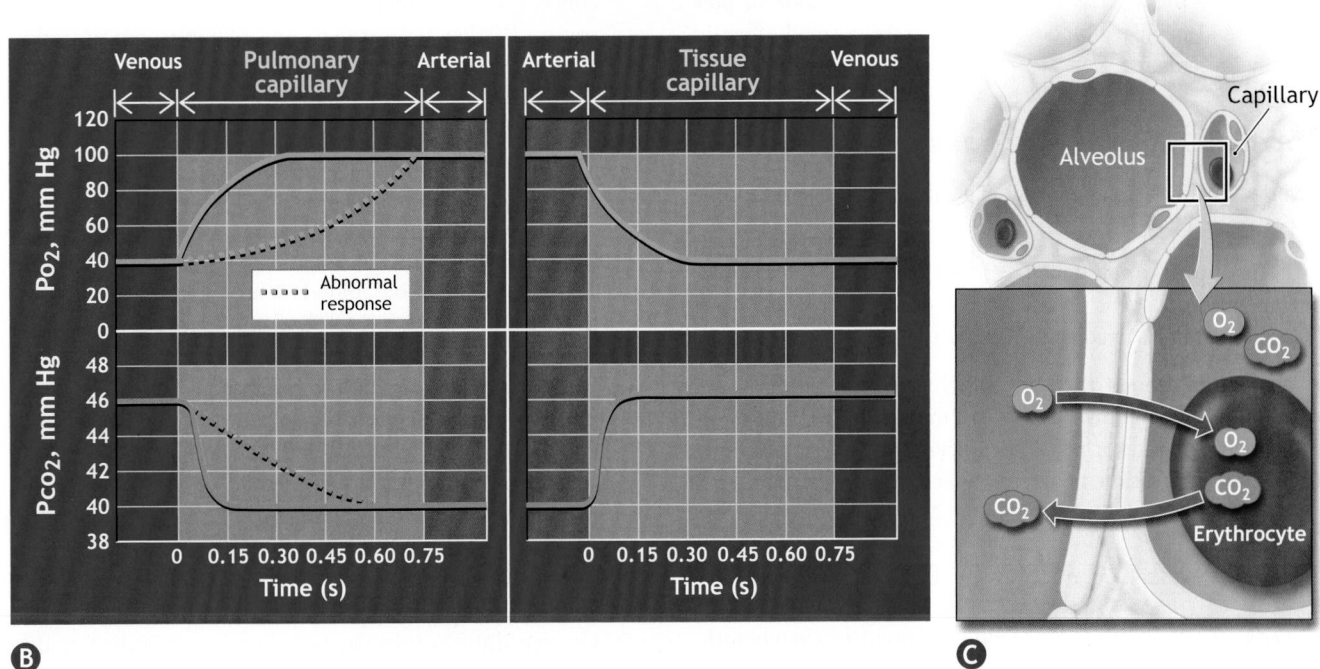

FIGURE 13.2 • Pressure gradients for gas transfer within the body at rest. **(A)** The P_{O_2} and P_{CO_2} of ambient, tracheal, and alveolar air and the gas pressures in venous and arterial blood and muscle tissue. Gas movement at the alveolar–capillary and tissue–capillary membranes always progresses from an area of higher partial pressure to lower partial pressure. **(B)** Time required for gas exchange. At rest, blood remains in the pulmonary and tissue capillaries for about 0.75 s. Pulmonary disease (*orange and blue dashed lines*) impairs the rate of gas transfer across the alveolar–capillary membrane, thus prolonging the time for equilibration of gases. Blood's transit time through the pulmonary capillaries during maximal exercise decreases to about 0.4 s, but this still remains adequate for complete aeration in the healthy lung. **(C)** Gas exchange (diffusion) between a pulmonary capillary and its adjacent alveolus.

in metabolic reactions, remains essentially unchanged in alveolar–capillary gas.

Gas exchange occurs so rapidly in the healthy lung that alveolar gas–blood gas equilibrium takes place in about 0.25 s, or within one-third of the blood's transit time through the lungs (Fig. 13.2B). Even in intense activity, a red blood cell's velocity through a pulmonary capillary generally does not exceed by more than 50% its velocity at rest. With increasing exercise intensity, the pulmonary capillaries increase the blood volume within them by about three times the resting value.[7] Accommodating a larger blood volume helps to maintain a relatively slow pulmonary blood flow velocity during physical activity. With complete aeration, the blood leaving the lungs contains oxygen at an average pressure of 100 mm Hg and carbon dioxide at 40 mm Hg. For most healthy people, these values vary little during vigorous physical activity.

 See the animation "Gas Exchange in Alveoli" on **http://thePoint.lww.com/mkk8e** for a demonstration of this concept.

The Po_2 of arterial blood usually remains slightly lower than alveolar Po_2 because some blood in the alveolar capillaries passes through poorly ventilated alveoli; also, the blood leaving the lungs mixes with venous blood from the bronchial and cardiac circulations. The term **venous admixture** defines this small amount of poorly oxygenated blood. Venous admixture reduces the arterial Po_2 slightly below the value in pulmonary end-capillary blood, and only exerts a small effect in healthy individuals.

Impaired Alveolar Gas Transfer

Two factors impair gas transfer capacity at the alveolar–capillary membrane:

1. Buildup of a pollutant layer that "thickens" the alveolar membrane
2. Reduction in alveolar surface area

Each factor extends the time before alveolar–capillary gas equilibrates. For individuals with impaired lung function, the added demand for rapid gas exchange in physical activity compromises aeration, negatively affecting performance.

 INTEGRATIVE QUESTION

Why do minute amounts of CO_2 and CO impurities in a breathing mixture exert such profound physiologic effects?

Gas Transfer in Tissues

In tissues, where energy metabolism consumes oxygen and produces an almost equal amount of carbon dioxide, gas pressures differ considerably from those recorded in arterial blood. At rest, the Po_2 in the fluid immediately outside a

muscle cell averages 40 mm Hg, and intracellular Pco_2 averages 46 mm Hg (Fig. 13.2A). In vigorous physical activity, oxygen pressure within muscle tissue falls toward 0 mm Hg, while the pressure of carbon dioxide approaches 90 mm Hg. *Pressure differences between gases in plasma and tissues establish diffusion gradients.* Oxygen leaves the blood and diffuses *toward* cells, while carbon dioxide flows *from* cells into the blood. Blood then passes into the venous circuit (venules and veins) for return to the heart and delivery to the lungs. Diffusion occurs rapidly as blood enters the dense pulmonary capillary network. The body does not attempt to rid itself completely of carbon dioxide. To the contrary, each liter of blood leaving the lungs with a Pco_2 of 40 mm Hg contains about 50 mL of carbon dioxide. As discussed in Chapter 14, this small "background level" of carbon dioxide provides the chemical basis for ventilatory control through its stimulating effect on the neurons of the pons and medullary centers of the brainstem. The term **respiratory center** describes this collection of neural tissue that controls ventilation.

Alveolar ventilation couples tightly to metabolic demands to keep alveolar gas composition remarkably constant. Stability in alveolar gas concentrations persists even during strenuous activity that increases oxygen consumption and carbon dioxide output 25 times the values at rest.

Summary

1. Gas molecules in the lungs and tissues diffuse down their concentration gradients from an area of higher concentration (higher pressure) to one of lower concentration (lower pressure).
2. The partial pressure of a specific gas in a mixture of gases varies directly with the concentration of the gas and the mixture's total pressure.
3. Henry's law states that pressure gradient and solubility determine how much gas dissolves in a fluid.
4. Oxygen, carbon dioxide, and nitrogen exhibit different solubilities in whole blood. Carbon dioxide dissolves most readily while oxygen and nitrogen show relatively low solubility.
5. Carbon dioxide solubility in plasma exceeds oxygen solubility by 25 times, allowing carbon dioxide to move into and from body fluids down a relatively small diffusion (pressure) gradient.
6. Maintaining a remarkably constant alveolar gas composition during rest and physical activity reflects fine adjustments in pulmonary ventilation. Alveolar ventilation maintains Po_2 at about 100 mm Hg and Pco_2 at 40 mm Hg.
7. Oxygen diffuses into the blood and carbon dioxide diffuses into the lungs because venous blood contains oxygen at lower pressure and carbon dioxide at higher pressure than alveolar gas.
8. Alveolar–blood gas exchange achieves equilibrium in the healthy lung at about the midpoint of the blood's transit through the pulmonary capillaries.
9. In intense exertion, blood flow velocity through the lungs generally does not compromise full loading of oxygen and unloading of carbon dioxide.

10. Diffusion gradients favor oxygen movement from the capillaries to the tissues and carbon dioxide from the tissues to the blood.
11. During physical activity, oxygen and carbon dioxide diffuse rapidly as their pressure gradients widen.

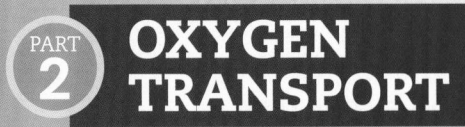

OXYGEN TRANSPORT IN BLOOD

The blood carries oxygen in two ways:

1. In physical solution dissolved in the fluid portion of blood
2. In loose combination with hemoglobin, the iron-protein molecule within the red blood cell

Oxygen in Physical Solution

Oxygen's relative insolubility in water keeps its concentration low within bodily fluids. At an alveolar Po_2 of 100 mm Hg, only about 0.3 mL of gaseous oxygen dissolves in each deciliter of blood (0.003 mL for each additional 1-mm Hg increase in Po_2). This equals 3 mL of oxygen per liter of blood. The blood volume of a 70-kg person averages about 5 L; thus, 15 mL of oxygen dissolves in the fluid portion of the blood (3 mL per L × 5). This small amount of oxygen would sustain life for about 4 s. Viewed from a different perspective, if oxygen in physical solution provided the sole oxygen source to the body, about 80 L of blood would need to circulate each minute to supply the resting oxygen requirements—a blood flow about twice the maximum ever recorded!

As with carbon dioxide, the small quantity of oxygen transported in physical solution serves several important functions. The random movement of dissolved oxygen molecules establishes the Po_2 of the plasma and tissue fluids. The pressure of oxygen in solution helps to regulate breathing, particularly at higher altitudes when ambient Po_2 decreases considerably; it also determines oxygen loading of hemoglobin in the lungs and subsequent release in tissues.

Oxygen Combined with Hemoglobin

Metallic compounds exist in the blood of many animal species to augment its oxygen-carrying capacity. FIGURE 13.3 illustrates the iron-containing globular protein pigment **hemoglobin** carried within the more than 25 trillion red blood cells of humans. The incomparable French physiologist Claude Bernard whom we chronicle in the introductory chapter

described hemoglobin's role in the blood. Derived from the words *heme* and *globin*, the term describes each subunit of hemoglobin as a globular protein with an embedded heme group containing one iron atom. In mammals, a single hemoglobin molecule contains four of these heme subunits. Normal hemoglobin concentration in blood carries 65 to 70 times more oxygen than normally dissolves in plasma. Thus, the approximately 280 million hemoglobin molecules temporarily "capture" and transport about 197 mL of oxygen in each liter of blood. Each of the four iron atoms in the hemoglobin molecule can loosely bind one oxygen molecule in the following reversible reaction:

$$Hb_4 + 4O_2 \leftrightarrow Hb_4O_8$$

The reaction requires no enzymes; it proceeds without a change in the valence of Fe^{2+} as in the more permanent oxidation process. *The partial pressure of oxygen dissolved in physical solution dictates the oxygenation of hemoglobin to oxyhemoglobin.*

Oxygen-Carrying Capacity of Hemoglobin

In males, each dL of blood contains about 15 g of hemoglobin. The value decreases 5 to 10% for females and averages nearly 14 g per dL of blood. This gender difference partly explains the lower aerobic capacity of women relative to men, even when considering differences in body mass and body fat. The reason for higher hemoglobin concentrations in men relates to the stimulating effects on red blood cell production of the "male" hormone testosterone.

Each gram of hemoglobin combines loosely with 1.34 mL of oxygen. Thus, if one knows the hemoglobin content of the blood, its oxygen-carrying capacity computes as follows:

Blood's oxygen capacity $(mL \cdot dL\ blood^{-1})$		Hemoglobin $(g \cdot dL\ blood^{-1})$		Oxygen capacity of hemoglobin
20 mL O_2	=	15	×	1.34 mL·g^{-1}

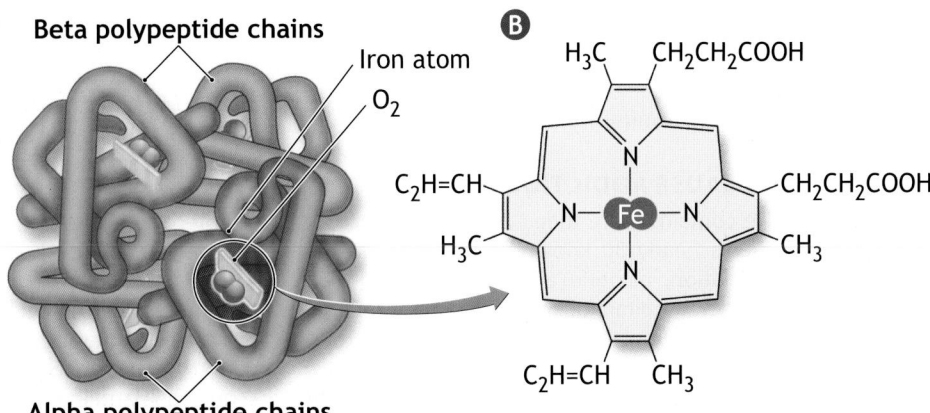

FIGURE 13.3 • The hemoglobin molecule **(A)** consists of the protein globin, composed of four subunit polypeptide chains. Each polypeptide **(B)** contains a single heme group with its single iron atom that acts as a "magnet" for oxygen.

IN A PRACTICAL SENSE

Factors that Contribute to the Smoking Habit

Research relating smoking habits to exercise performance remains meager, yet most endurance athletes avoid cigarettes for fear of hindering performance from a "loss of wind." Chronic cigarette smokers tend toward more sedentary lifestyles and have lower fitness levels than nonsmoking counterparts.[4,19,21] For some unknown reason, cigarette smoking increases one's dependence on carbohydrate for energy during rest and sustained exercise.[5] Smokers also have lower dynamic lung function that, if severe, manifests in chronic obstructive pulmonary disease. In adolescent smokers, chronic cigarette smoking obstructs the airways and slows normal lung function development, with greater deficits in girls than in boys.[10] Children who smoked had higher rates of asthma and wheezing and reduced dynamic lung function capacity in a dose–response relationship to their smoking habits. Female smokers who trained vigorously for 12 weeks improved aerobic capacity and endurance performance compared with smokers who remained sedentary.[1] The females who exercised and quit smoking made greater fitness improvements than counterparts who trained similarly but continued to smoke. Chapter 14 discusses the effects of cigarette smoking on the oxygen cost of breathing and the heart rate response to exercise.

Cigarette smoking represents the single greatest cause of death worldwide. Each year, more than 450,000 people in the United States die from smoking-related diseases—heart disease, cancer, stroke, aortic aneurysm, chronic bronchitis, emphysema, and peptic ulcers. Chronic cigarette smokers live an average of 18 years less than nonsmokers, and each cigarette smoked shortens life by 7 minutes!

WHY PEOPLE START SMOKING

People usually start smoking without realizing its detrimental effects. Cigarette smoking generally begins during the teen years or earlier. Health problems from smoking accrue quickly in young smokers. Three reasons generally explain why youths begin smoking:

1. Peer pressure
2. Desire to appear "grown up"
3. Rebellion against authority

CIGARETTES CAUSE ADDICTION

Tobacco smoke contains more than 1200 toxic chemicals; tar alone contains nearly 30 known carcinogens. Within seconds of inhalation, nicotine affects the central nervous system to act simultaneously as a tranquilizer and stimulant. Nicotine's stimulating effect produces a strong physiologic and psychologic dependency. Estimates place the physiologic addiction to nicotine at about six to eight times the addictive power of alcohol. Psychologic dependency develops over a longer time and associates with calming and pleasurable activities such as drinking coffee or alcohol, participating in social gatherings, relaxing after a meal, talking on the telephone, driving, reading, and watching television.

THE WHY-DO-YOU-SMOKE TEST

The **Why-Do-You-Smoke Test** (see table) identifies reasons for smoking, which provides the important first step in behavioral approaches to smoking cessation.

The test lists 18 statements about why people smoke. A score between 1 and 5 indicates the strength of agreement with the statement, with 5 representing the strongest agreement. The responses to each of the statements provide input about one of six factors most frequently related to a person's smoking behavior. The information obtained provides (1) insight as to why a person smokes and (2) possible behavioral substitutes to aid in cessation.

1. Stimulation ("cigarettes are stimulating"): You feel that they help wake you up, organize your energies, and keep you going. Choose a safe substitute—a brisk walk or moderate exercise.

2. Handling ("keep my hands busy"): Toy with a pen or pencil or doodle, play with a coin, piece of jewelry, or some other harmless object while quitting.

3. Accentuation of pleasure/pleasurable relaxation ("makes me feel good"): Substitute social and physical activities or other relaxing activities to accentuate pleasure.

4. Reduction of negative feelings/crutch ("gets me through the tough times"): Learning to handle stress helps with quitting.

5. Craving or dependence ("can't get through the day without them"): "Cold turkey" is the most effective way to quit; biofeedback has shown some success.

6. Habit ("don't even know when I'm smoking"): You need to break the habitual smoking pattern; being more aware of conditions and situations when smoking occurs aids in quitting.

Scores for each factor can vary between 3 and 15. A score of 11 or above indicates that for this factor smoking represents an important source of satisfaction. Scoring low (<7) on a factor indicates a greater likelihood of successful smoking cessation.

Enter the number you circled on the test questions in the spaces provided below, putting the number you circled to question A on line A, to question B on line B, etc. Add the three scores on each line to get a total for each factor. For example, the sum of your scores over lines A, G, and M give the score on "Stimulation"; lines B, H, and N give the score on "Handling," etc. Scores can vary between 3 and 15. Any score above 11 is high; any score 7 and below is low and indicates greater likelihood for successful smoking cessation.

Why-Do-You-Smoke Test

Question	Always	Frequently	Occasionally	Seldom	Never
A. I smoke in order to keep myself from slowing down.	5	4	3	2	1
B. Handling a cigarette is part of the enjoyment of smoking it.	5	4	3	2	1
C. Smoking is pleasant and relaxing.	5	4	3	2	1
D. I light up when I feel angry about something.	5	4	3	2	1
E. When I have run out of cigarettes, I find it almost unbearable until I can get them.	5	4	3	2	1
F. I smoke automatically without even being aware of it.	5	4	3	2	1
G. I smoke to stimulate myself, to perk myself up.	5	4	3	2	1
H. Part of the enjoyment of cigarettes comes from the steps I take to light up.	5	4	3	2	1
I. I find cigarettes pleasurable.	5	4	3	2	1
J. When I feel uncomfortable or upset about something, I light up.	5	4	3	2	1
K. I am very much aware of the act when I am not smoking.	5	4	3	2	1
L. I light up without realizing I still have one burning in the ashtray.	5	4	3	2	1
M. I smoke to give myself a "lift."	5	4	3	2	1
N. When I smoke, part of the enjoyment is watching the smoke as I exhale it.	5	4	3	2	1
O. I want a cigarette most when I am comfortable and relaxed.	5	4	3	2	1
P. When I feel "blue" or want to take my mind off cares and worries, I smoke.	5	4	3	2	1
Q. I get a real gnawing hunger for a cigarette when I haven't smoked for a while.	5	4	3	2	1
R. I've found a cigarette in my mouth and didn't remember putting it there.	5	4	3	2	1

Scoring

Enter the number you circled on the test questions in the spaces provided below, putting the number you circled to question A on line A, to question B on line B, etc. Add the three scores on each line to get a total for each factor. For example, the sum of your scores over lines A, G, and M give the score on "Stimulation"; lines B, H, and N give the score on "Handling," etc. Scores can vary between 3 and 15. Any score above 11 is high; any score 7 and below is low and indicates greater likelihood for successful smoking cessation.

A _____ + G _____ + M _____ = _____ Stimulation

B _____ + H _____ + N _____ = _____ Handling

C _____ + I _____ + O _____ = _____ Pleasure relaxation

D _____ + J _____ + P _____ = _____ Crutch: tension reduction

E _____ + K _____ + Q _____ = _____ Craving: psychologic addiction

F _____ + L _____ + R _____ = _____ Habit

From *A Self-Test for Smokers*. US Department of Health and Human Services, 1983.

With full oxygen saturation (i.e., when all hemoglobin converts to HbO_2) and with normal hemoglobin levels, hemoglobin carries nearly 20 mL of oxygen in each dL of whole blood.

Anemia Affects Oxygen Transport. Iron insufficiency is often observed among endurance athletes, particularly women involved in intense training.[2,6] The blood's oxygen transport capacity changes only slightly with normal variations in hemoglobin content. In contrast, a significant decrease in the iron content of red blood cells reduces the blood's oxygen-carrying capacity. Such **iron-deficiency anemia** diminishes a person's capacity to sustain even mild-intensity aerobic activity.[3,11]

TABLE 13.3 presents data from 29 iron-deficient anemic men and women with low hemoglobin levels. They formed two groups; one received intramuscular iron injections over an 80-day period, while the placebo group received similar intramuscular injections of a colored saline solution. A third group with normal hemoglobin levels served as controls. The researchers tested all groups during exercise prior to the experiment and after 80 days of either iron therapy or placebo treatment. The results clearly show that the anemic group given iron supplements improved in exercise response compared with their nonsupplemented counterparts. Peak heart rate during 5 min of stepping decreased from 155 to 113 $b \cdot min^{-1}$ for men and from 152 to 123 $b \cdot min^{-1}$ for women. This translates into an average of 15% more oxygen delivered per heartbeat.

Hemoglobin (Hb) Levels and Exercise Heart Rates of Normal and Anemic Subjects Prior to and Following Supplemental Iron Treatment

TABLE 13.3

Subjects	Hb (g per dL Blood)	Peak Exercise Heart Rate
Normal		
Men	14.3	119
Women	13.9	142
Iron-deficient men		
Pretreatment	7.1	155
Posttreatment	14.0	113
Iron-deficient women		
Pretreatment	7.7	152
Posttreatment	12.4	123
Iron-deficient men		
Preplacebo	7.7	146
Postplacebo	7.4	137
Iron-deficient women		
Preplacebo	8.1	154
Postplacebo	8.4	144

From Gardner GW, et al. Cardiorespiratory, hematological, and physical performance responses of anemic subjects to iron treatment. *Am J Clin Nutr* 1975;28:982.
Values represent group averages.

Po_2 and Hemoglobin Saturation

The term ***cooperative binding*** describes the union of oxygen with hemoglobin. The binding of an oxygen molecule to the iron atom in one of the four globin chains in FIGURE 13.3 progressively facilitates the binding of subsequent molecules. The cooperative binding phenomenon explains hemoglobin's sigmoid, or S-shaped, oxygen saturation curve.

The **oxyhemoglobin dissociation curve** (FIG. 13.4A) illustrates the saturation of hemoglobin with oxygen at various Po_2 values including alveolar–capillary gas at sea level (Po_2, 100 mm Hg). The right ordinate gives the quantity of oxygen carried in each deciliter of normal blood at a particular plasma Po_2 value. The term ***volume percent*** (**vol%**) describes blood's oxygen content. In this regard, volume percent refers to the milliliters of oxygen extracted (in a vacuum) from a deciliter sample of either whole blood (with plasma) or packed red blood cells (without plasma).

Physical chemists establish dissociation curves (oxygen content and percentage saturation) by exposing about 200 mL of blood in a sealed glass vessel called a tonometer to various pressures of oxygen at a given pH in a water bath of known temperature. Percentage saturation computes as follows:

$$\text{Percentage saturation} = \frac{O_2 \text{ combined with hemoglobin}}{O_2 \text{ capacity of hemoglobin}} \times 100$$

If an individual's hemoglobin oxygen-carrying capacity in whole blood equals 20 vol% and only 12 vol% oxygen actually combines with hemoglobin, then:

$$\text{Percentage saturation} = 12 \text{ vol\%} \div 20 \text{ vol\%} \times 100 = 60\%$$

One hundred percent saturation indicates that the oxygen combined with hemoglobin equals the oxygen-carrying capacity of hemoglobin.

FIGURE 13.4B depicts the **oxygen transport cascade** for oxygen partial pressure as oxygen moves from ambient air at sea level to the mitochondria of maximally active muscle tissue.

Po_2 in the Lungs

In the discussion about hemoglobin, the assumption has been that hemoglobin fully saturates with oxygen when exposed to alveolar gas. *This does not occur because at the sea-level alveolar Po_2 of 100 mm Hg, hemoglobin achieves only 98% oxygen saturation.* The right ordinate of Figure 13.4A shows that at a Po_2 of 100 mm Hg, the hemoglobin in each deciliter of blood leaving the lungs carries about 19.7 mL of oxygen. Clearly, any additional increase in alveolar Po_2 contributes little to how much more oxygen can combine with hemoglobin. In addition to the oxygen bound to hemoglobin, the plasma of each deciliter of arterial blood contains 0.3 mL of oxygen in solution. In healthy individuals who breathe ambient air at sea level, each deciliter of blood leaving the lungs carries approximately 20.0 mL of oxygen—19.7 mL bound to hemoglobin and 0.3 mL dissolved in plasma.

Figure 13.4 also shows that hemoglobin saturation with oxygen changes little until the pressure of oxygen declines to

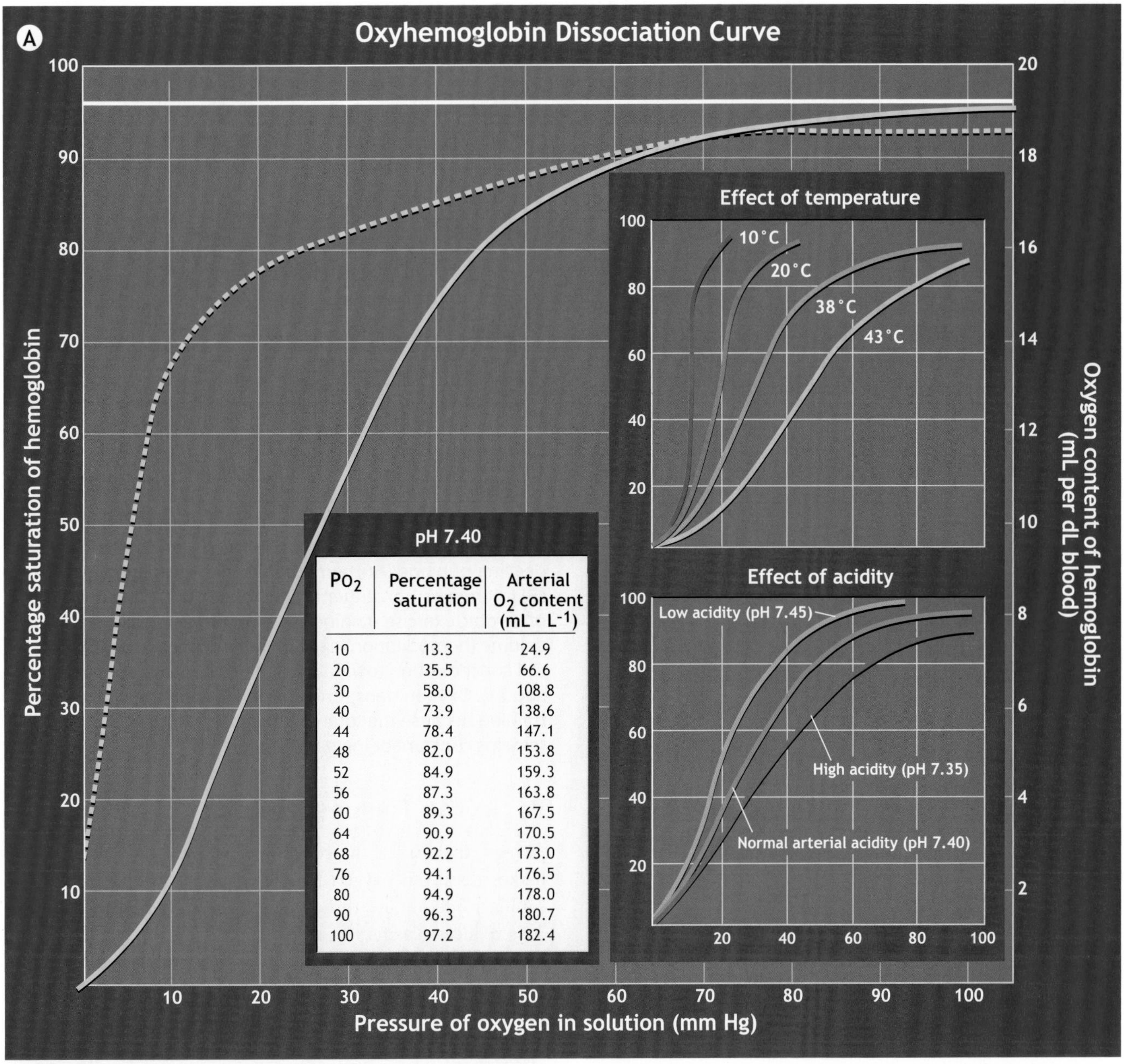

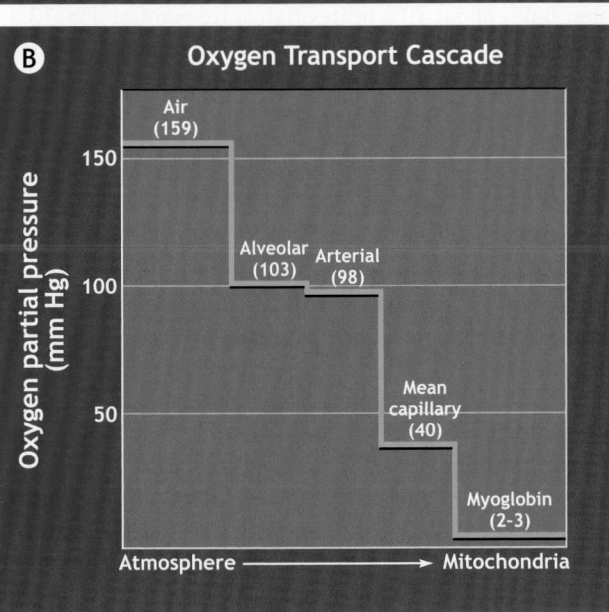

A Oxyhemoglobin Dissociation Curve

pH 7.40		
P_{O_2}	Percentage saturation	Arterial O_2 content (mL · L^{-1})
10	13.3	24.9
20	35.5	66.6
30	58.0	108.8
40	73.9	138.6
44	78.4	147.1
48	82.0	153.8
52	84.9	159.3
56	87.3	163.8
60	89.3	167.5
64	90.9	170.5
68	92.2	173.0
76	94.1	176.5
80	94.9	178.0
90	96.3	180.7
100	97.2	182.4

Effect of temperature

10°C 20°C 38°C 43°C

Effect of acidity

Low acidity (pH 7.45)
High acidity (pH 7.35)
Normal arterial acidity (pH 7.40)

Percentage saturation of hemoglobin

Oxygen content of hemoglobin (mL per dL blood)

Pressure of oxygen in solution (mm Hg)

B Oxygen Transport Cascade

Oxygen partial pressure (mm Hg)

Air (159)
Alveolar (103) Arterial (98)
Mean capillary (40)
Myoglobin (2-3)

Atmosphere ⟶ Mitochondria

FIGURE 13.4 • (A) Oxyhemoglobin dissociation curve. Lines indicate the percentage saturation of hemoglobin (*solid yellow line*) and myoglobin (*dashed yellow line*) in relation to oxygen pressure. The *right ordinate* shows the quantity of oxygen carried in each deciliter of blood under normal conditions. The *inset curves within the figure* illustrate the effects of temperature and acidity in altering hemoglobin's affinity for oxygen (Bohr effect). Inset box presents oxyhemoglobin saturation and arterial blood's oxygen-carrying capacity for different P_{O_2} values with hemoglobin concentration of 14 g · dL blood^{-1} at a pH of 7.40. The *white horizontal line* at the top of the graph indicates percentage saturation of hemoglobin at the average sea-level alveolar P_{O_2} of 100 mm Hg. **(B)** Partial pressures as oxygen moves from ambient air at sea level to the mitochondria of maximally active muscle tissue (*oxygen transport cascade*).

about 60 mm Hg. This flat upper portion of the oxyhemoglobin dissociation curve provides a margin of safety to ensure adequate saturation of arterial blood with oxygen despite considerable fluctuations in ambient Po_2. Even if alveolar Po_2 decreases to 75 mm Hg, as occurs in lung disease or at higher altitudes, the saturation of hemoglobin decreases by only about 6%. At an alveolar Po_2 of 60 mm Hg, hemoglobin still remains nearly 90% saturated with oxygen! Below this pressure, the quantity of oxygen combined with hemoglobin declines more rapidly.

On television, one frequently sees competitive athletes on the sidelines breathing a gas mixture of concentrated oxygen following strenuous physical activity. This makes no sense from an oxygen-transport perspective. The oxyhemoglobin dissociation curve shows little or no potential for increased hemoglobin loading from additional pressure of supplemental oxygen inhaled at sea level or at relatively low altitude. The topic of breathing hyperoxic gas mixtures and exercise performance is discussed in more detail in Chapter 23.

The Bohr Effect

The sigmoid, solid yellow line in Figure 13.4A represents the oxyhemoglobin dissociation curve under resting physiologic conditions at an arterial pH of 7.4 and tissue temperature of 98.6°F (37°C). The *inset curves* depict other important characteristics of hemoglobin's affinity for oxygen. Any increase in plasma acidity (including carbon dioxide concentration) and temperature causes the dissociation curve to shift downward and to the right. This phenomenon, called the Bohr effect for its 1891 discoverer, Danish physiologist Christian Bohr (1855–1911; father of Nobel physicist Niels Bohr [1885–1962]), indicates that hydrogen ions and carbon dioxide alter hemoglobin's molecular structure to decrease its oxygen-binding affinity. The reduced effectiveness of hemoglobin to hold oxygen occurs particularly in the Po_2 range between 20 and 50 mm Hg. The Bohr effect remains evident during intense exertion as more oxygen releases to tissues from associated increases in the following three factors:

1. Metabolic heat
2. Carbon dioxide
3. Acidity from blood lactate accumulation

At normal alveolar Po_2 the Bohr effect exerts almost no effect on pulmonary capillary blood (even during maximal exertion), so hemoglobin binds fully with oxygen as blood flows through the lungs.

FIGURE 13.5 shows the percentage composition of centrifuged whole blood for red blood cells (termed **hematocrit**) and plasma, including representative values for the quantity of oxygen carried in each component.

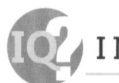

INTEGRATIVE QUESTION

Advise a coach who wants football players to breathe from an oxygen tank during time-outs or rest breaks to speed recovery.

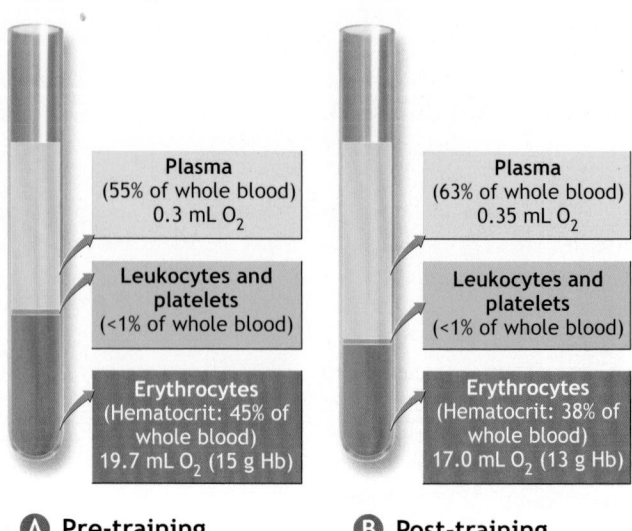

Centrifuged Whole Blood

A Pre-training   **B Post-training**

FIGURE 13.5 • **(A)** Major components of centrifuged whole blood, including the quantity of oxygen carried in each deciliter of blood (*Hb*, hemoglobin) in an untrained individual. **(B)** Changes in constituents of whole blood following 4 days of aerobic exercise training. Note that the increase in plasma volume (hemodilution) early in training decreases red blood cell concentration toward borderline anemia (see Chapters 2 and 21). Oxygen transport capacity does not decrease with training because the total erythrocyte mass of the blood remains constant or increases slightly.

Po_2 in the Tissues

At rest, the Po_2 in the cell fluids averages 40 mm Hg. This makes dissolved oxygen from the plasma diffuse across the capillary membrane through the tissue fluids into the cells. This reduces plasma Po_2 below the Po_2 in the red blood cell, causing hemoglobin to lower its oxygen saturation level. The released oxygen ($HbO_2 \rightarrow Hb + O_2$) moves out of the blood cells through the capillary membrane into the tissues.

At the tissue–capillary Po_2 at rest of 40 mm Hg, hemoglobin holds about 70% of its original oxygen (see Fig. 13.4). Thus, when blood leaves the tissues and returns to the heart, it carries about 15 mL of oxygen in each deciliter of blood, giving up 5 mL of oxygen to the tissues.

Arteriovenous Oxygen Difference

The **arterio-mixed-venous oxygen difference** (a-$\bar{v}O_2$ **difference**) describes the difference between the oxygen content of arterial blood and mixed-venous blood. The a-$\bar{v}O_2$ difference at rest normally averages 4 to 5 mL of oxygen per deciliter of blood. The large quantity of oxygen still attached to hemoglobin provides an "automatic" reserve so cells can immediately obtain oxygen should metabolic demands suddenly increase. Tissue Po_2 decreases as the cell's use of oxygen increases in physical activity. This causes hemoglobin to immediately release a larger amount of oxygen. During intense activity when extracellular Po_2 decreases to nearly 15 mm Hg, only about 5 mL of oxygen remains bound to hemoglobin.

This makes the a-$\bar{v}O_2$ difference increase to 15 mL of oxygen per 100 mL of blood (Fig. 13.6A and B). When active muscle Po_2 falls to 2 or 3 mm Hg during exhaustive exercise, the blood perfusing these tissues gives up virtually all its oxygen (Fig. 13.6 C).[20] Oxygen release from hemoglobin can occur without any increase in local tissue blood flow. The amount of oxygen released to the muscles increases almost three times above that normally supplied at rest—just by a more complete unloading of hemoglobin as it flows through the active muscles. *An active muscle's uncompromising capacity to use available oxygen in its large blood flow supports the position that oxygen supply (blood flow), not muscle oxygen use, limits aerobic capacity.*[17,23]

Red Blood Cell 2,3-DPG

A red blood cell derives its energy solely from the anaerobic reactions of glycolysis because they contain no mitochondria; this establishes the normal plasma lactate levels at rest. Red blood cells produce the compound **2,3-diphosphoglycerate** (**2,3-DPG**; also referred to as 2,3-biphosphoglycerate [2,3-BPG]) during glycolysis. 2,3-DPG binds loosely with subunits of the hemoglobin molecule, reducing its affinity for oxygen. This causes greater oxygen release to the tissues for a given decrease in Po_2.[8]

Increased levels of red blood cell 2,3-DPG occur in individuals with cardiopulmonary disorders and those who live at high altitudes. This compensatory adjustment facilitates oxygen release to the cells. During strenuous activity, 2,3-DPG also aids in oxygen transfer to muscles.[12] Conflicting results emerge in comparison of 2,3-DPG levels of trained and untrained subjects.[9,13,16] One study reported higher resting levels of 2,3-DPG in two groups of athletes than in untrained subjects.[221] The level of this metabolic intermediate increased by 15% for middle-distance runners following short-duration maximal effort. In contrast, prolonged steady-rate exercise in endurance athletes produced a small decrease in 2,3-DPG. These data support the proposition that increases in 2,3-DPG concentration with intense physical activity and perhaps training reflect an adaptive response that augments oxygen delivery to more metabolically active tissues. More than likely, the effort. of different types of activity on erythrocyte 2,3-DPG levels reflects the specific metabolic demands of exercise.

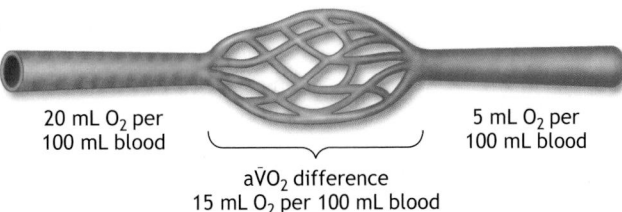

A Whole body at rest

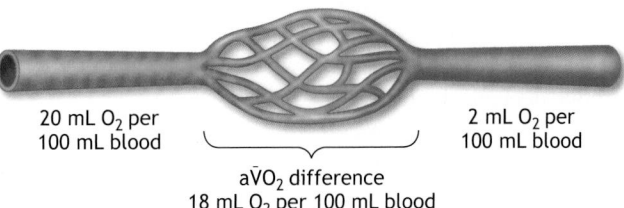

B Whole body during intense aerobic exercise

C Active skeletal muscle during intense aerobic exercise

FIGURE 13.6 • Average values for whole-body arteriovenous oxygen difference in skeletal muscle during (**A**) rest and (**B**) intense aerobic exercise, and in (**C**) active skeletal muscle during intense aerobic exercise.

Females have higher levels of red blood cell 2,3-DPG than males of similar fitness status and physical activity level. This gender difference might compensate for the lower hemoglobin levels in females.[15]

Myoglobin, the Muscle's Oxygen Storage

Myoglobin, an iron-containing globular protein in skeletal and cardiac muscle fibers with some 240 times greater affinity for oxygen than hemoglobin, provides intramuscular oxygen storage. Sir John C. Kendrew (1917–1997; 1962 Nobel Prize in Chemistry; http://www.nobelprize.org/nobel_prizes/chemistry/laureates/1962/) revealed myoglobin's structural details using x-ray crystallography in his studies of the structures of globular proteins. The molecule contains a peptide backbone embedded with the heme group and its metallic Fe^{2+}. Reddish muscle fibers have a high concentration of this respiratory pigment, whereas myoglobin-deficient fibers appear pale or white.[14] Myoglobin resembles hemoglobin because it also combines reversibly with oxygen but each molecule contains one iron atom while hemoglobin contains four. Myoglobin adds additional oxygen to the muscle in the following chemical reaction:

$$Mb + O_2 \rightarrow MbO_2$$

Oxygen Released at Low Pressures

Myoglobin facilitates oxygen transfer to the mitochondria when movement begins and during intense effort when cellular Po_2 declines rapidly and dramatically. The dissociation curve for myoglobin (Fig. 13.4; *dashed yellow line*) does not form an S-shaped line as does hemoglobin, but instead plots as a rectangular hyperbola. Compared with the oxygen saturation curve for hemoglobin, the curve for myoglobin shows that it much more readily binds and retains oxygen at low oxygen pressures. During rest and moderate physical activity, myoglobin maintains high oxygen saturation. For example, at a Po_2 of 40 mm Hg, myoglobin retains 95% of its oxygen. The greatest quantity of oxygen releases from MbO_2 when tissue Po_2 declines below 5 mm Hg.[18] Myoglobin's oxygen-binding affinity, unlike that of hemoglobin, is not affected by acidity, carbon dioxide, and temperature, so it does not exhibit a Bohr effect. Chapter 21 discusses the effects of aerobic training on the muscles' myoglobin content.

Summary

1. Hemoglobin, the iron-protein pigment in the red blood cell, increases the amount of oxygen carried in whole blood about 65 times that carried in physical solution in the plasma.
2. The small amount of oxygen dissolved in plasma exerts molecular movement and establishes the partial pressure of oxygen (Po_2) in the blood.
3. Plasma Po_2 determines the loading of hemoglobin at the lungs (oxygenation) and its unloading at the tissues (deoxygenation).
4. The blood's oxygen-transport capacity varies only slightly with normal variations in hemoglobin content. Iron-deficiency anemia lowers hemoglobin concentration, thus decreasing the blood's oxygen-carrying capacity and impairing aerobic exercise performance.
5. Hemoglobin saturation changes little until Po_2 declines below 60 mm Hg. The quantity of oxygen bound to hemoglobin falls sharply as oxygen moves from capillary blood to the tissues when metabolic demands increase.
6. Arterial blood releases only about 25% of its total oxygen content to the tissues at rest; the remaining 75% returns "unused" to the heart in venous blood.
7. The difference in oxygen content of arterial and venous blood under resting conditions indicates an automatic reserve of oxygen for rapid use should metabolism increase suddenly.
8. The Bohr effect reflects alterations in the molecular structure of hemoglobin from increased acidity, temperature, carbon dioxide concentration, and red blood cell 2,3-DPG that reduce its effectiveness to hold oxygen. Physical activity accentuates these factors to further facilitate oxygen's release to the tissues.
9. The iron-protein pigment myoglobin in skeletal and cardiac muscle provides an "extra" oxygen store to release oxygen at low Po_2. During intense activity, myoglobin facilitates oxygen transfer to the mitochondria when intracellular Po_2 in active skeletal muscle decreases dramatically.

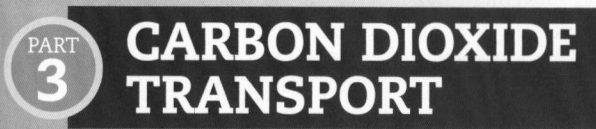

PART 3 — CARBON DIOXIDE TRANSPORT

CARBON DIOXIDE TRANSPORT IN THE BLOOD

Once carbon dioxide forms in the cell, diffusion and subsequent transport in the venous blood provides the only means for its "escape" through the lungs. The blood carries carbon dioxide in three ways:

1. A small amount in physical solution in plasma
2. Combined with hemoglobin within the red blood cell
3. As plasma bicarbonate

Figure 13.7 illustrates the three ways for transporting carbon dioxide from the tissues to the lungs.

Carbon Dioxide in Physical Solution

Approximately 5% of the carbon dioxide formed during energy metabolism moves into physical solution in the plasma as free carbon dioxide. *The random movement of this small quantity of dissolved carbon dioxide molecules establishes the Pco_2 of the blood.*

Carbon Dioxide Transport As Bicarbonate

Carbon dioxide in solution slowly combines with water to form carbonic acid in the following reversible reaction:

$$CO_2 + H_2O \longleftrightarrow H_2CO_3$$

Little carbon dioxide transport as carbonic acid would occur without **carbonic anhydrase**, a zinc-containing enzyme within the red blood cell. One mole of this catalyst tremendously accelerates the union of a mole of carbon dioxide and water to a rate of about 800,000 times a second (about 5000 times faster than without enzymatic action). The reaction attains equilibrium as the blood cell moves through the tissue's capillary.

Once carbonic acid forms in the tissues, most of it ionizes into hydrogen ions (H^+) and bicarbonate ions (HCO_3^-) as follows:

In tissues

$$CO_2 + H_2O \xrightarrow{\text{carbonic anhydrase}} H_2CO_3 \rightarrow H^+ + HCO_3^-$$

Buffering of the H^+ by the protein portion of hemoglobin maintains blood pH within relatively narrow limits (see "Acid-Base Regulation," Chapter 14). The HCO_3^- remains soluble so it diffuses from the red blood cell into plasma. There it exchanges for a chloride ion (Cl^-) that moves into the blood cell to maintain ionic equilibrium. This phenomenon, termed *chloride shift*, increases the Cl^- content of erythrocytes in venous blood more than in arterial red blood cells, particularly during exercise.

*Of the total carbon dioxide, 60 to 80% exists as **plasma bicarbonate**.* Bicarbonate forms in accordance with the law of mass action; carbonic acid formation accelerates as tissue Pco_2 increases. Plasma Pco_2 lowers as carbon dioxide leaves the blood via the lungs. This disturbs the equilibrium between carbonic acid and bicarbonate ion formation. The H^+ and HCO_3^- recombine to form carbonic acid. In turn, carbon dioxide and

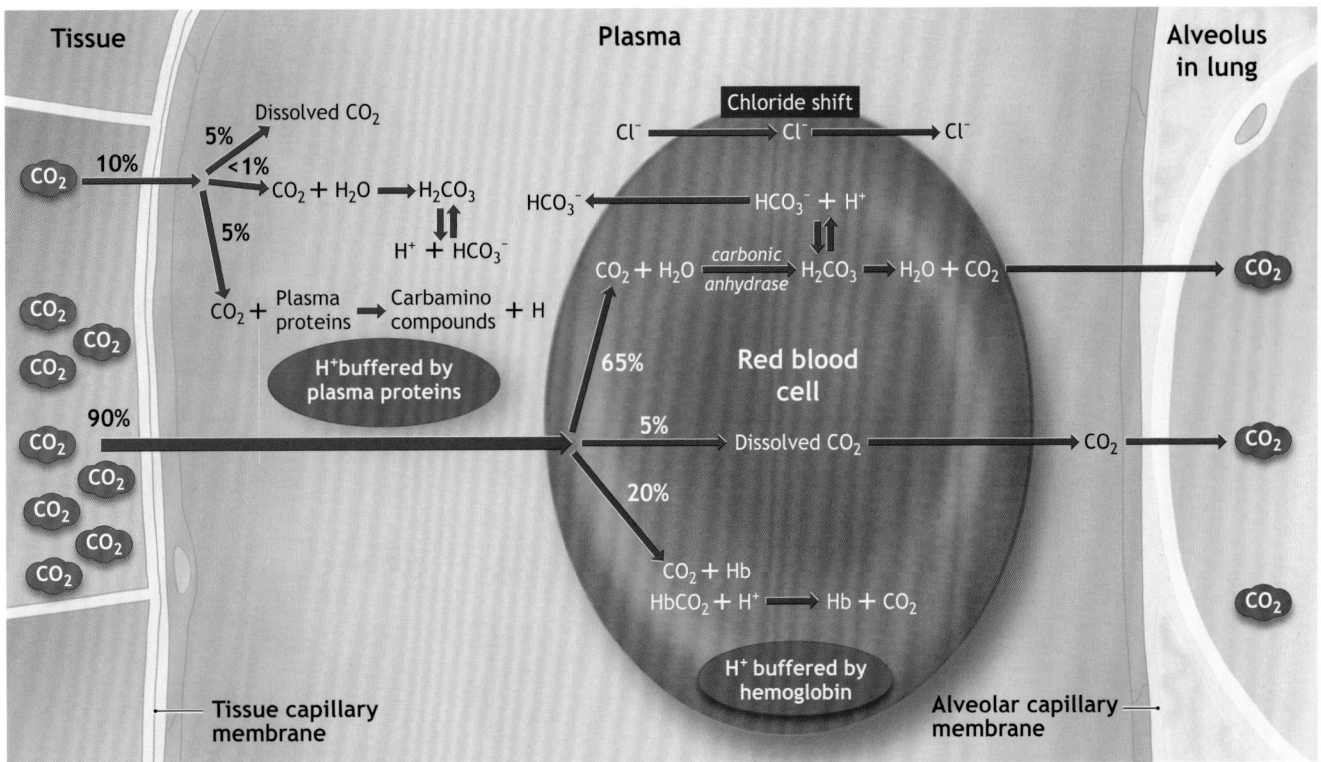

FIGURE 13.7 • Transport of carbon dioxide in the plasma and red blood cells as (1) dissolved CO_2, (2) bicarbonate, and (3) carbamino compounds. By far, the greatest amount of carbon dioxide combines with water to form carbonic acid.

water re-form and carbon dioxide exits through the lungs as follows:

In lungs

$$H^+ + HCO_3^- \rightarrow H_2CO_3 \xrightarrow{\text{carbonic anhydrase}} CO_2 + H_2O$$

The Cl^- moves from the red blood cell back into the plasma because plasma HCO_3^- decreases in the pulmonary capillaries.

Carbon Dioxide Transport as Carbamino Compounds

At the tissue level, carbamino compounds form when carbon dioxide reacts directly with the amino acid molecules of blood proteins. The globin portion of hemoglobin, which carries about 20% of the body's carbon dioxide, forms a carbamino compound as follows:

$$\begin{array}{ccc} CO_2 + & HbNH & \longrightarrow & HbNHCOOH \\ & \text{(Hemoglobin)} & & \text{(Carbaminohemoglobin)} \end{array}$$

A decrease in the plasma Pco_2 in the lungs reverses carbamino formation. This causes carbon dioxide to move into solution and enter the alveoli. Concurrently, oxygenation of hemoglobin reduces its ability to bind carbon dioxide. The interaction between oxygen loading and carbon dioxide release,

termed the **Haldane effect** after Scottish physiologist J. S. Haldane (1860–1936; inventor of the gas mask during World War I and developer of the first decompression tables for diving [see Chapter 26]), facilitates carbon dioxide removal in the lung.

Summary

1. About 5% of carbon dioxide travels in the plasma as free carbon dioxide in physical solution. Dissolved carbon dioxide establishes the Pco_2 of the blood, which modulates important physiologic functions.
2. The major quantity of carbon dioxide (80%) transports in chemical combination with water to form bicarbonate as follows:

$$CO_2 + H_2O \longrightarrow H_2CO_3 \longrightarrow H^+ + HCO_3^-$$

In the lungs, the reaction reverses and carbon dioxide exits the blood into the alveoli.

3. About 20% of the body's carbon dioxide combines with blood proteins, including hemoglobin, to form carbamino compounds.

thePoint References are available online at
http://thepoint.lww.com/mkk8e.

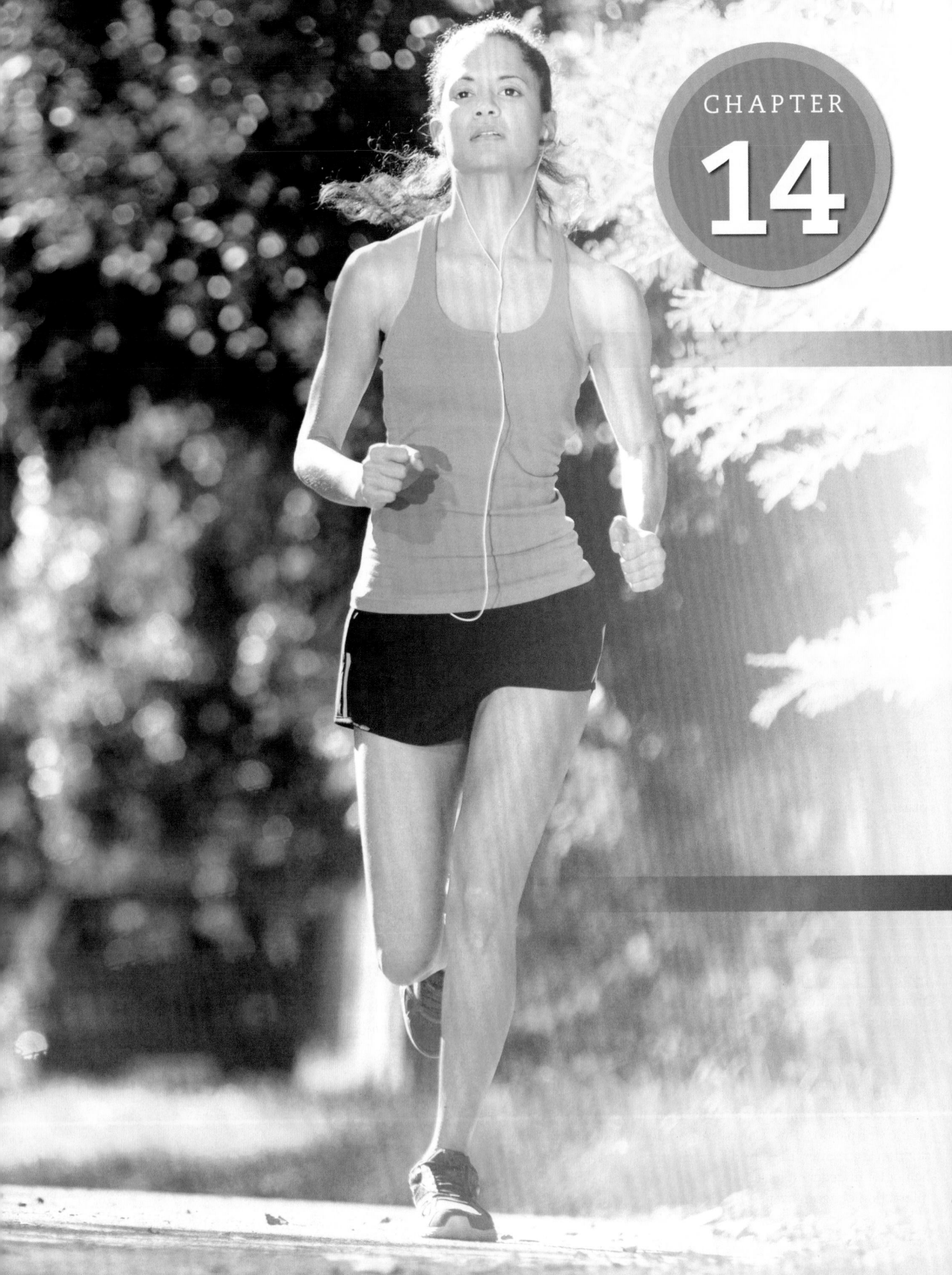

Dynamics of Pulmonary Ventilation

CHAPTER OBJECTIVES

- Describe how the hypothalamic neural command center controls pulmonary ventilation

- Explain how major chemical and nonchemical factors regulate pulmonary ventilation during rest and physical activity

- Describe how hyperventilation extends breath-holding time but also poses a danger in sport diving

- Outline the dynamic phases of minute ventilation at the onset, early phase, and late stage of moderate physical activity and recovery

- Graph the relationships among pulmonary ventilation, blood lactate, and oxygen consumption during incremental exercise, indicating the point of onset of blood lactate accumulation (OBLA)

- Explain the reasons for the increase in ventilatory equivalent during the transition from steady-rate to non–steady-rate activity

- Give the rationale for substituting the blood lactate threshold or OBLA for $\dot{V}O_{2max}$ to predict endurance performance

- Quantify the energy cost of breathing during rest and strenuous exertion in health and pulmonary disease

- Describe the acute effects of cigarette smoking on heart rate and energy cost of breathing during physical activity

- Outline endurance training adaptations in pulmonary ventilation during submaximal and maximal exercise

- Discuss pros and cons to the argument that pulmonary ventilation represents the "weak link" in oxygen supply during maximal activity

- Summarize how chemical and physiologic buffer systems regulate acid–base quality of body fluids during rest and physical activity

ANCILLARIES ⊙ at-a-Glance

Visit http://thePoint.lww.com/mkk8e to access the following resources.

- References: Chapter 14
- Interactive Question Bank
- Animation: Renal Function
- Focus on Research: Detecting the Onset of Anaerobic Metabolism

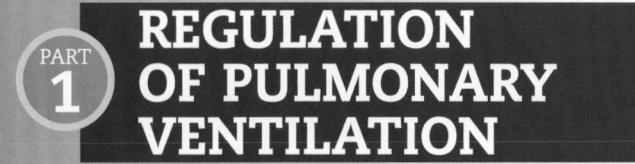

REGULATION OF PULMONARY VENTILATION

PART 1

and carotid artery chemoreceptors also mediate alveolar ventilation. In healthy individuals, these control mechanisms maintain relatively constant alveolar (and arterial) gas pressures throughout a broad range of exercise intensities. **FIGURE 14.1** presents a schematic view of the input for ventilatory control.

VENTILATORY CONTROL

Complex neural, humoral, and chemoreceptor mechanisms exquisitely adjust breathing rate and depth to the body's metabolic needs. Intricate neural circuits relay information from higher brain centers, lungs, and other sensors throughout the body to coordinate ventilatory control.[5,60] The gaseous and chemical states of the blood that bathe the medulla and aortic

Neural Factors

The inherent activity of inspiratory neurons with cell bodies located in the medial portion of the **medulla** governs the normal respiratory cycle. These neurons activate the diaphragm and intercostal muscles to cause the lungs to inflate. The inspiratory neurons cease firing because of self-limitations and inhibitory influence of expiratory neurons also located in the medulla. Inhibitory and excitatory signals from throughout the body influence the normal rhythm of medullary neurons. For example, lung inflation stimulates stretch receptors mainly in the bronchioles. These receptors act through afferent fibers to inhibit inspiration and stimulate expiration. Exhalation occurs as the inspiratory muscles relax, allowing for the passive recoil of the stretched lung tissue and raised ribs. This passive

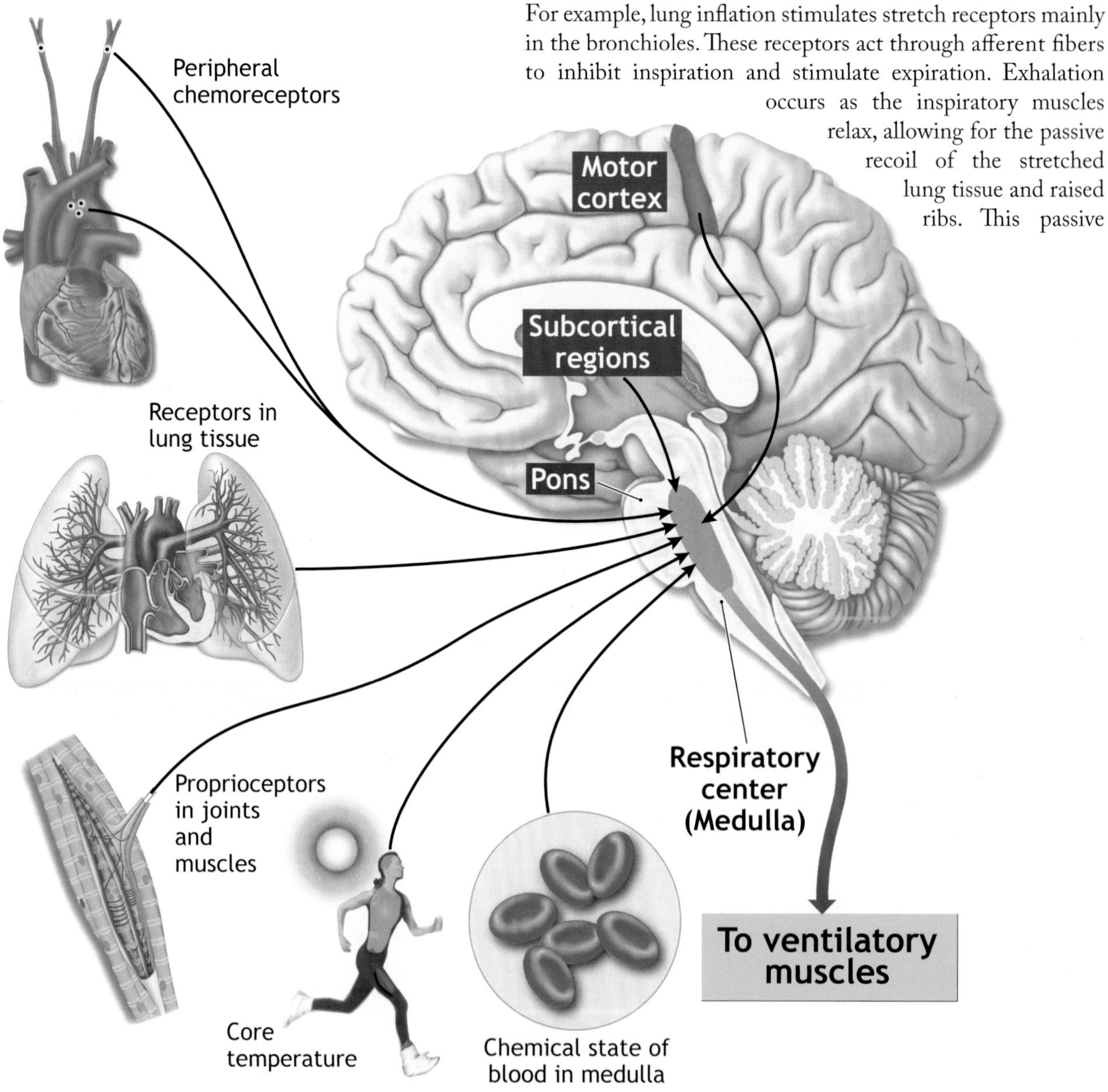

Peripheral chemoreceptors

Motor cortex

Subcortical regions

Pons

Receptors in lung tissue

Proprioceptors in joints and muscles

Respiratory center (Medulla)

Core temperature

Chemical state of blood in medulla

To ventilatory muscles

FIGURE 14.1 • Schematic representation of factors that affect medullary control of pulmonary ventilation. (Portions adapted and reprinted with permission from Moore, KL, Dalley, AF, Agur, AMR. *Clinically Oriented Anatomy*, 7th Ed., as used with permission from Agur, AMR, Dalley, AF, *Grant's Atlas of Anatomy*. 13th Ed. Baltimore: Wolters Kluwer Health, 2013.)

phase relies on synchronous activation of expiratory neurons and associated muscles that facilitate expiration. As expiration proceeds, the inspiratory center becomes progressively less inhibited and once again becomes active.

The inherent activity of the respiratory center alone cannot account for the smooth pattern of ventilatory adjustment to metabolic demands. The duration and intensity of the inspiratory cycle responds to the neural center in the hypothalamus that integrates input from descending neurons in the higher locomotor areas of the cerebral hemispheres, the pons, and other brain regions. During physical activity, ventilatory adjustments occur from mechanical and/or chemical changes within active muscles and its vasculature from ascending neural signals initiated to provide peripheral feedback control from the cerebellum to the respiratory center.

Humoral Factors

At rest, the chemical state of the blood exerts the greatest control of pulmonary ventilation. Variations in arterial Po_2, Pco_2, pH, and temperature activate sensitive neural units in the medulla and arterial system to adjust ventilation and maintain arterial blood chemistry within narrow limits.

Plasma Po_2 and Peripheral Chemoreceptors

Inhaling a gas mixture with 80% oxygen greatly increases alveolar Po_2 and reduces minute ventilation by 20%. Conversely, ventilation increases if inspired oxygen concentration decreases below ambient levels, particularly if alveolar Po_2 falls below 60 mm Hg. Hemoglobin saturation at this Po_2 begins to decrease considerably (see Fig. 13.4 in Chapter 13).

Sensitivity to reduced oxygen pressure does not reside in the respiratory center. Rather, peripheral **chemoreceptors** serve as the primary site to detect arterial hypoxia and reflexly initiate a ventilatory response. **Figure 14.2** shows these tiny specialized neurons located in the arch of the aorta and branching of the carotid arteries in the right and left sides of the neck. The strategic positioning of the **carotid bodies** monitors the state of arterial blood just before it perfuses the brain. Decreased arterial

Po_2, as occurs in pulmonary disease or ascent to high altitude, increases alveolar ventilation because of aortic and carotid chemoreceptor stimulation. These receptors *alone* protect the organism against reduced oxygen pressure in inspired air.

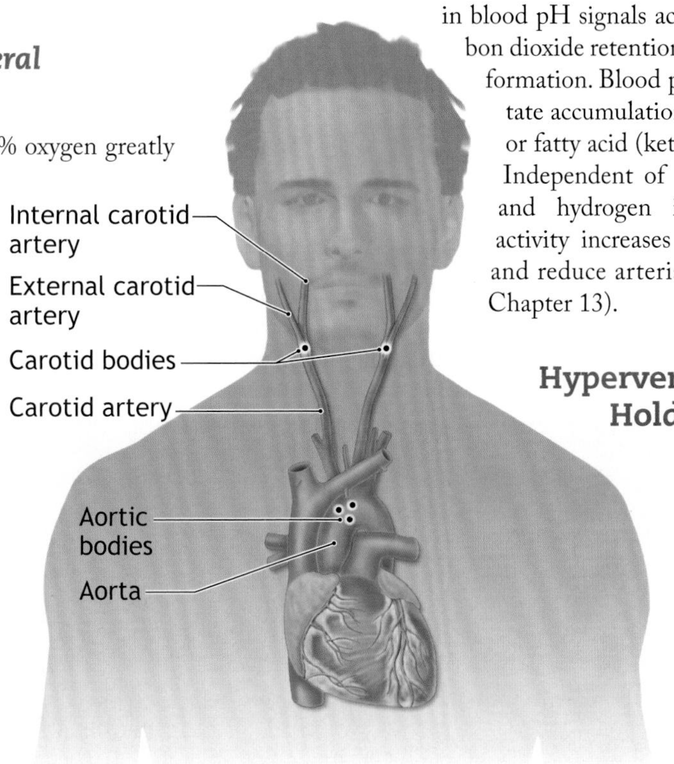

Peripheral chemoreceptor afferents also stimulate ventilation in physical activity, even though reductions in arterial Po_2 do not normally occur.[46,49] The stimulating effects of activity on carotid afferent chemoreceptor discharge mainly comes from increases in temperature, acidity, and carbon dioxide and potassium concentrations.[20,66]

Plasma Pco_2 and H^+ Concentration

At rest, carbon dioxide pressure in arterial plasma provides the most important respiratory stimulus. Small increases in Pco_2 in inspired air trigger large increases in minute ventilation. For example, the resting ventilation nearly doubles by increasing inspired Pco_2 to just 1.7 mm Hg (0.22% CO_2 in inspired air).

Molecular carbon dioxide per se does not mediate the ventilatory response to arterial Pco_2. Instead, plasma acidity, which varies directly with the blood's carbon dioxide content, exerts considerable command over minute ventilation. A fall in blood pH signals acidosis and usually reflects carbon dioxide retention and subsequent carbonic acid formation. Blood pH also can decrease from lactate accumulation in strenuous physical activity or fatty acid (ketone) accumulation in diabetes. Independent of cause, as arterial pH declines and hydrogen ions accumulate, inspiratory activity increases to eliminate carbon dioxide and reduce arterial levels of carbonic acid (see Chapter 13).

Hyperventilation and Breath Holding

Following a normal exhalation and then immediately holding ones breath, it takes approximately 40 s before the urge to breathe increases enough to initiate inspiration. The stimulus to breathe comes primarily from increased arterial Pco_2 and H^+ concentration, not decreased Po_2 in the breath-holding condition. The break point for breath holding corresponds to an increase in arterial Pco_2 to approximately 50 mm Hg.

If one consciously increases ventilation above normal level (**hyperventilation**) before breath holding, alveolar air composition

FIGURE 14.2 • The aortic arch and bifurcation of the carotid arteries contain cell bodies sensitive to reduced Po_2 and increased Pco_2 and H^+ and potassium concentrations in arterial blood. The peripheral chemoreceptors defend the body against arterial hypoxia in pulmonary disease and ascent to high altitude. The chemoreceptors also help to regulate exercise hyperpnea through the stimulating effects of increased arterial carbon dioxide and H^+ concentrations.

Labels in figure: Internal carotid artery; External carotid artery; Carotid bodies; Carotid artery; Aortic bodies; Aorta

becomes more like ambient air. Alveolar P_{CO_2} decreases from its normal value of 40 mm Hg to a low of 15 mm Hg. This creates a considerable diffusion gradient for carbon dioxide runoff into the alveoli from venous blood that enters the pulmonary capillaries. Consequently, a larger than normal quantity of carbon dioxide leaves the blood and arterial P_{CO_2} decreases. Hyperventilation extends breath-holding duration until arterial P_{CO_2} and/or H^+ concentration rises to levels that again stimulate the urge to breathe.

A Potentially Dangerous Maneuver

Swimmers and sport divers use hyperventilation and subsequent breath holding to improve performance. In sprint-swimming, for example, most sprinters hyperventilate on the starting blocks to prolong the breath-hold during the initial part of the swim and avoid taking a breath. In breath-hold diving, hyperventilation offers a similar effect—to extend breath-holding time. Tragedy while diving can occur with extended breath holding from hyperventilation. As the length and depth of a dive increase, the blood's oxygen content decreases to a critically low level before arterial P_{CO_2} rises enough to stimulate breathing and signal ascent. The diver, unfortunately, often loses consciousness before surfacing. Chapter 26 discusses hyperventilation and other factors important to sport diving.

REGULATION OF VENTILATION DURING PHYSICAL ACTIVITY

Chemical Control

Neither chemical stimulation nor any other single mechanism entirely accounts for the increase in ventilation (**hyperpnea**) during physical activity. For example, the classic feedback control of resting ventilation via oxygen- and carbon dioxide–mediated mechanisms does not adequately explain exercise hyperpnea. Inducing maximum changes in plasma acidity and inspired P_{O_2} and P_{CO_2} does not increase minute ventilation to values during vigorous exertion.

FIGURE 14.3 illustrates the relationships among oxygen consumption during graded exercise and venous and alveolar P_{CO_2} and alveolar P_{O_2}. As intensity increases, alveolar (arterial) P_{O_2} does not decrease to an extent that increases ventilation through chemoreceptor stimulation.[21] The large ventilatory volumes during intense physical activity cause alveolar P_{O_2} to rise *above* the average resting value of 100 mm Hg. Any increase in alveolar P_{O_2} in exercise hastens oxygenation of blood in the alveolar capillaries. Pulmonary ventilation during light and moderate activity closely couples with metabolism proportional to oxygen consumption and carbon dioxide production. Under these conditions, alveolar (and arterial) P_{CO_2} generally averages 40 mm Hg. During strenuous activity with its relatively large anaerobic component (lactate accumulation), increased carbon dioxide and subsequent H^+ concentrations provide an additional ventilatory stimulus. The resulting hyperventilation *reduces* alveolar and arterial P_{CO_2}, sometimes as low as 25 mm Hg. Any reduction in arterial P_{CO_2} decreases the ventilatory drive from carbon dioxide during exercise.

Nonchemical Control

The rapidity of the ventilatory response at the onset and cessation of movement suggests that input other than changes in arterial P_{CO_2} and H^+ concentration mediates these phases of exercise hyperpnea.

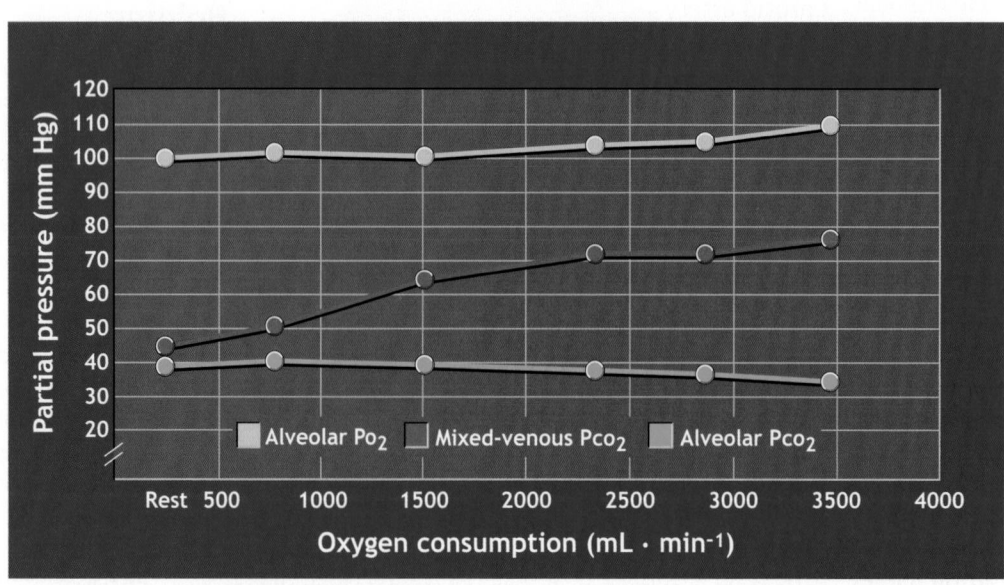

FIGURE 14.3 • Relationship between oxygen consumption during graded exercise and (1) values for P_{CO_2} in mixed-venous blood entering the lungs and (2) alveolar P_{O_2} and P_{CO_2}. Alveolar P_{O_2} and P_{CO_2} remain near resting levels throughout a broad range of exercise intensities, despite relatively large increases in mixed-venous P_{CO_2}.

Neurogenic Factors

Neurogenic factors for ventilatory control during physical activity include cortical and peripheral influences.

- *Cortical influence*: Neural outflow from regions of the motor cortex and cortical activation in anticipation of activity stimulate respiratory neurons in the medulla to initiate the abrupt increase in exercise ventilation.
- *Peripheral influence*: Sensory input from joints, tendons, and muscles influences the ventilatory adjustments throughout exercise. Experiments involving passive limb movements, electrical muscle stimulation, and voluntary movements with the muscle's blood flow occluded support the contribution of local mechanoreceptors and chemoreceptors to a reflex exercise hyperpnea.

Influence of Temperature

Except for extreme hyperthermia, an increase in body temperature exerts little effect on ventilatory regulation during physical activity. In most conditions, the rise in ventilation at activity onset and its decline during recovery occur too quickly to reflect control from core temperature changes.

Integrated Regulation

During Physical Activity

The combined and perhaps simultaneous effects of several chemical and neural stimuli initiate and modulate exercise alveolar ventilation. FIGURE 14.4 shows the dynamic phases of minute ventilation during moderate exercise and recovery. In **phase I ventilation** at the start of exercise, neurogenic stimuli from the cerebral cortex (**central command**), combined with feedback from the active limbs, stimulate the medulla to increase ventilation abruptly. Cortical and locomotor peripheral input continues throughout the activity period. After a short plateau (approximately 20 s), minute ventilation then rises exponentially in **phase II ventilation** to achieve a steady level related to the metabolic gas exchange demands. Central command input, including factors intrinsic to neurons of the respiratory control system, regulates this phase of exercise ventilation. Continued activity of respiratory neurons in the medulla causes short-term potentiation that augments their responsiveness to the same continuing stimulation. This brings minute ventilation to a new, higher level. In all likelihood, input from peripheral chemoreceptors in the carotid bodies also contributes to regulation during phase II ventilation.[66] The final phase III ventilation control involves fine-tuning of the steady-state ventilation through peripheral sensory feedback mechanisms. Central and reflex stimuli from the main byproducts of increased muscle metabolism—carbon dioxide and H^+ concentration—modulate alveolar gas pressures in this phase. These factors stimulate chemoreceptor group IV unmyelinated neurons that communicate with regions of the central nervous system to regulate cardiorespiratory function.[48] An additional stimulus to increase ventilation in strenuous activity occurs from the lactate anion itself, apart from lactic acidosis.[24]

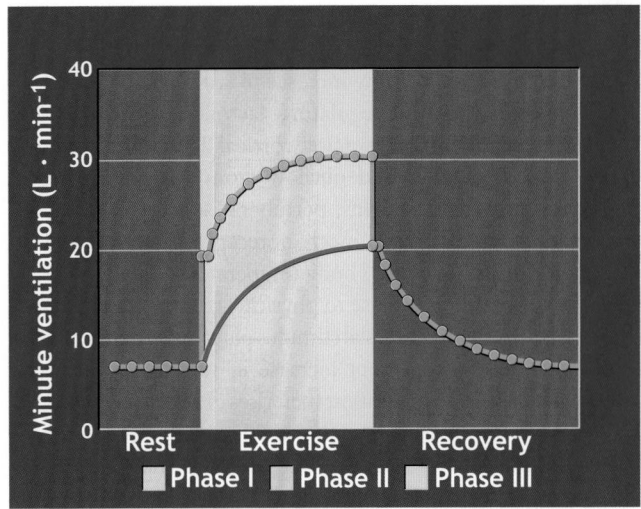

FIGURE 14.4 • Three phases of exercise hyperpnea. *Phase I*: rapid increase from rest and brief plateau from central command drive and input from active muscles. *Phase II*: Slower exponential rise begins approximately 20 s after exercise onset. Central command continues, along with feedback from active muscles plus the added effect of short-term potentiation of respiratory neurons. *Phase III*: Major regulatory mechanisms reach stable values; added input from peripheral chemoreceptors fine-tunes the ventilatory response. The *lower green curve* depicts only the contribution of central neuronal short-term potentiation and rising arterial H^+ concentration to the total respiratory response.

Reflexes related to pulmonary blood flow and mechanical movement of the lung and respiratory muscles also provide regulatory input during physical activity.

During Recovery

The abrupt decline in ventilation when physical activity ceases reflects removal of the central command drive and the sensory input from previously active muscles. More than likely, the slower recovery phase results from two factors:

1. Gradual diminution of the short-term potentiation of the respiratory center
2. Reestablishment of the body's normal metabolic, thermal, and chemical milieu

Summary

1. Inherent activity of neurons in the medulla regulates the normal respiratory cycle.
2. Input from higher brain centers, the lungs, and other sensors throughout the body interacts with medullary neural output to regulate ventilation.
3. Chemical factors that act directly on the respiratory center or modify its activity through peripheral chemoreceptors control alveolar ventilation at rest. Arterial P_{CO_2} and H^+ concentration are the most important regulatory factors.

4. Hyperventilation lowers arterial P_{CO_2} and H^+ concentration. This prolongs breath-holding time until levels of carbon dioxide and acidity increase to stimulate breathing.

5. Three nonchemical regulatory factors augment ventilatory adjustments to exercise: cortical activation in anticipation of activity and outflow from the motor cortex when movement begins, peripheral sensory input from chemoreceptors and mechanoreceptors in joints and muscles, and increased body temperature.

6. The ventilatory response to physical activity occurs in three phases. In Phase I, cortical stimulus plus feedback from active limbs causes the abrupt increase in ventilation as activity begins. Phase II ventilation then rises exponentially to reach a steady level related to the activity demands. Phase III ventilation involves fine-tuning of steady-state ventilation through peripheral sensory feedback mechanisms.

PART 2 PULMONARY VENTILATION DURING PHYSICAL ACTIVITY

VENTILATION AND ENERGY DEMANDS DURING PHYSICAL ACTIVITY

Physical activity affects oxygen consumption and carbon dioxide production more than any other physiologic stress. With exercise, oxygen diffuses from the alveoli into the venous blood as it returns to the lungs, while about the same quantity of carbon dioxide moves from the blood into the alveoli. Concurrently, increased alveolar ventilation maintains the proper gas concentrations to facilitate rapid gas exchange.

Ventilation in Steady-Rate Physical Acctivity

Figure 14.5 relates oxygen consumption and minute ventilation during increasing levels of exertion up to maximal oxygen consumption ($\dot{V}O_{2max}$) shown as final point at top right of figure. During light-to-moderate activity, ventilation increases *linearly* with oxygen consumption and carbon dioxide production, averaging between 20 and 25 L of air for each liter of oxygen consumed. Ventilation, in this case, increases mainly through increases in tidal volume; at higher intensities, breathing frequency takes on a more important role. Such ventilatory adjustments provide complete aeration of blood because alveolar P_{O_2} and P_{CO_2} remain near resting levels. Transit

time for blood in the pulmonary capillaries remains long enough for complete equilibration of the lung–blood gases (see Fig. 13.2 in Chapter 13).

The term ***ventilatory equivalent***, symbolized $\dot{V}_E/\dot{V}O_2$, describes the ratio of minute ventilation to oxygen consumption. Healthy young adults usually maintain this ratio at 25 (i.e., 25 L of air breathed per liter of O_2 consumed) during submaximal exercise up to approximately 55% of the $\dot{V}O_{2max}$. Higher ventilatory equivalents occur in children, with values averaging 32 L of air breathed per liter of O_2 consumed. Activity mode also affects the ventilatory equivalent. Prone swimming, for example, generates lower $\dot{V}_E/\dot{V}O_2$ ratios than running at all levels of energy expenditure. The restrictive nature of swimming on breathing lowers the ventilatory equivalent; this could constrain adequate gas exchange at maximal swimming velocities and partly explain the lower $\dot{V}O_{2max}$ during swimming than during running. The dynamics of pulmonary ventilation are highly adaptive to regular physical activity. Several weeks of aerobic training reduce the ventilatory equivalent during submaximal effort, which decreases the energy expended by the ventilatory musculature. Chapter 21 more fully discusses this adaptive ventilatory response.

Ventilation in Non–Steady-Rate Physical Activity

At higher levels of progressively more intense submaximal physical effort, minute ventilation moves sharply upward and increases disproportionately in relation to oxygen consumption. The ventilatory equivalent can attain values of 35 or 40 L of air breathed per liter of oxygen consumed.

Ventilatory Threshold

The term *ventilatory threshold* (Tvent) describes the point where pulmonary ventilation increases disproportionately relative to increases in oxygen consumption (i.e., there is a marked and precipitous increase in the $\dot{V}_E/\dot{V}O_2$ ratio) during graded exercise (see Fig. 14.5, *dashed white line* and "In a Practical Sense" later in this chapter). At this point, pulmonary ventilation no longer links tightly to oxygen demand at the cellular level. In fact, the "excess" ventilation comes directly from carbon dioxide's release from the buffering of lactic acid that begins to accumulate from increased glycolysis. Sodium bicarbonate in the blood buffers almost all of the lactic acid generated in anaerobic metabolism to sodium lactate in the following reaction:

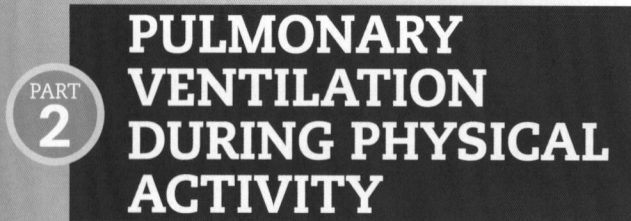

$$Lactic\ acid + NaHCO_3 \rightarrow Na\ Lactate + H_2CO_3$$
$$\Updownarrow$$
$$H_2O + CO_2$$

The excess carbon dioxide released in the buffering reaction stimulates pulmonary ventilation that disproportionately increases $\dot{V}_E/\dot{V}O_2$. Additional carbon dioxide exhaled from acid buffering causes the respiratory exchange ratio

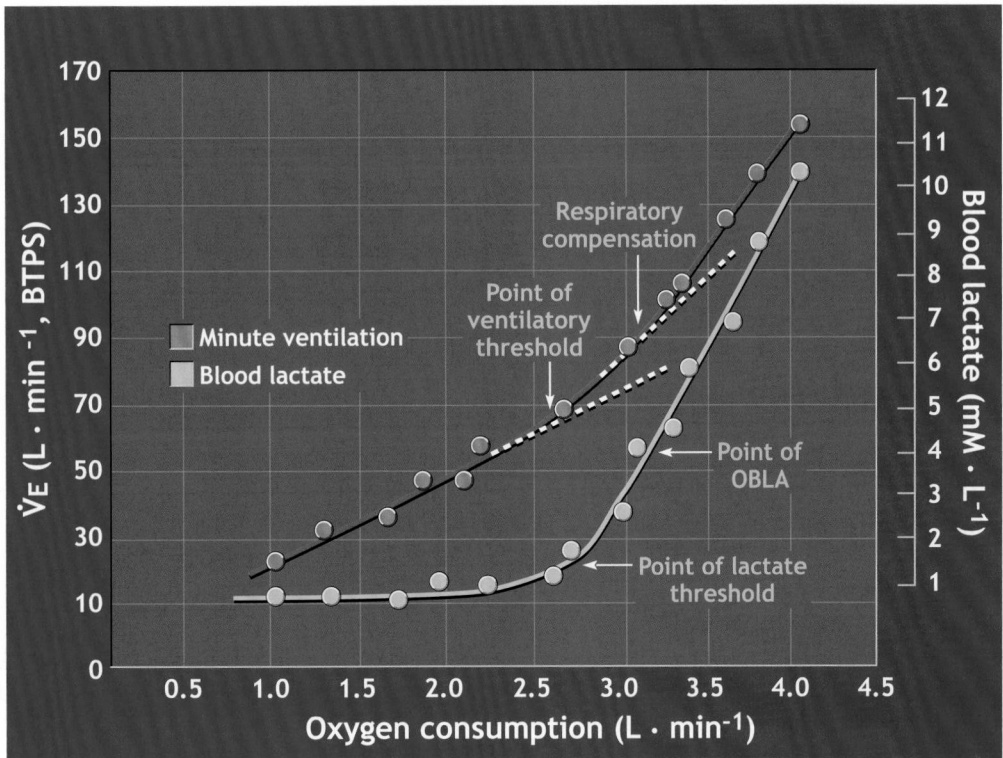

FIGURE 14.5 • Pulmonary ventilation, blood lactate concentration, and oxygen consumption during graded exercise to maximum. The *lower dashed white line* extrapolates the linear relationship between $\dot{V}_E$ and $\dot{V}O_2$ during submaximal effort. The lactate threshold (not necessarily the threshold for anaerobic metabolism) represents the highest exercise intensity (oxygen consumption) not associated with elevated blood lactate concentration. It occurs at the point at which the relationship between $\dot{V}_E$ and $\dot{V}O_2$ deviates from linearity, indicated as the *point of ventilatory threshold*. OBLA represents the point of lactate increase just above a 4.0-mM baseline. *Respiratory compensation* represents a further disproportionate increase in ventilation (indicated by deviation from *upper dashed white line*) to counter the decrease in plasma pH in intense physical activity.

$(R; \dot{V}CO_2/\dot{V}O_2)$ to exceed 1.00. Traditionally, researchers believed that the disproportionate increase in $\dot{V}_E$ and increase in R above 1.00 indicated that the oxygen demands of the active muscles exceeded mitochondrial oxygen supply with an increase in anaerobic energy transfer. They maintained that Tvent indicated the *threshold* for anaerobiosis and termed it the *anaerobic threshold*, or simply AT, to indicate increased reliance on anaerobic processes.

Attempts to validate a linkage between ventilatory changes and glycolytic events at the cellular level have proved elusive.

Onset of Blood Lactate Accumulation (OBLA)

During steady-rate physical activity, aerobic metabolism matches the energy requirements of the active muscles. Little or no blood lactate accumulates because any lactate production equals lactate disappearance. *The term **lactate threshold** describes the highest oxygen consumption or exercise intensity achieved with less than a 1.0 mM increase in blood lactate concentration above the pre-exercise level.*[63] By convention, blood lactate concentration is usually expressed in millimoles (mM) per liter of whole blood or as mg per deciliter

of whole blood, also termed volume percent (vol%); 1.0 mM equals 9.0 vol%. FIGURE 14.6 outlines possible underlying factors that relate to detecting the lactate threshold from pulmonary gas exchange dynamics during physical activity of progressively increasing intensity.

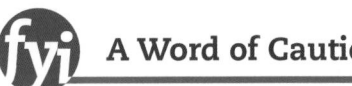 **A Word of Caution**

Early investigators linked the appearance of lactate in the blood to signal the onset of anaerobic conditions within active muscle, thus the term *anaerobic threshold*. Subsequent research using radioactive-labeled carbohydrate indicates that lactate's appearance in venous blood is more indicative of an imbalance between lactate production and lactate clearance within the muscle than the onset of anaerobic conditions. The fast-twitch fibers within active muscle that produce lactate "shuttle" this lactate to the muscle's slow-twitch oxidative fibers for use as aerobic energy substrate. The active muscles take up any lactate released into venous blood; other lactate-using organs like the heart and brain also catabolize lactate as an aerobic energy substrate.

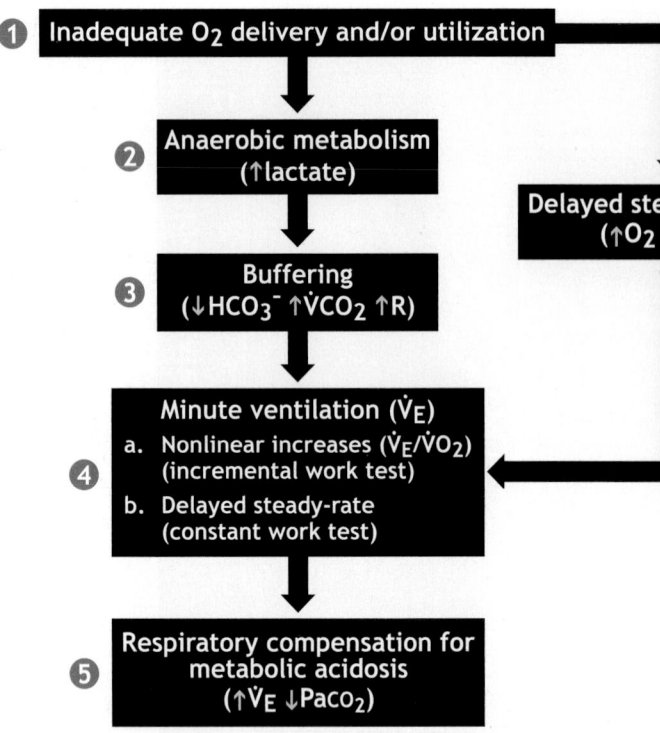

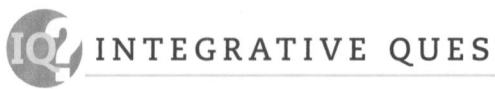

FIGURE 14.6 • Possible underlying factors that relate to detecting the lactate threshold from pulmonary gas exchange dynamics during physical activity of progressively increasing intensity. (Adapted with permission from Katch VL, McArdle WD, Katch FI, *Essentials of Exercise Physiology*. 4th Ed. Philadelphia: Wolters Kluwer Health, 2011.)

OBLA signifies when blood lactate concentration systematically increases to 4.0 mM.[12,53,63] Some researchers often use the terms *lactate threshold* and *OBLA* interchangeably, although each represents an operationally different precise point for intensity of effort and blood lactate level.

IQ INTEGRATIVE QUESTION

In what ways are the terms lactate threshold *and* onset of blood lactate accumulation *biochemically more precise than anaerobic threshold?*

The exact cause of OBLA remains controversial. Some researchers assume it represents a distinct point for the onset of muscle anaerobiosis even though blood lactate values do not always reflect lactate concentration in specific muscles. Lactate can accumulate not only from muscle anaerobiosis, but also from decreased total lactate clearance or increased lactate production in specific muscle fibers.

A threshold of lactate appearance could result from four factors:

1. Imbalance between the rate of glycolysis and mitochondrial respiration
2. Decreased redox potential (increased NADH relative to NAD$^+$)

3. Lower blood oxygen content
4. Lower blood flow to skeletal muscle

Caution should temper interpretations of the specific metabolic significance and cause of OBLA. However, it probably does signify initiation of an exponential accumulation of lactate in active muscle caused by physical activity.[32]

Blood lactate accumulation is reflected by plasma changes in pH, bicarbonate and H$^+$ concentrations, and carbon dioxide production via buffering, so these variables provide an indirect assessment of OBLA.[2,33,34,61] Changes in these measures do indeed relate to OBLA, but they probably cannot serve independently to establish the onset of anaerobic metabolism in muscle. However, they do provide practical information about exercise performance. "In a Practical Sense," on the next page, illustrates several common methods to indicate an imbalance between lactate formation and its clearance during physical activity.

Specificity of OBLA. Task specificity characterizes OBLA, as it does many measures of physiologic function and exercise performance. Differences in OBLA relative to the level of oxygen consumption occur in comparing bicycle, treadmill, and arm-crank exercise.[67] Variations in muscle mass activated in each activity form help to explain these differences. At a particular intensity or submaximal oxygen consumption, a higher metabolic rate per unit of active muscle mass exists for arm-crank and bicycle exercise than treadmill walking or running. OBLA therefore occurs at a lower level (oxygen consumption) during bicycling and arm-crank exercise. *Different activity modes cannot interchangeably define the point of OBLA during graded exercise testing. Each must be determined in its own exercise mode.*

Some Independence Between OBLA and $\dot{V}O_{2max}$. We previously indicated in Chapter 7 that blood lactate in trained individuals accumulates at higher submaximal oxygen consumptions and at higher percentages of $\dot{V}O_{2max}$ than in untrained individuals. For children and adults, endurance training often improves the exercise intensity at OBLA *without* concomitant increases in $\dot{V}O_{2max}$.[4,15,35,40] This suggests that different factors influence OBLA and $\dot{V}O_{2max}$. Muscle fiber type, capillary density, mitochondrial size and number, and enzyme concentrations play major roles in establishing the percentage of aerobic capacity sustainable without lactate accumulation.[11,30,62] In contrast, the functional capacity of the cardiovascular system for oxygen transport and the total muscle mass activated in exercise determine the $\dot{V}O_{2max}$.

OBLA and Endurance Performance. FIGURE 14.7 illustrates the major variables that contribute to oxygen transport and use. They ultimately determine the maximum intensity a person can maintain in prolonged physical activity. Two important factors influence endurance performance in a specific activity mode:

1. Maximum capacity to consume oxygen ($\dot{V}O_{2max}$)
2. Maximum level for steady-rate exercise (OBLA)

Most exercise physiologists apply $\dot{V}O_{2max}$ as a yardstick to gauge capacity for endurance activity. This measure generally relates to performance, but it does not fully explain success because one does not perform endurance activities at $\dot{V}O_{2max}$. *The exercise intensity at the point of OBLA consistently and powerfully predicts endurance performance of men and women.*[6,13,44,55] For race-walkers, race-walking velocity at the point of OBLA predicted 20-km times to within 0.6% of the actual time.[23] Similar results occurred in elite cyclists. Cycling power output at lactate threshold showed a strong relationship ($r = 0.93$) to average absolute power output maintained during a 1-hr ride in the laboratory.[14] The laboratory measurement accurately predicted performance in a 40-km road race. Improved endurance performance with training more closely relates to training-induced improvement in the exercise level for OBLA than $\dot{V}O_{2max}$ changes.[68]

 INTEGRATIVE QUESTION

Explain the rationale to measure pulmonary ventilation and gas exchange dynamics during graded exercise to indicate the onset of lactate buildup at the cellular level.

Racial Differences. The overwhelming dominance of African athletes in competitive endurance running between 3000 and 10,000 m has stimulated research into possible racial differences in resistance to fatigue, blood lactate accumulation, temperature regulation, and intramuscular oxidative enzyme capacity.[58] African and South African endurance runners consistently show greater resistance to fatigue at the same percentage of peak treadmill running velocity than Caucasian counterparts despite similar values for $\dot{V}O_{2max}$ and peak treadmill velocity.[10,64,65] The African athletes sustained a relatively higher percentage of maximal exercise capacity (i.e., superior fatigue resistance) from considerably higher oxidative enzyme profiles (citrate synthase and 3-hydroxyacyl-CoA dehydrogenase) and lower plasma lactate concentrations during sustained submaximal effort.[52] Greater running economy also probably contributes to superior endurance performance of elite African runners.[65] African runners perform better in high ambient temperatures than Caucasians due partly to their smaller size. This size "benefit" (larger surface-to-mass ratio) augments capacity to more readily transfer metabolic heat to the environment compared to the heavier Caucasian runners.[41]

 INTEGRATIVE QUESTION

Explain the biochemical rationale for measuring oxygen consumption and carbon dioxide production to infer the onset of metabolic anaerobiosis (lactate accumulation) during physical activity.

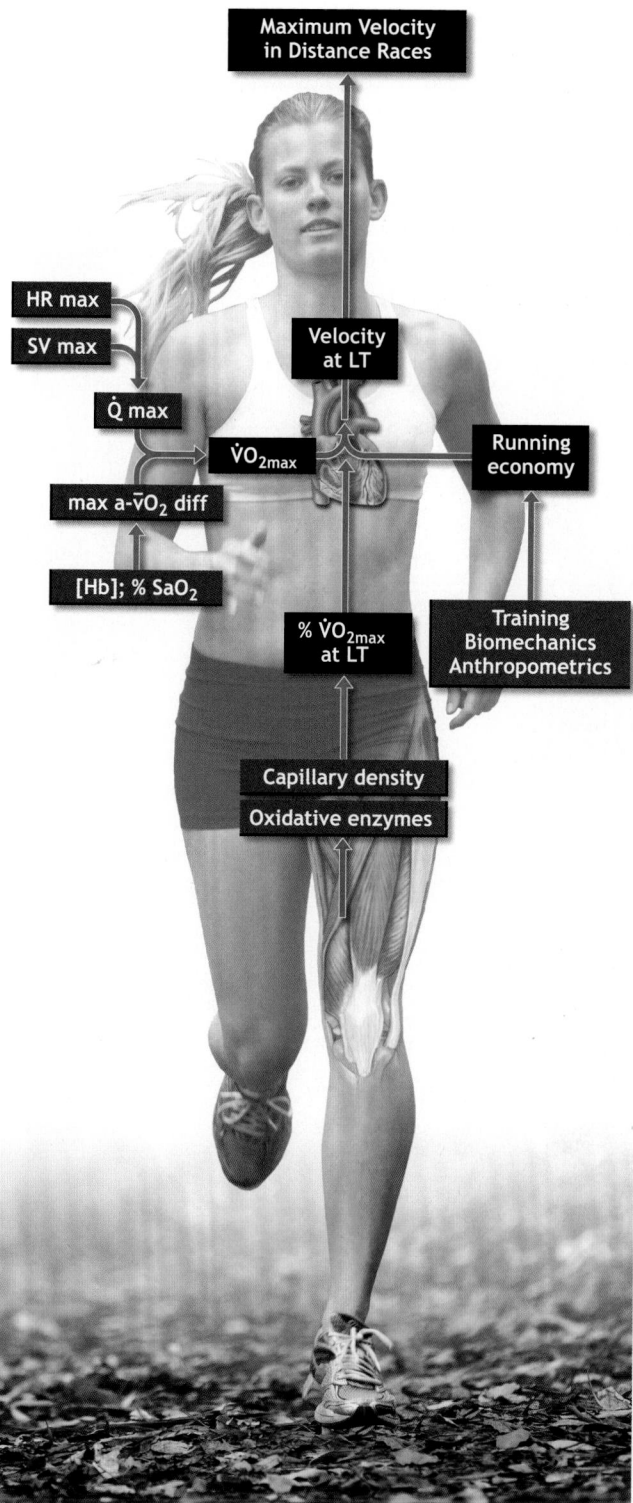

FIGURE 14.7 • Major variables related to maximal oxygen consumption, onset of blood lactate accumulation, and maximal running velocity during endurance exercise. $\dot{Q}$, cardiac output; [Hb], hemoglobin concentration; % SaO_2, percentage saturation with oxygen; max a-$\bar{v}O_2$ diff, maximum arteriovenous oxygen difference; LT, lactate threshold. (Adapted from Bassett DR Jr, Howley ET. Maximal oxygen uptake: "classical" versus "contemporary" viewpoints. *Med Sci Sports Exerc* 1997;29:591.) (Portions modified and reprinted with permission from Moore, KL, Dalley, AF, Agur, AMR. *Clinically Oriented Anatomy*, 7th Ed., as used with permission from Agur, AMR, Dalley, AF, *Grant's Atlas of Anatomy*. 13th Ed. Baltimore: Wolters Kluwer Health, 2013.)

IN A PRACTICAL SENSE

Determining the Lactate Threshold

Conceptually, the lactate threshold (LT) represents an exercise level (power output, $\dot{V}O_2$, or energy expenditure) where tissue hypoxia triggers an imbalance between lactate formation and its clearance, with a resulting increase in blood lactate concentration. All of the following terms refer essentially to the same LT phenomenon: *expiratory compensation threshold, anaerobic threshold, onset of blood lactate accumulation, optimal ventilatory efficiency, aerobic–anaerobic threshold, onset of plasma lactate accumulation, individual anaerobic threshold,* and *point of metabolic acidosis.*

The measurement of LT serves three important functions:

1. Provides a sensitive indicator of aerobic training status
2. Predicts endurance performance, often with greater accuracy than $\dot{V}O_{2max}$
3. Establishes an effective training intensity geared to the active muscles' aerobic metabolic dynamics

DIFFERENT INDICATORS OF LT

1. Fixed blood lactate concentration
2. Ventilatory threshold
3. Blood lactate–exercise $\dot{V}O_2$ response

Fixed Blood Lactate Concentration

During low-intensity, steady-rate physical activity, blood lactate concentration does not increase beyond normal biologic variation observed at rest. As intensity increases, blood lactate levels exceed normal variation. Exercise intensity (or $\dot{V}O_2$) associated with a fixed blood lactate concentration that exceeds normal resting variation denotes the LT. This often coincides with a 2.5-mM value. A 4.0-mM lactate value indicates the onset of blood lactate accumulation (OBLA). The top figure illustrates LT and OBLA computations from fixed blood lactate concentrations during incremental, 4-min exercise stages on a bicycle ergometer. Interpolation from a visual plot of power output ($\dot{V}O_2$) versus blood lactate determines the activity level associated with the fixed blood lactate concentrations.

The decision regarding stage duration, number of stages, and interval between stages becomes important. Stages 4 min or longer provide better predictability than shorter ones. For the data illustrated, LT occurred at a power output of 205 W; 225 W predicted the fixed blood lactate concentration for OBLA.

Ventilatory Threshold

Pulmonary minute ventilation ($\dot{V}_E$) during physical activity increases disproportionately in its relationship to oxygen consumption at about the same time blood lactate begins to accumulate. The ventilatory threshold (Tvent) predicts LT from the $\dot{V}_E$ response during graded exercise. The mechanistic link of lactate buffering by plasma bicarbonate to produce additional CO_2 (and respiratory stimulus unrelated to $\dot{V}O_2$) justifies the use of Tvent on a physiologic basis.

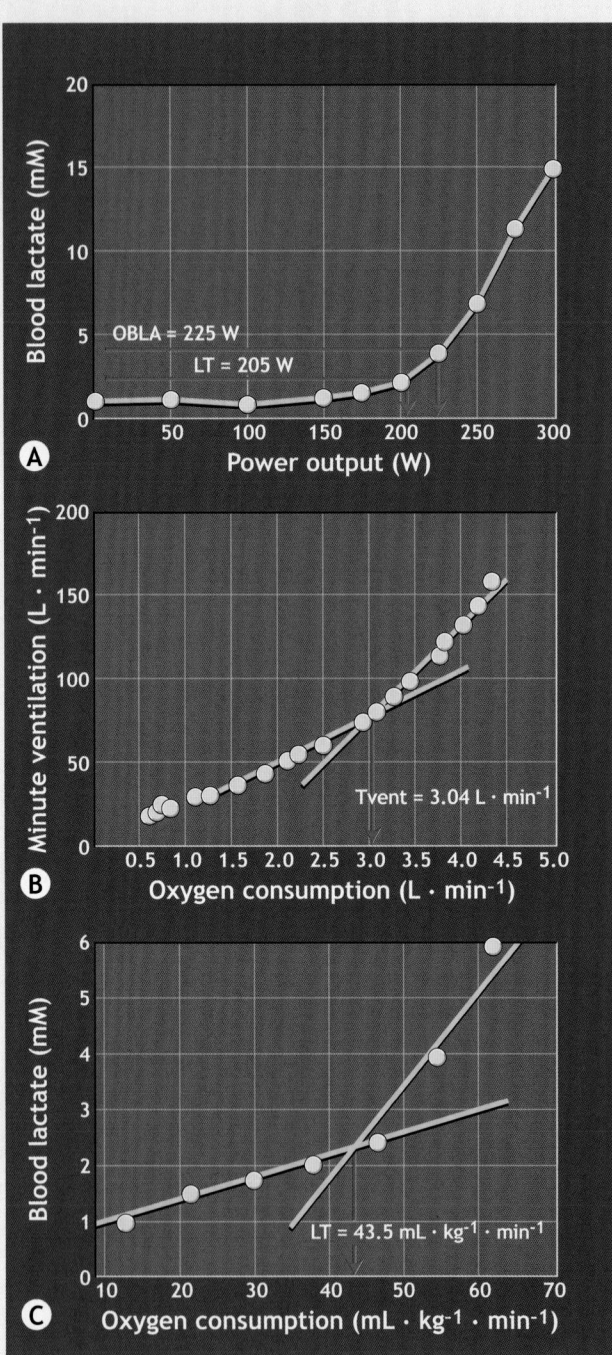

(A) Fixed blood lactate concentration method to determine lactate threshold (LT) and onset of blood lactate accumulation (OBLA). This example shows LT at a fixed blood lactate of 2.5 mM and OBLA at a fixed blood lactate of 4.0 mM. **(B)** Determination of LT from the relationship between pulmonary minute ventilation and oxygen consumption during incremental exercise. **(C)** Determination of LT from the relationship between blood lactate concentration and oxygen consumption during incremental exercise.

The test involves exercise with increments of short duration (a ramp test of 1- or 2-min increments) with continuous measurement of $\dot{V}_E$ (breath by breath or every 10, 20, or 30 s) to the point of fatigue (usually within 8 to 12 min). The point of nonlinear increase in $\dot{V}_E$ versus $\dot{V}O_2$ represents Tvent, expressed as a specific $\dot{V}O_2$ value rather than as running speed or power output common with the fixed blood lactate concentration method. The middle figure shows the relationship between $\dot{V}_E$ and $\dot{V}O_2$ during incremental exercise; Tvent occurs at an exercise $\dot{V}O_2$ of 3.04 L·min⁻¹. It is common to express the $\dot{V}O_2$ at LT as a percentage of $\dot{V}O_{2max}$ (71% in this example).

Blood Lactate–Exercise $\dot{V}O_2$ Response

This protocol plots blood lactate concentration versus either $\dot{V}O_2$ or exercise intensity in a manner similar to determination of fixed blood lactate concentration. The person exercises for 3- or 4-min increments on a bicycle ergometer or treadmill. With treadmill exercise, blood is sampled for lactate determination during a brief pause at the end of each stage, or without pause when using stationary cycling. The bottom figure plots blood lactate versus oxygen consumption throughout the test. A best-fitting straight line depicts the linear portion of the curve; a second line describes the upward-trending curve after it "breaks" from linearity. The intersection of the two lines represents LT.

ENERGY COST OF BREATHING

Figure 14.8 specifies the oxygen cost of breathing during whole-body graded exercise up to maximum. Figure 14.8A indicates the effects of increasing minute ventilation on the oxygen cost of breathing expressed as a percentage of the total exercise oxygen consumption. Figure 14.8B illustrates the influence of increasing minute ventilation on the oxygen cost per liter of air breathed per minute. The oxygen requirement of breathing remains relatively small at rest and during light-to-moderate activity with no differences observed between nonobese women and men.[39] For ventilations up to about 100 L·min⁻¹, oxygen cost averaged between 1.5 and 2.0 mL per liter of air breathed each minute. This represented from 3 to 5% of the total oxygen consumption in moderate activity and 8 to 11% for minute ventilations at $\dot{V}O_{2max}$ values typical for most individuals. Among highly trained endurance athletes with maximum minute ventilations of 150 L·min⁻¹ and higher, the cost of exercise hyperpnea can exceed 15% of the total oxygen consumption. At this level, the inspiratory muscles operate at 40 to 60% of maximum capacity to generate force.[1] The rate of blood flow to these muscles may equal that of limb locomotor muscles.[18]

Up to 15% of the total blood flow sustains the metabolic demands of respiratory muscles during maximal effort.[25,27] Evidence from healthy, fit individuals indicates a "competition" for blood flow and oxygen between respiratory and locomotor muscles during intense activity. For example, altering respiratory muscle work during maximal exercise to increase the energy cost of breathing vasoconstricts the locomotor muscles. Redirection of cardiac output to the respiratory musculature compromised perfusion of the active, nonrespiratory muscles. This reduced the total percentage of $\dot{V}O_{2max}$ used by the active locomotor muscles. Conversely, easing the work of breathing during maximal effort with an assist ventilator elicited a corresponding increase in oxygen consumption (greater %$\dot{V}O_{2max}$) of the active leg muscles.

Respiratory Disease

During even moderate physical activity, the healthy person rarely senses the effort to breathe. In respiratory disease, however, the work of breathing becomes an exhaustive effort in itself. In chronic obstructive pulmonary disease (COPD), the added expiratory resistance can triple the normal cost of breathing at rest; during light exercise, ventilatory cost may reach 10 mL of oxygen for each liter of air breathed. In severe pulmonary disease, the cost of breathing easily attains 40% of the total oxygen consumption. Competition between the oxygen–blood flow needs of locomotor and respiratory muscles encroaches on the oxygen available to the active, nonrespiratory muscle mass.[26] In COPD, the increased cost of breathing severely limits the exercise capacity of individuals with this debilitating medical condition. Unfortunately, exercise training produces only small improvements in pulmonary function parameters or disease status. Regular physical activity can, however, improve exercise capacity, reduce dyspnea, decrease ventilatory equivalents for oxygen, improve respiratory and peripheral muscle function, and enhance psychologic state.[8,16,47,54] Chapter 32 more fully discusses the role of regular physical activity in rehabilitating COPD patients.

Cigarette Smoking

Airway resistance at rest increases up to threefold in both chronic smokers and nonsmokers following 15 puffs on a cigarette during a 5-min period.[43] The added resistance to breathing lasts an average of 35 min; it probably exerts only a minor effect during light activity when breathing cost remains small. The residual smoking effect could prove detrimental during vigorous exercise because of the additional oxygen cost to move larger air volumes. Increased peripheral airway resistance with smoking comes mainly from two sources:

1. Vagal reflex—possibly triggered from sensory stimulation by minute particles in cigarette smoke
2. Stimulation of parasympathetic ganglia by nicotine

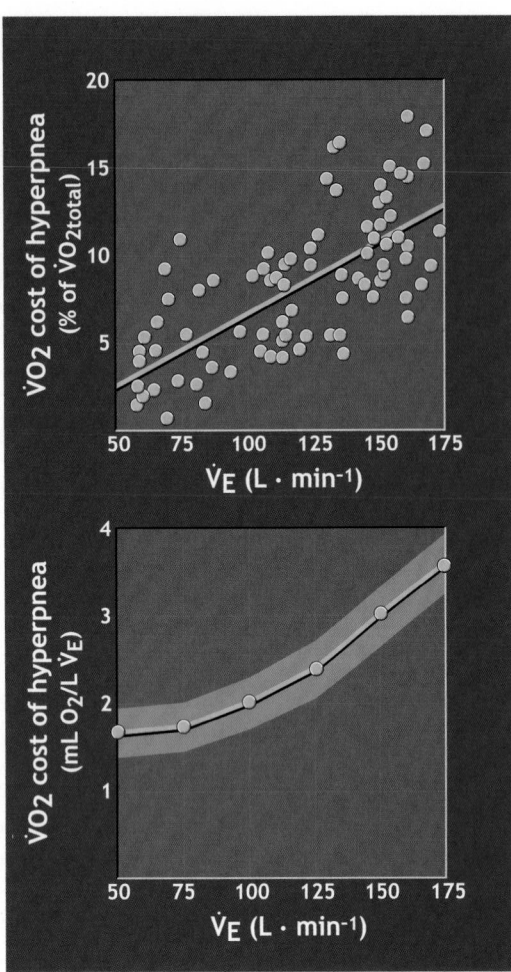

FIGURE 14.8 • Oxygen cost of breathing during whole-body graded exercise up to maximum. **(A)** Effects of increasing minute ventilation ($\dot{V}_E$) on the total oxygen cost of breathing expressed as a percentage of total exercise oxygen consumption. **(B)** Effects of increasing minute ventilation on the oxygen cost per liter air breathed per minute. (Adapted with permission from Dempsey JA, et al. Respiratory muscle perfusion and energetics during exercise. *Med Sci Sports Exerc* 1996;28:1123.)

Researchers determined the oxygen cost of breathing in six habitual smokers immediately after smoking two cigarettes and 1 day after tobacco abstinence. The subjects ran on a treadmill at a speed and grade requiring 80% of $\dot{V}_{O_{2max}}$. Two methods increased ventilation during the "smoking" and "nonsmoking" runs: (1) subjects voluntarily hyperventilated during the run (voluntary HV) and (2) researchers induced hyperventilation by increasing alveolar P_{CO_2} by having subjects breathe through a large-diameter tube that increased anatomic dead space by 1400 mL (dead space HV). The oxygen cost of the "extra" breathing equaled the difference between the normal oxygen consumption and that in the hyperventilation experiments.

Table 14.1 indicates that the oxygen cost of breathing decreased between 13 and 79% with smoking abstinence. The energy requirement of breathing during exercise averaged 14% of the total oxygen consumption after smoking, but only 9% in the nonsmoking trials for the heaviest smokers. Also, heart

rate averaged 5 to 7% lower during exercise following 1 day of cigarette abstinence; all subjects reported feeling better when they exercised in the nonsmoking condition. These findings indicate a substantial reversibility of the increased cost of breathing with smoking in chronic smokers with only 1 day of abstinence. *From a practical standpoint, an athlete who cannot eliminate smoking completely should at least abstain the day before a competition.* Additional research complements these findings; a 7-day smoking abstinence period by young men reduced submaximal exercise heart rate and enhanced time to exhaustion during graded treadmill testing.[28]

Cigarette Smoking Blunts Exercise Heart Rate Response

A paradox exists between the maximal exercise capacity of cigarette smokers and their submaximal heart rate response to exercise. Otherwise healthy chronic smokers exhibit significantly less endurance during graded exercise to maximum than nonsmokers.[28,36] Despite their poorer performance in maximal testing (i.e., shorter time to fatigue), the smokers spent more time to reach a heart rate of 130 b·min⁻¹ during a graded exercise test. This indicates a relatively *higher* fitness level (i.e., more exercise accomplished before reaching the submaximal heart rate value). An altered sensitivity in autonomic neural control from cigarette smoking may inhibit the heart rate response of smokers to submaximal effort.[37] This emphasizes the need to consider smoking status when evaluating fitness data from submaximal heart rate response to a standard step test or a heart rate prediction test. Failure to account for cigarette smoking would inflate fitness estimates because the blunted (lower) heart rate response of smokers erroneously implies higher aerobic fitness.

DOES VENTILATION LIMIT AEROBIC POWER AND ENDURANCE PERFORMANCE?

Aerobic training produces considerably less adaptation in pulmonary structure and function than in cardiovascular and neuromuscular adaptations. Interest concerns how the lack of pulmonary system "plasticity" affects aerobic performance, mainly at the high exercise levels routinely performed by elite endurance athletes.[17,19]

 INTEGRATIVE QUESTION

Advise a person who performs specific breathing exercises rather than endurance training to increase "wind" and eliminate "breathlessness" when running continuously for 20 to 30 min.

With inadequate breathing during graded exercise, the relationship between pulmonary ventilation and oxygen consumption would curve in a direction opposite to that indicated

TABLE 14.1 Oxygen Cost of Hyperventilation (HV) in "Smoking" and "Nonsmoking" Exercise at Approximately 80% of $\dot{V}O_{2max}$

	Smoking				Nonsmoking			
	Voluntary HV		Dead Space HV		Voluntary HV		Dead Space HV	
Subject	$\dot{V}_E$ (L·min⁻¹)	O₂ Cost (mL·L⁻¹)	$\dot{V}_E$ (L·min⁻¹)	O₂ Cost (mL·L⁻¹)	$\dot{V}_E$ (L·min⁻¹)	O₂ Cost (mL·L⁻¹)	$\dot{V}_E$ (L·min⁻¹)	O₂ Cost (mL·L⁻¹)
1	26.4	15.1	18.9	12.7	22.7	11.4	23.0	6.5
2	39.0	10.3	28.1	5.9	42.6	11.3	41.3	4.8
3	22.8	7.9	27.2	7.0	23.8	7.2	22.8	5.7
4	36.3	5.0	28.7	5.6	44.7	3.8	18.6	−1.6ᵃ
5	52.7	13.5	26.7	12.4	75.2	6.1	22.8	5.7
6	22.4	8.5	27.3	1.1	23.2	3.4	30.1	3.0
Average	32.6	10.1	26.2	7.4	38.7	7.2	26.5	4.0

Reprinted from Rode A, Shephard RJ. The influence of cigarette smoking upon the oxygen cost of breathing in near-maximal exercise. *Med Sci Sports Exerc* 1971;3:51.

ᵃ The implication of the "negative" cost of $\dot{V}_E$ in this subject is that the added dead space reduces the cost of the normal exercise ventilation.

in Figure 14.5 (i.e., decreased ventilatory equivalent). This common response in COPD patients indicates a *failure* of ventilation to keep pace with oxygen consumption[3]; in this case, one truly would "run out of breath." During strenuous effort, healthy individuals overbreathe at higher levels of oxygen consumption. The hyperventilation response generally decreases alveolar P_{CO_2} (see Fig. 14.3) and slightly increases alveolar P_{O_2}. Exercise conditions that trigger hyperventilation-induced reductions in arterial carbon dioxide restrict cerebral blood flow, which may compromise oxygen delivery to active brain areas and contribute to central fatigue.[45] Even during maximal activity, a considerable **breathing reserve** exists because minute ventilation at $\dot{V}O_{2max}$ equals only 60 to 85% of a healthy person's maximum voluntary ventilation (MVV). Most individuals have a 20 to 40% MVV reserve during intense physical activity. *Pulmonary function does not form a "weak link" in the oxygen transport system of healthy individuals with average to moderately large aerobic capacities.*

An Important Exception

For endurance athletes, the pulmonary system lags behind their exceptional cardiovascular and aerobic muscular adaptations to training.[59] The potential for inequality in alveolar ventilation relative to pulmonary capillary blood flow (i.e., impaired ventilation–perfusion ratio) during intense activity may compromise arterial saturation and oxygen transport capacity—a condition termed ***exercise-induced arterial hypoxemia (EIH)***.[31,38,42,50] EIH among trained individuals remains variable. It sometimes occurs at exercise levels as low as 40% $\dot{V}O_{2max}$ at sea level and mild to moderate altitudes.[7,22,51] When highly trained endurance athletes exercised near $\dot{V}O_{2max}$ (>65 mL·kg⁻¹·min⁻¹; **Fig. 14.9**), pressure differentials between

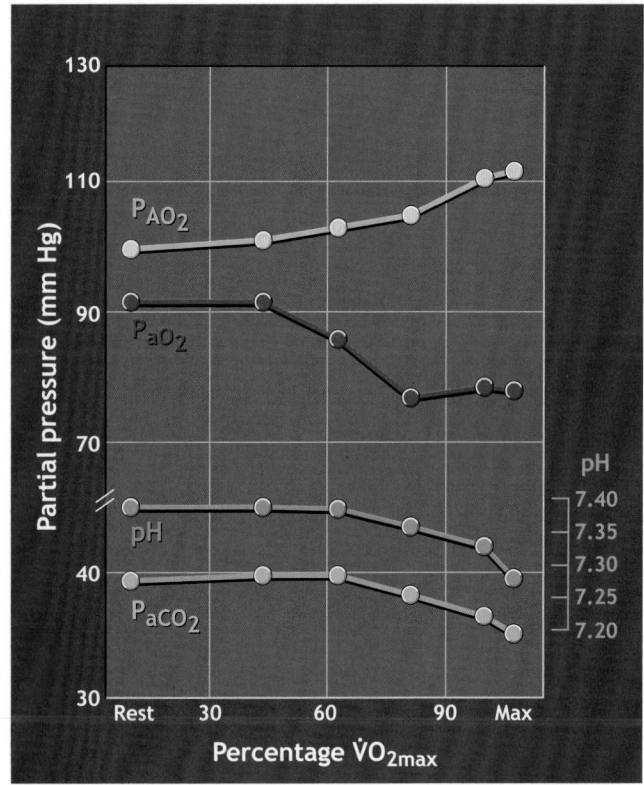

FIGURE 14.9 • Average values for blood gas pressures (Pao₂ and Paco₂), acid-base status (pH), and difference between alveolar (Pao₂) and arterial (Pao₂) oxygen pressure in eight male athletes during graded exercise up to $\dot{V}O_{2max}$. Note the widening of the (A-a)O₂ gradient and the fall in Pao₂ during maximal exercise. (Adapted with permission from Johnson BD, et al. Mechanical constraints on exercise hyperpnea in endurance athletes. *J Appl Physiol* 1992;73:874.)

alveolar and arterial oxygen widened to more than 30 mm Hg. This caused arterial oxygen saturation to fall below 90% with a corresponding arterial P_{O_2} below 75 mm Hg. Some elite endurance athletes cannot achieve complete aeration of the blood in the pulmonary capillaries in intense exercise; in this situation, arterial desaturation becomes more apparent as the duration of effort progresses. It does not appear that alterations in pulmonary structure at the alveolar–capillary interface produce EIH, although recruitment of intrapulmonary shunt vessels during exercise may contribute to the exercise-induced impairment in pulmonary gas exchange.[56,57]

Possible functionally based causes for arterial desaturation include:

1. Inequality in ventilation–perfusion ratio within the lungs or specific lung regions
2. Shunting of blood between venous and arterial circulations, thus bypassing areas for diffusion
3. Failure to achieve end-capillary equilibrium between alveolar oxygen pressure and pressure of oxygen in blood perfusing the pulmonary capillaries

 INTEGRATIVE QUESTION

Explain why pulmonary ventilation for most healthy persons does not limit aerobic exercise performance.

Summary

1. In light-to-moderate physical activity, pulmonary ventilation increases linearly with oxygen consumption so the ventilatory equivalent ($\dot{V}_E/\dot{V}O_2$) averages 20 to 25 L of air breathed per liter of oxygen consumed.
2. In non–steady-rate physical activity, ventilation increases disproportionately with increases in oxygen consumption, with ventilatory equivalents exceeding 35 L.
3. A disproportionately sharp rise in minute ventilation during incremental exercise provides a "bloodless" way to estimate the onset of blood lactate accumulation (OBLA).
4. OBLA provides a submaximal exercise measure of aerobic fitness that relates to the beginning of anaerobiosis in the active muscles.
5. OBLA occurs without significant metabolic acidosis or severe cardiovascular strain.
6. The oxygen cost of breathing for healthy individuals remains relatively small throughout a broad range of submaximal effort.
7. The work of breathing becomes excessive for individuals with respiratory disease, often producing inadequate alveolar ventilation.
8. Cigarette smoking causes airway resistance to rise considerably and increase the cost of breathing to adversely affect endurance performance.
9. Exercise training generally reduces the ventilatory equivalent in submaximal activity, which "conserves" oxygen during a particular task.

10. For individuals of average aerobic fitness, maximal physical activity does not tax pulmonary ventilation to a point that limits optimal alveolar gas exchange and arterial saturation.
11. Pulmonary function improvements for the endurance athlete can lag behind their exceptional adaptations in cardiovascular and muscle function, thereby compromising aeration of blood during maximal effort.

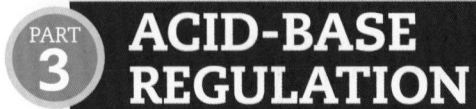

PART 3 **ACID-BASE REGULATION**

BUFFERING

Acids dissociate in solution and release H^+, whereas **bases** accept H^+ to form hydroxide ions (OH^-). The term **buffering** designates reactions that minimize changes in H^+ concentration; **buffers** refer to chemical and physiologic mechanisms that prevent this change.

The symbol **pH** designates a quantitative measure of acidity or alkalinity (basicity) of a liquid solution. Specifically, pH refers to the concentration of protons or H^+. Acid solutions have more H^+ than OH^- at a pH below 7.0, and vice versa for basic solutions whose pH exceeds 7.0. Chemically pure (distilled) water, considered neutral, has equal H^+ and OH^- and thus a pH of 7.0. The pH scale shown in **FIGURE 14.10**, devised in 1909 by Danish chemist Sören Sörensen (1868–1939; http://protomag.com/assets/soren-sorensen-pioneer-ph; known for his work in amino acid synthesis and enzyme reactions at Carlsberg laboratory in Copenhagen, Denmark), ranges from 1.0 to 14.0. An inverse relation exists between pH and H^+ concentration. The logarithmic nature of the pH scale means a one-unit change in pH produces a 10-fold change in H^+ concentration. For example, lemon juice and gastric juice (pH = 2.0) have 1000 times the H^+ concentration of black coffee (pH = 5.0), whereas hydrochloric acid (pH = 1.0) has approximately 1 million times the H^+ concentration of blood at a pH of 7.4.

The pH of bodily fluids ranges from a low of 1.0 for the digestive acid hydrochloric acid to a slightly basic pH between 7.35 and 7.45 for arterial and venous blood and most other bodily fluids. A decrease in H^+ concentration (increased pH or **alkalosis**) produces an increase in pH above the normal average of 7.4. Conversely, **acidosis** refers to increased H^+ concentration (decreased pH). The acid-base characteristics of bodily fluids fluctuate within narrow limits because metabolism remains highly sensitive to H^+ concentrations in the reacting medium. Three mechanisms regulate the pH of the internal environment:

1. Chemical buffers
2. Pulmonary ventilation
3. Renal function

Chemical Buffers

The chemical buffering system consists of a weak acid and salt of that acid. Bicarbonate buffer, for example, consists of the weak acid **carbonic acid** and its salt, **sodium bicarbonate**. Carbonic acid forms when bicarbonate binds H^+. When H^+ concentration remains elevated, the reaction produces the weak acid because excess H^+ ions bind in accord with the general reaction:

$$H^+ + Buffer \rightarrow H\text{-}Buffer$$

In contrast, when H^+ concentration decreases—as during hyperventilation, when plasma carbonic acid declines because carbon dioxide leaves the blood and exits through the lungs—the buffering reaction moves in the opposite direction and releases H^+:

$$H^+ + Buffer \leftarrow H\text{-}Buffer$$

Most of the carbon dioxide generated in energy metabolism reacts with water to form the relatively weak carbonic acid that dissociates into H^+ and HCO_3^-. Likewise, the stronger lactic acid reacts with sodium bicarbonate to form sodium lactate and carbonic acid; in turn, carbonic acid dissociates and increases the H^+ concentration of the extracellular fluids. Other organic acids such as fatty acids dissociate and liberate H^+, as do sulfuric and phosphoric acids generated during protein catabolism. Bicarbonate, phosphate, and protein chemical buffers provide the rapid first line of defense to maintain consistency in the acid-base character of the internal environment.

Bicarbonate Buffer

The bicarbonate buffer system consists of carbonic acid and sodium bicarbonate in solution. During buffering, hydrochloric acid (a strong acid) converts to the much weaker carbonic acid by combining with sodium bicarbonate in the following reaction:

$$HCl + NaHCO_3 \rightarrow NaCl + H_2CO_3 \leftrightarrow H^+ + HCO_3^-$$

The buffering of hydrochloric acid produces only a slight reduction in pH. Sodium bicarbonate in plasma exerts a strong buffering action on lactic acid to form sodium lactate and carbonic acid. Any additional increase in H^+ concentration from

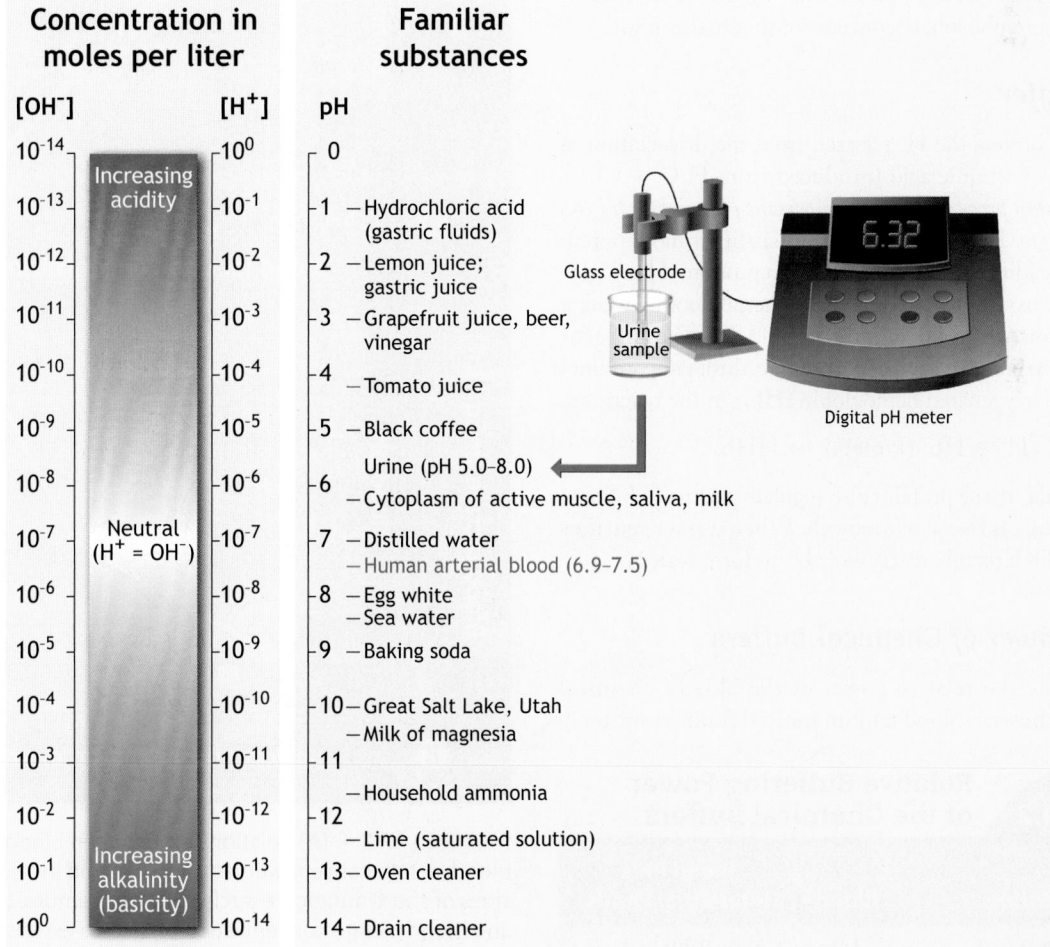

FIGURE 14.10 • The pH scale provides a quantitative measure of the acidity or alkalinity (basicity) of a liquid solution. Blood pH normally stabilizes at the slightly alkaline pH of 7.4. Values for blood pH rarely fall below pH of 6.9, even during the most strenuous physical activity, although values at the active muscle are lower. The digital pH meter accurately determines the pH of any substance. The example shows a pH of 6.32 for the urine sample.

carbonic acid dissociation causes the dissociation reaction to move in the opposite direction to release carbon dioxide into solution as follows:

Result of acidosis

$$H_2O + CO_2 \leftarrow H_2CO_3 \leftarrow H^+ + HCO_3^-$$

An increase in plasma carbon dioxide or H^+ concentration immediately stimulates ventilation to eliminate "excess" carbon dioxide.

Conversely, a decrease in plasma H^+ concentration inhibits the ventilatory drive and retains carbon dioxide that then combines with water to increase acidity (carbonic acid) and normalize pH.

Result of alkalosis

$$H_2O + CO_2 \rightarrow H_2CO_3 \rightarrow H^+ + HCO_3^-$$

Phosphate Buffer

The phosphate buffering system consists of phosphoric acid and sodium phosphate. These chemicals act similarly to the bicarbonate buffers. Phosphate buffer exerts an important effect on acid-base balance in the kidney tubules and intracellular fluids where phosphate concentration remains high.

Protein Buffer

Venous blood buffers the H^+ released from the dissociation of relatively weak carbonic acid (produced from $H_2O + CO_2$). *By far, hemoglobin provides the most important H^+ acceptor for this buffering function.* Hemoglobin is almost six times more potent in regulating acidity than the other plasma proteins. Hemoglobin's release of oxygen to the cells makes hemoglobin a weaker acid, thereby increasing its affinity to bind H^+. The H^+ generated when carbonic acid forms in the erythrocyte combines readily with deoxygenated hemoglobin (Hb^-) in the reaction:

$$H^+ + Hb^- \text{ (Protein)} \rightarrow HHb$$

Intracellular tissue proteins also regulate plasma pH. Some amino acids possess free acidic radicals. When dissociated, they form OH^-, which readily reacts with H^+ to form water.

Relative Power of Chemical Buffers

TABLE **14.2** lists the relative power of the blood's chemical buffers with those in blood and interstitial fluids combined.

TABLE 14.2	Relative Buffering Power of the Chemical Buffers	
Chemical Buffer	**Blood**	**Blood Plus Interstitial Fluids**
Bicarbonate	1.0	1.0
Phosphate	0.3	0.3
Proteins (excluding Hb)	1.4	0.8
Hemoglobin	5.3	1.5

As a frame of reference, the buffering power of the bicarbonate system receives the value 1.00.

PHYSIOLOGIC BUFFERS

The pulmonary and renal systems present the second line of defense in acid–base regulation. Their buffering function occurs only when a change in pH has already occurred.

Ventilatory Buffer

When the quantity of free H^+ in extracellular fluid and plasma increases, it directly stimulates the respiratory center to immediately increase alveolar ventilation. This rapid adjustment

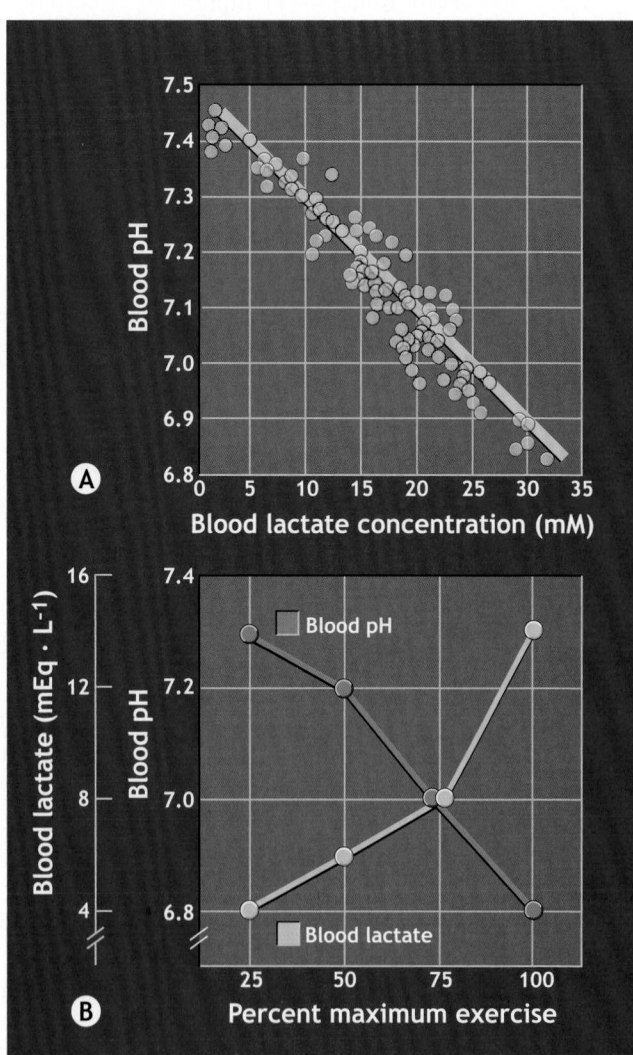

FIGURE 14.11 • (A) Relationship between blood pH and blood lactate concentration during rest and increasing intensities of short-duration exercise up to maximum. **(B)** Blood pH and blood lactate concentration related to exercise intensity expressed as a percentage of the maximum. Decreases in blood pH accompany increases in blood lactate concentration. (Adapted with permission from Osnes JB, Hermansen L. Acid-base balance after maximal exercise of short duration. *J Appl Physiol* 1972;32:59.)

reduces alveolar P_{CO_2} and causes carbon dioxide to be "blown off" from the blood. Reduced plasma carbon dioxide levels accelerate the recombination of H^+ and HCO_3^-, lowering free H^+ concentration in plasma. For example, doubling alveolar ventilation by hyperventilation at rest increases blood alkalinity and pH by 0.23 units, from 7.40 to 7.63. Conversely, reducing normal alveolar ventilation (hypoventilation) by one-half increases blood acidity by approximately 0.23 pH units. The potential magnitude of ventilatory buffering equals twice the combined effect of all the body's chemical buffers.

Renal Buffer

Chemical buffers only temporarily affect excess acid buildup. Excretion of H^+ by the kidneys, although relatively slow, provides an important longer-term defense that maintains the body's buffer reserve (alkaline reserve). To this end, the kidneys stand as the final sentinels. The renal tubules regulate acidity through complex chemical reactions that secrete ammonia and H^+ into the urine and then reabsorb alkali, chloride, and bicarbonate.

 See the animation "Renal Function" on **http://the Point.lww.com/mkk8e** for a demonstration of this process.

EFFECTS OF INTENSE PHYSICAL ACTIVITY

Increased H^+ concentration from carbon dioxide production and lactate formation during strenuous physcal activity makes pH regulation progressively more difficult. Acid–base regulation becomes exceedingly difficult during repeated, brief bouts of all-out effort that elevate blood lactate values to 30 mM (270 mg of lactate per dL of blood) or higher.[29] **FIGURE 14.11**

illustrates the inverse linear relationship between blood lactate concentration and blood pH. Blood lactate concentration in these experiments varied between 0.8 mM at rest (pH 7.43) and 32.1 mM during exhaustive exercise (pH 6.80). In active muscle, pH reaches even lower values than in blood, declining to 6.4 or lower at exhaustion.

The above data indicate that humans *temporarily* tolerate pronounced disturbances in acid-base balance during maximal physical effort, at least to an overall blood pH as low as 6.80—one of the lowest blood lactate values ever reported. A plasma pH below 7.00 does not occur without consequences; this level of acidosis produces nausea, headache, and dizziness, in addition to discomfort and pain that ranges from mild to severe within active muscles.

Summary

1. The chemical and physiologic buffer systems normally regulate the acid-base quality of bodily fluids within narrow limits.
2. The bicarbonate, phosphate, and protein chemical buffers provide the rapid first line of defense in acid-base regulation.
3. Chemical buffers consist of a weak acid and the salt of that acid. Their action during acidosis converts a strong acid to a weaker acid and a neutral salt.
4. The lungs and kidneys also contribute to pH regulation. Changes in alveolar ventilation rapidly alter free H^+ concentration in extracellular fluids. The renal tubules act as the body's final defense by secreting H^+ into the urine and reabsorbing bicarbonate.
5. Anaerobic exercise increases the demand for buffering, and makes pH regulation progressively more difficult.

thePoint References are available online at **http://thepoint.lww.com/mkk8e.**

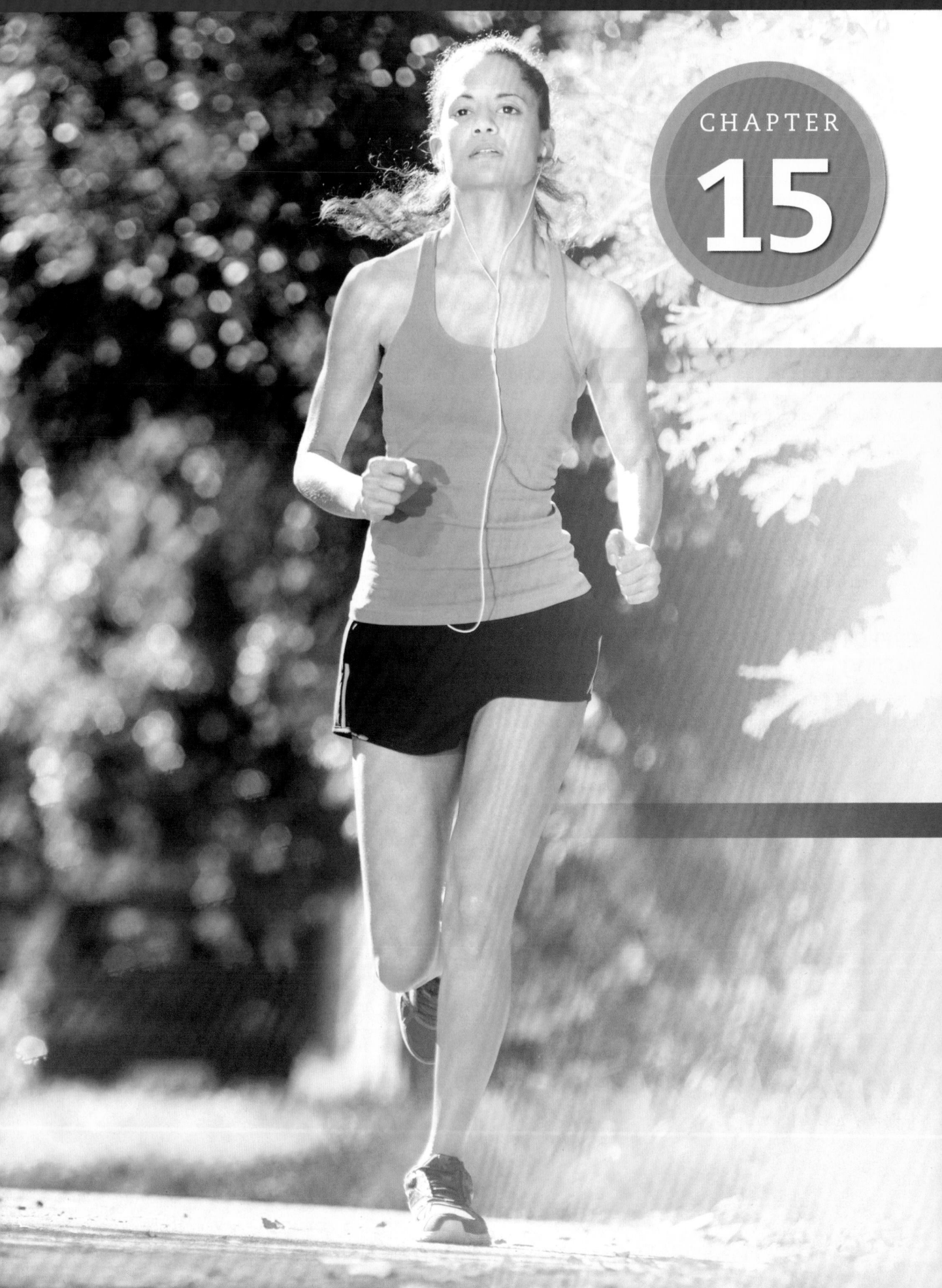

CHAPTER

15

The Cardiovascular System

- List four important cardiovascular system functions
- Describe the interactions among cardiac output, total peripheral resistance, and arterial blood pressure
- Explain the role of the venous system as an active blood reservoir
- Outline the structural differences in the various blood vessels of the body
- Explain how to measure blood pressure with the auscultatory method
- List typical systolic and diastolic blood pressures at rest, moderate, and intense aerobic physical activities

- Discuss how blood pressure responds during resistance exercise and upper-body exercise
- Explain why a "hypotensive response" might occur in recovery from physical activity
- Diagram the major vessels of the coronary circulation
- Describe the pattern of myocardial blood flow, oxygen consumption, and substrate use during rest and various intensities of physical exertion
- Explain the rate–pressure product, its meaning, and rationale for use in clinical exercise physiology

ANCILLARIES ⟨●⟩ *at-a-Glance*

Visit http://thePoint.lww.com/mkk8e to access the following resources.

- References: Chapter 15
- Appendix H: Supplemental Animations and Videos
- Interactive Question Bank
- Animation: Blood Circulation
- Animation: Cardiac Cycle
- Animation: Hypertension
- Animation: Measuring Blood Pressure
- Animation: Myocardial Blood Flow
- Focus on Research: Required Exercise Intensity to Improve Fitness

*The early "physiologists" during the time of Galen almost 2000 years ago (see the introduction to this text, "A View of the Past") proposed that the **cardiovascular system** integrates the body as a unit. For the contemporary exercise physiologist, one of the most important cardiovascular functions entails how well this highly integrated system provides active muscles with a continuous stream of nutrients and oxygen to sustain high levels of energy transfer and removal of metabolic byproducts from the tissues' active sites of energy release.*

Chapters 15, 16, and 17 explore the dynamics of circulation, particularly its role in oxygen delivery during physical activity. The maximum level for aerobic energy transfer during activity depends on oxygen transport and delivery, and most importantly, how muscles generate adenosine triphosphate (ATP) aerobically.

CARDIOVASCULAR SYSTEM COMPONENTS

The cardiovascular system consists of four components:

1. A pump that provides continuous linkage with the other three components
2. A high-pressure distribution circuit
3. Exchange vessels
4. A low-pressure collection and return circuit

If stretched in a line, the approximate 60,000 miles (100,000 km) of blood vessels of an average-sized adult would encircle the Earth about 2.4 times. **Figure 15.1** presents a schematic view of the cardiovascular system, including the major arteries. The table inset shows the distribution of blood in absolute and percentage terms. The small arteries, veins, and capillaries of the systemic circulation contain approximately 75% of the total blood volume, whereas the heart contains only 7%. Note that in the systemic circulation, the small veins account for the largest blood volume at any one time (46%), compared to the volume in the largest arteries (6%) and veins (18%).

 See the animation "Blood Circulation" on **http://thePoint.lww.com/mkk8e** for a demonstration of this process.

The Heart

The **heart** provides the impetus for blood flow. Situated in the midcenter of the chest cavity, about two thirds of its mass lies to the left of the body's midline. The four-chambered muscular organ weighs 11 oz for an average-sized adult male and 9 oz for an average-sized female and pumps about 2.4 oz, or 70 mL, on each beat. At rest, the heart's output of blood averages 1900 gallons daily, or 52 million gallons over a 75-year lifetime. For a person of average fitness status, the maximum output of blood from the heart in 1 min exceeds the fluid output from a household faucet turned wide open.

Figure 15.2 summarizes general functional and structural characteristics and mode of activation of the body's three types of muscle—skeletal, cardiac, and smooth. The heart muscle,

or **myocardium**, represents a homogenous form of striated muscle similar to the slow-twitch fibers in skeletal muscle with high capillary density and numerous mitochondria. In contrast to skeletal muscle, the multinucleated, individual cells or fibers interconnect in latticework fashion via **intercalated discs**. The stimulation or depolarization of one cell spreads the action potential through the myocardium to *all* cells to make the heart function as a unit.

Figure 15.3 shows the structural details of the heart as a pump.

 See the animation "Cardiac Cycle" on **http://thePoint.lww.com/mkk8e** for a demonstration of this process.

Functionally, one can view the heart as two separate pumps. The hollow chambers on the right side of the heart (right heart) perform two crucial functions:

1. Receives blood returning from throughout the body
2. Pumps blood to the lungs for aeration through the **pulmonary circulation**

The left side of the heart (referred to as the left heart) also performs two critical functions:

1. Receives oxygenated blood from the lungs
2. Pumps blood into the thick-walled, muscular aorta for distribution throughout the body in the **systemic circulation**

A thick, solid muscular wall or interventricular septum separates the heart's left and right sides. The **atrioventricular valves** within the heart provide one-way blood flow from the right atrium to the right ventricle via the **tricuspid valve**, and from the left atrium to the left ventricle through the **mitral** or **bicuspid valve**. The **semilunar valves**, located in the arterial wall just outside the heart, prevent blood from flowing back into the heart between contractions. The relatively thin-walled, saclike atrial chambers serve as primer or "booster" pumps to receive and store blood during ventricular contraction. Approximately 70% of the blood returning to the atria flows directly into the ventricles before the atria contract. The simultaneous contraction of both atria then forces the remaining blood into their respective ventricles directly below. Almost immediately after atrial contraction, the ventricles contract and propel blood into the arterial system. To learn more, visit **www.pbs.org/wgbh/nova/eheart/human.html**, which deals with important aspects of heart function.

As ventricular pressure builds, the atrioventricular valves snap closed. All heart valves remain closed for 0.02 to 0.06 s. This brief interval of rising ventricular tension, when heart volume and muscle fiber length remain unchanged, represents the heart's **isovolumetric contraction period**. Blood ejects from the heart when ventricular pressure exceeds arterial pressure. With each contraction, the spiral and circular arrangement of bands of cardiac muscle literally "wrings out" blood from the ventricles.

Body area	Blood volume	
	mL	Percentage
Heart	360	7.2
Lungs		
Arteries	130	2.6
Capillaries	110	2.2
Veins	200	4.0
Systemic		
Aorta, large arteries	300	6.0
Small arteries	400	8.0
Capillaries	300	6.0
Small veins	2300	46.0
Large veins	900	18.0
Total	5000	100.0

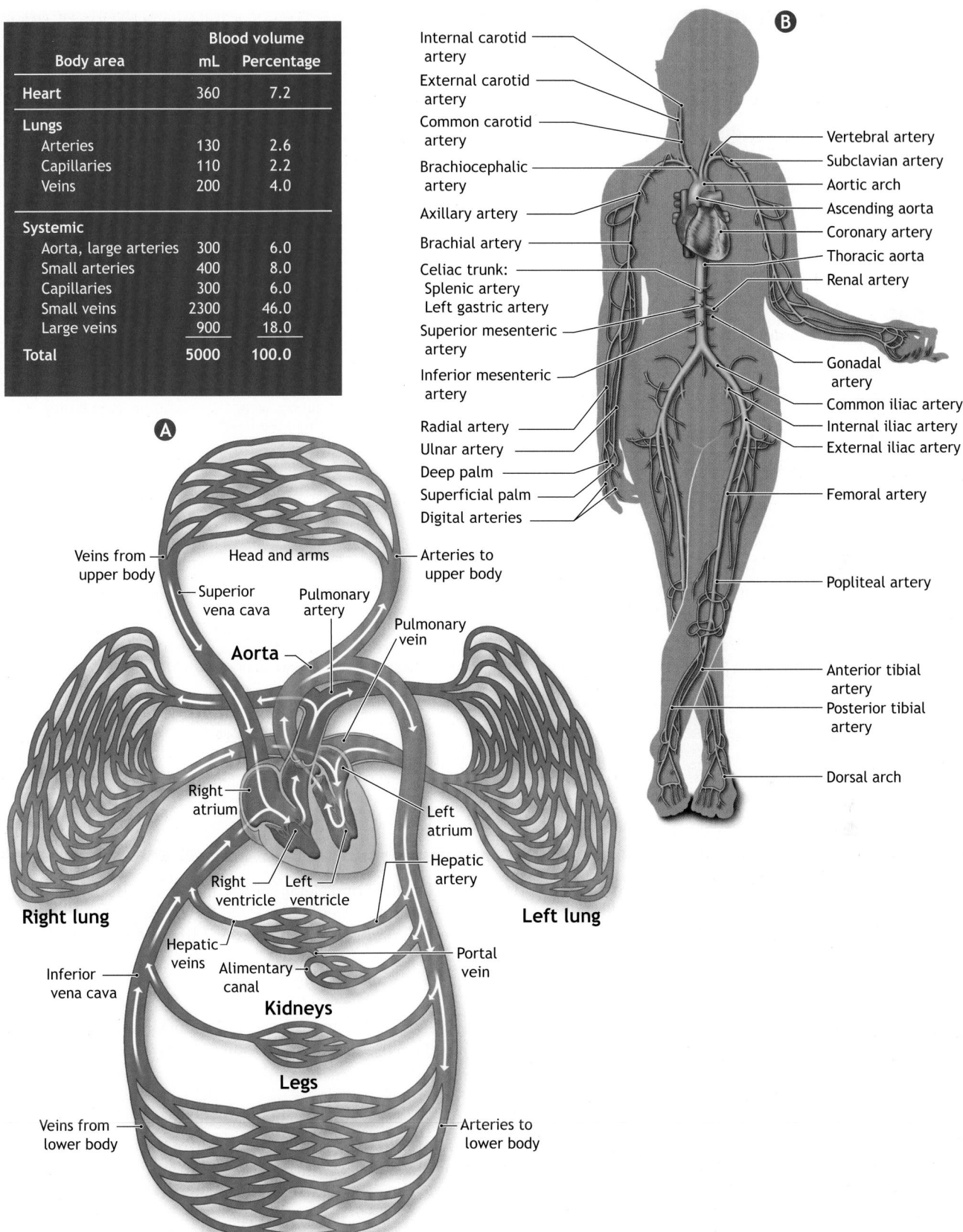

FIGURE 15.1 • (A) Schematic view of the cardiovascular system indicating the heart and pulmonary and systemic vascular circuits. *Red shading* depicts oxygen-rich arterial blood; *blue shading* denotes deoxygenated venous blood. The situation reverses in the pulmonary circuit; oxygenated blood returns to the heart in the right and left pulmonary veins. **(B)** Main arteries that compose the adult systemic circulation. The *inset table* at top left shows the absolute and percentage distribution of total blood volume in the pulmonary and systemic vascular circuits of a typical adult male at rest.

Muscle type	Location	Appearance	Type of activity	Stimulation
Skeletal ("striated" or "voluntary") muscle 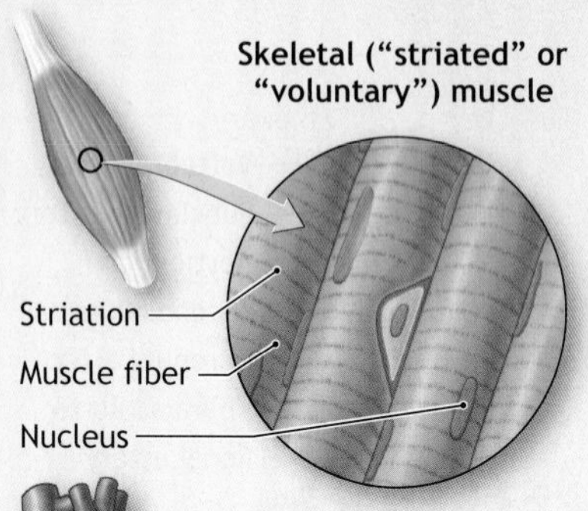 Striation Muscle fiber Nucleus	Named muscle (e.g., biceps of the arm) attached to the skeleton and fascia of limbs, body wall, and head/neck	Large, long, unbranched, cylindrical fibers with transverse striations (stripes) arranged in parallel bundles; multiple, peripherally located nuclei	Strong, quick intermittent (phasic) contraction above a baseline tonus; acts primarily to produce movement or resist gravity	Voluntary (or reflexive) by the somatic nervous system
Cardiac muscle 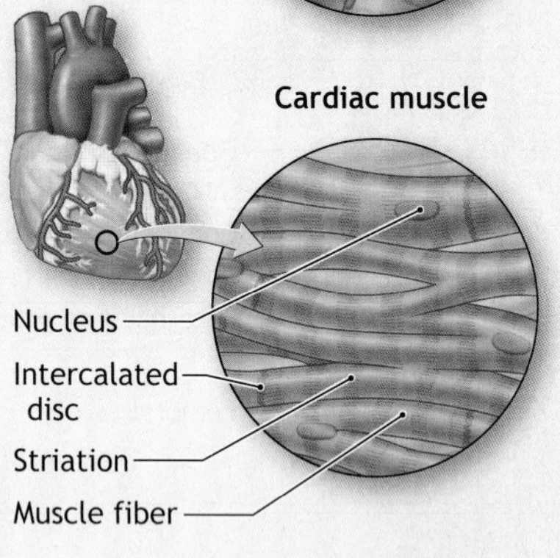 Nucleus Intercalated disc Striation Muscle fiber	Muscle of heart (myocardium) and adjacent portions of the great vessels (aorta, vena cava)	Branching and anastomosing shorter fibers with transverse striations (stripes) running parallel and connected end-to-end by complex junctions (intercalated discs); single, central nucleus	Strong, quick continuous rhythmic contraction; pumps blood from the heart	Involuntary; intrinsically (myogenically) stimulated and propagated; rate and strength of contraction modified by the autonomic nervous system
Smooth ("unstriated" or "involuntary") muscle 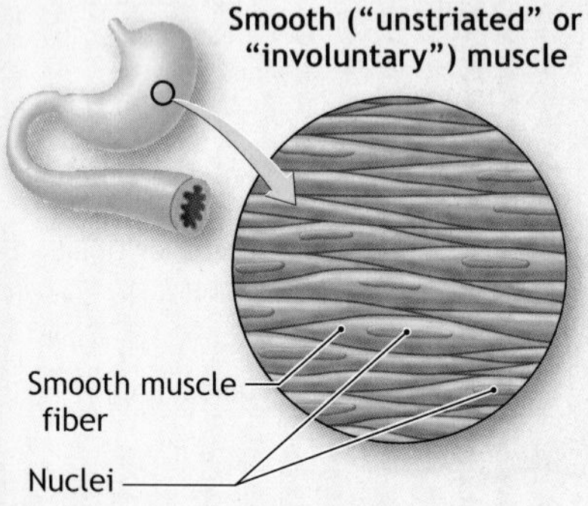 Smooth muscle fiber Nuclei	Walls of hollow viscera and blood vessels, iris, and ciliary body of eye; attached to hair follicles (arrector pili muscle of hair)	Single or agglomerated small, spindle-shaped fibers without striations; single, central nucleus	Weak, slow, rhythmic, or sustained tonic contraction; acts mainly to propel substances (peristalsis) and restrict flow (vasoconstriction and sphincteric activity)	Involuntary by autonomic nervous system

FIGURE 15.2 • Functional and structural characteristics and mode of activation of skeletal, cardiac, and smooth muscle. (Portions adapted with permission from Moore KL, Dalley AF, Agur AMR. *Clinically Oriented Anatomy*. 7th Ed. Baltimore: Wolters Kluwer Health, 2013 as adapted with permission from Agur, AMR, Dalley, AF. *Grant's Atlas of Anatomy*. 13th Ed. Baltimore: Wolters Kluwer Health, 2013.)

The Arterial System

The arteries compose the high-pressure tubing that propels oxygen-rich blood to the tissues. **FIGURE 15.4** illustrates that arteries shown on the right consist of layers of connective tissue and smooth muscle. No gaseous exchange takes place between arterial blood and surrounding tissues because of the thickness of these vessels. Blood pumped from the left ventricle into the highly muscular yet elastic **aorta** distributes in the body through an intricate and highly efficient network of arteries and smaller arterial branches called **arterioles**. The walls of arterioles contain circular layers of smooth muscle that either constrict or relax to regulate blood flow to the periphery. These "resistance vessels" dramatically alter their internal diameter to rapidly adjust blood flow through the vascular circuit. This redistribution function takes on added importance during physical activity because blood rapidly diverts to active muscles from areas that temporarily compromise their blood supply such as the splanchnic (visceral) and cutaneous tissues.[50,58] The inset table in Figure 15.4 lists average values for the diameter of blood vessels and corresponding velocities of blood flowing through them. Note that blood flowing through capillaries moves slowest (0.05-0.1 cm · s^{-1}) compared to any of the main arteries or veins.

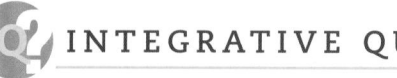 INTEGRATIVE QUESTION

What advantage does a "closed" circulatory system provide to the physically active individual?

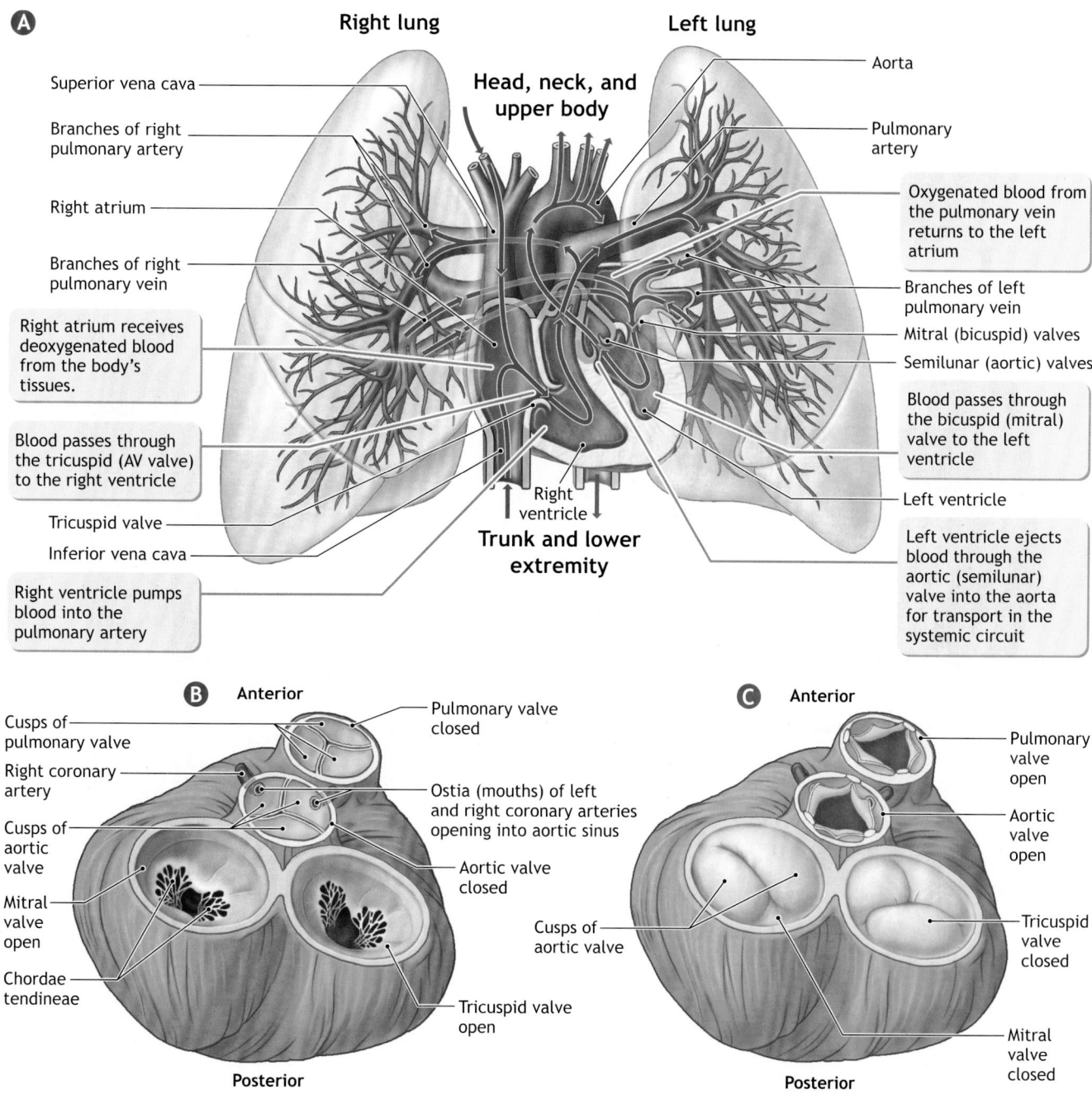

A

Right lung

Left lung

Head, neck, and upper body

Superior vena cava

Aorta

Branches of right pulmonary artery

Pulmonary artery

Right atrium

Oxygenated blood from the pulmonary vein returns to the left atrium

Branches of right pulmonary vein

Branches of left pulmonary vein

Right atrium receives deoxygenated blood from the body's tissues.

Mitral (bicuspid) valves

Semilunar (aortic) valves

Blood passes through the bicuspid (mitral) valve to the left ventricle

Blood passes through the tricuspid (AV valve) to the right ventricle

Left ventricle

Tricuspid valve

Right ventricle

Left ventricle ejects blood through the aortic (semilunar) valve into the aorta for transport in the systemic circuit

Inferior vena cava

Trunk and lower extremity

Right ventricle pumps blood into the pulmonary artery

B Anterior

Cusps of pulmonary valve

Pulmonary valve closed

Right coronary artery

Ostia (mouths) of left and right coronary arteries opening into aortic sinus

Cusps of aortic valve

Aortic valve closed

Mitral valve open

Chordae tendineae

Tricuspid valve open

Posterior

Diastole

C Anterior

Pulmonary valve open

Aortic valve open

Cusps of aortic valve

Tricuspid valve closed

Mitral valve closed

Posterior

Systole

FIGURE 15.3 • **(A)** The heart, its great vessels, and one-way blood flow through valves during the cardiac cycle, as indicated by the *arrows*. **(B)** In diastole, the aortic and pulmonary valves snap closed; shortly thereafter, the mitral and tricuspid valves open and blood flows into the ventricular cavities. **(C)** Initiation of systole and ventricular emptying closes the tricuspid and mitral valves, while the aortic and pulmonary valves open. When viewing the structural details of the figure, note that the right lung is shown on the left side and vice versa for the left lung. This is because when locating the structures, it's always done from the point of view of the person. Thus, the right lung appears on the left and the left lung on the right because this corresponds to the anatomical position of the person standing and facing forward. (Portions adapted with permission from Moore KL, Dalley AF, Agur AMR. *Clinically Oriented Anatomy*, 7th Ed., as used with permission from Agur AMR, Dalley AF. *Grant's Atlas of Anatomy*. 13th Ed. Baltimore: Wolters Kluwer Health, 2013.)

Blood Pressure

Each contraction of the left ventricle forces blood to surge through the aorta. Peripheral vessels do not permit blood to "run off" into the arterial system as rapidly as it ejects from the heart. Thus, the distensible aorta "stores" a portion of blood, which creates pressure within the entire arterial system, causing a pressure wave to travel down the aorta to remote branches of the arterial tree. The characteristic "pulse" in superficial arteries occurs from the stretch and subsequent recoil of the arteries during a cardiac cycle. In healthy individuals, identical values occur for pulse rate and heart rate. In essence, arteries

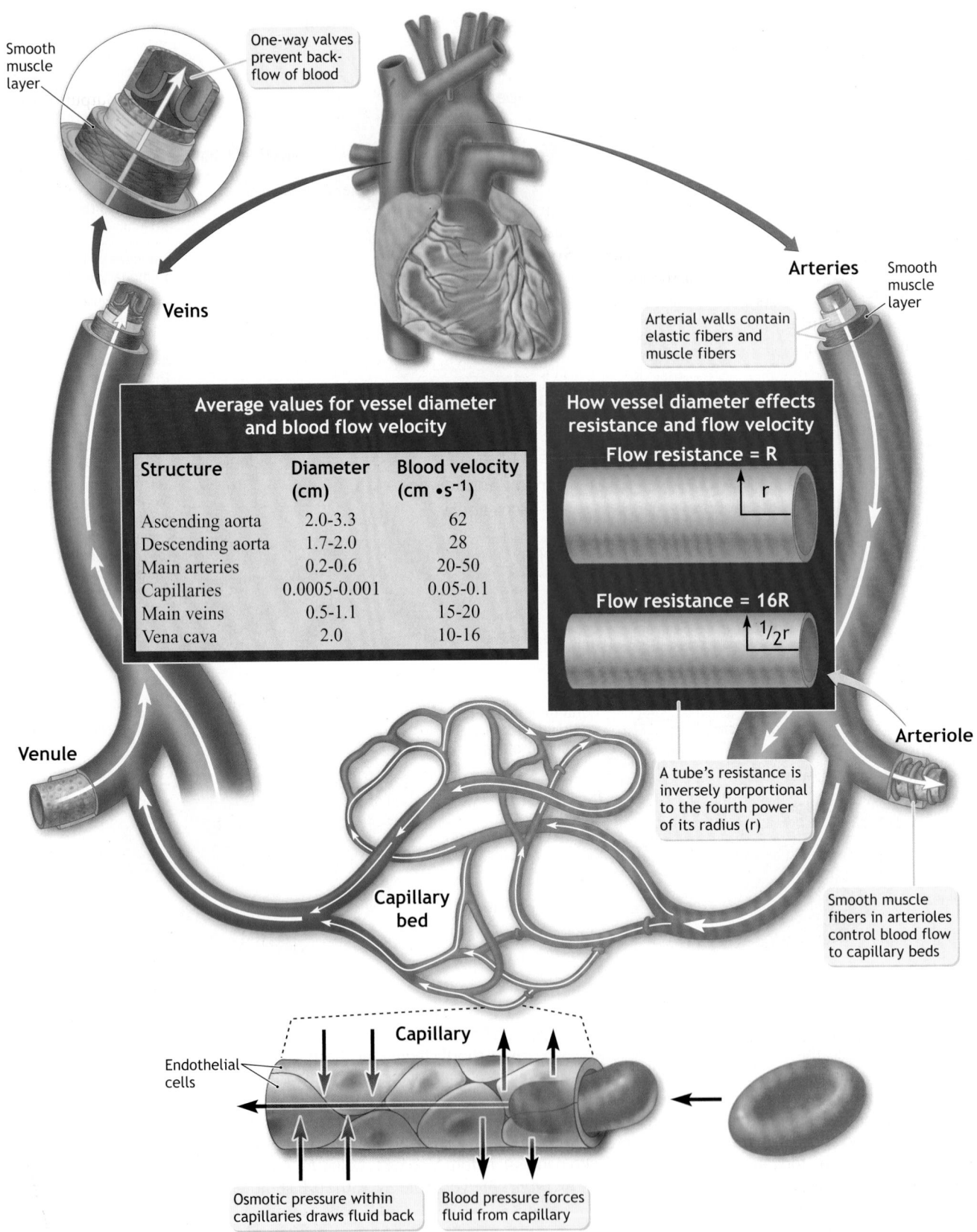

Smooth muscle layer

One-way valves prevent back-flow of blood

Veins

Arteries

Smooth muscle layer

Arterial walls contain elastic fibers and muscle fibers

Average values for vessel diameter and blood flow velocity

Structure	Diameter (cm)	Blood velocity (cm •s^{-1})
Ascending aorta	2.0-3.3	62
Descending aorta	1.7-2.0	28
Main arteries	0.2-0.6	20-50
Capillaries	0.0005-0.001	0.05-0.1
Main veins	0.5-1.1	15-20
Vena cava	2.0	10-16

How vessel diameter effects resistance and flow velocity

Flow resistance = R

r

Flow resistance = 16R

$^1/_2$r

Venule

A tube's resistance is inversely porportional to the fourth power of its radius (r)

Arteriole

Smooth muscle fibers in arterioles control blood flow to capillary beds

Capillary bed

Capillary

Endothelial cells

Osmotic pressure within capillaries draws fluid back

Blood pressure forces fluid from capillary

FIGURE 15.4 • The structure of the walls of the blood vessels. A single layer of endothelial cells lines each vessel. Fibrous tissue [wrap]ped in several layers of smooth muscle surrounds the arterial walls. A single layer of muscle cells sheaths the arterioles; [arte]ries consist of only one layer of rolled-up endothelial cells, often less than 1 micron (µm) thick, with a flat surface area of [about 1]200 µm². In the venule, fibrous tissue encases the endothelial cells; veins also possess a layer of smooth muscle. The *inset* [disp]lays the average values for vessel diameter and corresponding values for blood flow velocity. A vessel's resistance (R) to [bloo]ds on its radius. Decreasing vessel radius (r) by one-half increases resistance 16-fold.

pressure reflects the combined effects of arterial blood flow each minute (i.e., cardiac output) and resistance to that flow in the peripheral vasculature. The relationship can be expressed as:

Blood pressure = Cardiac output × Total peripheral resistance

Systolic Blood Pressure. At rest in normotensive individuals, the highest pressure generated by the heart averages 120 mm Hg during left ventricular contraction (termed *systole*). The brachial artery at the level of the right atrium usually serves as the point of reference for this measurement. **Systolic blood pressure** provides an estimate of the work of the heart and the force that blood exerts against the arterial walls during ventricular systole. During the heart's relaxation phase when aortic valves close, the natural elastic recoil of the arterial system maintains a continuous head of pressure. This provides a steady blood flow into the periphery until the next surge of blood.

Diastolic Blood Pressure. During the cardiac cycle's relaxation phase (termed *diastole*), arterial blood pressure decreases to 60 to 80 mm Hg. **Diastolic blood pressure** indicates peripheral resistance or the ease with which blood flows from the arterioles into the capillaries. With high peripheral resistance, pressure within the arteries after systole does not rapidly dissipate. Instead, it remains elevated for a larger portion of the cardiac cycle. "In a Practical Sense" illustrates the measurement of systolic and diastolic blood pressure by the common **auscultation method**.

Mean Arterial Pressure. Systolic blood pressure typically averages 120 mm Hg, and the diastolic pressure equals 80 mm Hg in young, healthy adults at rest. The average or **mean arterial pressure** (**MAP**) is slightly lower than the arithmetic average of systolic and diastolic pressures because the heart remains in diastole longer than in systole. MAP averages 93 mm Hg at rest; this represents the average force exerted by the blood against the arterial walls during a cardiac cycle. MAP computes as:

MAP = Diastolic BP + [0.333 (Systolic − Diastolic BP)]

For a person with a diastolic blood pressure of 89 mm Hg and a systolic pressure of 127 mm Hg, MAP equals 89 + [0.333 (127 − 89)] or 102 mm Hg.

Mean Arterial Pressure: Pulmonary Versus Systemic Circulations

Significant differences exist in blood pressure and vascular resistance in blood vessels of the lungs compared to vessels in the systemic circulation. For example, the mean arterial blood pressure in the pulmonary artery averages about 15 mm Hg while the pressure in the large systemic arteries averages about 95 mm Hg. With equivalent blood flow in both circulations, vascular resistance is lower in the pulmonary circuit. This accounts for the difference in blood vessel structure. Pulmonary arterial vessels are relatively thin walled with little smooth muscle compared to their thicker, more muscular systemic counterparts.

Cardiac Output and Total Peripheral Resistance. The hemodynamic equation that relates blood pressure to cardiac output and total peripheral resistance rearranges as follows to illustrate factors that determine either cardiac output or total peripheral resistance:

Cardiac output = MAP ÷ Total peripheral resistance

Total peripheral resistance = MAP ÷ Cardiac output

MAP (computed from systolic and diastolic blood pressures) and cardiac output estimate the change in total resistance to blood flow in the transition from rest to movement. Suppose systolic blood pressure at rest equals 120 mm Hg, diastolic pressure equals 80 mm Hg (MAP = 93.3 mm Hg), and cardiac output averages 5.0 L·min^{-1}. Substituting these values in the formula for total peripheral resistance yields 18.7 mm Hg per liter of blood flow (93.3 mm Hg ÷ 5.0 L·min^{-1}). Resistance to peripheral blood flow *decreases* dramatically during strenuous activity, when systolic pressure increases considerably more than diastolic pressure and cardiac output increases six or seven times the resting value in an elite endurance athlete. For example, if exercise cardiac output equals 35.0 L·min^{-1} and MAP equals 130 mm Hg (systolic = 210 mm Hg; diastolic = 90 mm Hg), then resistance to blood flow in the systemic circulation averages 3.71 mm Hg per liter per minute, or five times *less* than the resting value.

Capillaries

The arterioles branch and form smaller and less muscular vessels 10 to 20 microns (μm) in diameter called **metarterioles**. These vessels end in a meshwork of microscopically small blood vessels called **capillaries**, which generally contain 6% of the total blood volume. In skeletal muscle, with its widely varying oxygen requirements, each metarteriole interfaces with 8 to 10 capillaries. The average capillary diameter is 7 to 10 μm (approximately 1/100th of a mm). Figure 15.4 illustrates that the capillary wall usually consists of a single layer of rolled-up endothelial cells. Some capillaries are so narrow (about 3–4 μm in diameter) that only one blood cell at a time can squeeze through. In many instances, the extensive proliferation of capillaries causes their walls to abut the membranes of the surrounding cells. Capillary density varies throughout the body, depending on a particular tissue's location and function. Capillary density of human skeletal muscle averages between 2000 and 3000 capillaries per square millimeter of tissue. The density of capillaries is considerably greater in heart muscle where no cell lies farther than 0.008 mm from its nearest capillary.

Blood Flow in Capillaries

The **precapillary sphincter**, a ring of smooth muscle that encircles the vessel at its origin, controls capillary diameter. Sphincter constriction and relaxation provide an important local means of blood flow regulation within a specific tissue to meet metabolic requirements. Chapter 16 discusses specific factors for autoregulation of local blood supply.

IN A PRACTICAL SENSE

Blood Pressure Measurement, Classifications, and Recommended Follow-Up

Blood pressure represents the force exerted by blood against the arterial walls during a cardiac cycle. Systolic blood pressure, the higher of the two pressure measurements, occurs during ventricular contraction (systole) as the heart propels 70 to 100 mL of blood into the aorta. Following systole, the ventricles relax (diastole), the arteries recoil, and arterial pressure continually declines as blood flows into the periphery and the heart refills with blood. The lowest pressure attained during ventricular relaxation represents diastolic blood pressure. **Pulse pressure** refers to the difference between systolic and diastolic pressures. Systolic blood pressure in a typical adult varies between 110 and 140 mm Hg; diastolic pressure varies between 60 and 90 mm Hg, with slightly lower values among females. Elevated systolic or diastolic blood pressure (termed *hypertension*) refers to a resting systolic blood pressure above 140 mm Hg and diastolic pressure exceeding 90 mm Hg. Blood pressure readings that fall in the prehypertension range should be treated with lifestyle changes that include reducing excess weight, exercising more, quitting smoking, cutting back on salt, having no more than one or two alcoholic drinks a day, and eating more fruits, vegetables, and low-fat dairy products.

BLOOD PREASURE MEASUREMENT PROCEDURES

Blood pressure, measured indirectly by auscultation (listening to sounds; described in 1902 by Russian vascular surgeon Nikolai S. Korotkoff, 1874–1920; see, for example, http://circ.ahajournals.org/content/94/2/116.full), uses a stethoscope and sphygmomanometer consisting of a blood pressure cuff and either an aneroid or mercury column pressure gauge. A typical measurement sequence occurs as follows:

1. Subject, seated in a quiet room, exposes upper right arm.
2. Locate the brachial artery at the inner side of the upper arm, approximately 1 inch above the bend in the elbow.
3. Take the free end of the cuff, gently slide it through the metal loop (or wrap over exposed Velcro), and flap it back over so the cuff wraps around the upper arm at heart level. Align the arrows on the cuff with the brachial artery. Secure the Velcro parts of the cuff. To obtain accurate readings, fit the sphygmomanometer cuff snugly (but not tightly). Use appropriate-sized cuffs for children and obese persons.
4. Place the stethoscope bell below the antecubital space over the brachial artery.
5. The connecting tube from the sphygmomanometer bulb and gauge should exit the cuff toward the arm.
6. Before inflating the cuff, ensure that the air-release switch remains closed (turn the knob clockwise).
7. Inflate the cuff with quick, even pumps to 180 to 200 mm Hg.

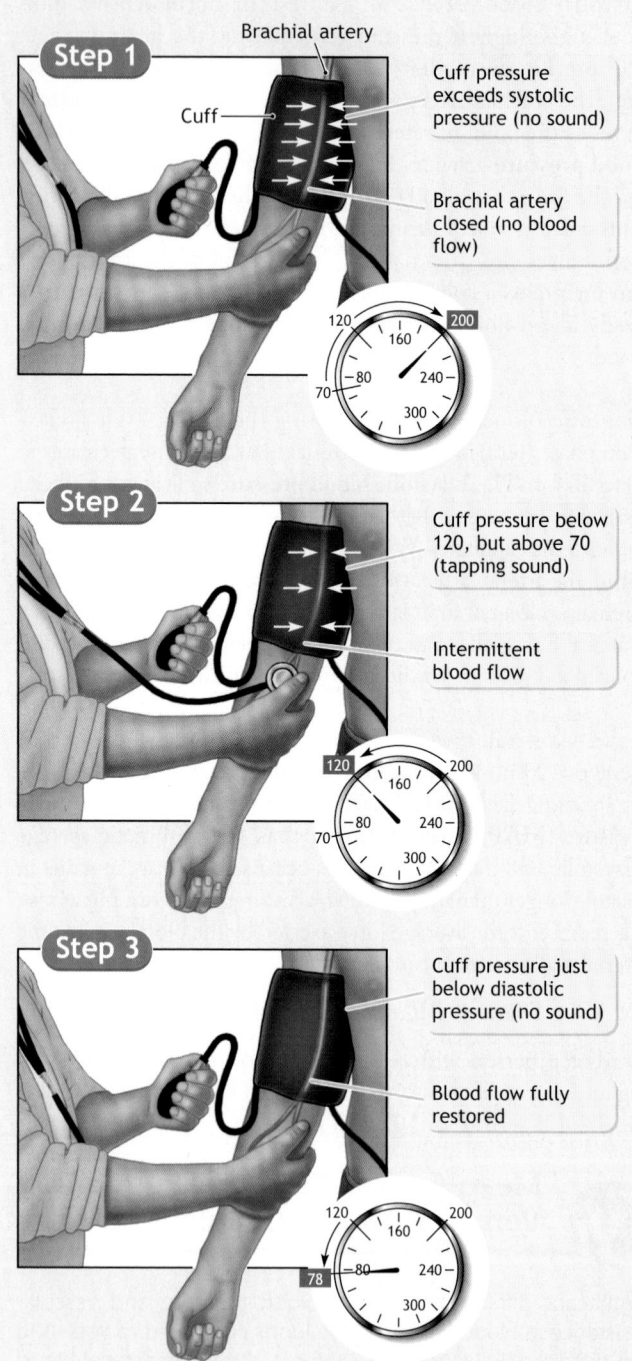

Step 1
Brachial artery
Cuff
- Cuff pressure exceeds systolic pressure (no sound)
- Brachial artery closed (no blood flow)

Step 2
- Cuff pressure below 120, but above 70 (tapping sound)
- Intermittent blood flow

Step 3
- Cuff pressure just below diastolic pressure (no sound)
- Blood flow fully restored

8. Gradually release cuff pressure (about 3–5 mm per s) by slowly opening the air-release knob (counterclockwise turn) and note the pressure when you hear the first sound. Turbulence from the sudden rush of blood produces the sound as the formerly closed artery briefly opens during the highest pressure in the cardiac cycle. The first appearance of sound represents systolic blood pressure.

IN A PRACTICAL SENSE *(continued)*

Classification and Recommended Follow-Up of Initial Blood Pressure Screening in Adults[a]

Systolic (mm Hg)	Diastolic (mm Hg)	Category	Follow-up
<120	<80	Optimal	—
<130	<85	Normal	Recheck in 2 y
130–139	85–89	High–normal	Recheck in 1 y
140–159	90–99	Stage 1 hypertension	Confirm within 2 months
160–179	100–109	Moderate (Stage 2) hypertension	Begin treatment within 1 month if blood pressure is consistently high
180–209	110–119	Severe (Stage 3) hypertension	Begin treatment within 1 week
≥210	≥120	Very severe (Stage 4) hypertension	Treat immediately

[a]Not taking antihypertensive drugs and not acutely ill. When systolic and diastolic blood pressure categories vary, the higher reading determines the blood pressure classification. For example, a reading of 152/82 mm Hg is classified as stage 1 hypertension.

Source: National Institutes of Health. The sixth report of the Joint National Committee on Detection, Evaluation, and Treatment of High Blood Pressure. NIH Pub. No. 98-4080, 1997.

9. Continue to reduce cuff pressure, noting when the sound muffles (fourth phase diastolic pressure) and when the sound disappears (fifth phase diastolic pressure). Clinicians usually record the fifth phase as diastolic blood pressure.

10. If the measured pressure exceeds 140/90 mm Hg, allow a 10-min period of quiet rest and repeat the procedure one or two more times and use the average of all measurements to represent the "true" blood pressure value.

See the following URL for a full explanation: http://www. nhlbi.nih. gov/guidelines/hypertension/express.pdf

 See the animation "Measuring Blood Pressure" on http://thePoint.lww.com/mkk8e for a demonstration of this process.

Classification of Blood Pressure (BP) for Adults

Classification	Systolic BP (mm Hg)	Diastolic BP (mm Hg)
Normal	<120	and <80
Prehypertension	120–139	or 80–89
Stage 1 Hypertension	140–159	or 90–99
Stage 2 Hypertension	≥160	or ≥100

Source: National Institutes of Health. The Seventh Report of the Joint National Committee on Prevention, Detection, Evaluation, and Treatment of High Blood Pressure. NIH Pub. No. 03-5233, 2003.

Figure 15.5 depicts a generalized view of the dynamics of capillary blood flow within muscle during rest (A) and physical activity (B). Fewer capillaries function at rest than are available. In this example for the gastrocnemius muscle at rest, blood flow each minute averages 5 mL for every 100 g of muscle tissue. For a muscle that weighs 600 g, approximately 30 mL of blood flows through it each minute. During activity, blood flow increases rapidly as previously "unused" capillaries open. Two factors trigger the relaxation of precapillary sphincters to open more capillaries:

1. Driving force of increased local blood pressure plus intrinsic neural control
2. Local metabolites produced in physical activity

Blood flow in active muscle increases almost linearly with exercise intensity and reaches peak values at maximal exertion. This occurs as a result of the combined effects of a small increase in perfusion pressure and with massive vasodilatation.[6] During strenuous activity, sustained local blood flow increases 15 to 20 times the resting value. For the gastrocnemius muscle, blood flow averages about 80 mL per 100 g of tissue per minute.

Branching of the capillary microcirculation increases its cross-sectional area to about 800 times the 1-inch diameter aorta. Blood flow velocity relates inversely to the vasculature's cross section.

$$\text{Velocity, } cm \cdot s^{-1} = \text{Volume of flow, } cm^3 \cdot s^{-1} \div \text{Cross-sectional area, } cm^2$$

Thus, velocity progressively decreases as blood moves toward and enters the capillaries. It takes approximately 1.5 s for a blood cell to pass through an average-sized capillary. The total surface area of the capillary walls exceeds by 100 times the external body surface of the average adult. *A huge surface area with a slow rate of blood flow of approximately 0.5 to 1.0 mm · s⁻¹ at rest provides a highly effective means of exchange between the blood and neighboring tissues.*

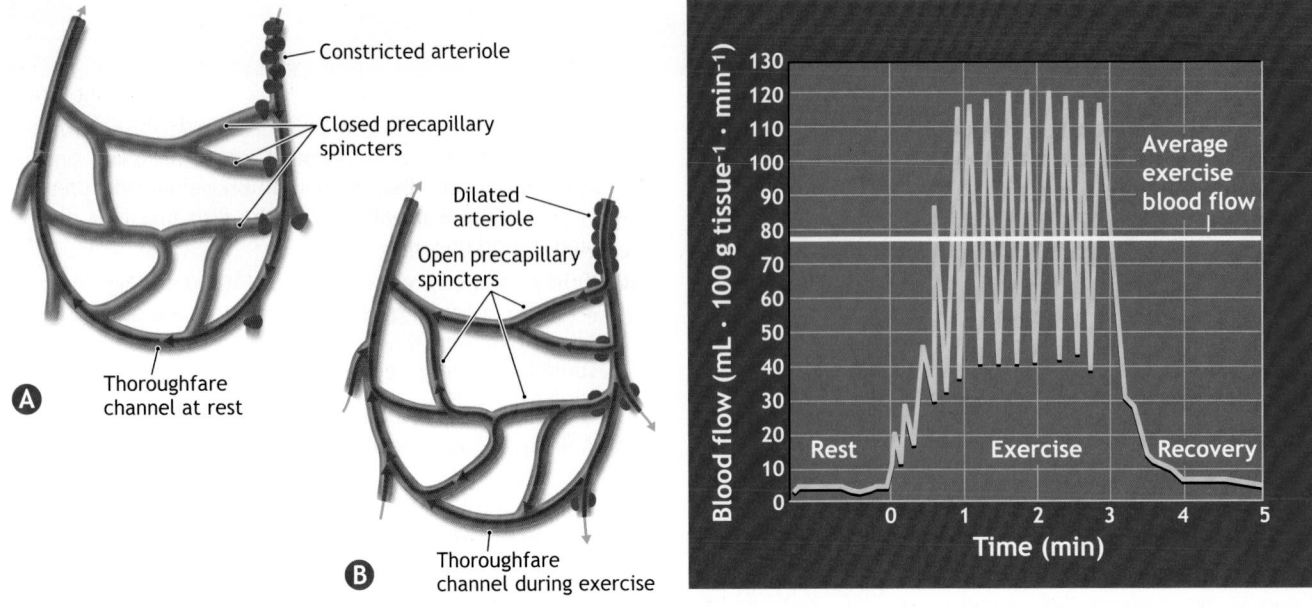

FIGURE 15.5 • Capillary blood flow during rest **(A)** and exercise **(B)**. Capillary diameter, red blood cell size, and blood viscosity all affect capillary blood flow. The position of the *dark red knobs* indicate closing or opening dormant capillaries. The right figure shows the pulsatile pattern of blood flow at rest, during exercise, and when exercise stops. Dilation of the active muscle's arterioles provides the major mechanism for augmenting local blood flow.

The Venous System

The continuity of the vascular system progresses as the capillaries feed deoxygenated blood at almost a trickle into the small veins or **venules** with which they merge. Blood flow velocity then increases because the cross-sectional area of the venous system is smaller than for capillaries. The smaller veins in the lower portion of the body eventually empty into the **inferior vena cava**, the body's largest vein (**Fig. 15.6**). This large vessel returns blood to the right atrium from the abdomen, pelvis, and lower extremities. Venous blood from tributary vessels in the head, neck, shoulder regions, thorax, and part of the abdominal wall flows into the 7-cm–long **superior vena cava** to join the inferior vena cava at heart level. The mixture of blood that drains the upper and lower body, called **mixed-venous blood**, then enters the right atrium. From there it flows forcefully downward through the tricuspid valve into the right ventricle for pumping through the pulmonary artery to the lungs. Gas exchange takes place in the alveolar–capillary network of the lungs; oxygenated blood then returns in the pulmonary veins to the left side of the heart to once again begin passage throughout the body.

Figure 15.7 shows how blood pressure and blood flow vary considerably in the systemic circulation. During the **cardiac cycle** (recall that cardiac activity is divided into two phases—systole and diastole), resting blood pressure fluctuates between 120 (systolic) and 80 (diastolic) mm Hg in the aorta and large arteries. The pressure then declines in direct proportion to the resistance encountered in the vascular circuit. Blood at the arteriole end of the capillaries, for example, exerts an average pressure of only 30 mm Hg. As blood enters the venules, it loses nearly all its impetus for forward movement. The pressure decreases to approximately 0 mm Hg by the time blood reaches the heart's right atrium. The venous system operates under relatively low pressure, so veins need much thinner and less muscular walls than the thicker-walled and less distensible arteries (see Fig. 15.4).

Venous Return

The low pressure of blood in the venous system poses a special problem that a unique structural characteristic of veins partly solves. **Figure 15.8** shows that thin, membranous, flap-like **valves** spaced at short intervals within veins allow blood to flow in only one direction toward the heart. This now seems logical, but in 1759 when William Harvey in England first proposed the idea to his colleagues during a medical lecture and demonstration (see, for example, www.nndb.com/people/269/000085014/), he was vilified for daring to contradict almost 2000 years of prior medical dogma since physician Galen (AD 129–c. 200/c. 216), one of the earliest medical practitioners, posited that blood simply "sloshed" back and forth through the heart and blood vessels (see section titled William Harvey in Introduction chapter).

The low pressure in the venous circuit means that the smallest muscular contractions, or even minor pressure changes within the thoracic cavity with breathing (**respiratory pump**), readily compress the veins.[22] The alternate compression and relaxation of veins, including the one-way action of their valves, provides a "milking" or wringing action that propels blood back to the heart. Without valves, blood would stagnate as it sometimes does in veins of the extremities. People would faint every time they stood up because of reduced venous return and cerebral blood flow.

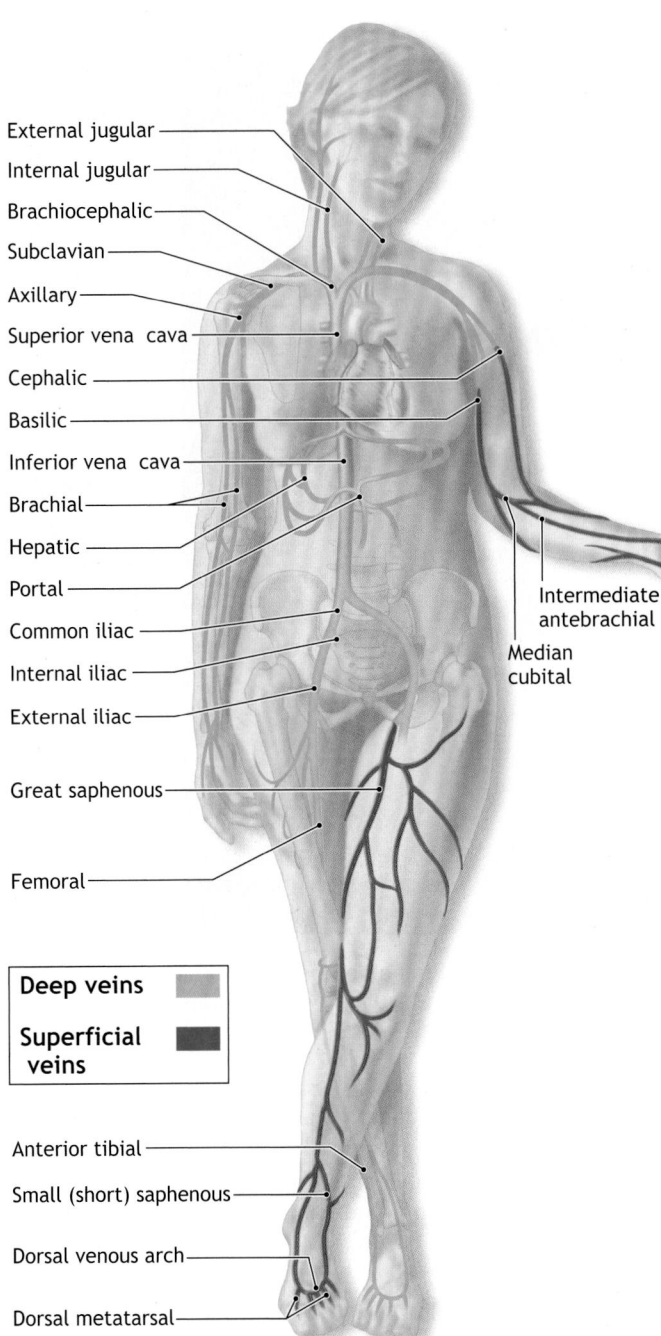

External jugular
Internal jugular
Brachiocephalic
Subclavian
Axillary
Superior vena cava
Cephalic
Basilic
Inferior vena cava
Brachial
Hepatic
Portal
Common iliac
Internal iliac
External iliac
Great saphenous
Femoral

Intermediate antebrachial
Median cubital

Deep veins
Superficial veins

Anterior tibial
Small (short) saphenous
Dorsal venous arch
Dorsal metatarsal

FIGURE 15.6 • Distribution of the superficial (*dark blue*) and deep (*light blue*) veins.

 The Physiology of Crucifixion

In ancient Rome, suspending people from a patibulum (crossbar) with rope or with nails that punctured the ends of the extremities to keep the body on the stipes (upright post), was the ultimate punishment. Death occurred mainly from blood pooling in the lower extremities, called hypovolemic shock, with accompanying pulmonary edema that resulted in asphyxia, not by excruciating physical torture as often assumed.[12]

A Question of an Active Vasculature

Contemporary physiologists have debated the role of the venous system as an active vasculature for mobilizing blood volume. At rest, the systemic venous vessels normally contain 65% of the total blood volume; the veins thus represent **capacitance vessels** that serve as blood reservoirs. This has led to speculation about the role of veins as an **active blood reservoir** to either retard or facilitate blood delivery to the systemic circulation. Physiologists who take this position maintain that any increase in tension or tone of the vessels' smooth muscle layer alters the diameter of the venous tree. If true, this would initiate rapid redistribution of blood from peripheral veins toward the central blood volume that returns to the heart. In contrast, physiologists who oppose this position believe that only the veins in the splanchnic and cutaneous regions are innervated richly enough to contribute to blood mobilization. They posit that skeletal muscle veins do not receive neural input, and whatever brief venoconstriction occurs in other regions would do little to contribute to blood redistribution. Current opinion maintains that the major contribution to blood mobilization in physical activity occurs by active muscle pump action and the passive effect of arterial vasoconstriction, not visceral venoconstriction, which reduces downstream venous pressure.[48]

Varicose Veins

Sometimes the valves within a vein fail to maintain their one-way blood flow, a defective condition termed *varicose veins*. This condition usually occurs in the surface veins of the lower extremities. Consequently, blood gathers in them so they become excessively distended and painful, which impairs circulation from the affected area. In severe cases, the venous wall becomes inflamed and progressively deteriorates—a condition called *phlebitis*. This necessitates vessel removal either surgically or nonsurgically by injecting solutions that irritate the vessel's surface membranes (a process termed *sclerotherapy*). This procedure and laser ablation cause a portion of the vein to collapse, fuse, and eventually shrivel up, thereby rerouting blood to the deeper veins.

Individuals with varicose veins should avoid static, straining-type exercises that accompany resistance training. During sustained, nonrhythmic muscle actions, the muscle and ventilatory "pumps" contribute little to venous return. Increased intrathoracic and abdominal pressures (Valsalva maneuver) with straining also impede venous return. These factors act to pool blood in the veins of the lower body, which can aggravate an existing varicose vein condition. Exercise training does not prevent varicose veins; however, regular and rhythmic physical activity can minimize complications because repeated muscle actions continually propel blood toward the heart.

Venous Pooling

The rhythmic action of muscular activity and consequent compression of the vascular tree (i.e., the muscle pump) contribute so much to venous return that many people faint

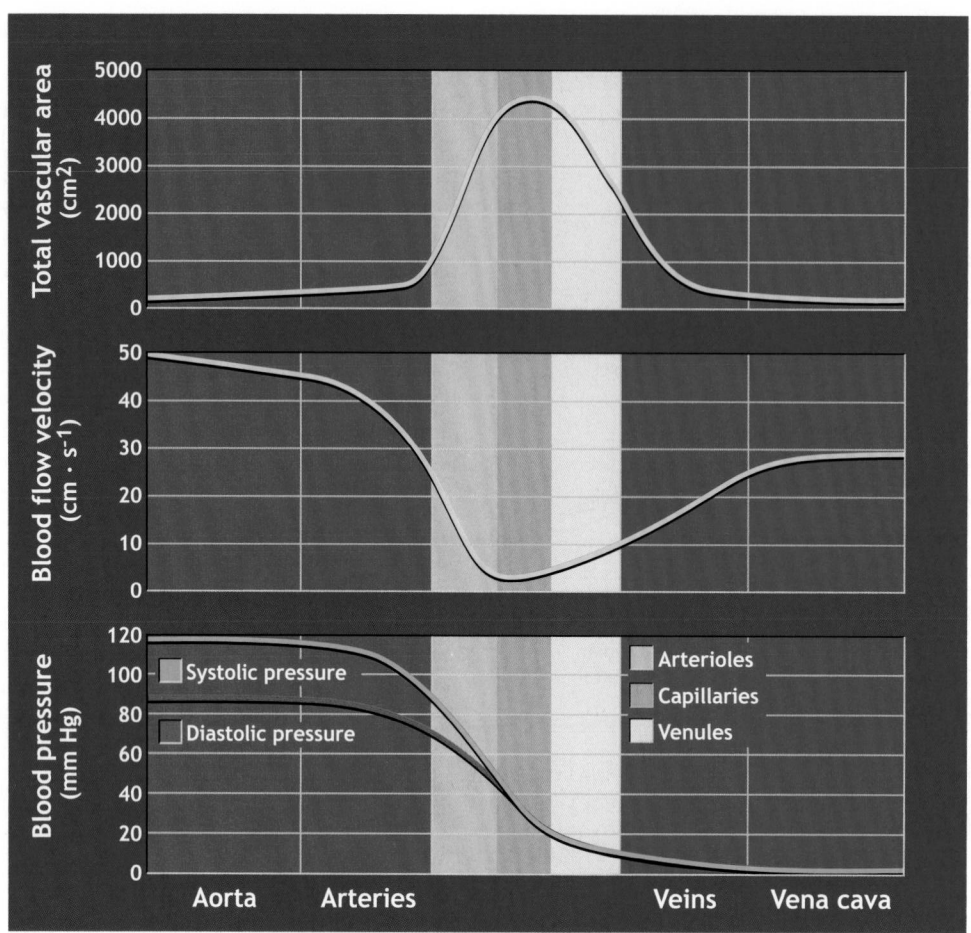

FIGURE 15.7 • Blood flow and blood pressure in the systemic circulation at rest. Note that blood pressure within each portion of the arterial system inversely relates to the total area (resistance) in that section of the vascular tree. For example, when total vascular area approaches 5000 cm², blood flow velocity is at its lowest level.

when forced to maintain an upright posture without movement. Examples include standing with minimal movement for long periods during any type of practice event, military or graduation ceremony, or on-the-job task, particularly in a hot, humid environment. The classic "tilt table" experiment demonstrates this point (www.mayoclinic.com/health/ **tilt-table-test**/MY01091; http://journals.lww.com/jnpt/ Pages/videogallery.aspx?videoId=48&autoPlay=true). A subject lies supine, secured on a table that pivots to different positions from the horizontal. Heart rate and blood pressure stabilize if the person remains horizontal. When the table tilts vertically, an uninterrupted column of blood exists from the heart to toes. This creates a hydrostatic force of 80 to 100 mm Hg that causes blood to pool in the lower extremities. Fluid backs up in the capillary bed and seeps into the surrounding tissues, causing them to swell (**edema**). Reduced venous return reduces cardiac output and arterial blood pressure; simultaneously, heart rate accelerates and blood mobilizes from the splanchnic region by upstream vasoconstriction (causing passive mobilization from downstream veins). Some active venoconstriction to counter the effects of venous pooling also may occur. Forcing the person to maintain the upright position induces fainting from insufficient cerebral blood supply (i.e., reduced cardiac output). Tilting the

person either horizontally or head down immediately restores circulation and consciousness. In Chapter 27, we discuss a variation of the tilt table experiment applied in microgravity research to induce symptoms and responses to weightlessness when subjects remain in a six-degree tilt-down position for weeks at a time.

The pressurized suits worn by test pilots of supersonic aircraft and special support stockings for individuals with varicose veins or poor venous return from swollen ankles reduce hydrostatic shifts of blood to the veins of the lower extremities in the upright position. A swimming pool provides a similar supportive effect in upright exercise because the water's external support facilitates venous return.

The Active Recovery "Cool-Down." The preceding discussion of venous pooling provides a sound rationale for continuing to walk or jog at a slow pace following strenuous activity. Moderate activity in recovery called "cooling down" facilitates blood flow through the vascular circuit, including myocardial vessels. In Chapter 7, we discuss how active recovery facilitates lactate removal from the blood. Continuation of mild physical activity in recovery also may blunt potential deleterious effects on cardiac function from the elevated catecholamines (epinephrine and norepinephrine) released during the activity.[9,10]

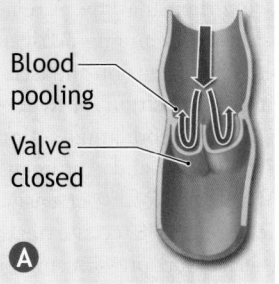
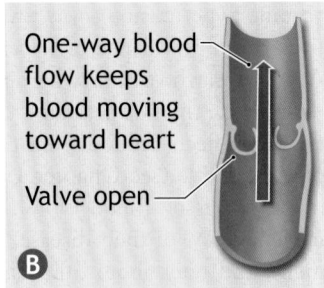

Blood pooling

Valve closed

A

One-way blood flow keeps blood moving toward heart

Valve open

B

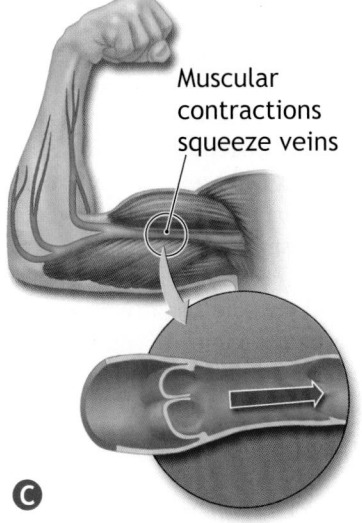
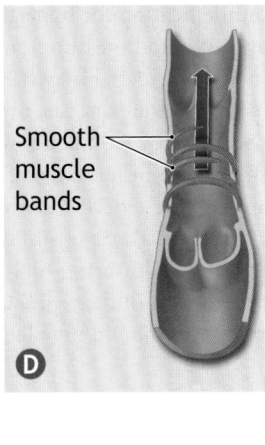

Muscular contractions squeeze veins

C

Smooth muscle bands

D

FIGURE 15.8 • The valves in veins **(A)** prevent the backflow of blood, but **(B)** do not hinder the normal one-way flow of blood. **(C)** Blood moves through veins by the action of nearby active muscle (muscle pump) or **(D)** contraction of smooth muscle bands within the veins.

 INTEGRATIVE QUESTION

The ancient Romans executed individuals by tying their arms and legs to a cross mounted in the vertical position. Discuss the physiologic responses that cause death under these circumstances.

HYPERTENSION

Systolic pressure at rest can exceed 300 mm Hg in individuals whose arteries exhibit the following characteristics:

1. "Hardening" with fatty materials deposited within their walls or because the vessel's connective tissue layer has thickened
2. Offer excessive resistance to peripheral blood flow because of neural hyperactivity or kidney malfunction

Diastolic pressure also can exceed 100 mm Hg under the above two conditions. Abnormally high blood pressure, termed *hypertension*, chronically strains the cardiovascular system and, left untreated, eventually damages arterial vessels and leads to arteriosclerosis, heart disease, stroke, and kidney failure.[29]

See the animation "Hypertension" on **http://thePoint.lww.com/mkk8e** for a demonstration of this process.

FIGURE 15.9 shows the percentages of the United States population with hypertension (systolic pressure >140 mm Hg; diastolic pressure >90 mm Hg) and its increased prevalence with age. The risk of becoming hypertensive increases with age such that the lifetime risk exceeds 80%. More than one-half of those 55 to 64 years old and three quarters of those 70 years and older are hypertensive.[8] An elevated systolic blood pressure provides a more reliable and accurate predictor of the risk associated with hypertension and need for treatment than diastolic blood pressure, particularly in middle age.[32]

A Prevalent Disorder

As America ages and continues to become more overweight and accumulate excess fat, the rate of hypertension increases to alarmingly high levels. The number of hypertensive Americans has increased to about 78 million from 50 million 15 years ago (see Fig. 15.9). Current estimates place nearly 35% of the adult U.S. population in the hypertensive category.[18] One of every three Americans and 1 billion people worldwide experience

 Lifestyle Choices That Lower Blood Pressure

Advice	Details	Drop in Systolic Blood Pressure
Lose excess weight	For every 20 lb reduced	5 to 20 mm Hg
Follow a DASH diet	Eat a lower-fat diet rich in vegetables, fruits, and low-fat dairy foods	8 to 14 mm Hg
Daily physical activity	Do 30 min a day of aerobic activity like brisk walking	4 to 9 mm Hg
Limit sodium	Eat no more than 2400 mg a day (1500 mg is better)	2 to 8 mm Hg
Limit alcohol	Consume no more than two drinks daily (men) and one drink daily (women) (*one drink = 12 oz. beer, 5 oz. wine, or 1.5 oz. 80-proof whiskey*)	2 to 4 mm Hg

Source: The Seventh Report of the Joint National Committee on Prevention, Detection, Evaluation, and Treatment of High Blood Pressure (**www.nhlbi.nih.gov/guidelines/hypertension**).

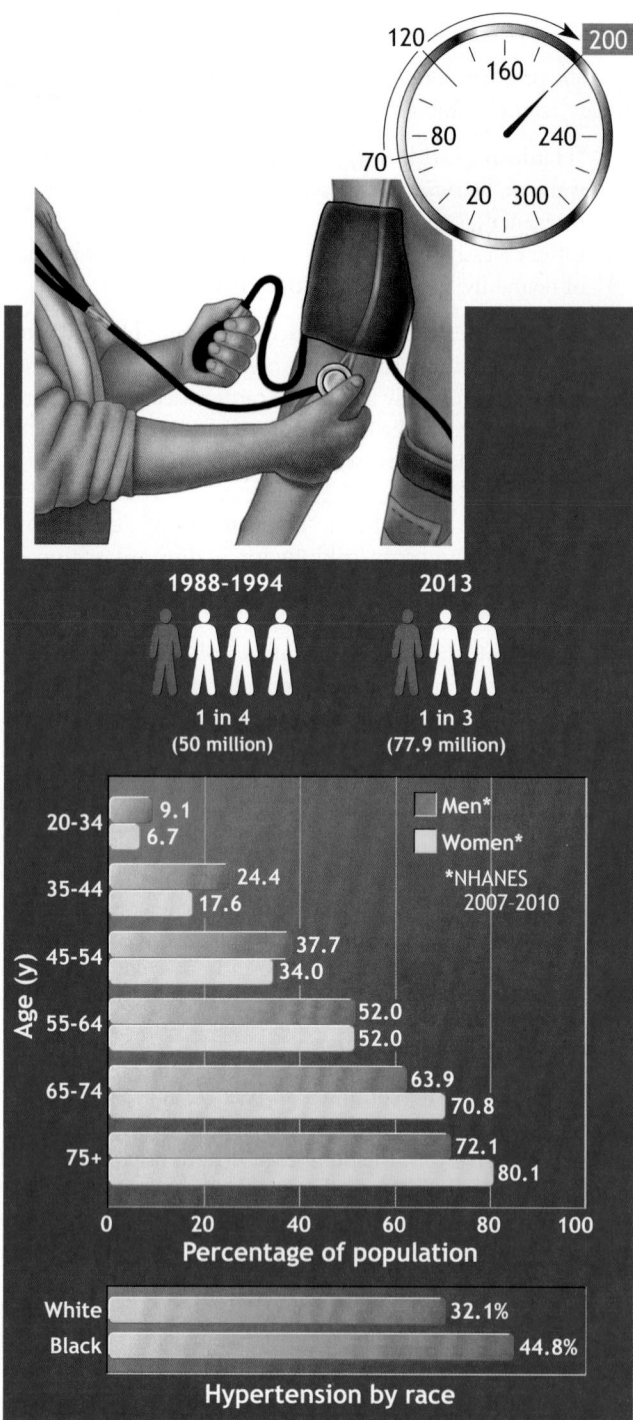

FIGURE 15.9 • Prevalence of hypertension in adults in the United States by age and gender. (Data from Centers for Disease Control and Prevention (CDC). National Center for Health Statistics (NCHS). National Health and Nutrition Examination Survey Data. Hyattsville, MD: U.S. Department of Health and Human Services, Centers for Disease Control and Prevention, [2007–2008][http://www.cdc.gov/nchs/nhanes/nhanes2007-2008/nhanes07_08.htm]; Go AS, Mozaffarian D, et al; on behalf of the American Heart Association Statistics Committee and Stroke Statistics Subcommittee. Heart disease and stroke statistics—2013 update: a report from the American Heart Association. *Circulation.* 2013; 127:143.)

chronic hypertension some time during their lifetime. A relatively high prevalence of hypertension exists among African Americans, who exhibit a higher risk of hypertension and ischemic stroke than Caucasians.[46] Their predisposition for hypertension reflects reduced sensitivity to the vasodilating action of nitric oxide (see Chapter 16, Nitric Oxide and Autoregulation of Tissue Blood Flow).[7,49] About 82% of hypertensive persons know of their disease, while about 75% receive treatment, and only about 50% have their blood pressure under control. Projections show that by 2030, prevalence of hypertension will increase 7.2% from 2013 estimates. An individual on medication for hypertension still classifies as hypertensive, even if blood pressure remains within the normal range.

Uncorrected hypertension often leads to congestive heart failure, kidney disease, myocardial infarction, or stroke. Blood pressure reduction, on the other hand, effectively prevents stroke and other vascular events including heart failure, even among the elderly.[4] Lowering systolic blood pressure 2 mm Hg reduces deaths from stroke by 6% and heart disease by 4%. In general, lowering high blood pressure also may reduce the progression of dementia and cognitive impairment, which are more common in people with hypertension.[44]

Effective Treatment Strategies

Preventing a chronic rise in blood pressure serves a crucial function. Even when elevated blood pressure normalizes through lifestyle changes or medication, the disease risk remains higher than if the person had never become hypertensive initially. Blood pressure should be checked periodically because hypertension often progresses unnoticed for years. Effective prevention strategies include lifestyle changes—regular physical activity consisting of daily exercise for at least 30 min at a moderate-to-vigorous level, modest weight loss for the overweight and obese, stress management, smoking cessation, reduced sodium and alcohol consumption, and adequate potassium, calcium, and magnesium intake.[1,2,27,41,57,60] Regular aerobic physical activity lowers systolic and diastolic blood pressure while more vigorous activity produces a greater lowering effect on diastolic pressure than more moderate physical activity.[52] Low cardiorespiratory fitness remains a significant predictor of hypertension risk, whereas the effect of body weight emerges only in the overweight range.[45]

In addition to lifestyle changes, hypertension treatment also combines medications that reduce either extracellular fluid volume or peripheral resistance to blood flow (Fig. 15.10). Lower odds of having to take medication for hypertension relate to both an increase in physical activity level and physical fitness level.[61] A prudent diet, weight control, and regular, moderate physical activity should precede pharmacologic treatment for **stage 1 hypertension** (140 to 159 mm Hg systolic; 90 to 99 mm Hg diastolic) and **stage 2 hypertension** (160 to 179 mm Hg systolic; 100 to 109 mm Hg diastolic). This is because of possible harmful side effects of drug therapy on other coronary artery disease risk factors.

IN A PRACTICAL SENSE

Understanding Hypertension: Effects on Bodily Systems

Effects in blood vessels
Damage to the interior arterial wall thickens it, thus reducing the space for transporting blood.

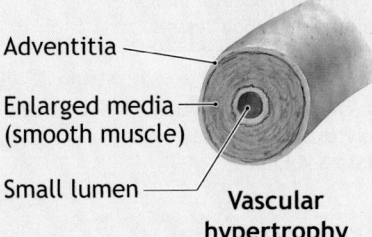

Adventitia

Enlarged media (smooth muscle)

Small lumen

Vascular hypertrophy

Adventitia

External elastic membrane

Media

Internal elastic membrane

Lamina propria

Endothilium

Lumen

Normal blood vessel

The arterial wall may dilate or bulge (aneurysm) and burst, causing blood loss, tissue damage, and death.

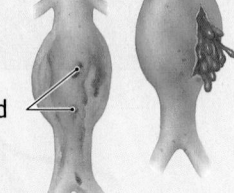

Blood clot

Fatty plaque develops in the damaged arterial wall, clogging blood flow and allowing clots to form and dislodge.

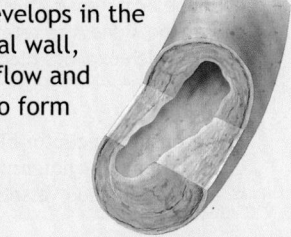

Atherosclerosis

Effects in brain
Blood clots can impair blood flow and cause strokes (and hemorrhage) from aneurysms that burst from increasing pressure.

Blood clot

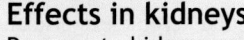

Aneurysm

Blood flow in heart
The right side of the heart receives blood from the body and delivers this deoxygenated blood to the lungs. The left side of the heart receives oxygen-rich blood from the lungs and pumps it to all body organs and tissues.

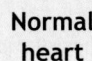

Normal heart

Aorta

Right ventricle

Left ventricle

Effects in heart
The left heart must pump more forcefully against a higher pressure from increased arterial resistance (increased preload), causing the left ventricle to enlarge and fail to effectively respond to the increased pressure.

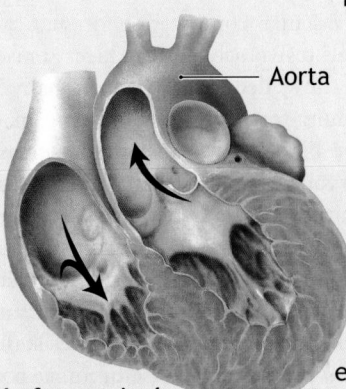

Left ventricular hypertrophy

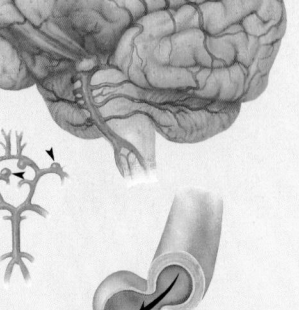

Effects in eye
Development of abnormal retinal vasculature.

Effects in kidneys
Damage to kidneys may cause hypertension from their failure to properly regulate salt and water balance.

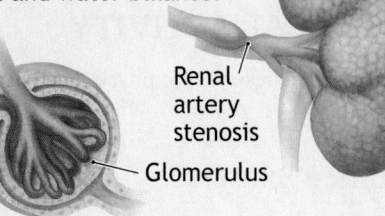

Renal artery stenosis

Glomerulus

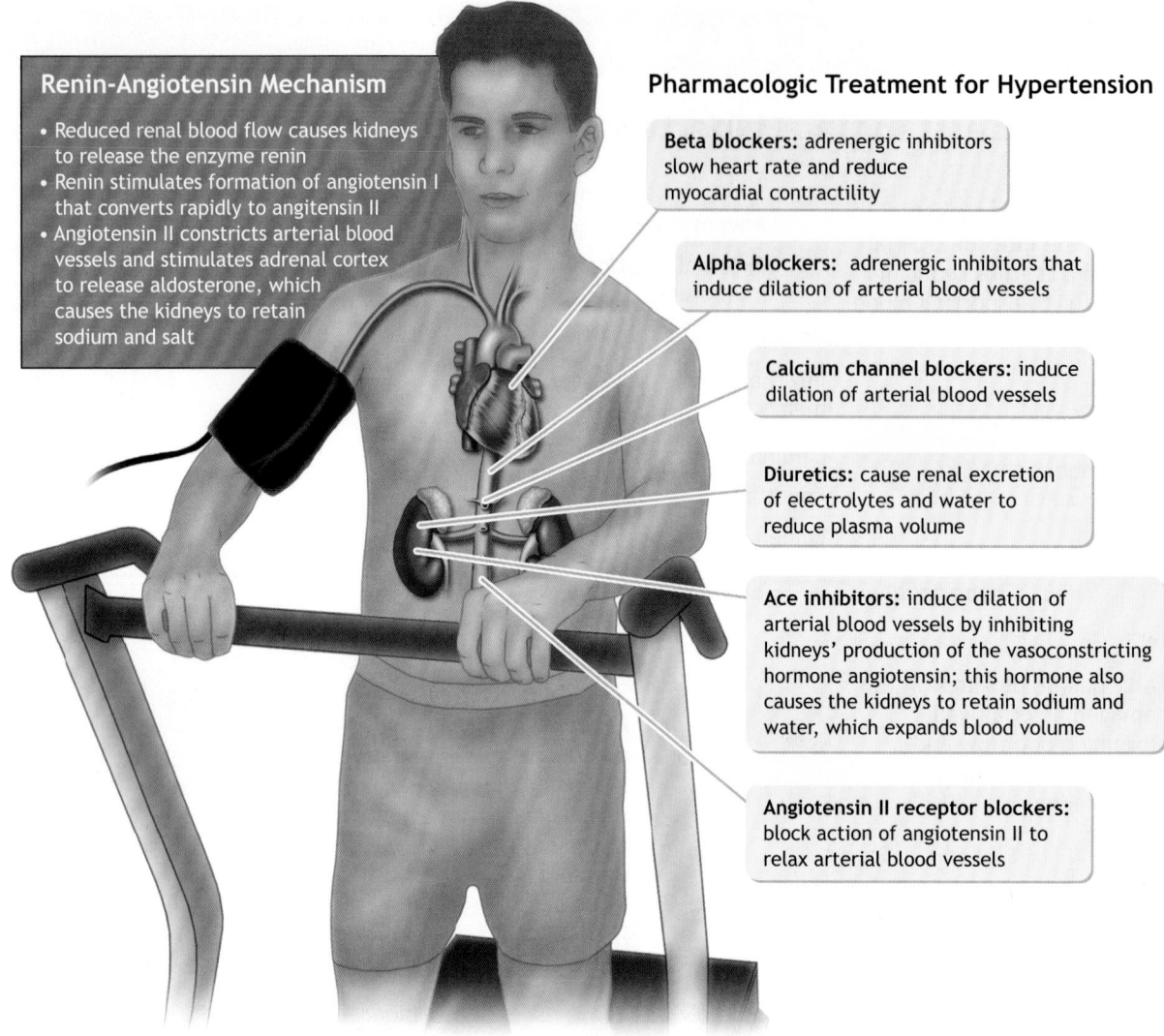

Renin-Angiotensin Mechanism

- Reduced renal blood flow causes kidneys to release the enzyme renin
- Renin stimulates formation of angiotensin I that converts rapidly to angitensin II
- Angiotensin II constricts arterial blood vessels and stimulates adrenal cortex to release aldosterone, which causes the kidneys to retain sodium and salt

Pharmacologic Treatment for Hypertension

Beta blockers: adrenergic inhibitors slow heart rate and reduce myocardial contractility

Alpha blockers: adrenergic inhibitors that induce dilation of arterial blood vessels

Calcium channel blockers: induce dilation of arterial blood vessels

Diuretics: cause renal excretion of electrolytes and water to reduce plasma volume

Ace inhibitors: induce dilation of arterial blood vessels by inhibiting kidneys' production of the vasoconstricting hormone angiotensin; this hormone also causes the kidneys to retain sodium and water, which expands blood volume

Angiotensin II receptor blockers: block action of angiotensin II to relax arterial blood vessels

FIGURE 15.10 • Recommended pharmacologic therapies for the treatment of hypertension if an initial 6 to 12 months of treatment with diet, weight loss, reduced alcohol intake, and regular physical activity proves ineffective. A chronically overactive renin–angiotensin mechanism also causes certain forms of high blood pressure (see Chapter 20).

The inset table in "In a Practical Sense" earlier in this chapter gives current classifications and recommended follow-up in initial blood pressure screening for adults. Chapter 32 discusses the role of regular aerobic exercise and resistance exercise to treat moderate hypertension.

BLOOD PRESSURE RESPONSE TO PHYSICAL ACTIVITY

The blood pressure response to physical activity varies with the activity mode.

Resistance Exercise

Straining muscle actions, particularly the concentric (shortening) and/or static phase of muscle actions, mechanically compresses the peripheral arterial vessels that supply active muscles. Arterial vascular compression dramatically increases total peripheral resistance and reduces muscle perfusion. Muscle blood flow decreases proportionally to the percentage of maximum force capacity exerted. In an attempt to restore muscle blood flow, substantial increases occur in sympathetic nervous system activity, cardiac output, and MAP. The magnitude of the hypertensive response relates directly to the intensity of effort and quantity of muscle mass activated.[16,24,39] Young and older healthy adults have similar short-term hemodynamic responses to resistance exercise.[36,37] For those who train regularly with resistance exercise, the elevated blood pressure response becomes considerably reduced.

A study from one of the authors' laboratories measured blood pressure of normotensive subjects directly with a

TABLE 15.1	Comparison of Peak Systolic and Diastolic Blood Pressure at Various Percentages of a Maximum Voluntary Contraction (MVC) During Isometric Exercise and Free-Weight and Hydraulic Bench Press Exercise							
	Isometric[a] (% MVC)				Free-Weight Bench Press[b] (% MVC)		Hydraulic Bench Press[c]	
Condition	**25**	**50**	**75**	**100**	**25**	**50**	**Slow**	**Fast**
Peak systolic, mm Hg	172	179	200	225	169	232	237	245
Peak diastolic, mm Hg	106	116	135	156	104	154	101	160

Values are averages for seven subjects. Data from Freedson PF, et al. Intra-arterial blood pressure during free weight and hydraulic resistive exercise. *Med Sci Sports Exerc* 1984;16:131 and unpublished data from the Human Performance Laboratory, Department of Exercise Science, University of Massachusetts, Amherst.
[a]Open glottis (no Valsalva maneuver); average of two trials; contraction time, 2 to 3 s; arm position that of bench-press exercise, with hands slightly above chest.
[b]The weight lifted was either 25 or 50% of previously determined isometric maximum action.
[c]Performed on Hydra-Fitness chest-press apparatus at dial setting 3 (slow) and 5 (fast) for 20 s of repeated maximal actions.

pressure transducer connected to a catheter inserted into the femoral artery. Measurements were made during three forms of exercise: (1) isometric bench press performed at 25, 50, 75, and 100% of the maximal voluntary contraction (MVC); (2) free-weight bench press performed at 25 and 50% of the isometric MVC; and (3) hydraulic resistance bench press exercise performed "all out" for 20 s at slow and fast speeds. The results, displayed in TABLE 15.1, show clearly that the three exercise modes substantially increased arterial blood pressure and the heart's corresponding workload (see "Rate–Pressure Product"). Other studies also show that movements that activate a large muscle mass and requires relatively great muscle strain elicit dramatic blood pressure increases.[14,30,35,40] As addressed in Chapter 16, this exacerbated blood pressure response results from the combined effect of:

1. Greater stimulation of the cardiovascular center by the active areas of the motor cortex
2. Large peripheral feedback to this center from the contracting muscle mass.

The acute cardiovascular strain with heavy-resistance exercise could prove harmful to individuals with heart and vascular disease, particularly individuals unfamiliar in this activity mode. FIGURE 15.11 presents generalized responses for blood pressure during rhythmic aerobic activity and resistance exercises that activate either a relatively small or relatively large muscle mass. In addition, intraocular pressure increases considerably during resistance exercise, which increases the risk for eye damage. Breath holding during the lift further magnifies the effect.[55,56]

Steady-Rate Physical Activity

During rhythmic muscular activity (e.g., jogging, swimming, bicycling), vasodilation in the active muscles reduces total peripheral resistance to enhance blood flow through large portions of the peripheral vasculature. Alternate muscle contraction and relaxation also provide an effective force to propel blood through the vascular circuit and return it to the heart. Increased blood flow during rhythmic, steady-rate

activities rapidly increases systolic pressure during the first few minutes. Blood pressure then levels off at 140 to 160 mm Hg for healthy men and women. As activity continues, systolic pressure gradually declines because the arterioles in the active muscles continue to dilate, further reducing peripheral resistance to blood flow. Diastolic blood pressure remains relatively unchanged throughout the activity period.

INTEGRATIVE QUESTION

Explain how regular resistance training that considerably elevates blood pressure during a two-arm curl with 80 lb in the early phase of training can ultimately blunt this blood pressure response as training progresses?

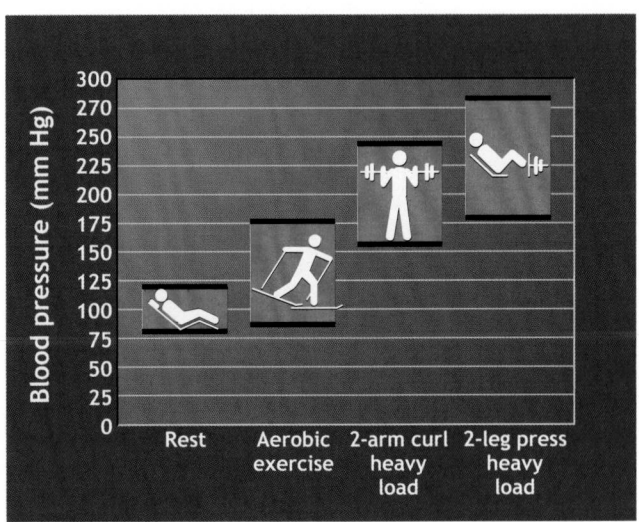

FIGURE 15.11 • Heavy-resistance exercise magnifies the exercise blood pressure response (higher with legs than arms) compared with rhythmic, continuous aerobic exercise. The height of the bar indicates pulse pressure.

Graded Exercise

Figure 15.12 illustrates the general pattern for systolic and diastolic blood pressures during continuous, graded treadmill walking and running. After an initial rapid rise from the resting level, systolic blood pressure increases linearly with exercise intensity, while diastolic pressure remains stable or decreases slightly at the higher activity levels. Healthy sedentary and endurance-trained men and women demonstrate similar blood pressure responses. During maximum exertion by trained individuals with high aerobic capacity, systolic blood pressure may increase to 200 mm Hg or higher, despite reduced total peripheral resistance.[39] This level of blood pressure most likely reflects the heart's large cardiac output.

Blood Pressure in Upper-Body Physical Activity

Physical activity with the arms produces considerably higher systolic and diastolic blood pressures and consequently greater cardiovascular strain than leg activity performed at a given percentage of $\dot{V}O_{2max}$ *in each form of exertion* (**Table 15.2**).[42,53] This occurs because the smaller arm muscle mass and vasculature offer greater resistance to blood flow than the larger leg mass and blood supply. Individuals with cardiovascular dysfunction should activate relatively large muscle groups (walking, bicycling, and running) in contrast to movements that engages a limited muscle mass as in shovelling, overhead hammering, or arm-crank exercise.[15,38] Chapter 17 focuses on the cardiovascular adjustments to upper-body physical activity.

Recovery From Physical Activity

Upon completion of a single bout of submaximal physical activity, blood pressure temporarily falls below pre-exercise

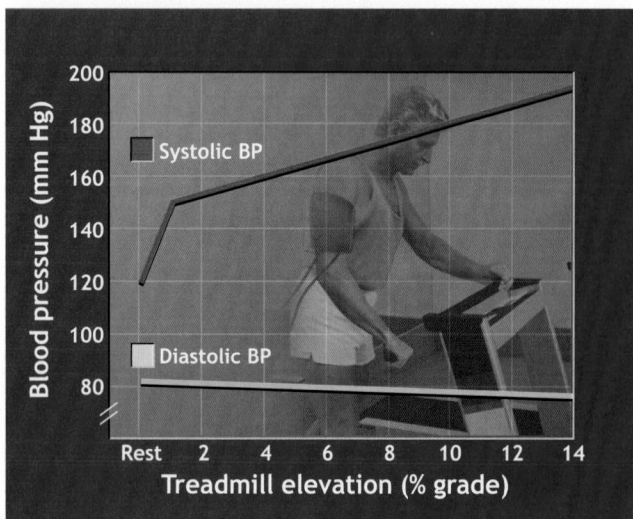

FIGURE 15.12 • Generalized response for systolic and diastolic blood pressures during continuous, graded treadmill exercise up to maximum.

	Systolic Pressure (mm Hg)		Diastolic Pressure (mm Hg)	
Percentage of $\dot{V}O_{2max}$	**Arms**	**Legs**	**Arms**	**Legs**
25	150	132	90	70
40	165	138	93	71
50	175	144	96	73
75	205	160	103	75

TABLE 15.2 — Comparison of Systolic and Diastolic Blood Pressure During Dynamic Arm and Leg Exercise at Similar Percentages of $\dot{V}O_{2max}$

From Åstrand PO, et al. Intraarterial blood pressure during exercise with different muscle groups. *J Appl Physiol* 1965;20:253.

levels for normotensive and hypertensive individuals from an unexplained peripheral vasodilation.[23,26,28,31,33] The **hypotensive response** to activity can last up to 12 hr. It occurs in response to either low- or moderate-intensity aerobic activity or resistance exercise.[34,42] One explanation for postexercise hypotension proposes that a considerable quantity of blood remains pooled in the visceral organs and/or skeletal muscle vascular beds during recovery.[11] The venous pooling effect reduces central blood volume, which in turn decreases atrial filling pressure and lowers systemic arterial blood pressure. A prolonged increase in splanchnic, renal, or cutaneous blood flow in recovery probably plays only a limited contributory role in the postexercise hypotensive response.[43,59] Independent of the mechanism, postexercise reductions in blood pressure further support moderate physical activity as a nonpharmacologic treatment for hypertension. *Relatively prolonged reductions in postexercise blood pressure justify recommending multiple periods of physical activity interspersed throughout the day.*[5]

THE HEART'S BLOOD SUPPLY

Each day, nearly 2000 gallons of blood flow through the heart's chambers—in one year, 730,000 gallons and in a lifetime of 72 years, 52.6 million gallons—all of it nonstop! None of the blood, however, passes directly into the myocardium because no direct circulatory channels lead from the chambers into the tissues. Instead, the heart muscle maintains its own intricate circulatory network. **Figure 15.13** shows that these vessels form a visible, crown-like network called the **coronary circulation** that arises from the top portion of the heart.

The right and left coronary arteries emerge from the upper part of the ascending aorta. Their openings form just above the semilunar valves at a point where oxygenated blood leaves the left ventricle. These arteries then curl around the heart's surface. The right coronary artery supplies predominantly the

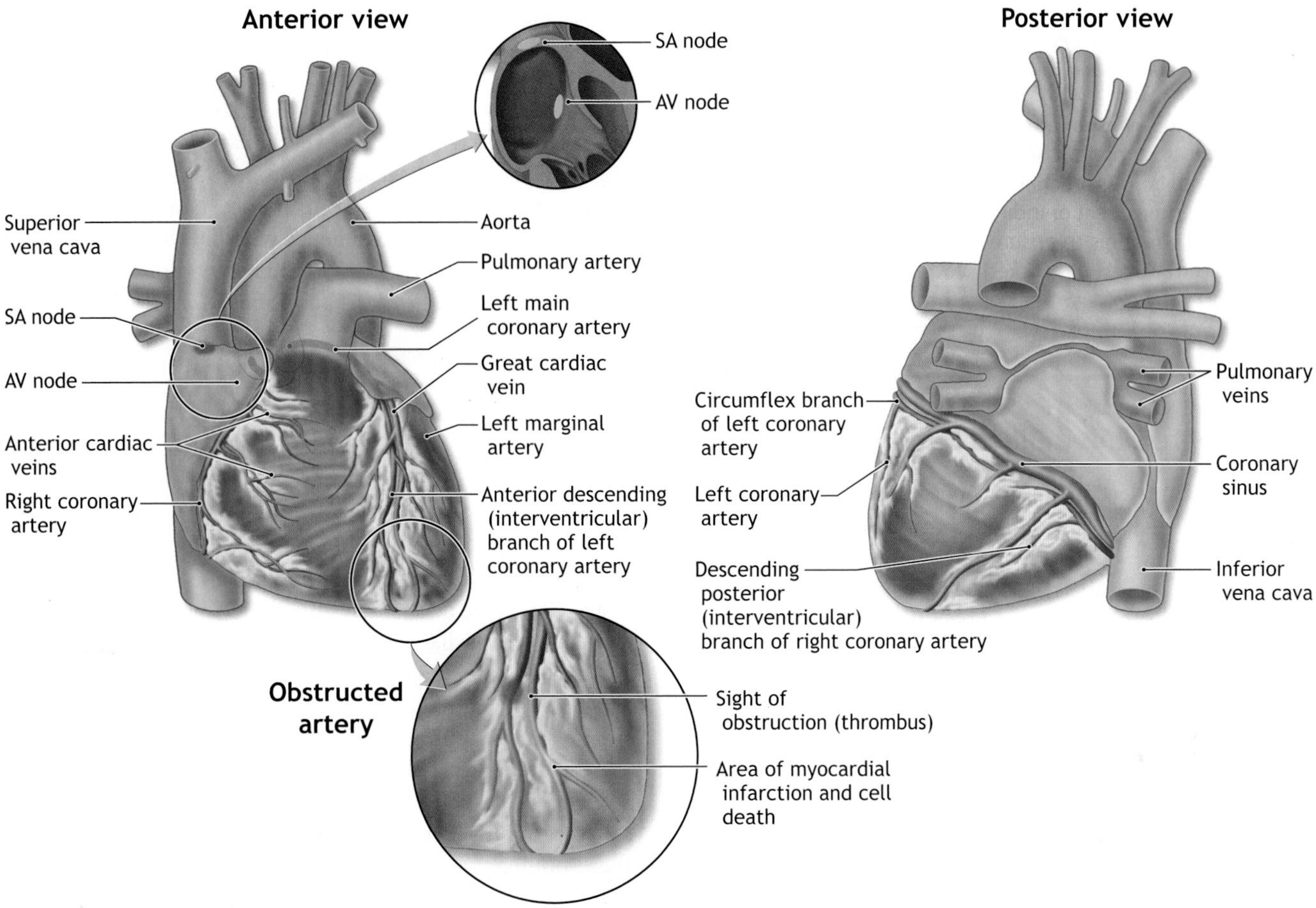

Anterior view

- SA node
- AV node

- Superior vena cava
- Aorta
- Pulmonary artery
- SA node
- Left main coronary artery
- AV node
- Great cardiac vein
- Anterior cardiac veins
- Left marginal artery
- Right coronary artery
- Anterior descending (interventricular) branch of left coronary artery

Obstructed artery

- Sight of obstruction (thrombus)
- Area of myocardial infarction and cell death

Posterior view

- Circumflex branch of left coronary artery
- Pulmonary veins
- Coronary sinus
- Left coronary artery
- Descending posterior (interventricular) branch of right coronary artery
- Inferior vena cava

FIGURE 15.13 • Anterior and posterior views of the coronary circulation including the SA and AV nodes (*upper inset*). Arteries are shaded *red* and veins *blue*, with the exception of the pulmonary circulation where colors reverse. The *lower inset* illustrates a myocardial infarction from the blockage of a coronary vessel.

right atrium and right ventricle. The greatest volume of blood flows in the left coronary artery to the left atrium and left ventricle and small sections of the right ventricle. These vessels divide and eventually form a dense capillary network within the myocardium. Blood leaves the tissues of the left ventricle through the **coronary sinus**; blood from the right ventricle exits via the **anterior cardiac veins**, which empty directly into the right atrium. The lower left inset figure illustrates the obstruction of a coronary vessel that ultimately leads to tissue death. This phenomenon of impaired coronary blood flow and/or arterial blockage and its resulting effects is more fully discussed in a subsequent section titled Effects of Impaired Blood Supply.

The driving force of each ventricular systole pushes some blood into the coronary arteries. Normal blood flow to the myocardium at rest equals 200 to 250 mL per minute; this represents approximately 5% of the heart's total output.

Myocardial Oxygen Supply and Use

At rest, the myocardium requires considerable oxygen relative to its blood flow; it extracts about 70 to 80% of the oxygen from the blood in the coronary vessels. The magnitude of myocardial oxygen extraction differs considerably from most other tissues, which use only about one-fourth of their available oxygen at rest. Consequently, a proportionate increase in coronary blood flow in physical activity essentially provides the sole mechanism to increase myocardial oxygen supply. During vigorous physical effort, coronary blood flow increases by as much as four times above the resting level. In general, coronary blood flow matches myocardial oxygen needs from increases in heart rate during physical activity. Coronary vessels dilate in exercise from the combined effects of feedforward mechanisms (mediated by sympathetic–adrenoceptor vasodilation) and feedback control mechanisms (possibly from vascular-stimulating adenine nucleotides released from erythrocytes) control mechanisms.[19,20,54] Arterial blood pressure also facilitates coronary blood flow. Increased aortic pressure during activity forces a proportionately greater volume of blood into the coronary circulation. The ebb and flow of blood in the coronary vessels consistently fluctuates with each phase of the cardiac cycle. On average, about 2.5 times more blood flows in the coronary vessels during diastole than systole.

 See the animation "Myocardial Blood Flow" on http://thePoint.lww.com/mkk8e for a demonstration of this process.

For Use in an Emergency

The heart muscle has an emergency "back-up" in case of compromised blood supply, achieved by a structural element called an **anastomosis.** This mechanism provides a natural communication link, either direct or indirect, between two blood vessels via collateral channels to ensure continuation of blood flow to an area with reduced or blocked blood supply. Some of these vessels currently exist in the body; others can develop under conditions of compromised blood supply.

Effects of Impaired Blood Supply

The myocardium depends on an adequate oxygen supply because, unlike skeletal muscle, it has limited anaerobic energy-generating capacity. Extensive vascular perfusion supplies at least one capillary to each of the heart's muscle fibers. Tissue hypoxia provides a potent stimulus to myocardial blood flow. Impaired coronary blood flow usually produces chest pains termed *angina pectoris*. More pronounced pain occurs during physical activity because the heart's energy requirements increase considerably. Fortunately, the stress of exercise provides an effective way to evaluate adequacy of myocardial blood flow. A blood clot or **thrombus** lodged in a coronary vessel usually impairs normal heart function (FIG. 15.14). This form of "heart attack," or more specifically **myocardial infarction**, may be mild; a more complete blockage severely damages the myocardium and causes death. Chapters 31 and 32 provide details about coronary heart disease, exercise stress testing, and the role of regular physical activity as preventative and rehabilitative medicine.

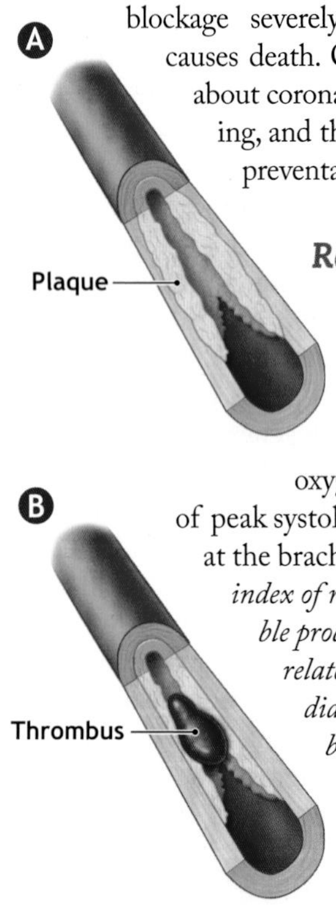

Rate–Pressure Product: An Estimate of Myocardial Work

One common estimate of myocardial workload (and resulting oxygen consumption) uses the product of peak systolic blood pressure (SBP), measured at the brachial artery, and heart rate (HR). *This index of relative cardiac work, termed the double product or **rate–pressure product (RPP)**, relates closely to directly measured myocardial oxygen consumption and coronary blood flow in healthy subjects over a wide range of exercise intensities.* RPP computes as follows:

$$RPP = SBP \times HR$$

FIGURE 15.14 • **(A)** Plaque. **(B)** Thrombus. (Adapted with permission from Moore KL, Dalley AF, Agur AMR. *Clinically Oriented Anatomy.* 7th Ed., as adapted with permission from Willis MC. *Medical Terminology: The Language of Health Care.* Baltimore: Lippincott Williams & Wilkins, 1995.)

Plaque

Thrombus

Changes in heart rate and blood pressure contribute equally to changes in RPP. Typical values for RPP range from 6000 at rest (HR = 50 b·min⁻¹; SBP = 120 mm Hg) to 40,000 (HR = 200 b·min⁻¹; SBP = 200 mm Hg) or above, depending on activity intensity and mode. Resistance training and upper-body physical activity produce substantially higher heart rate and blood pressure responses, hence higher RPPs, than more rhythmic movements with the lower body. This added myocardial work poses an unnecessary risk for coronary heart disease patients with compromised myocardial oxygen supply.

RPP, Physical Activity, and the Heart Disease Patient. Research with heart disease patients shows a physiologic correlation between RPP and onset of angina pectoris and electrocardiographic abnormalities during physical activity. The RPP thus provides an objective yardstick to evaluate the effects on cardiac performance of various clinical, surgical, or exercise interventions. The well-documented lowering of exercise heart rate and systolic blood pressure with lower RPP and myocardial oxygen requirement helps to explain the improved exercise capacity of cardiac patients before abnormal cardiac symptoms emerge following training. Prolonged, intense aerobic training also allows cardiac patients to achieve a higher exercise RPP.[13,21] In nine patients followed over a 7-year training period, RPP increased by 11.5% before ischemic symptoms appeared during graded exercise testing.[47] These findings provide indirect evidence for improved myocardial oxygenation, probably from greater coronary vascularization or reduced obstruction from the training adaptation.

 INTEGRATIVE QUESTION

Explain why a training-induced increase in the rate–pressure product before a patient experiences angina or electrocardiographic abnormalities during physical activity implies enhanced myocardial oxygenation.

the**Point** Appendix H, available online at http://thePoint.lww.com/mkk8e, provides a list of supplemental animations and videos on heart function, dysfunction, and treatment.

MYOCARDIAL METABOLISM

The myocardium relies almost exclusively on energy released in aerobic reactions; not surprisingly, then, myocardial tissue has a threefold higher oxidative capacity than skeletal muscle. Its muscle fibers contain the greatest mitochondrial concentration of all tissues, with exceptional capacity for long-chain fatty acid catabolism as a primary means for ATP resynthesis.

Figure 15.15 shows the specific substrate use on a percentage basis by the myocardium during rest and moderate and intense physical activity. Glucose, fatty acids, and lactate formed from glycolysis in skeletal muscle provide the energy

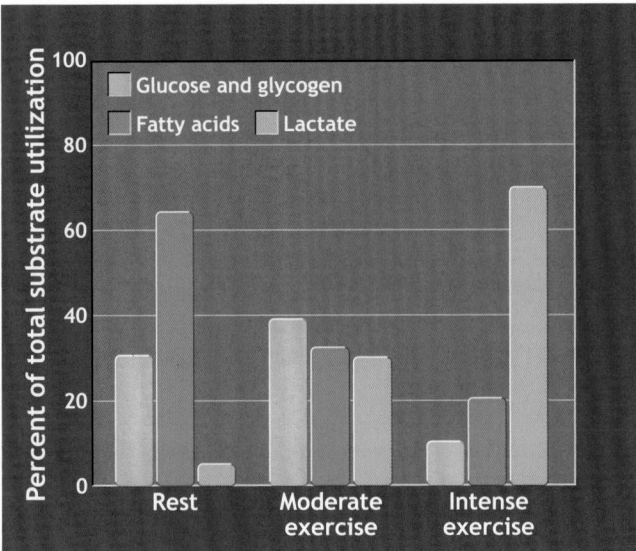

FIGURE 15.15 • Generalized pattern of myocardial substrate use at rest and in relation to exercise intensity.

for myocardial functioning.[3,25] At rest, these three substrates contribute to ATP resynthesis, with the most energy from free fatty acid breakdown (60 to 70%).[17,51] Following a meal, glucose becomes the preferred energy substrate. In essence, the heart uses for energy whatever substrate it "sees" on a physiologic level. During intense activity when lactate efflux from active skeletal muscle into the blood increases dramatically, the heart derives its major energy by oxidizing circulating lactate. In more moderate activity, equal amounts of fat and carbohydrate provide the energy fuel. In prolonged submaximal effort (not illustrated), myocardial metabolism of free fatty acids rises to almost 80% of the total energy requirement. Similar patterns of myocardial metabolism exist for trained and untrained individuals. An endurance-trained person, however, demonstrates considerably greater myocardial reliance on fat catabolism in submaximal exercise. This difference, similar to the effect for skeletal muscle, illustrates the "carbohydrate-sparing effect" of aerobic training.

Summary

1. Striated fibers of the myocardium interconnect to make portions of the heart contract in a unified manner.
2. The heart functions as two separate pumps: One pump receives blood from the body and pumps it to the lungs for aeration (pulmonary circulation); the other receives oxygenated blood from the lungs and pumps it throughout the systemic circulation.
3. Pressure changes created during the cardiac cycle act on the heart's valves to provide one-way blood flow in the vascular circuit.
4. The surge of blood with ventricular contraction and subsequent runoff of blood in relaxation creates pressure changes within the arterial vessels.
5. Ventricular contraction generates systolic blood pressure, the highest pressure during the cardiac cycle. Diastolic pressure represents the lowest pressure before the next ventricular contraction.
6. The dense capillary network provides a large and effective surface for exchange of chemicals between the blood and surrounding tissues. These minute-diameter blood vessels possess autoregulatory capacity to exquisitely adjust blood flow in response to the tissue's changing metabolic activity.
7. The venous tree contains the largest portion of central blood volume at rest, but an increase in venous tone (venoconstriction) probably contributes little to the redistribution of blood during physical activity.
8. Compression and relaxation of the veins by skeletal muscle action impart considerable energy to facilitate venous return. This "muscle pump" mechanism provides additional justification for active recovery immediately following vigorous effort.
9. Hypertension imposes a chronic cardiovascular stress that eventually damages arterial vessels and leads to arteriosclerosis, heart disease, stroke, and kidney failure. One of every three persons experiences chronic, abnormally high blood pressure sometime during their lifetime.
10. Systolic blood pressure increases in proportion to oxygen consumption and blood flow during graded exercise, whereas diastolic pressure remains relatively unchanged or decreases slightly.
11. At the same relative and absolute exercise levels, upper-body exercise produces a greater rise in systolic pressure than leg exercise.
12. Following physical activity, blood pressure decreases below the pre-exercise level and may remain lower for up to 12 hr.
13. During isometric, free-weight, and hydraulic resistance exercises, peak systolic and diastolic blood pressures mirror a hypertensive state.
14. Performing intense resistance exercises pose a risk to individuals with hypertension or heart disease.
15. At rest, the myocardium extracts approximately 80% of the oxygen flowing through the coronary arteries. An increase in coronary blood flow primarily provides for myocardial oxygen needs in physical activity.
16. The myocardium requires a continual and adequate oxygen supply. Coronary blood flow impairment initiates chest pains (angina); blockage of a coronary artery causes irreversible damage to the heart muscle (myocardial infarction).
17. The rate-pressure product (heart rate × systolic blood pressure) estimates myocardial workload.
18. The metabolism of glucose, fatty acids, and circulating lactate provides the energy to maintain myocardial function.
19. The percentage myocardial use of macronutrients for energy varies with the severity and duration of physical activity and the individual's training status.

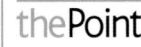 References are available online at
http://thepoint.lww.com/mkk8e.

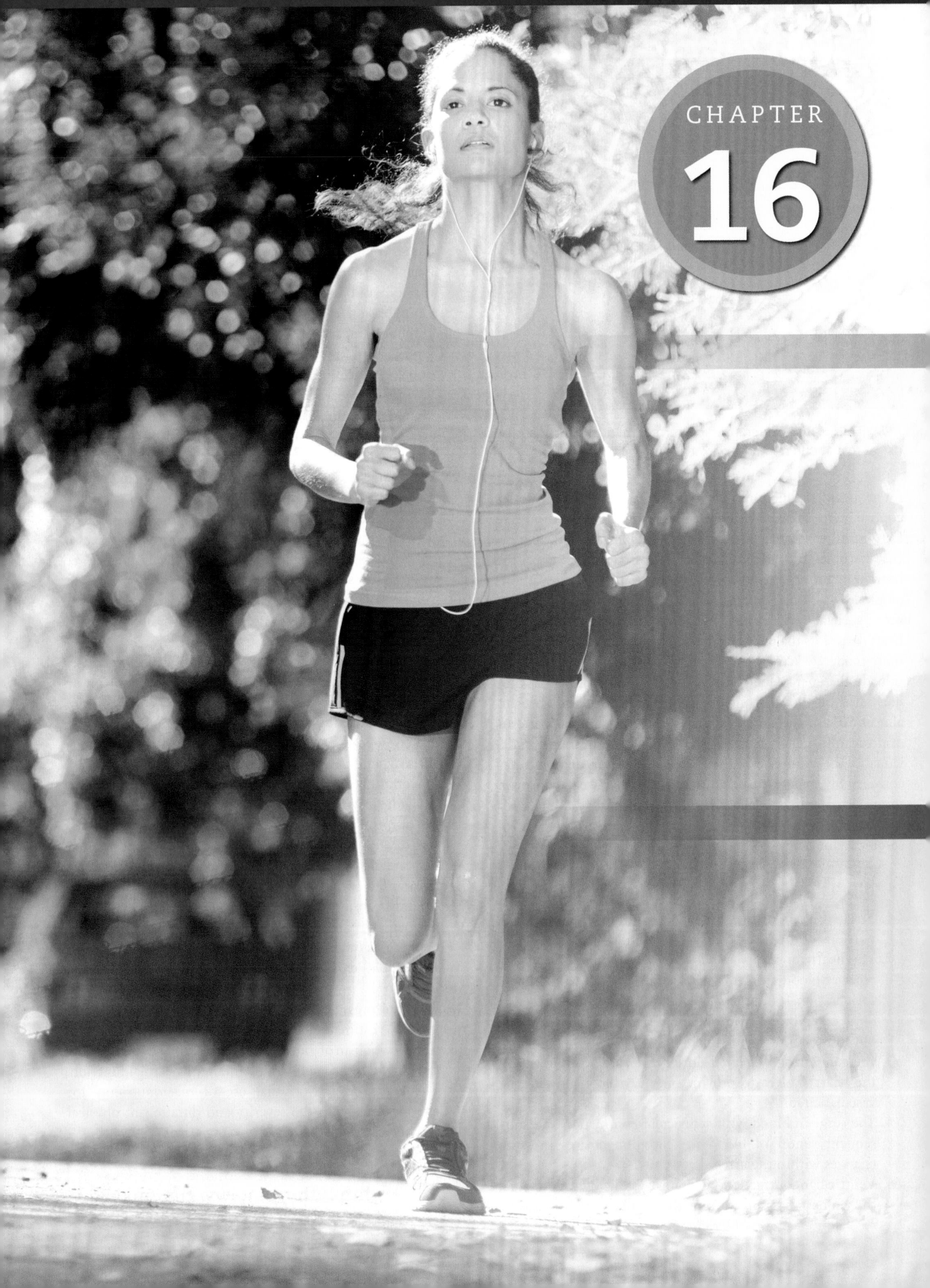

CHAPTER

16

Cardiovascular Regulation and Integration

- Explain how intrinsic and extrinsic factors regulate heart rate during rest and physical activity

- Draw a normal electrocardiogram (ECG) tracing and identify and describe its major components

- Describe how local metabolic factors regulate blood flow during rest and physical activity

- Explain the role of "central command" in cardiovascular regulation during exercise

- Describe the effects of aerobic training on neural regulation of heart rate

- Outline the contributions of chemoreceptors, mechanoreceptors, and the metaboreflex in cardiovascular regulation during physical activity

- List the physical factors that affect vasculature blood flow

- Indicate how each component of Poiseuille's law affects blood flow

- Summarize the dynamics of blood flow to diverse tissues at exercise onset and as exercise progresses in duration and intensity

- Describe the proposed mechanisms for nitric oxide's regulation of local blood flow

- Outline the heart transplant patient's cardiovascular response to physical activity

Visit http://thePoint.lww.com/mkk8e to access the following resources.

- References: Chapter 16
- Interactive Question Bank
- Animation: Cardiac Cycle
- Animation: Perform a Basic 12-Lead Electrocardiogram
- Animation: Renal Function
- Focus on Research: Age-Related Changes in Exercise-Induced Cardiovascular Function

Throughout the day, while awake or sleeping, complex mechanisms continually interact to dynamically balance systemic blood pressure and blood flow to different tissues. Neurochemical factors regulate heart rate and the internal diameter of blood vessels. Finely regulated cardiovascular responses provide rapid control of heart function and proper blood flow distribution throughout the body. At rest, the skin receives approximately 5% of the 5 L of blood pumped by the heart each minute. In contrast, during physical activity in a hot, humid environment, up to 20% of the total blood flow diverts to the body's surface for one major purpose—to dissipate heat. This "shunting" of blood and regulation of blood pressure occur only within a closed vascular system. This dynamic allows a near-immediate increase and redistribution of blood flow to meet changing metabolic and physiologic needs and environmental challenges in conditions of cold, heat, underwater, high altitudes, and zero gravity.

INTRINSIC REGULATION OF HEART RATE

Unlike other tissues, cardiac muscle maintains its own rhythm. If left to its inherent rhythmicity, the heart would beat steadily at about 100 b · min^{-1}. Situated within the posterior wall of the right atrium lies a small (3-mm wide and 1-cm long) mass of specialized muscle tissue called the **sinoatrial node** or **SA node**. This node spontaneously depolarizes and repolarizes to provide the innate stimulus for heart action. For this reason, the term *pacemaker* describes the SA node. FIGURE 16.1A shows the normal route for impulse transmission within the myocardium.

The Heart's Electrical Activity

Electrochemical rhythms originating at the SA node spread across the atria to another small knot of tissue situated close to the tricuspid valve known as the **atrioventricular node** or **AV node**. FIGURE 16.1B illustrates the time sequence of the propagation of the electrical impulse from the SA node throughout the myocardium.

An approximate 0.10-s delay occurs after the electrical impulse spreads through the atria to allow them to contract and propel blood into the ventricles below. The AV node gives rise to the 1-cm long **AV bundle**, also called the **bundle of His**, named after Swiss-born anatomist and cardiologist Wilhelm His, Jr. (1863–1934; http://circ.ahajournals.org/content/113/23/2775.full), who in 1893 first described this tissue. Later in his career, His advanced the idea that the heart's individual cells produced the heartbeat.

The AV bundle transmits the impulse rapidly through the ventricles over specialized conducting fibers referred to as the **Purkinje system** (named for Czech [Bohemian] anatomist/physiologist/biologist Jan Evangelista von Purkinje [1787–1869; http://circ.ahajournals.org/content/113/23/2775.full]). These fibers form distinct bundle branches that penetrate the right and left ventricles. Purkinje system fibers transmit the impulse about six times faster than normal

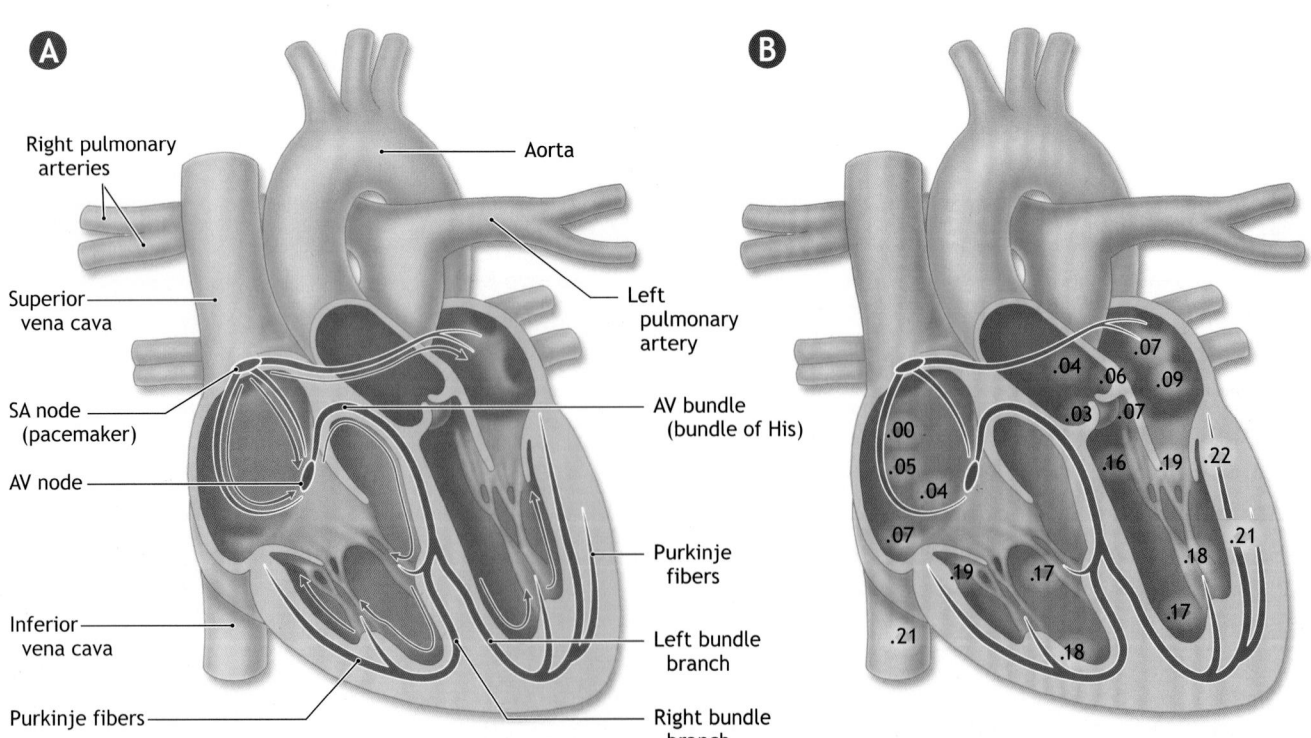

FIGURE 16.1 • **(A)** The red arrows denote the normal route for excitation and conduction of the cardiac impulse. The impulse originates at the SA node, travels to the AV node, and then spreads throughout the ventricular mass. **(B)** Time sequence in seconds for electrical impulse transmission from the SA node throughout the myocardium. Walter Gaskell (1847–1914) first demonstrated the specialized muscle fibers joining the atria and ventricles.

ventricular muscle fibers. The passage of the impulse into the ventricles stimulates each ventricular cell to allow a unified and simultaneous subsequent contraction of both ventricles. The transmission of the cardiac impulse flows as follows:

SA node → Atria → AV node → AV bundle
(Purkinje fibers) → Ventricles

 See the animation "Cardiac Cycle" on **http://thePoint. lww.com/mkk8e** for a demonstration of this process.

Electrocardiogram

Similar to all nerve and muscle tissue, the outer surface of the myocardial cells or fibers maintains a more positive electrical charge than the inside surface. Upon stimulation prior to contraction, polarity reverses and the myocardial cells' inside becomes more positive than its outside. During the diastolic phase of the cardiac cycle, the membranes repolarize to reestablish the normal resting membrane potential.

The myocardium's electrical activity creates an electrical field throughout the body. The salty bodily fluids provide an excellent conducting medium, so electrodes placed on the skin's surface readily detect voltage changes from the sequence of electrical events before and during each cardiac cycle. **Figure 16.2A** outlines the pathway of conduction of the electrical impulse as it spreads throughout the myocardium to produce the heart muscle's rhythmic contraction and dilation. **Figure 16.2B** graphically displays the normal cycle of the heart's electrical activity as recorded by an **electrocardiogram**, (**ECG**) (see also "In a Practical Sense"). Its important patterns of electrical deflection are referred to as P, QRS, and T waves, including the P-R and Q-T intervals and the S-T segment.

The **P wave** represents depolarization of the atria. It lasts approximately 0.15 s and heralds atrial contraction. The relatively large **QRS complex** follows the P wave; it signals electrical changes from ventricular depolarization. At this point, the ventricles contract. Atrial repolarization follows the P wave; it produces a wave so small that the large QRS complex usually obscures it. The **T wave** represents ventricular repolarization that occurs during ventricular diastole. The heart's relatively long depolarization period of 0.20 to 0.30 s prevents initiation of the next myocardial impulse (and subsequent contraction). This rest or brief time-out **refractory period** allows sufficient time for ventricular filling between beats.

The ECG Objectively Monitors Heart Rate During Physical Activity

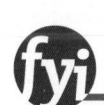

Radiotelemetry transmits the ECG while a person performs diverse sports and physical activity such as football, weightlifting, basketball, ice hockey, dancing, swimming, and extravehicular activity in space. The ECG can also detect contraindications to exercise, including previous myocardial infarction, ischemic S-T segment changes, conduction defects, and abnormal left ventricular enlargement (see Chapter 31).

 See the animation "Perform a Basic 12-Lead Electrocardiogram" on **http://thePoint.lww.com/mkk8e** for a demonstration of this process.

EXTRINSIC REGULATION OF HEART RATE AND CIRCULATION

Changes in heart rate occur rapidly through nerves that directly supply the myocardium and chemical "messengers" that circulate in blood. These **extrinsic controls** of cardiac function accelerate the heart in anticipation before physical activity begins, and then rapidly adjust to the intensity of physical effort. Extrinsic regulation can decrease heart rate to 25 to 30 b·min^{-1} under normal ambulatory conditions in highly trained endurance athletes and can increase it to 200 b·min^{-1} in maximal exertion in trained and untrained persons.[5]

Figure 16.3 illustrates neural mechanisms for cardiovascular regulation before and during activity. Input from the brain and peripheral nervous system continually bombards the cardiovascular control center in the **ventrolateral medulla**. This center regulates the heart's output of blood and blood's preferential distribution to all the body's tissues. The lower box of the figure describes the neural activation and response mechanisms during the pre-exercise "anticipatory" and exercise phases.

Sympathetic and Parasympathetic Neural Input

Neural influences can modulate and override the inherent myocardial rhythm. These influences originate in the cardiovascular center and flow through the **sympathetic** and **parasympathetic** components of the autonomic nervous system (see Chapter 19). These two divisions operate in parallel but act by distinctly different structural pathways and transmitter systems. **Figure 16.4** illustrates the distribution of sympathetic and parasympathetic nerve fibers within the myocardium. Numerous sympathetic and parasympathetic neurons innervate the atria, whereas the ventricles receive sympathetic fibers almost exclusively.

Sympathetic Influence

Stimulation of the sympathetic cardioaccelerator nerves releases the **catecholamines** epinephrine and norepinephrine. These neurohormones accelerate SA node depolarization, causing the heart to beat faster (the **chronotropic effect**). The term *tachycardia* describes heart rate acceleration, usually to rates that exceed 100 b·min^{-1} at rest. Catecholamines also increase myocardial contractility (the **inotropic effect**) to augment how much blood the heart pumps with each beat. The force of ventricular contraction nearly doubles under maximum sympathetic stimulation. Epinephrine, released into the blood from the medullary portion of the adrenal glands during general sympathetic activation, produces a similar but *slower*-acting tachycardia effect on cardiac function.

Sympathetic stimulation also profoundly impacts blood flow throughout the body to produce vasoconstriction, except in the coronary vasculature.[7,53] **Figure 16.5** schematically depicts

Ⓐ

Cardiac Conduction

Repeating electrical impulses travel through the heart to control the heart muscle's rhythmic contraction and dilation.

1. The impulse originates from the sinoatrial (S-A) node located in the right atrium, and spreads across the atria causing them to contract.

2. The impulse then passes to the atrioventricular (A-V) node, travels along the atrioventricular bundle into its' two branches, the right and left crus, and spreads into the ventricles causing them to contract.

3. Dissipation of the impulse causes the atria and ventricles to relax or dilate.

Sinoatrial (S-A) node 1.

Interatrial septum 2.

Atrioventricular 3.
(A-V) node

Atrioventricular bundle 4.
(bundle of His)

Right crus 5.

Left crus 6.

Interventricular 7.
septum

Purkinje's fibers 8.

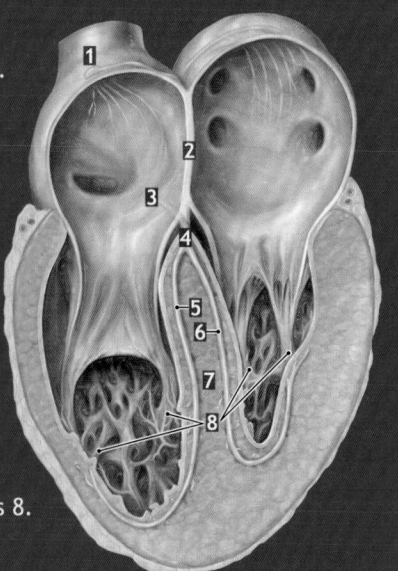

Ⓑ

Atrial Depolarization (P-wave)

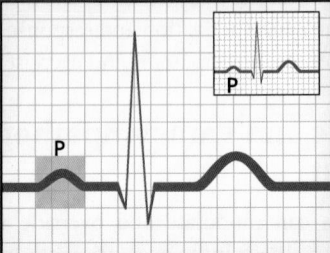

P-wave, the first ECG deflection, represents depolarization of both atria.

P-R Interval

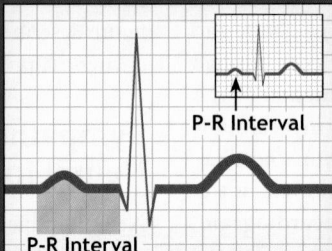

The electrical transmission from atria to ventricles includes the P-wave and P-R segment.

Ventricular Depolarization (QRS)

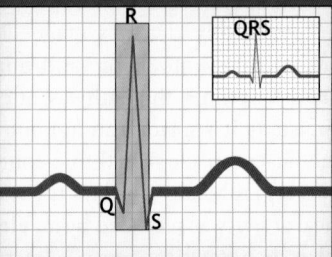

QRS complex indiates ventricular depolarization; R wave indicates the initial positive deflection; Q-wave the negative deflection before the R-wave; S-wave the negative deflection following the R-wave.

Ventricular Repolarization (S-T Segment)

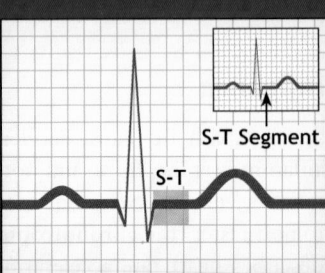

Earlier phase repolarization extends from end of the QRS to start of the T-wave. The J (junction) point represents where S-T segment joins the beginning of the T-wave.

Ventricular Repolarization (T-wave)

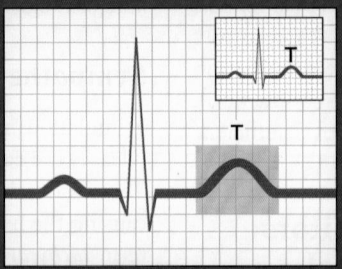

T-wave represents repolarization of both ventricles; S-T segment and T-wave provide sensitive indicators of the ventricular myocardium's oxygen demand-oxygen supply status.

Ventricular Depolarization and Repolarization (Q-T Interval)

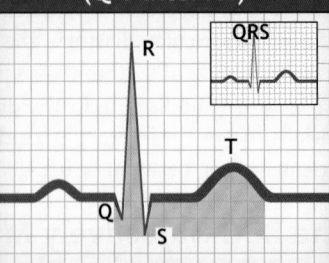

Q-T interval includes the QRS complex, S-T segment, and T-wave.

FIGURE 16.2 • **(A)** Normal transmission of the electrical impulse through the myocardium. **(B)** Different phases of the normal ECG from atrial depolarization (upper left) to ventricular repolarization (lower middle). (A, adapted with permission from Anatomical Chart Company.)

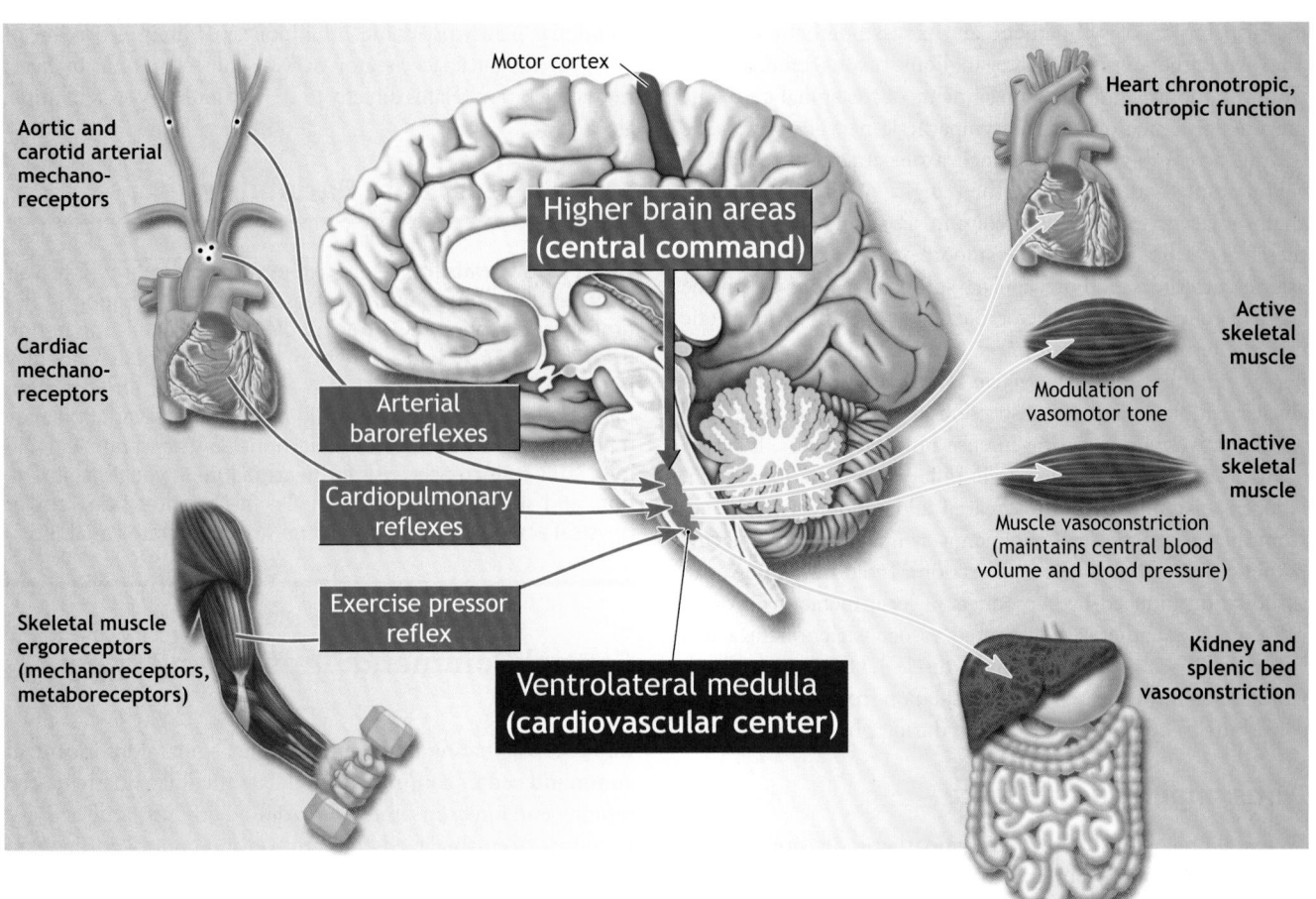

Condition	Activator	Response
Pre-exercise "anticipatory" response	Activation of central command from the motor cortex and higher areas of the brain causes an increase in sympathetic outflow and reciprocal inhibition of parasympathetic activity.	Acceleration of heart rate; increased myocardial contractility; vasodilation in skeletal and heart muscle (cholinergic fibers); vasoconstriction in other areas, especially skin, gut, spleen, liver, and kidneys (adrenergic fibers); increase in arterial blood pressure.
Exercise	Parasympathetic withdrawal at onset and during low-intensity exercise; progressive sympathetic stimulation in more intense exercise; reflex feedback from peripheral mechanical and chemical receptors that monitor muscle action; alterations in local metabolic conditions due to hypoxia, ↓pH, ↑P_{CO_2}, ↑ADP, ↑Mg^{2+}, ↑Ca^{2+}, and ↑temperature cause autoregulatory vasodilation in active muscle.	Further dilation of muscle vasculature.
	Continued sympathetic adrenergic outflow in conjunction with epinephrine and norepinephrine from the adrenal medulla.	Concomitant constriction of vasculature in inactive tissues to maintain adequate perfusion pressure throughout arterial system. Both muscle pump action and visceral vasoconstriction facilitate venous return and maintain central blood volume.

FIGURE 16.3 • Neural regulation of the cardiovascular system during physical activity. (Adapted with permission from Mitchell JH, Raven PB. Cardiovascular adaptation to physical activity. In: Bouchard C, et al., eds. *Physical Activity, Fitness, and Health.* Champaign, IL: Human Kinetics, 1994.)

the distribution of sympathetic and parasympathetic outflow. The sympathetic system's preganglionic axons emerge *only* from the thoracic and lumbar segments of the spinal cord. The preganglionic neurons of the sympathetic nervous system lie within the cord's gray matter. Their axons emerge through the ventral roots and synapse in the ganglia of the sympathetic chain adjacent to the spinal column. Postganglionic sympathetic nerve fibers end in the smooth muscle layers of small arteries, arterioles, and precapillary sphincters. Norepinephrine acts as a general vasoconstrictor released by specific sympathetic neurons termed *adrenergic fibers*. Some adrenergic constrictor nerves remain continually active. Thus, certain blood vessels always exhibit a state of constriction or **vasomotor tone** even within active muscle during intense physical activity. Dilation of blood vessels under adrenergic influence occurs more from reduced **vasomotor tone** (decreased adrenergic activity) than from increased activity of cholinergic sympathetic or parasympathetic dilator fibers (see next section). In addition, powerful vasodilation induced by byproducts of local metabolism overrides any sympathetically activated vasoconstriction in active tissue (see "Factors Within Active Muscle"). Humoral feedback from metabolites released to the circulation from active muscles contribute to heart rate acceleration during physical activity.[31]

Parasympathetic Influence

Preganglionic axons of the parasympathetic division emerge *only* from the brainstem and the cord's sacral segments. The parasympathetic and sympathetic systems thereby complement each other anatomically. The preganglionic parasympathetic neurons lie within brainstem tissue and the lower spinal cord. Their axons travel farther than sympathetic axons because their ganglia lie adjacent to or within target organs. Parasympathetic fibers distribute to the head, neck, and body cavities (except for erectile tissues of genitalia) and never emerge in the body wall and limbs. When stimulated, parasympathetic neurons release acetylcholine, which *retards* the rate of sinus discharge to slow the heart rate. A reduced heart rate, or **bradycardia**, results largely from stimulation of the pair of **vagus nerves** whose cell bodies originate in the medulla's cardioinhibitory center. The vagus nerves, the only cranial nerves that exit the head and neck region, descend to the thorax and abdominal regions. These nerves carry approximately 80% of all parasympathetic fibers. Vagal stimulation exerts no effect on myocardial contractility. Parasympathetic nerve fibers leave the brainstem and spinal cord to affect diverse body areas. Similar to sympathetic function, parasympathetic stimulation excites some tissues, including muscles of the iris, gallbladder and bile ducts, bronchi, and coronary arteries, and inhibits other tissues, including muscles of gut sphincters, intestines, and skin vasculature. Parasympathetic stimulation induces all glandular secretions except for those of the sweat glands.

At the start of and during low-to-moderate–intensity effort, heart rate increases by inhibition of parasympathetic stimulation largely through central command activation (explained in the next section). Heart rate in strenuous activity increases by additional parasympathetic inhibition and direct activation of sympathetic cardioaccelerator nerves. The magnitude of heart rate acceleration relates directly to activity intensity and duration.

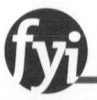

Heart Rate Variability

Heart rate variability refers to the variation in time intervals between heartbeats, usually measured as the variation in R-R time intervals on an ECG tracing over a particular time period (see Fig. 16.2). A wide variation in time intervals generally reflects a "healthy" balance between sympathetic and parasympathetic input to the myocardium, while little variation may reflect a dysfunctional autonomic input. Low heart rate variability relates to increased risk for heart failure, myocardial infarction, and sudden cardiac death. On the brighter side, regular physical activity promotes an increase in heart rate variability.

Central Command: Input from Higher Centers

Impulses originating in the brain's higher somatomotor **central command** center continually modulate medullary activity. The motor center recruits muscles required for physical activity. Impulses from the "feed-forward" central command descend via small afferent nerves through the cardiovascular center in the medulla. This neural input coordinates the rapid adjustment of the heart and blood vessels to optimize tissue perfusion and maintain central blood pressure. This type of neural control operates during the pre-exercise anticipatory period and during the early stage of exercise. Motor cortex stimulation of the medulla increases with the size of the muscle mass activated in physical activity. *Central command provides the greatest control over exercise heart rate.*[26,38,59]

FIGURE 16.6 shows the influence of the central command on heart rate when movement begins. In this experiment, radiotelemetry continuously monitored the heart rate of trained sprint runners at rest, at the starting commands, and during 60-, 220-, and 440-yard races. Heart rate averaged 148 b · min⁻¹ at the starting commands in anticipation of the 60-yard sprint; this represented 74% of the total heart rate adjustment to the run before the run even began. The longer sprint events elicited successively lower anticipatory heart rates. This pattern also occurred for longer-duration endurance events. For example, anticipatory heart rates of four athletes trained for the 880-yard run averaged 122 b · min⁻¹, whereas heart rates averaged 118 b · min⁻¹ during the starting commands of the 1-mile run and 108 b · min⁻¹ immediately before the 2-mile run. A high neural outflow from central command in anticipation of exercise and immediately at the start seems desirable for intense sprint activity to rapidly mobilize physiologic reserves. In contrast, "revving the body's engine" might prove wasteful before distance events. Interestingly, muscle blood flow also increases in anticipation of activity. The response demonstrates training specificity because the magnitude of the pre-exercise increases

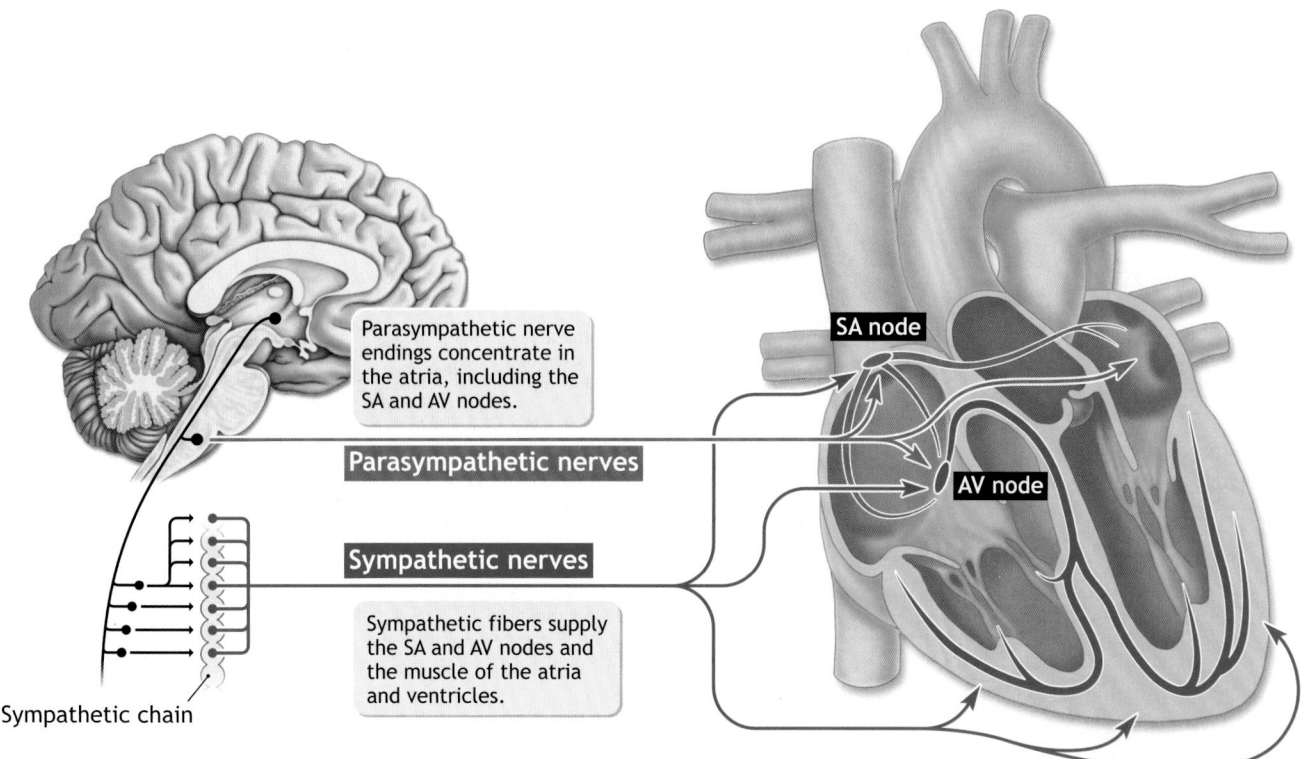

FIGURE 16.4 • Distribution of sympathetic and parasympathetic nerve fibers to the myocardium. Sympathetic nerve fiber endings secrete epinephrine. Sympathetic fibers supply the SA and AV nodes and the muscle of the atria and ventricles. Parasympathetic nerve endings secrete acetylcholine. These fibers concentrate in the atria, including the SA and AV nodes.

in mean arterial pressure and decreases in skeletal muscle vascular resistance varies with physical activity intensity, duration, and specific mode of prior training.[13]

The heart rapidly "turns on" during physical activity by decreasing parasympathetic inhibitory input and increasing stimulating input from the brain's central command. Activation of receptors in active joints and muscles also contributes to accelerator input when activity begins (refer to following section). The much slower contribution to heart rate increase from the sympathetic nervous system—triggered by reflex activity and *not* central command—does not occur until achieving moderate intensity. Even in so-called nonsprint events, heart rate reaches 180 b · min^{-1} within 30 s of 1- and 2-mile runs. Further heart rate increases progress gradually with several plateaus during the run. Almost identical results occur for heart rate measured by telemetry during competitive swimming events except for lower maximum heart rates during swimming.

Central command involvement in cardiovascular regulation also explains how variations in emotional state affect cardiovascular response. Such neural input creates difficulty obtaining "true" resting values for heart rate and blood pressure.

INTEGRATIVE QUESTION

Give a physiologic rationale for biofeedback and relaxation techniques to treat hypertension and stress-related disorders.

Peripheral Input

The cardiovascular center receives reflex sensory input (feedback) from peripheral receptors in blood vessels, joints, and muscles. **Chemoreceptors** and **mechanoreceptors** within muscle and its vasculature monitor the muscle's chemical and physical state. Afferent impulses from these receptors—slow-conducting, thin-fiber group III and IV afferents from pacinian corpuscles and unencapsulated nerve-ending receptors—provide rapid feedback. This input modifies either vagal (parasympathetic) or sympathetic outflow to initiate appropriate cardiovascular and respiratory responses to various physical activity intensities.[18,20,24,48] Activation of chemically sensitive afferents within the muscle's interstitium (interstitial space) helps to regulate sympathetic neural activation of muscle during submaximal effort. Metabolites produced primarily during the concentric phase of muscular activity stimulate this **metaboreflex**.[10] Three mechanisms continually assess the nature and intensity of physical activity and the mass of muscle activated:

1. Reflex neural input from mechanical deformation of type III afferents within active muscles
2. Chemical stimulation of type IV afferents within active muscles (referred to as the **exercise pressor reflex**)
3. Feed-forward outflow from the motor areas of the central command

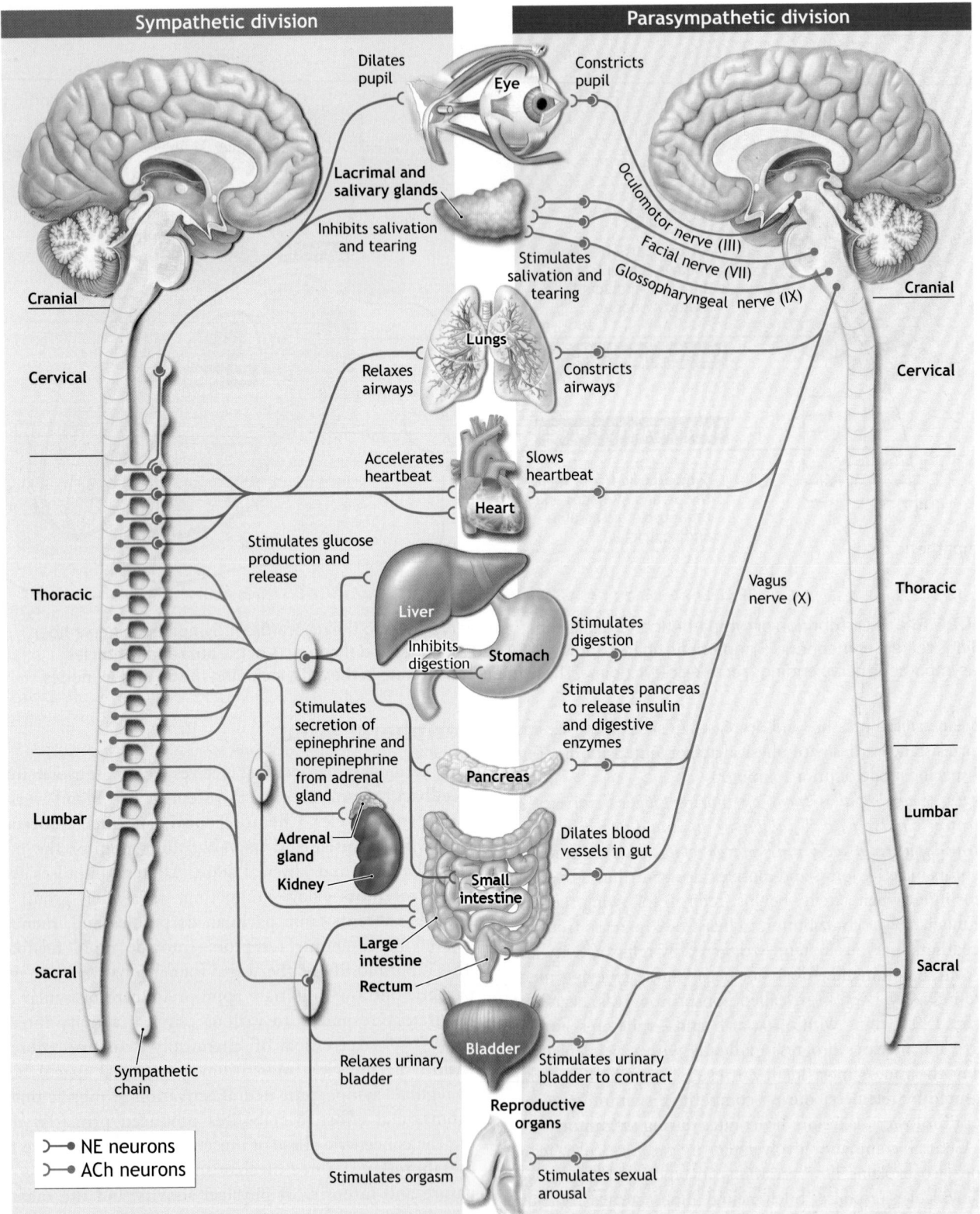

FIGURE 16.5 • Schematic view of the chemical, anatomic, and functional organization of the sympathetic and parasympathetic divisions of the autonomic nervous system. The preganglionic inputs of both divisions use acetylcholine (ACh; *red*) as the neurotransmitter. The postganglionic parasympathetic innervation to the visceral organs also uses ACh, but postganglionic sympathetic innervation uses norepinephrine (NE; *blue*), with the exception that ACh innervates sweat glands. The adrenal medulla receives preganglionic sympathetic innervation and secretes epinephrine into the bloodstream when activated. In general, sympathetic stimulation produces catabolic effects that prepare the body to "fight" or "flee," while parasympathetic stimulation produces anabolic responses that promote normal function and conserve energy. (Adapted with permission from Bear MF, et al. *Neuroscience: Exploring the Brain*. Baltimore: Lippincott Williams & Wilkins, 2006.)

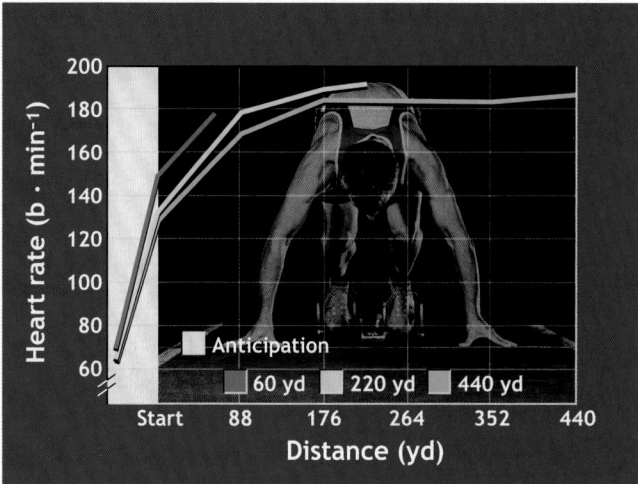

FIGURE 16.6 • Heart rate response of sprint-trained runners. The largest increase in anticipatory heart rate (HR immediately before exercising) occurred in the short-sprint events and was successively smaller before the longer sprints. (Adapted with permission from McArdle WD, et al. Telemetered cardiac response to selected running events. *J Appl Physiol* 1967;23:566.)

Specific mechanoreceptor feedback governs the central nervous system's regulation of blood flow and blood pressure during dynamic physical activity.[52] The aortic arch and carotid sinus contain pressure-sensitive **baroreceptors**, while cardiopulmonary mechanoreceptors assess mechanical activity in the left ventricle, right atrium, and large veins. These receptors function as negative feedback controllers to accomplish the following two functions:[45,60]

1. Inhibit sympathetic outflow from the cardiovascular center
2. Blunt an inordinate rise in arterial blood pressure

As blood pressure increases, stretching of arterial vessels activates baroreceptors to slow the heart reflexively and dilate the peripheral vasculature. This *decreases* blood pressure toward more normal levels. During physical activity, blood pressure remains effectively regulated but at higher levels. This

 **Exercise Pressor Reflex**

Neural signals generated from active muscle provide peripheral feedback to activate cardiovascular control centers in the brainstem (medulla oblongata) that initiate increases and adjustments in heart rate and blood pressure via sympathetic activation and parasympathetic withdrawal. These muscle-sensing mechanoreceptor organs, which are sensitive to stretch or pressure, including the muscle metabolite sensors called chemoreceptors, provide central command with a continual assessment of the mechanical and chemical state of the active muscle. Progressive increases in exercise intensity progressively increase activation of the exercise pressor reflex.

probably occurs from an override of the arterial baroreflex feedback mechanism or an upward resetting of its threshold and/or sensitivity (i.e., reduced baroreflex gain), partly from central command activation.[36,46] The baroreceptors more than likely serve as a brake, curtailing abnormally high blood pressure levels during activity. Regular physical activity improves cardiac baroreflex function and beneficially affects blood pressure regulation without negatively affecting cerebral autoregulation of blood flow. This positive effect is maintained into older age in individuals who exercise regularly.[1]

Carotid Artery Palpation

External pressure against the carotid artery sometimes slows the heart rate due to direct baroreceptor stimulation at the bifurcation of the carotid artery. The potential for bradycardia from **carotid artery palpation** is important to exercise specialists because this location is routinely used to determine heart rate during physical activity. Consistently low heart rate estimation with carotid artery palpation in susceptible individuals would push the person to a higher activity level—certainly an undesirable effect for cardiac patients.

Research in the late 1970s suggested that carotid artery palpation slowed postexercise heart rate and occasionally produced electrocardiographic abnormalities.[57] Subsequent reports indicated rather convincingly for healthy adults and cardiac patients that carotid artery palpation caused little or no heart rate alteration during rest or exercise and recovery.[41,50] Vascular disease can, however, negatively impact carotid sinus sensitivity and produce falsely low heart rate values. An excellent substitute location uses pulse rate measured at the radial artery (thumb side of wrist) or temporal artery at the side of the head at the temple; firm palpation of these vessels does not affect heart rate.

Local Factors

The byproducts of energy metabolism provide an autoregulatory mechanism within the muscle to augment perfusion during physical activity. We discuss the local control of circulation in the following sections.

DISTRIBUTION OF BLOOD

If fully dilated, the body's blood vessels could hold approximately 20 L of blood, four times more than the actual average total blood volume of 5 L. Thus, maintenance of blood flow and blood pressure, particularly during physical activity, requires a finely regulated balance between vascular dilation and vascular constriction. *The capacity of large portions of the vasculature to constrict or dilate provides rapid blood redistribution to meet metabolic requirements. It also optimizes blood pressure throughout the vascular circuit.*

Physical Factors Affect Blood Flow

Blood flows through the vascular circuit generally following physical laws of hydrodynamics applied to rigid, cylindrical vessels. The volume of flow in any vessel relates to two factors:

IN A PRACTICAL SENSE

Electrode Placement for Bipolar and 12-Lead ECG Recordings

Recording the heart's electrical activity began in 1841, when Italian physicist Carlo Matteuci (1811–1868) documented biologist Luigi Galvani's (1737–1798; www.corrosion-doctors.org/Biographies/GalvaniBio.htm) theory of the electrical properties of frog muscles. Seven years later, following considerable experiments also with frogs, world-renowned German electrophysiologist Emil Dubois-Reymond (1818–1868; www.informationphilosopher.com/solutions/philosophers/bois-reymond/) described the experimental setups, instruments, and frog preparations to explain the properties of electrical transmission through biologic tissues. In 1890, British physiologists Sir William Maddock Bayliss (1860–1924) and Ernest Starling (1866–1927) of University College, London, connected the terminals from a capillary electrometer to the subject's right hand and skin over the apex of the heart. This setup produced a pattern that showed a "triphasic variation accompanying, or rather preceding, each beat of the heart."

The electrocardiogram (ECG) represents a composite record of the heart's electrical events during a cardiac cycle. These events provide a way to monitor heart rate during different physical activities and exercise stress testing. A valid ECG tracing requires proper electrode placement. The term *ECG lead* indicates the specific placement of a pair of electrodes on the body that transmits the electrical signal to a recorder. The record of electrical differences across different ECG leads creates the composite electrical "picture" of myocardial activity.

SKIN PREPARATION

Proper skin preparation reduces extraneous electrical "noise" (interference and skeletal muscle artifact). Abrading the skin with fine sandpaper or commercially available pads and alcohol removes surface epidermis and oil; when done properly, the skin should appear red, slightly irritated, dry, and clean.

BIPOLAR (3-ELECTRODE) CONFIGURATION

The top figure shows the typical electrode placement for a 3-lead bipolar configuration. This positioning provides less sensitivity for diagnostic testing but proves useful for routine ECG monitoring in functional exercise testing and radiotelemetry of the ECG during physical activity. The ground (*green* or *black*) electrode attaches over the sternum; the positive (*red*) electrode attaches on the left side of the chest in the V_5 position (level of the fifth intercostal space adjacent to the midaxillary line); and the positive (*white*) electrode attaches on the right side of the chest just below the nipple at the level of the fifth intercostal space. Placement of the positive electrode can be altered to optimize the recording (e.g., third and fourth intercostal spaces, anterior portion of the right shoulder, or near the clavicle). Correct electrode placement can be remembered as follows: *white to right, green to ground, red to left.*

MODIFIED 12-LEAD (10-ELECTRODE TORSO-MOUNTED) CONFIGURATION FOR EXERCISE STRESS TESTING

The standard 12-lead ECG consists of three limb leads, three augmented unipolar leads, and six chest leads. For improved exercise ECG recordings, electrodes mounted on the torso (abdominal level) replace the conventional ankle (leg) and wrist electrodes. This "torso-mounted limb lead system"

(bottom figure) reduces electrical artifact introduced by limb movement during physical activity.

ELECTRODE POSITIONING FOR THE MODIFIED 10-ELECTRODE, TORSO-MOUNTED SYSTEM

1. RL (right leg): just above right iliac crest on midaxillary line
2. LL (left leg): just above left iliac crest on midaxillary line
3. RA (right arm): just below right clavicle medial to deltoid muscle
4. LA (left arm): just below left clavicle medial to deltoid muscle
5. V_1: on right sternal border in fourth intercostal space
6. V_2: on left sternal border in fourth intercostal space
7. V_3: at midpoint of a straight line between V_2 and V_4
8. V_4: on midclavicular line in fifth intercostal space
9. V_5: on anterior axillary line and horizontal to V_4
10. V_6: on midaxillary line and horizontal to V_4 and V_5

Source: Phibbs B, Buckels L. Comparative yields of ECG leads in multistage stress testing. *Am Heart J* 1985;90:275.

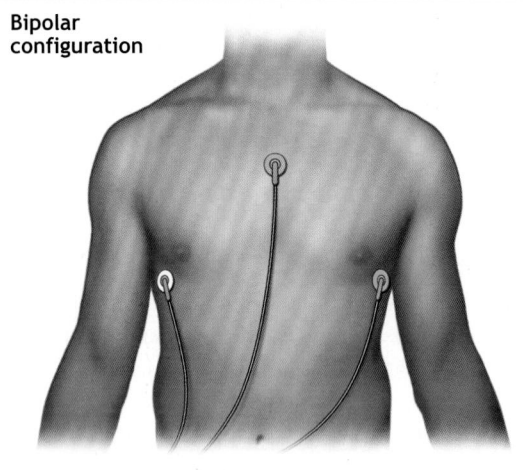

Bipolar configuration

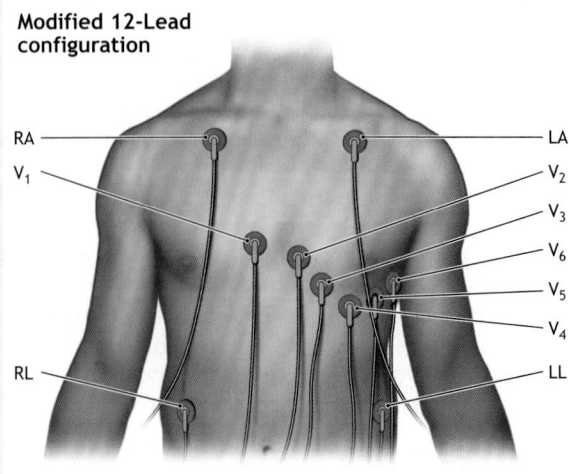

Modified 12-Lead configuration

RA — LA
V_1 — V_2
— V_3
— V_6
— V_5
— V_4
RL — LL

1. *Directly* to the pressure gradient between the two ends of the vessels, *not* to the absolute pressure within the vessel
2. *Inversely* to the resistance encountered to fluid flow

Friction between the blood and internal vascular wall creates resistance or force that impedes blood flow. Three factors determine resistance:

1. Blood thickness or viscosity
2. Length of the conducting tube
3. Blood vessel radius (probably the most important factor)

In 1838, French physician and physiologist Jean Louis Marie Poiseuille (1797–1869; http://mahi.ucsd.edu/guy/sio224/stokes-part2.pdf) derived an equation, later named **Poiseuille's law** in his honor, to express the general relationship among pressure differential, resistance, and flow. The *poise*, represents a standard unit of viscosity or resistance to flow. Poiseuille's law links the three determinants of resistance to flow listed above and pressure gradient to express the general relationship among pressure differential, resistance, and fluid flow through rigid cylindrical tubes as follows:

$$\text{Flow} = \text{Pressure gradient} \times \text{Vessel radius}^4 \div \text{Vessel length} \times \text{Fluid viscosity}$$

In the body, the transport vessel length remains constant, while blood viscosity varies only slightly under most conditions. The radius of the conducting tube affects blood flow the most because resistance to flow changes with the vessel's radius raised to the fourth power. For example, halving a vessel's radius decreases flow 16-fold. Conversely, doubling the radius increases volume 16-fold. With the pressure differential within the vascular circuit remaining constant, a small change in vessel radius dramatically alters blood flow. *Physiologically, constriction and dilation of the smaller arterial blood vessels provide the crucial mechanism to regulate regional blood flow.*

Exercise Effect

Any increase in energy expenditure requires rapid adjustments in blood flow that impact the entire cardiovascular system. For example, nerves and local metabolites act on smooth muscle bands of arteriole walls to alter their internal diameter almost instantaneously to meet the blood flow demands of an increased metabolism. Visceral vasoconstriction and muscle pump action divert a large flow of blood into the central circulation.

At movement onset, the vascular component of active muscles increases by dilation of local arterioles. These small-supply arteries to skeletal muscle normally possess well-developed flow-mediated and myogenic regulatory mechanisms. They require little modification through training to adequately supply the blood flow requirements of vigorous physical activity.[27] Concurrently, other vessels to tissues that can temporarily compromise their blood supply constrict, or "shut down." Two examples include the splanchnic and renal areas. Here, blood flow decreases in proportion to relative exercise intensity (i.e., %$\dot{V}O_{2max}$). Blood flow shifts from the abdominal viscera to active muscles even during relatively light exertion (HR ≤90 b · min⁻¹).[42] Two factors contribute to reduced blood flow to nonactive tissues:[33,34,37]

1. Increased sympathetic nervous system outflow (central and peripheral mechanisms)
2. Local chemicals that directly stimulate vasoconstriction or enhance the effects of other vasoconstrictors

The kidney vividly illustrates regional blood flow adjustment and conservation of bodily fluids via sympathetic vasoconstriction of its vasculature. Renal blood flow at rest normally averages 1100 mL per minute (20% of the total cardiac output), among the highest blood flow to any organ as either a percentage of cardiac output or relative to organ weight. During maximal effort, renal blood flow decreases to 250 mL per minute or only 1% of the total cardiac output. A large but temporary reduction in blood flow also occurs in the liver, pancreas, and gastrointestinal tract.[48]

 See the animation "Renal Function" on http://thePoint.lww.com/mkk8e for a demonstration of this process.

Factors Within Active Muscle

Skeletal muscle blood flow closely couples to metabolic demands. Regulation occurs from the interaction of neural vasoconstriction activity and locally derived vasoactive substances within active tissues' vascular endothelium and red blood cells.[12,15,49,58]

At rest, only one of every 30 to 40 capillaries in muscle tissue remains open. The opening of dormant capillaries during physical activity serves three important functions:

1. Increases total muscle blood flow
2. Delivers a large blood volume with only a minimal increase in blood flow velocity
3. Increases the effective surface for gas and nutrient exchange between blood and muscle fibers

Vasodilation occurs from local factors related to tissue metabolism that act directly on the smooth muscle bands of small arterioles and precapillary sphincters. This rapid response adjusts precisely to the muscle's force output and metabolic needs. Decreased tissue oxygen supply serves as a potent local stimulus for vasodilation in skeletal and cardiac muscle. Additionally, local increases in blood flow, temperature, carbon dioxide, acidity, adenosine, magnesium and potassium ions, and nitric oxide production by endothelial cells lining the blood vessels trigger the discharge of relaxing factors that enhance regional blood flow.[14,19,32] The venous system also may increase local blood flow by "assessing" increases in the metabolic needs of active muscle and releasing vasodilatory factors from venular endothelial cells that diffuse to and dilate the adjacent arteriole.[21] The **autoregulatory mechanisms** for blood flow make sense physiologically because they reflect elevated tissue metabolism and increased oxygen need.

Local regulation provides such strong control that it maintains adequate regional blood flow even in patients in whom the nerves to blood vessels have been surgically removed. Local metabolite stimulation of chemoreceptors also provides peripheral neural reflex input for medullary control of the heart and vasculature.

Nitric Oxide and Autoregulation of Tissue Blood Flow. **Nitric oxide (NO)** serves as an important signaling molecule that dilates blood vessels and decreases vascular resistance. This gas is a common, unstable industrial and automotive air pollutant formed when nitrogen burns. Most living organisms naturally produce this vascular gatekeeper from its precursor L-arginine. Stimuli from diverse signal chemicals (including neurotransmitters) and sheering stress and vessel stretch from increased blood flow through the vessel lumen provoke NO synthesis and release by the vascular endothelium. Formerly termed *endothelium-derived relaxing factor* by 1998 Nobel Prize in Physiology or Medicine corecipient Robert F. Furchgott (1916–2009; for discovering nitric oxide as a signaling molecule in the cardiovascular system; www.nobelprize.org/nobel_prizes/medicine/laureates/1998/furchgott-bio.html), NO rapidly spreads through underlying cell membranes to smooth muscle cells within the arterial wall. Here it binds with and activates *guanylyl cyclase*, an enzyme important in cellular communication and signal transduction. This initiates a cascade of reactions that attenuate sympathetic vasoconstriction and induce arterial smooth muscle relaxation to increase blood flow in neighboring blood vessels. NO exerts its potent vasodilator effect on skeletal muscle (including the diaphragm), spongelike vascular tissues, skin, and myocardial tissue (**Fig. 16.7**).[4,8,22,23,54]

NO mediates bodily functions as diverse as olfaction, inhibition of blood clot formation, and enhanced immune response regulation, and acts as an interneuron or signaling messenger. It also contributes to cutaneous active vasodilation during heat stress and rapidly dilates the coronary vasculature as an early adaptation to moderate exercise training.[28,29,57,55] Vascular wall receptors for NO contribute to blood pressure regulation in response to central cardiovascular stimulation during emotionally stressful situations including physical activity. Racial differences in resting blood pressure relate to a lower sensitivity to NO's dilating action in blacks than in whites.[9] In coronary artery disease, the endothelium produces less NO. Reduced NO bioavailability explains the potent beneficial effect of exogenous nitroglycerin treatment (which releases NO gas) to reverse chest discomfort or pain called angina pectoris from inadequate oxygen delivery brought about by coronary vessel disease.

Hormonal Factors

Sympathetic nerves terminate in the medullary portion of the adrenal glands. With sympathetic activation, this glandular tissue secretes large quantities of epinephrine and a smaller amount of norepinephrine into the blood. These hormonal chemical messengers induce a generalized constrictor response, except in blood vessels of the heart and skeletal muscles. Hormonal control of regional blood flow plays a relatively minor role during physical activity compared with the more local, rapid, and potent sympathetic neural drive.

INTEGRATIVE RESPONSE DURING PHYSICAL ACTIVITY

The neural command center above the medullary region initiates cardiovascular changes immediately before and at movement onset. Heart rate and myocardial contractility increase from feed-forward input from this center, which also suppresses parasympathetic activation. Concurrently, predictable alterations in regional blood flow occur in proportion to exercise severity. Modulation of vascular dilation and constriction optimizes blood flow to areas in need while maintaining blood pressure throughout the arterial system. As activity continues, reflex feedback to the medulla from peripheral mechanical and chemical receptors in active tissue appraises tissue metabolism and circulatory needs. Local metabolic factors act directly to dilate resistance vessels in active muscles. Vasodilation reduces peripheral resistance

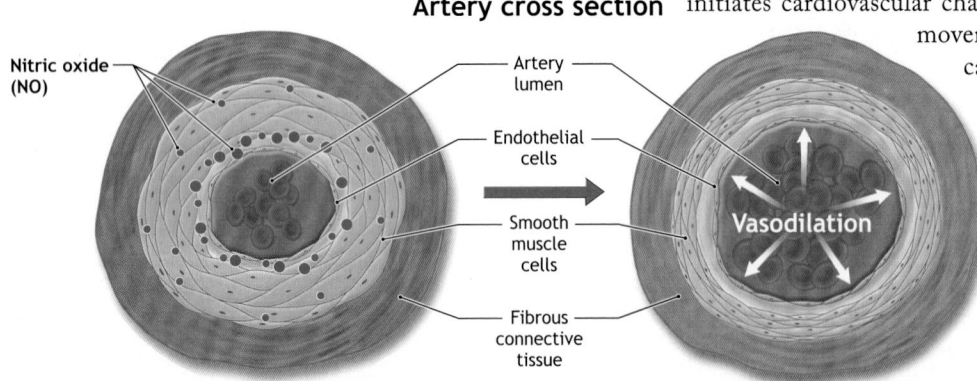

Artery cross section

Nitric oxide (NO) — Artery lumen — Endothelial cells — Smooth muscle cells — Fibrous connective tissue — Vasodilation

Role of Nitric Oxide

- Endothelial cells within blood vessels release nitric oxide (NO) gas, which initiates a cascade of events that attenuate sympathetic vasoconstriction and induce arterial smooth muscle relaxation to increase blood flow
- NO is either released by autonomic neurons and synthesized by the vascular endothelium or from drugs like Viagra or nitroglycerin (and related heart drugs), which cause vasodilation by stimulating NO gas release.
- Vasodilation occurs when NO penetrates smooth muscle cells.

FIGURE 16.7 • Mechanism for how nitric oxide regulates local blood flow.

for greater blood flow in these areas. Arterial blood flow through active muscles progresses in pulsatile oscillations that favor enhanced flow during eccentric (lengthening) muscle actions and/or the recovery phases of concentric (shortening) actions.[47] Centrally mediated constrictor adjustments also occur in the vasculature of inactive tissues, including skin, kidneys, the splanchnic region, and inactive muscle. Constrictor action maintains adequate perfusion pressure within active muscle while simultaneously increasing blood supply to meet metabolic demands.

 Venous Return Important

Factors that affect venous return are equally as important as those that regulate arterial blood flow. Muscle and ventilatory pump actions and visceral vasoconstriction immediately return blood to the right ventricle when exercise movement begins and continue to facilitate venous return as cardiac output increases. These adjustments balance venous return with cardiac output. In upright activity, gravity impedes return of blood from the extremities, thus making venous blood flow regulation crucial.

PHYSICAL ACTIVITY AFTER CARDIAC TRANSPLANTATION

Patients with left ventricular dysfunction—ejection fraction less than 20% referred to as *end-stage heart disease*—show poor long-term prognosis. For them, cardiac transplantation becomes their only hope of survival. From 1988 through 2012 approximately 32,000 heart transplants were performed in the United States. The yearly average of 2200 heart transplants range from newborns and children to the older elderly. Success with heart transplantation during the past decade has paved the way for multiple organ transplants—heart-lung, heart-kidney, and heart-liver. The 1-year survival of heart transplant patients averages close to 90% (www.uptodate.com/contents/heart-transplantation-beyond-the-basics).

Cardiac transplantation, also called **orthotopic transplantation**, illustrates the importance of extrinsic neural control of exercise heart rate. The procedure removes donor and recipient hearts by transection at the midatrial level—preserving the recipient's pulmonary venous connections of the posterior wall of the left atrium—and transection of the aorta just above the semilunar valves. Transplantation eliminates neural innervation of the myocardium, although hormonal feedback from circulating catecholamines largely from the adrenal medulla remains intact (**Fig. 16.8A**).

Improved Function but Altered Circulatory Dynamics

Following successful transplantation, patients generally report a favorable quality of life, and approximately 50% of individuals return to work. In general, a transplant patient demonstrates prolonged oxygen uptake kinetics, impaired exercise capacity, and diminished physiologic and hemodynamic function that rarely exceeds 45 to 70% of normal.[2,6,17,39,56] This does not necessarily represent the rule for younger, previously active patients who adhere to rehabilitation.[43] In general, heart transplant recipients can perform relatively intense training, and often achieve performance values of moderately trained healthy subjects.[11,25,40,44]

Figure 16.9A–C illustrates peak oxygen consumption ($\dot{V}O_{2peak}$) for an initial pool of 140 patients evaluated prior to transplantation and up to 9 years after the procedure. Cardiac transplantation produced an average 50% improvement in $\dot{V}O_{2peak}$ (Fig. 16.9A) from 14.2 mL·kg^{-1}·min^{-1} before to 21.4 mL·kg^{-1}·min^{-1} 11.2 months after surgery. The patients maintained improved aerobic capacity up to 9 years postsurgery (Fig. 16.9B). Figure 16.9C shows that younger patients exhibited the greatest improvement following transplantation.

Sluggish Circulatory Response

The short-term exercise response for transplant patients classifies as abnormal. These patients demonstrate limited cardiac output and oxygen consumption during exertion, with accompanying reduced left ventricular ejection capacity. Figure 16.9B reveals that circulatory sluggishness results from the denervated heart's inability to accelerate significantly with increasing physical demands, often it accelerates by only 20 to 40 b·min^{-1}.[3,16,35] The exercise response of the denervated transplanted heart does improve over the 12-month postsurgery period, yet the adaptations exert no meaningful effect on submaximal or peak oxygen consumption.

In healthy individuals, stroke volume increases up to approximately 50% of $\dot{V}O_{2max}$ and then plateaus; further increases in cardiac output come mainly from increases in heart rate. Transplant patients, in contrast, have no stroke volume plateau during graded exercise; instead, stroke volume progressively increases by the Frank-Starling mechanism (i.e., progressive increases in cardiac filling) throughout the exercise range. Chapter 32 discusses the effects of regular training for the heart transplant patient.

 INTEGRATIVE QUESTION

Explain the following statement: Task-specific, regular aerobic physical activity not only trains the cardiovascular system, but also "trains" the neuromuscular system to facilitate physiologic adjustments specific to the activity mode.

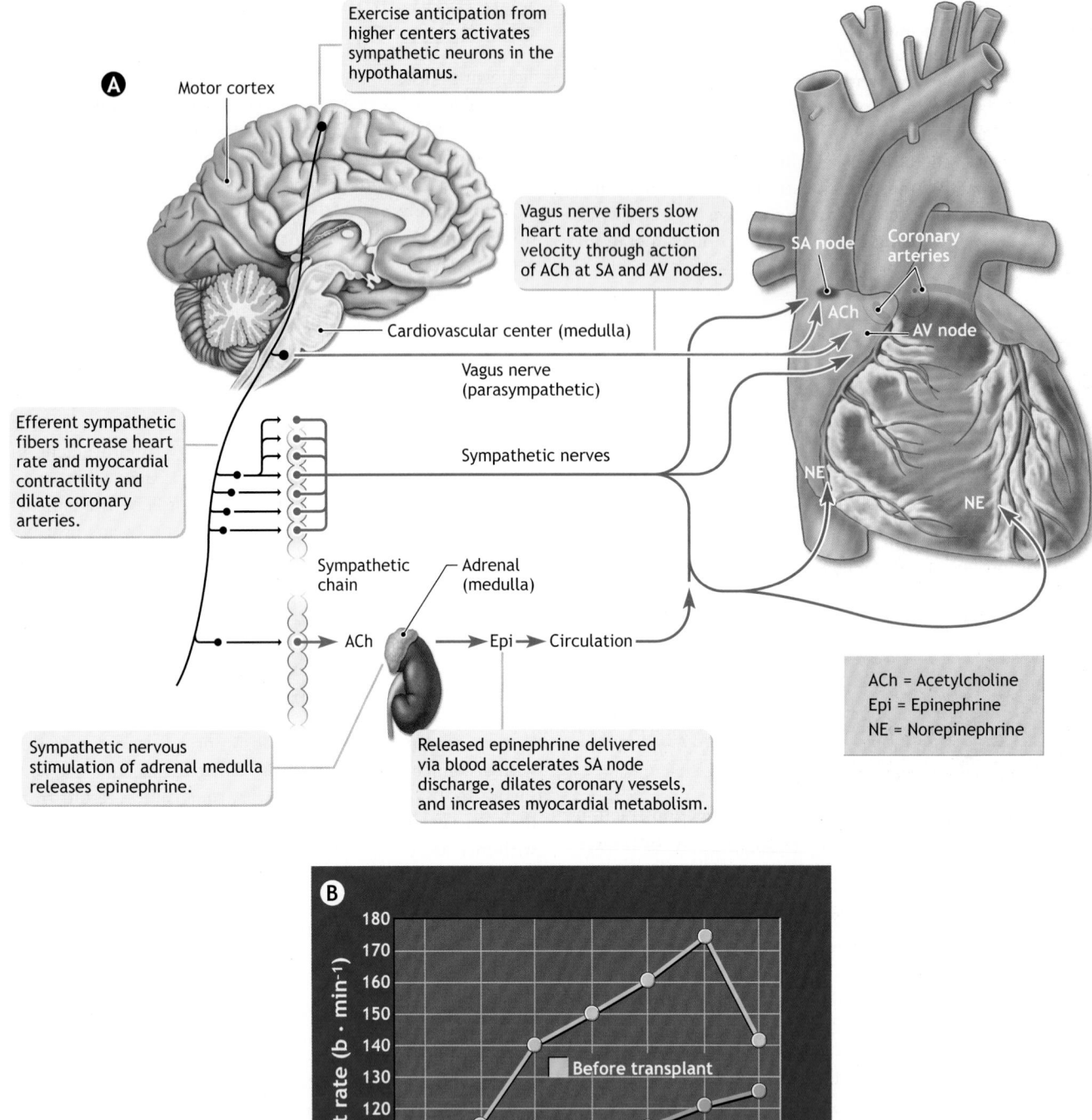

FIGURE 16.8 • **(A)** Regulation of heart rate under normal conditions. Heart transplantation produces cardiac denervation by removing vagal and sympathetic efferent stimulation to the myocardium. Circulating epinephrine from the adrenal medulla provides the primary mechanism to regulate exercise heart rate. **(B)** Heart rate response of a patient during graded exercise before and after orthotopic cardiac transplantation. Note the elevated resting heart rate and delayed and depressed heart rate response following transplantation. (B, adapted with permission from Squires RW. Exercise training after cardiac transplantation. *Med Sci Sports Exerc* 1991;23:686.)

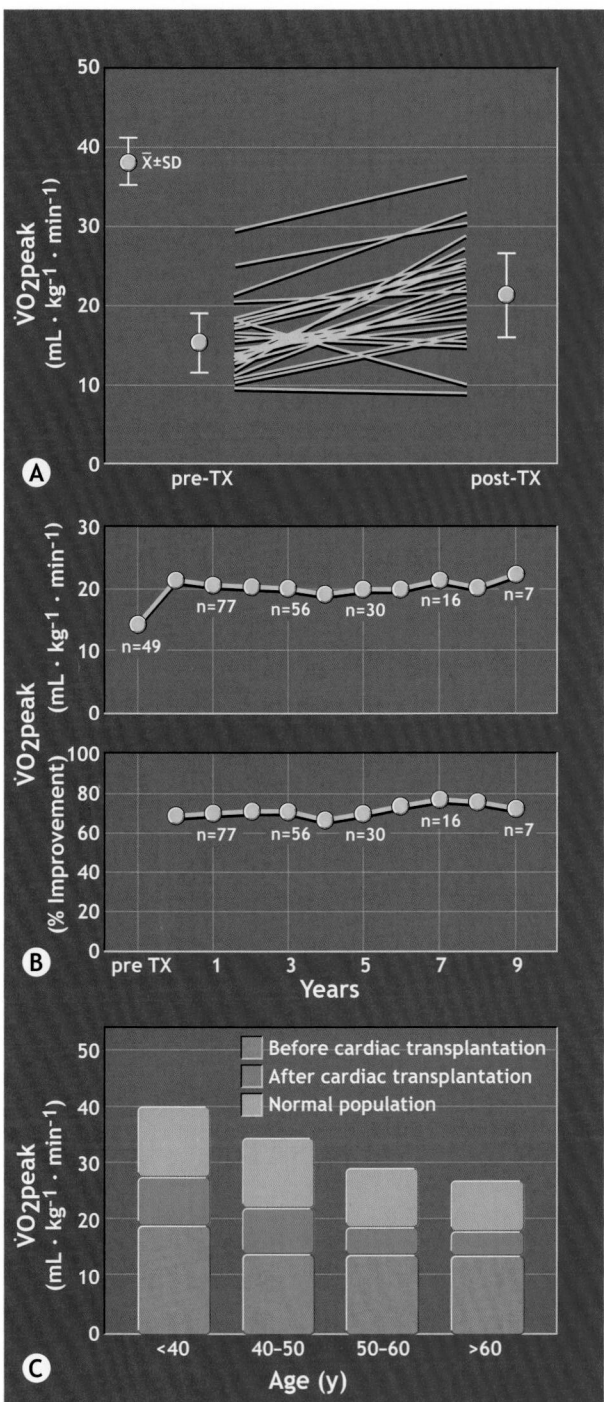

FIGURE 16.9 • Long-term effects of heart transplantation (TX) on aerobic functional capacity. **(A)** $\dot{V}O_{2peak}$ before and 11.2 months after cardiac transplantation in 43 patients who underwent testing at both intervals. Post-TX average is significantly higher than pre-TX. **(B)** Significant improvements in peak oxygen consumption ($\dot{V}O_{2peak}$) and percentage improvement occurred as early as 6 months after transplantation and remained improved up to 9 years after the transplant procedure. **(C)** Impact of age on improvement in $\dot{V}O_{2peak}$ in 43 patients who underwent exercise testing before and 1 year after cardiac transplantation. (Adapted with permission from Osada N, et al. Long-term cardiopulmonary exercise performance after heart transplantation. *Am J Cardiol* 1997;79:451.)

Summary

1. The cardiovascular system provides rapid heart rate regulation and effective distribution of blood through the vascular circuit (while maintaining blood pressure) in response to overall metabolic and physiologic needs.

2. The cardiac rhythm originates at the SA node. The impulse then travels across the atria to the AV node and, after a brief delay, spreads across the large ventricular mass. This conduction pattern initiates atrial and ventricular contractions to provide impetus for blood flow.

3. The electrocardiogram (ECG) records the sequence of the heart's electrical events during the cardiac cycle. The ECG detects various heart function abnormalities during rest and increasing intensity of effort.

4. Epinephrine and norepinephrine accelerate heart rate and increase myocardial contractility, while acetylcholine acts through the vagus nerve to slow heart rate.

5. The heart "turns on" in the transition from rest to physical activity from increased sympathetic and decreased parasympathetic activity integrated with central command input.

6. Cortical influence in anticipation before and during the initial stage of physical activity governs a substantial part of the heart rate adjustment to the activity.

7. Reflex sensory input from peripheral receptors in blood vessels, joints, and muscles provides the cardiovascular center with continual feedback about the physical and chemical state of active muscles.

8. Neural and hormonal extrinsic factors modify the heart's inherent rhythm.

9. The heart rate rapidly accelerates in anticipation of exercise and can reach about 200 b·min^{-1} in maximal effort.

10. Carotid artery palpation accurately accesses heart rate during and immediately after exercise in healthy individuals.

11. Nerves, hormones, and local metabolic factors act on the smooth muscle bands in blood vessels to alter the vessels' internal diameter and regulate blood flow to metabolic demands.

12. Blood flow changes with the vessels' radius raised to the fourth power in accord with Poiseuille's law.

13. Nitric oxide, an extraordinarily important and potent endothelium-derived relaxing factor, facilitates blood vessel dilation and decreases vascular resistance.

14. The kidneys and splanchnic regions dramatically compromise their blood flow in physical activity to augment delivery of blood to the muscles and maintain systemic blood pressure.

15. Patients who successfully undergo orthotopic transplantation have a depressed cardiovascular response to exercise; the denervated heart cannot accelerate rapidly to meet the increased demands of physical activity.

thePoint References are available online at **http://thepoint.lww.com/mkk8e.**

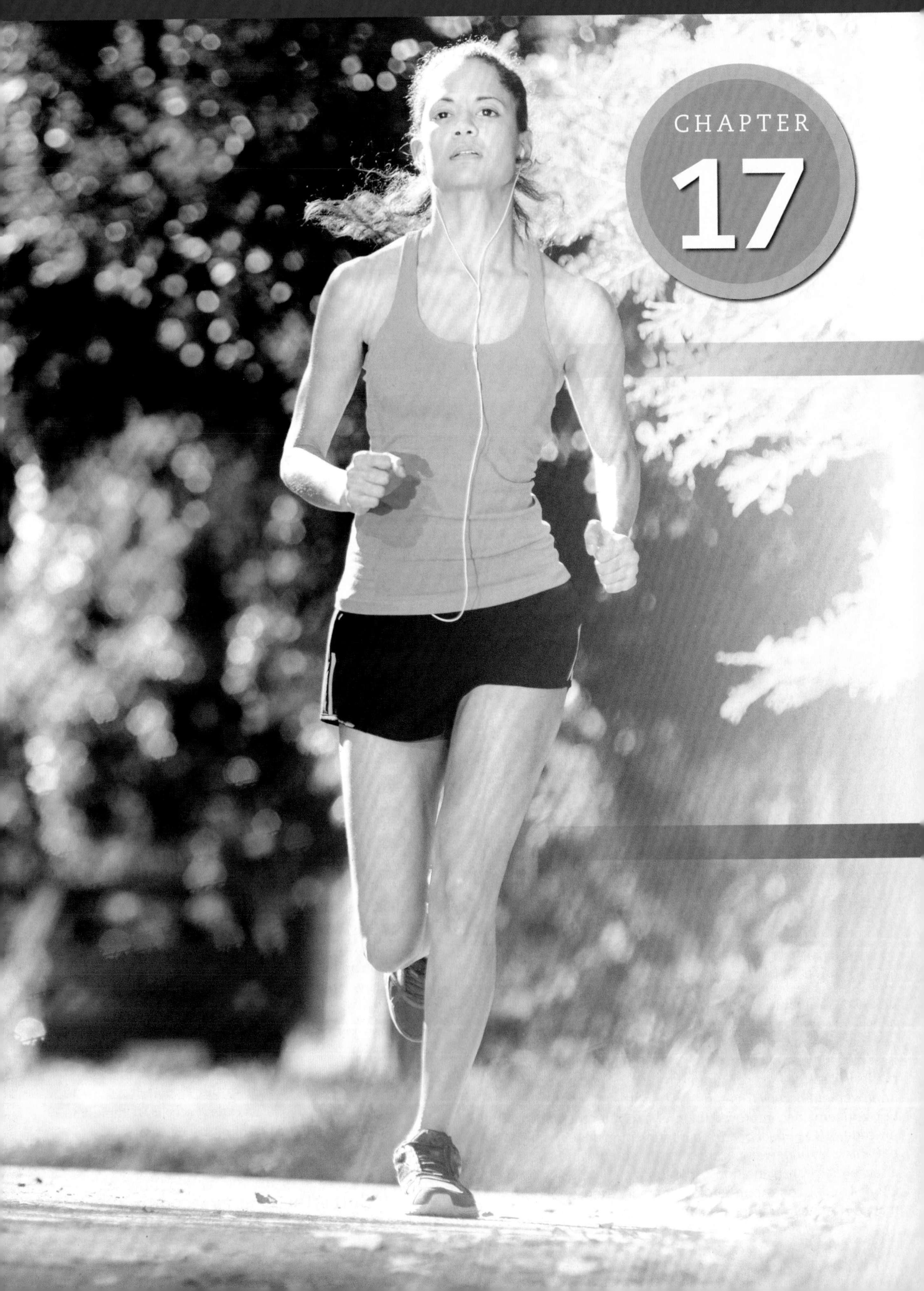

CHAPTER

17

Functional Capacity of the Cardiovascular System

CHAPTER OBJECTIVES

- Discuss advantages and disadvantages of the direct Fick, indicator dilution, and CO_2 rebreathing methods to measure cardiac output

- Compare cardiac output during rest and maximal effort for an endurance-trained and sedentary person

- Explain the influence of each component of the Fick equation on $\dot{V}O_{2max}$

- Discuss two physiologic mechanisms that influence exercise stroke volume

- Contrast the components of cardiac output during rest and maximal effort for sedentary and endurance-trained individuals

- Discuss the contribution of the Frank-Starling mechanism to augment cardiac output during different physical activity modes

- Outline the dynamics and proposed mechanisms for cardiovascular drift

- Outline cardiac output distribution to major body tissues during rest and intense aerobic physical activity

- Describe the relationship between maximal cardiac output and $\dot{V}O_{2max}$ among individuals who vary in aerobic fitness

- Give three factors that contribute to expanding the a-$\bar{v}O_2$ difference during graded exercise

- Contrast cardiovascular and metabolic dynamics during upper-body versus lower-body graded exercise

ANCILLARIES ◉ at-a-Glance

Visit http://thePoint.lww.com/mkk8e to access the following resources.

- References: Chapter 17
- Interactive Question Bank
- Animation: Blood Flow
- Animation: Myocardial Blood Flow
- Focus on Research: Consequences of Stopping Endurance Exercise Training

CARDIAC OUTPUT

Cardiac output ($\dot{Q}$ meaning quantity) expresses the amount of blood pumped by the heart during a 1-min period. The maximal value reflects the functional capacity of the cardiovascular system. Output from the heart, as with any pump, depends on its rate of pumping (**heart rate, HR**) and quantity of blood ejected with each stroke (**stroke volume, SV**). Cardiac output computes as follows:

Cardiac output = Heart rate × Stroke volume

 See the animation "Blood Flow" on **http://thePoint. lww.com/mkk8e** for a demonstration of this process.

Measuring Cardiac Output

The output from a hose, pump, or faucet is determined by opening the valve and collecting and measuring the volume of fluid ejected over a given time. To more fully understand cardiac output dynamics, we describe three common methods of measurement to assess the cardiac output of a closed circulatory system in humans:

1. Direct Fick
2. Indicator dilution
3. CO_2 rebreathing

Direct Fick Method

Two factors determine the output of fluid from a pump in a closed circuit:

1. Change in concentration of a substance between the outflow and inflow ports of the pump
2. Total quantity of that substance taken up or given off by the fluid in a given time

For cardiovascular dynamics, calculating cardiac output requires knowledge of two variables:

1. Average difference between the oxygen content of arterial and mixed-venous blood (a-$\bar{v}O_2$ difference)
2. Oxygen consumption during 1 min ($\dot{V}O_2$)

The question then becomes how much blood circulates during the minute to account for the observed oxygen consumption given the observed a-$\bar{v}O_2$ difference.

The **Fick equation**, published in 1870 by noted German mathematician/physiologist/physicist Adolph Gaston Fick (1829–1901; first to devise a technique to measure cardiac output), expresses the relationships among cardiac output, oxygen consumption, and a-$\bar{v}O_2$ difference. These variables could not be determined in humans until the perfection of cardiac catheterization as a clinical tool.

$$\text{Cardiac output} \atop (mL \cdot min^{-1})} = \frac{\dot{V}O_2\, mL \cdot min^{-1}}{\text{a-}\bar{v}O_2 \text{ difference} \atop (mL\, per\, 100\, mL\, blood)} \times 100$$

FIGURE 17.1 illustrates the use of the Fick principle to determine cardiac output. In this example, 250 mL of oxygen is consumed during 1 min at rest, and the a-$\bar{v}O_2$ difference during this time averages 5 mL of oxygen per 100 mL (deciliter [dL]) of blood. Cardiac output computes as follows by substituting these values in the Fick equation:

$$\text{Cardiac output} \atop (mL \cdot min^{-1})} = \frac{250\, mL\, O_2}{5\, mL\, O_2} \times 100 = 5000\, mL\, blood$$

Although straightforward in principle, the Fick method to determine cardiac output requires complex methodology usually performed in a hospital. Measuring oxygen consumption involves open-circuit spirometry methods (see Chapter 8). Measuring a-$\bar{v}O_2$ difference remains the more difficult task. A representative sample of arterial blood can come from any convenient systemic artery such as femoral, radial, or brachial. These arteries are easily located, but puncturing the artery with a needle confers risk, and sampling mixed-venous blood presents additional difficulties because the blood in each vein only reflects the metabolic activity of the specific area it drains. *An accurate estimate of the average oxygen content of all venous blood requires sampling from an anatomic "mixing chamber" such as the right atrium, right ventricle, or most accurately, the pulmonary artery.* Such sampling requires threading a small flexible catheter through the antecubital vein in the arm into the superior vena cava that drains into the right heart. Arterial and mixed-venous blood then are sampled simultaneously with measurement of oxygen consumption.

Studies of cardiovascular dynamics have applied the direct Fick method under various experimental conditions. The method generally serves as the criterion standard to validate other techniques for cardiac output measurement. The *invasive* nature of the Fick method can alter normal cardiovascular dynamics during the measurement period that may not reflect the person's usual cardiovascular response.

Indicator Dilution Method

The **indicator dilution method** involves venous and arterial punctures with a needle but does not require cardiac catheterization. A known quantity of an inert dye (e.g., indocyanine green) whose concentration curve can be measured in blood by light absorption is injected into a large vein. The indicator material remains in the vascular stream usually bound to plasma proteins or red blood cells. It then mixes in the blood as the blood travels to the lungs and returns to the heart before ejection throughout the systemic circuit. A photosensitive device continually assesses arterial blood samples. The area under the dilution–concentration curve obtained by repetitive sampling reflects the average concentration of indicator material in blood leaving the heart. Cardiac output computes as follows from the dilution of a known quantity of dye in an unknown quantity of blood:

$$\text{Cardiac output} = \frac{\text{Quantity of dye injected}}{\text{Average dye concentration in blood} \atop \text{for duration of curve} \times \text{Duration of curve}}$$

CO₂ Rebreathing Method

One can determine cardiac output by substituting CO_2 values for O_2 values in the Fick equation.[18,35] The same open-circuit spirometric method to determine oxygen consumption in the typical Fick technique determines CO_2 production in the rebreathing method. Using a rapid CO_2 gas analyzer and making reasonable assumptions about gas exchange provides valid estimates of mixed-venous and arterial CO_2 levels. This noninvasive or "bloodless" technique requires breath-by-breath CO_2 analysis, a technique common in today's exercise physiology laboratories. Values for CO_2 production and mixed-venous and arterial CO_2 concentrations, derived from expired CO_2 obtained during different times, provide the data to compute cardiac output in accordance with the Fick principle as follows:

$$\text{Cardiac output (mL} \cdot \text{min}^{-1}) = \frac{\dot{V}CO_2}{\bar{v}\text{-a } CO_2 \text{ difference}} \times 100$$

The CO_2 rebreathing method offers obvious advantages over the direct Fick and indicator dilution methods, particularly during physical activity. It does not require blood sampling or intense medical supervision and only minimally interferes with the subject during movement. One limitation of CO_2 rebreathing requires that subjects exercise under steady-rate aerobic metabolism. This restricts the method's use during maximal and "supermaximal" activities and in the transition from rest to exercise.

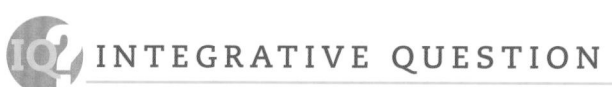

INTEGRATIVE QUESTION

In what way does the Fick equation fully explain the physiologic components that determine $\dot{V}O_{2max}$?

CARDIAC OUTPUT AT REST

An individual's cardiac output can vary considerably during rest. Influencing factors include emotional conditions that alter cortical outflow (central command) to the cardioaccelerator nerves and nerves that modulate arterial resistance

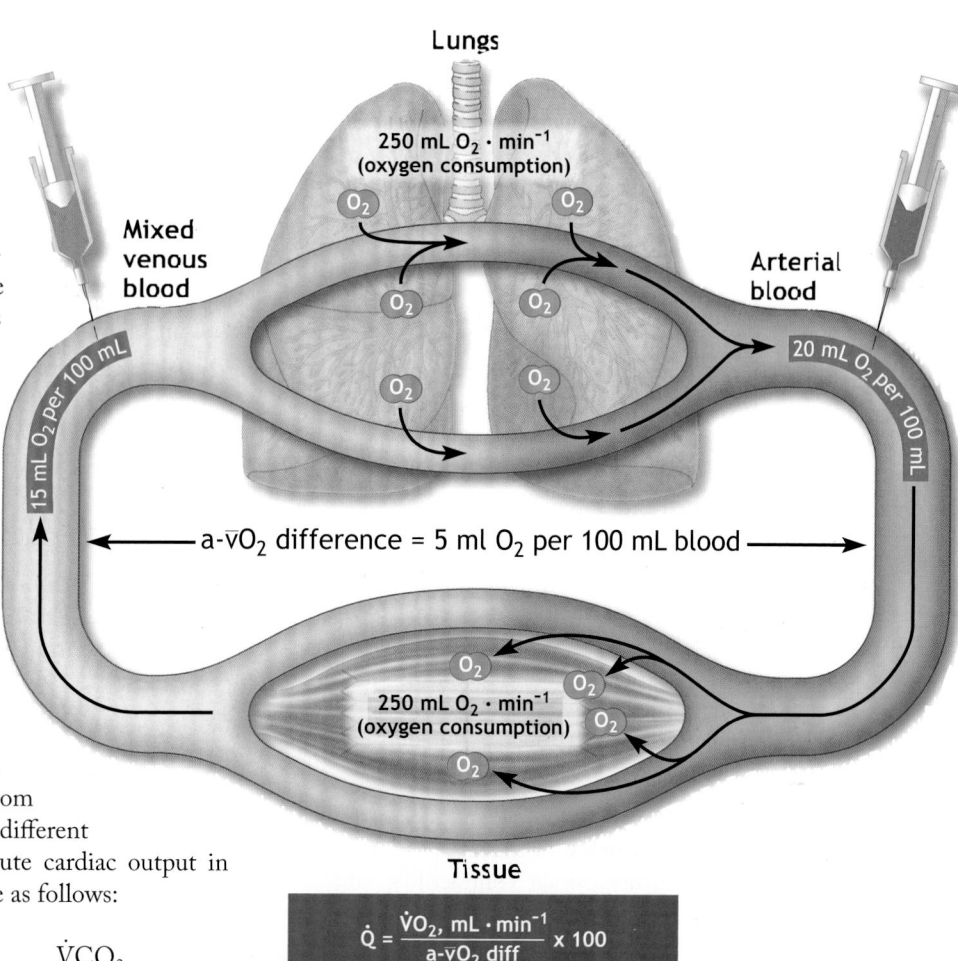

Lungs

250 mL $O_2 \cdot$ min⁻¹ (oxygen consumption)

Mixed venous blood   15 mL O_2 per 100 mL

Arterial blood   20 mL O_2 per 100 mL

a-v̄O_2 difference = 5 ml O_2 per 100 mL blood

250 mL $O_2 \cdot$ min⁻¹ (oxygen consumption)

Tissue

$$\dot{Q} = \frac{\dot{V}O_2, \text{mL} \cdot \text{min}^{-1}}{\text{a-v}O_2 \text{ diff}} \times 100$$

$$\dot{Q} = \frac{250}{5} \times 100$$

$$\dot{Q} = 5000 \text{ mL} \cdot \text{min}^{-1}$$

FIGURE 17.1 • The Fick principle to measure cardiac output per minute ($\dot{Q}$).

vessels. Each minute, the left ventricle pumps the entire 5-L blood volume of a representative 70-kg adult male. A 5-L cardiac output at rest represents an average value for trained and untrained males. Resting cardiac output for a representative 56-kg woman averages nearly 4.0 L · min⁻¹.

Untrained Individuals

For the typical sedentary person at rest, an average heart rate of 70 b · min⁻¹ usually sustains the 5-L cardiac output. Substituting this heart rate value in the cardiac output equation, the heart's calculated stroke volume equals 0.0714 L, or 71.4 mL ($SV = \dot{Q} \div HR$). Stroke volume and cardiac output for women average about 25% below values for men; in women, the stroke volume at rest averages 50 to 60 mL. This "gender difference" generally relates to the average woman's smaller body size.

Endurance Athletes

Endurance training brings the heart's sinus node under greater influence of acetylcholine, the parasympathetic hormone that slows heart rate. At the same time, resting sympathetic activity decreases. This longer-term training adaptation partially explains the low resting heart rates of many elite endurance athletes. Relatively brief training periods exert only a minimal lowering effect on resting heart rate.[1,39]

Heart rates in healthy endurance athletes generally average 50 b·min^{-1} at rest, although heart rates below 30 b·min^{-1} have been reported, but infrequently. The endurance athlete's resting cardiac output of 5 L·min^{-1} circulates with the relatively large stroke volume of 100 mL. The following summarizes average values for cardiac output, heart rate, and stroke volume for endurance-trained and untrained men at rest:

Rest

Cardiac output = Heart rate × Stroke volume

Untrained: 5000 mL·min^{-1} = 70 b·min^{-1} × 71 mL

Trained: 5000 mL·min^{-1} = 50 b·min^{-1} × 100 mL

Two factors help to explain the large stroke volume and low heart rate of endurance-trained athletes:

1. Increased vagal (parasympathetic) tone and decreased sympathetic drive, both of which slow the heart
2. Increased blood volume, myocardial contractility, and compliance (ability to distend in response to pressure; reduced cardiac stiffness) of the left ventricle, all of which augment the heart's stroke volume

CARDIAC OUTPUT DURING PHYSICAL ACTIVITY

Systemic blood flow increases directly with intensity of physical activity. Cardiac output increases rapidly during the transition from rest to steady-rate exercise. Thereafter, cardiac output rises gradually until it plateaus when blood flow meets the exercise metabolic requirements.

In sedentary, college-age males, cardiac output during maximal exertion increased four times above the resting level to 20 to 22 L·min^{-1}. Maximum heart rate for these young adults averaged 195 b·min^{-1}. Consequently, the stroke volume

generally ranged between 103 and 113 mL (20,000 mL·min^{-1} ÷ 195 b·min^{-1} = 103 mL·b^{-1}; 22,000 mL·min^{-1} ÷ 195 b·min^{-1} = 113 mL). In contrast, world-class endurance athletes achieve maximum cardiac outputs of 35 to 40 L·min^{-1}. This high value assumes greater significance when one considers that the trained person generally achieves a slightly lower maximum heart rate than a sedentary person of similar age. *The endurance athlete achieves a large maximal cardiac output solely through a large stroke volume.* For example, the cardiac output of an Olympic medal winner in cross-country skiing increased to 40 L·min^{-1} in maximum effort (almost eight times above rest); the stroke volume was 210 mL. This nearly doubled the maximum volume of blood pumped per beat by a sedentary counterpart. As a point of comparison among species, thoroughbred racehorses achieve cardiac outputs of 600 L·min^{-1} (accompanying a 120 to 150 mL·kg^{-1}·min^{-1} $\dot{V}O_{2max}$).[7,24]

The equation that follows summarizes average values for cardiac output, heart rate, and stroke volume for endurance-trained and untrained men during maximal physical activity:

Maximal Exercise

Cardiac output = Heart rate × Stroke volume

Untrained: 22,000 mL·min^{-1} = 195 b·min^{-1} × 113 mL

Trained: 35,000 mL·min^{-1} = 195 b·min^{-1} × 179 mL

The data in **TABLE 17.1** reveal the importance of stroke volume in differentiating among people with high and low $\dot{V}O_{2max}$. These data were obtained from three groups: athletes, healthy but sedentary men, and patients with mitral stenosis, a narrowing of the orifice of the mitral valve of the heart, restricting blood flow. The differences in $\dot{V}O_{2max}$ among groups closely relate to differences in maximal stroke volume. Patients with mitral stenosis had an aerobic capacity and maximum stroke volume half that of the sedentary subjects. The relationship also was apparent in comparisons between healthy subjects. The $\dot{V}O_{2max}$ of athletes averaged 62.5% larger than the sedentary group. This paralleled a 60% larger stroke volume. The maximal heart rates of all groups were similar, making the differences in cardiac output (and $\dot{V}O_{2max}$) almost entirely due to differences in maximal stroke volume.

TABLE 17.1		**Maximal Values for Oxygen Consumption, Heart Rate, Stroke Volume, and Cardiac Output in Three Groups with Very Low, Normal, and High Aerobic Capacities**		
Group	$\dot{V}O_{2max}$ **(L·min^{-1})**	**Max Heart Rate (B·min^{-1})**	**Max Stroke Volume (mL)**	**Max Cardiac Output (L·min^{-1})**
Mitral stenosis	1.6	190	50	9.5
Sedentary	3.2	200	100	20.0
Athlete	5.2	190	160	30.4

Adapted from Rowell LB. Circulation. *Med Sci Sports* 1969;1:15.

Enhancing Stroke Volume: Diastolic Filling Versus Systolic Emptying

Three physiologic mechanisms increase the heart's stroke volume during physical activity.[9,14,36]

1. The first, intrinsic to the myocardium, involves enhanced cardiac filling in diastole followed by a more forceful systolic contraction.
2. Neurohormonal influence governs the second mechanism that involves normal ventricular filling with a subsequent forceful ejection and emptying during systole.
3. Training adaptations that expand blood volume and reduce resistance to blood flow in peripheral tissues provides the third mechanism.

Ejection Fraction: A Measure of Ventricular Function

Clinicians often use ventricular **ejection fraction** as a measure of the heart's pumping ability and subsequent prognosis for cardiovascular health; those with significantly reduced ejection fractions typically have poorer prognosis. This measure is determined by the fraction of blood pumped from the left ventricle in relation to its end-diastolic volume. For example, if the ventricular end-diastolic volume equals 110 mL of blood and the heart's stroke volume equals 70 mL, the ejection fraction computes as 70 mL ÷ 110 or 0.64 or 64%. Healthy individuals usually have ejection fractions that range between 50% and 65%. Poor left-ventricular function often accompanies a depressed ejection fraction.

Enhanced Diastolic Filling

Any factor that increases venous return or slows the heart produces greater ventricular filling or **preload** during the cardiac cycle's diastolic phase. An increase in **end-diastolic volume** stretches myocardial fibers and initiates a powerful ejection stroke during contraction. This ejects the normal stroke volume plus any additional blood that entered the ventricles in diastole and stretched the myocardium.

Two researchers, German physiologist Otto Frank (1865–1944; investigated the isometric and isotonic contractile behavior of the heart) and British physiologist Ernest Henry Starling (1866–1927; first to use the term *hormone*), described the relationship between contractile force and the resting length of the heart's muscle fibers. This phenomenon, termed the **Frank-Starling law of the heart** (also known as *Starling's law* or the *Frank-Starling mechanism*) remains a fundamental principle of cardiac architecture. It states: *"Within physiological limits, the force of contraction is directly proportional to the initial length of the muscle fiber."* The principle operates during the cardiac cycle and applies to all of the heart's chambers. For years, physiologists taught that the Frank-Starling mechanism provided the modus operandi for *all* stroke volume increases during physical activity. They believed that venous return in exercise facilitated greater cardiac filling. The preload stretched the ventricles in diastole to produce a more forceful ejection stroke. More than likely, this response pattern for stroke volume operates during the transition from rest to activity or as a person moves from an upright to recumbent position. Enhanced diastolic filling also occurs in swimming because the body's horizontal position optimizes venous return. A more optimal arrangement of the sarcomere's myofilaments as the muscle fiber stretches enhances contractility.

The data in TABLE 17.2 illustrate the effect of body position on circulatory dynamics. The horizontal position produces the largest and most stable cardiac output and stroke volume. Stroke volume remains near maximum in this position at rest and increases only slightly during physical activity. In contrast, in the upright position, gravity counters the return flow of blood to the heart (decreased preload) to diminish stroke volume and cardiac output. During upright activity of increasing intensity, stroke volume approaches the maximum stroke volume in the supine position.

Greater Systolic Emptying

In most modes of upright physical activity, the heart does not fill to increase cardiac volume to the extent it does in the recumbent position. The progressive increase in stroke volume

TABLE 17.2 The Effect of Body Position on Cardiac Output, Stroke Volume, and Heart Rate at Rest and During Exercise in Physically Active Subjects[a]

	Rest		Moderate Exercise		Strenuous Exercise	
	Supine	Upright	Supine	Upright	Supine	Upright
Cardiac output, L · min^{-1}	9.2	6.6	19.0	16.9	26.3	24.5
Stroke volume, mL	141	103	163	149	164	155
Heart rate, beats · min^{-1}	65	64	115	112	160	159
Oxygen consumption, mL · min^{-1}	345	384	1769	1864	3364	3387

Data from Bevegard S, et al. Circulatory studies in well-trained athletes at rest and during heavy exercise, with special reference to stroke volume and the influence of body position. *Acta Physiol Scand* 1963;57:26.

during graded upright exercise in both children and adults results from the *combined effect* of enhanced diastolic filling and more complete emptying during systole.[5,12,23,33] Greater systolic ejection occurs despite increased resistance to blood flow in the arterial circuit from exercise-induced elevation of systolic blood pressure, called **afterload**.

Enhanced systolic ejection, with or without increased end-diastolic volume, occurs because the ventricles always contain a **functional residual blood volume**. At rest in the upright position, approximately 40% or 50 to 70 mL of the total end-diastolic blood volume remains in the left ventricle following systole. Catecholamine release in physical activity enhances myocardial contractile force to augment stroke power and facilitate systolic emptying.

Endurance training likely increases compliance of the left ventricle to facilitate acceptance of blood in the diastolic phase of the cardiac cycle.[19,43] Whether endurance training enhances the myocardium's innate contractile state remains unclear.[10,24] If this adaptation does occur, it too would contribute to a larger stroke volume effect.

Cardiovascular Drift: Reduced Stroke Volume and Increased Heart Rate During Prolonged Physical Activity

Submaximal physical activity performed for more than 15 min, particularly in the heat and accompanied with increases in core body temperature, produces progressive water loss through sweating and a fluid shift from plasma to tissues. A rise in core temperature also redistributes blood to the periphery for body cooling. Concurrently, the progressive fall in plasma volume decreases central venous cardiac filling pressure (preload) to reduce stroke volume. A reduced stroke volume initiates a compensatory progressive heart rate increase to maintain a nearly constant cardiac output as activity progresses and body temperature increases.[8] The term *cardiovascular drift* describes the gradual time-dependent downward "drift" in several cardiovascular responses, most notably stroke volume with concomitant heart rate increase during prolonged steady-rate exercise, particularly during high ambient temperatures.[15] At high ambient temperatures, a person must exercise at lower intensity than if the dynamics of cardiovascular drift did not occur.[3,11,41] A decrement in $\dot{V}O_{2max}$ accompanies the increased heart rate and reduced stroke volume in cardiovascular drift, which translates to a reduction in performance as evidenced by a decrease in maximal power output.[42]

One explanation for cardiovascular drift suggests the effects of a progressive increase in cutaneous blood flow as core temperature rises in prolonged physical activity. Increased redistribution of blood to the periphery for heat dissipation increases the skin's venous volume, ultimately reducing ventricular filling pressure and stroke volume. An alternative explanation exists for the stroke volume decline during cardiovascular drift in prolonged activity. FIGURE 17.2 illustrates responses for heart rate, stroke volume, and cutaneous blood flow (CBF) for seven active men during 60 min of submaximal cycling in a thermoneutral

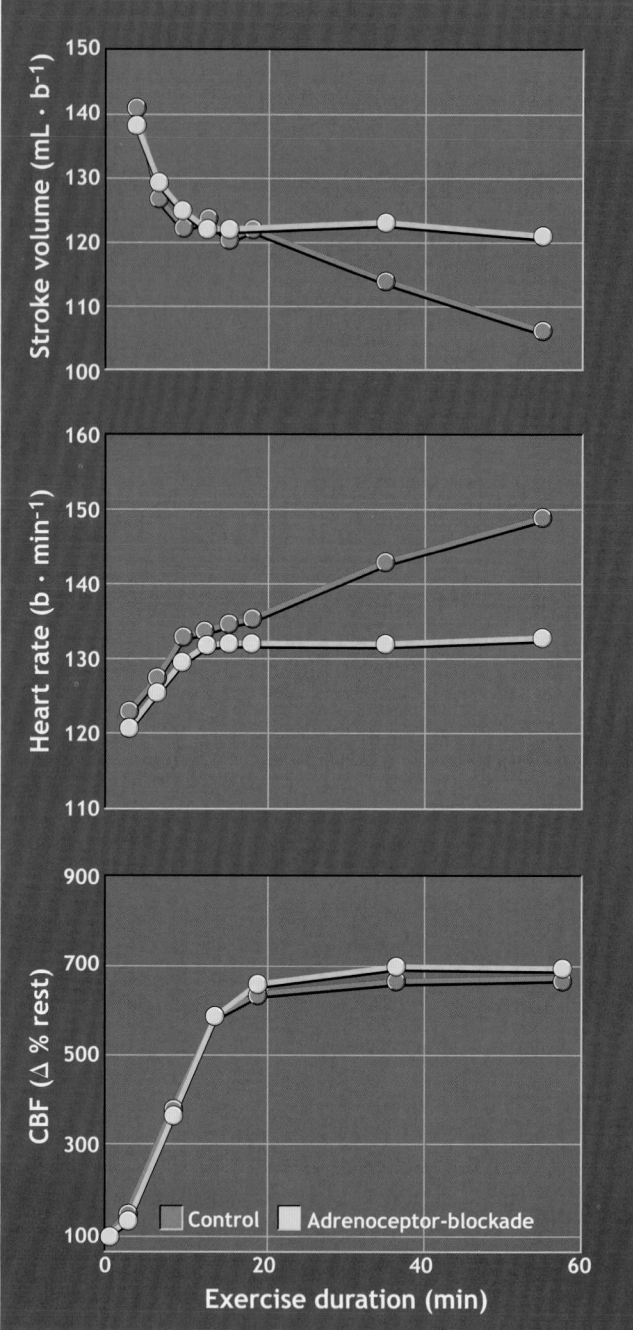

FIGURE 17.2 • Stroke volume, heart rate, and cutaneous blood flow (CBF) during 60 min of exercise under β_1-adrenoceptor blockade and control treatments. (Adapted with permission from Fritzsche RG, et al. Stroke volume decline during prolonged exercise is influenced by the increase in heart rate. *J Appl Physiol* 1999;86:799.)

environment. In one exercise trial, the men received a placebo; at the onset of exercise in the other trial, they received a small dose of a β_1-adrenoceptor blocker (atenolol) to prevent the heart rate increase or cardiovascular drift that normally occurs after 15 min of cycling. Fifteen minutes into activity, heart rate and stroke volume remained similar during control and β_1-adrenoceptor blockade conditions. From 15 to 55 min during the control trial, a 13% decrease in stroke volume accompanied an 11% heart rate increase, while cutaneous blood flow showed no increase from 20 to 60 min of cycling. In contrast, from 15 to 55 min of activity under blockade conditions when atenolol prevented a heart rate increase, stroke volume failed to decline compared with control conditions despite similar levels of cutaneous blood flow in both trials. Cardiac output remained stable at about 16 $L \cdot min^{-1}$ under both conditions. These observations confirm that a decline in stroke volume during prolonged physical activity in a thermoneutral environment primarily results from increased heart rate and not increased cutaneous blood flow as body temperature rises.[2] The progressive increase in heart rate with cardiovascular drift during exercise more than likely decreases the end-diastolic volume (i.e., less time for ventricular filling), thus reducing the heart's stroke volume.

INTEGRATIVE QUESTION

Increasing the blood's hemoglobin concentration increases $\dot{V}O_{2max}$ *during maximal physical activity at sea level. According to this effect, discuss what component of the Fick equation limits maximal oxygen consumption.*

CARDIAC OUTPUT DISTRIBUTION

Blood generally flows to tissues in proportion to their metabolic demands. Blood flow to the kidneys, skin, and splanchnic areas also varies with the metabolic demands of skeletal muscle during physical activity.

Blood Flow at Rest

At rest in a thermoneutral environment, the typical 5-L cardiac output generally distributes in the proportions shown in FIGURE 17.3A. Approximately one fifth of the cardiac output flows to muscle tissue, while the digestive tract, liver, spleen, brain, and kidneys receive major portions of the remaining blood.

Redistribution of Blood Flow During Physical Activity

FIGURE 17.3B illustrates the percentage distribution of cardiac output in an endurance athlete during intense physical activity. *Environmental stress, level of fatigue, and physical activity mode and intensity affect regional blood flow, but the major portion of the cardiac output diverts to active muscles.* Approximately 4 to 7 mL of blood flows each minute to each 100 g of muscle at rest. This flow increases steadily in graded exercise, with active muscle receiving up to 50 to 75 mL per 100 g of tissue each minute of maximal exertion.[28,29]

Blood flow within active muscle is highly regulated. The greatest quantity of blood diverts to the oxidative portions of the muscle at the expense of those areas with high glycolytic capacity.[4,16] Peak blood flow in a small portion of active quadriceps muscle reaches values as high as 300 to

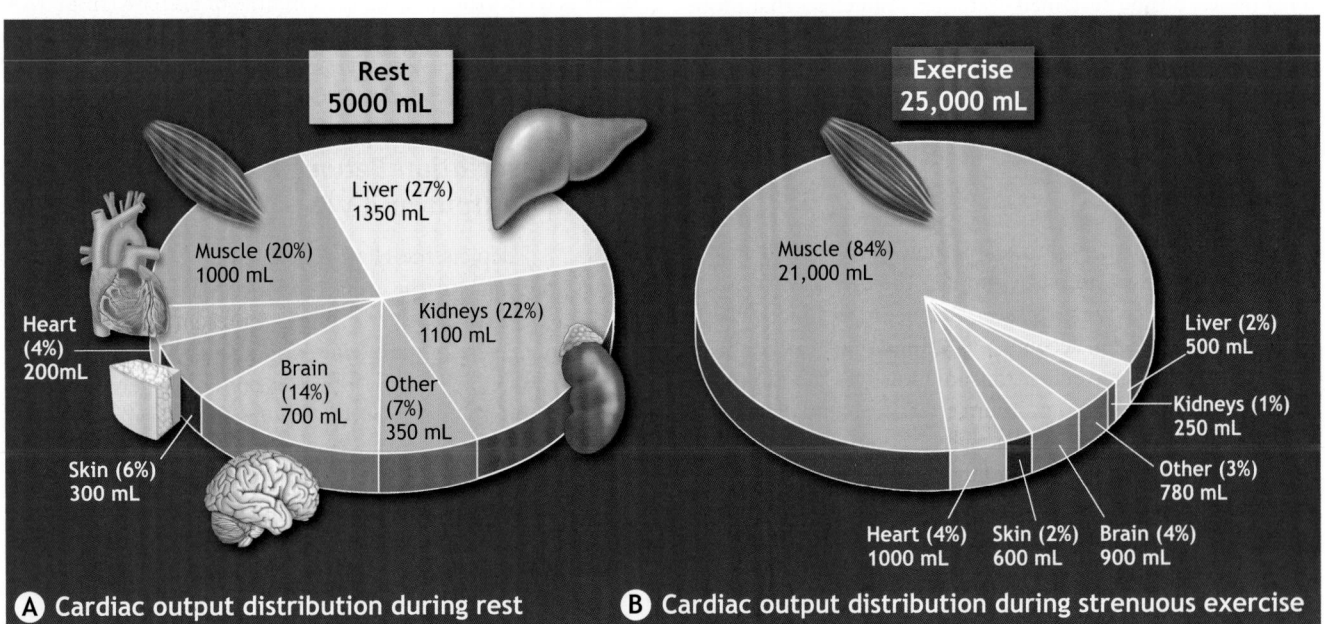

A Cardiac output distribution during rest

B Cardiac output distribution during strenuous exercise

FIGURE 17.3 • (A) Relative distribution of cardiac output during rest and **(B)** strenuous endurance exercise. The number in parentheses indicates percentage of the total cardiac output. The large absolute mass of muscle tissue at rest receives about the same quantity of blood as the much smaller kidneys. In strenuous physical activity, approximately 84% of the cardiac output diverts to the active musculature.

400 mL $\cdot$ 100 g^{-1} $\cdot$ min^{-1}.[26] During "big muscle" running and cycling at maximum intensity, muscle blood flow accounts for 80 to 85% of total cardiac output.[30]

Blood flow to muscle also increases disproportionately relative to flow to other tissues. For trained individuals, blood redistribution—from one organ to another by vasoconstriction in one and vasodilation in the other—begins in the anticipatory period just prior to movement.[4] Two factors, hormonal vascular regulation and local metabolic conditions, cause blood to route through active muscles from areas that temporarily tolerate compromised blood flow.[20] Blood redistribution among specific tissues occurs primarily during intense physical activity. For example, blood flow to the skin, the primary heat-exchange organ, increases during light and moderate activity in response to the rise in core temperature.[13,44] During near-maximal effort, the skin restricts its blood flow, redirecting it to active muscle, even in a hot environment.[27]

At rest, the kidneys and splanchnic tissues consume only 10 to 25% of the oxygen in their normal blood supply. These tissues can tolerate a considerably reduced blood flow before oxygen demand exceeds supply and compromises function.[22] Renal blood flow decreases by up to four fifths of its blood supply at rest. Increased oxygen extraction from the available blood supply generally maintains the oxygen needs of tissues with reduced blood flow. During intense effort, the visceral organs sustain a substantially reduced blood supply for more than 1 hr. Redistribution of 2 to 3 L of blood away from these tissues "frees" up to 600 mL of oxygen each minute for use by active muscles. Sustained blood flow reduction to the liver and kidneys may contribute to fatigue often experienced during prolonged submaximal effort. Regular aerobic training diminishes the typical vasoconstrictor response to splanchnic and renal tissues during sustained exercise,[20,34] an effect that probably contributes to improved endurance.

Blood Flow to the Heart and Brain

Heart and brain tissue cannot tolerate a compromised blood supply. At rest, the myocardium normally uses approximately 75% of the oxygen in the blood flowing through the coronary circulation. With such a limited margin of reserve, increased coronary blood flow primarily supplies the increased myocardial oxygen needed with exertion. A four- to fivefold increase in coronary circulation accompanies a similar increase in myocardial work during exercise; this amounts to a blood flow of about 1 L $\cdot$ min^{-1} during maximum effort. Cerebral blood flow also increases during physical activity by approximately 25 to 30% compared with the resting flow.[37]

CARDIAC OUTPUT AND OXYGEN TRANSPORT

Rest

Arterial blood carries about 200 mL of oxygen per liter in a person with a normal hemoglobin level (see Chapter 13). If resting cardiac output each minute equals 5 L, potentially 1000 mL of

oxygen becomes available to the body (5 L blood × 200 mL O_2). The resting oxygen consumption typically averages 250 to 300 mL $\cdot$ min^{-1}, allowing 750 mL of oxygen to return unused to the heart. This does not reflect an unnecessary waste of blood flow. Rather, the extra oxygen circulating above the resting requirement represents oxygen in reserve—a margin of safety when a tissue's metabolism increases dramatically, as would occur in the transition from rest to maximum physical effort.

 See the animation "Myocardial Blood Flow" on **http://thePoint.lww.com/mkk8e** for a demonstration of this process.

Physical Activity

A healthy, young adult with a maximum heart rate of 200 b $\cdot$ min^{-1} and stroke volume of 80 mL (0.08 L) generates a maximum cardiac output of 16 L $\cdot$ min^{-1} (200 × 0.08 L). Even during maximal activity, hemoglobin saturation with oxygen remains nearly complete, so each liter of arterial blood carries about 200 mL of oxygen. Consequently, 3200 mL of oxygen circulates each minute via a 16-L cardiac output (16 L × 200 mL $O_2 \cdot$ L^{-1}). Even if the tissues could extract all of the oxygen from all of the blood as it traveled throughout the body, the $\dot{V}O_{2max}$ could not exceed 3200 mL. This represents a purely theoretical value because the oxygen demands of the brain and skin tissues, for example, do not increase markedly with physical activity, yet they still require a substantial blood supply.

Based on the preceding example, increasing the heart's stroke volume from 80 to 200 mL while maintaining the maximum heart rate at 200 b $\cdot$ min^{-1} dramatically increases maximum cardiac output to 40 L $\cdot$ min^{-1}. This represents a 2.5-fold increase in oxygen circulated during each minute of exercise (from 3200 to 8000 mL). *An increase in maximum cardiac output clearly produces a proportionate increase in capacity to circulate oxygen and profoundly impacts an individual's maximal oxygen consumption.*

Close Association Between Maximum Cardiac Output and $\dot{V}O_{2max}$

FIGURE 17.4 depicts the close relationship between maximum cardiac output and the capacity for a high level of aerobic exercise metabolism. $\dot{V}O_{2max}$ values represent averages for the sedentary person and the elite endurance athlete. An unmistakable association exists—a low maximal oxygen consumption corresponds closely with a low maximum cardiac output, whereas a 5- or 6-L $\dot{V}O_{2max}$ invariably accompanies a 30- to 40-L cardiac output.

A 5- to 6-L increase in blood flow accompanies each 1-L increase in oxygen consumption above the resting value; this relationship remains essentially unchanged regardless of activity mode over a broad range of dynamic exercises. *High levels of maximal oxygen consumption and cardiac output provide distinguishing characteristics for preadolescent and adult endurance athletes.* An almost proportionate increase in maximum cardiac output accompanies increases in $\dot{V}O_{2max}$ with endurance training, as discussed in Chapter 21.

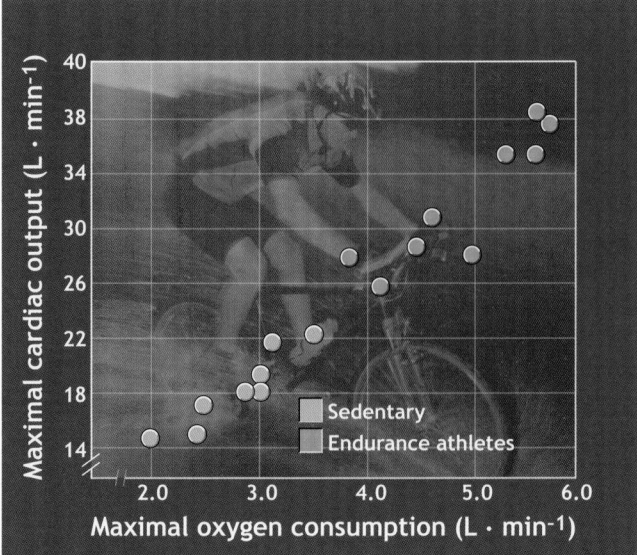

FIGURE 17.4 • Relationship between maximal cardiac output and maximal oxygen consumption ($\dot{V}O_{2max}$) in endurance-trained and untrained individuals. Maximal cardiac output relates to $\dot{V}O_{2max}$ in the ratio of about 6:1.

Cardiac Output Differences Among Men and Women and Children

Cardiac output and oxygen consumption remain linearly related during graded exercise for boys and girls and for men and women. Teenage and adult females generally exercise at any level of *submaximal* oxygen consumption with a 5 to 10% *larger* cardiac output than males.[25] The 10% *lower* hemoglobin concentration in women than in men explains this apparent gender difference in submaximal cardiac output. A proportionate increase in submaximal cardiac output compensates for this relatively minor decrease in the blood's oxygen-carrying capacity.

Higher heart rates in children compared to adults during submaximal treadmill and cycle ergometer exercise do not fully compensate for their smaller stroke volume. This produces a smaller cardiac output for children at a given submaximal oxygen consumption.[32,38] Consequently, the a-$\bar{v}O_2$ difference expands to meet the oxygen requirements. The biologic significance of this difference in central circulatory function between children and adults remains unclear. Comparisons of cardiac responses (stroke volume, aortic peak blood flow velocity, systolic ejection time) between prepubertal children and adults fail to demonstrate any age-related exercise impairment.[31]

Oxygen Extraction: The a-$\bar{v}O_2$ Difference

If only blood flow increased tissue oxygen supply, then increasing cardiac output from 5 L·min^{-1} at rest to 100 L·min^{-1} during maximum physical activity would achieve the 20-fold

oxygen consumption increase common among endurance athletes. Fortunately, strenuous activity does not require this large cardiac output. Instead, hemoglobin releases a considerable quantity of its "reserve" oxygen from blood that perfuses active tissues. Oxygen consumption during physical activity increases by two mechanisms:

1. Increased total quantity of blood pumped by the heart (i.e., increased cardiac output)
2. Greater use of the already existing large quantity of oxygen carried by the blood (i.e., expanded a-$\bar{v}O_2$ difference)

Rearranging the Fick equation summarizes the important relationship among cardiac output, a-$\bar{v}O_2$ difference, and $\dot{V}O_2$ as follows:

$$\dot{V}O_2 = \dot{Q} \times \text{a-}\bar{v}O_2 \text{ difference}$$

a-$\bar{v}O_2$ Difference During Rest

Resting metabolism consumes about 5 mL of oxygen from the 20 mL of oxygen in each deciliter of arterial blood (50 mL per liter) that passes through the tissue capillaries. This represents an a-$\bar{v}O_2$ difference of 5 mL of oxygen per deciliter of blood that perfuses the tissue-capillary bed. Thus, 15 mL of oxygen or 75% of the blood's original oxygen load still remains bound to hemoglobin.

 INTEGRATIVE QUESTION

Explain how factors that influence the a-$\bar{v}O_2$ difference in maximal physical activity account for the specificity of $\dot{V}O_{2max}$ improvement with different modes of aerobic training.

a-$\bar{v}O_2$ Difference During Physical Activity

FIGURE 17.5 shows a progressive expansion of the a-$\bar{v}O_2$ difference from rest to maximal effort for physically active men. A similar pattern emerges for women, except that arterial oxygen content averages 5 to 10% lower because of lower hemoglobin concentrations. The figure includes values for oxygen content of arterial and mixed-venous blood during different oxygen consumptions. Arterial blood oxygen content varies little from its value of 20 mL·dL^{-1} at rest throughout the full exercise intensity range. In contrast, mixed-venous oxygen content varies between 12 and 15 mL·dL^{-1} during rest to a low of 2 to 4 mL·dL^{-1} during maximal exertion. The difference between arterial and mixed-venous blood oxygen content at any discrete time (i.e., the a-$\bar{v}O_2$ difference) represents oxygen extraction from arterial blood as it circulates throughout the body.

The progressive expansion of the a-$\bar{v}O_2$ difference to at least three times resting value results from a reduced venous

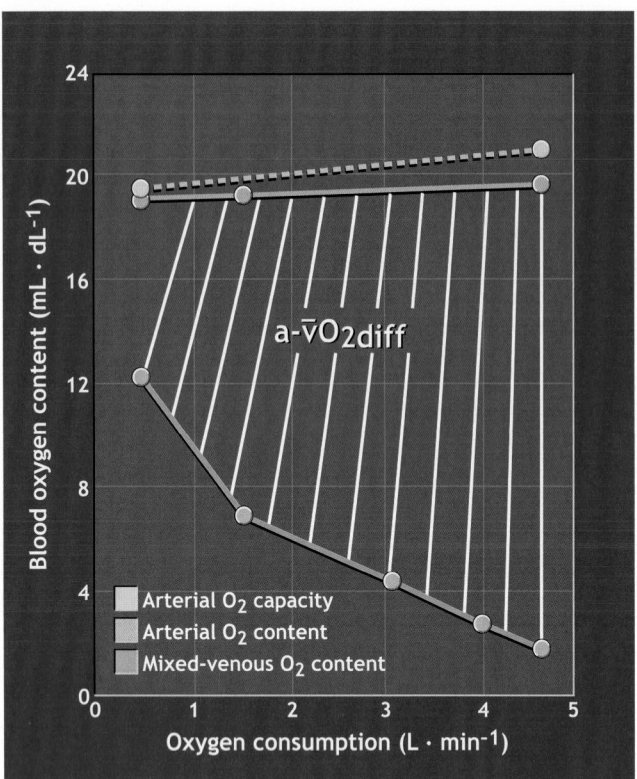

FIGURE 17.5 • Changes in a-$\bar{v}O_2$ difference from rest to maximal exercise in physically active men.

oxygen content, which in maximal effort approaches an a-vO_2 difference of 20 mL · dL^{-1} in active muscle. In this case, essentially all oxygen has been extracted. The oxygen content of a true mixed-venous sample from the pulmonary artery rarely falls below 2 to 4 mL · dL^{-1} because blood returning from active tissues mixes with oxygen-rich venous blood from metabolically less active regions.

Figure 17.5 also shows that capacity of each deciliter of arterial blood to carry oxygen (*yellow line*) increases during physical activity from an increased concentration of red blood cells known as *hemoconcentration*. Hemoconcentration results from the progressive movement of fluid from the plasma to the interstitial space by two mechanisms:

1. Increases in capillary hydrostatic pressure as blood pressure rises
2. Metabolic byproducts of exercise metabolism that osmotically draw fluid into tissue spaces from the plasma

Factors That Affect the a-$\bar{v}O_2$ Difference During Physical Activity

During physical activity, central and peripheral factors interact to increase oxygen extraction in active tissue. Diverting a large portion of the cardiac output to active musculature influences the magnitude of the a-$\bar{v}O_2$ difference in maximal effort. Some tissues temporarily decrease their blood supply

IN A PRACTICAL SENSE

Predicting $\dot{V}O_{2max}$ Using Walking and Swimming Tests

The 1-mile walk and the 12-min swim provide reliable and valid tests to predict $\dot{V}O_{2max}$. The tests, easily adapted depending on equipment availability, are effective for mass testing in schools and with recreational swimmers. We do not recommend these tests for unconditioned beginners, for men over age 40 and for women over age 50 without proper medical clearance, for symptomatic individuals, and for those with known disease or coronary heart disease risk factors. *The swim test assumes relatively high-level swimming skill.*

THE TESTS

1-Mile Walk Test

[**Reference:** Kline GM, Porcari JP, Hintermeister R, et. al. Estimation of $\dot{V}O_{2max}$ from a one mile track walk, gender, age, and body weight. *Med Sci Sports Exerc* 1987;19:253–259.]

1. Record *gender* and record *body weight* in lbs.
2. Testing site: a school track (each lap measures ¼ mile) or a premeasured 1-mile course.
3. Warm up for at least 3 min (easy stretching, mild calisthenics, and jogging in place).

4. Walk 1-mile distance as fast as possible. On a track, use the inside lane.
5. Record run time in min:s and convert to the nearest hundredth of a minute (e.g., if the time = 13 min 30 s, then the time converts to the nearest hundredth minute by dividing the seconds by 60—thus, the time records as 13.50 min).
6. Immediately upon crossing the 1-mile mark, record the 15 s heart rate (use radial or carotid pulse) and convert to beats/min by multiplying by 4.
7. Predict $\dot{V}O_{2max}$ using the following equation:

where
gender = 0 for women, and 1 for men
BM = body mass (pounds) in walking shoes
T = time to walk 1 mile (converted to nearest hundredth minute)
HR = immediate postexercise HR (beats/min)

8. Refer to TABLE 1.

Example Calculations:

Male (Body weight = 160 lbs; time to complete 1-mile walk = 13.50 min; heart rate = 1254 b/min [15 s HR = 41])

IN A PRACTICAL SENSE *(continued)*

TABLE 1 — Aerobic Fitness Categories for Men and Women

Age	Excellent	Very Good	Good	Average	Fair	Poor	Very Poor
Men							
18–20	>63	62–57	56–51	50–46	45–39	38–33	<33
21–25	>62	62–56	55–51	50–45	44–38	37–32	<32
26–30	>59	59–55	54–48	47–42	41–36	35–30	<30
Women							
18–20	>53	53–48	47–43	42–38	37–33	32–28	<28
21–25	>50	50–46	45–42	41–36	35–32	31–27	<27
26–30	>48	48–44	43–40	39–35	34–31	30–26	<26

Fitness Category $\dot{V}O_{2max}$ (mL · kg^{-1} · min^{-1})

Table derived from graphs in Shvartz E, Reibold RC Aerobic fitness norms for males and females aged 6 to 75 years: a review. *Aviat Space Environ Med* 1990;61:3–11.

$\dot{V}O_{2max}$ (mL · kg^{-1} · min^{-1}) = 88.768 + 8.892 (gender)
$\qquad$ − 0.0957 (BM lb) − 1.4537 (T)
$\qquad$ − 0.1194 (HR)

$\dot{V}O_{2max}$ (mL · kg^{-1} · min^{-1}) = 88.768 + 8.892 (1) − 0.0957 (160)
$\qquad$ − 1.4537 (13.5) − 0.1194 (124)

$\dot{V}O_{2max}$ (mL · kg^{-1} · min^{-1}) = 47.92

12-Minute Swim Test

Individuals swim as far as possible in 12 min, with distance measured in yards. *Differences in skill level, swim conditioning, and body composition greatly affect oxygen consumption (exercise economy), thus making VO_{2max} predictions less valid than those based on walking and running, which have a smaller variation in economy.*

1. Warm up for at least 3 min with easy stretching and mild calisthenics followed by several laps of easy swimming.

2. Swim as many laps as possible in 12 min; paced swimming is preferred to intervals of fast and slow effort.

3. Determine total distance swam in yards; if the test ends in the middle of the pool, estimate distance; find swim fitness and $\dot{V}O_{2max}$ prediction, easily adapted depending on equipment availability, in TABLE 2.

From Cooper KH. *The Aerobics Program for Total Well-Being*. New York: Bantam Books, 1982.

TABLE 2 — 12-Minute Swim Test Fitness Categories (Age 18–29 Years)

Distance (YD)	Fitness Category	Estimated $\dot{V}O_{2max}$ (mL · kg^{-1} · min^{-1}) Males	Females
>700	Excellent	>52.5	>41.0
500–700	Good	46.5–52.4	37.0–40.0
400–500	Average	42.5–46.4	33.0–36.9
200–400	Fair	36.5–42.4	29.0–32.9
<200	Poor	33.0–36.4	23.6–28.9

during physical activity by redistributing blood to make more oxygen available for muscle metabolism. Exercise training redirects a greater portion of the central circulation to active muscle.

Increases in skeletal muscle microcirculation also increase tissue oxygen extraction. Muscle biopsy specimens from the quadriceps femoris muscle show a relatively large ratio of capillaries to muscle fibers in individuals who exhibit large a-$\bar{v}$O$_2$ differences during intense activity. An increased capillary-to-fiber ratio reflects a positive endurance training adaptation that enlarges the interface for nutrient and metabolic gas exchange during exercise.

Individual muscle cells' ability to generate energy aerobically represents another important factor that governs oxygen extraction capacity. Increasing the size and number of mitochondria and augmenting aerobic enzyme activity improve a muscle's metabolic capacity in physical activity. Local vascular and metabolic improvements within muscle ultimately enhance its capacity to produce ATP aerobically.[40] These local training adaptations translate to an increased oxygen extraction capacity.

INTEGRATIVE QUESTION

Present a physiologic rationale to support the relative importance of (1) central circulatory factors (cardiac output) and (2) peripheral factors residing within the active muscle mass (a-$\bar{v}O_2$ differences) in limiting $\dot{V}O_{2max}$.

CARDIOVASCULAR ADJUSTMENTS TO UPPER-BODY EXERCISE

Upper-body exercise creates different metabolic and cardiovascular responses than does lower-body exercise, which requires predominantly leg musculature activation.

Maximal Oxygen Consumption

The highest oxygen consumption during arm exercise averages 20 to 30% lower than consumption during leg exercise. Similarly, arm exercise produces lower maximal values for heart rate and pulmonary ventilation. In large part, these differences relate to the relatively smaller muscle mass activated in arm exercise.

Submaximal Oxygen Consumption

Submaximal physical activity reverses the pattern for oxygen consumption between upper- and lower-body exercise observed during maximal effort. The dashed yellow line in FIGURE 17.6 reveals higher oxygen consumption values during arm cycling at all submaximal power outputs. The small

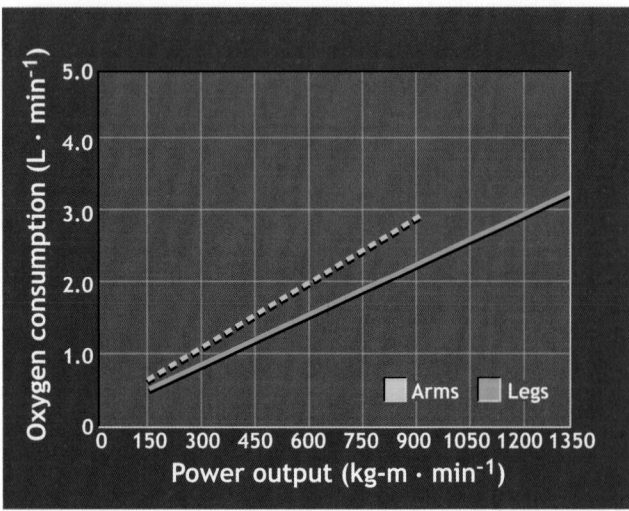

FIGURE 17.6 • Arm exercise requires greater oxygen consumption than leg exercise at any submaximal power output throughout the comparison range. The largest differences occur during intense exertion. Data represent averages for men and women. (From Laboratory of Applied Physiology, Queens College, Flushing, NY.)

differences during light exercise become progressively larger as intensity increases. Two factors produce this additional oxygen cost at higher intensities of arm cycling:

1. Lower mechanical efficiency in upper-body exercise from the additional energy requirement of static muscle actions that do not contribute to external work
2. Recruitment of additional musculature and hence energy requirement to stabilize the torso during arm exercise

Physiologic Response

Any level of submaximal oxygen consumption (or percentage $\dot{V}O_{2max}$) or power output with upper-body exercise provides greater physiologic strain than lower-body exercise. Specifically, submaximal arm exercise produces higher heart rates, pulmonary ventilations, and perceptions of effort than comparable intensities of leg exercise. This also applies to blood pressure during arm versus leg exercise (see Chapter 15).

The elevated heart rate response in submaximal arm exercise probably results from two factors:

1. Greater feed-forward stimulation from the brain's central command to the medullary control center
2. Increased feedback stimulation to the medulla from peripheral receptors in active tissue

Upper-body physical activities places a greater strain (i.e., greater force per unit muscle, greater percentage of maximum capacity, and more metabolic byproducts) on the relatively smaller upper-body musculature for any submaximum exercise level. Added strain augments peripheral feedback to the medulla, which increases heart rate and blood pressure. A smaller total muscle mass activated in maximal arm movements reduces input to the medullary cardiovascular control center from the motor cortex, with less peripheral feedback from the smaller upper-body muscle mass, which may account for the lower maximum heart rate in upper-body compared to lower-body activities.

Implications. *A standard submaximal exercise load (power output or oxygen consumption) with the upper body produces greater metabolic and physiologic strain than does leg exercise.* For this reason, exercise prescriptions based on running and bicycling do not apply to arm exercise. Low statistical correlations exist between $\dot{V}O_{2max}$ in arm versus leg exercise, so one should not expect to accurately predict aerobic capacity for arm exercise based on a test that uses the legs and vice versa.[6,17] This lack of strong association between the two activity modes further amplifies the specificity concept applied to aerobic fitness.

Summary

1. Cardiac output reflects the functional capacity of the cardiovascular system. Heart rate and stroke volume determine the heart's output capacity expressed as follows: Cardiac output = Heart rate × Stroke volume.

2. Several invasive and noninvasive methods measure cardiac output in humans. Each has specific advantages and disadvantages during physical activity.

3. Cardiac output increases proportionally with effort intensity, starting from approximately 5 $L \cdot min^{-1}$ at rest to a maximum of 20 to 25 $L \cdot min^{-1}$ in untrained, college-age men and 35 to 40 $L \cdot min^{-1}$ in elite male endurance athletes.

4. The large stroke volumes of endurance athletes explain the difference in maximum cardiac outputs compared with untrained persons.

5. Stroke volume increases during upright physical activity from the interaction between greater ventricular filling during diastole and more complete emptying during systole.

6. Sympathetic hormones augment systolic ejection by increasing stroke power during systole.

7. Blood flows to specific tissues in proportion to their metabolic activity.

8. Most of the cardiac output diverts to active muscles during exercise because the kidneys and splanchnic regions temporarily compromise blood supply to redistribute blood to the active muscles.

9. Maximum cardiac output and maximum a-$\bar{v}O_2$ difference determine maximal oxygen consumption.

10. A large cardiac output clearly differentiates endurance athletes from untrained counterparts.

11. Arm exercise generates 25% lower $\dot{V}O_{2max}$ than leg exercise.

12. Any level of submaximal oxygen consumption, %$\dot{V}O_{2max}$, or power output with upper-body exercise provides greater physiologic strain than lower-body exercise.

thePoint References are available online at http://thepoint.lww.com/mkk8e.

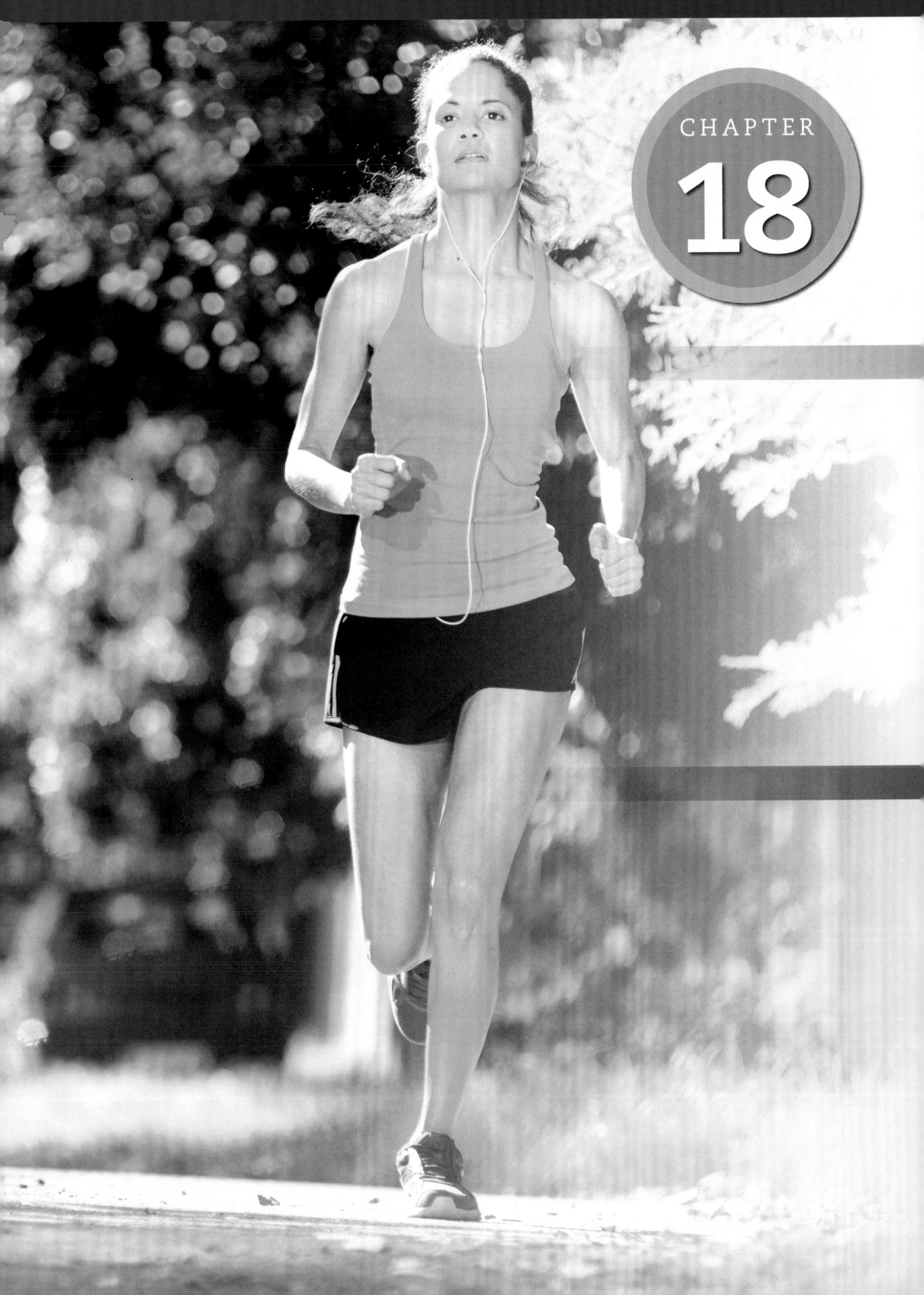
CHAPTER
18

Skeletal Muscle: Structure and Function

CHAPTER OBJECTIVES

- Outline five levels of organization in the gross structure of skeletal muscle

- List four major protein constituents of skeletal muscle and their functions

- Draw and label the structures that characterize a skeletal muscle fiber's striated appearance under the light microscope at low magnification

- Describe different arrangements of individual muscle fibers along the long axis of skeletal muscle and explain the biomechanical advantage of each

- Draw and label a skeletal muscle fiber's ultrastructural components

- Summarize the salient features of the sliding filament model of muscle contraction

- Outline the sequence of chemical and mechanical events during skeletal muscle excitation–contraction coupling and relaxation

- Discuss the function of the triad and T-tubule system

- Contrast slow-twitch and fast-twitch (including subdivisions) muscle fiber characteristics

- Outline distribution patterns of muscle fiber type among diverse groups of elite athletes

- Discuss modifications in muscle fibers and fiber types with specific exercise training

ANCILLARIES 👁 at-a-Glance

Visit http://thePoint.lww.com/mkk8e to access the following resources.

- References: Chapter 18
- Appendix H: Supplemental Animations and Videos
- Interactive Question Bank
- Animation: Muscle Contraction Type
- Animation: Sliding Filament Theory
- Focus on Research: A Tissue Response to Regular Exercise

Prior to the construction of compound microscopes in the 1600s by Dutch spectacle makers (notably Zacharias Jansen [1580–1638; http://micro.magnet.fsu.edu/optics/timeline/people/janssen.html] and Italian observational astronomer, physicist, and mathematician Galileo Galilei [1564–1642; http://inventors.about.com/od/gstartinventors/a/Galileo_Galilei.htm]), biologists had little insight about a muscle's internal structures.

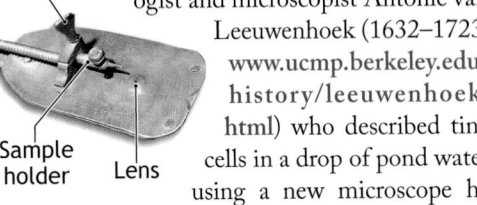

Focus knob
Sample translator
Sample holder
Lens

This was soon made easier by Dutch biologist and microscopist Antonie van Leeuwenhoek (1632–1723; www.ucmp.berkeley.edu/history/leeuwenhoek.html) who described tiny cells in a drop of pond water using a new microscope he perfected. Unlike the earlier Dutch microscopes that could magnify objects only six to nine times, van Leeuwenhoek's microscope included a single glass lens mounted in a flat brass or copper plate that magnified structures up to 250 times. The lens was held up to the eye, and the object for study was placed on the head of a movable pin on the other side of the lens. This breakthrough in microscope design spawned the development of more complex and powerful tools to explore the minute structural details of a muscle and other human and animal tissues. During the next century, tiny bits of muscle tissue observed under even more powerful microscopes showed faint light and dark areas along the tissue's length. We now know that the light and dark areas represent alternating bands of

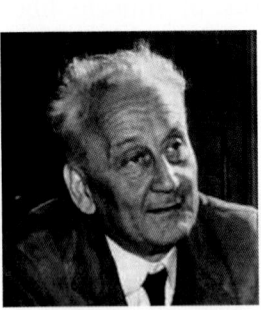

sarcomeres composed of thin and thicker substructures called filaments that "slide" past each other to alter fiber length and generate force. Albert Szent-Györgyi (1900–1900), awarded the 1938 Nobel Prize in Physiology or Medicine for discoveries of the biological combustion processes with reference to vitamin C and the breakdown of fumaric acid (www.nobelprize.org/nobel_prizes/medicine/laureates/1937/szent-gyorgyi-bio.html), also discovered the muscle proteins actin and myosin and their complex architecture. His crucial experiments led to a reproduction of the fundamental process of muscle contraction, which formed the basic foundation of muscle research in the following decades.

The following sections present the architectural organization of skeletal muscle with a focus on gross and microscopic structures. We also highlight the sequence of chemical and mechanical events in muscle action and relaxation assessed with the highly sophisticated scanning electron microscope profiled later in this chapter (http://legacy.mos.org/sln/SEM/sem.mov), including differences in muscle fiber characteristics among sedentary individuals and elite athletes in different sports.

 See the animation "Muscle Contraction Type" on http://thePoint.lww.com/mkk8e for a demonstration of this process.

 The Terms *Muscle Contraction* and *Muscle Action*

During the previous half-century, the term *muscle contraction* commonly referred to processes involving generation of muscular tension associated with muscle shortening. In striated muscle, three types of actions can occur while generating tension:

1. Muscle shortens (concentric action)
2. Muscle remains the same length (static action)
3. Muscle lengthens (eccentric action)

In this text, we use the terms *contraction* and *action* interchangeably to refer to the same event, although we acknowledge that *muscle action* may be preferable.

GROSS STRUCTURE OF SKELETAL MUSCLE

As illustrated in Chapter 15 (see Figure 15.2), humans possess three types of muscle—cardiac, smooth, and skeletal—each exhibiting distinct functional and anatomical differences. Cardiac muscle resides only in the heart. It shares several common features with skeletal muscle as both appear striated (striped) under low-magnification microscopic examination and both contract or shorten in a similar manner. Smooth muscle lacks a striated appearance but shares cardiac muscle's characteristic of nonconscious regulation under autonomic nervous system control. Skeletal muscle operates under *voluntary* control, as in curling a 25-lb barbell or smashing a golf ball. The individual can easily control the velocity of movement in the barbell curl, the range of motion during the lifting movement, and the number of repetitions completed. In golf, the player controls all aspects of the coordinated and hopefully perfectly timed movements of the arms, legs, and torso during the backswing and downswing. A different situation exists for both cardiac and smooth muscle tissue because activity of these tissues occurs *involuntarily*, although mediation from central centers can exert some influence. This means a general absence of conscious control as to how fast the heart beats, or how fast food moves through the digestive system, or how the miles of blood vessels contract and expand throughout the day.

Each of the body's approximately 600-plus skeletal muscles (depending on the source consulted) contains various wrappings of fibrous connective tissue. FIGURE 18.1 illustrates a cross section of skeletal muscle structures and arrangement of connective tissue wrappings, including the thousands of cylindrical wells called **fibers**.

thePoint Appendix H, available online at http://thePoint.lww.com/mkk8e, provides a list of supplemental animations and videos on this subject.

These long, slender, multinucleated fibers lie parallel to each other, with the force of action directed along the fiber's long axis. Their number probably remains largely fixed by the second trimester of fetal development. Individual fiber length varies from a few millimeters in the eye muscles to nearly 30 cm in the large antigravity leg muscles (with width reaching 0.15 mm).

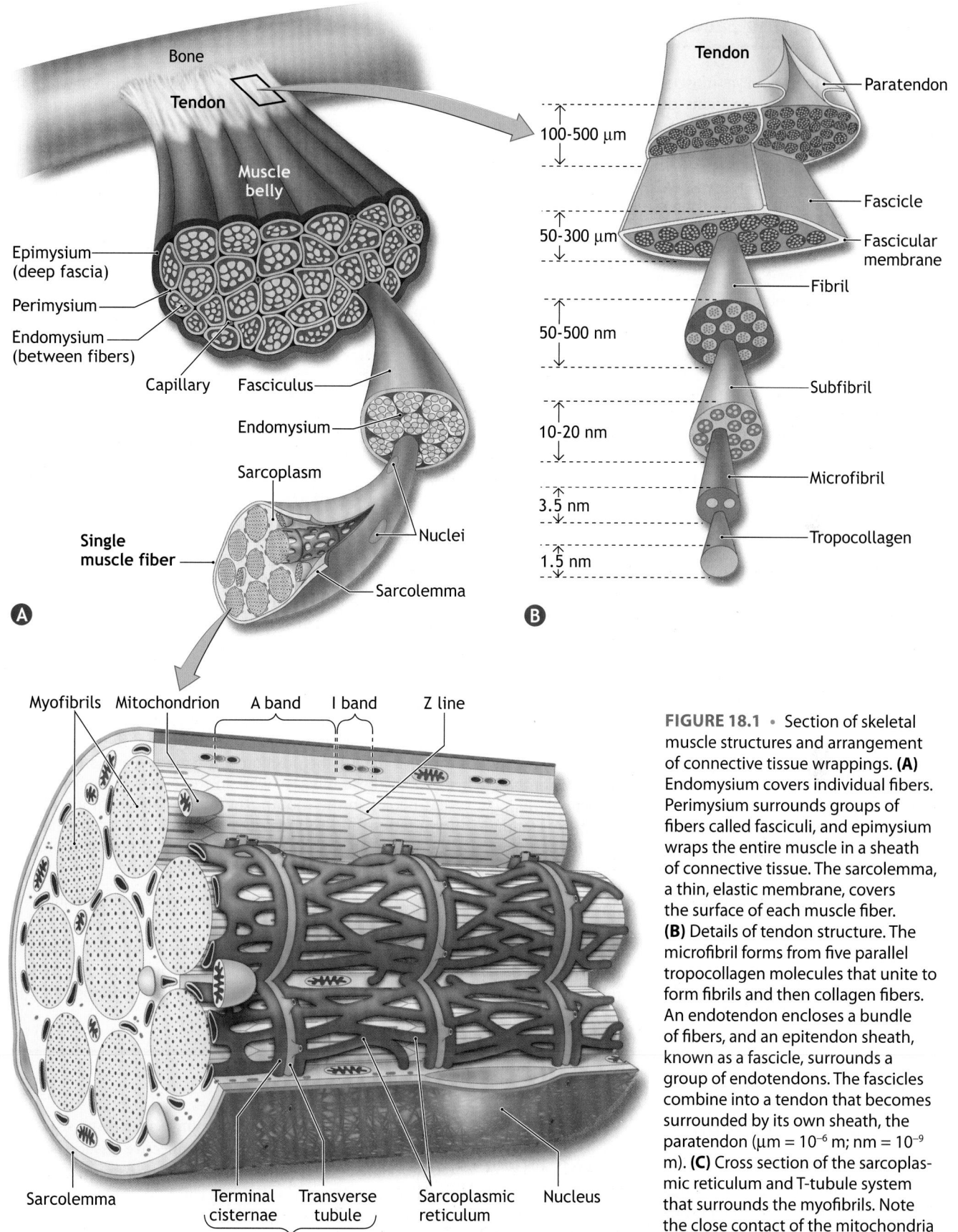

Bone

Tendon

Muscle belly

Epimysium (deep fascia)

Perimysium

Endomysium (between fibers)

Capillary   Fasciculus

Endomysium

Sarcoplasm

Single muscle fiber

Nuclei

Sarcolemma

A

Tendon

Paratendon

100-500 μm

Fascicle

50-300 μm

Fascicular membrane

Fibril

50-500 nm

Subfibril

10-20 nm

Microfibril

3.5 nm

Tropocollagen

1.5 nm

B

Myofibrils   Mitochondrion   A band   I band   Z line

Sarcolemma

Terminal cisternae

Transverse tubule

Sarcoplasmic reticulum

Nucleus

Reticulum triad

C

FIGURE 18.1 • Section of skeletal muscle structures and arrangement of connective tissue wrappings. **(A)** Endomysium covers individual fibers. Perimysium surrounds groups of fibers called fasciculi, and epimysium wraps the entire muscle in a sheath of connective tissue. The sarcolemma, a thin, elastic membrane, covers the surface of each muscle fiber. **(B)** Details of tendon structure. The microfibril forms from five parallel tropocollagen molecules that unite to form fibrils and then collagen fibers. An endotendon encloses a bundle of fibers, and an epitendon sheath, known as a fascicle, surrounds a group of endotendons. The fascicles combine into a tendon that becomes surrounded by its own sheath, the paratendon ($\mu m = 10^{-6}$ m; nm $= 10^{-9}$ m). **(C)** Cross section of the sarcoplasmic reticulum and T-tubule system that surrounds the myofibrils. Note the close contact of the mitochondria and network of intracellular membranes and tubules.

Interesting Facts About Muscles

External Eye Muscles: Eye muscles constantly move to readjust the eye's many positions during wakefulness. The eye blinks more than 100,000 times a day. When the head moves, the external muscles adjust eye position to maintain a steady fixation point. In 1 hr of continuous reading of this textbook, the eye muscles make about 10,000 coordinated movements to maintain focus. Yet these muscles are subject to fatigue. Frequently changing head position and focusing on different objects helps to dissipate eye muscle fatigue.

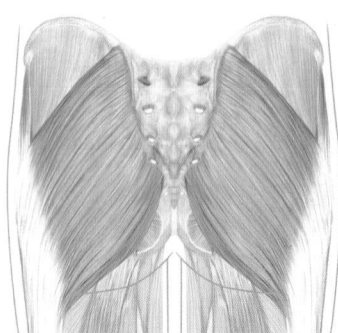

Gluteus Maximus: The main function of the gluteus maximus maximus muscle (from the Latin *musculus glutaeus maximus*), the largest and most powerful antigravity muscle in the body, helps to stabilize an erect posture. Without this muscle's almost continuous state of contraction, the body would collapse to the ground, unable to support the weight of the torso, arms, and head.

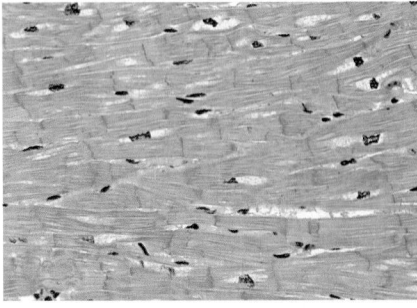

Cardiac Muscle: The heart represents the body's hardest working muscle. It pumps an amount of blood equal at a minimum to at least 2500 gallons or 9450 L daily. And this value only considers an average heart rate of 72 beats a minute. Under these conditions during a typical lifetime the heart beats nonstop over 3 billion times. And this does not consider the periods of physical activity interspersed throughout the day!

Masseter: One of the jaw muscles involved in chewing, the masseter called a masticatory muscle, represents the strongest muscle in the body in relation to its relatively small size in the jaw. With all the jaw muscles working together in chewing a piece of steak, for example, the teeth can close with a force of about 25 kg on the incisors or 91 kg on the molars. Chewing forces are estimated by use of electromyograms (EMGs), similar to determining the dynamic forces generated during a wide variety of physical activities.

Soleus: The soleus is located below and under the gastrocnemius muscle in the calf. Its major action is flexion of the ankle joint, particularly when the leg is bent at the knee, thereby extending the foot downward. It contracts with considerable force as it continually counters the force of gravity to keep the body upright during ambulation (e.g., walking, running, hiking).

Tongue: The tongue consists of a group of eight striated muscles. Its four intrinsic muscles act to change the shape of the tongue, and are not attached to any bone. The four extrinsic muscles change the position of the tongue, and are anchored to bone. These muscles work in the process of mixing foods that begins in the mouth. The tongue also contorts itself to form letters and sounds during speech. The tongue seldom "sleeps"; even during sleep it provides propulsive forces to maintain salivary flow down the throat.

Source: http://www.loc.gov/rr/scitech/mysteries/muscles.html

thePoint   Appendix H, available online at http://thepoint.lww.com/mkk8e, provides a list of supplemental animations and videos on this subject.

Levels of Organization

The **endomysium**, a fine layer of connective tissue, wraps each muscle fiber and separates it from neighboring fibers. Another layer of connective tissue, the **perimysium**, surrounds a bundle of up to 150 fibers called a **fasciculus**. A fascia of fibrous connective tissue, the epimysium, surrounds the entire muscle. This protective sheath tapers at its distal and proximal ends as it blends into and joins the intramuscular tissue sheaths to form the tendon's dense, strong connective tissue. **Tendons** connect both ends of the muscle to the **periosteum**, the bone's outermost covering. Tendinitis, a condition of tendon inflammation, most commonly occurs from trauma at the patellar tendon of the knee (common in basketball and volleyball athletes) and other body regions. These include the achilles region of the ankle (common in sports requiring high impact during lunging and jumping activities), or at the attachment of the rotator cuff muscles, a group of muscles and their tendons that act to stabilize the shoulder (common in sports that involve high-velocity baseball pitching, shotput, or discuss throwing). These injuries usually take months to heal, especially in older individuals. Tendinitis also can occur from overuse and putting limbs through extreme movements that exceed the joints' normal range of motion. In less severe tendon trauma, common therapies include nonsteroidal anti-inflammatory medicines (NSAIDs; http://www.nsaids-list.com), immobilization, ice, and rest, with gradual return to normal physical activities.

The tissues of the tendon intermesh with the collagenous fibers within bone. This forms a powerful link between muscle and bone that remains inseparable except during severe stress when the tendon can sever or literally pull away from the bone. When the tendon attaches to the end of a long bone, the bone adapts by enlarging at that end to create a more stable union. Depending on bone size, the term *tubercle*, *tuberosity*, or *trochanter* describes this overgrowth.

The force of muscle action transmits directly from the connective tissue harness to the tendons, which then pull on the bone at the point of attachment. The forces exerted on the tendinous attachments under muscular exertion range from 20 to 50 N (197 to 492 kg) per cm^2 of cross-sectional area—forces often larger than the muscle fibers themselves can tolerate. The muscle's **origin** refers to the location where the tendon joins a relatively stable skeletal part, generally the proximal or fixed end of the lever system or that nearest the body's midline; the point of distal muscle attachment to the moving bone represents the **insertion**. FIGURE 18.1B illustrates the tendon's ultra structural details. The protein collagen comprises about 70% of the tendon's dry mass.

Beneath the endomysium and surrounding each muscle fiber lies the **sarcolemma**, a thin, elastic membrane that encloses the fiber's cellular contents. It contains a plasma membrane (plasmalemma) and a basement membrane. The plasma membrane, a bilayer lipid structure, conducts the electrochemical wave of depolarization over the surface of the muscle fiber (see Chapter 19). The membrane also insulates one fiber from another during depolarization. Basement membrane proteins and strands of collagen fibrils fuse with the collagenous fibers in the outer covering of the tendon. Between the basement and plasma membranes lie myogenic stem cells known as **satellite cells**, the normally quiescent myoblasts that function in regenerative cellular growth provide possible adaptations to exercise training and recovery from injury.[18,39,52] Incorporation of satellite cell nuclei into existing muscle fibers seems a likely explanation for exercise-induced muscle fiber hypertrophy.[22]

The fiber's aqueous protoplasm or **sarcoplasm** contains enzymes, fat and glycogen particles, nuclei (approximately 250 per mm of fiber length) that contain the genes, mitochondria, and other specialized organelles. FIGURE 18.1C details the **sarcoplasmic reticulum**, an extensive longitudinal latticelike network of tubular channels and vesicles. This highly specialized system provides structural integrity to the cell. It allows the wave of depolarization to spread rapidly from the fiber's outer surface to its inner environment through the T-tubule system to initiate muscle action. The sarcoplasmic reticulum that surrounds each myofibril contains biologic "pumps" that take up Ca^{2+} from the fiber's sarcoplasm. This produces a calcium concentration gradient between the sarcoplasmic reticulum (higher $[Ca^{2+}]$) and the sarcoplasm surrounding the filaments (lower $[Ca^{2+}]$).

Muscles' Chemical Composition

Water constitutes approximately 75% of skeletal muscle mass while protein composes 20%. The remaining 5% contains salts and other substances, including high-energy phosphates;

Subcellular Systems and Muscle Function

According to researchers in the Department of Bioengineering and Orthopaedic Surgery at the University of California, San Diego (http://iem.ucsd.edu/centers/center-for-musculoskeletal-research), skeletal muscle function depends on efficient coordination patterns established among subcellular systems. A subset of tightly regulated genes encodes these protein-mediated systems. Even slightly altering system regulation can lead to disease, injury, and dysfunction. The researchers identified nine biologic networks critical to "normal" muscle function, which begin via the expression of proteins necessary to optimize neuromuscular junction function to initiate the muscle cell's action potential. That signal, transmitted to specialized proteins involved in excitation–contraction coupling, enables Ca^{2+} release, which activates contractile proteins to support actin and myosin crossbridge cycling. The forces generated by crossbridge action are then transmitted by cytoskeletal proteins through the sarcolemma to critical proteins that support the muscle extracellular matrix. Ultimately, muscle action requires "turning on" target-specific proteins that regulate energy metabolism. Inflammation, a common response to muscle injury, can alter many pathways within muscle. Muscle also possesses multiple pathways that regulate its mass through diminished size (*atrophy*) or enhanced size (*hypertrophy*). Different isoforms associated with "fast" muscle fibers and corresponding isoforms in "slow" muscle fibers perform highly specific functions. The different networks represent critical biological systems that affect skeletal muscle function. Analogous to a modern computer network, combining high-throughput systems analysis with advanced networking software can potentially study the interrelationships among network systems and muscle function.

Source: Smith LR, et al. Systems analysis of biological networks in skeletal muscle function. *Wiley Interdiscip Rev Syst Biol Med* 2013;5:55.

urea; lactate; the minerals calcium, magnesium, and phosphorus; various enzymes; sodium, potassium, and chloride ions; and amino acids, fats, and carbohydrates. The most abundant muscle proteins include titin, the largest protein in the body consisting of 27,000 amino acids (accounts for about 10% of muscle mass), myosin (approximately 60% of muscle protein), actin, and tropomyosin. Each 100 g of muscle tissue contains about 700 mg of the oxygen-binding, conjugated protein **myoglobin**.

Blood Supply

Arteries and veins that lie parallel to individual muscle fibers provide a rich vascular supply. These vessels divide into numerous arterioles, capillaries, and venules to form a diffuse network in and around the endomysium. Extensive branching of blood vessels ensures each muscle fiber an adequate oxygenated blood supply from the arterial system and rapid removal of carbon dioxide in the venous circulation. During vigorous physical activity for an elite endurance athlete, the muscle's oxygen uptake increases nearly 70 times to approximately 11 mL per 100 g per minute or a total muscle $\dot{V}O_2$ of 3400 $mL \cdot min^{-1}$. The local vascular bed delivers large quantities of blood through active tissues to accommodate this oxygen requirement. Blood flow distribution fluctuates in rhythmic running, swimming, cycling, and other similar activities. Flow decreases during the muscle's contraction phase and increases during relaxation to provide an auxiliary "milking action" that moves blood through the muscles and propels it via the venous system back to the heart. The rapid dilation of previously dormant capillaries complements the pulsatile blood flow. Between 200 and 500 capillaries deliver blood to each square millimeter of active muscle cross section, with up to four capillaries directly contacting each fiber. In endurance athletes, five to seven capillaries surround each fiber; this positive adaptation ensures greater local blood flow and adequate tissue oxygenation when needed (see next section).

Physical activities that require "straining" (i.e., exerting force against an immovable object) present a somewhat different picture for muscle blood flow. When a muscle generates about 60% of its force-generating capacity for several seconds, elevated intramuscular pressure occludes local blood flow during the contraction. With a sustained high-force contraction, the intramuscular high-energy phosphates and glycolytic anaerobic reactions provide the main energy source for muscular effort.

Capillarization

Trained muscles' increased capillary-to-muscle fiber ratio helps to explain improved exercise capacity with endurance training.[2,6] An enhanced capillary microcirculation expedites removal of heat and metabolic byproducts from active tissues in addition to facilitating delivery of oxygen, nutrients, and hormones. Electron microscopy reveals the total number of capillaries per muscle and capillaries per mm^2 of muscle tissue averages about 40% higher in endurance-trained athletes than untrained counterparts. This almost equals the 41% difference in $\dot{V}O_{2max}$ between the two groups. A positive association also exists between $\dot{V}O_{2max}$ and the average number of muscle capillaries.[42] Enhanced vascularization at the capillary level proves particularly beneficial during activities that require a high level of steady-rate aerobic metabolism. Vascular stretch and shear stress on the vessel walls from increased blood flow during exercise stimulate capillary development with intense aerobic training.[31]

SKELETAL MUSCLE ULTRASTRUCTURE

Highly technical and sophisticated techniques of electron microscopy, x-ray diffraction, histochemical staining, helium–neon laser diffraction, *in vitro* motility assays, single muscle fiber physiology, and optical tweezer technologies (see Chapter 33) reveal the detailed ultra structural details of skeletal muscle anatomy. **Figure 18.2A-F** shows the different levels of gross and subcellular organization within a skeletal muscle fiber. A single multinucleated muscle fiber contains smaller functional units that lie parallel to the fiber's long axis. These **fibrils** or **myofibrils**, approximately 1 μm (1 μm = 1/1000 mm) in diameter, contain even smaller subunits called **filaments** or **myofilaments** that lie parallel to the long axis of the myofibril. The myofilaments chiefly consist of ordered assemblages of the proteins actin and myosin that account for about 85% of the myofibrillar complex. Twelve to 15 other proteins either serve a structural function or affect protein filament interaction during muscle action. Six examples include the following:

1. Tropomyosin, located along the actin filaments (5%)
2. Troponin (which consists of troponin-1, T, C), located in the actin filaments (3%)
3. α-actinin, distributed in the Z-band region (7%)
4. β-actinin, found in the actin filaments (1%)
5. M protein, identified in the region of the M lines within the sarcomere (less than 1%)
6. C protein, which contributes to the sarcomere's structural integrity (less than 1%)

The Sarcomere

At low magnification, alternating light and dark bands along the length of the skeletal muscle fiber give it a characteristic **striated appearance**. **Figure 18.3A** illustrates structural details of this cross-striation pattern within a myofibril. The *I band* represents the lighter area and the *A band* represents the darker area. The *Z line* bisects the I band and adheres to the sarcolemma; it provides stability to the entire structure. Optical properties denote the specific bands. When polarized light passes through the I band, it moves at the same velocity in all directions (isotropic). Light passing through the A band does not scatter equally (anisotropic). The letter *Z* indicates "between" (from German, *zwischenscheibe*); the letter *M* (*mittelscheibe*) denotes "middle"; and the letter *H* (*hellerscheibe*) denotes "a clear disk or zone."

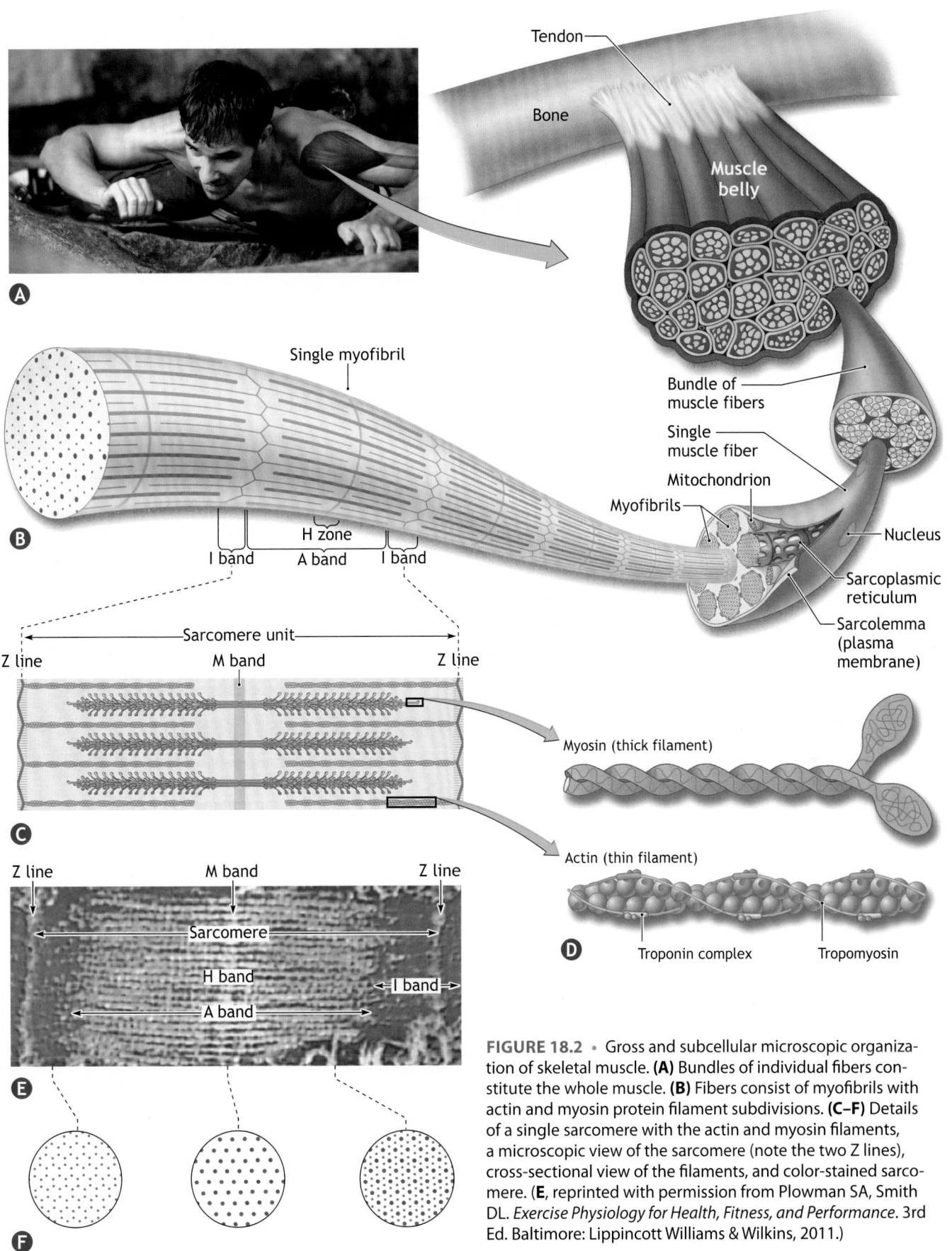

FIGURE 18.2 • Gross and subcellular microscopic organization of skeletal muscle. **(A)** Bundles of individual fibers constitute the whole muscle. **(B)** Fibers consist of myofibrils with actin and myosin protein filament subdivisions. **(C–F)** Details of a single sarcomere with the actin and myosin filaments, a microscopic view of the sarcomere (note the two Z lines), cross-sectional view of the filaments, and color-stained sarcomere. (**E**, reprinted with permission from Plowman SA, Smith DL. *Exercise Physiology for Health, Fitness, and Performance*. 3rd Ed. Baltimore: Lippincott Williams & Wilkins, 2011.)

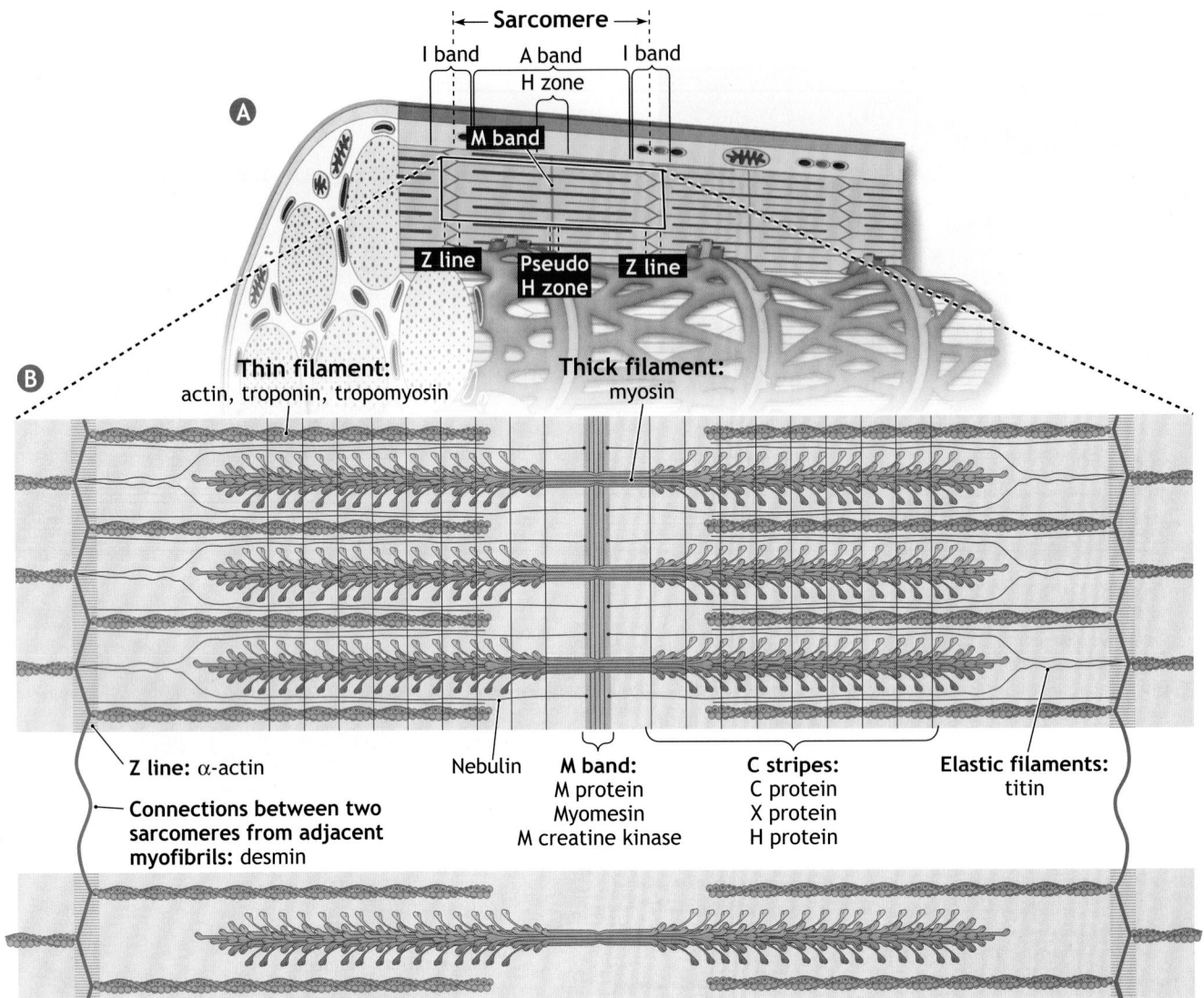

FIGURE 18.3 • **(A)** Structural position of the filaments in a sarcomere. The Z line bounds a sarcomere at both ends. **(B)** Detailed view of a sarcomere, including the proteins listed in Table 18.1.

The sarcomere consists of basic repeating units between two Z lines and comprises the functional unit of a muscle fiber. The actin and bipolar myosin filaments within the sarcomere contribute primarily to the mechanics of muscle contraction. Sarcomeres lie in series, and their filaments have a parallel configuration within a given fiber. At rest, the length of each sarcomere averages 2.5 μm. A myofibril 15-mm long contains about 6000 sarcomeres joined end to end. The sarcomere's length largely determines a muscle's functional properties.

The position of thin actin and thicker myosin proteins in the sarcomere creates an interdigitating overlap of the two filaments. The center of the A band contains the *H zone*, a region of lower optical density because this area has no actin filaments. The *M band* bisects the central portion of the H zone, which delineates the sarcomere's center. The M band consists of the protein structures that support the arrangement of the myosin filaments. **FIGURE 18.3B** shows a detailed view of a sarcomere and **TABLE 18.1** lists proposed functions of a sarcomere's proteins.

MUSCLE FIBER ALIGNMENT

The long axis of a muscle determines the arrangement of individual fibers from an imaginary line drawn through the origin and insertion, or the fiber angle relative to the force-generating axis. Differences in sarcomere alignment and length strongly affect a muscle's force- and power-generating capacity (**FIG. 18.4**). **Fusiform** or spindle-shaped fibers run parallel to the muscle's long axis (e.g., biceps brachii) and taper at the tendinous attachment. In contrast, **pennate** or fan-shaped fibers' fasciculi (bundles of fibers) lie at an oblique pennation angle that varies up to 30°. In the soleus muscle, for example, the pennation angle averages 25°, whereas for the vastus medialis it equals 5°; the sartorius muscle has no angle of pennation. Of functional significance, pennation characteristics directly impact sarcomere number per cross-sectional muscle area. No fibers run the full muscle length. In essence, pennation allows individual muscle fibers to remain short while the overall muscle may attain considerable length.

Lengthened Sarcomeres in Cerebral Palsy Patients

Patients with cerebral palsy (CP) often exhibit wrist contractures—muscles so highly shortened that the wrist gets "stuck" in the flexed position, as shown in the inset photo. Research has confirmed that muscle spasticity is neural in origin, yet spastic muscles are intrinsically abnormal.[a,b] Muscle fiber size and fiber type distribution are abnormal in cerebral palsy patients, suggesting altered myosin heavy-chain expression. Unfortunately, the muscle changes from spasticity are poorly understood. New procedures would be needed to restore muscle length to normal, or to permit fibers to shorten to more favorable lengths for active- and passive-force generation. Researchers[c] at the Muscle Physiology Laboratory at the University of California, San Diego, were surprised to discover that CP patients had *lengthened* sarcomeres in the cramped wrist flexors compared to patients without CP.

This finding, shown at right, using the sophisticated laser diffraction method (see Fig. 18.12), is unprecedented in the literature for any mammalian species including subhuman primates. The researchers hope to unravel the secrets of this unexpected (and as yet unexplained) muscle adaptation in the hope of developing treatment procedures to return sarcomere-fiber and muscle length to a more effective range.

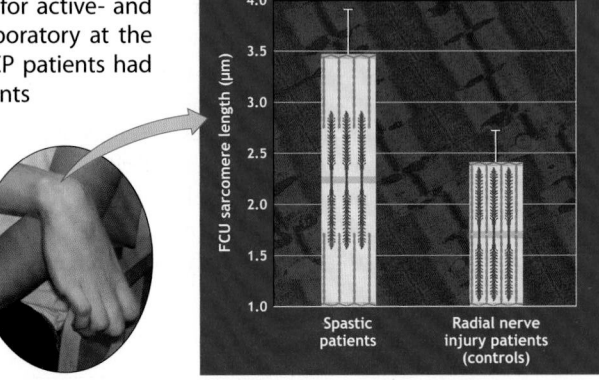

Sources:
[a]Katz RT, Rymer WZ. Spastic hypertonia: mechanisms and measurement. *Arch Phys Med Rehab* 1989;70:144.

[b]Lance JWB. Symposium synopsis. In: Feldman RG, et al., eds. *Spasticity: Disorder of Motor Control*. Chicago: Year Book, 1980:485.

[c]Lieber, RL, Friden, J. Spasticity causes a fundamental rearrangement of muscle–joint interaction. *Muscle Nerve* 2002;25:265.

Flexor carpi ulnaris (FCU) muscle sarcomere length measured during surgery in spastic muscle with the wrist fully flexed. Average FCU sarcomere length measured from six CP patients was 3.48 ± 0.44 µm; this was significantly longer (31%; $p < 0.001$) than the 2.41 ± 0.31 µm measured in 12 patients without CP but with radial nerve injury with the wrist fully flexed. Inset photo courtesy of RL Lieber.

TABLE 18.1	**Twelve Proteins Associated with a Muscle Fiber's Sarcomere and Their Proposed Functions**

Structure	Protein	Function
Thin filament	Actin	The main protein that interacts with myosin during excitation–contraction coupling
	Tropomyosin	Transduces the conformational change of the troponin complex to actin
	Troponin	Binds Ca^{2+} and affects tropomyosin; represents the "switch" that transforms the Ca^{2+} signal into a molecular signal that induces crossbridge cycling
	Nebulin	Presents adjacent to actin and believed to control the number of actin monomers joined to each other in a thin filament
Thick filament	Myosin	Splits ATP and responsible for the "power stroke" of the myosin head
C stripes	C protein	Holds the myosin thick filaments in a regular array; may hold the H protein of adjacent thick filaments at an even distance during force generation; may also control the number of myosin molecules in a thick filament
M line	M protein	Helps hold thick filaments in a regular array
	Myomesin	Provides a strong anchoring point for the protein titin
	M-CK	Provides ATP from phosphocreatine; located proximal to the myosin heads
Z line	α-actinin	Holds the thin filaments in place spatially
	Desmin	Forms the connection between adjacent Z lines from different myofibrils; helps to keep the sarcomeres in register to maintain their striated appearance. Can exhibit fiber-type shift from fast to slow isoforms of myosin heavy chain and significantly decreased sensitivity to insulin.[a]
Elastic filament	Titin	Helps keep the thick filament centered between two Z lines during contraction; believed to control the number of myosin molecules contained in the thick filament

[a]Meyer GA, et al. Role of the cytoskeleton in muscle transcriptional responses to altered use. *Physiol Genomics* 2013;45(8):321.

A fusiform fiber has no pennation, so the fiber's cross-sectional area represents the true anatomic cross section. In pennate muscle, the complex arrangement of connective tissue, tendons, and relatively short fibers creates a larger cross-sectional area than fusiform fibers because more sarcomeres "pack" into a given volume of muscle. The term *physiologic cross-sectional area* (**PCSA**) refers to the total cross-sectional areas of all fibers within a particular muscle. An unusually large pennation angle of 30° results in only a 13% loss in an individual fiber's force capacity; this makes for a huge increase in total fiber-packing ability.[33,45] Pennation per se allows packing of a large number of fibers into a smaller cross-sectional area. Pennate muscles tend to generate considerable power. **FIGURE 18.4B** illustrates the effect of pennation on fiber-packing and force-generating capacity.

Fusiform muscle fibers run parallel to a muscle's long axis. In this case, fiber length equals muscle length, and a fiber's force generation transmits directly to the tendon. *This arrangement facilitates rapid muscle shortening.* A unipennate fiber arrangement, where muscle fibers lie at an oblique angle to the tendon, produces a larger effective cross-sectional area than in fusiform muscle. *Other factors being equal, muscles with greater pennation, yet slower in contractile velocity, generate greater force and power than fusiform muscles because more sarcomeres contribute to muscle action.* A bipennate muscle has two sets of fibers that lie obliquely on both sides of a common tendon (e.g., gastrocnemius and rectus femoris muscles). The multipennate deltoid muscle contains more than two sets of fibers that converge at different angles and insert directly into tendons at both their ends. Pennate muscles differ from fusiform fibers in three ways:

1. They generally contain shorter fibers.
2. They possess more individual fibers.
3. They exhibit less range of motion.

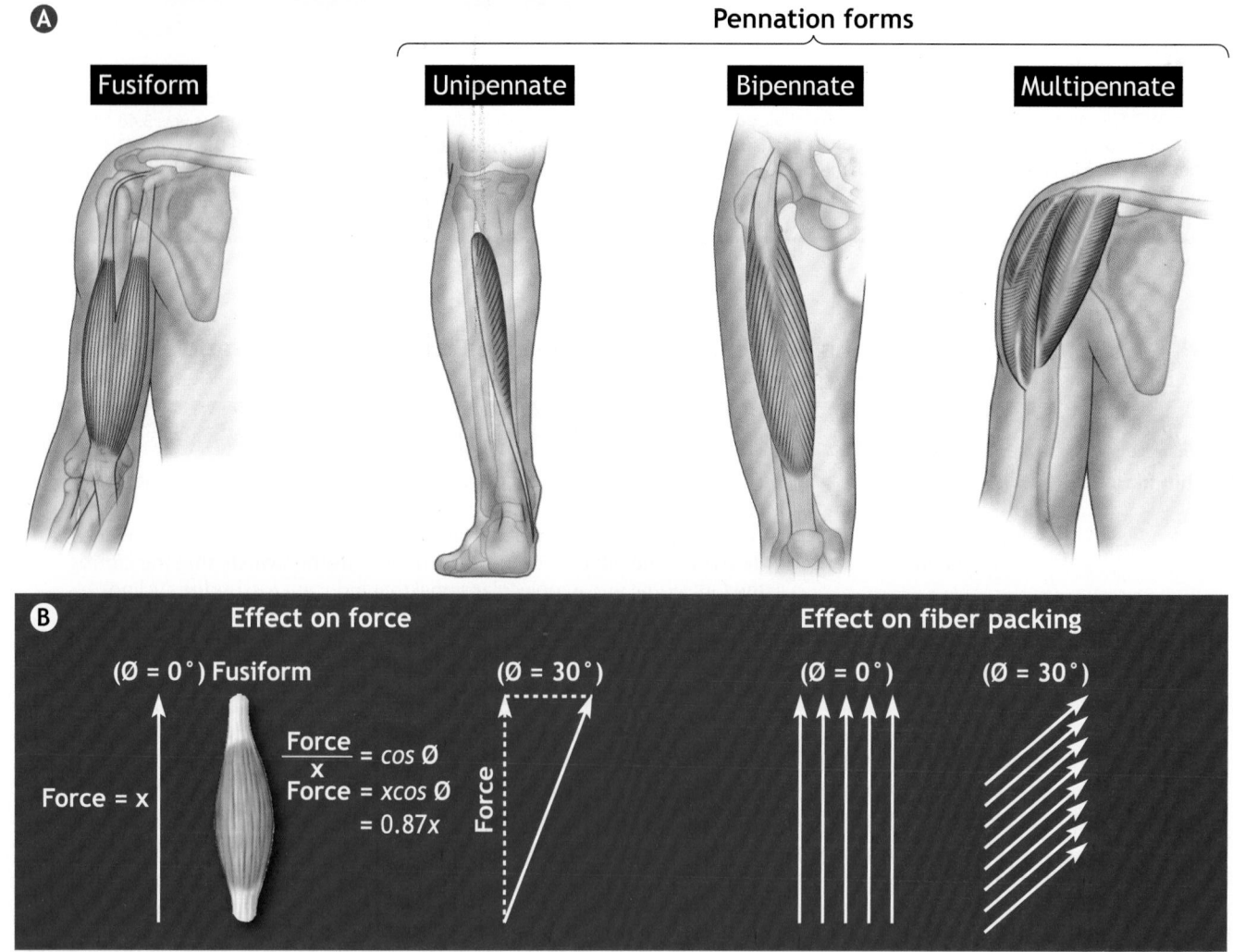

FIGURE 18.4 • **(A)** Various forms of fiber arrangement in human skeletal muscle. **(B)** Force development in a fusiform muscle with no angle of pennation (ø = 0°) and when ø = 30°. A 30° angle of pennation produces a 13% loss of each fiber's maximum force on the tendon, solely based on muscle mechanics. Pennation angle increases the number of fibers that pack into a given volume of muscle (*bottom right*). Muscle mass and the contractile capacity relate proportionally for a given muscle in comparisons among individuals. Because of the effect of pennation angle, it does not necessarily follow that muscle mass per se relates to an equivalent tension output among different muscle groups. (Adapted with permission from Lieber RL. *Skeletal Muscle Structure, Function, and Plasticity: The Physiological Basis of Rehabilitation.* 3rd Ed. Baltimore: Lippincott Williams & Wilkins, 2009.)

Complex Fusiform Arrangement

The **complex parallel muscle**, also called *series-fibered muscle*, features individual fibers that run parallel to the muscle's line of pull. Unlike simple fusiform arrangements where a fiber runs the entire muscle length, the complex parallel arrangement features muscle fibers that terminate in the muscle's midbelly and taper to interact with the connective tissue matrix or adjacent muscle fibers. This arrangement enables parallel packing of relatively short fibers within a long muscle (e.g., the 50-cm-long sartorius). This structural specialization with diverse intrafascicular terminations also creates lateral tension—either through connective tissue into tendon or through adjacent and series fibers into connective tissue—at strategic points along the fiber's surface.

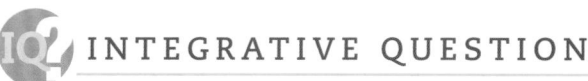 INTEGRATIVE QUESTION

List advantages of a skeletal muscle organ system composed of muscles whose fibers vary in architectural design.

Fiber Length–Muscle Length Ratio

The ratio of individual fiber length to muscle's total length usually varies between 0.2 and 0.6. This means that individual fibers in the longest muscles such as the upper and lower limbs remain shorter than the muscle's overall length. FIGURE 18.5A illustrates the architectural properties of four lower limb muscles. On average,

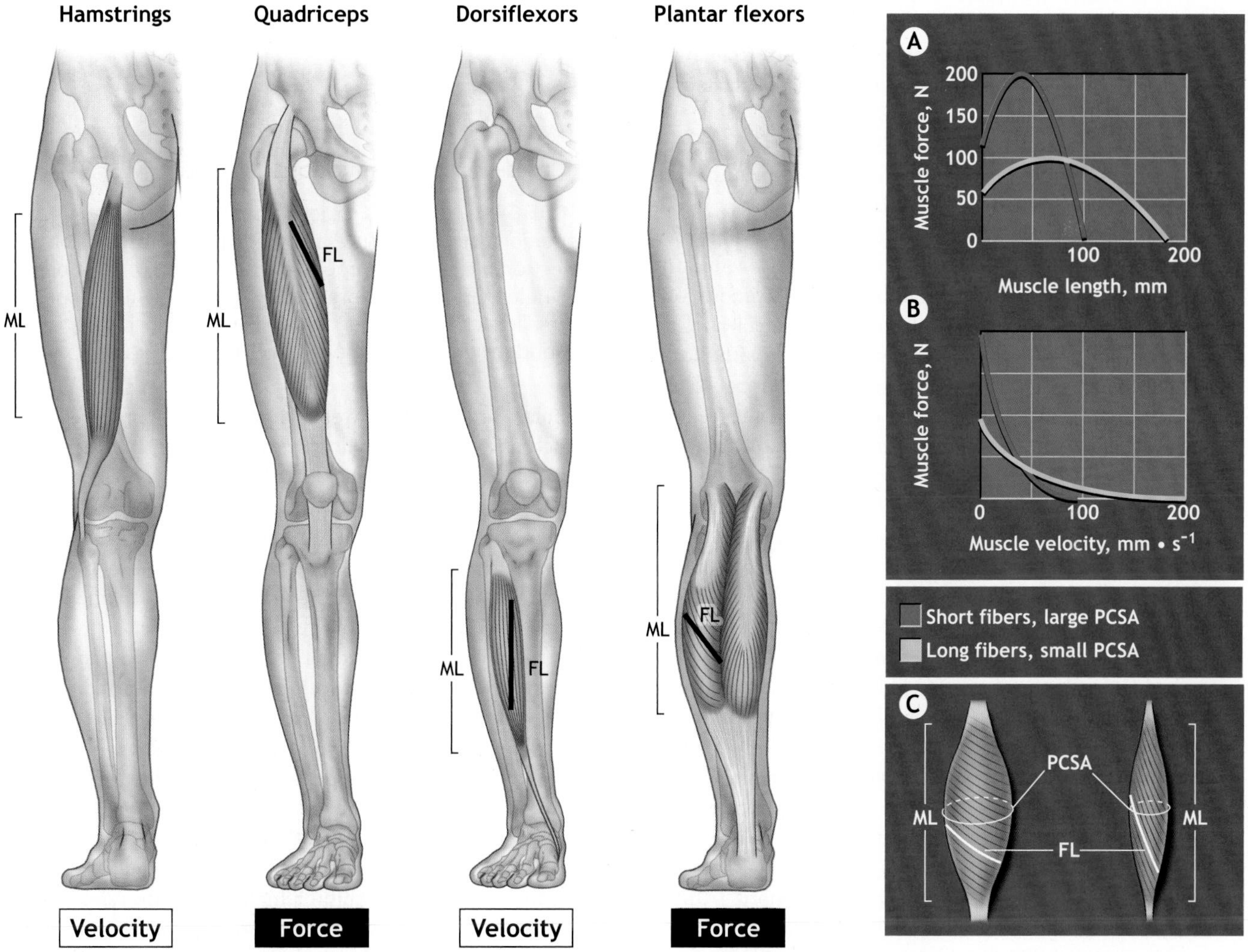

FIGURE 18.5 • Left Muscle architectural properties in the lower limb. The quadriceps and plantar flexors exhibit high force production from their low fiber length–to–muscle length (FL:ML) ratios and relatively large physiologic cross-sectional areas (PCSA). In contrast, the hamstrings and dorsiflexor muscles show architecture designed for high contractile velocity from their relatively high FL:ML and long FL. Hypothetical pennate (short fibers) muscles and fusiform (long fibers) muscles of the same length and same amount of contractile machinery. The muscle force–muscle length curve **(A)** shows the fusiform muscle with a longer working range and lower maximum force output than the pennate muscle. Lower force capacity (dorsiflexors and hamstrings) occurs because for a given change in muscle length, the individual sarcomeres lengthen less, with the change in muscle length distributed over more sarcomeres. A greater PCSA **(C)** produces a greater force output (quadriceps and plantar flexors). The muscle force–muscle velocity curve **(B)** shows that the fusiform muscle with longer fibers exhibits higher contractile velocity but a lower maximum force output. (Modified with permission from Lieber RL. *Skeletal Muscle Structure, Function, and Plasticity: The Physiological Basis of Rehabilitation.* 3rd Ed. Baltimore: Lippincott Williams & Wilkins, 2009.)

quadriceps muscle fibers maintain pennation angles that average 4.6°, a PCSA of approximately 21.7 cm², with a fiber length that averages about 68 mm. This contrasts with the biceps femoris (hamstring) muscle, with relatively long fibers (111 mm) and an intermediate PCSA (11.7 cm²). Quadriceps muscles exhibit approximately 50% greater force capacity than hamstrings, whose design allows for rapid shortening. These design differences suggest susceptibility of the hamstrings to tearing as often occurs in sprint-running when an abrupt force output imbalance occurs during maximal activation between the quadriceps and hamstrings. Part of the imbalance may be from a strength deficit between the hamstrings and quadriceps, which predisposes individuals to recurrent hamstring injuries and discomfort.[10] The hamstring-to-quadriceps strength ratio typically computes by dividing the maximal knee flexor (hamstring) moment by the maximal knee extensor (quadriceps) moment.[1] When sports trainers and physical therapists assess these ratios and detect larger-than-expected deficits during preseason screening, they can devise specific muscle training at preset velocities to improve hamstring-to-quadriceps deficits as an integral part of functional rehabilitation.[8,14,34]

Figure 18.5 A and B shows generalized muscle force–muscle length and muscle force–muscle velocity relationships for fusiform and pennate muscles with the same amount of contractile protein and identical muscle fiber type. In this hypothetical example, the muscle force–muscle length curve for fusiform muscle shows a longer working range and lower maximum force output because of longer individual fibers and a smaller PCSA (Fig. 18.5C). The opposite occurs for pennate muscle with shorter fibers and larger PCSA—these fibers generate about double the force of fusiform muscles. For the muscle force–muscle velocity curve, the fusiform muscle with longer fibers exhibits a higher contractile velocity but lower force–output capacity.

ACTIN–MYOSIN ORIENTATION

Thousands of myosin filaments lie along the line of a muscle fiber's actin filaments. FIGURE 18.6A illustrates sarcomere's resting length actin–myosin orientation. Figure 18.6B shows the hexagonal arrangement of myosin and actin filaments. Myosin filaments consist of bundles of molecules with polypeptide tails and globular heads. Actin filaments have two twisted chains of monomers bound by tropomyosin polypeptide chains. Six relatively thin actin filaments, each about 50 Å in diameter and 1 µm long, encircle the thicker myosin filament (150 Å in diameter and 1.5 µm long). This represents an extremely impressive substructural configuration. For example, a myofibril 1 µm in diameter contains approximately 450 thick filaments in the sarcomere's center and 900 thin filaments at each end. A muscle fiber 100 µm in diameter and 1 cm long contains approximately 8000 myofibrils; each myofibril consists of 4500 sarcomeres on average. In a single fiber, this arrangement consists of approximately 16 billion thick filaments and 64 billion thin filaments.

FIGURE 18.7 illustrates the spatial orientation of various components of contractile filaments. Projections or "**crossbridges**" spiral around the myosin filament in the region of overlap of the actin and myosin filaments. The crossbridges repeat at intervals of approximately 450 Å along the filament.

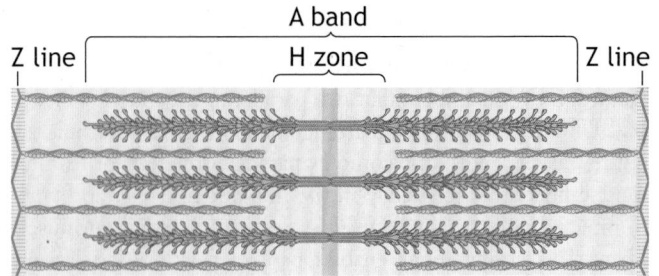

A Resting sarcomere

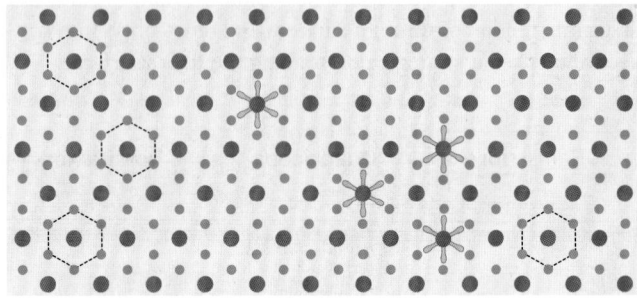

B Cross-section of myofibrils

FIGURE 18.6 • **(A)** Ultra structure of actin–myosin orientation within a resting sarcomere. **(B)** Representation of electron micrograph through a cross section of myofibrils in a single muscle fiber. Note the hexagonal orientation of the smaller actin and larger myosin filaments, including crossbridges that extend from a thick to thin filament.

Globular "lollipoplike" myosin heads extend perpendicularly to latch onto the thinner double-twisted actin strands to create structural and functional links between myofilaments. The unique feature of myosin's two heads concerns their opposite orientation at the ends of the thick filament. ATP hydrolysis activates the two heads, placing them in an optimal orientation to bind actin's active sites, pulling the thin filaments and Z lines of the sarcomere toward the middle.

Tropomyosin and troponin are two other important constituents of the actin helical structure. These proteins regulate make-and-break contacts between the myofilaments during muscle action. Tropomyosin distributes along the length of the actin filament in a groove formed by the double helix. Tropomyosin inhibits actin and myosin interaction (coupling) and prevents their permanent bonding. Troponin and its three-subunit proteins embedded at fairly regular intervals along the actin strands exhibit a high affinity for calcium ions (Ca²⁺), a mineral that plays a crucial role in muscle action and fatigue.[29] For example, Ca²⁺ and troponin trigger myofibrils to interact and slide past each other. During muscle fiber stimulation, troponin molecules undergo a conformational change that "tugs" on tropomyosin protein strands. Tropomyosin then moves deeper into the groove between two actin strands, "uncovering" actin's active sites so muscle action proceeds. Muscle fatigue relates to considerable reductions in Ca²⁺ concentration in the transverse tubules during intense exercise, in addition to intrinsic alterations in the contractile apparatus and sarcoplasmic reticulum function.[7,51]

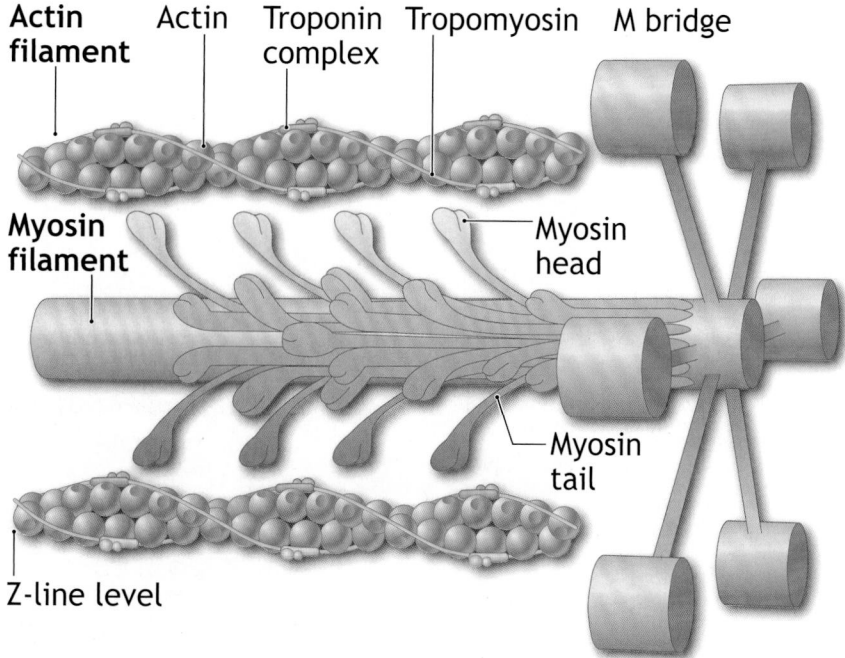

FIGURE 18.7 • Details of the thick and thin protein filaments including tropomyosin, troponin complex, and M bridge. The globular heads of the myosin contain myosin ATPase; this "active" head frees the energy from ATP for muscle action.

The M band consists of transversely and longitudinally oriented proteins that maintain myosin filament orientation within a sarcomere. As Figure 18.7 illustrates, the perpendicularly oriented M bridges interconnect in a hexagonal pattern with six adjacent myosin filaments.

An exciting area of muscle biochemistry, physiology, and mechanics involves the study of cytoskeletal proteins and structures that serve as an intermediate intracellular filament system.[36] The intracellular cytoskeleton provides the following:

1. Structural integrity in the inactive muscle cell
2. Lateral force transmission to adjacent sarcomeres through interaction with actomyosin during muscle action
3. Connections to the cell's surface membrane

A better understanding of the role of the cytoskeleton, its diverse proteins, and the myofibrillar lattice structure would enhance current understanding of muscle action, including processes in muscle injury, repair, and overload.

Intracellular Tubule Systems

Figure 18.8 illustrates the complex tubule system within a muscle fiber. The lateral end of each tubule channel terminates in a saclike vesicle that stores Ca^{2+}. Another network of tubules—the transverse tubule system or **T-tubule system**—runs perpendicular to the myofibril. T tubules lie between the most lateral part of two sarcoplasmic channels; vesicles of these structures abut the T tubule. The term *triad* describes this repeating pattern of two vesicles and a T tubule in each Z line region. Each sarcomere contains two triads, with the pattern repeated regularly along the myofibril's length.

The T tubules pass through the fiber and open externally from inside of the muscle cell. *The triad and T-tubule system function as a microtransportation network by spreading the action potential or wave of depolarization from the fiber's outer membrane inward to deeper cell regions.* Propagation of the action potential stimulates the triad sacs to release Ca^{2+}, which diffuses a short distance to "activate" the actin filaments. Muscle action begins when myosin filament crossbridges momentarily attach to active sites on the actin filaments. When electrical excitation ceases, Ca^{2+} concentration in cytoplasm decreases; this relates to muscle relaxation. To some extent, propagating an action potential depends on maintaining continued steep gradients of Na^+ and K^+ across the sarcolemma. Decreased chemical gradients of these electrolytes, including reduction in Na^+/K^+ pump activity, severely impacts muscle fiber excitability and consequent contractile performance of active muscles.[35]

CHEMICAL AND MECHANICAL EVENTS DURING MUSCLE ACTION AND RELAXATION

Electron microscopy, x-ray diffraction, and biochemical methods have unraveled many secrets of cellular structure and kinetics, providing testable hypotheses about chemical and mechanical events during muscle activation and relaxation. Many pieces of the puzzle remain unanswered, but considerable evidence supports the **sliding-filament model** to explain muscle action. Proposed over 60 years ago to explain molecular movements that underlie muscle action, the model still fits nicely with the ever-expanding details about muscle ultra structure and function.[21]

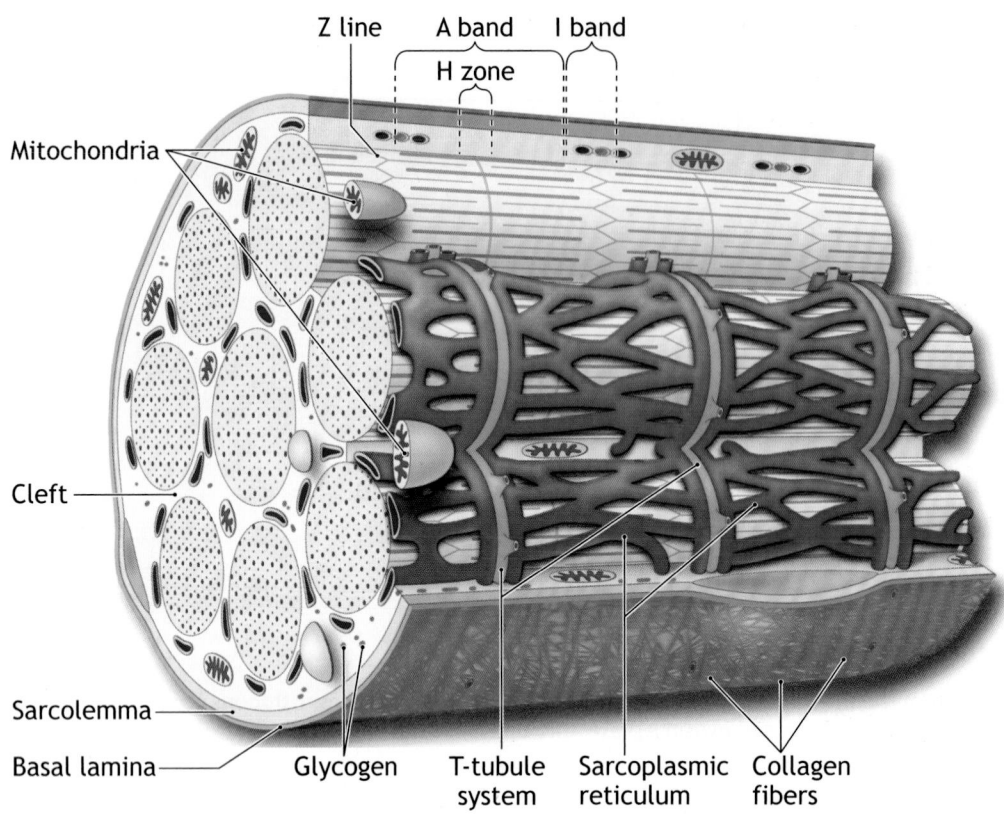

FIGURE 18.8 • The complex "highway" transportation tubule system within a muscle fiber.

 See the animation "Sliding Filament Theory" on http://thePoint.lww.com/mkk8e for a demonstration of this process.

Mechanics of Muscle Action: The Sliding-Filament Model

In the early 1950s, two British biologists, with the same last name but unrelated, and working independently, Hugh Esmor Huxley (1924–) and Sir Andrew Fielding Huxley (1917–2012; 1963 co-winner of the Nobel Prize in Physiology or Medicine for work on ionic mechanisms involved in excitation and inhibition in the peripheral and central portions of the nerve cell membrane), proposed a sliding-filament model of muscle contraction. A video lecture by Dr. Hugh Huxley provides salient details about his and others' research contributions to the sliding filament model of muscle contraction.

thePoint Appendix H, available online at http://thepoint.lww.com/mkk8e, provides a list of supplemental animations and videos on this subject.

In 1957, A. Huxley extended the theory to include specifics of crossbridge behavior.[22,23] *The theory proposes a muscle shortens or lengthens because thick and thin filaments slide past each other without changing length. The myosin crossbridges cyclically attach, rotate, and detach from the actin filaments with energy from ATP hydrolysis and provide the molecular motor to drive fiber shortening.*[13,40] This produces a major conformational change in relative size within the sarcomere's zones and bands and produces a force at the Z bands. FIGURE 18.9 shows the thin actin filaments move past the myosin myofilaments by translating over them by a preset amount and into the A band region during shortening and move out during the lengthening or relaxation phase.[4,5] The major structural rearrangement during shortening occurs in the region of the I band. This band decreases as the Z bands pull toward the center of each sarcomere. No change occurs in the width of the A band, while the H zone can disappear when the actin filaments make contact at the sarcomere center. A static or isometric muscle action generates force, but the fiber's length remains unchanged; the relative spacing of I and A bands remains constant. In this case, the same molecular groups interact continuously. The A band widens in an eccentric action as the fiber lengthens during force generation.

 ## Multimedia Muscle Action Videos

Links to a number of multimedia video animations presenting different aspects of muscle action processes can be found in Appendix H, available online at http://thepoint.lww.com/mkk8e. These videos, produced by students for students, are complementary to our presentation of muscle action dynamics.

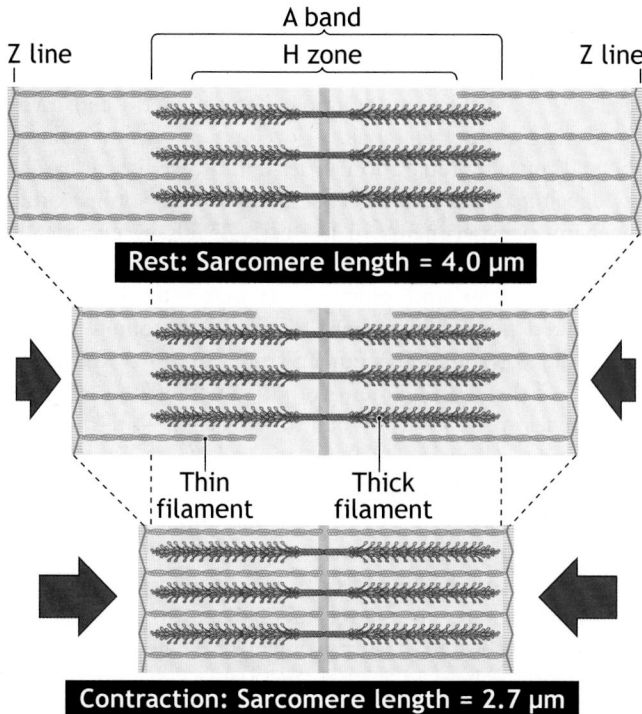

FIGURE 18.9 • Structural rearrangement of actin and myosin filaments at rest (sarcomere length, 4.0 μm) and during muscle shortening (contracted sarcomere length, 2.7 μm).

Mechanical Action of Crossbridges

Myosin plays both an enzymatic and structural role in muscle action.[50] The globular head of the myosin crossbridge, which contains an actin-activated ATPase in its actin-binding site, provides the mechanical power stroke for actin and myosin filaments to slide past each other. The cyclic, oscillating to-and-fro motion of crossbridges powered by ATP hydrolysis moves like oars *knifing* through water (FIG. 18.10). But unlike oars, crossbridges do not all move synchronously. If they did, muscle action would produce a series of uneven and jerky actions instead of finely graded, smoothly modulated movements and force outputs. During shortening, each crossbridge undergoes repeated but independent cycles of asynchronous movement.

thePoint Appendix H, available online at http://the point.lww.com/mkk8e, provides a list of supplemental animations and videos on this subject.

At any one time, approximately 50% of crossbridges make contact with actin filaments to form the protein complex **actomyosin**, which exhibits contractile properties. The remaining crossbridges move through other positions in their vibrating cycle. Figure 18.10 shows each crossbridge action contributes only a small longitudinal displacement to the filament's full sliding action. The process resembles movement of a person rope climbing. The arms and legs represent the crossbridges. Climbing progresses by first reaching with the arms; then grabbing, pulling, and breaking contact while the legs extend;

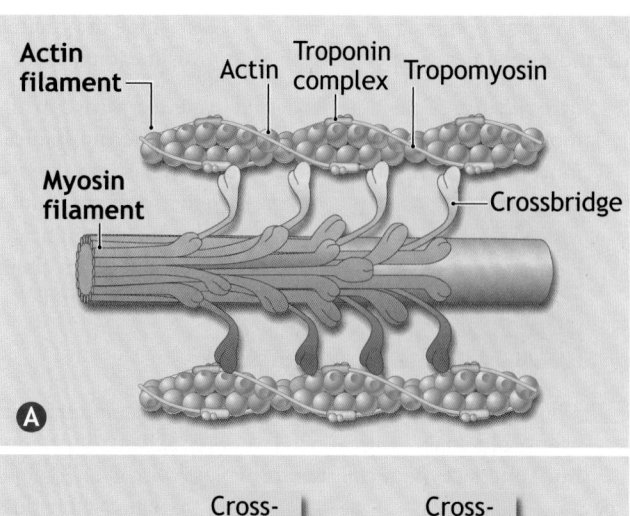

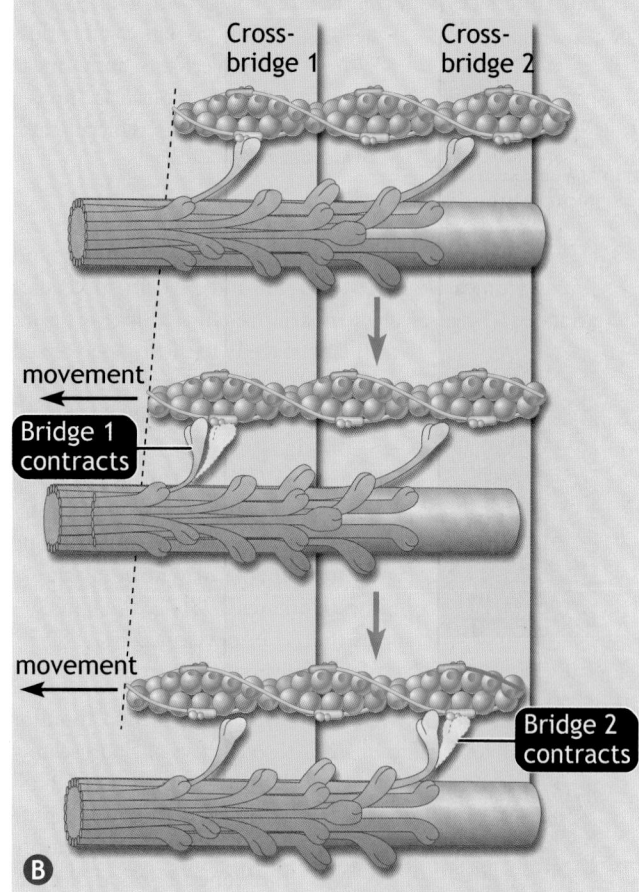

FIGURE 18.10 • **(A)** Relative positioning of actin and myosin filaments during crossbridge oscillation. **(B)** The action of each crossbridge contributes a small displacement of movement. For clarity, we show only one actin strand.

and then repeating this procedure throughout the climb as the person traverses from one point to the next point and so on.

The biochemical technique of *in vitro* motility assay (http://www.umass.edu/musclebiophy/techniques%20-%20 in%20vitro%20motility%20assay.html) can quantify the behavior of actin and myosin molecules.[11,29]

Careful experimentation has determined that myosin elicits a 1 to 10 piconewton (pN; 10^{-2} N) force, in which myosin movement ranges from 1 to 20 nanometers (nm; 10^{-9} m) over a

5 ms interval. Four elegant research tools determine the chemical and mechanical properties of the actomyosin complex:

1. *Microneedles.* A glass needle placed in contact with myosin molecules and an actin filament records the mechanical movements of the molecules.[53] Researchers then deduce the forces produced by the myosin heads as they slide along the actin strand.[24]

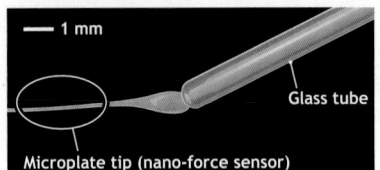

2. *Optical tweezers.* This technique (http://www.stanford.edu/group/blocklab/Optical%20Tweezers%20Introduction.htm) interfaces powerful laser technology with a microscope to isolate individual molecules and measure molecular movement one molecule at a time.[12]

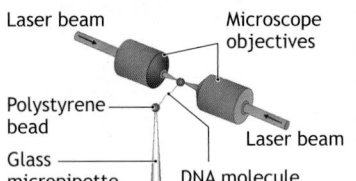

3. *Atomic force microscope* (AFM). The displacement and forces from a probe (with actin and myosin molecules attached; http://www.nanoscience.com/education/afm.html) interfaced with a specialized microscope yields quantitative data about actin–myosin interaction.[27] Gerd Binnig (1947-) and Heinrich Rohrer (1933-2013) won the 1986 Nobel Prize in Physics for developing the scanning tunneling microscope (www.nobelprize.org/nobel_prizes/physics/laureates/1986/), the precursor of the AFN developed in 1989 by Stanford University researchers.

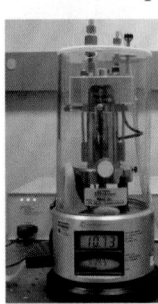

4. *Fluorescent probes.* Microscopy with the ability to monitor the physiologic state of a cell through use of flourescently labeled probes of high chemical sensitivity. Light-emitting probes quantify the kinetics of molecular binding and release between myosin and actin and how ATP releases energy when degraded to ADP and inorganic phosphate.[15] The technique reveals how actin rotates slightly as it moves along myosin and how the myosin heads function during their power stroke.[43]

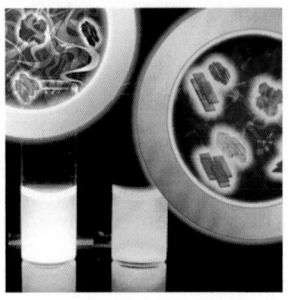

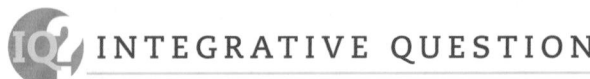

IQ² INTEGRATIVE QUESTION

Discuss the meaning of molecular motor to describe how myofilament crossbridges contribute to muscle fiber action.

Sarcomere Length—Isometric Tension Curve in an Isolated Fiber

FIGURE 18.11 displays interactions between actin and myosin during isometric tension development in an isolated skeletal muscle preparation. British and Swedish researchers developed this length–tension curve with sophisticated mechanical experiments in the early 1960s by electrically stimulating a single frog muscle fiber 8 mm long and 75 μm in diameter and plotting maximum tension output at selected muscle sarcomere lengths.[17] Sarcomere length along the horizontal axis ranged from 1.6 μm at maximum overlap of the actin filaments (approximately 70% of maximum tension) to 3.6 μm when fully relaxed. Note the crest of the upward curve for tension occurred at a sarcomere length between 2.0 and 2.25 μm; this length for maximal tension represents the region of maximum actin and myosin filament interaction. Interestingly, the difference of 0.2 μm at this part of the curve equals precisely the width of the region where no change takes place in actin–myosin interaction. The curve shifts downward when the sarcomere stretches beyond 2.2 μm, indicating a decline in peak tension. This decline occurs from reduced overlap between actin and myosin filaments; less overlap produces less cross-bridge interaction and diminished active tension development. Fibers fail to develop tension at the maximum point of stretch of 3.65 μm (maximum actin filament length, 2.0 μm; maximum myosin filament length, 1.65 μm). Cross-bridge interaction cannot take place at a sarcomere length of 3.65 μm and above.

Sarcomere Length—Isometric Tension Curve in Human Muscle Fibers in Vivo

An elegant technical procedure determines the range over which sarcomeres in intact human muscle operate along their length–tension curve. **FIGURE 18.12** illustrates sarcomere action during different wrist position angles in patients who undergo surgery to correct chronic lateral epicondylitis or "tennis elbow." The researchers compared length–tension characteristics of an animal preparation (Fig. 18.11) with those of human muscle *in vivo*. Figure 18.12 (*top right*) depicts the intraoperative helium–neon laser to quantify sarcomere length. The laser, positioned beneath the lateral end of the extensor carpi radialis brevis (ECRB) muscle, quantified sarcomere lengths at three different wrist positions: (1) full flexion to increase sarcomere length, (2) neutral, and (3) full extension to decrease sarcomere length. Figure 18.12 (*top left*) shows the laser diffraction pattern for computing sarcomere length. Biopsy specimens from the same muscle verified the laser determinations. An electron micrograph displayed behind the length–tension curve shows the actin and myosin filaments and A and I bands from a muscle biopsy sample. In this experiment, actin filament length equaled 1.30 μm, while the myosin filaments were 1.66 μm long. The thicker blue portion for the plateau and downward parts of the curve show the operating range

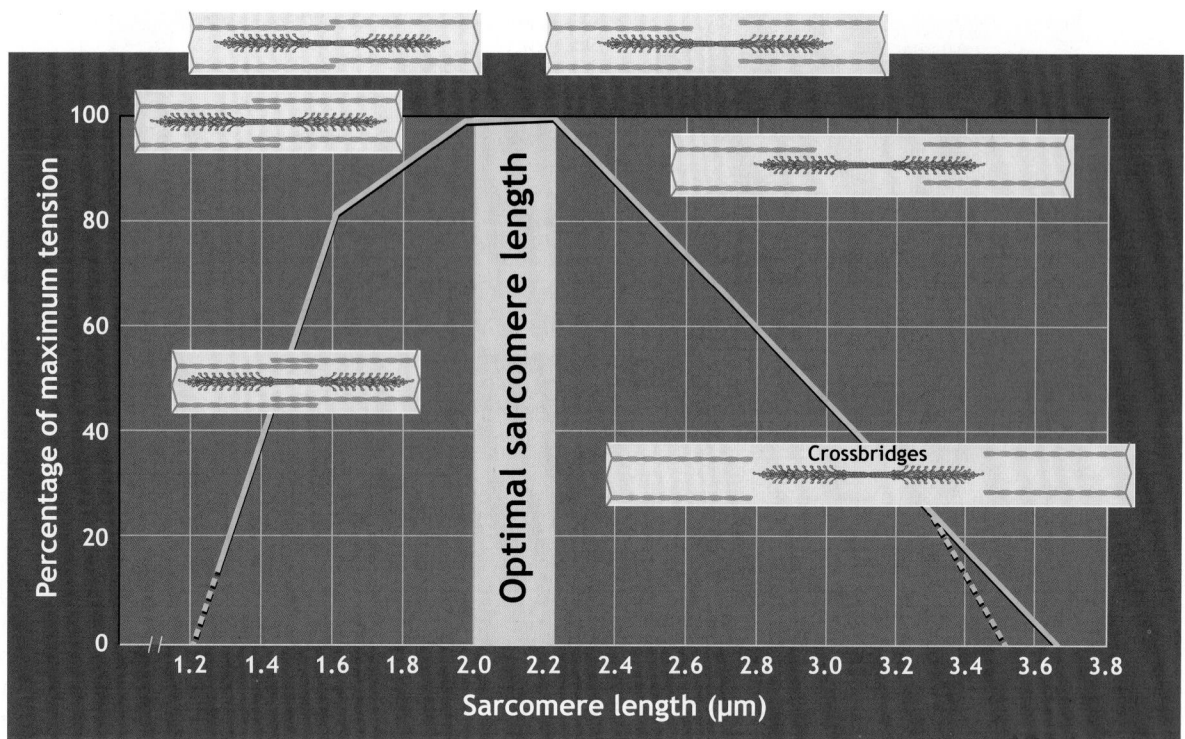

FIGURE 18.11 • Relationship between tension and sarcomere length in skeletal muscle during an isometric muscle action. Optimal sarcomere length (i.e., the one with the greatest interaction between actin and myosin filaments) occurs between 2.0 and 2.25 μm (*light blue vertical band*). Tension output decreases steadily as sarcomere length increases beyond the optimal length. Note the amount of overlap in the actin and myosin filaments at various regions of the tension–length curve and how tension output varies at different sarcomere lengths. Thin filament thickness equals 1.0 μm; thick filament thickness, 1.6 μm.

of ECRB sarcomeres during both passive (2.6–3.4 μm) and active (2.44–3.33 μm) muscle actions. These data objectify the intrinsic relation between sarcomere length and muscle fiber force capacity (length–tension curve) measured *in vivo* in human muscle.

Link Between Actin, Myosin, and ATP

The interaction and movement of the protein filaments during muscle action require that myosin crossbridges continually undergo oscillatory movements by combining, detaching, and recombining with new sites along the actin strands or the same sites in a static action. Myosin crossbridges detach from the actin filament when ATP molecules join the actomyosin complex. The myosin crossbridge in this chemical reaction returns to their original state ready to bind to a new active actin site. The dissociation of actomyosin occurs as follows:

$$Actomyosin + ATP \rightarrow Actin + Myosin\text{-}ATP$$

Energy from ATP hydrolysis transduces into mechanical force when ADP and inorganic phosphate end products form. One of the reacting sites on the globular head of the myosin crossbridge binds to an actin reactive site. The other myosin active site serves as the actin-activated enzyme **myofibrillar adenosine triphosphatase** (**myosin ATPase**). This enzyme splits ATP to yield energy for muscle action. The rate of ATP splitting remains relatively slow if myosin and actin continue apart; when they join, myosin ATPase reaction rates increase substantially. Energy released from ATP splitting activates crossbridges, causing them to oscillate. This course of energy transfer produces a conformational change in myosin's globular head so it interacts with the appropriate actin molecule. The actin filament slides forward from conformational change at multiple points of contact between myosin and actin.

Prior to muscle action, the elongated, pear-shaped, flexible myosin head literally bends around the energy-carrying ATP molecule and cocks like a spring. The myosin then interacts with the adjacent actin filament, splits a phosphate from ATP, and releases its stored mechanical energy as it straightens. This forces the sliding motion that generates muscle tension. Actin and myosin filaments slide past each other at speeds up to 15 μm · s⁻¹.[3]

Excitation–Contraction Coupling

Excitation–contraction coupling represents the physiologic mechanism whereby an electrical discharge at muscle initiates chemical

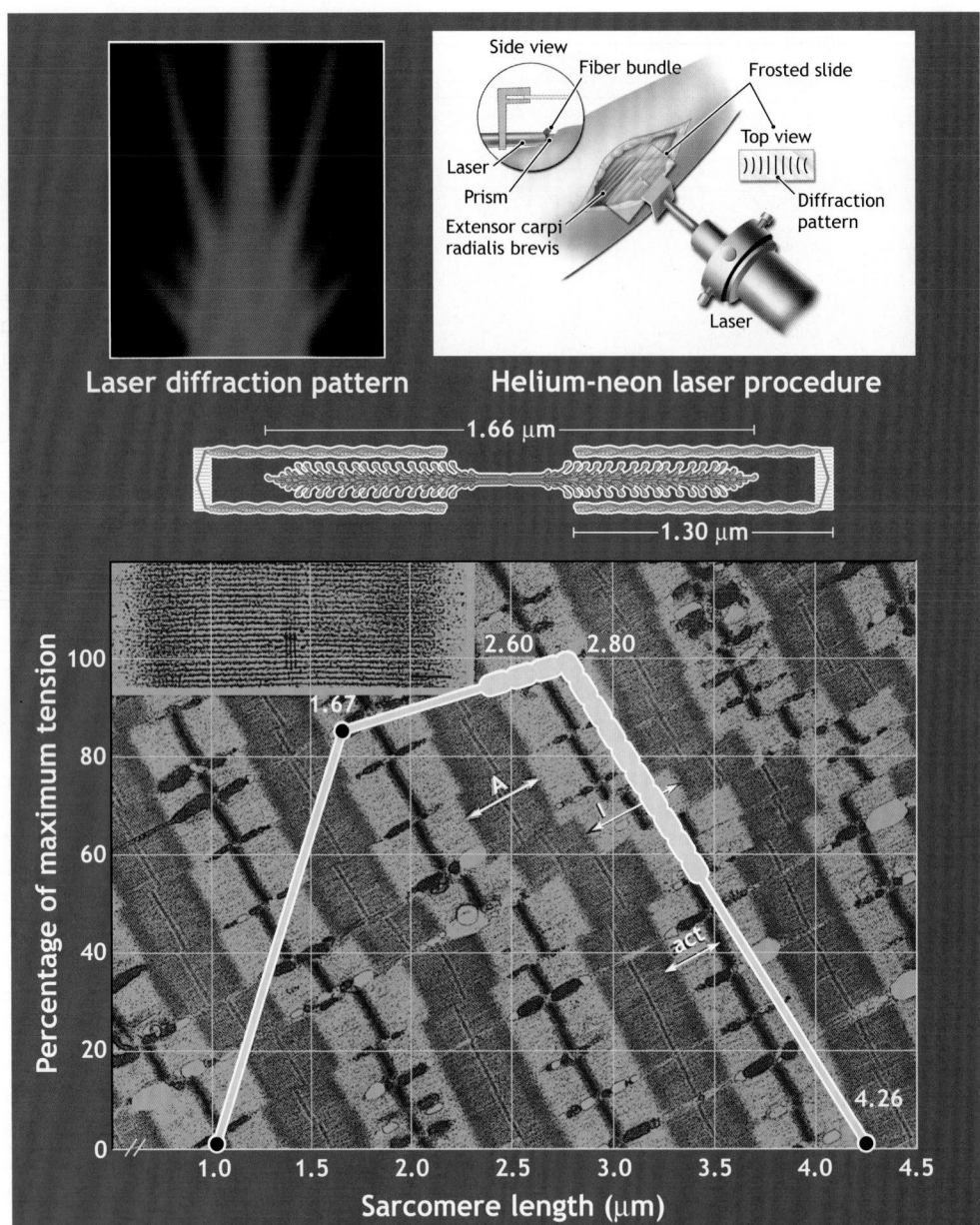

FIGURE 18.12 • Changes in the length–tension curve for sarcomeres *in vivo* during human wrist flexion and extension. The top insets illustrate the helium–neon laser procedure (and view of the illumination prism) used during the surgery. The electron micrograph depicted behind the length–tension curve shows the actin and myosin filaments and the A and I bands from biopsy samples of the extensor carpi radialis brevis muscle to verify sarcomere lengths. The *thickened yellow portion* of a hypothetical length–tension curve represents sarcomere length change during wrist flexion (causing sarcomere length increase) and wrist extension (causing sarcomere length decrease). The numbers over the curve represent the inflection points based on the measured filament lengths. (Adapted with permission from Lieber RL, et al. In vivo measurement of human wrist extensor muscle sarcomere length changes. *J Neurophysiol* 1994;71:874. Illustration of the experimental procedure, including the example of the laser diffraction pattern and electron micrograph courtesy of Dr. RL Lieber, Professor of Orthopaedics and Bioengineering, Biomedical Sciences Group, Muscle Physiology Laboratory, University of California, San Diego, CA; **http://muscle.ucsd.edu.**

events at the cell surface to release intracellular Ca²⁺ and ultimately produce muscle action.

Intracellular Ca^{2+} plays an intimate role in regulating a muscle fiber's contractile and metabolic activity. Ca^{2+} concentration within a nonactive muscle fiber remains relatively low compared with the extracellular fluid that bathes the cell. Muscle fiber stimulation causes an immediate, small increase in intracellular Ca^{2+}, which precedes contractile activity. Cellular Ca^{2+} increases when the action potential at the transverse tubules causes Ca^{2+} release from lateral sacs of the sarcoplasmic reticulum. The inhibitory action of troponin, which prevents actin–myosin interaction, rapidly dissipates when Ca^{2+} binds with this and other proteins in the actin filaments. In a sense, the muscle "turns on" for action.

$$Actin + Myosin\ ATPase \rightarrow Actomyosin + ATPase$$

Joining active sites on actin and myosin activates myosin ATPase to split ATP. The energy generated causes myosin crossbridge movement to produce muscle tension.

$$Actomyosin\ ATP \rightarrow Actomyosin + ADP + Pi + Energy$$

Crossbridges uncouple from actin when ATP binds to the myosin crossbridge. Coupling and uncoupling continue when Ca^{2+} concentration remains high enough to inhibit the troponin–tropomyosin system. When neural stimulation ceases, Ca^{2+} moves back into the lateral sacs of the sarcoplasmic reticulum. This restores the inhibitory action of troponin–tropomyosin, and actin and myosin stay apart, provided ATP concentration remains adequate. In **rigor mortis**, muscles stiffen and become rigid soon after death because muscle cells no longer contain ATP, and without ATP, myosin crossbridges and actin remain attached and do not separate. **Figure 18.13** illustrates the interaction between actin and myosin filaments, Ca^{2+}, and ATP in both a relaxed and shortened muscle fiber.

Stimulation produces a threefold rise in Ca^{2+} concentration and accompanying increase in the action potential in type II (fast-twitch) muscle fibers compared with type I (slow-twitch) muscle fibers in isolated muscle preparations. Such differences reflect faster Ca^{2+} transport through the sarcoplasmic reticulum and ultimately to the contractile proteins in type II fibers. During excitation–contraction coupling, electrochemical events occur within the cell membrane at the site of excitation. The common pathway for precisely targeting the chemical signal to the contractile proteins depends mostly on ion channel regulators. These relatively sophisticated microstructures serve as selective "gates" or "sensors" to modulate ion passage between intracellular and extracellular fluids prior to myofilament activation.

Relaxation

When muscle stimulation ceases, Ca^{2+} flow stops and troponin frees up to inhibit actin–myosin interaction. Recovery involves active pumping of Ca^{2+} into the sarcoplasmic reticulum where it concentrates in lateral vesicles. Retrieval of Ca^{2+} from the troponin–tropomyosin protein complex "turns off" active sites on the actin filament. Deactivation serves two purposes:

1. Prevents any mechanical link between myosin crossbridges and actin filaments
2. Inhibits myosin ATPase activity to curtail ATP splitting

Muscle relaxation occurs when actin and myosin filaments return to their original states.

Sequence of Events in Muscle Action

Figure 18.14 summarizes the main events in muscle activation, contraction, and relaxation..
The sequence begins with initiation of an action potential by the motor nerve. The impulse then propagates over the entire fiber surface or sarcolemma as it depolarizes. The following nine steps correspond to the numbered sequence in Figure 18.14:

Step 1: Generation of an action potential in the motor neuron causes the small, saclike vesicles within the terminal axon to release acetylcholine (ACh). ACh diffuses across the synaptic cleft and attaches to specialized ACh receptors on the sarcolemma. Almost perfect symmetry exists between the "imprint" of the presynaptic vesicles that contain ACh and the "imprint" of the postsynaptic receptors that capture ACh.

Step 2: The muscle action potential depolarizes the transverse tubules at the sarcomere's A–I junction.

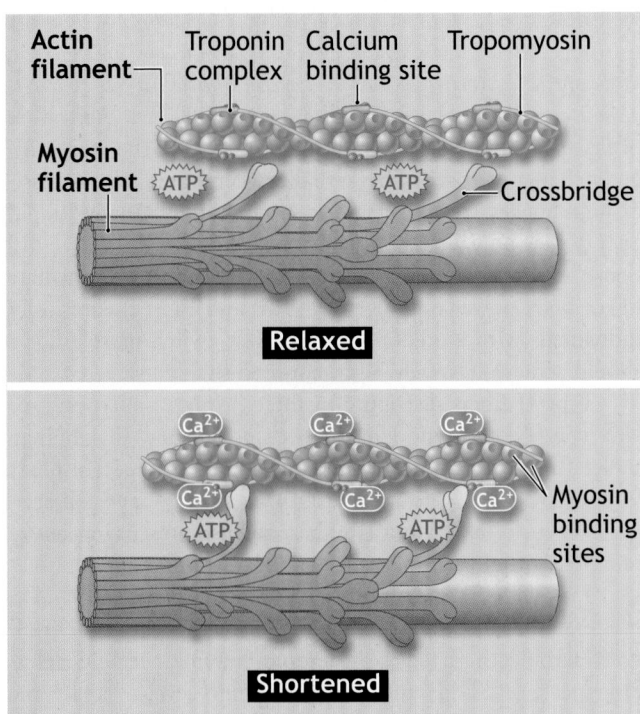

FIGURE 18.13 • Interaction among actin–myosin filaments, Ca^{2+}, and ATP in relaxed and shortened muscle. In the relaxed state, troponin and tropomyosin interact with actin, preventing the myosin crossbridge from coupling to actin. During muscle action, the crossbridge couples with actin from Ca^{2+} binding with troponin–tropomyosin.

Step 3: Depolarization of the T-tubule system causes Ca^{2+} release from lateral sacs (terminal cisternae) of the sarcoplasmic reticulum.

Step 4: Ca^{2+} binds to troponin–tropomyosin in actin filaments. This releases the inhibition that prevented actin from combining with myosin.

Step 5: During muscle action, actin combines with myosin–ATP. Actin also activates the enzyme myosin ATPase, which then splits ATP. The reaction's energy produces myosin crossbridge movement and creates tension.

Step 6: ATP binds to the myosin crossbridge; this breaks the actin–myosin bond and allows the crossbridge to dissociate from actin. The thick and thin filaments then slide past each other and muscle shortens.

Step 7: Crossbridge activation continues when Ca^{2+} concentration remains high enough from membrane depolarization to inhibit the troponin–tropomyosin system.

Step 8: When muscle stimulation ceases, intracellular Ca^{2+} concentration rapidly decreases as Ca^{2+} moves back into the lateral sacs of the sarcoplasmic reticulum through active transport that requires ATP hydrolysis.

Step 9: Ca^{2+} removal restores the inhibitory action of troponin–tropomyosin. In the presence of ATP, actin and myosin remain in the dissociated, relaxed state.

thePoint   Appendix H, available online at http://the point.lww.com/mkk8e, provides a list of supplemental animations and videos on this subject.

MUSCLE FIBER TYPE

Skeletal muscle does not simply contain a homogeneous group of fibers with similar metabolic and contractile properties. Rather, skeletal muscle contains two main types of fibers that differ in the primary mechanisms they use to produce ATP, the type of motor neuron innervation, and the type of myosin heavy chain expressed. The proportions of each muscle fiber type vary from muscle to muscle and from person to person.

A common technique to establish the specific muscle fiber type assesses myosin molecule's heavy chain that exists in three different forms or isoforms. Assessment evaluates a fiber's differential sensitivity to altered pH of the enzyme myosin ATPase (a measure of myosin phenotype).[28,30,37,38] The different characteristics of this enzyme determine the rapidity of ATP hydrolysis in the myosin heavy-chain region and the velocity of sarcomere shortening. More specifically, acid pH inactivates the activity of the specific myosin ATPase in fast-twitch fibers, but this enzyme remains fairly stable at an alkaline pH; these fibers stain *dark* for this enzyme. In contrast, specific myosin ATPase activity for slow-twitch fibers remains high at an acid pH but becomes inactive in an alkaline milieu;

these fibers stain *light* for myosin ATPase. Figure **18.15** illustrates serial cross sections of the human vastus lateralis muscle with identification of type I and type II muscle fibers and subdivisions. A special biopsy needle removes a small amount of tissue from an incision into the muscle belly after "numbing" the area with a local anesthetic. Table **18.2** lists different classification schemes for skeletal muscle fiber types on the basis of morphology, histochemistry and biochemistry, function, and contractility.

Fast-Twitch Fibers (Type II)

Fast-twitch muscle fibers exhibit the following four characteristics:

1. High capability for electrochemical transmission of action potentials
2. High myosin ATPase activity
3. Rapid Ca^{2+} release and uptake by an efficient sarcoplasmic reticulum
4. High rate of crossbridge turnover

These four factors determine this fiber's rapid energy generation for quick, powerful muscle actions. The fast-twitch fiber's intrinsic speed of shortening and tension development ranges three to five times faster than slow-twitch fibers (see following section). Fast-twitch fibers rely on a well-developed, short-term glycolytic system for energy transfer. *Fast-twitch fiber activation predominates in anaerobic -type sprint activities and other forceful muscle actions that rely almost entirely on anaerobic energy metabolism.*[3,16,26] Activation of fast-twitch fibers plays an important role in the stop-and-go or change-of-pace of basketball, soccer, water polo, lacrosse, or field hockey sports. These types of activities demand rapid energy that only anaerobic pathways generate. "In a Practical Sense" describes a popular jumping test to infer the immediate lower-body power output from ATP and PCr. Theoretically, individuals with a predominance of fast-twitch muscle fibers should achieve relatively high scores on such a test.

Type II fibers distribute in three primary subtypes: type IIa, type IIx, and type IIb. Recent studies show that human skeletal muscle contains type I, type IIa, and type IIx fibers (previously referred to as type IIb) and a new type IIb subtype.[46] Types IIa, IIx, and IIb fibers are also present in skeletal muscle of other mammals such as rodents and cats.

Type IIa fiber exhibits fast shortening speed and a moderately well-developed capacity for energy transfer from both aerobic (high level of aerobic enzyme succinic dehydrogenase, or SDH) and anaerobic (high level of anaerobic enzyme phosphofructokinase, or PFK) sources. These fibers represent the **fast–oxidative–glycolytic (FOG) fibers**. **Type IIb fiber** possesses the greatest anaerobic potential and most rapid shortening velocity; it represents the "true" fast-glycolytic (FG) fiber. A **type IIx fiber** falls midway between its a and b counterparts in physiologic and metabolic characteristics.

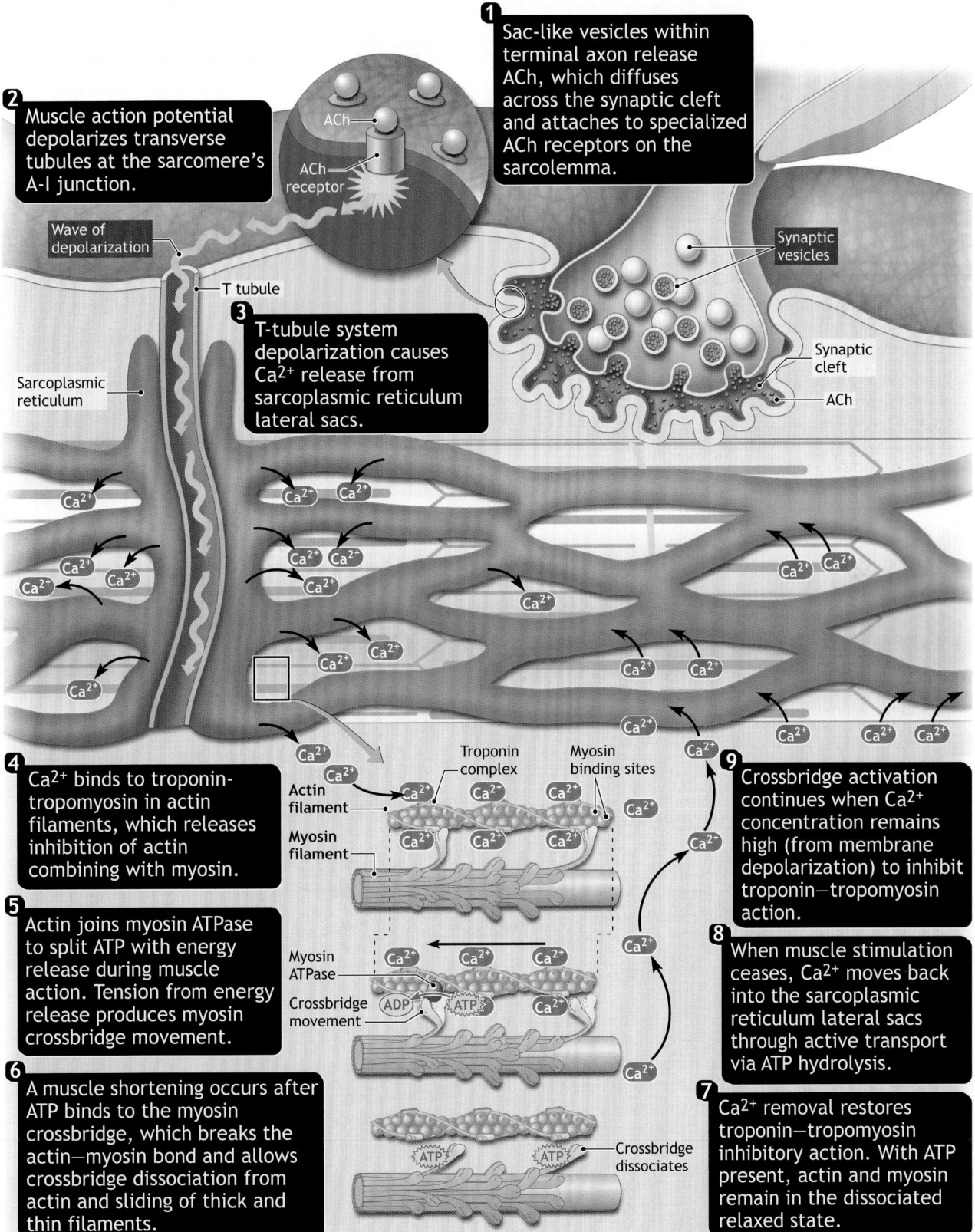

1 Sac-like vesicles within terminal axon release ACh, which diffuses across the synaptic cleft and attaches to specialized ACh receptors on the sarcolemma.

2 Muscle action potential depolarizes transverse tubules at the sarcomere's A-I junction.

3 T-tubule system depolarization causes Ca^{2+} release from sarcoplasmic reticulum lateral sacs.

4 Ca^{2+} binds to troponin-tropomyosin in actin filaments, which releases inhibition of actin combining with myosin.

5 Actin joins myosin ATPase to split ATP with energy release during muscle action. Tension from energy release produces myosin crossbridge movement.

6 A muscle shortening occurs after ATP binds to the myosin crossbridge, which breaks the actin–myosin bond and allows crossbridge dissociation from actin and sliding of thick and thin filaments.

7 Ca^{2+} removal restores troponin–tropomyosin inhibitory action. With ATP present, actin and myosin remain in the dissociated relaxed state.

8 When muscle stimulation ceases, Ca^{2+} moves back into the sarcoplasmic reticulum lateral sacs through active transport via ATP hydrolysis.

9 Crossbridge activation continues when Ca^{2+} concentration remains high (from membrane depolarization) to inhibit troponin–tropomyosin action.

FIGURE 18.14 • Schematic view of the nine main events in muscle contraction and relaxation. Numbers correspond to the sequence of nine steps outlined under "Sequence of Events in Muscle Action." The neurotransmitter acetylcholine (ACh), released from saclike vesicles within the terminal axon, initiates transmission at the myoneural junction. Here, the electrochemical signal "jumps" across the 0.05-μm cleft between neuron and muscle fiber. The electrical impulse, traveling at a velocity of 1 m · s⁻¹ or faster, spreads through the fiber's architecturally elegant tubule system to the myofibril's inner contractile "machinery."

IN A PRACTICAL SENSE

A Vertical Jump Test to Predict Peak Anaerobic Power Output

Peak anaerobic power output underlies success in many sports activities. The vertical jump test is often used to predict "explosive" peak anaerobic power output from the intramuscular high-energy phosphates.

VERTICAL JUMP TEST

The vertical jump test measures the highest distance jumped from a semicrouched position in the following protocol:

1. Establish standing reach height. The subject, standing with the preferred shoulder adjacent to a wall and feet flat on the floor, reaches as high as possible to touch the wall. The starting point (standing reach height) represents the distance from the wall mark (middle finger) to the floor, recorded in centimeters (cm) **(A)**.

2. Bend the knees to about a 90° angle while moving the arms back in a winged position **(B)**.

3. Thrust forward and upward, touching as high as possible on the wall **(C)**.

4. At a minimum, perform three trials of the jump test, using the highest score as the vertical height. An average of the last three trials of 10 provides a more dependable jump height.

5. Compute vertical jump height (cm) as the difference between standing reach height and vertical height achieved in the jump.

PREDICTING IMMEDIATE ANAEROBIC POWER OUTPUT

The following equation for males and females predicts peak anaerobic power output in watts (PAP_w) from vertical jump height in cm (VJ_{cm}) and body mass in kilograms (BM_{kg}):

$$PAP_w = 60.7\,(VJ_{cm}) + 45.3\,(BM_{Kg}) - 2055$$

EXAMPLE

A 21-year-old male weighing 78 kg records a vertical jump of 43 cm (standing reach height, 185 cm; vertical height, 228 cm); predict peak anaerobic power output in watts.

COMPUTATIONS

$$PAP_w = 60.7\,(VJ_{cm}) + 45.3\,(BM_{Kg}) - 2055$$

$$= 60.7\,(43\text{ cm}) + 45.3\,(78\text{ Kg}) - 2055$$

$$= 4.88.5\text{ W}$$

COMPARISONS

The average peak power output measured with this vertical jump protocol averages 4620.2 (SD = 822.5) W for males and 2993.7 (SD = 542.9) W for females.

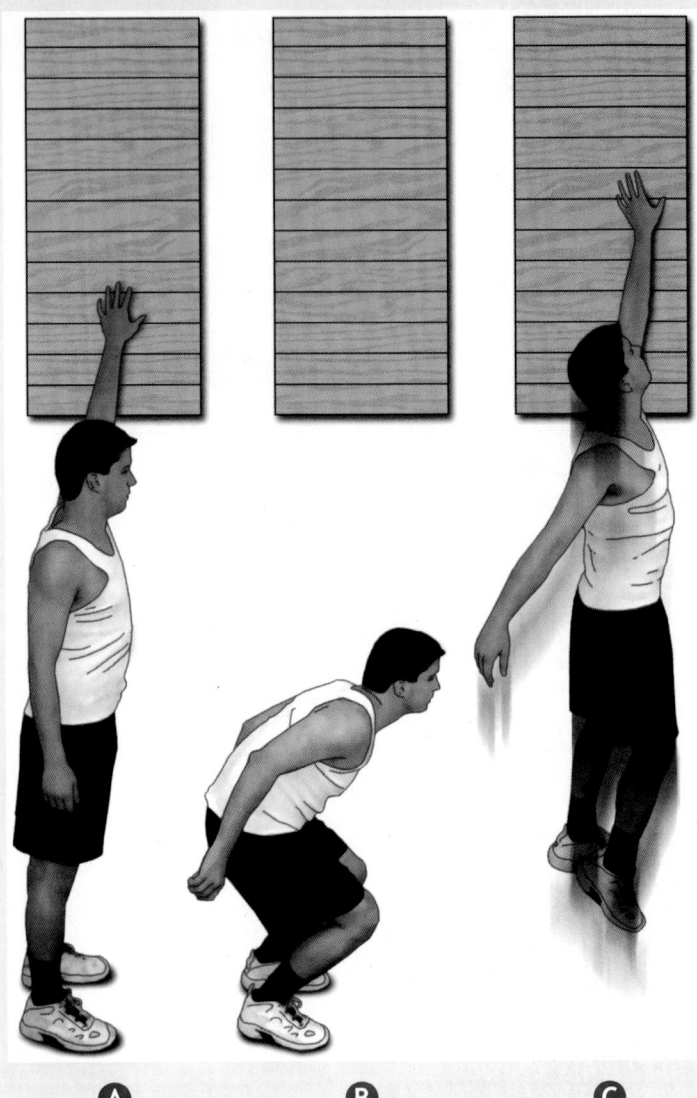

(A) Starting point (standing reach height), **(B)** just prior to jumping, and **(C)** final point in determining vertical jump height.

Sources:
Sayers S, et al. Cross-validation of three jump power equations. *Med Sci Sports Exerc* 1999;31:572.

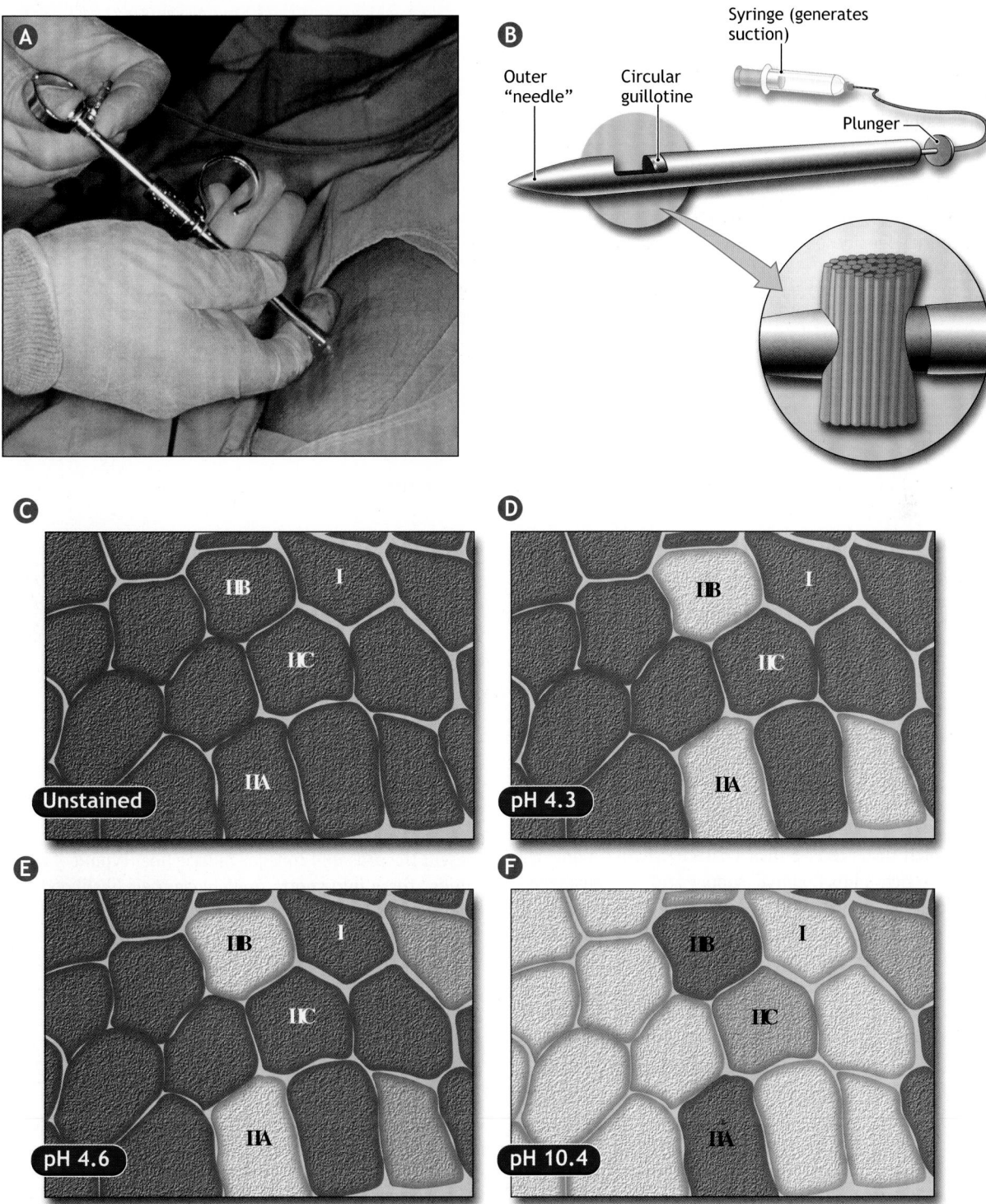

FIGURE 18.15 • Serial cross sections obtained by muscle biopsy of human vastus lateralis muscle (**A** and **B**) with identification of type I and type IIA, B, and C fiber subdivisions. The C fiber represents a former classification of a normally rare and undifferentiated subtype that may contribute to reinnervation and motor unit transformation. (**C**) Thick unstained section (40–50 μm) where all fibers appear similar. Three other panels indicate same fibers stained for myosin–ATPase activity at a preincubation pH of (**D**) 4.3 (highly acidic), (**E**) 4.6 (intermediate acidity), and (**F**) 10.4 (alkaline). (**A**, reprinted with permission from Plowman SA, Smith DL. *Exercise Physiology for Health, Fitness, and Performance*. 3rd Ed. Baltimore: Lippincott Williams & Wilkins, 2011.)

TABLE 18.2 Classification of Human Skeletal Muscle Fiber Types

Fiber Type	Type I Fibers	Type IIa Fibers	Type IIx Fibers	Type IIb Fibers
Contraction time	Slow	Moderately fast	Fast	Very fast
Size of motor neuron	Small	Medium	Large	Very large
Resistance to fatigue	High	Fairly high	Intermediate	Low
Activity used for	Aerobic	Long-term anaerobic	Short-term anaerobic	Short-term anaerobic
Maximum duration of use	Hours	<30 min	<5 min	<1 min
Force production	Low	Medium	High	Very high
Mitochondrial density	High	High	Medium	Low
Capillary density	High	Intermediate	Low	Low
Oxidative capacity	High	High	Intermediate	Low
Glycolytic capacity	Low	High	High	High
Major storage fuel	Triacylglycerol	Creatine phosphate, glycogen	Creatine phosphate, glycogen	Creatine phosphate, glycogen
Myosin-heavy chains, human genes	MYH7[a]	MYH2	MYH1	MYH4

[a]MYH7 is also known as myosin or myosin heavy chain 4 (http://ghr.nlm.nih.gov/gene/MYH7).

Slow-Twitch Fibers (Type I)

Slow-twitch fibers generate energy for ATP resynthesis predominantly through the aerobic system of energy transfer. Their four distinguishing characteristics include:

1. Low myosin ATPase activity
2. Slow calcium handling ability and shortening speed
3. Less well-developed glycolytic capacity than fast-twitch fibers
4. Large and numerous mitochondria

Slow-twitch fibers receive their characteristic red pigmentation from a rich mitochondrial supply and accompanying iron-containing cytochromes combined with high myoglobin levels. A high concentration of mitochondrial enzymes links closely to a slow-twitch fiber's enhanced aerobic metabolic machinery. *These characteristics make slow-twitch fibers highly fatigue resistant but ideally suited for prolonged aerobic physical activity.* The fibers have been labeled **SO**, or **slow-oxidative**, to describe their slow shortening speed and reliance on oxidative metabolism. Unlike fast-twitch fibers that fatigue readily, SO fibers (more precisely, motor units) are selectively recruited in aerobic activities.[25]

Muscle glycogen depletion patterns indicate that prolonged, intense aerobic activity demands almost exclusive reliance on slow-twitch muscle fibers. Even after exercising for 12 hr, the limited glycogen remaining in active muscle exists mostly in the relatively "unused" fast-twitch fibers. Differences in oxidative capacity between the two fiber types also determine the magnitude of blood flow through muscle, with slow-twitch fibers receiving the largest quantity.[31]

Most researchers classify slow-twitch fibers as **type I** and fast-twitch fibers (and proposed subdivisions) as **type II**. *Both slow and fast muscle fiber types contribute during near-maximum aerobic and anaerobic middle-distance running or swimming or basketball, field hockey, or soccer, which combine both high levels of aerobic and anaerobic energy transfer.*

 INTEGRATIVE QUESTION

Present the pros and cons for muscle fiber typing of children to "guide" them into sports to increase their likelihood of future success.

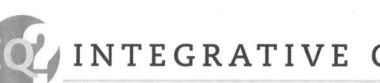 **Muscle Fiber Training Specificity**

Why do some highly trained athletes who switch to a sport requiring different muscle groups feel essentially untrained for the new activity? The answer is fairly straightforward—only the specific fibers activated in training adapt metabolically and physiologically to the specific exercise regimen. Swimmers or canoeists do not necessarily transfer their upper-body "fitness" to a running sport unless they specifically train the muscles required for that sport.

GENES THAT DEFINE SKELETAL MUSCLE PHENOTYPE

Several independent chemical signaling pathways regulate skeletal muscle fiber types in adult animals and most likely humans. These include pathways involved with the Ras/ mitogen-activated protein kinase (MAPK), calcineurin, calcium/ calmodulin-dependent protein kinase IV, and the peroxisome proliferator g coactivator 1 (PGC-1 α), a coactivator that promotes mitochondrial biogenesis, mitochondrial fatty acid oxidation, and hepatic gluconeogenesis. PGC-1 α also provides a direct link between external physiologic stimuli and the regulation of mitochondrial biogenesis, and serves as a major factor that regulates muscle fiber type determination. This pathway may also act in control of blood pressure, regulation of cellular cholesterol balance, and development of obesity. The Ras/MAPK signaling pathway links motor neurons and signaling systems, and coupling excitation and transcription regulation to promote nerve-dependent induction of muscle regeneration.

Mice that harbor an activated form of PGC-1 α display an "enduranced" phenotype, with a coordinated increase in oxidative enzymes and mitochondrial biogenesis and an increased proportion of slow-twitch muscle fibers. Functional genomics research (understanding the function of genes and other parts of the genome; http://www.ornl.gov/ sci/techresources/Human_Genome/research/function. shtml) reveals a signaling network to control skeletal muscle fiber-type transformation and metabolic profiles that protect against insulin resistance and obesity. Other pathways also influence adult muscle characteristics. For example, physical force generated within a muscle fiber may release the transcription factor serum response factor (SRF) from the structural muscle protein titin, leading to increased muscle growth. Titin acts as a "ruler" to control the relative positioning of the actin and myosin proteins, probably by calcium binding upon activation,[19] and regulates the "springiness" of the contracting muscle.[41,44] Titin also plays an important role in muscle force regulation, particularly for eccentric or active lengthening muscle actions. [20,32]

FIBER TYPE DIFFERENCES AMONG ATHLETIC GROUPS

Interesting observations concern muscle fiber type and the possible influence of specific training on fiber composition and metabolic capacity. Men, women, and children on average possess 45 to 55% slow-twitch fibers in their arm and leg muscles. The fast-twitch fibers probably distribute equally between type IIa and type IIb subdivisions. Although no gender differences exist in fiber distribution, large interindividual variation occurs. Generally, the trend in one's muscle fiber type distribution remains consistent among the body's major muscle groups.

Certain patterns of muscle fiber distribution appear in comparisons among highly proficient athletes.[47] Successful endurance athletes possess predominantly slow-twitch fibers in the major muscles activated in their sport. In contrast, fast-twitch fibers predominate for elite sprint athletes. FIGURE 18.16 illustrates fiber-type distribution for top Nordic competitors in different sports. Athletic groups with the highest aerobic and endurance capacities (e.g., distance runners and cross-country skiers) possess the highest percentage of slow-twitch fibers, often 90 to 95% in the leg's gastrocnemius muscle. Weightlifters, ice hockey players, and sprinters have more fast-twitch fibers and relatively lower aerobic capacities. As might be expected, men and women who perform in middle-distance events display approximately equal percentages of the two fiber types. The same distribution also occurs in power athletes—throwers, jumpers, and high jumpers.[9]

The relatively clear-cut distinctions between exercise performance and muscle fiber composition pertain mainly to elite athletes with prominence in a sport category. Even among this group, muscle fiber composition does not solely determine performance success. This seems reasonable because successful performance reflects blending of many

---

Decline in Skeletal Muscle Mass with Aging Mainly Attributed to Reduced Type II Muscle Fiber Size

Differences in leg muscle cross-sectional area (CSA) between young men and elderly men mainly reflect differences in muscle fiber size, and not the number of muscle fibers.

Quadriceps muscle CSA and type I and II muscle fiber size were initially measured in healthy young (n = 25; 23 years) and older (n = 26; 71 years) men. Older subjects then performed 6 months of resistance training, after which measurements were repeated. Pretraining differences in quadriceps muscle CSA were compared with differences in type I and II muscle fiber size. Quadriceps CSA was substantially smaller in older versus younger men (68 cm vs. 80 cm). Type II muscle fiber size was smaller in elderly compared to their young counterparts by 29%, with only a tendency for smaller type I muscle fibers. Type II muscle fiber size fully explained differences in quadriceps CSA between groups. Six months of resistance training in the elderly increased type II muscle fiber size by 24%, explaining 100% of the increase in quadriceps muscle CSA from 68 to 74 cm. These findings indicate that reduced muscle mass with aging results from a decrease in type II muscle fiber size that is unlikely accompanied by substantial muscle fiber loss.

Source: Nilwik R, et al. The decline in skeletal muscle mass with aging is mainly attributed to a reduction in type II muscle fiber size. *Exp Gerontol* 2013;48:492.

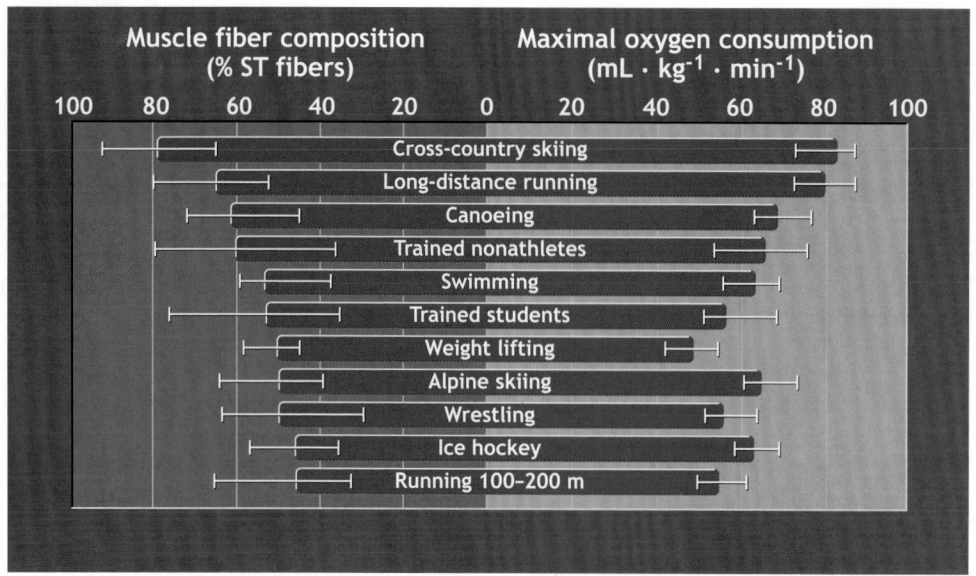

FIGURE 18.16 • Muscle fiber composition (% slow-twitch fibers, *left side*) and maximal oxygen consumption (*right side*) in athletes representing different sports. The *outer white bars* denote the range. (Reprinted with permission from Bergh U, et al. Maximal oxygen uptake and muscle fiber types in trained and untrained humans. *Med Sci Sports* 1978;10:151.)

physiologic, biochemical, neurologic, and biomechanical "support systems," not simply the single factor of muscle fiber type.

Endurance athletes have relatively normal-sized muscle fibers, with a tendency toward enlargement of the slow-twitch fibers. Conversely, weightlifters and other power athletes show definite enlargement in both fiber types, particularly fast-twitch fibers, which may exceed by 45% those of endurance athletes or sedentary persons of the same age.[48,49] Strength and power training induce enlargement of the fiber's contractile apparatus—specifically the actin and myosin filaments—and total glycogen content. *Larger muscle fibers in male athletes and a larger total muscle mass characterizes the principal gender differences in muscle morphology.* Chapter 22 discusses the potential for exercise training to alter metabolic and fiber-type characteristics and skeletal muscle size.

Summary

1. Various connective tissue wrappings that encase skeletal muscle blend into and join the tendinous attachment to bone. This harness enables muscles to act on bony levers to transform chemical energy of ATP into mechanical energy of motion.
2. A skeletal muscle fiber by weight consists of 75% water, 20% protein, and the remainder inorganic salts, enzymes, pigments, fats, and carbohydrates.
3. The muscle's oxygen consumption during vigorous physical activity increases up to 70 times the resting level.

Immediate adjustments and longer duration training adaptations that increase local vascular bed size support this elevated metabolic requirement.

4. The sarcomere represents the functional unit of the muscle fiber. It contains the contractile proteins actin and myosin. An average muscle fiber contains 4500 sarcomeres and 16 billion thick (myosin) and 64 billion thin (actin) filaments.
5. Myosin projections, or crossbridges, serve as structural links between thick and thin contractile filaments. During muscle action, tropomyosin and troponin regulate the make-and-break contacts between the filaments.
6. Tropomyosin inhibits actin and myosin interaction; troponin plus Ca^{2+} trigger the myofibrils to interact and slide past each other.
7. The triad and T-tubule system function as a micro-transportation network to spread the action potential from the fiber's outer membrane inward to deeper cell regions.
8. Muscle action takes place when Ca^{2+} activates actin; this causes the myosin crossbridges to attach to active sites on the actin filaments, while decreased Ca^{2+} concentration produces relaxation.
9. The sliding filament model proposes that a muscle shortens or lengthens because protein filaments slide past each other without altering their length. The excitation–contraction coupling mechanism links electrochemical and mechanical events to achieve muscle action.

10. Contractile and metabolic characteristics classify the two types of muscle fibers: fast-twitch (FT) fibers that generate energy predominantly anaerobically for quick, powerful actions and slow-twitch (ST) fibers that shorten relatively slowly and generate energy predominantly by aerobic metabolism. An intermediate, fast–oxidative–glycolytic (FOG) fiber also exists.

11. Several independent signaling pathways regulate skeletal muscle fiber-type phenotype in adult animals, including humans. Examples include the Ras/mitogen-activated protein kinase (MAPK), calcineurin, calcium/calmodulin-dependent protein kinase IV, and the peroxisome proliferator g coactivator 1 (PGC-1 α).

12. Genetic factors help to explain the variation in muscle fiber types, yet specific exercise training may produce some modification.

thePoint References are available online at **http://thepoint.lww.com/mkk8e.**

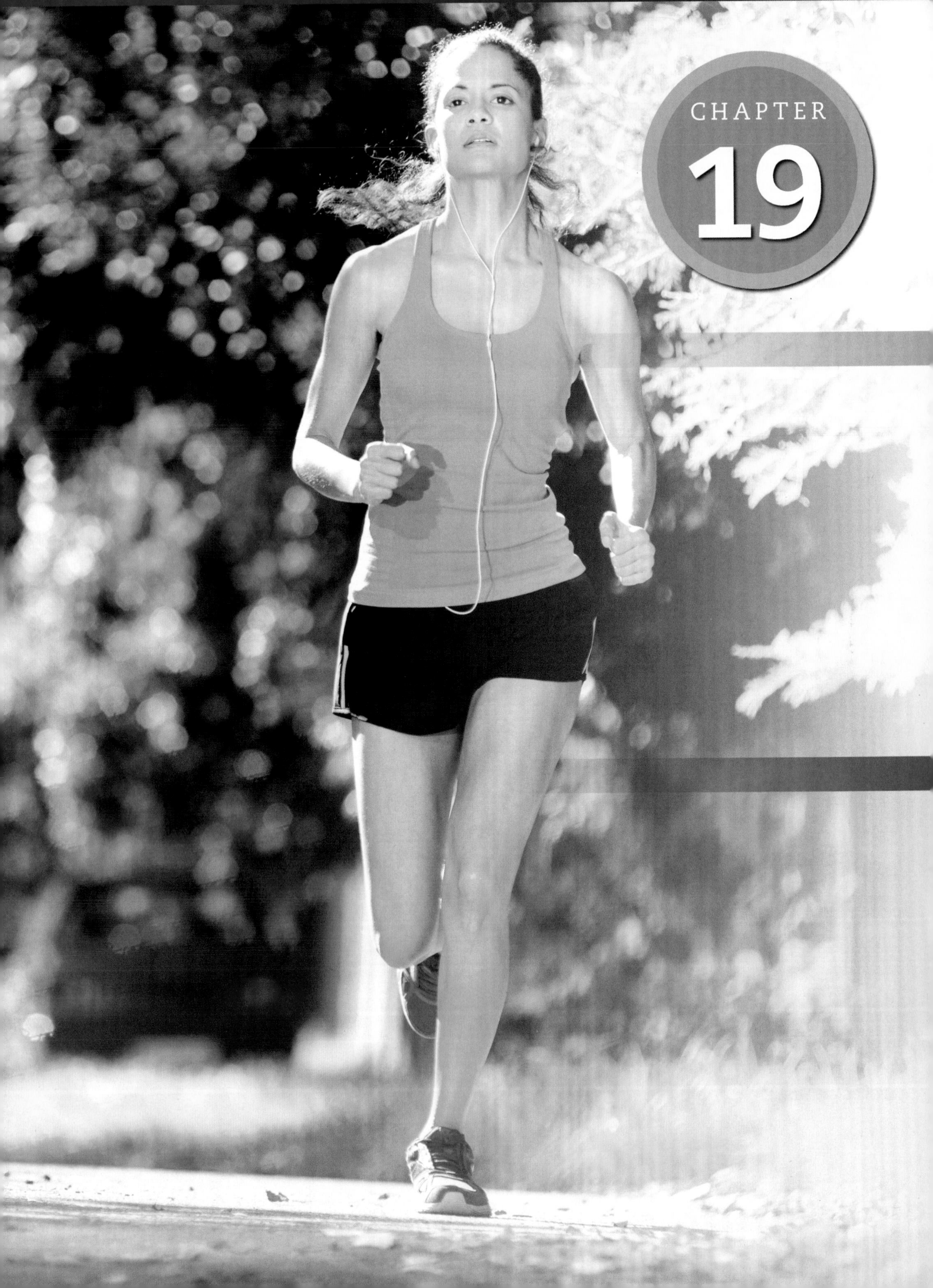

CHAPTER

19

Neural Control of Human Movement

The effective application of force during complex learned movements such as a tennis serve, shot put, golf swing, and back somersault off a diving board requires a series of precise, coordinated neuromuscular patterns and movements—not simply the strength of the muscles activated. The intricate sophisticated neural circuitry in the brain, spinal cord, and periphery functions in a manner somewhat similar to the most advanced "cloud" computer network. In response to changing internal and external stimuli, hundreds of millions of bits of sensory input automatically synchronize for near-instantaneous processing by central neural control mechanisms. This input must be properly organized, routed, and transmitted in fractions of nanoseconds with high efficiency to the effector organs, the skeletal muscles.[27]

NEUROMOTOR SYSTEM ORGANIZATION

The human nervous system consists of two major parts:

1. **Central nervous system (CNS)** consisting of the brain and spinal cord
2. **Peripheral nervous system (PNS)** consisting of nerves that transmit information to and from the CNS

FIGURE 19.1 presents an overview of these two subdivisions, including their functions in motor control.

Central Nervous System—The Brain

Over many thousands of years, the human **brain** has remained remarkably complex yet retains selective growth of different anatomic areas. From a comparative perspective, the size of the human brain exceeds that of most but not all mammals. Evolution of the cortex, particularly the frontal and temporal lobes, coincides with the unique human functions of spoken and written language, reasoning, and abstract thinking. Such differentiation frames the hypothesis that larger, more complex brains allow greater neural circuitry within the cortex and hence increased intellectual and higher center functioning.

For decades, conventional wisdom maintained that the number of brain cells remained fixed at birth, unlike the cells of other organ systems that continually renew themselves throughout life. Neurobiologists and the science community in general currently believe that brain cells, spinal neurons, and neural circuits are created throughout life, with elimination of unneeded or redundant synapses in developing neural tissues. From birth through late adolescence, the brain adds billions of new cells, literally constructing and reconstructing new circuits from these newly formed cells.[14] Following adolescence, the plasticity of neuronal addition and formation of new circuits slows but does not stop, even into older age. Regular physical activity contributes to the maintenance and development of optimal neural circuitry with aging.

FIGURE 19.2 shows the brain's six main areas: **medulla oblongata, pons, midbrain, cerebellum, diencephalon**, and **telencephalon**. Figure 19.2C depicts four lobes of the cerebral cortex and associated sensory areas. As a frame of reference, the body has roughly 10 million sensory (afferent) neurons, 50 billion central neurons, and 500,000 motor (efferent) neurons. This represents a ratio of about 20 to 1 between sensory and motor circuits.

Brainstem

The **brainstem** consists of the medulla, pons, and midbrain regions. The medulla, located immediately above the spinal cord, extends into the pons and serves as a neural bridge between the cerebellum's two hemispheres. The midbrain, only 1.5 cm long, attaches to the cerebellum and forms a connection between the pons and cerebral hemispheres. The midbrain contains tissues from the extrapyramidal motor system, specifically the red nucleus and substantia. The **reticular formation** integrates various incoming and outgoing signals that flow through it. These signals originate from the stretching of sensors in joints and muscles, from pain receptors in the skin, and as visual signals from the eye and auditory impulses from the ear. Once activated, the reticular system produces either inhibitory or facilitatory effects on other neurons. Twelve pairs of cranial nerves innervate predominantly the head region. Originally derived by the physician Galen about 1800 years ago (see "Exercise Physiology: Roots and Historical Perspectives," before Chapter 1), each cranial nerve has a name and associated number.

Mnemonic to Remember the 12 Cranial Nerves—Try It!

On **O**ld **O**lympus' **T**owering **T**op **A** **F**riendly **V**iking **G**rew **V**ines **A**nd **H**ops.

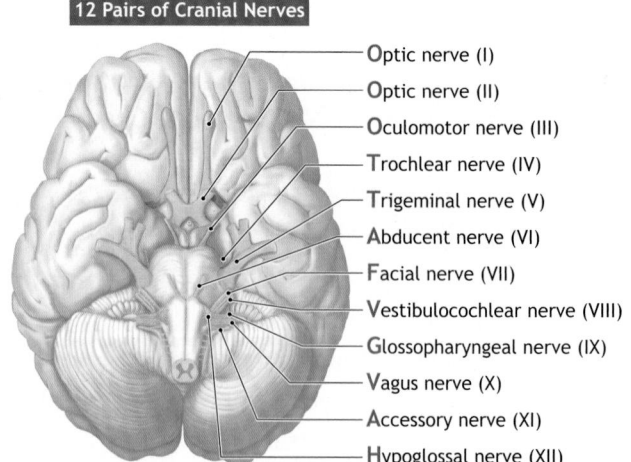

12 Pairs of Cranial Nerves

- Optic nerve (I)
- Optic nerve (II)
- Oculomotor nerve (III)
- Trochlear nerve (IV)
- Trigeminal nerve (V)
- Abducent nerve (VI)
- Facial nerve (VII)
- Vestibulocochlear nerve (VIII)
- Glossopharyngeal nerve (IX)
- Vagus nerve (X)
- Accessory nerve (XI)
- Hypoglossal nerve (XII)

Cerebellum

The cerebellum consists of two peach-sized mounds of folded tissue with lateral hemispheres and a central vermis. It functions by means of intricate feedback circuits to monitor and coordinate other areas of the brain and spinal cord involved in motor control. The cerebellum receives motor output signals from the central command in the cortex. This specialized brain tissue also obtains sensory information from peripheral receptors located in muscles,

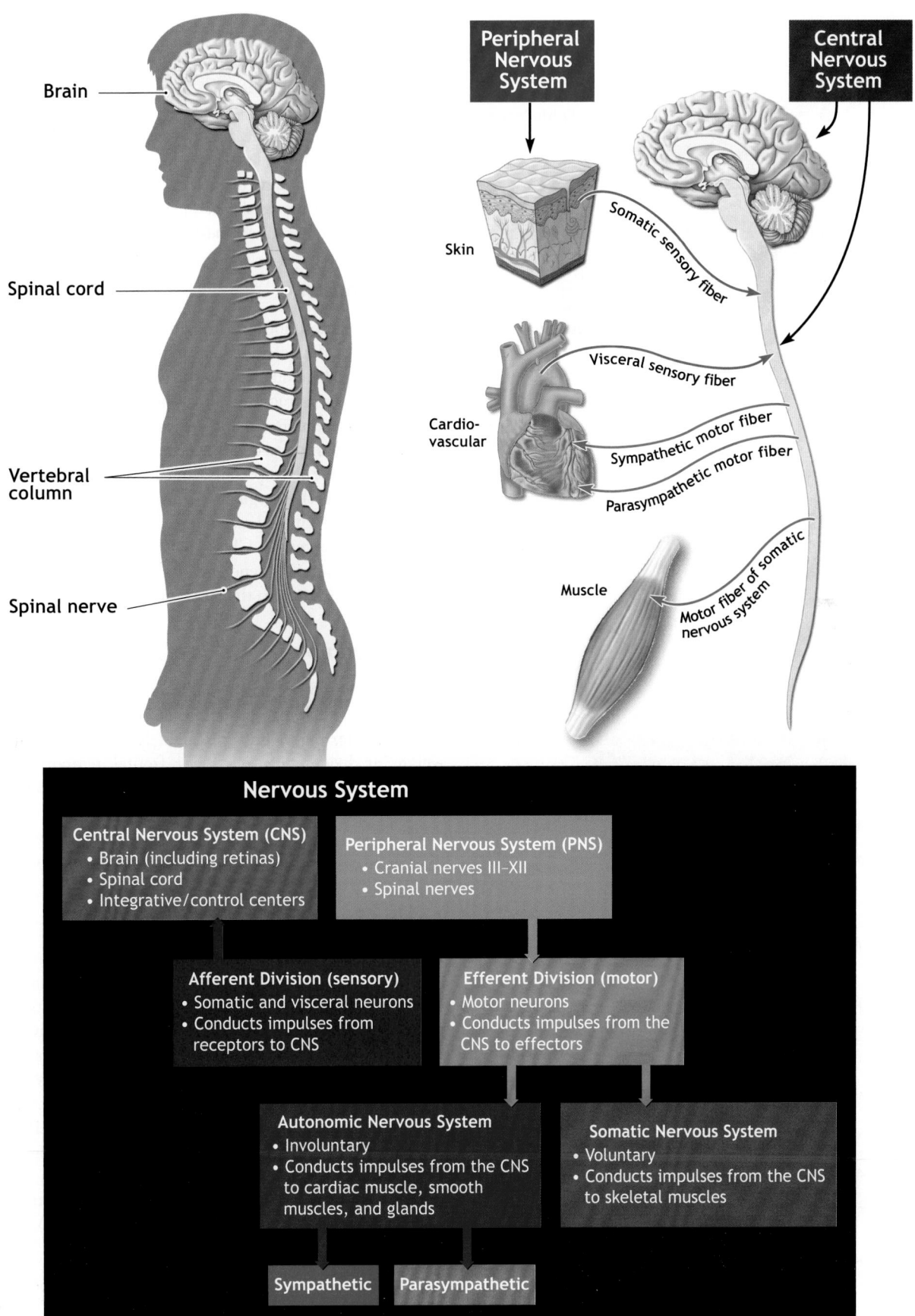

FIGURE 19.1 • The two divisions of the human nervous system. The central nervous system (CNS) contains the brain (including retinas), spinal cord, and integrating and control centers; the cranial nerves and spinal nerves compose the peripheral nervous system (PNS). The PNS further subdivides into the afferent (sensory) and efferent (motor) divisions. The efferent division consists of the somatic nervous system and autonomic nervous system (sympathetic and parasympathetic divisions).

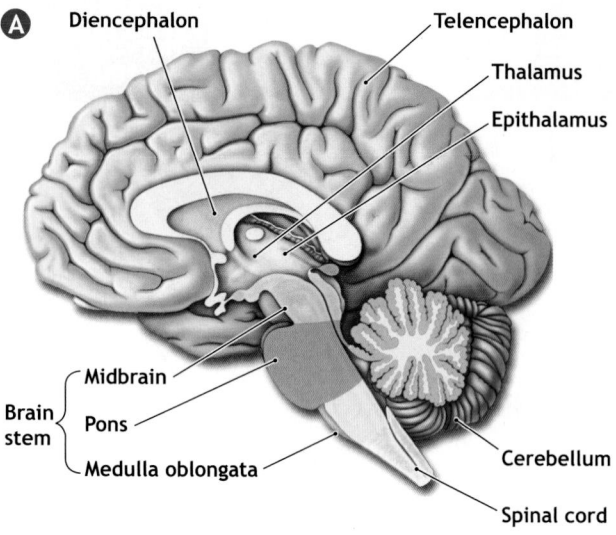

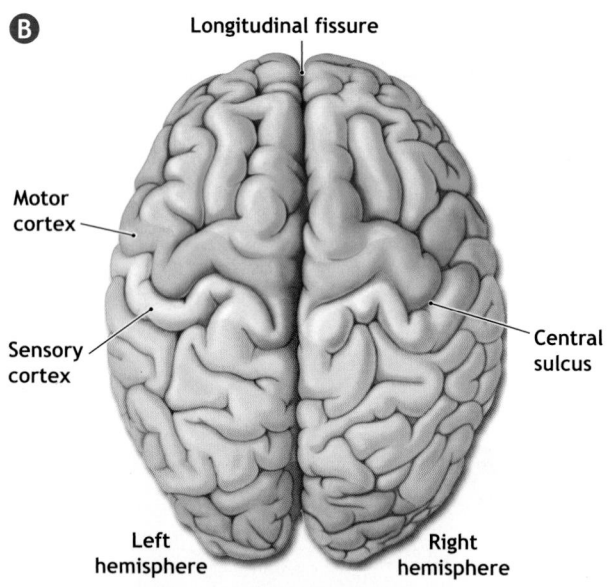

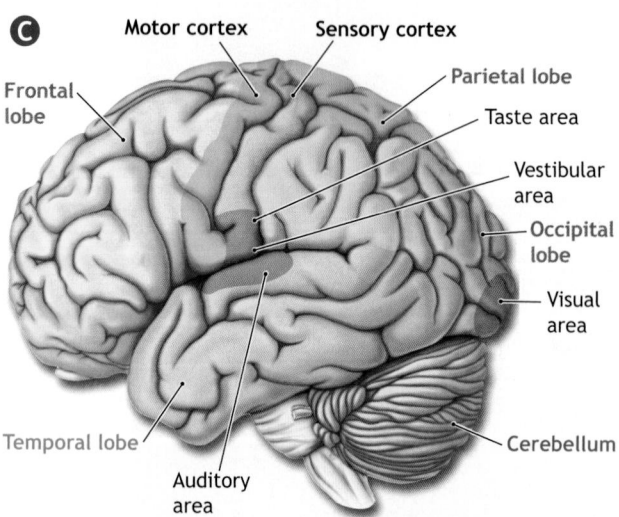

FIGURE 19.2 • **(A)** Side (medial) view of the brain and brainstem. **(B)** Superior view of the brain. **(C)** Four lobes of the cerebral cortex.

tendons, joints, and skin and from visual, auditory, and vestibular end organs. *The cerebellum functions as the major comparing, evaluating, and integrating center for postural adjustments, locomotion, maintenance of equilibrium, perceptions of speed of body movement, and other diverse reflex–related movement functions.* Movement tasks first learned by trial and error, like riding a bicycle or swinging a golf club at a particular cadence, remain coded as coordinated *patterns* in the cerebellar memory banks. In essence, this motor control center "fine-tunes" all forms of muscular activity.[29]

Diencephalon

The diencephalon, located immediately above the midbrain, forms part of the cerebral hemispheres. The thalamus, hypothalamus, epithalamus, and subthalamus compose the diencephalon's major structures. The hypothalamus, situated below the thalamus, regulates metabolic rate and body temperature. The **hypothalamus** also influences autonomic nervous system activity (see "Sympathetic and Parasympathetic Nervous Systems"); it receives regulatory input from the thalamus and limbic brain system and responds to the effects of diverse hormones (see Chapter 20). Changes in arterial blood pressure and blood gas tensions influence hypothalamic activity via peripheral receptors located in the aortic arch and carotid arteries.

Telencephalon

The telencephalon contains the two hemispheres of the **cerebral cortex**, including the corpus striatum and medulla. The cerebral cortex makes up approximately 40% of the total brain weight. It divides into four lobes: frontal, temporal, parietal, and occipital. Neurons in the cortex provide specialized sensory and motor functions. Beneath each cerebral hemisphere and in close association with the thalamus lie the basal ganglia, which play an important role in the control of motor movements.

Limbic System

In 1878, French anatomist, surgeon, neurologist, and anthropologist Paul Pierre Broca (1824–1880) described a group of areas on the medial surface of the cerebrum that were distinctly different from the surrounding cortex (see www.whonamedit.com/doctor.cfm/1982.html). Using the Latin word for "border" (*limbus*), Broca named the area the **limbic lobe** because its structures formed a ring or border around the brainstem and corpus callosum on the medial surface of the temporal lobe.[3] Broca also discovered the brain's speech center, now known as Broca's area, or the third circumvolution of the frontal lobe. Broca should be credited as the founder of modern brain surgery (http://www.muskingum.edu/~psych/psycweb/history/broca.htm).

Central Nervous System—The Spinal Cord

Figure 19.3 illustrates the **spinal cord**, about 45 cm in length and 1 cm in diameter, encased by 33 vertebrae (7 cervical, 12 thoracic, 5 lumbar, 5 sacral, and 4 coccygeal). The bony

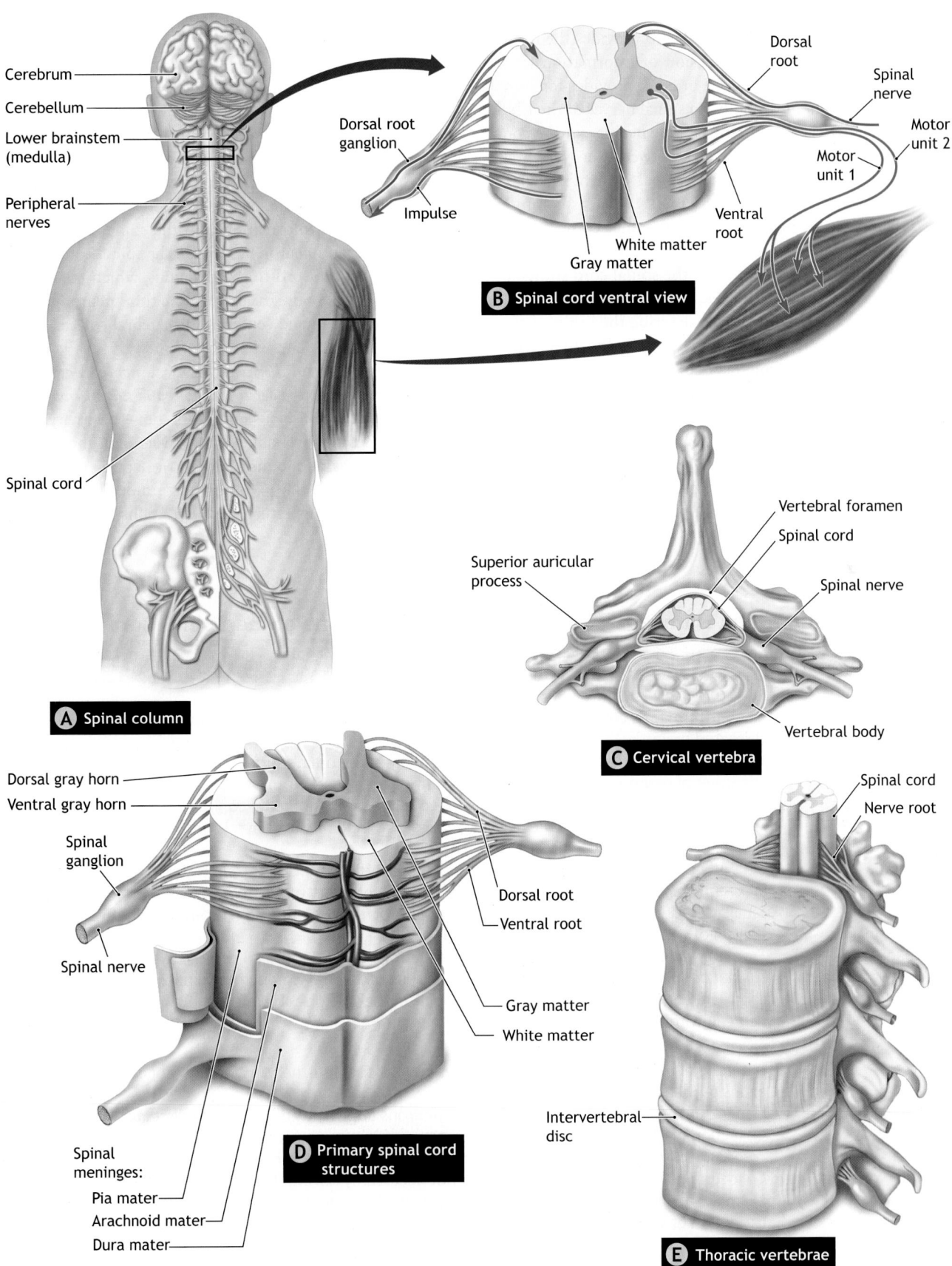

FIGURE 19.3 • Human central nervous system anatomy. **(A)** Spinal cord showing the peripheral nerves. **(B)** Ventral view of spinal cord section illustrates dorsal and ventral root neural pathways and nerve impulse direction. **(C)** Cross section through one cervical vertebra. **(D)** Primary spinal cord structures. **(E)** Enlarged view of the junction of three thoracic vertebral bodies.

vertebral column encases and protects the spinal cord, which attaches to the brainstem. The spinal cord provides the major conduit for the two-way transmission of information from the skin, joints, and muscles to the brain. It provides for communication throughout the body via spinal nerves of the PNS (see "Peripheral Nervous System"). These nerves exit the cord through small openings or notches between the vertebrae. Each spinal nerve connects to the spinal cord by the dorsal root and ventral root branches. TABLE 19.1 lists common names that describe the collections of spinal cord neurons and axons.

When viewed in cross section, the spinal cord shows an H-shaped core of gray matter (FIG. 19.4). The **ventral** (anterior) and **dorsal** (posterior) **horns** describe the limbs of this core. The spinal cord core contains principally three types of neurons: **motor neurons, sensory neurons**, and **interneurons**. The motor neurons (**efferent**) run through the ventral horn to supply the extrafusal and intrafusal skeletal muscle fibers (see "Receptors in Muscles, Joints, and Tendons," later in this chapter). Sensory (**afferent**) nerve fibers enter the spinal cord from the periphery by way of the dorsal horn. The white matter, containing the ascending and descending nerve tracts, surrounds the gray matter within the cord.

Ascending Nerve Tracts

Ascending nerve tracts in the spinal cord forward sensory information from peripheral receptors to the brain for processing. Three neurons typically form the sensory pathway. The dorsal root ganglion contains the cell body of the first neuron whose axon relays information into the spinal cord. The cell body of the second neuron lies within the spinal cord itself; its axon passes up the cord to the thalamus, which contains the third neuron's cell body. The axon of the third neuron traverses to the central command center in the cerebral cortex.

Sensory Receptors. *Peripheral sensory nerve endings serve as specialized receptors to detect conscious and subconscious sensory information.* The "conscious" receptors show sensitivity to kinaesthesia (detection of body position, weight, or movement of muscles, tendons, and joints) and proprioception (sense of the relative position of body parts and magnitude of effort applied in movement), temperature, and sensations of light, sound,

TABLE 19.1	Common Names Describing Neurons and Axons of the Spinal Cord
Name	**Description/Example**
Neurons	
Gray matter	Generic term for a collection of neuronal cell bodies in the CNS (neurons appear gray in a freshly dissected brain)
Cortex	Collection of neurons forming a thin sheet, usually at the brain's surface; example: *cerebral cortex*, the sheet of neurons found just under the surface of the cerebrum
Nucleus	Distinguishable mass of neurons, usually deep in the brain (not to be confused with the nucleus of a cell); example: *lateral geniculate nucleus*, a cell group in the brainstem relaying information from the eye to the cerebral cortex
Substantia	Related neurons deep within the brain, but with less distinct borders than those of nuclei; example: *substantia nigra*, a brainstem cell group involved in voluntary movement control
Locus (plural—loci)	Small, well-defined group of cells; example: *locus coeruleus*, a brainstem group of cells involved in control of wakefulness and behavioral arousal
Ganglion (plural—ganglia)	From the Greek term for "knot"; collection of neurons in the peripheral nervous system; example: *dorsal root ganglia* that contain the cell bodies of sensory axons entering the spinal cord in the dorsal roots; only one cell grouping, the basal ganglia, in the CNS goes by this name; the *basal ganglia* that lie deep within the cerebrum control movement
Axons	
Nerve	A bundle of axons in the peripheral nervous system; the optic nerve is the only collection of CNS axons termed *nerve*
White matter	Generic term for a collection of CNS axons (neurons appear white in a freshly dissected brain)
Tract	Collection of CNS axons having a common site of origin and a common destination; example: *corticospinal tract* that originates in the cerebral cortex and ends in the spinal cord
Bundle	Collection of axons running together but not necessarily having the same origin and destination; example: *medial forebrain bundle* that connects the brainstem with the cerebral cortex
Capsule	Collection of axons that connect the cerebrum with the brainstem; example: *internal capsule* that connects the brainstem with the cerebral cortex
Commissure	Any collection of axons that connect one side of the brain to the other side
Lemniscus	A tract that meanders through the brain in ribbonlike fashion; example: *medial lemniscus* that brings tactile information from the spinal cord through the brainstem

Reprinted with permission from Bear MF, et al. *Neuroscience: Exploring the Brain*. 3rd Ed. Baltimore: Lippincott Williams & Wilkins, 2006.

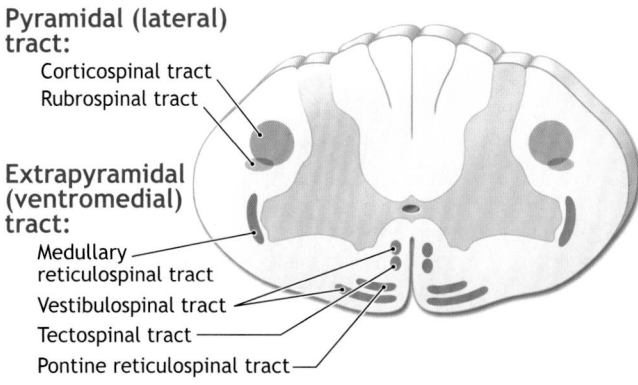

Pyramidal (lateral) tract:
- Corticospinal tract
- Rubrospinal tract

Extrapyramidal (ventromedial) tract:
- Medullary reticulospinal tract
- Vestibulospinal tract
- Tectospinal tract
- Pontine reticulospinal tract

FIGURE 19.4 • Descending spinal cord tracts from the brain. (Reprinted with permission from Bear MF, et al. *Neuroscience: Exploring the Brain.* 3rd Ed. Baltimore: Lippincott Williams & Wilkins, 2006.)

smell, taste, touch, and pain. Receptors also monitor subconscious changes in the body's internal environment; these include **chemoreceptors** that respond to changes in blood gas tension (P_{O_2}, P_{CO_2}) and pH and **baroreceptors** that react almost instantaneously to any change in arterial blood pressure. The term *mechanoreceptors* generally refers to the sensory receptors sensitive to mechanical stimuli of touch, pressure, stretch, and motion.

Descending Nerve Tracts

Axons from the brain move downward through the spinal cord along two major pathways, displayed in Figure 19.4. The **pyramidal (lateral) tract** activates the skeletal musculature in voluntary movement under direct cortical control. The other pathway, the **extrapyramidal (ventromedial) tract**, controls posture and muscle tone via the brainstem.

Pyramidal (Lateral) Tract. Neurons in the pyramidal tract including the corticospinal and rubrospinal tracts transmit impulses downward through the spinal cord. By means of direct routes and interconnecting neurons in the cord, these nerves eventually excite the **alpha (α) motor neurons** that control and modulate the fine and gross properties of skeletal muscles during all purposeful movements. The corticospinal tract, the longest and one of the largest CNS tracts, has two thirds of its axons originating from the brain's frontal lobe, collectively called the **motor cortex**.

Extrapyramidal (Ventromedial) Tract. The extrapyramidal neurons (reticulospinal, vestibulospinal, tectospinal tracts) originate in the brainstem and connect at all levels of the spinal cord. They control posture and provide a continual background level of neuromuscular tone.

Reticular Formation

The reticular formation provides an extensive and intricate neural network through the core of the brainstem that integrates the spinal cord, cerebral cortex, basal ganglia, and cerebellum. It receives a continuous flow of sensory data. Once activated, it either inhibits or facilitates other neurons. For example, the reticular formation helps to control posture by regulating the sensitivity of neurons to the antigravity muscles that maintain upright posture. Excitation of peripheral sensory neurons arouses the reticular nerve cells to excite the cerebral cortex. This initiates transmission of signals back to the reticular system to maintain appropriate cortical arousal and wakefulness. The reticular formation exerts a powerful regulating influence on cardiovascular and pulmonary functions.

Peripheral Nervous System

*The **peripheral nervous system** contains 31 pairs of spinal nerves and 12 pairs of cranial nerves.* **FIGURE 19.5** shows the distribution of the 12 pairs of cranial nerves numbered I through XII. Cranial nerves I and II serve visual and olfactory functions and are part of the CNS. Cranial nerves emerge through foramina, or fissures, in the skull or cranium. Cranial nerves, as do their spinal counterparts, contain fibers that transmit sensory and/or motor information. Their neurons innervate muscles or glands or transmit impulses from sensory areas into the brain. The spinal nerves consist of 8 pairs of cervical nerves, 12 pairs of thoracic nerves, 5 pairs of lumbar nerves, 5 pairs of sacral nerves, and 1 pair of coccygeal nerves. A specific letter and number identifies these nerves (e.g., C-1, first nerve from the cervical region; T-4, fourth nerve in the thoracic region). The exact location of the spinal nerves has been traced by mapping the tissues they innervate. This is fortuitous because an injury to a specific area of the spinal cord produces predictable neurologic damage.

The peripheral nervous system includes **afferent neurons** that relay sensory information from receptors in the periphery *toward* the CNS and **efferent neurons** that transmit information away from the brain to peripheral tissues. Two types of efferent neurons include **somatic** and **autonomic** nerves. Somatic nerve fibers, also called *motor neurons* or *motoneurons*, innervate skeletal muscle. Their firing above a threshold level always produces an excitatory response that activates muscle. The autonomic nerves, also called *visceral, involuntary,* or *vegetative nerves*, activate cardiac muscle, sweat and salivary glands, some endocrine glands, and smooth muscle cells, also called *involuntary muscle*, in the intestines and walls of blood vessels. Autonomic activity produces either an excitatory or inhibitory effect depending on the specific neurons activated.

Whereas tissues of the heart and viscera display considerable autonomic excitability, conscious control also affects these tissues. For example, individuals who practice yoga or meditation often control heart rate and blood flow "on command." Such conscious autonomic system control has some application as an alternative treatment in medicine (e.g., gastrointestinal disturbances, hypertension) and to enhance sports performance (e.g., lower heart rate and increase steadiness in target shooting). Competitors in archery and biathlon control

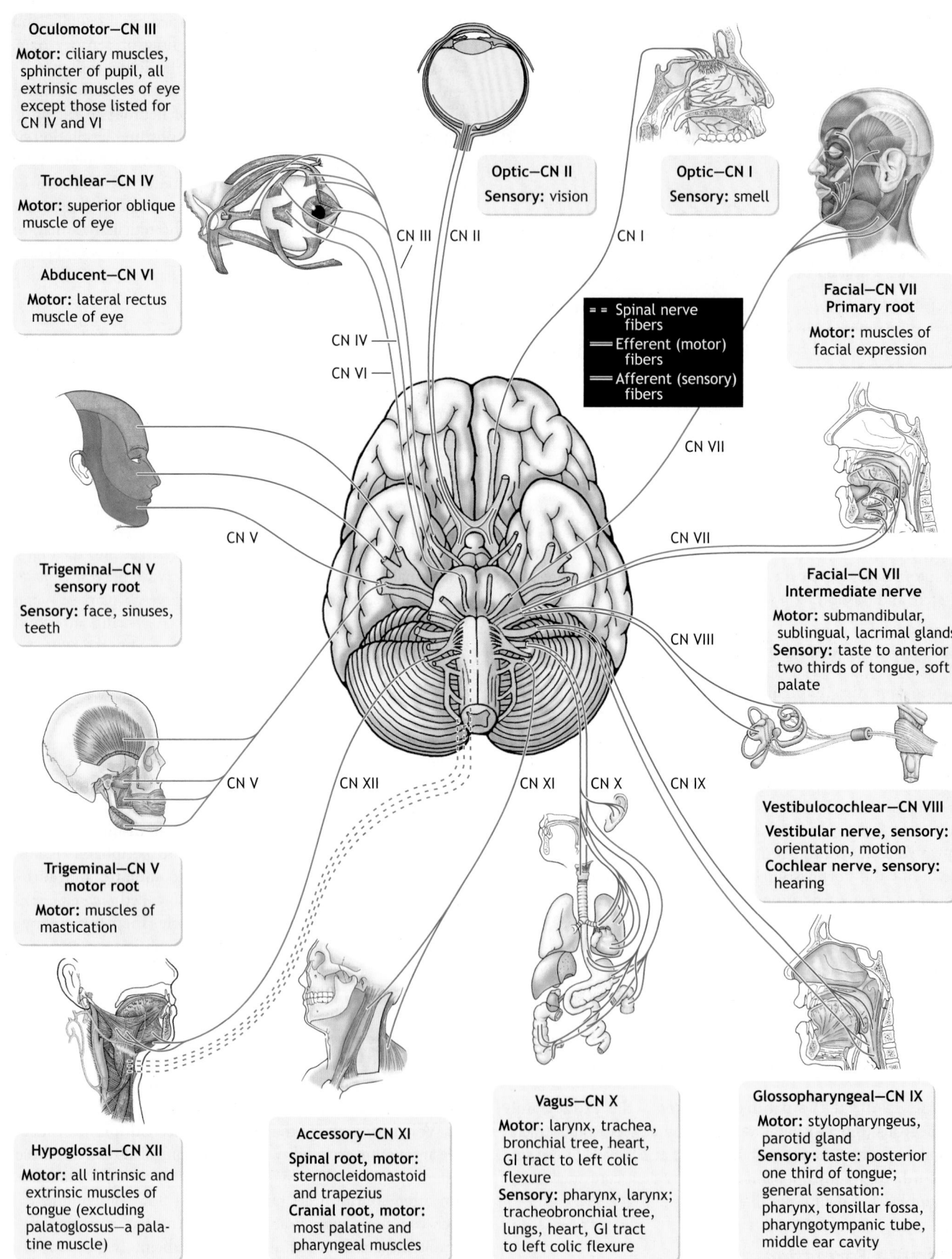

Oculomotor—CN III

Motor: ciliary muscles, sphincter of pupil, all extrinsic muscles of eye except those listed for CN IV and VI

Trochlear—CN IV

Motor: superior oblique muscle of eye

Abducent—CN VI

Motor: lateral rectus muscle of eye

Optic—CN II
Sensory: vision

Optic—CN I
Sensory: smell

= = Spinal nerve fibers
── Efferent (motor) fibers
── Afferent (sensory) fibers

Facial—CN VII
Primary root

Motor: muscles of facial expression

Trigeminal—CN V
sensory root

Sensory: face, sinuses, teeth

Facial—CN VII
Intermediate nerve

Motor: submandibular, sublingual, lacrimal glands
Sensory: taste to anterior two thirds of tongue, soft palate

Trigeminal—CN V
motor root

Motor: muscles of mastication

Vestibulocochlear—CN VIII

Vestibular nerve, sensory: orientation, motion
Cochlear nerve, sensory: hearing

Hypoglossal—CN XII

Motor: all intrinsic and extrinsic muscles of tongue (excluding palatoglossus—a palatine muscle)

Accessory—CN XI

Spinal root, motor: sternocleidomastoid and trapezius
Cranial root, motor: most palatine and pharyngeal muscles

Vagus—CN X

Motor: larynx, trachea, bronchial tree, heart, GI tract to left colic flexure
Sensory: pharynx, larynx; tracheobronchial tree, lungs, heart, GI tract to left colic flexure

Glossopharyngeal—CN IX

Motor: stylopharyngeus, parotid gland
Sensory: taste: posterior one third of tongue; general sensation: pharynx, tonsillar fossa, pharyngotympanic tube, middle ear cavity

CN III CN II CN I
CN IV CN VI CN VII CN V CN VII CN VIII CN V CN XII CN XI CN X CN IX

FIGURE 19.5 • Distribution of the 12 cranial nerves (CN). (Reprinted with permission from Moore KL, Dalley AF II, eds. *Clinically Oriented Anatomy*. 7th Ed. Baltimore: Lippincott Williams & Wilkins, 2013.)

cardiovascular activity and respiratory movements to temporarily halt the normal breathing cycle and slow heart rate during the crucial "steadiness" phase of the performance. The athlete triggers this maneuver immediately prior to releasing the bowstring or pulling the trigger to fire the rifle.

Sympathetic and Parasympathetic Nervous Systems

The **autonomic nervous system** subdivides into **sympathetic** and **parasympathetic** components. Based on anatomic and physiologic differences, these neurons operate in parallel but use structurally distinct pathways and differ in their transmitter systems. Figure 16.5 in Chapter 16 shows that axons of the sympathetic division emerge only from the middle third of the spinal cord in the thoracic and lumbar segments; in contrast, preganglionic axons of the parasympathetic division emerge only from the brainstem and lowest sacral spinal cord segments. The two systems operate independently in some functions and interact cooperatively in others.

Sympathetic fiber distribution, while displaying some overlap with parasympathetic fibers, supplies the heart, smooth muscle, sweat glands, and viscera. Parasympathetic nervous system fibers leave the brainstem and sacral segments of the spinal cord to supply the thorax, abdomen, and pelvic regions.

Regions of the medulla, pons, and diencephalon control the autonomic nervous system. Fibers that originate in the medullary region of the lower brainstem control blood pressure, heart rate, and pulmonary ventilation, whereas nerve fibers of upper hypothalamic origin regulate body temperature.

The Reflex Arc

FIGURE 19.6 diagrams the neural arrangement for a typical **reflex arc** in one of the 31 spinal cord segments. Afferent neurons that enter the spinal cord through the dorsal (sensory) root transmit sensory input from peripheral receptors. These neurons interconnect or **synapse** in the cord through **interneurons** that relay information to different cord levels. The impulse then passes over the **motor root pathway** via anterior motor neurons to the effector organ—the muscles.

 See the animation "Nerve Synapse" on http://thePoint.lww.com/mkk8e for a demonstration of this process.

An example of a simple reflex occurs when one suddenly but unexpectedly touches a hot object. Stimulation of pain receptors located in the skin of the fingers transmits sensory information over afferent fibers to the spinal cord. This activates efferent motor fibers to elicit an appropriate muscular response by immediately jerking the hand away. Concurrently, the signal transmits through interneuron activity up the cord to sensory areas in the brain, the area that actually "feels" the pain. These various levels of operation for sensory input,

processing, and motor output, including the reflex action just described, cause the hand to move quickly away from the hot object even before the outward perception of pain. Reflex actions in the spinal cord and other subconscious areas of the CNS control many muscle functions. Literally hundreds and sometimes thousands of hours of practicing a particular motor task "grooves" the neuromuscular movements to become automatic, no longer requiring conscious control. Unfortunately, improper practice also can automate a task to produce less than optimal neuromuscular actions. Most individuals who practice the golf swing, for example, do so by reinforcing poor habits. It starts with the grip and the first 6 inches of the takeaway in the backswing. Setting up in the stance with an improper grip followed by a rapid cocking of the wrists at the start of the backswing fuels a recipe for disaster. Instead of pounding one ball after another on the range—often hours on end—both aspiring and advanced golfers should purposely practice correct swing mechanics, hopefully under the eye of a proficient coach or teacher. The adage "practice makes perfect" should be amended to this five-word mnemonic—"*perfect* practice produces *perfect* performance." If one practices an incorrect movement pattern, no matter how simple or complex, that movement pattern becomes "learned" and "grooved"—in essence, perfecting poor mechanics and grooving improper movement sequencing produces just opposite the desired movement outcome!

NERVE SUPPLY TO MUSCLE

One nerve innervates at least one of the body's approximately 250 million muscle fibers. The typical individual possesses about 420,000 motor neurons; a single nerve usually supplies many individual muscle fibers. *The number of muscle fibers per motor neuron generally relates to a muscle's particular movement function.* Delicate and precise work of the eye muscles, for example, requires that a neuron control fewer than 10 muscle fibers. For less complex movements of the large muscle groups, a motor neuron may innervate as many as 2000 or 3000 fibers. During any muscular activity, the spinal cord represents the major processing and distribution center for motor control. The next sections examine how information processed in the CNS activates the muscles to trigger an appropriate motor response.

Motor Unit Anatomy

*The **motor unit** makes up the functional unit of movement; this anatomic unit consists of the anterior motor neuron and the specific muscle fibers it innervates.* The individual and combined actions of motor units produce specific muscle actions. Each muscle fiber generally receives input from only one neuron, yet a motor neuron may innervate many muscle fibers because the terminal end of an axon forms numerous branches. The **motor neuron pool** describes the collection of α-motor neurons that innervate a single muscle (e.g., triceps or biceps; FIG. 19.7). Different motor points exist within the muscle to allow neural stimulation throughout the muscle's length.[26]

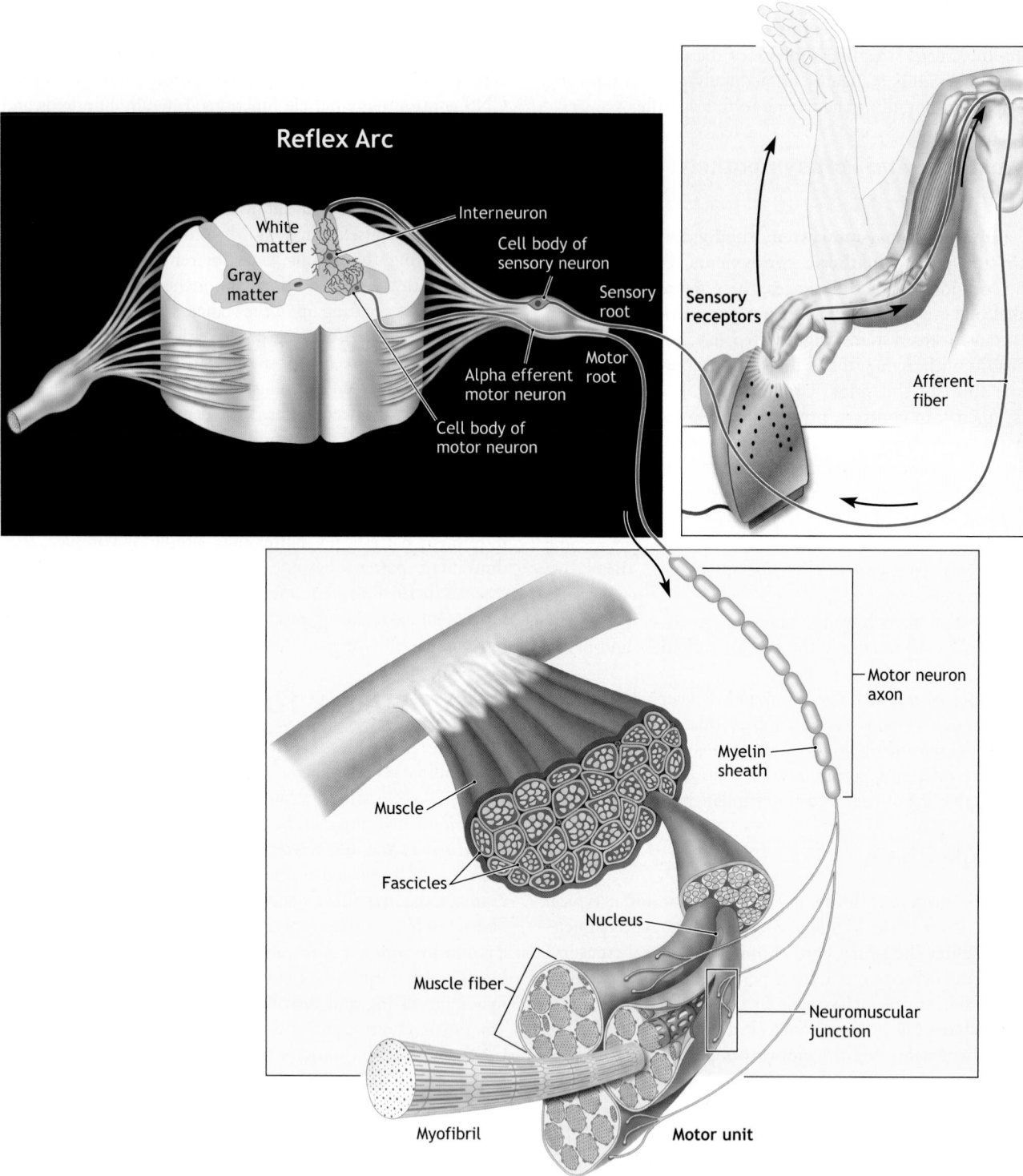

FIGURE 19.6 • Reflex arc showing afferent and efferent neurons plus an interneuron in a spinal cord segment. The darker shaded or gray matter contains the neuron cell bodies; longitudinal columns of nerve fibers make up the white matter. Stimulation of a single α-motor neuron activates up to 3000 muscle fibers. The motor neuron and the fibers it innervates collectively constitute the motor unit. The figure shows only one side of the spinal nerve complex.

Some motor units contain up to 1000 or more muscle fibers, whereas motor units of the larynx, fingers, or eyeball contain relatively few. For example, the first dorsal interosseous muscle of the finger contains 120 motor units that control 41,000 fibers; the medial gastrocnemius (calf) muscle contains 580 motor units and 1,030,000 muscle fibers. The ratio of muscle fibers to motor unit averages 340 for the finger muscle and about 1800 for the gastrocnemius muscle. Individual differences in muscle fiber–motor unit ratios probably contribute significantly to variation in sport skill performance.

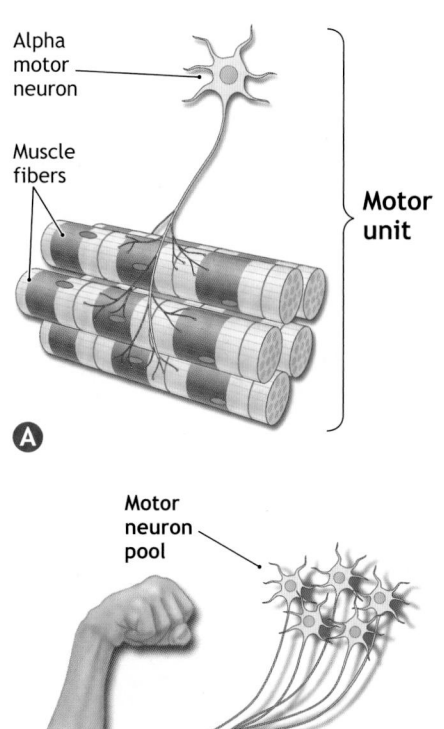

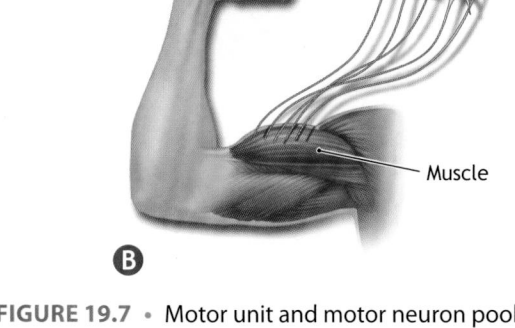

FIGURE 19.7 • Motor unit and motor neuron pool. **(A)** Motor unit represents an α-motor neuron and the fibers it innervates. **(B)** Motor neuron pool represents all the α-motor neurons that innervate one muscle.

 See the animation "Muscle Contraction" on http://thePoint.lww.com/mkk8e for a demonstration of this process.

The Anterior Motor Neuron

The anterior motor neuron illustrated in FIGURE 19.8 consists of a **cell body, axon**, and **dendrites**. Its unique biologic design allows transmission of an electrochemical impulse from the spinal cord to the muscle. The cell body houses the neuron's control center—the structures involved in genetic code replication and transmission. The spinal cord's gray matter contains the cell body of the motor neuron. The axon extends from the cord to deliver the impulse to the muscle; dendrites consist of short neural branches that receive impulses through numerous connections and conduct them toward the cell body. *Nerve cells conduct impulses in one direction only—down the axon away from the original stimulation point.*

The **myelin sheath**, a bilayer lipoprotein membrane that wraps around the axon over most of its length, encases larger nerve fibers. A large part of this sheath acts as an electrical insulator that envelops the axon akin to the plastic coating around a copper electrical wire. A specialized cell known as a **Schwann cell** covers the bare axon and then spirals around it, sometimes up to 100 times in the biggest fibers. A thinner

outermost membrane, the **neurilemma**, covers the myelin sheath. The **nodes of Ranvier** named for Paris physician and histologist Louis Antoine Ranvier (1835–1922; see www.whonamedit.com/doctor.cfm/3133.html), who also discovered the myelin sheath, interrupt the Schwann cells and myelin every 1 or 2 mm along the axon's length. Whereas myelin insulates the axon to the flow of ions, the nodes of Ranvier permit depolarization of the axon. This alternating sequence of myelin sheath and node of Ranvier at about 1-mm intervals allows impulses to "jump" from node to node, called *saltatory conduction* (from the Latin *saltare*, meaning to hop or leap), as the electrical current travels toward the terminal branches at the **motor endplate**. This type of conduction causes faster transmission velocities in myelinated fibers compared to unmyelinated fibers. *Conduction speed in a nerve fiber increases in direct proportion to a fiber's diameter and thickness of its myelin sheath.* Large, myelinated neurons conduct impulses at speeds that exceed 100 m · s^{-1} (224 mph).

 See the animation "Saltatory Conduction" on http://thePoint.lww.com/mkk8e for a demonstration of this process.

thePoint   Appendix H, available online at http://thepoint.lww.com/mkk8e, provides a list of supplemental animations and videos on this subject.

Four different nerve fiber groups exist based on size and thus transmission velocity:

1. A-alpha (A-α [13–20 μm; 80–120 m · s^{-1}])
2. A-beta (A-β [6–12 μm; 35–75 m · s^{-1}])
3. A-delta (A-δ [1–5 μm; 5–35 m · s^{-1}])
4. C-nerve (0.2–1.5 μm; 0.5–2.0 m · s^{-1})

Myelin insulation covers the A-α, A-β, and A-δ nerve fibers, whereas C nerve fibers remain unmyelinated. The thickness of a nerve fiber dictates the speed of neural transmission within the fiber—the thickest A-α fibers have the fastest transmission speed, while the smallest C fibers have the slowest transmission speed. These relatively tiny fibers relay information related to pain, temperature, and itch. To give some perspective about the speed of transmission, impulses in C-nerve fibers travel about 2.2 mph, slower than most people walk at about 2.4 mph. In contrast, the A-δ fibers conduct action potentials at the speed of the winning 100-m Olympic dash in just under 10 s, while the A-β fibers that relay information related to touch travel at speeds close to that of most propeller-driven aircraft that achieve speeds from 200 to 300 mph. As discussed in the section on proprioception, the γ-efferent fibers connect with special stretch sensors in skeletal muscle that detect minute changes in muscle fiber length.

All muscle action ultimately depends on three primary sources of input to α-motor neurons (motor units):

1. Dorsal root ganglion cells with axons that innervate specialized muscle spindle sensory units embedded within the muscle

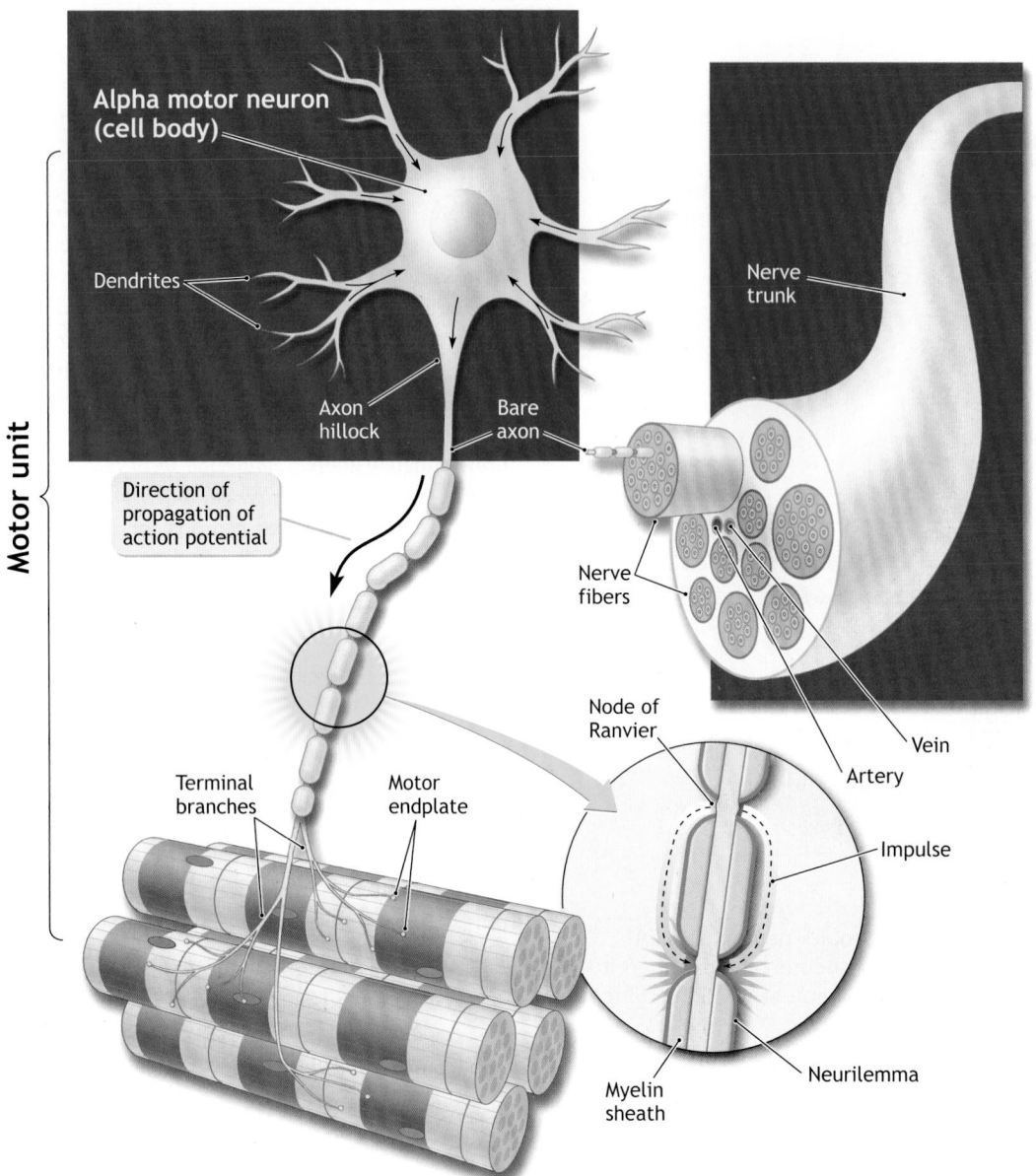

FIGURE 19.8 • (*Left*) The anterior (α) motor neuron consists of a cell body, axon, and dendrites. *Top right inset* shows a nerve trunk containing numerous individual nerve fibers, including a bare axon. *Bottom inset* shows a node of Ranvier on the bare axon, which permits impulses to jump from one node to another as the electrical current travels toward the terminal branches at the motor endplate.

2. Motor neurons in the brain, primarily in the cerebral cortex's precentral gyrus
3. Excitatory and inhibitory spinal cord interneurons, which make up the largest input

Neuromuscular Junction (Motor Endplate). The **neuromuscular junction** (**NMJ**) or **motor endplate** represents the interface between the end of a myelinated motor neuron and muscle fiber (**FIG. 19.9**). It transmits the nerve impulse to initiate muscle action. Each skeletal muscle fiber usually contains one NMJ.

Five common features describe the NMJ[5]:

1. Schwann cells are present.

2. Terminal section of the neuron contains the neurotransmitter substance acetylcholine (ACh).
3. Basement membrane lines the synaptic space.
4. Membrane across from the synaptic space (the postsynaptic membrane) contains ACh receptors.
5. Connector microtubules at the postsynaptic membrane transmit the electrical signal deep within the muscle fiber.

The terminal portion of the axon below the myelin sheath forms several smaller axon branches whose endings become the **presynaptic terminals**. This region possesses approximately 50 to 70 ACh-containing vesicles per square micrometer. They lie close to but do not come in contact

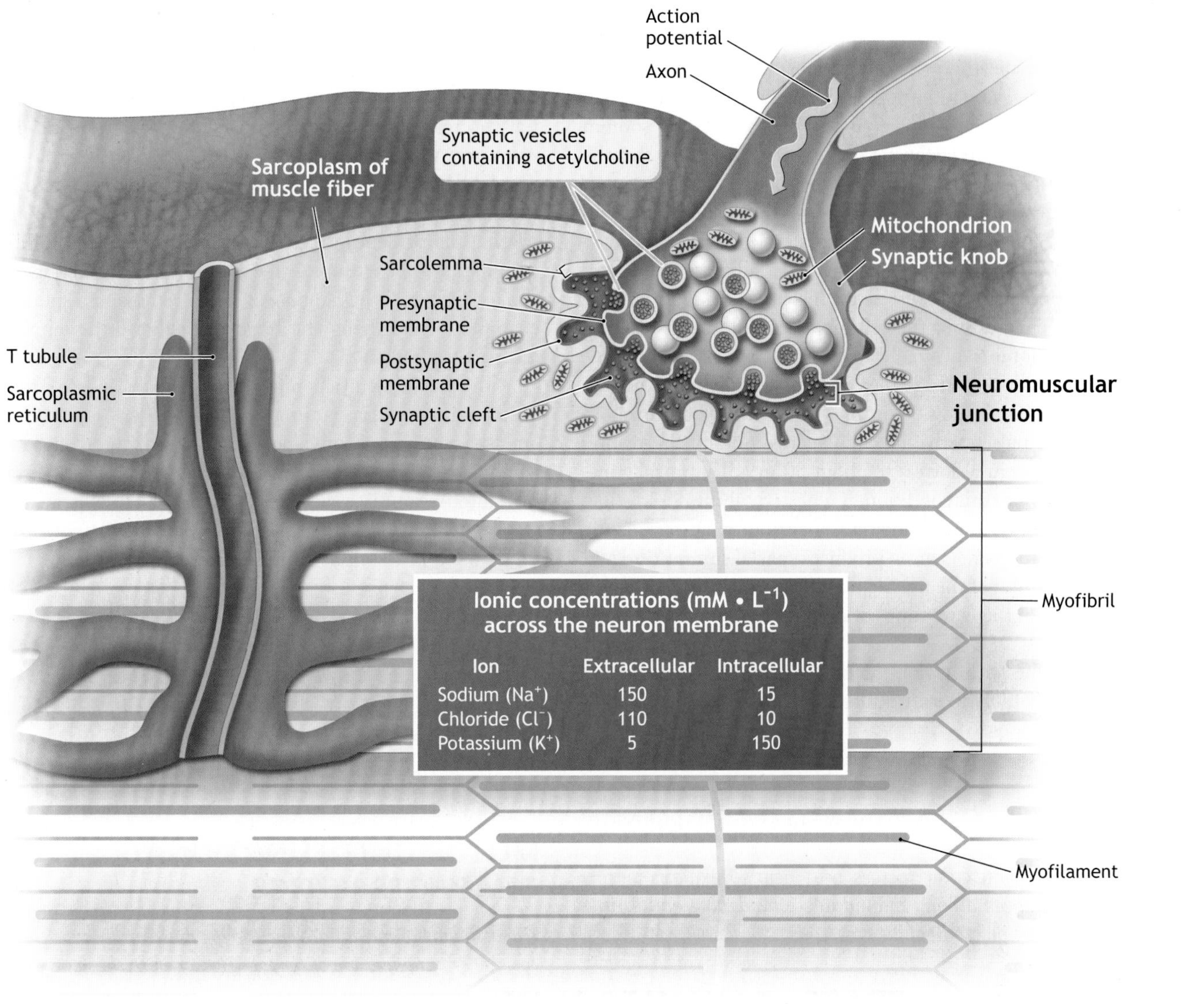

Action potential

Axon

Synaptic vesicles containing acetylcholine

Sarcoplasm of muscle fiber

Sarcolemma

Presynaptic membrane

Postsynaptic membrane

Synaptic cleft

T tubule

Sarcoplasmic reticulum

Mitochondrion
Synaptic knob

Neuromuscular junction

Myofibril

Ionic concentrations (mM • L^{-1}) across the neuron membrane		
Ion	Extracellular	Intracellular
Sodium (Na$^+$)	150	15
Chloride (Cl$^-$)	110	10
Potassium (K$^+$)	5	150

Myofilament

FIGURE 19.9 • Microanatomy of the neuromuscular junction, including details of the presynaptic and postsynaptic contact area between the motor neuron and the muscle fiber it innervates. *Inset* table shows representative values for ionic concentrations across the motor neuron membrane.

with the muscle fiber's sarcolemma. The invaginated region of the **postsynaptic membrane**, also called the *synaptic gutter*, has numerous infoldings that increase the membrane's surface area. The **synaptic cleft** between the synaptic gutter and the presynaptic terminal of the axon serves as the region for neural impulse transmission between nerve and muscle fiber.

Excitation. *Excitation normally occurs only at the NMJ.* When an impulse arrives at the NMJ, ACh releases from saclike vesicles in the terminal axons into the synaptic cleft. ACh, which changes a basically electrical neural impulse into a chemical stimulus, then combines with a transmitter–receptor complex in the postsynaptic membrane. The resulting change in electrical properties of the postsynaptic membrane elicits an **endplate potential** that spreads from the motor endplate to the extrajunctional sarcolemma of muscle. This causes an **action**

potential or wave of depolarization to travel the length of the muscle fiber, enter the T-tubule system, and spread to the inner structures of the muscle fiber to prime the contractile machinery for excitation.

 See the animations "Action Potential" and "Flipping the Membrane Potential" on **http://thePoint.lww. com/mkk8e** for a demonstration of this process.

The enzyme **cholinesterase**, concentrated at the borders of the junctional folds at the synaptic cleft, degrades ACh within 5 ms of its release from the synaptic vesicles. ACh hydrolysis by cholinesterase allows the postsynaptic membrane to repolarize rapidly. The axon resynthesizes the end products of cholinesterase action (composed of acetic acid and choline) to ACh so the entire process can perpetuate when another neural impulse arrives.

Facilitation. ACh release from synaptic vesicles excites the postsynaptic membrane of its connecting neuron. This changes membrane permeability so sodium ions diffuse into the stimulated neuron. An action potential generates if the *change* in transmembrane microvoltage (influx of extracellular sodium and/or efflux of intracellular potassium) reaches the **threshold for excitation**. The term *excitatory postsynaptic potential* (**EPSP**; www.ncbi.nlm.nih.gov/books/NBK11117/) describes this change in membrane potential at the junction between two neurons (**Fig. 19.10A**). The arrival of a subthreshold EPSP does not cause neuron to discharge. Instead, the migratory flow of positive charges into the cell increases to lower its **resting membrane potential** (usually an electrical potential of 65 mV between outside and inside the cell), temporarily increasing its tendency to "fire." The neuron fires when many subthreshold excitatory impulses arrive in rapid succession and the resting membrane potential lowers to about 50 mV. **Temporal summation** describes this condition of repeated subthreshold stimulation. Simultaneous stimulation of surrounding presynaptic terminals of the same neuron produces **spatial summation** and subsequent firing of the muscle fiber. This can induce an action potential from the "summing" of each individual effect.

 See the animation "Nerve Synapse" on http://thePoint.lww.com/mkk8e for a demonstration of this process.

 INTEGRATIVE QUESTION

Describe neuromuscular factors that help to explain performance differences among individuals who devote equal time practicing the volleyball spike.

The phenomenon of neural facilitation known as *disinhibition* affects neurons within the CNS rather than electrochemical events at the NMJ because the NMJ does not release inhibitory neurotransmitters. Three factors produce neuronal facilitation:

1. Decreased sensitivity of the motor neuron to inhibitory neurotransmitters
2. Reduced quantity of inhibitory neurotransmitter substance transported to the motor neuron
3. Combined effect of both mechanisms

Neural facilitation exerts an important influence under special, complex movement conditions. One of the basic tenets of topflight, all-out strength and power performance requires disinhibiting and maximally activating all motor neurons synchronously during the movement.[14,16,24] *Enhanced facilitation (disinhibition) leads to full activation of muscle groups during all-out effort and largely accounts for the rapid and highly specific strength increases during the early stages of resistance training.*[9,10,25,28] Chapter 22 discusses the potential for augmenting maximal strength performance through CNS facilitation with intense concentration or "psyching."

Inhibition. Some presynaptic terminals produce inhibitory impulses. The inhibitory transmitter substance increases the postsynaptic membrane's permeability to potassium and chloride ion efflux, increasing the cell's resting membrane potential to create an **inhibitory postsynaptic potential** (**IPSP**; www.ncbi.nlm.nih.gov/books/NBK11117/; Fig. 19.10B). The IPSP hyperpolarizes the neuron, making it more difficult to fire. A large IPSP prevents initiation of an action potential when a motor neuron receives both excitatory and inhibitory stimulation. For example, one usually can override or inhibit the reflex to pull the hand away when removing a splinter, for example, by steadying the hand to facilitate this unpleasant but necessary task.

The precise neurochemical that provokes an IPSP remains unknown, although gamma (γ)-aminobutyric acid (GABA) and the amino acid glycine exert inhibitory effects. Neural inhibition has protective functions and reduces the input of unwanted stimuli to achieve the goal of athletes at all skill levels—to execute a smooth, purposeful movement response on demand in the right sequence and tempo.

 INTEGRATIVE QUESTION

Explain how drugs that mimic neurotransmitters can affect physiologic response and physical performance.

MOTOR UNIT FUNCTIONAL CHARACTERISTICS

A motor unit contains only one specific muscle fiber type (type I or type II) or a subdivision of the type II fiber with the same metabolic profile. **TABLE 19.2** classifies motor units based on the following three physiologic and mechanical properties of the muscle fibers they innervate:

1. Twitch characteristics
2. Tension characteristics
3. Fatigue resistance

Twitch Characteristics

Early experiments in muscle/nerve physiology revealed that motor units developed high, low, or intermediate tension in response to a single electrical stimulus. Additionally, motor units with low force capacity exhibited a slow shortening time (and time to peak force) but remained fatigue resistant, whereas units with higher force capacity shortened rapidly but fatigued earlier. **FIGURE 19.11** illustrates the major characteristics for the three common motor unit categories:

1. Fast twitch, high force, and fast fatigue (type IIx)
2. Fast twitch, moderate force, and fatigue resistant (type IIa)
3. Slow twitch, low force, and fatigue resistant (type I)

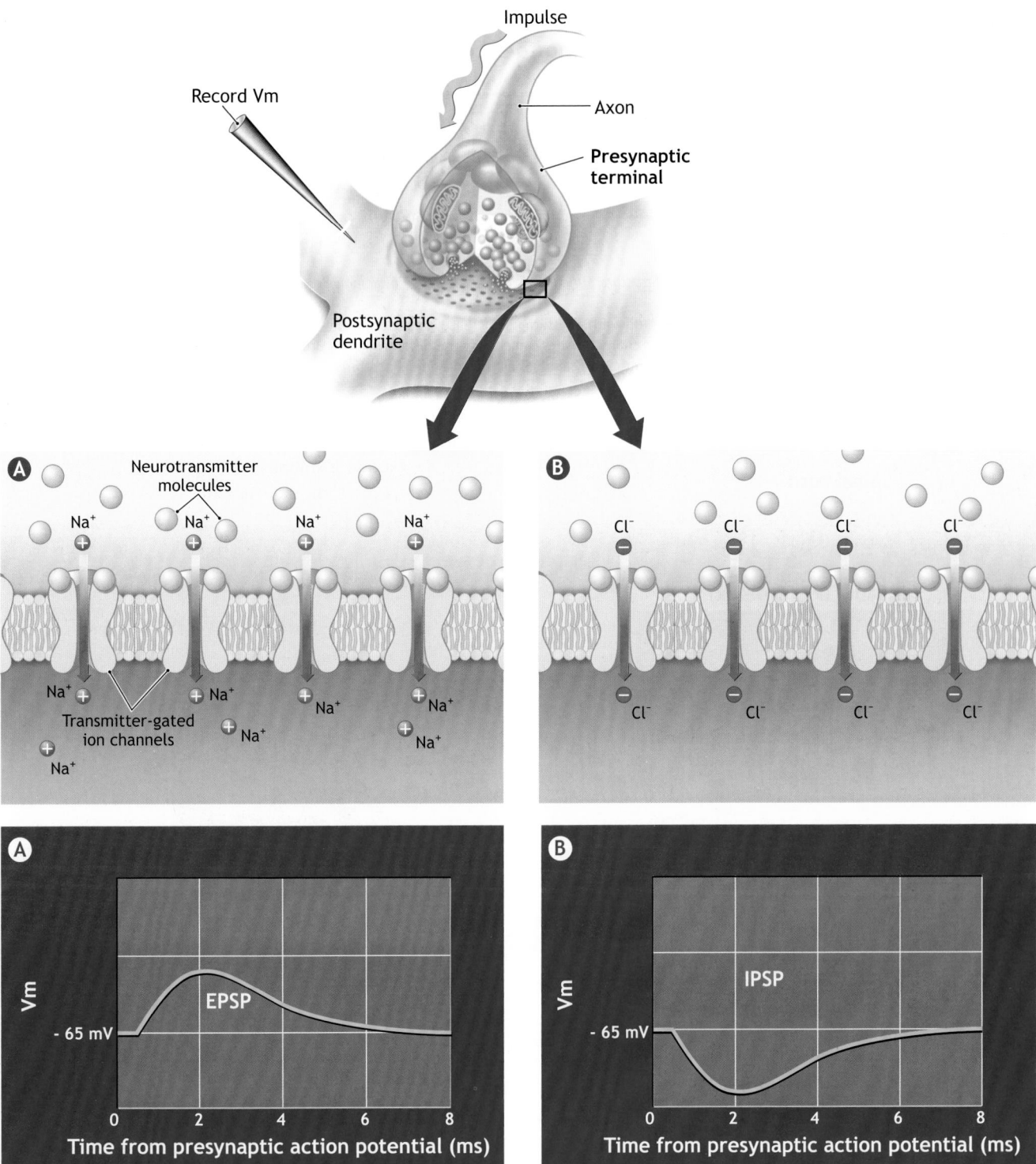

FIGURE 19.10 • **(A)** Generation of an excitatory postsynaptic potential (EPSP). An impulse arriving in the presynaptic terminal (*top inset*) causes neurotransmitter release. The molecules bind to transmitter-gated ion channels in the postsynaptic membrane. The membrane becomes hyperpolarized when Na^+ enters the postsynaptic cell through the open channels. The EPSP represents the resulting microvoltage (Vm) change in membrane potential recorded by a microelectrode in the cell. **(B)** Generation of an inhibitory postsynaptic potential (IPSP). An impulse arriving in the presynaptic terminal (*top inset*) causes neurotransmitter release. The molecules bind to transmitter-gated ion channels in the postsynaptic membrane. The membrane becomes hyperpolarized if Cl^- enters the postsynaptic cell through the open channels. The IPSP represents the resulting change in Vm recorded by a micro-electrode in the cell. (From Bear MF, et al. *Neuroscience: Exploring the Brain.* 3rd Ed. Baltimore: Lippincott Williams & Wilkins, 2006.)

TABLE 19.2	Characteristics and Correspondence Between Motor Units and Muscle Fiber Types					
Motor Unit Designation	**Force Production**	**Contraction Speed**	**Fatigue Resistance**	**Sag**[a]	**Muscle Fiber Type in the Motor Unit**	
Fast fatigable (FF—type IIx)	High	Fast	Low	Yes	Fast glycolytic (FG)	
Fast—fatigue-resistant (FR—type IIa)	Moderate	Fast	Moderate	Yes	Fast oxidative glycolytic (FOG)	
Slow (S—type I)	Low	Slow	High	No	Slow oxidative (SO)	

Adapted with permission from Lieber RL. *Skeletal Muscle Structure, Function, and Plasticity: The Physiologic Basis of Rehabilitation*. 3rd Ed. Baltimore: Lippincott Williams & Wilkins, 2009.

[a]Under repetitive stimuli, some motor units respond smoothly with a systematic increase in tension, while others first increase tension and then decrease or "sag" in response to the same tetanic stimulus. These sag characteristics can classify the different motor units. Only the slow motor units do not exhibit sag. This probably relates more to their diminished force-generating capabilities than fatigue characteristics.

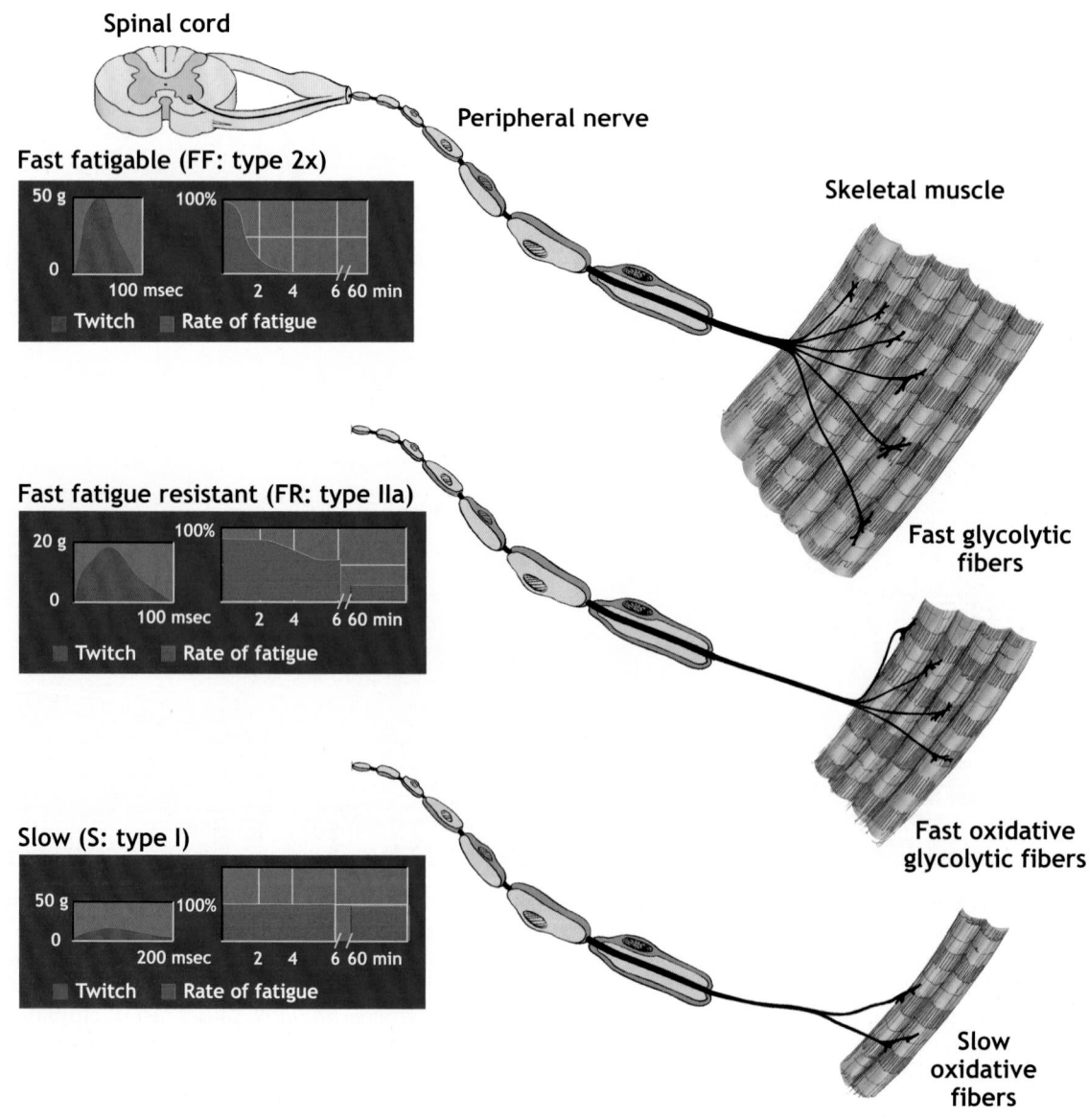

FIGURE 19.11 • Speed, force, and fatigue characteristics of motor units. "Phasic" motor neurons fire rapidly with short bursts; "tonic" motor neurons fire slowly but continuously.

Large motor neurons with fast conduction velocities innervate the two major subdivisions of fast-twitch muscle fibers. These motor units generally contain between 300 and 500 muscle fibers. The fast-fatigable (FF—type IIx) and fast–fatigue-resistant (FR—type IIa) units reach greater peak tension and develop it faster than slow-twitch (S—type I) motor units that receive innervation from smaller motor neurons with slow conduction velocities. The slower contracting units exhibit more fatigue resistance than the fast-twitch units. Specific training modifies the unique metabolic characteristics of each specific muscle fiber type. *With prolonged aerobic training, fast-twitch muscle fibers become almost as fatigue resistant as their slow-twitch counterparts* (see Chapter 22).

Motor neurons themselves have a trophic or stimulating effect on the muscle fibers they innervate in a way that modulates the fibers' properties and adaptive response to stimuli.[8] Surgically innervating fast-twitch muscle fibers with the neuron from a slow-twitch motor unit eventually alters the twitch characteristics of the fast-contracting fibers. Furthermore, application of long-term, low-frequency stimulation to intact fast-twitch motor units induces conversion of the muscle fibers to the slow-twitch type.[14,22] This neurotrophic effect suggests that the myoneural junction takes on much greater significance than just serving as the site of muscle fiber depolarization. It indicates a remarkable plasticity of skeletal muscle that may indeed be altered through long-term use.

Tension Characteristics

A stimulus strong enough to trigger an action potential in the motor neuron activates all of the accompanying muscle fibers in the motor unit to contract synchronously. A motor unit does not exert a force gradation—either the impulse elicits an action or it does not. After the neuron fires and the impulse reaches the NMJ, all fibers of the motor unit react simultaneously. This action embodies the principle of **"all or none"** that relates to the normal function of skeletal muscle.

Gradation of Force

The force of graded muscle action varies from slight to maximal via two mechanisms:

1. Increased *number* of motor units recruited
2. Increased *frequency* of motor unit discharge

A muscle generates considerable force when activated by all of its motor units. Repetitive stimuli that reach a muscle before it relaxes also increase the total tension. Blending recruitment of motor units and modification of their firing rate permits optimal patterns of neural discharge that allow a wide variety of graded muscle actions. These range from the delicate touch of the eye surgeon repairing a torn retina, to the maximal effort in throwing a baseball from deep centerfield on a straight line to throw out a runner charging home plate.

Control of Motor Function and Motor Unit Activity. Low-force muscle actions activate only a few motor units; a higher force requirement progressively enlists more motor units. **Motor unit recruitment** describes adding motor units to increase muscle force. As muscle force requirements increase, progressively larger axons recruit the required motor neurons. This exemplifies the **size principle**—an anatomic basis for the orderly recruitment of specific motor units to produce a smooth muscle action.

All of the motor units in a muscle do not fire at the same time (Fig. 19.12). If they did, it would be virtually impossible to control muscle force output. Consider the tremendous gradation of forces and speeds that muscles generate. When lifting a barbell, for example, specific muscles act to move the limb at a particular speed under a set rate of tension development. One can lift a light weight of 3 lb at a number of speeds. But as weight increases, say to 25 lb and then to 75 lb, the speed options decrease accordingly. When lifting a pencil, one generates just enough force to lift the pencil regardless of how fast or slowly the arm moves. When attempting to lift the heaviest weight possible, all of the available motor units require activation. *From the standpoint of neural control, the selective recruitment and firing pattern of the fast-twitch and slow-twitch motor units that control shoulder, arm, hand, and finger movements, and perhaps other stabilizing regions, provide the mechanism to produce the desired coordinated response.*

In accordance with the *size principle*, slow-twitch motor units with lower thresholds for activation are selectively recruited during light to moderate effort. Activation of slow-twitch units occurs during sustained jogging or cycling or slow swimming or slowly lifting a relatively light weight. More rapid, powerful movements progressively activate fast-twitch fatigue-resistant

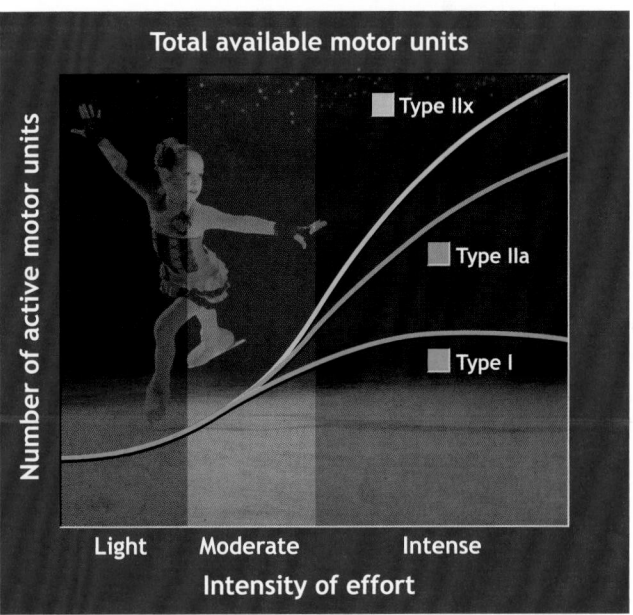

FIGURE 19.12 • Recruitment of slow-twitch (type I) and fast-twitch (type IIa and x) muscle fibers (motor units) in relation to exercise intensity. More intense exercise progressively recruits more fast-twitch fibers.

(type IIa) units up through the fast-twitch fatigable (type IIx) units at peak force. As a runner or cyclist reaches a hill during a distance race, selected fast-twitch units activate to maintain a fairly constant pace over varying terrain. Large single muscles with broad origins and/or insertions like the deltoid contain smaller, independently controlled "muscles within muscles" that activate depending on the segment's line of action and direction of the intended motion. Such an arrangement allows the CNS to offer flexibility to fine-tune skeletal muscle activity to meet the demands of the imposed motor task.[30]

The differential control of motor unit firing patterns represents a major factor that distinguishes skilled from unskilled performances and specific athletic groups.[6] Weightlifters generally exhibit a synchronous pattern of motor unit firing (i.e., many motor units recruited simultaneously during a lift), whereas the firing pattern of endurance athletes is more asynchronous as some motor units fire while others recover. The synchronous firing of fast-twitch motor units allows the weightlifter to mobilize forces quickly for the desired lift. In contrast, the asynchronous firing of predominantly slow-twitch, fatigue-resistant units for the endurance athlete serves as a built-in recuperative period so performance can continue with minimal fatigue. If this did not occur, the engaged muscles of the endurance athlete could not sustain high levels of force output for relatively long durations. In this situation, motor units share the burden of multiple movements and intensities during exercise.

INTEGRATIVE QUESTION

Explain how knowledge of neuromuscular exercise physiology can help enhance an athlete's (1) strength and power and (2) sports skill performance.

Fatigue Resistance

Fatigue represents the decline in muscle tension or force capacity with repeated stimulation or during a given time period. This definition also encompasses perceptual alterations of increased difficulty to achieve a desired submaximal or maximal outcome in physical activity. Many complex factors produce motor unit fatigue, each relating to specific activity demands that produce it.[1,13,15,17,18]

Voluntary muscle actions exhibit four main components listed in the following order of nervous system hierarchy:

1. Central nervous system
2. Peripheral nervous system
3. Neuromuscular junction
4. Muscle fiber

Fatigue occurs from disruption in the chain of events between the CNS and muscle fiber, regardless of the reason. Here are four examples:

1. Exercise-induced alterations in levels of CNS neurotransmitters serotonin, 5-hydroxytryptamine (5-HT), dopamine, and ACh in various brain regions, along with

the neuromodulators ammonia and cytokines secreted by immune cells, alter one's psychic or perceptual state to disrupt physical ability.[4,19]

2. Reduced glycogen content of active muscle fibers relates to fatigue during prolonged intense activity.[2,7] This "nutrient fatigue" occurs even with sufficient oxygen available to generate energy through aerobic pathways. Depletion of phosphocreatine (PCr) and a decline in total adenine nucleotide pool (ATP + ADP + AMP) also accompanies the fatigue state in prolonged submaximal effort.[2]

3. Lack of oxygen and increased level of blood and muscle lactate relate to muscle fatigue in short-term, maximal exertion. The dramatic increase in $[H^+]$ in the active muscle dramatically disrupts the intracellular environment.[12,23] Alterations in contractile function in anaerobic physical activity also relate to five factors:

   a. PCr depletion
   b. Changes in myosin ATPase
   c. Impaired glycolytic energy transfer capacity from reduced activity of the key enzymes phosphorylase and phosphofructokinase
   d. Disturbance in the T-tubule system for transmitting the impulse throughout the cell
   e. Ionic imbalances.[11] Downregulation in muscle Na^+, K^+, and Ca^{+2} release, distribution, and uptake alters the myofilament activity and impairs muscular performance,[16] even though nerve impulses continue to bombard the muscle fiber.

4. Fatigue occurs at the NMJ when an action potential fails to traverse from the motor neuron to the muscle fiber. The mechanism for this aspect of "neural fatigue" remains unknown.

As overall muscle function often declines during prolonged submaximal effort, additional motor-unit recruitment maintains the crucial force outputs required to maintain a relatively constant level of performance. During all-out exercise that presumably activates all motor units, a decrease in neural activity accompanies fatigue as measured by the electromyogram (EMG). Reduced neural activity supports the contention that failure in neural or myoneural transmission produces fatigue in maximal effort.

INTEGRATIVE QUESTION

From a neuromuscular perspective, discuss the validity of the adage "Perfect practice makes for perfect performance."

RECEPTORS IN MUSCLES, JOINTS, AND TENDONS: THE PROPRIOCEPTORS

Muscles and tendons contain highly specialized sensory receptors sensitive to stretch, tension, and pressure. These terminal end organs known as **proprioceptors** almost instantaneously

IN A PRACTICAL SENSE

How to Determine Upper-Arm Muscle and Fat

Girth measurements include bone surrounded by a mass of muscle tissue ringed by a layer of subcutaneous fat (FIG. A). Muscle represents the largest component of girth (except in obese and elderly persons), so girth indicates one's relative muscularity. The procedure for estimating limb muscle area assumes similarity between a limb and a cylinder, with subcutaneous fat evenly distributed around the cylinder (Fig. A).

MEASUREMENTS

Determine the following:
1. Upper-arm girth (relaxed triceps; G_{arm}): Measure with arm extended relaxed at the side (or parallel to the ground in an abducted position). Measure girth (cm) midway between the acromial and olecranon process (FIG. B).
2. Triceps skinfold (Sf_{tri}): Measure in decimeters (dm; mm ÷ 10) on the back of the arm over the triceps muscle as a vertical fold at the same level as the relaxed arm girth (FIG. C).

EXAMPLE

Data: Upper-arm girth (G_{arm}) in cm = 30.0; Sf_{tri} = 2.5 dm (25 mm).

COMPUTATIONS

1. Arm muscle girth, cm
$$= G_{arm} - (\pi Sf_{tri})$$
$$= 30.0 \text{ cm} - (\pi 2.5 \text{ dm})$$
$$= 30.0 - 7.854$$
$$= 22.1 \text{ cm}$$

2. Arm muscle area, cm^2
$$= [G_{arm} - (\pi Sf_{tri})] \div 4\pi$$
$$= (30.0 \text{ cm}) - (\pi 2.5 \text{ dm})^2 \div 4\pi$$
$$= 488.4 \div 12.566$$
$$= 38.9 \text{ cm}^2$$

3. Arm area (A), cm^2
$$= (G_{arm})^2 \div 4\pi$$
$$= (30.0 \text{ cm})^2 \div 4\pi$$
$$= 900 \div 12.566$$
$$= 71.6 \text{ cm}^2$$

4. Arm fat area, cm^2
$$= \text{arm area} - \text{arm muscle area}$$
$$= 71.6 \text{ cm}^2 - 38.9 \text{ cm}^2$$
$$= 32.7 \text{ cm}^2$$

5. Arm fat index, % fat area
$$= (\text{arm fat area} \div \text{arm area}) \times 100$$
$$= (32.7 \text{ cm}^2 \div 71.6) \times 100$$
$$= 45.7\%$$

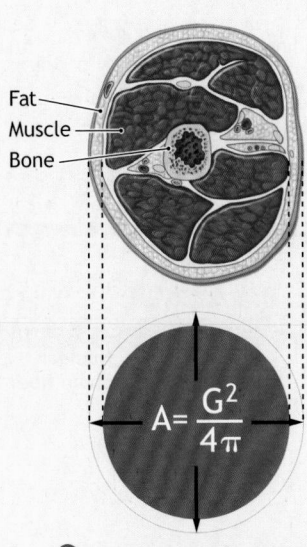

Fat
Muscle
Bone

$$A = \frac{G^2}{4\pi}$$

A Upper-arm composition and area

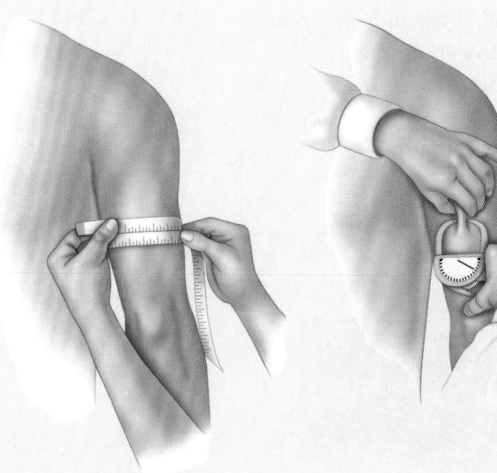

B Relaxed triceps arm girth, cm

C Triceps skinfold, mm

relay information about muscular dynamics and limb movement to conscious and subconscious portions of the CNS. Proprioception allows continual monitoring of the progress of any sequence of movements and serves to modify subsequent motor behavior.[20]

 See the animation "Proprioceptors" on **http://thePoint.lww.com/mkk8e** for a demonstration of this process.

Muscle Spindles

The **muscle spindles**, named for their similar shape to the spindle on a spinning wheel, provide mechano-sensory information about changes in muscle fiber length and tension. They primarily respond to any stretch of a muscle. Through reflex response, they initiate a stronger muscle action to counteract this stretch.

Structural Organization

Figure 19.13 shows a fusiform muscle spindle aligned in parallel to regular muscle fibers or **extrafusal fibers**. When the muscle stretches, the spindles also stretch. The number of spindles within a quantity of muscle varies depending on the muscle group. On a relative basis, muscles involved in complex movements contain more spindles per gram of muscle than muscles that perform gross movement patterns. The spindle, covered by a sheath of connective tissue, contains two specialized types of muscle fiber called **intrafusal fibers**. One type of intrafusal fiber, the fairly large **nuclear bag fiber**, contains numerous nuclei packed centrally through its diameter. Each spindle usually contains two nuclear bag fibers. The other type of intrafusal fiber, the **nuclear chain fiber**, contains many nuclei along its length. These fibers attach to the surface of the longer nuclear bag fibers. Each spindle usually contains four to five chain fibers. The ends of the intrafusal fibers contain actin and myosin filaments and exhibit shortening capability.

Two sensory afferent fibers and one motor efferent fiber innervate the spindles. A primary afferent nerve fiber, the **annulospiral nerve fiber,** composed of a set of rings in spiral configuration, entwines about the midregion of the bag fiber.

This fiber responds directly to the stretch of the spindle; its firing frequency or discharge rate increases in proportion to the stretch. A second group of smaller sensory nerve fibers, the **flower-spray endings**, makes connections mainly on the chain fibers but also attaches to the bag fibers. These endings show less sensitivity to stretch than annulospiral fibers. Activation of the annulospiral and flower-spray sensors relays impulses through the dorsal root into the cord to produce reflex activation of the motor neurons to the stretched muscle. This causes the muscle to act more forcefully and shorten, the end result of which reduces the stretch stimulus from the spindles.

The third type of spindle nerve fiber, the thin **γ-efferent fiber** that innervates the contractile, striated ends of the intrafusal fibers, serves a motor function. Higher centers in the brain activate these fibers to maintain optimal sensitivity of the spindle at all muscle lengths. Regardless of the muscle's overall length, γ-efferent stimulation activates the intrafusal fibers to regulate their length and sensitivity. This mechanism prepares the spindle for other lengthening actions, even when the muscle remains shortened. Adjustments in γ-efferent activation allow the spindle to continuously monitor the length of the muscles that contain them.

The Stretch Reflex

The muscle spindle detects, responds to, and modulates changes in the length of the extrafusal muscle fibers. This provides an important regulatory function for movement and maintenance of posture. Postural muscles continuously receive neural input to sustain their readiness to respond to conscious

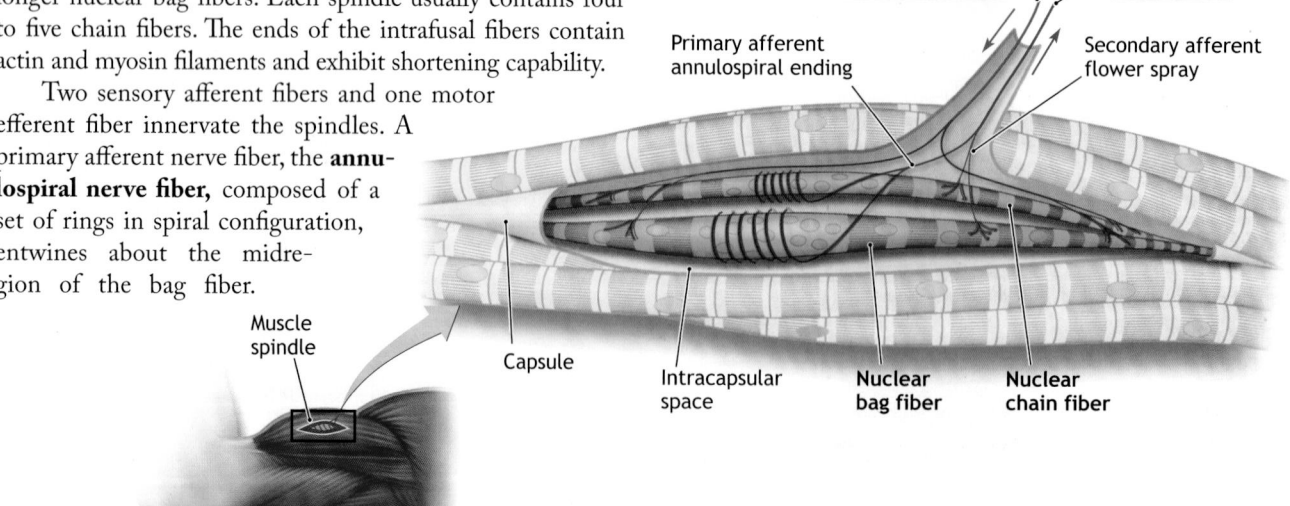

FIGURE 19.13 • Structural organization of the muscle spindle with an enlarged view of the equatorial region of the spindle.

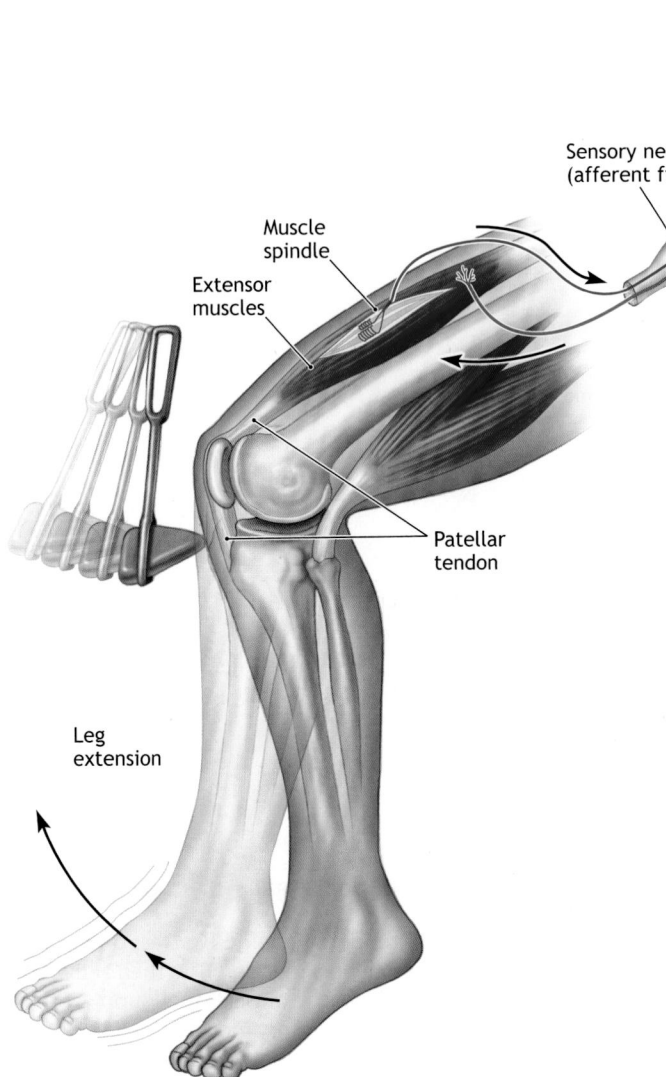

Dorsal horn
Ventral horn
White matter
Gray matter
Sensory neuron (afferent fiber)
Muscle spindle
Extensor muscles
Alpha motor neuron (efferent fiber)
Synapse
Patellar tendon
Leg extension

FIGURE 19.14 • The patella tendon stretch reflex (shows only one side of the spinal nerve complex).

elongate as the hammer strikes the patellar tendon. The spindle's sensory receptors fire when its intrafusal fibers stretch. This directs impulses through the dorsal root into the spinal cord to directly activate the anterior motor neurons. The gray matter contains neuron cell bodies; the white matter carries longitudinal columns of nerve fibers. Stimulation of a single α-motor neuron affects up to 3000 muscle fibers. The reflex also activates interneurons within the cord to facilitate the appropriate motor response. For example, excitatory impulses activate synergistic muscles that support the desired movement, while inhibitory impulses flow to motor units that normally counter the movement. In this way, the stretch reflex acts as a self-regulating, compensating mechanism. This salient feature allows the muscle to adjust automatically to differences in load and length without requiring immediate information processing through higher CNS centers.

Golgi Tendon Organs

In contrast to the muscle spindles that lie parallel to the extrafusal muscle fibers, the **Golgi tendon organs** (**GTOs**)—first identified in 1898 by Italian physician Camillo Golgi (1843–1926; see www.nobelprize.org/nobel_prizes/medicine/laureates/1906/golgi-bio.html) and named in his honor—connect up to 25 extrafusal fibers near the tendon's junction to the muscle. These fine-tuned sensory receptors detect differences in the tension generated by active muscle rather than muscle length. **FIGURE 19.15** shows that the GTOs respond as a feedback monitor to discharge impulses under either of two conditions:

1. Tension created in the muscle when it shortens
2. Tension when the muscle stretches passively

When stimulated by excessive tension, the GTO receptors transmit signals to the spinal cord to elicit *reflex inhibition* of the muscles they supply. This occurs from the overriding influence of the inhibitory spinal interneuron on the motor neurons supplying the muscle. Consider the GTOs as a *protective* sensory mechanism, much like a "governor" mechanism that sets the speed limit for motorized go-carts—no matter how "hard" you depress the gas pedal, the car only goes at a predetermined top speed. Excessive change in muscle tension increases the GTO sensor's discharge to depress motor neuron activity and reduces force output. GTO receptors remain relatively inactive and exert

voluntary movements. These muscles require continual subconscious activity to adjust to the pull of gravity in upright posture. Without this monitoring and feedback mechanism, the body would literally collapse into a heap from the absence of tension in neck muscles, spinal muscles, hip flexors, abdominal muscles, and large leg musculature. To this end, the stretch reflex provides a fundamental controlling mechanism.

The stretch reflex consists of three main components:

1. Muscle spindle that responds to stretch
2. Afferent nerve fiber that carries the sensory impulse from the spindle to the spinal cord
3. Efferent spinal cord motor neuron that activates the stretched muscle fibers

FIGURE 19.14 illustrates the patellar tendon stretch reflex or knee-jerk reflex, the simplest autonomic reflex arc that involves only one synapse called a monosynaptic synapse. The spindles lie parallel to the extrafusal fibers so they stretch when these fibers

little influence if muscle action produces little tension. *Ultimately, the GTOs protect the muscle and surrounding connective tissue harness from injury from a sudden, unaccustomed movement or an excessive load.*

Pacinian Corpuscles

Pacinian corpuscles are small, ellipsoidal bodies located close to the GTOs and embedded in a single, unmyelinated nerve fiber. These sensitive sensory receptors respond to quick movement and deep pressure. Deformation or compression by a mechanical force to the onion-like capsule transmits pressure to the sensory nerve ending within its core to change the electric potential of the sensory nerve ending. If this generator potential achieves sufficient magnitude, a sensory signal propagates down the myelinated axon that leaves the corpuscle and enters the spinal cord.

Pacinian corpuscles act as fast-adapting mechanical sensors; they discharge a few impulses at the onset of a steady stimulus and then remain electrically silent or they discharge a second volley of impulses when the stimulus ceases. They detect *changes* in movement or pressure rather than the magnitude of movement or the quantity of pressure applied.

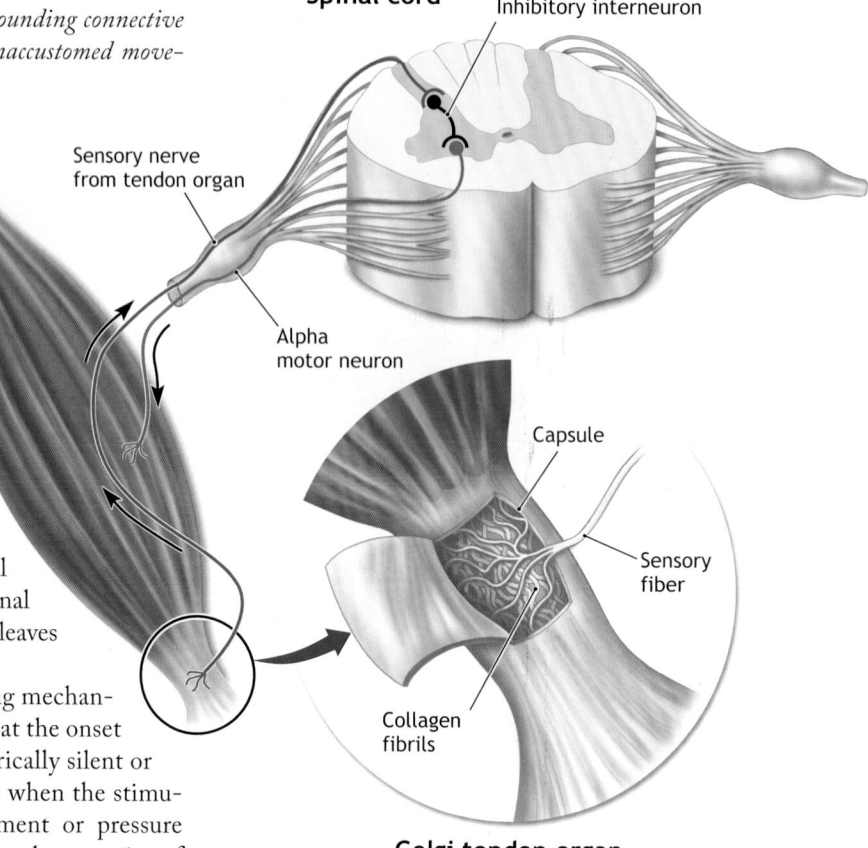

Golgi tendon organ

FIGURE 19.15 • Golgi tendon organs (GTOs) respond to excessive tension or stretch on a muscle. GTOs then activate to initiate a reflex inhibition of the muscles they supply. The GTOs function as a protective sensory mechanism to detect and subsequently inhibit undue strain within the muscle–tendon structure.

Summary

1. Neural control mechanisms located in the central nervous system (CNS) regulate human movement.
2. Skeletal muscles respond to internal and external stimuli where millions of bits of sensory input automatically are coded, routed, organized, and transmitted to the effector organ—the skeletal muscles.
3. Tracts of neural tissue descend from the brain to influence spinal cord neurons. Neurons in the extrapyramidal tract control posture and provide a continual background level of neuromuscular tone; the pyramidal tract neurons stimulate discrete muscular movements.
4. The cerebellum fine-tunes muscle activity through its function as the major comparing, evaluating, and integrating center.
5. The spinal cord and other subconscious areas of the CNS control many muscle functions. The reflex arc provides the basic mechanism to process "automatic" muscle actions.
6. The motor unit makes up the functional unit of movement. The number of muscle fibers in a motor unit depends on a muscle's movement function. Intricate movement patterns require a small fiber-to-neuron ratio; a single neuron can innervate 1000 muscle fibers for gross movements.

7. The anterior motor neuron, consisting of the cell body, axon, and dendrites, transmits electrochemical nerve impulses from the spinal cord to the muscle.
8. The dendrites receive impulses and conduct them toward the cell body; the axon transmits the impulse one way down the axon to the muscle.
9. The neuromuscular junction (NMJ) establishes the interface between the motor neuron and muscle fiber. Acetylcholine (ACh) release at the NMJ provides the chemical stimulus that activates the muscle fiber.
10. Stimulation of a muscle fiber progresses in the following six-step sequence: (a) action potential propagates down the motor neuron's axon; (b) calcium channels open at the end of the nerve terminal; (c) calcium moves into the nerve terminal; (d) ACh primes for release; (e) ACh traverses the synapse and binds to ACh receptors on the postsynaptic membrane at the sarcolemma; and (f) endplate potential generates and a depolarization wave spreads throughout the T-tubular network.
11. Excitatory and inhibitory impulses continually bombard the synaptic junctions between neurons. These impulses

alter a neuron's threshold for excitation by increasing or decreasing its tendency to fire.

12. During all-out power movements, a high degree of neural facilitation (disinhibition) proves beneficial because it maximally activates a muscle's motor units.

13. Motor units classify into three types depending on speed of muscle action, force generated, and fatigability: (a) fast twitch, high force, fast fatigue; (b) fast twitch, moderate force, fatigue resistant; and (c) slow twitch, low force, fatigue resistant.

14. Muscle force gradation progresses through the interaction of factors that regulate the number and type of motor units recruited and their discharge frequency. Low-intensity physical activity recruits slow-twitch motor units, followed by fast-twitch unit activation when requiring more-powerful forces.

15. Alterations in motor unit recruitment and firing pattern help to explain the rapid strength improvement during the early stages of resistance training.

16. Sensitive sensory receptors in muscles, tendons, and joints relay information about muscle dynamics and limb movement to specific portions of the CNS to provide important sensory feedback during physical activity.

17. Golgi tendon organ sensory receptors respond to quick movement and deep pressure, while pacinian corpuscles detect changes in movement or pressure.

the**Point** References are available online at
http://thepoint.lww.com/mkk8e.

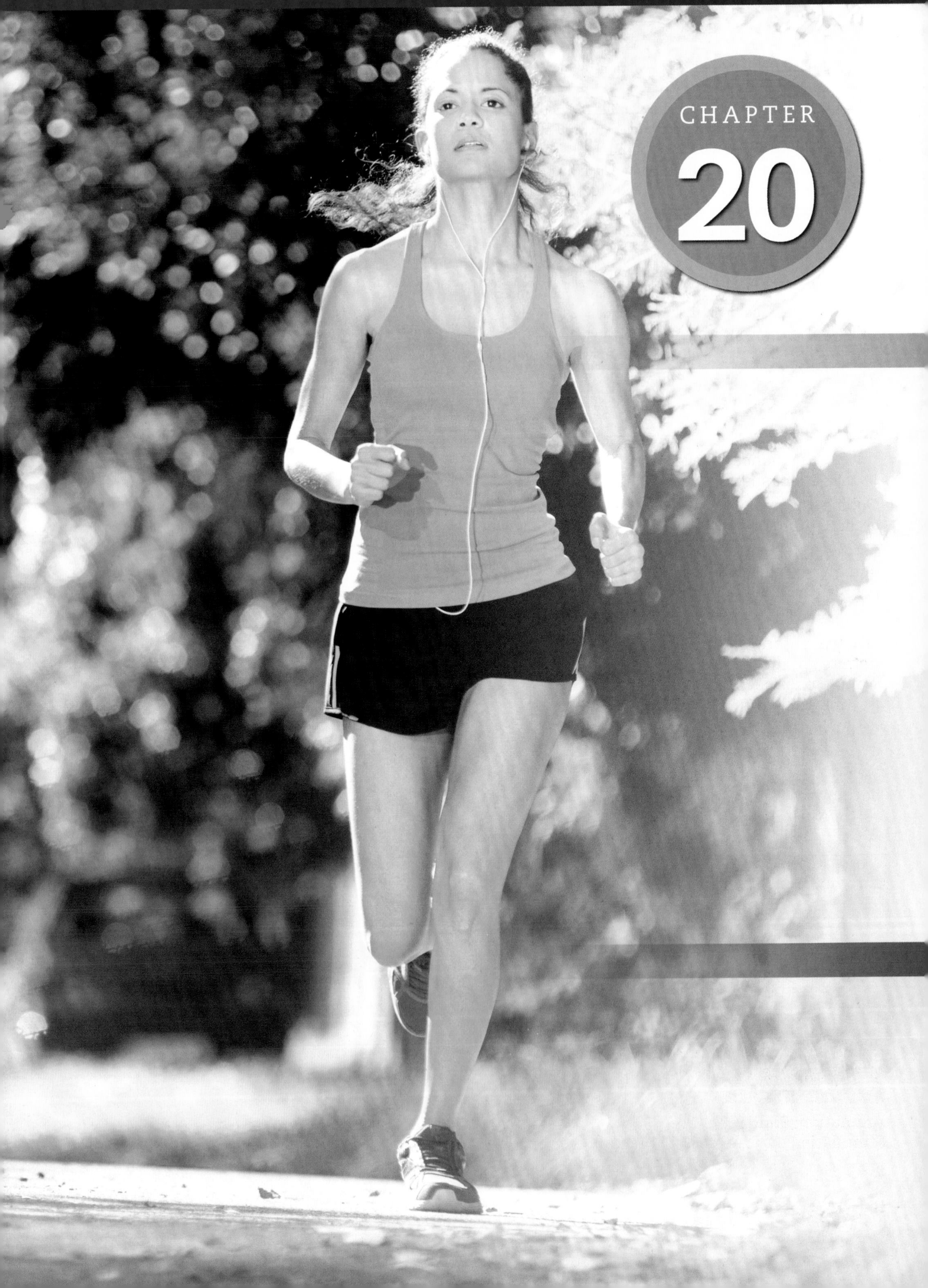

CHAPTER

20

The Endocrine System: Organization and Acute and Chronic Responses to Physical Activity

- Draw the locations of the body's major endocrine glands
- List the sequence of events to show how hormones affect specific "target cell" functions
- Outline the role of the intracellular messenger cyclic 3′, 5′-adenosine monophosphate (cyclic AMP)
- Explain how hormones affect enzyme activity and enzyme-mediated membrane transport
- Describe the influence of hormonal, humoral, and neural stimulation on endocrine gland activity
- List the anterior and posterior pituitary gland hormones, their functions, and how acute and chronic physical activity affects their release
- List the thyroid gland hormones, their functions, and how acute and chronic physical activity affects their release
- List the adrenal medulla and adrenal cortex hormones, their functions, and how acute and chronic physical activity affects their release
- List hormones of the α- and β-cells of the pancreas, their functions, and how acute and chronic physical activity affects their release

- Define type 1 and type 2 diabetes and the symptoms and effects of each disorder
- Describe three test options for diagnosing diabetes mellitus
- List the fasting blood glucose classification categories for type 2 diabetes
- List risk factors for type 2 diabetes and benefits of regular physical activity to prevent and treat this disease
- Outline how exercise training affects endocrine function
- Describe the effect of resistance training on testosterone and growth hormone release
- Characterize the functions of opioid peptides, their response to physical activity, and possible role in the "exercise high"
- Outline interactions among short-term, moderate, and exhaustive physical activity, training, susceptibility to illness, and immune function

Visit http://thePoint.lww.com/mkk8e to access the following resources.

- References: Chapter 20
- Interactive Question Bank
- Animation: Diabetes
- Animation: Endocrine Gland Stimulation

- Animation: Hormonal Control
- Animation: Immune Response
- Animation: Insulin Functions
- Focus on Research: Training Intensity Affects Growth Hormone Release

The endocrine system integrates and regulates bodily functions to stabilize the body's internal environment. Hormones produced by endocrine glands affect all aspects of human function; they activate enzyme systems, alter cell membrane permeability, trigger muscular contraction and relaxation, stimulate protein and fat synthesis, initiate cellular secretion, and determine how the body responds to physical and psychologic stress. The following sections provide a general overview of the endocrine system, its functions during rest and physical activity, and responses to acute exercise and training.

ENDOCRINE SYSTEM OVERVIEW

Small compared with other body organs, the combined weight of the endocrine organs averages 0.5 kg. FIGURE 20.1 illustrates the location of the six major endocrine organs—the pineal, pituitary, thyroid, parathyroid, thymus, and adrenal glands. Several other organs contain discrete areas of endocrine tissue that also produce hormones. These include the pancreas, gonads (ovaries and testes), hypothalamus, and adipose (fat) tissues (not shown). The hypothalamus also serves as a major organ of the nervous system; it functions as a **neuroendocrine organ**. Pockets of hormone-producing cells also form in the walls of the small intestine, stomach, kidneys, and myocytes in the heart's atria, yet these organs exert little influence on hormone production per se.

ENDOCRINE SYSTEM ORGANIZATION

The **endocrine system** *(endocrine means "hormone secreting") consists of a host organ (gland), minute quantities of chemical messengers (hormones), and a target or receptor organ.* Glands classify as either endocrine or exocrine. Some glands serve both endocrine and exocrine functions. Chinese and Arab physicians of antiquity observed bodily dysfunctions related to specialized "glands," but the written evidence relating to bodily disorders began in Egypt 3000 years before the Christian era with the Smith papyrus, the oldest medical text in existence (**www.annclinlabsci. org/content/40/4/386.full**). Housed in a vault in the library of the New York Academy of Medicine in New York City, the Smith papyrus details 48 medical case reports written on 15 feet of papyrus organized according to symptoms, diagnosis, treatment, and prognosis (**www.nlm.nih.gov/news/turn_ page_egyptian.html**; an app, *Turning the Pages*, allows users to virtually turn the pages of rare medical books from the collections of the U.S. National Library of Medicine; **http:// archive.nlm.nih.gov/proj/ttp/books.htm**). Centuries later, beginning in the Renaissance Period, many careful investigative studies and human surgeries began to unravel the structures and their functions, known formally as endocrine glands (**http://endocrinesurgery.ucla.edu/patient_ education_history.html**).

    Endocrine glands possess no ducts, referred to as *ductless glands*, and secrete substances directly into extracellular spaces around the gland. FIGURE 20.2 shows that secreted hormones diffuse into blood for transport throughout the body to bind

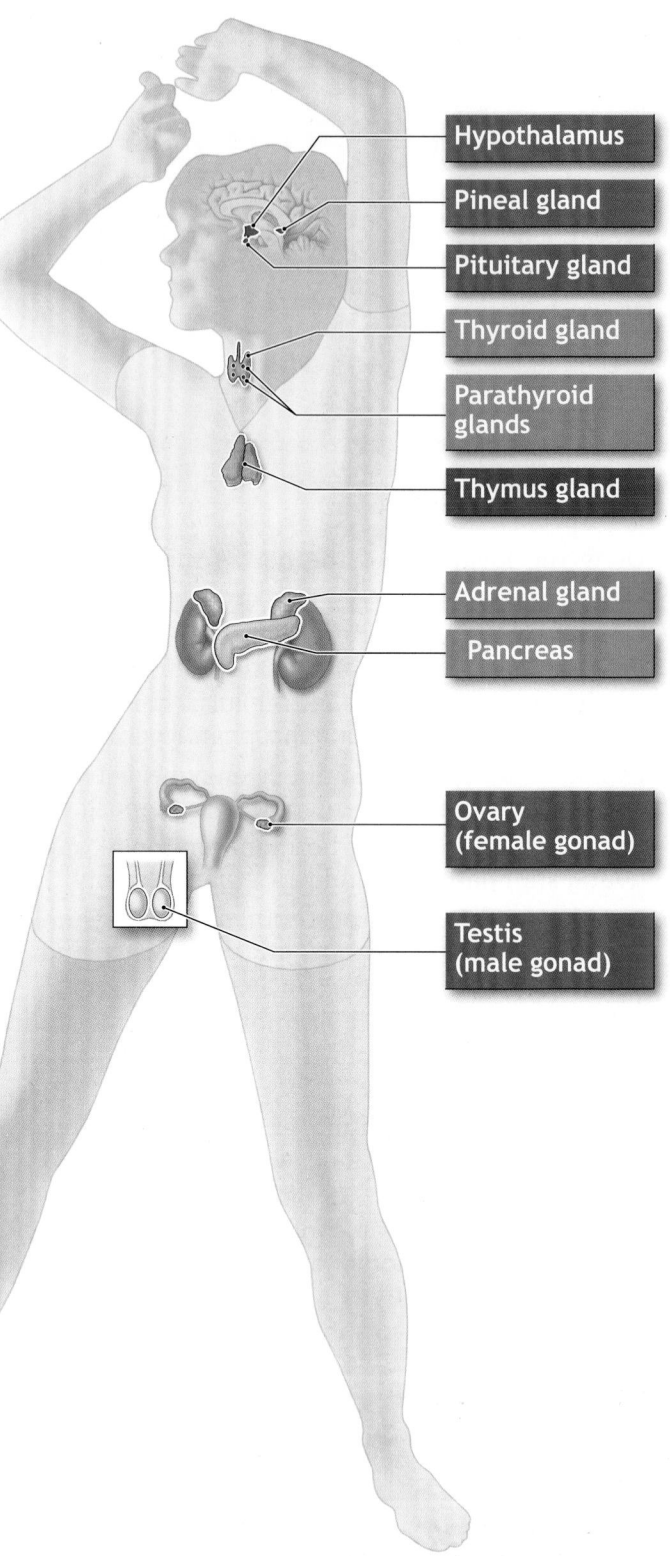

FIGURE 20.1 • Location of the hormone-producing endocrine organs.

with specific tissue receptors to fulfill their intercellular communication functions. **Exocrine glands**, in contrast, contain secretory ducts that carry substances directly to a specific compartment or surface. Examples of exocrine glands include sweat glands and glands of the upper digestive tract. The nervous system controls almost all exocrine glands.

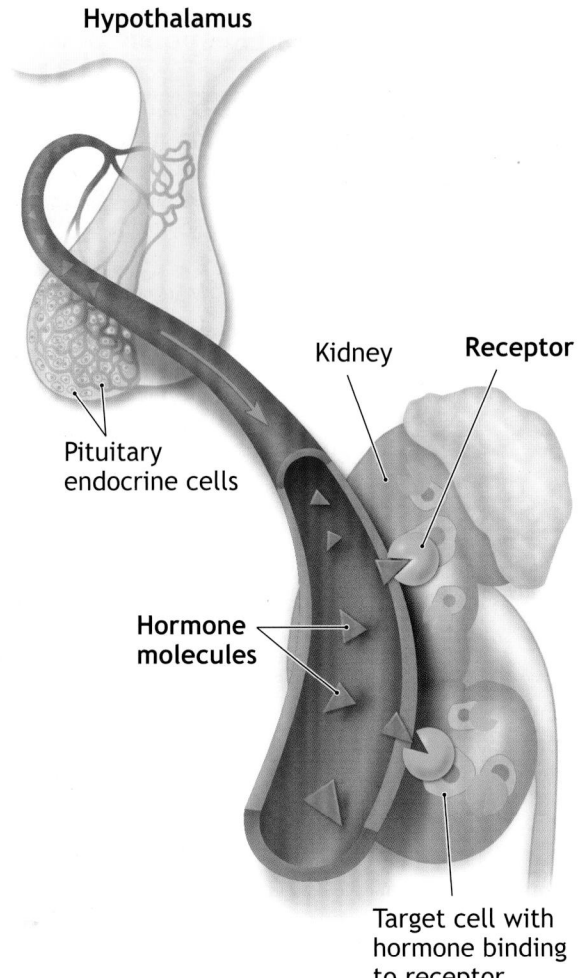

Hypothalamus

Kidney

Receptor

Pituitary endocrine cells

Hormone molecules

Target cell with hormone binding to receptor

FIGURE 20.2 • Hormones secreted from endocrine glands travel in the bloodstream to exert influence on body tissues.

 See the animation "Endocrine Gland Stimulation" on http://thePoint.lww.com/mkk8e for a demonstration of the functioning of endocrine glands.

Types of Hormones

Hormones, *chemical substances synthesized by specific host glands, enter the bloodstream for transport throughout the body.* Hormones generally fit into one of two categories: **steroid-derived hormones** and **amine** and **polypeptide hormones** synthesized from amino acids. In contrast to steroid hormones, amine and peptide hormones are soluble in blood plasma. This allows easy uptake at target sites. The term *half-life* describes the time required to reduce a hormone's blood concentration by one half. For example, epinephrine's half-life is slightly less than 3 min, while most orally consumed anabolic hormones such as testosterone have a half-life of approximately 3.5 hr. A hormone's half-life gives a good indication of how long its effect persists. TABLE 20.1 compares the storage, synthesis, release mechanism, transport medium, receptor location and receptor-ligand binding, and target organ response of the peptide, steroid, and amine hormones.

 ## The Term *Hormone* Enters the English Lexicon

The term *hormone* (from the Greek *hormao*, meaning "to excite" or "rapid motion toward") entered the English lexicon in 1905 when renowned British physiologists William Bayliss (1860–1924) and Ernest Starling (1866–1927) discovered *secretin*, a compound from the intestine that functioned as an active chemical messenger or signaller of cellular functions (www.britannica.com/EBchecked/topic/531937/secretin). The discipline of endocrinology emerged from these seminal discoveries.

TABLE 20.2 lists eight different hormones produced by organs other than the major endocrine glands. Of these, prostaglandins constitute a third chemical class of hormones; they represent biologically active lipids in the plasma membrane of nearly all cells. Erythropoietin, a glycoprotein, stimulates the bone marrow's production of red blood cells.

Most hormones circulate in the blood as messengers that affect tissues a distance from the specific gland. Other hormones (e.g., prostaglandins and the gastrointestinal hormone gastrin) exert local effects in their region of synthesis.

 See the animation "Hormonal Control" on http://thePoint.lww.com/mkk8e for a demonstration of hormone activity.

Hormone–Target Cell Specificity

Hormones alter cellular reactions of specific "target cells" in four ways:

1. Modify rate of intracellular protein synthesis by stimulating nuclear DNA
2. Change rate of enzyme activity
3. Alter plasma membrane transport via a second-messenger system
4. Induce secretory activity

A target cell's response to a hormone depends largely on the presence of specific protein receptors that bind the hormone in a complementary way. Target cell receptors occur either on the plasma membrane (up to 10,000 receptors per cell) or in the cell's interior switch as occurs for fat-soluble steroid hormones that pass through the plasma membrane. Hormone receptors exist in specific local areas or more diffusely throughout the body. For example, adrenal cortex cells contain receptors for adrenocorticotropic hormone (ACTH). In contrast, all cells contain receptors for thyroxine, the principal hormone that stimulates cellular metabolism.

Hormone–Receptor Binding

Hormone–receptor binding represents the first step in initiating hormone action. The extent of a target cell's activation by a hormone depends on three factors:

1. Hormone concentration in the blood
2. Number of target cell receptors for the hormone

TABLE 20.1	Storage, Synthesis, Release Mechanism, Transport Medium, Receptor Location and Receptor-Ligand Binding, and Target Organ Response of the Peptide, Steroid, and Amine Hormones			
			Amine Hormones	
	Peptide Hormones	**Steroid Hormones**	**Catecholamines**	**Thyroid Hormones**
Examples	Insulin, glucagon, leptin, IGF-1	Androgens, DHEA, cortisol	Epinephrine, norepinephrine	Thyroxine (T_4)
Synthesis and storage	Made in advance; stored in secretory vesicles	Synthesized on demand from precursors	Made in advance; stored in secretory vesicles	Made in advance; precursor stored in secretory vesicles
Release from parent cell	Exocytosis[a]	Simple diffusion	Exocytosis	Simple diffusion
Transport medium	Dissolved in plasma	Bound to carrier proteins	Dissolved in plasma	Bound to carrier proteins
Lifespan (half-life[b])	Short	Long	Short	Long
Receptor location	On cell membrane	Cytoplasm of nucleus; some have membrane receptors	On cell membrane	Nucleus
Response to receptor-ligand binding[c]	Activation of second messenger system; may activate genes	Activate genes for transcription and translation; may have nongenomic actions	Activation of second messenger system	Activate genes for transcription and translation
General target response	Modification of existing proteins and induction of new protein synthesis	Induction of new protein synthesis	Modification of existing proteins	Induction of new protein synthesis

[a]Process in which intracellular vesicles fuse with the cell membrane and release their contents into the extracellular fluid.
[b]Amount of time required to reduce hormone concentration by one half.
[c]A ligand (the molecule that binds to a receptor) binds to a membrane protein, which triggers endocytosis (process of how a cell brings molecules into the cytoplasm in vesicles formed from the cell membrane).

3. Sensitivity or strength of the union between hormone and receptor

Consider cell hormone receptors as dynamic structures that continually adjust to physiologic demands. **Up-regulation** describes the state whereby target cells form more receptors in response to increasing hormone levels to increase the hormone's effect. In contrast, prolonged exposure to high hormone concentrations desensitizes target cells to blunt hormonal stimulation. Such **down-regulation** also involves a loss of receptors to prevent target cells from overresponding to chronically high hormone levels to decrease the hormone's effect.

Cyclic AMP: The Intracellular Messenger. The binding of a hormone with its specific receptor in the plasma membrane alters the target cell's permeability to a particular chemical (e.g., insulin's effect on cellular glucose uptake) or modifies the target cell's ability to manufacture intracellular substances, primarily proteins. Such actions ultimately affect cellular function. **Figure 20.3** shows a schematic for a nonsteroid hormone (displayed as a triangle) as it binds to its receptor and penetrates the intracellular space through the bilayer plasma membrane., The binding hormone acts as **first messenger** to react with the enzyme **adenylate cyclase** in the plasma membrane to form the compound cyclic 3′5′-adenosine monophosphate (**cyclic AMP**) from an original ATP molecule

(www.ncbi.nlm.nih.gov/pmc/articles/PMC2720142/). Cyclic AMP then acts as a ubiquitous second messenger to activate a specific protein kinase, which then activates a target enzyme to alter cellular response.

Three factors establish the sequence of reactions set into motion by cyclic AMP:

1. Type of target cell
2. Specific enzymes contained in the target cell
3. Specific hormone that acts as first messenger

In thyroid cells, for example, cyclic AMP promotes thyroxine synthesis from the binding of thyroid-stimulating hormone. In bone and muscle, cyclic AMP produced via growth-hormone binding activates anabolic reactions to synthesize amino acids into tissue proteins.

Hormone Effects on Enzymes

Major hormone actions include altering enzyme activity and enzyme-mediated membrane transport. A hormone increases enzyme activity in one of three ways:

1. Stimulates enzyme production
2. Combines with the enzyme to alter its shape and ability to act, a chemical process known as **allosteric modulation**, and increases or decreases the enzyme's catalytic effectiveness

TABLE 20.2	Hormones Produced by Organs Other than the Major Endocrine Organs		
Hormone	**Composition**	**Source and Stimulus for Secretion**	**Target and Outcome**
Prostaglandins	20-carbon fatty acid synthesized from arachidonic acid	*Source:* plasma membrane of different body cells *Stimulus:* local irritation, different hormones	*Target:* multiple sites *Outcome:* controls local hormone response; stimulates arterioles to increase blood pressure; increases uterine contractions, HCl and pepsin secretion in stomach, platelet aggregation, blood clotting, constriction of bronchioles, inflammation, pain, and fever
Gastrin	Peptide	*Source:* stomach *Stimulus:* food	*Target:* stomach *Outcome:* release of HCl
Enterogastrin	Peptide	*Source:* duodenum *Stimulus:* food (especially lipids)	*Target:* stomach *Outcome:* inhibits HCl secretion and gastrointestinal motility
Secretin	Peptide	*Source:* duodenum *Stimulus:* food	*Target:* pancreas *Outcome:* release of bicarbonate-rich juice *Target:* liver *Outcome:* release of bile *Target:* stomach *Outcome:* inhibits secretion
Cholecystokinin	Peptide	*Source:* duodenum *Stimulus:* food	*Target:* pancreas *Outcome:* release of bicarbonate-rich juice *Target:* gallbladder *Outcome:* expulsion of bile *Target:* sphincter of Oddi *Outcome:* relaxes sphincter and allows bile to enter duodenum
Erythropoietin	Glycoprotein	*Source:* kidneys[a] *Stimulus:* hypoxia	*Target:* bone marrow *Outcome:* production of red blood cells
Active vitamin D_3	Steroid	*Source:* kidneys activate vitamin D from epidermal skin cells *Stimulus:* parathyroid hormone	*Target:* intestine *Outcome:* active transport of dietary Ca^+ across intestinal membranes
Atrial natriuretic hormone	Peptide	*Source:* atrium of heart *Stimulus:* atrial stretching	*Target:* kidneys *Outcome:* inhibits Na^+ reabsorption and renin release *Target:* adrenal cortex *Outcome:* inhibits secretion of aldosterone

[a]The kidneys release an enzyme that modifies a circulating blood protein to produce erythropoietin.

3. Activates inactive enzyme forms, increasing the total amount of active enzyme

In addition to altering enzyme activity, hormones either facilitate or inhibit uptake of substances by cells. Insulin, for example, facilitates glucose transport into the cell by combining with extracellular glucose and a glucose carrier within the plasma membrane. In contrast, epinephrine inhibits insulin release, slowing cellular glucose uptake.

Hormone action can exert potent although often indirect secondary effects. For instance, insulin release increases glucose uptake by muscle fibers (primary effect), which in turn increases muscle glycogen synthesis (secondary effect). This effect of insulin on glucose uptake and glycogen synthesis maintains fuel homeostasis during physical activity. In insulin-deficient individuals, depressed glucose metabolism impairs exercise performance. Inadequate cellular glucose uptake from chronic insulin deficiency abnormally increases blood glucose concentrations. In the extreme, glucose spills into the urine. We discuss the conditions of insulin insufficiency and/or insulin resistance in more detail later in this chapter.

Factors That Determine Hormone Levels

Hormone secretion rarely occurs at a constant rate. As with nervous system activity, hormone secretion usually adjusts rapidly to meet the demands of changing bodily conditions. For this reason, all protein hormones secrete in a pulsatile manner (see next section). Four factors determine plasma concentration of a particular hormone:

1. Quantity synthesized in the host gland
2. Rate of either catabolism or secretion into the blood
3. Quantity of transport proteins present (for some hormones)
4. Plasma volume changes

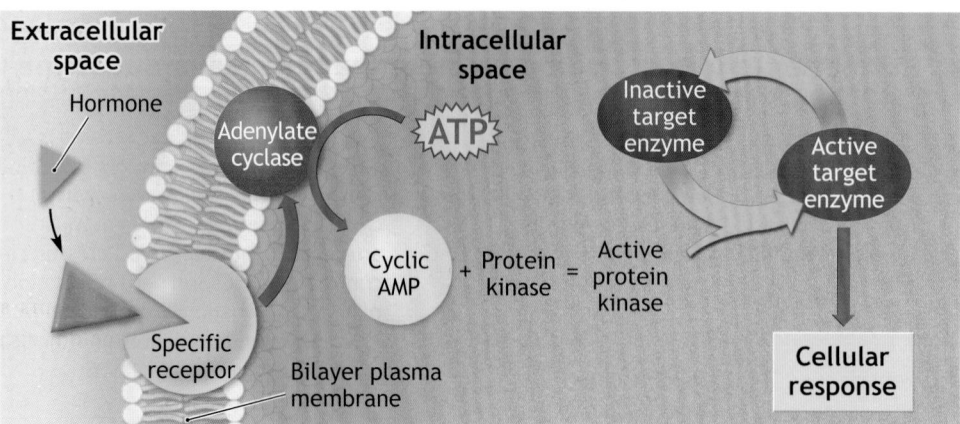

FIGURE 20.3 • Action of nonsteroid hormones. Circulating hormone (*first messenger*) binds to a specific receptor in the cell's plasma membrane to trigger production of cyclic AMP from ATP catalyzed by adenylate cyclase. Cyclic AMP then acts as second messenger to activate a protein kinase within the cell. This in turn activates an active target enzyme to elicit the cellular response.

Important Discoveries in Endocrinology

Though knowledge of the existence of exocrine and endocrine glands dates at least back to Galen's time (see "Exercise Physiology: Roots and Historical Perspectives," before Chapter 1), trying to understand their function began during the Renaissance. The function of the ductless glands remained a mystery until several investigators demonstrated that glandular extracts cured a variety of maladies; hypothyroidism, first treated with thyroid extract in 1891; Addison's disease (adrenocortical deficiency), first treated with adrenal extract in 1896; and diabetes mellitus (insulin deficiency), first treated successfully in 1922 with pancreatic extract. Other notable landmark discoveries in endocrinology include:

• Endocrine surgery most likely begins with the work of Swiss surgeon Emil Theodor Kocher (1841–1917; **www.nobelprize.org/nobel_prizes/medicine/laureates/1909/kocher-bio.html**) who pioneered pathology and surgical work on the thyroid gland, earning the 1909 Nobel Prize in Physiology or Medicine.
• 1893: English physicians George Oliver (1841–1915) and Edward Albert Schäfer (1850–1935) discovered that an extract from the adrenal gland medulla, when injected into the bloodstream, immediately raised an animal's blood pressure (**http://isccb12.webs.ull.es/ChromaffinCell/History.html**). Schäfer also proposed an active substance in the pancreas' islets of Langerhans he named *insulin*, almost a decade before its formal discovery.
• 1915: Walter Bradford Cannon (1871–1945; **http://hms.harvard.edu/departments/medical-education/student-services/academic-societies-hms/walter-bradford-cannon-society/walter-bradford-cannon**) uses the term *fight-or-flight response* to describe the mammalian reaction to physical threats.
• 1922: Two recipients of the 1923 Nobel Prize in Physiology or Medicine for their co-discovery of insulin, Sir Frederick Grant Banting and John James Rickard Macleod (1891–1941), were first to isolate insulin from canine (dog) and bovine (cow) pancreas (**www.nobelprize.org/nobel_prizes/medicine/laureates/1923/**).

• 1936: Hungarian endocrinologist Hans Hugo Bruno Selye (1907-1982; **www.princeton.edu/~achaney/tmve/wiki100k/docs/Hans_Selye.html**) builds upon Cannon's work and describes progression of the stress responses, now known as general adaptation syndrome (GAS). He posited that hormonal events underlying the stress response originate in the brain, and then involve the pituitary and adrenal glands in cascade fashion. Selye referred to this as the *hypothalamic–pituitary–adrenal axis*, a term still in use.
• 1934–1949: American chemist Edward Calvin Kendall (1886-1972), Polish-born Swiss chemist Tadeus Reichstein (1897–1996), and Philip Showalter Hench (1896–1965), winners of the 1950 Nobel Prize in Physiology or Medicine, isolate several steroid hormones from the adrenal cortex (**www.nobelprize.org/nobel_prizes/medicine/laureates/1950/kendall-facts.html**).
• 1952: American physician and physiologist Charles Brenton Huggins (1901–1997; 1966 Nobel Prize in Physiology or Medicine; **www.nobelprize.org/nobel_prizes/medicine/laureates/1966/huggins-bio.html**) discovers that hormones support the growth of certain cancers, and that surgical removal of the source of the hormones led to cancer regression.
• 1956–1971: French neurologist Roger Charles Louis Guillemin (1924–) and American endocrinologist Andrew Victor Schally (1926–; 1977 Nobel Prize in Physiology or Medicine, also shared with Rosalyn Yalow [1921–2011], for development of the radioimmunoassay technique) painstakingly isolate the brain's peptide hormones (**www.nobelprize.org/nobel_prizes/medicine/laureates/1977/guillemin-bio.html**). These small proteins, present in exceedingly tiny quantities, form the basis of the hypothalamic–pituitary–adrenal axis and other hormonal cascades and provide the link between consciousness and endocrine physiology.

Sources:
Welbourn RB, et al. *The History of Endocrine Surgery*. New York: Praeger, 1990.
Review: The history of endocrine surgery. *Ann Intern Med* 1991; 114:918.

Hormone secretion rate depends on the magnitude of chemical stimulatory or inhibitory input from more than one source. Insulin secretion from the pancreas, for example, responds directly to plasma changes in glucose and amino acids, norepinephrine (from sympathetic neurons) and circulating epinephrine, and acetylcholine released from parasympathetic neurons. Each of these chemical messengers supplies inhibitory or excitatory input that determines whether insulin secretion increases or decreases. Over an extended time, which differs for each hormone, hormone synthesis tends to equal hormone release. For a relatively short duration, however, hormone release can exceed its synthesis. The term **secreted amount** describes the plasma concentration of a hormone. In reality, this represents the sum of hormone synthesis and release by the host gland, in addition to its uptake by receptor tissues and removal by liver and kidneys.

Hormone concentration depends on its rate of secretion into the blood and/or the rate of its metabolism (i.e., it becomes inactive). Hormone inactivation takes place at or near receptors or in the liver or kidneys. Because blood flow to splanchnic and renal areas decreases during physical activity (blood distributes to active muscle), hormone inactivation rate decreases and plasma hormone concentration rises.

Changes in plasma volume also alter hormone concentrations, independent of the host organ's secretion rate. For example, decreased plasma volume during prolonged activity concurrently increases plasma hormone concentration, even without an absolute change in hormone amount.

FIGURE 20.4 shows how three factors—hormonal, humoral, and neural—stimulate endocrine activity for the pituitary, pancreas, and adrenal glands.

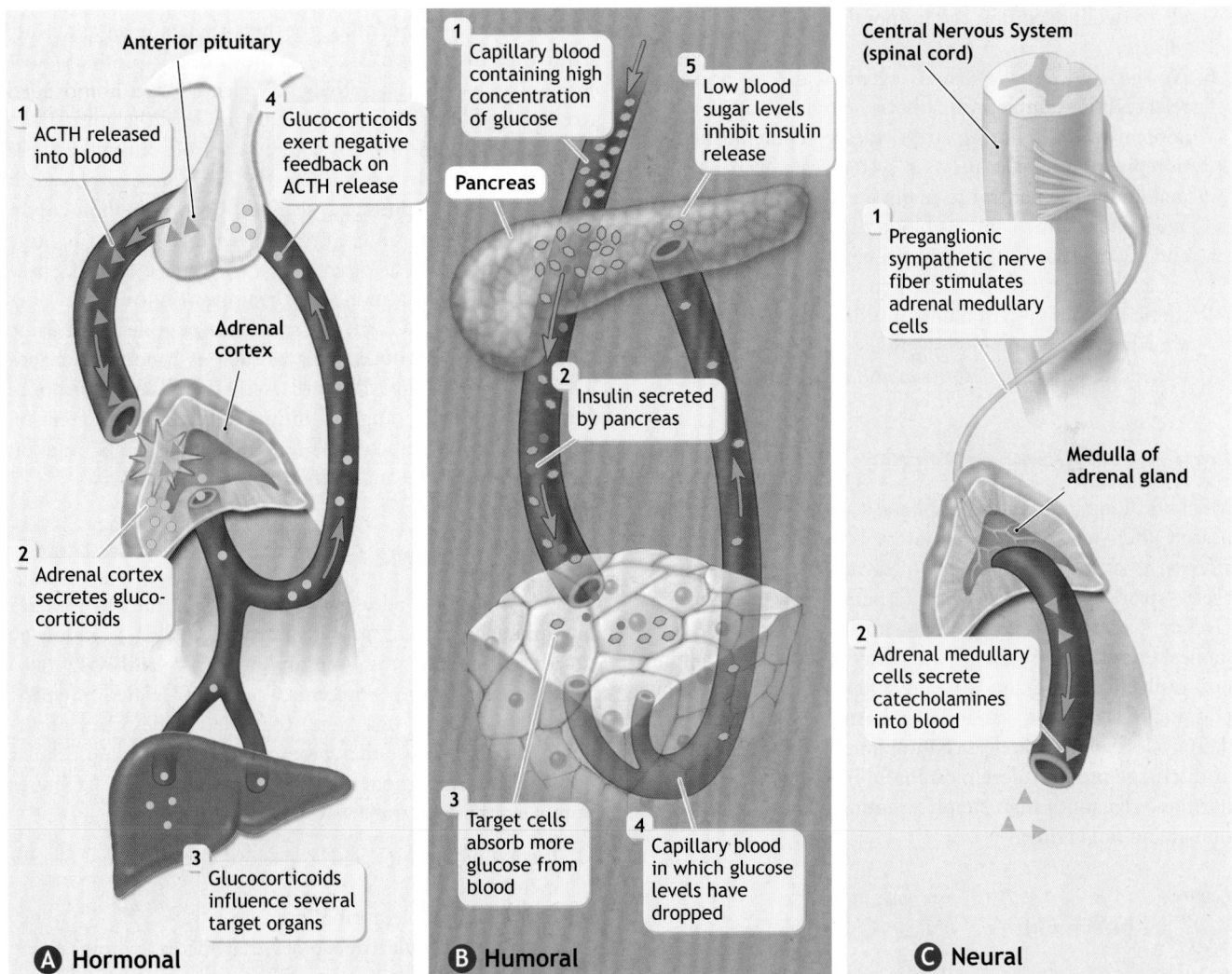

FIGURE 20.4 • Endocrine gland stimulation. **(A)** *Hormonal.* Adrenocorticotropic hormone (ACTH) stimulates release of glucocorticoid hormones by the adrenal cortex. **(B)** *Humoral.* High blood glucose concentrations trigger insulin release, causing rapid cellular glucose uptake. The subsequent decrease in blood glucose removes the stimulus for insulin release. **(C)** *Neural.* Sympathetic nervous system fibers trigger catecholamine release to blood. (Reprinted with permission from Marieb E, Hoehn K. *Human Anatomy and Physiology.* 7th Ed. Redwood City, CA: Benjamin/Cummings, 2007.)

1. *Hormonal stimulation.* Hormones influence secretion of other hormones. For example, release-inhibiting hormones produced by the hypothalamus regulate the secretion of most anterior pituitary hormones. Anterior pituitary hormones, in turn, stimulate other endocrine organs to release their hormones into the bloodstream. The increased blood levels of a hormone produced by the final target gland provide feedback to *inhibit* release of anterior pituitary hormones and ultimately their own release.

2. *Humoral stimulation.* Changing levels of ions and nutrients transported in blood, bile, and other body fluids stimulate hormone release. The term *humoral stimuli* describes these chemicals to distinguish them from bloodborne hormonal stimuli, which also are fluid-borne chemicals. For example, an increase in blood sugar concentration, which acts as the humoral agent, prompts the pancreas to release insulin. Insulin promotes glucose entry into cells, causing blood sugar levels to decline, ending the humoral stimulus for insulin release.

3. *Neural stimulation.* Neural activity affects hormone release. For example, sympathetic neural activation of the adrenal medulla during stress releases epinephrine and norepinephrine. The nervous system can override normal endocrine control to maintain homeostasis. Insulin action normally maintains blood sugar levels between 80 and 120 mg per 100 mL or 1 dL of blood. During physical activity, activation of the hypothalamus and sympathetic nervous system blunts insulin release to attenuate a further decline in blood sugar and ensure sufficient carbohydrate to fuel neural tissue and active muscle.

Patterns of Hormone Release

Most hormones respond to peripheral stimuli on an as-needed basis. Others release at regular intervals during a 24-hr cycle referred to as a **diurnal pattern** of secretion. Some secretory cycles span several weeks while others follow daily cycles. Cycling patterns are not confined to one category of hormones. Pulsatile hormone release patterns reveal information not available from a single blood sample that fails to show potentially significant variation in hormone levels during a daily cycle. Patterns of release and/or amplitude and frequency of discharge provide more meaningful information regarding hormone dynamics than simply examining mean concentration at any single time.

 **INTEGRATIVE QUESTION**

Explain the meaning of the following statement: Hormones act as silent messengers to integrate the body as a unit.

RESTING AND EXERCISE-INDUCED ENDOCRINE SECRETIONS

TABLE 20.3 lists the different endocrine host organs and nonglandular endocrine tissues, specific hormones secreted, hormone targets, and main effects. The following sections review these hormones, with special emphasis on their immediate response to exertion and adaptations to physical training.

Anterior Pituitary Hormones

FIGURE 20.5 illustrates the pituitary gland (also called the **hypophysis**), its secretions, and various target glands and their specialized hormone secretions. Located beneath the base of the brain, the pituitary secretes at least six specialized polypeptide hormones. Because of its widespread influence, the anterior pituitary gland was often called the *master gland.* Researchers now know that the hypothalamus controls anterior pituitary activity; thus, the hypothalamus should truly claim that distinction. Each of the primary pituitary hormones has its own hypothalamic-releasing hormone called a **releasing factor**. Neural input to the hypothalamus from anxiety, stress, and physical activity controls output of these releasing factors. In addition to the hormones displayed in Figure 20.5, the pituitary secretes **proopiomelanocortin (POMC;** www.eje-online.org/content/149/2/79**)**, a large precursor molecule of other active molecules. POMC provides the source of a number of neurotransmitters and hormones including ACTH, melanocortin peptides, and some of the naturally produced opiates such as β-endorphin (see "Opioid Peptides and Physical Activity"). These hormones exert a remarkable range of influence, including effects on pigmentation, adrenocortical function, food intake and fat storage, and nervous and immune system functions.

Growth Hormone

Growth hormone–releasing factor from the hypothalamus influences resting **growth hormone (GH)** secretion by directly stimulating the anterior pituitary gland. GH (also called **somatotropin**) represents a family of related polypeptides (derived from one gene) that exert widespread physiologic activity because they promote cell division and cellular proliferation throughout the body. In adults, GH facilitates protein synthesis in three ways:

1. Increasing amino acid transport through the plasma membrane
2. Stimulating RNA formation
3. Activating cellular ribosomes that increase protein synthesis

GH also slows carbohydrate breakdown and initiates subsequent mobilization and use of fat as an energy source.

TABLE 20.3 Endocrine Organs and Their Secretions, Targets, and Main Effects

Location	Gland or Cells	Chemical Type	Hormone	Target	Main Effect
Adipose tissue	Cells	Peptide	Leptin; adiponectin (resistin)	Hypothalamus, other tissues	Food intake, metabolism, reproduction
Adrenal cortex	Gland	Steroid	Mineralocorticoids (aldosterone)	Kidney	Stimulates Na^+ reabsorption and K^+ secretion
			Glucocorticoids (cortisol; corticosterone)	Many tissues	Promotes protein and fat catabolism; raises blood glucose levels; adapts body to stress
			Androgens (androstenedione; dehydroepiandro-sterone [DHEA]; estrone)	Many tissues	Promotes sex drive
Adrenal medulla	Gland	Amine	Epinephrine, norepinephrine	Many tissues	Facilitates sympathetic activity; increases cardiac output; regulates blood vessels; increases glycogen catabolism and fatty acid release
Gastrointestinal tract (stomach and small intestine)	Cells	Peptide	Gastrin; cholecystokinin (CCK); secretin; glucose-dependent insulinotropic peptide (GIP)	GI tract and pancreas	Assists digestion and absorption of nutrients; regulates gastrointestinal motility
Heart	Cells	Peptide	Atrial natriuretic peptide (ANP)	Kidney tubules	Inhibits sodium reabsorption
Hypothalamus	Clusters of neurons	Peptide	Trophic hormones (releasing and release-inhibiting hormones: corticotropin-releasing hormone [CRH]; thyrotropin-releasing hormone [TRH]; growth hormone-releasing hormone [GHRH]; gonadotropin-releasing hormone [GnRH])	Anterior pituitary	Releases or inhibits anterior pituitary hormones
Kidney	Cells	Peptide Steroid	Erythropoietin (EPO) 1,25 dihydroxy- vitamin D_3(calciferol)	Bone marrow Intestine	Red blood cell production Increases calcium absorption
Liver	Cells	Peptide	Angiotensinogen	Adrenal cortex, blood vessels, brain	Aldosterone secretion; increases blood pressure
			Insulin-like growth factors (IGF-1)	Many tissues	Growth
Muscle	Cells	Peptide	Insulin-like growth factors (IGF-1, IGF-II); myogenic regulatory factors (MRFs)	Many tissues	Growth
Pancreas	Gland	Peptide	Insulin	Many tissues	Lowers blood glucose levels; promotes protein, lipid, and glycogen synthesis
			Glucagon	Many tissues	Raises blood glucose levels; promotes glycogenolysis and gluconeogenesis
			Somatostatin (SS)	Many tissues	Inhibits secretion of pancreatic hormones; regulates digestion and absorption of nutrients by GI system

(Continued)

TABLE 20.3 Endocrine Organs and Their Secretions, Targets, and Main Effects *(Continued)*

Location	Gland or Cells	Chemical Type	Hormone	Target	Main Effect
Parathyroid	Gland	Peptide	Parathyroid hormone (PTH)	Bone, kidney	Promotes Ca^{2+} release from bone, Ca^{2+} absorption by intestine, and Ca^+ reabsorption by kidney; raises blood Ca^{2+} levels; stimulates vitamin D_3 synthesis
Pineal gland	Gland	Amine	Melatonin	Unknown	Controls circadian rhythms
Pituitary-anterior	Gland	Peptides	Growth hormone (GH)	Many tissues	Growth; stimulates bone and soft tissue growth; regulates protein, lipid, and CHO metabolism
			Adrenocorticotropic hormone (ACTH)	Adrenal cortex	Stimulates glucocorticoid secretion
			Thyroid-stimulating hormone (TSH)	Thyroid gland	Stimulates secretion of thyroid hormones
			Prolactin	Breast	Milk secretion
			Follicle-stimulating hormone (FSH)	Gonads	*Females:* stimulates growth and development of ovarian follicles and estrogen secretion; *Males:* sperm production by testis
			Luteinizing hormone (LH)	Gonads	*Females:* stimulates ovulation, secretion of estrogen and progesterone; *Males:* testosterone secretion by testis
Pituitary-posterior	Extension of hypothalamic neurons	Peptide	Oxytocin (OT)	Breast and uterus	*Females:* stimulates uterine contractions and milk ejection by mammary glands; *Males:* unknown function
			Antidiuretic hormone (ADH or vasopressin)	Kidney	Decreases urine output by kidneys; promotes blood vessel (arteriole) constriction
Placenta (pregnant female)	Gland	Steroid	Estrogens and progesterone	Many tissues	Fetal and maternal development
		Peptide	Chorionic somatomammotropin (CS)		Metabolism
			Chorionic gonadotropin (CG)		Hormone secretion
Skin	Cells	Steroid	Vitamin D_3	Intermediate hormone form	Precursor of 1,25 dihydroxy-vitamin D_3
Ovaries (female)	Glands	Steroid	Estrogens (estradiol)	Many tissues	Egg production; secondary sex characteristics
			Progestins (progesterone)	Uterus	Promotes endometrial growth to prepare uterus for pregnancy
		Peptide	Ovarian inhibin	Anterior pituitary	Inhibits FSH secretion
Testes (male)	Glands	Steroid	Androgen	Many tissues	Sperm production; secondary sex characteristics
		Peptide	Inhibin	Anterior pituitary	Inhibits FSH secretion
Thymus	Gland	Peptide	Thymosin, thymopoietin	Lymphocytes	Stimulates proliferation and function of T lymphocytes
Thyroid	Gland	Iodinated amines	Triiodothyronine (T_3); thyroxine (T_4)	Many tissues	Increases metabolic rate; normal physical development
		Peptide	Calcitonin (CT)	Bone	Promotes calcium deposition in bone; lowers blood calcium levels

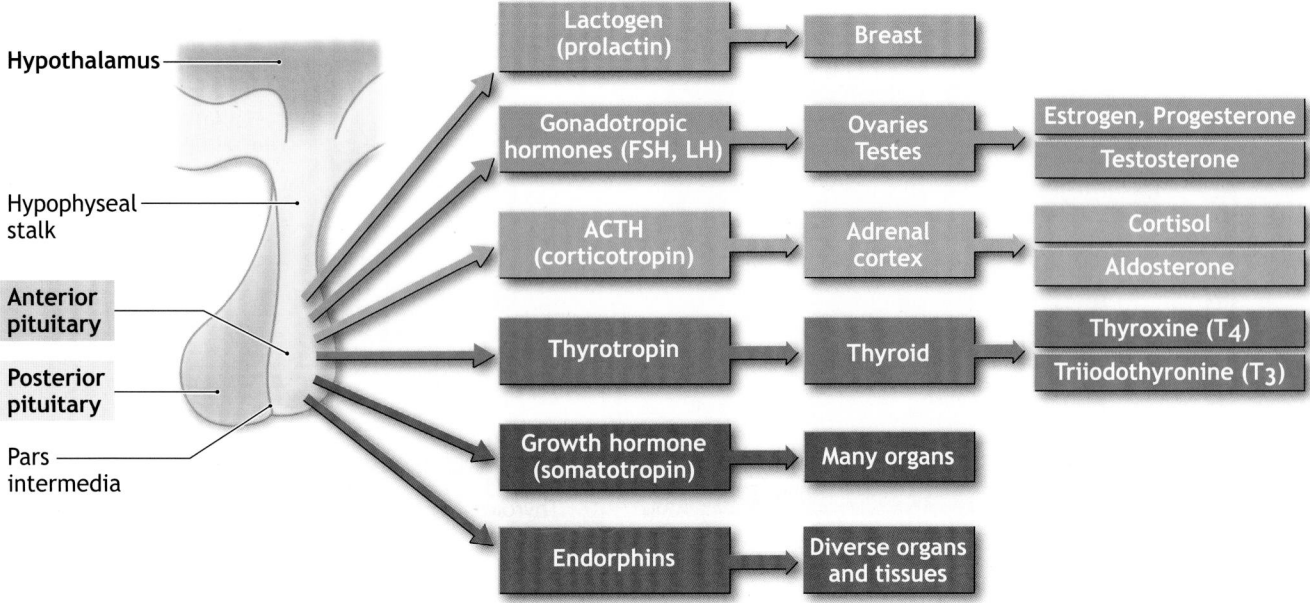

FIGURE 20.5 • The pituitary gland, its secretions, and targets.

Growth Hormone, Physical Activity, and Tissue Synthesis. Increased physical activity of relatively short duration stimulates a sharp rise in GH pulse amplitude and the amount of hormone secreted per pulse.[13,89,194] Perhaps more importantly, physical activity stimulates release of GH isoforms with extended half-lives, thereby extending GH's action on target tissues.[138] Augmented GH release benefits muscle, bone, and connective tissue growth and remodeling. It also optimizes the fuel mixture during physical activity, principally decreasing tissue glucose uptake, increasing free fatty acid mobilization, and enhancing liver gluconeogenesis. The net metabolic effect of increased exercise-induced GH production preserves plasma glucose concentration for central nervous system and muscle functions. Many of the growth-promoting effects of GH result from actions of intermediary chemical messengers on different target tissues, rather than a direct effect of GH itself. These peptide messengers, produced in the liver, are termed somatomedins, or **insulin-like growth factors (IGF-1 and IGF-II;** see next section) because of their structural similarity to insulin. These factors exert potent peripheral effects on motor units and other tissues.

How physical activity stimulates GH release to augment protein synthesis (and subsequent muscle hypertrophy), cartilage formation, skeletal growth, and cell proliferation remains unclear, although the total integrated growth hormone concentration increases with physical activity duration in men and women.[195] Concurrent measurements of circulating lactate, alanine, and pyruvate; blood glucose; and body temperature reveal no association with GH secretory patterns during exercise.[90] One hypothesis suggests that physical activity directly stimulates GH release (or release of somatomedins from the liver or kidneys), which in turn stimulates anabolic processes. Activity also may indirectly affect GH by stimulating cholinergic pathways to trigger GH release. Physical activity stimulates endogenous opiate production that facilitates GH release by inhibiting the liver's production of somatostatin, a hormone that blunts GH release.[189]

FIGURE 20.6 outlines the overall schema for GH's various direct and indirect metabolic actions; it modulates by feedback control the metabolic mixture during physical activity by stimulating fatty acid release from adipose tissue while simultaneously inhibiting cellular glucose uptake. This glucose-sparing action maintains blood glucose at relatively high levels to augment prolonged exercise performance.

Trained and sedentary individuals show similar increases in GH concentration with exercise to exhaustion. In contrast, the sedentary person maintains higher GH levels for several hours into recovery. During a standard bout of submaximal exertion, sedentary individuals have a greater GH response. The absolute submaximal activity level represents greater stress for the less fit person, allowing GH release to relate more to the *relative* strenuousness of physical effort.

Insulin-Like Growth Factors

IGFs (somatomedins) mediate many of GH's effects. In response to GH stimulation, liver cells synthesize IGF-I and IGF-II, a process that requires between 8 and 30 hr. IGFs travel in the blood attached to one of five types of binding proteins for release as free hormones to interact with specific receptors. The factors that influence IGF transport include binding proteins within muscle, nutritional status, and plasma insulin levels.

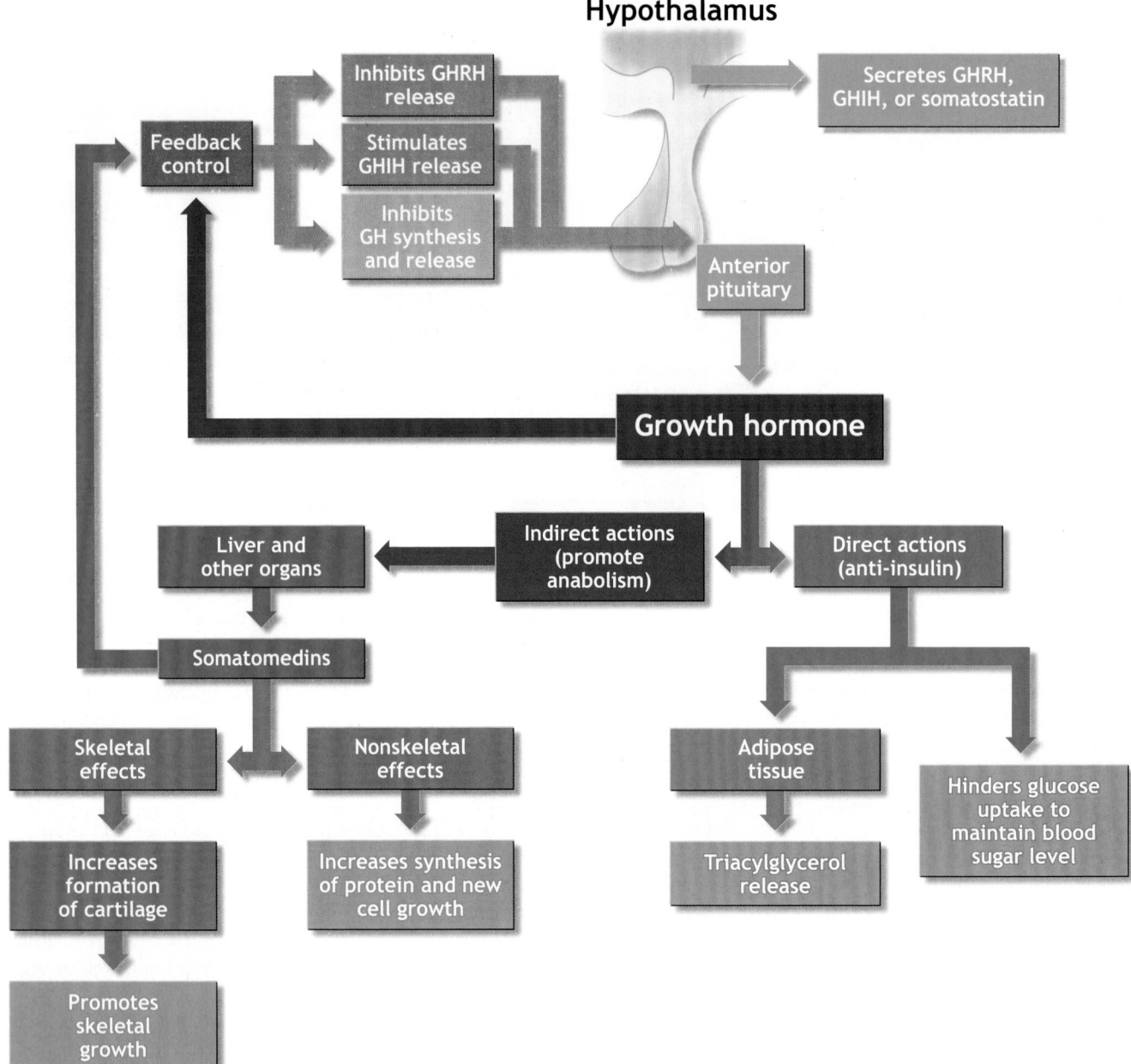

FIGURE 20.6 • Overview of growth hormone (GH) actions. GH stimulates breakdown and release of triacylglycerols from adipose tissue and hinders cellular glucose uptake (anti-insulin effect) to maintain a relatively high blood glucose level. Somatomedins mediate the indirect anabolic effects of GH. Elevated GH levels and somatomedins provide feedback to promote GH-inhibiting hormone (GHIH) release and depress hypothalamic release of GH-releasing hormone (GHRH); this further inhibits GH release by the anterior pituitary gland (**www.vivo.colostate.edu/hbooks/pathphys/endocrine/hypopit/gh.html**).

Thyrotropin

Thyrotropin, also known as **thyroid-stimulating hormone (TSH)**, controls hormone secretion by the thyroid gland. TSH maintains growth and development of the thyroid gland and increases thyroid cell metabolism. Considering the important role of thyroid hormones in regulating overall body metabolism, one would expect TSH output from the pituitary to increase during physical activity, but this response does not occur consistently.

Adrenocorticotropic Hormone

ACTH, also known as **corticotropin**, functions as part of the **hypothalamic–pituitary–adrenal axis** that regulates adrenal cortex output of hormones in a manner similar to TSH control of thyroid gland secretion. ACTH acts directly to enhance fatty acid mobilization from adipose tissue, increase gluconeogenesis, and stimulate protein catabolism. Owing to difficulty in assay methods and rapid disappearance of this hormone from the blood, data remain scarce concerning ACTH response during physical activity.[93]

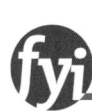

Elevated Thyroid Hormones Predict Metabolic Syndrome in Females

The existence of an association between thyrotropin (thyroid-stimulating hormone [TSH]) levels and metabolic syndrome in euthyroid subjects was confirmed in 2760 euthyroid young female volunteers (ages 18 to 39 y) with TSH levels in the normal range (0.3 to 4.5 mU·L⁻¹). The prevalence of metabolic syndrome (increased central obesity, hypertriglyceridemia, elevated systolic and diastolic blood pressure) was twofold greater in a subjects with higher levels of TSH (>2.5 mU·L⁻¹) compared to a counterparts with a TSH <2.5 mU·L⁻¹. Healthy young women with TSH levels > 2.5 mU·L⁻¹ should be assessed for the presence of metabolic syndrome, even if their TSH levels are within normal range.

Source: Oh JY, et al. Elevated thyroid stimulating hormone levels are associated with metabolic syndrome in euthyroid young women. *Korean J Intern Med* 2013;28:180.

ACTH concentrations may increase proportionately with intensity and duration of effort if intensity exceeds 25% of aerobic capacity.[42] Corticotropin-releasing hormone (CRH) and arginine vasopressin (AVP) mediate ACTH release. CRH exhibits a definite diurnal rhythm, with highest levels in early morning just after rising. As the day progresses, CRH levels decline, essentially blocking ACTH release. Factors that alter the normal ACTH rhythm by triggering CRH release include fever, hypoglycemia, and other stressors. CRH is both an ACTH regulator and a central nervous system neurotransmitter, and is often termed the *stress response integrator*. High-intensity physical activity favors AVP release while prolonged physical activity favors CRH release, both inhibiting ACTH.[78]

Prolactin

Prolactin (PRL) initiates and supports milk secretion from the mammary glands. PRL levels increase at high activity intensities and return toward baseline within 45 min during recovery. Owing to its important role in female sexual function, repeated exercise-induced PRL release may inhibit ovarian function and contribute to menstrual cycle alterations when females train intensely. Greater increases in PRL occur in women who run without wearing an undergarment support;[146] either fasting or consuming a high-fat diet enhances release of this hormone.[85] PRL concentration also increases in men following maximal physical effort.[30]

Gonadotropic Hormones

Gonadotropic hormones stimulate the male and female sex organs to grow and secrete their hormones at a faster rate.

The two gonadotropic hormones are **follicle-stimulating hormone (FSH)** and **luteinizing hormone (LH)**. FSH initiates follicle growth in the ovaries and stimulates these organs to secrete estrogen, one type of female sex hormone. LH complements FSH action to cause estrogen secretion and rupture of the follicle, which allows the ovum to pass through the fallopian tube for fertilization. In the male, FSH stimulates germinal epithelium growth in the testes to promote sperm development. LH also stimulates the testes to secrete testosterone.

Inconsistent reports describe short-term exercise-associated alterations in FSH and LH. LH release is normally pulsatile, making it difficult to separate any specific exercise-related change from the normal pulsatile pattern. Generally, LH concentration rises before movement begins and peaks during recovery.

Posterior Pituitary Hormones

The posterior pituitary gland forms as an outgrowth of the hypothalamus and resembles true neural tissue (see Fig. 20.5). This tissue, often called the **neurohypophysis**, stores **antidiuretic hormone (ADH, or vasopressin)** and **oxytocin**. The posterior pituitary does not synthesize its hormones. Instead, the hypothalamus produces these hormones and secretes them to the neurohypophysis for release as needed via neural stimulation. Damage or surgical removal of the posterior pituitary does not dramatically affect ADH or oxytocin production.

ADH influences water excretion by the kidneys. Its action limits production of large volumes of urine by stimulating water reabsorption in the kidney tubules. Oxytocin initiates muscle contraction in the uterus and stimulates ejection of milk during lactation.

Physical activity provides a potent stimulus for ADH secretion. Increased ADH release, probably stimulated by sweating, helps to conserve body fluids during hot-weather physical activity and accompanying dehydration. This water-conserving effect of ADH contributes to efficient modulation of the cardiovascular response to physical activity.[119] ADH release decreases with fluid overload to increase urine volume and produce more dilute urine (i.e., lighter-color urine). The effect of short-term physical activity on oxytocin release remains unknown.

Thyroid Hormones

The 15- to 20-g reddish brown thyroid gland, located nearer the first part of the trachea just below the larynx, comes under the influence of TSH produced by the anterior pituitary gland. In addition to secreting the calcium-regulating hormone **calcitonin**, the thyroid gland secretes two protein-iodine–bound hormones, **thyroxine (T_4)** and **triiodothyronine (T_3, the active form of thyroid hormone). These two hormones are often referred to as *major metabolic hormones*. More T_4 is secreted than T_3; although less abundant, T_3 acts several times faster than T_4. The majority of T_3 comes from the deiodination of T_4 in peripheral tissues, principally liver and kidney. Most receptor cells for T_4 metabolize it to T_3. T_3 and T_4 are not readily soluble in water, which means they bind to carrier proteins that circulate in blood. Thyroxine-binding globulin (glycoprotein synthesized in the liver) serves as the main transporter of thyroid hormones. This carrier protein (along with two others—transthyretin and albumin) permits a more consistent availability of thyroid hormones from which the active, free hormones release for target cell uptake.

Through its stimulating effect on enzyme activity, T_4 secretion raises metabolism of all cells except in the brain, spleen, testes, uterus, and thyroid gland itself. For example, abnormally high T_4 secretion raises basal metabolic rate (BMR) up to fourfold. This potent thermogenic effect produces large BMR deviations that often indicate thyroid gland abnormality (see Chapter 9). A person may lose weight rapidly with abnormally high thyroid activity. In contrast, depressed thyroid production blunts BMR, which usually leads to gains in body weight and body fat. *Fewer than 3% of obese persons show abnormal thyroid functions, so depressed thyroid activity cannot explain excessive body fat gain in most individuals.* For nervous system function, T_3 release facilitates neural reflex activity, whereas low T_4 levels cause sluggishness, often inducing people to sleep for up to 15 hr a day. Thyroid hormones provide important regulation for tissue growth and development, skeletal and nervous system formation, and maturation and reproduction. They also play a role in maintaining blood pressure by provoking an increase in adrenergic receptors in blood vessels.

Whole-body metabolism influences synthesis of thyroid hormones. Depressing the metabolic rate to some critical value directly stimulates hypothalamic release of TSH. This increases thyroid output and increases resting metabolism. Conversely, a chronic elevation in metabolism reduces TSH production, causing metabolism to slow. **Figure 20.7** illustrates this exquisitely regulated feedback system.

During physical activity, blood levels of *free T_4* (thyroxine not bound to plasma proteins) increase by approximately 35%. This increase could occur from an exercise-induced elevation in core temperature, which alters the protein binding of several hormones, including T_4. The importance of these transient exercise-induced alterations in thyroid hormone dynamics requires further study.

Thyroid Hormones Affect Quality of Life

Thyroid hormones are not essential for life but they do affect life's quality. In children, full expression of growth hormone requires thyroid activity. Thyroid hormones provide essential stimulation for normal growth and development, especially of nervous tissue. The actions of thyroid hormones become most noticeable in people who suffer from either hypersecretion or hyposecretion.

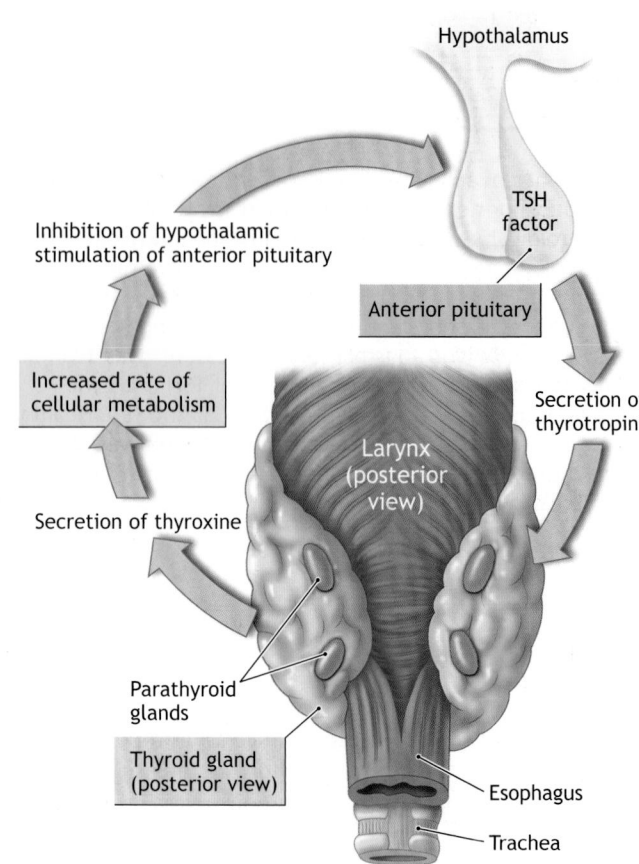

FIGURE 20.7 • Feedback system that controls thyroid hormone release.

Hypersecretion of thyroid hormones (**hyperthyroidism**) produces the following four effects:

1. Increased oxygen consumption and metabolic heat production during rest (heat intolerance is a common complaint)
2. Increased protein catabolism and subsequent muscle weakness and weight loss
3. Heightened reflex activity and psychological disturbances that range from irritability and insomnia to psychosis
4. Rapid heart rate (tachycardia)

Hyposecretion of thyroid hormones (**hypothyroidism**) produces the following four effects:

1. Reduced metabolic rate and cold intolerance from reduced internal heat production
2. Decreased protein synthesis produces brittle nails, thinning hair, and dry, thin skin
3. Depressed reflex activity, slow speech and thought processes, and feeling of fatigue (in infancy causes cretinism, marked by decreased mental capacity)
4. Slow heart rate (bradycardia)

Parathyroid Hormones

Four parathyroid glands, measuring 6-mm long, 4-mm wide, and 2-mm deep are embedded in the posterior aspect of the thyroid gland (see Fig. 20.7). As many as eight glands have been reported in some people, and glands have been found in other regions of the neck or in the thorax. **Parathyroid hormone** (**PTH**, or parathormone) controls blood calcium balance. A decrease in blood calcium levels triggers PTH release; increasing calcium concentrations inhibit its release. PTH's major effect increases ionic calcium levels by stimulating three target organs—bone, kidneys, and small intestine.

PTH release produces the following three effects:

1. Activation of bone-reabsorbing cells called osteoclasts digest some of the bone matrix to release ionic calcium and phosphate to the blood
2. Enhancement of calcium ion reabsorption and decreased retention of phosphate by the kidneys
3. Increased calcium absorption by intestinal mucosa

Plasma calcium ion homeostasis modulates nerve impulse conduction, muscle contraction, and blood clotting. Limited evidence suggests that physical activity increases PTH release in young, middle-age, and older individuals, an effect that contributes to the positive effects of mechanical forces from physical activity on bone mass accretion.[7,16,101]

Adrenal Hormones

The adrenal glands appear as flattened, caplike tissues situated just above each kidney (FIG. 20.8). The glands have two distinct parts: medulla (inner portion that secretes the catecholamines) and cortex (outer portion that secretes the mineralocorticoids, glycocorticoids, and androgens). Each part secretes different types of hormones; consequently, these two parts of the adrenal gland are generally considered two distinct glands.

Fatigue in Coronary Artery Disease Patients Associates with Lower Thyroid Axis Hormones and Cortisol Independent of Exercise Capacity

fyi

Coronary patients are encouraged to increase their level of physical activity to improve cardiovascular function. Often they experience extreme fatigue, usually attributable to a low fitness capacity. In a study of 65 men and 18 women with coronary artery disease who attended a rehabilitation program, fatigue and thyroid and adrenal hormones were assessed before and after a symptom-induced bicycle ergometer test. Results showed that lower morning cortisol and lower post-minus-pre-exercise cortisol values associated with fatigue after adjusting for age, gender, BMI, hypertension, previous myocardial infarction, depressive symptoms, and anxiety; lower free T3 concentrations remained associated with physical fatigue. Exercise capacity did not correlate with the endocrine factors.

Source: Bunevicius A, et al. Fatigue in patients with coronary artery disease: association with thyroid axis hormones and cortisol. *Psychosom Med* 2012;74:848.

Adrenal Medulla Hormones

The adrenal medulla makes up part of the sympathetic nervous system. It acts to prolong and augment sympathetic effects by secreting **epinephrine** and **norepinephrine**, hormones collectively called **catecholamines**. FIGURE 20.9 shows the chemical structure of epinephrine and norepinephrine and the role of each in substrate mobilization. Norepinephrine, a hormone in its own right, serves as an epinephrine precursor. It also acts as a neurotransmitter when released by sympathetic nerve endings. *Epinephrine represents 80% of adrenal medulla secretions, whereas norepinephrine provides the principle neurotransmitter released from the sympathetic nervous system.* An outflow of neural impulses from the hypothalamus stimulates the adrenal medulla to increase catecholamine release. These hormones affect the heart, blood

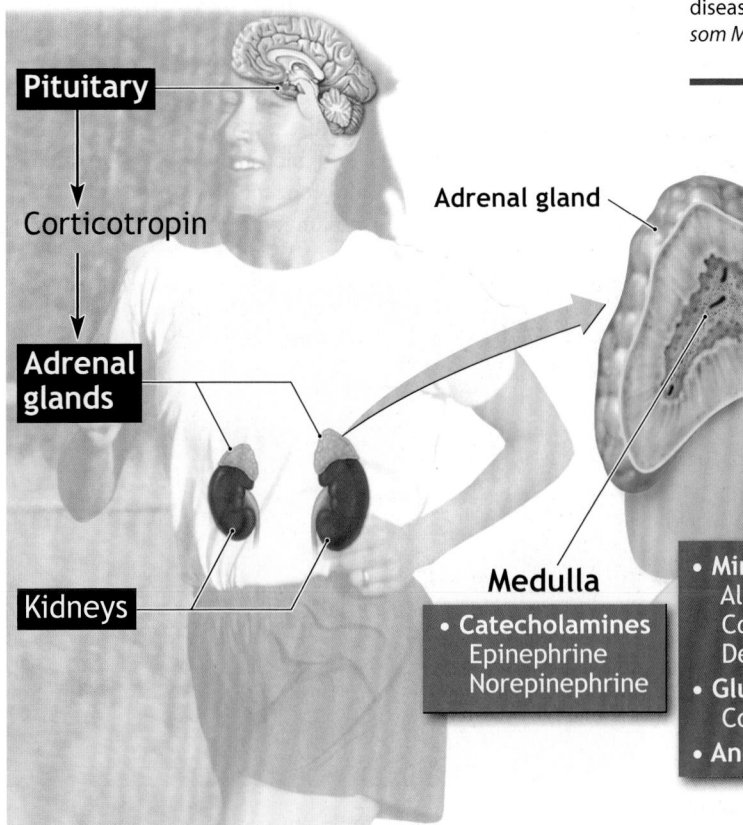

Pituitary
Corticotropin
Adrenal glands
Kidneys

Adrenal gland
Kidney
Cortex
Medulla

- **Catecholamines**
  Epinephrine
  Norepinephrine

- **Mineralocorticoids**
  Aldosterone
  Corticosterone
  Deoxycorticosterone
- **Glucocorticoids**
  Cortisol
- **Androgens**

FIGURE 20.8 • Adrenal gland secretions.

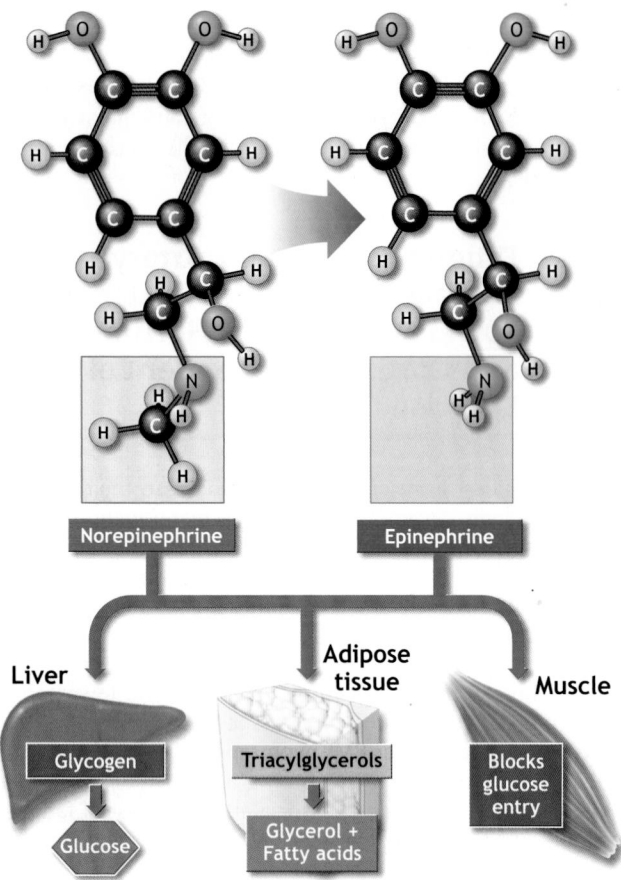

FIGURE 20.9 • Chemical structure of epinephrine and norepinephrine and their role in mobilizing glucose from the liver and free fatty acids from adipose tissue (and blunting glucose uptake by skeletal muscle). Norepinephrine serves as a hormone and as a precursor of epinephrine. It also functions as a neurotransmitter when released by sympathetic nerve endings.

vessels, and glands in the same, albeit slower-acting, way as direct sympathetic nervous system stimulation. Epinephrine's primary function in energy metabolism stimulates glycogenolysis (in the liver and active muscles) and lipolysis (in adipose tissue and active muscles); norepinephrine provides powerful lipolytic stimulation in adipose tissue.[44,120,170] Sympathetic nerve endings (including those to the adrenal gland) secrete both epinephrine and norepinephrine, so it is more appropriate to discuss the "sympathoadrenal" response to physical activity and training rather than the adrenal gland response. *The sympathoadrenal response to physical activity most closely relates to relative rather than absolute activity intensity.*

FIGURE 20.10 illustrates the catecholamine response at various cycling intensities (expressed as $\%\dot{V}O_{2max}$) in 10 male subjects. Norepinephrine increases markedly at intensities that exceed 50% $\dot{V}O_{2max}$, whereas epinephrine levels remain unchanged until cycling intensity exceeds the 75% level. At maximum effort, an approximate two- to sixfold increase in norepinephrine release takes place. More than likely, increased secretion occurs from sympathetic postganglionic nerve endings and relates to cardiovascular and metabolic

adjustments in active tissues. Physical activity also increases epinephrine output from the adrenal medulla, with the magnitude of increase related directly to effort intensity and duration.[26,98,121,171] Athletes involved in sprint–power training show greater sympathoadrenergic activation during maximal exertion than counterparts trained in aerobic activity.[168] This difference relates to the higher anaerobic contribution to maximal energy supply by sprint–power athletes. Age does not affect catecholamine response to physical activity among individuals equal in aerobic fitness.[91,113] The effects of increased adrenal medulla activity on blood flow distribution, cardiac contractility, and substrate mobilization all benefit the physical activity response.

Adrenocortical Hormones

The adrenal cortex, stimulated by corticotropin from the anterior pituitary, secretes adrenocortical hormones. These corticosteroid hormones, each produced in a different zone (layer) of the adrenal cortex, fit functionally into one of three groups:

1. **Mineralocorticoids**
2. **Glucocorticoids**
3. **Androgens**

Mineralocorticoids. As the name suggests, mineralocorticoids regulate the mineral salts sodium and potassium in the extracellular fluid. **Aldosterone**, the most physiologically important of the three mineralocorticoids, represents almost 95% of all mineralocorticoids produced.

FIGURE 20.11 shows four major controlling factors for aldosterone release from the adrenal cortex, ending with an increase in blood volume and blood pressure. Aldosterone secretion controls total sodium concentration and extracellular fluid volume. It stimulates sodium ion reabsorption along with

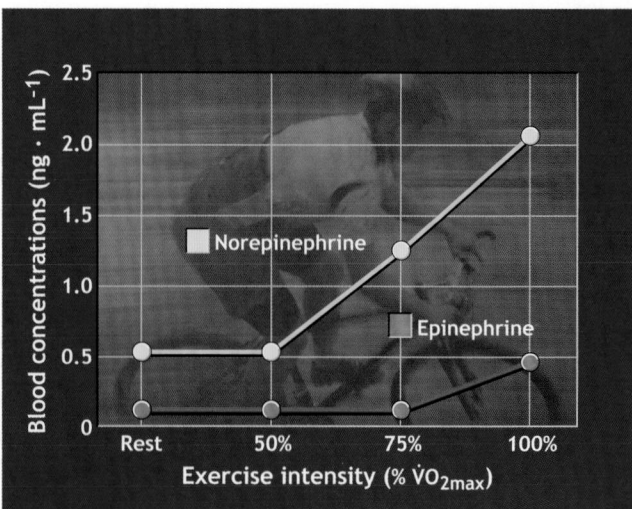

FIGURE 20.10 • Catecholamine response to cycling of increasing intensity in 10 male subjects. (Adapted with permission from Applied Physiology Laboratory, University of Michigan, Ann Arbor.)

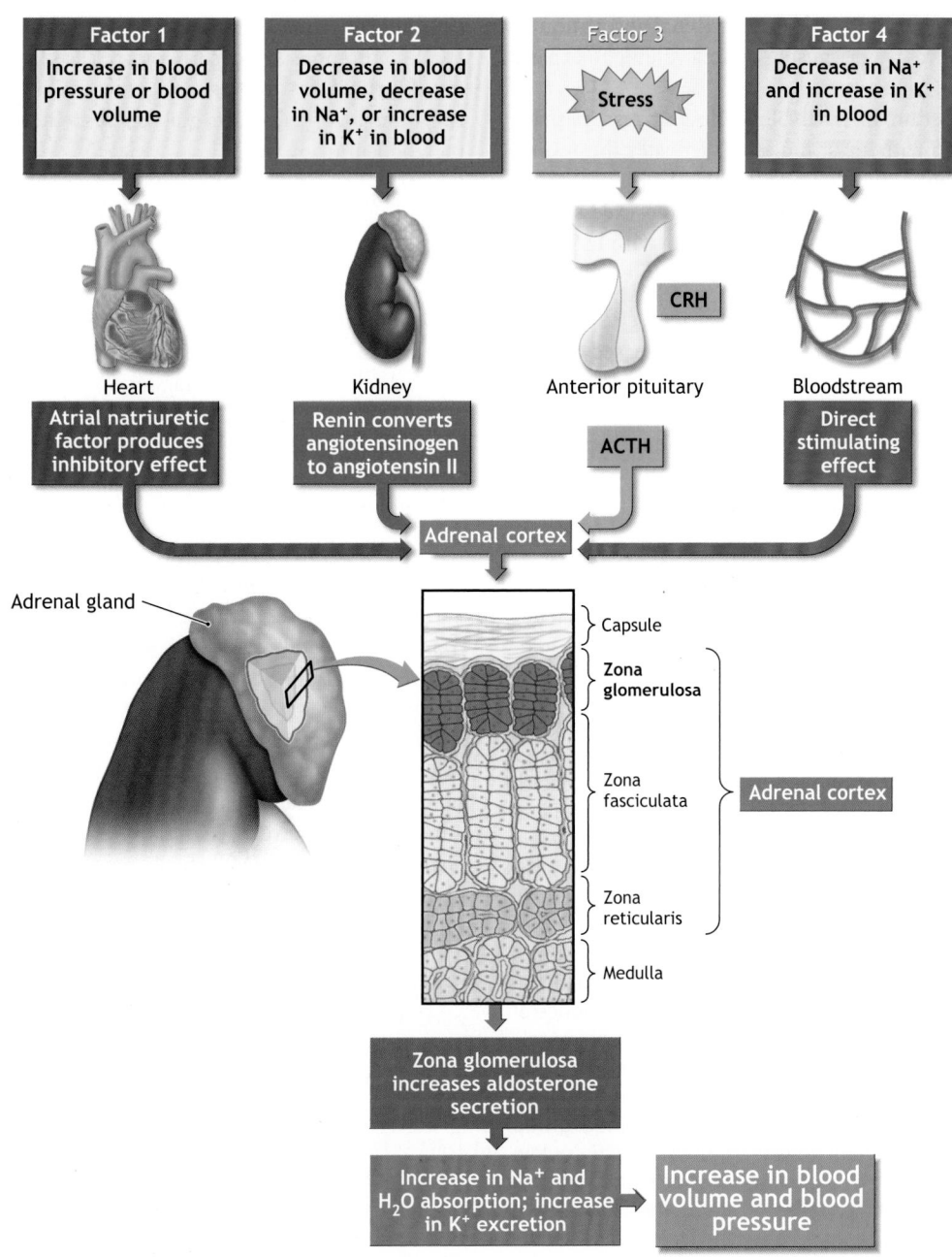

FIGURE 20.11 • Four major factors control aldosterone release from the adrenal cortex. *CRH*, corticotropin-releasing hormone; *ACTH*, adrenocorticotropic hormone.

fluid in the distal tubules of the kidneys by increasing synthesis of sodium transporter proteins by the epithelial cells of the tubules and collecting duct. Consequently, little sodium and fluid voids in the urine. Increases in cardiac output and arterial blood pressure also accompany increases in plasma volume with aldosterone secretion. In contrast, sodium and water literally flow into the urine when aldosterone secretion ceases. Aldosterone also helps to stabilize serum potassium and pH because the kidneys exchange either a K^+ or H^+ for each Na^+ reabsorbed. Proper mineral balance maintains nerve transmission and muscle function. As with all steroid hormones, cellular response to increased aldosterone production occurs

relatively slowly. It requires physical activity in excess of 45 min for aldosterone's effect to emerge; hence, its major effects occur during recovery.

Renin–Angiotensin Mechanism. Increased sympathetic nervous system activity during physical activity constricts blood vessels that serve the kidneys. Reduced renal blood flow stimulates the kidneys to release the enzyme renin into the blood. Increased renin concentration stimulates production of two kidney hormones, **angiotensin II** and **angiotensin III**. These hormones stimulate arterial constriction and adrenocortical secretion of aldosterone, which causes the kidneys to retain sodium and excrete potassium. Renal absorption of sodium also conserves water, causing plasma volume to expand and blood pressure to increase.

Chronic reduction in renal blood flow at rest, perhaps from abnormal sympathetic stimulation, activates the **renin–angiotensin system**. Hypertension occurs from prolonged overresponse of this mechanism with resulting excess aldosterone output. High blood pressure associated with increased aldosterone production often occurs in teenage obesity.[149] Teenage hypertension relates to three factors:

1. Decreased salt sensitivity (hence increased water retention)
2. Increased sodium intake
3. Decreased sensitivity to the effects of insulin (hyperinsulinemia)

Status of Cardiovascular Health of U.S. Adolescents

The most current estimates of cardiovascular health of US adolescents come from the 2005–2010 National Health and Nutrition Examination Prevalence Estimates Surveys representing approximately 33.2 million adolescents ages 12 to 19 years. Population prevalence of individual cardiovascular health behaviors and factors was estimated according to American Heart Association criteria for *poor*, *intermediate*, and *ideal* levels. Ideal blood pressure was most prevalent (males, 78%; females, 90%), whereas a dramatically low prevalence of ideal Healthy Diet Score was observed (males, <1%; females, <1%). Females exhibited a lower prevalence of ideal total cholesterol than males (65% vs. 72%, respectively) and ideal physical activity levels (44% vs. 67%, respectively), yet a higher prevalence of ideal blood glucose (89% vs. 74%, respectively). Approximately two thirds of adolescents exhibited ideal body mass index (males, 66%; females, 67%) and ideal smoking status (males, 66%; females, 70%). Less than 50% of the combined group exhibited five or more (total cholesterol, physical activity levels, blood glucose, body mass index) of the ideal cardiovascular health components (45%, males; 50%, females). Prevalence estimates according to sex were consistent across race/ethnic groups. It was concluded that the low prevalence of ideal cardiovascular health behaviors in U.S. adolescents, particularly physical activity and dietary intake, will likely contribute to a worsening prevalence of obesity, hypertension, hypercholesterolemia, and dysglycemia as the current U.S. adolescent population reaches adulthood.

Source: Shay CM. 2013. Status of cardiovascular health in us adolescents: Prevalence estimates from the National Health and Nutrition Examination Surveys (NHANES) 2005–2010. *Circulation* 2013;127:1369.

These interrelationships suggest a direct link between obesity as a disease and subsequent development of hypertension. Similar relationships occur in adults.[35,62]

Glucocorticoids. The stress of physical activity stimulates hypothalamic secretion of **corticotropin-releasing factor**,

causing the anterior pituitary to release ACTH. In turn, ACTH promotes glucocorticoid release by the adrenal cortex. **Cortisol** (hydrocortisone), the major glucocorticoid of the adrenal cortex, affects glucose, protein, and free fatty acid metabolism in six ways:

1. Promotes breakdown of protein to amino acids in all cells except the liver; the circulation delivers these "liberated" amino acids to the liver for synthesis to glucose via gluconeogenesis
2. Supports action of other hormones, primarily glucagon and GH in the gluconeogenic process
3. Serves as an insulin antagonist by inhibiting cellular glucose uptake and oxidation
4. Promotes triacylglycerol breakdown in adipose tissue to glycerol and fatty acids
5. Suppresses immune system function
6. Produces negative calcium balance

FIGURE 20.12 shows factors that affect cortisol secretion and its effects on target tissues, which includes adipose tissue, muscle tissue, and the liver. A strong diurnal pattern governs cortisol secretion. Secretions normally peak in the morning and subside at night. Cortisol secretion increases with stress, making it known as the "stress" hormone. Even though considered a catabolic hormone, cortisol's important effect counters hypoglycemia and is thus essential for life. Animals whose adrenal glands have been removed die if exposed to severe environmental stress. Cortisol, required for full activity of glucagon and the catecholamines, exerts a facilitating effect on these hormones.

Chronically high-serum cortisol levels initiate excessive protein breakdown, tissue wasting, and negative nitrogen balance. Cortisol secretion also accelerates fat mobilization for energy during starvation and intense, prolonged physical activity. With rapid and large increases in cortisol output, the liver splits mobilized fat into its simple ketoacid components. Excess ketoacid concentrations in the extracellular fluid can lead to the potentially dangerous condition of **ketosis** (a form of acidosis). Individuals who subsist on very-low-carbohydrate, low-calorie weight-loss diets (termed *ketogenic diets*; see Chapter 30) can experience ketosis, augmented by elevated cortisol secretion.

Cortisol turnover, the difference between its production and removal, provides a way to study cortisol response to physical activity. Cortisol turnover with physical activity exhibits considerable variability with intensity of effort, fitness level, nutritional status, and even circadian rhythm.[33,173] Most research indicates that cortisol output increases with activity intensity; this heightened output accelerates lipolysis, ketogenesis, and proteolysis. Extremely high cortisol levels occur following long-duration physical activity such as marathon running or other weight-bearing activity[159] and resistance training.[79,144]

Even during moderate physical activity, plasma cortisol concentration rises with prolonged duration. Data for cortisol turnover indicate that highly trained runners maintain a state of hypercortisolism that heightens before competition or

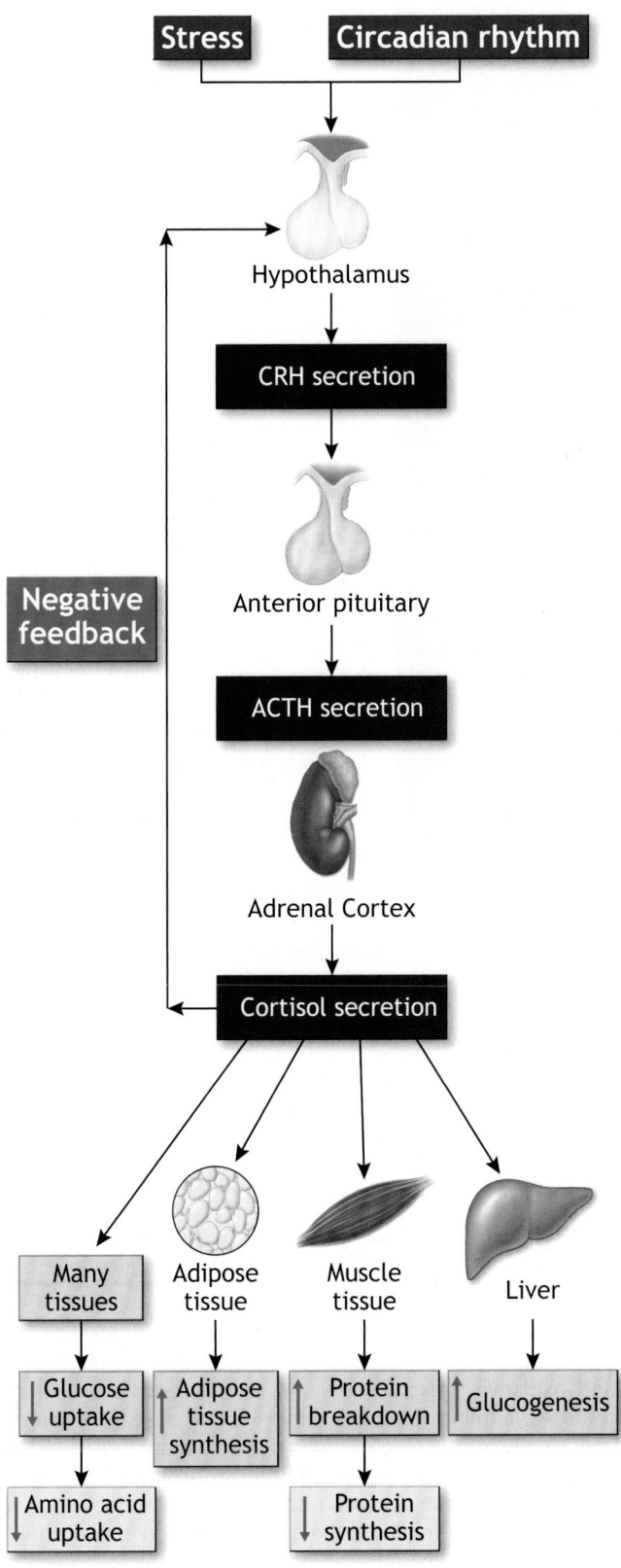

FIGURE 20.12 • Factors that affect cortisol secretion and its actions on target tissues. *CRH*, corticotropic releasing hormone; *ACTH*, adrenocorticotropic hormone.

intense training.[48,85] Cortisol levels also remain elevated for up to 2 hr following physical activity.[190] This suggests that cortisol plays a role in tissue recovery and repair. Unlike the direct, active metabolic effect of epinephrine and glucagon on fuel homeostasis during physical activity, cortisol exerts a more facilitating effect on substrate use.

Gonadocorticoids. The reproductive organs (gonads) provide the major source of the so-called sex steroids, but the adrenal cortex produces androgen hormones (gonadocorticoids) with similar actions. For example, the adrenal cortex produces **dehydroepiandrosterone**, which exerts effects similar to the dominant male hormone testosterone. Treatment with 50 mg of dehydroepiandrosterone in women with adrenal insufficiency over a 4-month trial improved well-being and sexual responsiveness as well as decreased depression and anxiety compared to placebo treatment. The adrenal cortex also produces small amounts of the "female" hormones estrogen and progesterone.

GONADAL HORMONES

The male testes and female ovaries are the respective endocrine reproductive glands. These glands produce hormones that promote sex-specific physical characteristics and initiate and maintain reproductive function. No distinctly "male" or "female" hormones exist, but rather general differences in hormone concentrations between the sexes. Testosterone is the most important androgen secreted by the interstitial cells of the testes. **Figure 20.13** shows that among its many functions testosterone initiates sperm production and stimulates development of male secondary sex characteristics, mainly an increase in facial, pubic, and body hair; vocal cord enlargement; and deepening of the voice. Testosterone's anabolic, tissue-building role contributes to male–female differences in muscle mass and strength that emerge at the onset of puberty. As noted in Chapter 2, testosterone conversion to estrogen in peripheral tissues, under control of the enzyme aromatase, provides the male with protection in maintaining bone structure throughout life.

The ovaries provide the primary source of estrogens, particularly **estradiol** and **progesterone**. Estrogens regulate ovulation, menstruation, and physiologic adjustments during pregnancy. Estrogen circulating in the bloodstream and generated locally in peripheral tissues also exerts effects on blood vessels, bone, lungs, liver, intestine, prostate, and testes through action on α- and β-receptor proteins. Progesterone contributes specific regulatory input to the female reproductive cycle, uterine smooth muscle action, and lactation. Controversy exists concerning the role of estrogen and progesterone in substrate metabolism during physical activity.[4,123] Estradiol-17β (biologically active estrogen synthesized from cholesterol) increases free fatty acid mobilization from adipose tissue and inhibits glucose uptake by peripheral tissues. In this way, the increases in estradiol-17β and GH during physical activity exert similar metabolic influences.

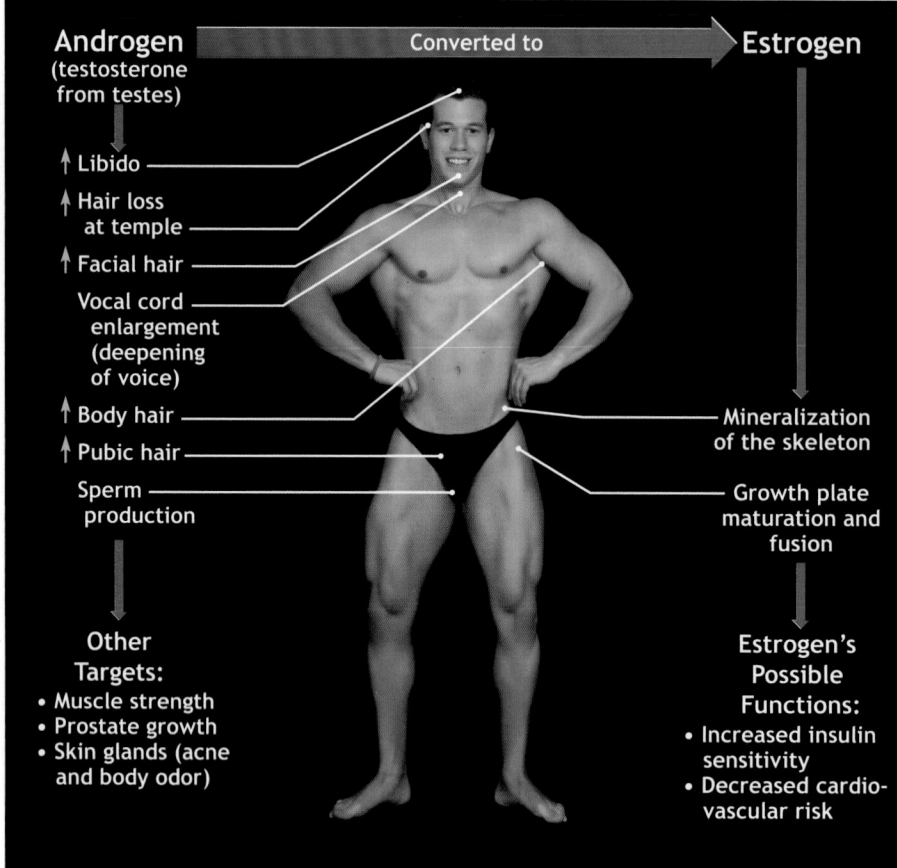

FIGURE 20.13 • Androgen's effects in men. Binding with special receptor sites in muscle and various other tissues, androgen (testosterone) contributes to male secondary sex characteristics and sex differences in muscle mass and strength that develop at the onset of puberty. Some androgen converts to estrogen in peripheral tissues and gives males a considerable edge over females in maintaining bone mass throughout life.

Physical activity also elevates estradiol and progesterone levels. In untrained males, resistance exercise and moderate aerobic activity increase serum and free testosterone levels after 15 to 20 min.[84] Findings remain equivocal concerning the effect of intense endurance exercise on testosterone levels.[144,179]

FIGURE 20.14 shows the pattern of plasma cortisol and testosterone 48 hr before swimming and immediately following 15 × 200-m freestyle at the swimmer's competitive velocity, with a 20-s rest between swims and 1 hr into recovery. Four 6-wk periods formed the training program, with careful monitoring of training volume. The results clearly show that postexercise cortisol (top left inset) and testosterone (bottom left inset) remain elevated. Values remained higher 1 hr after physical activity,, except for testosterone levels in training weeks 6 through 12 and 18 through 24. The generalized decrease in cortisol and testosterone concentrations when the swimmers "peaked" for the championships (weeks 18–24) indicates long-term adaptation for these hormones, not the immediate result of excess stress induced by overtraining and subsequent poor performance. The depressed performance during weeks 18 through 24 might indicate overtraining; this period corresponded to a large increase in training volume. Chapter 21 provides an in-depth discussion of overtraining and its related syndrome.

Testosterone

Plasma testosterone concentration commonly serves as a physiologic marker of anabolic status. In addition to its direct effects on muscle tissue synthesis, testosterone indirectly affects a muscle fiber's protein content by promoting GH release, leading to IGF synthesis and release from the liver. Testosterone also interacts with neural receptors to increase neurotransmitter release and initiate structural protein changes that alter the size of the neuromuscular junction. These neural effects enhance force-production capabilities of skeletal muscle.

Testosterone's effect on the cell nucleus remains controversial. More than likely, a transport protein (sex-hormone–binding globulin) delivers testosterone to target tissues, after which testosterone associates with a membrane-bound or cytosolic receptor. It subsequently migrates to the cell nucleus, where it interacts with nuclear receptors to initiate protein synthesis.

Plasma testosterone concentration in females, although only one tenth that in males, increases with physical activity.[112]

High Doses of Anabolic Steroids Cause Adverse Cardiovascular Side Effects, Including Endothelial Dysfunction

fyi

To investigate the effects of supra-physiological doses of testosterone on the endothelial production of nitric oxide (NO) and oxidative stress, *in-vitro* and *in-vivo* testosterone enanthate was administered as a single 500-mg dose to 27 healthy volunteers. *In-vivo* results showed that urinary NO level and antioxidative capacity were significantly decreased 2 days after testosterone administration. Also, the *in-vitro* studies showed that testosterone inhibited the gene expression of endothelial NO synthase (eNOS) after 48 hr. Supraphysiological doses of testosterone may induce endothelial cell dysfunction, which may partly explain the cardiovascular adverse side effects observed in anabolic androgenic steroid abusers.

Source: Skogastierna C. A supraphysiological dose of testosterone induces nitric oxide production and oxidative stress. *Eur J Prev Cardiol* 2013 Mar 7 [Epub ahead of print].

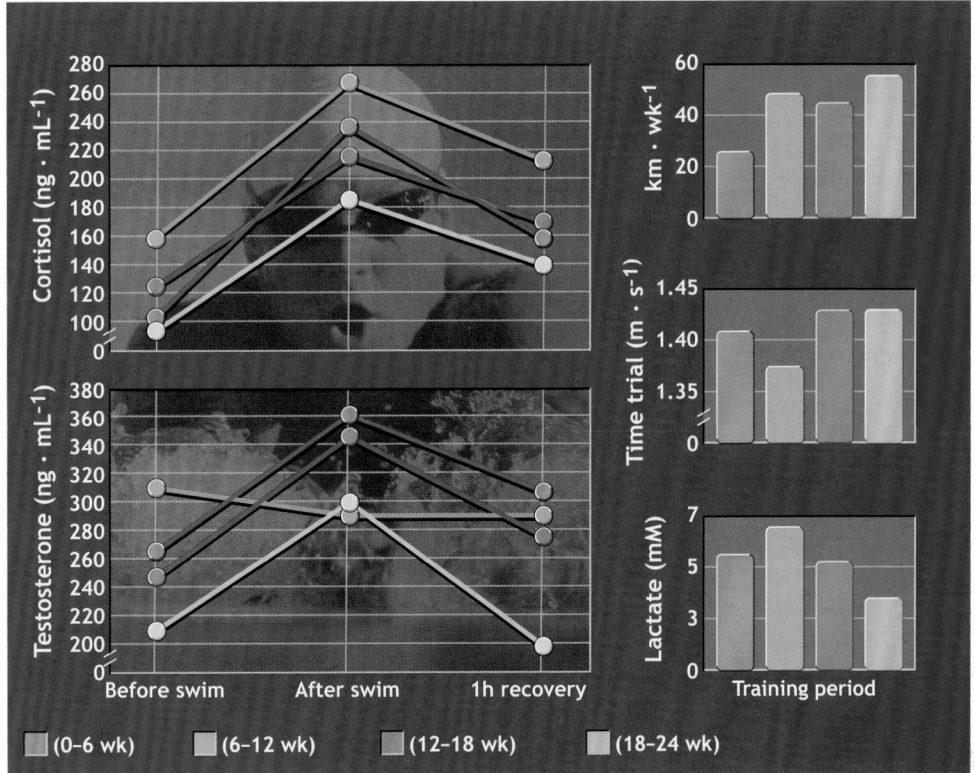

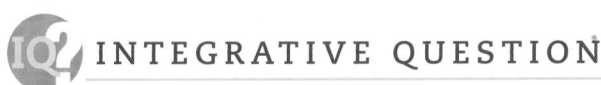

FIGURE 20.14 • Pattern of plasma cortisol and testosterone concentrations measured at three time intervals (4 hr before swimming, immediately after multiple sprint-swims, and after 1-hr recovery) over a 24-wk swim-training season. (Adapted with permission from Bonifazi M, et al. Blood levels of exercise during the training season. In: Miyashita M, et al., eds. *Medicine and Science in Aquatic Sports*. Basel, Switzerland: Karger, 1994.)

INTEGRATIVE QUESTION

Hormones play crucial roles in normal growth and development and the regulation of physiologic function. Give specific examples of why more is not necessarily better for these chemicals.

Pancreatic Hormones

The pancreas gland, approximately 14-cm long and weighing about 60 g, lies just below the stomach on the posterior abdominal wall. Two different types of tissues, **acini** and **islets of Langerhans**, named for German pathologist and anatomist Paul Langerhans (1847–1888; www.ncbi.nlm.nih.gov/pmc/articles/PMC1769627/), who first described this cluster of

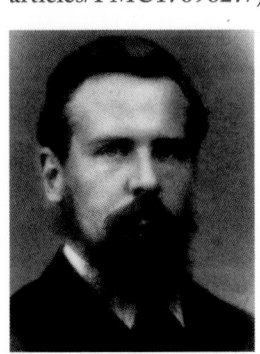

cells in 1869 (**Fig. 20.15**), compose the pancreas. The islets are comprised of about 20% α–cells that secrete glucagon and 75% β-cells that secrete insulin and a peptide called amylin. The remaining cells are somatostatin-secreting D cells and PP cells that produce pancreatic polypeptide. The acini serve an exocrine function and secrete digestive enzymes.

Insulin

Insulin regulates glucose entry into all tissues (primarily muscle and adipose) except the brain. Insulin's action mediates **facilitated diffusion**. In this process, glucose combines with a carrier protein on the cell's plasma membrane (see next section) for transport into cells. In this way, insulin regulates glucose metabolism. Any glucose not immediately catabolized for energy either stores as glycogen or synthesizes to triacylglycerol. Without insulin, only trace amounts of glucose enter the cells. **Figure 20.16A** illustrates that the anabolic functions of insulin promote glycogen, protein, and fat synthesis; Figure 20.16B outlines insulin's actions on most tissues including specific effects on adipose tissue and liver and muscle.

 See the animation "Insulin Functions" on http://thePoint.lww.com/mkk8e for a demonstration of insulin's activity.

Following a meal, insulin-mediated glucose uptake by cells (and correspondingly reduced hepatic glucose output) decreases blood glucose levels. In essence, insulin exerts a **hypoglycemic effect** by reducing blood glucose concentration. Conversely, with insufficient insulin secretion (or decreased insulin sensitivity), blood glucose concentration can increase from a normal level of about 90 mg·dL^{-1} to a

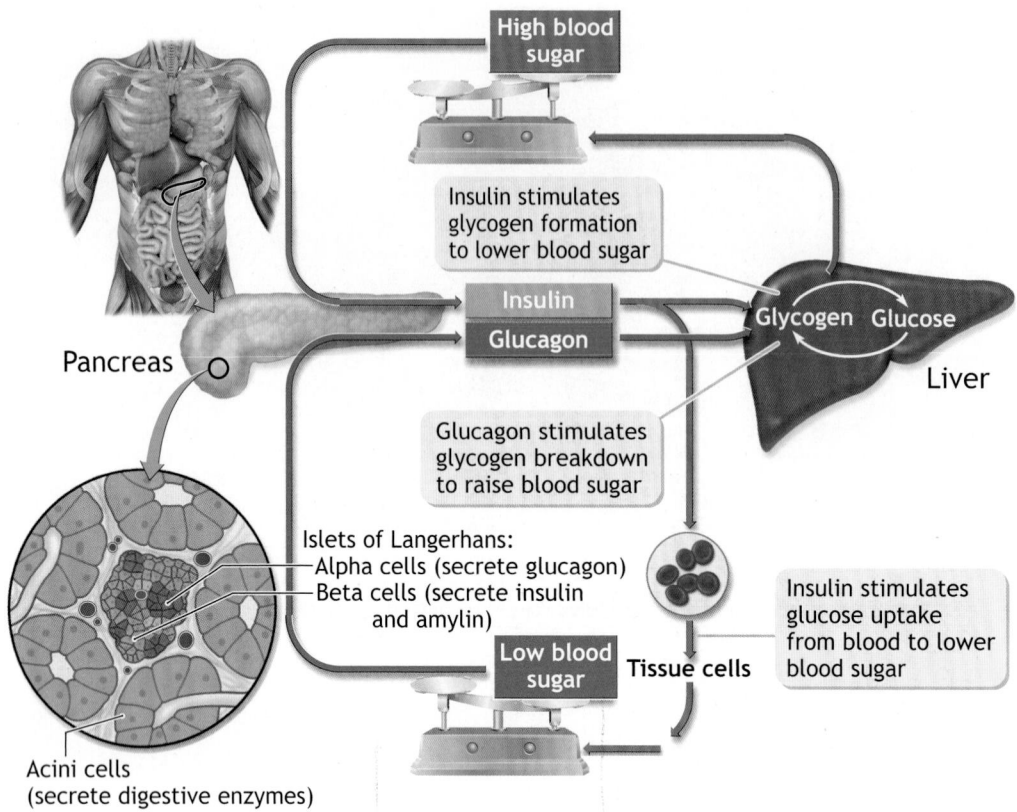

FIGURE 20.15 • The pancreas, its secretions, and their actions.

high of 350 mg·dL⁻¹. When blood glucose levels remain high, glucose ultimately spills into the urine. Without insulin, fatty acids metabolize as the primary energy substrate.

Insulin also exerts a pronounced effect on fat synthesis. A rise in blood glucose levels as normally occurs following a meal stimulates insulin release. This causes some glucose uptake by fat cells for synthesis to triacylglycerol. Insulin's action also triggers intracellular enzyme activity that facilitates protein synthesis. This occurs by one or all of the following three actions:

1. Increasing amino acid transport through the plasma membrane
2. Increasing cellular levels of RNA
3. Increasing protein formation by ribosomes

Insulin Transport of Glucose into Cells: Glucose Transporters. Cells possess different glucose transport proteins, termed **glucose transporters** or **GLUTs**, depending on the variation in insulin and glucose concentrations.[111,152] Muscle fibers contain GLUT-1 and GLUT-4, with most glucose entering by the GLUT-1 carrier during rest. With high blood glucose or insulin concentrations as occur after eating or during physical activity, muscle cells receive glucose via the insulin-dependent GLUT-4 transporter. GLUT-4 action is mediated through a second messenger, which permits migration of the intracellular GLUT-4 protein to the surface to promote glucose uptake. The fact that GLUT-4 moves to

the cell surface through a separate, insulin-independent mechanism coincides with observations that active muscles absorb glucose without insulin.

Glucose–Insulin Interaction. Blood glucose levels within the pancreas directly control insulin secretion. Elevated blood glucose levels cause insulin release. This, in turn, induces glucose entry into cells (lowers blood glucose), removing the stimulus for insulin release. In contrast, a decrease in blood glucose concentration dramatically lowers blood insulin levels to provide a favorable milieu to increase blood glucose. The interaction between glucose and insulin serves as a feedback mechanism to maintain blood glucose concentration within narrow limits. Rising levels of plasma amino acids also increase insulin secretion.

FIGURE **20.17** relates plasma insulin concentration to exercise duration for cycling at 70% $\dot{V}O_{2max}$. The inset graph shows plasma insulin response as a function of effort intensity (%$\dot{V}O_{2max}$). The decreased insulin concentration below rest values as duration extends or intensity increases results from inhibitory effects of an exercise-induced catecholamine release on pancreatic β-cell activity. Catecholamine suppression of insulin relates directly to physical activity intensity. *Physical activity inhibition of insulin output explains why no excessive insulin release (and possible rebound hypoglycemia) occurs with a concentrated glucose feeding during physical activity.* Prolonged physical activity derives progressively more energy from free fatty acids mobilized from the adipocytes from reduced insulin output and decreased carbohydrate reserves. Blood glucose

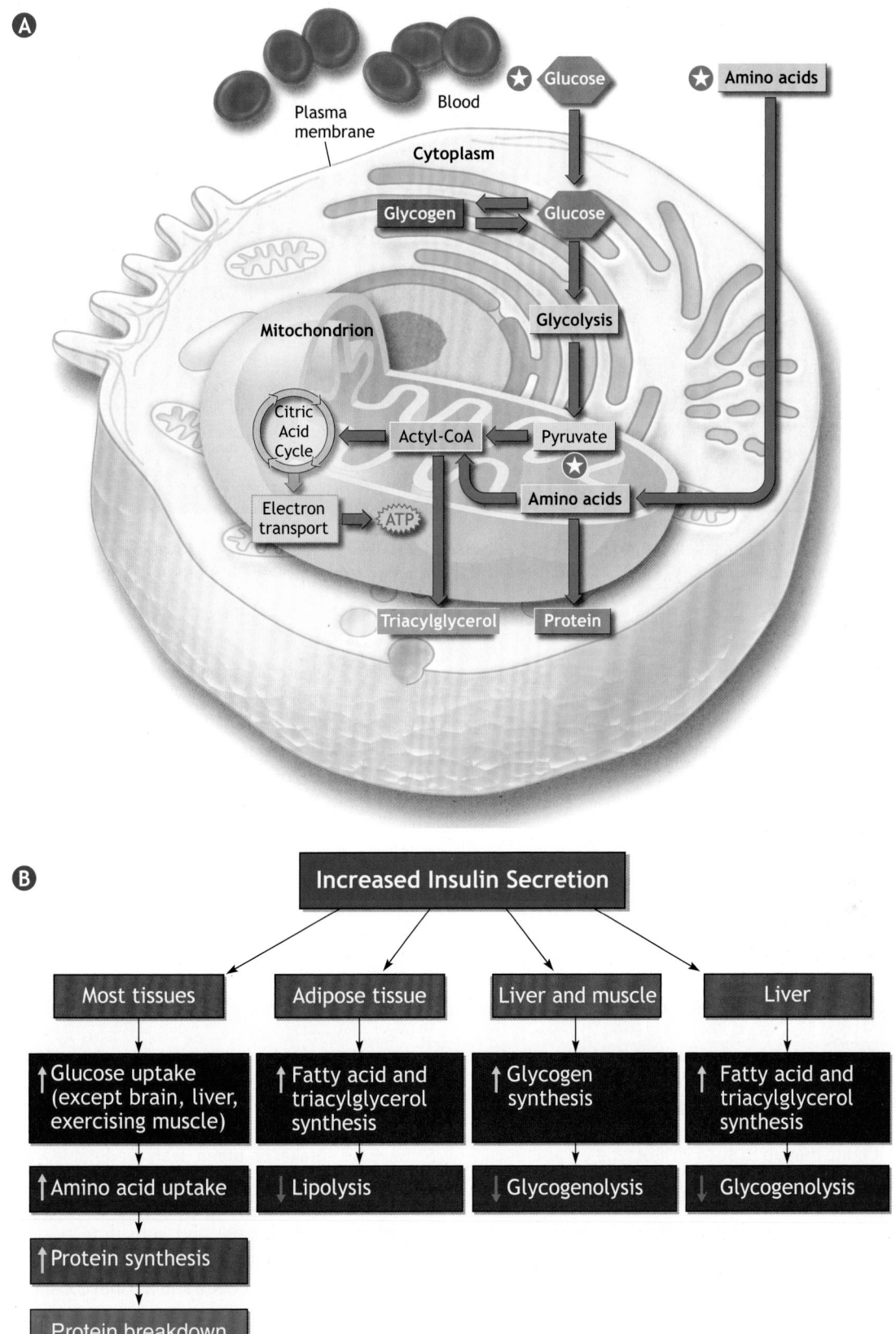

FIGURE 20.16 • **(A)** Primary functions of insulin in the body. The ⭐ show where insulin exerts its influence in metabolism. **(B)** Target tissues and specific metabolic responses to insulin's action. The anabolic functions of increased insulin promote glycogen, protein, and fat synthesis.

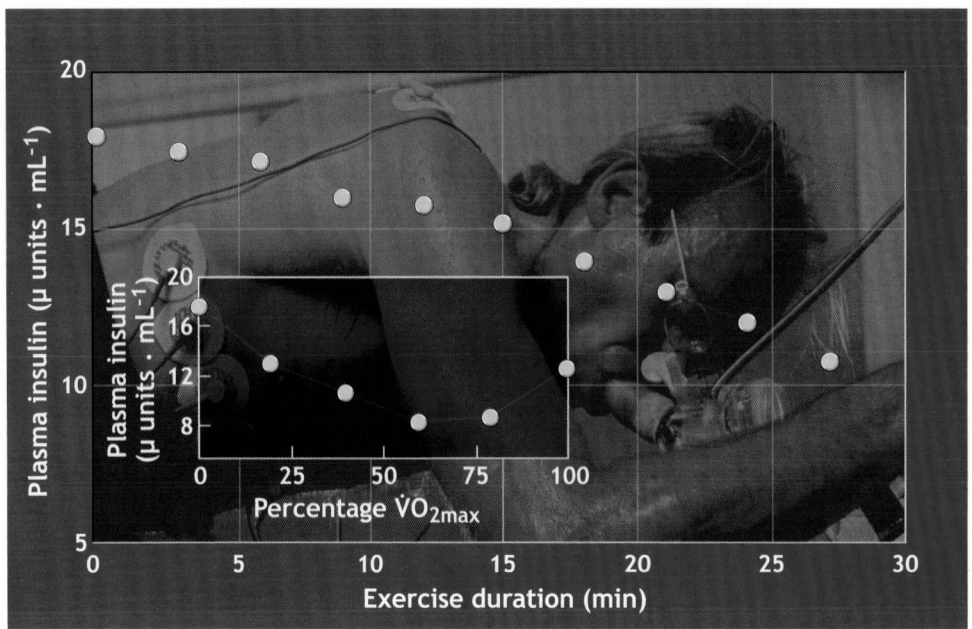

FIGURE 20.17 • Plasma insulin levels during 30 min of cycle ergometer exercise at 70% V̇O₂max. Inset, data show insulin concentrations related to cycling intensity (%V̇O₂max). (Adapted with permission from Applied Physiology Laboratory, University of Michigan, Ann Arbor.)

lowering with prolonged physical activity directly enhances hepatic glucose output and sensitizes the liver to the glucose-releasing effects of glucagon and epinephrine, whose actions help to stabilize blood glucose levels.

Diabetes Mellitus. Diabetes mellitus consists of subgroups of disorders with different pathophysiologies.

 See the animation "Diabetes" on **http://thePoint. lww.com/mkk8e** for an explanation of this disorder and its causes.

T ABLE **20.4** provides the latest published statistics regarding diabetes prevalence in the United States. They are staggering.

The costs of diabetes continue to spiral upward, as evidenced by data from the Centers for Disease Control and Prevention (CDC; March 6, 2013):

- $245 billion in total costs of diagnosed diabetes in the United States in 2012
- $176 billion for direct medical costs
- $69 billion in reduced productivity

IN A PRACTICAL SENSE

How to Reduce Diabetes Risk

Experts estimate that up to 80 to 90% of type 2 diabetes can be avoided by these seven dietary and lifestyle behavioral changes.

1. Lose excess weight; more than 80% of diabetics are overweight or obese, particularly those with abdominal fatness

2. Exercise regularly; regular physical activity reduces risk dramatically

3. Eliminate trans fats and increase intake of polyunsaturated fats and omega-3 fatty acids

4. Lower glycemic load; reduce intake of refined carbohydrates and sweet drinks and increase intake of fiber-rich, unrefined breads, cereals, and grains

5. Increase intake of green leafy vegetables and whole fruit

6. Curb intake of foods high in heme iron (e.g., red meats and processed meats) and substitute non-heme iron foods from plants and supplements

7. Maintain moderate coffee and alcohol consumption

Source: Reis JP, et al. Lifestyle factors and risk factors for new onset diabetes: a population-based cohort study. *Ann Intern Med* 2011;155:292.

TABLE 20.4   Data from the 2011 National Diabetes Fact Sheet

Total Prevalence - Diabetes	
Total	25.8 million children and adults in the United States—8.3% of the population—have diabetes.
Diagnosed	18.8 million people
Undiagnosed	7.0 million people
Prediabetes	79 million people In contrast to the 2007 National Diabetes Fact Sheet, which used fasting glucose data to estimate undiagnosed diabetes and prediabetes, the 2011 National Diabetes Fact Sheet uses both *fasting glucose and A1C levels* to *derive estimates for undiagnosed diabetes and prediabetes.* These tests were chosen because they are most frequently used in clinical practice.
New Cases	1.9 million new cases of diabetes are diagnosed in people age 20 years and older in 2010.
Under 20 years of age	215,000, or 0.26%, of all people in this age group have diabetes; about 1 in every 400 children and adolescents has diabetes
Age 20 years or older	25.6 million, or 11.3%, of all people in this age group have diabetes
Age 65 years or older	10.9 million, or 26.9%, of all people in this age group have diabetes
Men	13.0 million, or 11.8%, of all men age 20 years or older have diabetes
Women	12.6 million, or 10.8%, of all women age 20 years or older have diabetes

Race and Ethnic Differences in Prevalence of Diagnosed Diabetes

After adjusting for population age differences, 2007–2009 national survey data for people diagnosed with diabetes, diabetes age 20 years or older include the following prevalence by race/ethnicity:
- 7.1% of non-Hispanic whites
- 8.4% of Asian Americans
- 12.6% of non-Hispanic blacks
- 11.8% of Hispanics

Among Hispanics:
- 7.6% for Cubans
- 13.3% for Mexican Americans
- 13.8% for Puerto Ricans

Fact sheet was released January 26, 2011; published 2013. Available at http://www.diabetes.org/diabetes-basics/diabetes-statistics

- After adjusting for population age and sex differences, average medical expenditures among people with diagnosed diabetes were 2.3 times higher than what expenditures would be in the absence of diabetes.

The terms *type 1* (absolute insulin deficiency that develops early in life and represents 5 to 10% of the diabetic population) and *type 2* (relative insulin resistance and deficiency that develops later in life and associates with obesity, diet, and sedentary living) identify the two major diabetic subgroups.

Eleven diabetes symptoms include:

1. Presence of glucose in the urine (glycosuria)
2. Frequent urination (polyuria)
3. Excessive thirst (polydipsia)
4. Extreme hunger (polyphagia)
5. Unexplained weight loss
6. Increased fatigue
7. Irritability
8. Blurry vision
9. Numbness or tingling in the extremities (hands, feet)
10. Slow-healing wounds or sores
11. Abnormally high frequency of infection

 Calculating Your Diabetes Risk

Use the following Internet site to calculate your diabetes risk: www.diabetes.org/risk-test.jsp

Tests for Diabetes Mellitus. Different tests diagnose diabetes, including the laboratory-based glucose and insulin clamp methodology, an oral glucose-tolerance test, a simple 8-hr fasting plasma glucose test, and the hemoglobin A1c test.

- The clamp procedure involves maintaining insulin at a constantly above-normal blood concentration using infusion technology (termed *hyperinsulinemic clamp*). Once insulin stabilizes at the higher level, the body's use of glucose is measured by infusing a known amount of glucose into the patient's blood. A **euglycemic clamp** maintains blood glucose at near-normal concentration with insulin production measured. A **euglycemic–hyperinsulinemic**

clamp combines both clamp procedures. A large glucose uptake for a given insulin concentration reflects increased **insulin sensitivity**. Increased insulin release to a constant glucose condition relates to augmented **insulin responsiveness**. Decreased insulin sensitivity indicates inability of cells to adequately respond to insulin to increase glucose uptake. Type 2 diabetes commonly reflects inadequacies in either insulin receptors or cellular response to insulin binding (i.e., there is relative insulin resistance). Decreased insulin responsiveness indicates impaired β-cell function evident in some type 2 diabetics and is the primary cause of type 1 diabetes. [The term *impaired fasting glucose* (IFG) indicates fasting blood glucose values are ≥100 mg·dL^{-1} (5.6 mmol·L^{-1}), but <126 mg·dL^{-1} (7 mmol·L^{-1}).]

- **Oral glucose-tolerance test** evaluates blood sugar levels 2 hr after drinking 75 g of a concentrated glucose solution. Delayed removal of ingested glucose indicates diabetes. [The term *impaired glucose tolerance* (IGT) indicates a 2-hr glucose clearance between ≥140 mg·dL^{-1} (7.8 mmol·L^{-1}) but <200 mg·dL^{-1} (11.1 mmol·mL^{-1}).]
- **Fasting plasma glucose (FPG) test** measures plasma glucose following an 8-hr fast. The American Diabetes Association (www.diabetes.niddk.gov) currently recommends the FPG test as the first test for suspected type 2 diabetes.

Classification Categories for Fasting Blood Glucose

Category	Fasting Plasma Glucose
Normal	**<110 mg·dL^{-1}**
Impaired range	**110–125 mg·dL^{-1}**
Suspected diabetes	**>125 mg·dL^{-1}**

Considerable risks exist for impaired glucose homeostasis—probably a genetic trait that manifests itself in adolescence—in which blood glucose remains elevated, but not high enough for diabetic classification. Nondiabetic, middle-age men whose FPG falls in the upper range of normal show a higher risk of death from heart disease than those in the low–normal range.[8] Men with fasting blood glucose levels above 85 mg·dL^{-1} have a 40% higher risk of cardiovascular death than men with lower values, even after adjusting for age, smoking habits, blood pressure, and fitness status. The current plasma glucose cutoff for suspected diabetes is an FPG of 126 mg·dL^{-1}, down from the previous standard of 140 mg·dL^{-1} set in 1979. This lower cutoff acknowledges that patients can remain asymptomatic despite microvascular complications (damaged small blood vessels), with FPG values in the low- to mid-120 mg·dL^{-1} range. The *impaired range* represents a transition between normal and overt diabetes. In this situation, the body no longer responds properly to insulin and/or secretes inadequate insulin to achieve a more desirable blood glucose concentration.

- **The hemoglobin A1c test** (also called **HbA1c, glycated hemoglobin**, or **glycohemoglobin test**). When blood glucose becomes uncontrolled, the extra glucose enters red blood cells and links up (or glycates) with molecules of hemoglobin (http://diabetes.webmd.com/guide/glycated-hemoglobin-test-hba1c). The more excess glucose in blood, the more hemoglobin becomes glycated. In the body, red blood cells constantly form and die, but typically they live for about 3 months. The A1C test reflects the average of a person's blood glucose levels over the past 3 months. The A1C test results are reported as a percentage; the higher the percentage, the higher the blood glucose levels. A1C level between 5.7 and 6.4% suggests prediabetes. A1C levels below 5.7% are considered normal.

Metabolic Syndrome: A Dangerous Disease of Modern Civilization

Metabolic syndrome, first mentioned in the late 1980s, describes a common condition in which obesity, high blood pressure, high blood glucose, and dyslipidemia cluster together in one person. When these risk factors cluster, the chance of developing coronary heart disease, stroke, and diabetes are greater than when these risk factors develop independently.[10,46,105] Diet-induced insulin resistance/hyperinsulinemia often occurs before manifestations of metabolic syndrome appear.[5,126,163] Diagnosis of metabolic syndrome includes having three or more of the following five indicators:

1. Elevated blood glucose (fasting glucose ≥110 mg·dL^{-1})
2. Overweight with large waist girth (waist girth: men >102 cm [>40 in.]; women >88 cm [>35 in.])
3. High triacylglycerols (≥150 mg·dL^{-1})
4. Low levels of high-density lipoprotein cholesterol (men, <40 mg·dL^{-1}; women, <50 mg·dL^{-1})
5. Hypertension (>130/>85 mm Hg)

Individuals with metabolic syndrome exhibit high risk for cardiovascular disease, type 2 diabetes, Alzheimer's disease, and all-cause mortality.[104] Some researchers maintain that inappropriate food consumption (high levels of refined sugars), sedentary lifestyle, and poor levels of muscular strength and cardiorespiratory fitness not only associate with metabolic syndrome but represent features of this disease.[82,87,103,148] Estimates place the age-adjusted prevalence of metabolic syndrome in the United States at nearly 25%, or about 47 million men and women.[46] The age-adjusted prevalence is similar for men (24%) and women (23.4%). Mexican Americans have the highest age-adjusted prevalence of the syndrome (31.9%). The lowest prevalence occurs among whites (23.8%), African Americans (21.6%), and people reporting "other" for race or ethnicity (20.3%). Among African Americans, women exhibit a 57% higher prevalence than men; Mexican American women have a 26% higher prevalence.

Metabolic Syndrome: Organs Affected, Common Characteristics, Associated Medical Conditions, and Treatment

What is Metabolic Syndrome?

Metabolic syndrome afflicts 25% of adult Americans. This common condition includes **obesity, high blood pressure, high blood glucose ("blood sugar")**, and an **abnormal cholesterol profile (dyslipidemia)**. The chance of developing **coronary heart disease**, **stroke**, and **diabetes** increases when these risk factors cluster together significantly more than when risk factors develop independently.

Medical Conditions Associated with Metabolic Syndrome

Left untreated, metabolic syndrome increases risk of coronary heart disease, stroke, and type 2 diabetes.

Ⓐ Stroke

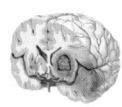

The term *stroke* refers to the sudden death of brain tissue from lack of oxygen. In ischemic stroke, blocked or reduced blood flow occurs in brain tissues. This blockage may result from atherosclerosis and blood clot formation.

Ⓑ Coronary Heart Disease

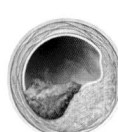

Narrowing of the coronary arteries can lead to a heart attack. Atherosclerosis, the buildup of plaque in the lining of the arteries, causes arterial narrowing; all of the metabolic syndrome risk factors can induce atherosclerosis. Heart attacks occur when blood fails to flow through narrowed coronary vessels, which results in ischemic myocardial tissue.

Ⓒ Type 2 Diabetes

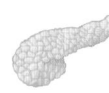

In type 2 diabetes, the pancreas produces little or no insulin and/or the body loses the ability to respond normally to insulin (called insulin resistance). Insulin transports glucose into the cells for use as energy; without insulin, body tissues have less access to essential nutrients for energy and storage. Diabetes requires proper management, and if left untreated, can lead to complications that impact the eyes, mouth, cardiovascular system, kidneys, nerves, and extremities.

Organs Affected by Untreated Metabolic Syndrome

Ⓐ Brain

Ⓑ Heart

Ⓒ Pancreas

High blood glucose: Sugar (glucose) builds up in bloodstream.

High blood pressure, if not treated causes damage to the lining of the arteries.

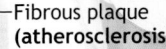
Fibrous plaque (atherosclerosis)

Common Characteristics
- Insulin resistance
- Glucose intolerance
- Dyslipidemia (high triglycerol, low HDL, high LDL)
- Stroke
- Upper-body obesity
- Type 2 diabetes
- Hypertension
- Coronary artery disease
- Reduced ability to dissolve blood clots

Treating Metabolic Syndrome

Metabolic syndrome requires long-term management of each risk factor. Poor nutrition and reduced physical activity represent underlying causes of these risk factors. Regular monitoring of blood pressure, cholesterol, and glucose are important for detecting the syndrome, even if an individual fails to experience outward disease symptoms.

- **Weight loss:** A weight loss of 5 to 10% of body weight improves insulin sensitivity.

- **Increased physical activity:** Increased physical activity reverses insulin resistance, reduces blood pressure, lowers "bad" cholesterol, raises "good" cholesterol, and reduces overall type 2 diabetes risk.

- **Eat a heart healthy diet:** Reduce saturated fat, cholesterol, and salt intake. Increase intake of high fiber fruits, vegetables, and grains.

| TABLE 20.5 | Thresholds of Percentage Body Fat (%BF) Corresponding to Established Body Mass Index Cutoffs Associated with Metabolic Syndrome Risk |

	%BF and Corresponding Percentiles									
	Men					Women				
BMI Cutoffs (kg·m⁻²)	Black		White			Black		White	
	Cutoff	Percentile	Cutoff	Percentile	Mean[a]	Cutoff	Percentile	Cutoff	Percentile
18.5	12.7	8.9	11.0	3.9	12	25.4	11.7	22.5	24
25	21.7	43.5	21.2	41.0	21	32.0	29.3	30.8	31
30	28.3	80.9	29.1	87.6	29	37.1	52.5	37.2	37
35	35.0	97.6	37.0	99.4	36	42.1	75.9	43.5	43

[a]Values were rounded.

From Zhu S, et al. Percentage body fat ranges associated with metabolic syndrome risk: results based on the third National Health and Nutrition Examination Survey (1988–1994). *Am J Clin Nutr* 2003;78:228.

Metabolic syndrome afflicts a large number of adults in Western industrialized countries, with it being more common in men than in women. Disease occurrence relates to genetic, hormonal, and lifestyle factors of obesity, physical inactivity, and nutrient excesses, including high intakes of saturated and trans-fatty acids. Characterized by the clustering of insulin resistance and hyperinsulinemia, dyslipidemia (atherogenic plasma lipid profile), essential hypertension, abdominal (visceral) obesity, and glucose intolerance, the syndrome also relates to abnormalities of blood coagulation, hyperuricemia, and microalbuminuria. Psychosocial stress, socioeconomic disadvantage, and abnormal psychiatric traits also link to the syndrome's pathogenesis.[9,10]

TABLE 20.5 provides percentage body fat ranges and associated risk equivalent to the traditional BMI cutoffs for metabolic syndrome for black and white men and women. Lifestyle modifications that include increased regular physical activity represent the cornerstone of national recommendations to prevent metabolic syndrome.[126,201]

Insulin Actions and Impaired Glucose Homeostasis

FIGURE 20.18 summarizes insulin's normal response and under insulin-resistant and type 2 diabetes conditions. The increase in blood glucose concentration following a meal induces insulin release from the β-cells in the islets of Langerhans. Insulin then migrates in the blood to target cells throughout the body, where it binds to receptor molecules on the cell surface. Insulin–receptor interaction triggers a series of events within the cell that enhance glucose uptake and subsequent catabolism or storage as glycogen and/or fat. A defect anywhere along the pathway for glucose uptake signals diabetes. Seven possible causes include:

1. Destruction of β-cells
2. Abnormal insulin synthesis
3. Depressed insulin release
4. Inactivation of insulin in the blood by antibodies or other blocking agents
5. Altered insulin receptors or a decreased number of receptors on peripheral cells
6. Defective processing of the insulin message within the target cells
7. Abnormal glucose metabolism

Type 1 Diabetes

Type 1 diabetes, formerly called juvenile-onset or child-onset diabetes, typically occurs in younger individuals and represents between 5 and 10% of all diabetes cases (**www.nlm.nih.gov/medlineplus/diabetestype1.html**). This diabetes form represents an autoimmune response, possibly from a single protein that renders the β-cells incapable of producing insulin and often other pancreatic hormones. Type 1 diabetic patients present a more severe abnormality for glucose homeostasis than individuals in the type 2 subgroup. Physical activity exerts more pronounced effects on the metabolic state in type 1 individuals, and the management of exercise-related problems requires greater attention (see "In a Practical Sense: Diabetes, Hypoglycemia, and Physical Activity"),

Type 2 Diabetes

Type 2 diabetes tends to occur after age 40, but a sharp increase now occurs in much younger individuals (often less than 10 years of age). This alarming new trend signals that type 2 diabetes may represent a "pediatric disease." Recent estimates indicate that diabetes has more than tripled in children over the last 3 to 5 years. Physicians consider the spiraling rate of childhood obesity—particularly among African Americans, Native Americans, and Hispanics (most notably children of Mexican descent)—as the predominant factor in the rising number of children with type 2 diabetes. Type 2 diabetes accounts for nearly 95% of all diabetes cases in the United States and represents the leading cause of death from the disease.

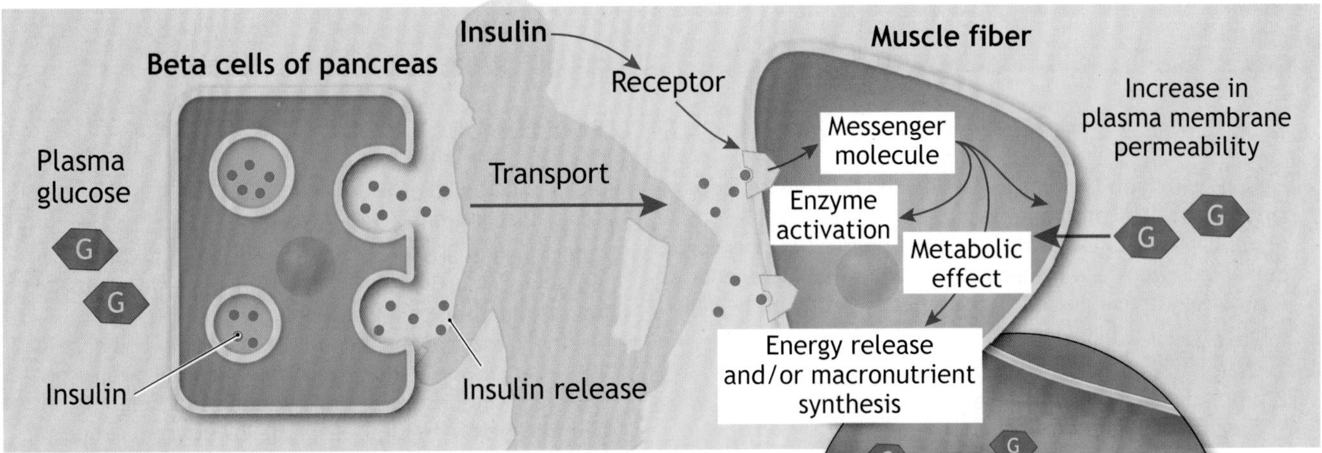

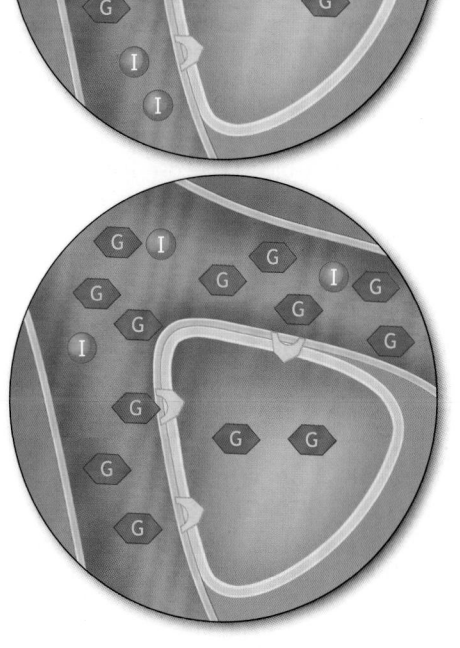

Beta cells of pancreas   Insulin   **Muscle fiber**

Plasma glucose

Receptor

Transport

Messenger molecule

Enzyme activation

Metabolic effect

Increase in plasma membrane permeability

Energy release and/or macronutrient synthesis

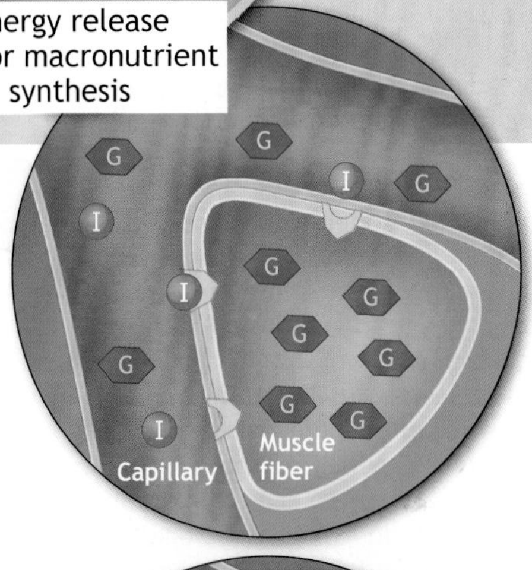

Insulin

Insulin release

Ⓐ Normal response

The rise in blood glucose Ⓖ after eating stimulates insulin Ⓘ release from the beta cells of the pancreas. Insulin mediates facilitated diffusion into the cell where glucose combines with a carrier on the plasma membrane of muscle and adipose tissue cells. Any glucose not immediately catabolized for energy stores as glycogen or synthesizes to fat for later use.

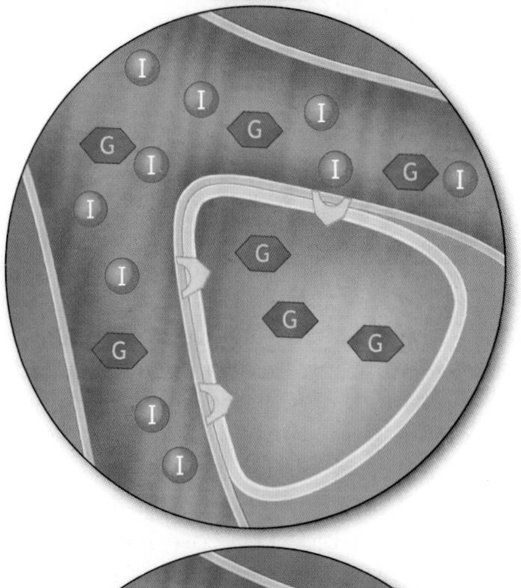

Ⓑ Insulin-resistant response

The pancrease overproduces insulin (abnormal output) in response to a rise in blood glucose as occurs from the rapid digestion and absorption of some dietary starches and simple sugars. Excess insulin production maintains blood glucose at the upper level of the normal range. Thus, the person does not classify as a type 2 diabetic. However, a chronic high insulin output in response to elevations in blood glucose after eating strongly relates to the metabolic syndrome of dyslipidemia, hypertension, upper-body obesity, and increased risk for heart attack and stroke.

Ⓒ Type 2 diabetes

The pancreas continues to secrete insulin. However, the severity of insulin resistance exceeds the pancreas' maximum insulin output to regulate blood glucose within the normal range. This results in the diagnosis of type 2 diabetes.

FIGURE 20.18 • **(A)** Normal insulin–glucose interaction, **(B)** with insulin resistance, and **(C)** with type 2 diabetes.

IN A PRACTICAL SENSE

Diabetes, Hypoglycemia, and Physical Activity

Persons with type 1 or type 2 diabetes should exercise regularly as part of a comprehensive treatment regimen. Hypoglycemia represents the major risk of physical activity for individuals who take insulin or oral hypoglycemic agents. A physically active diabetic person needs to pay particular attention to the following:

1. Warning signs of hypoglycemia
2. Immediate response to a hypoglycemic attack
3. Treatment of late-onset hypoglycemia

HYPOGLYCEMIA WARNING SIGNS

Symptoms of moderate and severe hypoglycemia (see Table) result from inadequate glucose supply to the brain. In general, hypoglycemic symptoms appear only after blood glucose concentration drops below 60 mg · dL^{-1}.

Symptoms of low blood glucose vary considerably. Some diabetic persons with autonomic neuropathy who lose the ability to secrete adrenalinelike hormones in response to hypoglycemia experience hypoglycemic unawareness. They require regular blood glucose monitoring during and after physical activity. Individuals who take β-blocker medication also have increased risk for hypoglycemic unawareness.

HYPOGLYCEMIA ATTACK: WHAT TO DO

1. Respond quickly: Hypoglycemic reactions appear suddenly and progress rapidly.
2. Stop exercising: Test blood glucose to confirm hypoglycemia.
3. Eat or drink carbohydrate: Immediately consume 10 to 15 g (2 to 3 ts) of simple sugar. A diabetic person should always carry high-glycemic carbohydrate while exercising (e.g., hard candy, sugar cubes, raisins, juice). Consuming ice cream or chocolates is a poor choice; their high fat content depresses the glycemic index and impedes glucose absorption.
4. Rest 10 to 15 min: This allows for intestinal absorption of glucose. Test blood glucose levels before resuming physical activity. If blood glucose registers below 100 mg · dL^{-1}, do not exercise but eat more sugar.
5. Remonitor during physical activity: After resuming physical activity, pay close attention to further signs of hypoglycemia. If possible, measure blood glucose within 30 to 45 min.
6. Replenish carbohydrate immediately after physical activity: Consume complex carbohydrates. If carbohydrate intake does not increase blood glucose concentration, be prepared to administer glucagon subcutaneously to boost glucose levels.

LATE-ONSET HYPOGLYCEMIA

Late-onset hypoglycemia describes the condition of excessively low blood glucose more than 4 hr (and up to 48 hr) after physical activity. It occurs more frequently in new exercisers or after a strenuous workout. Insulin sensitivity remains high for 24 to 48 hr after physical activity, so late-onset hypoglycemia poses a particular problem for many medicated diabetics. The following four precautions can guard against late-onset hypoglycemia:

- Adjust insulin dosage or other medication before starting physical activity. If needed, increase food intake before and during activity.
- If activity lasts beyond 45 min, monitor blood glucose at 2-hr intervals for 12 hr into recovery or until sleep. Consider reducing insulin or oral hypoglycemic agents until bedtime. Before retiring, eat some low-glycemic food to increase blood glucose levels.
- Use caution when initiating a physical activity program. Start slowly and gradually increase effort intensity and duration over a 3- to 6-wk period.
- If planning activity longer than 45 to 60 min, make sure to exercise with a friend who can assist in case of an emergency. Always carry snacks and important phone numbers (doctor, hospital, home) and wear a medical ID bracelet.

ADJUSTING INSULIN LEVELS

For intense physical activity, consider the following:

- Intermediate-acting insulin: Decrease dose by 30 to 35% on the day of exercise.
- Intermediate- and short-acting insulin: Omit dose if it normally precedes physical activity.
- Multiple doses of short-acting insulin: Reduce dose before exercise by 30% and supplement with carbohydrate-rich food.
- Continuous subcutaneous insulin infusion: Eliminate mealtime bolus or insulin increment that precedes or follows physical activity.
- Avoid exercising for 1 hr the muscles that receive the short-acting insulin injection.
- Avoid exercising in late evening.

Warning Signs of Hypoglycemia
Mild hypoglycemic reaction
• Trembling or shakiness
• Nervousness
• Rapid heart rate
• Palpitations
• Increased sweating
• Excessive hunger
Moderate hypoglycemic reactions
• Headache
• Irritability and abrupt mood changes
• Impaired concentration and attentiveness
• Mental confusion
• Drowsiness
Severe hypoglycemic reactions
• Unresponsiveness
• Unconsciousness and coma
• Convulsions

Type 2 Diabetes in Children: On the Rise and Not Easily Treated

Metaformin, the only drug approved for treating type 2 diabetes in children, is surprisingly ineffective among patients ages 10 to 17 years. This raises concern about this fast-growing and largely preventable disease among the nation's youth. In research that evaluated three drug-based regimens of treatment to control the disease, only about half of the participants successfully controlled their blood sugar levels despite relatively good compliance to the treatment. This suggests that type 2 diabetic children may require more than one oral medication or must resort to insulin injections for adequate blood glucose control. Once considered an adult disease, type 2 diabetes has increasingly emerged in children and adolescents in association with an increase in childhood obesity (see accompanying figure), which hinders the body's regulation of blood sugar. The CDC estimates the number of children in the United States with this disease to number in the tens of thousands with an increase of 3600 annually, with African American and Latino children at higher risk than white children, and girls at higher risk than boys. Such findings underscore the importance of early preventative measures through lifestyle intervention programs that emphasize healthy nutrition and regular physical activity for children at risk of becoming obese.

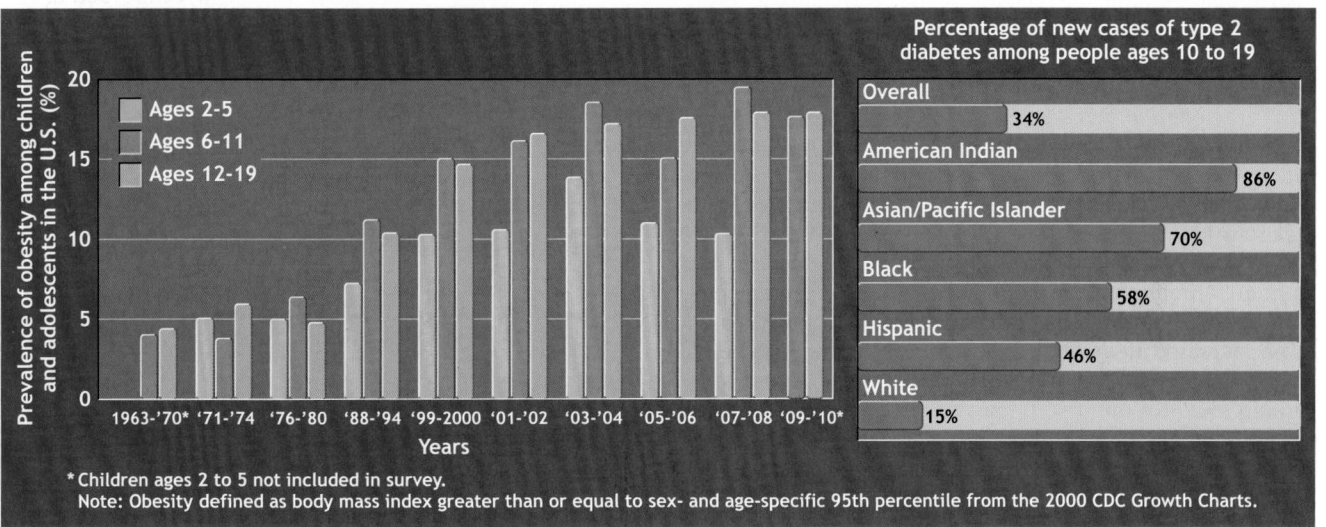

Sources:
Centers for Disease Control and Prevention, National Institute for Diabetes and Digestive and Kidney Diseases.
Zeitler P, et al. A clinical trial to maintain glycemic control in youth with type 2 diabetes. TODAY Study Group. *N Engl J Med* 2012;366:2247.

Three factors can produce high blood glucose levels in type 2 diabetes:

1. Inadequate insulin produced by the pancreas to control blood sugar (**relative insulin deficiency**)
2. Decreased insulin effects on peripheral tissue (**insulin resistance**), particularly skeletal muscle (Fig. 20.18)
3. Combined effect of factors 1 and 2

A dysregulation in glycolytic and oxidative capacities of skeletal muscle also relates to insulin resistance in type 2 diabetes.[74,162,172] The disease most likely results from the interaction of genes and lifestyle factors—physical inactivity, weight gain (up to 80% of type 2 diabetes are obese), aging, and possibly a high-fat diet. No doubt, these lifestyle factors have contributed to the 70% increase in the disorder among persons in their 30s during the last decade of the 20th century, and a 33% overall increase nationally. Also, the form of insulin resistance in type 2 diabetes has a strong genetic component. Diabetic-prone individuals possess a gene that directs synthesis of a protein that inhibits insulin's action in cellular glucose transport.

The Seven Leading Risk Factors for Type 2 Diabetes
1. Body mass exceeds 20% of ideal
2. First-degree relative with diabetes (genetic influence)
3. Member of a high-risk ethnic group (black, Hispanic American, Pacific Islander, American Indian, Asian)
4. Delivered a baby weighing more than 9 lb or developed gestational diabetes
5. Blood pressure at or above 140/90 mm Hg
6. HDL cholesterol level of 35 mg·dL^{-1} or below and/or a triacylglycerol level of 250 mg·dL^{-1} or above
7. Impaired fasting plasma glucose or impaired glucose tolerance on previous testing

Obesity, particularly upper-body fat distribution, and physical inactivity represent major risks for type 2 diabetes in adults and children.[187] An estimated 60 to 80 million Americans show insulin resistance but have not developed overt symptoms of type 2 diabetes. One-third of these individuals will eventually become full-blown diabetics, and many others are at heightened risk of cardiovascular disease.[59] Failure of insulin to exert its normal effect increases glucose conversion

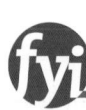

High Blood Sugar Linked to Dementia Independent of Diabetes

Individuals with diabetes have an increased risk of developing Alzheimer's disease and vascular dementia in their later years. What remained unknown was whether high blood sugar levels placed nondiabetic individuals at risk for dementia. For 7 years, researchers tracked 2067 members of a nonprofit HMO in Washington State. They used 35,264 clinical measurements of fasting and nonfasting blood glucose levels and 10,208 measurements of the more accurate long-term predictor glycated hemoglobin assay (HbA1C) from patients without dementia to examine the relationship between glucose levels and risk for developing dementia. Participants included 839 men and 1228 women whose mean age at baseline was 76 years; 232 participants currently had diabetes, and 1835 did not. Participants were categorized according to diabetes status, with adjustments for age, sex, study cohort, level of education, level of physical activity, blood pressure, and coronary and cerebrovascular diseases, atrial fibrillation, smoking, and hypertension treatment. Over 7 years' follow-up, dementia developed in 524 participants (74 with diabetes and 450 without). Among those without diabetes, higher average glucose levels within the preceding 5 years significantly related to an increased dementia risk ($p = 0.01$). This translated to an 18% greater risk in those whose blood glucose averaged 115 mg·dL⁻¹ (6.4 mmol·L⁻¹) than counterparts with an average 100 mg·dL⁻¹ (5.5 mmol·L⁻¹). In diabetics, higher average glucose levels (190 mg·dL⁻¹; 10.5 mmol·L⁻¹) related to a 40% increased risk of dementia compared with those who averaged 160 mg·dL⁻¹ (8.9 mmol·L⁻¹). The results suggest that higher blood glucose levels pose an additional risk factor for dementia, with the brain serving as a target organ for damage, even among persons without diabetes.

Source: Crane, PK et val. Glucose levels and risk of dementia. *N Engl J Med* 2013;369:540.

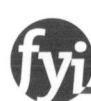

Characteristics of Type 1 and Type 2 Diabetes

Characteristics	Type 1 Diabetes	Type 2 Diabetes
Age at onset	Usually <20 y	Usually >40 y (but increasing in children)
Proportion of all diabetics	<10%	>90%
Appearance of symptoms	Acute or subacute	Slow
Metabolic ketoacidosis	Frequent	Rare
Obesity at onset	Uncommon	Common
β-cells	Decreased	Variable
Insulin	Decreased	Variable
Inflammatory cells in islets	Present initially	Absent
Family history	Uncommon	Common

glucose uptake, a diabetic person relies largely on fat catabolism for energy. This produces an excess of ketoacids and a tendency toward acidosis. In extreme situations, diabetic coma occurs as plasma pH falls as low as 7.0. Arteriosclerosis, small blood vessel and nerve disease, and susceptibility to infection occur at increased rates in type 2 diabetes. Obese diabetic women also face an almost threefold greater risk of endometrial cancer than diabetic women of normal weight, perhaps from their persistently high insulin levels (insulin insensitivity).[158]

Diabetes and Physical Activity Hypoglycemia remains the most common disturbance in glucose homeostasis during physical activity in diabetic persons who take exogenous insulin. Hypoglycemia most frequently occurs during prolonged, intense physical activity when hepatic glucose release does not match increased glucose use by active muscle. In addition, persons with type 2 diabetes often have reduced exercise tolerance independent of glycemic control. Contributing factors include genetics, undesirable lifestyle characteristics, excessive body fat, and poor physical fitness.[27,39]

INTEGRATIVE QUESTION

Explain the sweet-smelling breath of individuals who suffer from poorly regulated diabetes mellitus or malnutrition from starvation.

to triacylglycerol and storage as body fat. For the insulin-resistant individual, a diet high in simple sugars and refined carbohydrates with a relatively high glycemic index facilitates body fat accumulation.[49] Fat cell enlargement further exacerbates the situation because these cells exhibit insulin resistance from their reduced insulin receptor density. Interestingly, women with excess body fat and high cardiorespiratory fitness are more insulin sensitive than equally obese but sedentary counterparts.[50]

As with type 1 diabetes, adequate glucose fails to enter the cells of a person with type 2 diabetes. This triggers abnormally high levels of blood glucose that the kidney tubules filter and void in the urine (**glycosuria**). Excessive glucose particles in renal filtrate create an osmotic effect that diminishes water reabsorption, which results in loss of large amounts of fluid (**polyuria**). With decreased cellular

Muscle as an Endocrine Organ

In 2003, a humoral factor (a cytokine) was first identified as produced and released from contracting muscle cells that appeared to exhibit strong metabolic effects. This discovery of contracting muscle as a cytokine-producing organ opened a new paradigm that views skeletal muscle as an endocrine-secreting organ that influenced metabolism in other tissues and organs. These muscle-secreted cytokines (referred to as *myokines*) and other muscle-produced peptides, produced, expressed, and released by muscle fibers, exert autocrine, paracrine, or endocrine effects. Further research supports muscle as an active endocrine organ with the capacity to produce and express cytokines that belong to distinctly different families. The list currently includes IL-6, IL-8, IL-15, LIF, BDNF, follistatin-like 1, and FGF21. A muscle's contractile activity plays a role in regulating the expression of these cytokines.

Both type I and type II muscle fibers express the myokine *interleukin (IL)-6*, which subsequently exerts its effects both locally within the muscle (e.g., through activation of AMP-activated protein kinase [AMPK]), and when released into the circulation, peripherally in a hormonelike fashion. Specifically, in skeletal muscle, IL-6 acts in an autocrine or paracrine manner to signal through a gp130Rβ/IL-6Rα homodimer, resulting in activation of AMP kinase and/or phosphatidylinositol 3-kinase to increase glucose uptake and fat oxidation. For example, IL-6R in adipose tissue increases hepatic glucose production during physical activity or lipolysis. The insert figure illustrates the proposed biological role for interleukin (IL)-6R.

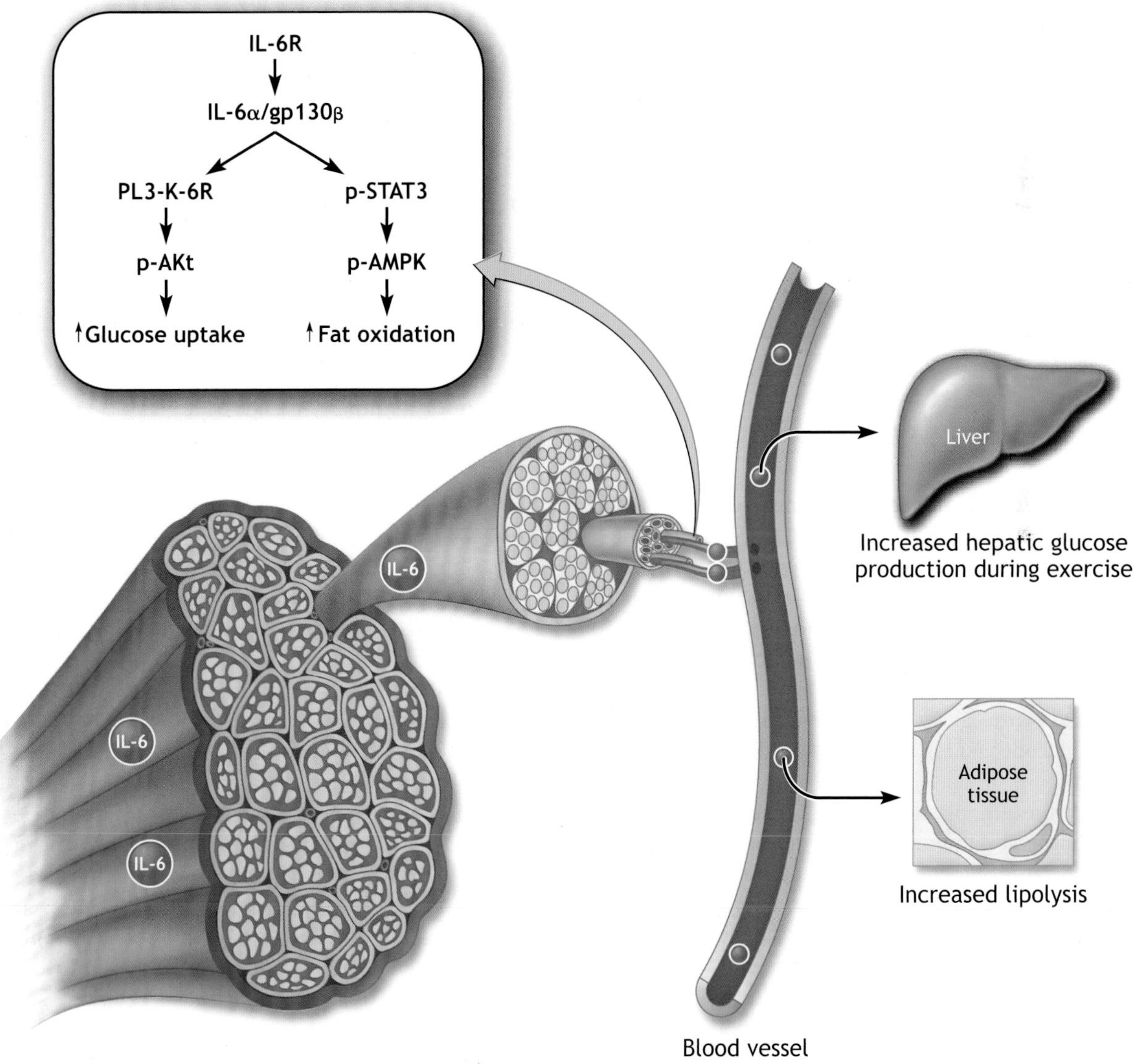

IL-6R
↓
IL-6α/gp130β
↙   ↘
PL3-K-6R   p-STAT3
↓   ↓
p-AKt   p-AMPK
↓   ↓
↑Glucose uptake   ↑Fat oxidation

Liver

Increased hepatic glucose production during exercise

IL-6

Adipose tissue

Increased lipolysis

Blood vessel

Sources:
Pedersen BK, Febbraio MA. Muscle as an endocrine organ: focus on muscle-derived interleukin-6. *Physiol Rev* 2008:88;1379.
Pedersen BK, Edward F. Adolph Distinguished Lecture: Muscle as an endocrine organ: IL-6 and other myokines. *J Appl Physiol* 2009: 107;1006.
Pedersen BK, Febbraio MA. Muscles, exercise and obesity: skeletal muscle as a secretory organ. *Nat Rev Endocrinol* 2012:8;457.

Adipose Tissue as an Endocrine Organ

Until recently adipose tissue has only been viewed as a principal energy supply depot of triacylglycerols. The last 10 to 15 years of research reveals that, in addition to energy storage, adipose tissue serves as an important endocrine organ. It is now widely accepted that adipose tissue secretes a number of peptide hormones, including leptin, which influences appetite (see Chapter 30); several cytokines; adipsin and acylation-stimulating protein (ASP); angiotensinogen; plasminogen activator inhibitor-1 (PAI-1); adiponectin, which increases insulin sensitivity and fatty acid oxidation in muscle; and resistin. Adipose tissue also produces steroid hormones. This secretory function of adipose tissue has shifted the view of adipose tissue in the direction of being at the heart of a complex network that influences energy homeostasis, glucose and lipid metabolism, vascular homeostasis, immune response, and even reproduction. Most known adipose secreted proteins are dysregulated when "normal" body fat becomes markedly altered—either increased in the overfat state or decreased in the underfat (lipoatrophy) state.

Sources:

Guerre-Millo M. Adipose tissue hormones. *J Endocrinol Invest* 2002;25:855.

Boscaro M, et al. Visceral adipose tissue: emerging role of gluco- and mineralocorticoid hormones in the setting of cardiometabolic alterations. *Ann N Y Acad Sci* 2012;1264:87.

Glucagon

The α-cells of the islets of Langerhans secrete glucagon, the "insulin antagonist" hormone. In contrast to insulin's effect in lowering blood sugar levels, glucagon primarily stimulates both glycogenolysis and gluconeogenesis by the liver and increases lipid catabolism (**Fig. 20.19**). The glucose generated by glucagon action then moves into the blood. Glucagon exerts its effect by activating adenylate cyclase. This enzyme stimulates cyclic AMP in liver cells and causes hepatic glycogen breakdown to glucose (glycogenolysis). Glucagon also stimulates gluconeogenesis by promoting the liver's uptake of amino acid.

As with insulin, plasma glucose concentration controls glucagon output by the pancreas. A decrease in blood glucose concentration from prolonged intense physical activity or food (or carbohydrate) restriction stimulates glucagon release.

Autonomic nervous stimulation does not mediate glucagon release, unlike its effects on insulin secretion. Also, no gender differences exist in the glucagon response to exercise when individuals exercise at the same percentage of aerobic capacity.[2,32,175] Glucagon release occurs later in exercise because this hormone exerts little influence in the early regulation of hepatic glycogenolysis. More than likely, it primarily contributes to blood glucose regulation as physical activity progresses and glycogen reserves deplete.

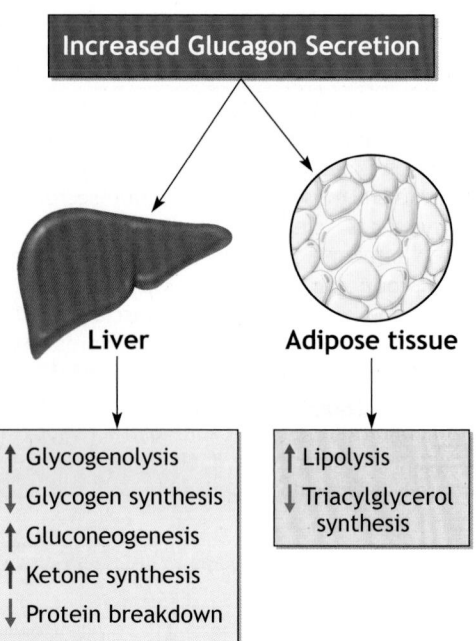

FIGURE 20.19 • Glucogen secretion and its action on target tissues.

Other Glands and Hormones

Other hormones also influence bodily functions. The liver secretes somatomedins, which affect growth of muscle, cartilage, and other tissues. The mucosal lining of the small intestine secretes **secretin**, **gastrin**, and **cholecystokinin** to promote and coordinate digestive processes. The hypothalamus itself constitutes an important endocrine gland that secretes stimulating or releasing hormones that activate or release anterior pituitary hormones. The hypothalamus also releases **somatoliberin**, which stimulates somatotropin secretion from the anterior pituitary gland.

EXERCISE TRAINING AND ENDOCRINE FUNCTION

TABLE 20.6 lists select hormones and their general response to exercise training. Only limited research has evaluated multiple hormone secretions and changes consequent to exercise training because of the complex interactions between endocrine secretions and the nervous system. *The magnitude of hormonal response to a standard exercise load generally declines with endurance training.* For example, when highly trained athletes perform at the same absolute activity level as sedentary subjects, hormonal responses remain lower in the athletes. Improved target tissue sensitivity and/or responsiveness to a given amount of hormone accounts for much of this lowered response.[29,75] A similar level of hormonal response occurs regardless of training state when subjects exercise at the same relative intensity of activity (i.e., same percentage of maximum [lower absolute load for the untrained]). With maximal exertion, trained subjects have an identical or somewhat greater hormonal response than untrained subjects.[20,37,63]

TABLE 23.6	Hormones and Their Responses to Endurance Training
Hormone	**Training Response**
Hypothalamus–pituitary hormones	
Growth hormone	No effect on resting values; less dramatic rise during exercise
Thyrotropin	No known training effect
ACTH	Increased exercise values
Prolactin	Some evidence that training lowers resting values
FSH, LH, and testosterone	Trained females have depressed values; reduced testosterone in males (testosterone levels may increase in males with long-term resistance training)
Posterior pituitary hormones	
Vasopressin (ADH)	Slightly reduced ADH at a given workload
Oxytocin	No research results available
Thyroid hormones	
Thyroxine (T_4)	Reduced concentration of total T_3 and increased free thyroxine at rest
Triiodothyronine (T_3)	Increased turnover of T_3 and T_4 during exercise
Adrenal hormones	
Aldosterone	No training adaptation
Cortisol	Slight elevation during exercise
Epinephrine and norepinephrine	Decreased secretion at rest and at the same absolute exercise intensity after training
Pancreatic hormones	
Insulin	Increased sensitivity to insulin; normal decrease in insulin during exercise greatly reduced with training
Glucagon	Smaller increase in glucose levels during exercise at absolute and relative workloads
Kidney enzyme and hormone	
Renin and angiotensin	No apparent training effect

Anterior Pituitary Hormones

Growth Hormone

GH stimulates lipolysis and inhibits carbohydrate breakdown, so some have argued that exercise training enhances GH secretion and conserves glycogen reserves. However, this does not occur. Compared with untrained counterparts, endurance-trained individuals show less rise in blood GH levels at a given physical activity intensity—a response attributed to reduced stress as training progresses and fitness improves.

Regardless of training status, women typically maintain higher GH levels at rest than men; this difference disappears during prolonged physical activity.[18] FIGURE 20.20A illustrates the training-induced depression of GH response of a representative subject from a group of six men during 20 min of constant-load, intense effort before and after 3 and 6 wk of endurance training. Integrated GH concentrations (exercise plus recovery) for the group averaged 45% lower than pretraining values at both training measures. Responses for plasma catecholamines (Fig. 20.20B and C) and blood lactate (Fig. 20.20D) paralleled the decrease in GH. Because the constant-load exercise test represented less physiologic demand after training (reflected by lower catecholamine and lactate levels), a similar release of GH after training probably requires higher absolute exercise intensity. The effect of training on GH release also may occur under nonexercise conditions.

ACTH (Adrenocorticotropic Hormone)

ACTH secreted by the posterior pituitary gland provides potent stimulation to the adrenal cortex and thus increases free fatty acid mobilization for energy. Training increases ACTH release during physical activity—a response that stimulates adrenal gland activity to promote fat catabolism and spare glycogen.[14,109] This effect would certainly benefit prolonged, high-intensity exercise performance.

PRL (Prolactin)

Little information exists concerning exercise-training changes in PRL. It does appear that resting PRL levels of male runners average below values for sedentary nonrunners.[61,192]

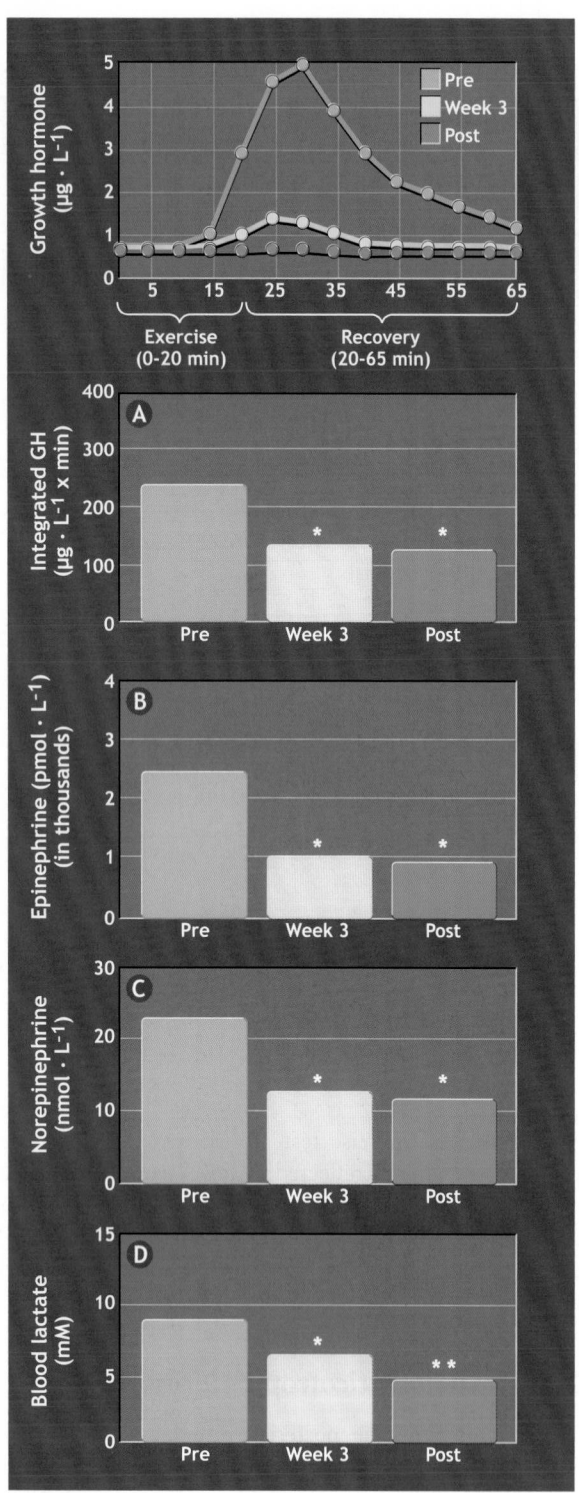

FIGURE 20.20 • *Top.* Serum growth hormone (*GH*) concentrations in a representative subject during 20 min of constant-load exercise and 45 min of recovery at pretraining, after 3 wk of training, and after 6 wk of training. *Bottom.* Effects of 6 wk of training on integrated GH concentration (**A**), and end-of-exercise concentrations of epinephrine (**B**), norepinephrine (**C**), and blood lactate (**D**) in response to constant-load cycle ergometry ($n = 6$, mean). Preweek 3, after 3 wk of training; Post, after 6 wk of training. $^*p < .05$ versus pretraining; $^{**}p < .05$ versus week 3. (Adapted with permission from Weltman A, et al. Exercise training decreases the growth hormone (GH) response to acute constant-load exercise. *Med Sci Sports Exerc* 1997;29:669.)

FSH (Follicle-Stimulating Hormone), LH (Leuteinizing Hormone), and Testosterone

Regular physical activity depresses reproductive hormone responses in women and men.[36,193] Male endurance athletes generally maintain resting testosterone levels between 60 and 85% of values for sedentary men.

Women. Women with a long history of physical activity participation have altered FSH and LH levels at different times in their menstrual cycles, which may contribute to menstrual dysfunction. For example, FSH levels remain depressed in trained females throughout an abbreviated anovulatory menstrual cycle, whereas LH and progesterone concentrations rise in the cycle's follicular phase. Variations in the menstrual cycle do not affect metabolic and hormonal responses to acute bouts of physical activity.[48,88]

Men. Endurance training affects a man's pituitary–gonadal function, including levels of testosterone and PRL. One study compared 46 male runners (average weekly running distance: 64 km) and 18 nonrunners matched for age, stature, and body mass.[192] The runners showed lower testosterone than nonrunners, with no differences in LH and FSH levels. Reduced testosterone concentration (both increased clearance and lower production) in endurance-trained men parallels the sex-steroid reductions observed in women who undergo endurance training and associated reductions in body fat.[169] No difference exists in LH and FSH levels between trained and untrained men; thus, impaired gonadotropin release from the anterior pituitary does not cause the lower testosterone levels during standard physical activity in the trained state.

Posterior Pituitary Hormones

ADH (Antidiuretic Hormone)

Intense physical activity to exhaustion or prolonged submaximal activity at the same relative intensity produces no difference in ADH levels between trained and untrained individuals. ADH concentration decreases with training when exercising at the same absolute submaximal intensity.

PTH (Parathyroid Hormone)

Endurance training enhances exercise-related increases in PTH in young and elderly adults.[137,176] The significance of a training-induced augmented rise in PTH for preserving bone mass with aging awaits further study.

Thyroid Hormones

Training produces a coordinated pituitary–thyroid response that reflects increased turnover of thyroid hormones. Increased thyroid turnover often reflects excessive hormonal action that ultimately leads to **hyperthyroidism** (i.e., overproduction of T_3 and T_4 hormones). However, no evidence indicates a higher incidence of hyperthyroidism in highly trained individuals. For example, inordinately high BMR levels and basal body temperatures rarely occur in the trained state. Consequently, the greater T_4 turnover that accompanies physical training occurs through a mechanism that differs from "normal" thyroid hormone dynamics.

Research on endurance-trained women yields interesting results regarding thyroid turnover. Changing from a baseline of relatively sedentary living to running 48 km per week produced a mild thyroid impairment reflected by decreased T_3 and T_4 levels.[15] In contrast, nearly doubling the weekly distance increased plasma hormone levels. To explain these apparent conflicting effects of regular physical activity, the researchers suggested that greater body fat loss with more intense training produced an exercise-induced increase in thyroid output. Six months of resistance training in men slightly reduced the concentrations of T_4 and plasma-free T_4, without change in TSH. However, the magnitude of the change was of no clinical or physiologic significance.[140]

Adrenal Hormones

Aldosterone

The renin–angiotensin–aldosterone system contributes to homeostatic control of body fluid volumes, electrolytes, and blood pressure, but training does not affect resting levels of these compounds or their normal response to physical activity.

Cortisol

Plasma cortisol levels increase less in trained subjects than in sedentary subjects who perform the same absolute level of submaximal exercise. Adrenal gland enlargement results from both cellular hypertrophy and hyperplasia with repeated bouts of intense training and correspondingly high cortisol output.

Epinephrine and Norepinephrine

Sympathoadrenal activity, principally norepinephrine release in response to an absolute submaximum workload, remains lower in trained than untrained individuals.[41] Epinephrine and norepinephrine output in standard exercise falls dramatically during the first several weeks of training. *The appearance of bradycardia and a smaller rise in blood pressure during submaximal activity represent the most familiar consequences of the sympathoadrenal training adaptation.* Reductions in heart rate and blood pressure reflect favorable adaptations because they lower myocardial oxygen demands during physical activity and possibly other forms of stress. For equivalent *relative* intensities of effort, a higher sympathoadrenal response occurs following aerobic training.[58]

Figure 20.21 illustrates norepinephrine and epinephrine response during physical activity at intensities that ranged between 60 to 85% of aerobic capacity by three adult men and six women prior to and following 10 wk of aerobic training that increased $\dot{V}O_{2max}$ by 20%. Plasma norepinephrine

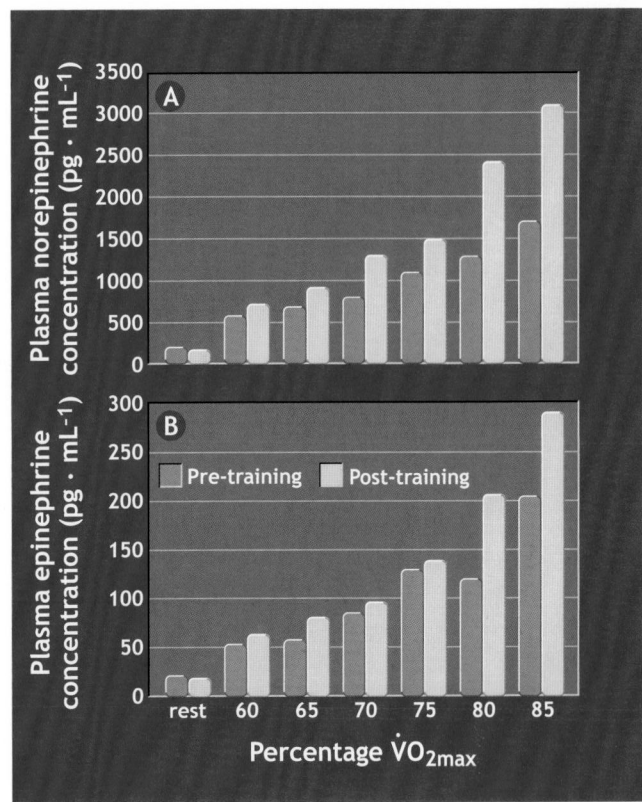

FIGURE 20.21 • Plasma norepinephrine **(A)** and epinephrine concentrations **(B)** at rest and after 15 min of exercise at the same relative exercise intensity (%$\dot{V}O_{2max}$) before and after 10 wk of endurance exercise training. (Adapted with permission from Greiwe JS, et al. Norepinephrine response to exercise at the same relative intensity before and after endurance training. *J Appl Physiol* 1999;86:531.)

levels (top inset) increased progressively with exercise intensity before and after training. Training produced higher plasma norepinephrine levels, particularly at higher intensities. Consistently higher epinephrine values also emerged following training (bottom inset), but the differences did not reach statistical significance. More than likely, greater catecholamine output at the same relative exercise intensity following training reflects three factors requiring greater sympathetic nervous system activation:

1. Greater absolute demand for substrate use via glycogenolysis and lipolysis
2. Increased overall cardiovascular response (e.g., cardiac output)
3. Larger muscle mass activation

Pancreatic Hormones

Endurance training maintains blood levels of insulin and glucagon during physical activity closer to resting levels. In essence, the trained state requires less insulin at any stage from rest through light to moderately intense physical activity. **Figure 20.22** shows plasma glucagon **(A)** and plasma insulin **(B)** responses in 10 young adults before and after 20 wk of

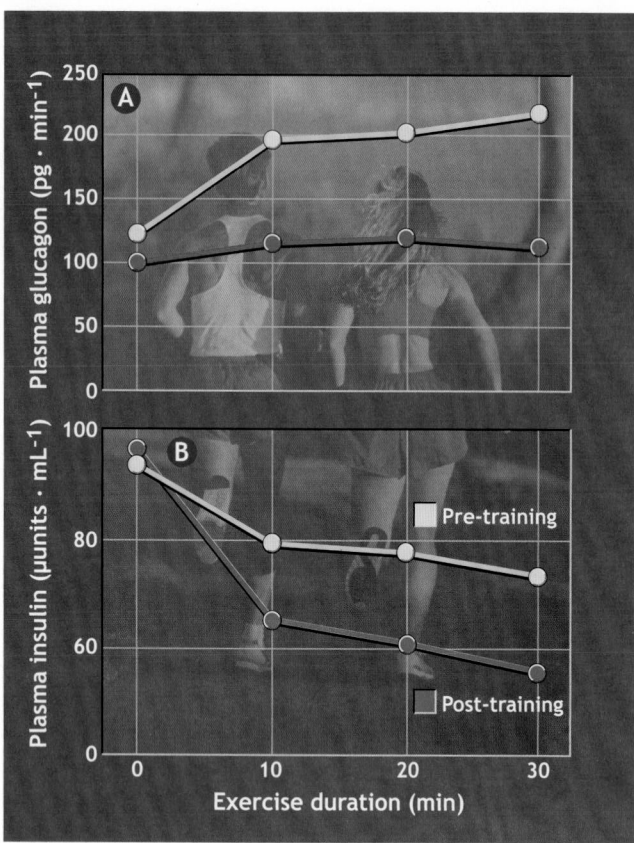

FIGURE 20.22 • Pre–post differences in plasma glucagon **(A)** and insulin **(B)** responses to exercise before and after 20 wk of an aerobic training program. (Adapted with permission from Applied Physiology Laboratory, University of Michigan.)

training at 60 to 80% $\dot{V}O_{2max}$. Aerobic training depressed the exercise response of both hormones, with glucagon showing the most pronounced reduction. These findings agree with previous reports for adults who trained by running and cycling.[60,108]

Regular Physical Activity and Type 2 Diabetes Risk

Cross-sectional, retrospective, prospective, and interventional epidemiologic research provide strong evidence that regular physical activity reduces type 2 diabetes prevalence in adolescents and adults with or without concomitant body composition changes.[3,17,69,99,185] (Refer to http://journals.lww.com/acsm-msse/Fulltext/2010 /12000/Exercise_and_Type_2_Diabetes__American_Col-lege_of.18.aspx for the ACSM position stand on physical activity and type 2 diabetes.) Those individuals at greatest risk for type 2 diabetes (obese, hypertensive, family history, sedentary lifestyle) gain the greatest benefit from regular physical activity.[1,115,141] For adult men and women, low fitness levels coincide with increased clustering of the metabolic abnormalities associated with metabolic syndrome (see "Metabolic Syndrome" section, earlier in this chapter), the "deadly quartet" of insulin resistance, glucose intolerance, abdominal obesity, and

dyslipidemia. For sedentary, middle-age men, aerobic physical activity plus weight loss lowers blood pressure and improves glucose and fat metabolism.[34,100] Resistance exercise also may provide benefits—every additional 10% increase in skeletal muscle mass associates with an 11% reduction in insulin resistance and a 12% lower risk of transitional, prediabetes, or diabetes. When researchers compared the one-quarter of participants with the most muscle mass with those at the bottom of the spectrum, those with the greatest muscle mass were 63% less prone to diabetes.[166]

Regular physical activity even may reduce the amount of antidiabetic medication a patient currently takes to control the disease.[197] A 6-year clinical trial evaluated the effects of diet and physical activity lifestyle interventions on the occurrence of type 2 diabetes in individuals with impaired glucose tolerance.[77] Men and women were randomly assigned to either control, diet-only, exercise-only, or diet-plus-exercise groups. Diet modification consisted of 25 to 30 kcal per kilogram of body mass (55 to 60% carbohydrate, 25 to 30% lipid, and 10 to 15% protein) for individuals with a BMI below 25. Those with a BMI above 25 maintained the same macronutrient mixture as the leaner group while gradually losing weight at a rate of 0.5 to 1.0 kg per month until their BMI decreased to 23. Physical activity intervention required a progressive increase in the quantity of mild-to-moderate regular physical activity. The diet–exercise intervention combined the major components of both diet and exercise treatments. Clearly, diet, physical activity, and combined diet–exercise interventions decreased incidence of diabetes after the 6-year intervention.

A large prospective study evaluated diabetes risk for a cohort of 70,102 female nurses ages 40 to 65 years without diabetes, cardiovascular disease, or cancer at baseline measurements in

 Resistance Training Reduces Risk of Type 2 Diabetes

Resistance training, either alone or combined with aerobic exercise, lowers diabetes risk in men. Strength training for at least 30 min a day, five times a week reduced the chance of developing type 2 diabetes by as much as 34%. Combining resistance training with diverse aerobic activities for a weekly total of 150 min reduced the risk by as much as 59%. A dose–response relationship emerged between an increasing amount of time spent on resistance training or aerobic activity and a lower diabetes risk.

Source: GrØntved A, et al. A prospective study of weight training and risk of type 2 diabetes mellitus in men. *Arch Intern Med* 2012;172:1306.

1986.[77] In agreement with previous prospective research on men, an 8-year follow-up found increased physical activity correlated with a substantially reduced relative risk for type 2 diabetes.

FIGURE 20.23 outlines the possible mechanisms of how exercise training—via its effects on skeletal muscle, pancreatic hormone output, adipose tissue, and liver—improves insulin action and blood glucose control in type 2 diabetes.

Physical Activity Benefits for Type 2 Diabetes. Regular physical activity provides considerable benefits for persons with type 2 diabetes.[67,145]

Glycemic Control. Skeletal muscle consumes the major amount of glucose transported in blood. Muscle, for example, generally clears between 70 and 90% of the glucose in an oral or intravenous glucose challenge. A single bout of moderate or intense physical activity abruptly decreases plasma glucose levels, an effect that persists for up to several days. Extending the duration of weekly physical activity from 115 min to 170 min produces the greatest increase in insulin sensitivity.[76] Most likely, the immediate effects of each activity session on increasing the active muscles' insulin sensitivity causes long-term improvement in glycemic control, not any exercise-induced chronic adaptations in tissue function. When resuming a sedentary lifestyle, the muscles' sensitivity to insulin decreases, which requires more insulin to clear a given quantity of blood glucose.[133] *Improved insulin sensitivity with regular physical activity provides type 2 diabetics with important "therapy" that ultimately lowers their insulin requirement.* Three factors account for the improved insulin sensitivity for glucose transport in skeletal muscle and adipose tissue after a bout of physical activity:

1. Translocation of the glucose transporter protein GLUT-4 from the endoplasmic reticulum to the cell surface
2. Increase in total quantity of GLUT-4
3. Increase in glycogen synthase activity and subsequent glycogen storage (independent of any effect on insulin signaling) [25,66,73,80,147]

The hyperinsulinemic patient who requires the largest insulin release for glucose regulation derives the greatest benefits from regular physical activity.[187] This observation supports the theory that regular physical activity acts by reversing insulin resistance (i.e., physical activity increases insulin sensitivity).

Combining resistance exercise and endurance training improves markers of insulin resistance and body composition for insulin-resistant individuals more than endurance training alone.[100,180] Benefits of resistance plus endurance training for hyperinsulinemia most likely come from the specific effects of activating a relatively larger muscle mass (than with endurance training alone) and additional caloric expenditure. *Improvements in blood glucose homeostasis with regular physical activity rapidly decrease once training ceases and completely dissipate within several weeks of inactivity.* Interestingly, reliance on intensive pharmacologic therapy to lower blood glucose levels in high-risk type 2 diabetics increased mortality but did not significantly reduce cardiovascular events compared with standard therapy.[177]

Cardiovascular Disease. Excess morbidity and mortality in type 2 diabetes results from coronary heart disease, stroke,

and peripheral vascular disease from accelerated atherosclerosis.[38] Disease risk factors that improve with regular physical activity include hyperinsulinemia, hyperglycemia, abnormal plasma lipoproteins, some blood coagulation parameters, and hypertension.[151]

Weight Loss. Weight loss and accompanying reduction in body fat and its distribution enhance glucose tolerance and insulin sensitivity.[6,99] The beneficial effects of physical activity on fat loss often are underestimated because body weight changes per se with exercise do not necessarily reflect the even more favorable, exercise-induced body composition changes (fat loss and muscle gain). Combining diet and regular physical activity reduces body fat in diabetic persons more effectively than either treatment alone.

Psychologic Profile. Improved exercise capacity in diabetic persons relates to decreased anxiety, improved mood and self-esteem, increased sense of well-being and psychologic control, enhanced socialization, and improved quality of life.[122,178]

Occurrence of Type 2 Diabetes. Regular physical activity contributes to delaying and even preventing the onset of insulin resistance and type 2 diabetes in persons at high risk for developing this disease. Physical activity benefits are particularly pronounced for obese individuals and perhaps all persons with increased abdominal fat deposition.

Physical Activity Risks for Type 2 Diabetics. FIGURE 20.24 lists 12 potential adverse effects of physical activity in type 2 diabetics on the systemic circulation, cardiovascular and metabolic functions, and musculoskeletal maladies. One can minimize these risks by properly screening patients before they start an activity program and carefully monitoring them during activity when the program begins.

Physical Activity Guidelines for Type 1 Diabetes. The clinical usefulness of regular physical activity to improve glucose control in type 1 diabetes remains uncertain. To complicate matters for type 1 diabetics, physical activity can trigger a potentially dangerous dual response:

1. Enhanced glucose uptake by active muscles
2. Greater than anticipated exogenous insulin distributed by more rapid circulation that accompanies physical activity

These two factors could worsen the imbalance between glucose supply and use, increasing the risk of serious complications from hypoglycemia. "In a Practical Sense:, Diabetes, Hypoglycemia, and Physical Activity" offers guidelines for the diabetic patient, including those with well-controlled type 1 diabetes who wish to perform prolonged and strenuous physical activity while minimizing the principal risk of hypoglycemia.

RESISTANCE TRAINING AND ENDOCRINE FUNCTION

Muscle remodeling in resistance training reflects a complex process of cell receptor interaction with different hormones and DNA-mediated production of new contractile proteins. The specific response to muscular overload initially

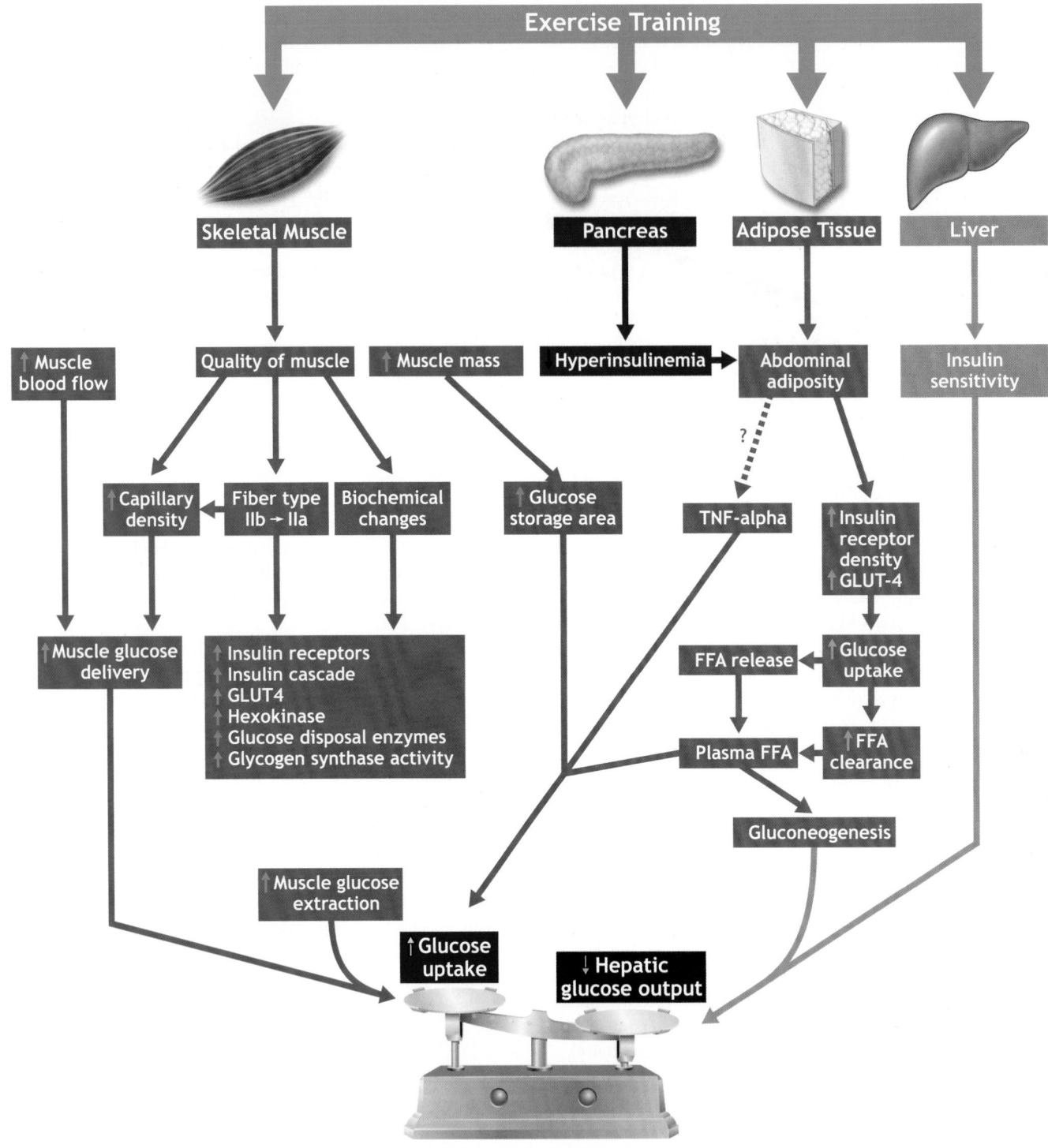

FIGURE 20.23 • Possible mechanisms of how regular physical activity improves insulin action and blood glucose homeostasis in type 2 diabetes. *TNF-alpha*, tumor necrosis factor-alpha, a hormonelike substance released from active adipocytes in the abdominal region, which may depress insulin-regulated glucose transport. (Adapted with permission from Ivy JL, et al. Prevention and treatment of noninsulin-dependent diabetes mellitus. *Exerc Sport Sci Rev* 1999;27:1.)

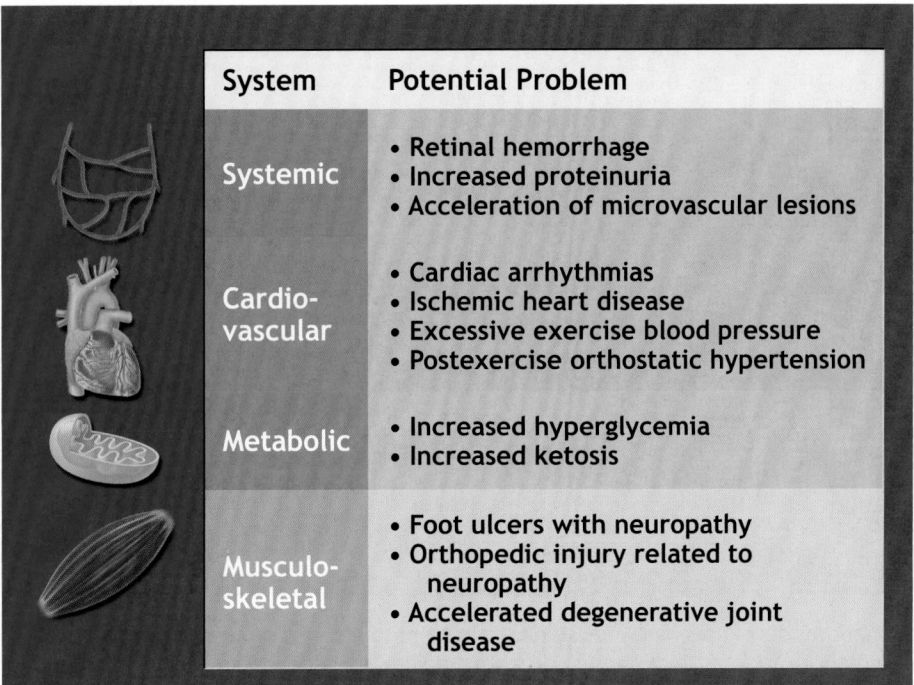

System	Potential Problem
Systemic	• Retinal hemorrhage • Increased proteinuria • Acceleration of microvascular lesions
Cardio-vascular	• Cardiac arrhythmias • Ischemic heart disease • Excessive exercise blood pressure • Postexercise orthostatic hypertension
Metabolic	• Increased hyperglycemia • Increased ketosis
Musculo-skeletal	• Foot ulcers with neuropathy • Orthopedic injury related to neuropathy • Accelerated degenerative joint disease

FIGURE 20.24 • Twelve potential physical and physiologic problems and problem areas faced by type 2 diabetics who begin a physical activity program.

links to configuration of the exercise stimulus—intensity, frequency, volume, sequence, mode, and recovery interval. **FIGURE 20.25** proposes how heavy resistance training improves overall muscular size, strength, and power. Hormonal factors responsible for training-induced changes in muscle size and function include these three factors:

1. Changes in hepatic and extrahepatic hormone clearance rates
2. Differential rates of hormone secretion with accompanying fluid shifts around the receptor sites
3. Altered receptor-site activation via neurohumoral control

In general, early-phase adaptations to resistance training reflect a hormonal response that mediates neuromuscular system adaptations that improve muscle strength.

Testosterone and GH are two primary hormones that affect adaptations to resistance training.[157,191] Testosterone augments GH release and interacts with nervous system function to increase muscle force production. These roles may be more important than any direct anabolic effect of testosterone per se. A single session of resistance training generally elicits a short-term rise in serum testosterone and decrease in cortisol, with a greater response in men than women.[32,56,96] Concurrently, catecholamine release from the adrenal medulla increases with the acute stress of high-force and high-power exercise protocols.[19]

Resistance training in men increases frequency and amplitude of testosterone and GH secretion, thereby creating a favorable hormonal environment for muscular growth (hypertrophy). In contrast, most studies fail to demonstrate changes in testosterone and GH concentrations with training in females. Gender differences in hormone output with resistance training may ultimately explain variations in responsiveness of muscle strength and size to prolonged muscular overload.

Testosterone response to resistance exercise reveals several factors that increase its release. Most effective include intense activation of large-muscle groups with dead lifts, power cleans, and squats, and other forms of heavy resistance exercise (i.e., 85 to 95% 1-RM) or high-volume (total quantity) training with multiple sets and/or physical activity with less than 1-min rest intervals.[97] Long-term resistance training in men increases resting testosterone levels, which correlates with the pattern of strength improvement over time.[64]

OPIOID PEPTIDES AND PHYSICAL ACTIVITY

Scientists who studied the pain-relieving effects of opioid peptides such as morphine on brain function in the 1970s reported these substances exhibited neurotransmitter effects and targeted specific opioid brain receptor sites. With this finding came the realization that perhaps the brain itself produced endogenous opioid, mood-altering substances. Evidence for existence of endogenous substances with opiate-like behavior first emerged with the isolation and purification of two opioid pentapeptides, methionine and leucine enkephalin (Greek, meaning "in the brain"). These opioids form part of a larger propiocortin precursor molecule produced in the anterior pituitary. Other opioid substances include β-lipotropin, β-endorphin, and dynorphin (the most potent of the opioid peptides).

The various endogenous opioids exert widespread effects with a range in function from neurohormones to neurotransmitters. Endogenous opiates strongly inhibit hormonal release from

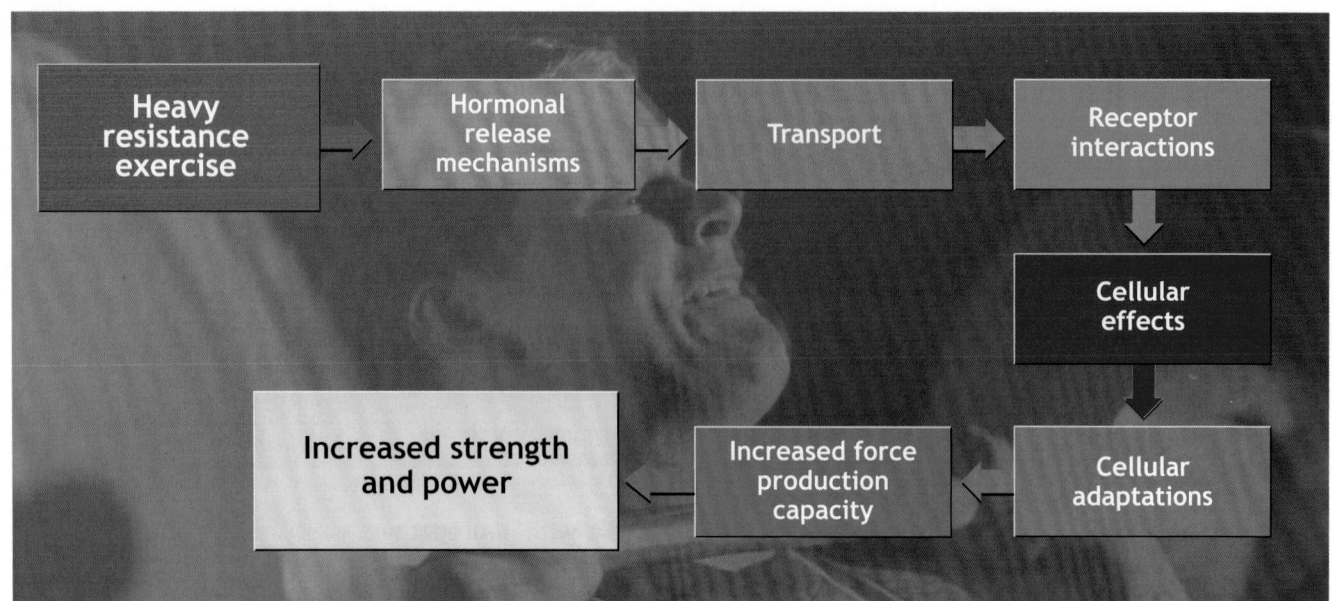

FIGURE 20.25 • Schematic model of how heavy resistance training produces favorable adaptations in muscle structure and maximal strength performance. (Adapted with permission from Kraemer WJ. Endocrine responses and adaptations to strength training. In: Komi PV, ed. *Strength and Power in Sport*. London: Blackwell Scientific, 1992.)

the anterior pituitary, principally LH and FSH release. This inhibition may play a key role in menstrual cycle disturbances observed among many physically active women—delay in menarche, dysfunctional uterine bleeding, secondary amenorrhea, and inadequacy of the luteal phase. In contrast to their inhibitory role, the opioid peptides stimulate GH and PRL release.

Endorphins also regulate other hormones including ACTH, the catecholamines, and cortisol. Serum concentrations of β-endorphin and/or β-lipotropin generally increase with physical activity similarly in men and women, although the response varies among individuals and varies inversely with activity intensity.[40,55,94] Physical activity increases β-endorphin up to five times the resting level and probably even more in the brain itself,[86] particularly region-specific effects in frontolimbic brain areas that are involved in the processing of affective states and mood.[12] With resistance exercise, β-endorphin release varies with the exercise protocol; longer duration (lighter resistance) and longer interset rest intervals elicit the greatest response.[95]

Evidence now links physical activity with decreases in mental depression, mediated through the endocannabinoid system's action on neurotrophins, such as **brain-derived neurotrophic factor** (**BDNF**). BDNF is considered a major candidate molecule for exercise-induced brain plasticity. Eleven healthy trained male cyclists intensely cycled for 60 min at 55% of maximum followed by 30 min at 75% maximum. Plasma levels of the endocannabinoids anandamide (AEA) and 2-arachidonoylglycerol (2-AG) were assessed and their possible link with serum BDNF evaluated. AEA levels increased during cycling and in 15 min of recovery, whereas 2-AG concentrations remained stable. BDNF levels increased significantly during cycling and then decreased during 15 min of recovery. Noteworthy, AEA and BDNF concentrations were positively correlated at the end of activity and after the 15-min recovery,

suggesting that AEA increases during exercise might be a factor involved in the exercise-induced increase in peripheral BDNF levels. AEA production during physical activity might be triggered by cortisol as positive correlations were observed between these two compounds and because corticosteroids are known to stimulate endocannabinoid biosynthesis. These findings provide evidence in humans that acute and strenuous physical activity presents a physiological stressor able to increase peripheral levels of AEA and that BDNF might be a mechanism by which AEA influences the neuroplastic and antidepressant effects of physical activity.[71]

The precise physiologic significance of the response of the various endogenous opioid peptides to physical activity remains unclear, but several noteworthy effects emerge. These include the postulated opioid effect in triggering the **exercise high**, a state described as euphoria and exhilaration, as the duration of moderate-to-intense aerobic activity increases. Endorphin secretion also may increase pain tolerance, improve appetite control, and reduce anxiety, tension, anger, and confusion. Interestingly, these effects generally reflect the documented psychologic benefits of regular physical activity.

The effect of training on endorphin response remains controversial. One study reported no significant change in β-endorphin response to prolonged effort following 8 wk of endurance training. Contrasting research showed that general physical conditioning augmented β-endorphin and β-lipotropin release in exercise.[22] Greater endorphin release also occurs with sprint-type training, suggesting that anaerobic factors also affect endorphin dynamics.[94]

Regular training can increase an individual's sensitivity to opioid effects, reducing the amount of hormone required to induce a specific effect. Regular physical activity causes the opioids produced during physical activity to degrade more slowly than in the pretraining condition. A slower rate of hormone disposal facilitates and prolongs an opioid response and possibly augments one's tolerance for extended physical activity. Taken in total, one could view the endogenous opioid response to regular physical activity as a form of "positive addiction."

 INTEGRATIVE QUESTION

List four supplements at your local health food store that claim to enhance exercise performance. Which supplements purport to stimulate hormone release? Based on hormonal regulation and function, explain whether these products can deliver on their claims.

PHYSICAL ACTIVITY, INFECTIOUS ILLNESS, CANCER, AND IMMUNE RESPONSE

"Don't exercise when fatigued or you'll get sick" reflects the common perception of parents, athletes, and coaches that excessive intense exercise increases susceptibility to certain illnesses. In contrast, some also believe that regular, more moderate physical activity improves health and reduces susceptibility to the common cold.

Studies as early as 1918 reported that most cases of pneumonia in boys in boarding school occurred among athletes, and respiratory infections seemed to progress toward pneumonia after intense sports training. Anecdotal reports also related the severity of poliomyelitis to participation in intense physical activity at the critical time of infection. Current epidemiologic and clinical findings from the field of **exercise immunology**— the study of the interactions of physical, environmental, and psychologic factors on immune function—support the contention that short-term, unusually strenuous physical activity affects immune function to increase susceptibility to illness, particularly upper respiratory tract infection (URTI). Repeated URTI may signal a state of overtraining (see Chapter 21).

The immune system comprises a highly complex and self-regulating grouping of cells, hormones, and interactive modulators that defend the body from invasion from outside microbes (bacterial, viral, and fungal), foreign macromolecules, and abnormal cancerous cell growth. This system has two functional divisions: (1) **innate immunity** and (2) **acquired immunity**. The innate immune system includes anatomic and physiologic components (skin, mucous membranes, body temperature, and specialized defenses such as natural killer cells, diverse phagocytes, and inflammatory barriers). The acquired immune system consists of specialized B- and T-lymphocyte cells. When activated these cells regulate a highly effective immune response to a specific infectious agent. If infection does occur, an optimal immune system diminishes the severity of illness and speeds recovery.

 See the animation "Immune Response" on http://thePoint.lww.com/mkk8e for a demonstration of this process.

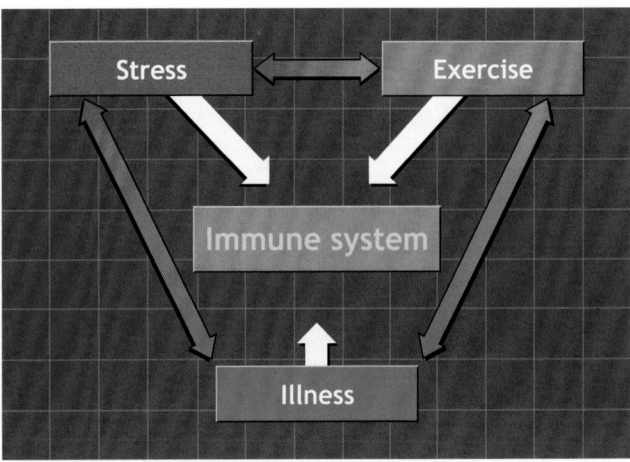

FIGURE 20.26 • Theoretical model of the interrelationships among stress, physical activity, illness, and the immune system. (Adapted with permission from MacKinnon LT. Current challenges and future expectations in exercise immunology: back to the future. *Med Sci Sports Exerc* 1994;26:191.)

FIGURE 20.26 proposes a theoretical model for the interactions of exercise, stress, illness, and the immune system. Within this framework, physical activity, stress, and illness interact, each exerting its separate effect on immunity. For example, physical activity affects susceptibility to illness, while certain illnesses clearly affect exercise capacity. Likewise, psychologic factors (via links between the hypothalamus and immune function) and other forms of stress, including nutritional deficiencies and acute alterations in normal sleep schedule, influence resistance to illness. Concurrently, physical activity can either positively or negatively modulate the response to stress. Each factor— stress, illness, and short- and long-term physical activity —exerts an independent effect on immune status, immune function, and resistance to disease.

Upper Respiratory Tract Infections

FIGURE 20.27 describes the general J-shaped curve relating exercise volume and/or intensity and risk to URTI.[54] Different immune function markers generally follow an *inverted J-shaped curve*.[139,200] Implications drawn from this relationship may be simplistic, but light to moderate physical activity offers more protection against URTI and possibly diverse cancers than a sedentary lifestyle.[110,114,160] Moderate physical activity does not exacerbate the severity and duration of illness when an infection occurs.[186] In contrast, a marathon run or intense training session provides an *"open window"* (3 to 72 hr) that decreases antiviral and antibacterial resistance and increases risk of URTI that manifests itself within 1 to 2 wk,[31,130] particularly for athletes prone to illness.[28] Approximately 13% of the participants in a Los Angeles marathon reported an episode of infectious URTI during the week following the race. For runners of comparable ability who did not compete for reasons other than illness, the infection rate approximated just 2%.[131]

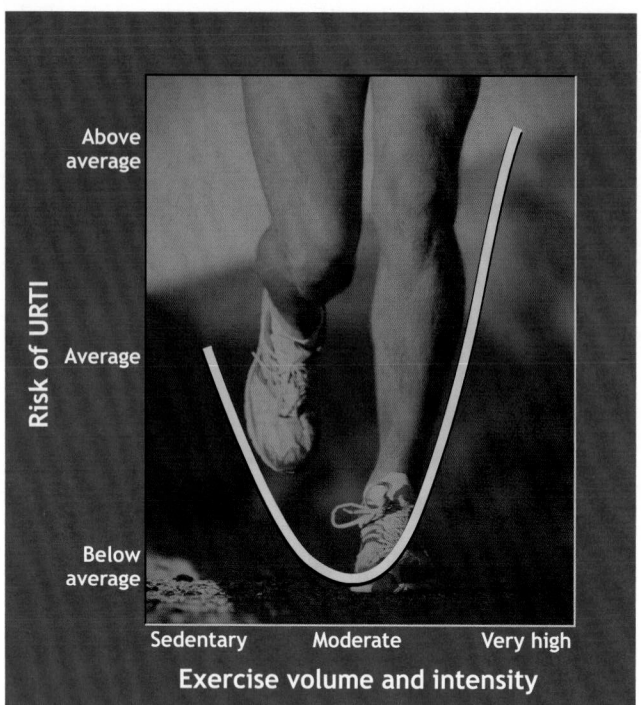

FIGURE 20.27 • General model showing the relationship between intensity of physical activity and susceptibility to upper respiratory tract infection (URTI). Moderate exercise reduces risk of URTI, whereas exhaustive competition or training places the participant at increased risk. (Adapted from Nieman DC. Exercise, upper respiratory tract infection, and the immune system. *Med Sci Sports Exerc* 1994;26:128.)

Short-Term Physical Activity Effects

Moderate activity. *Moderate physical activity boosts natural immune functions and host defenses for up to several hours.*[51] Noteworthy effects include increases in natural killer (NK) cell activity. These phagocytic lymphocyte subpopulations enhance the blood's cytotoxic capacity and provide the first line of defense against pathogens. The NK cell does not require prior or specific sensitization to foreign bodies or neoplastic cells. Rather, these cells demonstrate spontaneous cytolytic activity that ultimately ruptures and/or inactivates viruses and depresses the metastatic potential of tumor cells.

Exhaustive activity. *Prolonged exhaustive physical activity (and other forms of extreme stress or increased training) severely depresses the body's first line of defense against infection.*[92,106,128,142,188] Repeated cycles of unusually intense activity and sports participation further compound the risk.[198] Impaired immune function from strenuous exertion "carries over" to a second bout of exercise on the same day to augment negative changes in neutrophils, lymphocytes, and select CD cells.[153] Elevated temperature, cytokines, and various stress-related hormones (epinephrine, GH, cortisol, β-endorphins) in exhaustive effort may mediate the transient depression of innate (NK cell and neutrophil cytotoxicity) and depress adaptive immune defenses (T- and β-cell function).[168,174] Reduced immunity following strenuous physical activity remains in the mucosal immune system of the upper respiratory tract[53,125,183] and associates with increased URTI risk.[129] This negative effect on immune response clearly supports advising individuals with URTI symptoms to refrain from physical activity (or at least "go easy") to optimize normal immune mechanisms that combat infection. TABLE 20.7 summarizes components of the immune system that exhibit transient changes after prolonged intense exertion.

Long-Term Exercise Effects

Aerobic training positively affects natural immune functions in young and old individuals and obese persons during weight loss.[43,45,165] Areas of improvement include enhanced functional capacity of natural cytotoxic immune mechanisms (e.g., antitumor actions of NK cell activity) and diminished age-related decrease in T-cell function and associated cytokine production.[86] The cytotoxic T cells defend directly against viral and fungal infections and help regulate other immune mechanisms.

If exercise training enhances immune function, one might ask why trained individuals show increased susceptibility to

TABLE 20.7 — Immune System Components that Exhibit Negative Change after Prolonged, Intense Exercise

- High neutrophil and low lymphocyte blood counts, induced by high concentrations of plasma cortisol
- Increase in blood granulocyte and monocyte phagocytosis (engulfing of infectious agents and of breakdown products of muscle fiber); decrease in nasal neutrophil phagocytosis
- Decrease in granulocyte oxidative-burst activity (killing activity)
- Decrease in nasal mucociliary clearance (sweeping movement of cilia)
- Decrease in NK-cell cytotoxic activity (the ability to kill infected cells or cancer cells)
- Decrease in mitogen-induced lymphocyte proliferation (a measure of T-cell function)
- Decrease in the delayed-type hypersensitivity skin response (the ability of the immune system to produce hard red lumps after the skin is pricked with antigens)
- Increase in plasma concentrations of pro- and anti-inflammatory cytokines (e.g., interleukin-6 and interleukin-1 receptor antagonist)
- Decrease in *ex vivo* production of cytokines (interferon-8, interleukin-1, and interleukin-6) to mitogens and endotoxin
- Decrease in nasal and salivary IgA concentration (an important antibody)
- Blunted expression of major histocompatibility complex (MHC) II in macrophages (an important step in recognition of foreign agents by the immune system)

Source: Nieman DC. Immunity in athletes: current issues. *Sports Sci Exchange* 1998;11(2).

URTI after intense competition. The **open window hypothesis** maintains that an inordinate increase in training or competition exposes highly conditioned athletes to abnormal stress that transiently but severely depresses NK cell function. This period of immunodepression (open window) decreases natural resistance to infection. The inhibitory effect of strenuous physical activity on ACTH and cortisol's maintenance of optimal blood glucose concentrations may negatively affect the immune process. For individuals who are physically active regularly but *only* at moderate levels, the window of opportunity for infection remains "closed," thus maintaining the protective benefits of regular physical activity on immune function.

Resistance Training.

Nine years of prior resistance training did not affect resting NK cell activity or number compared to sedentary controls.[132] Comparisons also indicated that resistance training activated monocytes more than typically observed for aerobic training. Monocyte activation releases prostaglandins that down-regulate NK cells following physical activity, blunting the long-term positive effect of physical activity on NK cells. These researchers had previously reported a 225% increase in NK cells following a short-term bout of resistance exercise,[133] a response similar to the short-term effect of moderate aerobic activity.[47,184]

Perhaps a Role for Nutritional Supplements.

Nutrition may optimize immune system function with strenuous physical activity and training.[52,70,116,155]

Macronutrients. Consuming a high-fat diet (62% energy from lipids) negatively affected the immune system compared to a carbohydrate-rich diet (65% energy from carbohydrates). In general, endurance athletes who ingest carbohydrate during a race or prolonged trial experience lower disruption in hormonal and immune measures (indicating a diminished level of physiologic stress) than athletes not consuming carbohydrate.[156] Supplementing with a 6% carbohydrate beverage (0.71 L before; 0.25 L every 15 min during; 500 mL every hr throughout a 4.5-hr recovery) depressed cytokine levels in the inflammatory cascade after 2.5 hr of running at 77% $\dot{V}O_{2max}$.[127] Consuming carbohydrates (4 mL per kg of body mass) every 15 min during 2.5 hr of high-intensity running or cycling maintained higher plasma glucose levels in 10 triathletes during exercise than a placebo.[135] A blunted cortisol response and diminished pro- and anti-inflammatory cytokine responses accompanied the higher plasma glucose levels with supplementation in both forms of exercise. Similar benefits from carbohydrate ingestion for cortisol and select anti-inflammatory cytokines occur following marathon competition, regardless of age or gender.[136] *This suggests a carbohydrate-induced reduction in overall physiologic stress in prolonged intense physical activity.* In contrast, carbohydrate ingestion during 2 hr of intense resistance training produced no effect on immune changes compared to similar training with placebo ingestion.[137]

Micronutrients. Combined supplementation with antioxidant vitamins C and E produces more prominent immunopotentiating effects (enhanced cytokine production) in young, healthy adults than supplementation with either vitamin alone.[83] Also, a 200-mg daily vitamin E supplement enhanced several clinically relevant indices of T-cell–mediated function in healthy elderly subjects.[117] Long-term daily supplementation with a physiologic dose of vitamins and minerals or with 200 mg of vitamin E *did not lower* the incidence and severity of acute respiratory tract infections in noninstitutionalized persons aged 60 and older. For individuals with infections, those receiving vitamin E had *longer* total illness duration and restriction of activity.[57]

Daily supplementation with vitamin C benefits individuals engaged in intense physical activity, particularly those predisposed to frequent URTI.[68,143] Runners who received a 600-mg daily vitamin C supplement before and for 3 wk following a 90-km ultramarathon competition experienced fewer symptoms of URTI—running nose, sneezing, sore throat, coughing, fever—than runners given a placebo. Interestingly, infection risk inversely related to race performance; those with the fastest times suffered more symptoms. URTI also appeared most frequently in runners with strenuous training regimens. For these individuals, additional vitamin C and E and perhaps carbohydrate ingestion before, during, and after prolonged stressful exertion may boost immune mechanisms for combating this type of infection.[134] More than likely, other stressors—sleep deficit, mental stress, poor nutrition, or weight loss—magnify stress on the immune system from a single or repeated bout of exhaustive physical activity.

Glutamine and the Immune Response. The nonessential amino acid glutamine plays an important role in normal immune function. One protective aspect concerns glutamine's role as an energy fuel for nucleotide synthesis by disease-fighting cells, particularly lymphocytes and macrophages that defend against infection.[21,161,182] In humans, sepsis, injury, burns, surgery, and endurance exercise lower plasma and skeletal muscle glutamine levels. Lowered plasma glutamine levels most likely occur because glutamine demand by the liver, kidneys, gut, and immune system exceeds its supply from the diet and skeletal muscle. The lowered plasma glutamine concentration may contribute to the immunosuppression that accompanies extreme physical stress.[11,72,164] Glutamine supplementation might reduce susceptibility to URTI following prolonged competition or a bout of exhaustive training.

Marathoners who ingested a glutamine drink (5 g L-glutamine in 330 mL mineral water) at the end of a race and then 2 hr later reported fewer URTI symptoms than unsupplemented athletes.[23] In subsequent studies by the same researchers to determine a possible protective mechanism, glutamine's effect on postexercise infection risk did not relate to any change in blood lymphocyte distribution.[24] Appearance of URTI in athletes during intense training does not fluctuate with changes in plasma glutamine concentration. Pre-exercise glutamine supplementation does not affect the immune response following repeated bouts of intense physical activity.[102] Glutamine supplements taken 0, 30, 60, and 90 min after a marathon race prevented the drop in glutamine concentrations following the race but *did not influence* lymphokine-activated killer cell activity, proliferative responses, or exercise-induced changes in leukocyte subpopulations.[150] Based on current evidence, we cannot recommend glutamine supplements to reliably blunt immunosuppression from exhaustive activity.

A General Recommendation to Optimize Immunity

A lifestyle that emphasizes regular physical activity, maintenance of a well-balanced diet, reducing stress to a minimum, and obtaining adequate sleep generally optimizes immune function. For weight loss, we recommend a gradual approach because more rapid weight loss with accompanying severe caloric restriction suppresses immune function.[115] With prolonged intense activity, ingesting about $1 \text{ L} \cdot \text{hr}^{-1}$ of a typical carbohydrate-rich sports drink lessens negative changes in immune function from the stress of physical activity and accompanying carbohydrate depletion. In general, endurance athletes who consume carbohydrate during a race experience a lower disruption in hormonal and immune measures than athletes who do not consume carbohydrate.

The Physical Activity–Cancer Connection

Epidemiologic studies generally demonstrate a protective association between regular physical activity and risk of breast, colon, lung, and prostate cancers (see Chapter 31).[107,118] Long-term enhancement of other natural immune functions may contribute to the cancer-protective effect of regular physical activity in addition to its beneficial effect on NK cell activity. Upgraded defenses include augmented phagocytic capacity of the monocyte–macrophage lineage combined with more robust cytotoxic and intracellular killing capacities (T-cell activity) that inhibit tumor growth and destroy cancer cells.[199] Other potential effects of regular physical activity on aspects of cancer development include beneficial changes in the body's antioxidant functions; endocrine profiles; prostaglandin metabolism; body composition; and, in the case of colon cancer, a beneficial increase in intestinal transit time. A recent meta-analysis using seven prospective cohort studies that included more than 5000 patients concluded that regular physical activity significantly associated with reduced colorectal cancer-specific mortality and all-cause mortality.[81] In Chapter 31, we review the role of physical activity in the prevention and treatment of different cancers.

Summary

1. The endocrine system consists of a host organ, a transmitted substance (hormone), and a target or receptor organ. Hormones consist of steroids or amino acid (polypeptide) derivatives.

2. Hormones alter rates of cellular reactions by acting at specific receptor sites to enhance or inhibit enzyme function.

3. The amount of hormone synthesized, the amount released or taken up by the target organ, and the removal rate from the blood influence blood hormone concentration.

4. Most hormones respond to peripheral stimulus on an as-needed basis; others release at regular intervals. Some secretory cycles span several weeks; others pattern on a 24-hr cycle.

5. The anterior pituitary secretes at least six hormones: PRL, the gonadotropic hormones FSH and LH, corticotropin, TSH, and GH.

6. GH promotes cell division and cellular proliferation. IGFs (or somatomedins) mediate many of GH's effects.

7. TSH controls the amount of hormone secreted by the thyroid gland; ACTH regulates output of hormones from the adrenal cortex; PRL affects reproduction and development of secondary sex characteristics of females; FSH and LH stimulate the ovaries to secrete estrogen in females and the testes to secrete testosterone in males.

8. The posterior pituitary secretes ADH, which controls water excretion by the kidneys. It also secretes oxytocin, an important hormone in birthing and lactation.

9. PTH controls blood calcium balance. It increases ionic (free) calcium levels by stimulating three target organs: bone, kidneys, and the small intestine.

10. TSH stimulates metabolism of all cells and increases carbohydrate and fat breakdown in energy metabolism.

11. The medulla of the adrenal gland secretes epinephrine and norepinephrine. The adrenal cortex secretes mineralocorticoids (regulate extracellular sodium and potassium levels), glucocorticoids (stimulate gluconeogenesis and serve as insulin antagonists), and androgens (control male secondary sex characteristics).

12. Male testes produce testosterone and female ovaries produce the estrogens estradiol and progesterone.

13. Moderate aerobic and resistance exercise increases testosterone in untrained males; for females, plasma testosterone and estrogen levels increase during moderate physical activity.

14. Insulin increases glucose transport into cells to control blood glucose levels and carbohydrate metabolism.

15. Total lack of insulin or decreased sensitivity or increased resistance to this hormone produces diabetes mellitus.

16. The β-cells of the pancreas secrete glucagon, an insulin antagonist that raises blood sugar levels.

17. Regular physical activity exerts differential effects on resting and exercise-induced hormone production and release.

18. Trained persons have elevated hormone response during physical activity for ACTH and cortisol, and depressed values for GH, PRL, FSH, LH, testosterone, ADH, thyroxine, catecholamines, and insulin. No training response occurs for aldosterone, renin, and angiotensin.

19. Exercise-induced elevation of β-endorphins and other opioid-like hormones contributes to euphoria, increased pain tolerance, "exercise high," and altered menstrual function.

20. Unusually intense physical activity increases susceptibility to URTI. Moderate physical activity upgrades immune responses to protect against URTI.

21. Regular physical activity positively affects natural immune functions. An enhanced immune profile protects against URTI and various cancers.

thePoint References are available online at http://thepoint.lww.com/mkk8e.

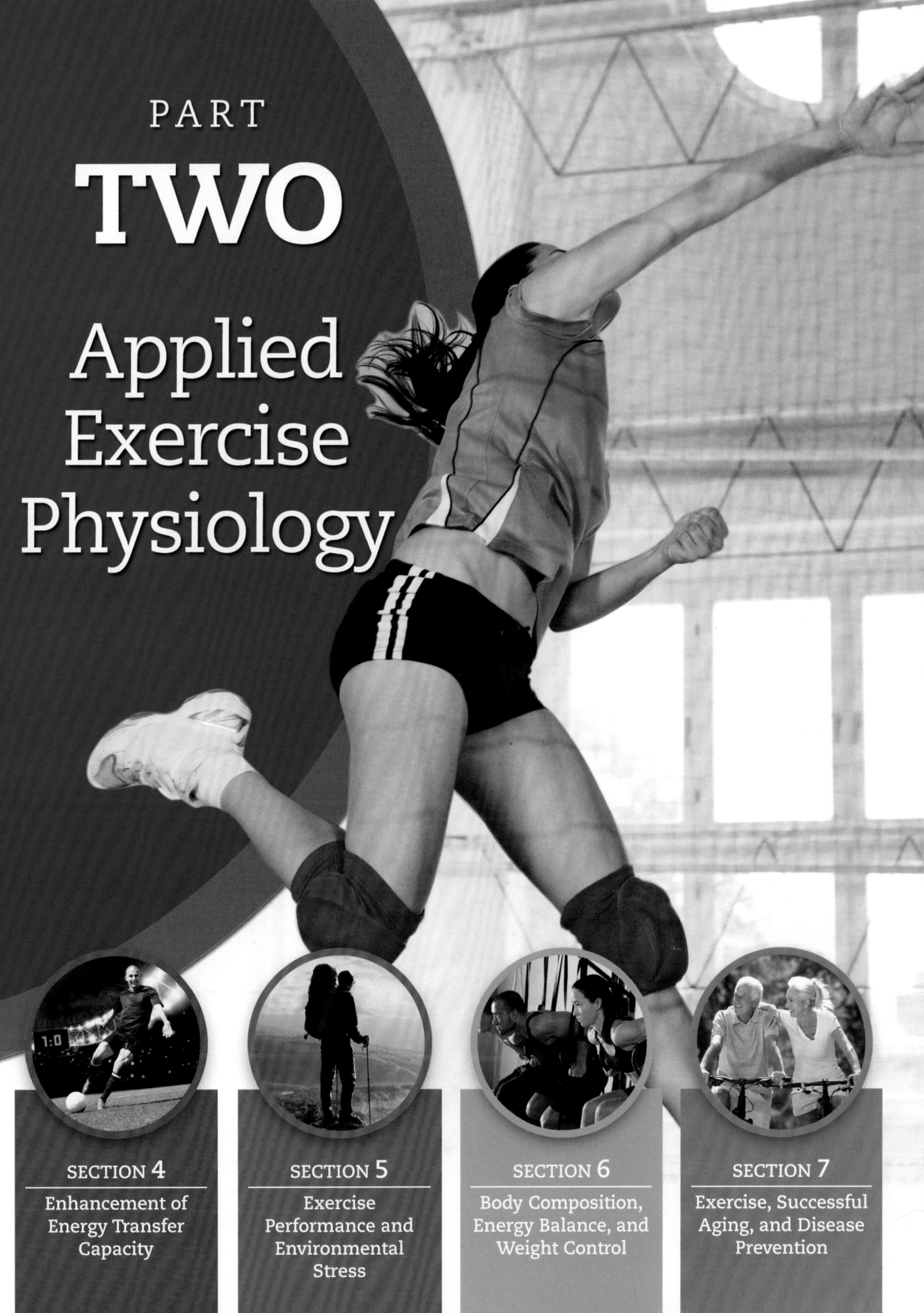

PART
TWO

Applied Exercise Physiology

SECTION 4

Enhancement of Energy Transfer Capacity

SECTION 5

Exercise Performance and Environmental Stress

SECTION 6

Body Composition, Energy Balance, and Weight Control

SECTION 7

Exercise, Successful Aging, and Disease Prevention

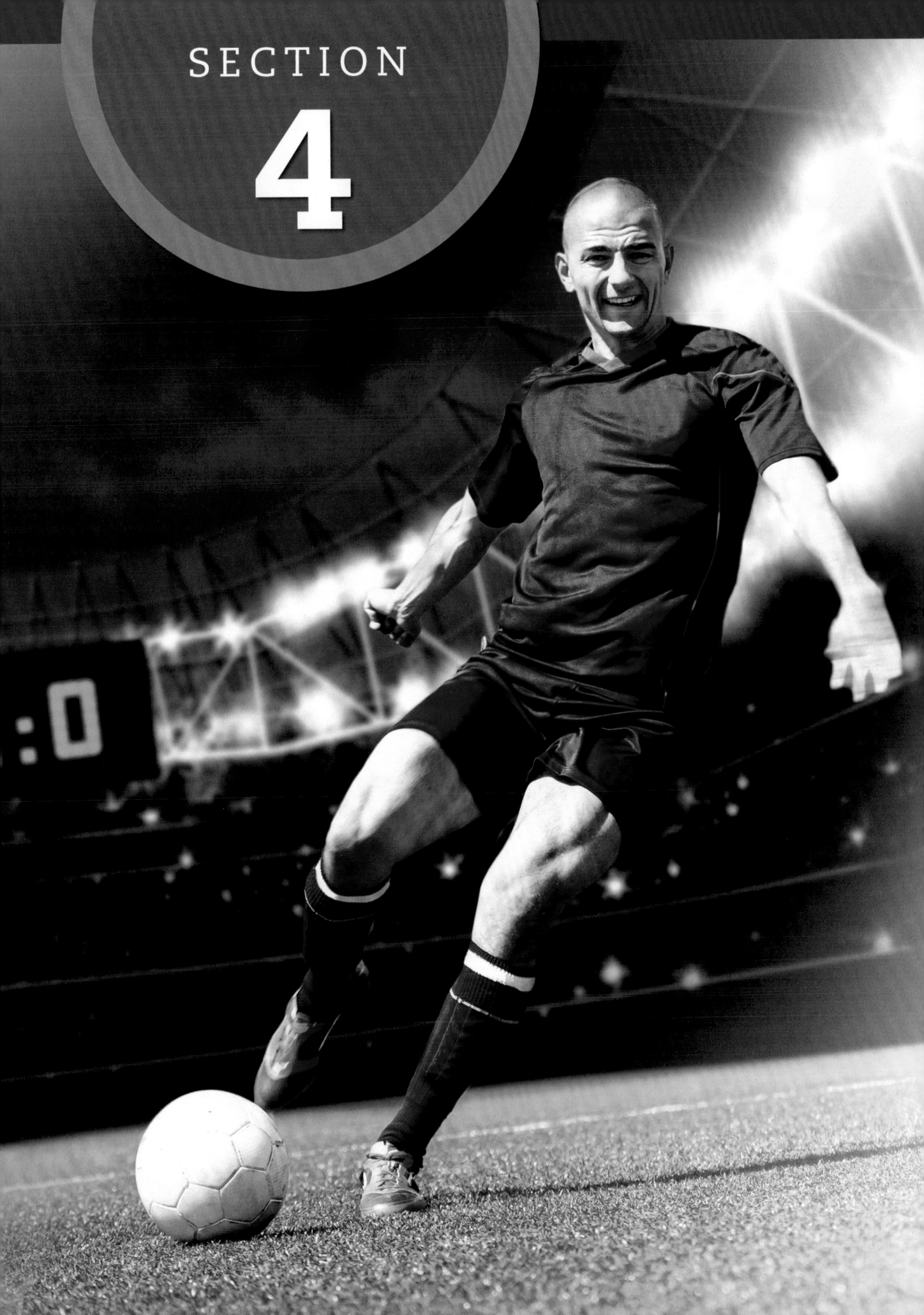

SECTION

4

Enhancement of Energy Transfer Capacity

OVERVIEW

Throughout this book, we emphasize that different physical activities, depending on duration and intensity, activate highly specific energy transfer systems. We acknowledge difficulty in placing certain activities into one category. For example, as a person increases aerobic fitness, an activity previously classified as anaerobic may become aerobic. In many cases, all three energy-transfer systems—adenosine triphosphate–phosphocreatine (ATP–PCr) system, lactic acid system, and aerobic system—operate predominantly at different times during physical activity, but each remains functional throughout the activity. Their relative contributions to the energy continuum directly relate to the duration and intensity (power output) of a specific activity.

Brief power activities for up to 6 s duration rely almost exclusively on "immediate" energy generated from the breakdown of stored intramuscular high-energy phosphates, ATP and PCr. Consequently, power athletes (e.g., sprinters, football players, shot putters, pole vaulters) must gear training toward improving this energy-transfer capacity. This includes the force-generating capacity of targeted muscles that power their sport. As all-out movement progresses to 60 s in duration and power output decreases, most of the energy for movement still arises through fast and slow anaerobic pathways. These metabolic reactions also involve the glycolytic short-term energy system with subsequent lactate accumulation. As exercise intensity diminishes and duration extends to 2 to 4 min, reliance on energy from the intramuscular phosphagens and anaerobic glycolysis decreases, making aerobic ATP production increasingly more important. As prolonged exercise duration increases, aerobic metabolism generates more than 99% of the total energy requirement. Clearly, an efficient training program allocates a proportionate commitment to targeted training of specific energy and physiologic systems activated in the activity. The chapters in this section discuss anaerobic and aerobic conditioning (Chapter 21), including procedures for training muscles to become stronger (Chapter 22), with emphasis on principles, methods, and short-term responses and longer-term training adaptations. In the final chapter (Chapter 23), we explore the safety and efficacy of diverse chemical, nutritional, and physiologic aids to enhance exercise training and physical performance.

INTERVIEW WITH
Bengt Saltin

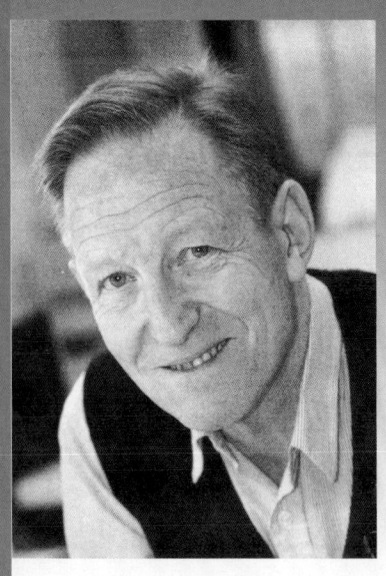

Education: Södertälje Gymnasium (1955); Medical School, Karolinska Institute, Stockholm (1956–62); Thesis in physiology, Karolinksa Institute, Stockholm (1964)

Current Affiliation: Director, Copenhagen Muscle Research Centre at Rigshospitalet and the University of Copenhagen; Adjunct Professor, August Krogh Institute, University of Copenhagen

Honors, Awards, and ACSM Honor Award Statement of Contributions: See Appendix C, available online at http://thepoint.lww.com/mkk8e

Research Focus: Exploration of integrative cardiovascular and metabolic response to physical exercise, including studies on skeletal muscle in humans by direct needle biopsy.

Memorable Publication: Saltin B, et al. Response to exercise after bed rest and after training: a longitudinal study of adaptive changes in oxygen transport and body composition. *Circulation* 1968;38(suppl 7):79.

➤ *What first inspired you to enter the exercise science field? What made you decide to pursue your advanced degree and/or line of research?*

In January 1958, I had my oral examination in physiology as part of my medical studies. The examiner was Professor Ulf von Euler 🔵 (later winning the 1970 Nobel Prize in Physiology or Medicine for discoveries concerning humoral transmitters in the nerve terminal and the mechanisms for their storage, release, and inactivation). At the end of the examination I was asked whether I would be interested in staying on as a student instructor. My answer was yes. As I had an interest in orienteering (a common sport in Scandinavia), I wanted to be associated with exercise-related research. Professor Euler called Erik Hohwü-Christensen, who was the professor of physiology at the Royal School of Gymnastics. The week after I met with Professor Hohwü-Christensen in the summer of 1958, I started to work with him on a project that evaluated energy demands in intermittent exercise. During the semesters, I helped with teaching while at the same time continuing my medical studies. In the fall of 1961, I decided to go for a doctoral thesis in physiology, which I defended in May 1964.

➤ *Who were the most influential people in your career, and why?*

Two people played a very important role in my scientific career. I would like to acknowledge Professor Erik Hohwü-Christensen and Professor Per-Olof Åstrand. Professor Hohwü-Christensen had been a student of Johannes Lindhard, the first Docent of the equivalent of an endowed Chair in Anatomy, Physiology, and Theory of Gymnastics at the University of Copenhagen, and had also done cooperative research with 1920 Nobel Prize winner August Krogh 🔵. Professor Per-Olof Åstrand at the Karolinska Institute was the equivalent of my PhD dissertation research advisor. My projects were concerned with trying to better understand maximal oxygen uptake in human subjects and its determinants under different

physiological and pathophysiological conditions, particularly thermal stress and dehydration. The knowledge and passion of these two pioneer scientists encouraged a younger generation of researchers-to-be to focus on human integrative physiology.

➤ *What has been the most interesting/enjoyable aspect of your involvement in science? What was the least interesting/enjoyable aspect?*

This is a difficult question to answer. I have been very fortunate to work with many scientists from all over the world. For example, in 1965, I spent 1 year in the Department of Medicine at the University of Texas in Dallas. Later, I worked for 5 months at the John B. Pierce Institute and Department of Physiology at Yale University. In 1972, I spent 2 months in the Department of Medicine at the University of California, San Francisco, and then in 1976, I spent 3 months working with David Costill in the Human Performance Laboratory at Ball State University. I also spent 4 months at Cumberland College and the Department of Physiology at New South Wales University in Sydney, Australia. For my interest in high-altitude physiology and temperature regulation, I was fortunate to spend from 1 to 5 months between the years of 1960 and 1989 in laboratories in northern Norway studying the physical profile and health of Nomadic Lapps, and at the following locations studying high-altitude physiology: Mt. Evans (Colorado), Mexico City, the Andes and Himalayan mountains, and Kenya. I also had a wonderful experience studying the physiological responses to exercise in racing camels in the Arabian desert.

➤ *What is your most meaningful contribution to the field of exercise science, and why is it so important?*

To try to better understand, not only to describe, basic phenomena concerned with physiological responses to exercise under various environmental conditions. Exercise science was a key area in science in the latter part of the 19th century and in the first three decades of the 20th century. There are many reasons for the lack of major contributions since then. One reason could be that the majority of exercise scientists describe a phenomenon, but they do not try hard enough to penetrate the mechanisms and thereby contribute to the fundamental understanding of the phenomenon.

> ### ➤ What advice would you give to students who express an interest in pursuing a career in exercise science research?

Become very focused and learn basic techniques. Today, exercise science is to a large extent the study of acute and chronic adaptations. Thus, one route I would highlight is to identify the exercise stimulus and the intracellular signaling of genes of importance for muscle adaptation. In an article in *Scientific American* (September 2000), we pointed out that Olympic athletes depend on how well their muscles adapt to the stress of high-intensity aerobic, anaerobic, and resistance training. However, recent research suggests that the ratio of fast- to slow-twitch muscle fibers depends on inherited characteristics. Unfortunately, future genetic technologies could change even that as athletes experiment with methods to enhance muscle performance.

> ### ➤ What interests have you pursued outside your professional career?

I have been heavily involved in the sport of orienteering, both as a runner and administrator. From 1982 to 1988, I served as a Board Member and President of the International Orienteering Federation. I am a theater freak and have an interest in literature. Ibsen and Strindberg are my favorites, but most classical plays from antique Greece onward will bring me to the theater. Throughout life my "reading companions" have been Katherine Mansfield, Albert Camus, Joseph Brodsky, and to name a Dane, J. P. Jacobsen.

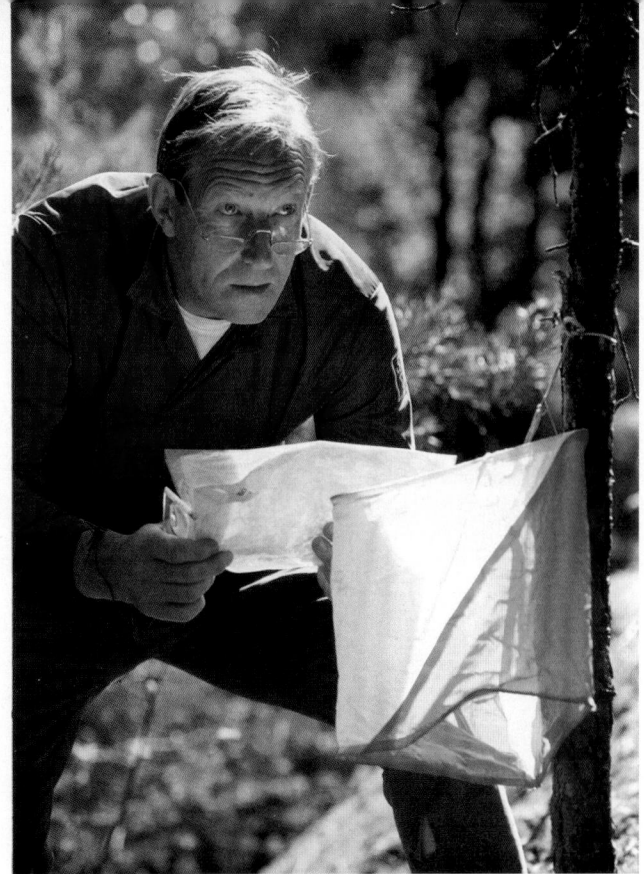

> ### ➤ You have the opportunity to give a last lecture. Describe its primary focus.

I have given my "last" lecture. It focused on how young exercise physiologists could best serve an area in research and also make a major contribution to science. A major point was to identify an important phenomenon. If there are ample methods to study it, then stay with it until it has been solved. In other words, be mechanistic, carefully explain the phenomena, and then do whatever you can to understand it.

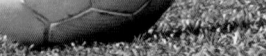

CHAPTER

21

Training for Anaerobic and Aerobic Power

CHAPTER OBJECTIVES

- Discuss and provide examples of the exercise training principles of overload, specificity, individual differences, and reversibility

- Outline the metabolic adaptations to anaerobic exercise training

- Outline the metabolic, cardiovascular, and pulmonary adaptations to aerobic exercise training

- Discuss factors that expand the a-$\bar{v}O_2$ difference during graded exercise, and how endurance training affects each component

- Explain the effects of endurance training on regional blood flow

- Explain the term *athlete's heart*; contrast structural and functional characteristics of the heart of an endurance athlete versus a resistance-trained athlete

- Describe the influence of initial fitness level, genetics, training frequency, training duration, and training intensity on the aerobic training response

- Discuss the rationale for using heart rate to establish intensity for aerobic training

- Discuss the term *training-sensitive zone*, including its rationale, advantages, limitations, and applications for men and women of different ages

- Give the reason for adjusting the training-sensitive zone for swimming and other forms of upper-body physical activity

- Justify the "rating of perceived exertion" to establish intensity for aerobic activities

- Outline advantages of training at the lactate threshold

- Contrast continuous and intermittent aerobic training and advantages and disadvantages of each

- Summarize current recommendations by the American College of Sports Medicine concerning the quantity and quality of exercise to develop and maintain cardiorespiratory and muscular fitness and joint flexibility in healthy adults

- Outline applications of the overload principle to train the intramuscular high-energy phosphates and glycolytic energy system

- Summarize important factors about the exercise prescription for interval training

- Describe the most common form of overtraining syndrome and summarize interacting factors that contribute to overtraining in endurance athletes

- Summarize current recommendations for regular physical activity during pregnancy

ANCILLARIES ◉ *at-a-Glance*

Visit http://thePoint.lww.com/mkk8e to access the following resources.

- References: Chapter 21
- Appendix H: Supplemental Animations and Videos
- Interactive Question Bank
- Focus on Research: Highly Specific Nature of the Training Response

461

EXERCISE TRAINING PRINCIPLES

Stimulating structural and functional adaptations to improve performance in specific physical tasks remains a major objective of exercise training. These adaptations require adherence to carefully planned programs with focus on frequency and length of workouts; type of training; speed, intensity, duration, and repetition of the activity; rest intervals; and appropriate competition. Application of these factors varies depending on performance and fitness goals. *The basic approach to physiologic conditioning applies similarly to men and women within a broad age range; both respond and adapt to training in essentially similar ways.* FIGURE 21.1 illustrates the four energy-generating pathways and corresponding examples of physical performance related to each pathway; these comprise ATP (strength–power), ATP + PCr (sustained power), ATP + PC + lactic acid (anaerobic power–endurance), and electron transport-oxidative phosphorylation (aerobic endurance). The sections that follow discuss the principles of physiologic conditioning common to improving performance related to these activity classifications.

Overload Principle

Regular application of a specific exercise overload enhances physiologic function to induce a training response. Exercising at intensities greater than normal stimulates highly specific adaptations so the body functions more efficiently. *Achieving the appropriate overload requires either manipulating training frequency, intensity, and duration, or a combination of these factors.*

The concept of individualized and progressive overload applies to athletes, sedentary persons, disabled persons, and even cardiac patients. An increasing number in this latter group have applied appropriate exercise rehabilitation to walk, jog, and eventually run and compete in marathons and triathlons. As we discuss in Chapter 31, achieving health-related benefits of regular physical activity requires lower effort intensity (but greater volume) than required to only improve maximum aerobic fitness.[112,131,214]

Specificity Principle

Exercise training specificity refers to adaptations in metabolic and physiologic functions that depend on the intensity, duration, frequency, and mode of overload imposed. A specific intense overload of short duration (e.g., strength–power training) induces specific strength–power adaptations; specific endurance training elicits specific aerobic system adaptations—with only limited interchange of benefits between strength–power training and aerobic training. Nonetheless, the specificity principle extends beyond this broad demarcation. Aerobic training, for example, does not represent a singular entity that requires only cardiovascular overload. Aerobic training that relies on specific muscles in the desired performance most effectively improves aerobic fitness for swimming,[58] bicycling,[159] running,[135] or upper-body activities.[117] Some evidence even suggests a temporal specificity in training response such that indicators of training improvement peak when measured at the time of day when training regularly occurred.[84] Task-specific training that involves practicing the actual motor skill of avoiding a fall after loss of balance may positively affect biomechanical variables that prove effective among older individuals in

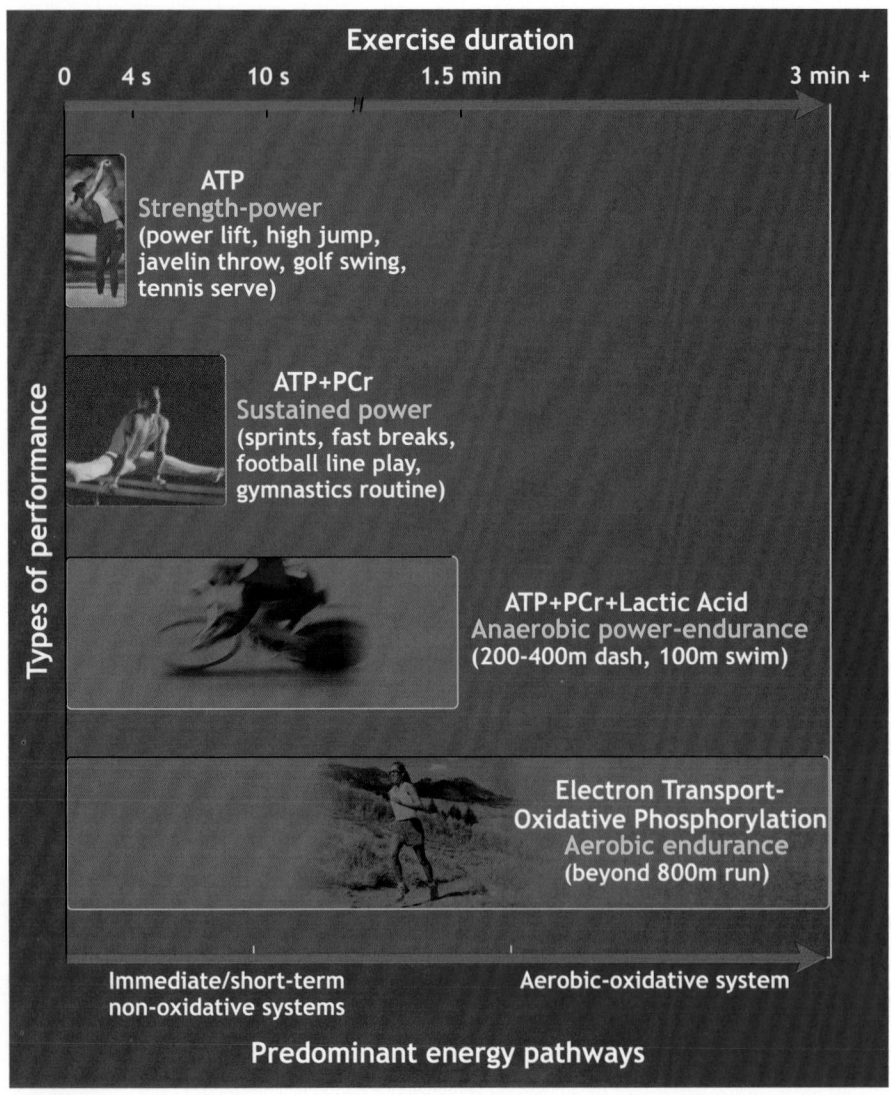

FIGURE 21.1 • Classification of physical activity based on duration of all-out effort and the corresponding predominant intracellular energy pathways.

avoiding a fall after a laboratory-induced trip.[65] The most effective evaluation of sport-specific performance occurs when the laboratory measurement most closely simulates the sport activity and/or uses the muscle mass and movement patterns required by the sport.[13,58,116] *Simply stated, specific exercise elicits specific adaptations to promote specific training effects that produce specific performance improvements.* Put in another easy-to-remember way: specificity refers to the **specific adaptations to imposed demands** (**SAID**) principle.

Specificity of $\dot{V}O_{2max}$

When training for specific aerobic activities such as cycling, swimming, rowing, or running, the overload must accomplish two objectives:

1. Engage the appropriate muscles required by the activity
2. Provide an intensity at a level sufficient to stress the cardiovascular system

Little improvement occurs when measuring aerobic capacity with dissimilar activities; the greatest improvement occurs when the test duplicates the training exercise. These results also apply in movement rehabilitation of patients with coronary artery disease.[152] Aerobic training induces a highly specific $\dot{V}O_{2max}$ improvement, whereas more general improvements take place in cardiac function. Ventricular contractility, for example, that improves with one mode of training also improves when exercising the untrained limbs.[216] Individuals apparently can train the myocardium per se with diverse "big-muscle" activity modes.

Specificity of Local Changes

Overloading specific muscle groups with endurance training enhances performance *and* aerobic power by facilitating oxygen transport and oxygen use at the local level of the trained muscles.[85,127] For example, the vastus lateralis muscle

 An Example of Aerobic Training Specificity

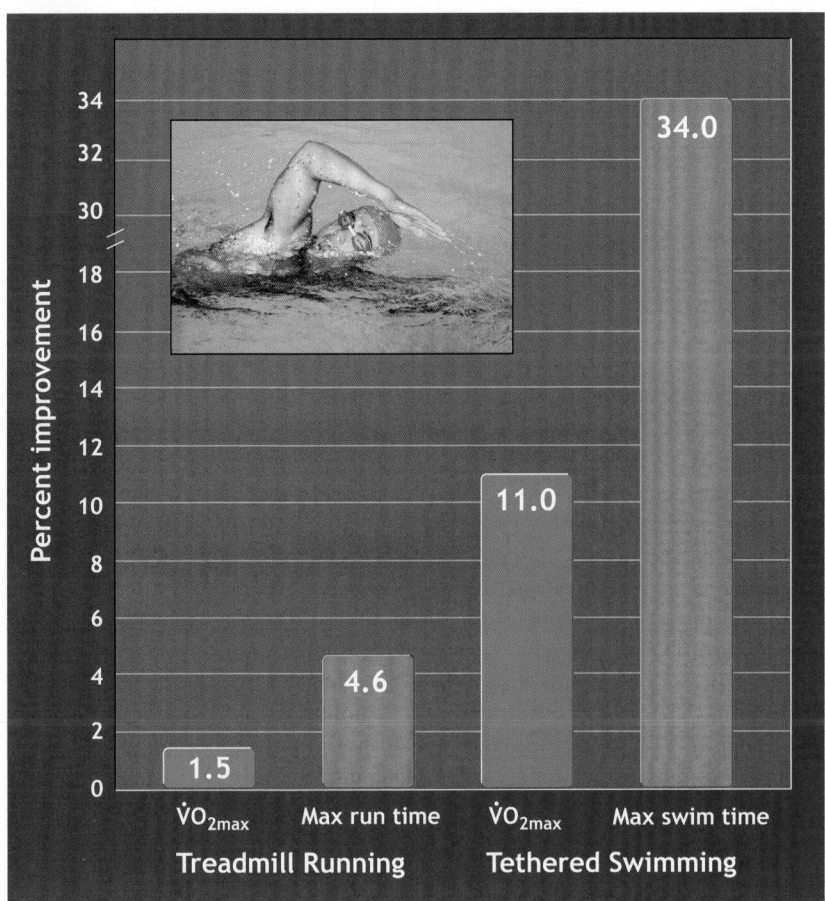

In an experiment in one of our laboratories on aerobic training specificity, 15 men swam 1 hr a day, 3 days a week, for 10 wk at heart rates between 85% and 95% of maximum (HR_{max}). $\dot{V}O_{2max}$ was measured during treadmill running and tethered swimming before and after training. Because vigorous swim training overloads the central circulation as reflected by high heart rates, we anticipated at least some transfer in aerobic power improvements from swim training to running. This did not occur; an almost total specificity accompanied the $\dot{V}O_{2max}$ improvement with swim training.

The accompanying figure illustrates that swim training improved $\dot{V}O_{2max}$ by 11% when measured during swimming, but only by 1.5% when measured during running. If only treadmill running had been used to evaluate swim training effects, we would mistakenly have concluded that there was *no training effect.* For maximum performance during testing, subjects improved 34% in swim time to exhaustion but only 4.6% in run time on the treadmill test.

These findings and other research studies strongly indicate that training for specific aerobic activities must provide an appropriate general level of cardiovascular stress *and* overload the *specific muscles* in a specific way required by the activity. Little improvement results when a dissimilar activity measures aerobic capacity or exercise performance. In contrast, considerable improvements emerge when the specific training mode evaluates the aerobic adaptations to training.

(Adapted with permission from Katch VL, McArdle WD, Katch FI, *Essentials of Exercise Physiology*. 4th Ed. Philadelphia: Wolters Kluwer Health, 2011.)

of well-trained cyclists has greater oxidative capacity than endurance runners; oxidative capacity in this muscle improves considerably following training on a bicycle ergometer. Such local metabolic adaptations increase the capacity of trained muscles to generate ATP aerobically before lactate accumulation onset. The specificity of aerobic improvement also may result from greater regional blood flow in active tissues from three factors:

1. Increased microcirculation
2. More effective redistribution of cardiac output
3. The combined effect of both factors

Regardless of the mechanism, these adaptations occur only in specifically trained muscles and *only* become apparent in physical activity that activates this musculature.

Individual Differences Principle

All individuals do not respond similarly to a given training stimulus. For example, a person's relative fitness level at the start of training exerts an influence. This subprinciple of **initial values** reveals that individuals with lower fitness deliver the greatest training improvement. This principle operates for healthy individuals as well as those with cardiovascular disease or at high risk for the disease.[19,176,236] When a relatively homogenous group begins a training regimen, one cannot expect each person to achieve the same state of fitness or exercise performance after only 10 or 12 wk. A coach should not insist that all athletes on the same team or even in the same event train the same way or at the same relative or absolute intensity of effort. *Optimal training benefits occur when exercise programs focus on the individual needs and capacities of participants.* Chapter 11 and the "Trainability and Genes" section of this chapter emphasize that genetic factors interact to impact the training response.

Reversibility Principle

Loss of physiologic and performance adaptations, termed *detraining*, occurs rapidly when a person terminates participation in regular physical activity. Only 1 or 2 wk of detraining reduces both metabolic and exercise capacity, with many training improvements fully lost within several months.[147] TABLE 21.1 shows the biologic consequences of various durations of short-term (<3 wk) and longer-term (3–12 wk) detraining in endurance-trained individuals. The data represent average responses reported in the literature. One research group confined five subjects to bed for 20 consecutive days.[191] VO_{2max} decreased by 25%. This decrease accompanied a similar decrement in maximal stroke volume and cardiac output, which decreased maximal aerobic power an average of 1% per day. Additionally, the number of capillaries within trained muscle decreased between 14 and 25% within 3 wk immediately following training.[190] For elderly subjects, 4 mo of detraining completely negated endurance training adaptations on cardiovascular functions and body water distribution.[165]

Among highly trained athletes, even the beneficial effects of many years of prior training remain transient and reversible. For this reason, most athletes begin a reconditioning program several months prior to the start of the competitive season, or at a minimum, maintain some moderate level of off-season, sport-specific training to slow the consequences of detraining.

HOW EXERCISE TRAINING IMPACTS THE ANAEROBIC SYSTEM

The following sections present a detailed listing of the diverse adaptations to anaerobic and aerobic exercise training responses outlined in TABLE 21.2.

ANAEROBIC SYSTEM CHANGES WITH TRAINING

FIGURE 21.2 summarizes responses for metabolic adaptations in anaerobic function that accompany anaerobic training. Consistent with the concept of training specificity, activities that demand a high level of anaerobic metabolism induce specific changes in the immediate and short-term energy systems with little concomitant increases in aerobic functions. Three important changes occur with anaerobic power training:

1. *Increased levels of anaerobic substrates.* Muscle biopsy specimens taken before and after resistance training (TABLE 21.3) show increases in the trained muscle's resting levels of ATP, PCr, free creatine, and glycogen, accompanied by a 28% improvement in muscular strength. Other studies have shown higher levels of ATP and total creatine content in trained muscles of sprint runners and track speed cyclists compared to distance runners and road racers.[151] Speed–power training also increases PCr content of the trained skeletal muscle.
2. *Increased quantity and activity of key enzymes that control the anaerobic (glycolytic) phase of glucose catabolism.* These changes do not achieve the magnitude for oxidative enzymes with aerobic training. The most dramatic increases in anaerobic enzyme function and fiber size occur in fast-twitch muscle fibers.
3. *Increased capacity to generate and tolerate high levels of blood lactate during all-out effort.* This adaptation probably results from (a) increased levels of glycogen and glycolytic enzymes and (b) improved motivation and tolerance to "pain" in fatiguing physical activity. Research has not yet demonstrated that training augments buffering capacity mechanisms. Motivational factors probably improve training-induced tolerance to elevated plasma acidity.

HOW TRAINING IMPACTS THE AEROBIC SYSTEM

FIGURE 21.3 shows four categories of diverse physiologic and metabolic factors related to oxygen transport and use: ventilation-aeration, central blood flow, active muscle metabolism, and peripheral blood flow *With adequate training, the positive*

TABLE 21.1 **Changes in Measures of Physiologic and Metabolic Function with Various Durations of Detraining[a]**

Variable	Trained	Detrained	Change, % Short-Term Detraining[b]	Change, % Longer-Term Detraining[c]
$\dot{V}O_{2max}$, mL·kg⁻¹·min⁻¹	62.2	57.3	−8	
	62.1	50.8		−18
$\dot{V}O_{2max}$, L·min⁻¹	4.45	4.16	−7	
Cardiac output, L·min⁻¹	27.8	25.5	−8	
	27.8	25.2		−10
Stroke volume, mL	155	139	−10	
	148	129		−13
Heart rate, b·min⁻¹	186	193	4	
	187	197		5
Oxygen pulse, mL·b⁻¹	12.7	10.9		−14
Sum 3-min recovery HR	190	237		25
Plasma volume, L	2.91	2.56	−12	
a-$\bar{v}O_2$diff, mL·100 mL⁻¹	15.1	15.4	−2 (NS)	
	15.1	14.1		−7
PCr, mM·(g wet wt)⁻¹	17.9	13.0		−27
ATP, mM·(g wet wt)⁻¹	5.97	5.08		−15
Glycogen, mM·(g wet wt)⁻¹	113.9	57.4		−50
Capillary density, cap·mm⁻²	511	476	−7	
	464	476		−2 (NS)
Oxidative enzyme capacity			−29	−32
Myoglobin, mg (g protein)⁻¹	43.3	41.0	−5 (NS)	
	43.3	40.7		−6
Insulin (rest)			17–120	
Norepinephrine/epinephrine (rest)			No change	
Norepinephrine/epinephrine (exercise)				65–100
Blood lactate			88	
Lactate threshold			−7	−18
Exercise lipolysis			−52	
Muscle glycogen synthesis			−29	−40
Time to fatigue, min			−10	
Swim power, W				−14
Elbow extension strength, ft-lb	39.0	25.5		−35

[a]Data represent an average computed from individual studies as cited in the following sources: McArdle WD, et al. *Essentials of Exercise Physiology*. 3rd Ed. Lippincott Williams & Wilkins, 2006, and Wilber RL, Moffatt RJ. Physiological and biochemical consequences of detraining in aerobically trained individuals. *J Strength Cond Res* 1994;8:110. Note that a change for heart rate represents a decline in functional capacity. Omitted values for trained and detrained excluded in original sources.
[b]Short term, 3 wk or less in primarily aerobically trained individuals.
[c]Long term, 3 to 12 wk in primarily aerobically trained individuals.
NS, not statistically significant.

adaptations in many of these factors remain independent of race, gender, age, and health status.[26,32,197,235]

Metabolic Adaptations

Aerobic training improves the capacity for respiratory control in skeletal muscle.

Metabolic Machinery

To some extent, mitochondrial potential and not oxygen supply limits the oxidative capacity of untrained muscle.[75] Endurance-trained skeletal muscle fibers contain *larger* and *more numerous* mitochondria than less active fibers. The enlarged mitochondrial structural machinery and enzyme

TABLE 21.2 Typical Metabolic and Physiologic Values for Healthy, Endurance-Trained and Untrained Men[a]

Variable	Untrained	Trained	Percentage Difference[b]
Glycogen, mM · (g wet muscle)$^{-1}$	85.0	120	41
Number of mitochondria, mmol^3	0.59	1.20	103
Mitochondrial volume, % muscle cell	2.15	8.00	272
Resting ATP, mM · (g wet muscle)$^{-1}$	3.0	6.0	100
Resting PCr, mM · (g wet muscle)$^{-1}$	11.0	18.0	64
Resting creatine, mM · (g wet muscle)$^{-1}$	10.7	14.5	35
Glycolytic enzymes			
Phosphofructokinase, mM · (g wet muscle)$^{-1}$	50.0	50.0	0
Phosphorylase, mM · (g wet muscle)$^{-1}$	4–6	6–9	60
Aerobic enzymes			
Succinate dehydrogenase, mM · (kg wet muscle)$^{-1}$	5–10	15–20	133
Max lactate, mM · (kg wet muscle)$^{-1}$	110	150	36
Muscle fibers			
Fast twitch, %	50	20–30	−50
Slow twitch, %	50	60	20
Max stroke volume, mL	120	180	50
Max cardiac output, L · min^{-1}	20	30–40	75
Resting heart rate, b · min^{-1}	70	40	−43
Max heart rate, b · min^{-1}	190	180	−5
Max a-$\bar{v}O_2$ diff, mL · dL^{-1}	14.5	16.0	10
$\dot{V}O_{2max}$, mL · kg^{-1} · min^{-1}	30–40	65–80	107
Heart volume, L	7.5	9.5	27
Blood volume, L	4.7	6.0	28
$\dot{V}_{Emax}$, L · min^{-1}	110	190	73
Percentage body fat	15	11	−27

[a]In some cases, approximate values are used. In all cases, trained values represent data from endurance athletes. Caution is advised in assuming that percentage differences between trained and untrained necessarily results from training because genetic factors exert a strong influence on many of these factors.

[b]Percentage difference: trained versus untrained.

activity adaptations with aerobic training, sometimes up to 50% increase in just a few weeks, greatly *increase* the capacity of subsarcolemmal and intermyofibrillar muscle mitochondria to generate ATP aerobically.[67,87,209,239] A nearly twofold increase in aerobic system enzymes within 5 to 10 days of training coincides with increased mitochondrial capacity to generate ATP aerobically.

Enzyme changes occur from increases in total mitochondrial material, not increased enzymatic activity per unit of mitochondrial protein. The increase in mitochondrial protein by a factor of two exceeds the typical 10 to 20% increases in $\dot{V}O_{2max}$ with endurance training. More than likely, enzymatic changes allow a person to sustain a higher percentage of aerobic capacity during prolonged effort without blood lactate accumulation.

Fat Metabolism. Endurance training increases the oxidation of fatty acids for energy during rest[157] and submaximal exercise, particularly as the duration of effort

extends (**FIG. 21.4**).[50,88,225] Enhanced fat catabolism becomes apparent at the same absolute submaximal workload without regard to fuel input (fed or fasted),[10,12,31] and the effect occurs within 2 wk of training.[212] Impressive increases also occur in trained muscle's capacity to use intramuscular triacylglycerols as the primary source for fatty acid oxidation.[132] Four factors contribute to a heightened training-induced increased lipolysis:

1. Greater blood flow within trained muscle
2. More fat-mobilizing and fat-metabolizing enzymes
3. Enhanced muscle mitochondrial respiratory capacity
4. Decreased catecholamine release for the same absolute power output

Enhanced fat catabolism in submaximal activity benefits endurance athletes because it conserves the glycogen reserves so important during prolonged, intense effort. Improved fatty acid β-oxidation and respiratory ATP production contribute to a cell's integrity and high level of function. This enhances endurance capacity independent of increases in glycogen reserves or aerobic power.

Carbohydrate Metabolism. Trained muscle exhibits enhanced capacity to oxidize carbohydrate during maximal exercise. Consequently, large quantities of pyruvate flow through aerobic energy pathways in this type of exercise, an effect consistent with increased mitochondrial oxidative capacity and enhanced glycogen storage within muscles. Reduced carbohydrate as fuel and increased fatty acid combustion in submaximal activity with endurance training results from the combined effects of the following three factors[31]:

1. Decreased muscle glycogen use
2. Reduced glucose production (decreased hepatic glycogenolysis and gluconeogenesis)
3. Reduced use of plasma-borne glucose

Training-enhanced hepatic gluconeogenic capacity provides further resistance to hypoglycemia during prolonged physical activity.[33,42]

Muscle Fiber Type and Size

Aerobic training elicits metabolic adaptations in each muscle fiber type. The basic fiber type probably does not "change" to any great extent; instead, all fibers maximize their already existing aerobic potential.

Selective hypertrophy occurs in the different muscle fiber types with specific overload training. Highly trained endurance athletes have larger slow-twitch (type I) fibers than fast-twitch (type II) fibers in the same muscle. Type II fibers are recruited less during aerobic training than type I counterparts, so their aerobic capacity does not appreciably change with this type of activity. With aerobic training, some type II fibers may undergo a transition to exhibit greater aerobic tendencies. This example of muscle "plasticity" probably occurs at the subcellular level.[99]

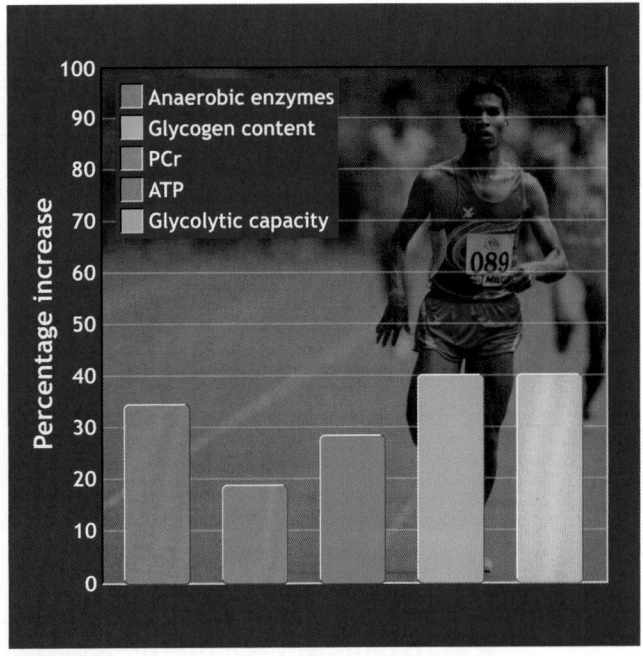

FIGURE 21.2. • Generalized potential for increases in anaerobic energy metabolism of skeletal muscle with short-term sprint–power training.

Myoglobin. Slow-twitch muscle fibers with high capacity to generate ATP aerobically contain relatively large quantities of myoglobin. Among animals, a muscle's myoglobin content relates to their level of physical activity. The leg muscles of hunting dogs, for example, contain more myoglobin than muscles of sedentary house pets; similar findings exist for grazing cattle compared with penned animals.[234] The effect of regular physical activity on myoglobin levels in humans remains undetermined, but any effect is likely negligible.

Cardiovascular Adaptations

FIGURE 21.5 summarizes important adaptations in cardiovascular function with aerobic training that increase oxygen delivery to active muscle.

TABLE 21.3	Changes in Resting Concentrations of PCr, Creatine, ATP, and Glycogen Following 5 Months of Heavy-Resistance Training in 9 Male Subjects		
Variable[a]	**Control**	**Posttraining**	**Percentage difference**[b]
PCr	17.07	17.94	+5.1
Creatine	14.52	10.74	+35.2
ATP	5.07	5.97	+17.8
Glycogen	113.90	86.28	+32.0

[a]All values are averages expressed in mM per gram of wet muscle.
[b]All percentage differences are statistically significant.
From MacDougall JD, et al. Biochemical adaptation of human skeletal muscle to heavy resistance training and immobilization. *J Appl Physiol* 1977;43:700.

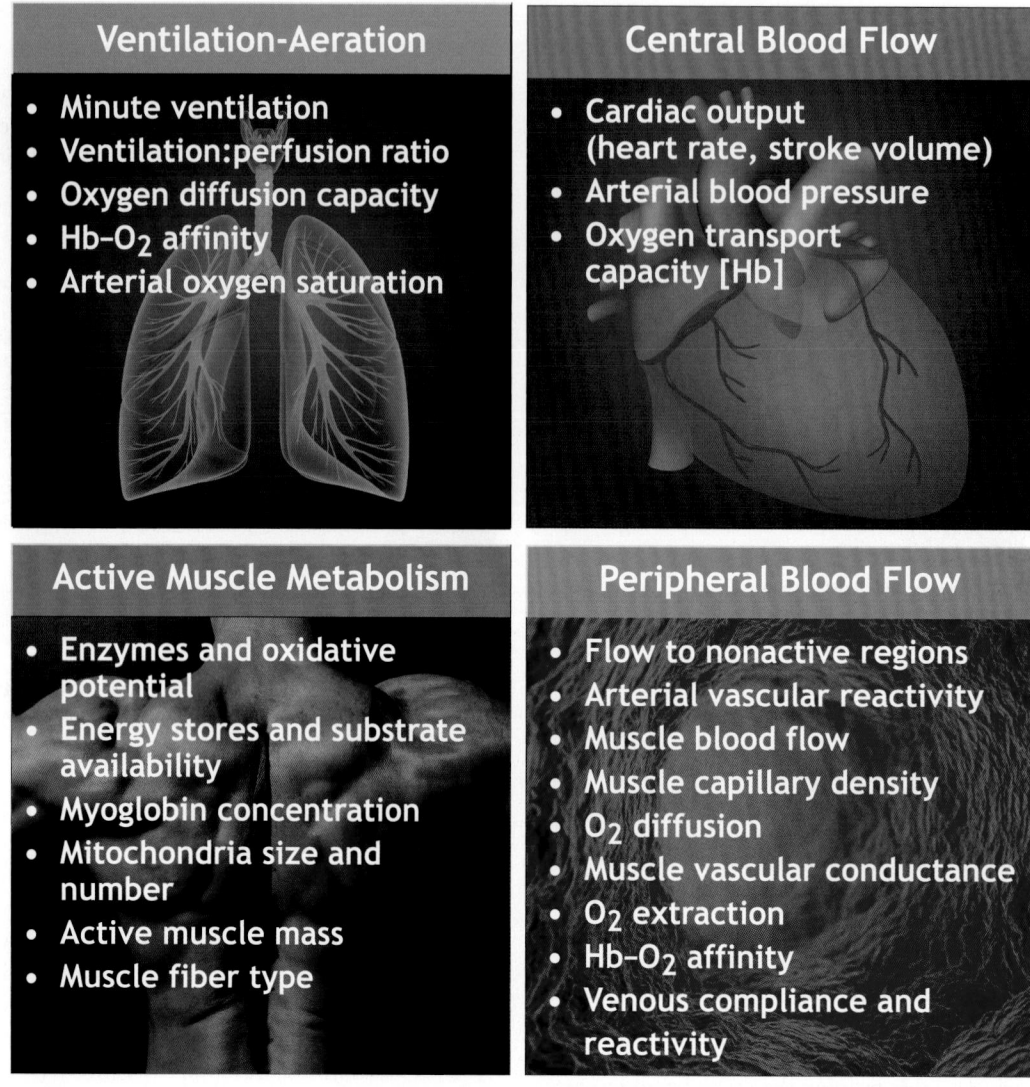

Ventilation-Aeration

- Minute ventilation
- Ventilation:perfusion ratio
- Oxygen diffusion capacity
- Hb-O_2 affinity
- Arterial oxygen saturation

Central Blood Flow

- Cardiac output (heart rate, stroke volume)
- Arterial blood pressure
- Oxygen transport capacity [Hb]

Active Muscle Metabolism

- Enzymes and oxidative potential
- Energy stores and substrate availability
- Myoglobin concentration
- Mitochondria size and number
- Active muscle mass
- Muscle fiber type

Peripheral Blood Flow

- Flow to nonactive regions
- Arterial vascular reactivity
- Muscle blood flow
- Muscle capillary density
- O_2 diffusion
- Muscle vascular conductance
- O_2 extraction
- Hb-O_2 affinity
- Venous compliance and reactivity

FIGURE 21.3 • Physiologic factors that limit $\dot{V}O_{2max}$ and aerobic exercise performance. *Hb*, hemoglobin.

Cardiac Hypertrophy: The "Athlete's Heart"

Long-term aerobic training generally *increases* the heart's mass and volume with greater left-ventricular end-diastolic volumes during rest and physical activity. Moderate cardiac hypertrophy secondary to longitudinal myocardial cell enlargement reflects a fundamental and normal training adaptation of muscle to an increased workload independent of age.[143] This enlargement is characterized by increased size of the left-ventricular cavity (**eccentric hypertrophy**) and modest thickening of its walls (**concentric hypertrophy**).

Regular training alters the contractile properties of cardiac muscle fibers that include increased sensitivity to activation by Ca^{2+}, changes in force–length relationship, and increased power output.[39] Myocardial overload stimulates greater cellular protein synthesis with concomitant reductions in protein breakdown. Increasing trained muscle's RNA content accelerates protein synthesis. Individual myofibrils thicken, while contractile filament number increases.

The heart volume of sedentary men averages about 800 mL. In athletes, increases in heart volume relate to the aerobic nature of the sport—endurance athletes average a 25% larger heart volume than sedentary counterparts. Researchers still would like to know if the larger heart volumes of endurance athletes reflect genetic endowment, training adaptations, or a combined effect.

Training duration affects cardiac size and structure. Several studies report no changes in cardiac dimensions with short-term training despite improvements in $\dot{V}O_{2max}$ and submaximal exercise heart rate response.[177,216] When endurance training increases left ventricular size, the enlargement does not reflect a permanent adaptation. Instead, heart size decreases to pretraining levels—without deleterious effects—as training intensity decreases.[38,83] **FIGURE 21.6** depicts the general trend for cardiac enlargement (reflected by left-ventricular mass) in untrained and strength–power- and endurance-trained male and female athletic groups.

Specific Nature of Cardiac Enlargement. The ultrasonic technique of echocardiography incorporates sound waves to "map" myocardial dimensions and heart chamber volume

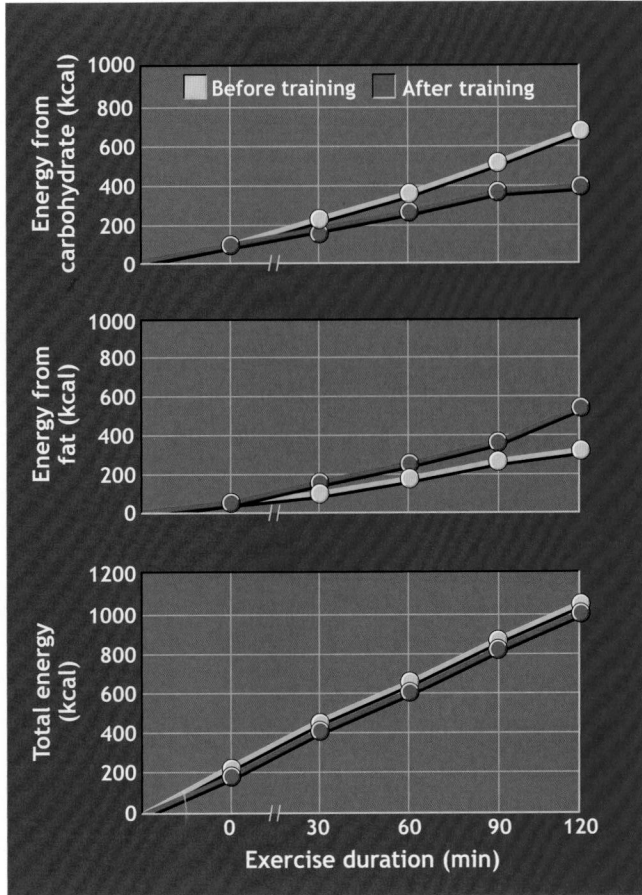

FIGURE 21.4 • Aerobic exercise training enhances fat catabolism in submaximal exercise. During constant-load, prolonged exercise, total energy derived from fat oxidation increases considerably following training. The carbohydrate-sparing adaptation results from facilitated release of fatty acids from adipose tissue depots (augmented by a reduced blood lactate level) and an increased amount of triacylglycerol within the endurance-trained muscle fibers. (Reprinted with permission from Hurley BF, et al. Muscle triglyceride utilization during exercise: effect of training. *J Appl Physiol* 1986;60:562.)

(see Chapter 32). This technique can evaluate the structural characteristics of hearts of male and female athletes (including other species of mammals) to determine how various training modes differentially affect cardiac enlargement.[160,210]

Cardiac dimensions of male swimmers, water polo players, distance runners, wrestlers, and shot putters were compared during their competitive seasons with untrained college men. The swimmers and runners represented athletes in "isotonic" or endurance events; the wrestlers and shot putters represented "isometric" or resistance-trained power athletes. TABLE 21.4 shows clear distinctions in structural characteristics of the hearts of healthy athletes and untrained individuals. Heart structural differences among athletes relate to the nature of exercise training. In swimmers, left-ventricular volume averaged 181 mL and mass equaled 308 g. In wrestlers, left-ventricular volume averaged 110 mL and mass averaged 330 g; the nonathletic controls averaged 101 mL for ventricular

volume and 211 g for ventricular mass. The resistance-trained athletes had thicker ventricular walls, whereas the heart walls of endurance athletes remained within a normal range. Cardiac morphologic and functional adaptations, including resting bradycardia, increased stroke volume, and enlarged ventricular internal dimensions, also occur in prepubertal children who undergo intense endurance training.[153]

One study showed the distribution of left-ventricular end-diastolic cavity dimensions in 1309 elite male and female Italian athletes ages 13 to 59 years. These dimensions ranged from 38 to 66 mm (average: 48.4 mm) in women and 43 to 70 mm (average: 55.5 mm) in men.[161] Ventricular cavity size of the majority of athletes remained within normal range, but 14% showed substantially enlarged dimensions.[189a] A large body surface area and participation in endurance cycling, cross-country skiing, and canoeing represented the major determinants of enlarged cavity dimension. The subjects remained free of heart problems over the 12-year study period. Other athletic groups also show an enlarged ventricular cavity (increased end-diastolic volume) with normal wall thickness,[139,180] with the effect less pronounced among females.[160]

Training-Induced Plasma Volume Provides a Possible Explanation. Myocardial structural and dimensional adaptations to regular physical activity generally reflect specific training demands.[158,168] As discussed in the upcoming section titled "Plasma Volume," a plasma volume increase within a day or two of the onset of endurance training contributes to intraventricular enlargement, or eccentric hypertrophy.[200] Increased plasma volume, coupled with a decreased heart rate and increased myocardial compliance, dilates or "stretches" the left-ventricular cavity, analogous to pumping water into a balloon.

In contrast to endurance athletes, male and female resistance-trained athletes possess the largest intraventricular septum, ventricular wall thickness, and ventricular mass, with little enlargement in the left ventricle's internal cavity.[57,115] These athletes do not experience volume overload with training. Instead, their training produces short-term episodes of elevated arterial blood pressure from high forces generated by a limited mass of skeletal muscle (see Chapter 15). An increase in ventricular wall thickness that generally falls within the normal range when expressed as ventricular mass per unit body size, particularly fat-free body mass,[160,161] compensates for additional afterload on the left ventricle without affecting ventricular cavity size. More than likely, considerable intraindividual variability exists for the heart's structural response to different forms of training. When changes do occur, the implications for myocardial blood supply and long-term cardiovascular health remain unknown. *No compelling scientific evidence indicates that specific modes of arduous physical activity and training damage a healthy heart.*[98] The same also pertains to cardiac patients who undergo a proper exercise-based cardiac rehabilitation program.[22]

Functional Versus Pathologic Cardiac Hypertrophy. Disease can induce considerable cardiac enlargement. In hypertension, for example, the heart chronically works against excessive resistance to blood flow called afterload. This stretches the heart muscle, which, in accord with the Frank-Starling

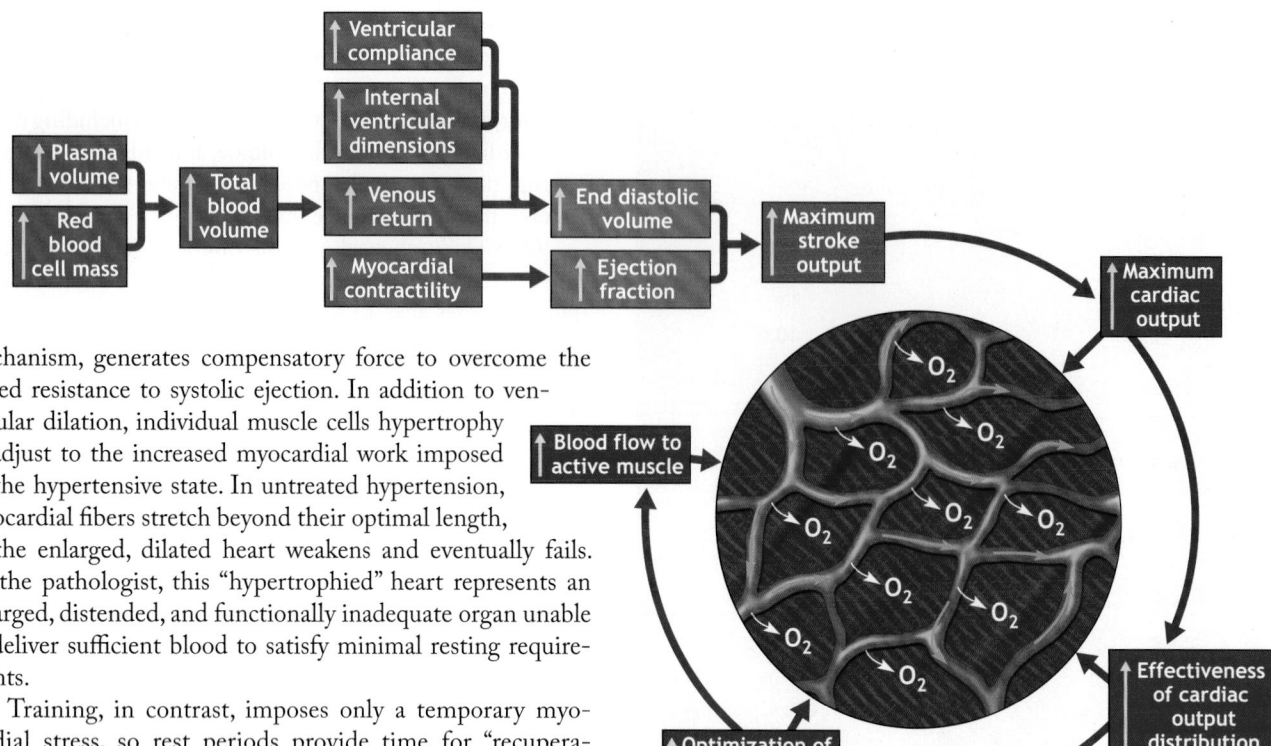

mechanism, generates compensatory force to overcome the added resistance to systolic ejection. In addition to ventricular dilation, individual muscle cells hypertrophy to adjust to the increased myocardial work imposed by the hypertensive state. In untreated hypertension, myocardial fibers stretch beyond their optimal length, so the enlarged, dilated heart weakens and eventually fails. To the pathologist, this "hypertrophied" heart represents an enlarged, distended, and functionally inadequate organ unable to deliver sufficient blood to satisfy minimal resting requirements.

Training, in contrast, imposes only a temporary myocardial stress, so rest periods provide time for "recuperation." Also, dilation and left ventricle weakening, a frequent response to chronic hypertension, does not accompany compensatory myocardial training adaptations. The enlarged heart size of elite athletes generally falls within the upper range of normal for either body size or increased end-diastolic volume. *The "athlete's heart" does not represent a dysfunctional organ. Rather, it demonstrates normal systolic and diastolic functions and superior functional capacity for stroke volume and cardiac output.* One possible exception concerns resistance-trained athletes who abuse anabolic steroids. An increase in both systolic and diastolic blood pressure, including exacerbation of the normal cardiac hypertrophy, occurs with prolonged steroid use.[66,73,96]

FIGURE 21.5 • Adaptations in cardiovascular function with aerobic training that increase oxygen delivery to active muscles.

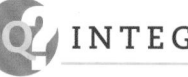 **INTEGRATIVE QUESTION**

Explain how cardiac hypertrophy with pressure overload training (e.g., resistance training) could affect oxygenation of myocardial tissues?

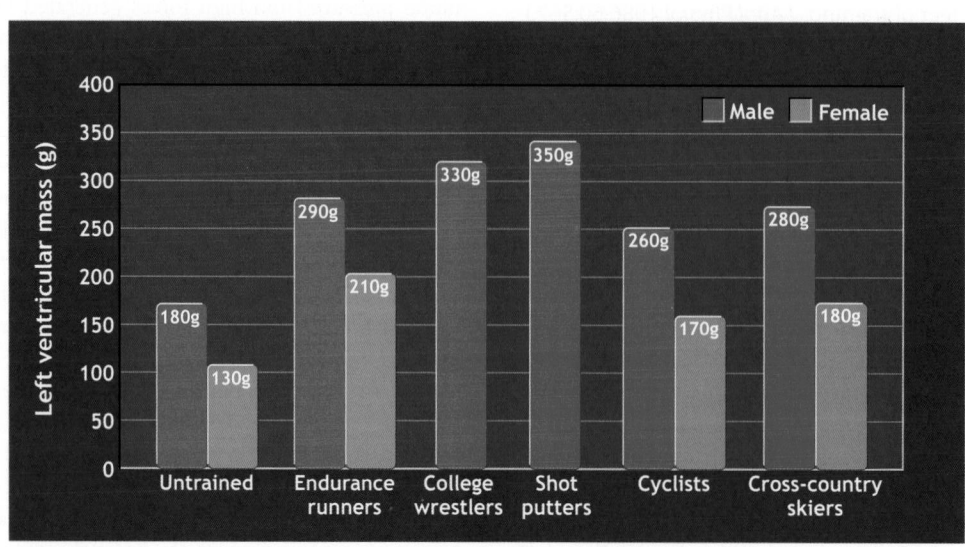

FIGURE 21.6 • General trend toward cardiac enlargement (left-ventricular mass) among the untrained and various groups of strength–power- and endurance-trained male and (where applicable) female athletes.

| TABLE 21.4 | Comparative Average Cardiac Dimensions in College Athletes, World-Class Athletes, and Normal Subjects |||||||

Dimension[a]	College Runners ($n = 15$)	College Swimmers ($n = 15$)	World-Class Runners ($n = 10$)	College Wrestlers ($n = 12$)	World-Class Shot Putters ($n = 4$)	Normals ($n = 16$)
LVID	54	51	48–59[b]	48	43–52[b]	46
LVV, mL	160	181	154	110	122	101
SV, mL	116	NR	113	75	68	NR
LV wall, mm	11.3	10.6	10.8	13.7	13.8	10.3
Septum, mm	10.9	10.7	10.9	13.0	13.5	10.3
LV mass, g	302	308	283	330	348	211

[a]LVID, left-ventricular internal dimension at end diastole; LVV, left-ventricular volume; SV, stroke volume; LV wall, posterobasal left-ventricular wall thickness; Septum, ventricular septal thickness; LV mass, left-ventricular mass.
[b]Range.
NR, Values not reported.
Reprinted from Morganroth J, et al. Comparative left-ventricular dimensions in trained athletes. *Ann Intern Med* 1975;82:521.

Plasma Volume

A 12 to 20% *increase* in plasma volume occurs after three to six aerobic training sessions, in the absence of changes in red blood cell mass. In fact, a measurable change occurs within 24 hr of the first exercise bout, with expansion of extracellular fluid volume requiring several weeks.[192] Intravascular volume expansion directly relates to increased synthesis and retention of plasma albumin.[141,149] A plasma volume increase enhances circulatory reserve and increases end-diastolic volume, stroke volume, oxygen transport, $\dot{V}O_{2max}$, and temperature-regulating ability during physical activity.[62,69] An expanded plasma volume returns to pretraining levels within 1 wk following training.[200,230] For endurance athletes in different sports, hemoglobin mass and blood volume averaged 35% higher than that of untrained subjects, with little difference in hemoglobin concentration among groups.[78]

Heart Rate

Endurance training creates an imbalance between tonic activity of sympathetic accelerator and parasympathetic depressor neurons in favor of greater vagal dominance—a response mediated primarily by increased parasympathetic activity and a small decrease in sympathetic discharge.[61,111] Training also decreases the intrinsic firing rate of sinoatrial (SA) nodal pacemaker tissue.[193] These adaptations contribute to the resting and submaximal exercise bradycardia in highly conditioned endurance athletes or previously sedentary individuals who train aerobically.

Exercise Heart Rate: Training Effects. Endurance training depresses submaximal heart rate for a standard physical task by 12 to 15 b·min⁻¹, while a much smaller decrease occurs for resting heart rate. Such heart rate reductions reflect the magnitude of training improvement because they generally coincide with increased maximum stroke volume and cardiac

output. FIGURE 21.7 illustrates the relationship between heart rate and oxygen consumption during graded exercise for athletes and sedentary students.[189] The group of six endurance athletes trained for several years; the other group consisted of three sedentary college students. The researchers evaluated the students' exercise responses before and after a 55-day training program designed to improve aerobic fitness. The lines relating heart rate and oxygen consumption remain essentially linear for both groups throughout the major portion of the oxygen consumption range. Whereas the untrained students' heart

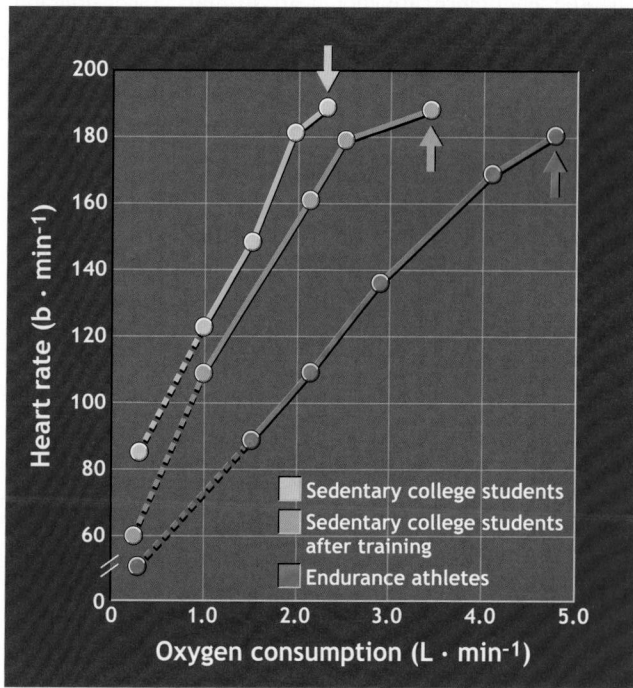

FIGURE 21.7 • Heart rate and oxygen consumption during upright exercise in endurance athletes (■) and sedentary college students before (■) and after (■) 55 days of aerobic training (⬆ = maximal values).

rates accelerate rapidly as oxygen consumption increases, the athletes' heart rates rise much less; that is, the slope, or rate of change, of the HR–$\dot{V}O_2$ lines differs considerably between trained and untrained persons. Consequently, an athlete or trained student performs more intense physical activity and achieves a higher oxygen consumption before achieving a specific submaximal heart rate than a sedentary student. At an oxygen consumption of 2.0 L·min⁻¹, the athletes' heart rate averaged 70 b·min⁻¹ less than for sedentary students. After 55 days of training, the difference in submaximal heart rate decreased to about 40 b·min⁻¹. In each instance, cardiac output remained essentially unchanged—an increase in stroke volume compensated for the lower heart rate.

Stroke Volume

Endurance training causes the heart's stroke volume to *increase* during rest and physical activity regardless of age or gender. Four factors produce this change[45,102,137]:

1. Increased internal left-ventricular volume (consequent to the training-induced plasma volume expansion) and mass
2. Reduced cardiac and arterial stiffness
3. Increased diastolic filling time (from training-induced bradycardia)
4. Possibly, improved intrinsic cardiac contractile function

Exercise Stroke Volume: Trained Versus Untrained. Figure 21.8 shows the stroke volume response during upright exercise for the men depicted in Figure 21.7. Five important training-related observations emerge:

1. The endurance athlete's heart exhibits a considerably larger stroke volume during rest and exercise than an untrained person of similar age.

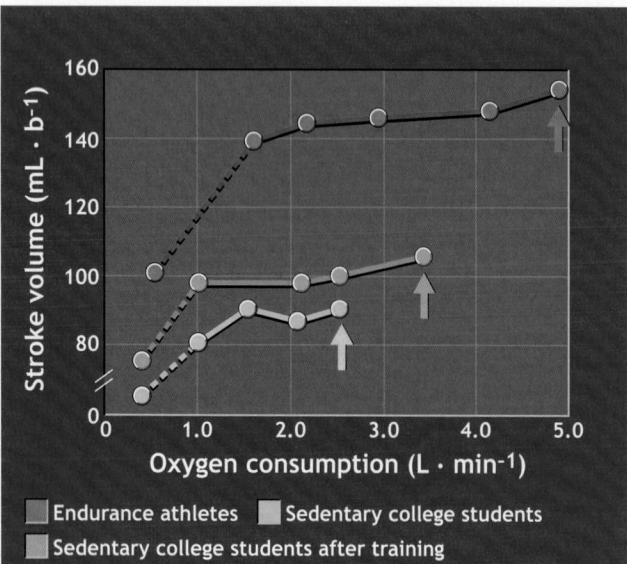

FIGURE 21.8 • Stroke volume and oxygen consumption during upright exercise in endurance athletes (■) and sedentary college students before (■) and after (■) 55 days of aerobic training (⬆ = maximal values).

2. The greatest stroke volume increase during exercise for trained and untrained persons occurs in transition from rest to moderate exercise. Only small increases in stroke volume accompany further increases in exercise intensity.
3. Maximum stroke volume generally occurs between 40 and 50% of $\dot{V}O_{2max}$ for untrained persons; this occurs at a heart rate of 110 to 120 b·min⁻¹ in young adults. Debate currently focuses on whether the stroke volume decreases, plateaus, or gradually increases during graded exercise to maximum, particularly among endurance athletes where the stroke volume may benefit from an enlarged plasma volume.[63,231] More than likely, endurance training minimizes the small decrease in stroke volume often observed during maximal effort. Even at near-maximal heart rates, sufficient time exists for the trained heart's ventricles to fill during diastole without reduction in stroke volume.[60,208,241] Improved ventricular filling with endurance training results in enhanced ventricular ejection via the Frank-Starling mechanism.
4. For untrained persons, only a small increase in stroke volume occurs during transition from rest to activity. Consequently, a cardiac output increase occurs from acceleration in heart rate. For endurance athletes, heart rate and stroke volume *both* increase to increase cardiac output; the athlete's stroke volume generally expands 60% above resting values. Relatively large stroke volume increases in transition from rest to exercise also occur in endurance-trained children and older men compared with healthy but untrained counterparts.[69,187]
5. Eight weeks of aerobic training by previously sedentary individuals substantially increases stroke volume, but these values remain below values for elite athletes.

Stroke Volume and $\dot{V}O_{2max}$. The data in Table 21.5 amplify the importance of stroke volume in differentiating persons with high and low $\dot{V}O_{2max}$ values. These data represent three groups: athletes, healthy but sedentary men, and patients with mitral stenosis, a valvular heart disease that causes inadequate emptying of the left ventricle. The differences in $\dot{V}O_{2max}$ among groups relate closely to differences in maximal stroke volume. Patients with mitral stenosis achieved an aerobic capacity and maximum stroke volume one half that of sedentary subjects. The importance of stroke volume also emerges in comparisons among healthy groups. Athletes achieved an average 62% larger $\dot{V}O_{2max}$ than sedentary subjects, almost entirely from the athletes' 60% larger stroke volume and cardiac output (see Figs. 21.8 and 21.9).

Cardiac Output

An increase in maximum cardiac output represents the most significant adaptation in cardiovascular function with aerobic training. Maximal heart rate generally decreases slightly with training; thus, increased cardiac output capacity results directly from improved stroke volume. A large maximum cardiac output (reflected by a larger stroke volume) distinguishes champion endurance athletes from other well-trained athletes and from untrained counterparts.

TABLE 21.5	Maximal Values for Oxygen Consumption, Heart Rate, Stroke Volume, and Cardiac Output in Three Groups with Low, Normal, and High Aerobic Capacities			
Group	$\dot{V}O_{2max}$ (L · min^{-1})	Max Heart Rate (B · min^{-1})	Max Stroke Volume (mL · B^{-1})	Max Cardiac Output (L · min^{-1})
Mitral stenosis	1.6	190	50	9.5
Sedentary	3.2	200	100	20.0
Athlete	5.2	190	160	30.4

Adapted from Rowell LB. Circulation. *Med Sci Sports* 1969;1:15.

FIGURE 21.9 illustrates the important role of cardiac output in achieving a high level of aerobic metabolism. In trained athletes and students, cardiac output increases *linearly* with oxygen consumption throughout the major portion of the exercise intensity range with the athletes achieving the highest values for both variables. A linear relationship between cardiac output and oxygen consumption in graded exercise also occurs in children and adolescents. For these young persons, increased stroke volume and proportionate increase in cardiac output closely matches the added oxygen requirement of physical activity during growth.[35]

Endurance Training and Submaximal Cardiac Output. Early reports showed that endurance training, while improving maximal cardiac output, reduced the heart's minute volume during moderate activity. In one study, average cardiac output of young men after 16 wk of aerobic training decreased by 1.1 and 1.5 L · min^{-1} at a specific submaximal oxygen consumption.[43] As expected, maximal cardiac output

increased 8%, from 22.4 to 24.2 L · min^{-1}. With reduced submaximal cardiac output, a corresponding increase in oxygen extraction in the active muscles achieves the exercise oxygen requirement. A training-induced reduction in submaximal cardiac output presumably reflects two factors:

1. More effective redistribution of blood flow
2. Trained muscles' enhanced capacity to generate ATP aerobically at a lower tissue Po_2

Oxygen Extraction (a-v̄O₂ Difference)

Endurance training *increases* the quantity of oxygen extracted (measured as arterio-venous oxygen differences, or a-v̄O₂ difference) from circulating blood.[194] An increase in the maximum a-v̄O₂ difference results from more effective cardiac output distribution to active muscles combined with enhanced capacity of trained muscle fibers to extract and process available oxygen. The a-v̄O₂ difference takes on even greater importance in contributing to improved aerobic capacity with training in older men and women because the elderly often show diminished capacity to improve cardiac output with training.[104,196]

FIGURE 21.10 compares the relationship between oxygen extraction (a-v̄O₂ difference) and exercise intensity for the

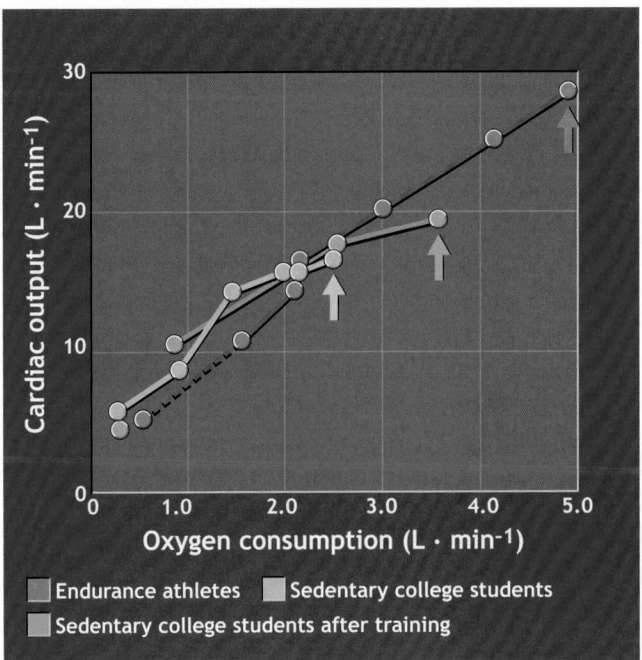

FIGURE 21.9 • Cardiac output and oxygen consumption during upright exercise in endurance athletes (■) and sedentary college students before (■) and after (■) 55 days of aerobic training (↑ = maximal values).

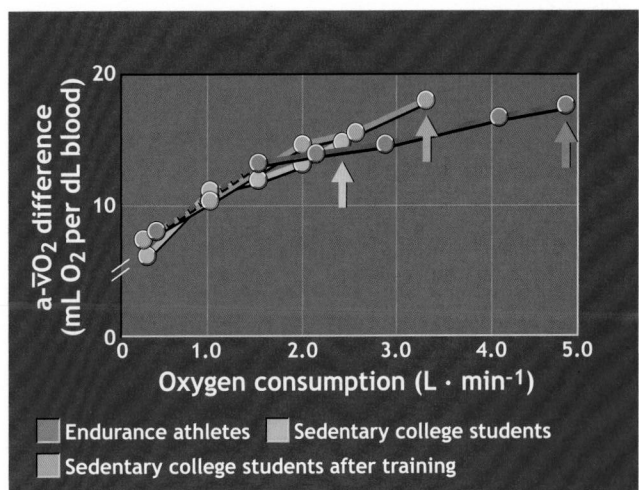

FIGURE 21.10 • The a-v̄O₂ difference and oxygen consumption during upright exercise in endurance athletes (■) and sedentary college students before (■) and after (■) 55 days of aerobic training (↑ = maximal values).

trained athletes and untrained students depicted in Figure 21.7. The a-$\bar{v}O_2$ difference for the students increases steadily during graded exercise to a maximum of 15 mL per deciliter of blood. Following 55 days of training, the students' maximum oxygen extraction increased 13% to 17 mL of oxygen. This means that during intense physical activity, arterial blood released approximately 85% of its oxygen content. Actually, the active muscles extract even more oxygen because the a-$\bar{v}O_2$ difference reflects an *average* based on sampling of mixed-venous blood, which contains blood returning from tissues that use much less oxygen during exercise than active muscle. The post-training value for maximal a-$\bar{v}O_2$ difference for the students equals the value of the endurance athletes. The students' lower cardiac output capacity explains the rather large difference in $\dot{V}O_{2max}$ that clearly differentiates athletes from students.

Blood Flow and Distribution

Submaximal Exercise. Trained persons perform submaximal exercise with a *lower* cardiac output (and unchanged or slightly lower muscle blood flow) than untrained persons. A relatively larger portion of submaximal cardiac output flows to high oxidative skeletal muscles composed primarily of type I fibers at the expense of blood flow to muscles with a large percentage of type IIb fibers with low oxidative capacity.[36] Two factors contribute to reduced muscle blood flow in submaximal exercise[108,215,229,237]:

1. Relatively rapid training-induced changes in vasoactive properties of large arteries and local resistance vessels within skeletal and cardiac muscle, mediated by the dilation effects of endothelium-derived nitric oxide
2. Changes within muscle cells that enhance oxidative capacity

Both adaptations support the principle of training specificity. As the muscle's ability to deliver, extract, and use oxygen increases, the active tissue's oxygen needs require proportionally less blood flow.

Maximal Exercise. Three factors affect how aerobic training increases total skeletal muscle blood flow during *maximal* exercise:

1. Larger maximal cardiac output.
2. Distribution of blood to muscle from nonactive areas that temporarily compromise blood flow during all-out effort
3. Enlargement of cross-sectional areas of large and small arteries (*arteriogenesis*) and veins, and 10 to 20% increase in capillarization per gram of muscle (*angiogenesis*).[80,178] This effect begins rapidly from increased vascular endothelial growth factors—produced by skeletal muscle cells to induce angiogenesis—following a single exercise bout in trained and untrained persons.[55,101,109]

Training-induced *decreases* in splanchnic and renal blood flow in physical activity occur from reduced sympathetic nervous system outflow to these tissues, which frees a relatively large quantity of blood for distribution to active muscles.[134]

Concurrently, training and accompanying exposure to elevated core temperatures produces heat loss adaptations via enhanced endothelium-dependent increases in skin blood flow for a given internal temperature.[92,103] Augmented cutaneous blood flow facilitates the endurance-trained person's capacity to dissipate the metabolic heat generated in physical activity.

The observation that oxygen extraction in skeletal muscle remains near maximal in intense activity supports the hypothesis that oxygen supply (i.e., blood flow), not oxygen use (extraction), limits the maximal respiratory rate of muscle tissue.[11,145,178]

Myocardial Blood Flow. For both normal persons and cardiac patients, structural and functional changes in the heart's vasculature, including modifications in mechanisms that regulate myocardial perfusion, parallel a modest training-induced myocardial hypertrophy.[72,106,107] Structural vascular modifications include increased cross-sectional area of the proximal coronary arteries, possible arteriolar proliferation and longitudinal growth, recruitment of collateral vessels, and increased capillary density. These adaptations provide adequate perfusion to support the increased blood flow and energy demands of the functionally improved myocardium.

Two mechanisms help explain how aerobic training increases coronary blood flow and capillary exchange capacity:

1. Ordered progression of structural remodeling that improves myocardial vascularization when new capillaries form and develop into small arterioles[106]
2. More effective control of vascular resistance and blood distribution within the myocardium[222,229]

The significance of vascular and cellular adaptations to the heart's functional capacity during physical activity remains unclear—mainly because the healthy, untrained heart does not suffer from reduced oxygen supply during maximal exertion. Training adaptations may provide some cardioprotection by enabling myocardial tissue to better tolerate and recover from transient episodes of ischemia (i.e., become more resistant to ischemic injury). The trained tissue also functions at a lower percentage of its total oxidative capacity during physical activity. Vascular adaptations do not accompany the myocardial hypertrophy that occurs with chronic resistance training.[143]

Blood Pressure

Regular aerobic training *reduces* systolic and diastolic blood pressure during rest and submaximal physical activity. The largest reduction occurs in systolic pressure, particularly in hypertensive subjects (Chapters 15 and 32 provide additional discussion about this topic).

Pulmonary Adaptations With Training

Aerobic training stimulates adaptations in pulmonary ventilation dynamics during submaximal and maximal effort. The adaptations generally reflect a breathing strategy that minimizes respiratory work at a given exercise intensity. This frees oxygen for use by the nonrespiratory active musculature.

Maximal Physical Activity

Maximal exercise ventilation increases from increased tidal volume and breathing rate as maximal oxygen consumption increases. This makes sense physiologically because any increase in $\dot{V}O_{2max}$ raises the body's oxygen requirement and corresponding need to eliminate additional carbon dioxide via alveolar ventilation.

Submaximal Physical Activity

Several weeks of aerobic training *reduce* the ventilatory equivalent for oxygen ($\dot{V}_E/\dot{V}O_2$) during submaximal physical activity and *lower* the percentage of the total oxygen cost attributable to breathing. Reduced oxygen consumption by the ventilatory musculature enhances endurance for two reasons:

1. Reduces fatiguing effects of physical activity on ventilatory musculature
2. Any oxygen freed from use by the respiratory musculature becomes available to active locomotor muscles

In general, training increases tidal volume and decreases breathing frequency. Consequently, air remains in the lungs for a longer time between breaths; this increases oxygen extraction from inspired air. For example, the exhaled air of trained individuals during submaximal exercise contains only 14 to 15% oxygen, whereas the expired air of untrained persons averages 18% at the same exercise intensity. This translates to the common observation that untrained persons ventilate proportionately more air to achieve the same submaximal oxygen consumption.

Substantial specificity exists for ventilatory responses relative to the activity mode and training adaptations. When subjects performed arm-only and leg-only exercise, consistently higher ventilatory equivalents occurred with the arms (Fig. 21.11). As expected, the ventilatory equivalent decreased in each mode with training. The reduction occurred only with exercise that used specifically trained muscles. For the group trained by arm-crank ergometry, the ventilation equivalent decreased only during arm effort and vice versa for the leg-trained group. The ventilatory training adaptation linked closely to a less pronounced rise in blood lactate and heart rate during the specific training exercise. This suggests that local adaptations in specifically trained muscles affect the ventilatory adjustment to training. In this regard, lower lactate levels with training remove the drive to breathe from any additional carbon dioxide produced from lactate buffering.

Training May Benefit Ventilatory Endurance

Prolonged, intense physical activity induces fatigue in the inspiratory muscles,[9,89,227] and reduces the abdominal muscles' capacity to generate maximal expiratory pressure.[52]

Exercise training allows for sustained, exceptionally high levels of submaximum ventilation.[20,91,204] Endurance training stabilizes the body's internal milieu during submaximal activity. Consequently, exercise causes less disruption in whole-body hormonal and acid-base balance that could negatively impact

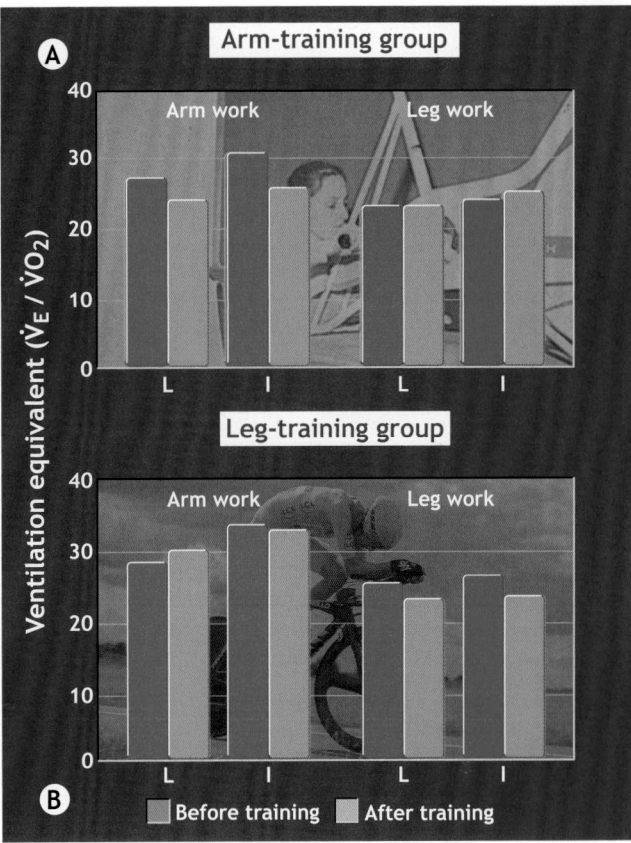

FIGURE 21.11 • Ventilation equivalents during light (L) and intense (I) submaximal arm and leg exercise before and after arm training **(A)** and leg training **(B)**. (Reprinted with permission from Rasmussen B, et al. Pulmonary ventilation, blood gases, and blood pH after training of the arms and the legs. *J Appl Physiol* 1975;38:250.)

inspiratory muscle function. The ventilatory muscles also benefit directly from training. For example, 20 wk of run training by healthy men and women improved ventilatory muscle endurance by approximately 16%, characterized by less lactate accumulation during standard breathing exercise. The training-induced increase in aerobic enzyme levels and oxidative capacity of the respiratory musculature contribute to enhanced ventilatory muscle function.[173,207] Training also increases inspiratory muscle capacity to generate force and sustain a given level of inspiratory pressure.[27] These adaptations benefit exercise performance in three ways:

1. Less respiratory work by ventilatory muscles reduces overall energy demands
2. Ventilatory muscles produce less lactate during intense, prolonged physical activity
3. Ventilatory muscles more efficiently metabolize circulating lactate as metabolic fuel

Blood Lactate Concentration

FIGURE 21.12 illustrates the generalized effect of endurance training in lowering blood lactate levels and extending physical

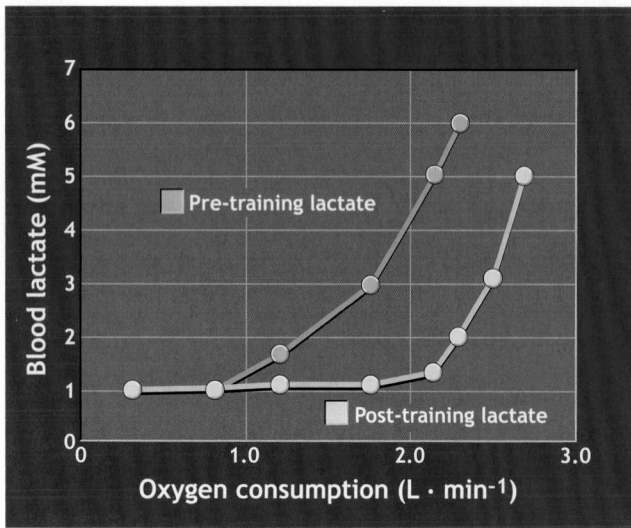

FIGURE 21.12 • Generalized response for pre- and posttraining lactate accumulation during graded exercise. (Plots based on data from the Applied Physiology Laboratory, University of Michigan, Ann Arbor.)

effort before onset of blood lactate accumulation (OBLA) during exercise of increasing intensity. The underlying explanation centers on three possibilities related to central and peripheral adaptations to aerobic training discussed in this chapter:

1. Decreased rate of lactate formation during physical activity
2. Increased rate of lactate clearance (removal) during physical activity
3. Combined effects of decreased lactate formation and increased lactate removal

Four Additional Aerobic Training Adaptations

1. *Body composition changes*: Regular aerobic activity for the obese or overweight person reduces body mass and body fat and augments a more favorable body fat distribution (see Chapter 30). Exercise only or combined with calorie restriction reduces body fat more than weight loss with dieting by promoting conservation of lean tissue.
2. *Body heat transfer*: Well-hydrated, trained individuals exercise more comfortably in hot environments because of a larger plasma volume and more responsive thermoregulatory mechanisms; in other words, they dissipate heat faster and more economically than sedentary individuals.
3. *Performance changes*: Enhanced endurance performance accompanies physiologic adaptations with training. FIGURE 21.13 depicts cycling performance prior to and following 10 wk of cycling training for 40 to 60 min, 4 days per week for 10 wk at 85% $\dot{V}O_{2max}$. In the performance test, subjects attempted to maintain a constant power output of 265 watts for 8 min. Training produced less dropoff from the initial rate in power output during the prescribed 8-min exercise test.

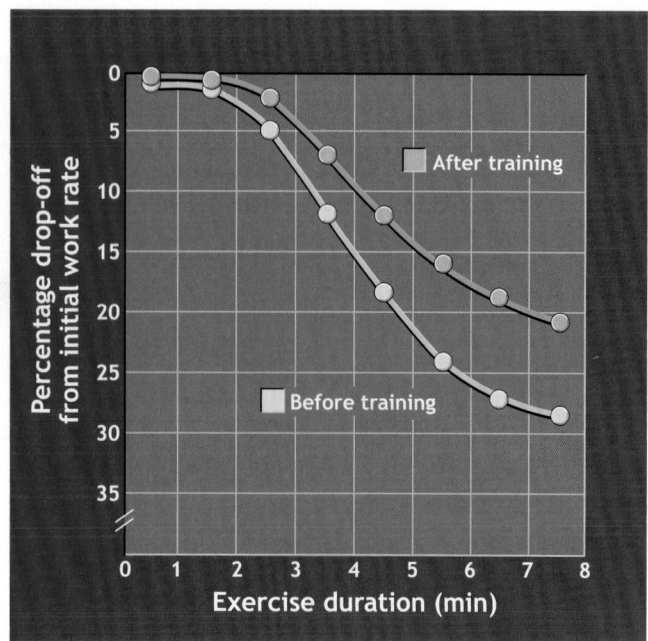

FIGURE 21.13 • Percentage dropoff from initial exercise intensity before and after 10 wk of endurance cycling training. (Reprinted with permission from the Applied Physiology Laboratory, University of Michigan, Ann Arbor.)

4. *Psychologic benefits*: Regular physical activity, regardless of age, creates important potential benefits on psychologic state. Adaptations often occur to a degree equal to that achieved with other therapeutic interventions, including pharmacologic therapy.[46,217]

Six Potential Psychologic Benefits From Regular Physical Activity

1. Reduction in state of anxiety (i.e., the level of anxiety at the time of measurement)
2. Decrease in mild-to-moderate depression
3. Reduction in neuroticism (long-term physical activity)
4. Adjunct to professional treatment of severe depression
5. Improvement in mood, self-esteem, and self-concept
6. Reduction in the various indices of psychologic stress

Summary View

FIGURE 21.14 summarizes adaptive changes in active muscle that accompany $\dot{V}O_{2max}$ improvements with endurance training and detraining. Aerobic capacity generally increases 15 to 25% over the first 3 mo of intensive training and may improve by 50% over a 2-year interval depending on initial fitness level. When training ceases, $\dot{V}O_{2max}$ rapidly decreases toward the pretraining level. Even more impressive training effects occur for aerobic enzymes of the citric acid cycle and electron-transport chain within the mitochondria of trained muscles. These enzymes increase rapidly and substantially throughout training in both fiber types and subdivisions. Conversely, 2 to 3 wk

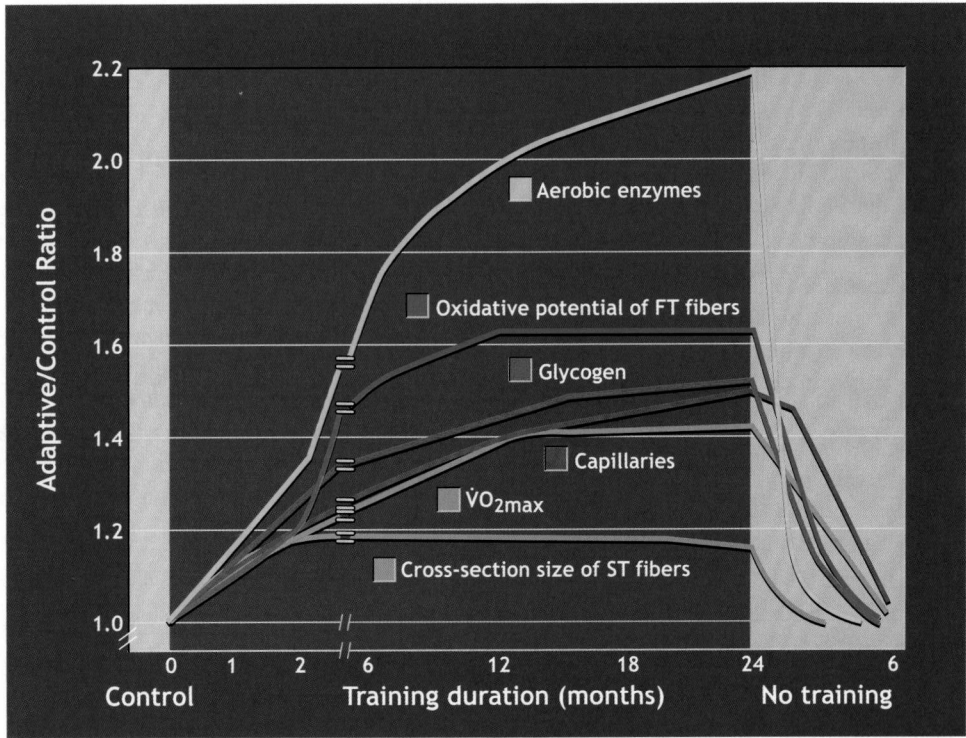

FIGURE 21.14 • Generalized summary of increase in aerobic capacity and muscle adaptations with endurance training. (Adapted with permission from Saltin B, et al. Fiber types and metabolic potentials of skeletal muscles in sedentary man and endurance runners. *Ann NY Acad Sci* 1977;301:3.)

of detraining substantially reduce a large portion of enzymatic adaptations. The number of muscle capillaries increases during training. When training ceases, this adaptation in blood supply probably decreases relatively slowly. The ultimate detraining occurs with aging. Regular physical activity slows but cannot halt the muscle atrophy, weakness, and fatigability that accompanies an increase in chronological age.[44]

Local metabolic improvement greatly exceeds improvements in capacity to circulate, deliver, and use oxygen, reflected by increases in $\dot{V}O_{2max}$ and cardiac output, during intense activity. With local training adaptations, a muscle's lactate flux remains at lower levels (lower production and/or greater removal rate) than similar submaximal effort before training. *These cellular adjustments account for how a trained person performs steady-rate exercise at a greater percentage of $\dot{V}O_{2max}$.*

FACTORS THAT AFFECT AEROBIC TRAINING RESPONSES

Four important factors influence the aerobic training response:

1. Initial level of aerobic fitness
2. Training intensity
3. Training frequency
4. Training duration

Initial Level of Aerobic Fitness

The magnitude of the training response depends on initial fitness level. *Someone who rates low at the start has considerable*

room for improvement. If capacity already rates high, the magnitude of improvement remains relatively small. Studies of sedentary, middle-age men with heart disease showed that $\dot{V}O_{2max}$ improved by 50%, while similar training in normally active, healthy adults improved 10 to 15%.[178] Of course, a relatively small improvement in aerobic capacity represents a crucial change for an elite athlete, where even a 1 to 2% performance change could be the difference between winning and losing, as a much larger increase in physiologic and performance capacity for a sedentary person. *As a general guideline, aerobic fitness improvements with endurance training range between 5 and 25%. Some of this improvement occurs within the first week of training.*

 INTEGRATIVE QUESTION

Respond to the question, "How long must I exercise to 'get in shape'?"

Training Intensity

Training-induced physiologic adaptations depend primarily on intensity of overload. At least seven different ways express the intensity of physical effort:

1. Energy expended per unit time (e.g., 9 kcal·min⁻¹ or 37.8 kJ·min⁻¹)
2. Absolute exercise level or power output (e.g., cycle at 900 kg-m·min⁻¹ or 147 W)

3. Relative metabolic level expressed as percentage of $\dot{V}O_{2max}$ (e.g., 85% $\dot{V}O_{2max}$)
4. Exercise below, at, or above the lactate threshold, or OBLA (e.g., 4 mM lactate)
5. Exercise heart rate, or percentage of maximum heart rate (e.g., 180 b·min⁻¹ or 80% HR_{max})
6. Multiples of resting metabolic rate (e.g., 6 METs)
7. Rating of perceived exertion (e.g., RPE = 14)

An example of absolute training intensity involves all individuals who perform at the same power output or energy expenditure (e.g., 9.0 kcal·min⁻¹) for 30 min. When everyone performs at the same intensity, the task can elicit considerable stress for one person yet fall short of training threshold for another, more fit person. For this reason, the *relative intensity* based on a person's physiologic systems usually establishes exercise intensity. The assigned relative intensity usually relates to some breakpoint for steady-rate exercise (e.g., lactate threshold, OBLA), some percentage of maximum physiologic capacity (e.g., %$\dot{V}O_{2max}$, or %HR_{max}), or maximum exercise capacity. General practice establishes aerobic training intensity via direct measurement (or estimation) of $\dot{V}O_{2max}$ or HR_{max} and then assigns an exercise level to correspond to some percentage of maximum.

Establishing training intensity from measures of oxygen consumption provides a high degree of accuracy, but its use requires sophisticated monitoring that renders this method impractical for general use. An effective alternative relies on *heart rate* to classify an activity for relative intensity when individualizing training programs. Exercise heart rate is convenient because %$\dot{V}O_{2max}$ and %HR_{max} relate in a predictable way regardless of gender, race, fitness level, activity mode, or age. Training does not affect a particular individual's heart rate at a given %$\dot{V}O_{2max}$. There is little need to frequently adjust the exercise prescription relative to training-induced changes in aerobic capacity as long as exercise occurs at the %HR_{max}.[203]

TABLE 21. 6 presents selected values for %$\dot{V}O_{2max}$ and corresponding %HR_{max}.[5,132] The error in estimating %$\dot{V}O_{2max}$ from %HR_{max}, or vice versa, equals approximately ± 8%. One need only monitor heart rate to estimate relative %$\dot{V}O_{2max}$, within the given error range. The relationship between %HR_{max} and %$\dot{V}O_{2max}$ remains the same for arm or leg activities among healthy subjects, normal-weight and obese persons, cardiac patients, and persons with spinal cord injuries.[49,86,138] *Importantly, arm (upper-body) exercise produces lower HR_{max} than leg exercise. One must consider this difference when formulating an individualized exercise prescription for different exercise modes* (see the "Running Versus Swimming and Other Forms of Upper-Body Exercise," section later in this chapter).

Train at a Percentage of HR_{max}

Aerobic capacity improves if effort intensity regularly maintains heart rate between 55 and 70% of maximum. During lower-body cycling, walking, or running, the increase heart rate equals about 40 to 55% of the $\dot{V}O_{2max}$. Consequently, for college-age men and women, training heart rate ranges from 120 to 140 b·min⁻¹.

An equally effective method to establish the training threshold, termed the ***Karvonen method*** after the researcher who pioneered its use, requires that subjects exercise at a heart rate equal to 60% of the difference between resting and maximum.[97] The Karvonen method computes training heart rate as follows:

$$HR_{threshold} = HR_{rest} + 0.60 \left(HR_{max} - HR_{rest}\right)$$

This approach to determining heart rate training threshold results in a *higher* value than simply computing threshold heart rate as 70% of HR_{max}.

Achieving positive training adaptations does not require strenuous physical activity. For most healthy persons, an heart rate of 70% HR_{max} represents "moderate activity" without discomfort. This training level, frequently referred to as moderate "**conversational exercise**," achieves sufficient intensity to stimulate a training effect yet does not produce a level of discomfort (e.g., lactate accumulation and associated hyperpnea) that would prevent talking during the activity. *A previously sedentary person need not exercise above this threshold heart rate to improve physiologic capacity.*

Figure 21.15 illustrates that as aerobic fitness improves, submaximal heart rate decreases 10 to 20 b·min⁻¹ at a given level of oxygen consumption. To keep pace with physiologic improvement, the activity level must increase periodically to achieve the desired heart rate. A person begins training by walking, then walks more briskly; jogging then replaces walking for periods of the workout; and eventually continuous running elicits the desired heart rate. *In each progression, exercise remains at the same "relative intensity."* If intensity progression does not increase with training improvements, the exercise essentially becomes a maintenance program for aerobic fitness.

Is Strenuous Training More Effective?

Generally, the higher the training intensity above threshold, the greater the training improvement for $\dot{V}O_{2max}$ when controlling for exercise volume.[64] A minimal threshold intensity exists below which no meaningful training effect occurs; a "ceiling" also may exist above which no further gains accrue. More fit men and women generally require higher threshold levels to stimulate a training response than less fit persons. The ceiling for training intensity remains unknown, although about 85% $\dot{V}O_{2max}$, corresponding to 90% HR_{max}, probably represents an upper limit. Regardless of the exertion level selected, more exercise does not necessarily produce greater or faster results. Excessive training intensity and abrupt increases in training volume

TABLE 21.6	Relationship Between Percentage Maximal Heart Rate and Percentage $\dot{V}O_{2max}$	
Percentage HR_{max}	**Percentage $\dot{V}O_{2max}$**	
50	28	
60	40	
70	58	
80	70	
90	83	
100	100	

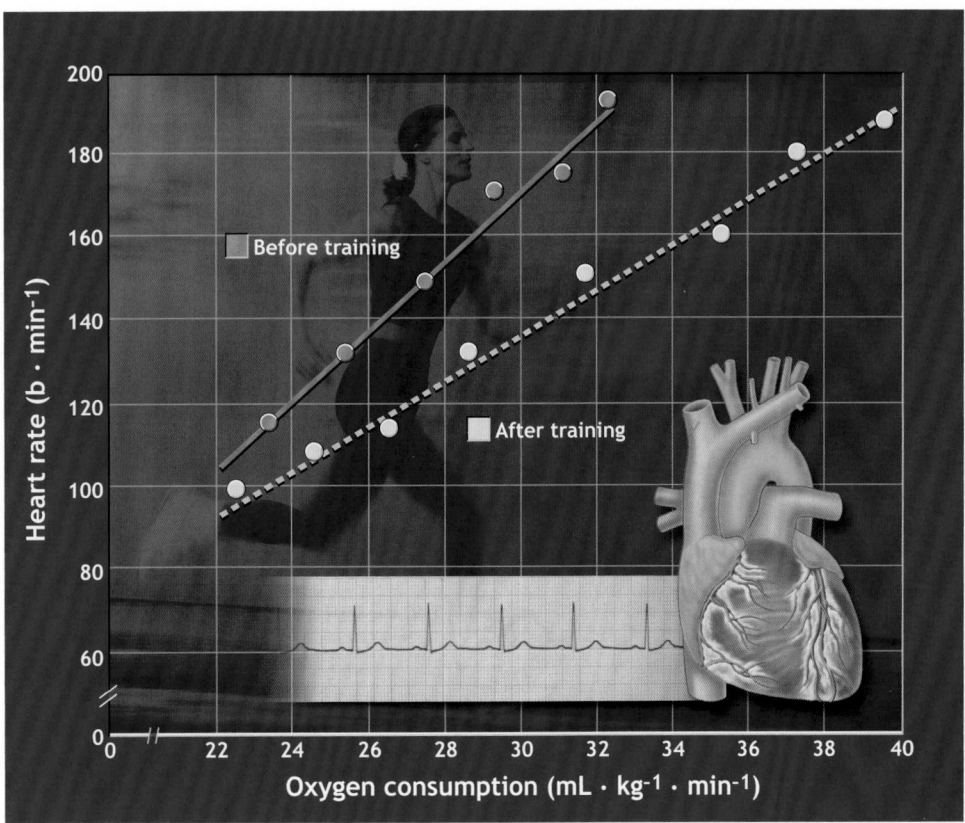

FIGURE 21.15 • Improvement in exercise heart rate response with aerobic training in relation to oxygen consumption. A reduction in exercise heart rate with training usually reflects enhanced stroke volume.

increase risk for injury to bones, joints, and muscles.[4,93] For men and women, the number of miles run each week represents the only variable consistently associated with running injuries. In preadolescent children, running excessive distances strains the articular cartilage, which could injure the bone's growth plate and adversely affect normal growth and development.

Determining the "Training-Sensitive Zone"

One can determine maximum heart rate immediately after several minutes of all-out effort. This intensity requires considerable motivation and stress—a requirement inadvisable for adults without medical clearance, particularly those predisposed to coronary heart disease. For most individuals, use **age-predicted maximum heart rates** presented in **FIGURE 21.16** based on averages in population studies.

While individuals of a given age have varying HR_{max} values, the inaccuracy from individual variation (± 10 b·min^{-1} standard deviation for any age-predicted HR_{max}) has little influence in establishing effective training for healthy persons. *Maximum heart rate has commonly been estimated as 220 minus age in years, with values independent of race or gender in children and adults.*[7,90,120]

$$HR_{max} = 220 - Age\,(y)$$

Perhaps a Modification Required. A longitudinal study of 132 persons measured an average of seven times over 9 years indicates a bias in the above prediction of HR_{max}. The bias overestimates this measure in men and women under the age of 40 years and underestimates it in those older than 40 years (**FIG. 21.17**).[56] This prediction equation, with a standard deviation of ± 5 to ± 8 beats per minute, independent of sex, BMI, and resting heart rate, is as follows:

$$HR_{max} = 206.9 - 0.67 \times Age\,(y)$$

For example, the above equation can estimate maximum heart rate for a 30-year-old man or woman:

$$HR_{max} = 206.9 - (0.67 \times 30)$$
$$= 206.9 - 20.1$$
$$= 187\ b·min^{-1}$$

This prediction agrees closely with prior research.[119,213]

These prediction formulae associate with a plus or minus error and should be used with caution. Each formula represents a convenient rule of thumb, and does not determine a specific person's maximum heart rate. For example, within normal variation limits and using the 220-minus-age formula, the actual maximum heart rate of 95% (± 2 standard deviations) of 40-year-old men and women ranges between 160 and 200 b·min^{-1}. Figure 21.17 also depicts the "training-sensitive zone" related to age.

Computing Lower- and Upper-Limit Target Heart Rates for Training

For men and women below the age of 60, the threshold stimulus or **lower-limit target heart rate (LL$_{THR}$)** for cardiovascular improvement ranges between 60% and 70% of HR$_{max}$, which represents about 50% to 60% of $\dot{V}O_{2max}$. The **upper-limit target heart rate (UL$_{THR}$)** equals about 90% of HR$_{max}$, which represents about 85% to 90% of $\dot{V}O_{2max}$. For those above age 60, LL$_{THR}$ equals 60% and UL$_{THR}$ equals 75% of HR$_{max}$.

METHOD 1: PERCENTAGE METHOD

This method calculates the lower-limit and upper-limit target heart rate as a simple percentage of the age-predicted HR$_{max}$.

1. Calculate LL$_{THR}$ as:

$$LL_{THR} = \text{Predicted HR}_{max} \times$$
$$\text{Lower-limit percentage for age}$$

where the lower-limit percentage = 70% for men and women ≤60 years and 60% for men and women >60 years.

2. Calculate UL$_{THR}$ as:

$$UL_{THR} = \text{Predicted HR}_{max} \times$$
$$\text{Upper-limit percentage for age}$$

where the upper-limit percentage = 90% for men and women ≤60 years and 80% for men and women >60 years.

Example
Data: Male, age 55 years

1. Calculate predicted HR$_{max}$

$$HR_{max} = 208 - (0.7 \times \text{Age, y}) = 170 \text{ b} \cdot \text{min}^{-1}$$
$$LL_{THR} = 170 \times \text{Lower-limit percentage for age}$$
$$= 170 \times 0.70$$
$$= 119 \text{ b} \cdot \text{min}^{-1}$$

2. Calculate UL$_{THR}$

$$UL_{THR} = HR_{max} \times \text{Upper-limit percentage for age}$$
$$= 170 \times 0.90$$
$$= 153 \text{ b} \cdot \text{min}^{-1}$$

METHOD 2: KARVONEN METHOD (HEART RATE RESERVE)

An alternate, equally effective method calculates the lower- and upper-limit target heart rates for training as a percentage of the difference between resting and maximum HR, termed **heart rate reserve** (**HRR**; also referred to as the **Karvonen method**, named after the Finnish physiologist who introduced this method). Karvonen's method produces somewhat higher values compared to heart rate computed as percentage of HR$_{max}$. The Karvonen method uses about 50% of HRR as LL$_{THR}$ and 85% of HRR as UL$_{THR}$ and computes as follows:

1. Calculate predicted HR$_{max}$:

$$HR_{max} = 208 - (0.7 \times \text{Age, y})$$

2. Calculate LL$_{THR}$:

$$LL_{THR} = \left[(HR_{max} - HR_{rest}) \times 0.50 \right] + HR_{rest}$$

3. Calculate UL$_{THR}$:

$$UL_{THR} = \left[(HR_{max} - HR_{rest}) \times 0.85 \right] + HR_{rest}$$

Example
Data: Male, age 55 years; HR$_{rest}$ = 60 b · min^{-1}

1. Calculate predicted HR$_{max}$:

$$HR_{max} = 208 - (0.7 \times \text{Age, y})$$
$$= 170 \text{ b} \cdot \text{min}^{-1}$$

2. Calculate LL$_{THR}$:

$$LL_{THR} = \left[(HR_{max} - HR_{rest}) \times 0.50 \right] + HR_{rest}$$
$$= \left[(170 - 60) \times 0.50 \right] + 60$$
$$= 115 \text{ b} \cdot \text{min}^{-1}$$

3. Calculate UL$_{THR}$:

$$UL_{THR} = \left[(HR_{max} - HR_{rest}) \times 0.85 \right] + HR_{rest}$$
$$= \left[(170 - 60) \times 0.85 \right] + 60$$
$$= 154 \text{ b} \cdot \text{min}^{-1}$$

Sources:

Davis JA, Convertino VA. A comparison of heart rate methods for predicting endurance training intensity. *Med Sci Sports Exerc* 1975;7:295.

Gellish RL, et al. Longitudinal modeling of the relationship between age and maximal heart rate. *Med Sci Sports Exerc* 2007;39:822.

Karvonen M, et al. The effects of training on heart rate. A longitudinal study. *Ann Med Exp Biol Fenn* 1957;35:307.

Tanaka H, et al. Age-predicted maximal heart rate revisited. *J Am Coll Cardiol* 2001;37:153.

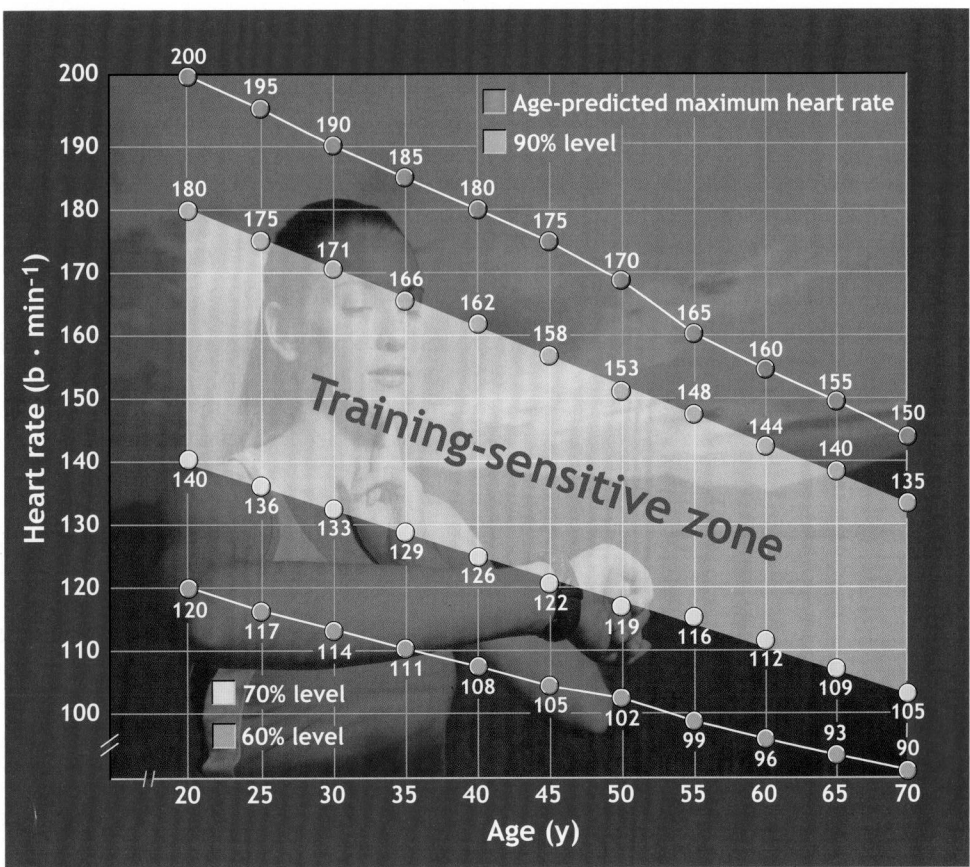

FIGURE 21.16 • Maximal heart rates and training-sensitive zone for aerobic training of men and women of different ages.

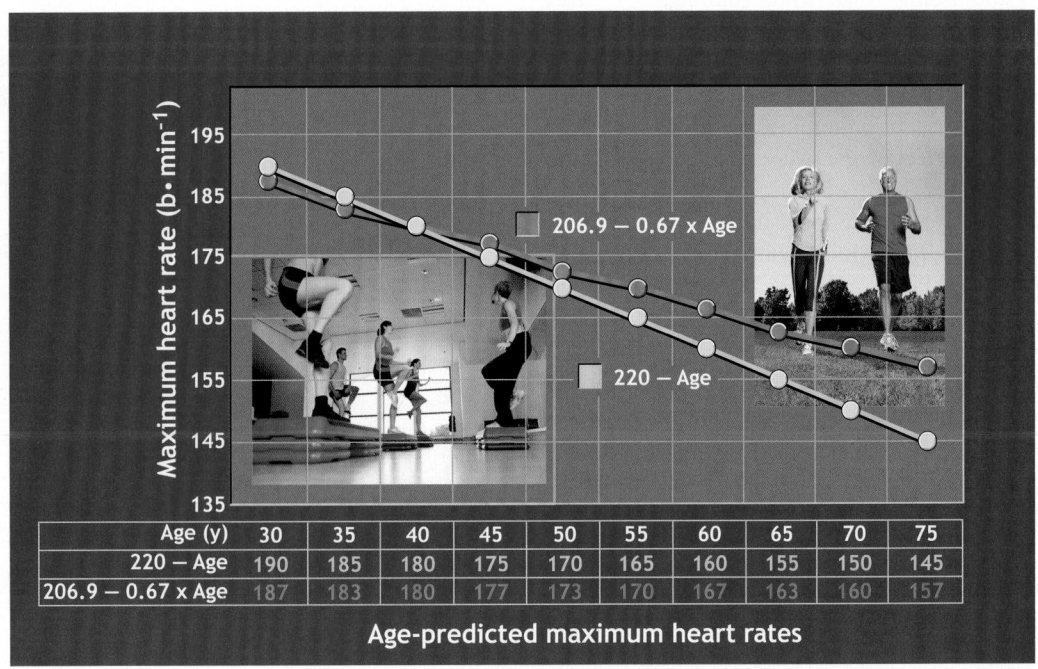

Age (y)	30	35	40	45	50	55	60	65	70	75
220 − Age	190	185	180	175	170	165	160	155	150	145
206.9 − 0.67 x Age	187	183	180	177	173	170	167	163	160	157

Age-predicted maximum heart rates

FIGURE 21.17 • Modified maximum heart rate versus age prediction compared with the commonly used equation of 220 − age. (Reprinted with permission from Gellish RL, et al. Longitudinal modeling of the relationship between age and maximal heart rate. *Med Sci Sports Exerc* 2007;39:822.)

A 40-year-old person who wants to train at moderate intensity but still achieve the threshold level would select a training heart rate of 70% of age-predicted HR_{max}. Using the 220-minus-age formula results in a target activity heart rate of 126 b·min⁻¹ (0.70 × 180). To increase training to 85% of maximum, intensity must increase to produce a heart rate of 153 b·min⁻¹ (0.85 × 180).

 ### Predicting Maximum Heart Rate in Overfat Individuals

For overfat men and women with percentage body fat levels ≥ 30%, HR_{max} predicts as:

$$HR_{max} = 200 - (0.5 \times \text{Age, y})$$

EXAMPLE

Calculate the HR_{max} for a 25-year-old female with a percentage body fat of 32%.

$$HR_{max} = 200 - (0.5 \times 25)$$
$$= 188 \text{ b} \cdot \text{min}^{-1}$$

Source: Miller WC, et al. Predicting max HR and the HR-VO₂ relationship for exercise prescription in obesity. *Med Sci Sports Exerc* 1993;25:1077.

Running Versus Swimming and Other Forms of Upper-Body Physical Activity. Estimation of HR_{max} requires an adjustment when swimming or performing other upper-body activities. Maximum heart rate during these activity modes averages about 13 b·min⁻¹ lower for trained and untrained men and women than while running.[49,58,135] This difference probably results from less feed-forward stimulation from the motor cortex to the medulla during swimming, in addition to less feedback stimulation from the smaller, active upper-body muscle mass. In swimming, the horizontal body position and cooling effect of the water also may contribute to a lower HR_{max}.

Establishing the appropriate intensity for swimming and other upper-body activities requires subtracting 13 b·min⁻¹ from the age-predicted HR_{max} in Figure 21.16. A 30-year-old person who chooses to swim at 70% HR_{max} should select a swimming speed that produces a heart rate of 124 b·min⁻¹ (0.70 × [190 − 13]). This would more accurately represent the proper threshold heart rate for swimming to induce a training effect. Without this adjustment, a prescription of upper-body activity based on %HR_{max} in leg effort *overestimates* the appropriate threshold training heart rate.

Can Less Intense Training be Effective?

The often-cited recommendation of 70% HR_{max} as a training threshold for aerobic improvement represents a *general guideline* for effective yet comfortable exertion. The lower limit may depend on the participant's initial exercise capacity and current state of training. In addition, older and less fit, including

sedentary, overweight men and women have training thresholds closer to 60% HR_{max} (corresponding to about 45% $\dot{V}O_{2max}$). Twenty to 30 min of continuous activity at 70% HR_{max} stimulates a training effect; exercise at the lower intensity of 60% HR_{max} for 45 min also proves beneficial. *Generally, longer exercise duration offsets lower exercise intensity in terms of benefits.*

Train at a Perception of Effort

The **rating of perceived exertion** (RPE) can also be applied to indicate intensity of physical activity.[16,156,183] With this psychophysiologic approach, the exerciser rates on a numerical scale perceived feelings relative to exertion level. Monitoring and adjusting RPE during activity provides an effective way to prescribe exercise from an individual's perception of effort that coincides with objective measures of physiologic/metabolic strain that includes %HR_{max}, %$\dot{V}O_{2max}$, and blood lactate concentration.

Physical activity that corresponds to higher levels of energy expenditure and physiologic strain produces higher RPE ratings. An RPE of 13 or 14 (feels "somewhat hard;" Fig. 21.18) coincides with about 70% HR_{max} during cycle ergometer and treadmill exercise; an RPE between 11 and 12 corresponds to exercise at the lactate threshold for trained and untrained individuals. The RPE establishes an exercise prescription for intensities that correspond to blood lactate concentrations of 2.5 mM (RPE ~ 15) and 4.0 mM (RPE ~ 18) during a 30-min treadmill run where subjects self-regulated the intensity of effort.[211] Similarly, a simple "talk test" that asks whether comfortable speech is

RPE Scale		Equivalent % HR_{max}	Equivalent % $\dot{V}O_{2max}$
6			
7	Very, very light		
8			
9	Very light		
10			
11	Fairly light	52-66	31-50
12			
13	Somewhat hard	61-85	51-75
14			
15	Hard	86-91	76-85
16			
17	Very hard	92	85
18			
19	Very, very hard		

FIGURE 21.18 • The Borg scale (and accompanying estimates of relative exercise intensity) for obtaining the RPE during exercise. (Adapted with permission from Borg GA. Psychological basis of physical exertion. *Med Sci Sports Exerc* 1982;14:377.)

possible produces intensities within accepted guidelines for exercise prescription using treadmill and cycle ergometer exercise.[162]

Train at the Lactate Threshold

Exercising at or slightly above the lactate threshold provides another effective aerobic training method. The higher intensity levels produce the greatest benefits, particularly for fit individuals.[118,231] FIGURE 21.19 illustrates how to determine the appropriate activity level by plotting intensity (e.g., running speed) related to blood lactate level. In this example, the running speed to produce a blood lactate concentration at the 4-mM OBLA represents the recommended training intensity. Many coaches use the 4-mM blood lactate level as the optimal aerobic training intensity, yet no convincing evidence exists to justify this particular blood lactate level as "ideal." Regardless of the specific blood lactate level chosen for endurance training, the blood lactate–exercise intensity relationship should be evaluated periodically, with activity intensity adjusted as fitness improves. If regular blood lactate measurement proves impractical, the heart rate at the initial lactate determination remains a convenient and relatively stable marker to set an appropriate predetermined level of intensity. During incremental activity, no systematic training-induced change occurs in the heart rate–blood lactate relationship.[47]

The RPE provides an effective tool to estimate blood lactate threshold when establishing training intensity for continuous physical activity. A change in the blood lactate concentration–RPE relationship does occur with repeated activity bouts. The relationship remains altered from a single bout, even after 3.5 hr of recovery.[233] This limits RPE to gauge effort intensity for a specific blood lactate concentration if repeated bouts of exercise occur during the same training session (e.g., during interval training; see "Interval Training," later in this chapter).

One important distinction between %HR$_{max}$ and lactate threshold for setting training intensity lies in the physiologic dynamics each method reflects. The %HR$_{max}$ method establishes a level of physiologic stress to overload the central circulation (e.g., stroke volume, cardiac output), whereas the capacity of the peripheral vasculature and active muscles to sustain steady-rate aerobic metabolism dictates exercise intensity adjustments based on lactate threshold.

Training Duration

No threshold duration per workout exists for optimal aerobic improvement. If a threshold exists, it likely depends on the interaction of total work accomplished (i.e., duration or training volume), intensity of effort, training frequency, and initial fitness level. For previously sedentary adults, a dose–response relationship may exist.[26] A 3- to 5-min daily activity period produces some improvements in poorly conditioned people, but 20- to 30-min sessions achieve more optimal results if intensity achieves at least the minimum threshold.

For training volume, more time devoted to workouts does not necessarily translate to greater improvements, particularly among physically active individuals. For collegiate swimmers, one group trained for 1.5 hr daily while another group performed two 1.5-hr exercise sessions daily.[34] Even when one group trained at twice the daily volume, *no differences* in swimming power, endurance, or performance time improvements emerged between groups.

Training Frequency

Do 2- and 5-day-a-week training produce different effects if duration and intensity remain constant for each training session? Unfortunately, the precise answer remains elusive. Some investigators report training frequency influences cardiovascular improvements, while others maintain this factor contributes considerably less than either intensity or duration of effort.[169] Studies with interval training show that training 2 days weekly produced $\dot{V}O_{2max}$ changes similar to training 5 days weekly.[48] In other studies that maintained a constant total exercise volume, *no differences* emerged in $\dot{V}O_{2max}$ improvement between training frequencies of 2 and 4 or 3 and 5 days a week.[202] More frequent training produces beneficial effects when training occurs at a lower intensity.

While the extra time invested to increase training frequency may not improve $\dot{V}O_{2max}$, the extra quantity of physical activity (e.g., 3 vs. 6 days a week) often represents a considerable caloric expenditure with concomitant improvements in well-being and health. *To produce meaningful weight loss through physical activity, each activity session should last at least 60 min at sufficient intensity to expend 300 kcal or more.* Training 1 day a week generally does not change anaerobic or aerobic capacity, body composition, or body weight.[6]

Typical aerobic training programs take place 3 days a week, usually with a single rest day separating workout days.

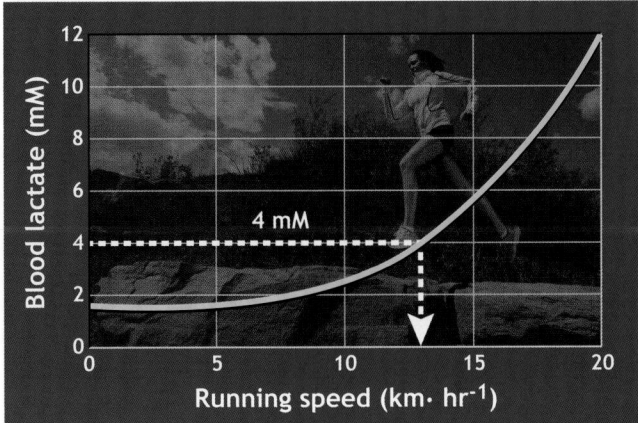

FIGURE 21.19 • Blood lactate concentration in relation to running speed for one subject. At a lactate level of 4.0 mM, the corresponding running speed was approximately 13 km·hr⁻¹. This speed establishes the subject's initial training intensity.

One could ask whether training on consecutive days would produce equally effective results. In an experiment regarding this question, nearly identical improvements in $\dot{V}O_{2max}$ occurred regardless of sequencing of the 3-days-per-week training schedule.[142] The stimulus for aerobic training probably links closely to effort intensity and total work accomplished, not to the sequencing of training days.

Exercise Mode

Maintaining constancy for exercise intensity, duration, and frequency produces a similar training response independent of training mode—provided the activity involves relatively large muscle groups. Bicycling, walking, running, rowing, swimming, in-line skating, rope skipping, bench-stepping, stair climbing, and simulated arm–leg climbing all provide excellent overload for the aerobic system.[21,126,228] Based on the specificity concept, the magnitude of training improvement varies considerably depending on training and testing mode. Individuals trained on a bicycle show greater improvement when tested on a bicycle rather than on a treadmill.[159] Likewise, individuals who train by swimming or arm cranking show the greatest improvement when measured during an upper-body activity.[58]

A Well-Rounded Overall Training Program

The primary goal of general physical activity for the adult population seeks to improve and maintain health.[7,76] The Centers for Disease Control (CDC) recently has updated the American College of Sports Medicine (ACSM) and American Heart Association (AHA) joint guidelines for a "well-rounded training program" for adults age 18 to 65 years (http://www.cdc.gov/physicalactivity/everyone/guidelines/adults.html) as well as for older adults (http://www.cdc.gov/physicalactivity/everyone/guidelines/olderadults.html). A combined program of aerobic training (150 min weekly of moderate-intensity activity or 75 min weekly of vigorous activity) and resistance training, which emphasizes all major muscle groups increases muscular strength and aerobic power, decreases body fat, and increases basal metabolic rate. Additional amounts of physical activity produce even greater health benefits. In contrast, singular-focus programs of either resistance *only* or aerobic training *only* produce singularly larger but more limited overall effects.[41,170] For older adults, emphasis should also focus on movements to increase joint flexibility and improve balance so as to reduce injury risk from slips and falls.[150]

 INTEGRATIVE QUESTION

Explain what factors account for differences in responsiveness of individuals to the same training program.

HOW LONG BEFORE IMPROVEMENTS OCCUR?

Improvements in aerobic fitness occur within several weeks. **FIGURE 21.20** shows absolute and percentage improvements in $\dot{V}O_{2max}$ for subjects who trained 6 days a week for 10 wk. Training consisted of stationary cycling for 30 min 3 days a week combined with running for up to 40 min on alternate days. The continuous week-to-week improvement in aerobic capacity indicates that training improvement in previously sedentary persons occurs rapidly and steadily. Adaptive responses eventually level off as subjects approach their "genetically predisposed" maximums. The exact time for this levelling off remains unknown, particularly for high-intensity training. The data presented in Figure 21.14 indicate that each physiologic and metabolic system responds in a unique and different way.

The data in **TABLE 21.7** complement those in Figure 21.20; they reveal the rapidity of maximum cardiovascular adaptations to aerobic training. Five young adult men and

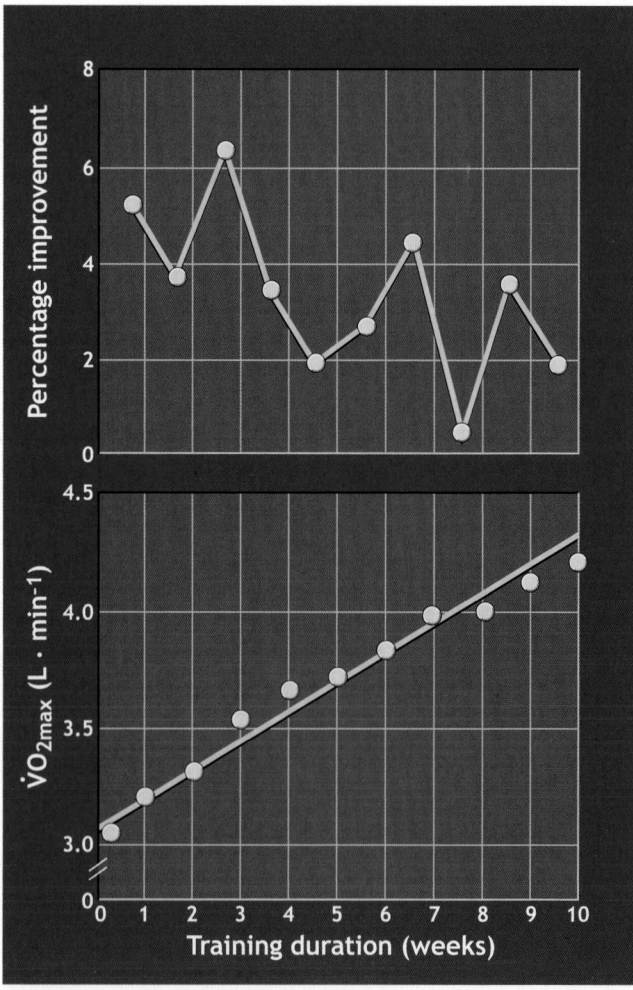

FIGURE 21.20 • Continuous improvements in $\dot{V}O_{2max}$ during 10 wk of high-intensity aerobic training. (Reprinted with permission from Hickson RC, et al. Linear increases in aerobic power induced by a program of endurance exercise. *J Appl Physiol* 1977;42:373.)

Variable	Pretraining	Posttraining
$\dot{V}O_{2peak}$, L·min^{-1}	2.54 ± 0.29	2.80 ± 0.32[a]
Cardiac output, L·min^{-1}	18.3 ± 1.3	20.5 ± 1.7[a]
Heart rate, b·min^{-1}	189 ± 2	184 ± 2[a]
Stroke volume, mL	97 ± 7	112 ± 9[a]
a-$\bar{v}O_2$ diff, mL·dL^{-1}	13.6 ± 0.8	13.4 ± 0.6
Plasma volume (rest), mL	2896 ± 175	3152 ± 220[a]

TABLE 21.7 Maximum Physiologic Responses During Peak Cycle Ergometer Exercises Before and After 10 Consecutive Days of Aerobic Training

[a]Statistically significant at the .05 level from pretraining value.
From Mier CM, et al. Cardiovascular adaptations to 10 days of cycle exercise. *J Appl Physiol* 1997; 83:1900.

five women trained daily for 10 consecutive days. Exercise consisted of 1 hr of cycling—10 min at 65% $\dot{V}O_{2peak}$, 25 min at 75% $\dot{V}O_{2peak}$, and the last 25 min of repeat five 3-min intervals at 95% $\dot{V}O_{2peak}$ followed by a 2-min recovery. This relatively brief 10-day training period induced a 10% increase in $\dot{V}O_{2peak}$ and a 12% increase in cardiac output, a 15% increase in stroke volume, and a slight decrease in peak heart rate. Resting plasma volume increased nearly 9% during the 10 days of training and correlated with the increases in exercise cardiac output and stroke volume. This means that cardiovascular adaptations occur with short-term training in young men and women. The stroke volume increases during physical activity reflect the *combined effects* of increased left-ventricular end-diastolic dimension and increased systolic ejection.

Trainability and Genes

A strenuous training program enhances a person's level of fitness regardless of genetic background. The limits for developing fitness capacity appear to link closely to natural endowment. Of two individuals in the same training program, one might show 10 times more improvement than the other. A genotype dependency exists for much of one's sensitivity in responding to maximal aerobic and anaerobic power training, including adaptations of most muscle enzymes.[18,40,70] Stated differently, identical twins generally show a training response of similar magnitude. **FIGURE 21.21** indicates a similarity in the response of $\dot{V}O_{2max}$ (both mL·kg^{-1}·min^{-1} and % improvement) among 10 pairs of male identical twins who participated in the same 20-wk aerobic training program. If one twin showed high responsiveness to training, a high likelihood existed that the other twin would also be a **responder**; similarly, the brother of a **nonresponder** to training generally showed little improvement. Presence of the muscle-specific creatine kinase gene provides one example of the possible contribution of genetic makeup to individual differences in responsiveness of $\dot{V}O_{2max}$ to endurance training.[181,182]

MAINTAINING GAINS IN AEROBIC FITNESS

An important question concerns optimal frequency, duration, and intensity of activity to *maintain* aerobic improvements with training. In one study, healthy young adults increased $\dot{V}O_{2max}$ 25% with 10 wk of interval training by bicycling and running for 40 min, 6 days a week.[81] They then joined one of two groups that continued to exercise an additional 15 wk at the same intensity and duration but at reduced *frequency* to either 4 or 2 days a week. Both groups maintained their gains in aerobic capacity despite up to two-thirds reduction in training frequency.

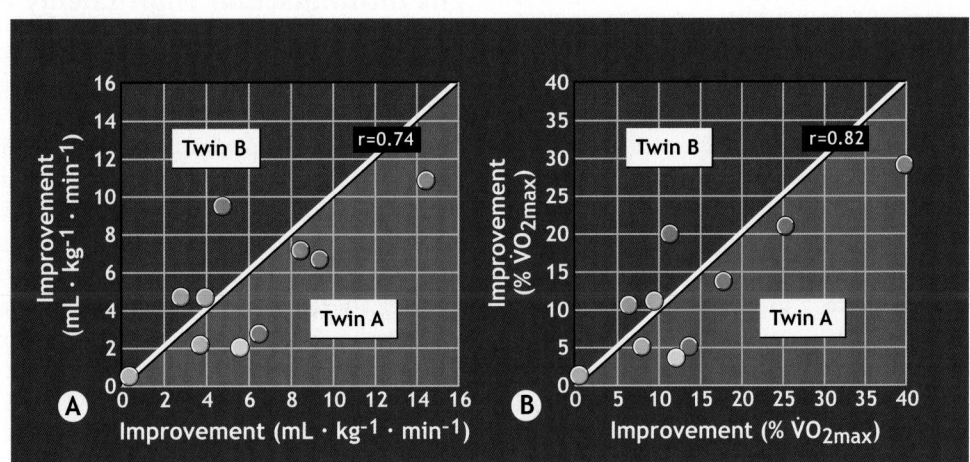

FIGURE 21.21 • Responsiveness of $\dot{V}O_{2max}$ (**A,** mL·kg^{-1}·min^{-1}; **B,** % improvement) of 10 pairs of identical twins to a 20-wk program of aerobic exercise training. *r*, Pearson product–moment correlation coefficient. Each of the 10 colored data points represents a twin pair. (Reprinted with permission from Bouchard C. Heredity, fitness, and health. In: Bouchard C, et al., eds. *Physical Activity, Fitness, and Health.* Champaign, IL: Human Kinetics, 1990.)

A similar study evaluated reduced training duration on maintenance of improved aerobic fitness.[82] Upon completion of the same protocol outlined previously for the initial 10 wk of training, subjects continued to maintain intensity and frequency of training for an additional 15 wk, but at reduced training *duration* from the original 40-min sessions to either 26 or 13 min per day. They maintained almost all $\dot{V}O_{2max}$ and performance increases despite a two-thirds reduction in training duration. Importantly, if training intensity decreased and frequency and duration remained constant, even a one-third reduction in intensity reduced the $\dot{V}O_{2max}$.[83]

Aerobic capacity improvement involves different training requirements than its maintenance. *With intensity held constant, the frequency and duration of activity required to maintain a certain level of aerobic fitness remain lower than required to induce improvement.* In contrast, a small decline in intensity of effort reduces $\dot{V}O_{2max}$. This indicates that intensity plays a principal role in maintaining the increase in aerobic capacity achieved through training.

Components Other Than $\dot{V}O_{2max}$

Fitness components other than $\dot{V}O_{2max}$ more readily suffer adverse effects of reduced training volume. Well-trained endurance athletes who normally trained 6 to 10 hr weekly reduced weekly training to one 35-min session over a 4-wk period.[130] $\dot{V}O_{2max}$ remained constant during this period of reduced training volume. However, endurance capacity at 75% $\dot{V}O_{2max}$ *decreased*; this performance decrement related to reduced pre-exercise glycogen stores and a diminished level of fat oxidation during activity. *A single measure such as $\dot{V}O_{2max}$ cannot adequately evaluate all of the factors that affect exercise training and detraining adaptations.*

Tapering for Peak Performance

Little improvement occurs in the aerobic systems *during* the competitive season. At best, athletes strive to prevent physiologic and performance deterioration as the season progresses. Before major competition, athletes often **taper** training intensity and/or volume, believing such adjustments reduce physiologic and psychologic stress of daily training and optimize competitive performance. The taper period and exact alterations in training vary by sport. A 1- to 3-wk taper that exponentially reduces training volume by 40 to 60%, while maintaining training intensity, provides the most efficient strategy to maximize performance gains.[17,219,220]

A 4- to 7-day taper should provide sufficient time for maximum muscle and liver glycogen replenishment, optimal nutritional support and restoration, alleviation of residual muscle soreness, and healing of minor injuries. In one study of competitive runners, a 1-wk taper period applied either no training (rest), low-intensity running (2 to 10 km daily at 60% $\dot{V}O_{2max}$), or high-intensity running while reducing training volume (five 500-m repeats on day 1, decreasing one repeat each day).[199] Measurements during the taper included blood volume, red blood cell mass, muscle glycogen content, muscle mitochondrial activity, and 1500-m race performance. Compared with rest and low-intensity exercise taper conditions, high-intensity taper produced the most benefit. An optimal taper should include progressive reductions in training volume while maintaining training intensity at a moderate-to-high level. With proper tapering, expected performance improvement usually ranges between 0.5 and 6.0%.[148] Tapering does not associate with substantial changes in exercise-induced oxidative stress.[226]

TRAINING METHODS

Performance improvements occur yearly in almost all athletic competitions. These advances generally relate to increased opportunities for participation: Individuals with "natural endowment" have opportunities to participate in different sports. Improved nutrition and health care, better equipment, and more systematic and scientific approaches to athletic training also contribute. The following sections present general guidelines for effective anaerobic and aerobic exercise training.

Anaerobic Training

Figure 21.1 showed that capacity to perform all-out exertion for up to 60 s largely depends on ATP generated by the immediate and short-term anaerobic systems for energy transfer.

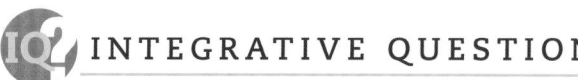

INTEGRATIVE QUESTION

In what specific ways would anaerobic training improve performance in all-out physical activity?

The Intramuscular High-Energy Phosphates

American football, weightlifting, and other brief sprint–power sport activities rely almost exclusively on energy derived from the intramuscular high-energy phosphates ATP and PCr. Engaging specific muscles in repeated 5- to 10-s maximum bursts of effort overloads energy transfer from this phosphagen pool. Only small amounts of lactate accumulate and recovery progresses rapidly. Activity can begin again after a 30-s rest period. The use of brief, all-out bursts of effort interspersed with recovery represents a highly specific application of interval training to anaerobic conditioning (see "Interval Training," later in this chapter).

Physical activities to enhance ATP–PCr energy transfer capacity must engage the sport-specific muscles at the movement speed and power output similar to performance of the sport itself. This strategy enhances metabolic capacity of specifically trained muscle fibers; it also facilitates recruitment and modulation of the neural firing sequence of appropriate motor units activated in the particular movement.

Lactate-Generating Capacity

Training must overload the short-term lactic acid energy system to improve this aspect of energy metabolism.

Training the glycolytic short-term energy system demands extreme physiologic and psychologic effort. Blood lactate rises to near-peak levels with a 1-min maximum bout of exercise. The individual repeats the same exercise bout after 3 to 5 min of recovery. Repetition of this sequence causes "lactate stacking," which produces a higher blood lactate level than just one all-out exhaustive effort. As with all training, one must activate the specific muscle groups that require enhanced anaerobic function. A backstroke swimmer trains by swimming the backstroke or use of an appropriate swim-bench ergometer; a cyclist should bicycle; and basketball, hockey, or soccer players rapidly perform various movements and direction changes specific to the sport requirement.

As discussed in Chapter 7, recovery requires considerable time when physical activity involves a large anaerobic component. For this reason, anaerobic power training of the short-term energy system should occur at the end of the conditioning session so fatigue does not hinder ability to perform subsequent aerobic training.

Aerobic Training

FIGURE 21.22 indicates two important factors in formulating regimens of aerobic training:

1. Cardiovascular demands must reach an intensity to sufficiently increase (overload) stroke volume and cardiac output.
2. Cardiovascular overload must activate sport-specific muscle groups to enhance local circulation and the muscle's "metabolic machinery."

Proper endurance training overloads all components of oxygen transport and use. This consideration embodies the specificity principle of aerobic training. Simply stated, runners must run, cyclists must bicycle, rowers must row, and swimmers must swim.

Relatively brief bouts of repeated activity, as well as continuous, long-duration efforts, enhance aerobic capacity, provided the activity attains sufficient intensity to overload the aerobic system. **Interval training**, **continuous training**, and **fartlek training** represent three common methods to improve aerobic fitness.

 INTEGRATIVE QUESTION

What information would you need to effectively improve aerobic capacity for the specific physical job performance requirements for (1) firefighters, (2) police officers, and (3) oil field workers?

Interval Training

With correct spacing of physical activity and rest intervals, one can perform extraordinary amounts of intense activity, not normally possible if activity progressed continuously. Repeated activity bouts (with brief rest periods or low-intensity relief intervals) typically vary from a few seconds to several minutes or longer depending on the desired training outcome.[79,108,110]

As little as six sessions of brief near all-out effort interval training over a 2-wk period increases skeletal muscle oxidative capacity and endurance performance.[59] The interval training prescription evolves from the following four considerations:

1. Intensity of activity interval
2. Duration of activity interval
3. Length of recovery (relief) interval
4. Number of repetitions of the exercise–relief interval

Consider the following example of performing a large volume of intense physical activity during an interval-training workout. Few people can maintain a 4-min-mile pace for longer than 1 min, let alone complete a mile in 4 min. Suppose running intervals were limited to only 10 s followed by a 30-s recovery. This scenario makes it reasonably easy to maintain the exercise–relief intervals and complete the mile in 4 min of actual running. This does not parallel a world-class performance but illustrates that a person can accomplish a considerable quantity of normally exhausting activity given proper spacing of rest and exercise intervals. This strategy of intense training interspersed with rest intervals would apply to treadmill, stair climbing, and bicycle ergometer exercise performed routinely in health clubs and training centers.

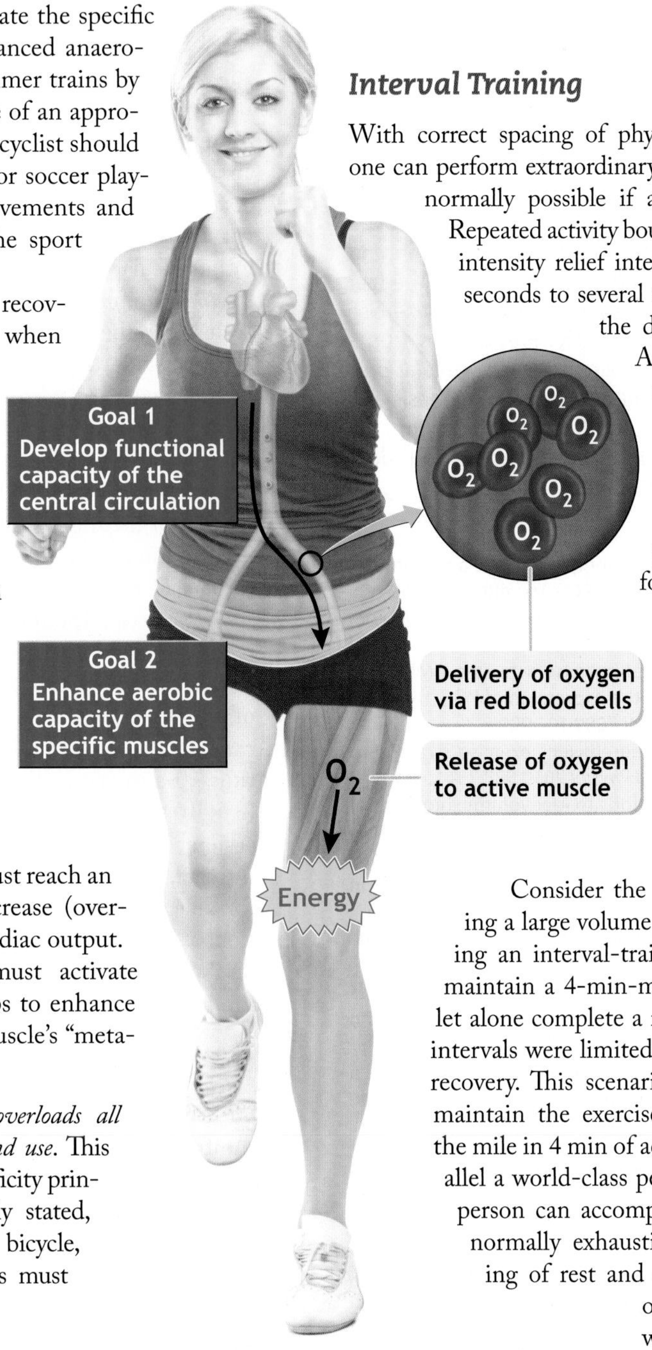

Goal 1
Develop functional capacity of the central circulation

Goal 2
Enhance aerobic capacity of the specific muscles

O_2 O_2 O_2 O_2 O_2 O_2 O_2

Delivery of oxygen via red blood cells

Release of oxygen to active muscle

O_2

Energy

FIGURE 21.22 • The two major goals of aerobic training: *Goal 1*, develop the capacity of the central circulation to deliver oxygen; *Goal 2*, enhance the capacity of the active musculature to supply and process oxygen.

One-Minute Bouts of Intense Physical Activity Improves Fitness and Health

Is the question really how much physical activity we need for improved health and fitness or rather how little is required? To answer the question, Canadian researchers studied several groups of volunteers consisting of sedentary but healthy middle-age men and women and the other composed of middle-age and older patients with diagnosed cardiovascular disease. Initial testing quantified their maximum heart rate and peak power output on a stationary bicycle. These values were not very high. Participants then trained using repetitive bouts of short bursts of high-intensity interval training (HIIT). This routine involved one-min exercise bouts at about 90% of maximum heart rate followed by 1 min of easy recovery with 10 total intervals of activity and recovery, for a total workout lasting only 20 min. Participants, particularly the cardiac patients, significantly improved overall health and cardiovascular fitness. The interesting finding was that all participants embraced the routine despite the fact that their ratings of perceived exertion during each exercise bout was 7 or higher on a 10-point scale. Previous investigations with HIIT have demonstrated increases in the cellular proteins involved in energy transfer (mitochondrial biogenesis and an increased capacity for glucose and fatty acid oxidation) via aerobic processes, improved insulin sensitivity, and blood sugar regulation, which reduced the risk of type 2 diabetes.

Sources:

Bartlett JD, et al. Matched work high-intensity interval and continuous running induce similar increases in PGC-1α mRNA, AMPK, p38 and p53 phosphorylation in human skeletal muscle. *J Appl Physiol* 2012;112:1135.

Gibala MJ, et al. Brief intense interval exercise activates AMPK and p38 MAPK signaling and increases the expression of PGC-1alpha in human skeletal muscle. *J Appl Physiol* 2009;106:929.

Gibala MJ, Little JP. Just HIT it!: A time-efficient exercise strategy to improve muscle insulin sensitivity. *J Physiol* 2010;588:3341.

Gibala MJ, et al. Physiological adaptations to low-volume, high-intensity interval training in health and disease. *J Physiol* 2012;590:1077.

Gillen JB, et al. Acute high-intensity interval exercise reduces the postprandial glucose response and prevalence of hyperglycaemia in patients with type 2 diabetes. *Diabetes Obes Metab* 2012;14:575.

Hood MS, et al. Low-volume interval training improves muscle oxidative capacity in sedentary adults. *Med Sci Sports Exerc.* 2011;43:1849.

Little JP, et al. Low-volume high-intensity interval training reduces hyperglycemia and increases muscle mitochondrial capacity in patients with type 2 diabetes. *J Appl Physiol* 2011;111:1554.

Little JP, et al. A practical model of low-volume high-intensity interval training induces mitochondrial biogenesis in human skeletal muscle: potential mechanisms. *J Physiol* 2010; 588:1011.

Rationale for Interval Training. Interval training regimens have a sound basis in physiology and energy metabolism. In the example of a continuous 4-min-mile run, anaerobic glycolysis generates a large portion of the energy requirement. Within a minute or two, the lactate level rises precipitously and the runner fatigues. For interval training, repeated 10-s exercise bouts permit completion of intense exercise without appreciable lactate buildup because intramuscular high-energy phosphates provide the primary energy source. Minimal fatigue develops during the predominantly short "alactic" exercise interval and recovery progresses rapidly. The exercise interval can then begin following only a brief rest.

In interval training, exercise intensity must activate the particular energy systems that require improvement. TABLE 21.8 provides practical guidelines to determine the appropriate exercise and recovery intervals for running and swimming different distances. Consider the following four examples:

1. *Exercise interval*: Generally *add* 1.5 to 5.0 s to the exerciser's "best time" for training distances between 55 and 220 yd (yards) for running and 15 and 55 yd for swimming.[48] If a person can run 60 yd from a running start in 8 s, the training time for each repeat equals 8 + 1.5, or 9.5 s. For an interval-training distance of 110 yd, add 3 s, and for a distance of 220 yd, add 5 s to the best running times. This particular type of interval training applies to training the intramuscular ATP–PCr energy system.

2. *Training distances* of 440 yd running or 110 yd swimming: Determine the exercise rate by *subtracting* 1 to 4 s from the best 440-yd part of a mile run or 110-yd part of a 440-yd swim. If a person runs a mile in 7 min (averaging 105 s per 440 yd), the interval time for each 440-yd repeat range is 104 s (105 − 1) to 101 s (105 − 4). For training intervals beyond 440 yd, *add* 3 to 4 s for each 440-yd portion of the interval distance. In running an interval of 880 yd, the 7-min miler runs each interval at about 216 s [(105 + 3) × 2 = 216].

3. *Relief interval*: The relief interval is either passive (rest–relief) or active (work–relief). A ratio of exercise duration to recovery duration usually formulates the duration of the relief interval. *The ratio 1:3 generally applies to training the immediate energy system.* For a sprinter who runs 10-s intervals, the relief interval equals about 30 s (3 × 10 s). For training the short-term glycolytic energy system, the relief interval averages twice the exercise interval, or a ratio of 1:2. These specific work–relief ratios for anaerobic training should ensure sufficient restoration of intramuscular phosphates and/or sufficient lactate removal so the next exercise bout can continue with minimal fatigue.

4. *The optimal exercise-to relief interval ratio usually is 1:1 or 1:1.5 to train the long-term aerobic energy system.* During a 60- to 90-s high-intensity exercise interval, oxygen consumption increases rapidly to a high level but remains inadequate to meet exercise energy requirements. The recommended relief interval causes the succeeding exercise interval to begin before complete recovery (before return to baseline oxygen consumption). This ensures that cardiovascular and aerobic metabolic stress attain near peak levels with repeated but relatively short exercise intervals. The duration of the rest interval takes on less importance with longer periods of intermittent exercise because sufficient time exists for the body to adjust metabolic and circulatory parameters during the activity.

TABLE 21.8	Guidelines for Determining Interval-Training Exercise Rates for Running and Swimming Different Distances	

Interval Training Distances (yd)		Work Rate for Each Exercise Interval or Repeat
Run	Swim	
55	15	1.5 s *slower* than best
110	25	3.0 times from a running (or *swimming*) start
220	55	5.0 for each distance
440	110	1 to 4 s *faster* than the average 440-yd run or 110-yd swim times recorded during a mile run or 440-yd swim
660–1320	165–320	3 to 4 s *slower* than the average 440-yd run or 100-yd swim times recorded during a mile run or 440-yd swim

Reprinted from Fox EL, Mathews DK. *Interval Training*. Philadelphia: WB Saunders, 1974.

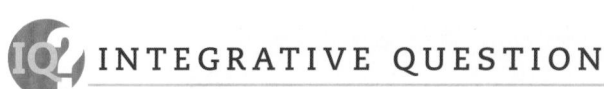

INTEGRATIVE QUESTION

A coach insists that a single activity mode improves aerobic capacity for all physical activities requiring a high level of aerobic fitness. Give your opinion regarding the potential effectiveness of single-mode exercise to produce generalized cross-training effects.

Sprint-Type Interval Training Affects Anaerobic and Aerobic Physiologic Systems. Figure 21.23 shows that relatively brief but intense sprint-type interval training increases parameters of both anaerobic and aerobic metabolic capacity. The 7-wk training program for 12 young adult men consisted of 30 s of maximum sprint effort (Wingate protocol) interspersed with 2 to 4 min of recovery performed three times a week. Week 1 began with four exercise intervals with 4 min recovery per interval and progressed to 10 exercise intervals with a 2.5-min recovery per exercise bout by week 7. Despite this relatively brief training stimulus in which exercise duration reached only 5 min per session during week 7, improvements occurred in $\dot{V}O_{2max}$, short-term power output, and maximal activity of key marker enzymes in the aerobic and anaerobic energy pathways. Healthy elderly persons also show positive clinical and cardiovascular adaptations to interval training.[3] High-intensity interval training in mice altered cardiac substrate utilization (36% increase in glucose oxidation and a concomitant reduction in fatty acid oxidation), improved cardiac efficiency by decreasing work-independent myocardial oxygen consumption, and increased cardiac maximal mitochondrial respiratory capacity. No such changes were observed for animals involved in distance-matched more moderate-intensity training.[68]

Continuous Training

Continuous or long, slow, distance (LSD) training involves steady-paced, prolonged activity at either moderate or high aerobic intensity, at between 60 to 80% $\dot{V}O_{2max}$. The exact pace can vary, but it must minimally meet a threshold intensity to ensure aerobic physiologic adaptations. Previously, we outlined the method to establish the training-sensitive zone that uses HR_{max} (see "Determining the 'Training-Sensitive Zone'," earlier in this chapter). Continuous training that exceeds 1 hr has become popular among fitness enthusiasts, including competitive triathletes and cross-country skiers. Many elite distance runners train twice daily and train by running 100 to 150 miles weekly to prepare for competition.

Because of its submaximal nature, continuous exercise training progresses in relative comfort. This contrasts with the potential hazards of high-intensity interval training for coronary-prone individuals and high level of motivation required for such vigorous effort. Continuous training ideally suits novices who wish to accumulate a large caloric expenditure for weight loss. When applied to athletic training, continuous training truly represents "overdistance" training, with most competitors training two to five times the actual distances of their events.

Continuous training allows endurance athletes to move at nearly the same intensity as actual competition. Specific motor unit recruitment depends on intensity of effort, making continuous training desirable to endurance athletes who desire adaptations at the cellular level. In contrast, interval training often places disproportionate stress on fast-twitch motor units, not slow-twitch units predominantly recruited in endurance competition.

Fartlek Training

Fartlek, a Swedish word meaning "speed play," represents a training method introduced to the United States in the 1940s

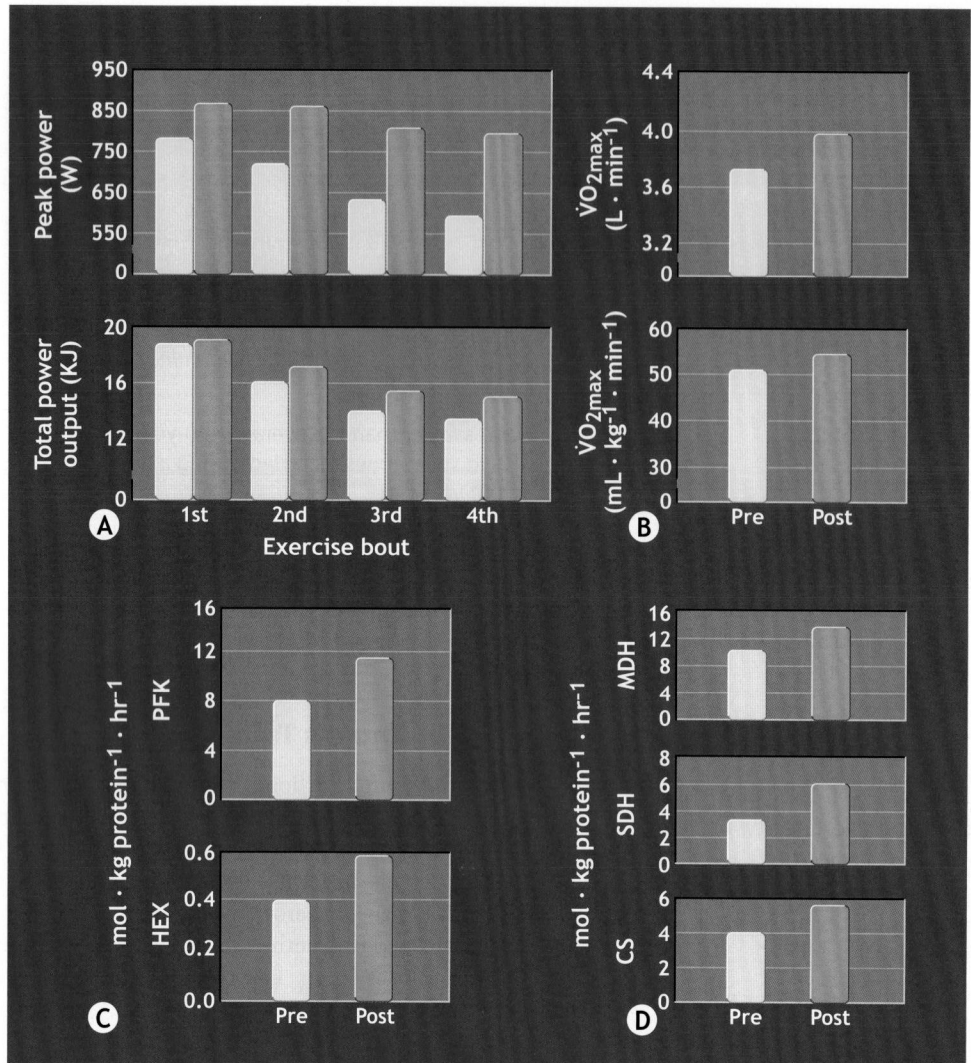

FIGURE 21.23 • Peak power output and total power output during four successive maximum 30-s efforts **(A)**; $\dot{V}O_{2max}$ **(B)**; maximal enzyme activity for phosphofructokinase (*PFK*) and hexokinase (*HEX*) **(C)**; and maximal enzyme activity for malate dehydrogenase (*MDH*), succinate dehydrogenase (*SDH*), and citrate synthase (*CS*) **(D)** before (*yellow bars*) and after (*orange bars*) 7 wk of sprint interval training. (Reprinted with permission from MacDougall JD, et al. Muscle performance and enzymatic adaptations to sprint interval training. *J Appl Physiol* 1998;84:2138.)

(http://www.newintervaltraining.com/fartlek-training.php) by former Swedish decathlete Gösta Holmér. This relatively unscientific blending of interval and continuous training has particular application to exercise out-of-doors over natural terrain. The system uses alternate running at fast and slow speeds over level and hilly terrain.

In contrast to the precise exercise-interval training prescription, fartlek training does not require systematic manipulation of exercise and relief intervals. Instead, the person determines the training schema based on "how it feels" at the time, similar to gauging effort intensity based on one's RPE. When properly applied, this method overloads one or all of the body's three energy systems. Fartlek training provides ideal general conditioning and off-season training strategies, yet it lacks the systematic and quantified approaches of interval

and continuous training. It also adds freedom and variety to workouts.

Insufficient evidence prevents proclaiming superiority of any specific training method to improve aerobic capacity and associated physiologic variables.[144] Each form of training produces success. One can probably use the various training methods interchangeably, particularly to modify training and achieve a more psychologically pleasing regimen of physical activity.

OVERTRAINING: TOO MUCH OF A GOOD THING

Ten to 20% of athletes experience **overtraining** or "staleness." The overtrained syndrome represents more than short-term inability to train hard or a slight dip in competition-level performance. Athletes can fail to endure and adapt to training so that normal performance deteriorates, and they encounter increasing difficulty fully recovering from a workout.[23,205,223] This takes on crucial importance for elite athletes where performance decrements of 1 to 3% can prevent a gold medalist from qualifying for competition. Overtraining also relates to increased incidence of infections, persistent muscle soreness, and general malaise and loss of interest in sustaining high-level training. Injuries occur more frequently in the overtrained state.[224]

Two clinical forms of overtraining have been described:

1. The less common **sympathetic form** (*basedowian* for thyroid hyperfunction patterns), characterized by increased sympathetic activity during rest and generally typified by hyperexcitability, restlessness, and impaired exercise performance. This form of overtraining may reflect excessive psychologic/emotional stress that accompanies the interaction among training, competition, and responsibilities of normal living.[113]

2. The more common **parasympathetic form** (*addisonoid* for adrenal insufficiency patterns), characterized by predominance of vagal activity during rest and physical activity. More properly termed *overreaching* in the early stages (within as few as 10 days), the syndrome qualitatively is similar in symptoms to the full-blown parasympathetic overtraining syndrome but of shorter duration. Excessive and protracted physical overload with inadequate recovery and rest leads to overreaching. Initially, maintaining exercise performance requires greater effort; this eventually leads to performance deterioration in training and competition. Short-term rest intervention of a few days up to several weeks usually restores full function. Untreated overreaching eventually leads to **overtraining syndrome**.

Parasympathetic overtraining syndrome involves chronic fatigue during workouts and recovery periods. Associated symptoms include sustained poor exercise performance, altered sleep patterns and appetite, frequent infections, persistent feelings of fatigue, altered immune and reproductive functions, acute and chronic alterations in systemic inflammatory responses, mood disturbances (anger, depression, anxiety), and general malaise and loss of interest in high-level training.

(fyi) Definitions of Terms Related to Overtraining Syndrome

- *Overload*: A planned, systematic, and progressive increase in training to improve performance.
- *Overreaching*: Unplanned, excessive overload with inadequate rest. Poor performance is observed in training and competition. Successful recovery should result from short-term (i.e., a few days up to 1 or 2 wk) interventions.
- *Overtraining syndrome*: Untreated overreaching that produces long-term decreased performance and impaired ability to train. Other associated problems may require medical attention.[175]

Figure 21.24 illustrates possible interactive factors that initiate parasympathetic-type overtraining syndrome. Interactions among chronic neuromuscular, neuroendocrine, psychologic, immunologic, and metabolic overload during long-term, high-volume training (with insufficient recuperation) eventually alter physiologic function and the stress response to produce the overtrained state.[71,128,184] Preexisting medical conditions; inadequate carbohydrate or dehydration; environmental stress of heat, humidity, and altitude; and psychosocial pressures (e.g., monotonous training, frequent competition, personal conflicts) often exacerbate training demands and increase the risk of developing overtraining syndrome.

Significant effects of a chronic imbalance of training load, competition, and nontraining stress factors in overtraining include the following:

1. Functional impairments in the hypothalamo–pituitary–gonadal and adrenal axes and sympathetic neuroendocrine system reflected by depressed urinary excretion of norepinephrine and a desensitization of the β_2-adrenergic system.[51,113,218]

2. Exercise-induced increases in adrenocorticotropic hormone and growth hormone and decreases in cortisol and insulin levels.[223]

In some ways, the syndrome reflects the body's attempt to provide the athlete with an appropriate recuperative period from intense training and competition. Despite the highly individualized specific symptoms of overtraining, those outlined in **Table 21.9** are most common. No simple method diagnoses overtraining in its earliest stages.[53,74] The best indications include deterioration in physical performance, alterations in mood, a relatively high cortisol/cortisone ratio, and possibly decreased nocturnal heart rate variability.[8,164,198] Conditions that cause some athletes to thrive in training initiate an overtraining response in others. Generally, rest can relieve the symptoms; if not, they can persist to thwart complete recovery that often requires weeks or months. No reliable strategy can determine the point of complete recovery from overtraining syndrome, but most athletes intuitively seem to know when they can successfully return to competition.

Coaches must allow adequate recuperation during the most intense training cycles or when an athlete attempts to regain peak form following a protracted layoff. Nutrition becomes important during intense training; special emphasis placed on glycogen replenishment, which requires sufficient recovery time, plus high levels of dietary carbohydrate and rehydration, reduce symptoms. Nevertheless, nutrition alone cannot prevent the syndrome's development.[1,175,201]

PHYSICAL ACTIVITY DURING PREGNANCY

Forty percent or more of women in the United States participate in different forms of physical activity during

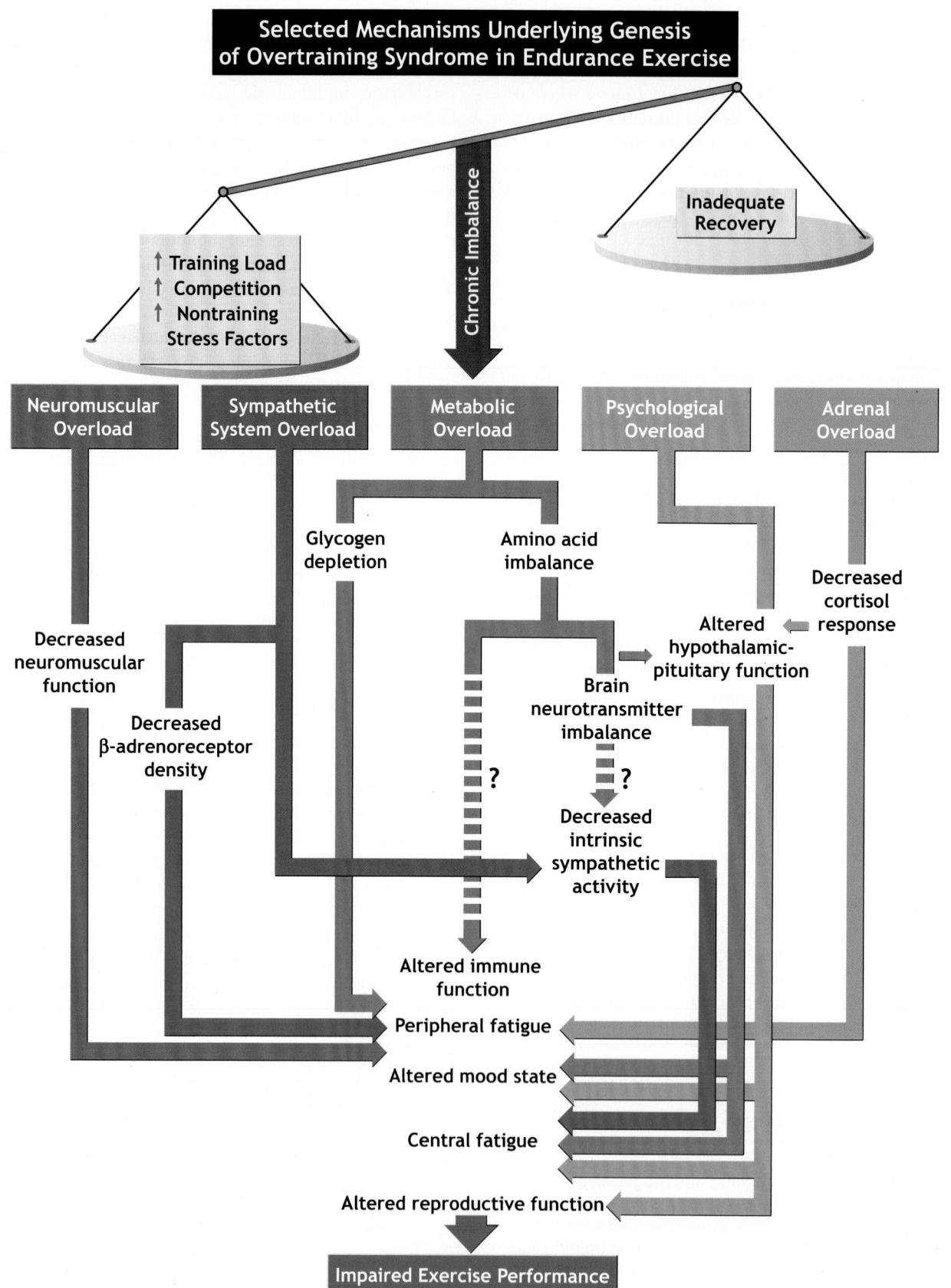

FIGURE 21.24 • Schematic overview of the genesis of overtraining syndrome in endurance sports requiring prolonged high-volume training. (Adapted with permission from Lehmann M, et al. Autonomic imbalance hypothesis and overtraining syndrome. *Med Sci Sports Exerc* 1998;30:1140.)

TABLE 21.9 **Overtraining Syndrome: Symptoms of Staleness**

- Unexplained and persistently poor performance and high fatigue ratings
- Prolonged recovery from typical training sessions or competitive events
- Disturbed mood states characterized by general fatigue, apathy, depression, irritability, and loss of competitive drive
- Persistent feelings of soreness and stiffness in muscles and joints
- Elevated resting pulse and increased susceptibility to upper respiratory infections (altered immune function) and gastrointestinal disturbances
- Insomnia
- Loss of appetite, weight loss, and inability to maintain proper body weight for competition
- Overuse injuries

pregnancy.[77,240] FIGURE 21.25 illustrates the prevalence and pattern of different activities during pregnancy among pregnant and nonpregnant women. Nonpregnant women were more likely than pregnant women to meet the moderate or vigorous physical activity recommendations. For both groups, walking represented the most common activity (52% for pregnant and 45% for nonpregnant). Pregnant women who engaged in either moderate or vigorous physical activity were generally younger, non-Hispanic white, unmarried, more educated,

nonsmokers, and had higher incomes than less physically active counterparts.

Physical Activity Effects on the Mother

Maternal cardiovascular dynamics follow normal response patterns; moderate physical activity offers no greater physiologic stress to the mother other than the additional weight gain and possible encumbrance of fetal tissue. In fact, regular physical activity during pregnancy can reduce maternal weight gain by an average 3.1 kg (6.8 lb) compared to women who are not regularly active.[105]

Pregnant women showed similar capacity as postpartum women to perform 40 min of cycling at 70 to 75% VO_{2max}. The physiologic responses to this weight-supported activity remained largely independent of gestation.[122] Pregnancy does not compromise the absolute value for aerobic capacity $(L \cdot min^{-1})$.[123] The increase in maternal body mass and changes in coordination and balance as pregnancy progresses adversely affect movement economy; this adds to effort with weight-bearing physical activity. Pregnancy, particularly in the last trimester, also increases pulmonary ventilation at a given submaximal level of effort.[122] The direct stimulating effects of progesterone and increased chemoreceptor sensitivity to carbon dioxide contribute to maternal exercise "hyperventilation."[238] Regular, moderate activity during the second and third trimesters reduces submaximal ventilatory demands and RPE.[154] This training adaptation increases the mother's ventilatory reserve and possibly inhibits exertional dyspnea. TABLE 21.10 summarizes the important maternal metabolic and cardiorespiratory adaptations during pregnancy.

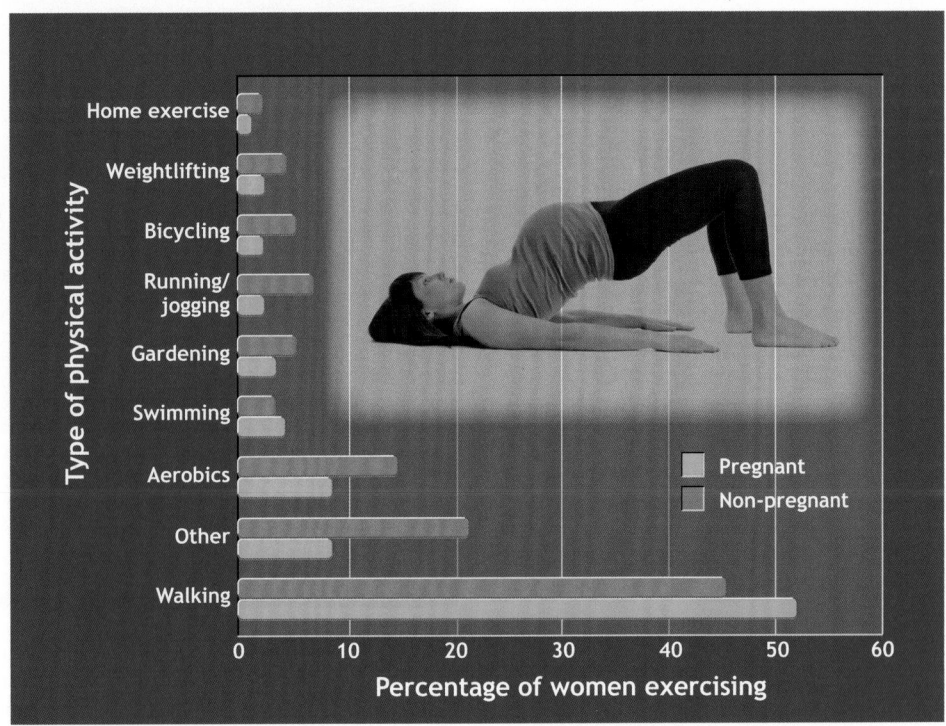

FIGURE 21.25 • Common physical activities among pregnant and nonpregnant women (1994, 1996, 1998, and 2000 data combined). (Reprinted with permission from Petersen AM, et al. Correlates of physical activity among pregnant women in the United States. *Med Sci Sports Exerc* 2005;37:1748.)

TABLE 21.10	Important Metabolic and Cardiorespiratory Adaptations During Pregnancy

- Blood volume increases 40 to 50%; hemodilution reduces hemoglobin concentration
- Increase in blood volume dilates the left ventricle
- Slight increase in oxygen consumption during rest and submaximal, weight-supported exercise such as stationary cycling
- Substantial increase in oxygen consumption during weight-bearing exercise such as walking and running
- Increased heart rate during rest and submaximal exercise
- No change in $\dot{V}O_{2max}$ (L·min⁻¹)
- Increased ventilatory response—largely progesterone induced—during rest and submaximal exercise
- Possible magnified hypoglycemic response during exercise, especially late in pregnancy
- Possible depressed sympathetic nervous system response to exercise in late gestation

Adapted from Wolfe LA, et al. Maternal exercise, fetal well-being and pregnancy outcome. *Exerc Sport Sci Rev* 1994;22:145.

Physical Activity Effects on the Fetus

Performing physical activity during pregnancy requires adherence to prudent guidelines and recommendations.[5] Epidemiologic evidence indicates that exercise during pregnancy does not increase risk of fetal deaths or low birth weights, and may significantly reduce the risk of preterm births.[94,155,174,195] A moderate program of weight-bearing exercise or recreational activity early in pregnancy through term enhances fetoplacental growth and reduces preeclampsia risk.[30,188] A study of middle-class women evaluated the effects of daily low-to-moderate physical activity (<1000 kcal·wk⁻¹), more intense activity (>1000 kcal·wk⁻¹), or no physical activity on timely delivery and the safety and potential benefits of regular activity during pregnancy.[77] No association emerged between low-to-moderate physical activity and gestation length. A positive finding indicated that higher volume weekly activity lowered rather than raised the risk of preterm birth; among births after the projected term, women who performed more intense physical activity delivered faster than nonexercisers.

Three potential risks of intense maternal exercise that could alter fetal growth and development include the following:

1. Reduced placental blood flow and accompanying fetal hypoxia
2. Fetal hyperthermia
3. Reduced fetal glucose supply

Any factor that might temporarily compromise fetal blood supply raises concern in counseling pregnant women about physical activity.

Neonates born to physically active mothers exhibit a neurobehavioral profile as early as the fifth day after birth, earlier than neonates from more sedentary counterparts.[29]

Active mothers either ran, performed aerobics, swam, or used stair-climbing activities at least three times weekly for more than 20 min at 55% of aerobic capacity or above. The women in the control group led active lives that did not include regular, sustained physical activity. Figure 21.26 shows data for five behavioral clusters of the Brazelton Neonatal Assessment Scales (http://www.brazelton-institute.com/intro.html) for the offspring of 34 women who exercised regularly and 31 sedentary women. No significant differences emerged between neonates born to physically active women and sedentary controls for clusters of factors to assess motor organization, autonomic stability, and range of state behaviors. Neonates born to physically active women scored higher in orientation behavior and ability to regulate state (i.e., more alert and interested in their surroundings and less demanding of their mothers). The inset table indicates that axial length and head circumference remained similar between groups, with the offspring of the active women lighter and leaner than offspring from the control group. The findings support the concept that continuing regular physical activity throughout pregnancy modifies neonatal behavior by positively affecting early neurodevelopment.

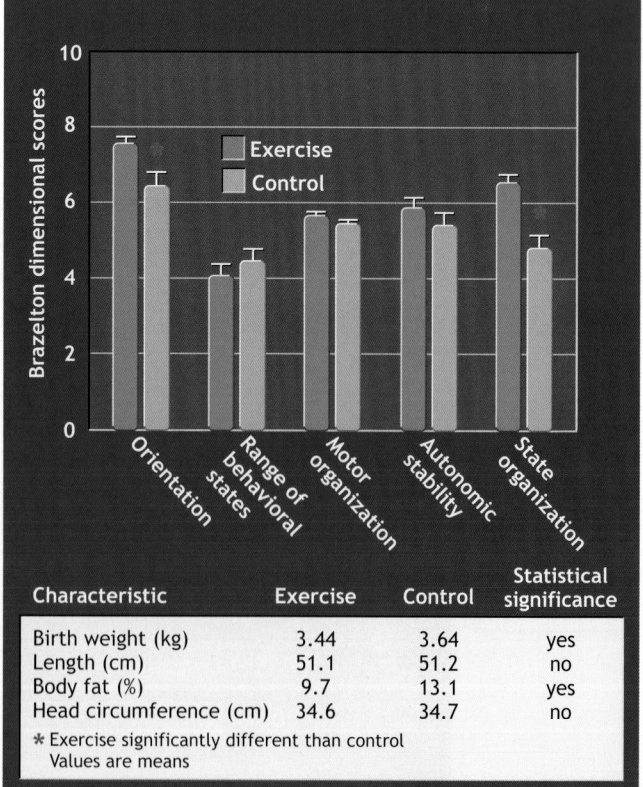

Characteristic	Exercise	Control	Statistical significance
Birth weight (kg)	3.44	3.64	yes
Length (cm)	51.1	51.2	no
Body fat (%)	9.7	13.1	yes
Head circumference (cm)	34.6	34.7	no

* Exercise significantly different than control
Values are means

**FIGURE 21.26 • ** Behavioral constellation scores of neonates in exercise and nonexercise control groups on Brazelton Neonatal Behavioral Assessment Scales. *Asterisks* indicate statistical significance at the .01 level. Insert table presents neonatal morphometric values. (Reprinted with permission from Clapp JF III, et al. Neonatal behavioral profile of the offspring of women who continue to exercise regularly throughout pregnancy. *Am J Obstet Gynecol* 1999;180:91.

INTEGRATIVE QUESTION

What weight control advantage during pregnancy would a daily walking program offer compared with stationary cycling if each program remained at the same initial intensity level (i.e., constant walking speed or cycling power output), frequency, and duration?

Current Opinion Regarding Physical Activity and Pregnancy

Conservative, prudent recommendations apply during a normal pregnancy despite examples of extreme physical activity for well-trained women without apparent negative effect on maternal or fetal health.[10,95,129] *Thirty to 40 min of moderate aerobic activity daily for a previously active, healthy, low–risk woman during an uncomplicated pregnancy does not compromise fetal oxygen supply*

IN A PRACTICAL SENSE

Exercise Prescription During Pregnancy

Pregnancy alters normal physiology, necessitating some modification in exercise prescription. Pregnant women should consult their physician before initiating a physical activity program (or modifying an existing program) to rule out possible complications. This pertains particularly to women of low fitness status and little exercise experience prior to pregnancy.

Physical activity during pregnancy should heighten awareness about heat dissipation, adequate caloric and nutrient intake, and knowing when to reduce the intensity of effort. For a normal, uncomplicated pregnancy, light-to-moderate activity does not negatively affect fetal development; the benefits of properly prescribed regular activity during pregnancy generally outweigh the potential risks.

PHYSICAL ACTIVITY GUIDELINES

Activity mode: Avoid exercise in the supine position, particularly after the first trimester. Supine exercise impairs venous return (mass of the fetus compresses inferior vena cava), which could affect cardiac output and uterine blood flow. Non–weight-bearing activity (e.g., cycling, swimming) minimizes the effect of gravity and the added weight associated with fetal development. Low-impact, weight-bearing activity in moderation should not pose a risk.

Activity frequency: Exercise 3 days a week, emphasizing continuous, steady-rate effort. Reduce the intensity of more frequent activities.

Activity duration: Exercise 30 to 40 min, depending on how the person feels.

Activity intensity: Pregnancy alters the relationship between heart rate and oxygen consumption, making it difficult to establish guidelines from heart rate. An effective alternative establishes exercise intensity based on RPE, which should range between 11 ("fairly light") to 13 ("somewhat hard").

Rate of progression: Exercise on a regular basis; moderate aerobic activity maintains cardiovascular fitness and often produces a small training effect. Most women should not strive to induce training effects, but rather maintain cardiorespiratory fitness, muscle mass, and physician-recommended weight gain. The combined effects of pregnancy per se and regular physical activity often produce improved fitness after delivery.

WHEN TO STOP EXERCISE AND SEEK MEDICAL ADVICE

Discontinue exercise immediately under the following conditions:

- Any signs of vaginal bleeding
- Any gush of fluid from the vagina (premature rupture of membranes)
- Sudden swelling of ankles, hands, or face
- Persistent, severe headaches and/or disturbances in vision; unexplained lightheadedness or dizziness
- Elevated pulse rate or blood pressure that does not rapidly return to normal following exercise
- Excessive fatigue, palpitations, or chest pain
- Persistent uterine contractions (more than 6 to 8 per hr)
- Unexplained or unusual abdominal pain
- Insufficient weight gain (<1.0 kg per month during the last two trimesters)

Contraindications to physical activity during pregnancy:

- Pregnancy-induced hypertension
- History of two or more spontaneous abortions
- Preterm rupture of membranes
- Preterm labor during the prior or current pregnancy
- Incompetent cervix
- Excessive alcohol intake
- Persistent second to third trimester bleeding
- History of premature labor
- Intrauterine growth retardation
- Anemia
- Type 1 diabetes
- Significant obesity
- Multiple pregnancy
- Smoking

Reprinted from Exercise during Pregnancy: Current Comment from the American College of Sports Medicine, August 2000. www.Americanpregnancyhealth/exerciseguidelines.html; http://www.acsm.org/docs/current-comments/exerciseduringpregnancy.pdf

or acid-base status, induce heart rate signs of fetal distress, or produce other adverse effects to mother or fetus.[2,37,121,146,206] Performed on a regular basis, such activity maintains cardiovascular fitness, promotes a training effect, and inhibits undesirable excessive weight gain for the mother, and is associated with resting fetal heart rate effects similar to a trained resopnse.[54,133,163,166,171,172,186] Four other positive maternal effects are:

1. Shorter labor and delivery times
2. Faster recovery after delivery
3. Decreased pregnancy discomforts
4. Fewer complications during pregnancy

Hormonal action via the sympathetic nervous system during strenuous effort probably diverts some blood from the uterus and visceral organs for preferential distribution to active muscles. This could pose a hazard to a fetus with restricted placental blood flow. "In a Practical Sense" (earlier in this chapter) outlines guidelines for formulating an exercise prescription during pregnancy. This prudent approach dictates that a pregnant woman (in consultation with her health care provider) should exercise in moderation, especially if the pregnancy is compromised. In addition, physical activity late in pregnancy can magnify the normal maternal hypoglycemic response by increasing glucose consumption by maternal skeletal muscle; in the extreme, this response could adversely affect fetal glucose supply.[15,28]

Pregnant women should avoid supine exercise, contact sports, high-altitude exertion, hot tub immersion, and scuba diving. A decrease in uterine blood flow or elevation in maternal core temperature with extended-duration activity during environmental heat stress can compromise heat dissipation from the fetus through the placenta.[136] Hyperthermia negatively affects fetal development (e.g., increased risk of neural tube defect), particularly in the first trimester,[140] so women should exercise during warm weather in the cool part of the day for shorter intervals while maintaining regular fluid intake. Within this framework, aquatic exercise serves as an ideal form of maternal physical activity.

Current fitness level and previous physical activity patterns should guide a woman's exercise behavior throughout an uncomplicated pregnancy and postpartum. Regular aerobic activity during pregnancy plays an important role to maintain functional capacity and general well-being. It also optimizes overall weight gain during the later stages of pregnancy[28] and may reduce risk for cesarean delivery in women who have never borne children.[24] Controversy remains about whether extremes of maternal physical effort benefit either mother or fetus or whether physical activity during pregnancy benefits labor, delivery, birth weight, and general outcome.[14,167] Beginning regular exercise 6 to 8 wk postpartum produces no deleterious effect on volume or composition of lactation and improves aerobic fitness without impairing immune function.[37,121,125] Fitness and strength declines in the early postpartum period relative to prepregnancy performance generally return by 27 wk following delivery.[221] Combining moderate physical activity with a reduced energy intake of about 500 kcal daily allows overweight lactating women to safely lose 0.5 kg per week without adverse affects on infant growth.[124]

Summary

1. Physical activities generally classify by the specific energy transfer system predominantly activated.
2. An effective conditioning program trains the appropriate energy system(s) to improve a desired physiologic function or performance goal.
3. Physical conditioning based on sound principles optimizes improvements. The four primary training principles include overload, specificity, individual differences, and reversibility.
4. Exercise training initiates cellular adaptations and gross physiologic changes that enhance functional capacity and physical performance.
5. Anaerobic training increases resting levels of intramuscular anaerobic substrates and key glycolytic enzymes. Adaptations usually accompany concomitant increases in maximal performance.
6. Aerobic training adaptations increase mitochondrial size and number, quantity of aerobic enzymes, muscle capillarization, and fat and carbohydrate oxidation. These improvements contribute to enhanced aerobic ATP production.
7. A linear relationship exists between heart rate and oxygen consumption from light to moderately intense physical activity in trained and untrained individuals. Improved stroke volume with aerobic training shifts this line to the right to decrease heart rate at any submaximal level of effort.
8. Aerobic training induces functional and dimensional changes in the cardiovascular system to decrease resting and submaximal heart rate, enhance stroke volume and cardiac output, and expand the a-$\bar{v}O_2$ difference.
9. Cardiac hypertrophy represents a fundamental biologic adaptation to increased myocardial workload imposed by training. Cardiac enlargement with endurance training increases left-ventricular volume and enhances stroke volume.
10. Structural and dimensional changes in the left ventricle vary with training modes. Regular physical activity does not harm normal cardiac function.
11. Exercise intensity is the most crucial factor that affects the magnitude of training improvements; other factors include initial fitness level, training frequency, exercise duration, and training mode.
12. Training intensity can be applied on either an absolute basis for exercise load or relative to a person's physiologic response. The most practical approach sets exercise intensity to a percentage of HR_{max}. Training levels between 60 and 90% HR_{max} induce meaningful changes in aerobic fitness.
13. Training duration and intensity interact to affect the training response. Generally, 30-min exercise sessions are practical and effective. Extending duration compensates for reduced intensity.

14. Two to 3 days a week represents the minimum frequency for aerobic training. Optimal training frequency remains undetermined.

15. Similar aerobic improvements occur when intensity, duration, and frequency remain constant, regardless of activity mode when training involves large muscle groups, and the evaluation process remains mode specific.

16. Training frequency and duration to maintain improved aerobic fitness are lower than those required to improve it. Small decreases in exercise intensity reduce $\dot{V}O_{2max}$.

17. Interval, continuous, and fartlek training improve the capacity of the different energy transfer systems.

18. Interval training most effectively improves the immediate and short-term anaerobic energy systems.

19. Aerobic training must overload both cardiovascular function and metabolic capacity of specific muscles. Peripheral adaptations in trained muscle profoundly enhance endurance performance.

20. Prolonged and intense endurance training can precipitate the syndrome of overtraining or staleness, with associated alterations in neuroendocrine and immune functions.

21. The overtraining syndrome includes chronic fatigue, poor exercise performance, frequent infections, and general loss of interest in training. Symptoms generally persist until the athlete relinquishes training, possibly for several days to months.

22. Approximately 40% of American women exercise during pregnancy, with walking the most common form of physical activity (42%), followed by swimming (12%) and aerobics (12%).

23. The most serious potential physical activity risks during pregnancy include reduced placental blood flow and accompanying fetal hypoxia, fetal hyperthermia, and reduced fetal glucose supply.

24. For previously active, healthy women, moderate aerobic activity does not compromise fetal oxygen supply.

thePoint References are available online at
http://thepoint.lww.com/mkk8e.

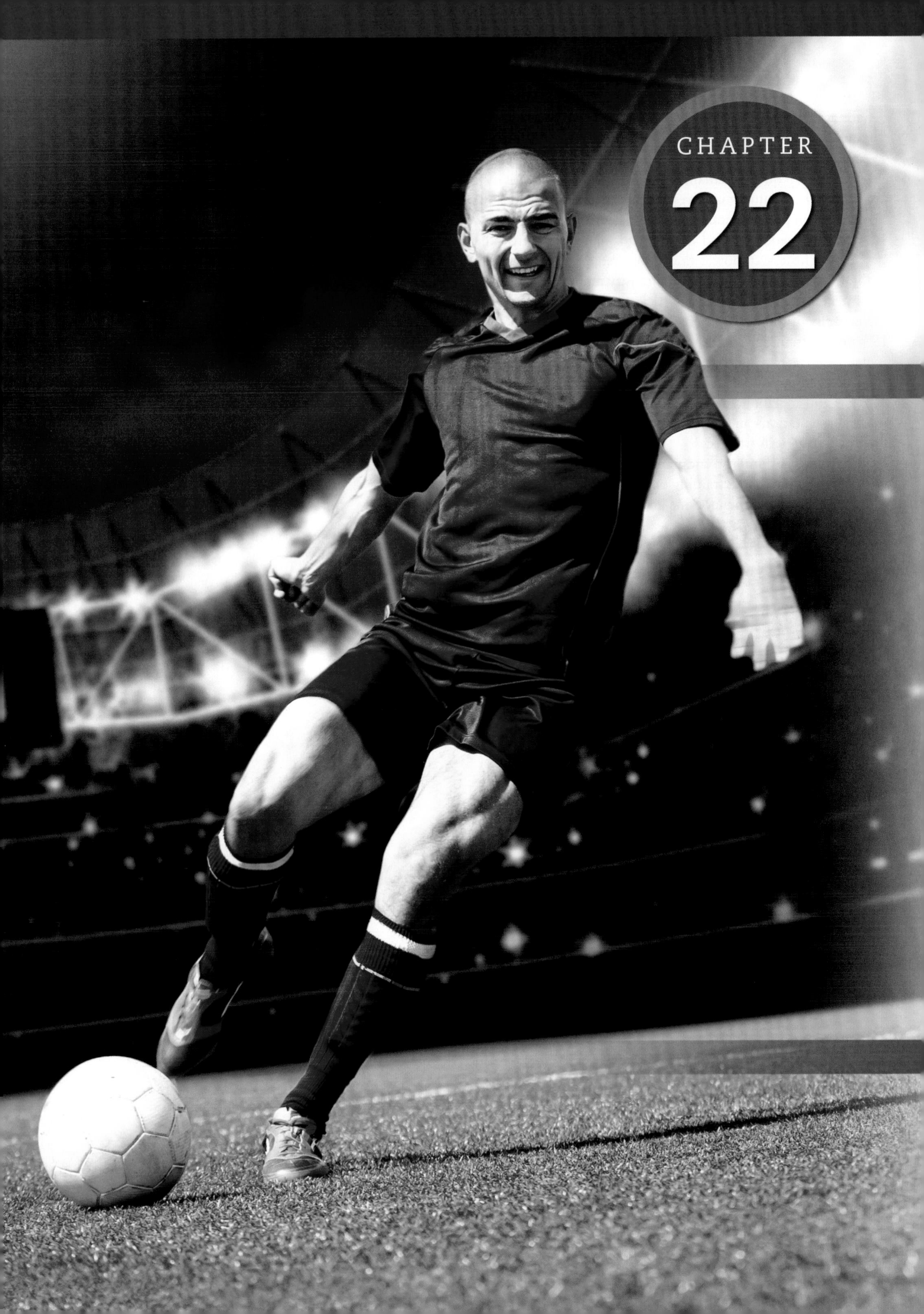
CHAPTER
22

Muscular Strength: Training Muscles to Become Stronger

CHAPTER OBJECTIVES

- Describe the following four methods to assess muscular strength: cable tensiometry, dynamometry, one-repetition maximum (1-RM), computer-assisted isokinetic dynamometry

- Outline a procedure to assess 1-RM for trained and untrained individuals

- Describe how to ensure test standardization and fairness to evaluate muscular strength

- Compare absolute and relative upper- and lower-body muscular strength in men and women

- Describe allometric scaling to "equalize" individuals when comparing physical and exercise performance characteristics

- Define concentric, eccentric, and isometric muscle actions and give examples of each

- Discuss the advisability of resistance training for children and adolescents

- Summarize main research findings on optimal number of sets and repetitions, and frequency and relative intensity of progressive-resistance training

- Outline the model for strength-training periodization

- Discuss specificity of strength-training related to sports and occupational tasks

- Differentiate between resistance training goals of competitive athletes and untrained middle-age and elderly persons

- Respond to the following question: Which is better for strength improvement—progressive resistance weight training, isometric training, or isokinetic training?

- Describe advantages and disadvantages of plyometric training for power athletes

- Describe how "psychologic" factors and "muscular" factors influence maximum strength capacity and training responsiveness

- List physiologic adaptations with chronic resistance training

- Summarize current opinion concerning resistance training's effect on muscle fiber type and number

- Outline a circuit resistance training program for middle-age men and women to improve muscular strength and aerobic fitness

- Discuss whether specific resistance training can "shape" a muscle's appearance

- Review the type of exercise most frequently associated with delayed-onset muscle soreness (DOMS), the best way to minimize DOMS when initiating training, and significant cellular alterations with DOMS

- Explain "core strength" development and its role in physical performance

ANCILLARIES ◉ at-a-Glance

Visit http://thePoint.lww.com/mkk8e to access the following resources.

- References: Chapter 22
- Interactive Question Bank
- Appendix D: The Metric System and Conversion Constants in Exercise Physiology
- Animation: Muscle Contraction Type
- Animation: RICE Method
- Animation: Stretch Shortening Cycle
- Focus on Research: Develop Strength by Increasing Load, Not Repetitions

PART 1

STRENGTH MEASUREMENT AND RESISTANCE TRAINING

Weightlifting in America in the early 1840s became a spectator sport practiced by "strongmen" who showcased their prowess in traveling carnivals and sideshows. As pointed out in the text's "Introduction: A View of the Past," the military evaluated the strength of conscripts during the Civil War; strength measurements also provided the basis for routine fitness assessments in the prototype college and university physical education programs.

Much of the early "science" of strength development can be attributed to Pehr Henrik Ling (1776–1839), a Swedish physical therapist, teacher of medical-gymnastics, and considered the father of "Swedish Gymnastics." In 1813, he founded the current Swedish School of Sport and Health Sciences under the name of the Royal Central Institute of Gymnastics, Stockholm. He and his son Hylmar (1820–1886) both were influential writers. Their many disciples became experts in physical education in Sweden and the rest of Europe. Their influential techniques of strength development migrated to the British Isles and eventually in the early 1800s to the United States. Teachers were trained not only as physical education instructors in the schools but also for government work as military gymnastics instructors and physiotherapists. Figure 22.1 shows examples of late 19th century "strength and exercise machines" popularized by Swedish physician Gustav Zander (1835–1920; www.retronaut.com/2011/07/vintage-exercise-machines/), which were strongly influenced by the Lings' Swedish Gymnastic movement. Zander's methods for treating patients and the common person included standard gymnastic exercise regimens, combined with calisthenics, balance, and core trunk and limb movements. Workouts on his mechanical exercise machines served double duty for general strength development and "mechanical gymnastic treatments" for morbid disorders and diseases of the heart, nerves, respiratory and abdominal organs, obesity, gout, and rheumatism of the articulations including scoliosis. Dr. Zander's many successful treatment clinics in the 1890s that featured his machines provided a new vista and attitude toward self-enhancement through exercise for fitness and health. During this period in the United States, measuring muscular strength became popular to evaluate physical fitness and body development, particularly in schools, colleges, physiotherapy centers, and local gymnasia and training centers. An 1897 meeting of American

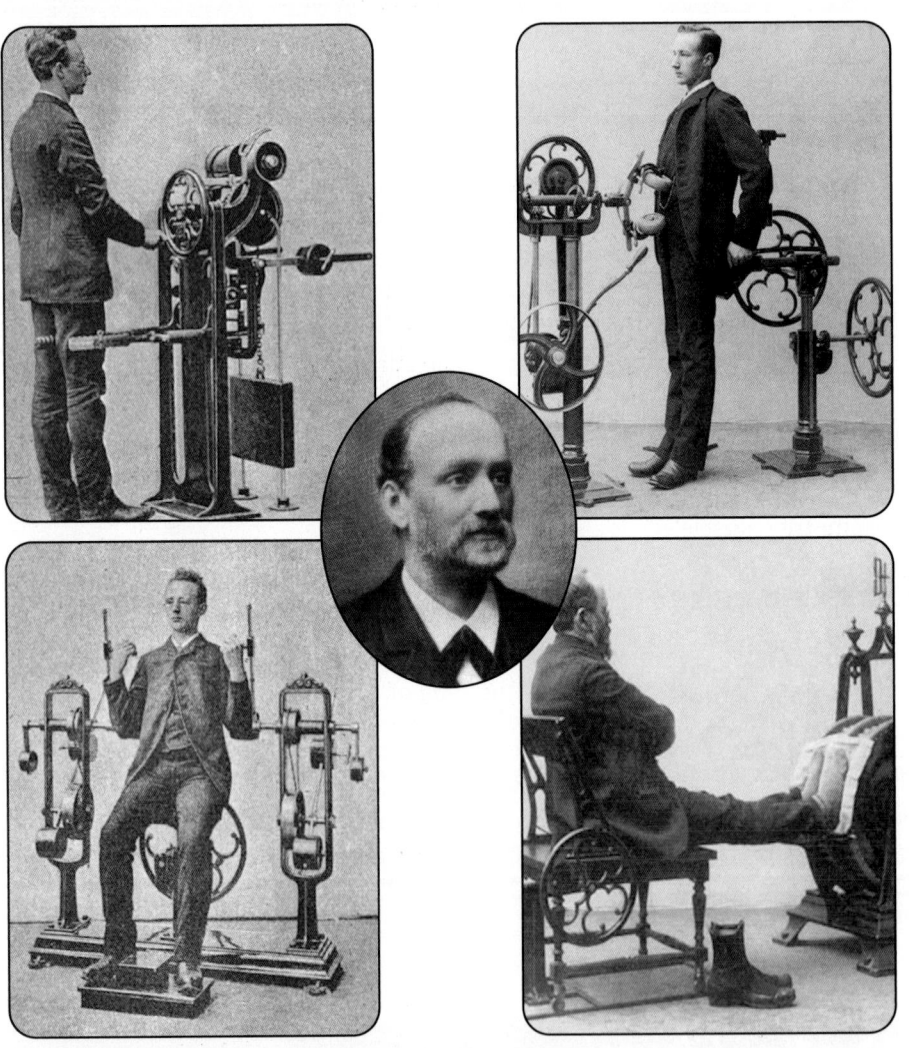

FIGURE 22.1 • Four examples of late 19th century "strength machines" popularized by Swedish physician Gustav Zander (1835–1920), who produced 27 mechanical apparatus that became prototypes of common equipment now ubiquitous in physical fitness gyms and training centers worldwide. Perhaps serendipitously (or not), the successful Nautilus line of exercise equipment was remarkably similar in design to many of the Zander machines (http://studioumanyc.com/zander.html). Photos used with permission from Levertin, A. *Dr. G. Zanders Medico-Mechanical Gymnastics. It's Method, Importance and Application.* P.A. Norstead & Sonner. Printers to the King. Stockholm. 1893. (Adapted with permission from Katch VL, McArdle WD, Katch FI, *Essentials of Exercise Physiology.* 4th Ed. Philadelphia: Wolters Kluwer Health, 2011.)

College Gymnasium Directors (Dr. D. A. Sargent, committee chair from Harvard University) established strength contests to determine overall body strength based on back, leg, arm, and chest strength measurements. The first six college participants included Amherst College, Columbia University, Harvard University, the University of Minnesota, Dickinson College, and Wesleyan College. Harvard was the overall winner of the competition, followed closely by Columbia.

By the mid-1900s, physical culture specialists, body builders, competitive weightlifters, field-event athletes, and some wrestlers used traditional weightlifting exercises, not the passive methods of massage and electrical vibration that also flourished during this time. Research in the late 1950s and early 1960s dispelled the myth that traditional muscle-strengthening exercises reduced movement speed or range of joint motion. Instead, the opposite usually occurred; elite weightlifters, body builders, and "muscle men" had exceptional joint flexibility without limitations in general limb movement speed. For untrained healthy individuals, heavy-resistance exercises increased the speed and power of muscular effort without impairing subsequent sports performance.

In the sections that follow, we explore the underlying rationale for resistance training and physiologic adaptations that occur when training muscles to become bigger, faster, and stronger. The discussion centers on different methods to measure muscular strength, gender differences in strength, and resistance-training programs to increase muscle strength (including a discussion of "core" strength) and power.

Muscular Strength Development: Its Roots in Antiquity

The inclusion of strength development programs as part of athletic training regimens is not new; it prepared men for warfare in ancient China, Japan, India, Greece, and Rome. When the ancient Olympic games first began in 776 BC, athletes trained nearly year-round and incorporated muscle-strengthening exercises into their training regimens (www.olympic.org/ancient-olympic-games). The scientific foundations for strength training for athletes began with the

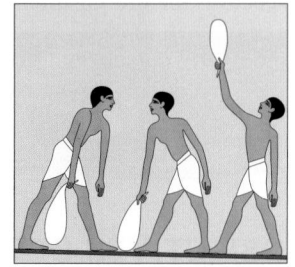

 Early Strongmen Who Popularized Body Building and Strength Training

Eugen Sandow (below *left*), born Frederick Mueller (1867–1925), emerged as one of the first successful muscular vaudeville strong-

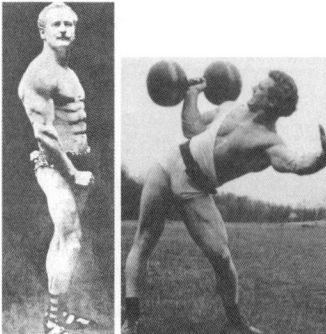

man in the early 1890s, who legendary showman Florenz Ziegfeld billed as "The Most Perfect Man." Sandow helped to design a physical fitness training program for the British military, inspiring a future generation of bodybuilders.[40] Sandow published popular magazines, promoted exercise equipment he used (mainly barbells), and was one of the first to also promote special foods for training. John Grimek (*right*), achieved notoriety as a member of the United States 1936 Olympic weightlifting team, two-time Mr. America (1940, 1941), 1948 Mr. Universe, and undefeated in body-building competition. Most authorities believed Grimek epitomized the "best-built human" of the first half of the 20th century.

In the late 1890s, Daniel L. Dowd (1854–1897) advertised strength equipment for home gym use.

Dowd was first to advertise his wall-fixed equipment

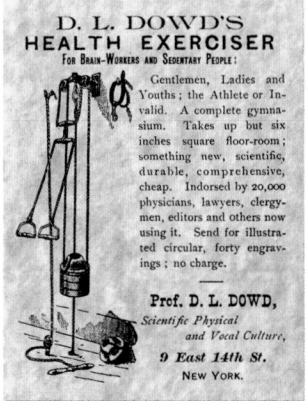

by showing "before" and "after" photographs of himself, which were prepared for self-help books published in 1878 devoted to physical culture, body building, and strength development (http://www.sandowplus.co.uk/Library/BB-dec%2053-dowd/dowd.htm). This engraving is of Dowd, published in his 1889 book, *Physical Culture for Home and School; Scientific and Practical* (New York: Fowler &Wells, 1889; http://www.starkcenter.org/static/igh/articles/igh9.3.20.pdf). Dowd weighed only 138 lb prior to training but 4 years later gained what he considered added muscle mass, now tipping the scales at 163 lb, ample evidence he believed of the value of his equipment. Dowd advocated large numbers of repetitions

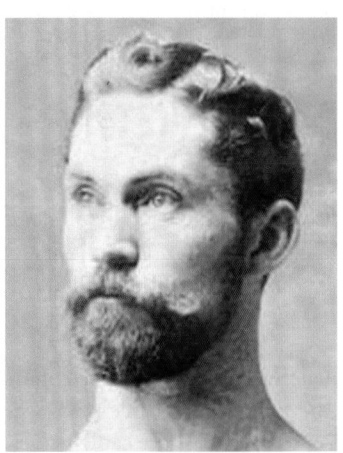

with light resistance to sculpt the perfect physique. His book contains numerous exercises for developing the musculature of the neck, trunk, and extremities. By the mid- to late 1800s, rowing machines and various strengthening devices became commonplace, eventually leading to studies of their effectiveness in the private American colleges of Harvard and Amherst in the 1890s.

Chinese in 3600 BC During the Chou dynasty (1122–249 BC) conscripts had to pass weightlifting tests before becoming soldiers. Weight training also took place in ancient Egypt and India; sculptures and illustrations depict athletes training with heavy stone weights.

Women also practiced weight training. Wall mosaics recovered from Roman villas showed young women exercising with handheld weights. During the "Age of Strength" in the 6th century, weightlifting competitions often took place between soldiers and athletes. Galen, the famous early Greek physician (see Exercise Physiology: Roots and Historical Perspectives, before Chapter 1) referred to Greek pentathletes 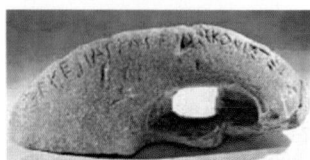 exercising with 1.5- to 2.0-kg (3.3- to 4.4-lb) handheld weights made of stone or lead (called halteres and shown at left) during jumping events.[171]

OBJECTIVES OF RESISTANCE TRAINING

Strength development through resistance training applies to six main areas:

1. Weightlifting and powerlifting competitions
2. Body building to maximize muscular development for aesthetic goals
3. General strength training for fitness and health enhancement
4. Physical therapy for rehabilitation from injury or disease
5. Sport-specific resistance training to maximize sport performance
6. Muscle physiology to understand structure, function, adaptations, and practical applications

MEASUREMENT OF MUSCLE STRENGTH

One of the following four methods commonly assesses **muscle strength** or, more precisely, maximum force or tension output generated by a single muscle or related muscle groups:

1. Cable tensiometry
2. Dynamometry
3. One-repetition maximum
4. Computer-assisted, electromechanical, and isokinetic methods

Cable Tensiometry

FIGURE 22.2A shows a **cable tensiometer** to assess knee extension muscle force. Increasing the force on the cable depresses the riser shown in the inset circle over which the cable passes. This deflects the pointer and indicates the subject's strength score. The instrument measures muscle force in a static or isometric muscle action that elicits little or no change in the muscle's external length. The tensiometer—lightweight, portable, and easy to use—provides the advantage of versatility for recording force measurements at virtually all angles about a specific joint's range of motion (ROM). Standardized cable-tension strength-test batteries can assess static force capacity of all major muscle groups.

Dynamometry

English mathematician and avid inventor Charles Babbage (1791–1871; http://mikes.railhistory.railfan.net/r062.html) was first to invent a dynamometer to record the forces over time exerted on a railway car. The ever-inventive Babbage devised a way to track data on a moving roll of paper to record the pulling force of the engine, plot the path of the railroad car carriage, and the vertical shake of the carriage. In the fields of kinesiology, ergonomics, physical medicine, and physical therapy, dynamometers routinely assess muscular force output of specific muscles before, during, and following physical training and rehabilitation regimens. The use of simple recording dynamometry in clinical medicine began in England in 1952 and continued in medical practice to test patients diagnosed with polio, rheumatic conditions, myasthenia gravis, focal cerebral lesions that affect downstream musculature, and various motor dysfunctions.[198]

FIGURES 22.2B AND C illustrate hand-grip and leg and back-lift **dynamometers** for static strength measurement based on the compression principle. An external force applied to the dynamometer compresses a steel spring and moves a pointer. The force required to move the pointer a given distance determines the external force applied to the dynamometer.

One-Repetition Maximum

A dynamic procedure for measuring muscular strength applies the **one-repetition maximum (1-RM) method**. 1-RM refers to the maximum amount of weight lifted *one time* using proper form during a standard weightlifting movement. To assess 1-RM for any muscle group, the tester makes a reasonable guess at an initial weight close to, but below, the person's maximum lifting capacity. Weight is progressively added to the exercise device on subsequent attempts until the person reaches maximum lift capacity. The weight increments usually range between 1 and 5 kg depending on the force-output capacity of the muscle group evaluated. Rest intervals of 1 to 5 min usually provide sufficient recuperation before attempting a lift at the next heavier weight.

Estimate the 1-RM

Impracticality and/or potential risk in performing 1-RM with preadolescents, the elderly, hypertensives, cardiac patients, and other special populations require an estimate of 1-RM from submaximal effort. Different equations are necessary because resistance training alters the relationship between submaximal performance (7- to 10-RM) and maximal lift capacity (1-RM). Generally, the weight that one can lift for

7- to 10-RM represents about 68% of the 1-RM score for the untrained person and 79% of the new 1-RM after training.[31] The following equations apply to untrained and resistance-trained young adults:

Untrained

$$1\text{-RM (kg)} = 1.554 \times 7\text{- to } 10\text{-RM weight (kg)} - 5.181$$

Trained

$$1\text{-RM (kg)} = 1.172 \times 7\text{- to } 10\text{-RM weight (kg)} + 7.704$$

For example, estimate 1-RM bench press score for a trained person whose 10-RM bench press equals 70 kg as follows:

$$1\text{-RM (kg)} = 1.172 \times 70\text{(kg)} + 7.704$$
$$= 89.7 \text{ kg}$$

Computer-Assisted, Electromechanical, and Isokinetic Methods

Microprocessor technology rapidly quantifies forces, torques, accelerations, and velocities of body segments in numerous movement patterns. Force platforms measure the external application of muscle force by a limb, as in jumping. Other electromechanical devices assess forces generated during all phases of an activity (e.g., cycling) or primarily arm (supine bench press) or leg (leg press) movements.

 ## Definition of Selected Terms Associated with Resistance Training

1. **Cheating.** Breaking from strict form when performing an exercise (e.g., rather than maintaining an erect upper body when performing a standing arm curl, a slight body swing at the start of the movement allows the person to lift a heavier weight or the same weight more times). Cheating increases injury risk if performed improperly.

2. **Circuit resistance training (CRT).** Series of resistance training exercises performed in sequence with minimal rest between exercises. More frequent repetitions with less resistance (usually 40 to 50% of 1-RM) stimulate the cardiovascular system to produce an aerobic training effect.

3. **Concentric action.** Muscle shortening during force application.

4. **Dynamic constant external resistance (DCER) training.** Resistance training where external resistance or weight does not change; joint flexion and extension occurs with each repetition. Formerly (but incorrectly) referred to as "isotonic" exercise.

5. **Eccentric action.** Muscle lengthening occurs during force application.

6. **Exercise intensity.** Muscle force expressed as a percentage of muscle's maximum force-generating capacity or some level of maximum.

7. **Isokinetic action.** Muscle action performed at constant angular limb velocity.

8. **Isometric action.** Muscle action without noticeable change in muscle length.

9. **Maximal voluntary muscle action (MVMA).** Maximal force generated in one repetition (1-RM), or performing a series of submaximal actions to momentary failure.

10. **Muscular endurance.** Sustaining maximum (or submaximum) force; often determined by assessing maximum number of exercise repetitions at a percentage of maximum strength.

11. **Overload.** A muscle acting against a resistance normally not encountered (unaccustomed stress).

12. **Periodization.** Variation in training volume and intensity over a specified time period; goal to prevent staleness while peaking physiologically for competition.

13. **Plyometrics.** Resistance training involving eccentric-to-concentric actions performed quickly so a muscle stretches slightly prior to the concentric action; utilizes stretch reflex to augment the muscle's force-generating capacity.

14. **Power.** Rate of performing work (Force × Distance ÷ Time, or Force × Velocity). Power applied to weightlifting relates to the mass lifted times the vertical distance it moves, divided by the time to complete the movement. If 100 lb moves vertically 3 ft in 1 s, then the power generated = 100 lb × 3 ft ÷ 1 s or 300 ft-lb·s⁻¹.

15. **Progressive overload.** Incrementally increasing the stress placed on a muscle to produce greater force or greater endurance.

16. **Range of motion (ROM).** Maximum range of movement through an arc of a joint.

17. **Repetition.** One complete exercise movement, usually consisting of concentric and eccentric muscle actions or one complete isometric muscle action.

18. **Repetition maximum (RM).** Greatest force generated for one repetition of a movement (1-RM), or predetermined number of repetitions (e.g., 5-RM or 10-RM).

19. **Set.** Preestablished number of repetitions performed.

20. **Sticking point.** Region in an exercise movement (against a set resistance) that provides the greatest difficulty to complete the movement.

21. **Strength.** Maximum force-generating capacity of a muscle or group of muscles.

22. **Suspension training.** Leveraging a person's body weight during exercise (without reliance on externally fixed weights, pulleys, or cams) by increasing or decreasing the suspension coordinates, the height of ropes, pulleys, slings, or bungee cords, relative to the suspension point.

22. **Torque.** Force that produces a turning, twisting, or rotary movement in any plane about an axis (i.e., movement of bones about a joint); commonly expressed in newton-meters (Nm).

23. **Training volume.** Total work performed in a single training session.

24. **Variable resistance training.** Training with equipment that uses a lever arm, cam, hydraulic system, or pulley to alter the resistance to match the increases and decreases in a muscle's capacity throughout a joint's ROM.

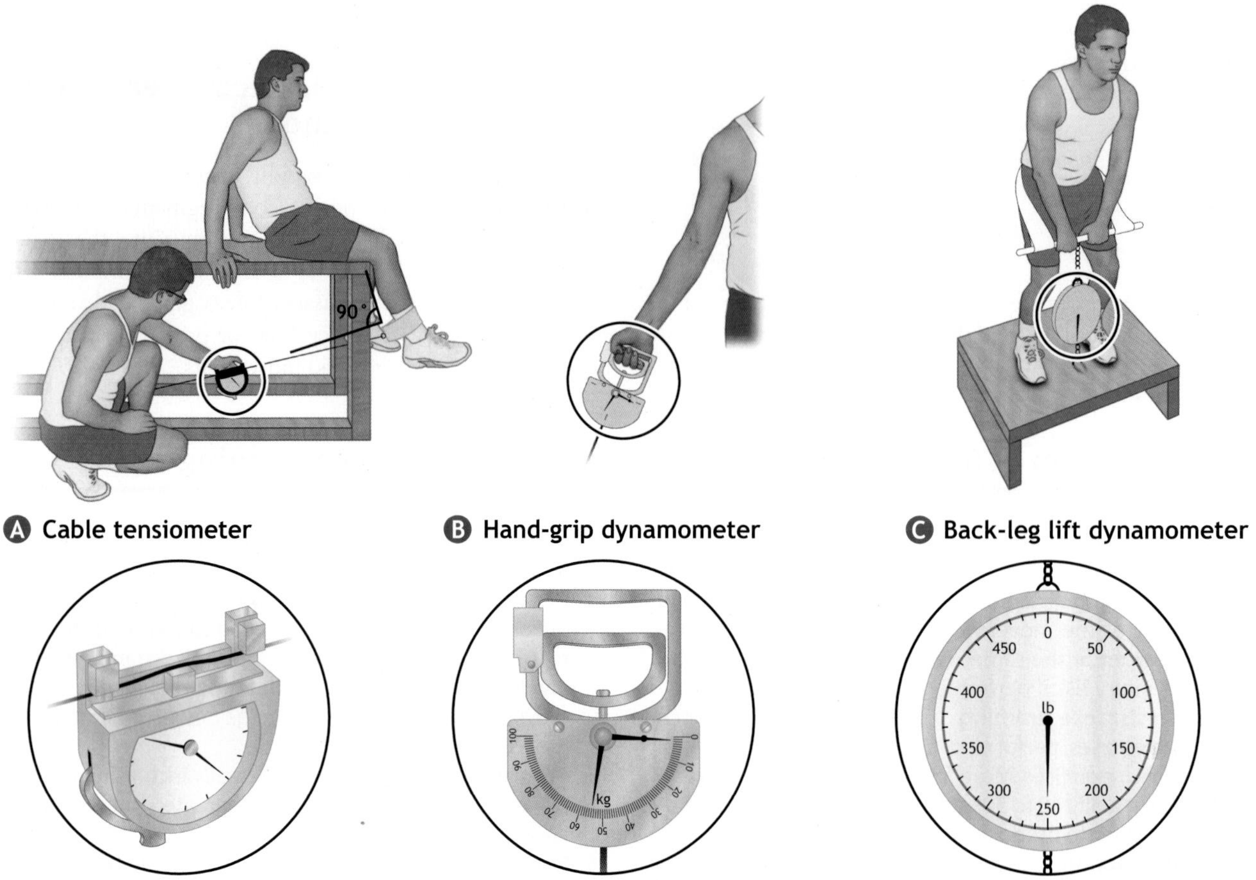

A Cable tensiometer   **B** Hand-grip dynamometer   **C** Back-leg lift dynamometer

FIGURE 22.2 • Measurement of static strength with **(A)** cable tensiometer, **(B)** hand-grip dynamometer, and **(C)** back–leg lift dynamometer.

An electromechanical accommodating resistance instrument, termed an *isokinetic dynamometer*, contains a speed-controlling mechanism that accelerates to a preset, constant velocity with force application. Once attaining this speed, the isokinetic loading mechanism adjusts automatically to provide a counterforce to variations in force generated by muscle as movement continues throughout the "strength curve." *Thus, maximum force (or any percentage of maximum effort) generates throughout the full ROM at a pre-established velocity of limb movement.* This allows training and measurement under a continuum from high-velocity (lower-force) to low-velocity (higher-force) conditions. A microprocessor within the dynamometer continuously monitors the immediate level of applied force. An electronic integrator in series with a monitor displays the average or peak force generated during any interval for almost instantaneous feedback about performance (e.g., force, torque, work). FIGURE 22.3 shows an example of a popular electromechanical accommodating resistance dynamometer.

The interface of microprocessor technology with mechanical devices provides the exercise scientist with valuable data to evaluate, train, and rehabilitate individuals. The argument in support of isokinetic strength measurement maintains that muscle strength dynamics involve considerably more than just the final outcome of 1-RM. For example, two individuals with identical 1-RM scores could exhibit dissimilar force curves throughout the movement. Individual differences in force dynamics (e.g., time to peak tension) throughout the full ROM may reflect an entirely different underlying neuromuscular physiology that 1-RM fails to assess. FIGURE 22.4 illustrates the differences between conventional 1-RM knee extension (**A**, highest force score during five lifts represents *only* total weight lifted) and a microprocessor-controlled, isokinetic resistance device that can produce a force curve throughout the ROM (**B**, force related to movement duration). In this example with an early-generation isokinetic device, note that peak torque occurs in the early phase of movement at the most advantageous angle in the ROM and then declines rapidly; the lowest torque occurs at full knee extension. TABLE 22.1 lists international system (SI) units for various expressions of muscular performance during linear and angular movements.

 INTEGRATIVE QUESTION

Explain why many resistance-trained athletes have their spotters during a free-weight bench press apply external force (to make the lift more difficult) in the early phase of the lift and provide assistance toward its completion.

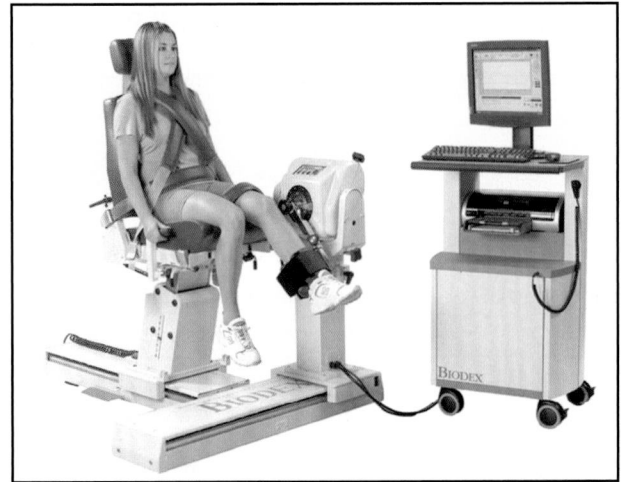

FIGURE 22.3 • Biodex advanced isokinetic electromechanical dynamometer. (Photo courtesy of Biodex; www.biodex.com/physical-medicine/products/dynamometers/system-4-quick-set).

Resistance-Training Equipment Categories

Resistance training typically uses one of four types of exercise equipment to manipulate movement speed and/or resistance throughout the ROM.

1. Free weights and barbells, common weightlifting equipment that does not control for or measure speed of movement of the resistance throughout the ROM
2. a. Isokinetic equipment that provides constant speed and variable resistance
   b. Isokinetic, hydraulic equipment that provides constant speed and variable resistance, where the individual controls movement speed
3. Cam devices and concentric–eccentric apparatus where movement speed varies and resistance remains constant

Strength-Testing Considerations

Seven important considerations exist for muscle strength testing regardless of measurement method:

1. Standardize instructions prior to testing.

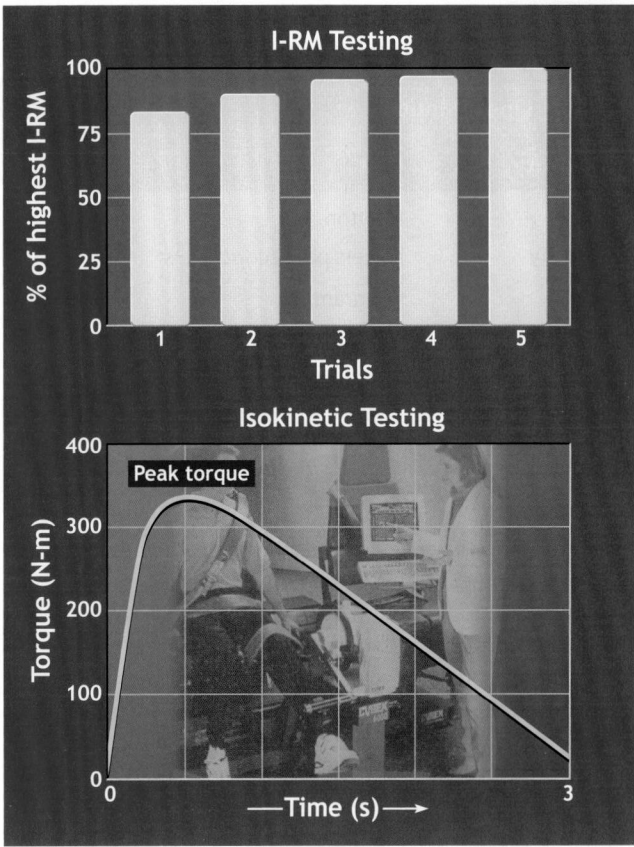

FIGURE 22.4 • **(A)** Conventional 1-RM testing. The heaviest weight lifted constitutes the 1-RM. If 150 kg (100%) is the maximum lifted, then 150 kg equals the 1-RM. **(B)** Force curve obtained during an isokinetic test performed at an angular velocity of $30° \cdot s^{-1}$ over a 3-s interval. Peak torque in this example equals 342 N-m. Average torque is the force-time integral, or impulse divided by time. Impulse equals 602 N-m $\cdot s^{-1}$, and average torque equals 200.7 N-m (602 N-m ÷ 3). Work equals the product of average torque × distance moved (90°, or 1.57 radians). Using the data for average torque and distance, work equals 174 N-m × 157 radians = 273 N-m, or 273 joules (J). Power is work per unit time, or 273 J ÷ 3.0 s = 91 W.

2. Ensure uniformity in duration and intensity of the warm-up.
3. Provide adequate practice prior to testing to minimize "learning" that could compromise initial results.

 Exercise Equipment to Overload Skeletal Muscle

Category	Speed	Resistance	Equipment Example
(I)	Variable	Variable	Barbells (resistance varies through ROM even though absolute weight remains constant)
(II)	Constant	Variable	Hydraulic (person controls speed)
	Constant	Variable	Computer-regulated (movement speed controlled by computer)
(III)	Variable	Constant	CAM-adjusted equipment and concentric–eccentric apparatus
(IV)	Constant	Constant	None available

TABLE 22.1	International System (SI) of Units for Expressing Muscular Strength and Power During Linear and Angular Motions[a]			
Linear Motion			**Angular Motion**	
Quantity	**Unit**		**Quantity**	**Unit**
Force	Newton, N		Torque, T	Newton meter, N-m
Velocity	Meters per second, $m \cdot s^{-1}$		Velocity, v	Radians per second, $rad \cdot s^{-1}$
Mass	Kilogram, kg		Moment of inertia, I or J	Kilogram meters squared, $kg\text{-}m^2$
Acceleration	Meters per second squared, $m \cdot s^{-2}$		Acceleration, a	Radians per second squared, $rad \cdot s^{-2}$
Displacement	Meter, m		Displacement, θ	Radian, rad
Time	Second, s		Time, t	Second, s

[a]Appendix D, available online at **http://thepoint.lww.com/mkk8e**, provides additional information about SI units, including interconversions.

4. Ensure consistency among subjects in the angle of limb measurement and/or body position on the test device.

5. Predetermine a minimum number of trials (repetitions) to establish a criterion strength score. For example, if administering five repetitions of a test, what score represents the individual's strength score? Is the highest score best, or should one use the average? In most cases, an average of several trials provides a more representative (reliable) strength or power score than a single measure.

6. Select test measures with high test score reproducibility. This crucial but often overlooked aspect of testing evaluates the variability of the subject's responses on repeated efforts. Lack of test score consistency (unreliability) can mask an individual's representative performance on the measure or change in performance when evaluating strength improvement.

7. Recognize individual differences in body size and composition when evaluating strength scores among individuals and groups.

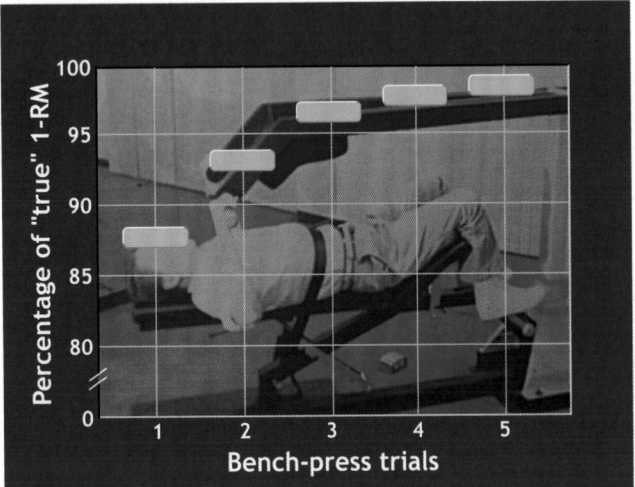

FIGURE 22.5 • Five repeated determinations of maximal force (1-RM) for the supine bench press with an electromechanical dynamometer. Strong verbal encouragement was provided on each attempt. (From F. Katch, Human Performance Laboratory, University of Massachusetts, Amherst.)

For example, consider the "fairness" of comparing absolute muscular strength of a 120-kg football lineman with the strength of a 62-kg distance runner. No clear-cut answer resolves this dilemma; in the section "Allometric Scaling," later in this chapter, we present alternatives for comparing strength scores relative to body size.

Learning Factors Affect Strength Measurements

In Chapter 19, we emphasized that initial gains in muscular strength with resistance training result largely from neural factors instead of structural changes within muscle *per se*. FIGURE 22.5 presents data for repetition-by-repetition performance improvements in maximal force (1-RM) at an angular velocity of $5° \cdot s^{-1}$ during a supine bench press with a 5-s interval between maximal effort repetitions. The amount of improvement averaged 11.4% between maximal force on attempt 1 and attempt 5 and 2.1% between the last two attempts. Strength "improvement" with repeated testing indicates the necessity for at least three attempts before maximum force scores begin to stabilize or plateau. Importantly, use of only one or two 1-RM attempts underestimates the "true" 1-RM by as much as 11%. If a single 1-RM trial preceded a 15-wk strength-training program, then any strength gains attributable to training would include the 11% "learning" improvement simply from familiarization, regardless of a true training effect!

GENDER DIFFERENCES IN MUSCLE STRENGTH

Several approaches determine whether a true gender difference exists in muscle strength. These evaluations relate to four factors:

1. Muscle cross-sectional area
2. Absolute muscle strength as total force exerted
3. Relative muscle strength indexed to estimates of body composition
4. Muscle strength indexed to allometric scaling

Muscle Cross-Sectional Area

Human skeletal muscle regardless of gender generates a maximum of between 16 and 30 newtons (N) of force per square centimeter of muscle cross section. *In the body, force-output capacity varies depending on the arrangement of the bony levers and muscle architecture* (see Chapter 18). Applying the value of 30 N as a representative force capacity per cm^2 of muscle tissue indicates that a muscle with a cross-sectional area of 5.0 cm^2 develops maximal force of 150 N. If all of the body's muscles became maximally activated simultaneously (with force applied in the same direction), the resulting force would equal 168 kN. This estimation assumes a muscle total cross section of 0.56 m^2.

FIGURE 22.6A compares the absolute arm flexor strength of men and women related to the flexor muscle's total cross-sectional area (MCSA). Clearly, individuals with the largest MCSA (10 to 20 cm^2) generate the greatest absolute force (30 to 40 kg). The near-linear relation between strength and muscle size indicates little difference in arm flexor strength for the same size muscle in men and women. FIGURE 22.6B further demonstrates this point when expressing the strength of the men and women per unit area of MCSA. In addition, women and men matched for absolute muscular strength show similar fatigability of the elbow flexor muscles during sustained low-level isometric contraction.[110]

Absolute Muscle Strength as Total Force Exerted

Comparisons of muscular strength on an *absolute* score basis (i.e., total force in lb or kg) indicate that men possess considerably greater strength than women for all muscle groups tested. Women score about 50% lower than men for upper-body strength and about 30% lower for leg strength. This gender disparity exists independent of the measuring system and generally coincides with gender-related difference in muscle mass distribution. Exceptions to these general findings usually emerge for strength-trained female track-and-field athletes and bodybuilders who have strength-trained for years.

A unique set of data exists on gender differences in weightlifting competitions in which men and women of identical body mass participated in the same weightlifting categories. FIGURE 22.7 displays the percentage differences in maximum weight lifted in the combined snatch and clean-and-jerk lifts during national championship competitions. These comparisons do not "equate" or "adjust" performance scores on the basis of the well-documented gender difference in body composition. The six body weight categories shown in the inset table range from 52 to 82.5 kg. The lighter-weight categories produced the smallest gender difference in strength, with the effect most pronounced in the heavier weight categories. Women of 75- and 82.5-kg body mass lift only about 60% of the maximal weight lifted by similar-weight male counterparts. This represents a more pronounced gender difference than other comparisons that matched male

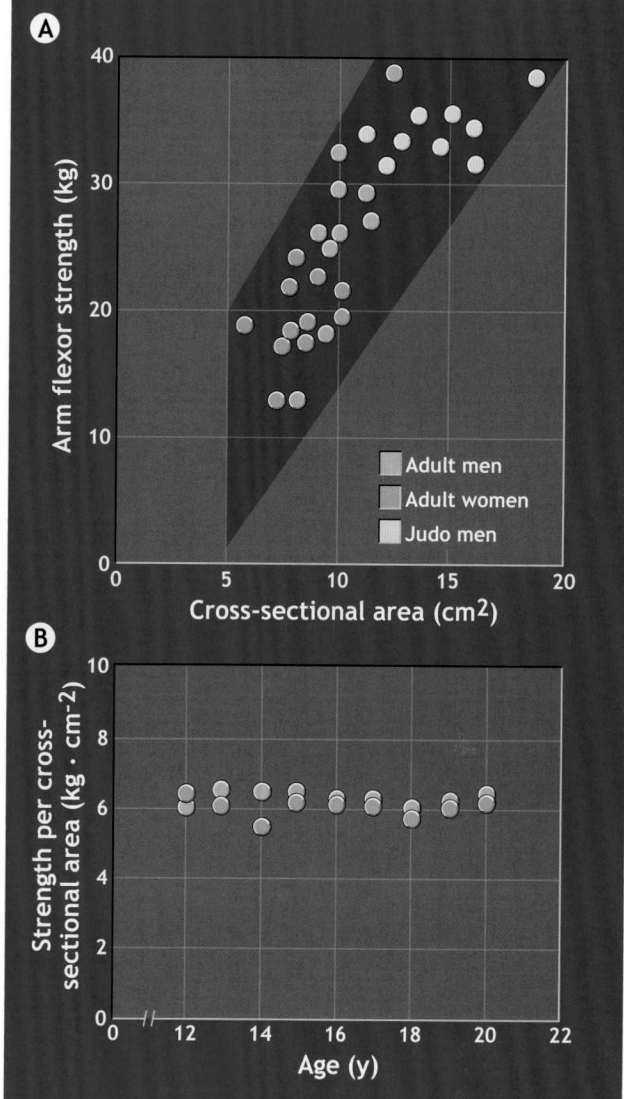

FIGURE 22.6 • **(A)** Variability of upper-arm flexion strength of men and women related to the flexor muscle's total cross-sectional area. **(B)** Strength per unit muscle cross-sectional area in males and females age 12 to 20 years. (Adapted with permission from Ikai M, Fukunaga T. Calculation of muscle strength per unit cross-sectional area of human muscle by means of ultrasonic measurements. *Arbeitsphysiologie* 1968;26:26.)

and female competitors for body composition, not just body mass. In such comparisons, it is impossible to determine what role if any anabolic steroid use impacted gender differences.

 INTEGRATIVE QUESTION

What performance would you expect in maximum weightlifting tests comparing (1) an average-size man and average-size woman, (2) a man and woman of equivalent training history and identical body mass, and (3) a man and woman of equivalent training history and identical fat-free body mass?

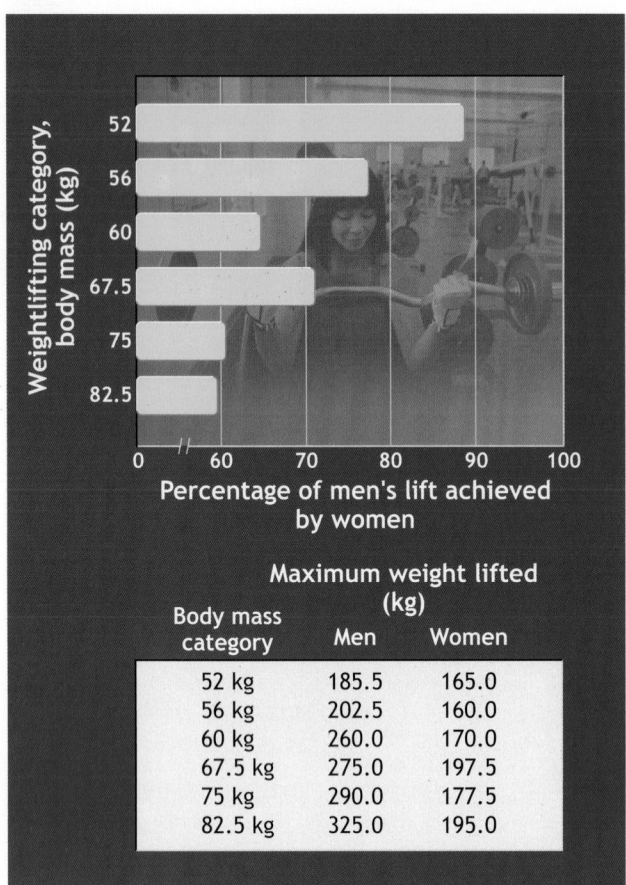

FIGURE 22.7 • Difference in maximum weight lifted between men and women in the same body mass categories during a national weightlifting competition. The *inset* shows the absolute weight lifted for each body mass category.

Relative Muscle Strength Indexed to Estimates of Body Composition

Relative strength comparisons among individuals involve creating a comparative ratio score by dividing a strength measurement (e.g., kg weight lifted or force exerted) by a reference measurement such as body mass, FFM, MCSA, or limb volume or girth. In general, such strength ratio scores based on body mass or FFM considerably reduce (if not eliminate) the large absolute strength differences usually observed between genders.[39]

Consider the following example. A male who weighs 95 kg bench-presses 114 kg; a 60-kg woman bench-presses only 70 kg (62% of the man's lift). Who is "stronger"? In absolute terms, we would conclude the male, by 61.3%. However, the bench-press score divided by body mass yields a much different conclusion. For the male, the strength ratio (114 kg ÷ 95 kg) equals 1.20; the ratio for the woman is 1.17 (70 kg ÷ 60 kg), which reduces the percentage difference in bench-press strength to only 2.5%! This alternative result would support the argument that little difference exists in muscle "quality" between men and women; rather, any observed gender difference in absolute muscle strength would reflect differences

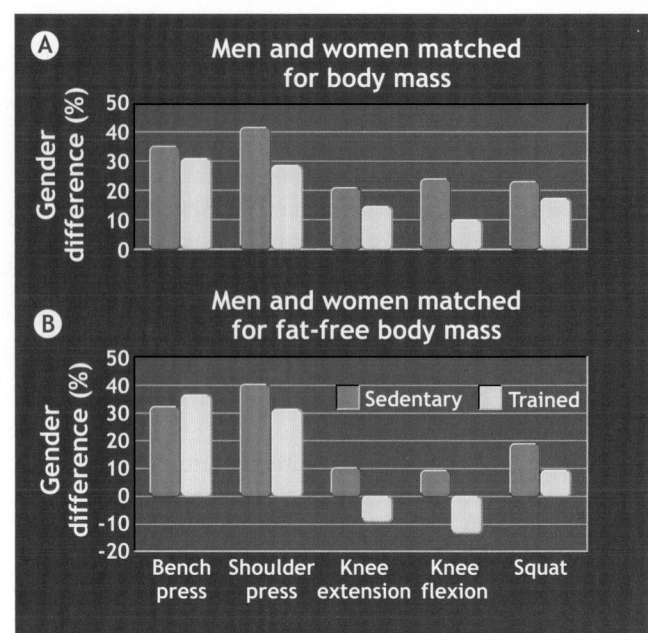

FIGURE 22.8 • Men and women matched for body mass **(A)** and fat-free body mass **(B)** for five measures of muscle strength. Above the zero line indicates the percentage by which values for men exceed values for women. (Data courtesy of Keller B. *The influence of body size variables on gender differences in strength and maximum aerobic capacity.* Unpublished doctoral dissertation, University of Massachusetts, Amherst, 1989.)

in muscle quantity (cross-sectional area). Men and women generally do not differ significantly in either upper- or lower-body strength when comparisons are made applying ratios with FFM (or MCSA) as the divisor.

We must emphasize that this traditional ratio adjustment may not equalize women and men on the basis of the underlying physiology. As with aerobic capacity (discussed in Chapter 11), a fair way to evaluate a potential gender difference in a criterion trait such as muscular strength or aerobic capacity includes one of two strategies:

1. Comparing men and women who do not differ in body size variables such as body mass or FFM and who exhibit similar training status
2. Adjusting for these variables through appropriate statistical control

These solutions preclude the need to create a ratio score because men and women in essence become equalized for body size and/or body composition. Using this approach, researchers assessed five measures of muscular strength for men and women, using 1-RM concentric (shortening) muscle actions for the bench press and squat and isokinetic dynamometry to assess maximum force during knee flexion and extension and seated shoulder press. FIGURE 22.8 shows that men and women matched for body mass produced larger gender differences in the sedentary group (44.0% for the shoulders and 25.1% for knee flexion) than in the trained group (33.0% for the bench press and 10.7% for knee flexion). The percentage differences decreased (but were not eliminated) for both groups by matching subjects for FFM. The shoulder press (39.4%) and bench press (31.2%) produced the largest gender differences in the sedentary group, while the corresponding differences for the trained group were 30.6% (shoulder press) and 35.4% (bench press).

These results differ from prior studies that used the traditional ratio score approach to express the strength of women and men. Without doubt, ratio scoring supports the argument that few gender differences exist in muscle quality, at least reflected by voluntary force output capacity. In contrast, matching men and women for body size, body composition, and training status before testing yields higher upper- and lower-body strength scores for men.[182] In a latter study of 2061 male and 1301 female military personnel, mean lift capacity averaged 51% greater in men despite a regression, ratio, or exponential mathematical adjustment in the strength score based on interindividual differences in FFM.

 INTEGRATIVE QUESTION

Based on gender-related differences in physical fitness components, devise a physical test that (1) minimizes and (2) maximizes performance differences between men and women.

Muscle Strength Indexed Using Allometric Scaling

Allometric scaling represents another mathematical procedure to try to establish a proper relationship between a body size variable (usually stature, body mass, or FFM) and some factor of interest such as muscular strength, aerobic capacity, power output, jumping height, or running speed.[24,55,207] The technique provides a statistical adjustment to evaluate the relative contribution of diverse independent variables (e.g., gender, maturation, habitual physical activity) on the dependent measure of interest (e.g., muscular strength, $\dot{V}O_{2max}$, pulmonary function). Allometric scaling, a well-accepted and valid statistical approach, also is applied in diverse areas of the biological sciences.[122,167,238,239–241]

FIGURE 22.9 illustrates the relationship between body mass and several different expressions of muscular strength. The top left graph (A) plots the total weight lifted versus body mass for Olympic weightlifters. Each point represents body mass of the top weightlifters in each weight category. Importantly, total weight lifted and body mass do not relate linearly but curvilinearly. Weightlifting strength relates proportionally to body mass raised to the exponent 0.7 (the slope of the line). The bottom six curves (B) depict the relationship between maximal grip strength and body mass in college-age men (*orange*) and women (*green*). The top graphs illustrate the simple relationship between body mass and grip strength without adjustment for body size. A positive relationship emerges ($r = 0.51$ for males and $r = 0.33$ for females). The middle graphs depict

the relationship with grip strength indexed to body mass (i.e., strength divided by body mass in kg). The bottom graphs illustrate the relationship between strength and allometric scaling of body mass. The resulting correlations between strength and body mass with the appropriate allometric scaling fall essentially to zero ($r = 0.013$ for males and $r = 0.03$ for females). This satisfies one of the basic tenets of allometry—the correlation between the scaled variable (muscular strength) and the scaling factor (body mass) must equal zero. The inset table (C) presents percentile norms for the grip strength adjusted to allometric-scaled body mass exponent (grip strength per $kg^{0.51}$) for college-age men and women.

 INTEGRATIVE QUESTION

You have a list of the names of young adult men with their corresponding body weights. Justify your selection of just two people to complete these tasks: one must push a vehicle stuck in the mud while the other must move hand-over-hand on a rope strung across a ravine. Hint: Consider absolute and relative strength requirements of each task and association between body mass and absolute and relative muscular strength.

TRAINING MUSCLES TO BECOME STRONGER

A muscle strengthens when trained near its current maximal force-generating capacity. Standard weightlifting equipment, pulleys or springs, immovable bars, resistance bands, or a variety of isokinetic and hydraulic devices provide effective muscle overload. Importantly, overload intensity (level of tension placed on muscle), not the type of device that applies the overload, generally governs strength improvements. Certain approaches, however, lend themselves to precise and systematic overload applications. **Progressive-resistance weight training**, **isometric training**, and **isokinetic training** represent three common systems to train muscles to become stronger. These systems rely on shortening or concentric, lengthening or eccentric (where muscle maintains tension as muscle lengthens), and static or isometric muscle actions, the types of muscle actions illustrated in **FIGURE 22.10A,B**.

Different Muscle Actions

Neural stimulation of a muscle causes the contractile elements of its fibers to attempt to shorten along the longitudinal axis. The terms *isometric* and *static* describe muscle activation without observable change in muscle fiber length.

 See the animation "Muscle Contraction Type" on **http://thePoint.lww.com/mkk8e** for a demonstration of the common types of muscle contraction.

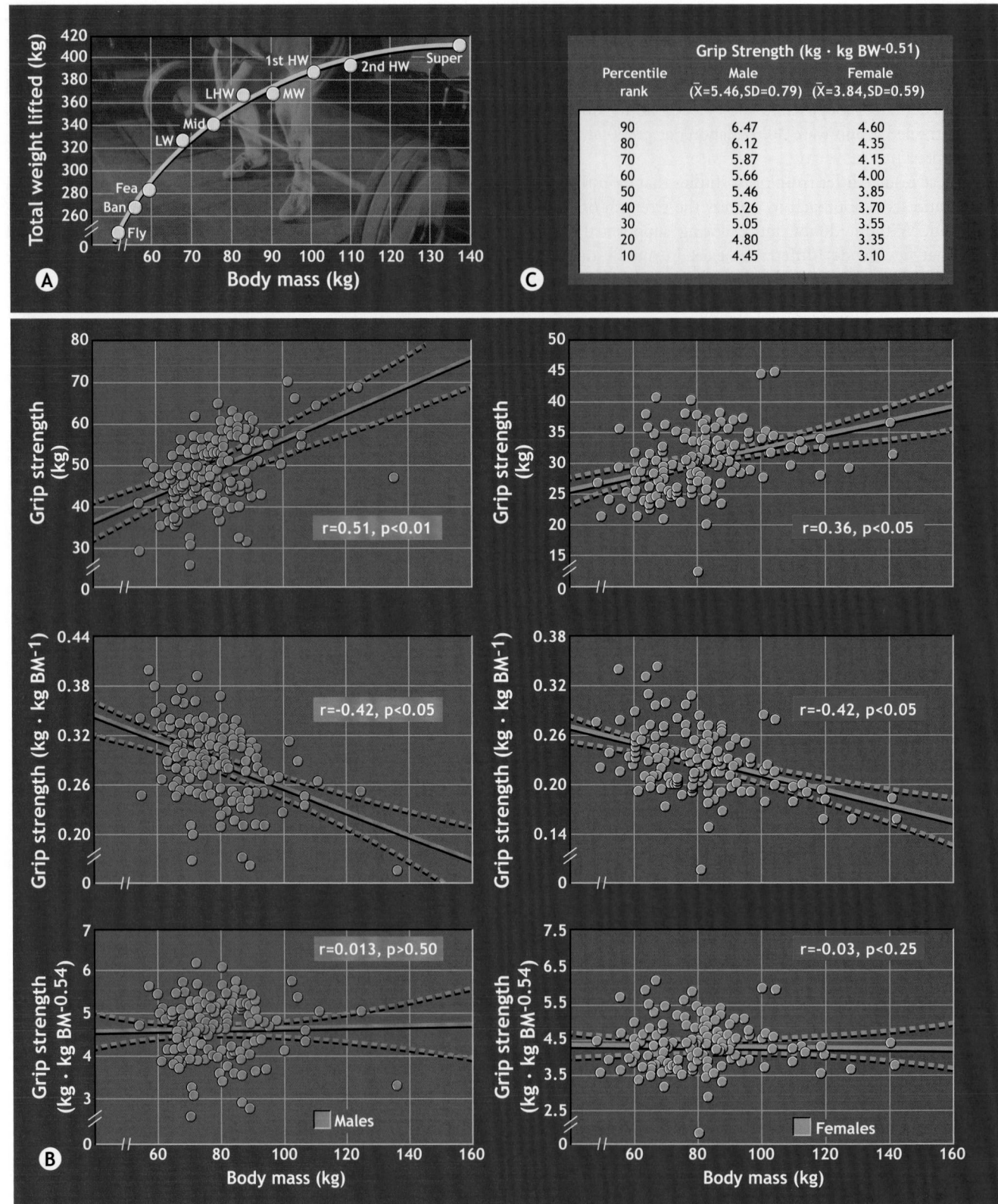

FIGURE 22.9 • Relationship between body mass and different expressions of muscular strength. **(A)** Total weight lifted in two events as a function of body mass of Olympic weightlifters (1980 Olympic Games). Each point represents the body mass of the top six male weightlifters in each of the following weight categories: *Fly*, flyweight; *Ban*, bantamweight; *Fea*, featherweight; *LW*, lightweight; *Mid*, middleweight; *LHW*, light-heavyweight; *MW*, middle-heavyweight; *1st HW*, first heavyweight; *2nd HW*, second heavyweight; and *Super*, superheavyweight. (Adapted with permission from Lathan and cited by Titel K, Wutscherk H. In: Komi PV, ed. Stength and power in sport. Oxford, UK: Blackwell Scientific, 1993.) **(B)** Maximal absolute grip strength, relative grip strength, and strength scaled allometrically to body mass of 100 men (orange) and 105 women (green) of college age. **(C)** Percentile norms for grip strength scaled to body mass. (Data courtesy of Dr. Paul Vanderburgh, University of Dayton.)

Isometric action (Fig. 22.10B): This action occurs when a muscle generates force and attempts to shorten but cannot overcome the external resistance. From a physics standpoint, this type of muscle action does not produce external work. An isometric (static) action can generate considerable force despite the lack of noticeable lengthening or shortening of muscle sarcomeres and subsequent joint movement.

A *dynamic* muscle action produces movement of a skeletal body part such as trunk or upper or lower limb. Concentric and eccentric actions represent the two types of dynamic muscle actions (Fig. 22.10A).

Concentric action: This occurs when the muscle shortens and joint movement occurs as tension develops. The example shows raising a dumbbell from the extended to the flexed elbow position.

Eccentric action: In this type of action, the muscle lengthens while it develops tension. The weight slowly lowers against the force of gravity. The muscle fibers (more specifically the sarcomeres) of the upper-arm muscles lengthen in an eccentric action to prevent the weight from crashing to the surface. In weightlifting, muscles frequently act eccentrically as the weight slowly returns to the starting position to begin the next concentric (shortening) action. Eccentric muscle action during this "recovery" phase adds to the total work and effectiveness of the exercise repetition.

Some coaches and trainers still refer to muscle actions as isotonic, derived from the Greek word *isotonos* (*iso* meaning "the same" or "equal," *tonos* meaning "tension" or "strain"), because concentric and eccentric muscle actions produce joint movement. However, this term lacks precision when applied to most dynamic muscle actions that involve movement; the muscle's effective force-generating capacity continually varies as the joint angle changes throughout the ROM.

Resistance Training

The most popular form of resistance training involves raising and lowering an external weight. In most cases, the weight lifted remains constant (e.g., raising and lowering the same 10-kg barbell); this application is known as **dynamic constant external resistance training** (**DCER**). With appropriate and progressive manipulation of training volume, intensity, and frequency to optimize dose response, this method selectively strengthens specific muscles to overcome a fixed initial or changing resistance. This resistance typically takes the form of a barbell, dumbbell, or weight plates on a pulley- or cam-type machine. As with cardiovascular training, muscular strength improvements vary inversely on a continuum with initial training status. Generally, improvements average 40% for the untrained, 20% in the moderately trained, 15% in the trained,

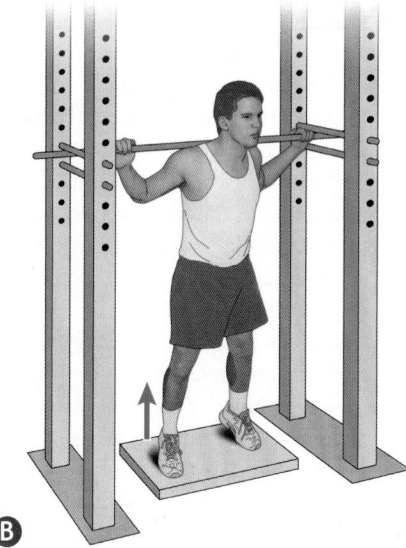

FIGURE 22.10 • **(A)** Muscle force generated during concentric (shortening) and eccentric (lengthening) muscle actions. **(B)** Isometric (static) muscle actions.

10% in the advanced, and 2% in elite athletes who achieve a high level of competitive success.[4]

Progressive Resistance Exercise

The **progressive resistance exercise** (**PRE**) training method provides a practical application of the overload principle and forms the basis of most resistance-training programs. Physical therapists in a rehabilitation hospital in the late 1940s and early 1950s devised weight-training regimens to improve the strength of previously injured limbs of soldiers returning from World War II. The procedure involved three sets of exercises, each set consisting of 10 repetitions done consecutively without resting. The first set required one half the maximum weight that could be lifted 10 times, or ½ 10-RM; the second set used ¾ 10-RM, and the final 10-RM required maximum weight. As patients trained, the muscles of the exercised limbs became stronger, so the 10-RM resistance increased periodically to maintain continued strength improvements. Similar improvements occurred even when reversing the intensity progression, so that patients performed the 10-RM as the first set.

Variations of PRE. The following summarizes 13 general findings from research studies on the optimal number of sets and repetitions, including frequency and relative intensity of PRE training for optimal strength improvement:

1. Eight- to 12-RM proves effective in novice training, whereas 1- to 12-RM effectively loads for intermediate training. This can then increase to more intense loading using 1- to 6-RM.

2. Rest 3 min between sets of an exercise at moderate movement velocity (1 to 2 s concentric; 1 to 2 s eccentric).

3. For PRE at a specific RM load, increase load 2 to 10% when the individual performs one to two repetitions above the current workload.

4. Performing one exercise set induces only slightly less strength improvement in recreational weightlifters than performing two or three sets.[38,97] For those who desire to maximize muscle strength and size gains, higher volume, multiple-set paradigms emphasizing 6- to 12-RM at moderate velocity with 1- to 2-min rests between sets prove most effective.

5. Single-set programs generally produce most of the health and fitness benefits of multiple-set programs. These "lower-volume" programs also produce greater compliance and reduce financial cost and time commitment.

6. Novices and intermediates should train 2 to 3 days a week, whereas the advanced can train 3 to 4 days a week. Such a generalization is not without a potential downside. High training frequency extends the transient activation of inflammatory signaling cascades, concomitant with persistent suppression of key mediators of anabolic responses, which could blunt the training response.[48]

7. Training twice every second day produces overall superior results compared with daily training.[94] This may occur from the effects of low muscle glycogen content (with training twice every second day) on enhanced transcription of genes involved in training adaptations.[216]

8. If training includes multiple exercises, 4 or 5 days per week may produce less improvement than training two or three times a week because near-daily training of the same muscles impairs muscle recuperation between training sessions. Inadequate recovery retards progress in neuromuscular and structural adaptations and strength development.

9. A fast rate of moving a given resistance generates more strength improvement than moving at a slower rate. Neither free weights (barbells, weight plates, dumbbells) nor an array of exercise machines shows inherent superiority for developing muscle strength.

10. Exercise should sequence to optimize workout quality by engaging large before small muscle groups, multiple-joint exercises before single-joint exercises, and higher-intensity exercise before lower-intensity exercise.

11. Combined resistance-training concentric and eccentric muscle actions augment effectiveness; include both single-joint and multiple-joint exercises to potentiate a muscle's strength and fiber size.[50,118,195,210,229]

12. Overload training that includes eccentric muscle actions preserves strength gains better during a maintenance phase than concentric-only training.[50]

13. Power training should apply the strategy to improve muscular strength plus include lighter loads (30 to 60% of 1-RM) performed at fast contraction velocity. Use 2- to 3-min rest periods between sets. Emphasize multiple-joint movements that activate larger muscle groups.

TABLE 22.2 summarizes the major recommendations of the American College of Sports Medicine position stand on progression in resistance training for healthy adults.

Periodization. In 1972, Russian scientist Leonid Matveyev introduced the concept of *strength-training periodization*;[155] it has since become incorporated in various forms into the training regimens of novice and champion athletes involved in resistance training.[32,117,133] Conceptually, periodization varies training intensity and volume to ensure that peak performance coincides with major competition. It also proves effective for achieving recreational and rehabilitative goals. Periodization subdivides a specific resistance-training period such as 1 year (*macrocycle*) into smaller periods or phases (*mesocycles*), with each mesocycle again separated into weekly *microcycles*. In essence, the training model progressively decreases training volume and increases intensity as duration of the program progresses to maximize gains in muscular strength and power. Fractionating the macrocycle into components allows multiple ways to manipulate training intensity, volume, frequency, sets, repetitions, and rest periods to prevent overtraining. It also provides a way to alter workout variety. Periodization variation can reduce negative overtraining or "staleness" effects so athletes achieve peak performance at competition. FIGURE 22.11 depicts the generalized design for periodization and a typical macrocycle's four distinct phases. As competition approaches, training volume gradually decreases while training intensity concurrently increases. Consider the following four phases:

Phase 1. **Preparation phase** emphasizes modest strength development with *high-volume* (3 to 5 sets, 8 to 12 reps), *low-intensity* workouts (50 to 80% 1-RM plus flexibility and aerobic and anaerobic training).

Phase 2. **First transition phase** emphasizes strength development with workouts of *moderate volume* (3 to 5 sets, 5 to 6 reps) and *moderate intensity* (80 to 90% 1-RM plus flexibility and interval aerobic training).

Phase 3. **Competition phase** lets the participant peak for competition. Selective strength development is emphasized with *low-volume, high-intensity* workouts (3 to 5 sets, 2 to 4 reps at 90 to 95% 1-RM plus short periods of interval training that emphasize sport-specific movements).

Phase 4. **Second transition phase** (**active recovery**) emphasizes recreational activities and low-intensity workouts that incorporate different activity modes. For the upcoming competition, the athlete repeats the periodization cycle.

Periodization structures an inverse relation between training volume and training intensity through the competition phase; it then decreases both aspects during the second transition or recuperation period. Note the increase in time devoted to technique training as competition approaches, with training volume at the periodization cycle's lowest point. The bottom

TABLE 22.2 Summary of Resistance Training Recommendations: an Overview of Different Program Variables Needed for Progression with Different Fitness Levels

	Muscle Action	Selection	Order	Loading	Volume	Rest Intervals	Velocity	Frequency
Strength			*For Nov, Int, Adv:*			*For Nov, Int, Adv:*		
Nov.	ECC & CON	SJ & MJ ex.	Large < small	60–70% of 1RM	1–3 sets, 8–12 reps	2–3 min for core	S, M	2–3×/wk
Int.	ECC & CON	SJ & MJ ex.	MJ < SJ	70–80% of 1RM	Mult. sets, 6–12 reps	1–2 min for others	M	2–IX/wk
Adv.	ECC & CON	SJ & MJ ex.—emphasis: MJ	HI < LI	1RM—PER	Mult. sets 1–12 reps—PER		US-F	4–6 X/wk
Hypertrophy			*For Nov, Int, Adv:*					
Nov.	ECC & CON	SJ & MJ ex.	Large < small	60–70% of 1RM	1–3 sets, 8–12 reps	1–2 min	S, M	2–3×/wk
Int.	ECC & CON	SJ & MJ ex.	MJ < SJ	70–80% of 1RM	Mult. sets, 6–12	1–2 min	S, M	2–IX/wk
Adv.	ECC & CON	SJ & MJ	HI < LI	70–100% of 1RM with emphasis on 70–85%—PER	Mult. sets 1–12 reps with emphasis on on 6–12 reps—PER	2–3 min—VH; 1–2 min—L-MH	S, M, F	4–6X /wk
Power		*For Nov, Int, Adv:*	*For Nov, Int, Adv:*	*For Nov, Int, Adv:*		*For Nov, Int, Adv:*		
Nov.	ECC & CON	Mostly MJ	Large < small	Heavy loads (>80%)—strength; Light (30–60%)—velocity—PER	Train for strength	2–3 min for core	M	2–3×/wk
Int.	ECC & CON		Most complex < least complex		1–3 sets, 3–6 reps	1–2 min for others	F	2–4X /wk
Adv.	ECC & CON		HI < LI		3–6 sets, 1–6 reps—PER		F	4–6×/wk
Endurance			*For Nov, Int, Adv:*			*For Nov, Int, Adv:*		
Nov.	ECC & CON	SJ & MJ ex.	Variety in sequencing recommended	50–70% of 1RM	1–3 sets, 10–15 reps	1–2 min for high-rep sets	S—MR	2–3X /wk
Int.	ECC & CON	SJ & MJ ex.		50–70% of 1RM	Mult. sets, 10–15 reps or more	<1 min for 10–15 reps	M—HR	2–4X /wk
Adv.	ECC & CON	SJ & MJ		30–80% of 1RM—PER	Mult. sets, 10–25 reps or more—PER			4–6×/wk

ECC, eccentric; CON, concentric; Nov, novice; Int, intermediate; Adv, advanced; SJ, single-joint; MJ, multiple-joint; ex., exercises; HI, high intensity; LI, low intensity; 1RM, 1-repetition maximum; PER, periodized; VH, very heavy; L-MH, light-to-moderately heavy; S, slow; M, moderate; US, unintentionally slow; F, fast; MR, moderate repetitions; HR, high repetitions.

From ACSM position stand on: Progression models in resistance training for healthy adults. *Med Sci Sports Exerc* 2002;34:364.

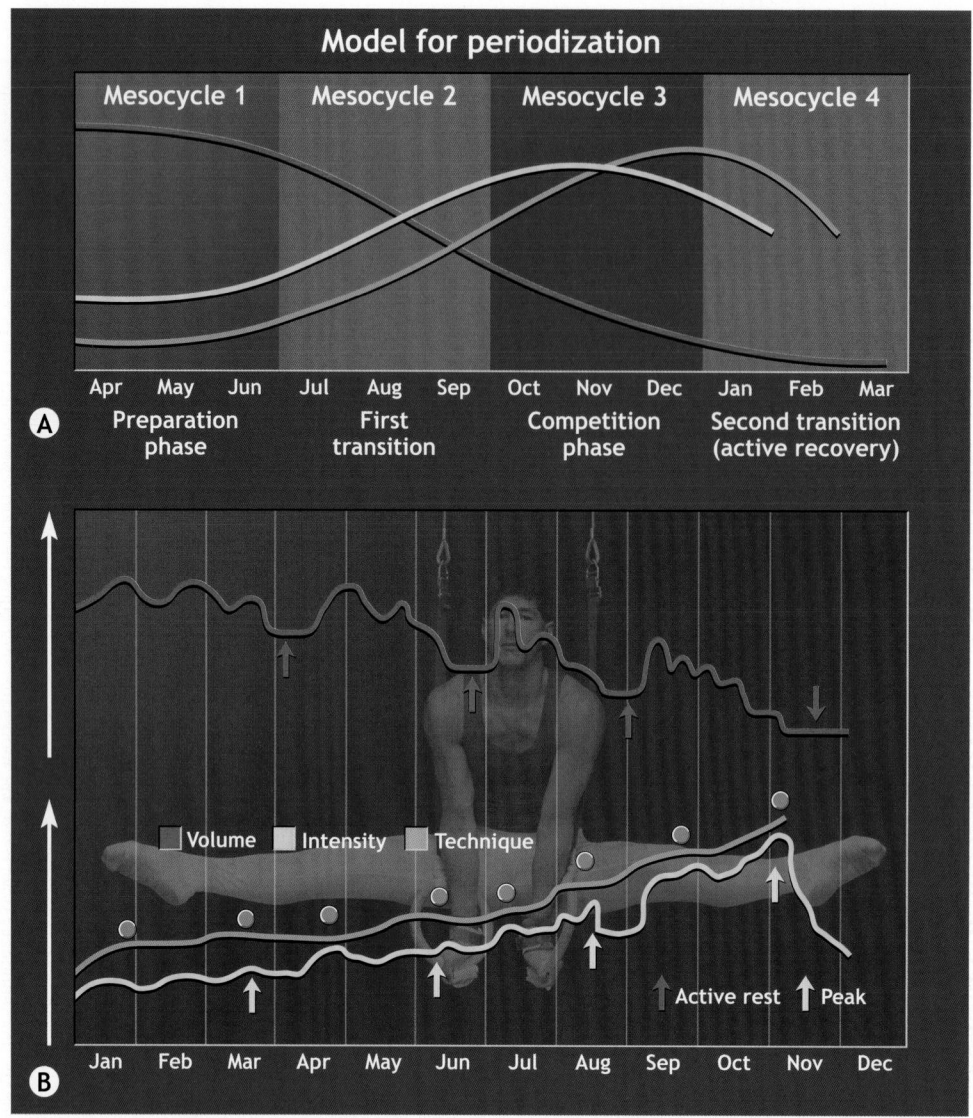

FIGURE 22.11 • **(A)** Periodization subdivides a macrocycle into distinct phases or mesocycles. These in turn separate into weekly microcycles. The general plan provides modifications, but mesocycles typically include four parts: (1) preparation phase, (2) first transition phase, (3) competition phase, and (4) a second transition or active recovery phase. **(B)** Example of periodization for an elite athlete (gymnast) preparing for competition. Competitions took place throughout the yearly training program so periodization focused on achieving peak performance at the end of each macrocycle. Periodization places training into context for intensity, duration, and frequency of strength–power workouts. The major purpose of this focus attempts to avoid overtraining (staleness), minimize injury potential, and reduce training monotony, while progressing toward peak competition performance (filled circles).

of Figure 22.11 illustrates how training volume (shown in *red*) and intensity (shown in *yellow*) interact within a mesocycle for an athlete in a specific sport.

Sport-specific training principles usually apply in periodization to design a training regimen based on a sport's distinct *strength*, *power*, and *endurance* requirements. A detailed analysis of metabolic and technical requirements of the sport also frames the training paradigm. The concept of periodization makes intuitive sense, yet limited data exist for the superiority of this training approach.

Researchers have studied shorter mesocycles to determine what combination of factors optimizes performance

improvements. One study that equated training volume and intensity among three approaches to periodization (linear periodization, undulating periodization, and a nonperiodized time interval) found each training method equally effective.[16] The training groups made similar gains in muscular strength (25% squat, 13.1% bench press) and muscular power (7.6% vertical jump). Without equating training volume and intensity, it is impossible to evaluate differences in training effects reported previously.[255]

A critical review of the studies of periodized strength training concluded that this approach produced greater improvements in muscular strength, body mass, and FFM, and reductions in percentage body fat than nonperiodized multi-set and single-set training programs.[77] Additional research must further assess how periodization interacts with fitness status,[172] age, gender,[61] and specific sports (motor) performance.[184,187] Studies must equate participants on various fitness parameters and then manipulate different linear and nonlinear training protocols to account for factors that affect training response. In essence, program evaluation must consider the following four factors, either singly or in combination:

1. Biomechanical and motor control sequences in the targeted sport skill
2. Changes in segmental and whole-body composition
3. Biochemical and ultrastructural tissue adaptations
4. Transfer of newly acquired strength to subsequent sport performance measures

 INTEGRATIVE QUESTION

Discuss the statement "There is no one best system of resistance training."

Resistance Training Guidelines for Sedentary Adults, the Elderly, and Cardiac Patients: Benefits for Health Enhancement and Disease Prevention

Currently, the American College of Sports Medicine (www.acsm.org), American Heart Association (www.americanheart.org), Centers for Disease Control and Prevention (www.cdc.gov), American Association of Cardiovascular and Pulmonary Rehabilitation (www.aacvpr.org), and the U.S. Surgeon General's Office (www.surgeongeneral.gov) consider regular resistance exercise an important component of a comprehensive, health-related physical fitness program.[3,78,192] Resistance training goals for competitive athletes focus on optimizing muscular strength, power, and hypertrophy (high-intensity with 1-RM to 6-RM training loads). *In contrast, goals for most middle-age and older adults focus on maintenance (and possible increase) of muscle and bone mass and muscular strength and muscular endurance to enhance the overall health and physical-fitness profile.* Adequate muscular strength in midlife maintains a margin of safety above the necessary threshold to prevent injury in later life.[28] Among 45- to 68-year-old men, hand-grip strength accurately predicted functional limitations and disability 25 years later.[194A] Men in the lowest one third for grip strength showed the greatest risk; those in the middle one third showed intermediate risk; and men in the top one third experienced the least disability risk at the 25-year follow-up. The resistance-training program recommended for middle-age and older men and women classifies as "moderate intensity." In contrast to the multiple-set, heavy-resistance approach of younger athletes, the program uses single sets of diverse exercises performed between 8- and 15-RM a minimum of twice weekly. **TABLE 22.3**

presents guidelines from different groups and health organizations for prudent resistance training of older men and women and cardiac patients.

 Impressive Resistance Training Results for Seniors

A meta-analysis that systematically examined the overall value of resistance exercise for muscular strength and lean body mass outcomes among healthy aging adults reported these individuals added 2.4 pounds of lean muscle and increased overall strength by 25 to 30% following an average of 18 to 20 wk of training. The amount of weight lifted and the frequency and duration of the training sessions interacted in a dose–response manner to affect improvement. Such an effect would counter the normal 0.4-lb muscle loss a year generally observed for individuals of this age.

Peterson MD, Gordon PM. Resistance exercise for the aging adult: clinical implications and prescription guidelines. *Am J Med* 2011;124:194.

Does Resistance Training Plus Aerobic Training Equal Less Strength Improvement?

Debate concerns whether concurrent resistance and aerobic training yields less muscular strength and power improvement than training for strength only.[15,21,132,161,259] This has caused many strength and power athletes and bodybuilders to refrain from including endurance activities in the belief they diminish strength improvements. Advocates for abstaining from aerobic training when attempting to optimize gains in muscle size and strength maintain that the added energy (and perhaps protein) demands of intense endurance training limit a muscle's growth and metabolic responsiveness to resistance training. Some data support this position. For example, different modes of exercise induce antagonistic molecular level, intracellular signaling mechanisms that could exert a negative impact on the muscle's adaptive response to resistance training.[177] Endurance training may also inhibit signaling to the muscles' protein-synthesis machinery, which would definitely be counterproductive to the goals of resistance training.[27,126,147,260]

A short-term bout of intense endurance activity also inhibits performance in subsequent muscular strength activities.[144] Further research must determine whether this acute effect on maximal force output limits ability to overload skeletal muscle optimally to a degree that impairs strength development with concurrent strength and endurance training. If it does, then a 20- to 30-min recovery between aerobic and strength-training components might enhance the quality of the subsequent strength workout. These considerations should not deter those who desire a well-rounded conditioning program that offers specific fitness and health benefits from incorporating *both* training modes.

TABLE 22.3	Strength-Training Guidelines for Sedentary Adults, Elderly Persons, and Cardiac Patients				
Guideline	Sets	Repetitions[a]	Number of Exercises	Frequency (Days/Week)
Healthy sedentary adults				
1990 ACSM Position Stand[b]	1	8–12	8–10[c]	2
1995 ACSM Guidelines[d]	1	8–12	8–10	2
1996 Surgeon General's Report[e]	1–2	8–12	8–10	2
Elderly persons				
Pollock et al.,[f] 1994	1	10–15	8–10	2
Cardiac patients				
1995 AHA Exercise Standards[g]	1	10–15	8–10	2–3
1995 AACVPR Guidelines[h]	1	10–15	8–10	2–3

ACSM, American College of Sports Medicine; AHA, American Heart Association; AACVPR, American Association of Cardiovascular and Pulmonary Rehabilitation.

[a]For healthy persons under age 50, weight should be sufficient to induce volitional fatigue with the number of repetitions listed. For older persons, lighter loads may be used.

[b]American College of Sports Medicine. The recommended quantity and quality of exercise for developing and maintaining cardiorespiratory and muscular fitness in healthy adults. *Med Sci Sports Exerc* 1990;22:265.

[c]Minimum one exercise per major muscle group (e.g., chest press, shoulder press, triceps extension, biceps curl, pull-down [upper back], lower back extension, abdominal crunch/curl-up, quadriceps extension, leg curls [hamstrings], calf-raise).

[d]American College of Sports Medicine. *Guidelines for Exercise Testing and Prescription.* 5th Ed. Baltimore: Williams & Wilkins, 1995; also included low-risk diseased populations.

[e]U.S. Department of Health and Human Services. Physical activity and health: a report of the surgeon general. Atlanta, GA: U.S. Department of Health and Human Services, Centers for Disease Control and Prevention, National Center for Chronic Disease Prevention and Health Promotion, 1996.

[f]Pollock ML, et al. Exercise training and prescription for the elderly. *South Med J* 1994;87:S88.

[g]Fletcher GF, et al. Exercise standards: a statement for health care professionals from the American Heart Association. *Circulation* 1995;91:580.

[h]American Association of Cardiovascular and Pulmonary Rehabilitation. *Guidelines for Cardiac Rehabilitation Programs.* 2nd Ed. Champaign, IL: Human Kinetics, 1995.

fyi Resistance Exercise May Enhance Molecular Signaling of Mitochondrial Biogenesis in Skeletal Muscle Induced by Endurance Exercise

Recent research has tested the hypothesis that molecular signaling of mitochondrial biogenesis after endurance exercise is impaired by a subsequent bout of resistance exercise (concurrent training). Muscle biopsies were obtained before and after either endurance exercise only (1 hr of cycling at ~65% $\dot{V}O_2$max) or endurance exercise followed by resistance exercise (6 sets of leg presses at 70 to 80% 1-RM) with an analysis of the mRNA of genes related to muscle biogenesis and substrate regulation. In contrast to the hypothesis tested, the results demonstrated that resistance exercise performed after endurance exercise *amplified* the adaptive signaling response of mitochondrial biogenesis compared with single-mode endurance exercise, thus suggesting that concurrent training may benefit the adaptation of muscle oxidative capacity.

Source: Wang L, et al. Resistance exercise enhances the molecular signaling of mitochondrial biogenesis induced by endurance exercise in human skeletal muscle. *J Appl Physiol* 2011;111:1335.

Resistance Training for Children

Many exercise physiology textbooks do not focus on the benefits and possible risks of resistance training for preadolescents, largely because of limited data in the literature. Obvious concern arises regarding the potential for injury from excessive musculoskeletal loading that includes epiphyseal fractures, ruptured intervertebral disks, lower back bony disruptions, and acute lower back trauma. A child's hormonal profile also lacks full development—particularly the tissue-building hormone testosterone (refer to Chapter 20). One might question whether resistance training in children could even induce meaningful strength improvements.

Supervised resistance training using concentric-only muscle actions with relatively high repetitions and low resistance improves muscular strength of children and adolescents without adverse effect on bone, muscle, or connective tissue,[189] including children with disabilities and disease[30,80,125] and obesity.[59,66]

More than likely, learning and enhanced neuromuscular activation rather than substantial increases in muscle size account for children's relatively rapid strength improvements. The guidelines in TABLE 22.4 provide prudent recommendations for initiating resistance exercise training for children and adolescents.

TABLE 22.4	Guidelines for Resistance-Exercise Training and Progression in Children and Adolescents
Age (y)	**Considerations**
7 or younger	Introduce child to basic exercises with little or no weight; develop the concept of a training session; teach exercise techniques; progress from body weight calisthenics, partner exercises, and lightly resisted exercises; keep volume low.
8–10	Gradually increase the number of exercises; practice exercise technique in all lifts; start gradual progressive loading of exercises; keep exercises simple; gradually increase training volume; carefully monitor toleration to the exercise stress.
11–13	Teach all basic exercise techniques; continue progressive loading of each exercise; emphasize exercise techniques; introduce more advanced exercises with little or no resistance.
14–15	Progress to more advanced youth programs in resistance exercise; add sport-specific components; emphasize exercise techniques; increase volume.
16 or older	Move child to entry-level adult programs after all background knowledge has been mastered and a basic level of training experience has been gained.

Reprinted from Kraemer WJ, Fleck SJ. *Strength Training for Young Athletes.* Champaign, IL: Human Kinetics, 1993.
Note: If a child of any age begins a program without previous experience, start the child at lower levels and move to more advanced levels as exercise toleration, skill, amount of training time, and understanding permit.

Isometric Strength Training

Research in Germany during the mid-1950s showed that isometric strength increased about 5% weekly by performing a daily single, maximum isometric muscle action of only 1-s duration, or a 6-s action at two-thirds maximum.[106] Repeating this action 5 to 10 times daily produced greater gains in isometric strength.

Isometric Training Limitations

Isometric exercise provides muscle overload and improves strength yet offers limited benefits for functional sports training. Without movement, one cannot readily evaluate the overload level and/or training progress. Also, isometric strength development fosters a high degree of muscle specificity adaptations. A muscle trained isometrically clearly improves strength primarily when the muscle acts isometrically, particularly at the training joint angle and body position. This means that isometric training to develop "strengths" for a particular movement probably necessitates training at many specific angles through the ROM. This becomes time-consuming, particularly given the availability of conventional dynamic weight training and isokinetic and other functional resistance training methodologies.

Isometric Training Benefits

The isometric method benefits muscle testing and rehabilitation. Isometric techniques can detect specific muscle weakness at a particular angle in the ROM, thus forming a basis for optimizing muscle overload at an appropriate joint angle.

Which Method is Better: Static or Dynamic?

Static and dynamic resistance training methods each increase muscle "strengths." An individual's specific needs determine the optimal resistance training method governed by the specificity of the training response.[173,268]

Specificity of Isometric Training Response

An isometrically trained muscle shows greatest strength improvement when measured isometrically; similarly, a dynamically trained muscle tests best when evaluated in resistance activities that require movement. Isometric strength developed at or near one joint angle does not readily transfer to other angles or body positions that must rely on the same muscles.[252] In dynamic activities, muscles trained through movement over a limited ROM show the greatest strength improvement when measured in that ROM.[19,88] Even *body position specificity* exists; muscular strength of ankle plantar and dorsiflexors developed in the standing position with concentric and eccentric muscle actions showed no transfer with the same muscles evaluated in the supine position.[193] Resistance training specificity makes sense because strength improvement blends adaptations in two factors:

1. The muscle fiber and connective tissue harness itself
2. Neural organization and excitability of motor units that power discrete patterns of voluntary movement

A muscle's maximal force output depends on neural factors that effectively recruit and synchronize firing of motor units, not just muscle fiber type and cross-sectional area.

A 3-mo study of young adult men and women emphasized the highly specific nature of resistance-training adaptations.[68] One group trained the adductor pollicis muscle isometrically with 10 daily actions of 5-s duration at a frequency of 1 per minute. The other group trained the same muscle dynamically with 10 daily 10-repetition bouts of weight movement at one-third maximal strength. The untrained muscle served as the control. To eliminate any training influence from psychologic factors and central nervous system adaptations, a supermaximal electrical stimulation applied to the motor nerve evaluated the force capacity of the trained muscle. The results were clear—both training groups improved maximal force capacity and peak rate of force development. The improvement in maximal force for the isometrically trained group nearly doubled the improvement for the dynamically trained group. Conversely, improvement in speed of force development averaged about 70% greater in the group trained with dynamic muscle actions. Such findings provide strong evidence that resistance training per se does not induce all-inclusive (*general*) adaptations in muscle structure and function. Rather, a muscle's contractile properties (maximal force, velocity of shortening, rate of tension development) improve in a manner highly specific to the muscle action in training. Both static and dynamic training methods produce strength increases, yet no one system rates consistently superior to the other in how best to assess muscle function. The crucial consideration concerns the intended purpose of the newly acquired strength.

Practical Implications. The complex interaction between nervous and muscular systems helps to explain why leg muscles strengthened in squats or deep knee bends fail to show equivalent improved force capability in other leg movements such as jumping or leg extension that require activation of the same musculature. Low relationships emerge between dynamic measures of leg extension force at any speed and vertical jumping height. A muscle group strengthened and enlarged by dynamic resistance training does not demonstrate equal improvement in force capacity when measured isometrically or isokinetically. Strengthening muscles for a specific athletic or occupational activity (e.g., golf, tennis, rowing, swimming, football, firefighting, package handling) demands more than just identifying and overloading the muscles generally involved in the movement. It requires neuromuscular training specifically in the important movements that necessitate improved strength. A more appropriate name for this type of training is **functional strength training** or **functional resistance movement training**.[7,9,49] Increasing leg muscle "strength" through general weightlifting will not necessarily improve performance in a variety of subsequent leg movements.[160] *Newly acquired strength seldom transfers fully to other types of strength movements, even those that activate the same trained muscles.* A standard program of weight training for leg extension increased leg extension strength by 227%. Evaluating leg extension peak torque of the same leg with an isokinetic dynamometer detected only a 10 to 17% improvement![62,79] *To improve a specific physical performance through resistance training, one must train the muscle(s) in movements that mimic the movement requiring force–capacity improvement, with focus on force, velocity, and power requirements rather than simply an isolated joint or muscle.*

Physical Testing in the Occupational Setting: The Role of Specificity

A comprehensive review outlines the development of physical tests and professionally and legally defensible validation strategies for pre-employment occupational testing requiring diverse physical abilities or specific fitness characteristics.[119] The high specificity of components of physical performance and physiologic function (e.g., muscular strength and power, joint flexibility, aerobic fitness) combined with the specific nature of the training response casts serious doubt that broad *constructs* of physical fitness exist to any important extent. Clearly, no single measure exists to quantify overall muscular strength or aerobic fitness. *Instead, an individual expresses an array of muscular strengths, powers, and aerobic "fitnesses."* These expressions of muscle function and exercise performance often relate poorly to each other if at all. Likewise, testing a person for aerobic fitness produces different fitness scores depending on the activity. For example, it would be undesirable to administer the 12-min run test (a test purporting to assess aerobic capacity) in the occupational setting to infer aerobic capacity for firefighting or lumbering (both requiring considerable upper-body aerobic function), or measuring static-grip or leg strength with tests to assess diverse dynamic strengths and powers required in these occupations.

Measurements applied in the occupational setting should closely resemble the actual requirements of the job (i.e., functional tests), not only for specific tasks but also in a manner that reflects the intensity, duration, and pace (i.e., physiologic demands) of the job. If such "content testing" remains impractical, one must substantiate alternative testing based on carefully conducted validation studies.

 INTEGRATIVE QUESTION

Advise a candidate for a firefighter's job about the most effective way to train for a physical test that requires 7 min of a series of job-related tasks (e.g., stair climb with equipment, hose drag, ladder raise, forcible entry with sledge hammer, simulated rescue dummy drag).

Isokinetic Resistance Training

Isokinetic resistance training combines the positive features of isometric exercise and dynamic weightlifting. It provides muscle overload at a preset constant speed while the muscle mobilizes its force-generating capacity throughout the full ROM. Any effort during the movement encounters an opposing force to that applied to the mechanical device; this represents **accommodating-resistance exercise**. Theoretically, isokinetic-type training activates the largest number of motor units to overload muscles consistently—even at the relatively "weaker" joint angles—as the bone–muscle–lever mechanics produce variations in force capacity throughout the ROM. Maintaining a constant movement speed remains a negative aspect of isokinetic resistance training because functional exercises rarely approximate a fixed speed of movement.

Isokinetics Versus Standard Weightlifting

An important distinction exists between a muscle overloaded isokinetically and one overloaded with a standard weightlifting movement. FIGURE 22.12 shows that the force capacity of a single muscle or group of muscles varies with the bony lever configuration (joint angle) as the joint moves through its ROM of approximately 40 to 160 degrees during flexion and 160 to 40 degrees extension movements. During weight training, the external weight lifted usually remains fixed at the greatest load that allows completion of the movement for the desired number of repetitions. *Resistance cannot exceed the maximum force generated at the weakest point in the ROM*. If it did not, then one could not complete the movement. The term *sticking point* describes this area in the ROM.

That muscles do not generate the same absolute maximum force through all movement phases represents a major limitation of weightlifting. For this reason, professional body builders and top athletes perform many variations of the same exercise but with different emphasis on movement patterns. For the biceps dumb-bell curl, for example, one set of exercises might be done without supinating or pronating the hand that holds the weight. Another set might be done with alternating hand pronation or supination during the curl, while a third set might engage lateral movements of the upper arm during the curling movement. These variations of the basic exercise target a different force-generating aspect of the movement. Additional variations can include changes in the speed of the movement from controlled slow to moving as fast as possible with good form. The most obvious variation changes the weight lifted

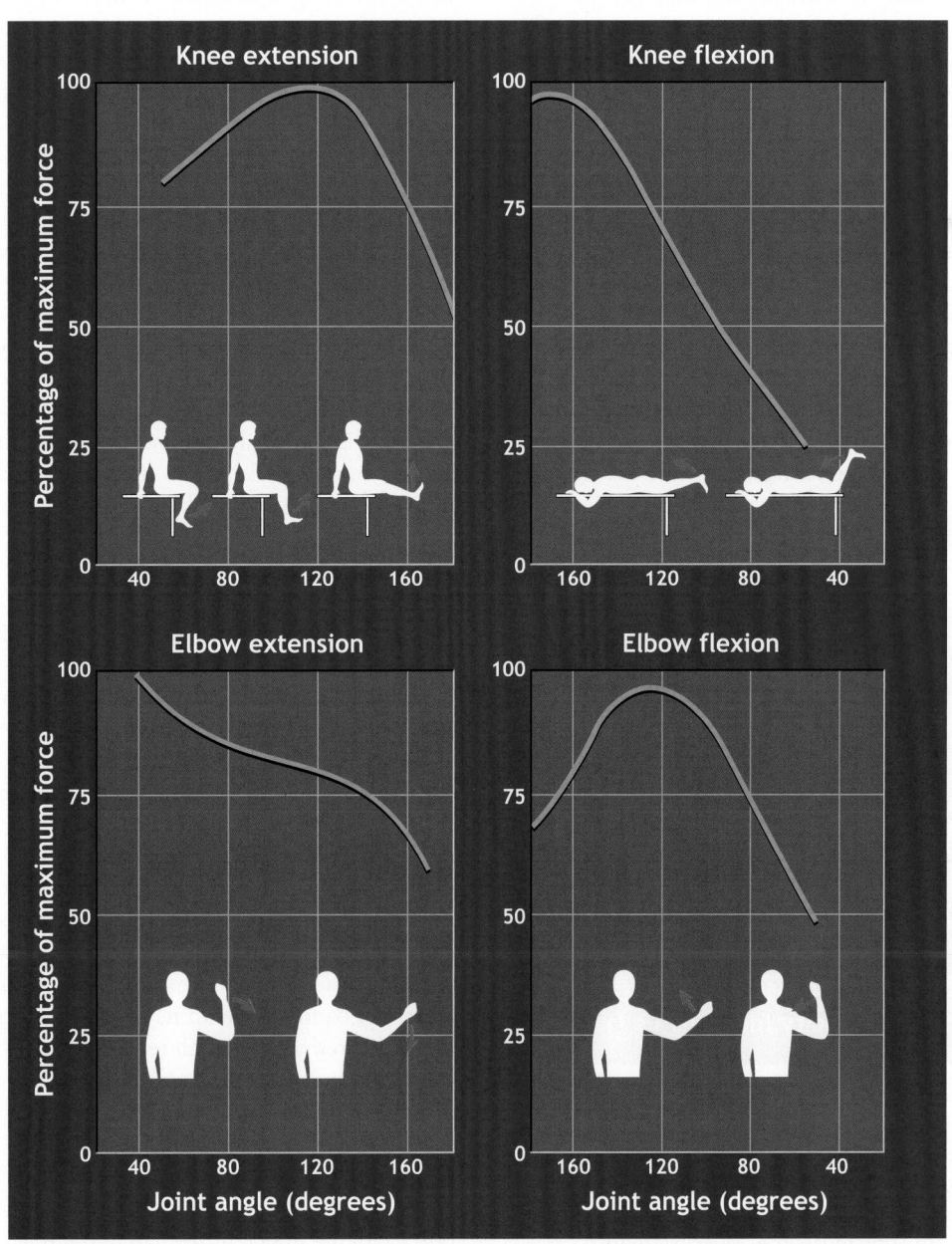

FIGURE 22.12 • Muscle force-generating capacity varies with joint angle in flexion and extension throughout the ROM.

from a light weight (can be lifted easily through the ROM) to a heavier weight that requires a slower movement rate. To help alleviate such variations, manufacturers have devised **variable-resistance training equipment** that adjusts resistance with the generalized lever characteristics of a particular joint movement. This equipment still represents a classic mode of weightlifting except the *relative resistance* offered to the muscle theoretically remains fairly constant with respect to muscle capacity at a particular shortening velocity throughout the ROM. With an isokinetically loaded muscle, the desired movement speed occurs almost instantaneously with maximum force application, allowing the muscle to generate peak power output *throughout* the ROM at a controlled shortening velocity.

Isokinetic Training Experiments

Experiments with isokinetic exercise have explored the force–velocity patterns in various movements related to muscle fiber type composition. Figure 22.13 shows the progressive decline in peak torque output with increasing angular velocity of knee extensor muscles in power- and endurance-trained groups who differ in their sports training regimens and predominant muscle fiber type. For movement at $180° \cdot s^{-1}$, maximal torque decrement averaged about 55% of maximal isometric ($0° \cdot s^{-1}$) force. The two curves in Figure 22.13 differ in peak torque depending on the group's muscle fiber composition. Peak force at zero velocity (isometric force) remained similar for athletes with relatively high (power athletes) or low (endurance athletes) percentages of fast-twitch muscle fibers; this indicated activation of *both* fast- and slow-twitch motor units in maximal isometric knee extension. As movement velocity increased, individuals with higher percentages of fast-twitch fibers exerted greater torque per unit body mass. This indicates the desirability of possessing a high percentage of fast-twitch fibers

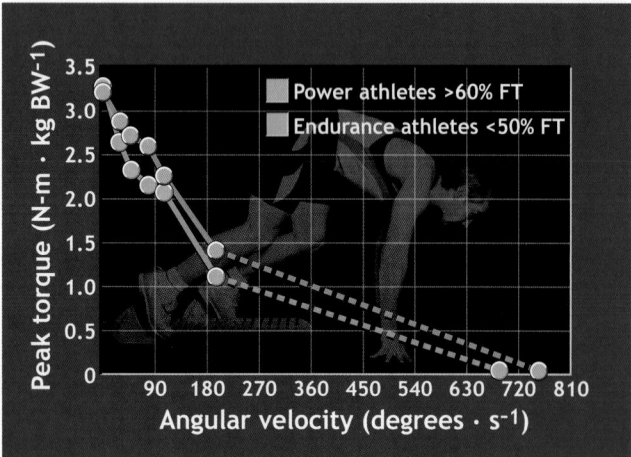

FIGURE 22.13 • Peak torque (per unit body mass) related to angular velocity of joint movement in two groups of athletes with different predominance of muscle-fiber type. The torque–velocity curves were extrapolated (*dashed line*) to the approximated maximal velocity for knee extension. (Adapted with permission from Thorstensson A. Muscle strength, fiber types, and enzyme activities in man. *Acta Physiol Scand* 1976(suppl):443.)

for power activities, where success largely depends on capacity to generate considerable torque at the most rapid movement velocities, as in throwing the discus, shot-put, and javelin.

Fast- Versus Slow-Speed Isokinetic Training

Studies of strength and power improvement with isokinetic training at slow and fast limb speeds further support the specificity of exercise performance and training response. For example, strength and power gains from slow-speed isokinetic training relate specifically to the angular velocity of the movement in training. In contrast, exercising at fast speeds facilitates more general improvement; power output increased at fast *and* slow movement speeds, although values at the fast angular velocity in training improved the most.[191] Muscle hypertrophy generally occurs from fast-speed training and mainly in the fast-contracting muscle fibers.[53] Muscle fiber hypertrophy may account for the greater generality of strength improvement with fast-speed training. Concentric muscle actions produce greater power increases and type II fiber hypertrophy from training than eccentric training at equivalent relative power levels.[157]

The attractiveness of isokinetic training allows muscular overload through a full ROM at many shortening velocities. Applications remain limited, however, because the most rapid speed of movement of the current isokinetic dynamometers approximates $400° \cdot s^{-1}$. Even this relatively "fast" movement speed does not approach limb speeds during sports activities. In baseball pitching, where upper-limb extension velocity exceeds $2000° \cdot s^{-1}$ in professional pitchers, even the relatively "slow" hip rotators move at $600° \cdot s^{-1}$ during a pitch.[35] Also, the present generation of isokinetic dynamometers cannot simultaneously overload eccentric muscle actions that serve important functions in limb deceleration and "braking" control in normal movements.

Plyometric Training

For sports that require powerful, propulsive movements—football, volleyball, sprinting, high jump, long jump, and basketball—athletes apply a special form of training termed **plyometrics**, or explosive jump training.[76,236,257] Plyometric movements require various jumps in place or rebound jumping (drop jumping from a preset height) to mobilize the inherent stretch–recoil characteristics of skeletal muscle and its modulation via the stretch or myotatic reflex. Stated somewhat differently, plyometric movement involves rapid stretching followed by shortening of a muscle group during a dynamic movement. Think of plyometrics when you stretch a rubber band; the stretch creates stored energy within the band that releases when the band returns to its "resting" position. Stretching in a muscle produces a stretch reflex and elastic recoil within the muscle. When combined with a vigorous muscle contraction, plyometric actions greatly increase the force that overloads the muscles, thereby augmenting increases in absolute strength and power.[258] Plyometric training ranges in difficulty from calf jumps off the ground to multiple one-leg jumps to and from boxes ranging in height from one foot to six feet.

The basic principle for all jumping and plyometric exercises is to absorb the shock with the arms or legs and then immediately contract the muscles. For example, when doing a series of squat jumps, jump again as quickly into the air as possible after you land, while at the same time thrusting both heels up toward the buttocks. Quicker jumps provide greater overload to the muscles. In essence, "fast" dynamic plyometric movement "trains" the nervous system to respond quickly to rapidly activate muscles.

Plyometric maneuvers avoid the disadvantage of having to decelerate a mass in the latter part of the joint ROM during a fast movement; this provides for maximal power production. FIGURE 22.14 compares a traditional bench press movement to achieve maximal power output with a ballistic bench throw

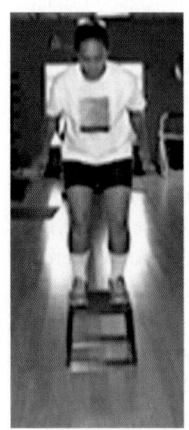

that attempts to maximize power output by projecting the barbell from the hands. The results were unequivocal. During a bench press, deceleration begins at about 60% of the bar position relative to the total concentric movement distance (*orange line*). In contrast, velocity during the bench throw (*yellow line*) continues to increase throughout the ROM and remains higher at all bar positions after movement begins. This translates into greater average force, average power, and peak power outputs. Achieving a faster average and peak velocity throughout the ROM produces greater power output and muscle activation (assessed by EMG) than the traditional weightlifting movement. The throw condition produced greater muscle activity for the pectoralis major (+19%), anterior deltoid (+34%), triceps brachii (+44%), and biceps brachii (+27%).

Allowing the athlete to develop greater power at the end of the movement more closely simulates the projection phase of throwing an object (ball or implement), maximal effort jumping movements, or impact in striking movements. In this form of training, called **ballistic resistance training**,

the person moves the weight or projectile as fast as possible while trying to produce maximal force before releasing it. Sports performance examples include shot-put, overhead soccer throw, javelin and discus throws, push away from the pole vigorously in the pole vault, takeoff jump for a volleyball spike, positioning and jumping for a basketball rebound, multiple punches in boxing, and takeoff in the high jump.

Plyometric movement overloads a muscle to provide forcible and rapid stretch (eccentric or stretch phase) immediately before the concentric or shortening phase of action. Recent reviews summarize that the **stretch-shortening cycle (SSC)** represents an important concept that describes how skeletal muscles function most efficiently in unrestricted, diverse human locomotor activities from soccer play[170,261] to simple sprinting performance.[200]

> See the animation "Stretch Shortening Cycle" on http://thePoint.lww.com/mkk8e for a demonstration of this process.

When the muscle spindles of the gastrocnemius muscle suddenly become stretched, their sensory receptors fire with impulses traveling through the dorsal root into the spinal cord (to activate the anterior motor neurons) and trigger the stretch reflex (see Chapter 19), the timing of which relies on the speed of movement.[54,116] The sequence of stretching and shortening muscle fibers as in the contact phase of running serves a fundamental purpose—to enhance the final pushoff phase. In many sports situations, the rapid lengthening phase in the **SSC** produces a more powerful subsequent movement from two main factors[115,143,146, 196]:

Factor 1. Attainment of a higher active muscle state (greater potential energy) before the concentric, shortening action
Factor 2. Stretch-induced evoking of segmental reflexes that potentiate subsequent muscle activation

These two effects form the basis for the speed–power benefits of this training mode.[248,262] More than likely, improvement occurs from changes in the mechanical properties of the muscle–tendon complex rather than changes in muscle activation strategies.[135] FIGURE 22.15 shows the sledge ergometer to (1) quantify force-generating capacity when affected by the stretch-shortening cycle, (2) train under such conditions, and (3) evaluate stretch reflex sensitivity and muscle stiffness under fatiguing physical activity.

Practical Application of Plyometrics

A plyometric drill uses body mass and gravity for the important rapid prestretch, or "cocking," phase of the SCC to activate the muscle's natural elastic recoil elements. Prior stretch augments the subsequent concentric muscle action in the opposite direction. Forcibly dropping the arms to the side before vertical jumping produces an eccentric prestretch of the quadriceps muscle group and exemplifies a natural plyometric movement. Lower-body plyometric drills include a standing jump, multiple jumps, repetitive jumping in place, depth jumps or drop jumping from a height of about 1 m,

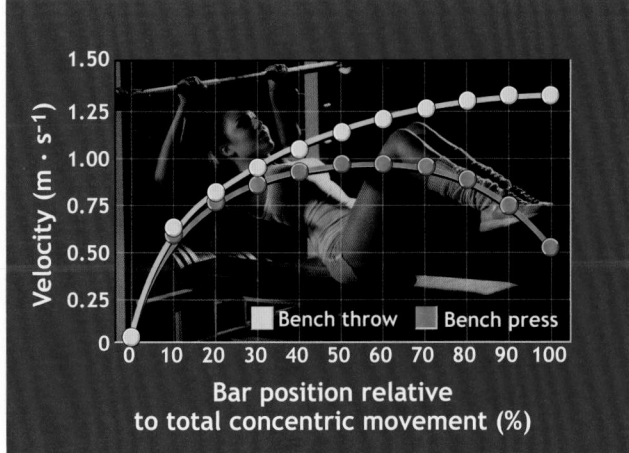

FIGURE 22.14 • Mean bar velocity in relation to total concentric bar movement for bench throw and traditional bench press performed rapidly. (Data from Newton RU, et al. Kinematics, kinetics, and muscle activation during explosive upper-body movements. *J Appl Biomech* 1996;12:31.)

single- and double-leg jumps, and various modifications. Proponents believe that repetitive plyometric actions serve as neuromuscular training to enhance power output of specific muscles and sport-specific power performances as in jumping.[136,162,266]

Testimonials tout the benefits of plyometric training, yet limited controlled experiments exists concerning both benefits and possible orthopedic risks of such workouts. Concern for musculoskeletal injury stems partly from the estimation that drop jumping generates external skeletal loads equal to up to 10 times body mass. Research must quantify the appropriate role of plyometric drills in a complete strength–power training program, particularly for children and older recreational athletes as well as for those in the initial phase of exercise training. A position paper from the National Strength and Conditioning Association (www.nsca-lift.org) suggests that athletes first achieve lifts of 1.5 times body weight in the squat exercise before initiating high-intensity plyometric training.[258] This practical guideline requires validation. FIGURE 22.16 shows the rebound jumping technique in plyometric training along with four examples of plyometric exercise drills described in the three purple inset boxes.

Body Weight–Loaded Training

Body weight–loaded training using **closed-kinetic chain exercise** to enhance sports performance[26,149] has gained popularity and research support, including such training in job-related functions[148] and treatment of pelvic pain following pregnancy.[224,225] Many different systems of body weight–loaded exercises have been developed over the past several centuries. Modern methods to develop muscular strength usually include some variation of free weights, barbells, mechanical systems for adjusting the load, cams, and pulleys. For historical perspective, the Ling system referred to previously (see "Strength Measurement and Resistance Training" section) devised progressive exercises to strengthen total body musculature. The method of progressive

sling suspension training was pioneered in Sweden beginning in the 1840s. Between 1914 and 1918 more advanced suspension and sling exercise and training methods were developed by physiotherapists working in English hospitals and rehabilitation facilities during and after World War I. Norwegian sling suspension training methods developed in the early 1990s also complemented physical therapy applications and supports strength development and general and specific fitness training. The sling suspension methodologies leverage the person's body weight as resistance increases or decreases by altering the suspension coordinates, the height of the slings, or the body position relative to the suspension point without reliance on externally fixed weights, pulleys, or cam-based devices. In weight-supported exercise, the distal segment bears the full body weight or a fraction of the body weight. This type of exercise activates both agonist and antagonist muscles about a joint, including other muscle groups along the kinetic chain.[219] Such training is often considered more functional compared to exercises where the distal segment is non–weight bearing, as in conventional weightlifting (where agonists and synergists are activated). In addition, body weight–loaded exercise, as employed with the sling-system apparatus, introduces the added component of instability to further challenge neuromuscular control of trunk and back musculature.[220,234,237] The role of adding perturbation during relatively simple and/or complex movements may play a key activating role in "training" the sophisticated signaling patterns involved in neuromuscular control of human movements.[73,154,233,235]

Studies using body weight–supported movements in the sling and rope system during functional performance training for soccer,[223] golf,[205] team handball,[204] and

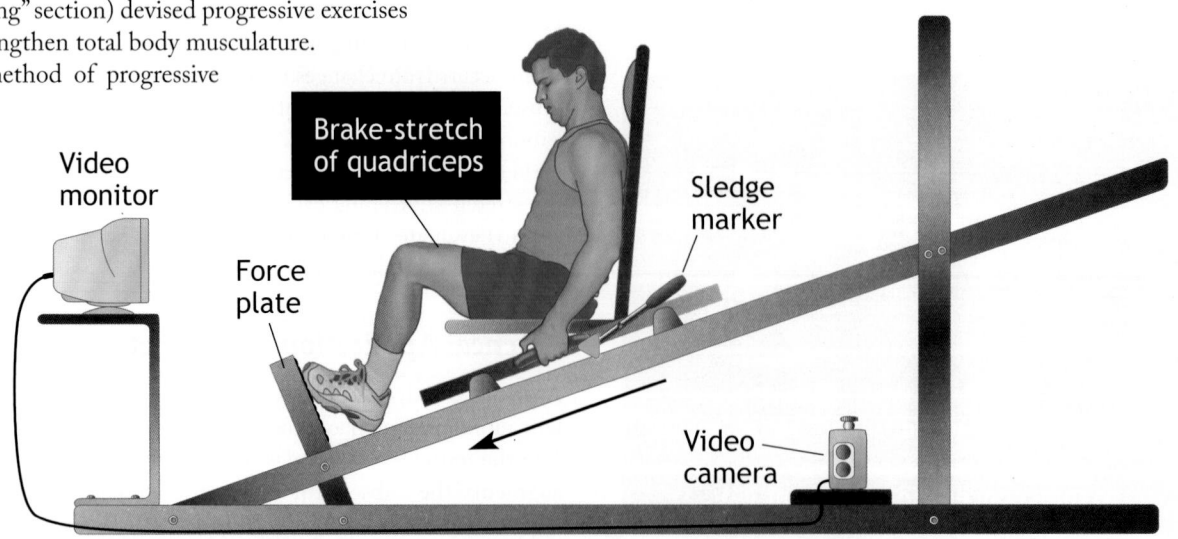

FIGURE 22.15 • The sledge ergometer for plyometric (stretch-shortening cycle) exercise, training, and research protocols. Illustration shows braking phase (and subsequent muscle stretch) just prior to maximal activation of leg and foot extensor muscles. (Adapted with permission from Strojnik V, Komi PV. Fatigue after submaximal intensive stretch-shortening cycle exercise. *Med Sci Sports Exerc* 2000;32:1314.)

softball[206] show improvements in functional sport movements that range from 3 to 5% in velocity of limb movement, increased golf club head velocity and hence distance, and static and dynamic balance and shoulder stabilization.

Concept of the Core

The last 10 years have seen a resurgence of "**core training**"—also referred to as lumbar stabilization, core strengthening, dynamic stabilization, neutral spine control, trunk stabilization, abdominal strength, core "pillar" training, and core-functional strength training.

The core concept does not simply refer to muscles that cross the midsection of the body and form the "six-pack" abdominals so commonly portrayed in magazine advertisements. Rather, the core represents a four-sided muscular frame with abdominal muscles in front, paraspinals and gluteals in back, the diaphragm at the top,

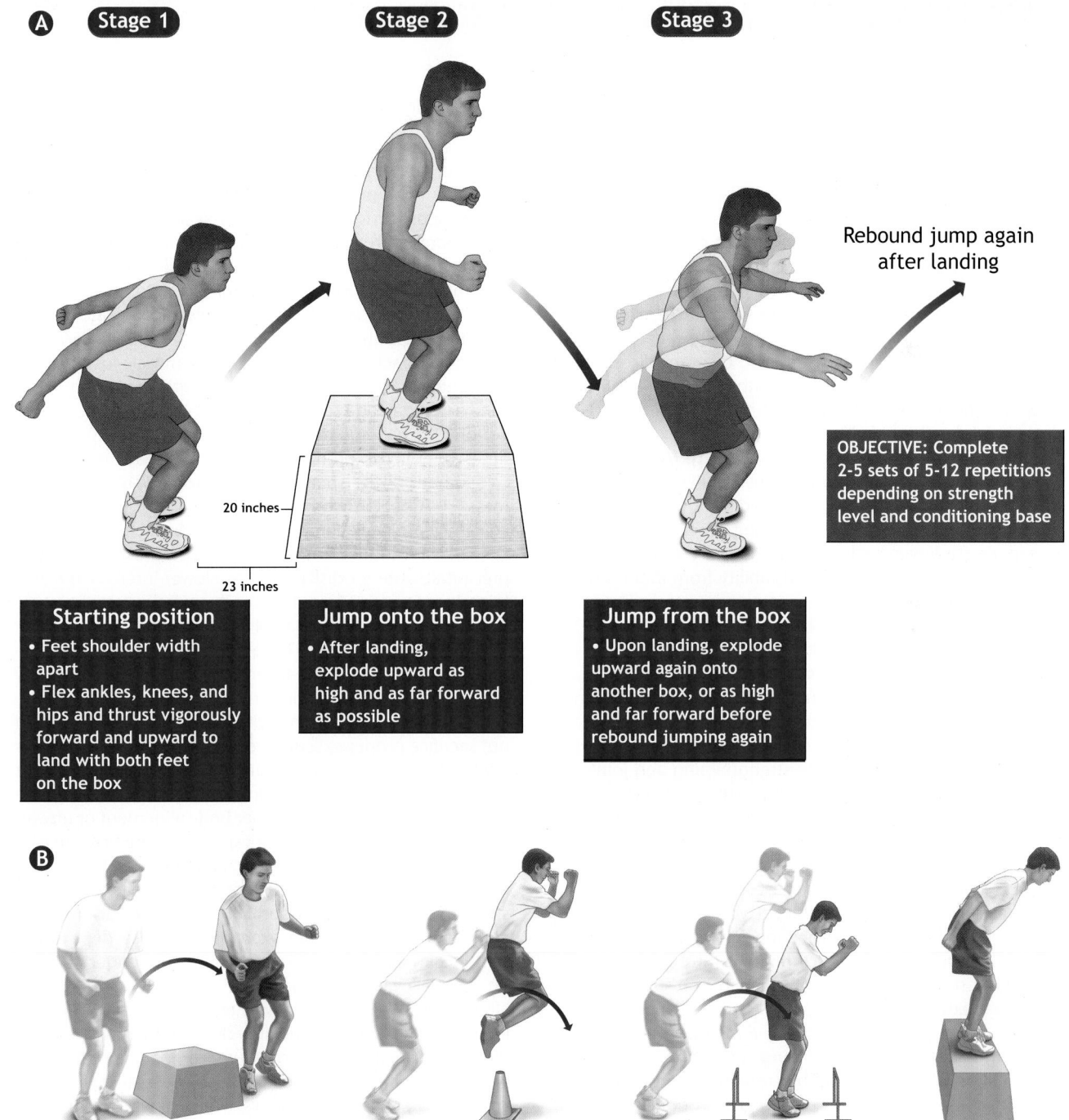

Stage 1

Stage 2

Stage 3

Rebound jump again after landing

20 inches

23 inches

OBJECTIVE: Complete 2-5 sets of 5-12 repetitions depending on strength level and conditioning base

Starting position
• Feet shoulder width apart
• Flex ankles, knees, and hips and thrust vigorously forward and upward to land with both feet on the box

Jump onto the box
• After landing, explode upward as high and as far forward as possible

Jump from the box
• Upon landing, explode upward again onto another box, or as high and far forward before rebound jumping again

FIGURE 22.16 • **(A)** Rebound jumping technique in plyometric training. **(B)** Four examples of plyometric exercise drills: (1) Box jump. (2) Cone hop. (3) Hurdle hop. (4) Long jump from box. (Examples of plyometric jumps courtesy of Dr. Thomas D. Fahey, California State University at Chico.)

and the pelvic floor and hip girdle musculature framing the bottom. This region includes 29 pairs of muscles that hold the trunk steady, and balance and stabilize the bony structures of the spine, pelvis, thorax, and other kinetic chain structures activated during most movements.[89] The totality of these spine-frame structures without adequate "strength and balance" would become mechanically unstable. A properly functioning core provides these four benefits[123,164]:

1. Appropriate force distribution
2. Optimal control and movement efficiency
3. Adequate absorption of ground-impact forces
4. Absence of excessive compressive, translation, and shearing forces on kinetic chain joints

IN A PRACTICAL SENSE

Strengthening The Lower Back

According to the Bone and Joint Decade Monitor Project and the World Health Organization (WHO) (**www.ota.org/downloads/ bjdExecSum.pdf**), the total costs in the United States related to musculoskeletal disability exceeds $250 billion yearly. Of this amount, direct costs account for $88.7 billion. Thirty-eight percent was spent on hospital admissions, 21% on nursing home admissions, 17% on physician visits, and 5% on administrative costs. Indirect costs account for 58% of the total ($126.2 billion), which include lost wages through morbidity or premature mortality. Musculoskeletal diseases include approximately 150 different diseases and syndromes typically associated with pain or inflammation. Back injuries account for one fourth of all work-related injuries and one third of all compensation costs, which, according to the Bureau of Labor Statistics (**http://www.bls.gov/spotlight/2009/health_care/**), cost the government in excess of $90 billion yearly in related health costs. Estimates indicate that at least 32 million adult Americans frequently experience lower back pain, the primary cause for workplace disability.[138] Workplace disability from injuries to the lower back region also occurs in common tasks like refuse collection and other manual handling and lifting tasks.[62,67,128]

Muscular weakness, particularly in the abdominal and lower lumbar back regions, lumbar spine instability, and poor joint flexibility in the back and legs represent primary external factors related to low back pain syndrome.[215]

Prevention of and rehabilitation from chronic low back strain commonly use muscle-strengthening and joint-flexibility exercises.[23,72,163] Continuing normal activities of daily living (within limits dictated by pain tolerance) yields more rapid recovery from acute back pain than bed rest. Maintaining normal physical activity facilitates greater recovery than specific back-mobilizing exercises performed after pain onset.[153] Prudent use of resistance-type training isolates and strengthens the abdomen and lower lumbar extensor muscles that support and protect the spine through its full range of motion. Patients with low back pain who strengthen the lumbar extensors with the pelvis stabilized experience less pain, fewer chronic symptoms, and improved muscular strength and endurance and range of motion.[37]

Golfers with poor initial hip rotation during the downward phase of the swing often exhibit poor hip and spinal rotation, primarily from weak (or deactivated) gluteus medius muscle action. Reactivating this key muscle with closed kinetic chain movements combined with vibration may help to alleviate the inefficient slide phase during the golf swing to restore effective hip rotation. Biomechanical analysis of the golf swing has provided insight into the rudiments of golf mechanics and injury incidence and disability in amateur and professional golfers.[71,85,142,245]

Improper performance of a typical resistance-exercise movement (with a relatively heavy load and the hips thrust forward with arched back) creates considerable compressive force on the lower spine. For example, pressing and curling exercises with back hyperextension create unusually high shearing stress on the lumbar vertebrae, often triggering low back pain accompanied by muscle instability in this region.[13,99,104] Compressive forces with heavy lifting also can hasten damage to the disks that cushion the vertebrae. Performing half squats with barbell loads from 0.8 to 1.6 times body mass produces compressive loads on the L3–L4 segment of the spine equivalent to 6 to 10 times body mass.[36,45] A person who weighs 90 kg and squats with 144 kg can create peak compressive forces in excess of 1367 kg (13,334 N)! A sudden amplification of compressive force can precipitate anterior disk prolapse; a lower-intensity but sustained compressive force that produces fatigue can increase posterior bulging of the lamellas in the posterior annulus.[6] In national-level male and female powerlifters, average compressive loads on L4–L5 reached 1757 kg (17,192 N).[165] At the practical level, during sports training with resistance methods (i.e., functional training with free weights), one should not sacrifice proper execution of an exercise to lift a heavier load or "squeeze out" additional repetitions. The extra weight lifted through improper technique does not facilitate muscle strengthening; instead, improper body alignment or unwarranted muscle substitution during force production can trigger debilitating injury where surgery unfortunately becomes the option of choice. This fact of life should encourage proper strengthening of "core" abdominal and lower back muscles (with lower back and hip exercises, as those depicted in this "In a Practical Sense", to avoid either prolonged reliance on pain-relieving drugs or potentially debilitating surgical alternatives. Wearing a relatively stiff weightlifting belt during heavy lifts (squats, dead lifts, clean-and-jerk maneuvers) reduces intra-abdominal pressure compared with lifting without a belt.[84,95,137] The belt reduces potentially injurious compressive forces on spinal disks during near-maximal lifting, including most Olympic and powerlifting events and associated training. In one study, nine experienced weightlifters lifted barbells up to 75% body weight under three conditions: (1) while inhaling and wearing a belt, (2) inhal-

IN A PRACTICAL SENSE *(continued)*

ing and not wearing a belt, and (3) exhaling and wearing a belt.[129] Measurements included intra-abdominal pressure, trunk muscle EMG, ground reaction forces, and kinematics. The belt reduced compression forces by about 10%, but only when inhaling before lifting. The authors concluded that wearing a tight and stiff-back belt while inhaling before lifting reduces spinal loading during the lift.

A person who normally trains wearing a belt should generally refrain from lifting without one. Further recommendations include performing at least some submaximal resistance training without a belt to strengthen the deep abdominal and pelvic stabilizing muscles. This also develops the proper pattern of muscle recruitment to generate high intra-abdominal pressures when not wearing a belt. Wearing a back belt to increase intra-abdominal pressure to ameliorate low back injuries in the workplace does not provide a clear-cut biomechanical advantage.[190] A 2-year prospective study of nearly 14,000 material-handling employees in 30 states evaluated the effectiveness of using back belts to reduce back injury worker's compensation claims and reports of low back pain.[250] Neither frequent back belt use (usually once a day, once or twice a week) nor a store policy that required the use of these belts reduced injury or reports of low back pain. Researchers continue to probe for answers about the etiology of low back pain syndrome and how to minimize its severity and reduce its occurrence.[121,209,254] Studies have focused on numerous contributing factors that include intradisk pressure[166]; facet loads and disk fiber strains[211]; lumbar disk height and cross-sectional area[179]; compressive follower loads[188]; spinal joint force distribution[43]; ligament strain, disk shear, and facet impingement[81]; and prediction models to estimate spinal compression and shear forces.[90,124]

The following 12 exercises provide general strengthening of the abdomen, pelvic region, and lower back, and improve hamstring and lower back flexibility for individuals with no apparent lower back and spinal injuries. Symptomatic individuals (including athletes) require specific back exercises.[194,206]

I. Lower back stretches (hold each exercise for 30 to 60 s)
  1. Knees-to-chest stretch: Lie supine and pull the knees into the chest while keeping the lower back flat on the surface.

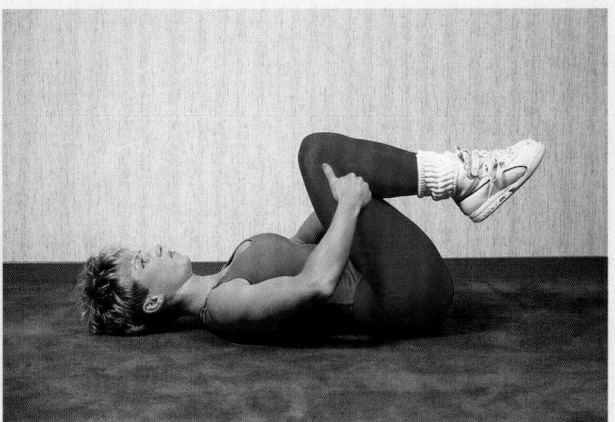

  2. Cross-leg stretch: Cross the legs and pull one 90°-flexed knee toward the chest.

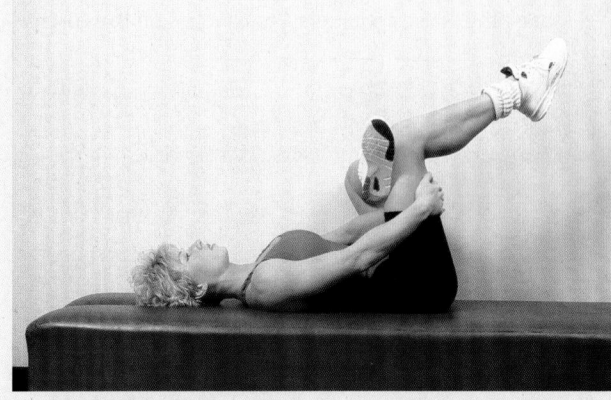

  3. Hamstring stretch: Wrap a strap over the foot, keeping lower back flat; pull leg upward toward the head.

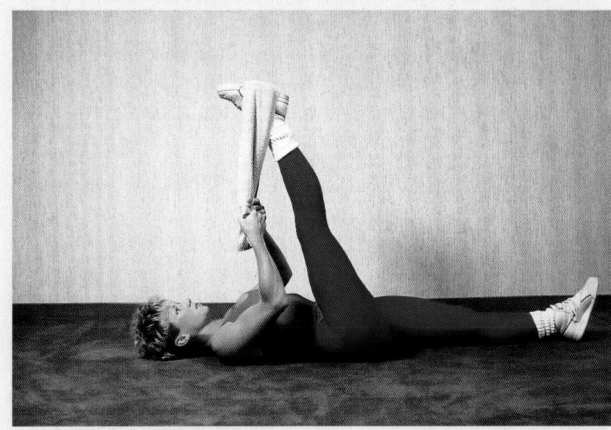

  4. Frog stretch: Sit, buttocks on bilateral heels; move hands as far as possible forward along the surface.

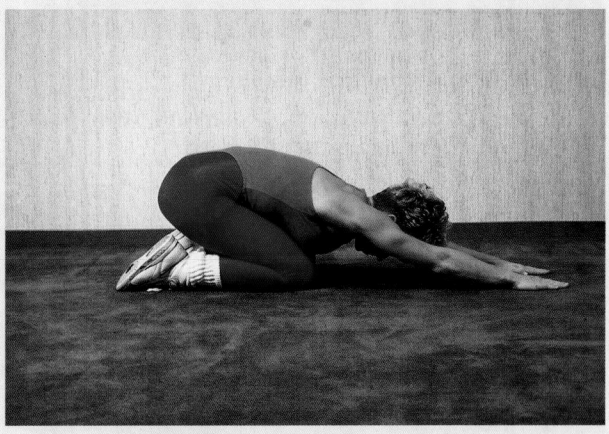

(Continued)

II. Abdominal exercises

5. Bent-knee sit-up: Keep hands low on neck (or across chest) with the head positioned over the shoulders. Roll up slowly, engaging one row of the abdominals at a time. Raise shoulders 4 to 6 inches off the surface.

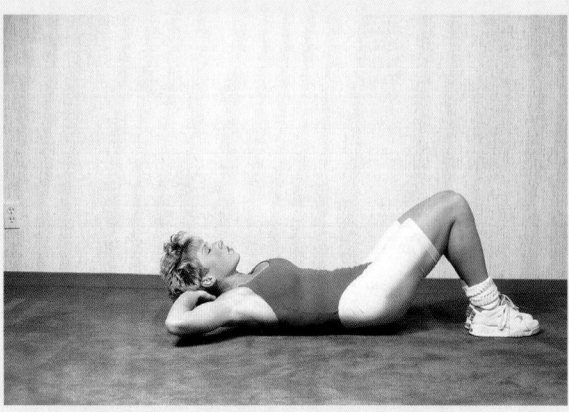

6. Dying bug: Flex the pelvis to flatten lower back against the surface. Over one side bring an extended arm and flexed knee together. On opposing side, extend arm straight overhead and leg straight backward. Maintain pelvic flexion while exchanging opposing arms and legs in this position.

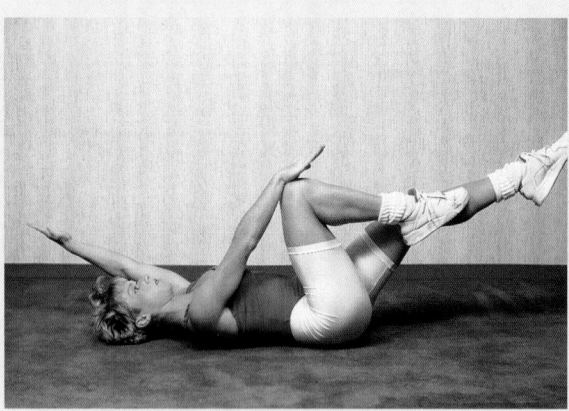

III. Prone lumbar extension exercises

7. Dry-land swimming: Lying prone with pelvic flexion, alternately lift opposite arm and leg.

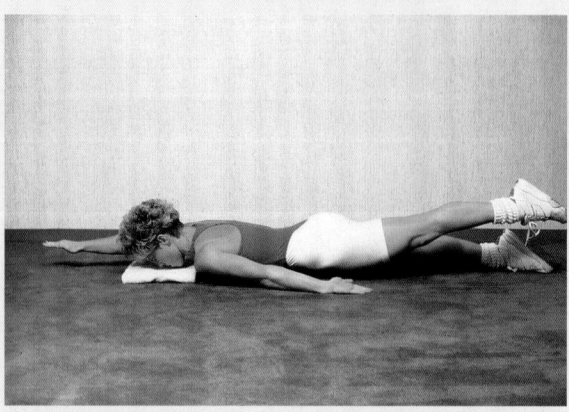

8. Both legs up: Lie prone with pelvic flexion, and lift both legs simultaneously while keeping the head on the floor.

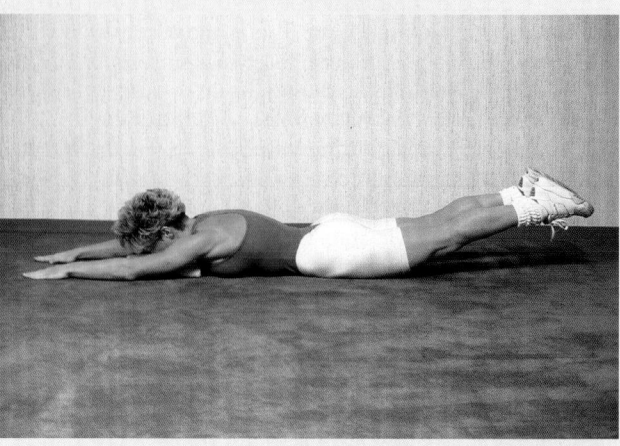

9. Upper-body up: Lying prone with pelvic flexion and arms outstretched or behind the back, lift upper torso while keeping legs on the floor.

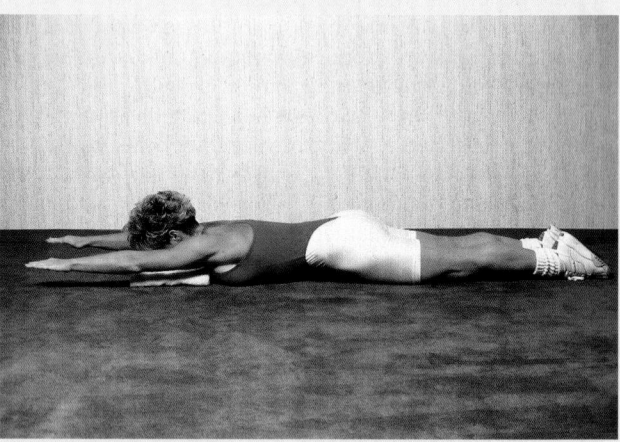

10. Pointer (bird dog): Start with hands and knees on the floor. Flex pelvis into a counter position. Exchange by pointing opposite arm and leg while keeping the torso level.

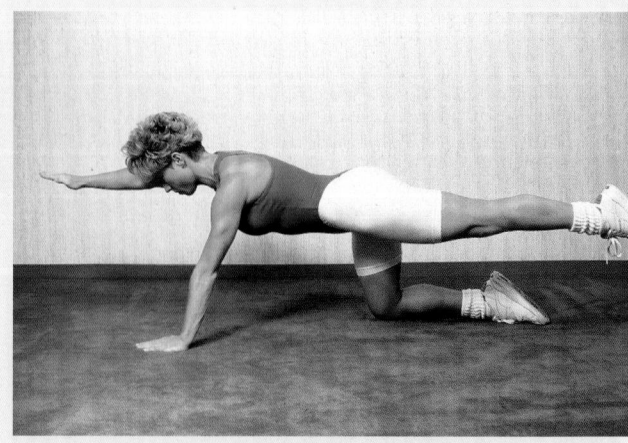

IV. Supine pelvic-flexion exercises

11. Leg pointer: Lie supine on the floor and flex pelvis with lower abdominals to flatten the lower back into the surface. Extend one arm upward and one leg outward while keeping quadriceps level.

12. Prone cobra push-up: Keep pelvis on the floor while pressing up with arms to produce lower back extension.

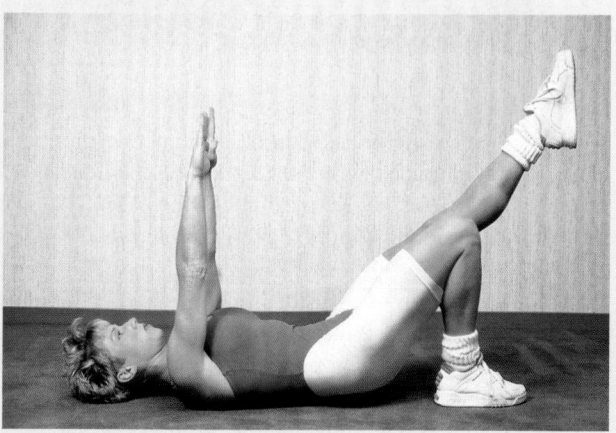

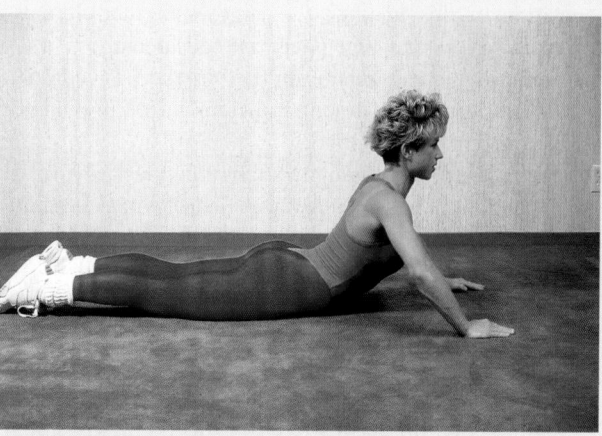

Photos courtesy of Dr. Bob Swanson, Santa Barbara Back and Neck Care, Santa Barbara, CA.

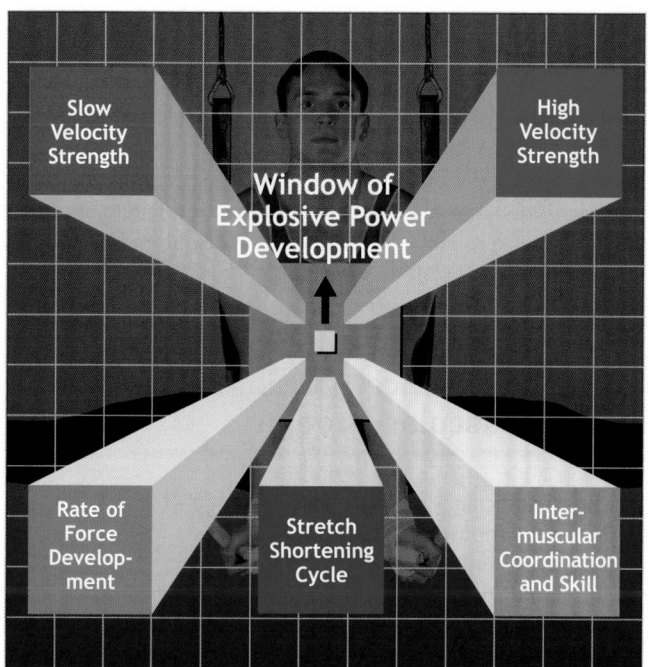

FIGURE 22.17 • Five components that contribute to explosive power development. (Adapted with permission from Dr. William J. Kraemer, Human Performance Laboratory, University of Connecticut, Storrs; Adapted with permission from Kraemer WJ, Newton RU. Training for muscular power. *Phys Med Rehabil Clin* 2000;11:341.)

Window for Explosive Power Development

FIGURE 22.17 lists five components that contribute to the **window of explosive power development**. In this model, each component makes important neuromuscular contributions to maximal power training. The window of adaptation opportunity shrinks for an athlete with already well-developed components and expands for components in need of considerable improvement. As an athlete approaches his or her high-velocity strength potential, that component's contribution to overall maximal power development diminishes. Athletes must focus on training their *least-developed* components. Stated somewhat differently, maximal power performance improves more readily when targeting specific training routines to improve the weakest links because these have the largest adaptation window to develop superior explosive power.

Summary

1. Tensiometry, dynamometry, 1-RM testing with weights, and computer-assisted force and work-output determinations including isokinetic-type measurements provide the most common methods to measure muscular performance.

2. Human skeletal muscle generates a maximum force of about 30 N per cm^2 of muscle cross section, regardless of gender. On an absolute basis, men generally exert greater

maximal force than women for any given muscular movement pattern.

3. The traditional method to evaluate gender differences in muscle strength creates a ratio score for strength (either strength per unit body mass, FFM, limb volume, and girth).

4. When considering measures of body size and/or composition in this manner, the large strength differences between men and women decrease considerably.

5. Allometric scaling offers another method to compare physiologic variables among individuals differing in body size and body composition.

6. Optimal overload training to strengthen muscles involves three factors: increasing resistance (load) to muscle action, increasing speed of muscle action, or combining increased load and speed of movement.

7. An overload between 60 and 80% of a muscle's force-generating capacity induces strength gains.

8. Three major strength-training systems include progressive resistance weight training, isometrics, and isokinetic training. Each produces strength gains highly specific to the type of training.

9. Isokinetic training offers potential to generate maximum force throughout the full ROM at different angular velocities of limb movement.

10. Closely supervised resistance training programs that use relatively moderate concentric muscle actions improve children's strength without adverse effects on bone, muscle, or connective tissue.

11. Periodization divides a distinct period or macrocycle of training into smaller training mesocycles; these subdivide into weekly microcycles.

12. Compartmentalization of training minimizes staleness and overtraining effects to maximize peak performance that coincides with competition.

13. Resistance training for competitive athletes optimizes muscular strength, power, and hypertrophy.

14. Training goals for middle-age and older adults aim to modestly improve muscular strength and endurance, maintain muscle and bone mass, and enhance overall health and fitness.

15. Concurrent training for muscular strength and aerobic capacity inhibits the magnitude of strength improvement compared with training only for muscular strength.

16. Plyometric training emphasizes the inherent stretch–recoil characteristics of the neuromuscular system to facilitate muscle power development.

17. Specificity of physiologic and performance measures and their response to training casts doubt on the efficacy of *general* fitness measures to predict ability to perform specific tasks or occupations.

18. Functional movement training via body weight–supported sling exercise offers a unique approach to sports training.

19. Core training remains an integral part of sports training and physical conditioning to improve muscular balance, muscular strength, and trunk stabilization and reduce injury risk.

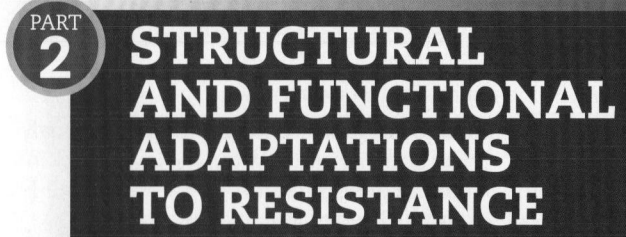

PART 2 STRUCTURAL AND FUNCTIONAL ADAPTATIONS TO RESISTANCE TRAINING

Muscle tissues exist in a dynamic state where proteins are alternately synthesized with a net *deposition* of amino acids and degraded with a net *release* of amino acids. FIGURE 22.18 lists six factors that develop and maintain muscle mass. Without a doubt, genetic factors provide the governing frame of reference that modulates each of the other factors that increase muscle mass and strength.[197] Muscular activity contributes little to tissue growth without appropriate nutrition, particularly amino acid availability, to provide essential building blocks. Similarly, specific hormones (e.g., testosterone, growth hormone, cortisol, and, most importantly, insulin and systemic and local insulinlike growth factors), including neural system innervation, help to pattern and reinforce the appropriate training response. Without tension overload, each of the other factors cannot effectively produce the desired training response.

FACTORS THAT MODIFY THE EXPRESSION OF HUMAN STRENGTH

FIGURE 22.19 shows that factors broadly characterized as psychologic (neural) and muscular influence the expression of human strength. A resistance-training program modifies many components of these factors; other factors remain training resistant, probably determined by natural endowment or established early in life.

 ### Six Neural Adaptations to Resistance Training That Increase Muscular Strength

1. Greater efficiency in neural recruitment patterns
2. Increased motor neuron excitability
3. Increased central nervous system activation
4. Improved motor unit synchronization and increased firing rates
5. Lowering of neural inhibitory reflexes
6. Inhibition of Golgi tendon organs

Psychologic–Neural Factors

Adaptive alterations in nervous system function that elevate motor neuron output largely account for the rapid and large strength increases observed early in training, often without an increase in

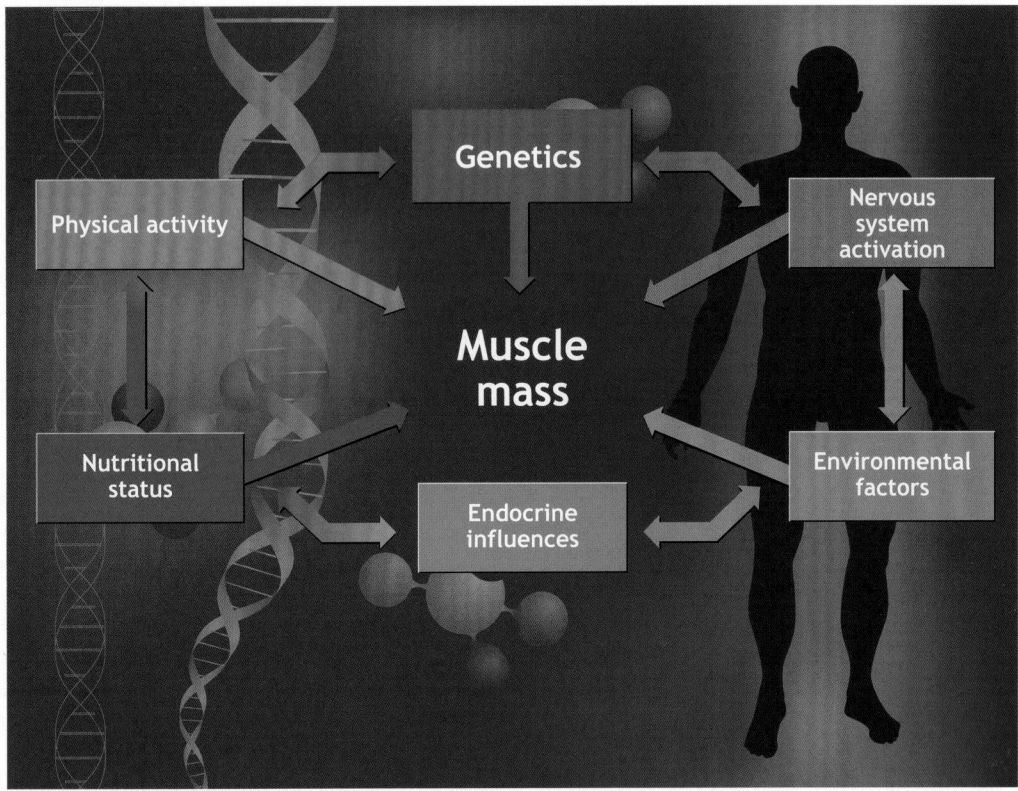

FIGURE 22.18 • Interaction of six factors that develop and maintain muscle mass.

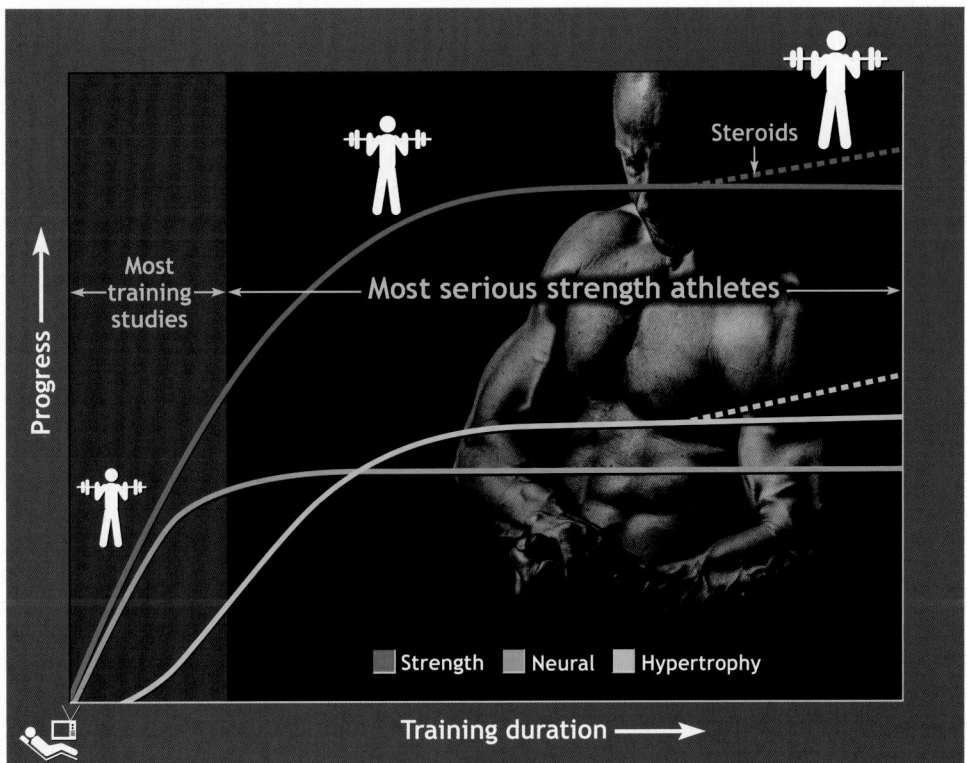

FIGURE 22.19 • Relative roles of neural and muscular adaptations in strength improvement with resistance training. Note that neural adaptations predominate in the early phase of training (this phase encompasses the duration of most research studies). Hypertrophy-induced adaptations place the upper limit on longer-term training improvements. This tempts many athletes to use anabolic steroids and/or human growth hormone (*dashed line*) to induce continual hypertrophy if training alone fails. (Adapted with permission from Sale DG. Neural adaptation to resistance training. *Med Sci Sports Exerc* 1988;20:135.)

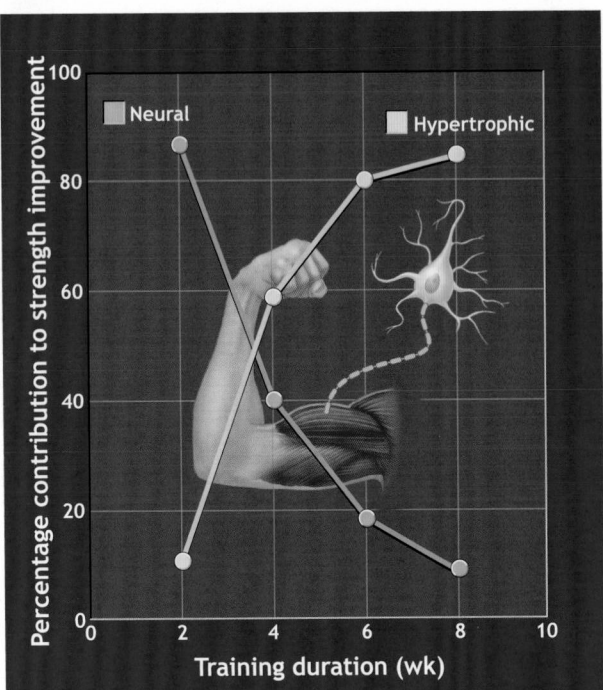

FIGURE 22.20 • Generalized response curve for gains in muscle strength with resistance training from neural (*orange*) or muscular (*yellow*) factors. During a typical 8-wk training period, neural factors account for approximately 90% of the strength gained over the first 2 wk. In the subsequent 2 wk, between 40 and 50% of the strength improvement still relates to nervous system adaptation. Thereafter, muscle fiber adaptations become progressively more important to strength improvement. Experiments of this type generally evaluate neural factors from integrated EMG recordings of the muscle groups trained.

muscle size and cross-sectional area.[1,201] Neural adaptations play a particularly important role in the dramatic muscular strength and power improvements of the elderly with resistance training.[92] **FIGURE 22.20** shows the generalized resistance training response curve for gains in muscle strength from neural facilitation and muscle hypertrophy.

Research has considered the effects of training on structural changes associated with the neuromuscular junction (NMJ). In one study with rats, endurance training improved the ratio of nerve terminal area to muscle fiber size by reducing fiber diameter without altering nerve terminal size.[246] In humans, high- and low-intensity training differentially affected the size of the NMJ.[64] Less-intense, prolonged workouts produced a more expansive NMJ area, whereas intense effort produced greater dispersion of synapses. Aging also interferes with the ability of the NMJ to adapt to training. Clearly, considerable complexity exists in the coordination of synaptic responses among different muscles, and different fiber types within muscles.[65]

A unique series of classic experiments illustrates the importance of psychologic factors in expressing muscular strength in humans.[113] The researchers measured arm strength in college-age men under (1) normal conditions, (2) immediately after a loud noise, (3) while the subject screamed loudly at the time of exertion, (4) under the influence of alcohol and amphetamines ("pep pills"), (5) and under hypnosis (told they possessed considerable

strength and should not fear injury). Each of the alterations generally increased strength above normal levels; hypnosis, the most "mental" of all treatments, produced the greatest increments. The investigators theorized that temporary modifications in central nervous system function accounted for strength improvements under the various experimental treatments. They argued that most persons normally operate at a level of neural inhibition, perhaps via protective reflex mechanisms that constrain the expression of strength capacity. Three factors—muscle cross-section, fiber type, and mechanical arrangement of bone and muscle—explain strength capacity. Neuromuscular inhibition can come from unpleasant past experiences with physical activity, an overly protective home environment, or fear of injury. Regardless of the reason, the person usually cannot reach maximum strength capacity. The excitement of intense competition or influence of disinhibitory drugs or hypnotic suggestion often induces a "supermaximal" performance from greatly reduced neural inhibition and optimal motor neuron recruitment.

Highly trained athletes often create an almost self-hypnotic state by intensely concentrating or "psyching" before competition. It sometimes takes years of training to perfect the "blockout" of extraneous stimuli (e.g., crowd noise) so the muscle action relates directly to the performance. This practice has been perfected in powerlifting competition where success depends on precise, coordinated movements *with* maximal muscle tension output within a specific, brief time frame. Enhanced arousal level and accompanying neural disinhibition or facilitation fully activate muscle groups. Increased

Superhuman Feats of Strength

In their book on strength training, Zatsiorsky and Kraemer describe three broad factors that limit an athlete's lifting potential. The highest potential, called *absolute strength*, represents the theoretical maximum force that muscle fibers, tendons, and bony structures can develop under neuromuscular-controlled, precise movement patterns. This value can never be exceeded or reached. The lowest maximum force value, termed *maximum strength*, represents the most one can lift under typical conditions that involve conscious effort, which equals about two thirds of their theoretical absolute strength. For someone who can lift 200 lb, for example, the theoretical maximum lift would equal 300 lb—a maximum tolerable amount that could be sustained by the body's tissues and bony structures. On the other hand, for experienced weightlifters who routinely train close to maximum during weekly workouts, their maximum lift capacity exceeds the two-thirds typical limit to about 80% before the muscular system would experience undue strain. The third type of lifting potential occurs when weightlifters set a world record at a competitive meet or when heroic efforts are performed under extreme duress. Under such conditions, other physiological mechanisms besides conscious control come into play, such as the "fight-or-flight" arousal response that immediately precedes and accompanies an emotionally charged condition (**http://learn.genetics.utah.edu/content/begin/cells/fight_flight/**).

Source: Zatsiorsky VM, Kraemer W. *Science and Practice of Strength Training*. 2nd Ed. Champaign, IL: Human Kinetics, 2006.

neurologic arousal also may account for "unexplainable" feats of strength and power during highly charged emergency and rescue situations (e.g., a relatively small person lifting an extremely heavy object off an injured person).

Muscular Factors

Psychologic disinhibition and learning factors greatly modify muscle strength in the early phase of training. Ultimately, anatomic and physiologic factors within the joint–muscle unit determine strength capacity. TABLE 22.5 lists the physiologic and performance changes associated with long-term resistance training. Most of these components adapt to training, with some modifications occurring within several weeks. Resistance training's effects on muscle fibers generally relate to adaptations in the contractile structures; these usually accompany substantial increases in muscular force and power through a given ROM.

Muscle Hypertrophy

An increase in muscular tension (force) with training provides the primary stimulus to initiate the process of skeletal muscle growth or hypertrophy. Changes in muscle size become detectable after only 3 wk of training, and the remodeling of muscle architecture precedes gains in muscle cross-sectional area. Two fundamental adaptations necessary for muscle hypertrophy (increased protein synthesis and satellite cell proliferation) are mobilized during the initial phases of resistance training.[208,267] Mechanical stress on components of the muscular system triggers signaling proteins to activate genes that translate messenger RNA and stimulate protein synthesis in excess of protein breakdown. Accelerated protein synthesis, particularly when combined with the effects of insulin and adequate amino acid availability, increases muscle size during resistance training.[127] *Muscle hypertrophy reflects a fundamental biologic adaptation to increased workload independent of gender and age.* As mentioned previously, improving muscular strength and power does not necessarily require muscle fiber hypertrophy because important neurologic factors initially affect the expression of human strength. The later, slower-occurring strength improvements generally coincide with noticeable alterations in a muscle's subcellular molecular architecture.

Overload training enlarges individual muscle fibers with subsequent muscle growth. The fast-twitch fibers of weightlifters average about 45% larger than fibers of healthy sedentary persons and endurance athletes. The hypertrophic process couples directly to increased mononuclear number and synthesis of cellular components, particularly protein filaments (myosin heavy chain and actin) that constitute the contractile elements.[17,98] Resistance training creates more efficient translation of mRNA that mediates stimulation of myofibrillar protein synthesis.[253] Muscle growth occurs from repeated muscle fiber injury (particularly with eccentric actions) followed by overcompensation of protein synthesis to produce a net anabolic effect. The cell's myofibrils thicken and increase in number, and additional sarcomeres form from accelerated protein synthesis and corresponding decreased protein breakdown. Intramuscular ATP, PCr, and glycogen also increase considerably. These anaerobic energy stores contribute to the rapid energy transfer required in resistance training. Body-build characteristics also help to explain individual differences in responsiveness to resistance training. The greatest increases in muscle mass occur for individuals with the largest relative FFM corrected for stature and body fat before training begins.[243] Age also impacts the hypertrophic response to resistance training. Cross-sectional areas of type I and type II muscle fibers increased less in older (61 y) compared to younger (26 y) men following 21 wk of progressive resistance training. The difference in fiber-size enlargement associates with lower protein and energy intake and greater increases in myostatin gene expression in the older men compared to the younger men.[168]

System/Variable	Response
TABLE 22.5 — Physiologic Adaptations to Resistance Training	
Muscle fibers	
Number	Equivocal
Size	Increase
Type	Unknown
Strength	Increase
Mitochondria	
Volume	Decrease
Density	Decrease
Twitch contraction time	Decrease
Enzymes	
Creatine phosphokinase	Increase
Myokinase	Increase
Enzymes of glycolysis	
Phosphofructokinase	Increase
Lactate dehydrogenase	No change
Aerobic metabolism enzymes	
Carbohydrate	Increase
Triglyceride	Not known
Basal metabolism	Increase
Intramuscular fuel stores	
Adenosine triphosphate	Increase
Phosphocreatine	Increase
Glycogen	Increase
Triglycerides	Not known
Aerobic capacity	
Circuit resistance training	Increase
Standard resistance training	No change
Connective tissue	
Ligament strength	Increase
Tendon strength	Increase
Collagen content of muscle	No change
Body composition	
Percent body fat	Decrease
Lean body mass	Increase
Bone	
Mineral content and density	Increase
Cross-sectional area	Increase

Adapted with permission from Fleck SJ, Kraemer WJ. Resistance training: physiological responses and adaptations (part 2 of 4). *Phys Sportsmed* 1988;16:108.

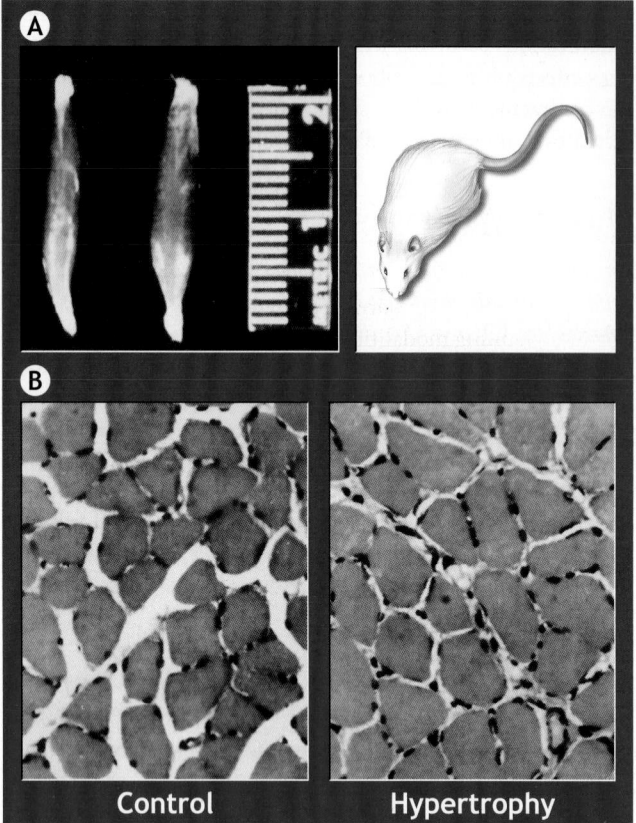

FIGURE 22.21 • **(A)** Control (*left*) and hypertrophied (*right*) rat soleus muscle. **(B)** Cross sections of control and hypertrophied muscles shown in A. The average diameter for 50 fibers of the hypertrophied muscle was 24 to 34% greater than for controls; the average number of nuclei in hypertrophied muscle averaged 40 to 52% greater than controls. (Reprinted with permission from Goldberg AL, et al. Mechanism of work-induced hypertrophy of skeletal muscle. *Med Sci Sports* 1975;3:185.)

FIGURE 22.21 shows the change in muscle fiber size that accompanies training-induced hypertrophy. Figure 22.21A compares trained and nontrained rat soleus muscle. Figure 22.21B, includes a typical cross section of untrained and hypertrophied muscles. Hypertrophied muscle diameter averages 30% larger and the fibers contain 45% more nuclei, which increase relative to fiber size. These compensatory changes relate to marked increases in DNA synthesis and proliferation of connective tissue cells and small, mononucleated satellite cells located beneath the basement membrane adjacent to the muscle fibers. The satellite cells, rich among type II muscle fibers, facilitate growth, maintenance, and repair of damaged muscle tissue.[93,100] Connective tissue cellular proliferation thickens and strengthens muscle's connective tissue harness to improve the structural and functional integrity of tendons and ligaments (cartilage lacks sufficient circulation to stimulate growth).[131] Such adaptations protect joints and muscles from injury and justify including resistance training in preventative and rehabilitative orthopedic programs.

Resistance-trained muscle fibers have increased total contractile protein and energy-generating compounds that occur *without* the following three components:

1. Parallel increases in vascular capillarization
2. Total volume of mitochondria
3. Mitochondrial enzymes

Absence of these factors decreases the ratio of mitochondrial volume and/or enzyme concentration to myofibrillar (contractile protein) volume. This training response does not hinder performance in strength and power activities because of the anaerobic nature of such efforts. It does, however, impede endurance in prolonged activity by reducing the fiber's aerobic capacity per unit of muscle mass.

Specificity of the Hypertrophic Response

One should not assume that a single form of resistance training creates uniform strength improvement or the hypertrophic response in the muscle(s) activated.[8] For example, biceps curls performed at close to 1-RM do *not* produce equal strength gains from the muscle's origin to its insertion. If they did, then the maximal force-generating capacity of the muscle would show similar percentage improvements throughout its ROM. This does not occur. Electrical activity measured by surface or needle EMG or MRI to assess a muscle's cross-sectional area does not produce a homogeneous response within the entire muscle during maximal activation. [169,202] A single muscle compartmentalizes into distinct regions. This indicates that the muscle's different areas respond differentially to the imposed adaptive stress. In essence, skeletal muscle remodels its internal architecture, potentially reconfiguring external orientation and hence its shape. The overall lack of homogeneity in skeletal muscle's response to overload, coupled with intramuscular differences in fiber type and composition, governs the training adaptation to specific resistance exercise.

Significant Metabolic Adaptations Occur

Elite sport performance success requires optimization of muscle fiber distribution. The relatively fixed nature of muscle fiber type suggests an obvious genetic predisposition for exceptional performance. Considerable *plasticity* exists for metabolic potential because specific training enhances the anaerobic and aerobic energy transfer capacity of both fiber types.

The heightened oxidative capacity of fast-twitch fibers with endurance training brings them to a level nearly equal to the aerobic capacity of the slow-twitch fibers of untrained counterparts. Endurance training induces some conversion of type IIb fibers to the more aerobic type IIa fibers.[264] The well-documented increase in mitochondrial size and number, and corresponding increase in total quantity of citric acid cycle and electron transport enzymes, accompanies these fiber subdivision changes. Only the specifically trained muscle fibers adapt to regular training; this helps to explain why trained athletes who change to a sport that requires different muscle groups, or different portions of the same muscle, often feel untrained. Within this framework, swimmers or canoeists with well-trained upper-body musculature do not necessarily transfer upper-body strength and performance to a running sport that relies predominantly on a highly conditioned lower-body musculature.

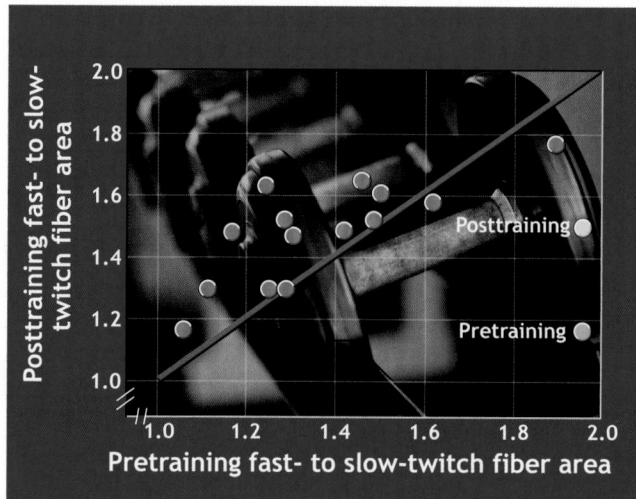

FIGURE 22.22 • Individual changes for 14 men in the ratio of fast- to slow-twitch muscle fiber area after 8 wk of resistance training. *Orange circle on right* indicates average pretraining FT:ST area ratio; *yellow circle* represents the posttraining average. (Adapted with permission from Thorstensson A. Muscle strength, fiber types, and enzyme activities in man. *Acta Physiol Scand* 1976(suppl):443.)

Metabolic characteristics of specific fibers and fiber subdivisions undergo modification within 4 to 8 wk of targeted resistance training. This occurs despite the lack of dramatic changes in inherent muscle fiber type. A decrease in the percentage of type IIx and corresponding increase in type IIa fibers denotes one of the more prominent and rapid training adaptations.[5] Furthermore, the volume of the trained fast-twitch fibers increases. FIGURE 22.22 clearly illustrates this increase for the relative areas of the fast- and slow-twitch muscle fibers before and after training. Considerable hypertrophy, predominantly of the fast-twitch fibers, occurs in power and Olympic-type lifters who train diligently over many years with progressive resistance

training.[226,228] This makes sense within the framework of exercise specificity because near-maximal resistance exercise that requires high levels of anaerobic power primarily recruits fast-twitch motor units. Resistance training also improves glucose transport in normal and insulin-resistant skeletal muscle by enhancing activation of the insulin signaling cascade and increasing GLUT-4 protein concentration. These training-induced alterations improve the quality of the skeletal muscle and occur independent of increases in skeletal muscle mass.[265]

TABLE 22.6 summarizes changes in skeletal muscle with specific training modalities. Generally, physical activity recruits both fiber types; however, certain activities require activation of a much greater proportion of one fiber type than another.

Muscle Cell Remodeling: Current Thinking

Skeletal muscles represent dynamic tissues whose cells do not remain as fixed populations throughout life. Rather, muscle fibers undergo regeneration and remodeling to diverse functional demands (e.g., resistance or endurance training) to alter their phenotypic profile.[101] Activation of muscle via specific types and intensities of long-term use stimulates otherwise dormant **myogenic stem cells** (**satellite cells**) situated under a muscle fiber's basement membrane to proliferate and differentiate to form new fibers. Fusion of satellite cell nuclei and incorporation into existing muscle fibers allow the fiber to synthesize more protein to form additional myofibril contractile elements. This process does not create new muscle fibers per se, but it does contribute directly to muscular hypertrophy and may stimulate transformation of existing fibers from one type to another.

A variety of extracellular signal molecules, primarily peptide growth factors (e.g., insulin-like growth factor [IGF], fibroblast growth factors, transforming growth factors, and hepatocyte growth factor) govern satellite cell activity and possibly training-induced muscle fiber proliferation and differentiation.

TABLE 22.6	Effects of Specific Types or Training on Skeletal Muscle				
	Slow-Twitch Fibers		**Fast-Twitch Fibers**		
	Type of Training				
Muscle Factor	**Strength**	**Endurance**	**Strength**	**Endurance**	
Percentage composition	0 or ?	0 or ?	0 or ?	0 or ?	
Size	+	0 or +	++	0	
Contractile property	0	0	0	0	
Oxidative capacity	0	++	0	+	
Anaerobic capacity	? or +	0	? or +	0	
Glycogen content	0	++	0	++	
Fat oxidation	0	++	0	+	
Capillary density	?	+	?	? or +	
Blood flow during exercise	?	? or +	?	?	

0, no change; ?, unknown; +, moderate increase; ++, large increase.

Figure 22.23 proposes a model for muscle cell remodeling that involves satellite cell incorporation into an existing muscle fiber. A specific set of genes (gene A in the figure within the preexisting nucleus) is expressed within the fiber. Chronic activation from physical activity stimulates satellite cell proliferation, with some cells differentiating and fusing with preexisting muscle fibers. The new muscle nuclei alter gene expression in the adapting muscle depicted by gene B within the myofibril.

Muscle fiber-type transformation may occur with specific training. In one study, four athletes trained anaerobically for 11 wk followed by 18 wk of aerobic training. Anaerobic training increased the percentage of type IIc fibers (a previous subclassification) and decreased the percentage of type I fibers; the opposite occurred during the aerobic training phase.[120] Similarly, 4 to 6 wk of sprint training increased the percentage of fast-twitch fibers, with a commensurate decrease in slow-twitch fiber percentage.[60] Increasing daily training duration also increases the fast- to slow-twitch shift in myosin heavy-chain phenotype in rat hind limb muscles.[63] Specific training (and perhaps inactivity) may convert different physiologic characteristics of type I to type II fibers (and vice versa).[212,226,227] Available evidence does not permit definitive statements concerning the fixed nature of a muscle's fiber composition. *One's genetic code more than likely exerts a large influence on fiber-type distribution.* The major direction of a muscle's fiber composition probably becomes fixed before birth or during the first few years of life.

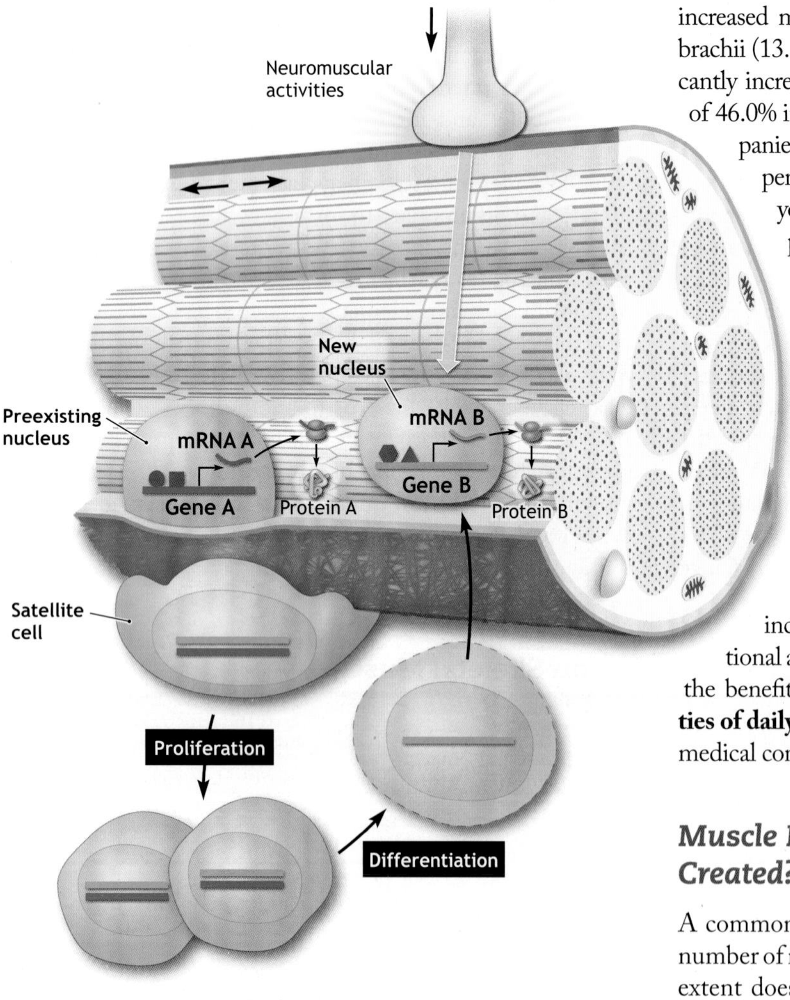

Benefits Regardless of Gender or Age

Muscles and tendons, highly adaptable tissues, respond favorably to chronic changes in loading independent of age or gender.[12,134,178] A study of five active, older, healthy men (average age 68 y) demonstrates the remarkable plasticity of human skeletal muscle (**Fig. 22.24**). The men trained for 12 wk using heavy-resistance isokinetic and free-weight exercises. Training significantly increased muscle volume and cross-sectional area of the biceps brachii (13.9%) and brachialis (26.0%), while hypertrophy significantly increased by 37.2% in the type II muscle fibers. Increases of 46.0% in peak torque and 28.6% in total work output accompanied cellular adaptations. Similarly, older men experience percentage improvements in these variables similar to younger counterparts in response to a rapid, high-power periodized resistance-training program.[180] Preserving muscle structure and function as one ages may provide a physical reserve capacity above the critical threshold required for independent living at old age.[2,263]

Equally impressive training responses occur for persons 80 years and older. One hundred nursing home residents (average age 87.1 y) trained for 10 wk with intense resistance exercise.[74] For the 63 women and 37 men who participated, muscle strength increased an average of 113%. Strength increases paralleled improved function, reflected by an 11.8% increase in normal gait velocity and 28.4% increase in stair-climbing speed; thigh muscle cross-sectional area increased by 2.7%. Other studies also have verified the benefits of functional strength training to improve **activities of daily living** (**ADL**), including countering the devastating medical consequences of slips and falls in the older elderly.[33]

FIGURE 22.23 • A model for skeletal muscle adaptation that involves satellite cells. A specific set of genes (*gene A*) is expressed in the preexisting myonuclei. Upon stimulation from increased neuromuscular activity, the satellite cells proliferate, and some of them differentiate and fuse with the preexisting myofibers. These myonuclei may alter gene expression (*gene B*) in the adapting muscle because they undergo altered differentiation from increased neuromuscular activities. (Adapted with permission from Yan Z. Skeletal muscle adaptation and cell cycle regulation. *Exerc Sport Sci Rev* 2000;1:24.)

Muscle Hyperplasia: Are New Muscle Fibers Created?

A common question concerns whether training increases the number of muscle cells (**hyperplasia**). If this does occur, to what extent does it contribute to muscle enlargement in humans? Chronic overload of skeletal muscle in various animal species stimulates new muscle fiber development from satellite cells or by longitudinal splitting.[10] Under conditions of (1) stress, (2) neuromuscular disease, and (3) muscle injury, the normally dormant satellite cells develop into new muscle fibers (see Fig. 22.23). With **longitudinal splitting**, a relatively large muscle fiber splits into two or more smaller individual daughter cells through lateral budding. These fibers function more efficiently than the large single fiber from which they originated.[11]

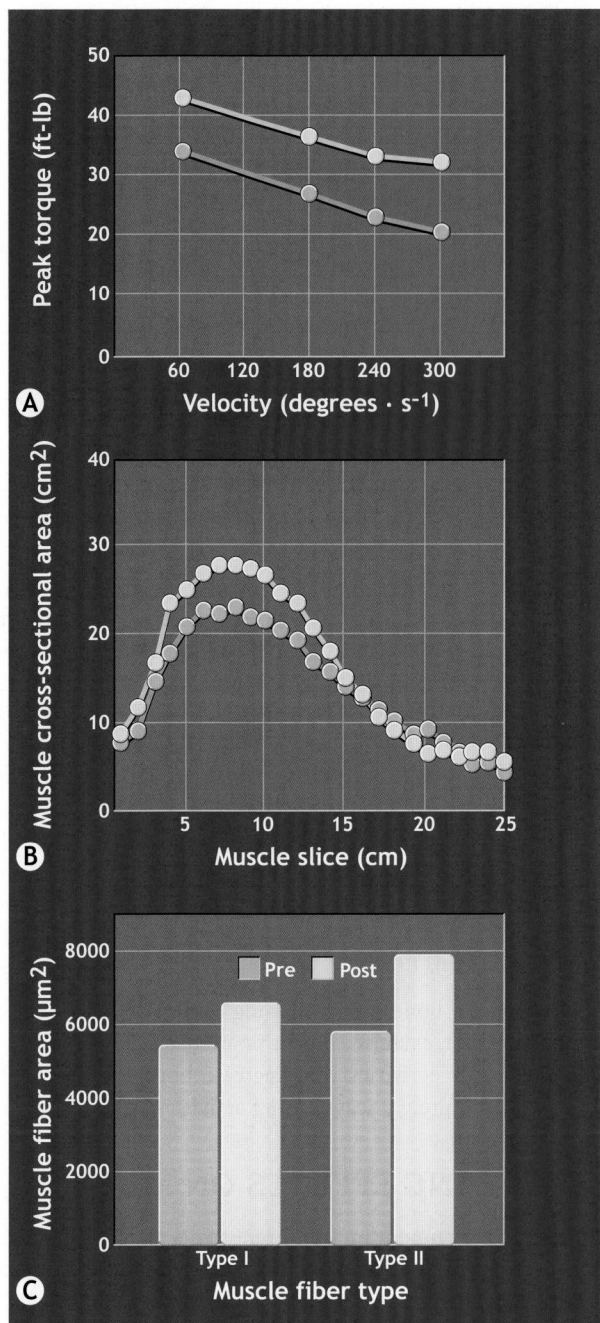

FIGURE 22.24 • Plasticity of aging muscle. Data from five men, 68 years of age, pre (*orange*) and post (*yellow*) 12 wk of heavy-resistance training. (**A**) Peak torque of elbow flexors. (**B**) Plot of flexor cross-sectional area computed from MRI scans from proximal (*right*) to distal (*left*) end of muscle. (**C**) Average for type I and type II fiber areas. (Adapted with permission from Roman WJ, et al. Adaptations in the elbow flexors of elderly males after heavy-resistance training. *J Appl Physiol* 1993;74:750.)

Generalizing findings from research on animals to humans poses a problem. The massive cellular hypertrophy observed in humans with resistance training does not occur in many animal species. In cats, for example, muscle fiber proliferation (hyperplasia) often reflects the primary compensatory adjustment to overload. Some evidence supporting hyperplasia in humans does exist. For example, autopsy data from young, healthy men who died accidentally show that muscle fiber counts of the larger and stronger leg (leg opposite the dominant hand) contained 10% more muscle fibers than the smaller leg.[213] Cross-sectional studies of bodybuilders with relatively large limb circumferences and muscle masses failed to show they possessed above-normal size individual muscle fibers.[151,152,227] Some of the bodybuilders may have inherited an initially large number of small muscle fibers (that "hypertrophied" to normal size with resistance training), yet the findings suggest hyperplasia with certain modes of resistance training. Muscle fibers may adapt differently to the high-volume, high-intensity training practiced by bodybuilders than the typical low-repetition, heavy-load system favored by strength and power athletes. *Even if other human studies replicate a training–induced hyperplasia (and even if the response reflects a positive adjustment), enlargement of existing individual muscle fibers represents the greatest contribution to increased muscle size from overload training.*

Changes in Muscle Fiber Type With Resistance Training

Research has evaluated the effects of 8 wk of resistance exercise on muscle fiber size and fiber composition for the leg extensor muscles of 14 men who performed three sets of 6-RM leg squats three times weekly.[231] Biopsy specimens from the vastus lateralis muscle before and after training showed *no change* in percentage distribution of fast- and slow-twitch muscle fibers. This finding agrees with previous short-term resistance and endurance-type training studies and indicates that several months of resistance training in adults *does not alter* the basic fiber composition of skeletal muscle. It remains unclear whether specific training early in life or for prolonged durations practiced by elite athletes alters a muscle fiber's inherent twitch (speed of shortening) characteristics. Some progressive fiber-type transformation may occur with longer-duration, specific training (see Chapter 18). Current thinking posits that genetic factors largely determine one's predominant muscle fiber type distribution.

COMPARATIVE TRAINING RESPONSES IN MEN AND WOMEN

Women now participate successfully in just about all sports and physical activities. Women generally had not incorporated resistance training during workouts to avoid developing overly enlarged muscles similar to men. This hesitation was unfortunate because specific strength acquisition enhances performance in tennis, golf, skiing, dance, gymnastics, and most other sports, including the physically demanding occupations of firefighting and construction work. The question often arises whether muscular strength acquisition differs between men and women and, if so, what factors might be responsible?

 INTEGRATIVE QUESTION

If women respond to resistance training essentially the same way as men, explain the disparity between the upper-arm girth of male and female bodybuilders.

Muscular Strength and Hypertrophy

The absolute amount of muscle hypertrophy with resistance training represents a primary gender difference. Computed axial tomography (CAT; see Chapter 28) scans for direct evaluation of muscle cross-sectional area show that men and women respond similarly in hypertrophic response to resistance training. Without doubt, men experience a greater absolute change in muscle size because of their larger initial muscle mass, but muscular enlargement on a *percentage* basis remains similar between genders.[56,109,249] Comparisons between elite male and female bodybuilders also indicate substantial muscular hypertrophy in females with many years of resistance training.[217,218,222] Gender-related differences in hormonal response to resistance exercise (e.g., increased testosterone and decreased cortisol for men) may determine any ultimate gender differences in muscle size and strength adaptations with prolonged training.[140] This intriguing area requires longitudinal research for a richer description of gender differences in how skeletal muscle responds to resistance training.

Does Muscle Strength Relate to Bone Density?

A positive relationship exists between muscular strength and bone mineral density.[46,58,156] Men and women who participate in strength and power activities have as much or more bone mass than endurance athletes.[199,203,262] The lumbar spine and proximal femur bone mass of elite teenage weightlifters[51] and in adolescent boys and girls[251] exceed representative values for fully mature bone of reference adults.

A linear relation exists between increases in bone mineral density (BMD) and total and exercise-specific weight lifted during a 1-year strength-training program.[57] Such findings have raised speculation about the possible positive relationship between muscular strength and bone mass. Laboratory experiments have documented greater maximum flexion and extension dynamic strength in postmenopausal women without osteoporosis than in osteoporotic counterparts.[221] For female gymnasts, BMD correlated moderately with maximal muscle strength and serum progesterone.[105] For adolescent female athletes, absolute knee extension strength moderately associated with total body, lumbar spine, femoral neck, and leg BMD.[69] **FIGURE 22.25** shows chest flexion and extension strength in normal and osteoporotic women. Women with normal BMD (measured by dual-photon absorptiometry in the lumbar spine and femur neck) exhibited 20% greater strength in 11 of 12 test comparisons for flexion; 4 of 12 comparisons for extension showed 13% higher strength values for women with normal bone density. Subsequent data complement these findings; they indicate that regional lean tissue mass (often an indication of muscular strength) accurately predicts bone mineral density.[181] Such findings suggest that differences in maximum dynamic strength among postmenopausal women may serve a clinically useful role in osteoporosis screening.

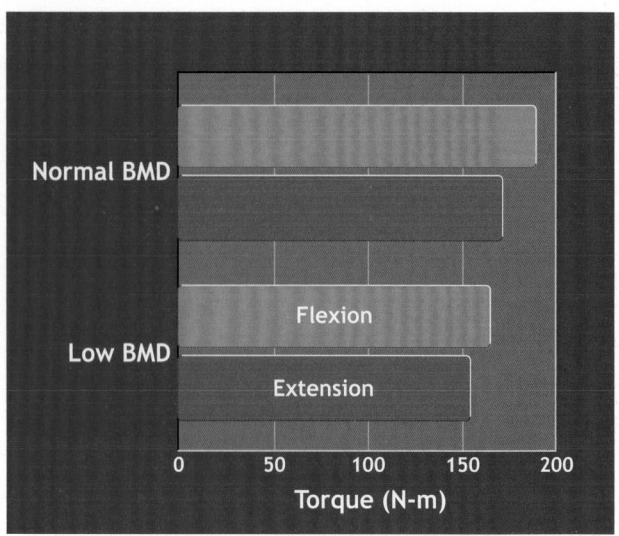

FIGURE 22.25 • Comparison of chest press extension and flexion strength in age- and weight-matched postmenopausal women with normal and low bone mineral density (BMD). Women with low BMD scored significantly lower on each measure of muscular strength than a reference group. (Adapted with permission from Stock JL, et al. Dynamic muscle strength is decreased in postmenopausal women with low bone density. *J Bone Miner Res* 1987;2:338; Janey C, et al. Maximum muscular strength differs in postmenopausal women with and without osteoporosis. *Med Sci Sports Exerc* 1987;19:S61.)

Women at risk for osteoporosis or with osteoporosis can attenuate their *factor of risk* (ratio of the load on bone to the bone's failure load) for fracture in one of two ways:[176]

1. Strengthen bone by increasing bone mineral density through diet, exercise, and/or pharmacologic therapy
2. Avoid risky activities that increase bone load or spinal compression (e.g., heavy lifting activities)

DETRAINING EFFECTS ON MUSCLE

Limited data document muscle strength decrements and associated factors with cessation of resistance training. Discontinuing training for 2 wk caused male power lifters to lose 12% of their isokinetic eccentric muscle strength and 6.4% of their type II muscle fiber area, without loss in type I fiber area.[107] Another study evaluated knee extensor muscle strength, muscle volume, and muscle quality in elderly women with a 12-wk strength training program followed by a similar period of detraining.[52] No effect of time occurred on muscle quality, yet strength increased 33% and muscle volume increased 26% from baseline to post-training. After detraining, the knee extensor strength remained 12% higher compared to baseline values, while the gains in muscle mass returned to baseline values. The authors concluded that muscular strength gains and losses from resistance training and detraining could not solely be determined by changes in muscle mass.

Abstaining for a short period of resistance training in previously sedentary men caused loss of strength gains within several weeks, most likely from reversal of training-induced neuromuscular and hormonal adaptations.[50] Some athletes and coaches encourage their athletes to "taper" their normal routines, including psychological parameters,[214] to allow for sufficient recovery before an upcoming competition.[174] The concept of a taper is a fruitful area for future research, as only limited quantitative data exists for athletes in training.[230] Reducing training frequency to only one or two weekly sessions provides sufficient stimulus to *maintain* training-induced strength gains.[87]

METABOLIC STRESS OF RESISTANCE TRAINING

Resistance training produces no improvement in $\dot{V}O_{2max}$ or submaximal exercise heart rate and stroke volume.[111] Lack of cardiovascular improvement with standard resistance training probably results from the relatively low "whole body" metabolic and circulatory demands and high anaerobic metabolic requirements of such training. This is reflected by the potent stimulation of glucose uptake and lactate release by the active muscle.[70] Data from young men during maximal isometric and 8- to 10-RM weightlifting exercises indicate that such activity elicits only light-to-moderate heart rate response (generally less than 130 b·min⁻¹) and oxygen consumption (3 to 4 METs).[158]

Resistance training places considerable localized stress on specific muscles. The brief activation period and typically small muscle mass activated in such training creates lower heart rates and aerobic metabolic demands than dynamic big-muscle running, hiking, climbing, swimming, or cycling. A person may devote an hour or more to complete a strength-training workout, yet the total time devoted to exercising does not usually exceed 8 min per hour. Traditional resistance-training workouts should *not* constitute the major portion of a program designed for cardiovascular improvement and weight control.

CIRCUIT RESISTANCE TRAINING

Modifying the traditional approach to resistance training increases the caloric cost of such exercise to improve several important fitness aspects. **Circuit resistance training (CRT)** deemphasizes the brief intervals of heavy, local-muscle overload in standard resistance training. It provides more general conditioning that improves body composition, muscular strength and endurance, and cardiovascular fitness.[8,22,83,175]

With CRT, a person lifts a weight between 40 and 55% of 1-RM as many times as possible with good form for 30 s. After a 15-s rest, the participant moves to the next resistance exercise station and so on to complete the circuit, usually composed of 8 to 15 different exercises. A modification that produces similar CRT energy expenditure uses exercise-to-rest ratios of 1:1, with either 15- or 30-s exercise periods.[18] The circuit repeated several times allows for 30 to 50 min of continuous exercise, not just the 6 to 8 min of the traditional resistance-training workout. As strength increases, a new 1-RM determined for each exercise provides the basis to increasing the resistance.

The CRT modification of standard resistance training offers an attractive alternative to those who desire a more general conditioning program. Medically supervised CRT programs effectively train coronary-prone, cardiac, and spinal cord–injured patients for a well-rounded fitness program.

CRT supplements off-season conditioning for sports that require high levels of strength, power, and muscular endurance.

Specificity of Aerobic Improvement With CRT

Some research indicates that CRT produces nearly 50% less aerobic fitness improvement than bicycle or run training.[82] Importantly, CRT usually involves substantial upper-body exercise, but assessment of aerobic benefits from this training relied on treadmill or bicycle tests that predominantly activate lower-body musculature. To compensate for this limitation, one study assessed CRT effects on aerobic capacity with treadmill running and arm-crank ergometry tests.[96] Aerobic capacity increased 8% with treadmill testing and 21% with arm-crank testing, thus confirming the training specificity principle. These findings take on added significance because they occurred without negative effects in a group of borderline hypertensives. The program also increased muscular strength, decreased blood pressure, and modestly improved body composition.

Energy Cost of Different Resistance-Exercise Methods

TABLE 22.7 displays energy expenditures for exercise performed using free weights, Nautilus (eccentric), Universal Gym (concentric/eccentric), Cybex (isokinetic), and Hydra-Fitness (hydraulic-concentric). Energy expenditure for hydraulic exercises averaged 9.0 kcal·min⁻¹; this averaged 35% higher than exercise with free weights, 29.4% higher than Nautilus exercise, and 11.5% more than CRT using Universal Gym equipment. The energy expenditure values for hydraulic exercise averaged about 6.4% less than slow- and fast-speed isokinetic

TABLE 22.7	Energy Expenditure for Different Modes of Resistance Exercise Compared with Walking[a]		
Mode	**Sex**	**kJ·min⁻¹**	**kcal·min⁻¹**
Nautilus, circuit	M	29.7	7.1
	F	24.3	5.8
Nautilus, circuit	M	22.6	5.4
Universal, circuit	M	33.1	7.9
	F	28.5	6.8
Isokinetic, slow	M	40.2	9.6
Isokinetic, fast	M	41.4	9.9
Isometric and free-weight	M	25.1	6.0
Hydra-Fitness, circuit	M	37.7	9.0
Walking on level	M	22.6	5.4

[a]Based on body weight of 68 kg.
Data from Katch FI, et al. Evaluation of acute cardiorespiratory responses to hydraulic resistance exercise. *Med Sci Sports Exerc* 1985;17:168.

circuit exercise. For comparison, the last line lists the energy expenditure for walking at a normal pace on a level surface.

MUSCLE SORENESS AND STIFFNESS

Following an extended layoff from exercise, or performing unaccustomed exercise, most persons experience soreness and stiffness in the exercised joints and muscles. Temporary soreness may persist for several hours immediately following such unaccustomed exercise, whereas residual **delayed-onset muscle soreness** (**DOMS**) appears later and can last for 3 or 4 days. Any one of the following seven factors can produce DOMS:

1. Minute tears in muscle tissue or damage to its contractile components with accompanying release of creatine kinase (CK), myoglobin (Mb), and troponin I, the muscle-specific marker of muscle fiber damage
2. Osmotic pressure changes that produce fluid retention in the surrounding tissues
3. Muscle spasms
4. Overstretching and tearing of portions of the muscle's connective tissue harness
5. Acute inflammation
6. Alteration in the cell's mechanism for calcium regulation
7. Combination of the above factors

Eccentric Actions Produce Muscle Soreness

The precise cause of muscle soreness remains unknown, although the degree of discomfort, muscle disturbance, and loss of strength depends largely on the intensity and duration of effort and type of movement performed.[91,103,112,232] The magnitude of active strain imposed on a muscle fiber (rather than absolute force) precipitates muscle damage and soreness.[145] *Eccentric muscle actions trigger the greatest postexercise discomfort*, particularly magnified in older individuals.[25,242,247] Existing muscle damage or soreness from previous activity does not exacerbate subsequent muscle damage or impair the repair process.[183]

In one study, subjects rated muscle soreness immediately after exercise and 24, 48, and 72 hr later. Greater soreness occurred from exercise that involved repeated intense strain during active lengthening in eccentric actions than from concentric and isometric actions. Soreness did not relate to lactate buildup because high-intensity, level running (concentric actions) produced no residual soreness despite significant elevations in blood lactate. In contrast, downhill running (eccentric actions) caused moderate-to-severe DOMS without lactate elevation during exercise.

TABLE **22.8** highlights muscle soreness and CK activity following an exercise circuit of either concentric-only or

TABLE 22.8 Acute Effects of Concentric-Only and Concentric-Eccentric Exercise on DOMS 25 Hours After Exercise[a]

| Site | Soreness Ratings | | Site | Soreness Ratings | |
	Concentric X̄	Concentric–Eccentric X̄		Concentric X̄	Concentric–Eccentric X̄
Chest	2.3	5.1	Forearm (front)	1.7	3.4
Back (upper)	2.6	2.8	Forearm (back)	1.7	2.9
Shoulders (front)	2.2	3.6	Back (lower)	1.7	2.9
Shoulders (back)	1.9	3.6	Buttocks	1.8	2.5
Biceps (mid)	1.9	4.3	Quadriceps (mid)	2.0	4.1
Biceps (lower)	1.8	3.5	Quadriceps (lower)	2.1	3.8
Triceps (mid)	1.9	3.4	Hamstrings (mid)	2.1	3.5
Triceps (lower)	1.9	3.0	Hamstrings (lower)	2.1	3.0

| | CK Activity (mU · mL^{-1}) | |
Sample Time	Concentric X̄	Concentric–Eccentric X̄
Pre	86.7	126.9
5 h post	344.8	232.0
10 h post	394.3	368.5
25 h post	288.0	482.2

X̄ = mean
[a]All differences between groups were statistically significant.
Reprinted from Byrnes WC. Muscle soreness following resistance exercise with and without eccentric muscle actions. *Res Q Exerc Sport* 1985;56:283.

concentric and eccentric muscle actions. Group 1 performed three sets of eight exercises (concentric–eccentric) at 60% of 1-RM on Universal Gym equipment: one set equaled 20 s of exercise followed by 40 s of rest; total exercise time was 24 min. Group 2 followed the same exercise protocol, but they exercised maximally for each repetition on resistance devices powered by hydraulic cylinders that produced concentric-only actions. Blood samples and ratings of perceived muscle soreness took place before exercise and 5, 10, and 25 hr after exercise. The major difference in soreness ratings between exercise groups occurred 25 hr postexercise; the concentric–eccentric workout produced higher perceived ratings of soreness for the major muscle groups exercised. The magnitude of increase in serum CK remained the same between groups from 5 to 25 hr postexercise. Both exercise modes elevated serum CK, but the concentric-only muscle actions did not cause DOMS.

Cell Damage

Running downhill at a 10° slope for 30 min produced considerable DOMS 42 hr after running.[34] Corresponding increases also occurred in serum levels of Mb and the muscle-specific enzyme CK, both common markers of muscle injury. Acute inflammation also augments greater mobilization of leukocytes and neutrophils. Subject testing also took place after 3, 6, and 9 wk. FIGURE 22.26 shows the perceived soreness rating for the leg muscles related to elapsed postexercise time for the three study durations. For the 3- and 6-wk comparisons, differences between exercise bouts reached statistical significance, with diminished DOMS noted in the second trial (orange). Similar patterns emerged for perception of muscle soreness and CK and Mb levels. Interestingly, peak soreness ratings at 48 hr did not relate to absolute or relative CK or Mb changes. Individuals who reported the greatest DOMS did not necessarily have the highest CK and Mb values. The first bout of repetitive, high-force exercise probably disrupts the integrity of the sarcolemma to produce mitochondrial swelling and temporary ultrastructural muscle damage in a pool of stress-susceptible or degenerating muscle fibers. This response occurs with an increase in blood markers such as protein carbonyls that reflect oxidative stress.[44,139]

The early mechanical damage to the myocytes (reflected by increased CK release) 24 hr postexercise does coincide with acute inflammatory cell infiltration within the muscle.[29] The subsequent decrease in muscle performance for several days following eccentric injury primarily stems from failure in excitation–contraction coupling and increased myofibrillar proteolysis.[114,256] The fast-twitch fibers with low oxidative capacities show particular vulnerability, with more extensive damage several days after exercise than in the immediate postexercise period. Single bouts of preconditioning eccentric exercise of at least 20% of maximal eccentric contraction and isometric exercise at a long muscle length provide a protective effect against maximal eccentric contraction–induced muscle damage.[41,42] Resistance to muscle damage in succeeding physical activity may result from an eccentric exercise–induced increase in muscle fiber sarcomeres connected in series.[150] Such adaptations support the wisdom of initiating a training program with

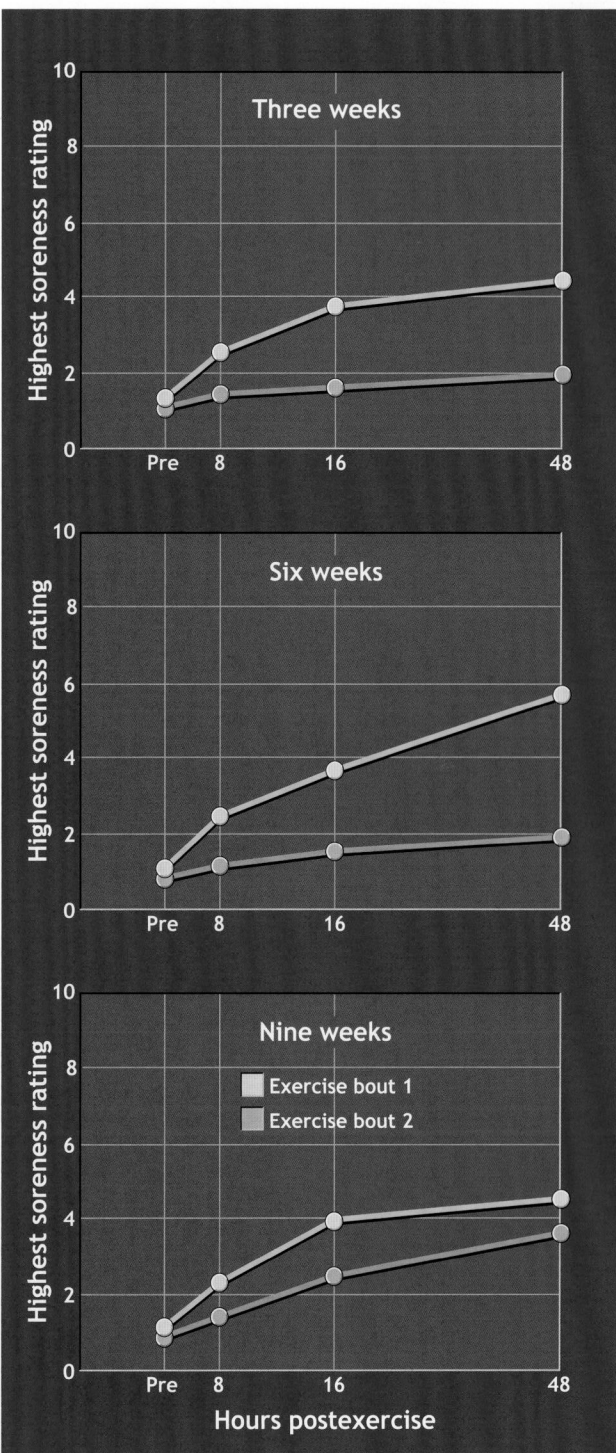

FIGURE 22.26 • Highest soreness rating before and 8, 16, and 48 hr after exercise bout 1 (*yellow*) and a subsequent exercise bout (bout 2, *orange*) performed either 3, 6, or 9 wk later. CK and Mb showed similar results. (Adapted with permission from Byrnes WC, et al. Delayed onset muscle soreness following repeated bouts of downhill running. *J Appl Physiol* 1985;59:710.)

light activity to protect against the muscle soreness that almost always follows an initial intense exercise bout that includes an eccentric component.[81] Intense concentric movements performed just prior to strenuous eccentric exercise does not magnify muscle damage. It may prepare the muscle to respond more effectively to the next eccentric exercise stress. Even prior lower-intensity exercise of specific muscles does not fully protect from DOMS with more intense movements.

Altered Sarcoplasmic Reticulum

Four factors produce major alterations in sarcoplasmic reticulum structure and function with unaccustomed physical activity:

1. Changes in pH
2. Changes in intramuscular high-energy phosphates
3. Changes in ionic balance
4. Changes in temperature

These effects depress the rates of Ca^{2+} uptake and release and increase free Ca^{2+} concentration as the mineral rapidly moves into the cytosol of the damaged fibers. Intracellular Ca^{2+} overload contributes to the autolytic process within damaged muscle fibers that degrades the contractile and noncontractile structures. Topographical mapping techniques to investigate sensory and EMG outcomes of DOMS have been investigated 24 hr and 48 hr following eccentric exercise in multiple locations of the quadriceps muscle. Greater DOMS occurred in the distal region of the quadriceps, indicating a greater tendency of this region to further injury following the eccentric exercise along with reduced force capacity.[102]

Vitamin E supplementation, and perhaps vitamin C and selenium, protects against cellular membrane disruption and enzyme loss following muscle damage from resistance exercise (see Chapter 2).[86,159] Postexercise protein supplementation also may protect against muscle soreness in severely exercise-stressed individuals.[75] In contrast, supplementing daily with either fish oil (high in omega-3 and omega-6 fatty acids) or isoflavones (soy isolate) for 30 days prior to and during the week of testing to reduce the inflammatory response produced no benefit to DOMS (strength, pain ratings, limb girth, and blood measures related to muscle

damage, inflammation, and lipid peroxidation) compared with placebo treatment.[141] Supplementation with 750 mg per day of phosphatidylserine for 10 days did not afford additional protection against DOMS and markers of muscle damage, inflammation, and oxidative stress that follow prolonged downhill running.[130] Similarly, taking a protease supplement had no effect on pain perception associated with DOMS or blood markers of muscle damage.[20]

 See the animation "RICE Method" on **http://thePoint.lww.com/mkk8e** for a demonstration of this process.

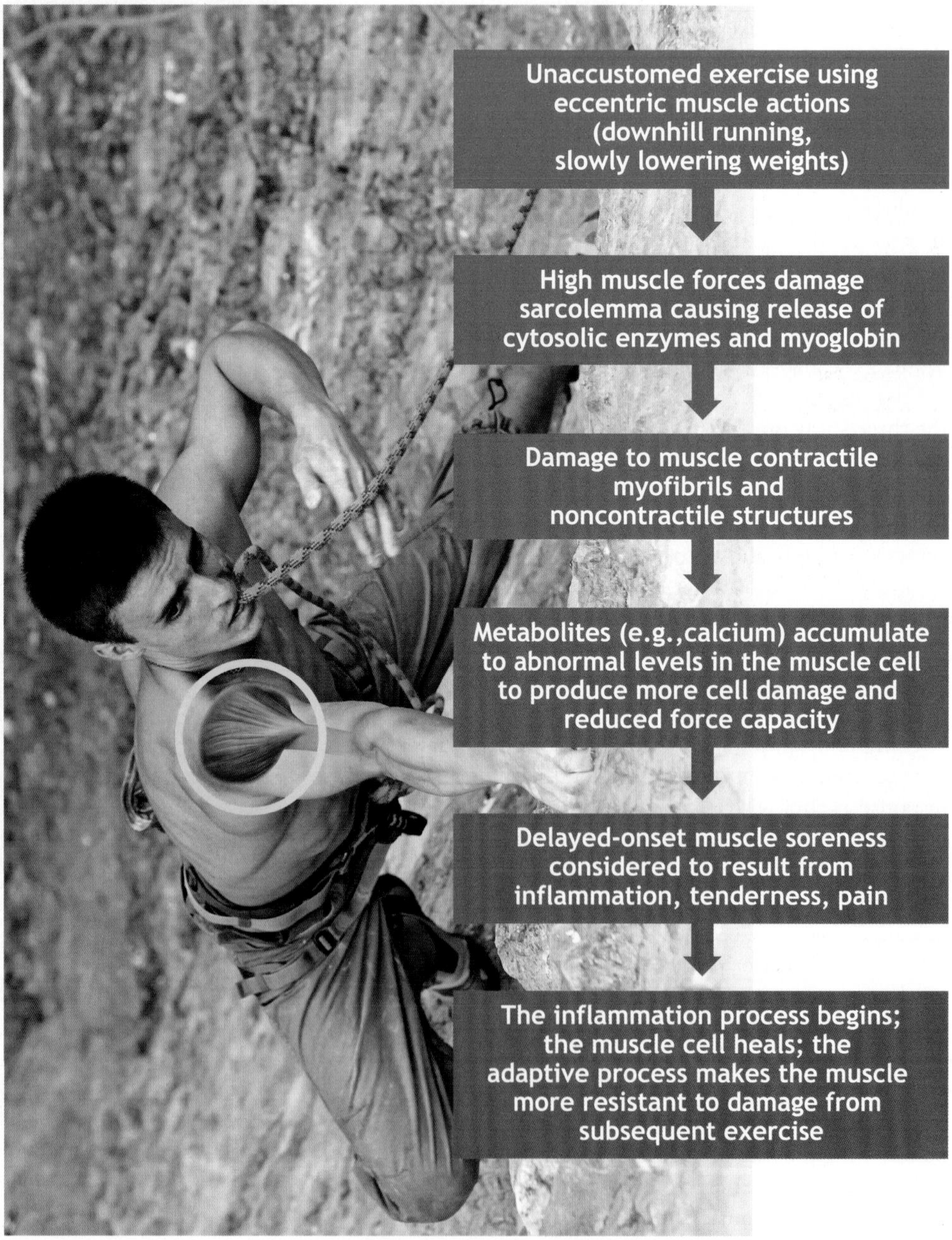

Unaccustomed exercise using eccentric muscle actions (downhill running, slowly lowering weights)

↓

High muscle forces damage sarcolemma causing release of cytosolic enzymes and myoglobin

↓

Damage to muscle contractile myofibrils and noncontractile structures

↓

Metabolites (e.g., calcium) accumulate to abnormal levels in the muscle cell to produce more cell damage and reduced force capacity

↓

Delayed-onset muscle soreness considered to result from inflammation, tenderness, pain

↓

The inflammation process begins; the muscle cell heals; the adaptive process makes the muscle more resistant to damage from subsequent exercise

FIGURE 22.27 • Proposed sequence of six phases for delayed-onset muscle soreness following unaccustomed exercise. Cellular adaptations to short-term exercise provide enhanced resistance to subsequent damage and pain.

Current DOMS Model

FIGURE 22.27 diagrams the probable six phases in DOMS development and subsequent recuperation.

 INTEGRATIVE QUESTION

Respond to the following: "I run and work out with free weights regularly, yet every spring my muscles are sore a day or two after a few hours of yard work."

Summary

1. The size and type of muscle fibers and the anatomic lever arrangement of bone and muscle (physiologic factors) largely govern the upper limit to human muscular strength.

2. Central nervous system influences activate the prime movers in a specific action to affect maximal force capacity.

3. Six factors—genetic, exercise, nutritional, hormonal, environmental, and neural—interact to regulate skeletal muscle mass and corresponding strength development with resistance training.

4. Three factors contribute to increased muscle strength with resistance training: improved capacity for motor unit recruitment, changes in motor neuron firing pattern efficiency, and alterations within the muscle fibers' contractile elements.

5. Muscular overload increases strength and selectively stimulates muscle fiber hypertrophy.

6. Muscle hypertrophy includes increased protein synthesis with myofibrillar thickening, connective tissue cell proliferation, and an increase in the number of satellite cells around each fiber.

7. Muscle hypertrophy entails structural changes within the contractile apparatus of individual fibers, particularly fast-twitch fibers and increased anaerobic energy stores.

8. The genetic code exerts the greatest influence on muscle fiber-type distribution; a muscle's fiber composition is largely fixed before birth or during the first few years of life.

9. Human muscle fibers adapt to increased functional demands via action of myogenic stem cells (satellite cells) that proliferate and differentiate to remodel the muscle.

10. Relatively brief periods of resistance training generate similar strength improvements (on a percentage basis) for women and men.

11. Muscle weakness in the abdominal and lower lumbar back regions (core), including poor flexibility in the lower back and legs, represent primary factors related to low back syndrome.

12. Core muscle-strengthening, flexibility, and balance exercises effectively protect against and rehabilitate low back syndrome.

13. Women at risk for osteoporosis or with the disease reduce fracture risk by increasing bone density and avoiding activities that increase spinal compression and bone stress.

14. Conventional resistance training does not improve aerobic fitness. These workouts do not affect weight loss because of their relatively low caloric cost.

15. Circuit resistance training, by using lower resistance and higher repetitions performed in a continuous manner, effectively combines the muscle-training benefits of resistance exercise with the cardiovascular, calorie-burning benefits of continuous dynamic exercise.

16. Eccentric muscle actions induce greater DOMS than concentric-only or isometric actions. Serum markers of muscle damage (CK and Mb) increase with each form of muscle action.

17. A single exercise bout protects against DOMS and muscle damage from subsequent exercise. The protection mechanism supports the wisdom when beginning a training program that requires application of considerable muscular force of progressing gradually at a lower intensity to minimize eccentric actions.

18. The body initiates a series of adaptive cellular events, basically an inflammation response, to unaccustomed physical activity that produces DOMS.

thePoint References are available online at http://thepoint.lww.com/mkk8e.

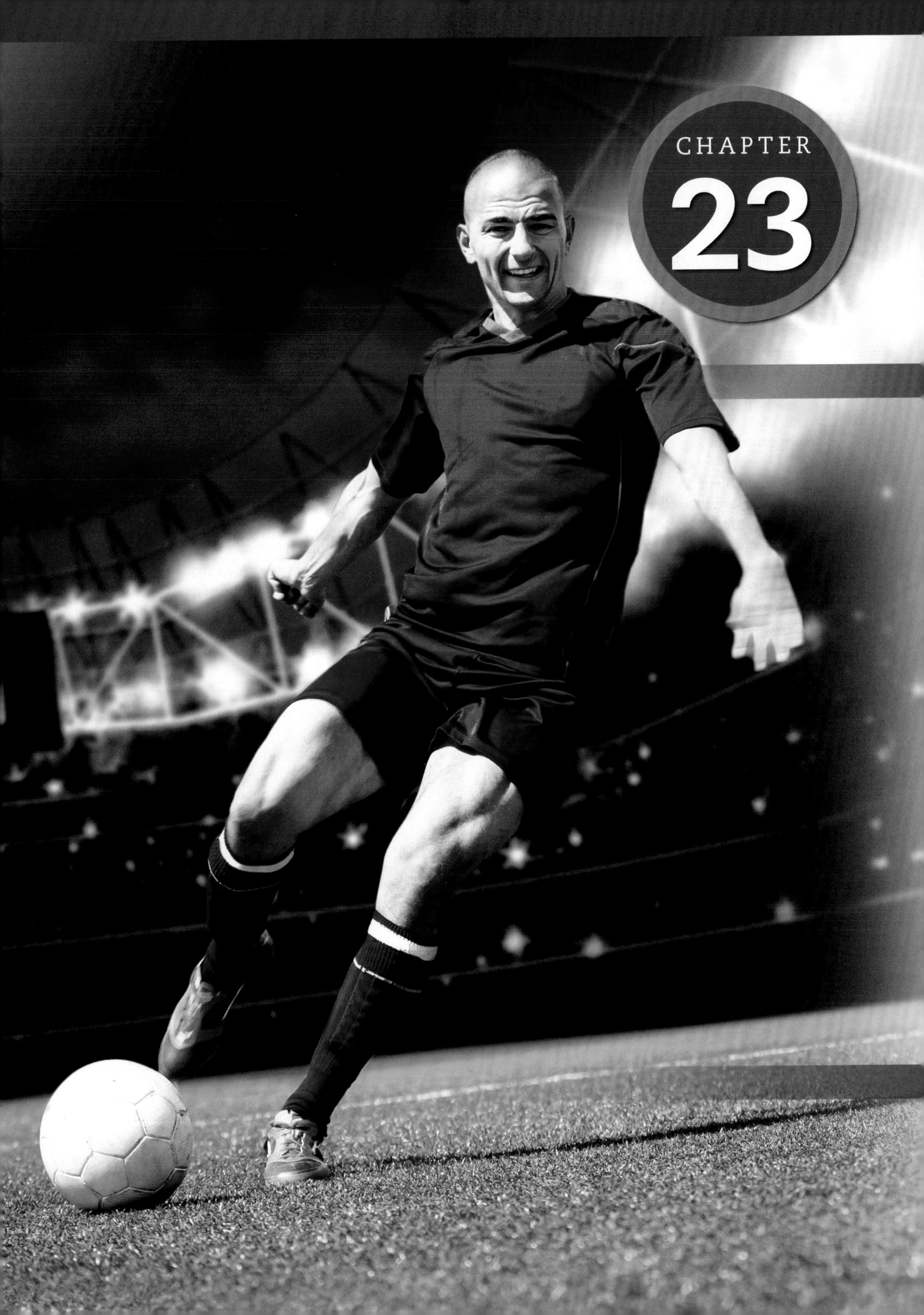
CHAPTER
23

Special Aids to Exercise Training and Performances

CHAPTER OBJECTIVES

- Define ergogenic aids and outline possible mechanisms for their purported effects
- Outline the procedure for formulating a randomized, double-blind, placebo-controlled research study and give the benefits of such a design
- List the eleven categories of substances currently banned by the International Olympic Committee
- Give five examples of substances or procedures with alleged ergogenic benefits
- Discuss the mode of action of anabolic steroids, their effectiveness, and risks when used by males and females
- Summarize the ACSM's "Position Stand on Use of Anabolic Steroids"
- Give positive and negative findings from research on animals of the effect of clenbuterol and other β_2-adrenergic agonists
- Discuss the medical use of human growth hormone and potential dangers for healthy athletes
- Outline the general trend for endogenous dehydroepiandrosterone (DHEA) production during a lifetime
- Discuss the rationale for DHEA as an ergogenic aid and its potential risks
- Summarize the controversy about androstenedione as a benign nutritional supplement or a harmful drug
- Discuss the effects of oral supplements of amino acids, carbohydrate-protein, and carbohydrate on hormone secretion, resistance-training responsiveness, and physical performance
- Summarize the general research findings about ergogenic benefits and risks of amphetamines, caffeine, buffering solutions, chromium picolinate, L-carnitine, glutamine, and β-hydroxy-β–methylbutyrate
- Describe the typical time course for red blood cell reinfusion and its mechanism for ergogenic effects on endurance performance and $\dot{V}O_{2max}$
- Discuss the medical use of erythropoietin and two potential dangers for healthy athletes
- Define *general warm-up* and *specific warm-up* and the potential benefits of each
- Describe possible cardiovascular benefits of moderate warm-up prior to extreme physical effort
- Give an example where breathing hyperoxic gas mixtures enhance endurance performance; quantify its potential to increase tissue oxygen availability
- Outline the classic carbohydrate-loading procedure and modified-loading procedure to augment glycogen storage
- Describe the theoretical role for an ergogenic effect of creatine supplements, and two physical activities that benefit from supplementation
- Summarize the research and rationale for consuming medium-chain triacylglycerols to enhance endurance performance
- Discuss the effects of pyruvate supplementation on endurance performance and body fat loss

ANCILLARIES ◉ at-a-Glance

Visit http://thePoint.lww.com/mkk8e to access the following resources.

- References: Chapter 23
- Appendix I: United States Olympic Committee (USOC) National Anti-Doping Policy Statement of Prohibited Substances and Methods
- Interactive Question Bank
- Focus on Research: Ergogenic Benefits of Caffeine

Considerable literature exists about **ergogenic aids** and athletic performance—*ergogenic referring to the application of a nutritional, physical, mechanical, psychologic, or pharmacologic procedure or aid to improve physical work capacity or athletic performance.* This literature includes studies of potential performance benefits of alcohol, amphetamines, ephedrine, hormones, carbohydrates, amino acids, fatty acids, additional red blood cells, caffeine, carnitine, creatine, phosphates, oxygen-rich breathing mixtures, massage, wheat-germ oil, vitamins, minerals, ionized air, music, hypnosis, and even marijuana and cocaine! Athletes routinely use only a few of these aids, and only a few evoke real controversy. Specific concern focuses on the use of anabolic steroids, human growth hormone, dehydroepiandrosterone (DHEA), and other exogenous hormones and prohormones, some nutritional supplements, amphetamines, and "blood doping." Warm-up and breathing hyperoxic gas are common procedures, so we include these in our discussion of the effectiveness and practicality of ergogenic aids for exercise training and performance. We also discuss nutritional requirements for macro- and micronutrients for active individuals in the specific sport chapters dealing with these nutrients.

The indiscriminate use of ergogenic substances increases the likelihood of adverse side effects that range from benign physical discomfort to life-threatening episodes. Many of these compounds fail to conform to labeling requirements to correctly identify the strength of the product's ingredients and contaminents.[113,139] For example, supplements available through the Internet and at retail often contain steroids and stimulants prohibited for use in elite sport competition.[137]

AN INCREASING CHALLENGE TO FAIR COMPETITION

Examples of ergogenic use by athletes date to antiquity. Many of the early "sports medicine" physicians encouraged Roman and Greek athletes to eat raw meat before competing to enhance their "animal competitiveness." In more modern times, the winner of the marathon in the 1904 Summer Olympic Games (officially known as the Games of the III Olympiad held in St. Louis, MO), Thomas John Hicks, a Briton running for the United States (see www.olympic.org/st-louis-1904-summer-olympics), consumed a small quantity of brandy and a nervous system stimulant—strychnine sulphate (a common rat poison)—administered by his physician several times during the race, designed to improve his performance.[290] Of the 279 medals won by the top ten nations, the host nation United States won 239 medals (78 gold, 82 silver, 79 bronze). Over the next 60 years of Olympic competition, a huge reversal occurred in the medal count, primarily because of better training methods, but also from the introduction of performance enhancing substances. For example, in the early 1960s, Soviet and American weightlifters used anabolic steroids just prior to competition, and this trend spread rapidly to most strength athletes in weightlifting and track and field. This was a time before steroids were banned, when world records were changing rapidly,[91] and accomplished world-class athletes admitted to steroid use (e.g., Harold Connolly, 1956 Olympic champion in the hammer throw; Dallas Long, 1964 Olympic shotput winner; Randy Matson, 1968 Olympic shotput champion; and Russ Hodge, world decathlon record holder). In the 1970s, Olympic athletes

were encouraged by their "personal nutritionists" to consume high-carbohydrate foods before competitions held in and around the city of Olympia (http://www.perseus.tufts.edu/Olympics/site_1q.html) to decrease muscle fatigue. Even this type of nutritional manipulation was not a unique phenomenon, having been practiced by Greek athletes in the ancient Olympic Games (776 B.C.–394 A.D.; http://www.olympic.org/ancient-olympic-games). Extreme examples included organotherapy (the eating of animal and human organs) to improve vigor, vitality, and performance in athletic contests.[10]

The incorporation of ergogenic aids including illegal drugs to improve competitive achievement in almost all sports has been making headlines for the past 60 years. Unfortunately, the prohibited use of performance-enhancing drugs (PEDs) has not abated, and present-day cycling competitions (including the high-profile disqualification of Lance Armstrong for admitted drug use in the 2012 Tour de France), track and field, car racing, boxing, mixed martial arts, cricket, weightlifting and bodybuilding, National Basketball Association, Major League Baseball, National Football League, and Major League Soccer have not been immune to such practices (http://www.ncbi.nlm.nih.gov/pmc/articles/PMC1859606/).

thePoint   Appendix I, available online at http://thepoint.lww.com/mkk8e, provides the United States Olympic Committee (USOC) National Anti-Doping Policy Statement of Prohibited Substances and Methods.

The Price of Lying and Cheating: The Rise, Fall, and Dishonor of Cyclist Lance Armstrong

On June 12, 2012, the US Anti-Doping Agency (USADA), a quasi-governmental agency that polices anti-doping in sports in the United States, brought formal doping charges against elite cyclist Lance Armstrong. The accusations alleged that the USADA collected blood samples from him in 2009 and 2010 that were "fully consistent with blood manipulation including EPO (erythropoietin) use and/or blood transfusions." The charges also alleged that "multiple riders with firsthand knowledge" will testify that Armstrong used the blood booster EPO, blood transfusions, testosterone, and masking agents, and that he distributed and administered drugs to other cyclists from 1998 to 2005. In addition to the specific accusations against Armstrong, the charges maintained that his cycling teams engaged in a "doping conspiracy" that involved "team officials, employees, doctors, and elite cyclists of the United States Postal Service and Discovery Channel cycling teams." In June 2012, the USADA formally charged Armstrong with having used performance-enhancing drugs and in August they announced disqualification from all his race results since August 1998 (including all seven Tour de France titles) and a lifetime ban from competition, which applies in all sports that follow the World Anti-Doping Agency code. In the words of the USADA's chief executive: "It's a heartbreaking example of win at all costs overtaking the fair and safe option. There is no success in cheating to win." On October 22, 2012, the Union Cycliste Internationale (http://www.uci.ch/), the cycling sports governing body, endorsed the USADA's verdict and confirmed both the lifetime ban and the stripping of his titles.

Urine Testing for Steroids

The primary "gold-standard" method for detecting illicit drug use in athletes involves urine testing. Testing consists of two steps, the first being the screening test. If the first screen turns out positive for traces of performance-enhancing drugs, a second step, known as the confirmation test, is then applied to samples that test positive during the screening test. Screening tests are usually done by immunoassay methods. The confirmation test in most laboratories (and all testing labs certified by SAMHSA—Substance Abuse and Mental Health Services Administration—a branch of the US Department of Health and Human Services; http://www.samhsa.gov), is performed using mass spectrometry. This precise analytical methodology assesses the mass-to-charge ratio of charged particles in a particular chemical substance. The sample, after being vaporized, creates charged particles after bombardment by an electron beam, and further analyzed into the precise amount of the chemical present. The distinct pattern or "signature" made by the molecules in the chemical deflected by the field is compared with known patterns of chemicals. Besides the detection of steroids, other banned substances can include alcohol, amphetamines, methamphetamine, MDMA (Ecstasy), barbituates, phenobarbital, benzodiazepines, cannabis, cocaine, cotinine (breakdown product of nicotine), morphine, tricyclic antidepressants (TCA), lysergic acid diethylamide (LSD), methadone, and phencyclidine (PCP, angel dust, supergrass). Testing time to obtain confirmation results can range from 1 day for barbituates to 3 to 30 days for steroids (http://www.deadiversion.usdoj.gov/drugs_concern/pcp.htm).

Unfortunately, highly celebrated and idolized but now disgraced Olympians were required by the International Olympic Committee (IOC; www.olympic.org/ioc) to return their medals for illegal doping during the last four Olympiads. High-profile track star Marion Jones, who won five medals (gold in the 100-m, 200-m, and 1600-m relay and bronze in the long jump and 40-m relay), pleaded guilty to two counts of lying to investigators about her doping abuse and served 6 mo in federal prison and 2 years' probation and community service.

Levels of Evidence

The National Heart, Lung and Blood Institute (NHLBI; www.nhlbi.nih.gov, part of the National Institutes of Health [NIH; www.nih.gov]) issued guidelines to consider when judging the strength of research evidence. The evidence guidelines presented in TABLE 23.1 indicate that the strongest and most conclusive evidence comes from randomized, double-blind, placebo-controlled studies published in peer-reviewed journals. But even the results of the best-designed research may not be enough. Reproducible results become an important part of the evaluation process such that strongest evidence emerges from the cumulative body of scientific literature and not simply the results of one study. Clearly, it is highly desirable that research evidence be strong before making recommendations about a given ergogenic aid. This, however, is not always possible, and recommendations are made supported only by fair or limited evidence, often anecdotal in nature. We maintain that until strong evidence supports use of a purported ergogenic substance, athletes and those involved in training, coaching, and advising these individuals should understand the relative strength of available research in this area, as presented in Table 23.1.

TABLE 23.1   Levels of Evidence on Which to Judge Research Findings

Evidence Category	Source of Evidence	Definition and Comment
I	Randomized controlled trials (RCTs) involving a rich body of data	Evidence from end points of well-designed RCTs (or trials that depart only minimally from randomization) that provide a consistent pattern of findings in the population for which the recommendation is made. Requires substantial number of participants. Very high confidence in findings.
II	RCTs involving a limited body of data	Evidence from endpoint of intervention studies that include only a limited number of RCTs, post hoc or subgroup analysis of RCTs, or meta-analysis of RCTs. In general this line of evidence is less convincing than level I because of some inconsistency in the results between studies.
III	Nonrandomized trials and observational studies	Evidence derived from outcomes of uncontrolled or nonrandomized trials or from observational studies.
IV	Panel consensus judgment	Expert judgment derived from experimental research described in the literature and/or derived from the consensus of panel members based on clinical experience or knowledge that does not meet the above listed criteria on other levels. This category is used only in cases where the provision of some guidance was deemed valuable but an adequately compelling clinical literature addressing the subject of the recommendation was deemed insufficient to justify placement in one of the other categories (I or III).

IN A PRACTICAL SENSE

A Need to Critically Evaluate the Scientific Evidence

Companies expend considerable money and effort to show a beneficial effect of an "aid." Often, however, a **placebo effect**, not the "aid," improves performance from psychological factors—the individual performs at a higher level because of the suggestive power of believing that a substance or procedure works. Those in the exercise sciences must evaluate the scientific merit of articles and advertisements about products and procedures. To separate marketing "hype" from scientific fact, we pose five areas for questioning the validity of research claims concerning the efficacy of chemical, pharmacologic, and nutritional ergogenic aids: justification; subjects; research sample and design; and dissemination of findings.

JUSTIFICATION

- *Scientific rationale:* Does the study represent a "fishing expedition" or is there a sound rationale that the specific treatment should produce an effect? For example, a theoretical basis exists to believe that ingesting creatine elevates intramuscular creatine and phosphocreatine to possibly improve short-term power output capacity. In contrast, no rationale exists to hypothesize that hyperhydration, breathing hyperoxic gas, or ingesting medium-chain triacylglycerols should enhance 100-m dash performance.

SUBJECTS

- *Animals or humans:* Many diverse mammals exhibit similar physiologic and metabolic dynamics, yet significant species differences exist, which often limit generalizations to humans. For example, the models for disease processes, nutrient requirements, hormone dynamics, and growth and development often differ markedly between humans and different animal groups.
- *Sex:* Sex-specific responses to the interactions between physical activity, training, and nutrient requirements and supplementation limit generalizability of findings to the sex studied.
- *Age:* Age often interacts to influence the outcome of an experimental treatment. Effective interventions for the elderly may not apply to growing children or young and middle-age adults.
- *Training status:* Fitness status and training level can influence the effectiveness (or ineffectiveness) of a particular diet or supplement intervention. Treatments that benefit the untrained (e.g., chemicals or procedures that enhance neurologic disinhibition) often have little effect on elite athletes who practice and compete routinely at maximal arousal levels.
- *Baseline level of nutrition:* The research should establish the subjects' nutritional status prior to experimental treatment. Clearly, a nutrient supplement administered to a malnourished group typically improves physical performance and training responsiveness. Such nutritional interventions fail to demonstrate whether the same effects occur if subjects received the supplement with their baseline nutrient intake at recommended levels. It should occasion little surprise, for example, that

supplemental iron enhances aerobic fitness in a group with iron-deficiency anemia. Yet one must not infer that iron supplements provide such benefits to all individuals.
- *Health status:* Nutritional, hormonal, and pharmacologic interventions profoundly affect the diseased and infirm yet offer no benefit to those in good health. Research findings from diseased groups should not be generalized to healthy populations.

RESEARCH SAMPLE AND DESIGN

- *Random assignment or self-selection:* Apply research findings only to groups similar to the sample studied. If subject volunteers "self-select" into an experimental group, does the experimental treatment produce the results, or did a change occur from the individual's motivation to take part in the study? For example, desire to enter a weight loss study may elicit behaviors that produce weight loss independent of the experimental treatment per se. Great difficulty exists in assigning truly random samples of subjects into an experimental group and a control group. When subjects volunteer to take part in an experiment, they must be randomly assigned to a control or experimental condition, a process termed **randomization**. When all subjects receive the experimental supplement and the placebo treatment (see below), supplement administration is counterbalanced, and half the subjects receive the supplement first, while the other half takes the placebo first.
- *Double-blind, placebo-controlled:* The ideal experiment to evaluate performance-enhancing effects of an exogenous supplement requires that experimental and control subjects remain unaware, or "blinded" to, the substance administered. To achieve this goal, subjects should receive a similar quantity and/or form of the proposed aid. In contrast, control group subjects receive an inert compound or placebo. The placebo treatment evaluates the possibility of subjects performing well or responding better simply because they receive a substance they believe should benefit them (psychological or placebo effect). To further reduce experimental bias from influencing the outcome, those administering the treatment and recording the response must not know which subjects receive the treatment or placebo. In such a **double-blinded** experiment, both investigator and subjects remain unaware of the treatment condition. The figure illustrates the design of a double-blind, placebo-controlled study with an accompanying crossover where treatment and placebo conditions are reversed.
- *Control of extraneous factors:* Under ideal conditions, experiences should be similar for both experimental and control groups, except for the treatment variable. Random assignment of subjects to control or experimental groups goes a long way to equalize control factors that could influence the study's outcome.
- *Appropriateness of measurements:* Reproducible, objective, and valid measurement tools must evaluate research outcomes. For example, a step test to predict aerobic

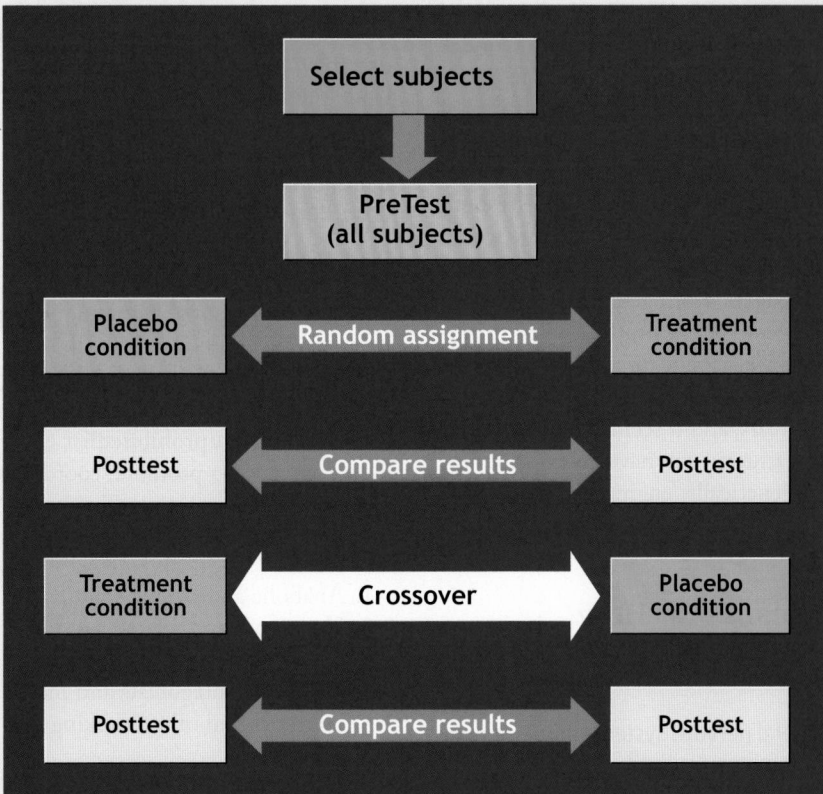

Example of a randomized, double-blind, placebo-controlled, crossover study. Following appropriate subject selection, participants are pretested and then randomly assigned to either the experimental (treatment) or control (placebo) group. Following treatment a posttest is administered. Participants then cross over into the opposite group for the same time period as in the first condition. A second posttest follows. Comparisons of the posttests determine the extent of a "treatment effect."

capacity, or infrared interactance to evaluate components of body composition, represents an imprecise tool to answer meaningful questions about the efficacy of a proposed ergogenic aid.

CONCLUSIONS

- *Findings should dictate conclusions:* The conclusions of a research study must logically follow from the research findings. Frequently, investigators who study ergogenic aids extrapolate conclusions beyond the scope of their data. The implications and generalizations of research findings must remain within the context of the measurements made, the subjects studied, and the magnitude of the response. For example, increases in anabolic hormone levels in response to a dietary supplement reflect just that; they do not necessarily indicate an augmented training responsiveness or an improved level of muscular function. Similarly, improvement in brief anaerobic power output capacity with creatine supplementation does not justify the conclusion that exogenous creatine improves overall "physical fitness."

- *Appropriate statistical analysis:* Appropriate inferential statistical analysis must be applied to quantify the potential that chance caused the research outcome. Other statistics must objectify averages, variability, and degree of association between variables.

- *Statistical versus practical significance:* The finding of statistical significance of a particular experimental treatment

only means a high probability exists that the result did not occur by chance. One must also evaluate the magnitude of an effect for its real impact on physiology and/or performance. A reduced heart rate of 3 beats per minute during submaximal effort may reach statistical significance yet confer little practical effect on aerobic fitness or cardiovascular function.

DISSEMINATION OF FINDINGS

- *Published in peer-reviewed journal:* High-quality research withstands the rigors of critical review and evaluation by colleagues with expertise in the specific area of investigation. **Peer review** provides a measure of quality control over scholarship and interpretation of research findings. Publications in popular magazines or quasi-professional journals do not undergo the same rigor of evaluation as peer review. In fact, self-appointed "experts" in sports nutrition and physical fitness pay eager publishers for magazine space to promote their particular viewpoint. In some cases, the expert owns the magazine!

- *Findings reproduced by other investigators:* Findings from one study do not necessarily establish scientific fact. Conclusions become stronger and more generalizable when support emerges from the laboratories of other independent investigators. Consensus reduces the influence of chance, flaws in experimental design, and investigator bias.

ON THE HORIZON

The day may be near when individuals born lacking certain "lucky" genes that augment growth and development and exercise performance will simply add them, doping undetectably with DNA, not drugs. In these instances, the use of "**gene doping**" misappropriates the medical applications of gene therapy that treats atherosclerosis, cystic fibrosis, and other potentially debilitating and deadly diseases. Gene doping offers the promise to increase the size, speed, and strength of healthy humans. Genes that cause muscles to enlarge would be ideal for sprinters, weightlifters, and other power athletes. Endurance athletes would benefit from genes that boost red blood cell production (e.g., gene for erythropoietin) or stimulate blood vessel development (e.g., gene for vascular endothelial growth factor). The world of sports doping has changed dramatically in the past 20 years, and it seems that thrust will continue, but this time the athletes will have access to a new arsenal of "magic bullet" genetically engineered drugs and treatments.

 ## Six Mechanisms for How Ergogenic Aids Might Work

1. Act as a central or peripheral nervous system stimulant (e.g., caffeine, choline, amphetamines, alcohol)
2. Increase storage and/or availability of a limiting substrate (e.g., carbohydrate, creatine, carnitine, chromium)
3. Act as a supplemental fuel source (e.g., glucose, medium-chain triacylglycerols)
4. Reduce or neutralize performance-inhibiting metabolic byproducts (e.g., sodium bicarbonate or sodium citrate, pangamic acid, phosphate)
5. Facilitate recovery (e.g., high-glycemic carbohydrates, water)
6. Enhance resistance-training responsiveness (anabolic steroids, human growth hormone, carbohydrate/protein supplements immediately postexercise)

PART 1 — PHARMACOLOGIC AGENTS FOR ERGOGENIC EFFECTS

Athletes go to great lengths to promote all aspects of their health: they train hard; eat well-balanced meals; consume the latest sports drink with megadoses of vitamins, minerals, and amino acids; and seek and receive medical advice for various injuries (no matter how minor). Yet ironically, they will ingest synthetic agents, many of which precipitate adverse effects

 ## Diuretics to Mask Drug Use

Diuretics facilitate urine production by the kidneys. In clinical use they are prescribed to control hypertension and reduce water retention or edema via a reduction in blood volume and total body water. For the athlete wishing to escape detection for illicit drug use, the increased production of urine with a diuretic may reduce the urine's concentration of the banned drug, decreasing the likelihood of its discovery.

ranging from nausea, hair loss, itching, and nervous irritability, to severe consequences such as sterility, liver disease, drug addiction, and even death caused by liver and blood cancer.

The World Anti-Doping Agency (WADA; www.wadaama.org/en/prohibitedlist.ch2)—an independent foundation created to promote, coordinate, and monitor the war against drugs in sport worldwide—currently bans the following 11 categories of substances:

1. Anabolic androgenic steroids
2. Hormones and related substances
3. Beta 2 agonists
4. Hormone antagonists and modulators
5. Diuretics and other masking agents
6. Stimulants
7. Narcotics
8. Cannabinoids
9. Glucocorticosteroids
10. Alcohol (in particular sports)
11. Beta-blockers (in particular sports)

Current information (2013) can be found at http://www.wadaama.org/en/Resources/Q-and-A/2013-Prohibited-List/.

Anabolic Steroids

Anabolic steroids gained prominence in the early 1950s for medical purposes, to treat patients deficient in natural androgens or with muscle-wasting diseases. Other legitimate steroid uses include treatment of osteoporosis and severe breast cancer in women, and countering the excessive decline in lean body mass and increase in body fat often observed in elderly men, people with HIV, and individuals who undergo kidney dialysis.

 ## INTEGRATIVE QUESTION

A student maintains that a chemical compound added to his diet produced profound improvements in weightlifting performance. Your review of the research literature indicates no ergogenic benefits for this compound. How would you reconcile the discrepancy?

Structure and Action

Anabolic steroids function in a manner similar to the chief male hormone testosterone. By binding with receptor sites on muscle and other tissues, testosterone contributes to male secondary sex characteristics. This includes gender differences in muscle mass and strength that develop at puberty onset. Testosterone production takes place mainly in the testes (95%), with the adrenal glands producing the remainder. Synthetically manipulating the steroid's chemical structure to increase muscle growth from anabolic tissue building and nitrogen retention reduces the hormone's androgenic or masculinizing effects. A masculinizing effect of synthetically derived steroids still exists, particularly for females.

Athletes typically combine multiple steroid preparations in oral and injectable form, a practice called **stacking**, because they believe that the various androgens differ in physiologic action. They also progressively increase drug dosage, a practice called **pyramiding**, usually in 6- to 12-wk cycles. The drug quantity far exceeds the recommended medical dose, often by 40-fold. The athlete then progressively reduces drug dosage in the months before competition to lower the chance of detection during drug testing.

A Drug with a Considerable Following

One often pictures steroid abusers as extremely muscular bodybuilders, but abuse also occurs among competitive athletes in road cycling, tennis, track and field, American collegiate and professional football, canoeing, auto racing, swimming, and other highly competitive sport activities. Surveys of United States Powerlifting Team members indicate that up to two thirds used androgenic-anabolic steroids.[68] Many athletes obtain steroids on the black market. Unfortunately, misinformed individuals often take massive and prolonged dosages without medical monitoring and suffer harmful alterations in physiologic function.

Steroid abuse among adolescents and its accompanying risks, including extreme virilization and premature cessation of bone growth, remains particularly worrisome. Boys and girls as young as 11 years of age use anabolic-androgenic steroids.[90] Teenagers cite improved athletic performance as the most common reason for taking steroids, yet many acknowledge enhanced appearance as a main reason. In this regard, a body image disturbance may contribute to anabolic steroid abuse among teenagers and adults.[101,197,288] A literature review summarizes the use and abuse of anabolic steroids and growth hormone among athletes.[123]

Effectiveness Questioned

Much of the confusion about the ergogenic effectiveness of anabolic steroids stems from variations in experimental design, lack of control groups, specific drugs and dosages, treatment duration, accompanying nutritional supplementation, training intensity, evaluation techniques, previous experience of subjects, and individual differences in responsiveness to a drug's effectiveness. The relatively small residual androgenic effect of the steroid facilitates central nervous system activation to make the athlete more aggressive (so-called *roid rage*), competitive, and fatigue resistant. Such facilitatory effects allow the person to train harder for a longer time or to believe that augmented training effects have actually occurred. Abnormal mood alterations and psychiatric dysfunction sometimes accompany androgen use.[58,100]

Research with animals suggests that anabolic steroid treatment combined with exercise and adequate protein intake stimulates protein synthesis and increases muscle protein content for myosin, myofibrillar, and sarcoplasmic factors.[223] In contrast, other research revealed that steroid treatment did not benefit leg muscle weight of rats subjected to functional overload by surgical removal of the synergistic muscle.[171] Treatment with anabolic steroids did not complement functional overload to stimulate additional muscular development.

The situation with humans is difficult to interpret. Some studies show that steroid use by men who train augments body mass gains and reduces body fat, while other studies show no effect on strength and power or body composition, despite sufficient energy and protein intake to support an anabolic effect.[95] When steroid use produces body weight gains, the compositional nature remains unclear for gains in water, muscle, and fat.

Patients receiving dialysis and those infected with HIV commonly experience malnutrition, decreases in muscle mass, and chronic fatigue. Dialysis patients given 6 mo of supplementation with the anabolic steroid nandrolone decanoate increased lean body mass and level of daily function.[136] In men with HIV, a moderately supraphysiologic androgen regimen that included the anabolic steroid oxandrolone increased lean tissue accrual and strength gains from resistance training substantially more than physiologic testosterone replacement alone.[251]

Steroid Dosage Important

The difference between dosages used in research studies and those used by athletes contributes to the credibility gap between scientific findings (often, little effect of steroids) and what most in the athletic community "know" to be true through trial-and-error self-experimentation. One study focused on 43 healthy men with some resistance-training experience.[14a] Experimental controls accounted for diet (energy and protein intake) and physical activity (standard weightlifting, three times weekly) with steroid dosage (600 mg of testosterone enanthate injected weekly or placebo) exceeding values in previous studies with humans. The men who received the hormone for 10 wks while continuing to train gained about 0.5 kg of lean tissue weekly with no increase in body fat. The group receiving the drug without training also increased muscle mass and strength compared with men receiving the placebo. Notably, their increases averaged less than men who trained while taking testosterone. The researchers emphasized they did not design the study to justify or endorse steroid use for athletic purposes because of the health risks (see next section). These data did, however, indicate a potential for medically supervised anabolic steroid treatment to restore and enhance muscle mass in individuals suffering from tissue-wasting diseases.

Risks Do Exist

Whether anabolic steroid use by athletes carries health risks remains controversial because research on risk generally has involved medical observations of hospitalized patients treated for anemia, renal insufficiency, impotence, or pituitary gland dysfunction. Some athletes take steroids on and off for years at dosages of 50 to 200 mg·d^{-1} versus the usual therapeutic dosage of 5 to 20 mg·d^{-1}. Prolonged high dosages of steroids can lead to prolonged impairment of normal testosterone endocrine function. In male power athletes, for example, 26 wk of steroid administration reduced serum testosterone to less than one half the level when the study began, with the effect lasting throughout a 12- to 16-wk follow-up.[95] Infertility, reduced sperm concentrations (azoospermia), and decreased testicular volume pose additional concerns for the steroid user.[104] Gonadal function usually returns to normal within several months after cessation of steroid use. Other hormonal alterations during steroid use by males include a sevenfold increase in estradiol concentration, the major female hormone. The higher estradiol level represented the average value for normal females; this possibly explains the **gynecomastia** (usually irreversible, excessive development of the male mammary glands, sometimes secreting milk) often reported when taking anabolic steroids.

Steroid use with training may damage connective tissue to decrease tendon tensile strength and elastic compliance.[160] Steroids also cause the following negative effects:[6,75,96,109,141]

1. Chronic stimulation of the prostate gland (with possible size increase)
2. Injury and alterations in cardiovascular function and myocardial cell cultures
3. Alterations in cardiac structure and function that include diminished cardiac diastolic motion and exacerbation of normal cardiac hypertrophy with resistance training; alterations in normal thyroid gland function and hormone action
4. Increased blood platelet aggregation, which could compromise cardiovascular system health and function and possibly increase risk of stroke and myocardial infarction

Steroid Use and Life-Threatening Disease. TABLE 23.2 lists adverse effects and medical risks of anabolic steroid use. Concern centers on possible links between androgen abuse and abnormal liver function. Because the liver almost exclusively metabolizes androgens, it becomes susceptible to damage from long-term steroid use and toxic excess. The development of localized blood-filled lesions, a serious medical condition with potentially fatal consequences called **peliosis hepatitis**. In the extreme, the liver eventually fails and the patient dies.

Steroid Use and Plasma Lipoproteins. Anabolic steroid use (particularly the orally active 17-alkylated androgens) by healthy men and women reduces high-density lipoprotein cholesterol (HDL-C) levels, elevates both low-density lipoprotein cholesterol (LDL-C) and total cholesterol levels, and reduces the HDL-C:LDL-C ratio.[60] Weightlifters who take anabolic steroids averaged an HDL-C level of 26 mg·dL^{-1} compared with 50 mg·dL^{-1} for weightlifters not taking this drug![140] Reducing HDL-C to this level increases a steroid user's risk of coronary artery disease. The dramatically low HDL-C levels among weightlifters remain low, even after they abstain for at least 8 wk between consecutive steroid cycles.[228] The long-term effects remain unknown of steroid use on cardiovascular morbidity and mortality.

| TABLE 23.2 | Side Effects and Medical Risks of Anabolic Steroid Use |

Males		Females	
Increase	**Decrease**	**Increase**	**Decrease**
Testicular atrophy	Sperm count	Voice change (deepening)	Breast tissue
Gynecomastia	Testosterone levels	Facial hair	
		Menstrual irregularities	
		Clitoral enlargement	

Males and Females		
Increase	**Decrease**	**Possible**
LDL-C	HDL-C	Hypertension
LDL-C/HDL-C		Connective tissue damage
Potential for neoplastic liver disease		Myocardial damage
Aggressiveness, hyperactivity, irritability		Myocardial infarction
Withdrawal and depression when steroid use stops		Impaired thyroid function
Acne		Altered myocardial structure
Peliosis hepatitis		

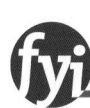

American College of Sports Medicine: Position Stand on Use of Anabolic Steroids[5]

Based on a comprehensive survey of the world literature and a careful analysis of the claims made for and against the efficacy of anabolic-androgenic steroids in improving human physical performance, it is the position of the American College of Sports Medicine (ACSM; www.acsm.org/) that:

- Anabolic-androgenic steroids in the presence of an adequate diet and training can contribute to increases in body weight, often in the lean muscle mass compartment.
- The gains in muscular strength achieved through high-intensity exercise and proper diet can occur by the increased use of anabolic-androgenic steroids in some individuals.
- Anabolic-androgenic steroids do not increase aerobic power or capacity for muscular exercise.
- Anabolic-androgenic steroids have been associated with adverse effects on the liver, cardiovascular system, reproductive system, and psychologic status in therapeutic trials and in limited research on athletes. Until further research is completed, the potential hazards of the use of the anabolic-androgenic steroids in athletes must include those found in therapeutic trials.
- The use of anabolic-androgenic steroids by athletes is contrary to the rules and ethical principles of athletic competition as set forth by many of the sports governing bodies. The American College of Sports Medicine supports these ethical principles and deplores the use of anabolic-androgenic steroids by athletes.

Specific Risks for Females. Testosterone levels normally range 20 to 30 times lower in females than in males, raising additional concerns about synthetic anabolic steroid abuse among females. Medical risks include virilization (more apparent than in men), disruption of normal growth pattern by premature closure of the plates for bone growth (also for boys), altered menstrual function, dramatic increase in sebaceous gland size, acne, hirsutism (excessive body and facial hair), and generally irreversible deepening of the voice, decreased breast size, enlarged clitoris, and hair loss. Serum levels of LH, FSH, progesterone, and estrogens also decline. These may negatively affect follicle formation, ovulation, and menstrual function. The long-term effects require further clarification on reproductive function, including possible sterility.

Clenbuterol and Other β₂-Adrenergic Agonists

Extensive, random testing of competitive athletes for steroid use has ushered in a number of steroid "substitutes." These have appeared on the health food, mail order, and "black market" drug network as competitors try to circumvent detection. One such drug, the sympathomimetic amine **clenbuterol** (brand names Clenasma, Monores, Novegan, Prontovent, Ventipulmin, and Spiropent) has become popular among athletes because of its purported tissue-building, fat-reducing benefits.

When a bodybuilder discontinues steroid use before competition to avoid detection and possible disqualification, the athlete substitutes clenbuterol to retard loss of muscle mass and facilitate fat burning to achieve the desirable "cut" look, particularly in the abdominal and back regions. Clenbuterol has particular appeal to female athletes because it does not produce the androgenic side effects of anabolic steroids.

Clenbuterol, one of a group of chemical compounds classified as β₂-adrenergic agonists (albuterol [salbutamol], bitoleraol, salmeterol, metaproterenol, perbuterol, terbutaline, and formoterol) facilitates responsiveness of adrenergic receptors to circulating epinephrine, norepinephrine, and other adrenergic amines (http://livertox.nlm.nih.gov/Beta2Adrenergic-Agonists.htm). A review of the available animal studies (to our knowledge, no human exercise studies have been conducted) indicates that when fed to sedentary, growing livestock in dosages in excess of those prescribed in Europe for human use for bronchial asthma, clenbuterol increases skeletal and cardiac muscle protein deposition and slows fat gain via enhanced lipolysis. It also increases FFM and decreases fat mass when administered long term at therapeutic levels to thoroughbred racehorses.[143] Clenbuterol has been used experimentally in animals to counter the effects on muscle of aging, immobilization, malnutrition, and pathologic tissue-wasting conditions. Under these conditions, β₂-agonists show specific growth-promoting actions on skeletal muscle.[79,291] For rats, clenbuterol altered muscle fiber type distribution, inducing enlargement and increased proportion of type II muscle fibers.[67] A decrease in protein breakdown and increase in protein synthesis accounted for the animals' increased muscle size.[2,26]

Potential Negative Effects on Muscle, Bone, and Cardiovascular Function (Animal Studies)

Female rats treated with clenbuterol ($2 \text{ mg} \cdot \text{kg}^{-1}$) injected subcutaneously versus controls sham-injected with the same volume of fluid carrier each day for 14 days increased muscle mass, absolute maximal force-generating capacity, and hypertrophy of fast- and slow-twitch muscle fibers.[76] A negative finding indicated hastened fatigue during short-term, intense muscle actions. In contrast, regular exercise combined with clenbuterol decreased muscular dystrophy progression in mice, reflected by increased muscle force-generating capacity.[291] The group receiving clenbuterol experienced increased muscle fatigability and cellular deformities not noted in the exercise-only group. This negative effect may explain findings that clenbuterol treatment negated the beneficial effects of training on endurance performance, despite increased muscle protein content.[127] Clenbuterol treatment induced muscular hypertrophy in young male rats but also inhibited longitudinal bone growth.[148] Negative effects of clenbuterol and salbutamol affected mechanical properties and microarchitecture of trabecular bone of animals. An increase of muscle mass with enhanced bone fragility increases fracture risk when treated with β₂-agonists as part of a doping regimen.[33,34] The negative effect on bone contraindicates its use for prepubescent and adolescent humans.

Echocardiographic evaluations of Standard-bred mares showed that chronic clenbuterol administration even at low therapeutic levels alters the heart's structural dimensions, which negatively affects cardiac function.[238] Effects occurred whether the animals exercised or remained inactive. Clenbuterol also caused aortic enlargement after physical activity to a degree that indicated increased risk of aortic rupture and sudden death. Clenbuterol treatment when combined with aerobic training blunts the normal training-induced increase in plasma volume in Standard-bred mares; this effect accompanied decreased aerobic performance and ability to recover.[142]

Clenbuterol: Not Approved for Human Use in the United States

Clenbuterol, commonly prescribed in other countries, functions as an inhaled bronchodilator to treat obstructive pulmonary disorders. Reported short-term side effects in humans who accidentally "overdosed" from eating clenbuterol-tainted meat include skeletal muscle tremor, agitation, palpitations, dizziness, nausea, muscle cramps, rapid heart rate, and headache. Despite these negative side effects, clenbuterol may benefit humans when used to treat muscle wasting in disease, forced immobilization, and aging. Unfortunately, no data exist for potential toxicity level or its efficacy and long-term safety. Clearly, clenbuterol use cannot be justified or recommended as an ergogenic aid.

Other Adrenergic Agonists

Research has focused on possible strength-enhancing effects of sympathomimetic β_2-adrenergic agonists other than clenbuterol. Men with cervical spinal-cord injuries took 80 mg of metaproterenol daily for 4 wk in conjunction with physical therapy. Increases occurred in estimated muscle cross-sectional area and elbow flexor and wrist extensor strength compared with a placebo condition.[237] Albuterol administration (16 mg·d^{-1} for 3 wk) without training improved muscular strength 10 to 15%.[168] Therapeutic doses of albuterol also facilitated isokinetic strength gains from slow-speed concentric–eccentric isokinetic training.[49] The acute administration of either low- or high-dose salbutamol produced no beneficial effect on aerobic capacity in normal subjects.[24]

Training State Makes a Difference

Animals. Untrained skeletal muscle of animals responds to the effects of β_2-adrenergic agonists. The increase in muscle mass with clenbuterol treatment plus training is more pronounced in animals without prior training experience than in trained animals that continue training and then receive this drug.[187]

Humans. Some research with humans shows improved muscle power output with albuterol administration.[236] No ergogenic effect occurred from salbutamol on short-term performance in two 10-min cycling trials.[62] Similarly, no effect occurred in power output during a 30-s Wingate test in non-

asthmatic trained cyclists who received 360 µg (twice the normal dose administered by inhaler in four measured doses of 90 µg each) 20 min before testing.[156] For men without asthma, acute therapeutic (200 µg) or supratherapeutic (800 µg) doses of inhaled salbutamol had no effect on quadriceps strength, fatigue, and recovery.[70] In other research, twice the recommended dose of salbutamol (albuterol: 400 µg administered in four inhalations 20 min before exercising) did not enhance anaerobic power output, endurance performance, ventilatory threshold, or dynamic lung function of trained endurance cyclists.[189] The researchers maintained that competitive athletes should not be prohibited from these compounds because they provide no ergogenic benefit, yet "normalize" individuals with obstructive pulmonary disorders. Differences in training status may explain discrepancies among studies concerning albuterol's effect on short-term power output.

Muscle Receptor's Sensitivity Changes with Training

Albuterol's ergogenic benefit supposedly comes from its stimulating effects on skeletal muscle β_2-receptors to increase muscle force and power. With exercise training, the muscle β_2-receptors undergo downregulation (i.e., become less sensitive to a given stimulus) from chronic exposure to training-induced elevations in blood catecholamine levels. This makes the trained athlete *less responsive* to a sympathomimetic drug than an untrained counterpart.

Growth Hormone: Genetic Engineering Now Common in Sports

Human growth hormone (**GH** or **hGH**), also known as *somatotropin*, currently competes with anabolic steroids in the illicit market of alleged tissue-building, performance-enhancing drugs. The adenohypophysis of the pituitary gland produces GH, a potent anabolic and lipolytic agent in tissue-building processes and growth. Specifically, GH stimulates bone and cartilage growth, enhances fatty acid oxidation, and reduces glucose and amino acid breakdown. Reduced GH secretion accounts for some of the decrease in FFM and increase in fat mass that accompanies aging. This condition reverses somewhat with exogenous recombinant GH supplements produced by genetically engineered bacteria. Healthy elderly men who received GH supplements increased FFM (4.3%) and decreased fat mass (13.1%).[195] *Supplementation did not reverse the negative effects of aging on functional measures of muscular strength and aerobic capacity.* Men receiving the supplement also experienced hand stiffness, malaise, arthralgias, and lower-extremity edema. One of the largest studies to date determined the effects of exogenous GH over a 6-mo period on changes in body composition and functional capacity of healthy men and women aged mid-60s to late 80s.[31] Men who took GH gained 7 lb of lean body mass and reduced a similar amount of fat mass. Women gained about 3 lb of lean body mass and lost 5 lb of body fat compared with counterparts receiving a placebo. Unfortunately, serious side effects afflicted between 24 and 46% of the subjects. These included swollen feet and ankles, joint pain, carpal tunnel syndrome (swelling of tendon sheath over a nerve in the wrist), and development of a diabetic or prediabetic condition. As in prior research, no effects occurred for GH treatment on measures of muscular strength or endurance capacity despite increases in lean body mass.

Excessive GH production during skeletal growth produces **gigantism**, an endocrine and metabolic disorder characterized by abnormal size or overgrowth of the entire body or any of its parts. Excessive hormone production following growth cessation produces the irreversible disorder **acromegaly** that presents as enlarged hands, feet, and facial features. Children who suffer from kidney failure or who produce insufficient GH receive thrice-weekly biosynthetic GH injections until adolescence to help them achieve near-normal size. In young adults with hypopituitarism, GH replacement therapy improves muscle volume, isometric strength, and exercise capacity.

 ## A New Test Now Available

GH occurs naturally in the body, making ready detection as an ergogenic substance difficult. Scientists and international anti-doping officials have endorsed a new blood test (with WADA approval) that can detect the use of GH for up to 21 days.[152] This extends the detection window from the previous "isoform" test (first used in 2004), which only identifies the drug's use going back 12 to 72 hr. This new biomarker test scans for the effects of exogenous growth hormone via chemicals produced by the body after its use. In addition to its applicability in the testing of Olympic and other international sport competitors, the test would also be useful for the National Football League, whose players' union has yet to agree to any GH testing because it questions its safety and reliability. No positive tests have been reported for Olympic athletes since the beginning of testing for GH in 2004, Nevertheless, eight positive tests have been reported in sports outside of the Olympics. A two-time Olympic cross-country skiing champion was banned for three years in August 2011 for a positive test by the sport's governing body. On January 10, 2013, the day after Hall of Fame voters denied entry to the superstars from the steroid era, Major League Baseball and the Players Association announced an unprecedented step to begin blood tests of players during the regular season to detect GH use. Also agreed upon was an expanded effort to detect abnormally high levels of testosterone by using a WADA-accredited laboratory in Montreal to maintain a baseline level of every player to compare with any abnormal urine samples.

No Unanimity Among Researchers

At first glance, GH use seems appealing to strength and power athletes because at physiologic levels, this hormone stimulates amino acid uptake and muscle protein synthesis while enhancing fat breakdown and conserving glycogen reserves. Unfortunately, few well-controlled studies have examined how GH supplements affect healthy subjects who undertake exercise training. In one study, six well-trained men maintained a high-protein diet while taking either biosynthetic GH or a placebo.[66] During 6 wk of standard resistance training with GH, percentage body fat decreased and FFM increased. No changes in body composition occurred for the group training with the placebo. Subsequent investigations failed to replicate these findings. For example, 16 previously sedentary young men who participated in a 12-wk resistance training program received recombinant human GH supplements $(40 \ \mu g \cdot kg^{-1} \cdot d^{-1})$ or a placebo.[289] FFM, total body water, and whole-body protein synthesis increased more in the GH recipients. No significant differences emerged between groups in fractional rate of protein synthesis in skeletal muscle, torso and limb circumferences, or muscle function in dynamic and static strength measures (**TABLE 23.3**). The authors attributed the greater increase in whole-body protein synthesis in the GH group to a possible increase in nitrogen retention in lean tissue other than skeletal muscle—for example, connective tissue, fluid, and noncontractile protein.

Nonprescription GH only can be obtained on the black market and most likely in an adulterated form. Human cadaver–derived GH (used until May 1985 by U.S. physicians to treat children of short stature) greatly increases risk for contracting Creutzfeldt-Jakob disease, an infectious, incurable, and fatal brain-deteriorating disorder (http://www.ninds.nih.gov/disorders/cjd/detail_cjd.htm). A synthetic form of GH (Protropin and Humatrope), produced by genetic engineering, currently treats GH-deficient children. Undoubtedly, child athletes who receive GH believing they gain a competitive edge will suffer increased incidence of gigantism, while adults will develop acromegalic syndrome. Additional, less obvious side effects include insulin resistance that leads to type 2 diabetes, water retention, and carpal tunnel compression syndrome created by induced bone growth. Any potential benefits of GH must be weighed against potential adverse effects. Claims that growth hormone enhances physical performance are not supported by the scientific literature. The limited available evidence suggests that growth hormone increases lean body mass, but it may not improve strength; in addition, it may worsen physical capacity and increase adverse events. More research will conclusively determine the effects of growth hormone on athletic performance.[162,175]

DHEA

Dehydroepiandrosterone (**DHEA** and its sulfated ester DHEA sulfate or DHEAS, the most common hormone in the body) is a weak steroid hormone synthesized primarily from cholesterol by the adrenal cortex of primates. The body produces more DHEA than all other known steroids. This "mother hormone" has a chemical structure that closely resembles testosterone and estrogen; a small amount of DHEA and related **prohormones**—intermediate substances in the hormone-building process—are naturally derived precursors to testosterone or other anabolic steroids. Athletes consume these products believing they will lead to endogenous testosterone

TABLE 23.3 **Maximal Force Production of Knee Extensor and Flexor Muscle Groups Before and After Training With or Without Growth Hormone Supplements**

	Exercise plus Placebo			Exercise plus GH		
	Initial	Final	% Change	Initial	Final	% Change
Concentric						
Knee extensors	212 ± 13^a	248 ± 10	17	191 ± 11	214 ± 9	12
Knee flexors	137 ± 11^a	158 ± 7	15	122 ± 12	143 ± 6	17
Isometric						
Knee extensors	220 ± 13^a	252 ± 13	14	198 ± 15	207 ± 7	5
Knee flexors	131 ± 8^a	158 ± 8	20	127 ± 13	140 ± 16	10

Reprinted from Yarasheski KF, et al. Effect of growth hormone and resistance exercise on muscle growth in young men. *Am J Physiol* 1992;262:E261.

[a]Values are mean ± SE. Maximum force (N • m) determined using a Cybex dynamometer. Concentric force measured at $60° • s^{-1}$ angular velocity. Isometric force measured at 135° of knee extension. The maximum concentric force production of knee flexor and extensor muscles increased significantly in both groups ($p < .05$), but these increments and the increments in maximum isometric force production were not greater in the exercise plus GH group.

secretion. **Figure 23.1** outlines the major pathways for synthesizing DHEA, androstenedione, and related compounds. The red directional arrows signify one-way and two-way conversions, including intermediate compounds. Those illustrated in **bold** serve as DHEA-precursor products currently available on the market. For example, androstenedione, the popular 19-carbon steroid hormone produced in gonads and adrenal glands serves as an intermediary step that eventually forms testosterone, estrone, and estradiol. These conversions require specialized enzymes (e.g., 17β-hydroxysteroid dehydrogenase for testosterone, and aromatase for estrone and estradiol). Many of these prohormone compounds only can be purchased with a medical prescription, and in the case of androstenedione, may produce undesirable estrogenic side effects (breast enlargement or tenderness, ankle and leg swelling, appetite loss, water retention, vomiting, abdominal cramping, and bloatedness).

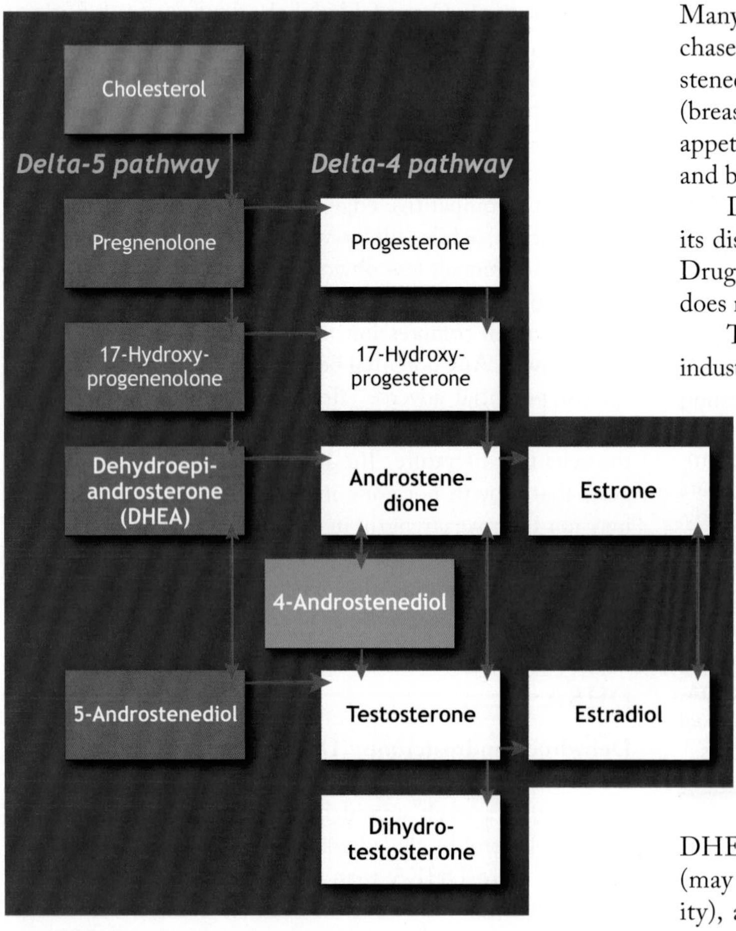

DHEA occurs naturally, curtailing the FDA's control of its distribution or claims for its action and effectiveness. The Drug Enforcement Administration (www.usdoj.gov/dea/) does not consider DHEA an anabolic steroid.

The lay press and mail-order, Internet, and health food industry and advertisements tout DHEA as a "superhormone"—

a Holy Grail that increases testosterone production; protects against cancer, heart disease, diabetes, and osteoporosis; bolsters the immune system; preserves youth; invigorates sex life; decreases joint pain and fatigue; facilitates lean tissue gain and body fat loss; enhances mood and memory and generally counters the debilitating effects of aging; and extends life. The hormone's detractors consider it the "snake oil" of the 21st century, and WADA has banned DHEA at zero-tolerance levels.

Figure 23.2 illustrates the generalized trend for plasma DHEA levels during a lifetime, with six common claims by manufacturers of supplements. Boys and girls have substantial levels of DHEA at birth, which then decline sharply (not shown). DHEA production increases steadily from age 6 to 10 years (may contribute to the beginning of puberty and sexuality), and then rises sharply with peak production (higher in males than in females) between ages 20 and 25 years. In contrast to the glucocorticoid and mineralocorticoid adrenal steroids whose plasma levels remain relatively high with aging, DHEA levels undergo a steady decline after age 30. By age 75, the plasma level averages only about 20% of that

FIGURE 23.1 • Outline of metabolic pathways for dehydroepiandrosterone (DHEA), androstenedione, and related compounds. Directional arrows signify one-way and two-way conversions. Compounds in **bold** are DHEA-precursor products currently available on the market.

in young adults. This low level means that plasma DHEA levels might serve as a biochemical marker of biologic aging and disease susceptibility.

Popular reasoning concludes that supplementing with DHEA blunts the negative effects of aging by raising plasma levels to more "youthful" concentrations. Individuals supplement with this "natural" hormone just in case it proves beneficial—typically without considering the potential for biologic harm.

An Unregulated Compound with Uncertain Safety

Appropriate DHEA dosage for humans remains uncertain. Concern exists about possible harmful effects on blood lipids, glucose tolerance, and prostate gland health, particularly because medical problems associated with hormone supplementation often do not appear until years after initiation of drug use.

With humans, cross-sectional observations relating DHEA levels to risk of death from heart disease provided early indirect evidence for a beneficial effect. A high DHEA level conferred protection in men; for women, however, elevated DHEA increased heart disease risk. Subsequent research showed only a moderate protective association for men and no association for women. Studies suggest that DHEA supplements may provide cardioprotection during aging (more beneficial in men than in women),[133] decrease abdominal fat and improve insulin sensitivity among the elderly to help prevent and treat metabolic syndrome,[271] boost immune function in disease,[269] and provide some antioxidant protection.[7]

In additional research on humans, eight men and eight women ages 50 to 65 years received either 100 mg of DHEA or a placebo daily for 3 mo and the other treatment for the next 3 mo.[185] All subjects showed a 1.2% increase in lean body mass during DHEA supplementation. Fat mass decreased in men but increased slightly in women. Chemical markers indicated improved immune function. These findings suggest some positive effects of exogenous DHEA on muscle mass and immune function in middle-age men and women. Subsequent research evaluated short-term ingestion of 50 mg of DHEA

daily on serum steroid hormones and 8 wk supplementation (150 mg daily) on resistance-training adaptations in young men.[36] Short-term supplementation rapidly increased serum androstenedione (see next section) concentrations but exerted *no effect* on serum testosterone and estrogen concentrations. Long-term DHEA supplementation elevated serum androstenedione levels but did *not* affect anabolic hormones, serum lipids, liver enzymes, muscular strength, and lean body mass, compared with a placebo for men undergoing similar training. These and similar results verify that relatively low dosages of DHEA do not increase serum testosterone levels, enhance muscular strength, change muscle and fat cross-sectional areas, or facilitate positive adaptations to resistance training.[199,278]

Concern exists about the effect of unregulated long-term DHEA supplementation on bodily function and overall health, particularly at or above 50-mg daily. Converting DHEA into potent androgens such as testosterone promotes facial hair growth in females and alters normal menstrual function. Like exogenous anabolic steroids, DHEA lowers HDL-C levels to increase heart disease risk. Conflicting data center on its effects on breast cancer risk. Also, clinicians have expressed fear that elevating plasma DHEA by supplementation might stimulate the growth of otherwise dormant prostate gland tumors or cause benign prostate gland hypertrophy. If cancer exists, DHEA may accelerate its growth. *Despite its popularity among fitness enthusiasts, no data support an ergogenic effect of exogenous DHEA on young adult men and women.*

Androstenedione: Benign Prohormone Nutritional Supplement or Potentially Harmful Drug?

The over-the-counter prohormone supplement **androstenedione,** popular in the strength training culture (in addition to norandrostenediol and norandrostenedione, which convert to the steroid nandrolone), supposedly has these four effects:

1. Stimulates production of endogenous testosterone or forms androgenlike derivatives
2. Enables more intense training
3. Builds muscle mass
4. Rapidly repairs tissue injury

Found naturally in meat and some plant extracts, androstenedione is promoted as a prohormone metabolite only one step away from the biosynthesis of

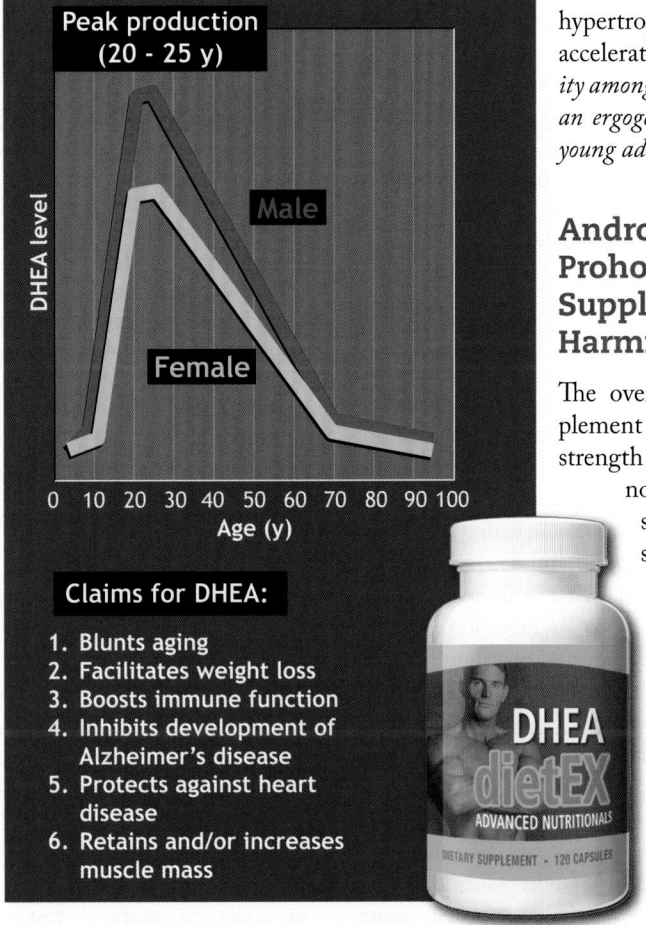

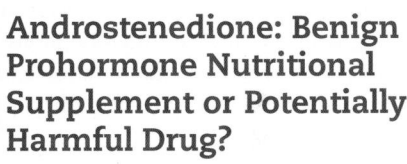

Claims for DHEA:

1. Blunts aging
2. Facilitates weight loss
3. Boosts immune function
4. Inhibits development of Alzheimer's disease
5. Protects against heart disease
6. Retains and/or increases muscle mass

FIGURE 23.2 • Generalized trend for plasma levels of DHEA for men and women over a lifetime. (Adapted with permission from McArdle WD, Katch FI, Katch VL. *Sports and Exercise Nutrition.* 4th Ed. Philadelphia: Wolters Kluwer Health, 2013.)

testosterone. The National Football League, National Collegiate Athletic Association, Men's Tennis Association, and WADA ban its use because they believe it provides unfair competitive advantage and may endanger health.

INTEGRATIVE QUESTION

Respond to this question: If testosterone, growth hormone, and DHEA occur naturally in the body, what harm could exist in supplementing with these "natural" compounds?

By calling the substance a supplement and avoiding any claims of medical benefit, savvy marketers created a lucrative business for androstenedione, mostly via Internet sales and over-the-counter at health food stores. The public can purchase androstenedione-containing chewing gum and steroid lozenges that dissolve under the tongue at grocery and pharmacy stores.

Androstenedione, an intermediate precursor hormone between DHEA and testosterone, aids the liver in synthesizing other biologically active steroid hormones. Androstenedione is normally produced by the adrenal glands and gonads and converted to testosterone enzymatically by 17β-hydroxysteroid dehydrogenase found in the body's diverse tissues. It also serves as an estrogen precursor.

Taking exogenous androstenedione raises testosterone levels. Daily oral treatment with 200 mg of 4-androstene-3,17-dione or 200 mg of 4-androstene-3β,17β-diol increased peripheral plasma total and free testosterone concentrations compared with a placebo.[80] Androstenedione dosages up to 300 mg daily elevated testosterone levels by 34%.[155] Chronic androstenedione administration also elevates serum estradiol and estrone in men and women, perhaps offsetting any potential anabolic effect.

Little scientific evidence supports claims of androstenedione's ergogenic effectiveness or anabolic qualities. One study systematically evaluated whether short- and long-term androstenedione supplementation elevates blood testosterone concentrations or enhances muscle size and strength gains during resistance training.[146a] In one phase of the investigation, young adult men received either a single 100-mg dose of androstenedione or a placebo containing 250 mg of rice flour. Serum androstenedione rose 175% during the first 60 min following ingestion and then increased further to about 350% above baseline values between minutes 90 and 270. Short-term supplementation did *not* affect serum concentrations of either free or total testosterone.

In the experiment's second phase, 20 young, untrained men received 300 mg of androstenedione daily ($N = 10$) or 250 mg of a rice flour placebo ($N = 10$) during weeks 1, 2, 4, 5, 7, and 8 of an 8-wk total-body resistance-training program. Serum androstenedione levels increased 100% in the androstenedione-supplemented group and remained elevated throughout training. Serum testosterone levels remained higher in the androstenedione-supplemented group than in the placebo group before and following supplementation. Free and total testosterone levels remained unaltered for both groups. Serum estradiol and

estrone concentrations only increased during training for the supplemented group, suggesting increased aromatization of the ingested androstenedione to estrogens. Resistance training increased muscle strength and lean body mass and reduced body fat for both groups, but *no* synergistic effect emerged for the group supplemented with androstenedione. The supplement produced a 12% HDL-C *reduction* after only 2 wk, which remained lower for the 8 wk of training and supplementation. Serum liver enzyme concentrations stayed within normal limits for both groups throughout the experiment.

Research to date verifies that prohormone nutritional supplements (DHEA, androstenedione, androstenediol, and other prohormone compounds) do not produce anabolic or ergogenic effects, despite heavily promoted marketing and advertising claims. Research findings show *no effect* of androstenedione supplementation on basal serum concentrations of testosterone or training response for muscle size and strength and body composition. The potential negative effects of the HDL-C reduction on overall heart disease risk and the elevated serum estrogen levels on risk of gynecomastia and possibly pancreatic and other cancers cause concern. Findings must be viewed within the context of this specific study because subjects took smaller amounts of androstenedione than the 500 to 1200 mg per day routinely consumed for ergogenic purposes.

Summary of Research Findings Concerning Androstenediones

- Conflicting findings about elevation of plasma testosterone concentrations
- No favorable effect on muscle mass
- No favorable effect on muscular performance
- No favorable alterations in body composition
- Elevates a variety of estrogen subfractions
- No favorable effect on muscle protein synthesis or tissue anabolism
- Impairs blood lipid profile in healthy men
- Increases likelihood of a positive steroid test result

Modified Versions of Androstenedione Available

Norandrostenedione and norandrostenediol represent norsteroid compounds available over the counter in the United States. They are chemically similar to androstenedione and androstenediol with only slight chemical modification without converting to testosterone, but do convert to the steroid nandrolone. These modifications should theoretically confer anabolic effects via the compounds' direct activation of skeletal muscle's androgen receptors. To test this hypothesis, research evaluated 8 wk of low-dose norsteroid supplementation on body composition, girth measures, muscular strength, and mood states of young adult, resistance-trained men.[263] Each subject did resistance training 4 days weekly for the duration of the study.

Norsteroid supplementation provided *no additional effect* on any of the body composition or exercise performance variables.

Competitive Athletes Beware

Elite athletes who take androstenedione can fail a urine screening test for the banned anabolic steroid nandrolone because the supplement often contains contaminates with trace amounts of 19-norandrosterone, the standard marker for nandrolone use. Many androstenedione preparations are grossly mislabeled. Analysis of nine different brands of 100-mg doses indicate wide fluctuations in overall content ranging from 0 to 103 mg of androstenedione, with one brand contaminated with testosterone.[52]

 INTEGRATIVE QUESTION

Outline the points you would make in a talk to a high school football team concerning whether they should consider using performance-enhancing chemicals and hormones.

Amino Acid Supplementation

An emerging trend involves using nutrition as a "legal" alternative to activate the body's normal anabolic mechanisms. Highly specific dietary changes supposedly create a hormonal milieu that facilitates protein synthesis in skeletal muscle. Weightlifters, bodybuilders, and fitness enthusiasts routinely consume amino acid supplements, believing they boost the body's natural production of testosterone, GH, insulin, or insulin-like growth factor I (IGF-I) to improve muscle size and strength and decrease body fat. The rationale for nutritional ergogenic stimulants comes from the clinical use of amino acid infusion or ingestion to regulate anabolic hormones in deficient patients.

Research on healthy subjects *does not* provide convincing evidence for an ergogenic effect of a generalized *regular dietary intake* of amino acid supplements above the recommended protein intake on hormone secretion, training responsiveness, or physical performance. In studies with appropriate design and statistical analysis, oral supplements of arginine, lysine, ornithine, tyrosine, and other amino acids, either singly or in combination, produced no positive effect on GH levels,[61,154] insulin secretion,[38,94] diverse measures of anaerobic power,[93] or all-out running performance at $\dot{V}O_{2max}$.[248] Elite junior weightlifters who regularly supplemented with all 20 amino acids did not improve physical performance or change resting or exercise levels of testosterone, cortisol, or GH.[100] Regular intake of amino acids in the quantities recommended in commercial supplements does not benefit the hormonal profile, body composition and muscle size, or physical performance. Indiscriminate consumption of amino acid supplements at dosages considered pharmacologic rather than nutritional raises the possibility of direct toxic effects or the creation of an amino acid imbalance.

Specific Timing of Nutrient Intake Can Stimulate an Anabolic Effect

Manipulation and timing of intake of nutritional variables in the immediate pre- and postexercise periods can affect responsiveness to resistance training (see "In a Practical Sense: Nutrient Timing to Optimize Muscle Response to Resistance Training"). This occurs via mechanisms that alter nutrient availability, enzyme activity, circulating metabolites and hormonal secretions, interactions with receptors on target tissues, and gene translation and transcription.[85,146,259] Resistance training stimulates protein synthesis and protein degradation in exercised muscle fibers. Muscle hypertrophy occurs when a *net increase* in protein synthesis results from a shift in the body's normal dynamic state of synthesis and degradation. The normal hormonal milieu of insulin and GH levels in the period following resistance exercise stimulates the muscle fiber's anabolic processes while inhibiting muscle protein degradation. Dietary modifications immediately prior to physical activity and/or in the recovery period that increase amino acid transport into muscles, raise energy availability, or increase anabolic hormones, particularly insulin, should theoretically increase the rate of anabolism and/or depress catabolism. Either effect would create a positive body protein balance to improve muscle growth and strength.

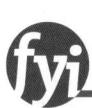 ## Four Goals for Optimizing Postexercise Recovery with Nutritional Strategies

1. Minimize activity-induced muscle cell damage and protein breakdown
2. Facilitate protein synthesis by muscle in the recovery period
3. Replenish fuel reserves for energy and tissue synthesis depleted by previous exercise
4. Provide nutrients to protect against inflammation and suppression of the immune system

Carbohydrate–Protein-Creatine Supplementation in Recovery Augments Hormonal Response to Resistance Exercise. Studies of hormonal dynamics and protein anabolism indicate a transient but potential ergogenic effect of up to a fourfold increase in protein synthesis[210] of carbohydrate and/or protein supplements consumed *prior to*[43,258,287] or *immediately following*[29,129,177] a resistance exercise workout. Supplementation in the immediate postexercise period also can enhance repair and synthesis of muscle proteins following aerobic activity.[17,157,184] Protein sources producing a slow amino acid release when consumed immediately before resistance exercise are as effective as rapidly digested proteins in promoting postexercise muscle protein synthesis.[43]

In one study, drug-free male weightlifters with at least 2 years of training experience consumed carbohydrate and protein supplements immediately after a standard workout.[53] Treatment included either (1) placebo of pure water or a supplement of (2) carbohydrate (1.5 g per kg body mass),

(3) protein (1.38 g per kg body mass), or (4) carbohydrate–protein (1.06 g carbohydrate plus 0.41 g protein per kg body mass) consumed immediately following and then 2 hr after the training session. Each nutritive supplement produced a hormonal environment including elevated plasma insulin and GH concentrations during recovery more conducive to protein synthesis and muscle tissue growth than the placebo condition. Subsequent research showed that protein–carbohydrate supplementation before and immediately following resistance training altered the metabolic and hormonal responses to 3 consecutive days of heavy resistance training.[150] Changes in the immediate recovery period included increased concentrations of glucose, insulin, GH, and IGF-I and decreased blood lactate concentration. Such data provide indirect evidence for a possible training benefit. This translated to enhanced glycogen and protein synthesis in recovery from increased carbohydrate and/or protein intake immediately following a workout.

Research compared the effects of the strategic consumption of protein and carbohydrate before and/or after each workout compared with supplementation in the hours not close to the workout on muscle fiber hypertrophy, muscular strength, and body composition. Resistance-trained men matched for strength were placed in one of two groups; one group consumed a supplement (1 g per kg body weight) containing protein–creatine–glucose immediately before and after resistance training, while the other group received the same supplement dose in the morning and late evening of the workout day. Measurements of body composition by dual energy x-ray absorptiometry (DXA; see Chapter 28), strength (1-RM), muscle fiber type, cross-sectional area, contractile protein, creatine, and glycogen content from vastus lateralis muscle biopsies took place the week prior to and immediately after a 10-wk training program. Supplementation in the immediate pre/post exercise period produced a significantly greater increase in lean body mass and 1-RM strength in two of three measures (**Fig. 23.3**). Body composition changes were supported by greater increases in muscle cross-sectional area of the type II muscle fibers and their contractile protein content. These findings indicate that supplement timing provides a simple but effective strategy to enhance the desired adaptations from resistance training.

Postexercise Glucose Augments Protein Balance After Resistance-Training. Research with postexercise glucose ingestion complements the previously described studies of carbohydrate–protein supplementation following resistance training. Healthy men familiar with resistance training performed 8 sets of 10 repetitions of unilateral knee extensor exercise at 85% of maximum strength in a placebo-controlled, randomized, double-blind trial. Immediately after the exercise session and 1 hr later, subjects received either a glucose supplement (1.0 g per kg body mass) or a placebo of Nutrasweet. Measurements consisted of urinary 3-methylhistidine excretion (3-MH) as a marker of muscle protein degradation, vastus lateralis muscle incorporation rate for the amino acid leucine (L-[l-^{13}C]leucine) to indicate protein synthesis,

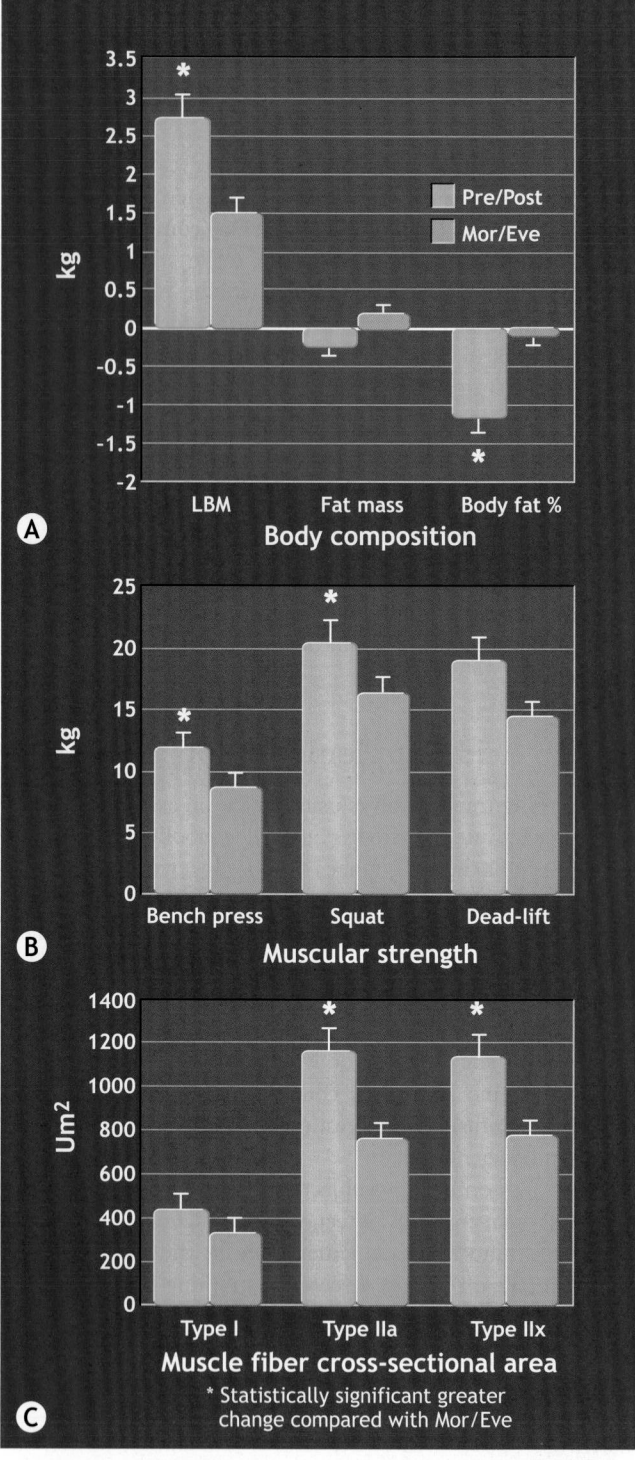

FIGURE 23.3 • Effects of receiving a supplement (1 g per kg of body weight) of protein, creatine, and glucose immediately before and after resistance (**Pre/Post**) exercise training or in the early morning (Mor) or late evening (Eve) of the training day on changes in (**A**) body composition, (**B**) 1-RM strength, and (**C**) muscle cross-sectional area (Adapted with permission from Cribb PJ, Hayes A. Effects of supplement timing and resistance exercise on skeletal muscle hypertrophy. *Med Sci Sports Exerc* 2006;38:1918.)

and urinary nitrogen excretion to reflect protein breakdown. **FIGURE 23.4A AND B** shows that glucose supplementation significantly reduced myofibrillar protein breakdown as reflected by decreased excretion of 3-MH and urinary nitrogen. While not statistically significant, glucose supplementation also increased the rate of leucine incorporation into the vastus lateralis over the 10-hr postexercise period (**FIG. 23.4C**). These alterations indicated that the supplemented condition produced a more positive body protein balance after exercise. The beneficial effect of a postexercise high-glycemic glucose supplementation most likely occurred from increased insulin release with glucose intake, which should enhance muscle protein balance in recovery.

One should view the effects of immediate postexercise carbohydrate and/or protein supplementation in perspective. The question awaiting answer concerns the degree that any transient yet positive change in hormonal milieu favoring anabolism and net protein synthesis caused by postexercise dietary maneuvers contributes to long-term muscle growth and strength enhancement. In this regard, no effect occurred from immediate postexercise ingestion of an amino acid–carbohydrate mixture on muscular strength or size gains of older men who did 12 wk of knee extensor resistance training.[106] Differences in study population, criterion variables, specific amino acid mixtures, overall diet composition, and subjects' age may account for future discrepancies in research findings.

Dietary Lipid May Affect Hormonal Milieu. The diet's lipid content can modulate resting neuroendocrine homeostasis to modify tissue synthesis and training responsiveness. Research evaluated the effects of an intense resistance-exercise bout on postexercise plasma testosterone. In agreement with prior research, testosterone levels increased 5 min postexercise. A more impressive finding was a close association between the macronutrient composition of the individual's regular diet and resting testosterone levels. **TABLE 23.4** shows that the quantity and percentage of dietary macronutrients correlated with pre-exercise testosterone concentrations. Dietary lipid and saturated and monounsaturated fatty acid levels best predicted testosterone concentrations at rest—lower levels of each of these dietary components accompanied lower resting levels of testosterone. These findings support prior studies that showed that a ~20% low-fat diet produced *lower* testosterone levels than a diet with higher ~40% lipid content.[208,256] The diet's protein percentage correlated inversely with resting testosterone levels—*higher* dietary protein related to *lower* testosterone levels (see Table 23.4). Many resistance-trained athletes consume considerable dietary protein, so the implications of this association for the training response remain unresolved. If a low dietary lipid intake decreases resting testosterone levels, then individuals who typically consume low-fat diets (e.g., vegetarians, dancers, gymnasts, wrestlers) may experience a diminished training response. Athletes who show low plasma testosterone levels from overtraining may benefit from changing their diet's macronutrient composition to lower protein and higher fat.

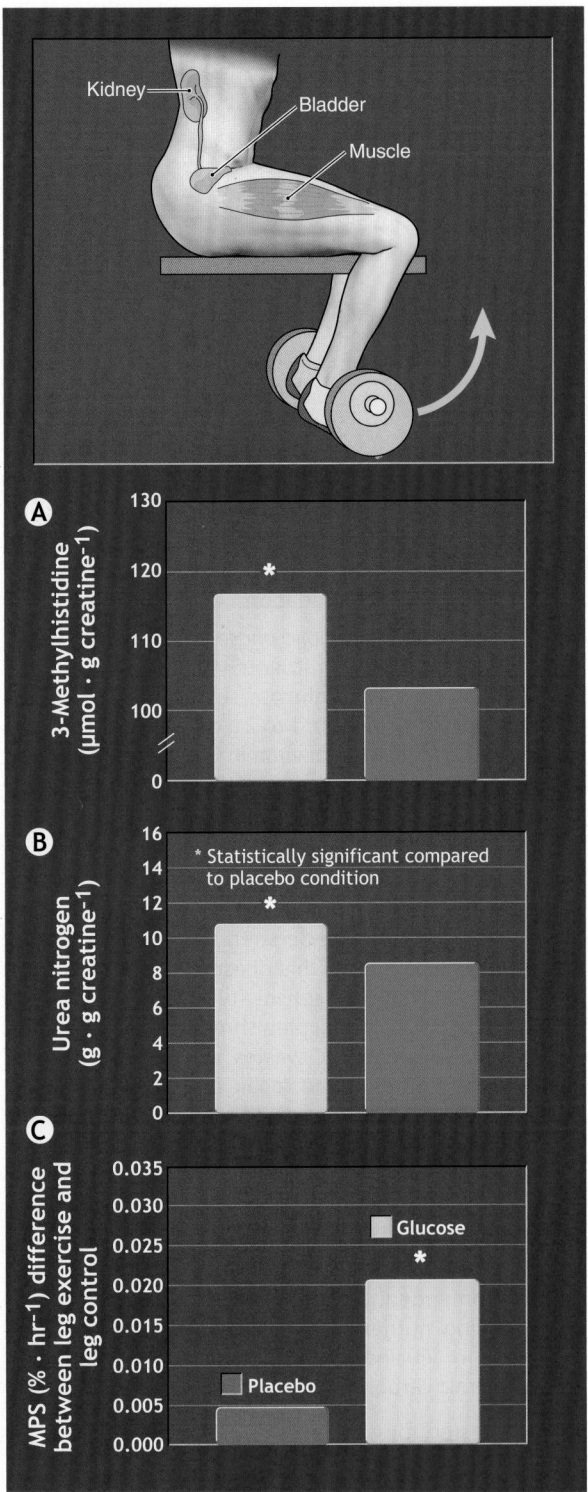

FIGURE 23.4 • Effects of glucose (1.0 g per kg body mass) versus Nutrasweet placebo, ingested immediately after exercise and 1 hr later, on protein degradation reflected by 24-hr urinary output of **(A)** 3-methylhistidine, **(B)** urinary urea nitrogen, and **(C)** rate of muscle protein synthesis (MPS) measured by vastus lateralis muscle incorporation of leucine (L-[I-¹³C]). *Bars* for MPS indicate difference between exercise and control leg for glucose and placebo conditions. (Adapted with permission from Roy BD, et al. Effect of glucose supplement timing on protein metabolism after resistance training. *J Appl Physiol* 1997;82:1882.)

IN A PRACTICAL SENSE

Nutrient Timing to Optimize Muscle Response to Resistance Training

An evidence-based nutritional approach can enhance the quality of resistance training and facilitate muscle growth and strength development. This easy-to-follow new dimension to sports nutrition emphasizes not only the specific type and mixture of nutrients but also the timing of nutrient intake. Its goal—to blunt the catabolic state (release of hormones glucagon, epinephrine, norepinephrine, cortisol) and activate the natural muscle-building hormones (testosterone, growth hormone, IGF-1, insulin) to facilitate recovery from physical activity and maximize muscle growth. Three phases for optimizing specific nutrient intake comprise the following:

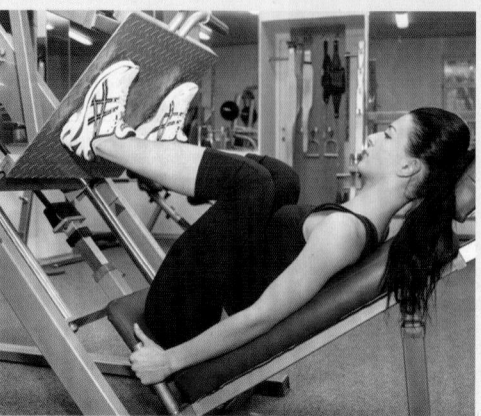

Phase 1. The ***energy phase*** enhances nutrient intake to spare muscle glycogen and protein, enhance muscular endurance, limit immune system suppression, reduce muscle damage, and facilitate recovery in the postexercise period. Consuming a carbohydrate–protein supplement in the immediate pre-exercise period and during exercise extends muscular endurance; the ingested protein promotes protein metabolism, reducing demand for amino acid release from muscle. The carbohydrates consumed during physical activity suppress release of cortisol. This blunts the suppressive effects of exercise on immune system function and lessens the use of branched-chain amino acids (leucine, isoleucine, valine) generated by protein breakdown for energy.

The recommended energy phase supplement contains the following nutrients: 20 to 26 g of high-glycemic carbohydrates (glucose, sucrose, maltodextrin), 5 to 6 g of whey protein (rapidly digested, high-quality protein separated from milk in the cheese-making process), 1 g of leucine; 30 to 120 mg of vitamin C, 20 to 60 IU of vitamin E, 100 to 250 mg of sodium, 60 to 100 mg of potassium, and 60 to 220 mg magnesium. Ingestion of the more slowly digested whole protein casein after an activity bout produces similar increases in muscle protein net balance and a short-term net muscle protein synthesis compared with whey protein. Casein and whey protein are often combined as supplements to provide both faster- and slower-acting protein sources for the recovery process.

Phase 2. The ***anabolic phase*** consists of a 45-min postexercise metabolic window—a period of enhanced insulin sensitivity for muscle glycogen replenishment and repair and synthesis of muscle tissue. This shift from catabolic to anabolic state occurs largely by blunting the action of the catabolic hormone cortisol and increasing the anabolic, muscle-building effects of the hormone insulin by consuming a standard high-glycemic carbohydrate–protein supplement in liquid form (e.g., whey protein and high-glycemic carbohydrates). In essence, the high-glycemic carbohydrate consumed postexercise serves as a nutrient activator to stimulate insulin release, which, in the presence of amino acids, increases muscle tissue synthesis and decreases protein degradation.

The recommended *anabolic phase* supplement profile contains the following nutrients: 40 to 50 g of high-glycemic carbohydrates (glucose, sucrose, maltodextrin), 13 to 15 g of whey protein, 1 to 2 g of leucine; 1 to 2 g of glutamine, 60 to 120 mg of vitamin C, and 80 to 400 IU of vitamin E.

Phase 3. The ***growth phase*** extends from the end of the anabolic phase to the beginning of the next workout. It represents the time period to maximize insulin sensitivity and maintain an anabolic state to accentuate gains in muscle mass and muscle strength. The first several hours (*rapid segment*) of this phase is geared to maintaining increased insulin sensitivity and glucose uptake to maximize glycogen replenishment. It also speeds elimination of metabolic wastes via increased blood flow and stimulates tissue repair and muscle growth. The next 16 to 18 hr (*sustained segment*) maintains a positive nitrogen balance. This occurs with a relatively high daily protein intake of between 0.91 and 1.2 g of protein per pound of body weight that fosters sustained but slower muscle tissue synthesis. An adequate carbohydrate intake emphasizes glycogen replenishment.

The recommended *growth phase* supplement contains the following nutrients: 14 g of whey protein, 2 g of casein, 3 g of leucine, 1 g of glutamine, and 2 to 4 g of high-glycemic carbohydrates.

Products tested for banned substances and certified by independent laboratories are marked with a "Tested and True" seal.

Sources:

Ivy J, Portman R. *Nutrient Timing: The Future of Sports Nutrition.* Laguna Beach, CA: Basic Health Publications, 2004.

Crigg PJ, Hayes A. Effects of supplement timing and resistance exercise on skeletal muscle hypertrophy. *Med Sci Sports Exerc* 2006; 38:1918.

Zoorob R, et al. Sports nutrition needs: before, during, and after exercise. *Prim Care* 2013;40:475.

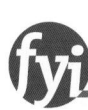

Potential Ergogenic Role of the Branched-Chain Amino Acids Leucine, Isoleucine, and Valine

- *Leucine*: an amino acid for anabolic signaling in muscle
- *Leucine*: serves as a fuel source for active muscle, especially with low carbohydrate reserves
- *Branched-chain amino acids*: decrease muscle soreness and structural damage caused by physical activity
- *Branched-chain amino acids*: reduce central nervous system fatigue in physical activity by competing with the brain's uptake of tryptophan

Amphetamines

Amphetamines, or "pep pills," comprise a group of pharmacologic compounds that exert powerful stimulating effects on central nervous system function. Amphetamine (Benzedrine) and dextroamphetamine sulfate (Dexedrine) have frequently been used by athletes. Amphetamines exert sympathomimetic effects—their action mimics epinephrine and norepinephrine (sympathomimetic)—to increase blood pressure, heart rate, cardiac output, breathing rate, metabolism, and blood glucose. Five to 20 mg of amphetamine usually exerts its

TABLE 23.4 Relationships Between Pre-exercise Testosterone Concentration and Selected Nutritional Variables

Nutrient	Correlation with Testosterone[a]
Energy, kJ	−0.18
Protein, %[b]	−0.71*
CHO, %[b]	−0.30
Lipid, %[b]	0.72*
SFA, g 1000 kcal^{-1}·d^{-1}	0.77†
MUFA, g 1000 kcal^{-1}·d^{-1}	0.79‡
PUFA, g 1000 kcal^{-1}·d^{-1}	0.25
Cholesterol, g 1000 kcal^{-1}·d^{-1}	0.53
PUFA/SFA	−0.63‡
Dietary fiber, g 1000 kcal^{-1}·d^{-1}	−0.19
Protein/CHO	−0.59‡
Protein/lipid	0.16
CHO/lipid	0.16

Reprinted from Volek JS, et al. Testosterone and cortisol in relationship to dietary nutrients and resistance exercise. *J Appl Physiol* 1997;82:49.
[a] Pearson product–moment correlations.
[b] Nutrient percentage values expressed as percentage of total energy per day.
*$p \leq .01$; †$p \leq .005$; ‡$p \leq .05$.
SFA, saturated fatty acids; MUFA, monounsaturated fatty acids; PUFA, polyunsaturated fatty acids; CHO, carbohydrate.

effect for 30 to 90 min after ingestion, although its influence often persists for longer. Amphetamines increase alertness, wakefulness, and capacity to perform work by depressing the sensation of muscle fatigue. The deaths of two famed cyclists in the 1960s during competitive road racing were attributed to amphetamine use. In one of these deaths in 1967, British Tour de France rider Tom Simpson overheated and suffered a fatal heart attack during the ascent of Mont Ventoux in Provence, France.

Dangers of Amphetamines

Amphetamine use in athletics makes little sense for the following five reasons:

1. Regular use can lead to either physiologic or emotional drug dependency. This causes a cyclical reliance on "uppers" (amphetamines) or "downers" (barbiturates)—the barbiturates reduce or tranquilize the "hyper" state brought on by amphetamines.
2. General side effects include headache, tremulousness, agitation, fever, dizziness, and confusion, all of which negatively affect sports performance that requires rapid reaction and judgment and a high level of steadiness and mental concentration.
3. Larger doses are required to achieve the same effect because drug tolerance increases with prolonged use; this can aggravate and precipitate cardiovascular disorders.
4. Inhibition or suppression of the body's normal mechanisms for perceiving and responding to pain, fatigue, or heat stress jeopardizes health and safety.
5. Effects of prolonged intake of high doses remain unknown.

Amphetamine Use and Exercise Performance

TABLE 23.5 summarizes the results of seven experiments on amphetamines and physical performance. In general, amphetamines did not affect physical capacity or performance of simple psychomotor tasks.

Athletes take amphetamines to "get up" for the event and keep psychologically ready to compete. The day or evening before a contest, competitors often become nervous and irritable and have difficulty relaxing. Under these circumstances, a barbiturate induces sleep. The athlete then regains the hyper condition by popping an "upper" prior to competition. WADA and international sport-governing groups disqualify athletes for amphetamine use. Ironically, most research indicates that amphetamines do *not* enhance physical performance. Perhaps their greatest influence lies in the psychologic realm; a placebo containing an inert substance often produces similar results believed by athletes to enhance athletic performance!

Caffeine

Caffeine represents a possible exception to the general rule against taking stimulants to promote ergogenic effects. Caffeine's

TABLE 23.5 Effects of Amphetamines on Athletic Performance

Study	Dose (mg)	Experiment	Effect of Amphetamines
(1)	10–20	Two all-out treadmill runs with 10-min rest between runs	None
		Consecutive 100-yd swims with 10-min rest intervals	None
		220–440-yd swims for time	None
		220-yd track runs for time	None
		100-yd to 2-mile track runs for time	None
(2)	10	Bench stepping to fatigue carrying weights equal to one-third body mass, three times with 3-min rest intervals	None
(3)	5	100-yd swim for speed	None
(4)	15	All-out treadmill runs	None
(5)	10	Stationary cycling at work rates of 275–2215 kg-m · min⁻¹ for 25–35 min followed by a treadmill run to exhaustion	None on submaximal or maximal $\dot{V}O_2$, heart rate, ventilation volume, or blood lactate; time on the bicycle and treadmill increased significantly
(6)	20	Reaction and movement time to a visual stimulus	None; subjective feelings of alertness or lethargy unrelated to reaction or movement time
(7)	5	Psychomotor performance during a simulated airplane flight	Enhanced performance and lessened fatigue; if preceded by secobarbital (barbiturate), performance decreased

1. Karpovich PV. Effect of amphetamine sulfate on athletic performance. *JAMA* 1959;170:558.
2. Foltz EE, et al. The influence of amphetamine (Benzedrine) sulfate and caffeine on the performance of rapidly exhausting work by untrained subjects. *J Lab Clin Med* 1943;28:601.
3. Haldi J, Wynn, W. Action of drugs on efficiency of swimmers. *Res Q* 1959;17:96.
4. Golding LA, Barnard RJ. The effects of d-amphetamine sulfate on physical performance. *J Sports Med Phys Fitness* 1963;3:221.
5. Wyndham CH, et al. Physiological effects of the amphetamines during exercise. *S Afr Med J* 1971;45:247.
6. Pierson WR, et al. Some psychological effects of the administration of amphetamine sulfate and meprobamate on speed of movement and reaction time. *Med Sci Sports* 1961;12:61.
7. McKenzie RE, Elliot LL. Effects of secobarbital and D-amphetamine on performance during a simulated air mission. *Aerospace Med* 1965;36:774.

classification and prior regulatory status depend on its use as either a drug (over-the-counter for migraine headaches), food (in coffee and soft drinks), or dietary supplement (alertness products). The most widely consumed behaviorally active substance in the world, caffeine belongs to a group of lipid soluble purines (proper chemical name: 1,3,7-trimethylxanthine) found naturally in coffee beans, tea leaves, chocolate, cocoa beans, and cola nuts and often added to carbonated beverages and nonprescription medicines (TABLE 23.6). Depending on preparation, one cup of brewed coffee contains between 60 and 150 mg of caffeine, instant coffee about 100 mg, brewed tea between 20 and 50 mg, and caffeinated soft drinks about 50 mg. For comparison, 2.5 cups of percolated coffee contain 250 to 400 mg, or generally between 3 and 6 mg per kilogram of body mass.

The intestinal tract absorbs caffeine rapidly; peak plasma concentration is reached within 1 hr. It also clears from the body relatively quickly, taking about 3 to 6 hr for blood caffeine concentrations to decrease by one half, compared with about 10 hr for the stimulant methamphetamine.

Ergogenic Effects

Drinking 2.5 cups of regularly percolated coffee up to 1 hr before exercising often extends endurance in strenuous aerobic activities; it also improves higher-intensity, shorter-duration effort and muscular strength and power in prolonged activity and enhances fatigue resistance, cognitive performance, and complex cognitive ability, and team sport performance.[71,77,124,180,209,240]

Elite distance runners who consumed 10 mg of caffeine per kilogram of body mass immediately before a treadmill run to exhaustion improved performance time compared with placebo or control conditions.[98] Ergogenic effects during exhaustive exercise at 80% $\dot{V}O_{2max}$ that follows a 5-mg · kg⁻¹ caffeine dose are maintained 5 hr later in a subsequent exercise challenge.[19] No need exists to ingest an additional dose to maintain high blood caffeine levels and ergogenic effects during subsequent activity within 5 hr. Caffeine ingestion does not impede glycogen resynthesis with carbohydrate supplementation after extreme depletion of muscle glycogen.[16] From a health perspective, drinking either caffeinated or decaffeinated coffee

Clandestine Caffeine—New Energy-Packing Foods

In 2007, there were 10,088 energy-drink-related emergency room visits—doubling to 20,783 visits in just 4 years (2011)—and 16 deaths linked to these beverages since 2004. The doubling of emergency visits can be attributed partly because the Food and Drug Administration does not currently limit the amount of caffeine in popular beverage drinks or "shots." These beverages contain caffeine in varying amounts, including small quantities of taurine, guarana, ginseng, sucrose, B vitamins, glucuronolactone, inositol, and/or other components. Herbal sources of caffeine found in some energy drinks include guarana, yerba mate, kola nut, and green tea extract, 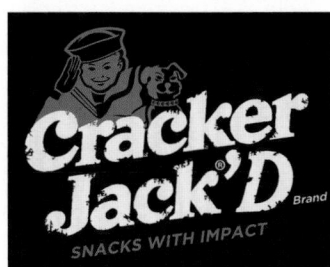 with the amount of caffeine ranging from 50 to 505 mg per can or bottle. For the more than 70 products marketed as "energy shots," each 2- to 3-oz can or bottle contains B vitamins—thiamin, riboflavin, niacin, vitamin B6, folic acid, vitamin B_{12}, and pantothenic acid—and varying amounts of caffeine and taurine. They also contain herbs and botanicals (e.g., royal jelly, ginseng, gotu kola, green tea, guarana, and ginger), and they have less sugar (and calories) than the regular caffeinated drinks. By comparison, an 8 oz cup of coffee contains about 100 mg of caffeine, which could rise to 300 mg or more per serving for some commercial coffee shops. For cola-type beverages the FDA established the maximum allowable caffeine limit at 0.02% caffeine (71 mg per 12 oz serving; http://www.fda.gov/Food/DietarySupplements/). Unfortunately, no allowable limits exist for the caffeine content permitted in foods. Popular caffeine-containing snack foods include cookies, gums, popcorn, marshmallows, hot sauce, jerky, jelly beans, waffles, maple syrup, and even popular candies such as Snickers Charged (60 mg of caffeine per 1.83 oz bar), Butterfinger Buzz (80 mg of caffeine per 2.1 oz bar), Hershey's Buzz Bites (100 mg of caffeine per piece!), and Frito-Lay's Cracker Jack D (70 mg of caffeine per 2 oz pack).

In 2008 when energy foods hit $1.1 billion in sales, the number of new caffeine-containing foods proliferated and sales jumped $500 million to $1.6 billion in 2012. The American public can expect more of these clandestine caffeine-laced foods to hit the marketplace, and with different marketing strategies—unfortunately aimed at a younger demographic. Only the FDA can implement legislation to place limits on the amount of caffeine in foods (as it now does for cola-type beverages); such legislation would take the responsibility out of the hands of the companies that produce these products to determine their safety.

(up to 6 cups a day) in a dose–response relationship inversely related with total and all-specific mortality (i.e., the greater the coffee intake the lower the risk of heart disease, respiratory disease, stroke, injuries and accidents, diabetes, and infections, but not deaths from cancer).[97]

Early research showed that subjects performed on average 90.2 min of exercise with caffeine (green triangle, bottom data line) and 75.5 min without it (orange diamond, bottom data line; Fig. 23.5). Consuming caffeine before exercise increased fat catabolism and reduced carbohydrate oxidation during exercise. The ergogenic effect of caffeine also applies to physical activity performed at high ambient temperatures.[59]

Caffeine also benefits maximal swimming performance. In a double-blind, crossover research design, seven male and four female competitive distance swimmers (<25 min for 1500 m) consumed caffeine (6 mg per kg body mass) 2.5 hr before swimming 1500 m. Figure 23.6 shows that split times improved with caffeine for each 500-m of the swim. Swim time averaged 1.9% faster with caffeine than without it (20:58.6 vs. 21:21.8). Enhanced performance with caffeine associated with a lower plasma potassium concentration before exercise and higher blood glucose levels at the end of the trial. These responses suggest a possible caffeine effect on electrolyte balance and glucose availability.

No Dose–Response Relationship. FIGURE 23.7 illustrates the effects of manipulating pre-exercise caffeine dosage on endurance time of nine trained male cyclists. Subjects received a placebo or a capsule containing 5, 9, or 13 mg of caffeine per kilogram of body mass 1 hr before cycling at 80% of maximal power output on a $\dot{V}O_{2max}$ test. All caffeine trials showed a 24% improvement in performance with no additional benefit from caffeine quantities above 5 mg per kg body mass.

Proposed Mechanism for Ergogenic Effect

A precise explanation for the ergogenic boost from caffeine remains elusive. The ergogenic effect of caffeine (or related methylxanthine compounds) in intense endurance activity has generally been attributed to facilitated fat use as an energy fuel, sparing carbohydrate reserves. In the quantities usually administered to humans, caffeine probably affects metabolism in either of two ways:

1. Directly on adipose and peripheral vascular tissues
2. Indirectly by stimulating epinephrine release from the adrenal medulla

Epinephrine then acts as an antagonist of the adenosine receptors on adipocyte cells, which normally repress lipolysis. Caffeine's inhibition of adenosine receptors increases cellular levels of the second-messenger cyclic 3′,5′-adenosine monophosphate or cyclic AMP (see Chapter 20). Cyclic AMP then activates hormone-sensitive lipases to promote lipolysis; this effect causes the release of free fatty acids (FFAs) into the plasma. Elevated FFA levels increase fat oxidation, thus conserving liver and muscle glycogen to benefit intense endurance performance.

Caffeine's ergogenic effects also appear unrelated to hormonal or metabolic changes. This suggests a possible direct action of caffeine on specific tissues, including the nervous

TABLE 23.6

Caffeine Content (mg) of Some Common Foods, Beverages, and Over-the-Counter and Prescription Medications

Substance	Caffeine content (mg)	Substance	Caffeine content (mg)
Beverages and Foods		**Frozen Desserts**	
Coffee[a]		Ben and Jerry's no-fat coffee fudge frozen yogurt, 1 cup	85
Coffee, Starbucks, decaf, 12 oz	10	Starbucks coffee ice cream, assorted flavors, 1 cup	40–60
Coffee, Starbucks, grande, 16 oz	550	Haagen-Dazs coffee ice cream, 1 cup	58
Coffee, Starbucks, tall, 12 oz	375	Haagen-Dazs coffee frozen yogurt, fat-free, 1 cup	42
Coffee, Starbucks, short, 8 oz	250	Haagen-Dazs coffee fudge ice cream, low-fat, 1 cup	30
Caffe, Starbucks, Americano, grande, 16 oz	105	Starbucks frappuccino bar, 1 bar (2.5 oz)	15
Caffe, Starbucks, Americano, tall, 12 oz	70	Healthy Choice cappuccino, chocolate chunk, or cappuccino mocha fudge ice cream, 1 cup	8
Caffe, Starbucks, Americano, short, 8 oz	35		
Caffe, Starbucks, latte or cappuccino, grande, 16 oz	70	**Over-the-Counter Products**	
Caffe, Mocha, Starbucks, short (8 oz) or tall (12 oz)	35	**Cold remedies**	
Espresso, Starbucks, 8 oz	280	Dristan, Coryban-D, Triaminicin, Sinarest	30–31
Brewed, drip method	110–150	Excedrin	65
Brewed, percolator	64–124	Actifed, Contac, Comtrex, Sudafed	0
Instant	40–108	**Diuretics**	
Expresso	100	Aqua-ban	200
Decaffeinated, brewed or instant; Sanka	2–5	Pre-Mens Forte	100
Coffe Frappuccino, Starbucks, grande, 16 oz	170	**Pain remedies**	
Tea, 5 oz cup[a]		Vanquish	33
Brewed, 1 min	9–33	Anacin; Midol	32
Brewed, 3 min	20–46	Aspirin, any brand; Bufferin, Tylenol, Excedrin P.M.	0
Brewed, 5 min	20–50	**Stimulants**	
Nestea Sweetened Lemon Ice Tea	20	Vivarin tablet, NoDoz maximum strength caplet, Caffedrine	200
Iced tea, 12 oz; instant tea	12–36	NoDoz tablet	100
Green tea, 8oz	30	Enerjets lozenges	75
Chocolate		**Weight control aids**	
Baker's semi-sweet, 1 oz; Baker's chocolate chips, ¼ cup	13	Dexatrim, Dietac	200
Cocoa, 5 oz cup, made from mix	6–10	Prolamine	140
Milk chocolate candy, 1 oz	6	**Pain drugs[b]**	
Sweet/dark chocolate, 1 oz	20	Cafergot	100
Baking chocolate, 1 oz	35	Migrol	50
Chocolate bar, 3.5 oz	12–15	Fiorinal	40
Jello chocolate fudge mousse	12	Darvon	32
Ovaltine	0		
Soft Drinks (12 oz.)			
7-Eleven Big Gulp Cola, 64 oz	190		
Jolt	100		
Sugar Free Mr. Pibb	59		
Mellow Yellow, Mountain Dew	53–54		
Tab	47		
Coca Cola, Diet Coke	46		
Shasta-Cola, Cherry Cola, Diet Cola	44		
Dr. Pepper, Mr. Pibb	40–41		
Dr. Pepper, sugar free	40		
Pepsi Cola	38		
Diet Pepsi, Pepsi Light, Diet RC, RC Cola, Diet Rite	36		
Red Bull, 8 oz	80		

Data from product labels and manufacturers, and National Soft Drink Association, 1997.

[a]Brewing tea or coffee for longer periods slightly increases the caffeine content.

[b]Prescription, 1 oz; 30 mL.

system. Caffeine and its metabolites readily cross the blood–brain barrier to produce analgesic effects on the central nervous system, potentially reducing the perception of effort during physical activity. Caffeine enhances motoneuronal excitability to facilitate motor unit recruitment. The stimulating effects of caffeine do not occur from its direct action on the central nervous system. Instead, caffeine acts indirectly by blocking the receptors for adenosine (discussed earlier) that also serve a neuromodulator function to calm brain and spinal cord neurons. The following four factors probably interact to produce caffeine's facilitating effect on neuromuscular activity:

1. Lower threshold for motor unit recruitment
2. Alter excitation–contraction coupling
3. Facilitate nerve transmission
4. Increase ion transport within the muscle

Inconsistent Effects Relate to Diet and Habitual Caffeine Use. Prior nutrition partly accounts for why individual differences exist in exercise response after consuming caffeine. Those who normally consume a high-carbohydrate diet show a depressed effect for caffeine on FFA mobilization.[280] Individual differences in caffeine sensitivity, tolerance, and hormonal response from short- and long-term patterns of caffeine consumption also affect this drug's ergogenic qualities. The ergogenic effects of caffeine occur less for caffeine in coffee than in capsule form.

An athlete should consider "caffeine tolerance" rather than assume that caffeine provides a consistent benefit to everyone. *From a practical standpoint, the athlete should omit caffeine-containing foods and beverages 4 to 6 days before competition to optimize pre-exercise caffeine's potential for ergogenic effects.*

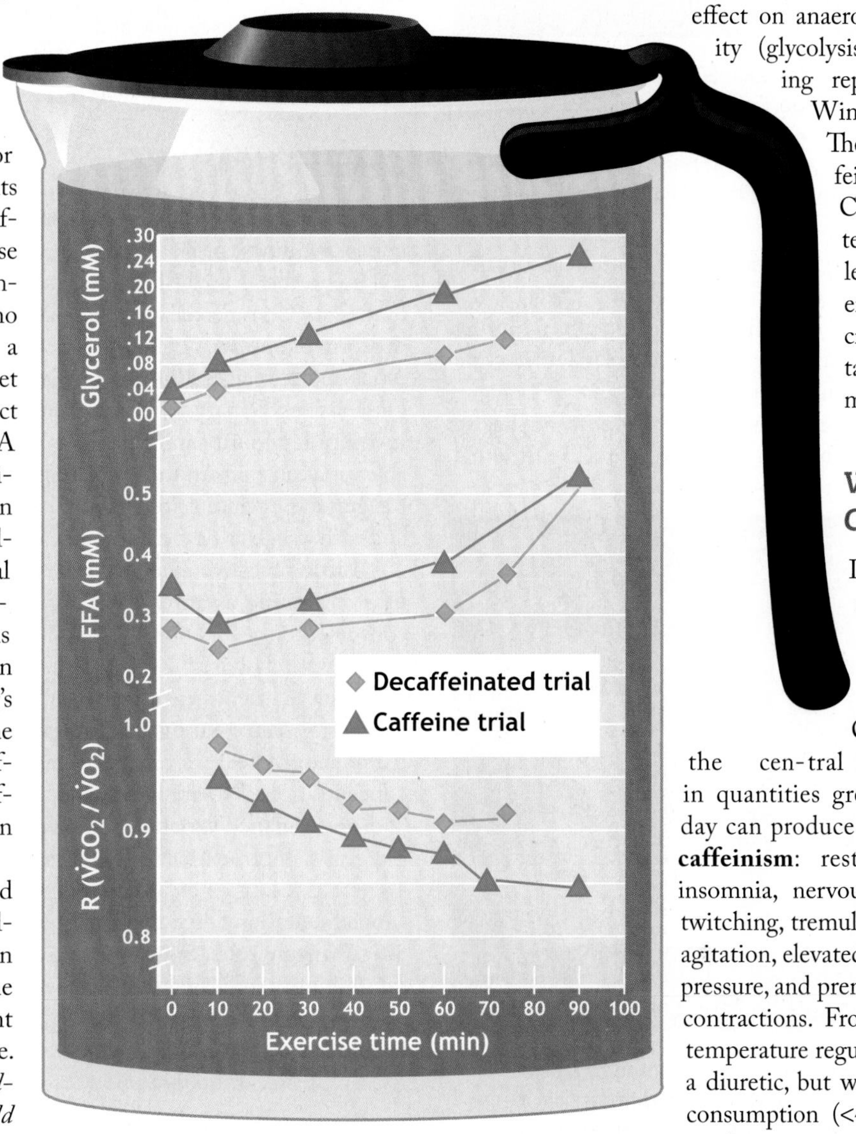

Effects on Muscle

Caffeine acts directly on muscle to enhance physical capacity, particularly repeated submaximum muscle actions.[179,226] A double-blind research design evaluated voluntary and electrically stimulated muscle actions under "caffeine-free" conditions and following oral administration of 500 mg of caffeine.[163] Electrically stimulating the motor nerve allowed the researchers to remove central nervous system control and quantify caffeine's direct effects on skeletal muscle. Caffeine produced no effect on maximal muscle force during voluntary or electrically stimulated muscle actions. For submaximal effort, caffeine increased force output for low-frequency electrical stimulation before and after muscle fatigue. Pre-exercise caffeine administration also increased by 17% repeated submaximal isometric muscular endurance.[200] Caffeine exerts no ergogenic effect on anaerobic metabolic capacity (glycolysis) as measured during repeated high-intensity Wingate exercise tests.[114] The section "Stop Caffeine When Using Creatine" of this chapter discusses caffeine's lessening effect on the ergogenic benefits of creatine supplementation on short-term muscular power.

Warning About Caffeine

Individuals who normally avoid caffeine may experience adverse effects when they consume it. Caffeine stimulates the central nervous system and in quantities greater than 1.5 g per day can produce typical symptoms of **caffeinism**: restlessness, headaches, insomnia, nervous irritability, muscle twitching, tremulousness, psychomotor agitation, elevated heart rate and blood pressure, and premature left-ventricular contractions. From the standpoint of temperature regulation, caffeine acts as a diuretic, but with moderate caffeine consumption (<456 mg) it does not produce water–electrolyte imbalances or reduced exercise heat tolerance.[8] Caffeine's effect on fluid loss lessens when consumed during physical activity because catecholamine release in activity greatly reduces renal blood

FIGURE 23.5 • Average values for plasma glycerol, free fatty acids (FFA), and the respiratory exchange ratio (R) during endurance exercise trials after ingesting caffeine and decaffeinated liquids. (Adapted with permission from Costill DL, et al. Effects of caffeine ingestion on metabolism and exercise performance. *Med Sci Sports* 1978;10:155.)

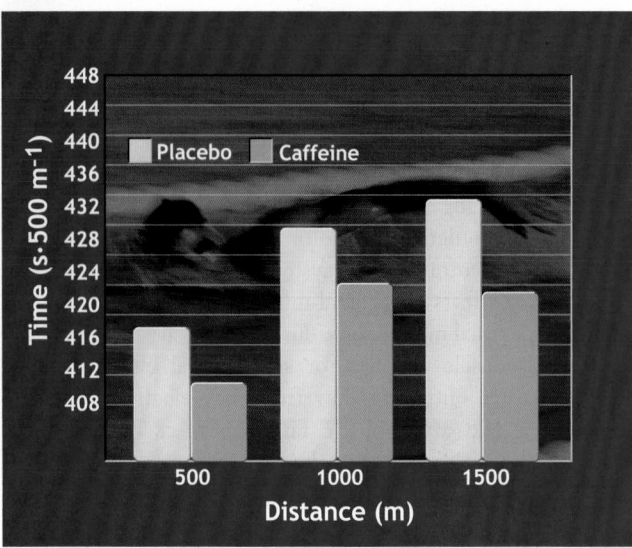

FIGURE 23.6 • Split times for each 500 m of a 1500-m time trial with caffeine and placebo. Caffeine produced significantly faster split times. (Adapted with permission from MacIntosh BR, Wright BM. Caffeine ingestion and performance of a 1500-metre swim. *Can J Appl Physiol* 1995;20:168.)

flow and physical activity enhances renal solute reabsorption and consequently water conservation (osmotic effect). Caffeine ingestion at a dose that elicits ergogenic effects during exertion has no detrimental effect on blood platelet function in young healthy individuals.[282]

The effects of excess caffeine generally pose no health risk, yet a caffeine overdose can be lethal. The LD_{50} or lethal oral dose required to kill 50% of the population for caffeine is about 10 g (150 mg per kg body mass) for a 70-kg person. A 50-kg woman has an acute health risk with a caffeine intake of 7.5 g. Moderate caffeine toxicity exists for small children who consume 35 mg per kilogram of body mass. Such observations provide clear indication of the inverted U-shaped relationship between certain exogenous chemicals and health and safety and probably exercise performance. Ingesting even small quantities of caffeine usually produces desirable effects—consuming an excess can wreak havoc.

Ginseng and Ephedrine

Ginseng and ephedrine have been commonly marketed as nutritional supplements to "reduce tension," "revitalize," "burn calories," and "optimize mental and physical performance," particularly during fatigue and stress. Ginseng also plays a role as an alternative therapy to treat diabetes and male impotence and stimulate immune function.

Ginseng

The ginseng root (*Panax ginseng*, C. A. Meyer), often sold as Panax or Chinese or Korean ginseng, serves no recognized medical use in the United States except as a soothing agent in skin ointments. Commercial ginseng root preparations generally take the form of powder, liquid, tablets, or capsules; widely marketed foods and beverages also contain various types and amounts of ginsenosides. Dietary supplements need not meet the same quality control for purity and potency as pharmaceuticals. Considerable variation exists in the concentrations of marker compounds for ginseng, including potentially harmful levels of impurities and toxins such as pesticides and heavy metals.[117]

Little objective evidence exists to support the effectiveness of ginseng as an ergogenic aid. For example, volunteers consumed either 200 or 400 mg of the standardized ginseng concentrate daily for 8 wk in a double-blind research protocol.[86] Neither treatment affected submaximal or maximal exercise performance, ratings of perceived exertion, or physiologic parameters of heart rate, oxygen consumption, or blood lactate concentrations. No ergogenic effects occurred for physiologic and performance variables following 1-wk treatment with a ginseng saponin extract administered in doses of either 8 or 16 mg per kilogram of body mass.[183] Similarly, 8 wk of ginseng supplementation failed to affect performance or recovery from 30-s Wingate tests. Supplementation had no effect on mucosal immunity indicated by changes in secretory IgA at rest or following intense physical activity.[87] When effectiveness has been demonstrated, the research failed to use adequate controls, placebos, or double-blind testing protocols.

Ephedrine

Unlike ginseng, Western medicine recognizes the potent amphetamine-like alkaloid compound ephedrine with sympathomimetic physiologic effects present in several species of the plant ephedra (dried plant stem called ma huang

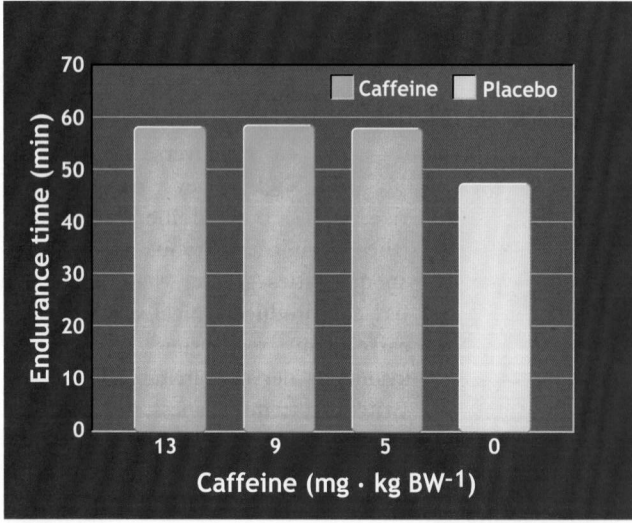

FIGURE 23.7 • Endurance performance (time to fatigue) following pre-exercise doses of caffeine in different concentrations. Cycling time (min) represents the average for nine male cyclists. All caffeine trials produced significantly better performance than the placebo condition. No dose–response relationship emerged between caffeine concentration and endurance performance. (Adapted with permission from Pasman WJ, et al. The effect of different dosages of caffeine on endurance performance time. *Int J Sports Med* 1995;16:225.)

[ma wong; *Ephedra sinica*]). The ephedra plant contains two major active components, first isolated in 1928: ephedrine and pseudoephedrine. The medicinal role includes treatment of asthma, symptoms of the common cold, hypotension, and urinary incontinence, and as a central stimulant to treat depression. Physicians in the United States discontinued ephedrine as a decongestant and asthma treatment in the 1930s in favor of safer medications. The milder pseudoephedrine remains common in nonprescription cold and flu medications and clinically treats mucosal congestion that accompanies hay fever, allergic rhinitis, sinusitis, and other respiratory conditions. This drug has been removed from the banned substance list by the IOC and placed on the monitoring program because of lack of convincing evidence for an ergogenic effect.

Ephedrine exerts central and peripheral effects, with the latter reflected in increased heart rate, cardiac output, and blood pressure. Ephedrine produces bronchodilation in the lungs owing to its β-adrenergic effect. High ephedrine dosages produce hypertension, insomnia, hyperthermia, and cardiac arrhythmias. Other side effects include dizziness, restlessness, anxiety, irritability, personality changes, gastrointestinal symptoms, and difficulty concentrating.

Despite the legal and scientific categorizations of ephedrine as a potent drug, one can legally sell it as a dietary supplement. Its claim for accelerated metabolism and enhanced exercise performance greatly increased ephedrine's popularity as a nutritional supplement. Many commercial weight-loss products have contained high-dosage combinations of ephedrine and caffeine designed to speed up metabolism, yet no credible evidence exists that any initial weight loss lasts beyond 6 mo, and the combination may produce adverse side effects.[167,234]

The potent physiologic effects of ephedrine have led researchers to investigate its potential as an ergogenic aid. No effect of a 40-mg dose of ephedrine occurred on indirect indicators of physical performance or ratings of perceived exertion (RPE).[73] The less concentrated pseudoephedrine also produced no effect on $\dot{V}O_{2max}$, RPE, aerobic cycling efficiency,[121,252] anaerobic power output (Wingate test), time to exhaustion on a bicycle and a 40-km cycling trial,[105] or physiologic and performance measures during 20 min of running at 70% of $\dot{V}O_{2max}$ followed by a 5000-m time trial.[55]

In contrast, a series of double-blind, placebo-controlled studies by the Canadian Defense and Civil Institute of Environmental Medicine using a pre-exercise ephedrine dosage (0.8 to 1.0 mg per kg body mass), either alone or combined with caffeine, produced small but statistically significant effects on endurance performance[18,20,22] and anaerobic power output during the early phase of the Wingate test.[21] An ergogenic effect of a relatively high dosage of pseudoephedrine (2.5 mg per kg body mass) enhanced runners' times by 2.1% in a 1500-m time trial.[122] Ephedrine supplementation also increased muscular endurance during the first set of traditional resistance-training exercise.[132] Whether central mechanisms that increase arousal and tolerance to discomfort, peripheral mechanisms that influence substrate metabolism and muscle function, or the combined effect of both account for any ergogenic effect remains undetermined.

Not Without Risk

An evaluation of more than 16,000 adverse reactions showed "five deaths, five heart attacks, 11 cerebrovascular accidents, four seizures, and eight psychiatric cases as 'sentinel events' associated with prior consumption of ephedra or ephedrine."[234] In general, the cardiovascular toxic effects of ephedra (increased heart rate and blood vessel constriction) are not limited to massive doses but rather to the amount recommended by the manufacturer. Most sports organizations now ban ephedrine, and the National Football League was the first professional sports league to do so. Professional baseball discourages ephedrine use, but it does not ban it. Based on analysis of existing data, the Food and Drug Administration banned ephedra on December 31, 2003, the first time this federal agency banned a dietary supplement.

Buffering Solutions

Maximal exertion for 30 to 120 s dramatically alters the chemical balance between intra- and extracellular fluids because the active muscle fibers rely predominantly on anaerobic energy transfer. Lactate accumulates with a concurrent fall in intracellular pH. Increased acidity ultimately inhibits energy transfer and contractile dynamics in the active muscle fibers, and physical performance deteriorates.

The bicarbonate aspect of the body's buffering system mentioned in Chapter 14 provides a rapid first line of defense against intracellular increases in H^+ concentration. Maintaining extracellular bicarbonate at a high level facilitates H^+ efflux from the cell, which reduces intracellular acidosis. Increasing the bicarbonate reserve before short-term anaerobic exercise might enhance performance by delaying the fall in intracellular pH associated with exhaustive effort. Variations in pre-exercise dosage of sodium bicarbonate and type of exercise to evaluate pre-exercise alkalosis have produced conflicting results about the ergogenic effectiveness of buffering agents.[231,249,265]

To improve experimental design, one study investigated the effects of acute metabolic alkalosis on exhaustive effort that increased anaerobic metabolites. Six trained middle-distance runners ran an 880-m race under control conditions and following alkalosis induced by ingesting a sodium bicarbonate solution (300 mg per kg body mass) or a calcium carbonate placebo of similar concentration. Table 23.7 shows that the alkaline drink raised pH and standard bicarbonate level before exercise. Subjects ran on average 2.9 s faster under alkalosis and exhibited higher postexercise blood lactate, pH, and extracellular H^+ concentration than in the placebo condition. Augmented anaerobic energy transfer and/or delayed onset of intracellular acidification during intense effort most likely explains the ergogenic effect of pre-exercise alkalosis.[30,206,213] The addition of β-alanine to the pre-exercise bicarbonate supplement, hypothesized to delay muscular fatigue onset, provided no added ergogenic effect.[23] Increased extracellular

TABLE 23.7	Performance Time and Acid-Base Profiles for Subjects Under Control, Placebo, and Induced Pre-exercise Alkalosis Conditions Before and After an 800-M Race				
Variable	**Condition**	**Pretreatment**	**Pre-exercise**	**Postexercise**
pH	Control	7.40	7.39	7.07
	Placebo	7.39	7.40	7.09
	Alkalosis	7.40	7.49[a]	7.18[b]
Lactate	Control	1.21	1.15	12.62
(mmol · L⁻¹)	Placebo	1.38	1.23	13.62
	Alkalosis	1.29	1.31	14.29[b]
Standard HCO_3^-	Control	25.8	24.5	9.90
(mEq · L⁻¹)	Placebo	25.6	26.2	11.00
	Alkalosis	25.2	33.5[a]	14.30[b]

	Control	**Placebo**	**Alkalosis**
Performance time (min:s)	2:05.8	2:05.1	2:02.9[c]

Reprinted from Wilkes D. et al. Effects of induced metabolic alkalosis on 800-m racing time. *Med Sci Sports Exerc* 1983;15:277.
[a]Pre-exercise values significantly higher than pretreatment values.
[b]Alkalosis values significantly higher than placebo and control values after exercise.
[c]Alkalosis time significantly faster than control and placebo times.

buffering from pre-exercise sodium bicarbonate ingestion facilitates H⁺ efflux from active muscle fibers during exercise in a dose-dependent manner.[78] This delays the fall in intracellular pH and its subsequent negative effects on muscle function. An improvement of 2.9 s in 800-m race time represents a dramatic performance improvement—a distance of 19 m at race pace brings a last-place finisher to first place in most 800-m races!

The ergogenic effect of pre-exercise alkalosis (use not banned by WADA) also occurs for women (**FIG. 23.8**). Physically active women performed one bout of maximal cycling for 60 s on separate days under three conditions in a double-blind research design: (1) control, no treatment; (2) sodium bicarbonate dose of 300 mg per kg body mass in 400 mL of low-calorie flavored water 90 min before testing; and (3) placebo of equimolar dose of sodium chloride (to maintain

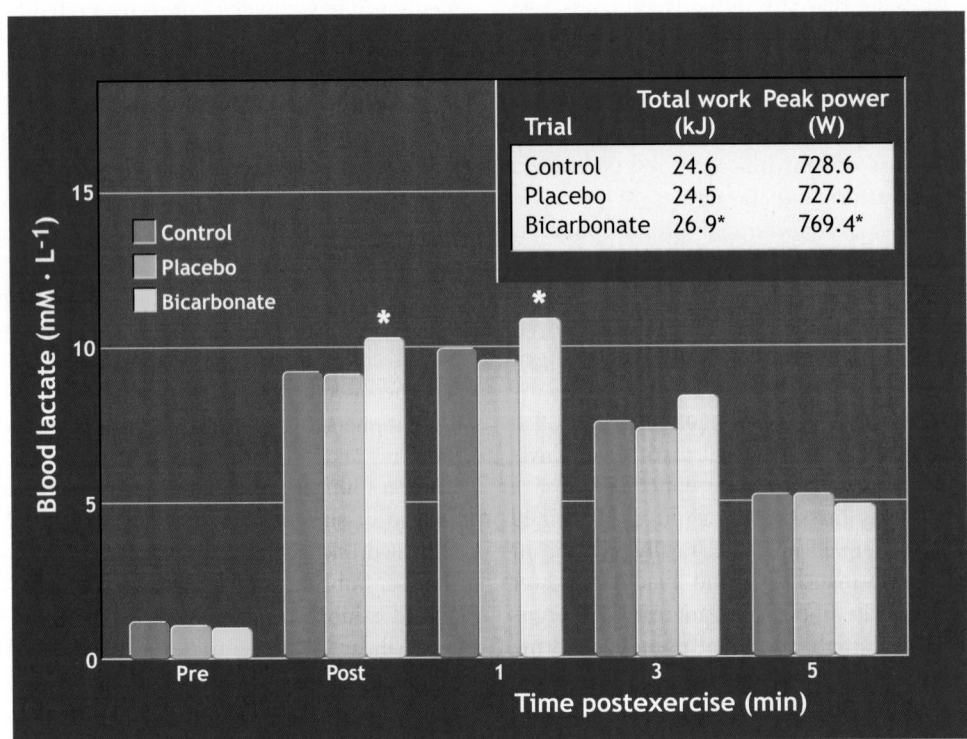

FIGURE 23.8 • Effects of bicarbonate loading on total work, peak power output, and postexercise blood lactate levels in moderately trained women. *Significantly higher than either control or placebo. (Adapted with permission from McNaughton LR, et al. Effect of sodium bicarbonate ingestion on high intensity exercise in moderately trained women. *J Strength Cond Res* 1997;11:98.)

intravascular fluid status similar to bicarbonate condition) administered like the bicarbonate treatment. Cycling capacity represented total work accomplished in the 60-s ride. The figure's *inset box* shows that total work (kJ) and peak power output (W) reached higher levels with pre-exercise bicarbonate treatment than under either control or placebo conditions. The bicarbonate treatment produced a significantly higher blood lactate level in the immediate and 1-min postexercise period; the effect explains the greater work capacity attained in the short-term, anaerobic exercise trial.

Effect Related to Dosage and Degree of Anaerobiosis

Bicarbonate dosage and the cumulative anaerobic nature of physical activity interact to influence the potential ergogenic effect of pre-exercise bicarbonate loading. Doses of at least 0.3 g per kilogram of body mass facilitate H⁺ efflux from the cell and enhance a single 1- to 2-min maximal effort and longer-term arm or leg exercise that exhausts within 6 to 8 min.[169,174,220] No ergogenic effect emerges for performance typical of heavy-resistance training, perhaps because of the lower absolute anaerobic metabolic load than in supramaximal whole-body running or cycling.[204] Bicarbonate loading with all-out effort of less than 1 min exerts an ergogenic effect with repetitive (intermittent) exercise.[65]

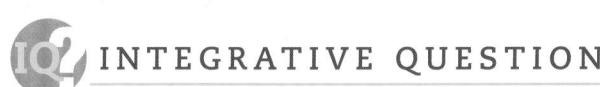

INTEGRATIVE QUESTION

Advise an Olympic-caliber weightlifter who plans to bicarbonate load because the competitive event requires all-out effort of an anaerobic nature.

High-Intensity Endurance Performance

Pre-exercise-induced alkalosis does not benefit low-intensity aerobic activity because pH and lactate remain at near-resting levels, but it may enhance aerobic activity of higher intensity. Intense endurance exercise, while predominantly aerobic, increases blood lactate and decreases pH, which negatively affects performance. Eight trained male cyclists consumed sodium citrate (0.5 g per kg body mass) before a 30-km time trial.[205] Race times were faster and plasma pH and lactate concentrations higher after sodium citrate ingestion than with the placebo. Despite the relatively·small anaerobic component in intense aerobic exercise compared with short-term, maximal exercise, ingesting a buffer before such exercise facilitates lactate and hydrogen ion efflux and improves muscle function.[173] Individuals who bicarbonate load often experience abdominal cramps and diarrhea about 1 hr after ingestion.[242] This adverse effect would surely minimize any potential ergogenic effect. Substituting sodium citrate (0.4 to 0.5 g per kg body mass) for sodium bicarbonate reduces or eliminates adverse gastrointestinal effects while still providing ergogenic benefits.[159,172]

Anticortisol Compounds: Glutamine and Phosphatidylserine

The hypothalamus normally secretes corticotrophin-releasing factor in response to emotional stress, trauma, infection, surgery, and physical exertion. This releasing factor stimulates the anterior pituitary gland to release adrenocorticotropic hormone (ACTH), which induces the adrenal cortex to discharge the glucocorticoid hormone **cortisol** (hydrocortisone). Cortisol decreases amino acid transport into the cell; this depresses anabolism and stimulates protein breakdown to its building-block amino acids in all cells except the liver. The circulation delivers these "liberated" amino acids to the liver for glucose synthesis (gluconeogenesis). Cortisol also serves as an insulin antagonist by inhibiting cellular glucose uptake and oxidation.

A prolonged, elevated serum concentration of cortisol—usually from therapeutic exogenous glucocorticoid intake in drug form—leads to excessive protein breakdown, tissue wasting, and negative nitrogen balance. The potential catabolic effect of cortisol has convinced many strength and power athletes to use supplements thought to inhibit normal cortisol release. They believe that depressing cortisol's normal rise following physical activity augments muscular development by attenuating catabolism. In this way, muscle tissue synthesis progresses unimpeded in recovery. Glutamine and phosphatidylserine are two supplements used to produce an anticortisol effect.

Glutamine

The nonessential amino acid **glutamine**, the most abundant amino acid in plasma and skeletal muscle, accounts for more than half of the muscles' free amino acid pool. Glutamine exerts many regulatory functions, one of which provides an anticatabolic effect that augments protein synthesis. From a clinical perspective, glutamine supplementation effectively counteracts the decline in protein synthesis and muscle wasting from repeated glucocorticoid use.[120] Infusing glutamine following physical activity promotes muscle glycogen accumulation, perhaps by serving as a gluconeogenic substrate in the liver.[269]

The potential anticatabolic and glycogen synthesizing effects of glutamine have promoted speculation that supplementation might benefit resistance training effects. Daily glutamine supplementation (0.9 g per kg lean tissue mass) during 6 wk of resistance training in healthy young adults did not affect muscle performance, body composition, or muscle protein degradation compared with a placebo.[47]

Glutamine and the Immune Response. Glutamine plays an important role in normal immune function. One protective aspect concerns glutamine's use as metabolic fuel by infection-fighting cells, particularly lymphocytes and macrophages. Glutamine plasma concentration decreases following prolonged intense physical activity, so glutamine deficiency has been linked to immunosuppression from strenuous physical effort (see Chapter 7).[32,225]

Glutamine supplementation might lessen increased susceptibility to upper respiratory tract infection (URTI) following prolonged competition or a bout of strenuous training. Marathoners who consumed a glutamine drink (5 g L-glutamine in 330 mL mineral water) at the end of a race and then 2 hr later reported fewer URTI symptoms than unsupplemented athletes.[50] More specifically, 65% more athletes reported no symptoms of infection than did a placebo group. The mechanism for glutamine's effect on postexercise infection risk remains elusive. For example, subsequent studies by the same researchers showed *no effect* of glutamine supplementation on changes in the blood's disease-fighting white blood cell lymphocyte distribution.[51] Dietary glutamine supplementation did *not* benefit lymphocyte metabolism or immune function with more moderate exercise training in rats.[235] Research with humans indicates that pre-exercise glutamine supplementation does *not* affect the immune response following repeated bouts of intense effort.[215,279] Supplements of nine equal doses of 100 mg of L-glutamine per kg of body mass taken 30 min before the end of exercise, at the end of exercise, and 30 min into recovery abolished the postexercise decline in glutamine following a race but did *not* impact immune function.[214]

Phosphatidylserine

Phosphatidylserine (PS) is a glycerophospholipid typical of a class of natural lipids that compose the structural components of the internal layer of the plasma membrane that surrounds all cells. Through its potential for modulating functional events in the plasma membrane (e.g., number and affinity of membrane receptor sites), PS might modify the neuroendocrine response to stress. In one study, healthy men consumed 800 mg of PS derived from bovine cerebral cortex daily for 10 days.[182] Three 6-min intervals of cycle ergometer exercise of increasing intensity induced physical stress. Compared with the placebo condition, PS treatment diminished ACTH and cortisol release without affecting growth hormone release. These results confirmed that a single intravenous PS injection counteracted hypothalamic–pituitary–adrenal axis activation with exercise.[181] A 750 mg per day supplement of PS for 10 days did not protect against delayed-onset muscle soreness or markers of muscle damage, inflammation, and oxidative stress following a bout of prolonged downhill running.[147]

β-Hydroxy–β-Methylbutyrate

β-Hydroxy–β-methylbutyrate (HMB), a bioactive metabolite generated in the breakdown of the essential branched-chain amino acid leucine, decreases protein loss during stress by inhibiting protein catabolism. In rats and chicks, less protein breakdown and slight increase in protein synthesis occurred in muscle tissue (*in vitro*) exposed to HMB.[150] An HMB-induced increase occurred in fatty acid oxidation in mammalian muscle cells exposed to HMB.[54] Depending on the quantity of HMB in food (relatively rich sources include catfish, grapefruit, and breast milk), humans synthesize between 0.3 and 1.0 g of HMB daily, with about 5% from dietary leucine catabolism.

HMB supplements are taken by fitness enthusiasts because of their potential nitrogen-retaining effects to prevent or slow muscle damage and inhibit muscle breakdown (proteolysis) with intense physical effort.

Four Ways HMB Might Work as an Ergogenic Aid

1. Serves as substrate for cholesterol synthesis in muscle (skeletal muscle depends on cholesterol synthesis for proper functioning; increased cell membrane integrity with improved cholesterol synthesis)
2. Serves as an anticatabolic agent, particularly as related to muscle protein degradation
3. Stimulates protein synthesis in muscle by augmenting the mTOR—mammalian target of rapamycin—pathway
4. Reduces exercise-induced muscle cell disruption and increased sarcolemmal integrity

Research has studied the effects of exogenous HMB on skeletal muscles' response to resistance training. In part one of a two-part study (**Fig. 23.9**), young adult men participated in two randomized trials. In the first study, 41 subjects received 0, 1.5, or 3.0 g of HMB daily at two protein levels, either 117 g or 175 g daily, for 3 wk. The men resistance-trained during this time for 1.5 hr, 3 days a week. In the second study, 28 subjects consumed either 0 or 3.0 g of HMB daily and resistance-trained for 2 to 3 hr, 6 days a week, for 7 wk. In the first study, HMB supplementation depressed the exercise-induced rise in muscle proteolysis (reflected by urinary 3-methylhistidine and plasma creatine phosphokinase [CPK] levels) during the first 2 wk of training. These biochemical indices of muscle damage were 20 to 60% lower in the HMB-supplemented group. In addition, the supplemented group lifted more total weight during each training week (Fig. 23.9A), with the greatest effect in the group receiving the largest HMB supplement. Muscular strength increased 8% in the unsupplemented group and more in the HMB-supplemented groups (13% for the 1.5-g group and 18.4% for the 3.0-g group). Added protein (not indicated in graph) did not affect any of the measurements; one should view this lack of effect in proper context—the "lower" protein quantity (115 g·d^{-1}) equaled twice the RDA.

In the second study, individuals who received HMB supplementation had higher FFM than the unsupplemented group at 2 and 4 to 6 wk of training (Fig. 23.9B). However, at the last measurement during training, the difference between groups decreased and failed to differ from the difference between pre-training baseline values. Subsequent research shows that HMB supplementation augments the response to resistance training to a greater extent when compared to unsupplemented controls. Supplementation increased resting and exercise-induced testosterone and resting GH concentrations and reduced pre-exercise cortisol concentrations.[151] Compared to controls, the supplemented group showed greater training-induced changes in lean body mass and muscle strength and power, including beneficial hormonal responses and markers of muscle damage.

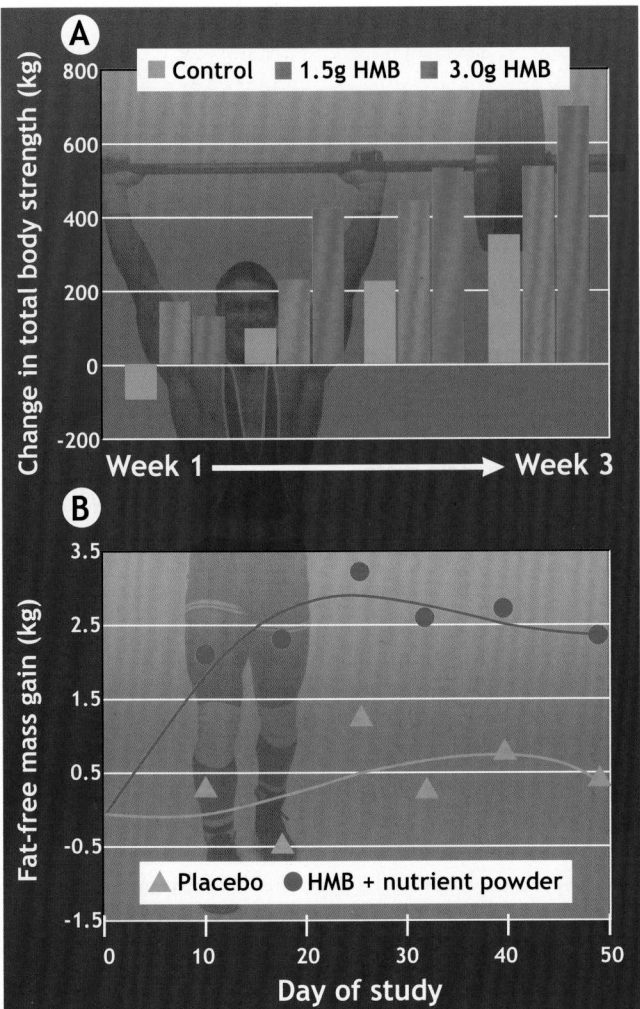

FIGURE 23.9 • (A) Change in muscle strength (total weight lifted in upper- and lower-body exercises) during study 1 (week 1 to week 3) in subjects who supplemented with HMB. Each group of bars represents one complete set of upper- and lower-body workouts. **(B)** Total body electrical conductivity-assessed change in FFM during study 2 for a control group that received a carbohydrate drink (*placebo*) and a group that received 3 g of Ca-HMB each day mixed in a nutrient powder (*HMB + nutrient powder*). (Reprinted with permission from Nissen S, et al. Effect of leucine metabolite β-hydroxy–β-methylbutyrate on muscle metabolism during resistance-exercise training. *J Appl Physiol* 1996;81:2095, as adapted with permission from McArdle WD, Katch FI, Katch VL. *Sports and Exercise Nutrition*. 4th Ed. Philadelphia: Wolters Kluwer Health, 2013.)

The mechanism for any HMB effect on muscle metabolism, strength improvement, and body composition remains unknown. Perhaps this metabolite inhibits normal proteolytic processes that accompany intense muscular overload. The results demonstrate an ergogenic effect for HMB supplementation, but it remains unclear just what component of the FFM (protein, bone, water) HMB affects. The data in Figure 23.9B indicate potentially transient body composition benefits of supplementation that tend to revert toward the unsupplemented state as training progresses.

Not all research shows beneficial effects of HMB supplementation with resistance training. One study evaluated the effects of variations in HMB supplementation (approximately 3 vs. 6 g·d[-1]) on muscular strength during 8 wk of whole-body resistance training in untrained young adult men.[102] The study's primary finding indicated that HMB supplementation, regardless of dosage, produced *no difference* in most of the strength data (including 1-RM strength) compared with the placebo group. In contrast to the findings presented in Figure 23.9A, increases in training volume remained similar among groups. In both HMB-supplemented groups, lower CPK levels in recovery indicated some potential effect of HMB to inhibit muscle breakdown. The group that consumed the lower HMB dosage increased more in FFM than the other two groups. Inferences from these findings are limited because skinfolds assessed body composition changes. HMB supplementation with a daily dosage as high as 6 g·d[-1] during 8 wk of resistance training does not adversely affect hepatic enzyme function, blood lipid profile, renal function, or immune function.[103] Age does not affect responsiveness to HMB supplementation.[275] HMB supplementation may prove most effective among untrained individuals with a greater potential for muscle mass and muscular strength accretion than more highly trained counterparts.[191,193,284]

PART 2 NONPHARMACOLOGIC APPROACHES FOR ERGOGENIC EFFECTS

Athletes often use physical, mechanical, physiologic, and nutritional means to potentiate ergogenic effects.

Red Blood Cell Reinfusion—Blood Doping

Red blood cell reinfusion, often called induced *erythrocythemia*, *blood boosting*, or *blood doping*, gained public prominence as a possible ergogenic technique during the 1972 Munich Olympics, when relatively unknown "dark horse" Finnish runner Lasse Artturi Virén (1949–), allegedly used this procedure prior to his two gold medal–winning 5000- and 10,000-m runs, and two more gold medals won at the 1976 Montreal Olympics.

How It Works

Red blood cell reinfusion involves withdrawing 1 to 4 units (1 unit = 450 mL of whole blood) of a person's blood, immediately reinfusing the plasma, and placing the packed red blood cells in frozen storage for later infusion (**autologous transfusion**). **Homologous transfusion** infuses a type-matched donor's blood. To prevent dramatic reductions in blood-cell concentration, each unit of blood withdrawal takes place at 3- to 8-wk intervals because it takes this time to reestablish normal red blood cell levels. Stored blood cells are then infused 1 to 7 days before an endurance event; this increases red blood cell count and hemoglobin levels from 8 to 20%.

Hemoconcentration translates to an average hemoglobin increase for men from a normal 15 g·dL^{-1} of blood to 19 g·dL^{-1}, increasing the hematocrit 40 to 60%. Hematologic parameters remain elevated for at least 14 days. Theoretically, the added blood volume contributes to a larger maximal cardiac output, while red blood cell packing increases the blood's oxygen-carrying capacity. Enhanced oxygen transport and delivery to active tissues provides meaningful performance benefits to endurance athletes.

An ergogenic effect occurs with infusion of 900 to 1800 mL of freeze-preserved autologous blood. Each 500-mL infusion of whole blood, equivalent to 275 mL of packed red blood cells, adds about 100 mL of oxygen to the blood's total oxygen-carrying capacity—each 100 mL of whole blood carries about 20 mL of oxygen. An elite endurance athlete's total blood volume circulates five to six times each minute in intense activity, so the potential "extra" oxygen available to the tissues from red blood cell reinfusion averages 500 mL (0.5 L). Autologous blood transfusion to boost the blood's hemoglobin/oxygen-carrying capacity to improve athletic performance cannot be detected; nonetheless, it is possible to track an athlete's blood constituents over time to note unreasonable changes based on cut-points for an overly dramatic response.[27,81,161,164]

Blood doping might also produce effects opposite to those intended. For example, a large red blood cell infusion and increase in blood cell concentration could increase blood viscosity, or "thickness," and thus *decrease* cardiac output, blood flow velocity, and peripheral oxygen supply—effects that reduce aerobic capacity and endurance performance. Any increase in blood viscosity could also compromise blood flow through narrowed, atherosclerotic vessels of individuals with artery disease to increase their risk for heart attack or stroke.

Does Blood Doping Work?

A theoretical basis for blood doping exists and experimental evidence justifies its use for physiologic reasons. Early research in this area noted a rapid increase in $\dot{V}O_{2max}$ following infusion of whole blood.[83] One study reported a 23% overnight increase in exercise performance and a 9% increase in $\dot{V}O_{2max}$.[84] Subsequent investigations support previous findings and show physiologic and performance improvements with red blood cell reinfusion.[219,241]

Differences in results among various studies of exercise performance following red blood cell reinfusion largely result from variations in blood storage methods. Freezing red blood cells permits storage for more than 6 wk without significant cell loss. With storage at 39.2°F (4°C) used in some earlier studies, substantial hemolysis occurs after only 3 wk. This represents an important difference because it usually takes a person 5 to 6 wk to reestablish blood cells lost after withdrawal of 2 units of whole blood (Fig. 23.10).

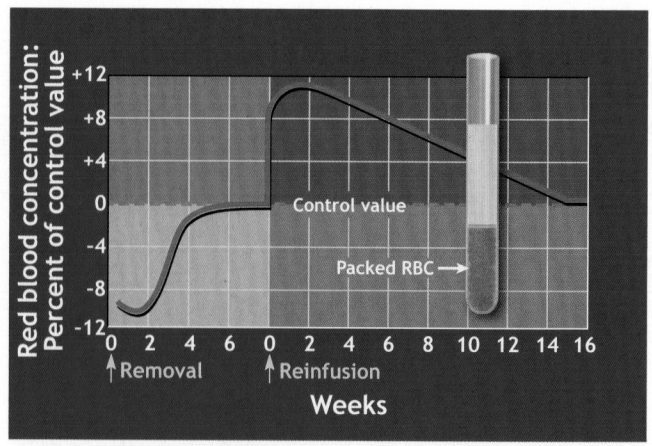

FIGURE 23.10 • Time course of hematologic changes after removal and reinfusion of 900 mL of freeze-preserved blood. (Adapted with permission from Gledhill N. Blood doping and related issues: a brief review. *Med Sci Sports Exerc* 1982;14:183.)

With appropriate blood storage methods, red blood cell reinfusion elevates hematologic parameters of men and women. This in turn translates to a 5 to 13% increase in aerobic capacity, decreased heart rate and blood lactate during submaximal effort, and augmented endurance at sea level and altitude. In addition, red blood cell reinfusion benefits thermoregulatory response during physical activity in the heat (reduced body heat storage and improved sweating response). Increased oxygen content in arterial blood in the infused state likely "frees" blood for delivery to the skin for heat dissipation during exertional heat stress while adequately supplying active tissues. TABLE 23.8 illustrates hematologic, physiologic, and performance responses for five adult men during submaximal and maximal activity before and 24 hr after infusion of 750 mL of packed red blood cells. These response patterns generally represent the current thinking in this area.

A New Twist: Hormonal Blood Boosting

Endurance athletes now use epoetin, a synthetic form of **erythropoietin** (**EPO** or recombinant human EPO [rHuEPO]), to eliminate the cumbersome and lengthy blood doping process. This hormone, produced by the kidneys in response to reduced oxygen pressure in arterial plasma, regulates red blood cell production within the marrow of the long bones, but also is essential in the synthesis and proper functioning of several erythrocyte membrane proteins, particularly those facilitating lactate exchange.[9,37,63] Medically, exogenous recombinant human EPO, commercially available since 1988, has proved useful in combating anemia in patients undergoing chemotherapy or with severe renal disease. Normally, a decrease in red blood cell concentration or decline in the pressure of oxygen in arterial blood—as in severe pulmonary disease or on ascent to high altitude—releases this hormone to stimulate erythrocyte production. The 12% increase in hemoglobin and hematocrit that typically follows 6-wk EPO treatment greatly improves endurance exercise performance.[227,257] Unfortunately,

TABLE 23.8	Physiologic, Performance, and Hematologic Characteristics Before and 24 Hours After Reinfusion of 750 mL of Packed Red Blood Cells			
Variable	**Preinfusion**	**Postinfusion**	**Difference**	**Difference, %**
Hemoglobin, g · dL blood^{-1}	13.8	17.6	3.8[b]	+ 27.5[b]
Hematocrit,[a] %	43.3	54.8	11.5[b]	+ 26.5[b]
Submaximal $\dot{V}O_2$, L · min^{-1}	1.60	1.59	−0.01	−0.6
Submaximal HR, b · min^{-1}	127.4	109.2	18.2[b]	−14.3[b]
$\dot{V}O_{2max}$, L · min^{-1}	3.28	3.70	0.42[b]	+12.8[b]
HR_{max}, b · min^{-1}	181.6	180.0	−1.6	−0.9
Treadmill run time, s	793	918	125[b]	15.8[b]

[a]Hematocrit expressed as the percentage (%) of 100 mL (1 dL) of whole blood occupied by red blood cells.
[b]Difference statistically significant.
Reprinted from Roberston RJ, et al. Effect of induced erythrocythemia on hypoxia tolerance during exercise. *J Appl Physiol* 1982;53:490.

self-administration in an unregulated and unmonitored manner—simply injecting the hormone requires much less sophistication than blood-doping procedures—can increase hematocrit more than 60%. This dangerously high hemoconcentration (and corresponding increase in blood viscosity) increases the likelihood for stroke, heart attack, heart failure, and pulmonary edema. Other side effects include increased platelet adhesion, arterial hypertension, headache, muscle cramps, upper respiratory tract infection, and posttreatment anemia.

EPO use has become particularly prevalent in cycling competition and allegedly contributed to at least 18 deaths among competitive cyclists, mainly from heart attack. While EPO use can be detected in urine, the blood hematocrit serves as a surrogate marker. The International Cycling Union has set a hematocrit threshold of 50% for males and 47% for females; the International Skiing Federation uses a hemoglobin concentration of 18.5 g · dL^{-1} as the threshold for disqualification. Hematocrit cutoff values of 52% for men and 48% for women (roughly 3 standard deviations above the mean) represent "abnormally high" or extreme values in triathletes.[192] Use of hematocrit level cutoff raises the unanswered question of the number of disqualified "clean" cyclists. Estimates place this number between 3 and 5% due to factors that affect normal variation in hematocrit such as genetics, posture, altitude training, and hydration level.

 ### Iron Anomaly Among Elite Cyclists

Current concern centers on an anomaly in iron metabolism frequently observed among high-level international cyclists. Many have serum iron levels above 500 ng · L^{-1} (normal: 100 ng · L^{-1}), with some values as high as 1000 ng · L^{-1}. The elevated iron level results from their regular injections of supplemental iron to support increased synthesis of red blood cells induced by repeated EPO use. Such chronic iron overload increases risk of liver dysfunction among these athletes.

The enhancement of oxygen availability to muscles by EPO analog and mimetics constitutes one of the main challenges to doping control. The concern of sports governing bodies has now shifted from simple red blood cell reinfusion to concern about transfection to an athlete's genes that code for erythropoietin and its subsequent impact on exercise performance. Sports authorities have incorporated such "gene doping" among the prohibited practices.

Other Means to Enhance Oxygen Transport

New classes of substances may emerge to enhance aerobic performance. These doping threats include perfluorocarbon emulsions and solutions formulated from either bovine or human hemoglobin that improve oxygen transport and delivery to muscle. Despite their potential benefits in clinical use, these substances exhibit potentially lethal side effects that include increased systemic and pulmonary blood pressure, renal toxicity, and impaired immune function.

Warm-Up (Preliminary Exercise)

Coaches, trainers, and athletes at all levels of competition generally recommend engaging in some type of physical activity or warm-up prior to vigorous physical effort. Conventional wisdom maintains that preliminary exercise helps the performer prepare physiologically or psychologically and reduces the likelihood of joint and muscle injury.[229] With animals, injuring a "warmed-up" muscle requires more force and greater muscle length than injuring a muscle in the "cold" condition.[229] The warming-up process stretches the muscle–tendon unit to allow greater length and less tension on exposure to a given external load.

Warm-up generally fits into one of two categories, although overlap exists:

1. **General warm-up** uses body movements or "loosening-up" activities unrelated to the specific neuromuscular actions of the anticipated performance. Examples include calisthenics and stretching.
2. **Specific warm-up** applies big-muscle, rhythmic movements that provide skill rehearsal in the activity. Examples

include swinging a golf club, throwing a baseball or football, tennis practice, basketball shooting and movements, and preliminary lead-up in the high jump or pole vault.

Psychologic Considerations

Competitors at all levels generally believe that performing some prior skill-related activity prepares them mentally to focus on the upcoming performance. A specific warm-up related to the intended activity also may improve the necessary skill and coordination requirements. Consequently, sports that require accuracy, timing, and precise movements generally benefit from some type of specific or "formal" preliminary practice.

The notion also exists that prior exercise before strenuous effort gradually prepares a person to go "all out" without fear of injury. The ritual warm-up of baseball pitchers exemplifies this belief. Is it conceivable that a pitcher would enter a game, throwing at competitive speeds, without previously warming up? Would any athlete begin competition without first stretching and engaging in a particular form, intensity, or duration of warm-up? Most performers would respond with a definite no, yet objective support for this response remains elusive. One reason is the difficulty of designing a well-controlled experiment with top-flight athletes to determine the necessity of warming up and whether it improves subsequent performance with reduced injury risk. For pre-exercise stretching, research with army recruits indicates that a typical muscle-stretching protocol in the pre-exercise warm-up produces *no* clinically meaningful reductions in risk of exercise-related injury compared with subsequent exercise without warm-up.[203] Strength loss, loss of motion, soreness, or markers of muscle damage from eccentric movements were no different between groups that received pre-exercise passive warm-up with short-wave diathermy, active warm-up with concentric muscle actions, or no warm-up.[89]

Certain sport-related situations require peak performance with little time for warming up. A reserve player entering the last few minutes of a game has no time for stretching, vigorous calisthenics, or taking practice shots; the player must go all out and achieve optimal performance without warm-up except that done before the game or at intermission. Do more injuries occur in such cases? Does physical performance (e.g., shooting, rebounding, or basketball defense) deteriorate during the first few minutes of this "unwarmed" condition from that proceeded by a warm-up? Future research must address such questions.

Psychologic factors, including an athlete's ingrained belief in the importance of warming up, establish a definite bias when comparing maximum performance with and without warm-up. It is difficult if not impossible to obtain a maximum effort without warm-up if a subject believes in the importance of preliminary exercise.

Physiologic and Performance Effects

One study evaluated the effect of warm-up on 2-min sprint-cycling performance at 120% of the power output at $\dot{V}O_{2max}$.

Warm-up produces a higher muscle temperature, increased local muscle oxygen availability and oxygen uptake, lower blood lactate level, and higher oxygen consumption during the early phase of activity than the no-warm-up condition.[72,218] Warm-up performed at moderate- and high-intensity improved intense cycling performance by 2 to 3%.[44] A pre-exercise warm-up irrespective of intensity enhanced a 3- to 4-min (3-km) cycling time trial. This effect likely resulted from an acceleration of oxygen uptake kinetics from augmented blood flow at exercise onset.[115] An active warm-up 5 min prior to a 30-s maximal sprint on a bicycle ergometer produced less blood and muscle lactate than equivalent effort without a physical warm-up.[109] Differences in muscle temperature with an active warm-up could not account for the ergogenic effect because exercise in the control condition also involved passively heating the muscle to the same temperature. These findings suggest a decreased reliance on anaerobic sources of energy during the activity period preceded by a physical warm-up.

Five mechanisms explain why warm-up "should" improve physical performance and exercise capacity because of subsequent increases in blood flow and muscle and core temperature:

1. Faster muscle contraction and relaxation
2. Greater economy of movement from lowered viscous resistance within active muscles
3. Facilitated oxygen delivery and use by muscles because hemoglobin releases oxygen more readily at higher temperatures (Bohr effect)
4. Facilitated nerve transmission and muscle metabolism because increased temperature accelerates bodily processes; a specific warm-up may also enhance required motor unit recruitment
5. Increased blood flow through active tissues as the local vascular bed dilates from increased metabolism and higher muscle temperature

Clinical Considerations: Warm-Up Prior to Sudden Strenuous Physical Activity

Sudden exertion can trigger the onset of myocardial infarction, particularly in sedentary persons and those with latent coronary artery disease.[39,178] With this in mind, consideration of possible benefits from warming up takes on clinical significance. Several studies have evaluated the effects of preliminary exercise on the cardiovascular response to sudden, strenuous effort. The findings provide an essentially different physiologic framework to justify warm-up that relates importantly to adult fitness and cardiac rehabilitation programs and occupations and sports that require sudden bursts of physical effort.

In one study, 44 men free of overt symptoms of coronary artery disease ran on a treadmill at high intensity for 10 to 15 s without prior warm-up.[13] Evaluation of postexercise ECGs revealed that 70% of the subjects displayed abnormal changes attributable to inadequate myocardial oxygen supply unrelated to age or fitness level. To evaluate the effect of a warm-up, 22 of the men with an abnormal ECG from the treadmill run jogged in place for 2 min before treadmill running at moderate intensity (heart rate, 145 b·min^{-1}). With this warm-up, 10 men now showed normal tracings during sudden exertion, while another 10 men displayed improved ECG responses; only two subjects showed significant abnormalities. In a subsequent study, the exercise blood pressure response also improved with prior warm-up.[14] For seven men with no warm-up, systolic blood pressure averaged 168 mm Hg immediately after the 15-s treadmill run. This decreased to 140 mm Hg when the 2-min jog-in-place warm-up preceded exercise.

Coronary blood flow does not adjust instantaneously to a sudden increase in myocardial work; transient myocardial ischemia (poor oxygen supply) can occur in apparently healthy and fit individuals. *Prior warm-up (at least 2 min of easy jogging) benefits the subsequent ECG and blood pressure responses to vigorous physical activity to indicate a more favorable relationship between myocardial oxygen supply and demand.* Warming up before strenuous effort is particularly important for individuals with limited myocardial blood flow from coronary artery disease. A brief warm-up provides more optimal blood pressure and hormonal adjustments at the onset of subsequent strenuous exercise. The warm-up serves two beneficial purposes under these conditions:

1. Reduces myocardial workload and thus the myocardial oxygen requirement
2. Augments blood flow through the coronary arteries

Oxygen Inhalation (Hyperoxia)

Athletes breathe oxygen-enriched or **hyperoxic gas mixtures** during time-outs, at half-time, or following strenuous activity. They believe this procedure enhances the blood's oxygen-carrying capacity to facilitate oxygen transport to active or recovering muscles, when it does not. The fact remains that when healthy persons breathe ambient air at sea level, hemoglobin in blood leaving the lungs normally remains 95 to 98% saturated with oxygen (see Chapter 13). In physiologic terms, consider these two factors:

1. Breathing air with a higher than normal oxygen concentration increases oxygen transport by hemoglobin to only a small extent—by about 1 mL of extra oxygen for every deciliter of blood (10 mL O_2 per liter).
2. Oxygen that dissolves in plasma when breathing a hyperoxic mixture also increases by about 0.4 mL per deciliter of blood (4.0 mL O_2 per liter), or from the normal 0.3 mL per deciliter (3.0 mL per liter) to about 0.7 mL per deciliter (7.0 mL per liter) of blood.

Based on these two factors, the blood's oxygen-carrying capacity under hyperoxic conditions potentially increases by only about 14 mL of oxygen for every liter of blood—10 mL "extra" attached to hemoglobin and 4 mL "extra" dissolved in plasma.

Pre-exercise Oxygen Breathing

Blood volume for a 70-kg person averages about 5000 mL (5.0 L). Breathing hyperoxic gas adds about 70 mL of oxygen to the total blood volume (5.0 L of blood × 14 mL "extra" O_2 per liter of blood). Despite any potential psychologic benefit for the athlete who believes that pre-exercise oxygen breathing helps subsequent performance, this procedure confers only a trivial physiologic advantage from any additional oxygen per se. This small benefit emerges only if subsequent exercise takes place without breathing ambient air in the interval between hyperoxic breathing and exercise. This occurs because ambient air's lower oxygen pressure than its pressure in hyperoxic blood causes any additional oxygen in the blood to exit the body.

The athlete who breathes an oxygen-rich mixture on the sideline before returning to the competition does not gain a competitive edge from physiologic benefits. This is particularly ironic in football because metabolic reactions that do not require oxygen generate almost all of the energy to power each play.

Oxygen Breathing During Exercise

Breathing hyperoxic gas during submaximal and maximal aerobic activity enhances endurance performance. Oxygen breathing during vigorous exertion accelerates oxygen consumption at the onset of exercise (smaller oxygen deficit in repeated bouts of intense effort); reduces blood lactate, heart rate, and pulmonary ventilation in submaximal effort; and increases $\dot{V}O_{2max}$ and training intensity.[166,198,216] In one study, subjects performed a 6.5-min endurance ride on a bicycle ergometer at an exercise level equal to 115% of $\dot{V}O_{2max}$ while breathing either room air or 100% oxygen.[281] Tanks of compressed gas supplied both air and oxygen to mask a subject's knowledge of the breathing mixture. **Figure 23.11A** shows superior endurance (less dropoff in pedal revolutions) while breathing 100% oxygen during cycling compared to breathing room air. **Figure 23.11B** shows that the hyperoxic condition produced significantly higher oxygen consumptions throughout the 6-min intense activity period.

Figure 23.12 shows that oxygen consumption of the quadriceps muscle of seven trained subjects during maximum knee-extension movement varied with the level of inspired oxygen, averaging lower in hypoxia (12% O_2) than in normoxia (21% O_2) and higher in hyperoxia (100% O_2) than normoxia. The figure also includes confirmatory results (*dashed yellow line*) from a previous study of cycle ergometry under comparable conditions.[149] Cycle ergometry produced lower muscle-specific $\dot{V}O_{2peak}$ values than knee-extension exercise. The slopes of the lines relating oxygen delivery to peak muscle oxidative metabolism were remarkably similar for both activity modes. For maximal knee-extension exercise, oxygen content of venous blood leaving the active muscles remained essentially equal among conditions averaging 4 mL·dL^{-1}. Oxygen delivery in arterial blood increased from 17.3 to 19.5 to 21.8 mL·dL^{-1} with increasing levels of oxygen inhalation. The hyperoxic condition during maximal

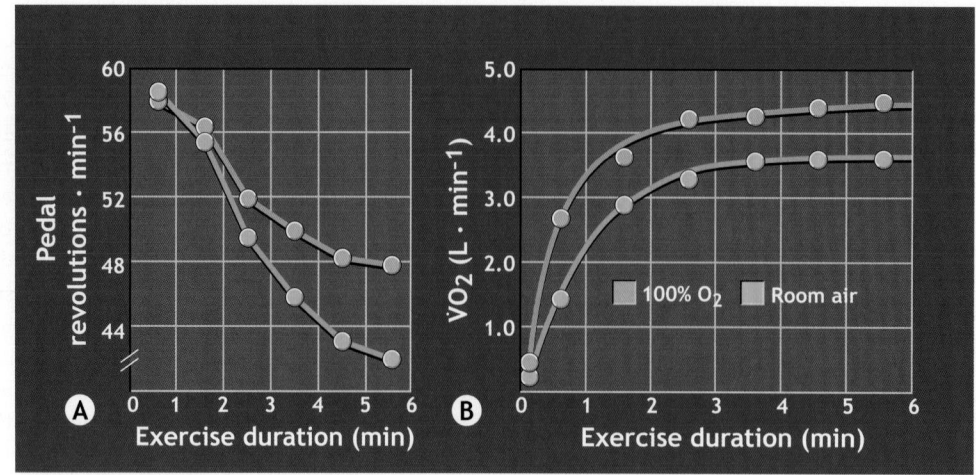

FIGURE 23.11 • **(A)** Endurance (measured by pedal revolutions each minute) while breathing 100% oxygen or ambient air. **(B)** Oxygen consumption curves during the endurance rides show enhanced oxygen consumption while breathing oxygen. (Data from Weltman A, et al. Effects of increasing oxygen availability on bicycle ergometer endurance performance. *Ergonomics* 1978;21:427.)

effort produced the largest skeletal muscle a-vO₂ difference and $\dot{V}O_{2peak}$. Similarly, maximal exercise intensity decreased 25% when breathing 12% inspired oxygen and increased 14% under 100% inspired oxygen compared with normoxic conditions. *Oxygen delivery to active muscles in the circulation, not its use via mitochondrial metabolism, limits aerobic exercise performance.*

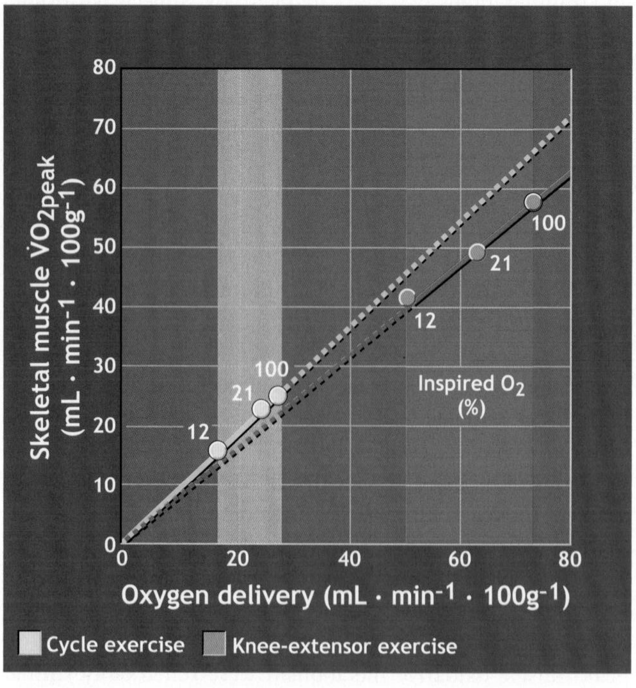

Breathing hyperoxic gas does not increase maximal cardiac output; an expanded a-vO₂ difference must account for the increased exercise oxygen consumption. The small increases in arterial hemoglobin saturation and dissolved plasma oxygen with hyperoxic breathing increase total oxygen availability as blood volume circulates four to seven times each minute in strenuous effort. The additional but relatively small 14 mL of oxygen in each 1 L of blood from breathing hyperoxic gas represents considerable extra oxygen when exercising at a 20- to 30-L cardiac output. If the muscles metabolized the added oxygen during physical activity, $\dot{V}O_{2max}$ would increase by 5 to 10%. The increased partial pressure of oxygen in solution from breathing hyperoxic gas also facilitates its diffusion across the tissue–capillary membrane into the mitochondria, which may account for the higher oxygen consumption at the onset of activity. Breathing hyperoxic mixtures *during* endurance activity offers positive ergogenic benefits, but offers limited practical sports application. The "legality" of using an appropriate breathing system during actual competition seems unlikely.

Oxygen Breathing During Recovery

Breathing hyperoxic mixtures does not facilitate recovery from exercise or improve performance in a subsequent exercise bout (FIG. 23.13). Following 1 min of all-out cycling, subjects recovered while breathing either room air or 100% oxygen for 10 or 20 min. They then repeated the all-out bicycle ride. No significant differences emerged in cumulative revolutions (*inset A*) and 6-s × 6-s revolutions (*inset B*) for the 1-min ride after breathing room air or 100% oxygen during recovery from previous effort. Breathing either room air or oxygen yielded similar blood lactate levels in the 10- or 20-min recovery periods. This indicated that breathing oxygen in recovery did not

FIGURE 23.12 • Relationship between skeletal muscle $\dot{V}O_{2peak}$ and oxygen delivery per 100 g of muscle during conventional maximal cycle ergometry exercise (*yellow*) and knee-extension exercise (*green*) under hypoxia, normoxia, and hyperoxia. (Adapted with permission from Richardson RS, et al. Evidence of O₂ supply–dependent $\dot{V}O_{2max}$ in exercise-trained human quadriceps. *J Appl Physiol* 1999;86:1048.)

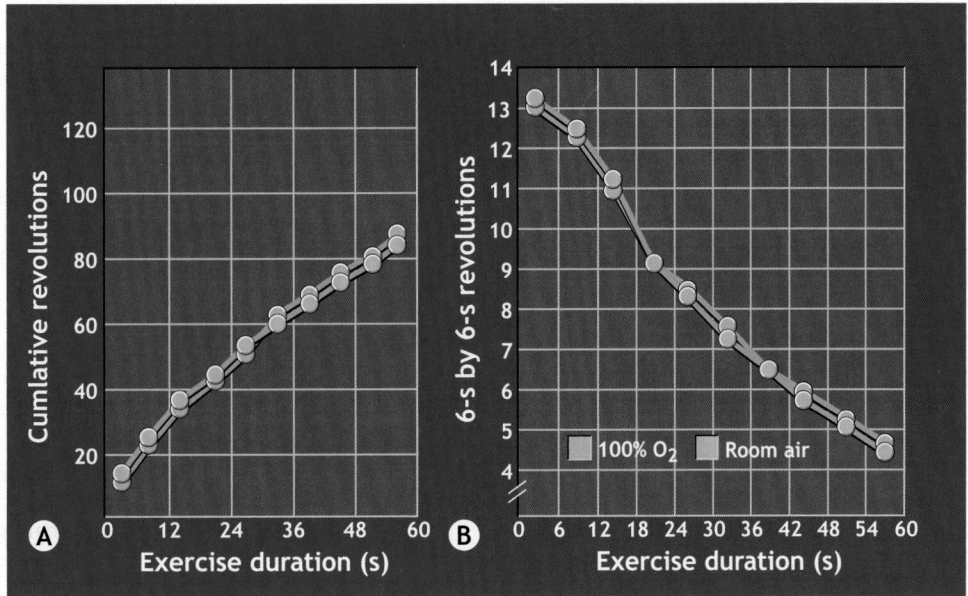

FIGURE 23.13 • Cumulative **(A)** and absolute **(B)** 6-s pedal revolutions on a bicycle ergometer during 1 min of maximal exercise after breathing either 100% oxygen or ambient air during recovery from a previous maximal exercise bout. (Adapted with permission from Weltman A, et al. Exercise recovery, lactate removal, and subsequent high-intensity exercise performance. *Res Q* 1977;48:786.)

facilitate lactate removal. Subsequent research supports these findings; breathing oxygen after short intervals of submaximal and maximal physical effort did not affect recovery kinetics for minute ventilation, heart rate, or serum lactate or the level of ensuing exercise performance.[217,285]

Modification of Carbohydrate Intake

Increased carbohydrate intake before and during intense aerobic physical activity, including periods of strenuous training, is a sound macronutrient manipulation that benefits performance, lowers ratings of perceived exertion, and improves psychologic state (see Chapter 3).[1,261] Vigilance and mood also improve with a carbohydrate beverage administered during a day of sustained aerobic activity interspersed with rest periods.[158] One of the more popular nutritional exercise modifications used by endurance athletes to augment glycogen reserves involves **carbohydrate loading**, or **glycogen supercompensation**. The procedure produces considerably higher "packing" of muscle glycogen than simply maintaining a high-carbohydrate diet. Normally, each 100 g of muscle contains about 1.7 g of glycogen; carbohydrate loading packs up to 4 to 5 g of glycogen.

Nutrient-Related Fatigue in Prolonged Physical Activity

Glycogen stored in the liver and active muscle supplies most of the energy for intense aerobic activity. Prolonging such activity reduces the body's glycogen reserves. This allows fat catabolism—from adipose tissue and liver fatty acid mobilization and intramuscular fat stores—to supply a progressively greater percentage of energy. A substantially lowered muscle glycogen level precipitates fatigue, yet active muscle maintains

sufficient oxygen with an almost unlimited potential energy from fat. Consuming a glucose and water solution near the point of fatigue allows exercise to continue, but for all practical purposes, "the muscles' fuel tank reads empty." Reliance on fat catabolism decreases power output from the considerably slower mobilization and breakdown of fat than carbohydrate. Marathon runners use the term ***hitting the wall***, while endurance cyclists use the term *bonking* to describe sensations of fatigue and muscle pain associated when exercising with severe glycogen depletion. The important role of carbohydrate as an energy substrate during 1 to 2 hr of intense exercise has led researchers to search for additional ways to increase pre-exercise glycogen reserves.

Classic Loading Procedure

TABLE 23.9 presents the classic procedure for achieving the supercompensation effect. The first phase involves reducing the muscle's glycogen content with prolonged exercise about 6 days before competition. Glycogen supercompensation occurs only in the specific muscles depleted by exercise, so athletes must engage the muscles activated in their sport. Preparing for marathon running, endurance swimming, or bicycling requires 90 min of moderately intense submaximal effort in the specific activity. The athlete then maintains a low-carbohydrate diet (about 60 to 100 $g \cdot d^{-1}$) for several days to further deplete glycogen stores. Note that glycogen depletion increases intermediate forms of the glycogen-storing enzyme **glycogen synthase** within the depleted muscle fibers. Moderate training continues during this time. Then, 3 days before competing, the athlete switches to a high-carbohydrate diet (400 to 700 $g \cdot d^{-1}$) and maintains this intake up to the precompetition meal. The supercompensation diet should also contain adequate daily

TABLE 23.9 Two-Stage Dietary Plan to Increase Muscle Glycogen Storage

Stage 1—Depletion
Day 1: Exhausting exercise to deplete muscle glycogen in specific muscles
Days 2, 3, 4: Low-carbohydrate intake (60–100 g · d⁻¹; high percentage of protein and lipid in daily diet)

Stage 2—Carbohydrate loading
Days 5, 6, 7: High-carbohydrate intake (400–700 g · d⁻¹; normal percentage of protein in daily diet)

Competition day
High-carbohydrate precompetition meal

protein, minerals and vitamins, and abundant water. Supercompensated muscle glycogen levels remain stable for at least 3 days during a maintenance phase (in a nonactive individual) if the diet contains 60% of calories as carbohydrate.[107]

If an athlete decides to supercompensate after weighing the pros and cons (see "Nutrient-Related Fatigue in Prolonged Physical Activity" and FYI "Negative Aspects of Carbohydrate Loading"), the new food regimen should proceed in stages during training, not for the first time before competition. For example, the athlete should start with a long run followed by a high-carbohydrate diet. A detailed log should record how the dietary manipulation affects performance. A record of subjective feelings should include exercise depletion

and replenishment phases. With positive results, the athlete can try the entire series—depletion, low-carbohydrate diet, and high-carbohydrate diet—but maintain the low-carbohydrate diet for only 1 day. With no adverse effects, the low-carbohydrate diet can gradually extend to a maximum of 4 days.

Sample Diets to Achieve the Supercompensation Effect. TABLE 23.10 provides a sample meal plan for carbohydrate depletion (stage 1) and carbohydrate loading (stage 2) preceding an endurance event.

Limited Applicability. *Carbohydrate loading's benefits to performance apply only to intense aerobic activities lasting longer than 60 min. Activities lasting less than 60 min require only normal carbohydrate intake and glycogen reserves.*[165,194] For example, carbohydrate loading did not benefit trained runners in a 20.9-km (13-mile) run compared with a run following a low-carbohydrate diet. Similarly, no ergogenic effect emerged for time trial performance, heart rate, and RPE for endurance-trained cyclists in a 100-km trial that simulated continuous changes in cycling intensity typical of competition.[42]

For sports competition and training, a daily diet that contains about 60 to 70% of calories as carbohydrates provides adequate muscle and liver glycogen reserves. This diet ensures about twice as much muscle glycogen as a typical diet of 45 to 50% carbohydrate. For well-nourished athletes, the supercompensation effect remains relatively small. During intense training, athletes who do not upgrade daily calorie and carbohydrate intakes to meet energy demands can experience chronic muscle fatigue and staleness.

TABLE 23.10 Sample Meal Plan for Carbohydrate Depletion and Carbohydrate Loading Preceding an Endurance Event

Meal	Stage 1 Depletion	Stage 2 Carbohydrate Loading
Breakfast	0.5 cup fruit juice 2 eggs 1 slice whole-wheat toast 1 glass whole milk	1 cup fruit juice 1 bowl hot or cold cereal 1–2 muffins 1 tbsp butter
Lunch	6 oz hamburger 2 slices bread Salad (normal size) 1 tbsp mayonnaise and salad dressing 1 glass whole milk	2–3 oz hamburger with bun 1 cup juice 1 orange 1 tbsp mayonnaise Pie or cake (one 8-in slice) 1 cup yogurt, fruit, or cookies
Snack	1 cup yogurt	1–1.5 pieces of chicken, baked
Dinner	2–3 pieces of chicken, fried 1 baked potato with sour cream 0.5 cup vegetables Iced tea (no sugar) 2 tbsp butter	1 cup vegetables 0.5 cup sweetened pineapple Iced tea (sugar) 1 tbsp butter 1 glass chocolate milk with 4 cookies
Snack	1 glass whole milk	

During stage 1, the intake of carbohydrate approaches 60 g or 240 kcal; in stage 2, the carbohydrate intake increases to 400–700 g or about 1600–2800 kcal.

Gender Differences in Glycogen Storage and Catabolism During Physical Activity

Gender-related differences in muscle glycogen supercompensation remain controversial. One study reported a relatively small 13% increase in the muscle glycogen content of women when they switched from a mixed diet to a high-carbohydrate diet.[276] Other research indicated that women do not increase glycogen storage when dietary carbohydrate increases from 60 to 75% of total caloric intake.[254] Importantly, this increase in carbohydrate intake as a percentage of total calories represents *considerably less total carbohydrate intake* relative to lean body mass (body composition component responsible for considerable glycogen storage) for women than for men. **FIGURE 23.14** illustrates that equalizing daily carbohydrate intake for endurance-trained men and women at 12 g per kilogram of lean body mass for 3 consecutive days produced no gender differences in glycogen loading. *These and other findings show that men and women possess an equal capacity to accumulate muscle glycogen when fed comparable amounts of carbohydrate relative to lean body mass.*[253,255] Women oxidize more lipid and less carbohydrate and protein compared with men during endurance activity.[99,125] The increase in fat oxidation is associated with higher intramyocellular lipid content and use as well as greater adipocyte lipolysis. The greater fat oxidation for women during submaximal endurance effort seems to

occur partly through a sex hormone–mediated enhancement of lipid-oxidation pathways.[253]

Glycogen Supercompensation Enhanced by Prior Creatine Supplementation

A synergy exists between glycogen storage and creatine supplementation. For example, preceding glycogen loading with a 5-day creatine loading protocol (20 g daily) produced 10% greater glycogen packing in the vastus lateralis muscle than achieved with only glycogen loading.[222] More than likely, increases in creatine and cellular volume with creatine supplementation facilitate subsequent storage of muscle glycogen.

Modified Loading Procedures

A less stringent **modified loading procedure** displayed in **FIGURE 23.15** eliminates many potential negative aspects of the classic glycogen-loading sequence. The protocol increases glycogen synthase activity without requiring dramatic glycogen depletion with exercise as with the classic loading procedure; it increases glycogen storage to nearly the same level. The 6-day protocol does not require prior exhaustive physical effort. Rather, the athlete trains at about 75% of $\dot{V}O_{2max}$ (85% HR_{max}) for 1.5 hr (*red line*) and then, on successive days, gradually reduces (tapers) exercise duration. During the first 3 days, carbohydrates represent about 50% of total calories (*blue line*). Three days before competition, the diet's carbohydrate content increases to 70% of total energy intake.

 INTEGRATIVE QUESTION

What advice would you give to a sprint athlete who plans to carbohydrate-load for competition?

Rapid Loading Procedure: A One-Day Requirement. The 2 to 6 days required to achieve supranormal muscle glycogen levels represents a limitation of typical carbohydrate-loading procedures. The desired loading effect can also occur with a shortened duration that combines a brief bout of intense activity with only 1 day of high-carbohydrate intake. Endurance-trained athletes cycled for 150 s at an intensity of 130% $\dot{V}O_{2max}$ followed by 30 s of all-out cycling. In the recovery period, the men consumed 10.3 g per kg body mass of high glycemic carbohydrate foods. Biopsy data presented in **FIGURE 23.16** indicated that glycogen in the vastus lateralis muscle increased from a 109.1 mmol · kg^{-1} preloading average to 198.3 mmol · kg^{-1} postloading after only 24 hr. This 82% increase in glycogen storage equaled or exceeded values reported by others using a 2- to 6-day regimen. The short-duration loading procedure benefits individuals who do not wish to disrupt normal training with the time required and potential negative aspects of longer loading protocols.[233]

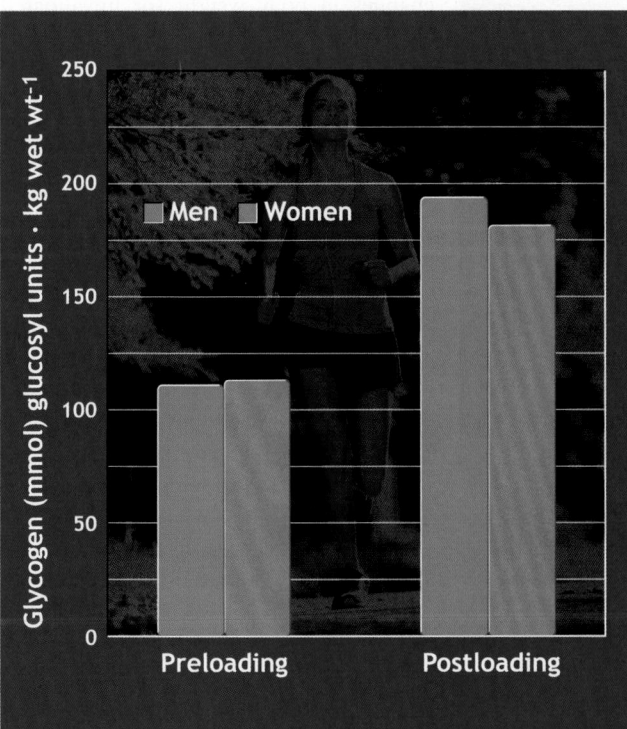

FIGURE 23.14 • Muscle glycogen concentrations pre- and post-carbohydrate loading (12 g carbohydrate per kg lean body mass) in exercise-trained men and women. (Adapted with permission from James AP, et al. Muscle glycogen supercompensation: absence of a gender-related difference. *Eur J Appl Physiol* 2001;85:533.)

Negative Aspects of Carbohydrate Loading

The addition of 2.7 g of water with each gram of glycogen makes it a heavy fuel compared with equivalent energy stored as fat. Athletes often feel "heavy" and uncomfortable with this added water weight; any extra load also directly adds to the energy cost of weight-bearing activities. The extra weight may negate any potential benefits from increased glycogen storage. On the positive side, water liberated during glycogen breakdown aids in temperature regulation, which benefits exercise in hot environments.

The classic model for supercompensation may pose potential negative consequences for individuals with specific health problems. A severe chronic carbohydrate overload, interspersed with periods of high lipid and/or high protein intake, can increase blood cholesterol and urea nitrogen levels. High lipid intake often causes gastrointestinal distress plus poor recovery from the exercise-depletion sequence of the loading procedure. During the low-carbohydrate phase of loading, marked ketosis can occur in individuals who exercise while carbohydrate depleted. Failure to eat a balanced diet also produces mineral and vitamin deficiencies, particularly of the water-soluble vitamins. The glycogen-depleted state reduces the ability to train, possibly leading to a detraining effect during portions of the loading sequence. Dramatically reducing dietary carbohydrate for 3 or 4 days also could set the stage for lean tissue loss because muscle protein serves as gluconeogenic substrate to maintain blood glucose levels in the glycogen-depleted state.

Chromium

The trace mineral chromium serves as a cofactor (as trivalent chromium) for a low–molecular-weight protein that potentiates insulin function, yet its precise mechanism of action remains unclear. Insulin promotes carbohydrate transport into cells, augments fatty acid catabolism, and triggers cellular enzyme activity that facilitates muscle protein synthesis. Chronic chromium deficiency can increase blood cholesterol and decrease the body's sensitivity to insulin, thus raising the risk for type 2 diabetes.

Numerous Alleged Benefits

Touted in popular muscle development magazines as a "fat burner" and "muscle builder," chromium is one of the most hyped minerals in the health food–fitness literature. Supplemental intake of chromium, usually as **chromium picolinate**, often reaches 600 µg daily compared to 50 to 200 µg of chromium, considered the estimated safe and adequate daily dietary intake (ESADDI). This chelated picolinic acid combination supposedly yields better chromium absorption than the inorganic salt chromium chloride. Millions of Americans believe the unsubstantiated claims of health food faddists, television infomercials, and exercise zealots that additional chromium promotes muscle growth, curbs appetite, fosters body fat loss, and even lengthens life. Advertisers target chromium to bodybuilders and other resistance-trained athletes as a safe alternative to anabolic steroids to favorably change body composition. Chromium supplements supposedly potentiate insulin action to increase amino acid anabolism in skeletal muscle. This belief persists despite data that chromium supplements exert no effect on glucose or insulin concentrations in nondiabetic individuals.[4]

Generally, studies suggesting beneficial effects of chromium supplements on body fat and muscle mass infer body composition changes from changes in body weight (or unvalidated anthropometric measurements). One study observed that supplementing daily with 200 µg (3.85 mmol) of chromium picolinate for 40 days produced a small increase in FFM estimated from skinfold thickness and decrease in body fat in young men who resistance-trained for 6 wk.[88] The researchers provided no data to show increased muscular strength. Another study reported increases in body mass without changes in strength or body composition in previously untrained female college students (no change in males) who received a daily 200-µg chromium supplement during 12 wk of resistance training compared with unsupplemented controls.[119]

Other research evaluated the effects of a chromium supplement of 200 µg daily on muscle strength, body composition, and chromium excretion in 16 untrained males during

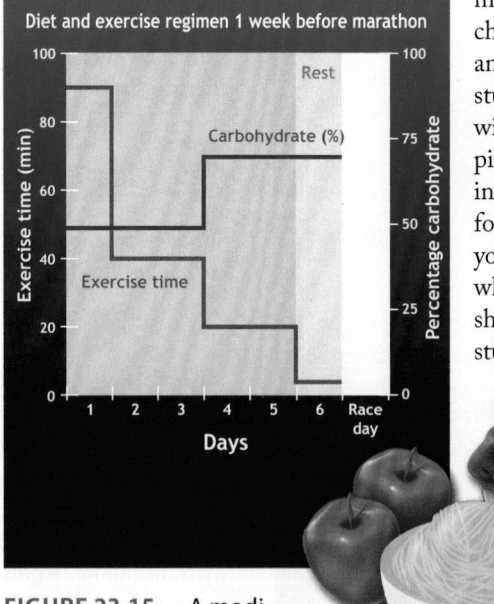

FIGURE 23.15 • A modified approach to carbohydrate loading. Recommended combination of diet and exercise for overloading muscle glycogen stores in the week before an endurance contest. Exercise time is gradually reduced during the week, while the diet's carbohydrate content increases for the last 3 days. (Reprinted with permission from Sherman WM, et al. Effect of exercise-diet manipulation on muscle glycogen and its subsequent utilization during performance. *Int J Sports Med* 1981;2:114, as adapted with permission in McArdle WD, Katch FI, Katch VL. *Sports and Exercise Nutrition*. 4th Ed. Philadelphia: Wolters Kluwer Health, 2013.)

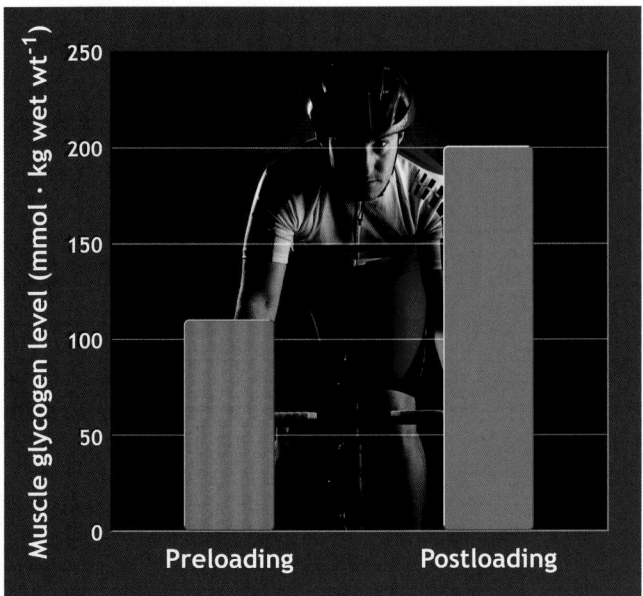

FIGURE 23.16 • Muscle glycogen concentration of the vastus lateralis before (preloading) and after 180 s of near-maximal intensity cycling followed by 1 day of high- carbohydrate intake (postloading). (Reprinted with permission from Fairchild TJ, et al. Rapid carbohydrate loading after short bout of near maximal-intensity exercise. *Med Sci Sports Exerc* 2002;34:980, as adapted with permission in McArdle WD, Katch FI, Katch VL. *Sports and Exercise Nutrition*. 4th Ed. Philadelphia: Wolters Kluwer Health, 2013.)

12 wk of resistance training.[116] Muscular strength improved 24% for the supplemented group and 33% for the placebo group during training. No changes occurred in any of the body composition variables. The group receiving the supplement did show higher chromium excretion than controls after 6 wk of training. The researchers concluded that chromium supplements provided *no ergogenic effect* on any measured variable. Supplementing with 800 μg of chromium picolinate (plus 6 mg of boron) proved no more effective than a malto-dextrin placebo to enhance lean tissue gain or promote fat loss during resistance training.[3] Daily supplementation with 400 μg of chromium picolinate for 9 wk did not promote weight loss in sedentary obese women; it actually caused weight gain during the treatment period.[110]

In support of chromium supplementation, greater body fat loss (no increase in FFM) occurred in subjects "recruited from a variety of fitness and athletic clubs" who consumed 400 μg of chromium daily over 90 days than in subjects who received a placebo.[138] Hydrostatic weighing and DEXA techniques assessed body composition. Body compositional data from hydrostatic weighing do not appear in the report, and the DEXA-derived analysis indicated average body fat values of 42% for both control and experimental subjects, an extraordinary level of obesity for members of fitness clubs. Collegiate football players who received daily 200-μg supplements of chromium picolinate for 9 wk showed no changes in body composition and muscular strength from intense weight

training compared with controls receiving a placebo.[57] Similar findings of no benefit on body composition and physical performance emerged from a 14-wk study of NCAA Division I wrestlers that compared combined chromium picolinate supplementation with a typical preseason training program with identical training without supplementation.[277]

Loss of muscle mass commonly affects older individuals, so potential ergogenic effect on muscle from chromium supplementation should emerge readily in this age group. This did not occur for older men involved in intense resistance training; a high chromium picolinate dosage (924 μg·d⁻¹) did not augment muscle size, strength, or power or FFM accretion above the unsupplemented condition.[46] Obese personnel enrolled in the United States Navy's mandatory remedial physical-conditioning program who consumed an additional 400 μg of chromium picolinate daily showed no greater loss in body weight or percentage body fat or increase in FFM than a group receiving a placebo.[260]

A comprehensive double-blind study examined the effects of a daily chromium supplement (3.3 to 3.5 μmol as either chromium chloride or chromium picolinate) or a placebo for 8 wk during resistance training in 36 young men. For each group, dietary intakes of protein, magnesium, zinc, copper, and iron equaled or exceeded recommended levels during training; subjects also maintained adequate baseline dietary chromium intakes. Supplementation increased serum chromium concentration and urinary chromium excretion equally regardless of its ingested form. TABLE 23.11 shows that compared with placebo treatment, chromium supplementation did not affect training-related changes in muscular strength, FFM, or muscle mass.

Excess Chromium Poses Potential Risks

Chromium competes with iron for binding to transferrin, the plasma protein that transports iron from ingested food and damaged red blood cells for delivery to tissues in need. The chromium picolinate supplement for the group whose data appear in Table 23.11 reduced serum transferrin (a measure of adequacy of current iron intake) compared with chromium chloride or placebo treatments. Conversely, other researchers observed that giving middle-age men 924 μg of supplemental chromium daily as chromium picolinate for 12 wk did not affect hematologic measures or indices of iron metabolism or iron status.[45] We are unaware of studies that have evaluated the safety of long-term chromium supplementation or the ergogenic efficacy of supplementing in individuals with suboptimal chromium status. Concerning the bioavailability of trace minerals in the diet, excessive dietary chromium inhibits zinc and iron absorption. At the extreme, this could induce iron-deficiency anemia, blunt the ability to train intensely, and negatively affect performance requiring high-level aerobic metabolism.

Creatine

Meat, poultry, and fish provide a rich source of creatine, containing 4 to 5 g of creatine per kilogram of food. The body

TABLE 23.11

Effects of Two Different Forms of Chromium Supplementation on Average Values for Anthropometric, Bone, and Soft-Tissue Composition Measurements Before and After Resistance Training

	Placebo		Chromium Chloride		Chromium Picolinate	
	Pre	Post	Pre	Post	Pre	Post
Age (y)	21.1	21.5	23.3	23.5	22.3	22.5
Stature (cm)	179.3	179.2	177.3	177.3	178.0	178.2
Weight (kg)	79.9	80.5[a]	79.3	81.1[a]	79.2	80.5
$\Sigma 4$ skinfold thickness (mm)[b]	42.0	41.5	42.6	42.2	43.3	43.1
Upper-arm girth (cm)	30.9	31.6[a]	31.3	32.0[a]	31.1	31.4
Lower-leg girth (cm)	38.2	37.9	37.4	37.5	37.1	37.0
FFMFM (kg)[c]	62.9	64.3[a]	61.1	63.1[a]	61.3	62.7[a]
Bone mineral (g)	2952	2968	2860	2878	2918	2940
Fat-free body mass (kg)	65.9	67.3[a]	64.0	65.9[a]	64.2	66.1[a]
Fat (kg)	13.4	13.1	14.7	15.1	14.7	14.5
Body fat (%)	16.4	15.7	18.4	18.2	18.4	17.9

Reprinted from Lukaski HC, et al. Chromium supplementation and resistance training: effects on body composition, strength, and trace element status of men. *Am J Clin Nutr* 1996;63:954.
[a]Significantly different from pretraining value.
[b]Measured at biceps, triceps, subscapular, and suprailiac sites.
[c]Fat-free, mineral-free mass.

synthesizes only about 1 g of this nitrogen-containing organic compound daily from the nonessential amino acids arginine, glycine, and methionine in the kidneys, liver, and pancreas. The animal kingdom contains the richest creatine-containing foods, placing vegetarians at a distinct disadvantage for ready sources of exogenous creatine. Skeletal muscle contains approximately 95% of the body's total 120 to 140 g of creatine.

Creatine sold in supplemental form as **creatine monohydrate (CrH₂O)** comes as a powder, tablet, capsule, and stabilized liquid. Creatine can be purchased over-the-counter or mail order as a nutritional supplement (but without guarantee of purity). Ingesting a liquid suspension of creatine monohydrate at the relatively high dosage of 20 to 30 g per day for 2 wk increases intramuscular concentrations of free creatine and PCr up to 30%. These levels remain high for weeks after only a few days of supplementation.[126,170] Sports-governing bodies do not consider creatine an illegal substance.

Important Component of High-Energy Phosphates

Creatine passes through the digestive tract's intestinal mucosa unaltered for absorption into the bloodstream. Just about all ingested creatine incorporates into skeletal muscle (average concentration, 125 mM [range 90 to 160 mM] per kg dry muscle). About 40% exists as free creatine; the remainder combines readily with phosphate to form PCr. Type II, fast-twitch muscle fibers store about four to six times more PCr than ATP. As emphasized in Chapter 5, PCr serves as the cells' "energy reservoir" to provide rapid phosphate-bond energy to resynthesize ATP (more rapid

than ATP regenerated in glycogenolysis) in the reversible reaction:

$$PCr + ADP \xrightarrow{\text{creatine kinase}} Cr + ATP$$

PCr also shuttles intramuscular high-energy phosphate between the mitochondria and muscle filament cross-bridge sites

Quercetin Fails the Test

The popular polyphenolic flavinoid quercetin (QS) occurs naturally in many fruits, vegetables, and beverages. Some human and animal studies have reported health and performance benefits from its antioxidant and anti-inflammatory activity, including increases in mitochondrial biogenesis. Aside from alleged health benefits, marketers have included QS in many products heavily marketed for ergogenic benefits on endurance performance and maximal oxygen uptake (e.g., **http://www.stopagingnow.com/QCT/Quercetin-Capsules-with-Bromelain?gclid=Clio7_6ljrUCFcpdpQod9GEAyg**). To evaluate these claims, researchers performed a meta-analysis of available research on this topic (seven published studies that included 288 subjects). The conclusion, based on the totality of the evidence in the authors' own words: "This meta-analysis indicates that QS is unlikely to prove ergogenic for aerobic-oriented exercises in trained and untrained individuals."

Source: Pelletier DM, et al. Effects of quercetin supplementation on endurance performance and maximal oxygen consumption: a meta-analysis. *IJSENM* 2013;23:73.

that initiate muscle action. Maintaining a high sarcoplasmic ATP:ADP ratio by energy transfer from PCr plays an important role in maximum effort lasting up to 10 s. This duration places high demands on ATP resynthesis that exceed energy transfer from intracellular macronutrient breakdown. Improved energy transfer capacity from PCr also lessens reliance on energy from anaerobic glycolysis with associated increase in intramuscular H^+ and decrease in pH from lactate accumulation.[12] Because of limited intramuscular PCr, it seems reasonable that any PCr increase should accomplish the following:

1. Accelerate ATP turnover to maintain power output during short-term muscular effort.
2. Delay PCr depletion.
3. Diminish dependence on anaerobic glycolysis and decrease subsequent lactate formation.
4. Facilitate muscle relaxation and recovery from repeated bouts of intense, brief effort via faster ATP and PCr resynthesis; rapid recovery allows continued higher-level power output.

Documented Benefits in Humans

Creatine supplementation received notoriety as an ergogenic aid when British sprinters and hurdlers used it in the 1992 Barcelona Olympic Games. Creatine supplementation at recommended levels exerts the following three effects:

1. Improves performance in muscular strength and power activities
2. Augments short bursts of muscular endurance
3. Provides for greater muscular overload to augment training effectiveness

No serious adverse effects from creatine supplementation for up to 4 years have been reported.[232] Anecdotes indicate a possible association between creatine supplementation and cramping in multiple muscle areas during competition or lengthy practice in American football players. This effect may result from (1) altered intracellular dynamics because of increased levels of free creatine and PCr, (2) osmotically induced enlarged cell volume (greater cellular hydration)

TABLE 23.12	Selected Studies Showing Increases in Exercise Performance Following Creatine Monohydrate Supplementation		
Reference	**Exercise**	**Protocol**	**Exercise Performance**
d	Isokinetic, unilat, knee extensions ($180° \cdot s^{-1}$)	5 bouts of 30 ext, w/1-min rest periods	Less decline in peak torque production during bouts 2, 3, and 4
e	Running	4–300 m w/4-min rest periods 4–1000 m w/3-min rest periods	Improved time for final 300- and 1000-m runs Improved total time for 4–1000-m runs; reduction in best time for 300- and 1000-m runs
a	Cycle ergometry (140 rev $\cdot min^{-1}$)	Ten 6-s bouts w/1-min rest periods	Better able to maintain pedal frequency during second 4-6 s of each bout
f	Cycle ergometry (140 rev $\cdot min^{-1}$)	Five 6-s bouts w/30-s recovery followed by one 10-s bout	Better able to maintain pedal frequency near end of 10-s bout
b	Cycle ergometry (80 rev $\cdot min^{-1}$)	Three 30-s bouts w/4-min rest periods	Increase in peak power during bout 1 and increase in mean power and total work during bouts 1 and 2
c	Bench press	1-RM bench press and total reps at 70% 1-RM	Increase in 1-RM; increase in reps at 70% of 1-RM
g	Bench press	5 sets bench press w/2-min rest periods	Increase in reps completed during all 5 sets
g	Jump squat	5 sets jump squat w/2-min rest periods	Increase in peak power during all 5 sets

Reprinted from Volek JS, Kraemer WJ, Creatine supplementation: its effect on human muscular performance and body composition. *J Strength Cond Res* 1996;10:200.
[a]Balsom PD, et al. Creatine supplementation and dynamic high-intensity intermittent exercise. *Scand J Med Sci Sports* 1995;3:143.
[b]Birch R, et al. The influence of dietary creatine supplementation on performance during repeated bouts of maximal isokinetic cycling in man. *Eur J Appl Physiol* 1994;69:268.
[c]Earnest CP, et al. The effect of creatine monohydrate ingestion in anaerobic power indices, muscular strength and body composition. *Acta Physiol Scand* 1995;153:207.
[d]Greenhaff PL, et al. Influence of oral creatine supplementation on muscle torque during repeated bouts of maximal voluntary exercise in man. *Clin Sci* 1993;84:565.
[e]Harris RC, et al. The effect of oral creatine supplementation on running performance during maximal short-term exercise in man. *J Physiol* 1993;467:74P.
[f]Soderlund K, et al. Creatine supplementation and high-intensity exercise: influence on performance and muscle metabolism. *Clin Sci* 1994;87(suppl):120.
[g]Volek JS, et al. Creatine supplementation enhances muscular performance during high-intensity resistance exercise. *J Am Diet Assoc* 1997;97:765.

from the muscle fibers' increased creatine content, and (3) inadequate whole-body hydration. Gastrointestinal tract disturbances (nausea, indigestion, and difficulty absorbing food) have been linked to exogenous creatine ingestion.

Creatine monohydrate supplements substantially increase muscle creatine content and performance in intense physical activity, particularly repeated muscular effort (TABLE 23.12).[211,212,273] FIGURE 23.17 illustrates the ergogenic effects of creatine supplementation on total work accomplished during repetitive sprint cycling performance. Physically active but untrained males performed sets of maximal 6-s bicycle sprints interspersed with various recovery periods (24, 54, or 84 s) to simulate sport conditions. Performance evaluations took place under creatine-loaded (20 g per day for 5 days) or placebo conditions. Supplementation increased muscle creatine (48.9%) and PCr (12.5%), which produced a 6% increase in total work accomplished (251.7 kJ presupplement vs. 266.9 kJ creatine loaded) compared to the placebo group (254.0 kJ pretest vs. 252.3 kJ placebo). Creatine supplements have benefited an on-court "ghosting" routine of simulated positional play of competitive squash players.[224]

One research study evaluated a creatine dose of 30 g daily for 6 days in trained runners under two conditions: (1) four repeated 300-m runs with a 4-min recovery and (2) four 1000-m runs with a 3-min recovery.[118] Compared with placebo treatment, creatine supplementation improved performance under both conditions, with the most impressive gains in repeated 1000-m runs. Supplementing with 20 g of creatine daily for 4 days also benefited anaerobic capacity in three 30-s Wingate tests with a 5-min rest between trials. For Division I football players, creatine supplementation with resistance training increased body mass, lean body mass, cellular hydration, and muscular strength and performance.[25] Similarly, supplementation augmented muscular strength and size increases during 12 wk of resistance training.[282] The enhanced hypertrophic response with supplementation and resistance training possibly results from accelerated myosin heavy-chain synthesis. For resistance-trained men classified as "responders" to creatine supplementation (i.e., a creatine increase ≥32 mmol $\cdot$ kg dry wt muscle^{-1}), 5 days of supplementation increased body weight and FFM, and peak force and total force during repeated maximal isometric bench presses.[145] For men classified as "nonresponders" to supplementation (i.e., creatine increase ≤21 mmol $\cdot$ kg dry wt muscle^{-1}), no ergogenic effect occurred. Research also indicates that creatine supplementation plus resistance training may retard production of the protein myostatin, which inhibits muscle growth, to facilitate muscle mass accretion and reduce the markers of muscle damage after intense endurance effort.[15,230]

FIGURE 23.18 outlines possible mechanisms for enhanced performance and training response by elevating intramuscular free creatine and PCr. Consuming a high dose of creatine increases pre-exercise intramuscular Cr and PCr availability to power short-term effort and helps replenish muscle creatine in recovery. This metabolic "preloading" and "reloading" reduces reliance on glycolytic energy-releasing

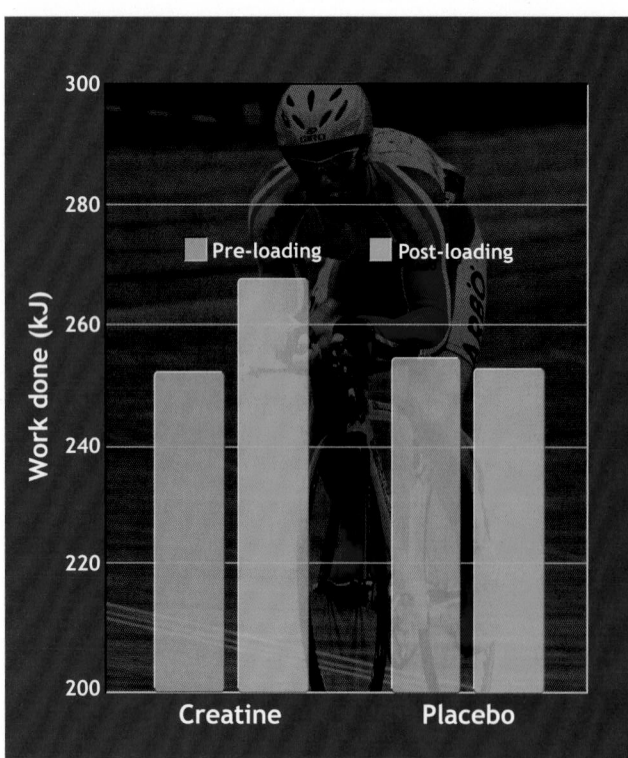

FIGURE 23.17 • Effects of creatine loading versus placebo on total work accomplished during long-term (80 min) repetitive sprint-cycling performance. (Adapted with permission from Preen CD, et al. Effect of creatine loading on long-term sprint exercise performance and metabolism. *Med Sci Sports Exerc* 2001;33:814.)

 ### Potential Risks of Creatine Supplementation

Potential dangers of short-term creatine supplementation have been studied in healthy individuals, particularly on cardiac muscle and kidney function (creatine degrades to creatinine before excretion in urine). Creatine consumed 20 g a day for 5 consecutive days produced no detrimental effect on blood pressure, insulin action, plasma creatine, plasma CK activity, or renal function, measured by glomerular filtration rate, kidney permeability, and total protein and albumin excretion rates.[153,176,292] Only limited information exists about the effects of long-term, high-dose supplementation with creatine. For healthy subjects, no differences in plasma contents and urinary excretion rates for creatinine, urea, and albumin emerged between control subjects and individuals who consumed creatine for up to 5 years.[201] Glomerular filtration rate, tubular reabsorption, and glomerular membrane permeability also remained normal with long-term creatine use. Individuals with suspected renal malfunction should refrain from creatine supplementation because of the potential for exacerbating the disorder.[207]

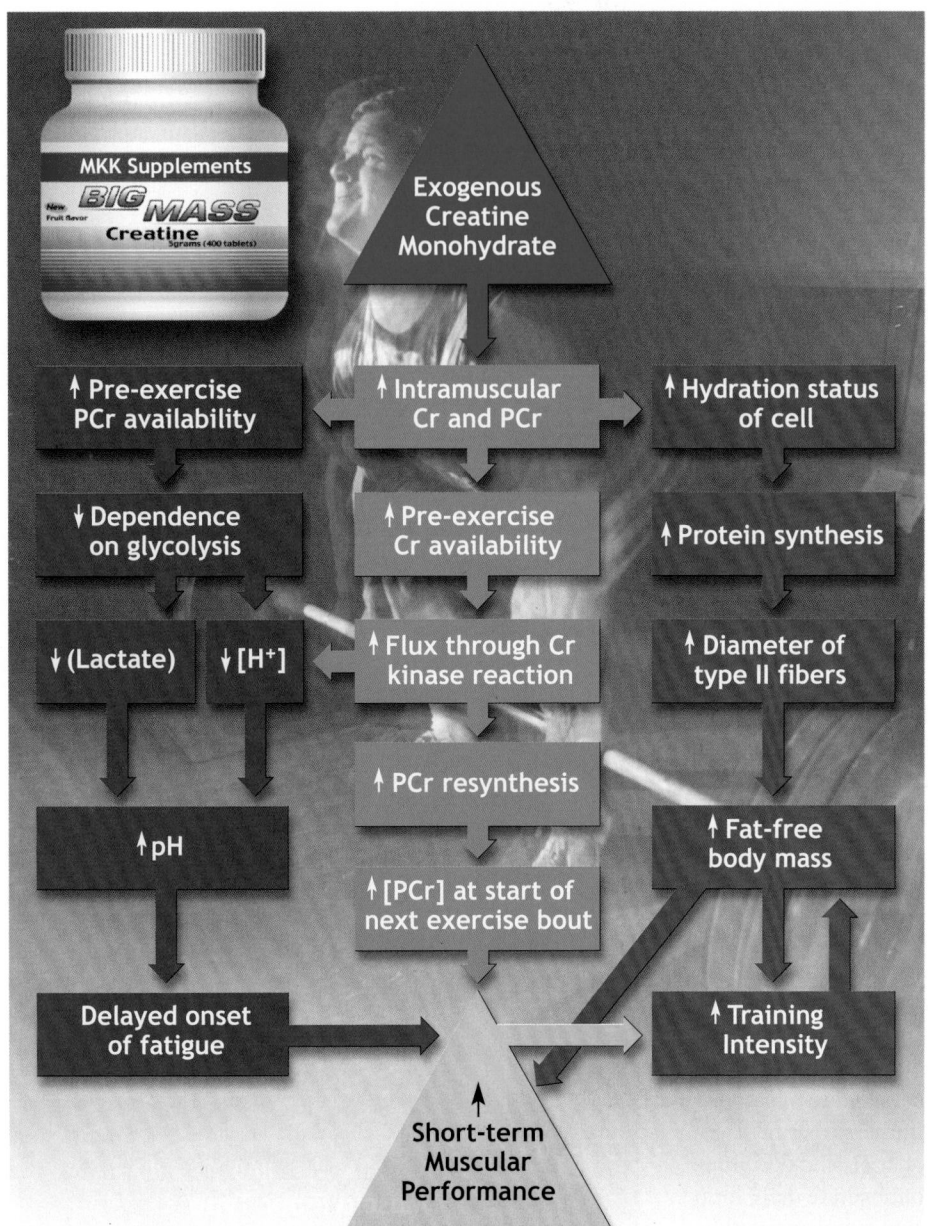

jumping, football, and volleyball. Oral creatine supplementation combined with resistance training affects cellular processes in a manner that increases protein deposition within the muscle's contractile mechanism.[283] This response could explain any increase in muscle size and strength associated with creatine supplementation.

Creatine supplementation does not improve cardiovascular and metabolic responses during continuous incremental treadmill running or performance that requires a high level of aerobic energy transfer.[11,112]

Age Effects Uncertain

Whether creatine supplementation augments the training response in older individuals remains equivocal. For 70-year-old men, a creatine supplementation loading phase (0.3 g per kg body mass for 5 days) followed by a daily maintenance phase (0.07 g per kg body mass) increased lean tissue mass, leg strength, muscular endurance, and average power of the legs during resistance training to a greater extent than a placebo.[56] Creatine supplements also benefit muscular performance in normally active older men.[108] In contrast, no enhancement in resistance-training response to creatine ingestion occurred among sedentary and weight-trained older adults, perhaps due to an age-related decline in creatine transport efficiency.[28] Short-term creatine supplementation per se, without resistance training, does not increase muscle protein synthesis or FFM.[196]

FIGURE 23.18 • Mechanisms to explain why increased intracellular creatine (*Cr*) and phosphocreatine (*PCr*) might enhance intense, short-term exercise performance and the exercise-training response. (Adapted with permission from Volek JS, Kraemer WJ. Creatine supplementation: its effect on human muscular performance and body composition. *J Strength Cond Res* 1996;10:200.)

Effects on Body Mass and Body Composition

Increases in body mass between 0.5 and 5.2 kg often accompany creatine supplementation, independent of changes in testosterone or cortisol concentrations.[130,274] How much of the weight gain occurs from the anabolic effect of creatine on muscle tissue synthesis, retention of intracellular water from increased creatine stores, or other factors remains unclear.

Resistance-trained men matched for physical characteristics and maximal strength randomly received a placebo or creatine supplement. Supplementation consisted of

processes (and accompanying lactate formation) and helps replenish muscle creatine following intense physical activity and promotes recovery of muscle contractile capacity, enabling athletes to maintain repeated efforts of intense exercise and training. A facilitated rate of muscle relaxation may also contribute to the ergogenic action of creatine supplementation.[264] Besides benefiting weightlifting and bodybuilding, improved immediate anaerobic power output capacity aids sprint running, swimming, kayaking, cycling,

25 g daily followed by maintenance at 5 g daily. Both groups engaged in heavy resistance training for 12 wk. **Figure 23.19A** shows a greater training-induced increase occurred in body mass and FFM for the creatine-supplemented group compared with controls. The same was true for maximum bench press and squat strength increases in the creatine group than in controls (**Fig. 23.19B**). Creatine supplementation induced greater muscle fiber hypertrophy with resistance training, indicated by greater enlargement in types I (35 vs. 11%), IIA (36 vs. 15%), and IIAB muscle fiber cross-sectional areas (35 vs. 6%; **Fig. 23.19C**). The larger volume of weight lifted during weeks 5 to 8 by the creatine supplement group suggests that higher-quality training sessions mediated more favorable adaptations in FFM, muscle morphology, and strength performance.

Creatine Loading

Many creatine users pursue a loading phase by ingesting 20 to 30 g of creatine daily for 5 to 7 days. Individuals who consume vegetarian-type diets show the greatest increase in muscle creatine levels because of their low dietary creatine content. Particularly large increases characterize individuals with normally low basal levels of intramuscular creatine.[40,48] A maintenance phase follows the loading phase. During this time, the athlete supplements with as little as 2 to 5 g of creatine daily.

Practical questions for the athlete desiring to elevate intramuscular creatine levels concern the magnitude and time course of intramuscular creatine increase with supplementation, dosage needed to maintain the creatine increase, and rate of creatine loss or "washout" when supplementation ceases. To provide insight into these questions, researchers studied two groups of men. In one experiment, six men ingested 20 g of creatine monohydrate (approximately 0.3 g per kg of body mass) for 6 consecutive days and then stopped the supplementation. Biopsies assessed muscle creatine levels before supplement ingestion and at days 7, 21, and 35. Similarly, nine men took 20 g of creatine monohydrate daily for 6 consecutive days. Instead of discontinuing supplementation, they reduced dosage to 2 g daily (approximately 0.03 g per kg body mass) for an additional 28 days. **Figure 23.20A** shows that total muscle creatine concentration increased approximately 20% (from 122 to 146 mM · kg dm^{-1}) after 6 days. Without continued supplementation, muscle creatine content gradually declined to near baseline in 35 days. The group that continued to supplement with reduced creatine intake for an additional 28 days maintained muscle creatine at the higher level (**Fig. 23.20B**).

For both groups, the increase in total muscle creatine content during the initial 6-day supplementation period averaged about 23 mmol per kg of dry muscle; this represented about 20 g (17%) of total creatine ingested. A similar 20% increase in total muscle creatine concentration occurred with only a 3-g daily supplement (not shown). The increase occurred more gradually and required 28 days rather than 6 days with the 6-g supplement.

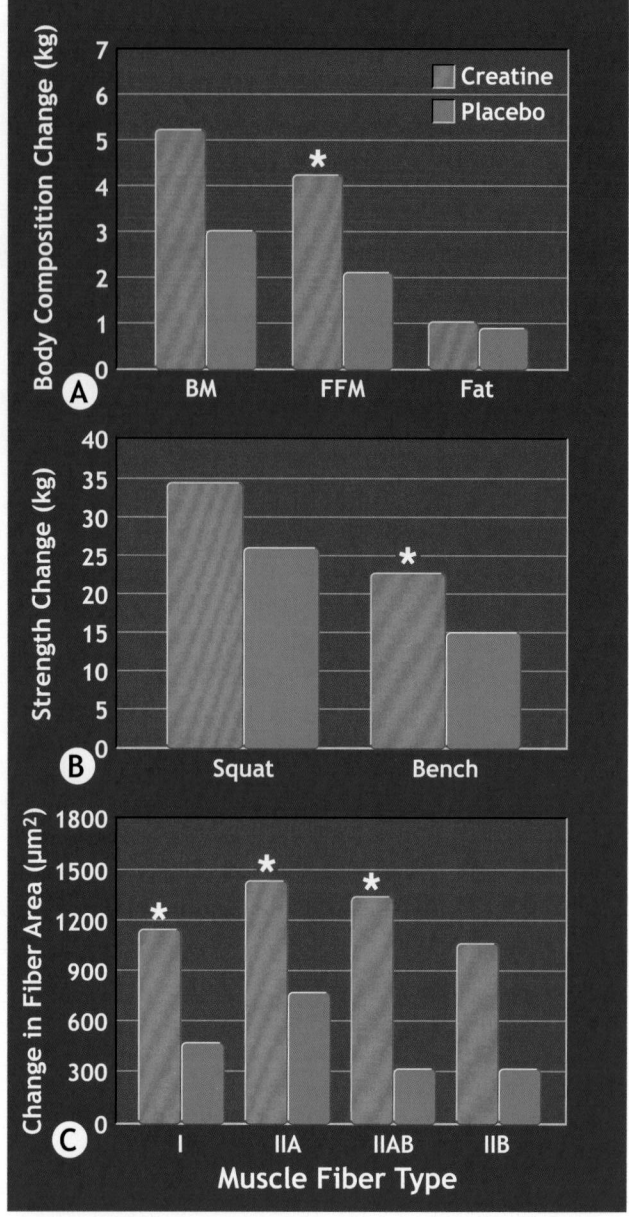

FIGURE 23.19 • Effects of 12 wk of creatine supplementation plus heavy-resistance training on changes in (A) body mass (BM), fat-free body mass (FFM), and body fat; (B) muscular strength in the squat and bench press; and (C) cross-sectional areas of specific muscle fiber types. The placebo group did identical training and received an equivalent quantity of powdered cellulose in capsule form. *Change significantly greater compared to the placebo group. (Reprinted with permission from Volek JS, et al. Performance and muscle fiber adaptations to creatine supplementation and heavy-resistance training. *Med Sci Sports Exerc* 1999;31:1147, as adapted with permission from McArdle WD, Katch FI, Katch VL. *Sports and Exercise Nutrition.* 4th Ed. Philadelphia: Wolters Kluwer Health, 2013.)

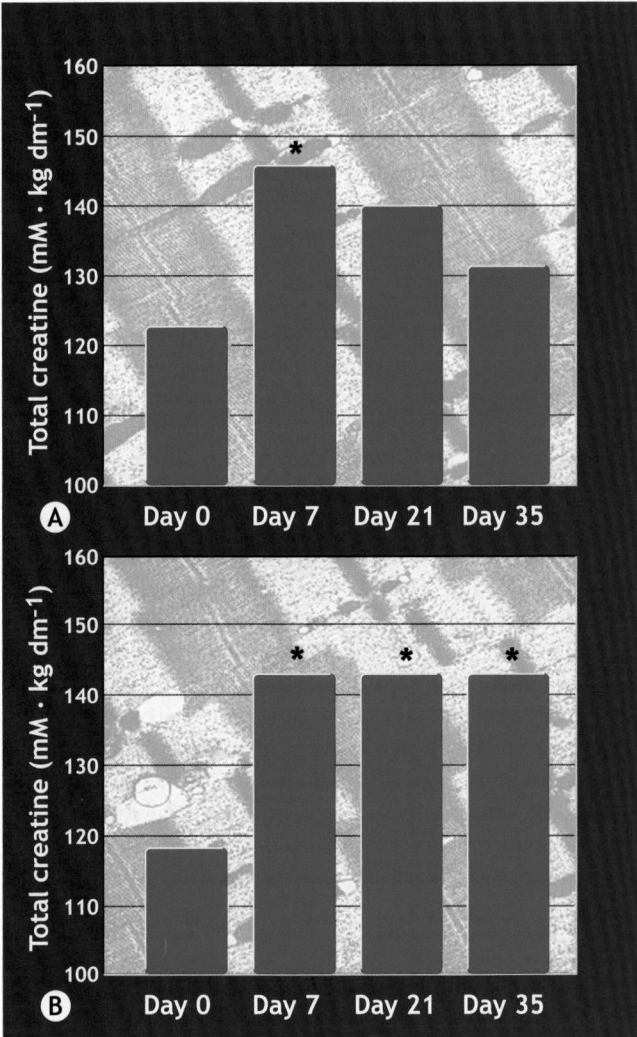

FIGURE 23.20 • **(A)** Total muscle creatine concentration in six men who consumed 20 g of creatine for 6 consecutive days and then stopped the supplement. Muscle biopsies done before ingestion (day 0) and on days 7, 21, and 35. **(B)** Total muscle creatine concentration in nine men who ingested 20 g of creatine for 6 consecutive days and then ingested 2 g of creatine daily for the next 28 days. Muscle biopsies taken before ingestion (day 0) and on days 7, 21, and 35. Values refer to averages per dry mass (dm). *Significantly different from day 0. (Adapted with permission from Hultman E, et al. Muscle creatine loading in men. *J Appl Physiol* 1996;81:232.)

 Rapid Way to Creatine-Load

A rapid way to creatine-load skeletal muscle requires ingesting 20 g of creatine monohydrate daily for 6 days; switching to a reduced 2-g per day dosage keeps these levels elevated for up to 28 days. If rapidity of loading is of little concern, supplementing with 3 g daily for 28 days achieves the same high levels.

Carbohydrate Ingestion Augments Creatine Loading. Consuming creatine with a sugar-containing drink increases creatine uptake and storage in skeletal muscle (**Fig. 23.21**).[239] For 5 days, subjects received either 5 g of creatine four times daily or a 5-g supplement followed 30 min later by 93 g of a high-glycemic simple sugar four times daily. The creatine-only group increased muscle PCr (7.2%), free creatine (13.5%), and total creatine (20.7%). Much larger increases occurred for the creatine-plus-sugar–supplemented group (14.7% for PCr, 18.1% for free creatine, and 33.0% for total creatine). Creatine supplementation alone did not affect insulin secretion, whereas adding sugar elevated plasma insulin levels. More than likely, augmented creatine storage with a creatine-plus-sugar supplement resulted from insulin-mediated glucose transport into skeletal muscle, which facilitated creatine transport into muscle fibers.

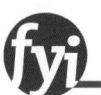 **Stop Caffeine When Using Creatine**

Caffeine negates the ergogenic effect of creatine supplementation. To evaluate the effect of pre-exercise caffeine ingestion on intramuscular creatine stores and intense exercise performance, subjects consumed either a placebo, a daily creatine supplement (0.5 g per kg body mass), or the same daily creatine supplement plus caffeine (5 mg per kg body mass) for 6 days.[262] Under each condition, subjects performed maximal intermittent knee-extension movements to fatigue on an isokinetic dynamometer. Creatine supplementation, with or without caffeine, increased intramuscular PCr (evaluated by nuclear magnetic resonance spectroscopy) between 4 and 6%. Dynamic torque production also increased 10 to 23% with creatine compared with the placebo. Consuming caffeine totally negated creatine's ergogenic effect. *To optimize creatine's benefits, athletes should abstain from caffeine-containing foods and beverages for several days prior to and during creatine loading, training, and competition.*

Some Research Shows No Benefit

Not all research confirms positive effects of creatine supplementation. Ergogenic effects may not emerge under the following seven conditions, but the reason for the discrepancies remains unknown:

1. In untrained subjects performing a single 15-s bout of sprint cycling[64]
2. In trained subjects performing bouts of sport-specific physical activities such as swimming, cycling, and running[41,92]
3. In trained and untrained older adults[131,286]
4. In resistance-trained individuals[250]
5. In trained rowers[74]
6. During rapid weight loss[190]
7. When short-term supplementation does not increase muscle PCr[92,186]

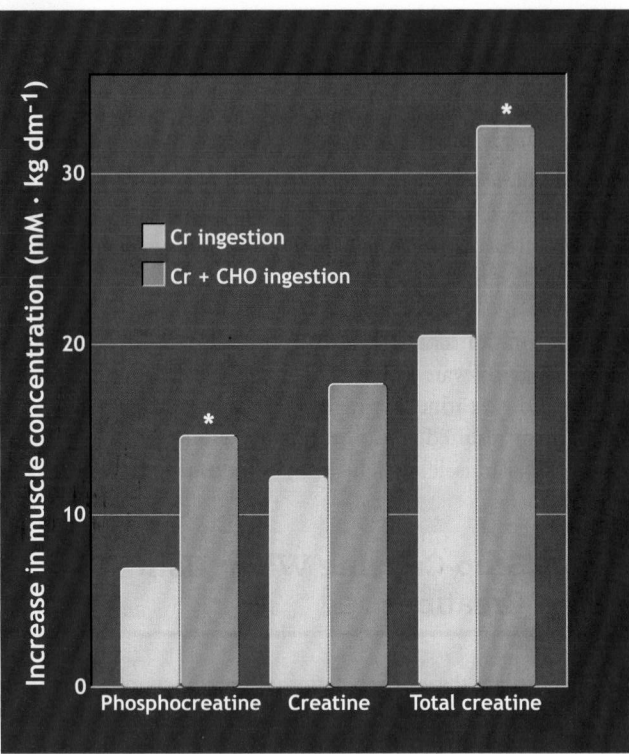

FIGURE 23.21 • Increases in dry muscle (dm) concentrations of phosphocreatine (PCr), creatine (Cr), and total creatine in one group after 5 days of Cr supplementation and in another group after 5 days of Cr and carbohydrate (CHO) supplementation. Values represent averages. *Significantly greater than creatine-only supplementation. (Adapted with permission from Green AL, et al. Carbohydrate ingestion augments skeletal muscle creatine accumulation during creatine supplementation in humans. *Am J Physiol* 1996;271:E821.)

Lipid Supplementation with Medium-Chain Triacylglycerols

Do high-fat foods or lipid supplements elevate plasma fatty acid levels to increase energy availability from fat during prolonged aerobic physical activity? Several factors affect the answer to this question. First, consuming triacylglycerols composed of predominantly 12 to 18 carbon long-chain fatty acids delays gastric emptying. This negatively affects the rapidity of fat availability and slows fluid and carbohydrate replenishment, both crucial factors in intense endurance activity. Second, after digestion and intestinal absorption (normally 3 to 4 hr), long-chain triacylglycerols reassemble with phospholipids, fatty acids, and a cholesterol shell to form fatty droplets called *chylomicrons*. These substances travel slowly to the systemic circulation via the lymphatic system. They eventually empty into the systemic venous blood in the neck region by way of the thoracic duct. Through the action of the enzyme lipoprotein lipase that lines capillary walls, chylomicrons in the bloodstream readily hydrolyze to provide free fatty acids and glycerol for use by peripheral tissues.

The relatively slow rate of gastric emptying and subsequent digestion, absorption, and assimilation of long-chain triacylglycerols makes this energy source an undesirable supplement to augment energy metabolism during physical activity.

Medium-chain triacylglycerols (MCTs) provide a more rapid source of fatty acid fuel. MCTs are processed oils, frequently produced for patients with intestinal malabsorption and tissue-wasting diseases. Marketing for the sports enthusiast hypes MCTs as "fat burners," "energy sources," "glycogen sparers," and "muscle builders." Unlike longer-chain triacylglycerols, MCTs contain saturated fatty acids with 8 to 10 carbon atoms along the fatty acid chain. During digestion, lipase in the mouth, stomach, and intestinal duodenum hydrolyzes MCTs to glycerol and medium-chain fatty acids (MCFAs). Their water solubility allows MCFAs to move rapidly across the intestinal mucosa directly into the bloodstream (portal vein) without first being transported as chylomicrons by the lymphatic system as long-chain triacylglycerols require. Once at the tissues, MCFAs move readily through the plasma membrane where they diffuse across the inner mitochondrial membrane for oxidation—they enter the mitochondria largely independent of the carnitine–acyl-CoA transferase system. The speed of cellular uptake and mitochondrial oxidation contrasts with the relatively slower transfer and oxidation rate of long-chain fatty acids. MCTs do not usually store as body fat because of their relative ease of oxidation. Ingesting MCTs rapidly elevates plasma FFAs, making it plausible that these lipids might spare liver and muscle glycogen during aerobic exercise.

Inconclusive Exercise Benefits of MCTs

Consuming MCTs does not inhibit gastric emptying, as does common fat, but conflicting research supports their use prior to physical activity.[268,272] In early studies, subjects consumed 380 mg of MCT oil per kilogram of body mass 1 hr before exercising at 60 to 70% of $\dot{V}O_{2max}$ for 1 hr.[69] Plasma ketone levels generally increased, but the exercise metabolic mixture did not change compared with a placebo trial or a trial after subjects consumed a glucose polymer. Catabolism of 30 g of MCTs (estimated maximal amount tolerated in the gastrointestinal tract) consumed before exercising contributed only 3 to 7% to the total energy requirement.[134]

 INTEGRATIVE QUESTION

Discuss the importance of the psychologic or "placebo" effect to evaluate claims for the effectiveness of particular nutrients, chemicals, or procedures as ergogenic aids.

Subsequent research investigated possible metabolic and ergogenic effects of consuming 86 g of MCT (surprisingly well tolerated). Six endurance-trained cyclists rode for 2 hr at 60% of $\dot{V}O_{2peak}$ while ingesting 2 L of 4.3% MCT emulsion,

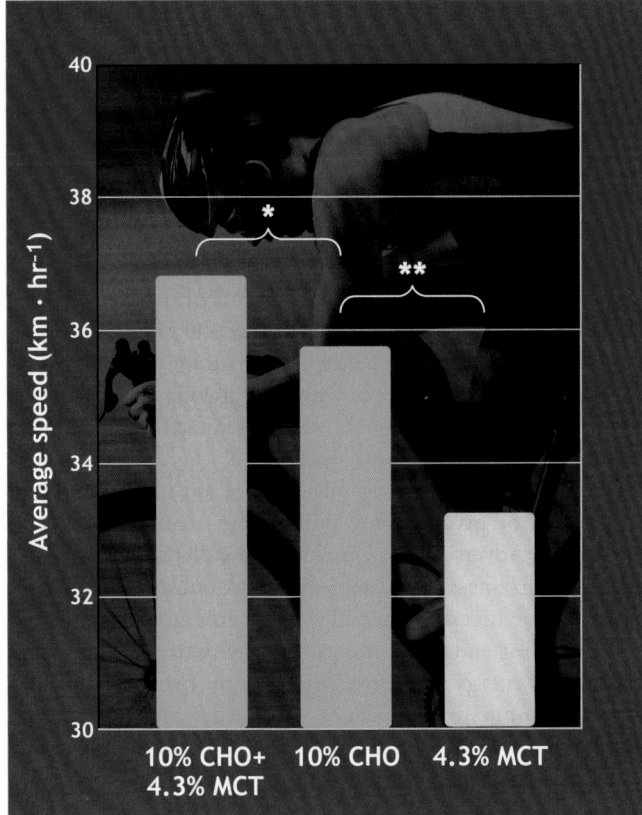

FIGURE 23.22 • Effects of carbohydrate (CHO; 10% solution), medium-chain triacylglycerol (MCT; 4.3% emulsion), and carbohydrate 1 MCT (10% CHO 1 4.3% MCT) ingestion during cycling on simulated 40-km time-trial cycling speeds after 2 hr of exercise at 60% of $\dot{V}O_{2peak}$. *Significantly faster than 10% CHO trials; **Significantly faster than 4.3% MCT trials. (Adapted with permission from Van Zyl CG, et al. Effects of medium-chain triglyceride ingestion on fuel metabolism and cycling performance. *J Appl Physiol* 1996;80:2217.)

10% glucose plus 4.3% MCT emulsion, or a 10% glucose solution during exercise. They then performed a simulated 40-km cycling time trial. **FIGURE 23.22** shows the effects of the different beverages on average speed in the time trials. Replacing the carbohydrate beverage with only MCTs produced an 8% decrement in performance (in agreement with another study), but the combined carbohydrate plus MCT solution consumed throughout the activity produced only a 2.5% improvement in cycling speed compared with the two other conditions. This ergogenic effect occurred with reduced total carbohydrate oxidation at a given level of oxygen consumption, higher final circulating FFA and ketone levels, and lower final glucose and lactate concentrations.

The small ergogenic enhancement by MCT supplementation probably occurred because this exogenous source of fatty acids contributes relatively little to the total energy expenditure (and total fat oxidation) during sustained effort.[135] MCT ingestion does not stimulate release of bile, the gall bladder's fat-emulsifying agent. Consequently, cramping and diarrhea

often accompany excess intake of this lipid. It provides little ergogenic effect.

Pyruvate

Ergogenic effects have been extolled for pyruvate, the three-carbon end product of the cytoplasmic breakdown of glucose in glycolysis. Exogenous pyruvate, as a partial replacement for dietary carbohydrate, supposedly augments endurance performance and promotes fat loss. Pyruvic acid, a relatively unstable chemical, causes intestinal distress, so various forms of the salt of this acid that includes sodium, potassium, calcium, or magnesium pyruvate are manufactured in capsule, tablet, or powder form.

Dosage recommendations range between a total of 2 and 5 g of pyruvate spread throughout the day and taken with meals. One capsule usually contains 600 mg pyruvate. The calcium form of pyruvate also contains approximately 80 mg of calcium with 600 mg of pyruvate. Some advertisements recommend dosage of one capsule per 20 lb of body weight. Manufacturers also combine creatine monohydrate and pyruvate; 1 g of creatine pyruvate provides about 80 mg of creatine and 400 mg of pyruvate. Recommended pyruvate dosages range from 5 to 20 g per day. Pyruvate content in the normal diet ranges from 100 to 2000 mg daily. The largest dietary amounts occur in fruits and vegetables, particularly red apples (500 mg each), with smaller quantities in dark beer (80 mg per 12 oz) and red wine (75 mg per 6 oz).

Endurance Performance

Reports indicate beneficial effects of exogenous pyruvate on endurance performance. Two double-blind, crossover studies by the same laboratory showed that 7 days of daily supplementation of a 100-g mixture of pyruvate (25 g) plus 75 g of dihydroxyacetone (DHA, another three-carbon compound of glycolysis) increased upper- and lower-body aerobic endurance by 20% compared with exercise with a 100-g supplement of an isocaloric glucose polymer.[244,245] The pyruvate–DHA mixture increased cycle ergometer time to exhaustion of the legs by 13 min (66 vs. 79 min), while upper-body arm-cranking time increased by 27 min (133 vs. 160 min). Exercising with the pyruvate–DHA mixture reduced local muscle and overall body ratings of perceived exertion compared with the placebo condition.[221]

Proponents of pyruvate supplementation maintain that elevated extracellular pyruvate augments glucose transport into active muscle. Enhanced "glucose extraction" from the blood provides the important energy source to sustain high-intensity aerobic effort while conserving intramuscular glycogen stores.[128] When the individual's diet contains a normal level of carbohydrate (approximately 55% of total energy intake), pyruvate supplementation also increases pre-exercise muscle glycogen levels.[245] Both of these effects—higher pre-exercise glycogen levels and facilitated glucose uptake and oxidation by active muscle—benefit endurance similarly as pre-exercise carbohydrate loading and glucose feedings during exercise exert ergogenic effects.

Body Fat Loss

Subsequent research by the same investigators who showed ergogenic effects of pyruvate supplementation indicates that exogenous pyruvate intake augments body fat loss when accompanied by a low-calorie diet. Overfat women in a metabolic ward maintained a liquid 1000-kcal daily energy intake (68% carbohydrate, 22% protein, 10% lipid). Adding 20 g of sodium pyruvate plus 16 g of calcium pyruvate (13% of energy intake) daily for 3 wk induced greater weight loss (13.0 vs. 9.5 lb) and fat loss (8.8 vs. 5.9 lb) than a control group on the same diet who received an equivalent amount of extra energy as glucose.[246] These findings complement the researchers' previous study with obese subjects that showed that adding DHA and pyruvate (substituted as equivalent energy for glucose) to a severely restricted low-energy diet facilitated body weight and fat loss (without increased nitrogen loss).[247] Consuming pyruvate may stimulate small increases in futile metabolic activity where metabolism does not couple to ATP production with a subsequent wasting of energy.

Adverse side effects of a 30- to 100-g daily pyruvate intake include diarrhea and gastrointestinal gurgling and discomfort. *Until studies from independent laboratories reproduce existing findings for physical performance and body fat loss, one should view the effectiveness of pyruvate supplementation with caution.*[82]

Summary

1. The term *ergogenic aid* describes substances or procedures that improve physical work capacity, physiologic function, or athletic performance.
2. The strongest research studies apply a randomized, double-blind, placebo-controlled design.
3. Different levels of evidence permit grading the strengths of research studies.
4. Anabolic steroids compose a group of pharmacologic agents frequently used for ergogenic purposes. These drugs function like the hormone testosterone; they increase muscle size, strength, and power with resistance training in some individuals.
5. The β_2-adrenergic agonists clenbuterol and albuterol increase skeletal muscle mass and slow fat gain in animals to counter aging, immobilization, malnutrition, and tissue-wasting pathology. A negative finding showed hastened fatigue during short-term, intense muscle actions.
6. Debate exists about whether administration of growth hormone to healthy individuals augments muscular hypertrophy when combined with resistance training. Health risks exist for those who abuse this chemical.
7. Dehydroepiandersterone (DHEA), a relatively weak steroid hormone synthesized from cholesterol by the adrenal cortex, steadily decreases throughout adulthood, prompting individuals to supplement, hoping to counteract the effects of natural aging. DHEA does not produce an ergogenic effect.
8. Research indicates no effect of androstenedione supplementation on basal serum concentrations of testosterone or training response for muscle size and strength and body composition.
9. No ergogenic effects exist for healthy subjects from chronic oral amino acid supplements on hormone secretion, training responsiveness, or physical performance.
10. Hormonal dynamics from carbohydrate and/or protein supplementation immediately following a resistance-exercise workout suggests an ergogenic effect on training responsiveness.
11. Amphetamines, or pep pills, do not aid physical performance or psychomotor skills, other than by a placebo effect. Adverse effects include drug dependency, headache, dizziness, confusion, and gastrointestinal distress.
12. Caffeine ingestion typically exerts an ergogenic effect by extending endurance in aerobic activity from increased fat use for energy and conservation of glycogen reserves.
13. No compelling evidence supports ginseng supplementation to benefit physiologic function or exercise performance. Significant health risks accompany ephedrine use.
14. Concentrated buffering solutions consumed before physical activity improve anaerobic performance.
15. Further research must determine the benefits and risks of glutamine, phosphatidylserine, and β-hydroxyl–β-methylbutyrate to provide a "natural" anabolic boost with resistance training.
16. The additional blood volume and increased red cell mass and concentration from red blood cell reinfusion contribute to a larger maximum cardiac output and an increase in the blood's oxygen-carrying capacity and $\dot{V}O_{2max}$.
17. A physiologic rationale for why warm-up should enhance exercise performance includes benefits on muscle-shortening velocity and efficiency, enhanced oxygen delivery and use, and facilitated transmission of nerve impulses.
18. Moderate warm-up proves beneficial immediately before sudden, strenuous exertion by reducing myocardial work and augmenting coronary blood flow when activity begins.
19. Breathing hyperoxic gas during physical activity extends endurance by increasing oxygen consumption, reducing blood lactate, and lowering pulmonary ventilation, but provides no ergogenic effect before or after exercise.
20. Carbohydrate loading augments endurance in prolonged submaximal effort. Athletes should be well informed about this procedure because of potential negative effects.
21. A modification of the classic loading procedure provides the same high level of glycogen storage without dramatic alterations in the diet and exercise routine.

22. No benefits emerge from chromium supplements on training-related changes in muscular strength, physique, or muscle mass for individuals with adequate dietary chromium intake.

23. Creatine supplements increase intramuscular creatine and PCr, enhance brief anaerobic power output capacity, and facilitate recovery from repeated bouts of intense effort.

24. Medium-chain triacylglycerols (MCTs) enhance fat oxidation and conserve glycogen during endurance activity.

This procedure does enhance performance by an additional 2.5%.

25. Pyruvate supplementation purportedly augments endurance performance and promotes fat loss, but a definitive conclusion concerning its effectiveness requires research verification.

thePoint References are available online at **http://thepoint.lww.com/mkk8e.**

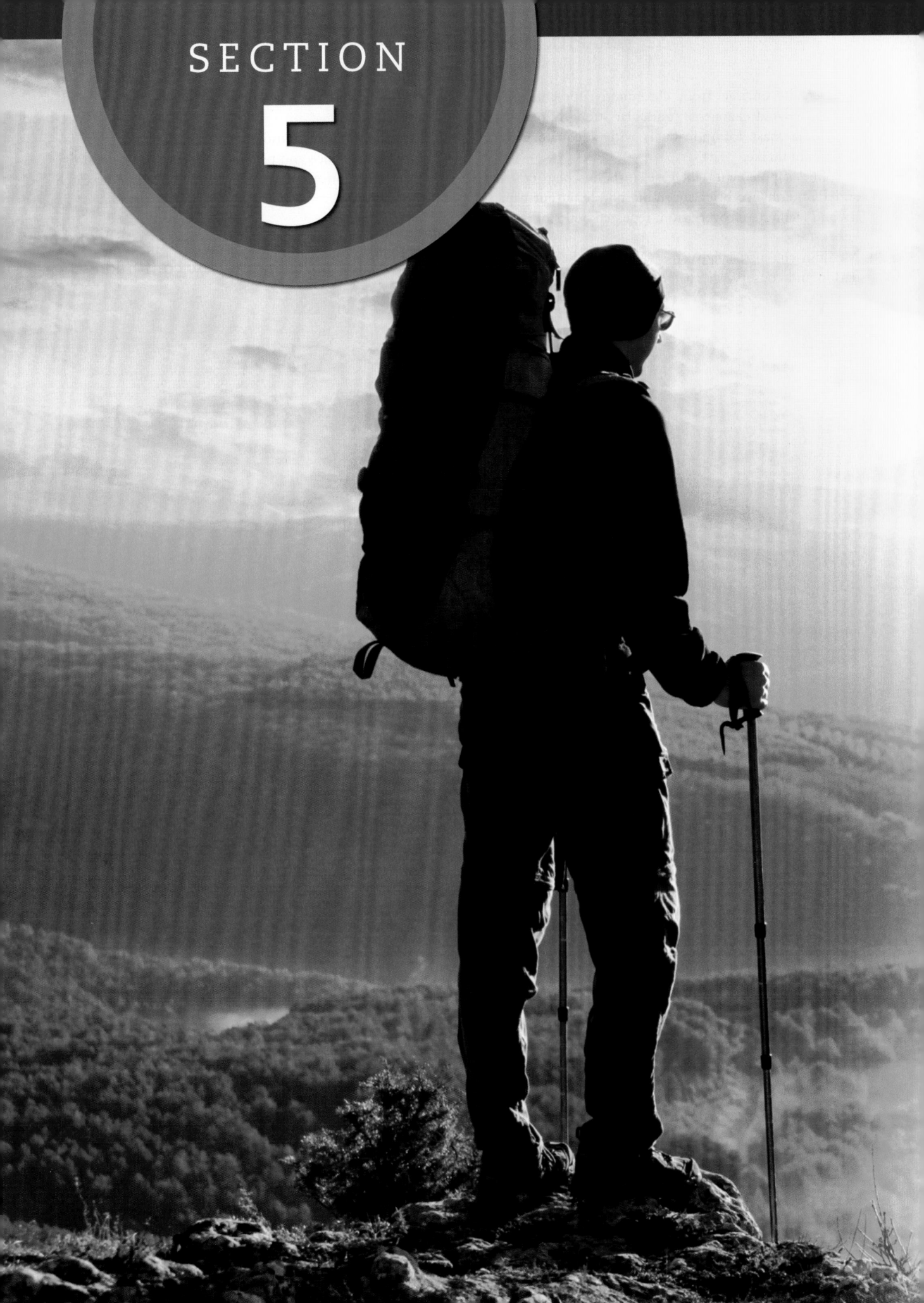

Exercise Performance and Environmental Stress

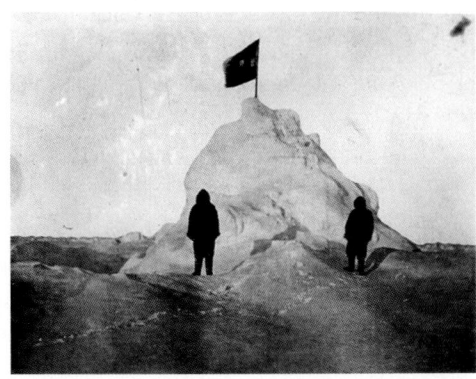

"The true explorer does his work not for any hopes of reward or honor, but because the thing he has set for himself to do is a part of his being, and must be accomplished for the sake of the accomplishment. And he counts lightly hardships, risks, obstacles, if only they do not bar him from his goal."

—Rear Admiral Robert E. Peary (1856–1920), polar explorer who discovered the North Pole

Image from www.history.navy.mil/bios/peary_roberte.htm

OVERVIEW

Sport activities often take place at terrestrial elevations that impair oxygenation of blood flowing through the lungs and severely limit aerobic energy metabolism for exercise. At the other extreme, exploration beneath the water's surface poses a different challenge. Divers must transport their sea-level environment as a gas mixture compressed in a scuba tank carried on the back. Some diving enthusiasts use no external assistance, and the length of an underwater excursion becomes limited by two factors:

1. Quantity of air inhaled into the lungs just before the dive
2. Buildup of arterial carbon dioxide during the dive

In both breath-hold diving and scuba diving, the environment provides unique challenges and dangers for the participant, often independent of the stress of exercise. Consideration also must focus on the thermal quality of the environment. On land, exercising in a hot, humid environment or extreme cold imposes severe stress. These environmental demands impair exercise capacity and pose a severe threat to health and safety. Space exploration and accompanying short- and long-term exposures to near-zero gravity present a unique set of environmental stressors that impinge on physiologic function, structural mass, and exercise capacity both during flight and upon return to Earth. The extent that each environmental stressor deviates from neutral conditions and the duration of the exposure determine the total impact on the body. The effect of several simultaneous environmental stressors, as for example, extreme cold and exposure at high altitude, may exceed the simple additive consequence of each stressor imposed separately.

In the four chapters that follow, we explore the specific problems encountered at altitude, during exercise in hot and cold environments, and from prolonged exposure to microgravity. We also discuss the immediate physiologic adjustments and long-term adaptations as the body strives to maintain internal consistency despite an environmental challenge. The chapter on sport diving considers the unique problems associated with this increasingly popular form of sport and recreation.

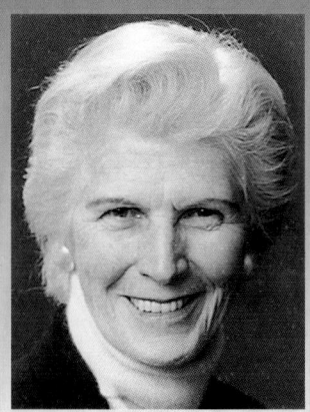

INTERVIEW WITH
Barbara Drinkwater

Education: BS (Douglass College, Rutgers University, New Brunswick, NJ); MEd (University of North Carolina, Greensboro, NC); PhD (Purdue University, West Lafayette, IN).

Current Affiliation: Retired May 1, 2000. Previously, Research Physiologist, Department of Medicine, Pacific Medical Center, Seattle, WA.

Honors, Awards, and ACSM Honor Award Statement of Contributions: See Appendix C, available online at http://thepoint.lww.com/mkk8e

Research Focus: The response of women to exercise as mediated by environmental factors and aging. Special areas of interest have been the female athlete, her physical performance under environmental stressors such as heat and altitude, the effect of exercise-associated amenorrhea on bone health, and the role of exercise, calcium, and exercise in preventing osteoporosis.

Memorable Publication: Drinkwater BL. Bone mineral content of amenorrheic and eumenorrheic athletes. *N Engl J Med* 1984;311:277.

What first inspired you to enter the exercise science field? What made you decide to pursue your advanced degree and/or line of research?

➤ In 1965, I was teaching a methods course in track and field to physical education majors. One of them asked me why women weren't allowed to compete in the marathon and were restricted to running twice around the track. I decide to investigate the scientific rationale and found instead that myths and prejudice, not science, limited women's participation in sports. Several years later I had the opportunity to join the Institute of Environmental Stress at the University of California, Santa Barbara. The Institute, established in February 1965, was an interdepartmental organization providing broad coverage of the borderline fields that relate human function to the complex and changing environments to which humans and other organisms are continuously exposed. With the encouragement of the director, Steven M. Horvath, PhD, I began the series of studies that would demonstrate clearly that women of all ages could attain high levels of aerobic power and that cardiovascular fitness, not gender, accounted for the previous notion that women could not tolerate exercise in the heat.

What influence did your undergraduate education have on your final career choice?

➤ My undergraduate degree was in physical education. I had an excellent program that emphasized science as well as sports skills and teaching methods. However, none of the female faculty members had a doctorate degree, and graduate education was never mentioned. The assumption in those days was that we "majors" would go directly into teaching. However, I'm sure it was my love for sport and the excellent courses I had in physiology and kinesiology that later led me into the exercise science field.

Who were the most influential people in your career, and why?

➤ Oddly enough, the most influential individual in my career was Ben Winer, PhD, who taught the statistics courses I took in the doctoral program at Purdue. He was an outstanding teacher, and the skills and knowledge of experimental design that I gained in his classes led to my unofficial role of statistician and advisor on study designs at the Institute of Environmental Stress. Obviously, I owe a great deal to Steve Horvath as well, who gave me the opportunity to work at the Institute. A career encompasses not only your research and teaching, but your professional contributions as well. Individuals such as Charles Tipton, John Sutton, Carl Gilsolfi, Peter Raven, Chris Wells, Toby Tate, and a multitude of others all enhanced that aspect of my career. Their support and encouragement had a tremendous impact on my career and me.

What has been the most interesting/enjoyable aspect of your involvement in science? What was the least interesting/enjoyable aspect?

➤ The most enjoyable aspect of my scientific career has been the opportunity to encourage and "open some doors" for younger women on the road toward their own careers. That, plus the opportunity to speak to a wide variety of audiences about topics of importance to their health and well-being, have given me a great deal of satisfaction. The least enjoyable aspect has been the constant need to search for funds to keep the research program going.

What is your most meaningful contribution to the field of exercise science, and why is it so important?

➤ I would like to think that my most meaningful contribution to the field of exercise science has been to stimulate interest of other investigators in evaluating women's response to exercise, environmental stress, and aging. In terms of a specific area of research, I would have to select the area of the Female Athlete Triad, which demonstrates that the amenorrhea experienced by many female athletes can lead to irreversible bone loss. Until our 1984 paper in the *New England Journal of Medicine*, amenorrhea was assumed to be a benign—and welcome—condition by the athletes. When additional studies confirmed our results, athletes and those responsible for their health began to take the Triad seriously.

What advice would you give to students who express an interest in pursuing a career in exercise science research?

➤ My advice to an undergraduate student would be to select as many science courses as possible in areas related to exercise science and work hard to get good grades. Your selection to the better graduate programs will depend largely on your grade point average and the recommendations of your professors. If you are not a serious student, you are not going to have a successful career in research. In selecting a doctoral program, investigate thoroughly before applying. Not only will you be spending 4 to 5 years of your life in that department, but you will be depending on the reputation of that program and the faculty to secure a postdoctoral position. Among the factors to consider are the publications of the faculty and graduate students, ongoing research in your area of interest, laboratory facilities and equipment, success of graduates in obtaining postdoctoral positions, and the requirements for the PhD. If possible, talk with some recent graduates of the program and get their honest appraisal of their experience.

What interests have you pursued outside of your professional career?

➤ Sports, aviation, and animals. I've been active in a number of sports, but am now totally involved with golf—playing several times a week and even taking my clubs over to Australia to play when not at an Olympic venue. When I was in Santa Barbara, I found time to get a commercial pilot's license, an instrument rating, and an instrument instructor's rating. I spent many hours in the air on trips throughout California and the Southwest. When I moved to Vashon in 1982, I had two dogs and one cat. Within 6 months, a puppy found at the dump and another six cats that had come out of the woods joined the family. At that point, I decided the island needed a humane society, so I started one. Sixteen years later, the program is going strong and now includes a low-cost spay neuter program, a lost-and-found hotline, an adoption service, education programs in the schools, and medical–surgical help as well.

Where do you see the exercise science field (particularly your area of greatest interest) heading in the next 20 years?

➤ The exercise science field is so diverse that it may be impossible to make a general statement regarding future directions. I do believe there will be increasing interest in the

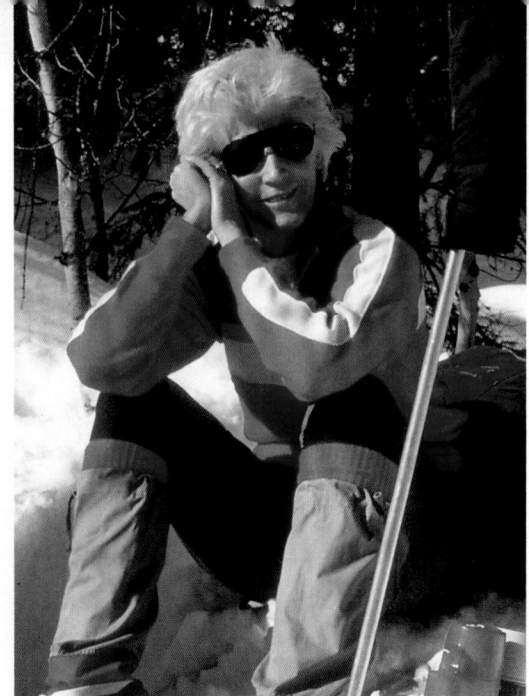

interaction of exercise and health. As our population continues to age, the rising cost of medical care will force an emphasis on lifestyle and other preventative measures. The Surgeon General's Healthy People 2000 Report has made physical activity and fitness the number one priority for health promotion and disease prevention. The responsibility for providing data-based evidence that physical activity does indeed prevent or ameliorate disease states, as well as defining the optimum exercise program for each segment of the population, will be the responsibility of the exercise scientist who is challenged by studying integrated physiological systems.

You have the opportunity to give a "last lecture." Describe its primary focus.

➤ I can't even conceive of accepting an invitation to give a "last lecture"! The actual final lecture I give will be one that I probably accepted to give 6 months earlier, and in the interim I've decided I've said enough, I have nothing new to say, and it's time to leave the stage to younger professionals with new and exciting data and insights. I hope I have the good sense to recognize that time when it comes.

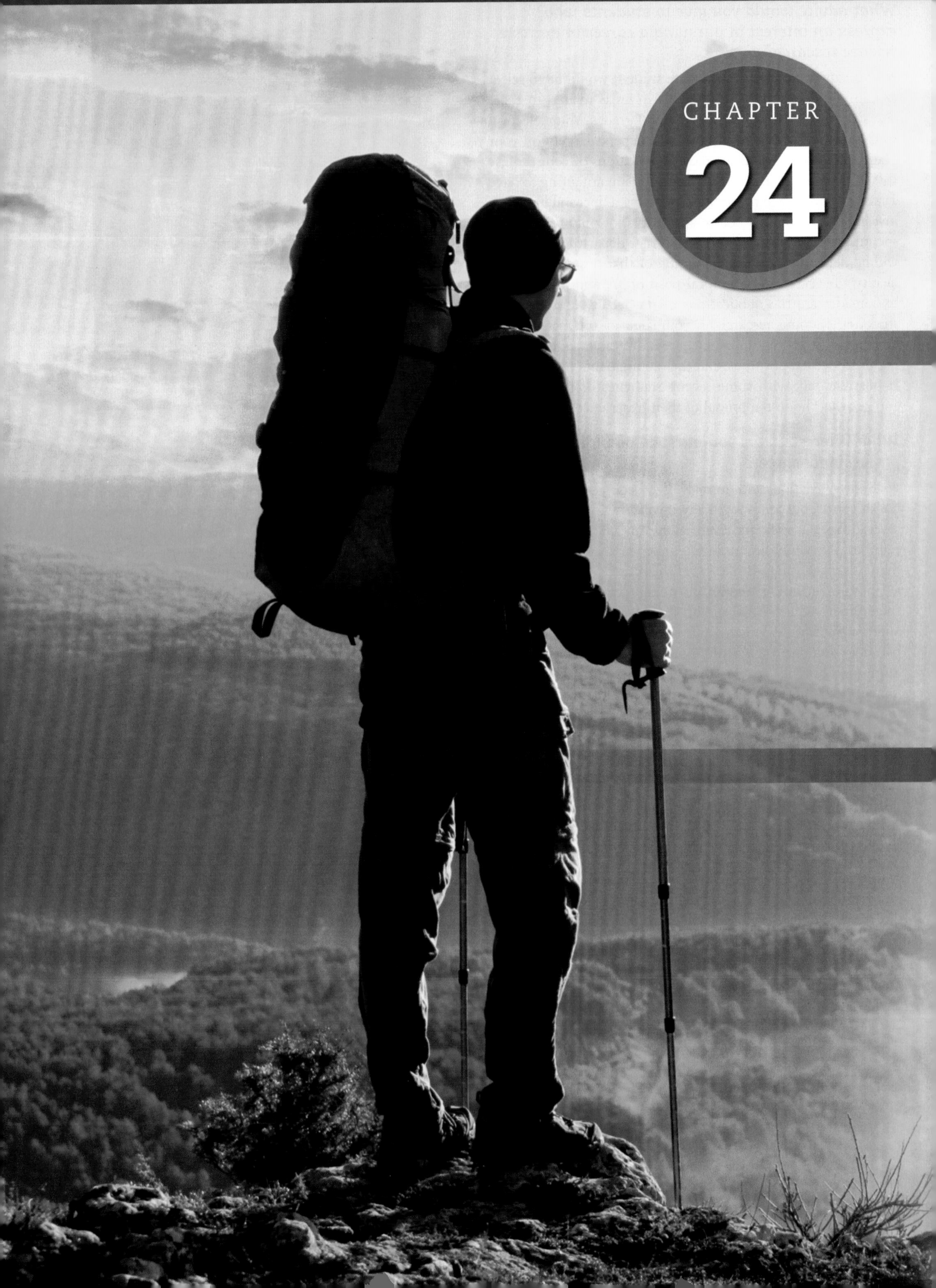

CHAPTER

24

Physical Activity at Medium and High Altitude

CHAPTER OBJECTIVES

- Outline the effects of increasingly higher altitudes on these three factors: partial pressure of oxygen in ambient air, oxygen saturation of hemoglobin in pulmonary capillaries, and $\dot{V}O_{2max}$

- Describe and quantify the oxygen transport cascade at sea level and 4300 m (14,108 ft)

- Discuss immediate and longer-term physiologic adjustments to altitude exposure

- Give symptoms, possible causes, and treatment for acute mountain sickness, high-altitude pulmonary edema, and high-altitude cerebral edema

- Describe the "lactate paradox" and possible causes for its occurrence

- Summarize factors that affect the time course for altitude acclimatization

- Graph the relationship between increasing altitude exposure and the decrease in $\dot{V}O_{2max}$ (% sea-level value)

- Discuss alterations in circulatory function that offset the benefits of altitude acclimatization on oxygen transport capacity

- Discuss whether altitude training produces greater improvement than sea-level training on sea-level exercise performance

- Describe the training concept of "living high, training low"

ANCILLARIES 👁 at-a-Glance

Visit http://thePoint.lww.com/mkk8e to access the following resources.

- References: Chapter 24
- Interactive Question Bank
- Focus on Research: High Altitude—A Hostile Environment

More than 40 million people live, work, and recreate at terrestrial elevations between 3048 m (10,000 ft) and 5486 m (18,000 ft) above sea level. Based on the Earth's topography, these elevations encompass the range generally considered **high altitude**. High-altitude natives inhabit permanent settlements up to 5486 m in the Andes and Himalayas. Prolonged exposure of an unacclimatized person to this altitude causes death from the ambient air's subnormal oxygen pressure (**hypoxia**), even if the person remains physically inactive. The physiologic challenge of even medium-altitude exposure becomes readily apparent during physical activity.[11] In the United States, in excess of 1 million people a year ascend Pikes Peak, Colorado (4300 m; 14,108 ft), the most visited mountain peak in North America and second most visited in the world, by train, car, or railroad, and thousands of others do so by climbing, cycling, and running. Millions more throughout the world ascend to high altitudes for mountaineering, trekking, tourism, business, and scientific and military excursions. Many newcomers to altitude do not take sufficient time to acclimatize to the physiologic challenge of the reduced partial pressure of oxygen (Po_2) in ambient air.

THE STRESS OF ALTITUDE

Altitude's physiologic challenge comes directly from decreased ambient Po_2, not from reduced total barometric pressure per se or any change in the relative concentrations (percentages) of gases in inspired (ambient) air. FIGURE 24.1 illustrates the barometric pressure, pressures of the respired gases, and percentage saturation of hemoglobin at various terrestrial elevations from Denver, CO to Mt. Everest. The dashed line shows the upper limit for permanent residence, the highest being about 4572 m (15,000 ft) in the mountainous region of Aguada Quilcha, Chile, a sparsely populated region with only 26 inhabitants per mile (http://www.satelliteview.co/?lid=3874233_CL_HSPNG_03). Compared to sea level ambient barometric pressure of 760 mm Hg, the ambient pressure at Aguada Quilcha is reduced by nearly one-half. FIGURE 24.2 shows changes that occur in oxygen availability (reflected by Po_2) in ambient air, alveolar air, and arterial and mixed-venous blood as one ascends from sea level to Pikes Peak. The **oxygen transport cascade** refers to the progressive change in the environment's oxygen pressure and in various body areas.

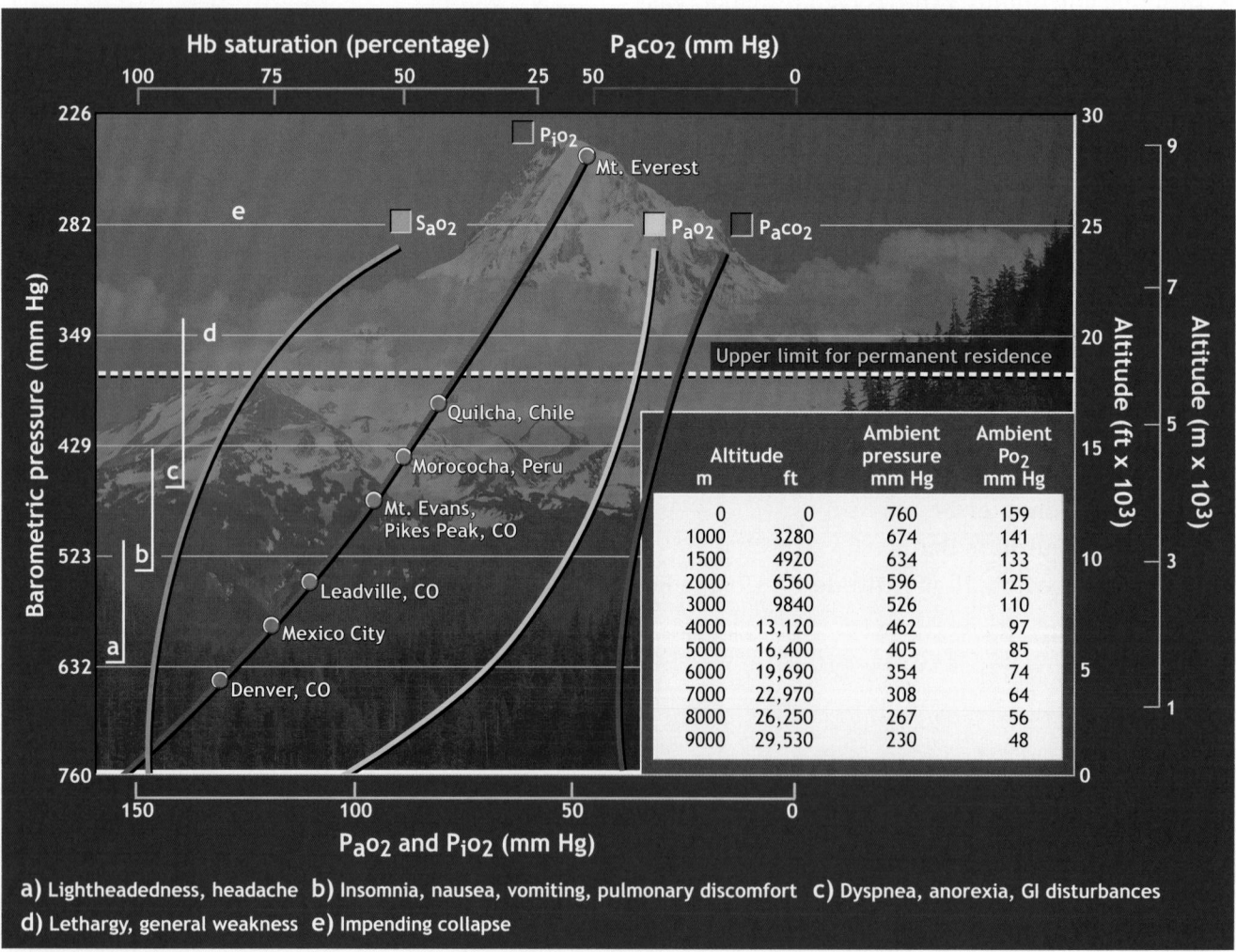

Altitude		Ambient pressure	Ambient Po_2
m	ft	mm Hg	mm Hg
0	0	760	159
1000	3280	674	141
1500	4920	634	133
2000	6560	596	125
3000	9840	526	110
4000	13,120	462	97
5000	16,400	405	85
6000	19,690	354	74
7000	22,970	308	64
8000	26,250	267	56
9000	29,530	230	48

a) Lightheadedness, headache **b)** Insomnia, nausea, vomiting, pulmonary discomfort **c)** Dyspnea, anorexia, GI disturbances
d) Lethargy, general weakness **e)** Impending collapse

FIGURE 24.1 • Changes in environmental and physiologic variables with progressive elevations in altitude (P_aO_2, partial pressure of arterial oxygen; P_aCO_2, partial pressure of arterial carbon dioxide; P_iO_2, partial pressure of oxygen in inspired air; S_aO_2, oxygen saturation of hemoglobin).

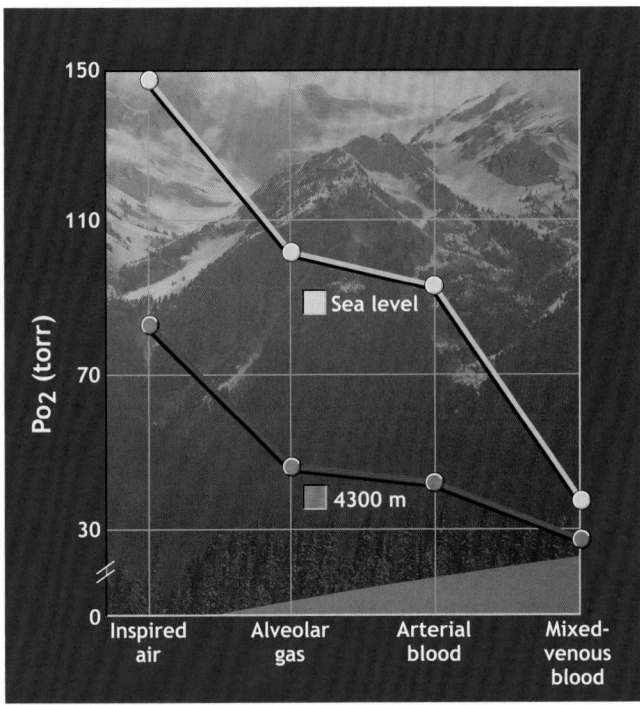

FIGURE 24.2 • Oxygen transport cascade from sea level to 4300 m (14,108 ft).

Air density decreases progressively with ascent above sea level. For example, barometric pressure at sea level averages 760 mm Hg; at 3048 m (10,000 ft), the barometer drops to 510 mm Hg. At an elevation of 5486 m (17,999 ft), the pressure of a column of air at the Earth's surface equals about one half of its sea-level pressure. Dry ambient air at sea level and altitude contains 20.93% oxygen, while the Po_2 (density of the oxygen molecules) of air decreases directly with the fall in barometric pressure upon ascending to higher elevations ($Po_2 = 0.2093 \times$ barometric pressure). Thus, ambient Po_2 at sea level averages 150 mm Hg, but only 107 mm Hg at 3048 m (10,000 ft). At the summit of Mt. Everest (8848 m; 29,028 ft), ambient air pressure usually ranges between 251 and 253 mm Hg with a concomitant alveolar Po_2 of about 25 mm Hg (ambient air Po_2 between 42 and 43 mm Hg).[110] This equals only about 30% of the oxygen available in air at sea level. *Arterial hypoxia that accompanies the reduction in Po_2 precipitates both the immediate physiologic adjustments to altitude and the longer-term process of acclimatization.* Following the recommendation of the International Union of Physiological Sciences (www.iups.org), **acclimatization** refers to adaptations produced by changes in the natural environment, whether through a change in season or place of residence. In contrast, **acclimation** concerns adaptations produced in a controlled laboratory environment (in specialized chambers) that simulate high altitude or microgravity, hypoxic environments, and extremes of thermal stress.

Oxygen Loading at Altitude

The S-shaped nature of the oxyhemoglobin dissociation curve (see Fig. 13.4, Chapter 13) indicates that only a small change occurs in hemoglobin's percentage saturation with oxygen until an altitude of about 3048 m (10,000 ft). At 1981 m (6500 ft), for example, alveolar Po_2 decreases from its sea-level value of 100 mm Hg to 78 mm Hg, yet hemoglobin remains 90% saturated with oxygen. This relatively small arterial desaturation exerts little effect on a person during rest or performance of mild physical activity but severely curtails performance in vigorous aerobic activities. The poorer performances of men and women in middle-distance and distance running and swimming during the 1968 Olympics in Mexico City (altitude 2300 m; 7546 ft) resulted from the small reduction in oxygen transport at this altitude. No new world records were established in events lasting longer than 2.5 min. Altitude does *not* impair the short-term anaerobic energy system at moderate altitude (e.g., glycogen storage, pathways of glycolysis, and corresponding phosphorylase and phosphofructokinase enzyme activity) or success in sprint–power activities such as sprint-running, speed skating, track cycling, jumping, and discus.[29,33] Performance in single bouts of such activities often improves because lower air density reduces air resistance or drag force more at altitude than at sea level. The lessened air resistance from a 24% reduction in air density at 2300 m (7546 ft) should also improve performance in the shot-put, hammer throw, and javelin. Impaired performance has been reported for *repeated intervals* of short-term power output (15-s training intervals) in elite athletes.[14]

In the transition from moderate altitude to higher elevations, values for alveolar (arterial) Po_2 position on the steep part of the oxyhemoglobin dissociation curve. This dramatically reduces hemoglobin oxygenation and oxygen transport capacity and negatively affects even mild-intensity aerobic activities. At high elevations in the Andes and Himalayas, oxygen loading of hemoglobin decreases dramatically, and physical activity becomes at best difficult to sustain. Any small change in inspired Po_2 (i.e., barometric pressure) greatly affects aerobic capacity at the summit of Mt. Everest. For well-acclimatized mountain climbers, breathing ambient air with a Po_2 of 48.5 mm Hg produces a $\dot{V}O_{2max}$ of 1450 mL · min^{-1}. This declines to 1070 mL · min^{-1} with only a 6-mm Hg decrease in inspired Po_2—a decrease of 63 mL · min^{-1} in $\dot{V}O_{2max}$ for each 1-mm Hg drop in inspired Po_2.[109,110]

Sudden exposure to an altitude of 4300 m (14,197 ft) reduces aerobic capacity by 32% compared with sea-level values.[119] Permanent living becomes nearly impossible at altitudes above 5182 m (17,000 ft) and mountain climbing at that altitude frequently requires the aid of hyperoxic breathing mixtures. At 5486 m (18,000 ft), arterial Po_2 averages 38 mm Hg, and hemoglobin maintains only 73% oxygen saturation. Amazingly, reports describe acclimatized mountaineers who lived for weeks at 6706 m (22,000 ft) breathing only ambient air.[45] In fact, members of two Swiss expeditions to Mt. Everest remained at the summit for 2 hr without breathing equipment![74] This represents an impressive feat considering that arterial Po_2 averaged only 25 mm Hg with a corresponding arterial blood oxygen saturation of 58%. An unacclimatized person becomes unconscious within 30 s under these conditions. For acclimatized men at simulated extreme altitudes that approach the summit of Mt. Everest (8848 m; 29,029 ft),

$\dot{V}O_{2max}$ decreases by 70%, from 4.13 to 1.17 L·min⁻¹, or from 49.1 to 15.3 mL·kg⁻¹·min⁻¹.[35] These low values reflect the sea-level aerobic capacity of a sedentary 80-year-old man. In addition to impairment in oxygen transport capacity, high-altitude exposure impairs the homeostatic regulation of immune balance; this potentially could favor long-term immunological alterations and increase the risk of infections.[27] In 2006, after 40 days of climbing, Mark Inglis became the first ever double amputee to scale Mount Everest. Although remarkable performances at high altitude reflect exceptions and not the rule, they demonstrate the enormous adaptive capability of humans to survive and even achieve extraordinary athletic performances without external support at extreme terrestrial elevations.

INTEGRATIVE QUESTION

Respond to this question: If altitude has such negative effects on the body, why are certain track and field records broken during competition at higher elevations?

ACCLIMATIZATION

During the many years that mountaineers attempted to climb the world's highest peaks, they knew it required weeks to adjust to successively higher elevations. *The term **altitude acclimatization** broadly describes adaptive responses in physiology and metabolism that improve tolerance to altitude hypoxia.* Each adjustment to a higher elevation proceeds progressively, and full acclimatization requires an appropriate time period. Successful adjustment to medium altitude affords only partial adjustment to a higher elevation. Residents of moderate altitudes, however, show less decrement in physiologic capacity

and physical performance than lowlanders when both groups travel to a higher altitude.[62]

TABLE 24.1 reveals that compensatory responses to altitude occur almost immediately, while other adaptations take weeks or even months. The rapidity of the body's response remains largely altitude dependent, yet considerable individual variability exists for both the rate and success of acclimatization. A person can retain many of the beneficial submaximal exercise responses with 16 days of acclimatization at 4300 m (14,108 ft) despite intermittent 8-day sojourns to sea level.[7] This suggests that certain aspects of acclimatization regress more slowly than their acquisition.

Immediate Responses to Altitude Exposure

Arrival at elevations of 2300 m (2546 ft) and higher initiates rapid physiologic adjustments to compensate for thinner air and accompanying reduction in alveolar Po_2. The two more important responses include:

1. Increase in the respiratory drive to produce hyperventilation
2. Increase in blood flow during rest and submaximal physical activity

Hyperventilation

Hyperventilation from reduced arterial Po_2 reflects the most important and clear-cut immediate response of the native lowlander to altitude exposure. Once initiated, this "hypoxic drive" increases during the first few weeks and can remain elevated for a year or longer during prolonged altitude residence.[53]

The aortic arch and branching of the carotid arteries in the neck contain peripheral chemoreceptors sensitive to

TABLE 24.1	Immediate and Longer-Term Adjustments to Altitude Hypoxia	
System	**Immediate**	**Longer Term**
Pulmonary acid-base	Hyperventilation Bodily fluids become more alkaline due to reduction in carbon dioxide (H_2CO_3) with hyperventilation	Hyperventilation Excretion of base (HCO_3^-) via the kidneys and concomitant reduction in alkaline reserve
Cardiovascular	Increase in submaximal heart rate Increase in submaximal cardiac output Stroke volume remains the same or decreases slightly Maximum cardiac output remains the same or decreases slightly	Submaximal heart rate remains elevated Submaximal cardiac output falls to or below sea-level values Stroke volume decreases Maximum cardiac output decreases
Hematologic		Decreased plasma volume Increased hematocrit Increased hemoglobin concentration Increased total number of red blood cells
Local		Possible increased capillarization of skeletal muscle Increased red blood cell 2,3-DPG Increased mitochondrial density Increased aerobic enzymes in muscle Loss of body weight and lean body mass

reduced oxygen pressure. Reduced arterial P_{O_2} that occurs at altitudes above 2000 m (6562 ft) progressively stimulates these receptors. This modifies inspiratory activity to increase alveolar ventilation, causing alveolar P_{O_2} to rise toward the level in ambient air. Even small increases in alveolar P_{O_2} with hyperventilation facilitate oxygen loading in the lungs and provide the rapid first line of defense against reduced ambient P_{O_2}. For females, variations in menstrual cycle phase do not affect ventilatory responses and performance decrements during short-term altitude exposure compared with at sea level.[8] Mountaineers who respond with a strong, hypoxic ventilatory drive to sudden but extreme altitude exposure perform physical tasks more effectively and reach higher altitude than climbers with a depressed hypoxic ventilatory response.[97]

 INTEGRATIVE QUESTION

From a physiologic perspective, what represents a safe altitude for flight in an airplane with a nonpressurized cabin?

Increased Cardiovascular Response

Resting systemic blood pressure increases in the early stages of altitude adaptation. In addition, submaximal heart rate and cardiac output can rise to 50% above sea-level values, while the heart's stroke volume remains unchanged. The increased submaximal blood flow at altitude largely compensates for arterial desaturation. For example, a 10% increase in cardiac output during rest or moderate physical activity offsets a 10% reduction in arterial oxygen saturation in terms of total oxygen transported through the body. **Figure 24.3** shows that the oxygen cost of submaximal effort at 100 watts on a bicycle ergometer at sea level and high altitude remains unchanged at about 2.0 L·min^{-1}, but the relative strenuousness of effort increases dramatically at altitude. In this example, submaximal exercise representing 50% of sea-level $\dot{V}O_{2max}$ equals 70% of $\dot{V}O_{2max}$ at 4300 m (14,108 ft).

Catecholamine Response

Sympathoadrenal activity progressively increases over time during rest and physical activity with altitude exposure.[63,66,67] Increased blood pressure and heart rate at altitude coincide with the steady rise in plasma levels and excretion rates of epinephrine. Norepinephrine levels peak in women and men after 6 days of high-altitude exposure and then remain stable.[65,117] Increased sympathoadrenal activity also contributes to regulation of blood pressure, vascular resistance, and substrate mixture (enhanced carbohydrate use)[13] during short- and long-term hypobaric exposures. **Figure 24.4** shows 24-hr urinary excretion of norepinephrine and epinephrine during control (sea-level) measurements and following 7 days of exposure to 4300-m (14,108 ft) altitude. Epinephrine changed little but norepinephrine excretion increased significantly by the fourth day and remained elevated through day 7. Urinary norepinephrine levels remain elevated for approximately 1 wk following return to sea level.

TABLE 24.2 shows metabolic and cardiorespiratory responses to moderate and maximal cycling in young men at

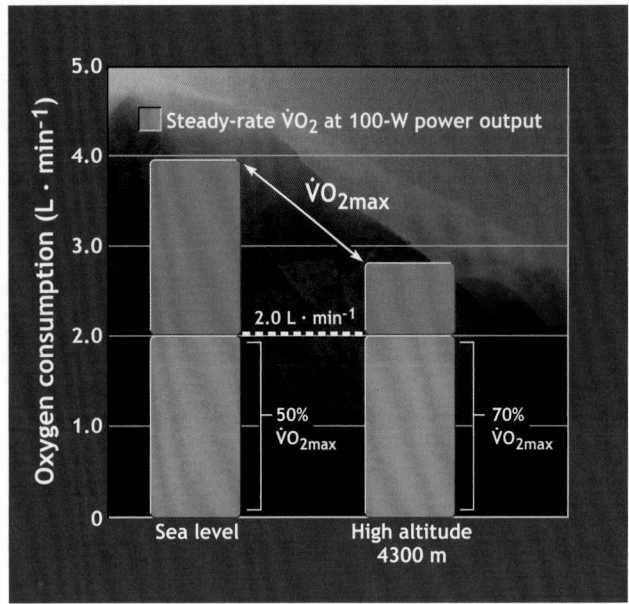

FIGURE 24.3 • Comparison of oxygen cost and relative strenuousness of submaximal exercise at sea level and high altitude.

sea level and during brief exposure to simulated altitude of 4000 m. Despite the increase in pulmonary ventilation during submaximal effort at "altitude," arterial oxygen saturation decreased from 96% at sea level to 70% during all cycling intensities. In submaximal exercise, increased cardiac output entirely compensated for the blood's reduced oxygen content. Greater blood flow occurred from a higher heart rate (stroke volume remained unchanged). With an increase in cardiac output, submaximal oxygen consumption remained essentially

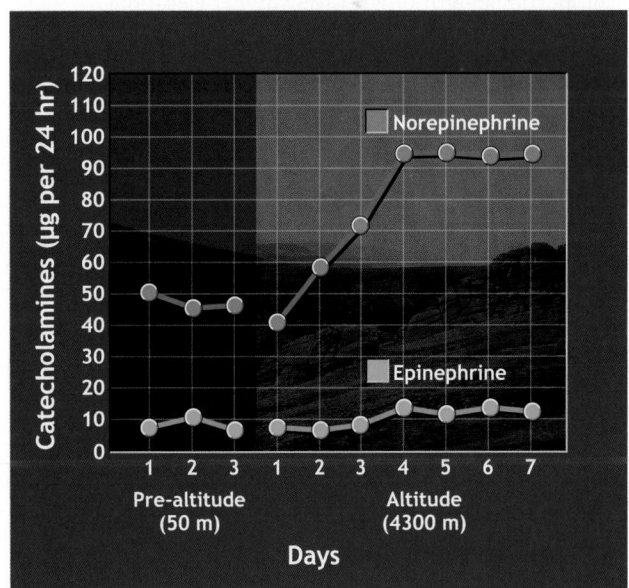

FIGURE 24.4 • Generalized response for a short stay at a high altitude (4300 m; 14,108 ft) on urinary norepinephrine and epinephrine in eight male sea-level residents. (Adapted with permission from Surks MJ, et al. Changes in plasma thyroxine concentration and metabolism, catecholamine excretion and basal oxygen uptake during acute exposure to high altitude [14,100 ft]. *J Clin Invest* 1966;45:1442.)

| TABLE 24.2 | Cardiorespiratory and Metabolic Response During Submaximal and Maximal Exercise at Sea Level and Simulated Altitude of 4000 m (13,123 ft) | | | | | | |

Exercise Level	$\dot{V}O_2$ (L·min^{-1})		$\dot{V}E$ (L·min^{-1} BTPS)		Arterial Saturation (%)	
Altitude, m	0	4000	0	4000	0	4000
600 kg-m·min^{-1}	1.50	1.56	39.6	53.7	96	71
900 kg-m·min^{-1}	2.17	2.23	59.0	93.7	95	69
Maximum	3.46	2.50	123.5	118.0	94	70

Exercise Level	$\dot{Q}$ (L·min^{-1})		HR (B·min^{-1})		SV (mL)		a-$\overline{v}O_2$ Diff (mL O_2·dL^{-1})	
Altitude, m	0	4000	0	4000	0	4000	0	4000
600 kg-m·min^{-1}	13.0	16.7	115	148	122	113	10.8	9.4
900 kg-m·min^{-1}	19.2	21.6	154	176	125	123	11.4	10.4
Maximum	23.7	23.2	186	184	127	126	14.6	10.8

Reprinted from Sternberg J, et al. Hemodynamic response to work at simulated altitude 4000 m. *J Appl Physiol* 1966;21:1589.
$\dot{Q}$, cardiac output; HR, heart rate; SV, stroke volume; a-$\overline{v}O_2$ Diff, arteriovenous oxygen difference.

identical at sea level and altitude. The greatest altitude effect on aerobic metabolism emerged during maximal exertion, when $\dot{V}O_{2max}$ decreased to 72% of the sea-level value.

With maximal effort during short-term altitude exposure (≤7 d), ventilatory and circulatory adjustments fail to compensate for the depressed arterial oxygen content. **FIGURE 24.5** illustrates the relationship between pulmonary ventilation and oxygen consumption (and exercise intensity expressed in W, top axis) up to maximum during cycling at sea level and simulated altitudes from 1000 to 4000 m (3280 to 13,123 ft). Each 1000-m (3280-ft) increase in altitude proportionately increased exercise ventilation volume. When oxygen consumption exceeded 2.0 L·min^{-1}, pulmonary ventilation increased disproportionately at progressively higher elevations.

Fluid Loss

Ambient air in mountainous regions remains cool and dry, allowing considerable body water to evaporate as inspired air becomes warmed and moistened in the respiratory passages. This fluid loss often leads to moderate dehydration and accompanying dryness of the lips, mouth, and throat. Fluid loss becomes pronounced for physically active people because of their large daily total sweat loss and exercise pulmonary ventilation volumes, and hence water loss. These individuals should have access to water at all times.

Sensory Functions. **FIGURE 24.6** shows the percentage deterioration in a variety of sensory and mental functions with decreases in arterial oxygen saturation with increasing altitude. Neurologic alterations range from a 5% decrease in sensitivity to light at 1524 m to a further 25% decrease in light sensitivity and 30% decrease in visual acuity when elevation doubles to 3048 m; at 6096 m, a 25% deterioration occurs in coding task performance and simple reaction time.

Myocardial Function. Individuals with normal electrocardiograms at sea level including patients with stable chronic heart failure generally show no adverse changes to indicate myocardial ischemia (e.g., arrythmias, angina, ECG abnormalities) at simulated high altitudes, even during maximal effort.[2,85,100] On Mt. Everest, the heart's contractile function remains stable despite considerable arterial hypoxia.[78] Little information exists about the effects of altitude on individuals with coronary artery disease, so such patients should avoid high-altitude exposure altogether.

Longer-Term Adjustments to Altitude

Hyperventilation and increased submaximal cardiac output provide a rapid and relatively effective counter to the short-term challenge of altitude exposure. Concurrently, other slower-acting adjustments occur during a prolonged altitude stay. Three important longer-term adjustments improve tolerance to the relative hypoxia of medium and high altitudes:

1. Regulation of acid-base balance of body fluids altered by hyperventilation
2. Synthesis of hemoglobin and red blood cells and accompanying changes in local circulation and aerobic cellular function
3. Elevated sympathetic neurohumoral activity reflected by increased norepinephrine that peaks within 1 wk

Acid–Base Readjustment

The beneficial effect of hyperventilation at altitude to increase alveolar Po_2 produces opposite effects on the body's carbon dioxide level. Ambient air contains essentially no carbon dioxide, so the increased breathing volumes at altitude dilute normal alveolar carbon dioxide concentrations. This creates a larger than normal gradient for diffusion ("washout") of carbon dioxide from the blood to the lungs, causing a considerable decrease in arterial Pco_2. For example, exposure to 3048 m decreases alveolar Pco_2 to about 24 mm Hg, in contrast to its usual 40 mm Hg sea-level value. Alveolar Pco_2 decreases to 10 mm Hg during a prolonged high-altitude stay.

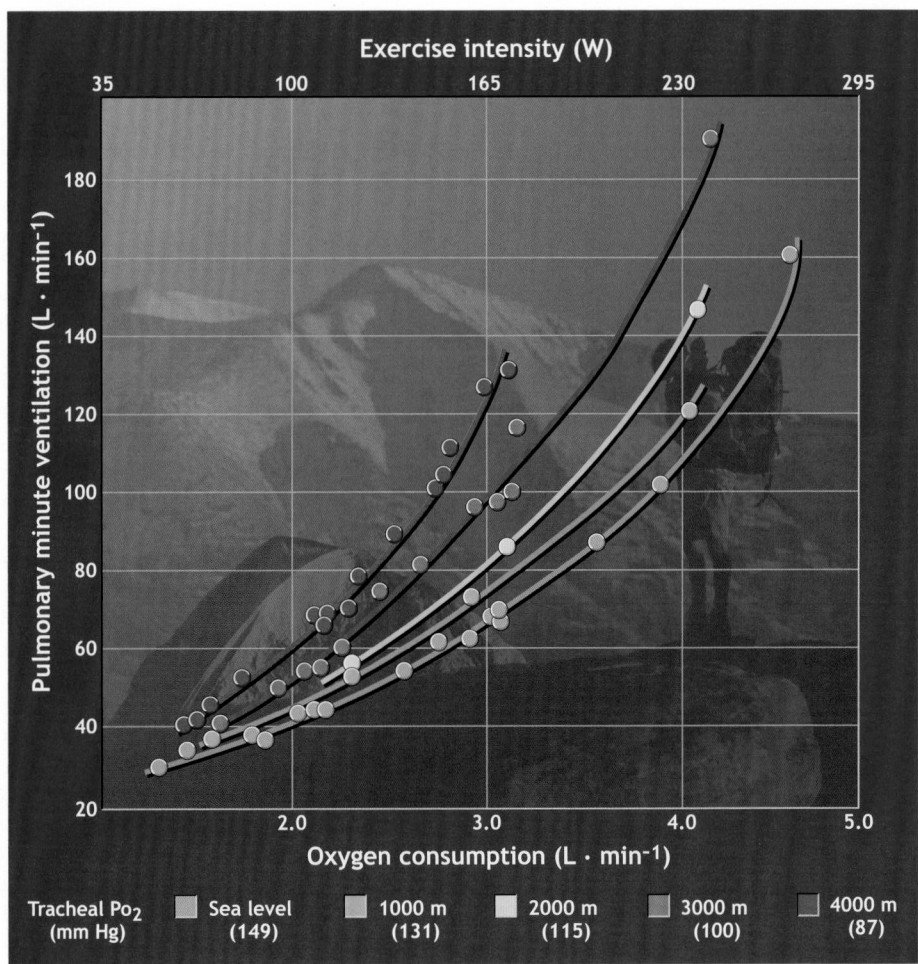

FIGURE 24.5 • Effects of a progressive increase in simulated altitude from sea level (tracheal P_{O_2} = 149 mm Hg) to 4000 m (13,123 ft) (tracheal P_{O_2} = 87 mm Hg) on the relationship between pulmonary ventilation and oxygen consumption during cycle ergometry. (Adapted with permission from Åstrand PO. The respiratory activity in man exposed to prolonged hypoxia. *Acta Physiol Scand* 1954;30:343.)

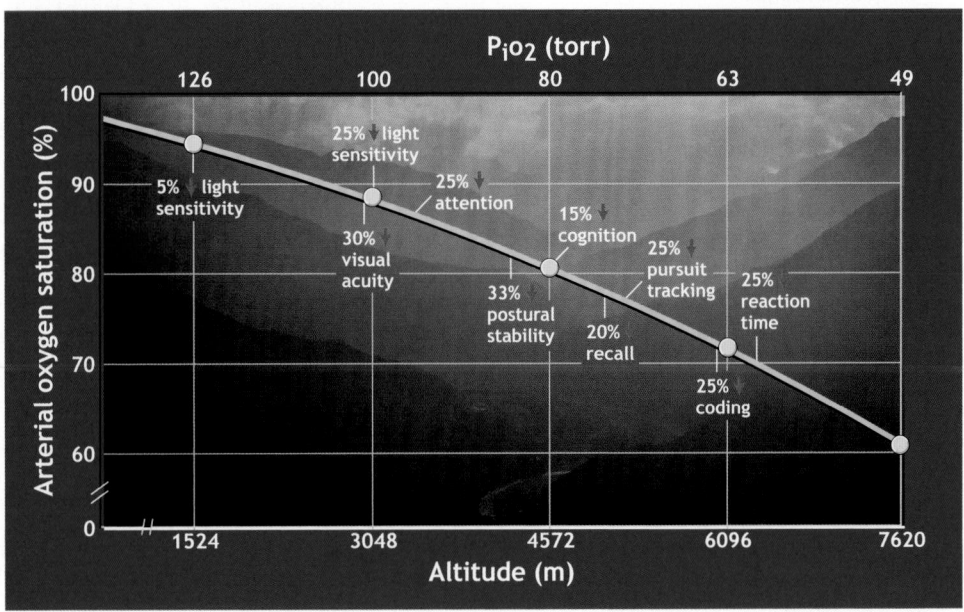

FIGURE 24.6 • Arterial desaturation as a function of increasing altitude and corresponding impairment (↓) in diverse sensory and mental functions. (Adapted with permission from Fulco CS, Cymerman A. Human performance and acute hypoxia. In: Pandolf KB, et al., eds. *Human Performance Physiology and Environmental Medicine at Terrestrial Extremes*. Carmel, IN: Cooper Publishing Group, 1988.)

IN A PRACTICAL SENSE

Identification and Treatment of Altitude-Related Medical Problems

Natives who live and work at high altitudes as well as newcomers risk a variety of medical problems associated with reduced arterial P_{O_2}. These problems usually remain mild and dissipate within several days, depending on the rapidity of the ascent and degree of exposure. Other medical complications compromise overall health and safety. Three medical conditions threaten those who ascend to high altitude:

1. *Acute mountain sickness (AMS)*, the most common malady
2. *High-altitude pulmonary edema (HAPE)*, which reverses if the person returns quickly to a lower altitude
3. *High-altitude cerebral edema (HACE)*, a potentially fatal condition if not diagnosed and treated immediately

ACUTE MOUNTAIN SICKNESS

Most people experience the discomfort of AMS during the first few days at altitudes of 2500 m (8202 ft) and above. Factors that predispose to AMS include individual susceptibility, rapid rate of ascent, and lack of prealtitude exposure.[96] Nonspecific symptoms include headache, nausea, dizziness,

fatigue, insomnia, and peripheral edema. This relatively benign condition, which becomes exacerbated by physical activity in the first few hours of exposure,[82] possibly results from acute reduction in cerebral oxygen saturation.[89] Maintenance of hydration and adequate sleep allowance may be critical performance requirements at altitude.[72] It occurs most frequently in those who ascend rapidly to a high altitude without benefiting from gradual and progressive acclimatization to lower altitudes. Symptoms (**TABLE 1**) usually begin within 4 to 12 hr and dissipate within the first week.[37,42,55] These symptoms are not exacerbated by exertion.[88] Headache, the most frequent symptom, probably results from increased cerebral hemodynamics from short-term hyperventilation.[46] Most symptoms become prevalent above 3000 m. Rapid ascent to 4200 m almost guarantees some form of AMS.

Decreased thirst sensation and severe appetite suppression occur during the early stages, often resulting in a 40% reduction in energy intake and consequent body mass loss. Diets low in salt and high in carbohydrates are well tolerated during the early stay at high altitude. A potential benefit of maintaining carbohydrate reserves through dietary intake lies in the liberation of more energy per unit oxygen with carbohydrate oxidation than with fat (5.0 kcal vs. 4.7 kcal per L of oxygen). Also, high blood lipid levels following a high-fat meal may reduce arterial oxygen saturation. Benefits of maintaining a high-carbohydrate diet include:

1. Enhanced altitude tolerance
2. Reduced severity of mountain sickness
3. Lessened physical performance decrements during the early stages of altitude exposure

Even moderate physical activity becomes intolerable for persons who suffer the effects of AMS. Symptoms subside and often disappear as acclimatization progresses. Acclimatizing slowly to moderate altitudes below 3048 m (10,000 ft), followed by a gradual progression to higher elevations (termed *staged ascent*), usually prevents AMS. Climbers should spend several nights at 2500 to 3000 m (8200 to 9800 ft) before going higher, and an extra night should be added for each additional 600 to 900 m (1968 to 2952 ft) climbed. Abrupt increases of more than 600 m in the altitude for sleeping should be avoided at 2500 m (8202 ft) or above ("climb high–sleep low"). If acclimatization proves ineffective, a 300-m (984-ft) descent usually alleviates symptoms; supplemental oxygen and the drug acetazolamide (Diamox) facilitate recovery.

HIGH-ALTITUDE PULMONARY EDEMA

For unknown reasons, about 2% of sojourners to altitudes above 3000 m (9842 ft) experience HAPE. Symptoms (Table 1) usually manifest within 12 to 96 hr following rapid ascent. Major predisposing factors for HAPE include level of altitude, rate of ascent, and individual susceptibility.[5,6] Changes in pulmonary function test variables after rapid ascent to high altitude fail to predict susceptibility to HAPE.[98]

TABLE 1	Altitude-Related Medical Conditions and Symptoms
Condition	**Symptoms**
Acute mountain sickness (AMS)	Severe headache, fatigue, irritability, nausea, vomiting, loss of appetite, indigestion, flatulence, generalized weakness, constipation, decreased urine output with normal hydration, sleep disturbance
High-altitude pulmonary edema (HAPE)	Debilitating headache and severe fatigue; excessively rapid breathing and heart rate; rales;[a] cough producing pink frothy sputum; bluish skin color (from low blood P_{O_2}); disruption of vision, bladder, and bowel functions; poor reflexes; loss of coordination of trunk muscles; paralysis on one side of the body
High-altitude cerebral edema (HACE)	Staggered gait, dyspnea upon exertion, severe weakness/fatigue, persistent cough with pulmonary infection, pain or pressure in substernal area, confusion, impaired mental processing, drowsiness, ashen skin color, loss of consciousness

For current information about physical/medical problems at altitude:
www.uptodate.com/contents/high-altitude-illness-including-mountain-sickness-beyond-the-basics

[a]Excess mucus in the lungs, diagnosed as clicking sounds heard through a stethoscope.

Fluid accumulates in the brain and lungs in this life-threatening condition.[3,81] At first, symptoms do not seem severe, but the syndrome progresses to pulmonary edema and fluid retention by the kidneys. Chest examination reveals wheezy, raspy sounds known as rales. Even in well-acclimatized individuals, HAPE can develop with severe exertion at elevations above 5486 m (18,000 ft), probably the result of increased pulmonary artery pressure with damage to the blood–gas barrier.[111]

TABLE 2 lists appropriate methods to avoid and treat HAPE. Treatment to prevent severe disability or even death requires immediate descent to lower altitude on a stretcher (or being flown to safety) because physical activity from

TABLE 2 — Prevention and Treatment of High-Altitude Pulmonary Edema

Prevention
1. Slow ascent for susceptible individuals (average increase in sleeping altitude of 300 to 350 m·d⁻¹ (984 to 1148 ft·d⁻¹) above 2500 m (8200 ft))
2. No ascent to higher altitude with symptoms of AMS
3. Descent when AMS symptoms do not improve after a day of rest
4. Under circumstances of high risk: Avoid vigorous activity when not acclimatized
5. Nifedipine: 20 mg slow-release formulation every 6 hr (or 30 to 60 mg sustained-release formulation once daily) for susceptible individuals when slow ascent is impossible

Treatment
1. Descent by at least 1000 m (3280 ft) (primary choice in mountaineering)
2. Supplemental oxygen: 2–4 L·min⁻¹ (primary choice in areas with medical facilities)
3. When #1 and/or #2 are not possible:
   - Administer 20 mg nifedipine slow-release formulation every 6 hr
   - Use a portable hyperbaric chamber (see Fig. 26.9)
   - Descend to low altitude immediately

walking potentiates complications. With proper treatment, symptoms subside within hours, with complete clinical recovery within days. HAPE poses no problem for healthy individuals who journey to and recreate without acclimatization at altitudes below 1676 m (5499 ft).

HIGH-ALTITUDE CEREBRAL EDEMA

HACE is a potentially fatal neurologic syndrome that develops within hours or days in individuals with AMS. HACE occurs in about 1% of persons exposed to altitudes above 2700 m (8858 ft); it involves increased intracranial pressure that causes coma and death if left untreated. The early symptoms (Table 1), similar to those of AMS and HAPE, progressively worsen as the altitude stay progresses. Cerebral edema probably results from cerebral vasodilation and elevations in capillary hydrostatic pressure that moves fluid and protein from the vascular compartment across the blood–brain barrier.[38] An enlarged cerebral fluid volume eventually distorts brain structures, particularly the white matter, which exacerbates symptoms and increases sympathetic nervous system activity. Tissue hypoxia caused by high-altitude exposure also initiates a series of local events that stimulate angiogenesis (new capillary vessel growth) in brain tissue.[118] Immediate descent to a lower elevation is mandatory because of the difficulty in adequately diagnosing HACE at high altitude.

OTHER CONDITIONS

Chronic mountain sickness (CMS), prevalent in a small number of altitude natives, can develop after months and years at altitude. CMS relates to excessive polycythemia, perhaps from a genetically linked variation in the EPO response to hypoxic stress.[73] CMS symptoms include lethargy, weakness, sleep disturbance, bluish skin coloring (cyanosis), and change in mental status. **High-altitude retinal hemorrhage (HARH)** affects virtually all climbers at altitudes above 6700 m (21,982 ft). HARH usually progresses unnoticed, with no specific treatment or means for prevention. Hemorrhage in the macula of the eye—the oval "yellow spot" region in the back of the eyeball close to the optic disc—produces irreversible visual defects. Retinal bleeding probably results from surges in blood pressure with exercise that cause blood vessels in the eye to dilate and rupture from increased cerebral blood flow.

Carbon dioxide loss from body fluids in a hypoxic environment creates a physiologic disequilibrium. In Chapter 13, we point out that carbonic acid (H_2CO_3) normally carries the largest quantity of carbon dioxide in the body. This relatively weak acid readily dissociates into H^+ and HCO_3^- that move to the lungs in the venous circulation. The H^+ and HCO_3^- recombine in the pulmonary capillaries to form H_2CO_3, which in turn forms carbon dioxide and water; carbon dioxide diffuses from the blood into the alveoli and leaves the body. A decrease in carbon dioxide level with hyperventilation increases the pH from loss of carbonic acid, making bodily fluids more alkaline.

Hyperventilation represents a sustained and beneficial response to altitude exposure, with physiologic adjustments proceeding during acclimatization to minimize the accompanying negative disruption in acid-base balance. Control of ventilatory-induced alkalosis advances slowly as the kidneys excrete base (HCO_3^-) through the renal tubules. In turn, restoration of normal pH increases the respiratory center's responsiveness to enable even greater hyperventilation with altitude hypoxia.

Reduced Buffering Capacity and the "Lactate Paradox." *Establishing acid-base equilibrium with acclimatization occurs at the expense of a loss of absolute alkaline reserve. The pathways of* anaerobic metabolism remain unaffected at altitude, yet the blood's capacity for buffering acid gradually decreases; this lowers the critical level for acid metabolite accumulation.

On immediate ascent to high altitude, a given submaximal exercise load increases blood lactate concentration compared with sea-level values. Greater reliance on anaerobic glycolysis with altitude hypoxia presumably increases lactate accumulation. Surprisingly, after several weeks of hypoxic exposure the same submaximal and maximal effort with large muscle groups produces *lower* lactate levels (**FIG. 24.7**).[20,112] This occurs despite a lack of increase in either $\dot{V}O_{2max}$ or regional blood flow in active tissues. A general depression in maximum lactate concentrations becomes apparent in maximal exertion above 4000 m (13,123 ft). A question arises concerning this apparent physiologic contradiction, termed the **lactate paradox**: *How is lactate accumulation reduced without a corresponding increase in tissue oxygenation, when the hypoxemia associated with high altitude should promote lactate accumulation?*[107]

Research to resolve the lactate paradox points to reduced output of epinephrine, the glucose-mobilizing hormone, during chronic high-altitude exposure.[10] Reduced glucose mobilization from the liver reduces capacity for lactate formation. Diminished intracellular ADP during long-term altitude exposure may also inhibit activation of the glycolytic pathway. In addition, depressed lactate formation during maximal exercise may partly reflect an overall reduced central nervous system drive, which reduces capacity for all-out physical effort.[64] Interestingly, lower blood lactate accumulation at high altitude does not relate to decreased buffering capacity with high-altitude acclimatization.[50]

Hematologic Changes

An increase in the blood's oxygen-carrying capacity provides the most important longer-term adjustment to altitude exposure. Two factors account for this adaptation:

1. Initial decrease in plasma volume, followed by
2. Increase in erythrocytes and hemoglobin synthesis

Initial Plasma Volume Decrease. During the first several days of altitude exposure, the body's fluid shifts from the intravascular space to the interstitial and intracellular spaces. The decrease in plasma volume within several hours of altitude exposure increases red blood cell concentration.[86] After a week at 2300 m (7545 ft), for example, plasma volume declines by about 8%, whereas red blood cell concentration (hematocrit) increases 4% and hemoglobin 10%. A 1-wk stay at 4300 m (14,107 ft) decreases plasma volume 16 to 25% along with increases in hematocrit (6%) and hemoglobin (20%) concentration.[39] The rapid plasma volume reduction (and accompanying hemoconcentration) increases the oxygen content of arterial blood above values observed on arrival at altitude. Increased urine output, termed *diuresis*, accompanies the fluid shift from plasma during acclimatization; this maintains balance in the fluid compartments despite a lower total body water content.

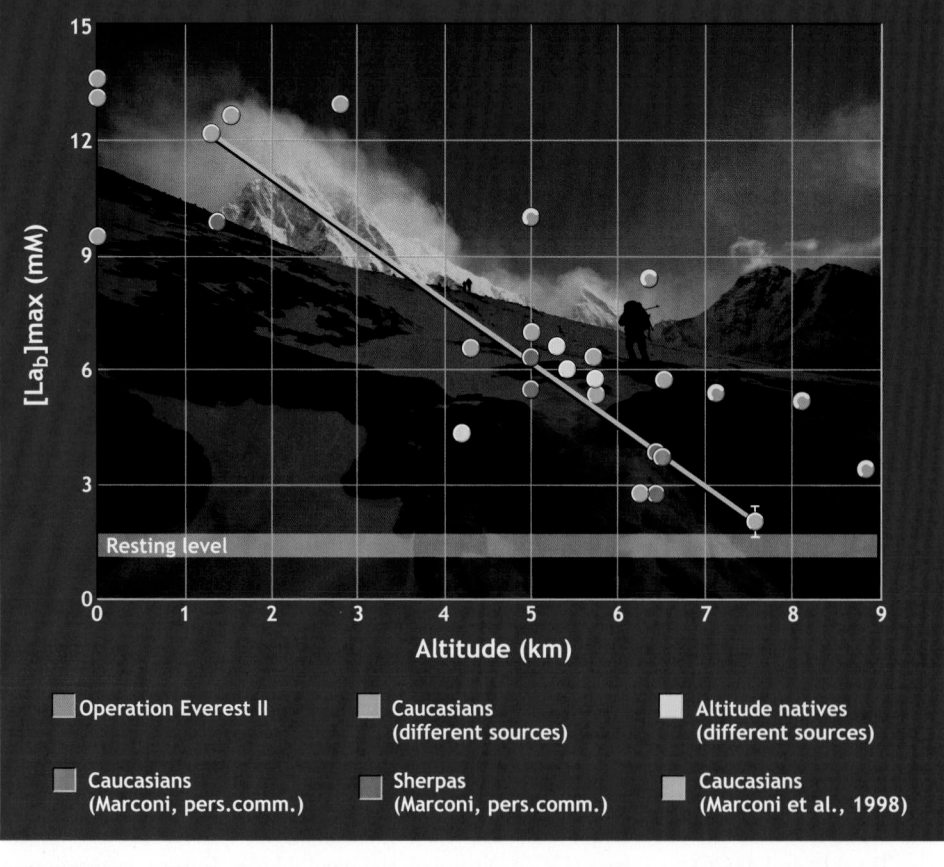

Operation Everest II **Caucasians (different sources)** **Altitude natives (different sources)**

Caucasians (Marconi, pers.comm.) **Sherpas (Marconi, pers.comm.)** **Caucasians (Marconi et al., 1998)**

FIGURE 24.7 • The lactate paradox: Less oxygen equals less (not more) lactate. Maximal blood lactate concentration ($[La_b]$max) as a function of altitude in both acclimatized lowlanders and high-altitude residents. The solid line of best fit includes all the points above an altitude of 1 km, except the four from Operation Everest II shown by I. (Adapted with permission from Ceretelli P, Samaja M. Acid–base balance at exercise in normoxia and in chronic hypoxia. Revisiting the "lactate paradox." *Eur J Appl Physiol* 2003;90:431; West JB. Point: The lactate paradox does/does not occur during exercise at high altitude *J Appl Physiol* 2007;102:2398.)

Red Blood Cell Mass Increases. Reduced arterial Po_2 at altitude stimulates an increase in total number of red blood cells, or **polycythemia**. The erythrocyte-stimulating hormone erythropoietin (EPO), synthesized and released primarily from the kidneys in response to localized arterial hypoxia, initiates red blood cell formation within 15 hr after altitude ascent. In the weeks that follow, erythrocyte production in the marrow of the long bones increases and remains elevated throughout the altitude stay.[36] The blood of a typical miner in the Andes contains 38% more erythrocytes than a lowlander. In some apparently healthy high-altitude natives, red blood cell count may reach levels 50% above normal—8 million cells per mm³ compared with 5.3 million for the native lowlander![61] Climbers acclimatized at 6500 m (21,325 ft) during a 1973 Mt. Everest expedition showed a 40% increase in hemoglobin concentration and a 66% increase in hematocrit.[19] Debate concerns the precise benefits of increased hematopoiesis with altitude exposure and whether an optimum exists for hemoglobin concentration at high altitude.[79,106] Clearly, extreme erythrocyte packing increases blood viscosity and restricts tissue blood flow and oxygen diffusion.

 INTEGRATIVE QUESTION

For their assault on Mt. Everest, elite mountaineers spend 3 mo at camps at 4877 m (16,600 ft), 5944 m (19,500 ft), 6492 m (21,300 ft), 7315 m (24,000 ft), and 7925 m (26,000 ft) before the final ascent. Explain the physiologic rationale for this "stage-ascent" approach to mountaineering.

In general, altitude-induced polycythemia translates directly to an increase in the blood's capacity to transport oxygen. For example, the oxygen-carrying capacity of blood in high-altitude residents of Peru averages 28% above sea-level values. The blood of well-acclimatized mountaineers carries 25 to 31 mL of oxygen per deciliter of blood compared with 20 mL for lowland residents.[75] Despite reduced hemoglobin oxygen saturation at altitude, the *quantity* of oxygen in arterial blood may approach or even equal sea-level values.[68] FIGURE 24.8A illustrates the general trend for increased hemoglobin and hematocrit during acclimatization for eight young women who lived and worked for 10 wk at the 4267-m (14,000-ft) summit of Pikes Peak. The researchers' previous work showed fewer hematologic changes during acclimatization in women than in men, possibly from inadequate iron intake. In this experiment, each woman received iron supplementation prior to, during, and on return from altitude. Red blood cell concentration increased rapidly upon reaching Pikes Peak. A reduced plasma volume within the first 24 hr at altitude produced hemoconcentration. Hemoglobin concentration and hematocrit continued to rise in the month that followed and then stabilized for the remainder of the stay. Prealtitude values reestablished within 2 wk after return to Missouri.

FIGURE 24.8B shows that iron supplementation progressively increased prealtitude values for hematocrit and hemoglobin. One might anticipate this finding because young women frequently suffer from mild dietary iron insufficiency with depressed iron reserves (see Chapter 2). Comparison of

the acclimatization curves for the iron-supplemented women and another group of women not given additional iron showed greater hematocrit increase in the supplemented group. Iron supplementation enhanced hematocrit increases at altitude to a level equivalent to men at the same location. Athletes with borderline iron stores may not respond to acclimatization as effectively as individuals who arrive at altitude with iron reserves adequate to sustain increased erythrocyte production.

Cellular Adaptations

Debate concerns whether extreme terrestrial hypoxia stimulates vascular and cellular adaptations in humans that improve local oxygen extraction and maximize oxidative functions.[34,41,43,69,102] Animals born and raised at high altitude show

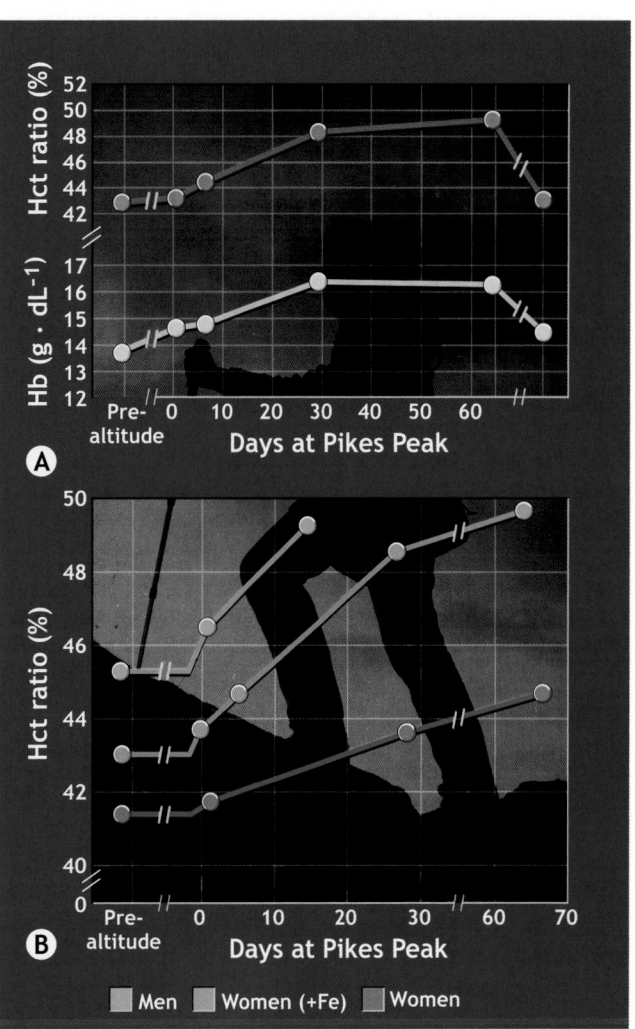

FIGURE 24.8 • **(A)** Effects of altitude on hemoglobin (Hb; *yellow line*) and hematocrit (Hct; *red line*) levels of eight young women from the University of Missouri (213 m [699 ft]) prior to, during, and 2 wk after exposure to 4267 m (13,999 ft) at Pikes Peak, Colorado. (Adapted with permission from Hannon JP, et al. Effects of altitude acclimatization on blood composition of women. *J Appl Physiol* 1968;26:540.) **(B)** Hematocrit response of young women receiving supplemental iron [+Fe] prior to and during altitude exposure compared with male and female subjects receiving no supplemental iron. (Courtesy of Dr. J. P. Hannon.)

more concentrated capillarization of skeletal muscle (number per mm^2) than sea-level counterparts.[105] Chronic hypoxia can initiate remodeling of capillary diameter and length, with formation of new capillaries to increase oxygen conductance to neural tissues.[12]

Human residents of sea level also increase tissue capillarization during an altitude stay.[70] A more prolific microcirculation reduces the oxygen diffusion distance between blood and tissues to optimize tissue oxygenation at altitude when arterial Po$_2$ decreases. Muscle biopsy specimens from humans living at altitude indicate that myoglobin increases up to 16% after acclimatization.[80] Additional myoglobin augments oxygen "storage" in specific fibers and facilitates intracellular oxygen release and delivery at a low-tissue Po$_2$. Researchers are unclear whether the small increase in mitochondrial number and concentration of aerobic energy transfer enzymes with prolonged exposure,[59] or when training under normobaric hypoxic versus normoxic conditions,[69] reflects training effects, the hypoxic environment, or the combination of both factors.[44,91]

High-altitude natives benefit from a slight shift to the right of the oxyhemoglobin dissociation curve at altitude. This effect decreases hemoglobin's affinity for oxygen to favor more oxygen release to tissues for a given cellular Po$_2$. Increased concentration of red blood cell 2,3-diphosphoglycerate (2,3-DPG; see Chapter 13) also facilitates oxygen release from hemoglobin with long-term altitude exposure. Increased 2,3-DPG coupled with more circulating hemoglobin and red blood cells favorably affects the long-term resident's capacity to supply oxygen to active tissue during physical activity.

Body Mass and Body Composition

Prolonged high-altitude exposure reduces lean body mass (muscle fibers atrophy by 20%) and body fat, with the magnitude of weight loss directly related to terrestrial elevation. Six men participated in a 40-day progressive decompression to an ambient pressure of 249 mm Hg in a hypobaric chamber to simulate ascent of Mt. Everest.[87] Daily caloric intake from depressed appetite decreased by 43% during the exposure period. Reduced energy intake reduced body mass 7.4 kg, predominantly from the muscle component of the fat-free body mass. In addition to depressed appetite and food intake during high-altitude exposure, efficiency of intestinal absorption decreases, compounding the difficulty in maintaining body weight.[16,25,113] Basal metabolic rate increases upon arrival at altitude to further affect the tendency to lose weight. To some extent, one can override an accelerated metabolic rate and minimize weight loss by consciously increasing energy intake while at altitude.[17]

Time Required for Acclimatization

The time required to acclimatize to altitude depends on terrestrial elevation. Acclimation to one altitude ensures only partial adjustment to a higher elevation. As a broad guideline, it takes about 2 wk to adapt to altitudes up to 2300 m (7545 ft). Thereafter,

each 610-m (2000-ft) altitude increase requires an additional week to fully acclimatize up to 4600 m (15,091ft). Athletes who desire to compete at altitude should begin intense training immediately during acclimatization. Rapid initiation of training minimizes detraining effects induced by the normal tendency to reduce physical activity in the first few days at altitude. Acclimatization adaptations dissipate within 2 or 3 wk after returning to sea level.

METABOLIC, PHYSIOLOGIC, AND EXERCISE CAPACITIES AT ALTITUDE

The stress of high altitude considerably restricts exercise capacity and physiologic function. Even at lower altitudes, exercise performance deteriorates because physiologic and metabolic adjustments do not fully compensate for the reduced ambient oxygen pressure. Stroke volume and maximum heart rate acclimatize in a direction that reduces oxygen transport capacity and $\dot{V}O_{2max}$.[31,90]

Maximal Oxygen Consumption

Figure 24.9A depicts the relationship between the decrease in $\dot{V}O_{2max}$ (% of sea-level value) and increasing altitude or simulated exposures (i.e., hypobaric chambers or normobaric hypoxic gas breathing) reported in diverse civilian and military studies. Disparities in experimental design and procedures and physiologic differences among subjects help to explain the variation in the points about the orange line that depict the relationship. Small declines in $\dot{V}O_{2max}$ become noticeable at an altitude of 589 m (1932 ft). *Thereafter, arterial desaturation decreases $\dot{V}O_{2max}$ by 7 to 9% per 1000-m (3280-ft) altitude increase to 6300 m (20,700 ft), where aerobic capacity declines at a more rapid, nonlinear rate.*[23,76] For example, aerobic capacity at 4000 m (13,123 ft) averages 75% of the sea-level value. At 7000 m (22,965 ft), $\dot{V}O_{2max}$ averages one half that at sea level. The $\dot{V}O_{2max}$ of relatively fit men atop Mt. Everest averages about 1000 mL · min^{-1};[74] this corresponds to an exercise power output of only 50 watts on a bicycle ergometer (equivalent to 0.72 kcal · min^{-1}; 0.14 L O$_2$ · min^{-1}; or less than 0.5 METS for a 72.6-kg person).

Physical conditioning prior to altitude exposure offers little protection because the endurance athlete experiences a slightly greater percentage reduction in $\dot{V}O_{2max}$ than an untrained person. In addition, large variability exists among individuals in the decrement in $\dot{V}O_{2max}$ with altitude exposure. Men experience the largest decrease, particularly those with (1) large lean body mass, (2) large sea-level aerobic capacity, and (3) low sea-level lactate threshold.[84] To some extent, arterial desaturation and decrease in $\dot{V}O_{2max}$ become more pronounced in individuals with a depressed hyperventilation response to exertion in a hypoxic environment.[30] Despite any unique effects of altitude exposure on aerobically fit individuals, a standard physical task at altitude at a given absolute amount of effort still provides relatively less stress for well-conditioned women and men because they perform it at a lower percentage of their $\dot{V}O_{2max}$.

No change in exercise economy occurs in response to 4 wk of intermittent altitude exposure.[104]

Exercise Performance

Seven days of intermittent (4 hr · d⁻¹) simulated altitude exposure, in combination with either rest or training, improves time-trial performance and induces physiologic adaptations during constant–work-rate exercise at 4300 m (14,107 ft), consistent with chronic exposure to this altitude.[9] Specific nonhematological adaptations to hypoxic exposure that improve sea-level performance include *improved* muscle efficiency at the mitochondrial level from a tighter coupling of intracellular bioenergetic and mitochondrial function, greater muscle buffering, and ability to tolerate lactic acid production.[32] FIGURE 24.9B illustrates the generalized trend in physical performance decrements primarily during competition for athletes at different altitude exposures. Altitude exerts *no* adverse effect on events lasting less than 2 min. For longer-duration events, poorer performance occurs at higher elevations than at sea level. The threshold for decrements appears at about 1600 m (5250 ft) for events of 2 to 5 min, while only a 600- to 700-m (1970 to 2300 ft) altitude induces poorer performance in events longer than 20 min. For the 1- and 3-mile runs, medium altitude (2300 m; 7546 ft) decreases performance by 2 to 13% for fit subjects.[28] This coincides with the 7.2% increase in 2-mile run times for highly trained middle-distance runners at the same altitude.[1] After 29 days of acclimatization, high-altitude exposure still increases 3-mile run time, compared with sea-level runs.[77] The small improvement in endurance during acclimatization, despite lack of concomitant increase in $\dot{V}O_{2max}$, relates to three factors:

1. Increased minute pulmonary ventilation (ventilatory acclimatization)
2. Increased arterial oxygen saturation and cellular aerobic functions
3. Blunted blood lactate response in physical activity (see the section "Reduced Buffering Capacity and the 'Lactate Paradox'")

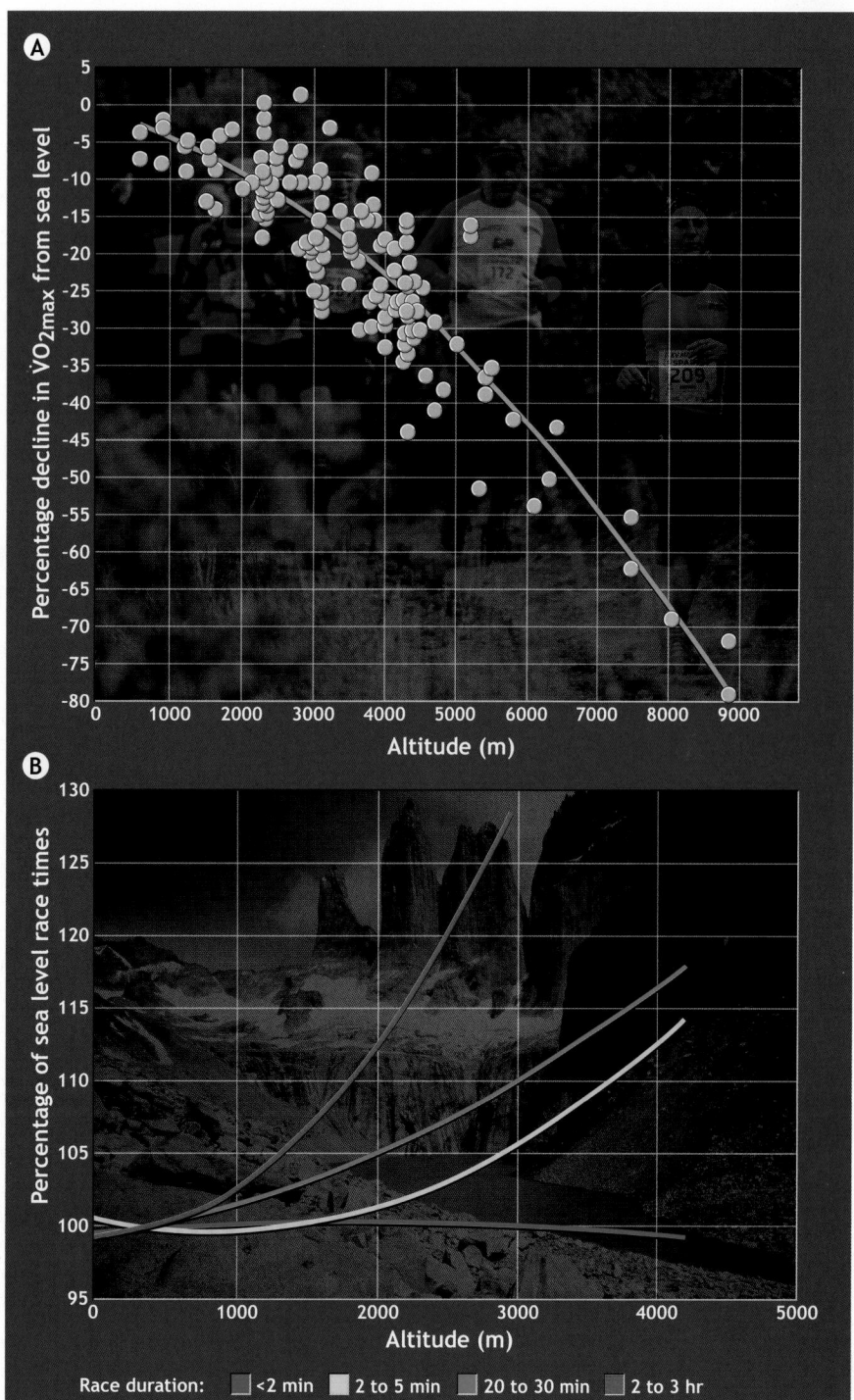

FIGURE 24.9 • (A) Reduction in $\dot{V}O_{2max}$ as a percentage of the sea-level value related to altitude exposure derived from 146 average data points from 67 different civilian and military investigations conducted at altitudes from 580 m (1902 ft) to 8848 m (29,021 ft). "Altitude" represents data from actual terrestrial elevations or simulated elevations with hypoxic chambers or hypoxic gas breathing. The orange curvilinear line is a database regression line drawn using the 146 points. **(B)** Generalized trend in performance decrements related to altitude exposure for runners and swimmers, primarily during competition. (Adapted with permission from Fulco CS, et al. Maximal and submaximal exercise performance at altitude. *Aviat Space Environ Med* 1998;69:793.)

Circulatory Factors

After several months of acclimatization to hypoxia, $\dot{V}O_{2max}$ at altitude still remains below sea-level values, even with relatively rapid and pronounced increases in hemoglobin concentration. This occurs because reduced circulatory capacity—combined effect of lowered maximum heart and stroke volume—offsets the hematologic benefits of acclimatization.

Submaximal Physical Activity

The immediate altitude response to physical activity increases submaximal cardiac output (Table 24.2), but this adjustment diminishes as acclimatization progresses and does not improve with prolonged exposure.[51] A progressive decrease in the heart's stroke volume (associated with diminished plasma volume) during the altitude stay reduces exercise cardiac output. With a lower cardiac output, submaximal oxygen consumption remains stable through an expanded a-vO_2 difference. To some extent, an increased submaximal heart rate offsets the decrease in stroke volume during submaximal effort.

Maximal Physical Activity

Maximum cardiac output decreases after about 1 wk above 3048 m and remains lower throughout one's stay. *Reduced blood flow during maximal effort results from the combined effect of decreases in maximum heart rate and stroke volume, both of which continue to decrease with the length and magnitude of altitude exposure.* This blunted cardiac response does not result from myocardial hypoxia as reflected by normal electrocardiographic and coronary blood flow measurements during vigorous activity at high altitudes.[40,90] Decreased plasma volume and increased total peripheral vascular resistance contribute to the reduced maximum stroke volume. Enhanced parasympathetic tone induced by prolonged altitude exposure reduces maximum heart rate.[93]

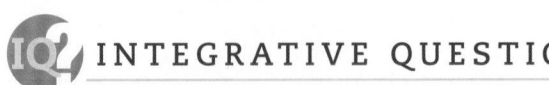 INTEGRATIVE QUESTION

If altitude acclimatization improves endurance performance at altitude, why doesn't it improve similar performance immediately upon return to sea level?

Aerobic Capacity on Return to Sea Level

Sea-level exercise performance does not improve after living at altitude when $\dot{V}O_{2max}$ serves as the improvement criterion.[47,57,70] An 18-day stay at 3100 m (10,500 ft) produced no change in the altitude-induced 25% reduction in aerobic capacity in young runners.[36] Also, $\dot{V}O_{2max}$ remained at the same prealtitude value on return to sea level. Even in studies that reported small improvements in $\dot{V}O_{2max}$ or physical performance at altitude and on return to sea level, the change often relates to the effects of training and/or repeated testing during altitude exposure.[24,52]

Possible Negative Effects

Several physiologic changes during prolonged altitude exposure negate adaptations that could improve physical performance on return to sea level. For example, the residual effects of muscle mass loss and reduced maximum heart rate and stroke volume do not enhance sea-level performance. Any reduction in maximum cardiac output at altitude offsets benefits from an increase in the blood's oxygen-carrying capacity. A depressed circulatory capacity returns to normal after a few weeks at sea level, but so also do potentially positive hematologic adaptations. Within a physiologic context, the controversial use of blood doping (see Chapter 23) mimics the hematologic benefits of altitude exposure without the negative effects on maximum cardiovascular dynamics and body composition.

ALTITUDE TRAINING AND SEA-LEVEL PERFORMANCE

Endurance training at altitude does not improve subsequent sea-level exercise performance. Altitude acclimatization improves capacity for physical activity at altitude, particularly high altitude. The effect of altitude training on aerobic capacity and endurance performance immediately on return to sea level remains unclear. Altitude adaptations in local circulation and cellular metabolism, combined with compensatory increases in the blood's oxygen-carrying capacity, should improve subsequent sea-level performance. Also, positive pulmonary adaptations and responses during prolonged hypoxic exposure do not regress immediately upon descent from altitude. If tissue hypoxia provides an important training stimulus, altitude plus training should act synergistically, making the total effect exceed similar training only at sea level. Unfortunately, much of the training–altitude exposure research contains experimental design flaws that limit assessment of this possibility.[58]

Researchers used equivalent groups to compare effectiveness of altitude training (2300 m; 7550 ft) and equivalent training at sea level.[1] Six middle-distance runners trained at sea level for 3 wk at 75% of sea-level $\dot{V}O_{2max}$. Another group of six runners trained an equivalent distance at the same percentage $\dot{V}O_{2max}$ at 2300 m (7550 ft). The groups then exchanged training sites (indicated by *red arrows*) and continued to train for 3 wk at the same relative intensity as the preceding group. Initially, 2-mile run times averaged 7.2% slower at altitude than at sea level. Run times improved 2.0% for both groups during altitude training, but postaltitude performance at sea level remained similar to the prealtitude sea-level runs. **FIGURE 24.10** shows that short-term altitude exposure decreased $\dot{V}O_{2max}$ 17.4% for both groups; it improved only slightly after 20 days of altitude training. When the runners returned to sea level after altitude training, aerobic capacity remained 2.8% *below* prealtitude sea-level values. Clearly, for these well-conditioned middle-distance runners, no synergistic effect emerged from combining aerobic training at medium altitude compared with equivalent sea-level training.

Other studies have duplicated these observations for $\dot{V}O_{2max}$ and endurance performance at moderate and higher altitudes in athletes from sea level.[26,54] Highly trained male track athletes flew to Nunoa, Peru (altitude 4000 m; (13,123 ft), where they continued to train and acclimatize for 40 to 57 days.[101] $\dot{V}O_{2max}$ decreased 29% below sea-level values after the initial 3 days at altitude; after 48 days it still remained 26% lower. The 440-yd, 880-yd, and 1- and 2-mile runs during a "track meet" with the altitude natives measured running performance after acclimatization. The times after acclimatization remained slower than prealtitude sea-level times, particularly for the longer runs. When the athletes returned to sea level, $\dot{V}O_{2max}$ and running performance did not differ from prealtitude measures. On no occasion did a runner improve his previous prealtitude run time. Running times in the longer events averaged 5% below prealtitude trials. In other studies, training in a hypobaric chamber provided no additional benefit to sea-level performance compared with similar training (albeit at a higher absolute exercise level) at sea level. As expected, the "altitude-trained" group achieved better performance at simulated altitude than sea-level residents.

Altitude Natives May Respond Differently

For endurance athletes native to moderate altitude, total hemoglobin and blood volume synergistically increase by training and altitude exposure compared to endurance athletes from sea level.[95] This adaptive response, unique to athletes born and living at altitude (e.g., Kenyan runners, Colombian cyclists, Mexican walkers), may contribute to their extraordinary endurance performance. Longer-term altitude acclimatized cyclists also show improved aerobic capacity and peak power output during sea-level exercise simulations.[15]

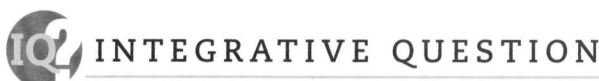 INTEGRATIVE QUESTION

Give your opinion (and rationale) about what effects a 2-wk exposure to 3000 m (9842 ft) would have on maximal exercise performance of 60-s duration.

Decrement in Absolute Training Level at Altitude

One must lower the absolute workload to perform aerobic activity at the same relative intensity at altitude as at sea level. If not, anaerobic metabolism provides a larger portion of the energy for exercise at altitude (see Fig. 24.3) and fatigue develops. Exposure to 2300 m (7545 ft) and above makes it nearly

impossible to train at the same absolute intensity as at sea level. TABLE 24.3 shows the reduction in intensity for training relative to sea-level standards for six college athletes. At 4000 m (13,123 ft), the runners could train only at the intensity equivalent to 39% of sea-level $\dot{V}O_{2max}$ compared with an intensity of 78% when training at sea level. The absolute training level at altitude may become so reduced that an athlete cannot maintain peak condition for sea-level competition. In this regard, elite athletes benefit from periodically returning from altitude to sea level for intense training to offset "detraining" during a prolonged altitude stay (see next section). Returning to a lower altitude intermittently does not interfere with acclimatization and might benefit altitude performance.[7,24,99] Independent of the training model, athletes who train at altitude should include high-intensity speed work to maintain muscle power.

COMBINE ALTITUDE STAY WITH LOW-ALTITUDE TRAINING

Research has focused on the optimal combination of high-altitude stay plus low-altitude training in competitive runners.

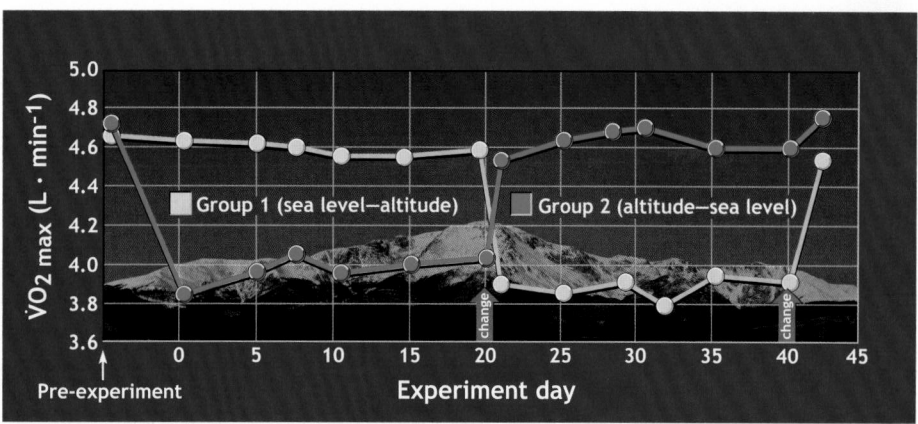

FIGURE 24.10 • Maximal oxygen consumption of two equivalent groups during training for 3 wk at altitude and 3 wk at sea level. Group 1 trained first at sea level and continued training for 3 wk at altitude. For group 2, the procedure reversed; they trained first at altitude and then at sea level. *Red arrows* indicate change in training site. (Adapted with permission from Adams WC, et al. Effects of equivalent sea-level and altitude training on $\dot{V}O_{2max}$ and running performance. *J Appl Physiol* 1975;39:262.)

TABLE 24.3	Effect of Altitude on Training Exercise Intensity for Six Collegiate Athletes			
	Altitude			
	300	**2300**	**3100**	**4000**
Intensity of workout (%$\dot{V}O_{2max}$ at 200 m)	78	60	56	39

Reprinted from Kollias J, Buskirk ER. Exercise and altitude. In: Johnson WR, Buskirk ER, eds. *Science and Medicine of Exercise and Sports.* 2nd Ed. New York: Harper & Row, 1974.

Athletes who lived at 2500 m but returned regularly to lower altitudes (1000 to 1250 m; 3280 to 4100 ft) to train at near–sea-level intensity (i.e., **live high–train low**) showed greater average increases in $\dot{V}O_{2max}$ and 5000-m run performance than athletes who lived and trained only at 2500 m or those who lived and trained only at sea level.[56,108] Strategies that combine altitude acclimatization and maintenance of sea-level training intensity provide *synergistic benefits* to sea-level endurance performance. Regular training exposure to a near–sea-level environment prevents the impaired systolic function (i.e., reduced maximum stroke volume and cardiac output) typically observed during altitude training. Muscular and systemic capacity for maintaining pH and K^+ balance during intense effort remained unchanged after a 4-wk exposure to this training protocol.[71] Such an approach to training also improves running economy and the hypoxic ventilatory drive of elite distance runners, along with the benefits of the hypoxia-induced increases in serum erythropoietin (EPO) and accelerated erythropoiesis.[49,92,103,116] To remove the inconvenience and cost of the live high–train low strategy, a modification applies supplemental oxygen during training at altitude.[114] Compared with control trials, supplemental oxygen increases the following:

1. Arterial oxyhemoglobin saturation
2. Exercise oxygen consumption
3. Average power output during high-intensity workouts at moderate altitude.

This form of training allows athletes to live at altitude yet effectively "train low" with minimal travel expense and inconvenience, and without inducing additional free radical oxidative stress.[115]

Not all individuals benefit to the same degree from the living high, training low strategy.[41,83] Within a group that showed physiologic and performance increases with this protocol, some individuals were "responders," whereas others showed little positive adjustment.[21] The "nonresponders" displayed a smaller increase in plasma concentration of the erythrocyte-producing hormone EPO after 30 hr at altitude than the responders. Such individuals experience a depressed increase in hematocrit during acclimatization to altitude exposure. The benefit from combining altitude living and lower-altitude training depend on three prerequisites:

1. The elevation must be high enough to raise EPO concentrations to increase total red blood cell volume and $\dot{V}O_{2max}$.
2. The athlete must respond positively with increased EPO output.
3. Training must take place at an elevation low enough to maintain training intensity and exercise oxygen consumption at near–sea-level values.

 INTEGRATIVE QUESTION

Respond to a person who suggests that periodic breath-holding while exercising at sea level should produce physiologic adaptations similar to training at altitude.

At-Home Acclimatization

Application of the live high–train low training model poses considerable practical and financial hurdles. Unfortunately, some endurance athletes use the banned (and dangerous) practices of either blood doping or EPO injections to increase hematocrit and hemoglobin concentration without the potential negative effects of an altitude stay.

A more prudent approach makes use of the observation that altitude's beneficial effects on erythropoiesis and aerobic capacity may require relatively short-term exposures to hypoxia. For example, daily intermittent exposures of 3 to 5 hr for 9 days to simulated altitudes of 4000 to 5500 m (13,123 to 18,044 ft) in a hypobaric chamber increased endurance performance, red blood cell count, and hemoglobin concentration in elite mountain climbers.[18,86] This approach also decreases the rate of lactate appearance during intense effort.[22] These effects may be time and protocol dependent because a 4-wk regimen of intermittent normobaric hypoxia at rest (5:5 min hypoxia-to-normoxia ratio for 70 min, 5 days a week) did not improve endurance or augment erythropoietic markers in trained runners.[48] Intermittent hypoxic training under normobaric conditions provides an added bonus with clinical and cardioprotective implications—it augments training's effect on selected metabolic and cardiovascular risk factors.[4]

In the absence of a hypobaric chamber, three approaches create an "altitude" environment where an athlete, mountaineer, or hot-air balloonist living at sea level spends a large enough portion of the day to stimulate an altitude acclimatization response.

1. **Gamow Hypobaric Chamber.** A person rests and sleeps for about 10 hr each day. The chamber's total air pressure decreases to simulate the barometric pressure of a preselected altitude. Reduced barometric pressure proportionately reduces the inspired air's PO_2 to simulate altitude exposure and induce physiologic adaptations.
2. Simulate altitude at sea level by increasing the nitrogen percentage of the air within an enclosure. Increased nitrogen percentage correspondingly reduces the air's oxygen percentage, thus decreasing inspired air PO_2. Nordic skiers have applied this technique by living for 3 to 4 wk in a house that provides "air" with only 15.3% oxygen rather than its normal concentration of 20.9%. The system requires mixing nitrogen gas and carefully monitoring the breathing mixture. Interestingly, the Norwegian Olympic Organization has banned these "altitude houses" for its own athletes because they consider this practice "gray-zone" doping.
3. A suitcase-sized unit developed by two-time British Olympic cyclist Shaun Wallace continuously supplies air with an oxygen content of approximately 15% to simulate an altitude of 2500 m (**Hypoxico Altitude Tent, Fig. 24.11**). The 70-lb unit consists of a portable tent that fits over a normal bed. A "hypoxic generator" housed in an airline suitcase continually feeds altitude-simulating hypoxic air into the tent. The porosity of the tent's material limits the rate of diffusion of outside oxygen into the tent and maintains the 15% oxygen concentration. Equilibration of the tent's environment at the 15% oxygen level requires about 90 min.

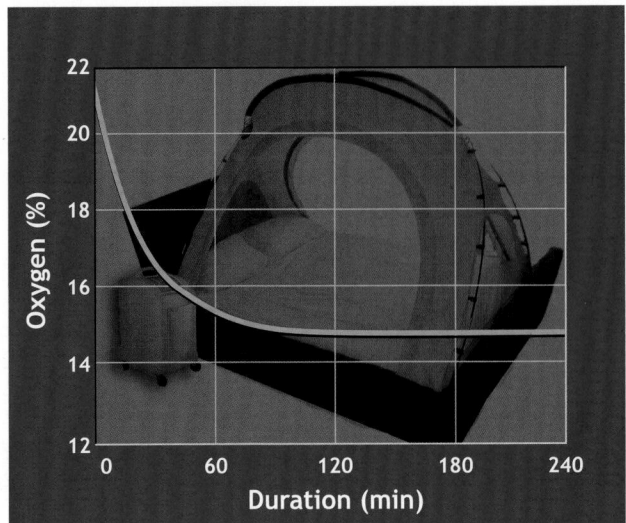

FIGURE 24.11 • The Hypoxico Altitude Tent fits over a double or queen-size bed or can be constructed for in-home use as a semipermanent cubicle. Patches of "breathable" nylon allow ambient oxygen (at higher Po_2) to diffuse into the tent (at lower Po_2) to maintain the percentage of oxygen within the tent at about 15%. A hypoxic generator (*left of tent*) continuously supplies air with oxygen content that equilibrates within the tent to near 15%. The graph shows the time course for equilibration of air within the tent to reach the 15% oxygen level. (Photo courtesy of Hypoxico Inc., **www.hypoxico.com**, Cardiff, CA.)

Summary

1. The progressive reduction in ambient Po_2 with increasing altitude produces inadequate hemoglobin oxygenation in arterial blood. Arterial desaturation impairs aerobic physical activities at altitudes of 2000 m (6561 ft) and above.

2. Altitude exposure does not adversely affect short-term (anaerobic) sprint and power performances that depend almost entirely on energy from intramuscular high-energy phosphates and glycolytic reactions.

3. Reduced Po_2 and accompanying hypoxia at altitude stimulate physiologic responses and adjustments that improve altitude tolerance during rest and exercise. Hyperventilation and increased submaximal cardiac output via elevated heart rate provide the primary immediate responses.

4. Medical problems ranging from mild to life-threatening —AMS, HAPE, and HACE—often emerge during altitude exposure. The potentially lethal conditions of HAPE and HACE require immediate removal to a lower altitude.

5. Acclimatization entails physiologic and metabolic adjustments that improve tolerance to altitude hypoxia. The main adjustments involve reestablishment of acid-base balance of the bodily fluids, increased synthesis of hemoglobin and red blood cells, and improved local circulation and cellular metabolism.

6. The rate of altitude acclimatization depends on the terrestrial elevation. Noticeable improvements occur within several days. The major adjustments require about 2 wk, but acclimatization to high altitudes requires 4 to 6 wk.

7. Alveolar Po_2 averages 25 mm Hg at the summit of Mt. Everest. For acclimatized men, this reduces $\dot{V}O_{2max}$ by 70% to about 15 mL $\dot{V}O_2 \cdot kg^{-1} \cdot min^{-1}$.

8. Even with acclimatization, $\dot{V}O_{2max}$ decreases about 2% for every 300 m (984 ft) above 1500 m (4921 ft). A decrement in endurance-related performance parallels reduced aerobic capacity.

9. Altitude-related declines in maximum heart rate and stroke volume offset any beneficial effects of acclimatization. This partly explains the inability to achieve sea-level $\dot{V}O_{2max}$ values at altitude, even after acclimatization.

10. Training at altitude provides no greater benefit to sea-level performance than equivalent training at sea level.

11. Athletes benefit from periodically returning from altitude to sea level for intense training to offset any "detraining" from lower levels of exercise during a prolonged altitude stay.

12. The Gamow hyperbaric chamber and Hypoxico tent system represent two approaches to creating an "altitude" environment under sea-level conditions.

thePoint References are available online at **http://thepoint.lww.com/mkk8e.**

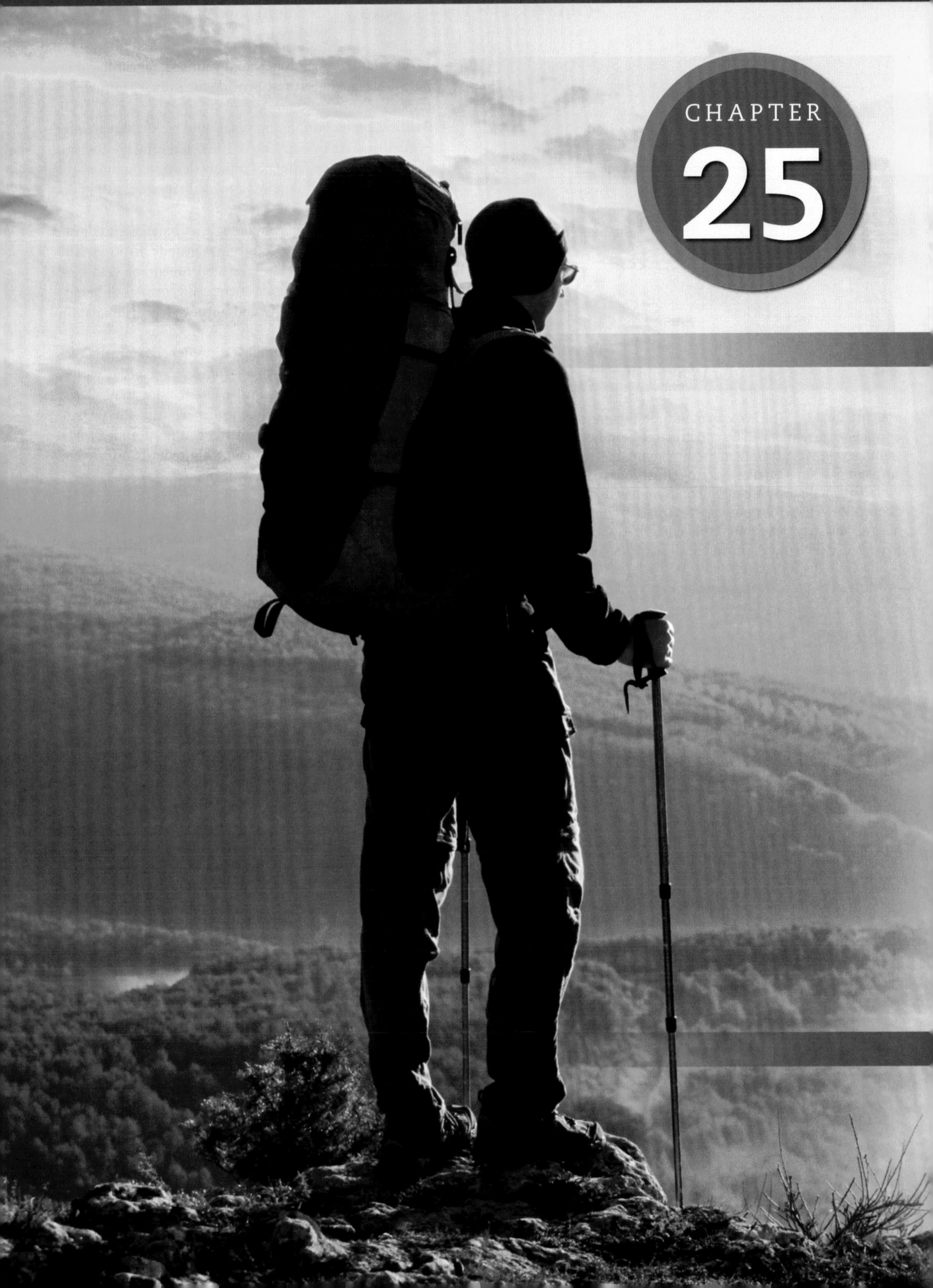

CHAPTER

25

Exercise and Thermal Stress

- Explain how the hypothalamus maintains thermal balance

- Explain the four physical factors that contribute to heat gain and heat loss

- Discuss how the circulatory system serves as a "workhorse" for thermoregulation

- List two desirable clothing characteristics for exercising in cold and warm weather

- List six factors that affect the insulation (clo) value of clothing

- Describe how football equipment and the cycling helmet affect heat dissipation and thermoregulation in physical activity

- Discuss factors that maintain cutaneous and muscle blood flow and blood pressure during exertion in the heat

- Describe the cardiac-output, heart-rate, and stroke-volume response during hot-weather physical activity

- Graph the relationship between core temperature and relative exercise intensity ($\%\dot{V}O_{2max}$)

- Quantify fluid loss during hot-weather exercise, and indicate the consequences of dehydration on physiology and performance

- Describe the purposes of fluid replacement and proposed benefits of pre-exercise hyperhydration and glycerol supplementation during physical activity in a hot environment

- Describe the volume and electrolyte characteristics of a rehydration beverage to restore water and electrolyte balance following prolonged effort in the heat

- Explain how acclimatization, training, age, gender, and body fat modify heat tolerance during physical activity

- Give symptoms, possible causes, and treatment for heat cramps, heat exhaustion, and exertional heat stroke

- Describe factors that constitute the WB-GT index and the relative importance of each factor

- List six factors that reduce the insulatory properties of clothing

- Summarize the American College of Sports Medicine WB-GT recommendations for endurance running and cycling

- Discuss immediate and possible longer-term physiologic adjustments to cold stress

- Explain the purpose of the wind-chill temperature index and factors that comprise it

Visit http://thepoint.lww.com/mkk8e to access the following resources.

- References: Chapter 25
- Interactive Question Bank
- Focus on Research: Heat Stress and Cardiovascular Dynamics in Exercise

Humans can tolerate a decline in deep body temperature of 10°C (18°F) but a body temperature increase of only half that of 5°C (9°F). **Temperature** technically represents the mean kinetic energy of a substance's atoms as they move. The potential for heat exchange between substances (e.g., blood to capillary walls) or objects (e.g., running surface to participant's body) reflects a functional definition of this term. Over the past 30 years, more than 100 American football players from high school, college, and professional have died from excessive heat stress during practice or competition, most of them unnecessarily. Corey Stringer (1974–2001), an All-American at The Ohio State University and first-round draft choice of the NFL Minnesota Vikings, died from complications of heat stroke during summer training camp. Stringer's death brought about major changes in how the NFL promoted heat stroke awareness and prevention during early-season practices. The National Center for Catastrophic Sport Injury Research (www.unc.edu/depts/nccsi/) prepares three annual reports about death and permanent disability sports injury data that involve brain and/or spinal cord injuries.

Hyperthermia and dehydration also contributed to the deaths of three apparently healthy collegiate wrestlers just before their competitive season,[140] with numerous accounts worldwide of heat-related deaths during marathon runs and other long-duration events. The people who organize and guide athletic events and physical activity programs bear most of the responsibility for helping to eradicate heat injuries. A proper understanding of thermoregulation and the best ways to support these mechanisms should prevent such tragedies.

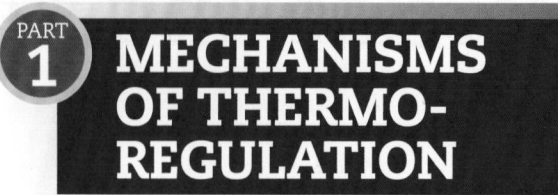

PART 1 · MECHANISMS OF THERMO-REGULATION

THERMAL BALANCE

FIGURE 25.1 shows that temperature of the deeper central tissues or **core** represents a dynamic equilibrium between factors that add and subtract body heat. Integration of mechanisms that alter heat transfer to the periphery (**shell**) regulates evaporative cooling and varies the body's heat production to sustain thermal balance. Core temperature rises when factors that promote heat gain exceed the mechanisms for heat loss, as readily occurs during vigorous physical activity in a warm, humid environment; in contrast, core temperature declines in the cold when the body's heat loss exceeds heat production.

TABLE 25.1 presents thermal data for heat production and heat loss via sweating during rest and maximal exertion. The chemical reactions of energy metabolism produce body heat gains that can reach considerable levels during muscular activity. From shivering alone, whole body metabolism increases three- to five-fold.[139] Metabolism in elite athletes often rises 20 to 25 times above the resting level, to about 20 kcal·min⁻¹ during intense aerobic activity; this theoretically can increase core temperature by 1°C (1.8°F) every 5 to 7 min. The body also absorbs heat from solar radiation and objects warmer than the body. Heat leaves the body via the physical mechanisms of radiation, conduction, and convection, and most importantly by water vaporization from the skin and respiratory passages. Under optimal conditions, evaporative cooling with maximal sweating accounts for a heat loss of about 18 kcal·min⁻¹.

Circulatory adjustments provide "fine-tuning" for

Body heat content

Heat loss
Radiation
Conduction
Convection
Evaporation

Daily variation
37°C

Heat gain
BMR
Muscular activity
Hormones
Thermic effect of food
Postural changes
Environment

FIGURE 25.1 • Contributing factors to heat gain and heat loss to regulate core temperature at about 37°C (98.6°F).

TABLE 25.1	Thermodynamics During Rest and Exercise	
Condition	**Rest**	**Maximal Exercise**
Body's heat production (1 L O$_2$ consumption = 4.82 kcal)	~0.25 L O$_2 \cdot$ min^{-1} ~1.2 kcal $\cdot$ min^{-1}	~4.0 L O$_2 \cdot$ min^{-1} ~20.0 kcal $\cdot$ min^{-1}
Body's capacity for evaporative cooling (Each 1 mL sweat evaporation = ~0.6 kcal body heat loss)	**Maximal sweating** ~30 mL $\cdot$ min^{-1} = 18 kcal $\cdot$ min^{-1}	
Core temperature increase	No increase	~1 °C every 5 to 7 min

temperature regulation. Heat conservation occurs when blood shunts rapidly to the deep cranial, thoracic, and abdominal cavities and portions of the muscle mass. This optimizes insulation from subcutaneous fat and other components of the body's shell. Conversely, increases in internal heat dilate peripheral vessels as warm blood flows to the cooler periphery. The drive to maintain thermal balance remains so strong that it readily triggers a sweating rate of 2.0 L $\cdot$ hr^{-1} in exercise in the heat, or an oxygen consumption of 1200 mL $\cdot$ min^{-1} from shivering in severe cold.

HYPOTHALAMIC TEMPERATURE REGULATION

*The **hypothalamus** contains the central coordinating center for temperature regulation.* This group of specialized neurons at the floor of the brain acts as a "thermostat"—usually set and carefully regulated at about 37°C ± 1°C (98.6°F ± 1.8°F)—that continually makes thermoregulatory adjustments to deviations from a temperature norm. Unlike the automatic home thermostat, the hypothalamus cannot "turn off" the heat; it only can initiate responses to protect the body from either a buildup or loss of heat.

Two ways activate the body's heat-regulating mechanisms:

1. Thermal receptors in the skin provide input to the central control center.
2. Changes in the temperature of blood that perfuses the hypothalamus directly stimulate this area.

FIGURE 25.2 shows the diverse structures embedded within the skin and subcutaneous tissue. The *inset* on the right depicts the transfer of heat produced by active muscles for cooling at the body surface via the dynamics of sweat evaporation when the water vapor pressure at the skin surface exceeds that of the surrounding air. Peripheral thermal receptors responsive to rapid changes in heat and cold exist predominantly as free nerve afferent endings in the skin. The more numerous cutaneous cold receptors generally exist near the skin surface. Cold receptors play an important role in initiating regulatory responses to a cold environment. The cutaneous thermal receptors act as an "early warning system" that relays sensory information to the hypothalamus and cortex. This direct line of communication evokes appropriate

heat-conserving or heat-dissipating physiologic adjustments, and the individual consciously seeks relief from any thermal challenge.

The central hypothalamic regulatory center plays the primary role in maintaining thermal balance. Cells in the anterior portion of the hypothalamus detect slight changes in blood temperature in addition to receiving peripheral input. These cells' heightened activity stimulates the posterior hypothalamus to initiate coordinated responses for heat conservation or the anterior hypothalamus to facilitate heat loss. The temperature of the blood that perfuses the hypothalamus provides the primary monitoring system to assess body warmth, in contrast to peripheral receptors that detect cold.

THERMOREGULATION IN COLD STRESS: HEAT CONSERVATION AND HEAT PRODUCTION

The normal heat transfer gradient flows from the body to the environment. Generally, core temperature regulation involves little or no physiologic strain. Nevertheless, excessive heat loss can occur in extreme cold, particularly at rest. The body's heat production in this case increases, while heat loss slows to minimize any decline in core temperature.

Vascular Adjustments

Stimulation of cutaneous cold receptors constricts peripheral blood vessels, which immediately reduces the flow of warm blood to the body's cooler surface and redirects it to the warmer core. For example, cutaneous blood flow averages 250 mL $\cdot$ min^{-1} in a thermoneutral environment, yet with severe cold stress this flow approaches zero.[60] Consequently, skin temperature declines toward ambient temperature to maximize the insulatory benefits of skin, muscle, and subcutaneous fat. A person with excessive body fat who is exposed to cold stress benefits from this heat-conserving mechanism. For a thinly clad person with normal body fat content, cutaneous blood flow regulation generally provides effective thermoregulation at ambient temperatures between 25 and 29°C (77 and 84°F).

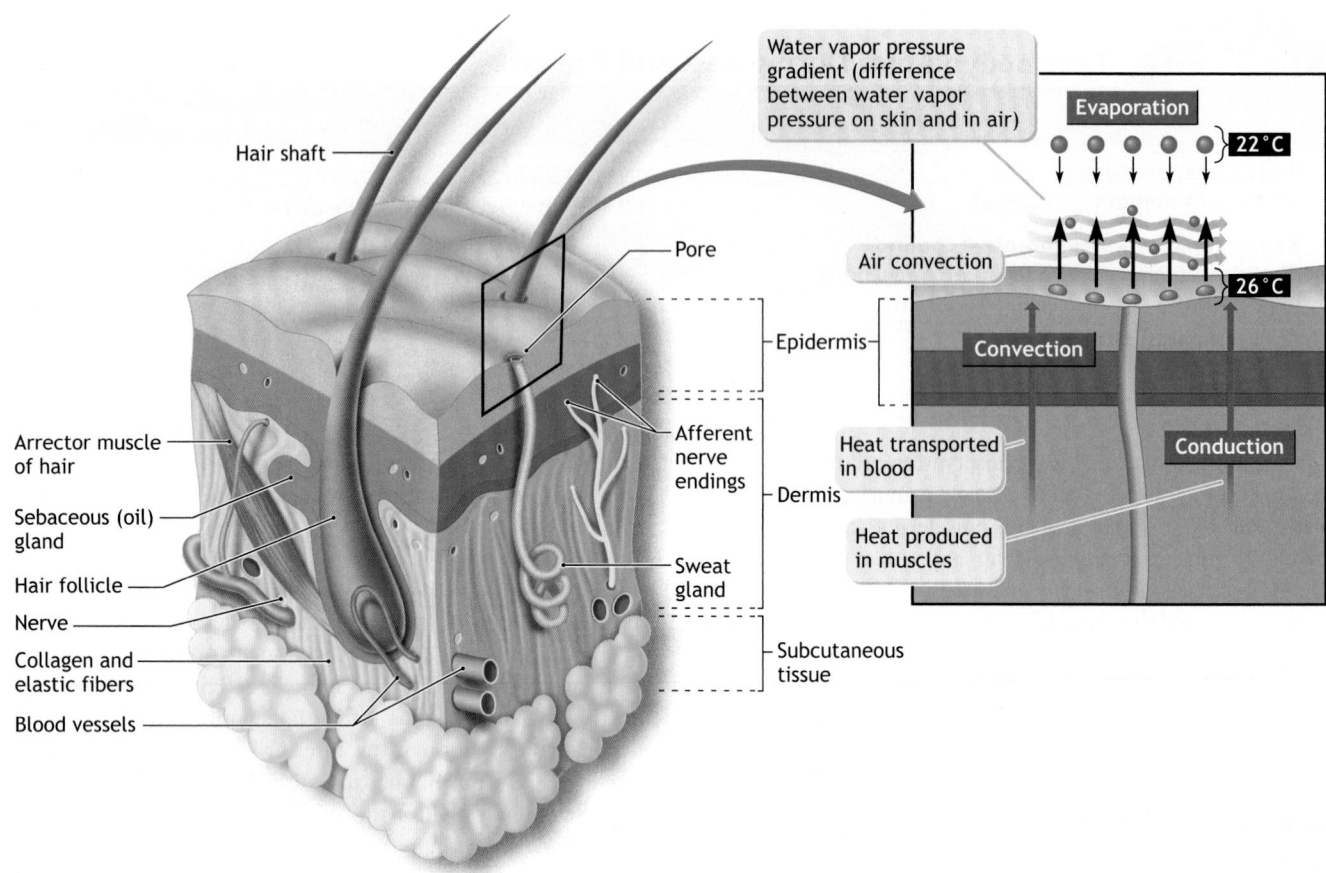

FIGURE 25.2 • *Right inset.* Schematic illustration of the skin and underlying structures. The inset enlargement of the skin surface shows the dynamics of conduction, convection, and sweat evaporation for heat dissipation from the body. Each 1 L of water evaporated from the skin transfers 580 kcal of heat energy to the environment.

Muscular Activity

Shivering generates metabolic heat, but physical activity provides the greatest contribution in defending against cold. Energy metabolism during movement sustains a constant core temperature in air as cold as −30°C (−22°F) without reliance on a heavy, restrictive clothing barrier. Internal temperature, not the body's heat production per se, mediates the thermoregulatory response to cold. Shivering still occurs during vigorous activity if the core temperature remains low. Cold stress often induces higher exercise oxygen consumptions from shivering compared to performing the same exercise in a warmer environment.

When metabolism decreases during physical activity (e.g., from fatigue), shivering alone may not prevent a decline in core temperature. To some extent, the variability among individuals in shivering response dictates the diverse outcomes for those caught unprepared for accidental wet–cold exposures. General muscle fatigue induced by prior strenuous exertion does not depress the shivering response.[137]

Hormonal Output

Two "calorigenic" adrenal medulla hormones, epinephrine and norepinephrine, increase heat production during cold exposure. Prolonged cold stress also stimulates release of thyroxine, the thyroid hormone that increases resting metabolism.

THERMOREGULATION IN HEAT STRESS: HEAT LOSS

The body's thermoregulatory mechanisms primarily protect against overheating. Dissipating heat efficiently becomes crucial during physical activity in hot weather, when inherent competition exists between mechanisms that maintain a large muscle blood flow and thermoregulatory mechanisms. **FIGURE 25.3** illustrates the factors that contribute to heat gain and heat loss during physical activity. Body heat loss occurs by four physical processes:

1. Radiation
2. Conduction
3. Convection
4. Evaporation

Heat Loss by Radiation

All objects, including humans, continually emit electromagnetic heat waves or radiant energy. The human body usually remains

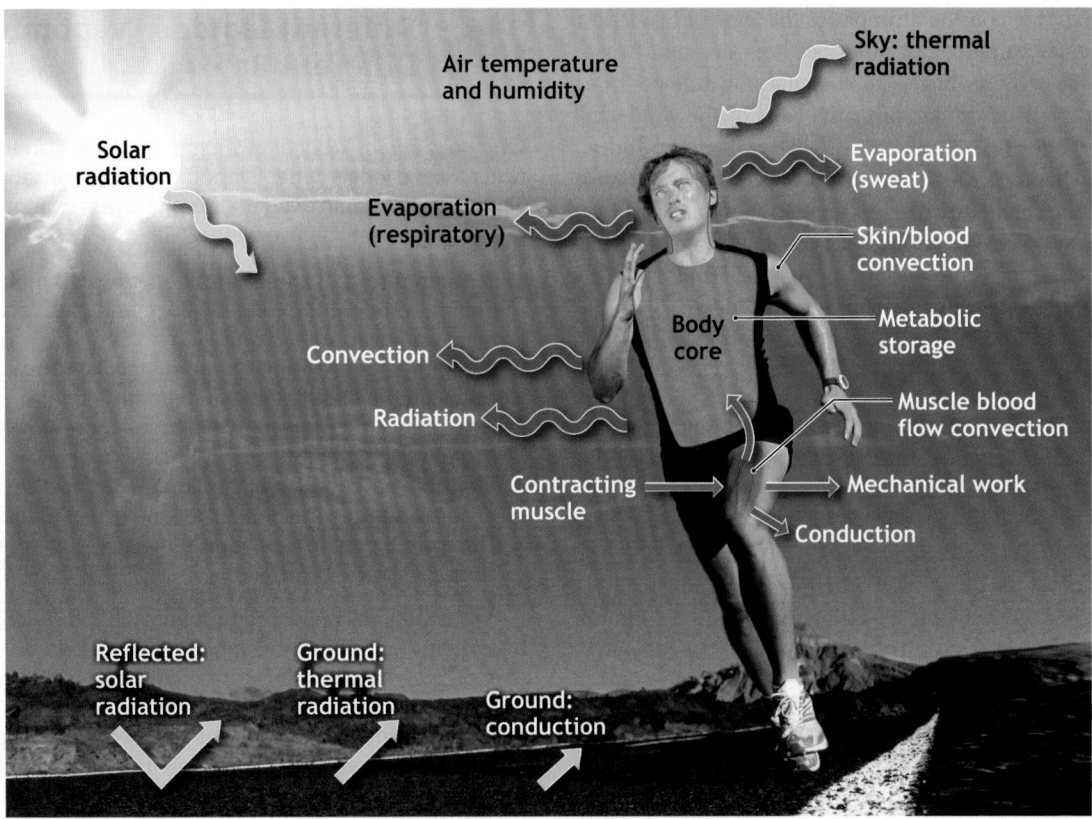

FIGURE 25.3 • Heat production within active muscle and its transfer from the core to the skin. Under appropriate environmental conditions, excess body heat dissipates to the environment to regulate core temperature within a narrow range. (Adapted with permission from Katch VL, McArdle WD, Katch FI. *Essentials of Exercise Physiology*. 4th Ed. Philadelphia: Wolters Kluwer Health, 2011, as adapted from Gisolfi CV, Wenger CB. Temperature regulation during exercise: old concepts, new ideas. *Exerc Sport Sci Rev* 1984;12:339.)

warmer than the environment, making the net exchange of radiant heat energy move through the air to solid, cooler objects in the environment. This form of heat transfer does not require molecular contact between objects; it provides the means for the sun's warming effect on the Earth. A person can remain warm by absorbing radiant heat energy from direct sunlight or by reflection from snow, sand, or water, even in subfreezing air temperatures. The body absorbs radiant heat energy from the surroundings when an object's temperature exceeds skin temperature.

Heat Loss by Conduction

Heat exchange by conduction involves direct heat transfer from one molecule to another through a liquid, solid, or gas. The circulation transports most body heat to the shell, but a small amount continually moves by conduction directly through the deep tissues to the cooler surface. Heat loss by conduction then involves warming air molecules and cooler surfaces that contact the skin.

The rate of conductive heat loss depends on two factors:

1. Temperature gradient between the skin and surrounding surfaces
2. Thermal qualities of the surfaces

For example, immersing the body in cool water can produce considerable heat loss. Placing one hand in room-temperature water clearly illustrates this phenomenon. Why does the hand in water feel much colder than the hand in air, even though the water and air have identical temperatures? The answer is straightforward: Water absorbs several thousand times more heat than air and conducts it away from the warmer body part. Sitting in an indoor swimming pool with water at 28°C (82.4°F) provides more discomfort than sitting on the pool deck at the same temperature. Hikers often gain considerable body heat when trekking in a warm environment. Lying on a rock shielded from the sun facilitates some body heat loss by conductance between the rock's cool surface and the hiker's warmer surface.

Heat Loss by Convection

The effectiveness of heat loss by conduction depends on how rapidly the air (or water) adjacent to the body exchanges once it warms. If air movement or convection proceeds slowly, the air next to the skin warms and acts as a "zone of insulation" that minimizes further conductive heat loss. Conversely, if cooler air continually replaces warmer air about the body on a breezy day, in a room with a fan, or when running, heat loss increases because convection continually replaces the zone of insulation. For example, air currents at 4 miles per hour are about twice as effective for body cooling as air currents at 1 mile per hour. The cooling effect of airflow forms the basis of the wind-chill temperature index (see "The Wind-Chill Temperature Index," later in this chapter). This index indicates the equivalent still-air temperature for a particular ambient temperature at different wind velocities. Convection also exerts an effect on thermal balance in water because the body loses heat more rapidly when swimming than when remaining motionless.

Heat Loss by Evaporation

Water vaporizing from the respiratory passages and skin surface continually transfers heat to the environment. Convective airflow that moves the moist, humidified air from the skin's surface continues to facilitate heat loss.[98] Each vaporized liter of water extracts 580 kcal from the body and transfers it to the environment.

The body's surface contains approximately 2 to 4 million sweat glands. During heat stress, these *eccrine glands*—controlled by cholinergic sympathetic nerve fibers—secrete hypotonic saline solution (0.2–0.4% NaCl). Evaporation of sweat from the skin exerts a cooling effect. The cooled skin in turn cools the blood diverted from interior tissues to the surface. In addition to heat loss through sweat evaporation, about 350 mL of insensible perspiration seeps through the skin each day and evaporates to the environment. Also, about 300 mL of water vaporizes daily from the moist mucous membranes of the respiratory passages. This manifests as "foggy breath" in cold weather.

Evaporative Heat Loss at High Ambient Temperatures

Evaporation provides the major defense against overheating. As ambient temperature increases, conduction, convection, and radiation decrease in their effectiveness to facilitate body heat loss. When ambient temperature exceeds body temperature, the body gains heat by these three thermal transfer mechanisms. In such environments, or when conduction, convection, and radiation cannot dissipate a large metabolic heat load, sweat evaporation from the skin and respiratory tract provide the only means for heat dissipation. Increases in ambient temperature generally induce proportionate increases in sweating rate.

 INTEGRATIVE QUESTION

A person walks along a beach on a cloudy day at a constant speed of 4 mph. The wind blows from the west at a steady 12 mph. The westerly portion of the walk feels cooler than the return walk to the east, which feels warmer. Give a possible reason for this discrepancy based on the physical principles of heat gain–heat loss.

 ## Different Liquids Evaporate at Different Rates

Why does liquids alcohol evaporate from the skin rapidly while water takes a longer time? Evaporation or vaporization continually occurs at a liquid's surface, but the rate of evaporation varies depending largely on five factors:

1. Temperature or average kinetic energy of its molecules, with higher temperature directly increasing molecular movement and evaporation rate
2. Magnitude of cohesion or intermolecular force of attraction between the liquid's molecular bonds
3. Heavier-weight molecules evaporate more slowly than molecules of less weight
4. Molecules escape from the liquid's surface; the larger the exposed surface the greater the molecular escape
5. The evaporation rate of liquids increases with the flow of air currents above its surface

Ethyl alcohol, known commonly as rubbing alcohol, evaporates nearly five times more rapidly as water because the molecular force of attraction is less than between the atoms of water molecules. When molecules with higher kinetic (heat) energy evaporate from a liquid, lower-kinetic energy, lower-temperature molecules remain, which accounts for the cooling effect on the skin of rapidly evaporating alcohol. Oils, in contrast, evaporate at a more "sluggish" rate than either alcohol or water.

Heat Loss During High Humidity

Three factors influence the total amount of sweat vaporized from the skin and/or pulmonary surfaces:

1. Surface exposed to the environment
2. Temperature and relative humidity of the ambient air
3. Convective air currents about the body

Relative humidity *represents the most important factor in determining the effectiveness of evaporative heat loss.* Relative humidity refers to the ratio of water in ambient air at a particular temperature compared to the total quantity of moisture that air could contain expressed as a percentage. For example, 40% relative humidity means that ambient air contains only 40% of the air's moisture-carrying capacity at that specific temperature. With high humidity, the ambient vapor pressure approaches that of moist skin of about 40 mm Hg. In this case, evaporation greatly diminishes even though large quantities of sweat bead on the skin and eventually roll off. This form of sweating represents useless water loss that can produce dehydration and overheating. A dangerous rise in core temperature can occur in athletes who compete in moderate- to high-intensity sports that exceed 30 min duration in environments above 35°C (95°F) and 60% relative humidity. "In a Practical Sense," that follows, describes how to assess the heat quality of the environment, with accompanying recommendations concerning physical activity related to ambient temperature, radiant heat, and relative humidity.

Continually drying the skin with a towel while sweating, as some tennis players do between games and sets, thwarts evaporative cooling. *Evaporation, not sweat, cools the skin.* Individuals can tolerate relatively high environmental temperatures provided relative humidity remains low. Most persons find hot, dry desert climates more comfortable than cooler but more humid tropical climates.

 INTEGRATIVE QUESTION

In deciding on the starting time for an upcoming summer marathon, what prior meteorologic information would be most valuable and why?

Integration of Heat-Dissipating Mechanisms

The mechanisms for heat loss remain the same whether the heat load originates internally from metabolic heat or externally from environmental heat.

Circulation

The circulatory system represents the "workhorse" to maintain thermal balance. At rest in the heat, heart rate and cardiac output increase, while superficial arterial and venous blood vessels dilate to divert warm blood to the body shell. This manifests as a flushed or reddened face on a hot day or during vigorous activity. With extreme heat stress, 15 to 25% of the cardiac output passes through the skin. Enhanced cutaneous blood flow greatly increases the thermal conductance of peripheral tissues. This favors radiative heat loss to the environment, particularly from the hands, forehead, forearms, ears, and tibial areas.

Evaporation

Sweating begins within several seconds of the start of vigorous activity. After about 30 min, it achieves equilibrium in direct relation to the exercise load. An effective thermal defense exists when evaporative cooling combines with a large cutaneous blood flow. The cooled peripheral blood then flows to the deeper tissues to absorb additional heat on its return to the heart.

Hormonal Adjustments

Sweating produces loss of water and electrolytes; this initiates hormonal adjustments to conserve salts and fluid. Fluid conservation makes urine more concentrated during heat stress. Concurrently, repeated days of exertion in the heat or just a single bout of activity stimulates adrenocortical release of the sodium-conserving hormone **aldosterone** to act on the renal tubules to increase sodium reabsorption. Aldosterone also reduces sweat's osmolality. This causes sweat sodium concentration to decrease during repeated heat exposure to further conserve electrolytes. At the same time, exercise and/or hypohydration stimulates **vasopressin**, also called *antidiuretic hormone*, release from the neurohypophysis of the hypothalamus. Vasopressin increases permeability of the collecting tubules of the kidneys to facilitate fluid retention. The magnitude of aldosterone and vasopressin release depends on hypohydration severity and physical activity intensity.[93]

EFFECTS OF CLOTHING ON THERMOREGULATION

Clothing insulates the body from its surroundings. It can reduce radiant heat gain in a hot environment or retard conductive and convective heat loss in the cold.

Clothing Insulations (Clo Units)

The United States military has made a strong research commitment to develop standards for the insulatory properties of clothing to meet environmental challenges. The clo unit represents an index of thermal resistance. It indicates the insulatory capacity provided by any layer of trapped air between the skin and clothing, including the clothing's insulation value. Assuming an environment with negligible air movement and body movement to disturb the insulatory layer of air about the body, a clo unit of 1 maintains a sedentary person at 1 MET indefinitely in an environment of 21°C (68.8°F) and 50% relative humidity.

An individual's metabolic rate at a given environmental temperature also affects the clo unit requirement. Data in TABLE 25.2 show six conditions of metabolic intensity from sleeping to heavy work expressed in MET units and three environmental temperatures (0°C, –20°C, –50°C [32°F, 4°F, –58°F]). Note the inverse relationship between metabolic intensity and the insulation requirement (more clothing required for less work). At rest (1 MET) at 0°C (32°F), the clo requirement is 5.4, but when temperature drops to –50°C (–58°F), the clo requirement increases by 130% to 12.4.

TABLE 25.2 clo Values Required to Maintain Core Temperature Related to Physical Activity Level and Ambient Temperature

Activity	Temperature, °C		
	0	–20	–50
Heavy work, 6.0 METs	1.0	1.6	2.2
Moderate work, 3.0 METs	1.6	2.8	4.2
Light work, 2.0 METs	2.6	4.0	6.2
Very light work, 1.5 METs	3.4	5.6	8.2
Rest, 1.0 MET	5.4	8.3	12.4
Sleep, 0.8 METs	6.7	10.6	15.5

IN A PRACTICAL SENSE

Assessing Heat Quality of the Environment: How Hot Is Too Hot?

Seven important factors determine the physiologic strain imposed by environmental heat:

1. Air temperature and relative humidity
2. Individual differences in body size and fatness
3. State of training
4. Degree of acclimatization
5. Environmental influences such as convective air currents and radiant heat gain
6. Intensity of physical activity
7. Amount, type, and color of clothing

Several football deaths from heat injury occurred with air temperature below 23.9°C (75°F) but with relative humidity above 95%. Prevention is the most effective control of heat-stress injuries. Most importantly, acclimatization minimizes the likelihood of heat injury. Another consideration requires evaluating the environment for its potential thermal challenge using the wet bulb–globe temperature (WB–GT) index. This index of environmental heat stress developed by the military provides important information to the National Collegiate Athletic Association to establish thresholds for increased risk of heat injury and physical performance decrements. The WB–GT index depends on ambient temperature, relative humidity, and radiant heat as related in the following equation:

WB − GT = 0.1 × DBT + 0.7 × WBT + 0.2 × GT

where DBT represents the dry-bulb temperature (air temperature) recorded by an ordinary mercury thermometer, and WBT equals the wet-bulb temperature recorded by a similar thermometer except that a wet wick surrounds the mercury bulb (**Fig. 1**). With high relative humidity, little evaporative cooling occurs from the wetted bulb, so this thermometer's temperature remains similar to the dry bulb. On a dry day, considerable evaporation occurs from the wetted bulb to maximize the difference between the two thermometer readings. A small difference between thermometer readings indicates high relative humidity, whereas a large difference indicates little air moisture and rapid evaporation. GT represents the globe temperature

recorded by a thermometer with a black metal sphere enclosing its bulb. The black globe absorbs radiant energy from the surroundings to measure this source of heat gain. Most industrial supply companies sell this relatively inexpensive thermometer. One can also assess ambient heat load from wet-bulb thermometer (WBT) because this reading reflects both air temperature and relative humidity.

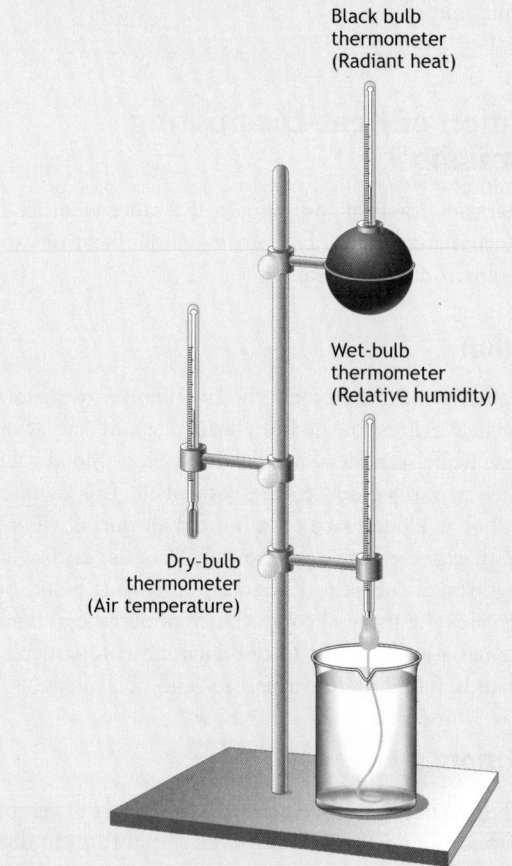

FIGURE 1 • Apparatus to measure wet bulb–globe temperature (WB–GT).

Six factors affect the insulation (**clo value**) of clothing:

1. *Wind speed*—Increased speed disturbs the zone of insulation.
2. *Body movements*—Pumping actions of arms and legs disturb the zone of insulation.
3. *Chimney effect*—Loosely hanging clothing ventilates the trapped air layers away from the body.
4. *Bellows effect*—Vigorous body movements increase ventilation of air layers that conserve body heat.
5. *Water vapor transfer*—Clothing resists the passage of water vapor and thus decreases heat loss by evaporative cooling.

6. *Permeation efficiency factor*—How well clothing absorbs liquid (sweat) by capillary action (wicking); wicking sweat away from the body surface reduces the cooling effect of evaporation, thus improving clothing's effectiveness for conserving body heat.

Table 25.3 presents clo values for common garments. To determine the total insulatory value of what a person wears, add the individual clo values for each garment. Without wind penetration or air movement around the clothing, the clo value for a given weight of clothes equals 0.15 times the

The American College of Sports Medicine proposes the following recommendations concerning risk for heat injury with continuous physical activity based on the WB–GT:

WB-GT RECOMMENDATIONS FOR CONTINUOUS ACTIVITIES SUCH AS ENDURANCE RUNNING AND CYCLING[2]

- *Very high risk*: Above 28°C (82°F)—Postpone race.
- *High risk*: 23 to 28°C (73–82°F)—Heat-sensitive individuals (e.g., obese, low physical fitness, unacclimatized, dehydrated, previous history of heat injury) should not compete.
- *Moderate risk*: 18 to 23°C (65–73°F)
- *Low risk*: Below 18°C (65°F)

Without the WBT, but knowing relative humidity (local meteorologic stations or media reports), the heat-stress index (Fɪɢ. 2) evaluates the relative heat stress. The index should rely on data close to the actual sport site to eliminate potential error from meteorologic data some distance from the event.

Relative humidity	\multicolumn{11}{c}{Air temperature (°F)}
	70	75	80	85	90	95	100	105	110	115	120
	\multicolumn{11}{c}{Heat sensation (°F)}
0%	64	69	73	78	83	87	91	95	99	103	107
10%	65	70	75	80	85	90	95	100	105	111	116
20%	66	72	77	82	87	93	99	105	112	120	130
30%	67	73	78	84	90	96	104	113	123	135	148
40%	68	74	79	86	93	101	110	123	137	151	
50%	69	75	81	88	96	107	120	135	150		
60%	70	76	82	90	100	114	132	149			
70%	70	77	85	93	106	124	144				
80%	71	78	86	97	113	136					
90%	71	79	88	102	122						
100%	72	80	91	108							

90°–105°F   Possibility of heat cramps
105°–130°F   Heat cramps or heat exhaustion likely, heat stroke possible
130°+   Heat stroke a definite risk

FIGURE 2 • The heat-stress index.

clothing weight in pounds. For example, wearing 10 pounds of clothes produces a clo value of 1.5 (0.15 × 10 lb).

Cold-Weather Clothing

In providing insulation from the cold, the mesh of the cloth fibers traps air that then warms. This establishes a barrier to heat loss because the cloth and air conduct heat poorly; insulation becomes more effective with a thicker zone of trapped air above the skin. For this reason, several layers of light clothing, or garments lined with animal fur, feathers, or synthetic fabrics with numerous layers of trapped air, provide better insulation than a single bulky layer. The clothing layer against the skin should also wick moisture from the body's surface to the next insulating clothing layer for subsequent evaporation. Wool or synthetics (e.g., polypropylene) that insulate well and dry quickly serve this purpose. A wool cap contributes considerably to heat conservation; nearly 30 to 40% of body heat dissipates through the highly vascularized head region that represents only about 8% of the body's total surface area. Conversely, cooling the head during physical activity in hot weather reduces symptoms of thermal discomfort. When clothing becomes wet, through either external moisture or condensation from sweating, it loses almost 90% of its insulating properties. This facilitates heat loss from the body because water conducts heat 25 times faster than air.

The thermoregulatory challenge when exercising in cold air arises not from inadequate insulation, but from metabolic heat dissipation through a thick air–clothing barrier. Cross-country skiers alleviate this problem by removing layers of clothing as the body warms. This practice maintains core temperature without reliance on evaporative cooling. *The ideal winter garment in cold, dry weather blocks air movement but also allows water vapor from sweating to escape through the clothing.*

Warm-Weather Clothing

Dry clothing, no matter how lightweight, retards heat exchange more than the same clothing fully wet. Switching to a dry tennis, basketball, or football uniform in hot weather makes little sense for temperature regulation. Evaporative heat loss occurs only when the clothing becomes wet. *A dry uniform simply prolongs the time lag between sweating and subsequent evaporative cooling.*

Different materials absorb water at different rates. Cottons and linens readily absorb moisture. In contrast, heavy sweatshirts and rubber or plastic clothing produce high relative humidity close to the skin. This retards vaporization of moisture from its surface, blunting or even preventing evaporative cooling. Warm-weather clothing should fit loosely to permit free circulation of air between the skin and environment to promote convection and evaporation from the skin. Moisture-wicking garments (e.g., polypropylene, CoolMax™, Dry-Lite™) optimally transfer heat and moisture from the skin to the environment, particularly during intense activity in hot weather. They also benefit the individual during physical activity in cold environments because dry clothing, in contrast to sweat-drenched clothing, reduces hypothermia risk Color

TABLE 25.3   clo Values for Some Common Garments[a]

Garment Description	clo	Garment Description	clo
Underwear, pants		**Coats, jacket, and overtrousers**	
Pantyhose	0.02	Coat	0.6
Panties	0.03	Down jacket	0.55
Briefs	0.04	Parka	0.7
Pants, long legs	0.1	**Accessories**	
Underwear, shirts		Socks	0.02
Bra	0.01	Ankle socks (thick)	0.05
Shirt, sleeveless	0.06	Long socks (thick)	0.1
T-shirt	0.09	Slippers, quilted fleece	0.03
Shirt with long sleeves	0.12	Shoes (thin soled)	0.02
Half-slip, nylon	0.14	Shoes (thick soled)	0.04
Shirts		Boots, gloves	0.05
Tube top	0.06	**Skirts, dresses**	
Short sleeve	0.09	Light skirt, 15 cm above knee	0.10
Lightweight blouse, short sleeves	0.15	Light skirt, 15 cm below knee	0.18
Lightweight blouse, long sleeves	0.20	Heavy skirt, knee-length	0.25
Normal, long sleeves	0.25	Light dress, sleeveless	0.25
Flannel shirt, long sleeves	0.3	Winter dress, long sleeves	0.4
Trousers		**Sleepwear**	
Shorts	0.06	Long gown, long sleeves	0.3
Walking shorts	0.11	Short gown, thin-strap	0.15
Lightweight trousers	0.20	Hospital gown	0.31
Normal trousers	0.25	Long pajamas, long sleeves	0.50
Flannel trousers	0.28	**Robes**	
Overalls	0.28	Long-sleeve, wrap, long	0.53
Sweaters		Long-sleeve, wrap, short	0.41
Sleeveless vest	0.12	**Coveralls**	
Thin sweater	0.2	Daily wear, belted, work	0.49
Turtleneck, long sleeves (thin)	0.26	Highly insulating multicomponent, filling coveralls	1.03
Sweater	0.28		
Thick sweater	0.35	Fiber-pelt	1.13
Turtleneck, long sleeves (thick)	0.37		
Jacket			
Vest	0.13		
Light summer jacket	0.25		
Jacket	0.35		

[a]Higher numbers indicate greater insulatory capacity.

also exerts an influence; dark colors absorb light rays and add to radiant heat gain, whereas lighter-colored clothing reflects heat rays away from the body.

Football Uniforms

Football uniforms and equipment present a considerable barrier to heat dissipation during environmental heat exposure.[86] Even with loose-fitting porous jerseys, the wrappings, padding with its plastic covering, helmet, and other objects of "armor" effectively seal off 50% of the body's surface from the benefits of evaporative cooling. The 6 or 7 kg of equipment, frequently transported over a hot artificial playing surface adds to the player's total metabolic load. The large size of many of the athletes further magnifies heat stress, particularly for offensive and defensive linemen with relatively small surface area–body mass ratio and higher body fat percentage than smaller teammates at the other skill positions.

FIGURE 25.4 depicts the metabolic and thermal stress provided by a football uniform. The experiment tested nine men who ran for 30 min at 25.6°C (78°F) and 35% relative humidity. In one test, the men wore only shorts; in another, they wore the complete football uniform including helmet and plastic padding. In a third series, they wore shorts and carried a backpack that contained 6.2 kg, the exact weight of the uniform and equipment.

Wearing football gear while exercising produced higher rectal and skin temperatures during exercise and recovery than the other exercise conditions. Skin temperature directly

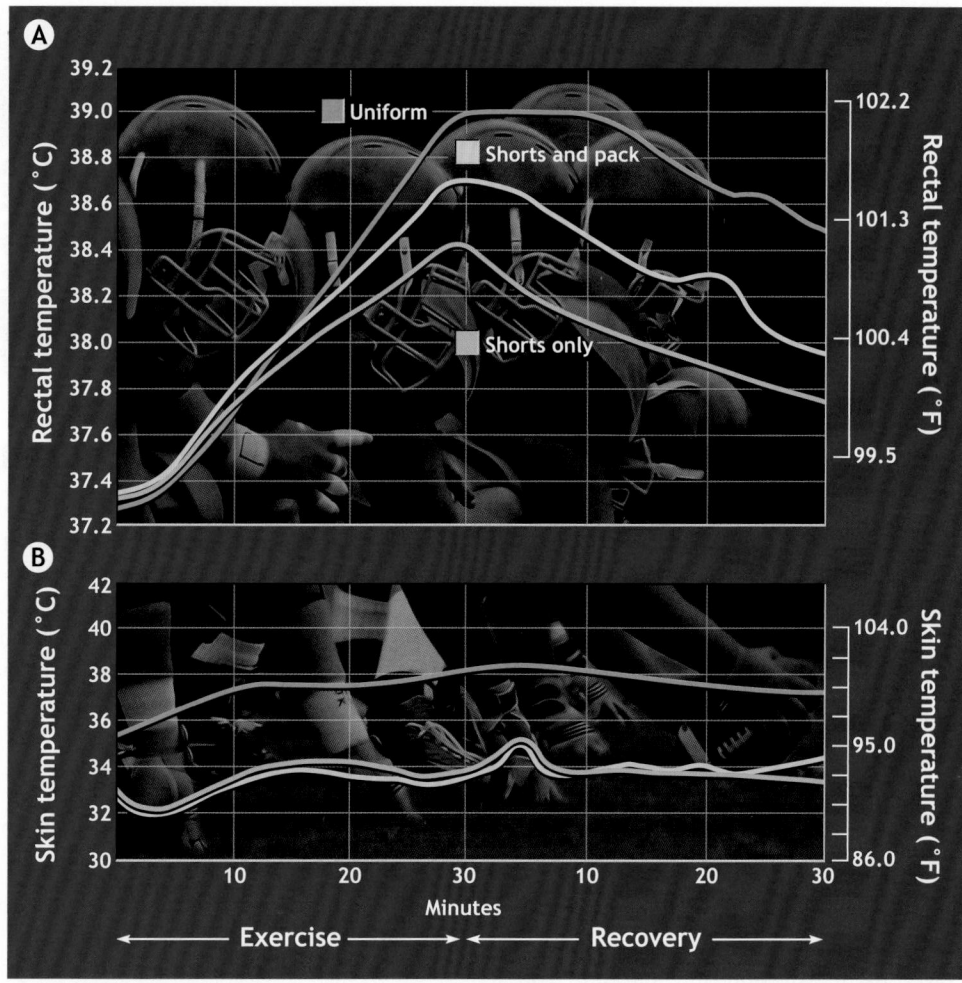

FIGURE 25.4 • Effects of full football uniform and its equivalent weight on **(A)** rectal temperature and **(B)** skin temperature during physical activity. Subjects ran at 9.6 km·hr⁻¹ for 30 min at 25.6°C (78°F) and 35% relative humidity. The uniform (*orange line*) caused the largest heat stress because of its effect in retarding evaporative cooling. This significantly elevated rectal and skin temperatures. (Adapted with permission from Mathews DK, et al. Physiological responses during exercise and recovery in a football uniform. *J Appl Physiol* 1969;26:611.)

beneath the padding averaged only 1°C (1.8°F) less than rectal temperature. This indicates that subcutaneous blood in these areas cooled by only about one fifth as much as blood near the skin surface directly exposed to the environment. Rectal temperature remained elevated in recovery with uniforms, so a rest period offers limited value in normalizing thermal status unless the athlete removes the uniform. The *yellow* line shows that the weight of the uniform accounts for a large portion of the heat load. Not wearing the uniform (*aqua* line in Fig. 25.4A and B) produced cooler skin temperatures and lower sweat rates. Without the uniform, evaporation from the skin progressed freely, whereas the uniform insulated the athlete and reduced the effective evaporative surface.

The Modern Cycling Helmet Does Not Thwart Heat Dissipation

For cyclists, wearing a commercially available helmet provides vital protection against possible head trauma, but does the cycling helmet impede thermoregulatory processes in a hot–dry or hot–humid environment? Because the head provides an important avenue for heat loss during exercise-induced hyperthermia, many competitive cyclists believe riding without a helmet reduces thermal strain and physical discomfort. This belief persists even though the design of the current commercial protective helmet retains aerodynamic and lightweight features with ventilation ports for convective and evaporative cooling. To evaluate physiologic and perceptual responses of wearing a helmet, 10 male and 4 female competitive cyclists pedaled for 90 min at 60% of $\dot{V}O_{2peak}$ in both hot–dry (35°C [95°F], 20% relative humidity) and hot–humid (35°C [95°F], 70% relative humidity) environments, with and without a protective helmet.[127] The results for oxygen consumption, heart rate, core, skin, and head skin temperatures, rating of perceived exertion, and perceived thermal sensations of the head and body revealed that cycling in a hot–humid environment produced greater thermal stress than cycling under thermoneutral conditions.

Wearing the helmet, however, did not increase the riders' heat strain or perceived heat sensation from the head or body.

Summary

1. Exposure to heat or cold stress initiates thermoregulatory mechanisms that generate and conserve heat at low ambient temperatures and dissipate heat at high temperatures.
2. The "thermostat" for temperature regulation resides in the brain's hypothalamus. This coordinating center initiates adjustments in response to input from thermal receptors in the skin and changes in the temperature of the blood that perfuses the hypothalamic region.
3. Heat conservation in cold stress results from vascular adjustments that shunt blood from the cooler periphery to the warmer deep tissues of the body's core.
4. If vascular mechanisms prove ineffective during cold stress, shivering provides input of metabolic heat. Prolonged cold stress stimulates release of hormones that elevate resting metabolism.
5. Heat stress diverts warm blood from the body's core to the shell. Four factors—radiation, conduction, convection, and evaporation—contribute to heat dissipation.
6. Evaporation provides the major physiologic defense against overheating at high ambient temperatures and intense physical activity.
7. Effectiveness of evaporative heat loss diminishes dramatically in warm, humid environments, making a person vulnerable to dehydration and spiraling core temperature.
8. Two practical heat-stress indices, the wet bulb–globe temperature index and the heat-stress index, use ambient temperature, radiant heat, and relative humidity to evaluate the environment's potential heat challenge.
9. Three factors influence sweat vaporization from the skin or pulmonary surfaces: surface exposure, ambient air temperature and relative humidity, and convective air currents.
10. Vigorous physical activity generates metabolic heat to maintain core temperature in cold air environments, even if the person wears little clothing.
11. The clo unit reflects thermal resistance from clothing—the insulatory capacity of air trapped between skin and clothing including the clothing's insulation value.
12. Wearing several layers of light clothing traps a zone of air against the skin; this provides more effective insulation from cold than a single thick layer of clothing.
13. Wet clothing loses its insulating properties; this greatly facilitates heat flow from the body.
14. Ideal warm-weather clothing is lightweight, loose fitting, and light colored. Even with these characteristics, heat loss slows until the clothing becomes wet and allows evaporative cooling.
15. Football uniforms impose a barrier to heat dissipation because they effectively shield about 50% of the body's surface from the beneficial effects of evaporative cooling.

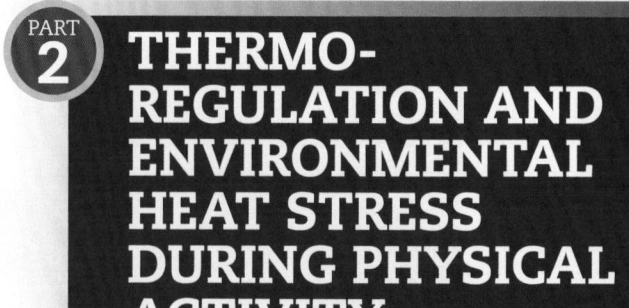

PART 2

THERMO-REGULATION AND ENVIRONMENTAL HEAT STRESS DURING PHYSICAL ACTIVITY

PHYSICAL ACTIVITY IN THE HEAT

The refrigerating mechanism of evaporative cooling dissipates metabolic heat during physical activity, particularly in hot weather. This places a demand on the body's fluid reserves and often produces relative hypohydration. Excessive sweating leads to more serious fluid loss and reduced plasma volume. This causes circulatory failure in the extreme, and core temperature rises to lethal levels.

Circulatory Adjustments

The body encounters two competitive cardiovascular demands when exercising in the heat:

1. Demand muscles require delivery of arterial blood (oxygen) to sustain energy metabolism.
2. Demand arterial blood diverts to the periphery to transport metabolic heat for cooling at the skin surface; this blood cannot deliver its oxygen to active muscle.

Submaximal effort produces similar cardiac outputs in hot and cold environments.[117] The heart's stroke volume usually remains lower in the heat in proportion to the fluid deficit and reduced blood volume created in physical activity.[44,96] This translates to *higher heart rates* at all submaximal levels of activity in the heat. In contrast, the reflex compensatory increase in heart rate in maximal effort fails to offset the stroke volume decrease, so maximal cardiac output decreases.

Vascular Constriction and Dilation

Maintaining adequate cutaneous and muscle blood flow during physical activity under heat stress requires other tissues to temporarily compromise blood supply. For example, during environmental heat stress, compensatory constriction of the splanchnic vascular bed and renal tissues rapidly counteracts active vasodilation of the subcutaneous vessels responsible for 80 to 95% of elevated skin blood flow.[59,83] A prolonged reduction in renal and visceral tissue blood flow probably contributes to liver and renal complications during exertional heat stress.

Maintenance of Blood Pressure

Vasoconstriction in the viscera increases total vascular resistance. A balance between dilation and constriction maintains arterial blood pressure during exercise in the heat. In intense effort, with accompanying dehydration, relatively less blood diverts to peripheral areas for heat dissipation. Reduced peripheral blood flow reflects the body's attempt to maintain cardiac output in the face of diminishing plasma volume caused by sweating. *Circulatory regulation and muscle blood flow take precedence over temperature regulation during physical activity in the heat.* When submaximal effort progresses without excessive physiologic strain, a greater dependence still exists on anaerobic metabolism than in cooler conditions.[148] This produces earlier accumulation of lactate, encroachment on glycogen reserves, and premature fatigue during prolonged moderate activity. Two factors increase blood lactate accumulation:

1. Decreased lactate uptake by the liver from reduced hepatic blood flow
2. Reduced muscle catabolism of circulating lactate because heat dissipation diverts a large portion of the cardiac output to the periphery

Core Temperature During Physical Activity

Heat generated by active muscles can raise core temperature to fever levels that would incapacitate a person if caused by external heat stress alone. Endurance runners, including champions, show no ill effects from rectal temperatures as high as 41°C (105.8°F) at the end of a 3-mile race.[13] Aerobically fit subjects perform longer in *uncompensably hot environments*, environments where thermoregulatory mechanisms are inadequate, and tolerate higher levels of hyperthermia than less fit subjects.[17] This ability of trained individuals to reach higher core temperatures than untrained counterparts may leave them more prone to experience heat-related problems.[97,99] An abnormally high core temperature for trained and untrained subjects impairs exercise performance. Fatigue generally coincides with core temperatures between 38 and 40°C (100–104°F). This temperature range

reflects a "critical" high body temperature that impairs muscle activation directly from a high brain temperature that decreases the central drive to exercise. In addition to the fatiguing effects of altered cerebral blood flow and depressed neuromuscular drive, a thermally induced exercise impairment may also result from reduced blood flow to specific regions of the gastrointestinal tract to produce gastrointestinal barrier dysfunction and increased permeability. This effect allows endotoxins to enter the internal environment and contribute to fatigue.[18,69]

Temperature Regulated at a Higher Level During Physical Activity

Within limits, the increase in core temperature with physical activity does not reflect a failure of the heat-dissipating mechanisms or contribute to early fatigue. To the contrary, it represents a well-regulated response even during exercise in the cold. **FIGURE 25.5A** illustrates the relationship between core temperature as measured in the esophagus and power output, expressed as oxygen consumption, for five men and two women of varying fitness levels during progressively more intense effort. Core temperature increases to a higher level for all subjects as intensity of effort increases, although considerable intersubject variation occurs in temperature response. Note that the lines move closer together in **FIGURE 25.5B**, which plots core temperature related to oxygen consumption expressed as a percentage of each person's $\dot{V}O_{2max}$. This indicates that relative workload (i.e., the percentage of capacity) determines the change in core temperature with exercise. *More than likely, a modest rise in core temperature represents a favorable adjustment that optimizes physiologic and metabolic functions.*

In general, physical effort at 50% $\dot{V}O_{2max}$ in a comfortable environment increases core temperature to a new steady level of about 37.3°C (99°F), whereas work at 75% of maximum elevates temperature to 38.5°C (101°F), regardless of the absolute oxygen consumption. This means that a fit person

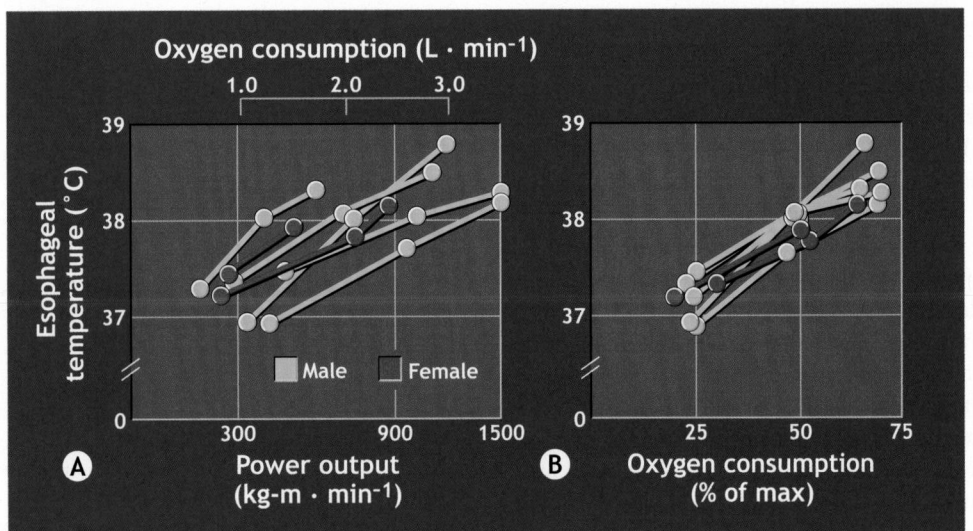

FIGURE 25.5 • Relationship between esophageal temperature and **(A)** oxygen consumption (absolute exercise intensity expressed as power output) and **(B)** oxygen consumption as a percentage of $\dot{V}O_{2max}$. (Adapted with permission from Saltin B, Hermansen L. Esophageal, rectal, and muscle temperature during exercise. *J Appl Physiol* 1966;21:1757.)

generates more total energy (heat) in physical activity than a less-fit person at the same percentage of $\dot{V}O_{2max}$, yet both maintain about the same core temperature. The extra metabolic heat for the trained person dissipates via a larger sweat output. The trained person exercises with a lower core temperature than the untrained person at identical exercise levels (i.e., same absolute $\dot{V}O_2$).

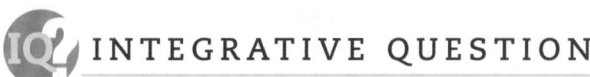

INTEGRATIVE QUESTION

What mechanisms explain how improved aerobic fitness increases exercise tolerance in a warm, humid environment?

Water Loss in the Heat: Dehydration

Dehydration refers to body water loss from a hyperhydrated state to euhydration or from euhydration downward to hypohydration. A moderate workout over 1 hr generally produces a sweat loss of 0.5 to 1.0 L. Greater water loss occurs from several hours of intense activity in a hot environment. Sweating still occurs in less challenging thermal environments such as cross-country skiing or swimming. For swimmers and divers, water immersion also stimulates fluid loss through increased urine production. Non–exercise-induced water loss occurs when wrestlers, boxers, weightlifters, and rowers aggressively attempt to "make weight" through rapid weight loss induced by common dehydration techniques—external heat exposure via sauna, steam room, hot whirlpool or shower, fluid and food restriction, diuretic and laxative use, and vomiting. Athletes often combine these techniques, hoping to accelerate weight loss. *The risk of heat illness greatly increases when a person begins physical activity in a dehydrated state.*

Fluid deficits in the intracellular and extracellular compartments (*hypovolemia*) with hypohydration can rapidly reach levels that reduce the body's ability to dissipate heat and increase the rate of heat storage and cardiovascular strain owing to reductions in sweating rate and skin blood flow for a given core temperature. Reduced heat tolerance severely compromises cardiovascular function and physical capacity with intense exertion in hot environments.[95,124] Sweat remains hypotonic to other body fluids, so the hypovolemia from sweating correspondingly increases plasma osmolality.

For physical performance, rapid weight loss through dehydration does not impair muscular strength or a single bout of anaerobic power performance up to 60-s duration, although the effects on muscular endurance remain equivocal.[19,45,94,143] Losing body water rapidly before a short-duration activity even improves muscular power and strength on a relative basis (per kg body mass).[57] When intense effort lasts longer than 1 min, dehydration profoundly impairs physiologic function and optimal ability to train and compete. A moderate hypohydration equivalent to 1.5% body mass produced poorer intermittent all-out performance than similar effort in the euhydrated state.[82] Dehydration associated with a 3% decrease in body weight also slows gastric emptying rate, increasing epigastric cramps and feelings of nausea.

Magnitude of Fluid Loss

For an acclimatized person, water loss by sweating reaches a peak of about 3 L·hr⁻¹ during intense physical activity in the heat and totals nearly 12 L on a daily basis. Several hours of intense sweating can produce sweat-gland fatigue that ultimately interferes with core temperature regulation. Elite marathon runners frequently experience fluid loss in excess of 5 L during competition, a loss equivalent to 6 to 10% of body mass. For a slower-paced ultramarathon, the average fluid loss rarely exceeds 500 mL per hour. Even in a temperate climate of 10°C (50°F), soccer players lose an average of 2 L during a 90-min game.[79] *Acclimatized humans sustain their exceptional potential for evaporative cooling only with adequate fluid replacement.* **TABLE 25.4** provides the predicted sweating rates

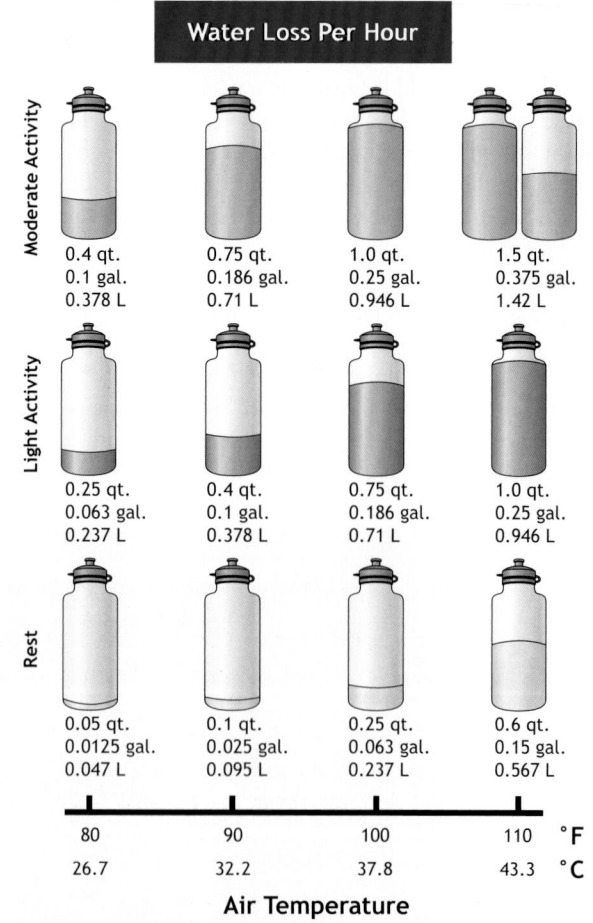

Water Loss Relates to Activity Intensity and Ambient Temperature

Average water loss per hour for a typical adult caused by sweating at various air temperatures during rest and light and moderate physical activity. (Reprinted with permission from Katch VL, McArdle WD, Katch FI, *Essentials of Exercise Physiology.* 4th Ed. Philadelphia: Wolters Kluwer Health, 2011.)

| TABLE 25.4 | Predicted Sweating Rates (L·hr⁻¹) for Running at 8.5 to 15.0 km·hr⁻¹ in Cool/Temperate (TDBᵃ = 18°C) and Warm (TDB = 28°C) Weather | | | | |

Body Weight (kg)	Climate	8.5 km·hr⁻¹ (5.3 mph)	10 km·hr⁻¹ (6.3 mph)	12.5 km·hr⁻¹ (7.9 mph)	15 km·hr⁻¹ (9.5 mph)
50	Cool/temperate	0.43	0.53	0.69	0.86
	Warm	0.52	0.62	0.79	0.96
70	Cool/temperate	0.65	0.79	1.02	1.25
	Warm	0.75	0.89	1.12	1.36
90	Cool/temperate	0.86	1.04	1.34	1.64
	Warm	0.97	1.15	1.46	1.76

ᵃTDB, temperature of dry bulb thermometer.

Reprinted from Montain SJ, et al. Exercise-associated hyponatremia: quantitative analysis for understanding the aetiology. *Br J Sports Med* 2006;40:98.

for individuals of different body weights running at various speeds in cold/temperate and warm weather conditions.

Sports other than distance running induce a large sweat output and accompanying fluid loss. Football, basketball, lacrosse, soccer, and hockey players lose large quantities of fluid during competition. Before a change in certification standards, high school wrestlers often lost 9 to 13% of preseason body weight prior to certification; the greatest portion of this weight loss came from voluntarily reducing water intake and excessive sweating just prior to the weigh-in. Collegiate wrestlers, excluding heavyweights, regained an average of 3.7 kg during the 20 hr between weigh-in and competition.[126] In their desire to "make weight," high school and collegiate wrestlers usually competed in a dehydrated state, with reduced blood and plasma volumes.[1,147] Transient, reversible mood alterations and impaired short-term memory also accompanied rapid weight loss in collegiate wrestlers.[21]

Significant Consequences of Dehydration

Almost any dehydration impairs physiologic function and thermoregulation. Even a modest fluid loss of 2% body mass adversely affects exercise performance.[29,32,92,141] As dehydration progresses and plasma volume decreases, peripheral blood flow and sweating rate diminish, making thermoregulation progressively more difficult. Pre-exercise dehydration equivalent to 5% of body mass increases rectal temperature and heart rate and decreases sweating rate, $\dot{V}O_{2max}$, and exercise capacity; it also attenuates multiset-multirepetition resistance exercise performance compared with exercise under normal hydration.[61,122,129] Reduced central blood volume lowers ventricular filling pressure and helps to explain the elevated heart rate and 25 to 30% stroke volume reduction in the dehydrated state. An increase in heart rate does not offset the reduced stroke volume; consequently, cardiac output and arterial blood pressure decline.

Fluid loss becomes most apparent during physical activity in hot, humid environments because the high vapor pressure of ambient air thwarts evaporative cooling. FIGURE 25.6 shows the linear dependency between sweating rate during rest and activity) and the air's moisture content reflected by wet-bulb temperature (see "In a Practical Sense," earlier in this chapter). Ironically, excessive sweat output in high humidity contributes little to cooling because of minimal evaporation.

Physiologic and Performance Decrements

Physiologic mechanisms contributing to dehydration-mediated physical performance degradation include augmented hyperthermia, increased cardiovascular strain, altered metabolic and central nervous system functions, and increased perception of effort.[123] Reduced peripheral blood flow and increased core temperature in activity relate closely to dehydration level. A fluid loss equivalent to only 1% of body mass increases rectal temperature compared with the same exercise and normal hydration. For each liter of sweat-loss dehydration, exercise heart rate increases 8 b·min⁻¹, with a corresponding 1.0 L·min⁻¹ decrease in cardiac output.[22] A large portion of water lost through sweating comes from blood plasma, so circulatory capacity progressively

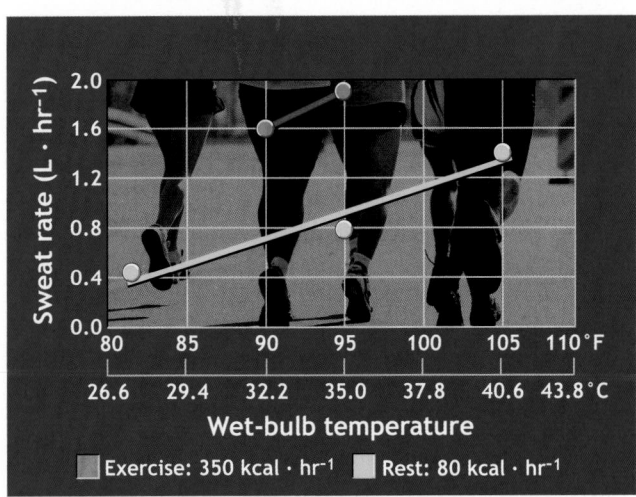

FIGURE 25.6 • Effect of humidity (wet-bulb temperature) on sweat rate during rest and exercise in the heat. Ambient dry-bulb temperature was 43.4°C (110°F). (Adapted with permission from Iampietro PF. Exercise in hot environments. In: Shephard RJ, ed. *Frontiers of Fitness.* Springfield, IL: Charles C. Thomas, 1971.)

decreases as sweat loss progresses. Fluid loss coincides with the following five factors:

1. Decreased plasma volume
2. Reduced skin blood flow for a given core temperature
3. Reduced stroke volume
4. Increased near-compensatory heart rate
5. General deterioration in circulatory and thermoregulatory efficiency in exercise

Impact of Weather on Running Performance

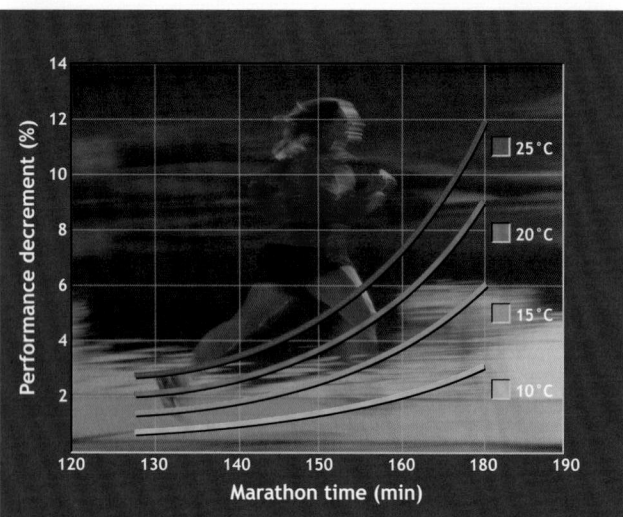

A progressive slowing of marathon running performance of men and women as the wet bulb–globe temperature (WB-GT) increased from 10 to 25°C (50 to 77°F) with performance more negatively affected for slower runners. (Adapted with permission from Ely MR, et al. Impact of weather on marathon-running performance. *Med Sci Sports Exerc* 2007;39:487.)

In terms of performance, dehydration equal to 4.3% of body mass reduced walking endurance by 48%; concurrently, $\dot{V}O_{2max}$ decreased by 22%.[23] These same experiments showed decreased endurance performance (−22%) and $\dot{V}O_{2max}$ (−10%) when dehydration averaged only 1.9% of body mass. Clearly, even modest dehydration imposes adverse thermoregulatory effects during physical activity that relate to progressive deterioration in sports skill performance.[6,7]

Diuretics

Diuretic-induced dehydration draws a greater percentage of water from the plasma than body water lost through sweating. In addition, drugs that cause diuresis markedly impair neuromuscular function; this does not occur with comparable fluid loss through physical activity. Chemicals that induce vomiting and diarrhea for sudden weight loss trigger dehydration and promote excessive mineral loss with accompanying muscle weakness and impaired neuromuscular function.

MAINTAINING FLUID BALANCE: REHYDRATION AND HYPERHYDRATION

Fluid replacement must focus on maintaining plasma volume so circulation and sweating progress at optimal levels. Ingesting fluid during physical activity increases blood flow to the skin for more effective cooling, independent of any change in plasma volume. Such fluid replacement during activity also reverses the sustained postexercise hypotension frequently observed in trained athletes.[40] Prevention of dehydration and its consequences, especially hyperthermia, occurs only with an adequate and strictly observed water replacement schedule.[125] Combined use of intravenous infusion plus oral rehydration methods may prove even more effective than the single approach of oral rehydration.[87] Meeting this requirement often presents difficulties because some coaches and athletes believe that ingesting water hinders performance. Left on their own, most individuals voluntarily replace only about half of the water lost in physical activity (<500 mL·hr^{-1}).

Optimal Goals for Fluid Intake During Physical Activity

- *Goal of prehydrating:* Start the activity euhydrated and with normal plasma electrolyte levels. This should be initiated when needed, at least several hours before the activity to enable fluid absorption and allow urine output to return to normal levels.
- *Goal of drinking during activity:* Prevent excessive dehydration (>2% body weight loss from water deficit) and excessive changes in electrolyte balance to avert compromising performance and health. During activity, consuming beverages containing electrolytes and carbohydrate generally provide benefits over water alone.

Source: American College of Sports Medicine Position Stand. Exercise and fluid replacement. *Med Sci Sports Exerc* 2007;39:377.

Adequate hydration provides the most effective defense against heat stress. The ideal hydration protocol requires balancing water loss with water intake, not pouring water over the head or body. No evidence indicates that restricting fluid intake during training in some way makes an athlete better able to adjust to subsequent work in the heat. *A well-hydrated athlete always functions at a higher level than one who exercises in a dehydrated state.*

Ingesting "extra" water (**hyperhydration**) before exercising in the heat offers thermoregulatory protection. Hyperhydration delays hypohydration from inadequate fluid replacement during exercise, increases sweating during exercise, and produces a smaller rise in core temperature in **uncompensable heat stress**, where evaporative cooling is inadequate to maintain thermal balance.[70] Three practical ways to promote acute pre-exercise hyperhydration involve the following:

1. Consume at least 500 mL of water before sleeping the night before exercising in the heat.

2. Consume another 500 mL upon awakening.
3. Consume an additional 400 to 600 mL of cold water 20 min before exercise.

An extended, systematic regimen of hyperhydration ($4.5 \text{ L} \cdot \text{d}^{-1}$) 1 wk before soccer competition by elite young soccer players in Puerto Rico increased body water reserves (despite greater urine output) and improved temperature regulation during a soccer match in warm weather.[111] The structured sequence of pre-exercise hyperhydration produced a 1.1 L greater total body fluid volume than with the athletes' normal daily 2.5-L fluid intake.

Pre-exercise hyperhydration does not replace the need for continual fluid replacement during activity. In this regard, fluid temperature may play an augmenting role. Compared with fluid at body temperature of 37°C, ingesting a cold drink (4°C) before and during exercise in the heat attenuated the increase in rectal temperature and reduced physiologic strain during exercise, which resulted in a 23% improved endurance capacity.[73] The benefits of hyperhydration usually subside if the individual remains euhydrated during exercise. In distance running, for example, matching fluid loss with fluid intake becomes virtually impossible because only 800 to 1000 mL of fluid empty from the stomach each hour. This rate of stomach emptying does not match a water loss that can average nearly 2000 mL per hour. Under these conditions, pre-exercise hyperhydration proves beneficial.

Does Exogenous Glycerol Provide a Benefit?

The three-carbon glycerol molecule achieved clinical notoriety (along with mannitol, sorbitol, and urea) for its role in producing osmotic diuresis. The capacity to influence water movement within the body makes glycerol effective in reducing excess fluid accumulation (edema) in the brain and eye.

When consumed with 1 to 2 L of water, glycerol facilitates intestinal water absorption and extracellular fluid retention, mainly in the plasma and interstitial fluid compartments.[39,142] An expanded body fluid volume potentially sets the stage for fluid excretion from increased renal filtrate and urine flow. Because proximal and distal kidney tubules reabsorb large amounts of glycerol, much of the fluid portion of the increased renal filtrate is also reabsorbed; this averts marked diuresis and promotes hyperhydration.

Proponents of glycerol supplementation maintain that its hyperhydration effect reduces overall heat stress in physical activity as reflected by increased sweating rate; this leads to a lower exercise heart rate and body temperature and enhanced endurance performance. Reducing heat stress with augmented hyperhydration before exercise using glycerol plus water supplementation increases the safety of the participant. One gram of glycerol per kilogram of body mass with 1 to 2 L of water is the typical recommended pre-exercise glycerol dose; its hyperhydration effect lasts up to 6 hr.

Not all research demonstrates meaningful thermoregulatory benefits from glycerol hyperhydration over pre-exercise hyperhydration with plain water.[70] For example, exogenous glycerol diluted in 500 mL of water consumed 4 hr before exercise failed to promote fluid retention or ergogenic effects.[54] No cardiovascular or thermoregulatory advantages result from consuming glycerol with small volumes of water during activity.[101] Side effects of exogenous glycerol ingestion include headache, nausea, dizziness, bloating, and light-headedness. A definitive conclusion about thermoregulatory benefits of exogenous glycerol awaits further research.

Adequacy of Rehydration

Changes in body weight indicate water loss and adequacy of rehydration during and following participation in physical activity. Voiding small volumes of dark yellow urine with a strong odor qualitatively indicates inadequate hydration. Well-hydrated individuals typically produce large volumes of light-colored urine without a strong smell.

The ideal condition replaces water losses from sweating during physical activity at a rate close to or equal to sweating rate. Athletes can be weighed before and after practice. Each pound of weight lost represents 450 mL (15 fl oz) of dehydration. Periodic water breaks during activity deter fluid depletion. Coaches and trainers must urge athletes to rehydrate because the thirst mechanism imprecisely monitors dehydration or the body's fluid needs (see "American College of Sports Medicine Clarifies Indicators for Fluid Replacement" [www.acsm-msse.org]). The elderly generally require a longer time to rehydrate after dehydration.[64] If a person relied entirely on thirst for rehydration, it could take several days to reestablish fluid balance following severe dehydration. Alcohol-containing beverages generally impede restoration of fluid balance, particularly if the rehydration fluid contains 4% or more alcohol.[130,131]

 ## Optimize Hydration

PRE-ACTIVITY
1. Drink approximately 17 to 20 oz 2 to 3 hr before activity
2. Consume another 7 to 10 oz after warm-up (10 to 15 min before exercise).

DURING ACTIVITY
1. Drink approximately 28 to 40 oz every hour of exercise (7 to 10 oz every 10 to 15 min).
2. Rapidly replace lost fluids (sweat and urine) within 2 hr after activity to enhance recovery by drinking 20 to 24 oz for every pound of body weight lost through sweating.

Electrolyte Replacement: Added Sodium May Benefit Rehydration

Restoration of water and electrolyte balance in recovery occurs more rapidly by adding moderate-to-high amounts of sodium (between 20 and 60 $\text{mmol} \cdot \text{L}^{-1}$) to the rehydration drink or combining solid food with appropriate sodium content with plain water.[80,118] Adding 2 to 5 mmol · L^{-1} of potassium may enhance water retention in the intracellular space and reestablish any extra potassium excretion that accompanies sodium retention by the kidneys.[24,121] The ACSM recommends that sports drinks contain 0.5 to 0.7 g of sodium per liter of fluid consumed during activity lasting more than 1 hr. A beverage that tastes good to the individual also contributes to voluntary rehydration during physical activity and recovery.[113,146]

The volume of ingested fluid following physical activity must exceed by 25 to 50% the exercise sweat loss to restore fluid balance because the kidneys continually form some urine regardless of hydration status. Pure water absorbed from the gut rapidly dilutes plasma sodium. In turn, decreased plasma osmolality stimulates urine production and blunts the normal sodium-dependent stimulation of the thirst mechanism. These responses counter the goal of rehydration. Without sufficient sodium in the beverage, excess fluid intake merely increases urine output without fully benefiting rehydration.[132] *Maintaining a relatively high plasma sodium concentration by adding sodium to ingested fluid sustains the thirst drive, promotes retention of ingested fluids (lower urine output), and restores lost plasma volume more rapidly.*

FIGURE 25.7 illustrates the effect of a rehydration beverage with added sodium on ingested fluid retention in recovery. Six healthy men exercised in a warm, humid environment until sweating produced a 1.9% weight loss. They then ingested one of four test drinks (2045 mL) with sodium concentrations of either 2, 26, 52, or 100 mmol · L^{-1} (typical "sports drinks" contain 10–25 mmol sodium; normal plasma sodium concentration ranges between 138 and 142 mmol)

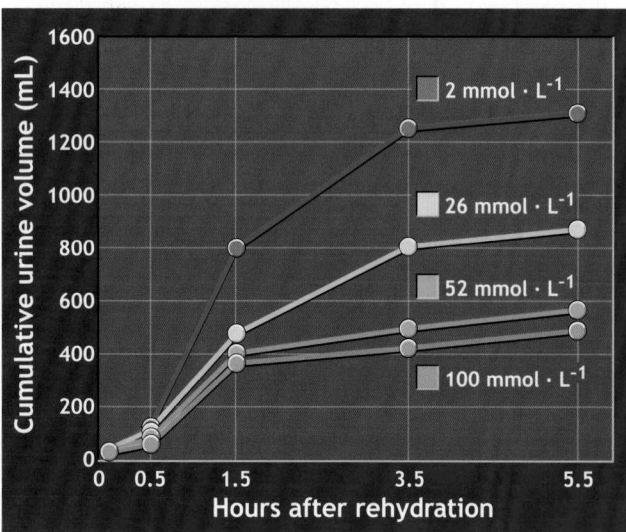

FIGURE 25.7 • Cumulative urine output during recovery from exercise-induced dehydration. The oral rehydration beverages were four test drinks (equivalent to 1.5 times body weight loss, or 2045 mL) containing sodium (and matching anion) in a concentration of either 2, 26, 52, or 100 mmol · L^{-1}. (Adapted with permission from Maughan RJ, Leiper JB. Sodium intake and post-exercise rehydration in man. *Eur J Appl Physiol* 1995;71:311.)

over a 30-min period beginning 30 min after stopping exercise. From the 1.5-hr urine sample onward, urine volume inversely related to the rehydration beverage's sodium content. At completion of the study period, a difference in total body water content of 787 mL existed between trials using drinks with the lowest and highest sodium content. The drink containing 100 mmol sodium contributed to the greatest fluid retention.

With prolonged effort in the heat, sweat loss can deplete the body of 13 to 17 g of salt (2.3–3.4 g · L^{-1} of sweat) daily, about 8 g more than typically consumed. It seems prudent in this deficit situation to replace the lost sodium by adding about one-third teaspoon of table salt to 1 L of water. Moderate activity generally produces a negligible potassium loss in sweat. Even at competitive physical activity levels, potassium loss in sweat ranges between 5 and 18 mEq, which poses little or no immediate danger.[24] With heavy sweating, increasing the intake of potassium-rich citrus fruits and bananas replaces most potassium losses. *Minor adjustments in food intake and electrolyte conservation by the kidneys adequately compensate for mineral loss through sweating.*

Whole-Body Precooling

"Cold treatments" that periodically apply cold towels to the forehead and abdomen during exercise or a cold shower before exercising in the heat improve heat transfer at the body's surface only slightly above the same activity without skin wetting. Whole-body precooling (core temperature decrease of 0.7°C [1.26°F]) with up to 60 min immersion in water at 23.5°C (74°F), on the other hand, increases subsequent endurance in a hot, humid environment. Time to exhaustion inversely related to initial body temperature (lowered via precooling) and directly related to the rate of heat storage.[43] Precooling with cold-water immersion facilitated postexercise recovery, enhanced the rate of heat storage, and caused less thermoregulatory strain—attenuated rise in skin and rectal temperatures and heart rates—during activity.[11,34,108,145] In addition, whole-body precooling of the skin by 5 to 6°C (9–10.8°F) without reduction in core temperature reduced thermal strain and increased distance cycled in 30 min under warm, humid conditions.[62] In contrast, whole-body precooling provided no thermoregulatory benefit during a simulated triathlon[9] or on the physiologic responses to a 90-min soccer-specific activities protocol under normal environmental conditions.[31]

FACTORS THAT MODIFY HEAT TOLERANCE

Five factors interact to improve physiologic adjustments and exercise tolerance during environmental heat stress:

1. Acclimatization
2. Training status
3. Age
4. Gender
5. Body fat level

Acclimatization

Relatively easy tasks performed in cool weather become taxing if attempted on the first hot day of spring. The early stages of preseason training for warm-weather sports often pose the greatest hazards for heat injury because thermoregulatory mechanisms have not adjusted to the dual challenge of physical activity and environmental heat. Repeated exposure to hot environments when combined with physical activity improves exercise capacity, with less discomfort upon subsequent heat exposure.[105,122]

*The term **heat acclimatization** describes the collective physiologic adaptive changes that improve heat tolerance.* The major portion of acclimatization occurs during the first week of heat exposure, with full acclimatization thereafter. The process requires only 2 to 4 hr of daily heat exposure. The first several sessions in the heat should include 15 to 20 min of light-intensity physical activity. Exercise sessions then should increase in duration and intensity.

 INTEGRATIVE QUESTION

Your Maine, U.S.–based soccer team competes in Hawaii in early spring. Discuss how you would prepare the team to compete in this hot–humid environment making all precompetition preparations (1) at your school or (2) elsewhere, if time, money, and travel were not considerations.

TABLE 25.5 summarizes the main physiologic adjustments during heat acclimatization. *Optimal acclimatization requires adequate hydration.* During exercise, larger quantities of blood flow to cutaneous vessels to facilitate heat transfer from the core to periphery. A more effective cardiac output distribution also helps stabilize blood pressure during exertion. A lowered threshold for sweating complements these "circulatory

acclimatizations." Consequently, cooling begins before core temperature increases appreciably. Sweating capacity, the most significant factor for heat acclimatization, increases early and nearly doubles after 10 days of heat exposure; sweat also becomes more dilute (less salt lost) and distributes more evenly over the skin surface, which does not seem to occur in exercise training without acclimatization.[48] Concurrently, heat acclimatization reduces sodium loss from the kidneys. Adjustments in circulation and evaporative cooling enable the heat-acclimatized person to exercise with lower skin and core temperatures and heart rates. A lower exercise core temperature requires diversion of less blood to the skin, freeing a larger percentage of the cardiac output for active muscles. Acclimatization also reduces carbohydrate use in physical activity, a response consistent with acclimatization-induced plasma epinephrine reduction.[38] The major benefits of acclimatization dissipate within 2 to 3 wk after returning to a more temperate environment.

Training Status

Exercise-induced "internal" heat stress in a cool environment induces adjustments in peripheral circulation and evaporative cooling qualitatively similar to training in hot ambient temperatures. These training adaptations facilitate elimination of metabolic heat generated by exercise and generally occur with an 8- to 12-wk training period at an intensity above 50% of aerobic capacity. This makes well-conditioned men and women living in a temperate climate respond more effectively to sudden, severe heat stress than sedentary counterparts.[5] Training increases the sensitivity and capacity of the sweating response so that sweating begins at a lower core temperature, hence producing larger volumes of more-dilute sweat, which thus conserves a variety of minerals.[20] This results partly from intrinsic adaptations in the sweat glands. Concurrently, a training-induced adjustment in cutaneous circulation provides greater skin blood flow at a given internal temperature or percentage of $\dot{V}O_{2max}$, independent of age.[59] Plasma and extravascular

TABLE 25.5	Physiologic Adjustments During Heat Acclimatization	
Acclimatization Response	**Effect**
• Improved cutaneous blood flow	• Transports metabolic heat from deep tissues (core) to shell
• Effective distribution of cardiac output	• Appropriate circulation to skin and muscles to meet demands of metabolism and thermoregulation; greater blood pressure stability during exercise
• Lowered threshold for start of sweating	• Evaporative cooling begins early in exercise
• More effective distribution of sweat over skin surface	• Optimum use of effective body surface for evaporative cooling
• Increased sweat output	• Maximizes evaporative cooling
• Lowered salt concentration of sweat	• Dilute sweat preserves electrolytes in extracellular fluid
• Lower skin and core temperatures and heart rate for standard exercise	• Frees greater proportion of cardiac output to the active muscles
• Less reliance on carbohydrate catabolism during exercise	• Carbohydrate sparing

fluid volumes also increase during the initial stages of aerobic training.[75,81] Enhanced physiologic fitness also sustains better blood flow to the gastrointestinal tract. This maintains the normal barrier to endotoxin movement from the gut lumen into the plasma, blunting the potential for endotoxin-induced fever that could aggravate exercise hyperthermia.[120] The thermoregulatory benefit for training occurs provided the individual remains fully hydrated during the activity.[122]

Exercise "heat conditioning" in cool weather offers fewer benefits than acclimatization from similar hot weather training. *A physically active person cannot achieve full heat acclimatization without exposure to environmental heat stress.* Athletes who train and compete in hot weather have a distinct thermoregulatory advantage over athletes who train in cool climates and only periodically compete in hot weather.

Age

Debate concerns the effects of aging on tolerance and acclimatization to moderate heat stress. An early study exposed men and women ages 60 to 93 years to 70 min of heat stress during exercise at intensities that ranged from 2 to 5 METs. **FIGURE 25.8** shows the relationship between heart rate and exercise intensity in the heat for these older subjects and young men and women. The less-fit elderly subjects exercised at higher heart rates than young adults of the same gender. Environmental heat imposed no greater physiologic strain for the older groups because body temperature increased an average of only 0.3°C (0.54°F), compared with 0.2°C (0.36°F) for the younger group. Testing elderly subjects in the spring and fall evaluated their extent of natural heat acclimatization during the summer months. By fall, all subjects had lower heart rates during the standard thermal–exercise stress.

Comparisons between young and middle-age competitive runners indicate no age-related decrements in thermoregulation during marathon running.[115] Thermoregulatory function was not impaired in trained 50-year-old men compared with younger men.[107] Likewise, sweating capacity for men ages 58 to 84 years adequately regulated body temperature during prolonged desert walks.[27] *Research shows little or no age-related decrements in thermoregulatory capacity or heat-stress acclimatization with appropriate controls for body size and composition, aerobic fitness, hydration, degree of acclimatization, and chronological age.*

Age-Related Differences Do Exist

Several age-related factors affect thermoregulatory dynamics despite equivalence between young and older adults in capacity to regulate core temperature during heat stress. Aging delays the onset of sweating and blunts the magnitude of the sweating response in one of three ways[56,63]:

1. Modified sensitivity of thermoreceptors
2. Limited sweat gland output per se
3. Dehydration-limited sweat output with insufficient fluid replacement

Aging also alters the intrinsic structure and function of the skin and its vasculature.[51,55,66,78] Aging impairs the mechanisms that mediate cutaneous vasodilation, which results in an attenuated vasodilation response. Age-related vascular changes include depressed peripheral sensitivity that impairs cutaneous vasodilation from two factors:

1. Smaller release of vasomotor tone
2. Less active vasodilation once sweating begins

Older athletes show a 25 to 40% lower skin blood flow with increased core temperature than do younger athletes.[65] Contributing factors include the combined effects of a lower cardiac output and reduced blood distribution from the splanchnic and renal circulations.[90] Older adults do not recover from dehydration as readily as do younger counterparts because of a reduced thirst drive. This places elderly individuals in a chronic state of hypohydration with a less-than-optimal plasma volume, which could impair thermoregulatory dynamics. An altered thirst mechanism and shift in the operating point for body fluid volume and composition control also decrease total blood volume in older individuals.[25,77]

Children

Children sweat less and maintain higher core temperatures during heat stress than adolescents and adults, even though children possess a larger number of heat-activated sweat glands per unit skin area.[8,36] A reduced sweating response likely results from underdeveloped peripheral mechanisms, including the sweat glands and their surrounding tissues, rather than a depressed central drive for sweating.[128] The age difference in thermoregulation lasts through puberty; it generally does not limit physical capacity except during extreme environmental heat stress.[116] Sweat composition differs between children and adults; children's sweat shows higher sodium and chlorine concentrations and lower concentrations of lactate, H^+, and potassium.[36,89] *From a practical standpoint, intensity of effort should decrease for children exposed to a hot environment; they also require more time to acclimatize than older competitors.*

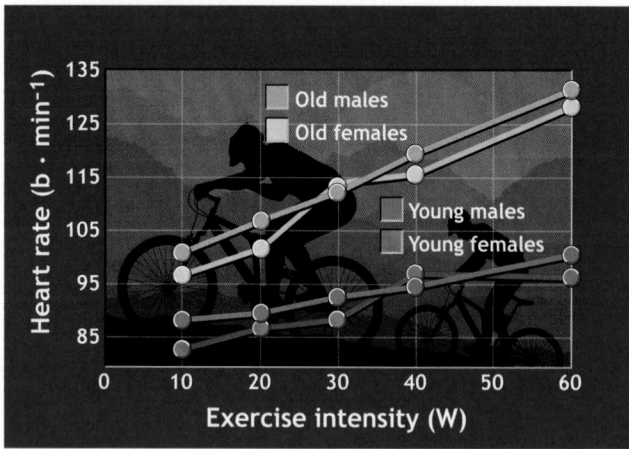

FIGURE 25.8 • Heart rate during moderate exercise in the heat in young and older men and women. Dry-bulb ambient temperature was 33.5°C (92.3°F) and wet-bulb was 28.5°C (83.3°F). (Adapted with permission from Henshel A. The environment and performance. In: Simonsen E, ed. *Physiology of Work Capacity and Fatigue.* Springfield, IL: Charles C. Thomas, 1971.)

Gender

Early comparisons of thermoregulation in men and women indicated that men exhibited greater tolerance to environmental heat stress during a standard bout of physical activity. A major flaw in this research required that women exercise at a higher percentage of aerobic capacity than men. Thermoregulatory differences became less pronounced when researchers controlled for this factor and compared men and women of equal fitness or exercised both at the same %$\dot{V}O_{2max}$.[30,53] *In essence, women tolerate the thermal stress of physical activity at least as well as do men of comparable aerobic fitness and level of acclimatization; both genders also acclimatize to the same degree.*

Sweating

Sweating represents a distinct gender difference in thermoregulation. Women sweat less prolifically than men, despite possessing more heat-activated sweat glands per unit skin area. Women start to sweat at higher skin and core temperatures and produce less sweat than men do with a comparable heat-exercise load, even after equivalent acclimatization.

Evaporative Cooling versus Circulatory Cooling. Women tolerate heat much like men of equal aerobic fitness at the same activity level, despite a lower sweat output. Women probably use circulatory mechanisms for heat dissipation, whereas men make greater use of evaporative cooling. Clearly, producing less sweat to maintain thermal balance protects women from dehydration during exertion at high ambient temperatures.

Ratio of Body Surface Area to Body Mass. The typically smaller female has a relatively large external surface per unit of body mass exposed to the environment. This factor conveys favorable dimensional characteristic for heat dissipation. Under identical conditions of heat exposure, women tend to cool faster than men. Children also possess a similar "geometric" advantage during heat stress from their larger ratio of surface area-to-mass than adults.

Menstruation. Phases of the menstrual cycle influence cutaneous vascular control that alters skin blood flow and sweating response during rest and physical activity.[16,136] For example, a higher core temperature threshold initiates sweating during the luteal phase at both 60% and 80% of aerobic capacity.[68] An upward resetting of the thermoregulatory setpoint for sweating occurs during the luteal phase and probably reflects a unique feature of hormone dynamics throughout the cycle.[50,136] An upward shift of approximately 0.4°C (0.72°F) in oral temperature persists for about 6 days during the luteal phase. The change in thermoregulatory sensitivity during this phase does *not* impair ability for intense activity.[76] No changes in the level of exercise performance, lactate threshold, or ventilatory threshold associate with the menstrual cycle in temperate environments.[133] Recent evidence suggests that in hot, humid conditions, exercise performance decreases during the luteal phase, perhaps the result of physiological and perceptual changes and a greater thermosensitivity at the onset of activity.[58]

Body Fat Level

Excess body fat represents a liability when exercising in the heat. Because the specific heat of fat exceeds muscle tissue, fat increases the insulatory quality of the body shell and retards heat conduction to the periphery. The large, overly fat person also has a smaller ratio of body surface area-to-body mass for effective sweat evaporation than a leaner, smaller person with less body fat.

Excess body fat and body weight directly adds to the metabolic cost of weight-bearing activities. A hot, humid environment places the overly fat person at a distinct disadvantage for temperature regulation and physical performance.[106] Additional compounding factors include the added weight of sports equipment as in American football, ice hockey, or lacrosse gear and intense competition. Fatal heat stroke occurs 3.5 times more frequently in excessively overweight young adults than in individuals of average body size (see next section). Recall from the introductory section of this chapter the heat-related death during football practice of NFL professional player Corey Stringer. At 6'4" and 335 pounds, this player was at great risk due to his excessively large body size, with a body mass index (BMI) of 40.8 that exceeds the most liberal standard for an excess of body weight.

 INTEGRATIVE QUESTION

Describe the ideal physical and physiologic characteristics that minimize heat injury risk while exercising in the heat.

COMPLICATIONS FROM EXCESSIVE HEAT STRESS

Approximately 400 people die yearly in the United States from excessive heat stress, and about half of these are men and women age 65 and older. If the normal signs of heat stress go unheeded—thirst, tiredness, grogginess, and visual disturbances—cardiovascular compensation begins to fail. This initiates a cascade of disabling complications collectively termed **heat illness.** Heat cramps, heat exhaustion, and heat stroke constitute the major heat illnesses in order of increasing severity. Heat-related disabilities occur more frequently among overweight, unacclimatized, and poorly conditioned individuals, including those who exercise when dehydrated.[2,14,109] No clear-cut demarcation exists between maladies because symptoms often overlap; exercise-induced heat injury frequently results from the cumulative effects of multiple adverse interacting stimuli.[135] TABLE 25.6 summarizes the salient features of the cardiovascular response patterns during three distinct stages of exercise hyperthermia. These stages—compensation, crisis, and failure—apply to heat exhaustion and heat stroke. The response patterns are broadly classified as either central circulatory, peripheral, or central nervous system effects. With serious heat illness, only immediate corrective action reduces heat stress until medical help arrives.[28]

| TABLE 25.6 | Cardiovascular Responses During the Three Stages of Exercise Hyperthermia |

	Central Circulation		Peripheral Circulation	Rectal Temperature	Central Nervous System Status
Compensation	↑ CO ↑ SV, ↑ HR ↓ PV Respiratory alkalosis	↓ Low SPBF ↓ PV	↓ Low TPVR ↑ Skin BF ↑ Muscle BF	37.0°C to 39.5°C	Premonitory signs Dizziness Headache Euphoria Psychoses
Crises	↑↓ CO ↑ MABP ↓ SV ↑↑ HR Tachycardia (180 b·min⁻¹) Metabolic acidosis	↑↓ SPBF ↓ PV Moderate CVP	↓ TPVR ↑↓ Skin BF	39.5°C 41.5°C	↓ Cerebral congestion ↓ Cerebral edema Intracranial hypertension
Failure	↓↓ CO ↓↓ MABP ↑ HR Tachycardia Metabolic acidosis	↑↑ SPBF (autoregulatory escape); high CVP but low if hypovolemic	↓ TPVR ↓ Low skin BF	41.5°C	↓ Coma, decreased cerebral perfusion ↓ Cerebral ischemia Neurologic damage, seizures

CO, cardiac output; SV, stroke volume; HR, heart rate; SPBF, splanchnic blood flow; PV, plasma volume; TPVR, total peripheral vascular resistance; BF, blood flow; MABP, mean arterial blood pressure; CVP, central venous pressure. ↑ = moderate increase; ↑↑ = strong increase; ↓ = moderate decrease; ↓↓ = strong decrease; ↑↓ = increase then decrease; ↓ = progressing to.
Data from Hubbard RW, Armstrong LE. The heat illnesses: biochemical, ultrastructural, and fluid-electrolyte considerations. In: Pandolf K et al., eds. *Human Performance Physiology and Environmental Medicine at Terrestrial Extremes*. Carmel, IN: Cooper Publishing Group, 1994; original data of Kielblock AJ, et al. Cardiovascular origins of heatstroke pathophysiology: an anesthetized rat model. *Aviat Space Environ Med* 1982;53:171.

Heat Cramps

Heat cramps—severe involuntary, sustained, and spreading muscle spasms—occur during or after intense physical activity, usually in the specifically active muscles. Core temperature often remains within normal range. An imbalance in the body's fluid level and electrolyte concentrations produces this form of heat illness. Crampers tend to have high sweat rates and/or high sweat sodium concentrations. With heat cramps, body temperature does not necessarily increase. Prevention involves two factors:

1. Providing sufficient water that contains salt
2. Increasing daily salt intake (e.g., adding salt to foods at mealtime) several days before heat stress

Sweating causes electrolyte loss during prolonged heat exposure. Failure to replenish these minerals often leads to muscle pain and spasm, most commonly in the abdomen and extremities. Drinking copious amounts of water and increasing daily salt intake several days before heat stress generally prevents this heat-related malady.[33]

Heat Exhaustion

Heat exhaustion can develop in unacclimatized persons during the first summer heat wave or with the first hard training session on a hot day. Exercise-induced heat exhaustion occurs from ineffective circulatory adjustments compounded by depletion of extracellular fluid, principally plasma volume from excessive sweating. Blood usually pools in the dilated peripheral vessels; this drastically reduces the central blood volume necessary to maintain cardiac output. Characteristics of heat exhaustion include a weak and rapid pulse, low blood pressure in the upright position, headache, dizziness, and general weakness. Sweating may decrease somewhat, but core temperature does not rise to dangerous levels of 40°C (104°F) or higher. A person who experiences symptoms of heat exhaustion should stop activity and move to a cooler environment. Intravenous therapy replenishes fluid most effectively.

Heat Stroke

Heat stroke, the most serious and complex of the heat-stress maladies, requires immediate medical attention. It reflects failure of the heat-regulating mechanisms from an excessively high core temperature and can affect seemingly healthy adults even in a relatively cool environment.[3,35,110,114] The *classic form* of heat stroke—core temperature exceeds 40.5°C (105°F), altered mental status, absence of sweating—usually occurs during heat waves. It affects young children, the elderly, and those with chronic diseases. In classic heat stroke, environmental heat overloads the body's heat-dissipating mechanisms. Severe heat stress also produces a continuum of potentially negative alterations in the immune system and in leukocyte adhesion and activation processes (unrelated to elevated catecholamine levels).[47] One in three individuals who survive a near-fatal case of classic heat stroke remains permanently disabled with multisystem organ dysfunction.[26]

Exertional heat stroke is a state of extreme hyperthermia from the interactive effects of two factors:

1. Metabolic heat load in physical activity
2. Challenge for heat dissipation from a hot, humid environment

When thermoregulation fails, sweating diminishes, the skin becomes dry and hot, and body temperature rises to 41.5°C (106.7°F) and above. This places an inordinate strain on cardiovascular function. The often subtle symptoms compound the complexity of emergency hyperthermia. With intense activity, usually by young, highly motivated individuals, sweating may progress but body heat gain overpowers the avenues for heat loss. Other predisposing factors for exertional heat stroke include poor fitness status, obesity, inadequate acclimatization, sweat gland dysfunction, dehydration, and infectious disease. If left untreated, the disability progresses rapidly and death ensues from circulatory collapse and damage to the central nervous system and other organ systems. While awaiting medical treatment, aggressive steps must be taken to lower core temperature because mortality relates to the magnitude and duration of hyperthermia. Immediate treatment includes fluid replacement and body cooling with alcohol rubs, application of ice packs to the neck area, and whole-body immersion in cold or even ice water, the "gold standard" for treating exertional heat stroke.[15,100,102] No attempt should be made to slow the respiratory rate because a rapid rate of breathing compensates for metabolic acidosis. Prudent treatment also includes specific drug therapy to counter possible endotoxin effects precipitated by heat stroke pathology.[46]

Oral Temperature Unreliable

Oral temperature inaccurately measures core temperature after strenuous exercise. Rectal temperature following a 14-mile race in a tropical climate averaged 39.7°C (103.5°F), while oral temperature surprisingly remained normal at 36.6°C (98°F).[119] Part of the discrepancy lies in the effects on oral temperature of evaporative cooling of the mouth and airways during high levels of exercise pulmonary ventilation.

Summary

1. Core temperature normally increases during physical activity; the relative stress of activity determines the magnitude of the increase.
2. A well-regulated temperature increase creates a more favorable environment for physiologic and metabolic functions.
3. Excessive sweating compromises fluid reserves to create a relative state of dehydration.
4. Sweating without fluid replacement decreases plasma volume, which leads to circulatory dysfunction and a precipitous rise in core temperature.
5. Physical activity in a hot, humid environment poses a considerable thermoregulatory challenge because the large sweat loss in high humidity contributes little to evaporative cooling.

6. Fluid loss of more than 4% of body weight impedes heat dissipation, compromises cardiovascular function, and diminishes exercise capacity.
7. Adequate fluid replacement maintains plasma volume so circulation and sweating progress optimally.
8. The ideal replacement schedule during physical activity matches fluid intake to fluid loss, a process effectively monitored by changes in body weight.
9. The small intestine can absorb about 1000 mL of water each hour. A small amount of electrolytes in the rehydration beverage facilitates fluid replacement more than drinking plain water.
10. The diet generally replaces minerals lost through sweating. With prolonged exercise in the heat, adding a small amount of salt to the replacement fluid (1 tsp · L^{-1}) facilitates sodium and fluid replenishment.
11. Repeated heat stress initiates thermoregulatory adjustments that improve physical capacity and reduce discomfort on heat exposure.
12. Ten days of heat exposure promotes full acclimatization.
13. Aging affects thermoregulatory functions but does not appreciably alter temperature regulation during exercise or acclimatization to moderate heat stress.
14. Women and men show equivalent thermoregulation during physical activity when controlled for levels of fitness and acclimatization. Women produce less sweat than men when exercising at the same core temperature.
15. Heat cramps, heat exhaustion, and heat stroke constitute the major heat illnesses. Heat stroke, a medical emergency, is the most serious and complex of these maladies.
16. Oral temperature after physical activity inaccurately measures core temperature because of evaporative cooling of the mouth and airways with high levels of pulmonary ventilation during activity and recovery.

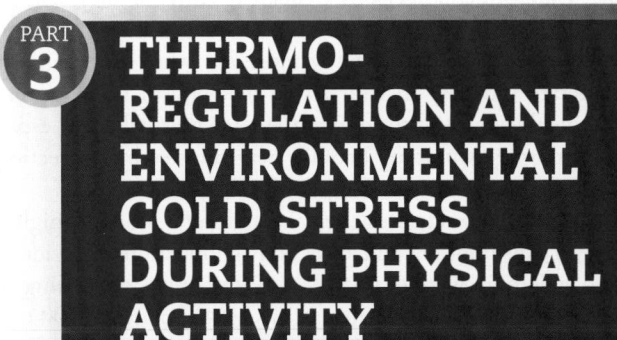

PART 3
THERMO-REGULATION AND ENVIRONMENTAL COLD STRESS DURING PHYSICAL ACTIVITY

PHYSICAL ACTIVITY IN THE COLD

Human exposure to extreme cold produces significant physiologic and psychologic challenges. Cold ranks high among the differing terrestrial environmental stressors for its potentially lethal consequences. Core temperature becomes further compromised during chronic exertional fatigue and sleep

TABLE 25.7 — Core Temperature and Associated Physiological Changes that Occur as Core Temperature Falls; Individuals Respond Differently at Each Level of Core Temperature

Stage	Core Temperature °F	Core Temperature °C	Physiological Changes
Normothermia	98.6	37.0	No noticeable effect
Mild hypothermia	95.0	35.0	Maximal shivering, increased blood pressure
	93.2	34.0	Amnesia; dysarthria; poor judgment; behavior change
	91.4	33.0	Ataxia; apathy
Moderate hypothermia	89.6	32.0	Stupor
	87.8	31.0	Shivering ceases; pupils dilate
	85.2	30.0	Cardiac arrhythmias; decreased cardiac output
	85.2	29.0	Unconsciousness
Severe hypothermia	82.4	28.0	Ventricular fibrillation likely; hypoventilation
	80.6	27.0	Loss of reflexes and voluntary motion
	78.8	26.0	Acid-base disturbances; no response to pain
	77.0	25.0	Reduced cerebral blood flow
	75.2	24.0	Hypotension; bradycardia; pulmonary edema
	73.4	23.0	No corneal reflexes; areflexia
	66.2	19.0	Electroencephalographic silence
	64.4	18.0	Asystole
	59.2	15.0	Lowest infant survival from accidental hypothermia
	56.7	13.7	Lowest adult survival from accidental hypothermia

Reprinted from American College of Sports Medicine Position Stand. Prevention of cold injuries during exercise. *Med Sci Sports Exerc* 2007;38:2012.

loss, inadequate nourishment, reduced tissue insulation, and a depressed shivering heat production.[149] TABLE 25.7 presents the physiologic changes associated with hypothermia that range from mild to severe.

Water provides an excellent medium to study physiologic adjustment to cold because it conducts heat about 25 times faster than air at the same temperature. Consequently, immersion in cool water of only 28° to 30°C (82–86°F) imposes a thermal stress that rapidly initiates an array of thermoregulatory adjustments. Persons frequently shiver if they remain inactive in a pool or ocean environment because of a large conductive heat loss to the water. Even when exercising at moderate intensity in cold water, metabolism often generates insufficient heat to counter the large thermal drain, especially during swimming because heat transfer by convection increases when water moves past the skin surface.

Light and moderate activity in cold water produces higher oxygen consumptions and lower body temperatures than identical activity in warmer water.[84,138] For example, swimming at a submaximal pace in a flume at 18°C (64°F) requires 500 mL of oxygen more per minute than swimming at the same speed in 26°C (79°F) water.[103] The additional oxygen consumption directly relates to the energy cost of shivering as the body combats heat loss in colder water. Shivering also serves an important role in recovering from hypothermia; it attenuates the typical postexercise decline in core temperature and facilitates core rewarming.[42] The body shows remarkable flexibility in oxidative fuel selection during sustained cold exposure, but shifts occur in shivering substrate from lipid to carbohydrate with intense cold stress.[49]

Body Fat, Physical Activity, and Cold Stress

Differences in body fat content among individuals influence physiologic function in the cold during rest and physical activity.[85,139] Successful ocean swimmers possess a larger amount of subcutaneous fat than highly trained non–ocean swimmers. The additional fat increases the effective insulation in cold water when peripheral blood diverts from the body's shell to the core. With this advantage, athletes with greater thermal insulation from fat accretion swim in cool ocean water with almost no decline in core temperature. For leaner swimmers, exercise does not generate sufficient heat to offset heat drain to the water, and the body's core cools.

Consider the stress from "cold" as highly relative. The physiologic strain from cold-water and cold-land environments depends on one's level of metabolism and the body fat's resistance to heat flow. A person with excess body fat who rests comfortably immersed to the neck in 26°C (78.8°F) water may sweat about the forehead during vigorous physical activity. For this person, 18°C (64.4°F) provides a more favorable water temperature for high-intensity effort. For a lean person, water at 18°C (64.4°F) proves debilitating during rest and activity. An optimum water temperature exists for each person and for each physical activity. For most persons, water temperatures between 26°C (78.8°F) and 30°C (86°F) allow effective heat dissipation in sustained exertion without compromising capacity from large deviations in core temperature. Even colder water may optimize performance in shorter-term, near-maximal effort, particularly for fatter people. For some as yet unexplained reason, older adults do not withstand the challenge of cold during rest and low-intensity activity as effectively as younger counterparts with similar aerobic capacities.[37] Age-related variations in body composition or hormonal functions may provide part of the explanation.

Children and Cold Stress

Cold water provides an exceptionally stressful thermoregulatory environment for children. A child's distinctly large ratio of body surface area-to-mass facilitates heat loss in a warm environment but becomes a liability during cold stress because body heat dissipates rapidly. During physical activity in the less stressful cold-air environment, children rely on two mechanisms to compensate for their relatively large body surface area[134]:

1. Augmented energy metabolism
2. More effective peripheral vasoconstriction in the limbs

COLD ACCLIMATIZATION

Humans possess much less capacity for adaptation to long-term cold exposure than to prolonged heat exposure. The basic response of Eskimos and Lapps involves avoiding the cold or minimizing its effects. Their clothing provides a near-tropical microclimate; the temperature inside an igloo typically averages 15.6°C (60°F) despite freezing outside temperatures with gale-force winds or freezing rain.

The Ama

Studies of the **Ama**, the women divers of Korea and southern Japan (**www.jpf.org.au/onlinearticles/hitokuchimemo/issue31.html**; see Chapter 26), indicate some human cold adaptation.[52] These women tolerate daily prolonged exposure to diving for food in cold water that in winter averages 10°C (50°F). During the summer, when water temperature rises to 25°C (77°F), the Ama perform three bouts of diving, each 45 min long. In winter, they perform only one 15-min dive daily. The women generally remain in the water until oral temperature declines to about 34°C (93.2°F). **Figure 25.9** shows skin and core (rectal) temperature responses of the Ama relative to total time in the water. Mean skin and mean body temperatures always remained lower during the winter dives. Earlier research described the relationship between water temperature and coldest water temperatures when at least 50% of the Ama and nondiving Korean women and men started shivering.[51a] The response curve (not shown) for the Ama shifted to the right, clearly indicating a blunted thermogenic response (higher shivering threshold) until water temperature reached about 28°C (82.4°F). An elevated resting metabolism may contribute to how the Ama tolerate extreme cold. In winter, resting metabolic rate increased by about 25% compared with nondiving women from the same country. Interestingly, the Ama and nondiving female counterparts had equivalent body fat percentages. This suggests that circulatory adaptations aid

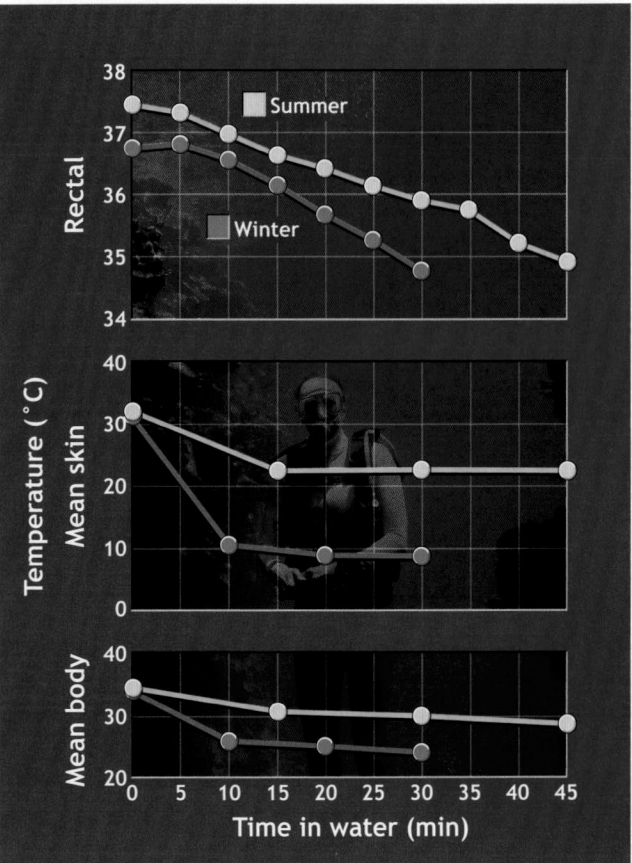

FIGURE 25.9 • Differences in rectal temperature, mean skin temperature, and mean body temperature related to water temperature during summer and winter in Ama divers upon resurfacing from a dive. (Adapted with permission from Kang DH, et al. Energy metabolism and body temperature of the Ama. *J Appl Physiol* 1965;18:483.)

the Ama by retarding heat transfer from the core to the skin during cold-water immersion.

Other Examples of Cold Adaptation

A type of general cold adaptation occurs with regular and prolonged cold-air exposure. In this situation, heat production does not balance heat loss, and the person regulates at a lower core temperature during cold stress. Some peripheral circulatory adaptations also reflect a form of acclimation with severe local cold exposure.[71,72,74] Repeated cold exposure of the hands or feet increases blood flow through these tissues during cold stress. This commonly occurs in fishermen who routinely handle nets and fish in cold water.[104] Local adaptations facilitate heat loss from the periphery but provide a self-defense because a vigorous circulation of warm blood in exposed tissue thwarts tissue damage from localized hypothermia. Long-term cold exposure may also blunt the typical depression of immune responses with acute cold stress.[67] Improved physical fitness (high aerobic capacity and relatively large muscle mass) enhances thermoregulatory defense against cold stress to produce a larger shivering response and earlier (more sensitive) onset of shivering with cold exposure.[9]

Acclimatization to Cold

The following three responses give some indication of a mild acclimatization to chronic cold exposure:

1. Shivering occurs at a lower body temperature because more heat is generated without shivering
2. Improved ability to sleep in the cold
3. Change in peripheral blood flow distribution that either conserves heat in the core or warms the extremities to prevent cold injury

HOW COLD IS TOO COLD?

Cold injuries from overexposure continue to rise because of increased participation by the general population in ice skating, ice fishing, Alpine and Nordic skiing, snowboarding, snowmobiling, and all-season walking, hiking, jogging, and cycling. Pronounced peripheral vasoconstriction during severe cold exposure causes dangerously low skin and extremity temperatures, particularly when compounded by marked increases in convective and conductive heat loss. Predisposing factors to frostbite include alcohol use, low physical fitness, fatigue, dehydration, and poor peripheral circulation.[112] Early warning signs of cold injury include tingling and numbness in the fingers and toes or a burning sensation in the nose and ears. Overexposure from failure to heed these warning signs leads to frostbite; in the extreme, irreversible damage occurs that requires surgical removal of the damaged tissue. From military operations and occupational perspectives, application of external heat to the torso during cold exposure can overcome the local effects of environmental cold and maintain fingers and toes at a relatively comfortable temperature for up to 3 hr with exposure to −15°C (5°F).[12]

INTEGRATIVE QUESTION

What information contributes to predicting an individual's survival time during extreme cold exposure?

In severe cold stress (e.g., near drowning in prolonged cold-water submersion), brain temperature significantly decreases, which reduces its oxygen needs. The central nervous system also benefits from a redistribution of blood from tissues that compromise their supply for relatively long periods. Other responses include potential benefits from the mammalian dive reflex (see Chapter 26, "Diving Reflex in Humans") and possibly cold-induced changes in neurotransmitter release.[41]

INTEGRATIVE QUESTION

Explain the greater likelihood for resuscitation and survival from cold-water drowning than from drowning in warmer water.

The Wind-Chill Temperature Index

One dilemma in evaluating the thermal quality of an environment relates to the inadequacy of ambient temperature alone to assess coldness. Many of us have experienced the chilling winds of a spring day even though air temperature remained well above freezing. In contrast, a calm subfreezing day may feel comfortable. *Wind makes the difference—air currents on a windy day magnify heat loss because the warmer insulating air layer surrounding the body continually exchanges with cooler ambient air.*

The **wind-chill temperature index**, presented in FIGURE 25.10, has been used by the National Weather Service since 1973 and then modified in 2001. Based on advances in science, technology, and computer modeling, the 2001 revised formula provides a more accurate, understandable, and useful way to understand the dangers from winter winds and freezing temperatures and provides frostbite threshold values.[91] For example, a −1°C (30°F) ambient air reading is equivalent to −12.7°C (9°F) with a wind speed of 25 mph, while a 12.2°C (10°F) reading equals −23.8°C (−11°F) at the same wind velocity. If a person runs, skis, or skates into the wind, the effective cooling increases directly with forward velocity. Running at 8 mph into a 12-mph headwind creates the equivalent of a 20-mph wind speed. Conversely, running at 8 mph with a 12-mph wind at one's back creates a relative wind speed of only 4 mph. The *white zone* in the left of the figure denotes relatively little danger from cold injury for a properly clothed person. In contrast, the *yellow-, orange-,* and *red-shaded zones* indicate frostbite threshold values; the danger to exposed flesh increases, especially for the ears, nose, and fingers, when moving to the right of the chart. In the *red-shaded zone*, the equivalent wind-chill temperatures pose serious risk of exposed flesh freezing within minutes.

Respiratory Tract During Cold-Weather Physical Activity

Cold ambient air generally poses no special danger of damaging respiratory passages. Even in extreme cold, incoming air warms to between 26°C (78.8°F) and 32°C (89.6°F) as it reaches the bronchi, with values as low as 20°C (68°F) observed with breathing large volumes of cold, dry air.[88] Warming an incoming breath of cold air greatly increases its capacity to hold moisture. Humidification of inspired cold air produces considerable water and heat loss from the respiratory tract with large ventilatory volumes during physical activity. Airway moisture loss during cold-weather physical activity contributes to mouth dryness, a burning

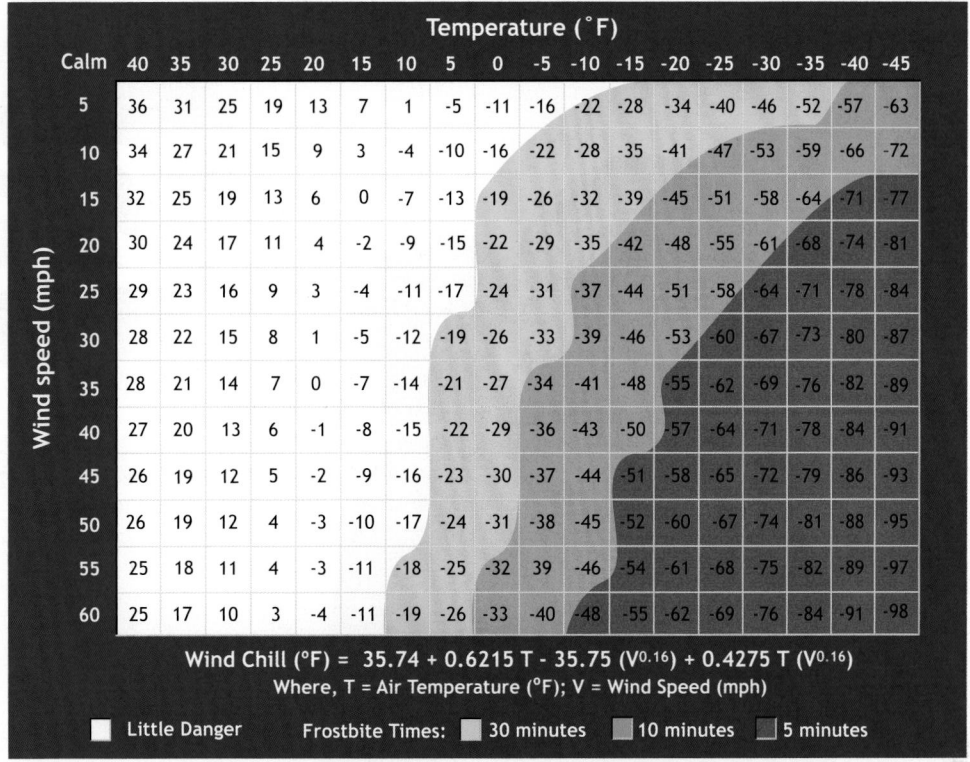

FIGURE 25.10 • The wind-chill temperature index. The proper way to evaluate the "coldness" of an environment. Figure shows the wind-chill temperatures for the relative risk of frostbite and the predicted times to freezing of exposed facial skin. Wet skin exposed to wind will cool even faster, and if the skin is wet and exposed to wind, the ambient temperature used for the wind-chill table should be 10°C (50°F) lower than the actual ambient temperature. (Reprinted with permission from American College of Sports Medicine Position Stand. Prevention of cold injuries during exercise. *Med Sci Sports Exerc* 2006;38:2012.)

sensation in the throat, irritation of the respiratory passages, and general dehydration. Wearing a scarf or cellulose mask-type baklava that covers the nose and mouth and traps the water in exhaled air, and warms and moistens the next incoming breath, helps minimize uncomfortable respiratory symptoms.

Summary

1. Water conducts heat about 25 times faster than air; immersion in water of only 28 to 30°C (82 to 86°F) provides considerable thermal stress that initiates rapid thermoregulatory adjustments.
2. Heat production from shivering and physical activity offsets heat flux to a cold environment. Shivering increases the metabolic rate by 3 to 6 METs.
3. Subcutaneous fat provides excellent insulation against cold stress. It greatly enhances the effectiveness of vasomotor adjustments, so individuals with excess body fat retain a large percentage of metabolic heat.
4. Individuals exhibit much less physiologic adaptation to chronic cold stress than to prolonged heat exposure.
5. Wearing appropriate clothing enables humans to tolerate some of the coldest climates on Earth.
6. Ambient temperature and wind influence the coldness of an environment. The wind-chill index determines the wind's cooling effect on exposed tissue.
7. Pronounced peripheral vasoconstriction during severe cold exposure causes dangerously low skin and extremity temperatures when compounded by marked increases in convective and conductive heat loss.
8. Considerable water loss occurs from the respiratory passages during physical activity on a cold day, but inspired air temperature generally does not pose a danger to respiratory tract tissues.
9. The Ama, the women divers of Korea and southern Japan, display cold adaptation from a blunted thermogenic response to prolonged diving that allows them to effectively tolerate extreme cold.

the**Point** References are available online at
http://thepoint.lww.com/mkk8e.

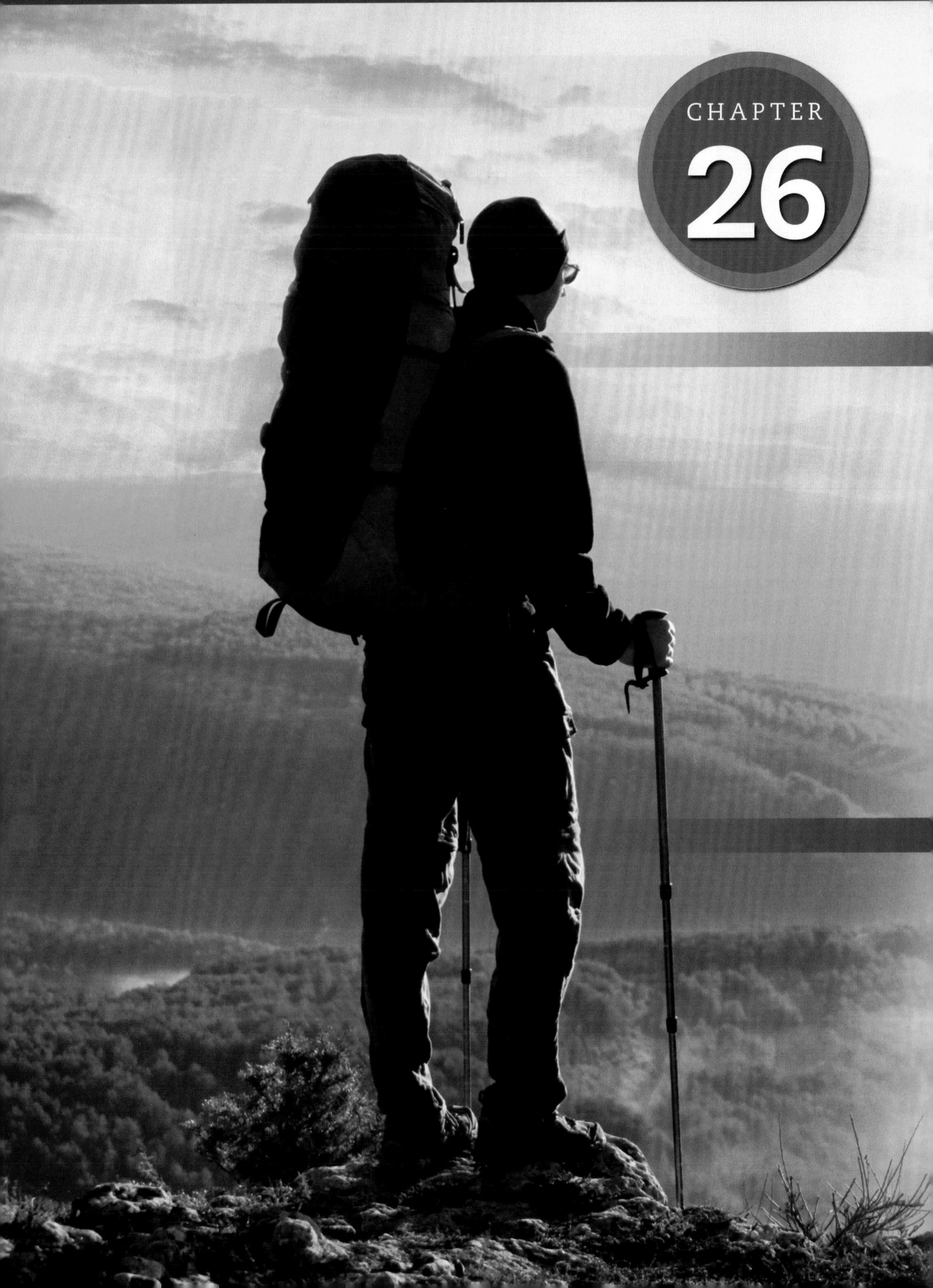

CHAPTER

26

Sport Diving

CHAPTER OBJECTIVES

- Quantify, with examples, the relationship between depth underwater and gas pressure and volume
- Discuss the rationale for snorkel size and underwater breathing depth
- Describe factors that limit the depth of a breath-hold dive
- Describe the effects of hyperventilation on breath-hold duration and potential risks before diving
- Outline evidence that supports a "diving reflex" in humans
- Contrast open-circuit and closed-circuit scuba systems
- List causes, symptoms, and treatment of air embolism, lung burst, pneumothorax, mask squeeze, aerotitis, nitrogen narcosis, decompression sickness, and oxygen poisoning
- Discuss the purpose and influencing factors of the decompression schedule for diving with compressed air
- Outline the rationale for saturation diving, and describe the environment where the diver lives for prolonged dives to exceptional depths
- Give reasons for breathing helium–oxygen mixtures at great depth and discuss limitations to deep diving with these mixtures
- Describe the closed-circuit, mixed-gas system used by the U.S. Navy in technical diving
- Describe the four free dive categories, and outline a general training strategy for free dive success

ANCILLARIES 👁 at-a-Glance

Visit http://thePoint.lww.com/mkk8e to access the following resources.

- References: Chapter 26
- Interactive Question Bank
- Appendix H: Supplemental Animation and Video Links
- Focus on Research: The Oxygen Cost of Swimming Underwater

An estimated 5.1 million individuals in the United States scuba dive for work or recreation, with an additional 510,000 divers trained each year. Unquestionably, safe diving requires thorough knowledge of diving physics and physiology. In this chapter we emphasize the relationships among diving depth, pressure, and gas volume and the potentially toxic effects of various gases breathed in diving at high pressures.[6,30,32]

DIVING HISTORY—ANTIQUITY TO THE PRESENT

Men and women have practiced breath-hold diving for centuries as they hunted for sponges and food, salvaged artifacts and treasures, repaired ships, observed marine life, and participated in military maneuvers. The 5th-century Greek historian Herodotus tells of the underwater exploits in 480 BC of the Greek patriot Scyllias and his daughter Hydna during the war against the Persians. When Scyllias, taken as prisoner aboard a ship, learned that Xerxes planned to attack a Greek flotilla, they escaped by jumping overboard. The Persians presumed they had drowned. To the contrary, Scyllias used a hollow reed as a snorkel and remained undiscovered, surfacing at night to cut each enemy ship loose from its moorings—saving the Greek Navy from sure disaster.

Understandably, each dive could last only a few minutes until the discovery that permitted dives for longer durations. Using longer "snorkels" did not work because the diver could not inhale against water pressure at depths greater than several feet (see "Snorkelng and Breath-Hold Diving"). Rebreathing from an air-filled bag submerged underwater also failed because the buildup of exhaled carbon dioxide caused the diver to react erratically and lose consciousness.

The first solutions to these problems took place in the 1530s with the invention of diving bells supplied with surface air. The bell, positioned a few feet from the surface, had its bottom open to water, with its top portion containing air compressed by water pressure. A diver in the bell with his head surrounded by air could then hold his breath, swim from the bell for a minute or two, and return for a short while, repeating the process until the air remaining in the bell became toxic.

In England and France in the 16th century, diving suits made of leather allowed descent to depths of 60 ft. Manual pumps delivered fresh air from the surface to the diver. Soon metal helmets could withstand greater water pressures, and divers could descend further. By the 1830s, perfection of the surface-supplied air helmet allowed extensive underwater salvage work.

Starting in the 19th century, two main avenues of investigation—one scientific and the other technologic—accelerated underwater exploration. Two scientists, French physiologist Paul Bert (1833–1886) and Scottish physiologist John Scott Haldane (1860–1936), explained the physiologic effects of water pressure on body tissues and also defined safe limits for compressed air diving using a decompression chamber and accompanying decompression tables he devised based on numerous animal experiments. Technologic improvements with compressed air pumps, carbon dioxide scrubbers, and demand-valve regulators allowed prolonged underwater explorations. The next section presents a timeline of selected events in diving history, highlighting the inventions and inventors over centuries of improvements in diving gear and technologies.

Chronology of Selected Events in Diving History

We present a brief chronology of selected events in diving history, rich in legend and scientific discovery. The Historical Diving Society offers more in-depth reading and references (www.hds.org).

4500 BC: Archeologists unearth shells in Mesopotamia dated to this period that must have originated from the sea floor.

3200 BC: Archeologists discover mother-of-pearl (abalone) shell ornaments dated to this period from the Egyptian Theban VI dynasty.

2500 BC: Greek divers make sponges widely available in commerce; *The Iliad* and *The Odyssey* mention diving and sponges.

550 BC: Pearl diving documented in India and Ceylon.

500 BC: Scyllias demonstrates the practical use of breath-hold diving in military exploits against the Persians.

100 BC: The Ama, Japan's women breath-hold divers of antiquity and modern times, gather pearl oysters, shellfish, and edible

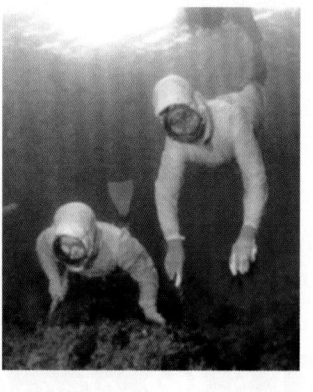

seaweed (see insert photo) (www.jpf.org.au/online articles/hitokuchimemo/issue31.html).

1500: Da Vinci designs the first "snorkel" device and dive fins for the hands and feet.

1530: Invention of the first diving bell by Italian Guglielmo de Lorena. From 1531 until 1535, de Lorena built a large "bell" that rested on the diver's shoulders with a tube running from the surface into the bell to supply fresh air during commercial sponge fishing and salvaging operations of ships and sunken treasure.

1650: First effective air pump developed by German scientist and inventor Otto Von Guericke (1602–1686), which physicist Robert Boyle (1627–1691) makes use of in compression and decompression experiments with animals.

1667: Robert Boyle makes first recorded observation of decompression sickness, or "bends," by documenting a gas bubble in the eye of a viper that had been compressed and then decompressed.

1690: Sir Edmund Halley (1656–1742; of comet fame) patents a practical diving bell consisting of lead-coated wood with a glass top to allow light to enter, 60 cubic ft (1.7 m³) in volume and connected by a pipe to weighted barrels of air replenished from the surface, which permitted dives to 60 ft for 90 min.

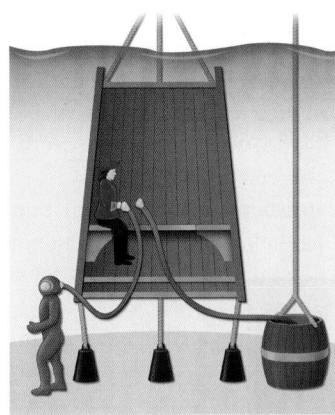

1715: John Lethbridge (1675–1759) constructs a "diving engine" or underwater "diving machine" built from an oak cylinder and supplied with compressed surface air. The diver remained submerged for 30 min at 60 ft; holes in the cylinder sealed by greased leather cuffs allowed his arms to protrude into the water for salvage work.

1776: First confirmed submarine battle depicted in artist David Bushnell's American *Turtle* against the HMS *Eagle* (British) in New York harbor (www.handshouse.org/turtle.html).

1788: John Smeaton's (1724–1792) popular diving bell uses a hand pump to supply fresh surface air and a one-way valve to prevent air from returning to the pump when it stops.

1808: Friedrich von Drieberg (1780–1856) invents a bellows-in-a-box device named Triton. Worn on the diver's back, it delivered compressed air from the surface.

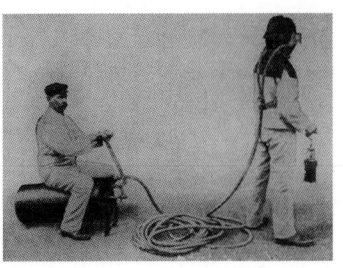

The device never worked successfully but nonetheless suggested compressed air could be used in diving, an idea conceived by Halley in the late 1690s.

1823: Charles Anthony Deane (1796–1848) patents the "smoke helmet" for fighting structural fires. Later modified for diving, the helmet fastened over the head with weights and received surface air through a hose.

In 1828, Charles Deane and his brother John market the helmet with a loosely attached "diving suit" so the diver could perform salvage work, but only in the full vertical position to prevent water from entering the suit.

1825: First prototype for "scuba" invented by Englishman William H. James incorporates a cylindrical belt (air reservoir) around the diver's trunk that supplies air to a helmet at 450 psi (lb per inch²) by a hand-operated valve and rubber tube. This 1873 newspaper illustration from a London paper shows a crewmember at the upper left tightening the wing nuts to secure the diver's helmet to the suit, while other crew members straighten the air hose.

The diver inhales through the nose and exhales through a mouthpiece connected by a short tube to an escape valve in the helmet's crown. With the reservoir charged to 30 atmospheres, James believed a diver would have enough air to last 60 min.

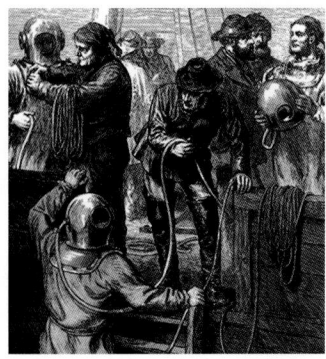

1837: Augustus Siebe (1788–1872), the father of diving, seals the Deane brothers' diving helmet to a waist-length jacket to create a full, watertight rubber suit that received surface air. This suit served as the forerunner for modern hardhat diving gear.

1839: Siebe's diving suit is used during salvage of the British warship HMS *Royal George*, sunk in 1782 to a depth of 65 ft; divers report the first symptoms of decompression sickness.

1843: From experience salvaging the HMS *Royal George*, the British Royal Navy establishes the first diving school.

1865: Benoît Rouquayrol (1826–1875) and Auguste Denayrouze (1837–1883) patent an underwater breathing apparatus called the "aerophore," which consisted of a steel tank of compressed air at 250 to 350 psi worn on the back and connected through an automatic demand valve to a mouthpiece (www.divinghelmet.nl/divinghelmet/1860_Rouquayrol_Denayrouze_2.html).

This forerunner of modern scuba enabled the diver to disconnect from a tether that supplied surface air and swim freely with the tank for several minutes.

1873: Dr. Andrew H. Smith, surgeon to the New York Bridge Company (the builders of the Brooklyn Bridge), reports about bends in workers who leave their pressurized caisson. Smith recommends chamber recompression for future projects but does not mention nitrogen bubbles as the cause of decompression sickness.

1878: Henry A. Fleuss, an engineer, develops the first self-contained diving apparatus by using compressed oxygen that employs the closed-circuit principle, not compressed air. Rope soaked in caustic potash absorbed carbon dioxide

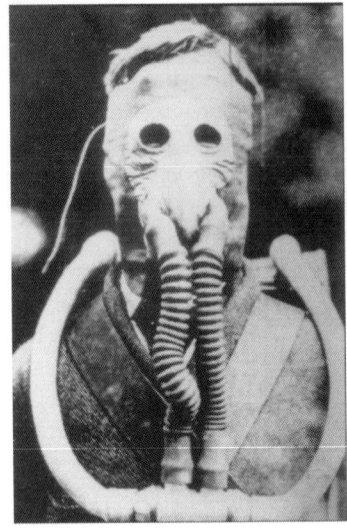

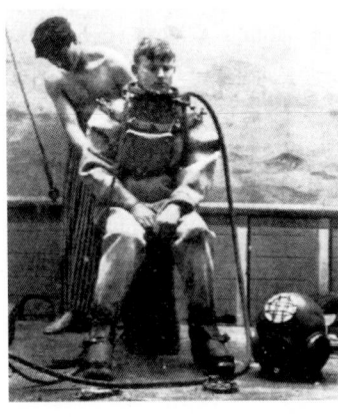

so the diver rebreathed exhaled air without bubbles entering the water. The apparatus provided divers up to 3 hr of "bottom time."

1878: Paul Bert (1833–1886), a French zoologist, physiologist, and politician, publishes *La Pression Barométrique*, which describes physiologic studies of pressure changes. Bert proves that nitrogen gas bubbles cause decompression sickness (the "bends" or caisson disease), while gradual ascent prevents the problem and recompression relieves pain. Deep sea pearl divers of that era experienced the bends.

1908: John Scott Haldane (1860–1936), Arthur Boycott, and Guybon Damant publish "The Prevention of Compressed-Air Illness," a landmark paper that describes staged decompression to combat decompression sickness. Based on this work, the British Royal Navy and United States Navy develop diving tables for compressed air diving up to 200 ft deep.

1910: English inventor Sir Robert Davis (1870–1965) patents the Davis Submerged Escape Apparatus (DSEA), essentially an oxygen rebreather. This equipment was the forerunner of devices that allowed British submarine crews about 30 min time to escape when their ship started to sink.

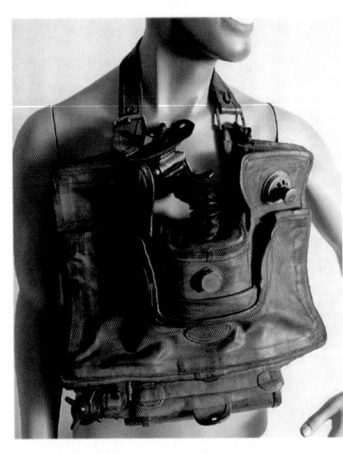

The DSEA rig shown in the inset figure at left contained a rubber breathing/buoyancy bag with a canister of barium hydroxide to scrub exhaled CO_2. The DSEA included a steel pressure cylinder with a control valve connected to the breathing bag that contained approximately 56 L of oxygen at a pressure of 120 ata. Opening the cylinder's valve admitted oxygen to the bag and charged it to the pressure of the surrounding water. The canister of CO_2 absorbent inside the breathing bag was connected to a mouthpiece by a flexible corrugated tube; breathing was done by mouth only (the nose being closed by a clip). Goggles were a standard part of the DSEA.

1917: The U.S. Bureau of Construction and Repair first introduces the Mark V diving helmet, which revolutionizes salvage operations in World War II.

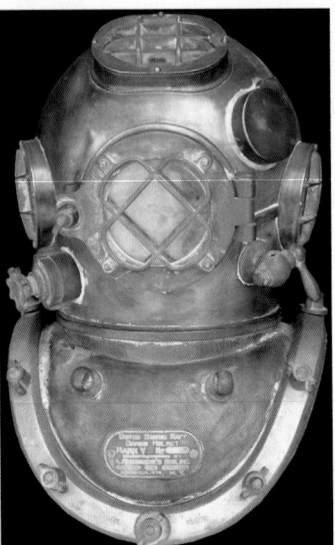

This "gold standard" in helmet design served five purposes: it sealed the whole of the diver's head from the water, it allowed the diver to see clearly underwater, it provided the diver with breathing gas, it protected the diver's head when doing heavy or dangerous work, and it provided voice communications with the surface during the dive. If a diver became incapacitated during a dive but was still breathing, the helmet remained in place and continued to deliver breathing gas until a rescue took place.

1920s: U.S. researchers experiment with helium–oxygen mixtures for deep dives.

1924: The U.S. Navy and Bureau of Mines conduct the first experiments with helium–oxygen mixtures.

1930: Dr. Charles William Beebe (1877–1962) and Lieutenant and submariner Otis Barton (1899–1992) descend 1426 ft in a 4′ 9″ bathysphere attached to a barge by a steel cable. In the photo, Bebe is on the left, Barton on the right (**https://sites.google.com/site/cwilliambeebe/Home/bathysphere**).

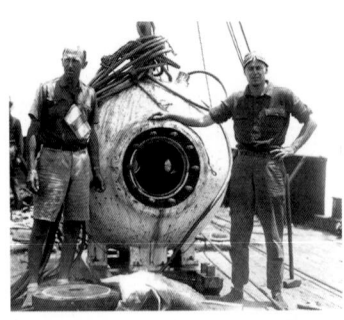

The bathysphere walls measured 1.5 ft thick and were made of a single casting. The vessel was tethered from a mother ship at the ocean's surface by a single, nontwisting cable 3500 ft long. The steel cable was 7/8-inch thick with a breaking strain of 29 tons. An additional 100 strands of cable were interwoven around the steel central core to ensure the cable would not rotate the sphere upon descent or on return to the ocean's surface. Electric lines for light and a telephone line were wrapped inside a rubber hose, which entered through a small hole at the top of the bathysphere. Oxygen tanks with automatic valves were installed. Trays of calcium chloride (to absorb moisture) were placed on racks alongside trays of soda lime to remove excess carbon dioxide. The two explorers were sealed inside using a 15-inch, 400-lb circular door put in place by a winch and then hand-tightened with 10 large bolts. The Bebe and Barton dive was one of the great exploration triumphs of the 1930s, for which they received worldwide notoriety. Bebe wrote a riveting account of the historic dive in his book (Bebe W. *Half Mile Down.* New York: Duell Sloan Pearce, 1951), which can be read online at **http://archive.org/stream/halfmiledown00beeb#page/n0/mode/2up** or downloaded as a PDF document.

1930s: American pilot and writer Guy Gilpatric (1896–1950) pioneers the use of rubber goggles with glass lenses for skin diving. He added putty to aviator goggles for eye protection from salt water. By the mid-1930s, face masks, fins (also called "swimming propellers"), and snorkels were in common use.

The famous female 1924 Olympic champion and competition swimmer Gertrude Ederle (1905–2003) broke

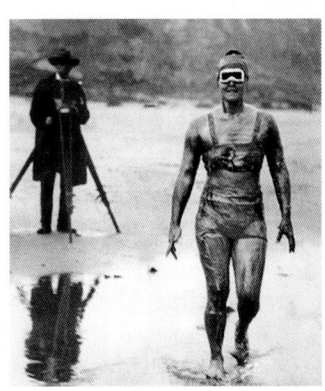

the prior men's Channel record on August 6, 1926, by 2 hr, becoming the first woman to swim the Channel and the first person (male or female) to swim the front crawl the whole way. What made her swim possible were the motorcycle goggles she waterproofed with a paraffin seal.

1933: French Navy captain Yves Le Prieur (1885–1963) modifies the Rouquayrol-Denayrouze "aerophore" by combining a new demand valve with a 1500 psi high-pressure air tank without a regulator, to eliminate restricting effects of hoses and lines. The diver breathes fresh air by opening a tap, while exhaled air escapes under the edge of the diver's mask.

1934: William Beebe and Otis Barton descend 3028 ft in their bathysphere near Bermuda, setting a depth record that remained until 1948.

1935: French Navy adopts Yves Le Prieur's "scuba" equipment.

1936: Le Prieur establishes the world's first scuba diving club, called the "Club of Divers and Underwater Life."

1938: Dr. Edgar End and Max Nohl make the first intentional saturation "dive" in a Milwaukee hospital hyperbaric chamber (27 hr at a 101-ft depth). Decompression takes 5 hr, and Nohl suffers the bends. End believes that helium can replace nitrogen to reduce nitrogen narcosis.

1939: A new diving bell, the McCann–Erickson Rescue Chamber, makes the first successful rescue of men aboard the submarine USS *Squalus,* a new 310-ft submarine sunk in 243 ft of water in the North Atlantic.

The chamber fit over the submarine's escape hatch, which four men at a time entered under one atmosphere of pressure. The rescue involved attaching salvage pontoons along the sides of the submarine with chains slung under the hull. The pontoons inflated to lift the boat off the bottom and moved

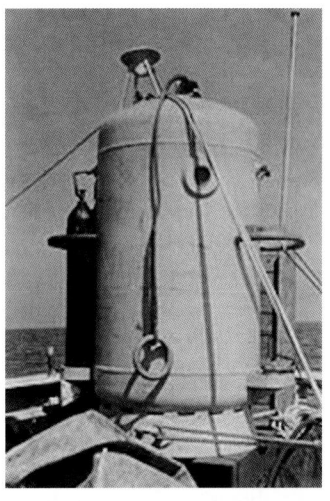

to shallower water where the pontoons were reset. The process was repeated until *Squalus* was shallow enough to enter the river at Portsmouth. The subsequent rescue and salvage operations ushered in several new technologies, including the use of the McCann Rescue Chamber and the first operational use of helium diving by the U.S. Navy. Dr. Albert Behnke (see Chapter 28, "Reference Man and Reference Woman") helped to supervise the successful rescue efforts (**www.cisatlantic.com/trimix/other/squalus.htm**) and provided operational support as one of the medical officers. (For further reading, see Maas P. *The Terrible Hours: The Man Behind the Greatest Submarine Rescue in History.* New York: Harper, 1999.)

1941–1944: Italian divers, working out of midget submarines during World War II, use closed-circuit scuba to place explosives under British naval and merchant marine vessels. The British adopt this technology to sink the German battleship *Tirpitz* on November 12, 1944 (**www.bismarckclass.dk/tirpitz/tirpitz_menu.html**).

1942–1943: Jacques-Yves Cousteau (1910–1997; French naval lieutenant) and Emile Gagnan (1900–1979; engineer for a Parisian natural gas company) redesign a car regulator

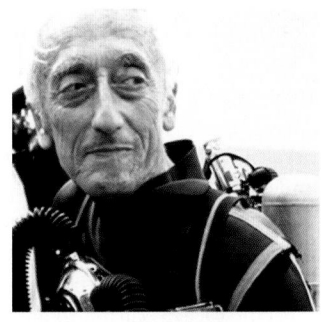

to supply compressed air to a diver in initiation of a breathing cycle. They attach their new demand valve regulator to hoses, a mouthpiece, and a pair of compressed air tanks, which they patent as the Aqua-Lung. Frederic Dumas (1913–1991) descends to 210 ft in the Mediterranean Sea and experiences *l'ivresse des grandes profondeurs* ("the rapture of the great depths"). Cousteau achieves worldwide acclaim for his underwater explorations, movies, books, and dedication to environmental causes (**www.cousteau.org**).

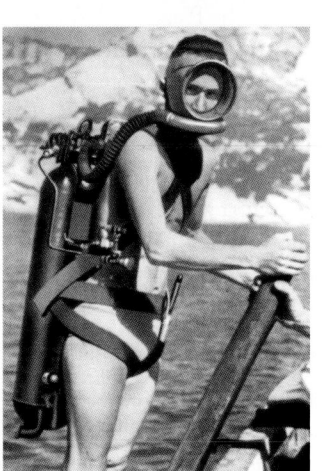

1947: Frederic Dumas uses the AquaLung and dives to 94 m (307 ft) in the Mediterranean Sea.

1948: Otis Barton (1899–1992) descends in a modified bathysphere to 1370 m (4500 ft) off the coast of California.

1950s: August Picard and Jacques Picard develop the Swiss-designed, Italian-built research bathyscaphe (deep boat; http://bjsonline.com/watches/articles/0022_3.shtml),

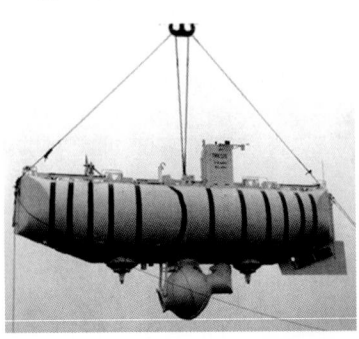

a completely self-contained vessel. In 1954 the bathyscaphe set a diving record of 4050 m (13,287 ft).

For submarine survival equipment, a British company pioneered the development of Submarine Escape technology in 1952 (www.rfdbeaufortmarine.com). Designed to provide protection for submariners from a stricken submarine,

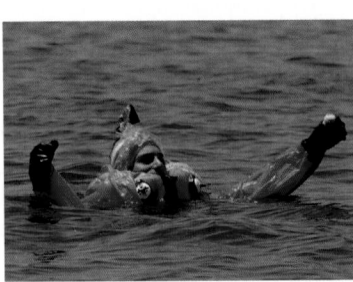

the products include single-skinned suits with integrated life rafts, escape jerkins, inflatable abandonment suits, external submarine life raft systems, and freeboard extenders. There are in excess of 30,000 units of submarine escape equipment in use, and 30 of the world's navies (including the U.S. Navy) use the latest Submarine Escape Immersion Equipment (SEIE) MK-11. The suit allows survivors to escape a disabled submarine at depths down to 600 ft (183 m), at a rate of eight or more men per hour.

1959: The YMCA begins the first nationally organized course for scuba certification.

1960: Jacques Picard and Don Walsh descend to approximately 10,916 m (35,820 ft, 6.78 miles; water pressure 16,883 psi, temperature 3°C [37.4°F]) in the August Picard–designed, Swiss-built, U.S. Navy–owned bathyscaphe *Trieste*, to the bottom of the Mariana Trench (deepest known seafloor depression on Earth) in the Pacific Ocean. Listen to a first-person account by Don Walsh of the Picard and Walsh 1960 dive to the deepest spot in the ocean floor (Mariana Trench), including a historical perspective of the dive and its accomplishments for science (http://spectrum.ieee.org/geek-life/profiles/don-walsh-describes-the-trip-to-the-bottom-of-the-mariana-trench#.UPGN6mMa4lg.mailto).

1960s: As accident rates for scuba divers climb, the first national agencies form to train and certify divers: the NAUI (National Association of Underwater Instructors) forms in 1960 and the PADI (Professional Association of Diving Instructors) forms in 1966.

1962: Albert Falco and Claude Wesley, in the first of three planned experiments called Conshelf (continental shelf) sought to establish that humans can live underwater for an extended period. Falco (Cousteau's lead diver) and Wesley

spent 7 days under 10 m (33 ft) of water in the open sea near Marseilles, France, in an underwater-living habitat named *Diogenes*.

They ate, worked, and slept in the vessel, breathing compressed air fed through pipes from the surface. TV monitors recorded their activities, and other divers, including

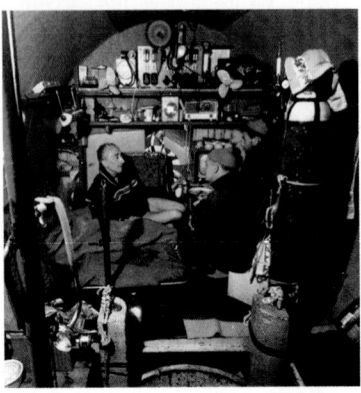

Jacques Cousteau, at left in the image, paid regular visits to the "oceanauts." No ill physiological effects occurred from that first sojourn.

1963–1965: Divers live and work in underwater habitats for a month at a time at 60 m.

1963: Whitey Stefens (*left*) and Bob Ratcliffe (*right*), commercial abalone divers from Santa Barbara, California, pose with the first prototype of a div-

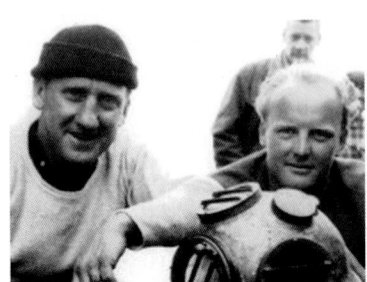

ing helmet converted for deep diving use by commercial construction and oilfield divers.

The DESCO commercial abalone helmet (www.descocorp.com/desco_abalone_divers_helmet.htm) had been fitted with a newly developed second-stage SCUBA breathing regulator, which conserved the expensive oxygen and helium breathing mixture required for ultra-deep (200-plus ft.) commercial construction and offshore oilfield diving.

1964: Abalone diver and young entrepreneur Danny Wilson (see "FYI: Santa Barbara, CA: The Historical Roots of Deepwater Diving") out of necessity to dive 250 to 500 ft

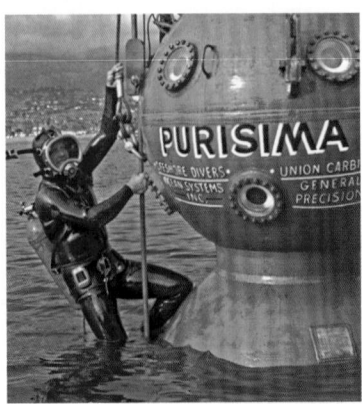

off the Santa Barbara channel without limitations of conventional heavy gear, built the Purisima diving bell shown in the photo at left with diver Bob Ratcliffe. This represented the world's first oxy–helium-equipped, deep capability commercial diver lockout bell.

Purisima's goal was to provide relatively short-duration "bounce" dives to the extreme depths that required an oxy–helium mixture.

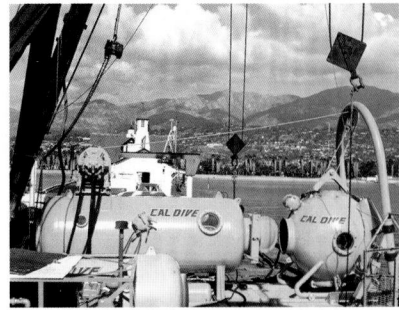

With the divers safely back in the diving bell upon completion of their task, a bell similar to the one shown at the right in the photo was quickly raised to the surface by an overhead hoist and carefully mated to the cylindrical, deck decompression chamber (photo *left*) for lengthy decompression to avoid the bends.

1968: John J. Gruener and R. Neal Watson dive to 133 m (436 ft), breathing compressed air.

1969: Following the commercial success of the Purisima diving bell, divers Bob Ratcliffe, Lad and Gene Handelman, and Ken Lengyel formed California Divers Inc. (known as Cal Dive), which later evolved into Oceaneering International Inc. (www.oceaneering.com), an acknowledged world leader in subsea engineering and applied technology.

1970s: Implementation of diving safety standards include the following: certification cards to indicate a minimum training level and as a requirement for tank refills, change from J-valve reserve systems to nonreserve K-valves, adoption of submersible pressure gauges, and use of the buoyancy compensator and single-hose regulators.

1980: Divers Alert Network is founded at Duke University as a nonprofit organization to promote safe diving (www.diversalertnetwork.org).

1981: Record 686-m (2250-ft) "dive" is made in a Duke Medical Center chamber. Stephen Porter, Len Whitlock, and Erik Kramer live in the 8-ft chamber for 43 days, breathing a nitrogen, oxygen, and helium mixture.

1983: Introduction of the first commercially available dive computer (Orca Edge).

1985: Oceanographer, Naval Intelligence Officer, and explorer Robert Ballard (Institute for Exploration at Mystic Aquarium, Mystic, CT; www.ife.org) and Ralph White use a remote-controlled camera to explore the wreck of the *Titanic* shown in

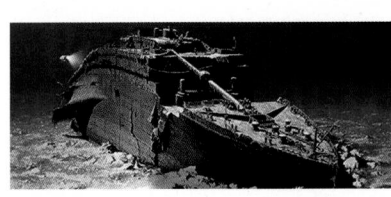

the inset (3810-m [12,500-ft] depth), located about 1000 miles due east of Boston.

In this brief video (http://video.nationalgeographic.com/video/specials/in-the-field-specials/ballard-underwater-nglive/), Ballard discusses his exploration of underwater wrecks, including his key discovery of deep-sea hydrothermal vents (massive formations that spew superheated fluids from the ocean floor). Ballard also discovered the wreck of the *Bismarck* and the USS *Yorktown* during his more than 135 expeditions.

1990s: An estimated 500,000 new scuba divers are certified yearly in the United States as this activity's popularity for recreational and commercial purposes increases.

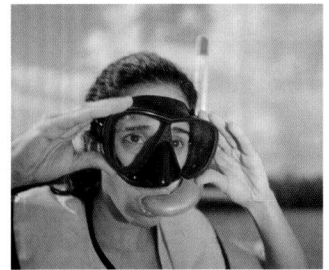

Numerous scientific experiments using submersibles explored worldwide deep-diving sites in the Atlantic and Pacific oceans. The journeys included probing deep-sea vulcanism, deep geology, and searching for artifacts from sunken vessels, including 2000-year-old shipwrecks in the Mediterranean Sea.

2003: Tanya Streeter, a world champion freediver, shatters the men's and women's variable ballast free diving world records

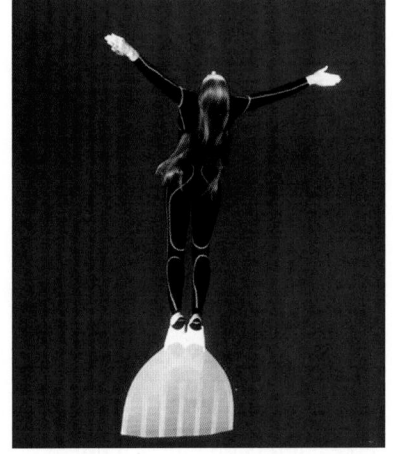

by descending 400 ft (122 m in 3 min 38 s) to capture the variable ballast record. Streeter becomes the first person to break all four deep free diving world records.

2004–2006: Expansion of technical diving by nonprofessionals who use mixed gases, new propulsion systems, full-face masks, underwater voice communication, and digital cameras.

2004–2013: World records continue to be set for the many types of breath-hold diving. Table 26.1 provides a summary of key achievements.

2012: Oceanographer and filmmaker James Cameron completes record-breaking Mariana Trench solo submersible dive of nearly 7 miles. Cameron achieved the milestone on March 25, 2012, descending to the deepest part of the world's oceans located in the western Pacific Ocean to the east of the Mariana Islands in a 12-ton submarine vessel called the *Deepsea Challenger* (www.guardian.co.uk/film/video/2012/mar/26/james-cameron-mariana-trench-video). The trench is about 255 0 km (1580 mi) long with an average width of 69 km (43 mi). The maximum-known depth is 10.911 km (10,911 ± 40 m) or 6.831 mi (36,069 ± 131 ft) at the Challenger Deep, a small slot-shaped valley in its floor. The dive was part of Deepsea Challenge (http://deepseachallenge.com), a scientific expedition by Cameron, the National Geographic Society, and Rolex to conduct deep-ocean research. Watch the videos of Cameron's exploration at http://video.nationalgeographic.com/video/news/environment-news/cameron-deepest-dive-record-vin/; http://deepseachallenge.com/the-latest/.

TABLE 26.1	Breadth-Hold Diving World Records as of August 2013	
MEN		**WOMEN**
Constant Weight Apnea Without Fins (CNF)		
101 m Name: William Trubridge (NZL) Date: 2010-12-16 Place: Long Island, Bahamas		**68 m** Name: Natalia Molchanova (RUS) Date: 2013-04-25 Place: Blue Hole, Dahab
Constant Weight Apnea (CWT)		
126 m Name: Alexey Molchanov (RUS) Date: 2012-11-20 Place: Long Island, Bahamas		**101 m** Name: Natalia Molchanova (RUS) Date: 2011-09-23 Place: Kalamata, Greece
Dynamic Apnea Without Fins (DNF)		
218 m Name: Dave Mullins (NZL) Date: 2010-09-27 Place: Naenae & Porirua, New Zealand		**182 m** Name: Natalia Molchanova (RUS) Date: 2013-06-27 Place: Belgrade, Serbia
Dynamic Apnea (DYN)		
281 m Name: Goran Čolak (CRO) Date: 2013-06-28 Place: Belgrade, Serbia		**234 m** Name: Natalia Molchanova (RUS) Date: 2013-06-28 Place: Belgrade, Serbia
Static Apnea (STA)		
11 min 35 sec Name: Stéphane Mifsud (FRA) Date: 2009-06-08 Place: Hyères, France		**9 min 02 sec** Name: Natalia Molchanova (RUS) Date: 2013-06-29 Place: Belgrade, Serbia
Free Immersion Apnea (FIM)		
121 m Name: William Trubridge (NZL) Date: 2010-04-10 Place: Long Island, Bahamas		**88 m** Name: Natalia Molchanova (RUS) Date: 2011-09-24 Place: Kalamata, Greece
Variable Weight Apnea (VWT)		
142 m Name: Herbert Nitsch (AUT) Date: 2009-12-07 Place: Long Island, Bahamas		**127 m** Name: Natalia Molchanova (RUS) Date: 2012-06-06 Place: Sharm el-Sheikh, Egypt
No Limits Apnea (NLT)		
214 m Name: Herbert Nitsch (AUT) Date: 2007-06-14 Place: Spetses, Greece		**160 m** Name: Tanya Streeter (USA) Date: 2002-08-17 Place: Turks & Caicos

Source: www.aidainternational.org/competitive/worlds-records

The Historical Roots of Deepwater Diving

Santa Barbara, CA

Santa Barbara, CA, can rightfully lay claim to a historic dive that revolutionized commercial diving and the expansion of deepwater oil exploration. On November 3, 1962, Santa Barbara abalone diver Hugh "Danny" Wilson (1931–2007), recognizing a need for the commercial use of mixed-gas diving techniques to support offshore petroleum exploration, modified his abalone diving helmet for use with an oxygen and helium mixture and dove to about 400 ft off the east end of Santa Cruz Island in the Santa Barbara Channel.

Prior to the 1960s and Wilson's historic dive, the depths of diving were severely limited by the narcotic effects of high pressures of nitrogen and the deleterious central nervous system toxicity of high pressures of oxygen in typical compressed air diving. The large support vessel and numerous support crew members required for the U. S.

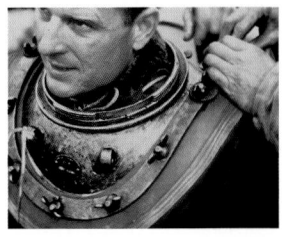

Navy's equipment and approach to deep water diving was neither cost effective nor practical for commercial construction or offshore oilfield diving. However, the Navy's helmet and procedures had been used successfully in 1939 in the salvage of the crew of the submarine *USS Squalus* off the coast of New Hampshire (see the chronicle of Dr. Albert Behnke, medical physician, and the successful rescue mission that saved 33 lives). The Navy system was largely viewed as impractical for the needs of deepwater commercial operations. Wilson conceived of the dive to emphasize a point to the executives of oil companies then drilling in the Santa Barbara Channel that a better way existed for dive operations.

Those companies and petroleum geologists were convinced that vast oil and gas reserves were available at depths

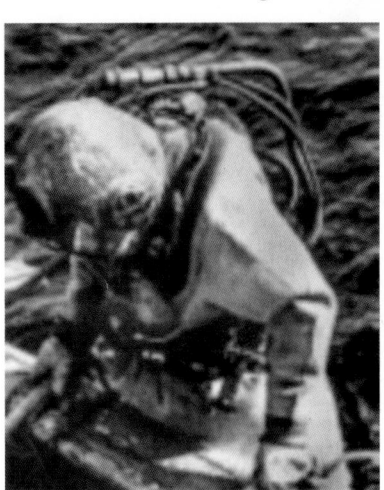

beyond 300 ft, yet they could not drill at those depths without better diving support in the form of workable, lightweight diving gear and appropriate gas mixtures. Wilson, hoping to enter the then "closed" cadre of divers who worked for the Associated Divers Company in the 1950s and 1960s, was told his proposed methods would not work. Now motivated to succeed and break domination of the market, he modified his open-circuit air free-flow abalone helmet into an open-circuit demand/free-flow system fed with a heliox mixture. Wilson did not publicize his final "test" dive, to avoid alerting competing local divers. When they later heard of the dive, they considered it foolish and dangerous because he dove using untried and unproven equipment and gas mixtures, and made the dive from a relatively small fishing boat that lacked space for a decompression chamber in the event he experienced the bends or other decompression problems.

Wilson, who had risked his life on the dive, successfully demonstrated the usefulness of the prototype helmet design that permitted working in deep water for 60 min without deleterious effects of nitrogen narcosis (mental torpidity or euphoria similar to altitude anoxia or alcoholic intoxication) that typically hinder such tasks. In the diving operations offered by competitor Associated Divers, the diver, while working at depth, could remain there for only about 25 min breathing ordinary compressed air.

As Barthelmess points out, "The David of diving had slain Goliath, as the eventual demise of Associated Divers had begun." Wilson's breakthrough demonstration dive using

his newly designed helmet—relying on a breathing mixture of 80% helium, 20% oxygen for descent, and a bottom mix of 90% helium and 10% oxygen—broke an important barrier in diving technology with a lasting economic impact. Wilson's contribution served as the forerunner to the modern-day open-circuit demand/free-flow helmets in use today (www. sbcc.edu/marinediving/website/whatsnew/workshops/ Helium_Rush%20HDSJDH.pdf; http://www.sbmm.org/ wp-content/uploads/2012/11/Wilson-SBNP3.pdf).[5a]

The Man and the Dive: Reflections of Bob Ratcliffe

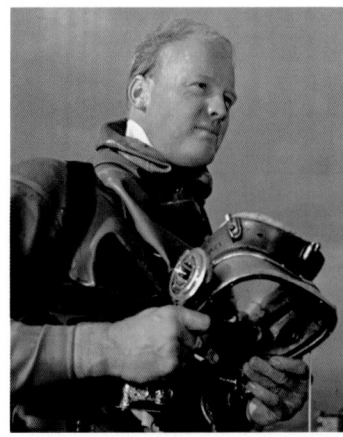

Bob Ratcliffe, inventor of the "Rat-Hat" diving helmet in use worldwide (www.divescrap.com/ DiveScrap_INDEX/ Oceaneering.html), and 2010 inductee into the Commercial Diving Hall of Fame, spent about a decade diving with Danny Wilson for abalone and participated with him in commercial oxy–helium diving along the California coast. He provides the following reflections on his experience:

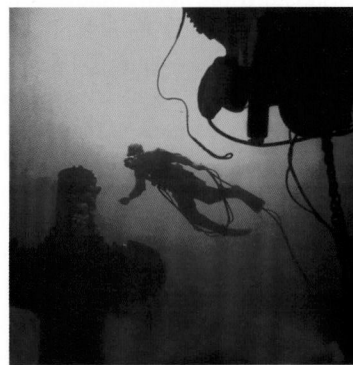

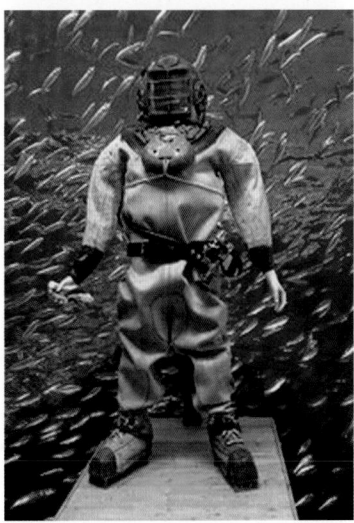

Oil companies that want to drill in deep water are not interested in paying commercial divers to descend to their sea floor equipment in 250 FSW (feet of salt water) to blow bubbles! They want the highly paid divers to perform the work on the sea floor assigned to them. Nitrogen narcosis severely reduces the amount of time of useful work that a diver can accomplish. Use of oxygen and helium mixtures for the diver's breathing gas allows the diver to perform the amount of work in very deep water comparable to what he could accomplish in very shallow water. He is as clear headed at depth as he is working in his own back yard. Dan Wilson's purpose was to allow him to break into oilfield diving (for lucrative pay) by being able to perform

more useful work in deep water as an inexperienced oilfield diver using oxy–helium than the experienced, excellent divers could accomplish breathing compressed air.

This was in fact what happened. The new oxy–helium divers accomplished much more for each dive, when calculated per dollar paid, than the compressed air divers. The inset photo (see the prior page) shows me leaving through the lower hatch of our diving bell Purisima, and swimming to a sub-sea wellhead (consisting of valves and pipes) on the sea floor in the Santa Barbara channel in the early 1960s. Wilson did this many times during contract work for oil companies, due in part to the effective use of oxy–helium mixtures during deep-water dives.

The inset photo at the bottom of the prior page shows a model of the diving suit and gear Wilson wore during his historic dive on November 3, 1962 (www.sbmm.org), that paved the way for future endeavors in commercial deep-sea diving.

The Salvage of the Squalus: A Historic Undersea Rescue

"When the submarine USS Squalus (SS 192) and her 59 crewmen sank off New Hampshire on May 23, 1939, the crew's struggle for survival and the courage of rescuers kept Americans close to their radio dials. Before television, before the Internet, the public was gripped by compelling events far beneath the sea in what became the greatest submarine rescue in U.S. history."

—Robert F. Dorr, February 18, 2010
(www.defensemedianetwork.com/stories/squalus-disaster-rescue-
gripped-a-nation-on-the-eve-of-war/)

The rescue of the submarine *Squalus* in 1939, the last Naval salvage operation prior to World War II, provided a unique opportunity for then Lieutenant Commander Albert R. Behnke, Jr. MC (U.S. Navy), to assist in the medical operations that saved 33 men when the submarine sank in 243 ft of water

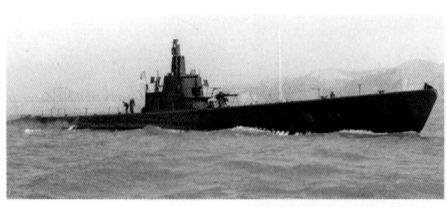

off the Isles of Shoals along the New Hampshire coast during a "crash" test requiring the rapid submersion of a vessel to avoid enemy detection.

During the initial dive, a valve that supplied air to the diesel engine apparently remained open. This caused immediate flooding of the aft torpedo room, both engine rooms, and the crew's quarters—forcing the submarine to sink to the ocean floor. It took the Navy rescue workers using the relatively untested Monson-McCann rescue chamber and four dives over 13 hr, including a full day, to reach the submarine and to rescue the 33 submariners (**www.history.navy.mil/photos/ sh-usn/usnsh-s/ss192-j.htm**).

As part of an invited Harvard Lecture about research related to the physiology of deep-sea diving and its risks, subsequently published in 1942 in the *Bulletin of the New York Academy of Sciences*, Behnke provided details about two rescue operations, each relating to how divers used breathing mixtures of helium and oxygen gases that permitted

them to work effectively at depths below 200 ft without experiencing the narcotic-like, intoxicating effects of submersion while breathing compressed air for extended periods. Behnke first discussed an ergometer test to assess the effects of working while breathing different gas concentrations, then provided details about practical applications during rescue missions.

The observations made in the laboratory soon governed field practice during diving operations in submarine disasters.
In 1939, divers breathing air at a depth of 240 ft in salvage work on the USS Squalus suffered lapses of memory, mental confusion, and occasionally loss of consciousness.

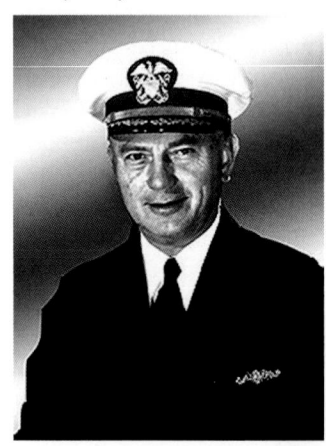

It proved to be not only dangerous but futile to work within a maze of hose and cables at a depth of 240 ft in an atmosphere of air.
As in the laboratory, so also in the field; the substitution of helium for nitrogen rendered the impairment in neuromuscular coordination negligible and enabled divers to work efficiently when under 7 atmospheres of pressure. The successful termination of the salvage operations was made possible only by the employment of helium.
In 1940 a second submarine disaster occurred in water 440 ft deep. Although the pressure at this depth was sufficient to crush the hull of the disabled craft, divers breathing a mixture of helium and oxygen reached the bottom and were able to survey the sunken vessel. These divers, in spite of subjection to a pressure of 14 atmospheres, felt well and had little difficulty in performing the work required in descent and ascent to a depth corresponding closely to the height of the Washington monument.[5b]

PRESSURE–VOLUME RELATIONSHIPS AND DIVING DEPTH

Diving Depth and Pressure

Water remains essentially noncompressible owing to its high density relative to air. Consequently, its pressure against a diver's body increases directly with the depth of the dive. Two forces produce increased external pressure (**hyperbaria**) in diving:

1. Weight of the column of water directly above the diver, called *hydrostatic pressure*
2. Weight of the atmosphere (*ata*, or *bar*) at the water's surface

TABLE 26.2 shows that a column of seawater exerts a force of 1 sea-level ata (760 mm Hg, or 14.7 psi) for each 10-m or 33-ft descent below the water's surface. Freshwater is less dense than seawater, so a depth of approximately 34 ft corresponds to 1 ata in freshwater diving. Thus, a dive to 33 ft in seawater exposes the diver to a pressure of 2 ata: 1 ata from the weight of ambient air at the surface and the other from the weight of the column of water itself. Diving from sea level to

TABLE 26.2 Relationship of Depth in Water to External Pressure, Lung Volume, and Inspired Gas Pressures

Depth		Pressure		Hypothetical Lung Volume	Inspired Air (mm Hg)	
ft	m	atm	mm Hg	mL	P_{O_2}	P_{N_2}
Sea level		1	760	6000	159	600
33	10	2	1520	3000	318	1201
66	20	3	2280	2000	477	1802
99	30	4	3040	1500	636	2402
133	40	5	3800	1200	795	3003
166	50	6	4560	1000	954	3604
200	60	7	5320	857	1113	4204
300	90	10	7600	600	1590	6006
400	120	13	9880	461	2068	7808
500	150	16	12,160	375	2545	9610
600	180	19	14,440	316	3022	11,412

20 m (66 ft) exposes a diver to an absolute external pressure of 3 ata; the pressure is 4 ata at 30 m (99 ft), and so on. Clearly, considerable external pressure builds up when diving relatively short distances below the surface.

Water constitutes a large portion of the body's tissues, so they too remain noncompressible and not particularly susceptible to increased external pressure during diving. The body also contains air-filled cavities—notably the lungs, respiratory passages, and sinus and middle ear spaces. Volume and pressure in these cavities change considerably with any increase or decrease in diving depth. The consequences, without adjustments to *equalize* the rapid and large changes in pressure that occur in a hyperbaric environment, can lead to pain, injury, and even death.

Diving Depth and Gas Volume

Boyle's law (formulated in 1662 by chemist/physicist Robert Boyle) *states that at constant temperature, the volume of a given mass of gas varies inversely with pressure*. When pressure doubles, volume halves; conversely, reducing pressure by one half expands any gas volume to twice its previous size. Figure 26.1 (and Table 26.2) shows that if divers fill their lungs with 6 L of air at the surface and then descend to 10 m (33 ft), the lung volume compresses to 3 L. Diving an additional 10 m to a depth of 20 m (65.6 ft; external pressure now 3 ata) reduces the original 6-L lung volume by two thirds, to 2 L. At 91 m (300 ft; 10 ata), the lung volume compresses to 0.6 L, simply from the compressive force of water against the air-filled thoracic cavity. The inset figure graphically illustrates the curvilinear relation between lung volume at the surface and depth in seawater. For most individuals, further increases in diving depth reduce the pulmonary air volume and seriously damage the chest wall and lung tissue. As the diver returns to the surface, the air volume reexpands to its *original* 6-L volume. For the scuba diver who

breathes pressurized air beneath the water, a 6-L lung volume at a 10-m depth expands to 12 L at the water's surface; this 6-L volume at 50-m depth occupies 36 L at sea-level pressure. Lung tissues will rupture during ascent from the powerful force of expanding gases if the "extra" air volume cannot escape through the nose or mouth.

SNORKELING AND BREATH-HOLD DIVING

Swimming at the water's surface with fins, mask, and snorkel provides a common form of recreation and sport for spear fishing and exploring shallow areas of clear water. A J-shaped tube or **snorkel** allows the swimmer to breathe continually with the face immersed in water. The swimmer periodically takes a full breath of air and dives to explore beneath the water's surface. After about 30 s, the carbon dioxide level in arterial blood builds up, causing the diver to sense the need to breathe and surface quickly. Snorkeling is essentially an extension of swimming, with diving limited entirely by the swimmer's breath-holding ability.

Limits to Snorkel Size

Novice skin divers often speculate that if they had a longer snorkel, they could swim deeper under the water and still breathe ambient air through the top of the snorkel. Some neophytes believe they can sit at a pool bottom and breathe through a garden hose extending to the pool deck! The idea of a longer snorkel seems intriguing, but two factors limit snorkel length and volume:

1. Increased hydrostatic pressure on the chest cavity as one descends beneath the water
2. Increased pulmonary dead space by enlarging the snorkel's volume

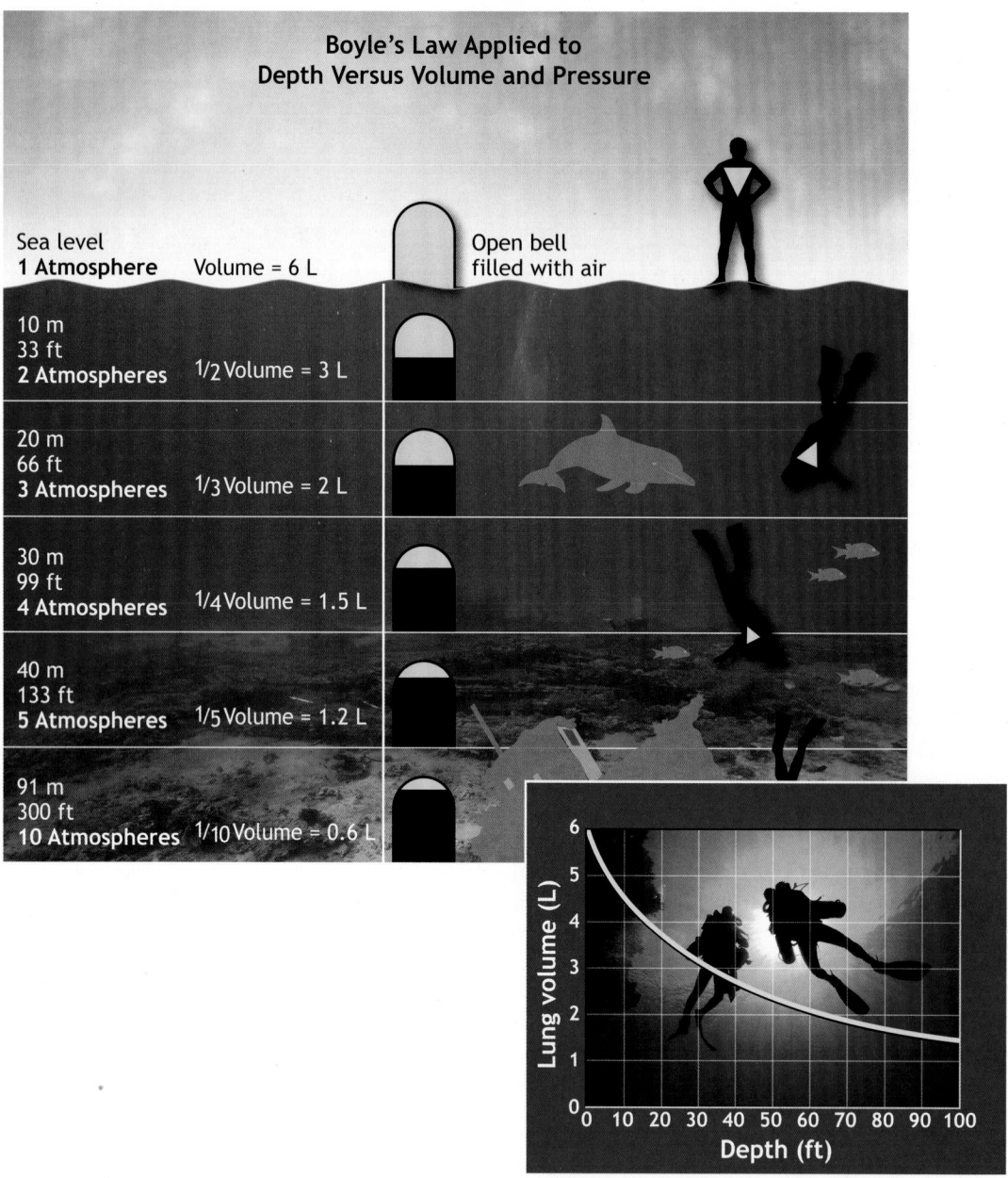

FIGURE 26.1 • Gas volume varies inversely with the pressure acting upon it. A 6-L volume, whether in an open bell or in the flexible thoracic cavity, compresses to 3 L in 33 ft (10 m) of seawater (fsw) because of a doubling of the external water pressure. At 99 fsw, or 4 ata, the gas decreases to 25% of original volume, or 1.5 L. The inset figure graphically illustrates the curvilinear relation between lung volume at the surface and depth in seawater. The volume change per unit depth change is greatest nearest the water's surface. The two scuba divers remain in close proximity to the free diver to provide safety and support.

Inspiratory Capacity and Diving Depth

When breathing through a snorkel, the diver inspires air at atmospheric pressure. At a depth of about 3 ft (1 m), the compressive force of water against the chest cavity becomes so large that the inspiratory muscles cannot overcome external pressure and expand thoracic dimensions. This makes inspiration impossible without external air at sufficient pressure to counter the compressive force of water at the particular depth. This reality forms the basis for the use of the scuba apparatus discussed in the section "Scuba Diving."

Snorkel Size and Pulmonary Dead Space

In Chapter 12, we explain that not all inspired air enters the alveoli. Approximately 150 mL of each breath fills the nose, mouth, and other non-diffusible portions of the respiratory tract. The snorkel, an extension of the airways, adds to the volume of the anatomic dead space. Consequently, the ideal snorkel averages about 15 inch (38 cm) in length, with an inside diameter of five eighths to three quarters of an inch to minimize the effects of added dead space and resistance to breathing.[36] Any further increase in snorkel size (or volume)

Training Regimen for Free Diving from a Free Dive Champion

Background: Free diving refers to diving underwater without relying on external breathing devices such as scuba; instead, the diver relies on the ability to breath-hold. Examples include attempts to breath-hold in a swimming pool, spear fishing, underwater photography, and the popular apneic diving where divers try to attain the deepest depth on a single breath. Two world associations govern competitive free diving: AIDA International (International Association for Development of Apnea; **www.aidainternational.org**) and CMAS (World Underwater Federation; **www.cmas.org**). AIDA has established the depth disciplines for the following free diving competitions:

1. **Constant Weight Apnea**: athlete dives to the depth following a guideline they cannot actively use during the dive. "Constant Weight" (French: "*poids constant*") means the athlete cannot drop any diving weights during the dive. The diver can use either bi-fins or a monofin for propulsion.

   - **Constant Weight Apnea Without Fins:** follows the identical rules as Constant Weight but without use of swimming aids (fins).
   - **Free Immersion Apnea:** uses a vertical guide rope to traverse down to depth and return to the surface.
   - **Variable Weight Apnea:** athlete uses a weighted sled for descent (see inset), and returns to the surface by pulling up along a line or swimming while using fins.

2. **No-Limits Apnea:** athlete can use any means of breath-hold diving to depth and return to the surface with a guideline to measure distance. Most divers use a weighted sled to dive down and an inflatable bag to return to the surface.

ANNELLE POMPE, SWEDISH CHAMPION FREE DIVER TRAINING REGIMEN

In addition to free diving, Annelle Pompe (1981-) is an accomplished mountain climber; in 2011 she became the first Swedish woman to climb the north side of Mt. Everest, Tibet (8848 m).

The best way to become a good climber and freediver is of course to climb and freedive. But sooner or later you will reach your limit within equalization, oxygen consumption, squeeze, physical or mental ability. Now it's only for you to determine: which one of these stops you from going higher and deeper?

—Annelle Pompe

Free Diving Competition Merits	Dive Personal Bests[a]	Physical Characteristics
1. New Swedish 72m CWT record 2007	CWT: 87 m	Age: 31
2. World team Champs 2006	FIM: 71 m	Stature: 164 cm
3. 2nd Triple Depth 1 2006 4th women	VAR: 126 m	Body mass: 56 kg ± 3 kg
4. Nordic Deep 2005 1st women	NLT: 102 m	Rest heart rate: 44 ± 3 bpm
5. World Champ individual 2nd	CNF: 42 m DYN: 131 m	Vital capacity: 4.2 L $\dot{V}O_{2max}$: 60.9 mL · kg^{-1} · min^{-1}
	STA: 5.25 min	

Source: http://www.anneliepompe.com/about.html
[a] CWT, Weight Apnea Constant; FIM, Free Immersion Apnea; VAR, Variable weight; NLT, No Limit Apnea; CNF, Constant Weight Apnea. Without Fins; DYN, Dynamic Apnea With Fins; STA, Static Apnea.

Specific Training

Purpose: Train free dive specific arm, trunk, and leg muscles, including the immediate, intermediate, and long-term energy systems. Continue yoga and flexibility training, with emphasis on breath-hold (hypoxic) training of the ventilatory musculature (to tolerate the highest levels of CO_2 possible), and general strengthening exercise as in basic training.

Basic Training

Purpose: Build general trunk and limb strength (basic dynamic strengthening exercises with free weights and closed-kinetic chain exercises), flexibility (yoga with general trunk and limb stretching), and cardio-vascular fitness (indoor and outdoor interval sprint and short distance training including cycling).

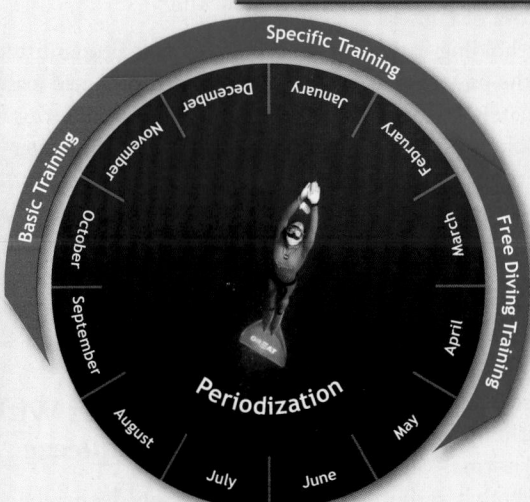

Periodization

Free Diving Training

Purpose: Train free dive specific arm, trunk, and leg muscles, concentrating on the specifics of the dive, particularly the ability to sustain holding one's breath similar to controlled dive conditions that require exquisite control of lung musculature. Continue strength training, including mental control during prolonged apneic overload and overload training of lung muscu-lature, and more specialized breathing control (pranayama yoga; www.freediving.biz/features/breathing.html).

Photos courtesy of and used with permission from Sebastian Naslund, **www.freediving.biz**; Annelie Pompe, **www.anneliepompe.com**

increases anatomic dead space volume, thus encroaching on alveolar ventilation.

Breath-Hold Diving

The duration and depth of a breath-hold dive depends on two factors:

1. Breath-hold duration until arterial carbon dioxide pressure reaches the breath-hold breakpoint
2. Relationship between a diver's total lung capacity (TLC) and residual lung volume (RLV)

A full inspiration of ambient air causes 1 L of oxygen to move into the respiratory passages and lungs. Upon breath hold, 650 mL of oxygen sustains metabolism before partial pressures of arterial oxygen (Po_2) and carbon dioxide (Pco_2) signal the need to renew breathing.[8] With some practice, most persons can breath-hold for up to 1 min, and 2 min represents a typical upper limit.

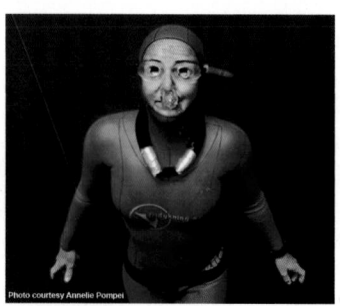

Photo courtesy Annelie Pompel

During this time, arterial Po_2 drops to 60 mm Hg, whereas Pco_2, the most important factor controlling breath holding, rises to 50 mm Hg, signaling an urgency to breathe. Physical activity greatly reduces breath-holding time because oxygen consumption and carbon dioxide production increase with exercise intensity.

Hyperventilation and Breath-Hold Diving: Blackout

Hyperventilation before breath-hold diving extends the breath-hold period; at the same time, the risk to the diver greatly increases. **Blackout** (including shallow water blackout [SWB]; you can read about this condition at **http://shallowwaterblack outprevention.org**) refers to a sudden loss of consciousness, which poses a serious danger in breath-holding activities; it usually afflicts those who try to extend the underwater duration beyond reasonable limits. Unfortunately, SWB also can occur regardless of water depth in any pool, lake, or even when body surfing. A critical reduction in arterial Po_2 (and lowered Pco_2 to the brain with prolonged hyperventilation) can cause blackout, a condition that contributes to a total relaxation of respiratory muscles.

The breakpoint for breath-holding corresponds to an increase in arterial Pco_2 to 50 mm Hg. Some persons can ignore this stimulus and continue breath-holding until arterial carbon dioxide reaches levels that cause severe disorientation and even blackout. When hyperventilation precedes breath hold, arterial Pco_2 decreases from its normal value of 40 mm Hg to 15 mm Hg. Lowering the body's carbon dioxide content before the dive extends the breath-hold duration until arterial Pco_2 increases to a level that stimulates

ventilation. For example, 342 s is the Guinness world record set by German free diver Tom Sietas on June 4, 2012. This represents the longest breath hold recorded while breathing air without prior hyperventilation (**www.dailymail.co.uk/ news/article-2154442/Free-diver-breaks-world-record-holding-breath-underwater-22-22-minutes.html**). Breath holds of 15 to 20 min routinely occur in free divers with hyperventilation followed by several deep breaths of pure oxygen.[22]

Combining hyperventilation, breath-holding, and exercise in the underwater environment poses serious risks. Consider the following scenario: A skin diver hyperventilates at the surface before a dive to reduce arterial Pco_2 to augment breath-hold duration. The diver now takes a full inhalation and descends beneath the water. Alveolar oxygen continually moves into the blood for delivery to active muscles. Owing to previous hyperventilation, arterial carbon dioxide levels remain low, freeing the diver from the urge to breathe. Concurrently, as the diver swims deeper, external water pressure compresses the thorax, increasing gas pressure within this cavity. Increased intrathoracic pressure maintains a relatively high alveolar Po_2. Even though absolute alveolar oxygen quantity decreases as oxygen moves into the blood during the dive, Po_2 continually loads hemoglobin as the dive progresses. When the diver senses the need to breathe from carbon dioxide buildup and begins to ascend, reversals occur in intrathoracic pressure. As water pressure on the thorax decreases with ascent, lung volume expands and alveolar Po_2 decreases to a level where no gradient exists for oxygen diffusion *into* arterial blood. This places the diver in a hypoxic state. Near the surface, alveolar Po_2 reaches levels so low that dissolved oxygen diffuses *from* venous blood returning to the lungs and flows into the alveoli; this causes the diver to suddenly lose consciousness before surfacing.

Additional Considerations. Two additional risks from hyperventilation preceding a breath-hold dive include the following:

1. A normal quantity of arterial carbon dioxide maintains the blood's acid-base balance, mediated by H^+ release as carbonic acid forms from the union of carbon dioxide and water. By reducing the blood's carbon dioxide content through hyperventilation, H^+ concentration decreases, thus increasing pH and alkalinity.
2. Normal arterial Pco_2 stimulates dilation of arterioles in the brain.[27,30] A decrease in arterial carbon dioxide with hyperventilation can reduce cerebral blood flow to produce dizziness or loss of consciousness.

Depths Limits With Breath-Hold Diving: Thoracic Squeeze

Progressing deeper beneath the water subjects the body's air cavities to tremendous compressive forces. Generally, when the lung volume compresses below 1.5 to 1.0 L

IN A PRACTICAL SENSE

Estimating Residual Lung Volume from Age, Stature, and Body Mass

In breath-hold diving, RLV plays a significant role by affecting the depth a diver can achieve without danger of lung squeeze. In fact, the diver's TLC–RLV ratio at the surface generally determines the critical diving depth before lung squeeze.

Laboratory techniques of helium dilution, nitrogen washout, or oxygen dilution routinely measure RLV (see Chapter 12). Each procedure requires complicated and expensive laboratory equipment. An alternative but less valid approach estimates RLV with gender-specific prediction equations based on age, stature, and body mass. The standard error of estimate for predicting RLV ranges between 325 and 500 mL.

RLV PREDICTION EQUATIONS

Variables: Age (y); St, stature (cm); BM, body mass (kg).

Normal-weight males

$$RLV (L) = (0.022 \times Age) + (0.0198 \times St) - (0.015 \times BM) - 1.54$$

Normal-weight females (only age and stature used)

$$RLV (L) = (0.007 \times Age) + (0.0268 \times St) - 3.42$$

Overweight males (%fat ≥25) *and females* (%fat ≥30)

$$RLV (L) = (0.0167 \times Age) + (0.0130 \times BM) + (0.0185 \times St) - 3.3413$$

EXAMPLES

1. Male: age: 21.0 y; body mass: 80 kg; stature: 182.9 cm
$$RLV (L) = (0.022 \times 21) + (0.0198 \times 182.9) - (0.015 \times 80) - 1.54$$
$$= 0.462 + 3.621 - 1.2 - 1.54$$
$$= 1.34 \, L$$

2. Female: age: 19 y; stature: 160.0 cm
$$RLV (L) = (0.007 \times 19) + (0.0268 \times 160.0) - 3.42$$
$$= 0.133 + 4.288 - 3.42$$
$$= 1.00 \, L$$

3. Overweight male: age: 35 y; body mass: 104 kg; stature: 179.5 cm
$$RLV (L) = (0.0167 \times 35) + (0.0130 3 104) + (0.0185 \times 179.5) - 3.3413$$
$$= 0.5845 + 1.352 + 3.321 - 3.3413$$
$$= 1.39 \, L$$

Sources:

Grimby G, Söderholm B. Spirometric studies in normal subjects, III: static lung volumes and maximum ventilatory ventilation in adults with a note on physical fitness. *Acta Med Scand* 1963;2:199.

Miller WCT, et al. Derivation of prediction equations for RV in overweight men and women. *Med Sci Sports Exerc* 1998;30:322.

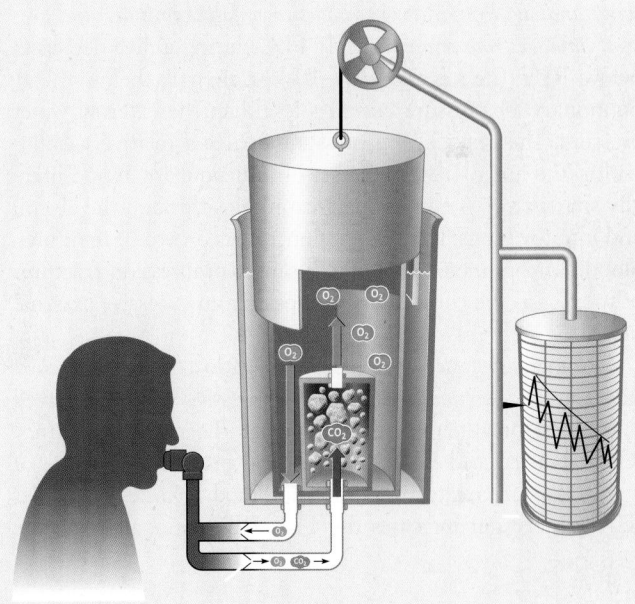

(i.e., to RLV), internal and external pressures fail to equalize and **lung squeeze** occurs. (The "In a Practical Sense: Estimating Residual Lung Volume from Age, Stature, and Body Mass" provides equations to estimate RLV from age, stature, and body mass.) Excessive hydrostatic pressure on pulmonary air volume causes extensive damage to pulmonary tissues.

Commercial breath-hold diving generally does not exceed depths of 100 feet of salt water (fsw), and lung squeeze generally occurs at depths between 150 and 200 fsw. However, individuals show considerable variability in the safe depth for breath-hold diving without danger of lung squeeze. New Zealander William Trubridge (1980-) in 2010 established a world record by swimming to a depth of 100 m (328 ft) on a single breath and with only hands and feet for propulsion. The world record for "no-limits" breath-hold diving depth following a single breath of air for men is an amazing 249.5 m (819 ft), a level below the typical cruising depth of nuclear submarines. The external water pressure against the diver's thoracic cavity at this depth compresses chest girth to less than 20 inches. Austrian Herbert Nitsch (1970-) achieved this remarkable physiologic feat on June 6, 2012, off the coast of the historic Greek island Santorini, but not without serious injury after his ascent. Unconscious, he was brought to the surface by rescue divers after reaching his record-breaking depth. For almost a year afterward no information emerged about the accident or Nitsch's condition. He fully recovered and continues his attempts at achieving an unthinkable "1000-foot dive."

Tanya Streeter (1973-) of the Cayman Islands in 2003 redefined the limits of achievement for a woman by setting the world record for no-limits breath-hold diving when she reached 524 fsw or 160 m. At this depth, the lungs compress to about 1/17th of their normal volume—a real threat to lung collapse. Of the six men and women who have dived to depths deeper than 160 m, two have died during sled diving (use of a weighed sled for descent and an inflatable bag to return to the surface), with four serious cases of decompression sickness (http://freediving.biz/nolimit/).

The ratio of the diver's TLC to RLV at the surface generally determines the critical diving depth before lung squeeze; this ratio typically averages 4:1 at the surface. For example, for a diver with a 6.0-L TLC and a 1.5-L RLV, Boyle's law predicts that TLC would compress to RLV at 30 m or 4 ata external pressure. *No danger from lung squeeze exists if lung volume remains greater than RLV because sufficient air remains in the lungs and rigid respiratory passages to equalize pressure and prevent damage from compression.* If TLC during a dive decreases below RLV (i.e., if the TLV–RLV ratio falls below 1.00), pulmonary air pressure becomes less than the external water pressure. The unequalized pressure creates a relative vacuum within the lungs. In severe cases of lung squeeze, blood literally spurts from the pulmonary capillaries through the alveoli and into the lungs. In this situation, divers drown in their own blood. Further increases in depth cause compression fractures of the ribs as the chest cavity collapses from excessive external pressure.

In many instances, the TLV–RLV ratio at the surface considerably *underestimates* the actual impressive depths achieved by trained breath-hold divers. Part of the explanation may relate to a reduced RLV as immersion progresses because of a shift toward greater intrathoracic blood volume. A smaller RLV underwater increases the TLV–RLV ratio, allowing the

individual to increase maximal depth before reaching the critical ratio.

Other Problems. If pressures within internal air spaces do not continually equalize with external hydrostatic pressures, problems other than lung squeeze limit the depth of a breath-hold dive. For example, if air at ambient pressure remains trapped within the middle ear from inflamed tissue or a mucous plug and cannot equilibrate with air in the lungs, external hydrostatic pressure forces the eardrum inward and it ruptures. A ruptured eardrum frequently occurs at relatively shallow depths.

The sinus cavities also present difficulty for skin divers. Air compressed in the lungs by the external force of water attempts to move into the paranasal sinuses. Sinuses inflamed and irritated from infection provide extremely narrow openings that hinder sinus space equilibration with pressure changes in the respiratory tract. Failure to equilibrate creates a relative vacuum in the sinus cavities that distorts their tissues' shape and causes intense sinus pain. With severe disequilibrium, fluid and blood move into the sinuses to fill the vacuum.

Diving Reflex in Humans

Physiologic responses to immersion, collectively termed the ***diving reflex***, enable diving mammals to spend considerable time underwater. These four responses include:

1. Bradycardia
2. Decreased cardiac output
3. Increased peripheral vasoconstriction
4. Lactate accumulation in underperfused muscle

A modified diving response also has been described for humans during face immersion, breath-hold face immersion, and dives to modest depths.[1,13,17,23] The research has primarily documented increased vagal activity that induces bradycardia in humans during face immersion and diving, particularly in cool and cold water. Elevated blood lactate concentration during breath-hold dives to 65 m at energy expenditures only slightly above rest also suggests a diving-mediated peripheral vasoconstriction that decreases blood flow (oxygen supply) to skeletal muscles and compromises performance.[12]

Some research has expanded findings on blood lactate concentration to include hemodynamic aspects of breath-hold diving in thermoneutral and cool water by elite divers to depths of 40 to 55 m. FIGURE 26.2A illustrates the responses for one diver during descent to 40 m, bottom stay, and ascent (depth indicated by *green line*) in water at 25°C and 35°C. The electrocardiographic tracing (FIG. 26.2B) shows the longest R–R interval recorded during the cool-water dive. After an initial tachycardia, bradycardia rapidly ensued and became most pronounced in cool water, where heart rate decreased to 16 b·min⁻¹ near the bottom. Because stroke volume did not change appreciably during the dive, lower heart rates reduced cardiac output (yellow line). Output decreased to a low of 3 L·min⁻¹ (25°C [77°F]) compared with the value of 6.4 L·min⁻¹ at the surface. A large number of diverse arrhythmic

Mammalian Adaptation to Deep-Depth Dives

Seals and whales that descend to great depths on a single breath of air have evolved special adaptations for survival. Based on sonar readings, the endangered sperm whale, with a length of up to 65 ft and a weight of 40 to 50 tons, reportedly dives to 3300 ft (1000 m) in about 27 min. At this depth, the pressure on the animal exceeds 3500 psi. Some estimates indicate that a typical dive lasts 90 min while the whale searches for about 900 kg of fish and squid daily, with extended breath-hold times to 120 min. Whales cruise the oceans at about 23 miles (37 km) per hour. Apparently, these aquatic mammals have more elastic chest cavities than humans; their lungs, even when reduced, do not separate from the chest wall, and their bodies adapt to use the oxygen in the bloodstream with high efficiency (**www.ftexploring.com/askdrg/askdrgalapagos2.html; www.britannica.com/EBchecked/topic/559395/sperm-whale**).

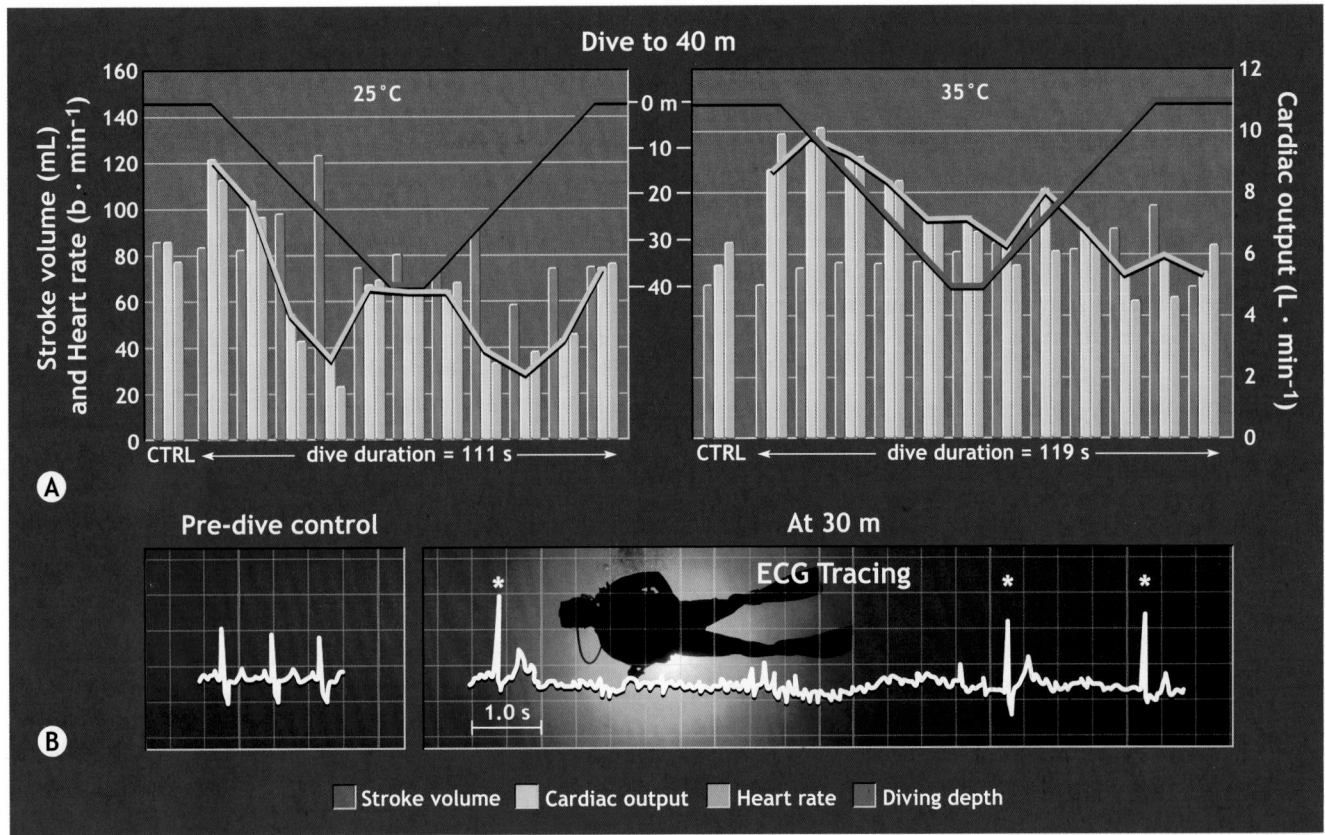

FIGURE 26.2 • **(A)** Heart rate, stroke volume, and cardiac output for an elite breath-hold diver throughout a dive to 40 m (131 ft) in warm (35°C [95°F]) and cool (25°C [77°F]) water. Green line, diving depth in relation to time; yellow line, cardiac output throughout the dive; CTRL, control measures prior to dive. **(B)** Electrocardiographic tracing (see Fig. 16.2 in Chapter 16) showing longest R-R interval during the dive in 25°C water. (*), QRS complex during the dive. (Adapted with permission from Ferrigno M, et al. Cardiovascular changes during deep breath-hold dives in a pressure chamber. *J Appl Physiol* 1997;83:1282.)

beats, often more frequent than true sinus beats, accompanied bradycardia, mainly in the cool-water dives. Arterial blood pressure increased suddenly and dramatically, reaching 280/200 and 290/150 mm Hg in two divers. This hypertensive response reflected overall peripheral vasoconstriction; the large increase in blood lactate concentrations reflected increased anaerobic metabolism.

The intense cardiovascular responses to breath-hold diving in elite divers resembles response patterns of diving mammals.[21,26] The occurrence of arrhythmias and large increases in blood pressure probably reflects species differences and less perfect human adaptation.

SCUBA DIVING

The discussion of snorkeling emphasized that at depths below 1 m, inspiratory muscle power cannot overcome the compressive force of water against the thoracic cavity. Air under pressure from an external source to promote inspiratory action counteracts the external hydrostatic force. The modern **self-contained underwater breathing apparatus (scuba)**, principally developed in 1943 by French oceanographer/ecologist/researcher Jacques-Yves Cousteau (1910–1997; www.cousteau.org) and Emile Gagnan (1915–2003; www.scubahalloffame.com/

hallmembers/2000/emilegagnan.html), represents the most common apparatus to supply air under pressure for complete independence from the surface. *Sport divers should use only this form of scuba*. The scuba system, strapped to the diver's chest or back, includes a tank of compressed air and a demand regulator valve that delivers air the diver needs at a particular depth with hose and mouthpiece or full face mask. Two basic scuba designs exist:

1. Common **open-circuit system**
2. **Closed-circuit system**, used primarily for clandestine military operations and special applications that require mixed gases

Underwater commercial operations frequently apply surface-demand diving techniques in operations below a 50-m depth. This approach supplies air directly from a compressor at the surface to the diver via a direct reinforced hose. German-born British engineer/inventor Augustus Siebe (1788–1872; www.divinghelmet.nl/divinghelmet/1839_Augustus_Siebe.html) provided the original design for this system in 1819. His design consisted of a copper helmet (hard hat) riveted to a leather jacket, with air delivered continuously from the surface. The excess supplied air and the diver's expired air bubbled out from the bottom of the jacket. If the diver moved substantially from the vertical position, water would rush in through the bottom of the jacket and fill the headpiece. Siebe modified this design in 1837 (Siebe's early diving suit is pictured in "Chronology of Selected Events in Diving History," earlier in this chapter); he constructed a full waterproof diving suit bolted to a breastplate and helmet that allowed a diver to work in any position because the suit encapsulated the entire body. Valves admitted air through the diver's helmet as needed, and expired air exited the helmet also through valves.[20] Siebe's "closed" diving helmet allowed divers to dive safely to depths previously impossible to attain.

Open-Circuit Scuba

Figure 26.3 illustrates the typical open-circuit scuba system for submerged swimming with neutral buoyancy in relatively shallow water. For most diving purposes, the steel or aluminum tanks (lightweight titanium that withstands high pressures is also used) contain 2000 L (70–80 ft³) of air compressed to about 3000 psi; deeper and longer exposures require 3500 L (120 ft³) of compressed air. One tank supplies enough air for a 0.5- to 1-hr dive to moderate depths. The start of inspiration creates a slight negative pressure. This opens the demand valve and releases air to the diver at a pressure nearly equal to the water's external pressure. The positive pressure created with exhalation closes the inspiratory valves and discharges the exhaled air into the water. The scuba gear contains gauges that continually monitor tank pressure and diving depth.

Open-circuit scuba presents several drawbacks. The air exhaled into the water generally contains approximately 17%

oxygen, so the open-circuit system "wastes" about 75% of the total oxygen in the tank. In addition, the diver requires a considerable mass of air at increased depths to provide tidal volume for adequate pulmonary ventilation. As an extreme example, inhalation of a 5-L volume at 300 fsw or 90 m requires the equivalent of 50 L of air at sea level!

This dramatic effect of pressure on air volume greatly limits the time one can remain at great depth before depleting the scuba tank's air. Factors that influence energy cost of swimming underwater and thus pulmonary ventilation include gender (lower in women than in men), gear and number of tanks (25% higher with two tanks), fin type (flexible fin lower than rigid fin), and diver's experience (lower in advanced divers).[29] Diving tanks contain moisture-free compressed air, making each breath produce heat and moisture loss as the inspired air warms and humidifies on its passage down the respiratory tract. This causes substantial body heat loss during prolonged diving. To counter heat loss, the diver breathes a *heated* gas mixture of compressed helium-oxygen to avoid hypothermia during deep diving (see "Helium-Oxygen Mixtures," later in this chapter).

Figure 26.4 shows the theoretical air time limits for a diver who performs similar work at various underwater depths. These time limits for "bottom time" (red dashed line) and time for descent plus time on the bottom (yellow solid line) assume a completely filled standard compressed air tank and ascent and descent at 60 ft per minute. For example, a single aluminum tank that contains 80 ft³ of air compressed to 3000 psi normally sustains an 80-min dive near the surface. At a depth of 10 m, this tank supplies enough air for about 40 min, whereas at 3 ata (20 m), dive duration decreases by one third, to 27 min. These time limits vary with the diver's body size, type and intensity of physical activity, fitness level, and diving experience, all of which affect exercise energy cost and ventilatory volumes.

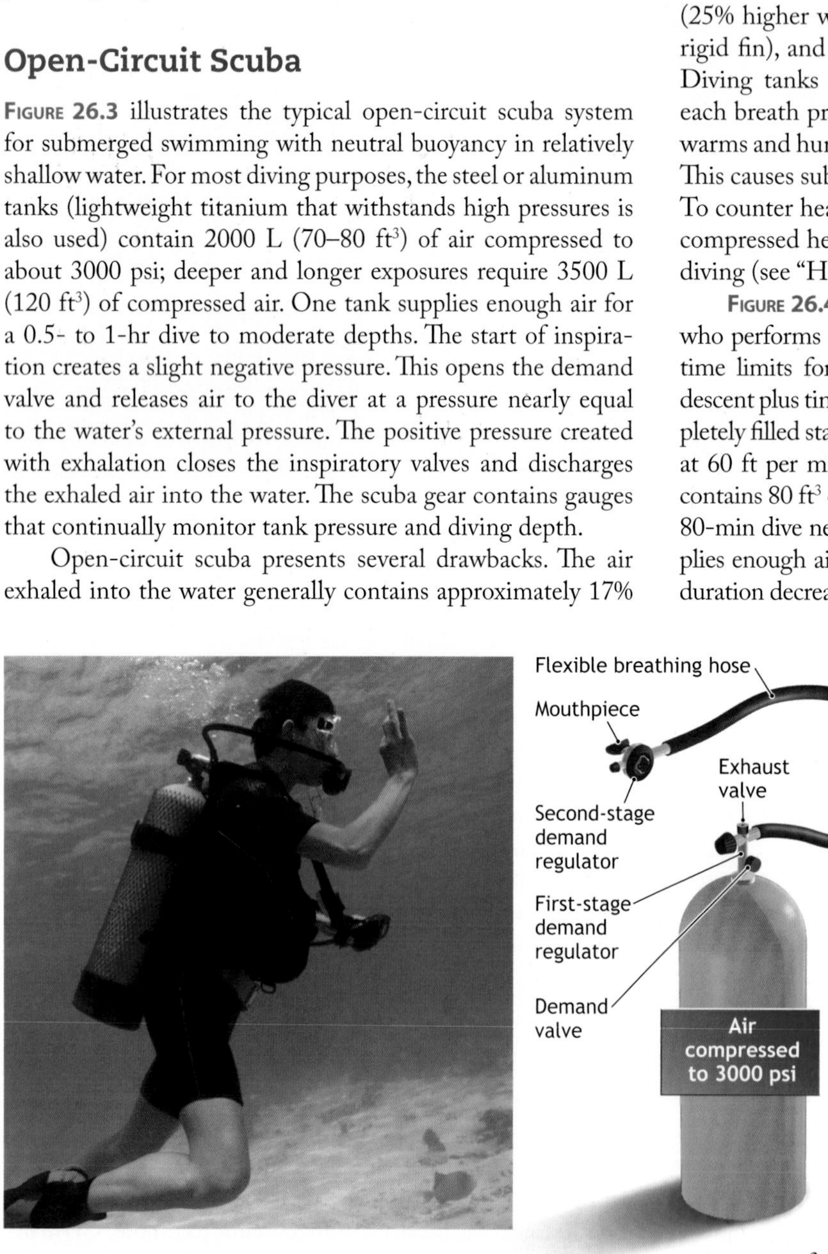

The **wet suit**, the most common protective garment worn by recreational scuba divers and surfers, counters cold stress during diving. This garment, constructed of air-impregnated rubber (usually foam neoprene), traps water against the diver's skin, which warms to body temperature to provide the insulatory boundary. The suit, filled with thousands of tiny gas bubbles, provides insulation. Wet suits generally furnish sufficient thermal protection for relatively short dives, even in ice water. For longer dives in moderately cold water (17–18.5°C [63–65°F]), a full wet suit offers insufficient thermal protection.[4] Compression of the wet suit as the diver descends progressively diminishes the suit's insulating properties.

The modern **dry suit**—made from foam neoprene, crushed neoprene, vulcanized rubber, or heavy-duty nylon with laminated waterproof materials, and often worn over insulating garments—maximizes protection from cold stress. This protective clothing ensemble keeps the diver dry; has

FIGURE 26.3 • General design of an open-circuit scuba unit. Compressed air flows through a two-stage regulator valve that reduces tank pressure to a near breathable pressure at a specific depth and releases air to the diver on demand at pressure equal to "ambient" so the diver breathes without difficulty.

Labels in figure:
Flexible breathing hose
Mouthpiece
Exhaust valve
Second-stage demand regulator
First-stage demand regulator
Demand valve
Air compressed to 3000 psi

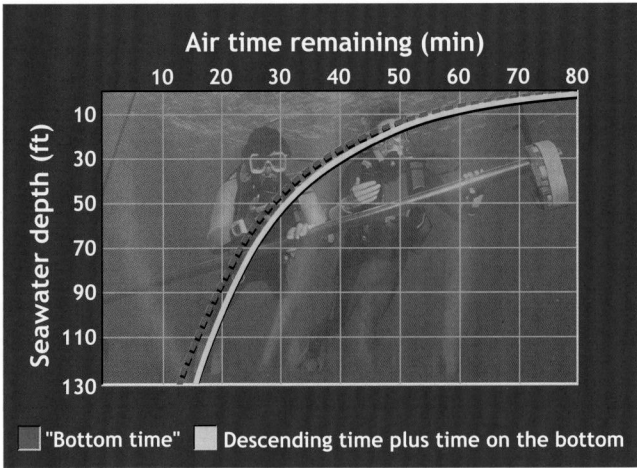

FIGURE 26.4 • Theoretical air time for a single tank containing 80 cubic ft of air. The yellow line includes the time spent descending at a rate of 60 ft · min⁻¹ plus time on the bottom; dashed line, only "bottom time."

seals at the neck, wrists, and ankles; and has a waterproof zipper to prevent water from entering the suit. Dry-suit underwear traps a layer of air between the diver and the water for additional insulation. Layering of underwear adjusts insulation to water temperature.

Closed-Circuit Scuba

The need for shallow diving maneuvers during World War II produced a new diving form that used rebreathing of pure oxygen and absorption of carbon dioxide within a closed system. The closed-circuit underwater breathing apparatus operates similarly to the closed-circuit spirometer described in Chapter 8. A small cylinder feeds pure oxygen into a bellows or bag from which the diver breathes. The breathing bag acts as a pressure regulator. Valves in the breathing mask direct the exhaled gas through a carbon dioxide–absorbing canister that contains soda lime; the carbon dioxide–free gas then passes back to the diver. The oxygen cylinder replenishes the oxygen consumed in energy metabolism, allowing the diver to continually rebreathe oxygen, the only gas removed from the breathing bag. A small oxygen cylinder sustains the submerged diver for 3 hr or longer. Because no expired air releases into the water, the system provides a near-silent and bubble-free operation for clandestine activities. **FIGURE 26.5** illustrates a closed-circuit scuba design currently used by the U.S. Navy that requires only a single cylinder of compressed oxygen shown in green. The other type of closed-circuit system uses mixed gas: one bottle of pure oxygen and a second bottle of a mixed gas containing helium and oxygen (**heliox**) or nitrogen and oxygen (**nitrox**; see "Dives to Exceptional Depths: Mixed-Gas Diving," later in this chapter).

The closed-circuit system requires a high level of proficiency for safe use. Two main problems exist with its use. First, a serious medical emergency occurs if carbon dioxide output exceeds its rate of absorption or if absorption fails altogether.

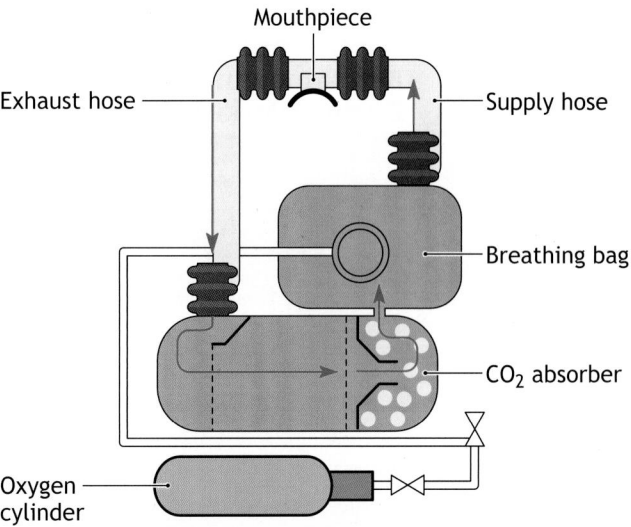

FIGURE 26.5 • General design of a closed-circuit scuba system used by the U.S. Navy. A small cylinder of pure oxygen feeds into a bellows or bag from which the diver breathes. The breathing bag acts as a pressure regulator. Valves in the breathing mask direct the exhaled gas through a CO_2- absorbing canister containing soda lime; the CO_2-free gas then passes back to the diver. The oxygen cylinder replenishes oxygen consumed in metabolism. *Arrows* indicate direction of airflow.

With a faulty rebreathing system, the diver may not receive warning symptoms, becoming anesthetized by arterial carbon dioxide buildup, with drowning as the end result. Second, high concentrations of inspired oxygen, particularly when breathed under high pressures beneath the water, produce a variety of adverse effects on physiologic functions, particularly those related to the central nervous system. These problems remain minimal if the depth–time limits do not exceed the recommendations in **TABLE 26.3**. Closed-circuit oxygen breathing generally should not exceed a maximum depth of 25 fsw and definitely should not exceed 50 fsw; at that point, oxygen poisoning produces a high risk of central nervous system seizures. Minimal risk usually exists in military diving because most clandestine operations require swimming underwater in relatively shallow depths to avoid detection at night. Decompression sickness does not pose a problem because no inert gas absorption occurs when rebreathing pure oxygen. The increased resistance to breathing and the generally large dead space common with the closed-circuit system limit intense physical work.

SPECIAL PROBLEMS WITH BREATHING GASES AT HIGH PRESSURES

Henry's law (first proposed in 1803 by English physician and chemist William Henry [1734–1816) states that the quantity of gas dissolved in a liquid at a given temperature varies directly with two factors:

1. Pressure differential between the gas and the liquid
2. Gas solubility in the liquid

TABLE 28.3 U.S. Navy–Recommended Depth-Time Limits Breathing Pure Oxygen During Working Dives[a]

Normal Operations		
Depth		
(ft)	(m)	Time (min)
10	3.0	240
15	4.6	150
20	6.1	150
25	7.6	75
Exceptional Operations		
Depth		
(ft)	(m)	Time (min)
30	9.2	45
35	10.7	20
40	12.2	10

[a]No symptoms of oxygen poisoning were noted at these depths and durations.

Underwater breathing systems must supply air, oxygen, or other gas mixtures at sufficient pressure to overcome the force of water against the diver's thorax. For example, at 3 ata (20-m depth) the respired gas requires delivery at approximately 2280 mm Hg (3 × 760 mm Hg), whereas gas delivery at 60 m requires a pressure of 5320 mm Hg. The material that follows considers the specific dynamics of breathing gases at high pressures and their effects on physiologic functions. We also examine the physical responses of a gas to abrupt changes in pressure. FIGURE 26.6 summarizes the main hazards of scuba diving posed by improper equalization of pressure within the body's air spaces and diving mask to changes in external pressure.

Air Embolism

An air volume breathed underwater expands in direct proportion to the reduction in external pressure as the diver ascends to the surface. Air breathed at a depth of 10 m doubles in volume if brought to the surface. If normal breathing continues during ascent, the expanding air vents freely through the nose and mouth. If a diver takes a full breath at 10 m but fails to exhale while ascending, the rapidly expanding gas eventually ruptures the lungs before the diver reaches the surface. **Lung burst** becomes a real possibility in scuba diving. Many inexperienced divers react to a perceived underwater danger by filling their lungs and then holding their breath while swimming rapidly to the surface. This particular diving hazard does not necessarily require a deep dive. Accidents caused by breath-hold ascent with scuba frequently occur in shallow dives; changes in pressure exert the greatest effect on the expanding lung volume near the water surface (see

inset box in Fig. 26.1). *Inhaling a full breath of compressed air in 6 ft of water causes serious overdistension of lung tissue if the diver fails to exhale during ascent.* Fatal air embolism can occur in swimming pools as shallow as 8 ft for an inexperienced scuba diver. Air embolism from pulmonary barotrauma ranks second only to drowning as a cause of death among recreational scuba divers.

If expansion of air in the respiratory tract causes lung tissue to rupture during ascent from underwater—from either breath-holding or pulmonary obstruction (bronchospasm, excessive pulmonary secretions, or bronchial inflammation)—air bubbles or **emboli** enter the pulmonary venous system (www.rightdiagnosis.com/a/air_embolism/intro.htm). Emboli then flow to the heart and enter the systemic circulation. The diver usually maintains a head-up, vertical position on ascent; consequently, the air bubbles move upward in the body. Eventually, they lodge in the small arterioles or capillaries and restrict blood supply to vital tissue. General symptoms of air embolism include confusion, weakness, dizziness, and blurred vision. Severe blockage of pulmonary, coronary, and cerebral circulation causes collapse, unconsciousness, and frequently death. Effective treatment for air embolism requires rapid decompression to reduce bubble size and force them into solution to open the plugged vessels. Even with rapid, expert treatment, 16% of air embolism victims die (www.encyclopedia.com/topic/Embolism.aspx).

Pneumothorax: Lung Collapse

Air forced through the alveoli when lung tissue ruptures sometimes migrates laterally to burst through the pleural sac that covers the lungs. In about 10% of cases of this form of pulmonary barotrauma, an air pocket forms in the chest cavity outside the lungs, between the chest wall and lung itself. Continued expansion of trapped air during ascent collapses the ruptured lung, a condition called *pneumothorax*. Pneumothorax treatment often requires surgical intervention with a syringe to extract the air pocket (www.muschealth.com/video/Default.aspx?videoId=10204&cId=38&type=rel).

To eliminate the danger of air embolism and pneumothorax, instructors teach divers to ascend slowly and breathe normally when using scuba gear (www.ncbi.nlm.nih.gov/pubmedhealth/PMH0001151/). The diver's lungs also must remain free from any disease that could lead to air trapping (e.g., chronic obstructive pulmonary disease). Air trapping creates difficulty equalizing alveolar pressure and external pressure during ascent.

Facemask "Squeeze"

Air in a facemask or goggles before a dive equals ambient air pressure at the surface. As the diver progresses deeper, a considerable pressure differential develops between the inside and outside of the mask to create a relative vacuum within the mask. For example,

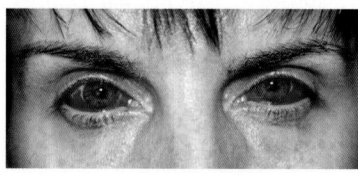

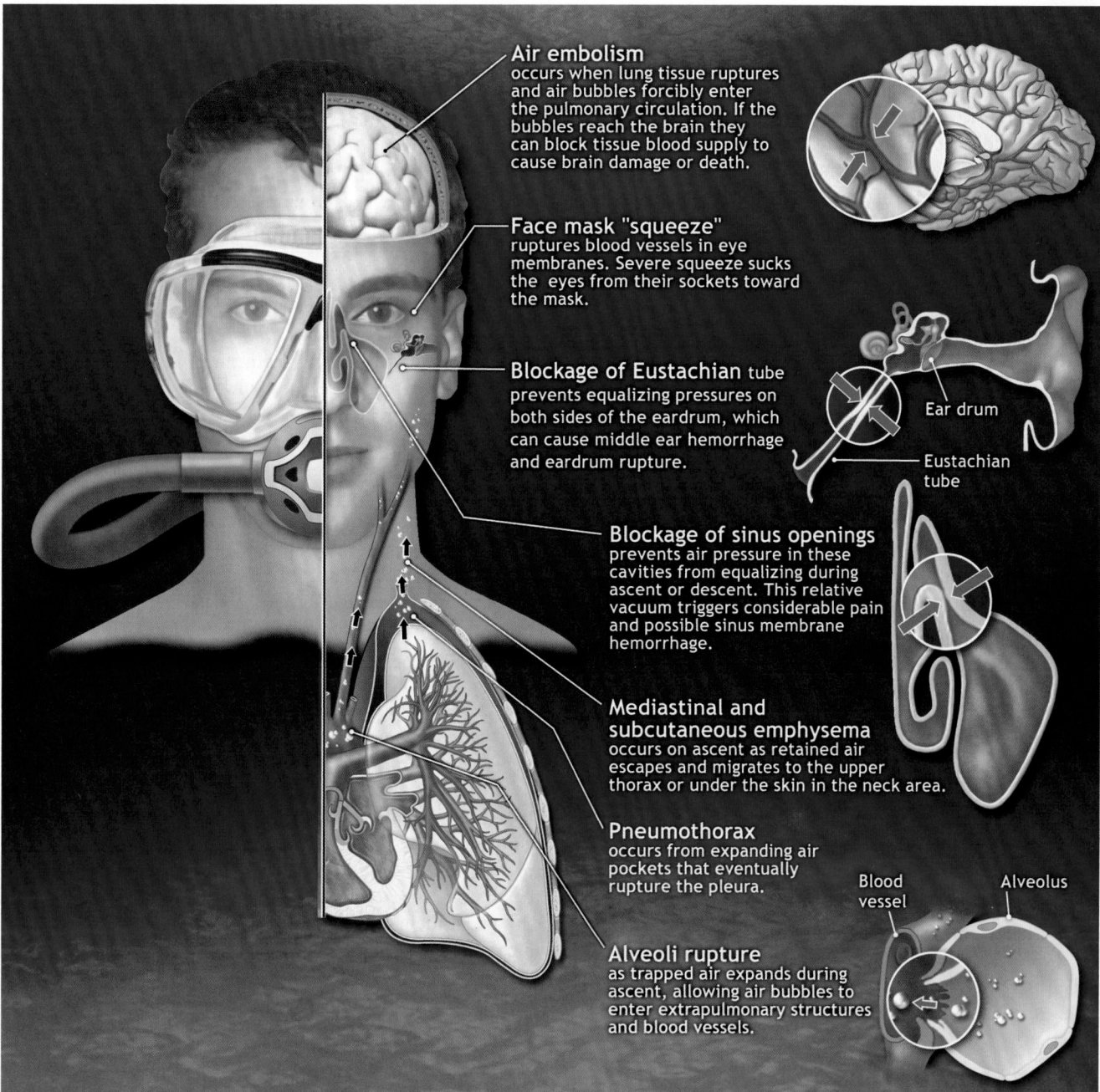

Air embolism
occurs when lung tissue ruptures and air bubbles forcibly enter the pulmonary circulation. If the bubbles reach the brain they can block tissue blood supply to cause brain damage or death.

Face mask "squeeze"
ruptures blood vessels in eye membranes. Severe squeeze sucks the eyes from their sockets toward the mask.

Blockage of Eustachian tube
prevents equalizing pressures on both sides of the eardrum, which can cause middle ear hemorrhage and eardrum rupture.

Ear drum

Eustachian tube

Blockage of sinus openings
prevents air pressure in these cavities from equalizing during ascent or descent. This relative vacuum triggers considerable pain and possible sinus membrane hemorrhage.

Mediastinal and subcutaneous emphysema
occurs on ascent as retained air escapes and migrates to the upper thorax or under the skin in the neck area.

Pneumothorax
occurs from expanding air pockets that eventually rupture the pleura.

Blood vessel

Alveolus

Alveoli rupture
as trapped air expands during ascent, allowing air bubbles to enter extrapulmonary structures and blood vessels.

FIGURE 26.6 • Scuba diving hazards from failure to equalize internal and external gas pressures.

wearing swimming goggles to improve vision and protect the eyes from irritants during a dive beneath the water can cause the eyes to bulge or squeeze from their sockets.

This leads to capillary rupture and hemorrhage of the eyes and surrounding soft tissue. The squeeze effect occurs because most goggles are constructed from rigid materials. Displacement of the eye and surrounding soft tissue into the air space between the eye and the goggles provides the only means to equalize the difference in air pressure between the goggle space and external water pressure during breath-hold diving (www.diversalertnetwork.org/medical/faq/Mask_Squeeze). As newer pools with separate diving areas reach depths of

14 ft (4.3 m), goggles pose a distinct risk to swimmers who dive to this depth.

Breath-hold diving with a facemask that covers the eyes and nose represents a somewhat different situation than diving with only swim goggles. Air pressure within the mask that covers the eyes and nose readily equalizes to external water pressure as air flows freely between the nasal passages and the lungs' relatively large air volume. In breath-hold diving, air in the lungs compresses and passes through the nose to equalize mask pressure. With scuba, inspired air automatically adjusts to the external water pressure. Periodically exhaling through the nose into the mask balances pressures on both sides of the facemask.

Blockage of Eustachian Tube: Middle-Ear Squeeze

Divers often encounter problems equalizing pressure within the air space of the Eustachian tubes (the passages that connect the middle ear with the back of the throat).[38] These relatively narrow, mucus-lined channels generally resist air flow. In healthy individuals, the tubes remain clear and changes in external pressure against the eardrum equalize by pressure changes transmitted from the lungs through the tubes. In skin and scuba diving (and air travel in nonpressurized aircraft), middle-ear pressure equalizes with external pressure by blowing gently against closed nostrils. Swallowing, yawning, or moving the jaws from side to side also helps to "pop" the ears.

thePoint   Appendix H, available online at http://thepoint. lww.com/mkk8e, provides a list of supplemental animations and videos on this subject.

In upper-respiratory tract infection, the Eustachian tube membranes swell and produce mucus that can plug cranial air passages. The greatest difficulty involves equalizing middle-ear pressure during descent because an equal force from the ear canal does not readily match the pressure change against the eardrum's outer surface. The magnitude of pressure changes in diving considerably exceed those experienced in air travel. Divers can suffer severe pain only a few feet underwater because the eardrum stretches and moves inward toward the plugged canal. Further pressure disequilibrium creates a relative vacuum in the middle ear that hemorrhages tissues. Complete blockage of the Eustachian tubes can rupture the eardrum, forcing water into the middle ear as pressure equalizes.

Never Use Earplugs. *WARNING—Never wear earplugs while diving!* During a dive, the external water pressure pushes the earplug deep into the external ear canal. A pocket of ambient air trapped between the plug and eardrum can rupture the eardrum outward during descent.

Aerosinusitis

Inflamed, congested sinuses prevent air pressure in these cavities from equalizing during diving. Sinus air pressure that does not equalize during descent remains at atmospheric pressure while external pressure increases. This relative vacuum creates "sinus squeeze," causing sinus membranes to bleed as blood occupies the space to equalize the pressure differential.[28]

Nitrogen Narcosis: "Rapture of the Deep"

The total pressure of the respired gas during diving increases in direct proportion to diving depth. Likewise, the partial pressure of each gas in the breathing mixture increases: at 10 m, the nitrogen partial pressure doubles the sea-level value to 1200 mm Hg. With each additional 10-m depth, nitrogen partial pressure increases by 600 mm Hg—inspired P_{N_2} equals 4200 mm Hg at a 60 m depth. At each successive depth, the gradient increases for the net flow of nitrogen across the alveolar membrane into the blood and eventually into all tissue fluids for equilibration. At 20 m, all tissues eventually contain three times more nitrogen as before the dive. Tissue perfusion, tissue solubility coefficients, body composition, and temperature all influence nitrogen uptake at the tissue level.

Three-hundred fsw is generally set as the limit for compressed air diving because dissolved nitrogen accumulation in the body's fluids and tissues renders all but the most experienced divers incapable of accomplishing meaningful work. The U.S. Navy sets the maximum operating depth at 190 fsw for breathing compressed air (www.ndc.noaa.gov/dp_forms.html). In 1935, Dr. Albert Behnke (see Chapter 28) and coworkers discovered for the first time that the increase in inspired nitrogen pressure while breathing compressed air during diving produced a narcotic effect characterized by a general state of euphoria similar to alcohol intoxication, termed *rapture of the deep*. Dissolved nitrogen at a depth of 30 m (98 ft) produces effects similar to those felt after consuming alcohol on an empty stomach. Divers often speak of "Martini's Law." This well-known dictum states that every 50 ft (15.2 m) of seawater produces effects equal to drinking 1 dry martini on an empty stomach. As a rough estimate, this would mean a diver at 200 ft (61 m) experiences intoxication from pressurized nitrogen equal to four martinis! Eventually, high nitrogen levels produce a numbing, anesthetic effect on the central nervous system.

The term **nitrogen narcosis**, or "inert gas narcosis," collectively describes these mimicking effects of intoxication. The term was first coined by Jacques Cousteau (1910–1997; www.cousteau.org) in his 1953 book, *The Silent World*. Cousteau's partner Frederic Dumas was diving to about 240 ft in the Mediterranean Sea. The following quote from Dumas was the first widely read description of the intoxicating effect of breathing nitrogen under pressure.

> I'm anxious about that line, but I really feel wonderful. I have a queer feeling of the beatitude. I am drunk and carefree. My ears buzz and my mouth tastes bitter. The current staggers me as though I had too many drinks. I [have] forgotten Jacques and the people in the boats. My eyes are tired. I lower on down, trying to think about the bottom, but I can't. I'm going to sleep, but I can't fall asleep in such dizziness.

At the extreme, mental processes deteriorate so that a diver may feel that the scuba serves little purpose and remove it or swim deeper instead of toward the surface (www.ndc.noaa.gov/dp_forms.html).

Nitrogen diffuses slowly into body tissues so the narcosis effect depends on dive depth and duration. Considerable individual variation exists for nitrogen sensitivity, but a mild narcosis usually appears after an hour or more at 30 to 40 m (98 to 131 ft)—the maximum recommended depth for recreational scuba divers. Treatment requires that the diver ascend to a shallower depth, where complete recovery usually occurs rapidly. The precise role of body fatness in nitrogen narcosis remains controversial.

Decompression Sickness

With rapid ascent, the external pressure against the diver's body decreases dramatically. Excess dissolved nitrogen in the body tissues begins to separate from the dissolved state; it eventually forms bubbles in the tissues, an effect not unlike the appearance of carbon dioxide bubbles when removing the cap from a carbonated beverage bottle. With the cap in place, gas remains dissolved under pressure. Removing the cap suddenly reduces pressure above the fluid, causing bubbles to form. *Decompression sickness occurs when dissolved nitrogen moves out of solution and forms bubbles in body tissues and fluids.* It results from ascending to the surface too rapidly following a deep, prolonged dive, often made possible with double and triple air tanks.

the**Point** Appendix H, available online at http://thepoint. lww.com/mkk8e, provides a list of supplemental animations and videos on this subject.

Nitrogen reaches equilibrium slowly in many tissues, particularly fatty tissues, so it leaves the body slowly.[18,40] This means that women (with greater average percentage body fat than men) and overfat men face greater risk for decompression sickness. FIGURE 26.7 compares nitrogen elimination after a simulated "dive" by two dogs differing in fat content. The dog with relatively high body fat content (*yellow line*) eliminated considerably more nitrogen over the 4-hr decompression than the dog with lower body fat.

The term *bends*, a synonym for decompression sickness, was coined during construction of piers for the Brooklyn Bridge (1869–1883) to reflect the bent-over position of limping workers who emerged from the pressurized caisson. The following poignantly describes the time course and fatal consequences of decompression sickness in an early history of this malady[39]:

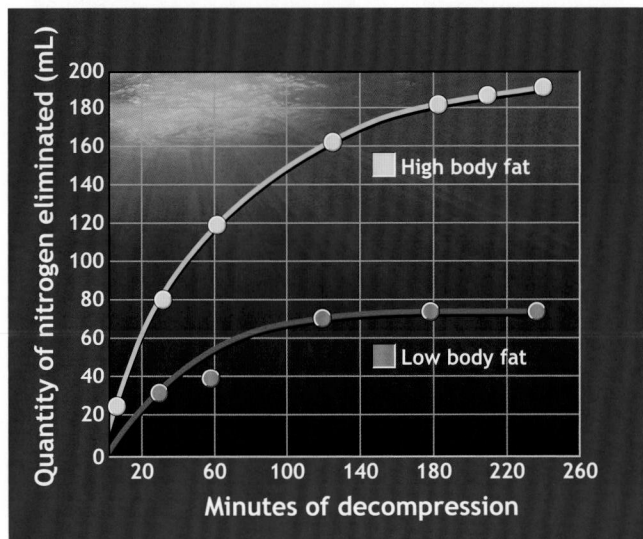

FIGURE 26.7 • Nitrogen elimination from body tissues of a relatively lean dog and one higher in body fat during decompression in a chamber. (Courtesy of Dr. A. R. Behnke.)

In 1900 ... a Royal Navy diver descended to 150 fsw in 40 minutes, spent 40 minutes at depth searching for a torpedo, and ascended to the surface in 20 minutes without apparent difficulty. Ten minutes later, he complained of abdominal pain and fainted. His breathing was labored, he was cyanotic, and he died after 7 minutes. An autopsy the next day revealed the organs to be healthy, but gas was present in the liver, spleen, heart, cardiac veins, venous, subcutaneous, and cerebral veins and ventricles.

Nitrogen Elimination: Zero Decompression Limits

Diving at a depth of 30 m (98 ft) for up to 30 min represents the time limit before sufficient nitrogen dissolves to pose danger from decompression sickness. About 18 min is the limit at 40 m (131 ft), and one can spend almost an hour at 20 m without danger from decompression sickness. If a diver exceeds the depth–duration recommendations for compressed air diving shown in FIGURE 26.8 in the area to the right of the yellow line, the ascent to the surface must progress in a preestablished manner. With this approach, a recreational or commercial diver ascends at a prescribed, relatively slow rate designed not to require stops. This rate of ascent enables all excess dissolved nitrogen to diffuse from the tissues into the blood and escape through the lungs without bubbles forming. Contrary to conventional wisdom, exercise before diving or during decompression does not increase the number of bubbles or magnify the risk of decompression sickness.[10] In fact, a period of mild continuous exercise (30% $\dot{V}O_{2max}$) during a 3-min decompression period may reduce postdive formation of gas bubbles.[9]

Stage decompression requires the diver to make one or more stops on ascent to the surface. The time required for the slowest tissue compartment to lose sufficient nitrogen to allow ascent to the next depth determines the duration of such pauses (termed *stage-decompression stops*). For example, a dive to 30 m (98 ft) for 50 min requires one 2-min decompression stop at 6 m (20 ft) and a 24-min stop at 3 m (10 ft). Surface stage decompression involves transfer of the diver from the water (after several in-water stops) to a decompression chamber at the surface. The judicious use of a hyperoxic breathing mixture facilitates recompression.

A conservative approach recommends that the sport diver not exceed a 20- to 25-m (66–82 ft) depth (30 m [98 ft] maximum). During single or repetitive dives, the diver should never approach the time limits indicated by the decompression tables. The recommendations in Figure 26.8 assume a single dive, with a minimum of 12 hr between dives. For repeated dives within 12 hr, the diver must consult the appropriate repetitive dive decompression schedules.[36,37] These recommendations account for the residual nitrogen remaining in the body at the start of the next dive if it occurs within the 12-hr period. Interestingly, air travel within 24 hr of scuba diving increases risk of decompression sickness because commercial airlines usually pressurize cabins to an equivalent altitude of 7000 ft. This further reduction in ambient atmospheric pressure may initiate bubble formation from excess nitrogen dissolved in body tissues during the prior preflight dive(s).[19]

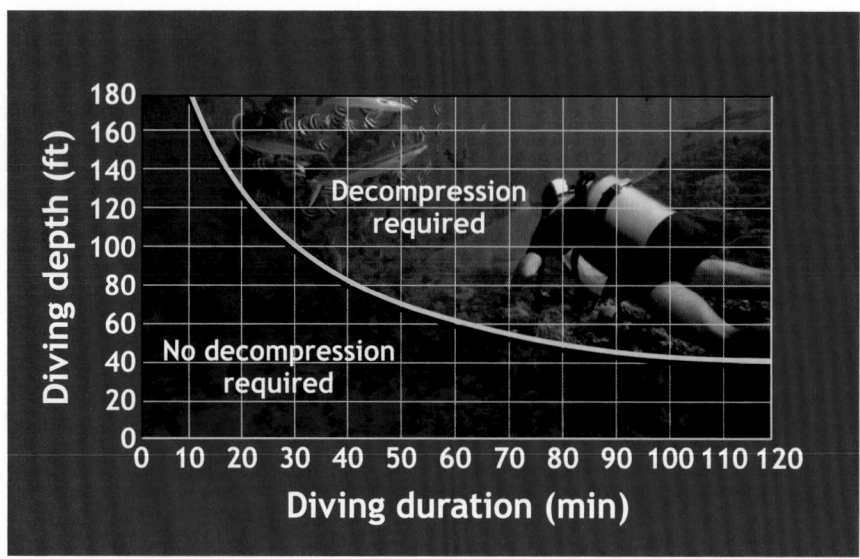

FIGURE 26.8 • Zero decompression limits. Any single dive that falls on the left side of the curve requires no decompression provided the rate of ascent does not exceed 60 ft per minute (m = ft × 0.34048). Dives on the right side of the line require the decompression period specified in standard decompression tables. (Reprinted from U.S. Navy Diving Manual, Vol. 5, Superintendent of Documents, U.S. Government Printing Office, Washington, DC 20402, 2008.)

Consequences of Inadequate Decompression

Bubbles within the vascular circuit initiate complications from decompression injury.[5,11,25] With the exception of bubbles in central nervous tissue that cause lesions in the brain and spinal cord and damage intravertebral disks,[14] the primary bubbles form in the venous and arterial vascular bed. Symptoms of decompression sickness usually appear within 4 to 6 hr following a dive. Severe violation of decompression procedures (e.g., diver runs out of air and ascends too rapidly) initiates symptoms immediately; these symptoms progress to paralysis within minutes. Indications of inadequate decompression include dizziness, itchy skin, and aching pain in the legs and arms, particularly in tight tissues such as ligaments and tendons (the classic and most common characteristic). The degree of injury depends on bubble size and where they form. Bubbles in the lungs cause choking and asphyxia; bubbles in the brain and coronary arteries block blood flow and deprive these vital tissues of oxygen and nutrients, to produce cellular damage and death. Central nervous system bends occurs with some frequency; failure to provide immediate treatment leads to permanent neural damage.

Treatment. Treatment for the bends involves lengthy recompression in a **hyperbaric chamber**. This specialized device elevates external pressure to force nitrogen gas back into solution. Gradual decompression then follows to provide time for the expanding gas to leave the body as the diver returns to the "surface." Immediate recompression offers the best chance for success; any delay decreases prognosis for complete recovery. **FIGURE 26.9** shows a collapsible, lightweight, transportable chamber for rapid deployment during transport of the diver

to an appropriate facility to treat decompression accidents. Chances are slim for a sport diver to have ready access to such a recompression chamber. This makes it imperative that divers adhere strictly to recommendations for diving depth and duration.

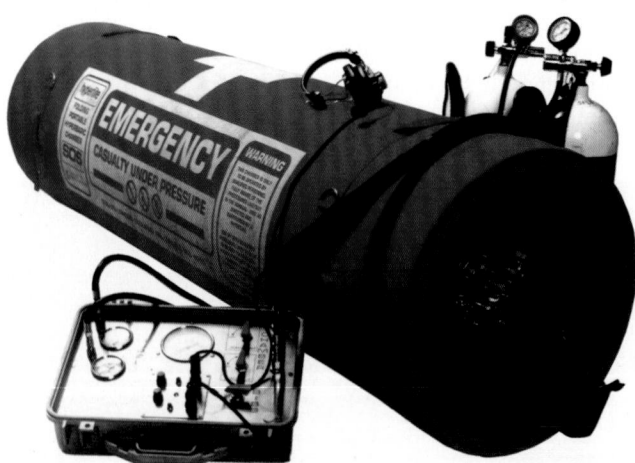

FIGURE 26.9 • Portable, collapsible recompression chamber (50 kg [110 lb]) for diving in remote locations. A compressed air cylinder provides a working pressure differential of 2.1 ata (bars), or 70 fsw, between the chamber environment and ambient conditions; the diver receives oxygen via a breathing mask. The tube is constructed from para-aramid fiber (like Kevlar) in a matrix of silicone rubber. This provides flexibility (can fold when not in use) and considerable strength under pressure (burst pressure approximately 14 ata differential pressure). (Manufactured by SOS Limited, London, England; photo courtesy of John Selby of SOS Hyperlite of Douglas, Isle of Man.)

Higher Prevalence with a Patent Foramen Ovale. Decompression sickness sometimes occurs after uneventful dives, without any reported errors in recommended decompression procedures. Divers with lesions localized in the high cervical spinal cord and brain areas show a higher prevalence of patent foramen ovale (PFO) of the myocardium than divers who experience decompression sickness that localizes in the lower spinal cord.[15] PFO consists of an interatrial septum channel that forms a functional valve between the right and left atria. This channel could cause localized decompression sickness because nitrogen bubbles that the pulmonary vasculature normally filters pass through the PFO into the arterial circulation. The bubbles then migrate preferentially into the carotid and/or vertebral arteries. Divers should be evaluated for PFO with unexplained decompression sickness but with symptoms suggesting cerebral or high spinal localization.[16]

Oxygen Poisoning

Inspiring a gas with a Po_2 above 2 ata (1520 mm Hg) greatly increases a diver's susceptibility to **oxygen poisoning**, particularly at elevated metabolic rates during physical activity.[2] For this reason, closed-circuit scuba that uses pure oxygen severely restricts both diving depth and duration (**TABLE 26.4**). At depths greater than 25 fsw (7.6 m), the diver should *not* rebreathe pure oxygen except in extraordinary circumstances. A decreased vital capacity strongly indicates impaired pulmonary function under hyperoxic conditions.[7]

Breathing high pressures of oxygen negatively affects bodily functions in three ways:

1. Irritates respiratory passages and eventually induces bronchopneumonia if exposure persists
2. Constricts cerebral blood vessels at pressures above 2 ata and alters central nervous system function
3. Depresses carbon dioxide elimination

For carbon dioxide elimination, an elevated inspired Po_2 may force sufficient oxygen into solution in the plasma to supply the diver's metabolic needs. In this case, oxygen

TABLE 26.4	Representative Depth-Time Limits for Closed-Circuit Diving with 100% Oxygen
Depth (fsw)	**Maximum Time (min)**
25	240
30	80
35	25
40	15
50	10

Adapted from U.S. Navy Diving Manual, Vol. 5, Superintendent of Documents, U.S. Government Printing Office, Washington, DC 20402, 2008.

remains combined with hemoglobin (called oxyhemoglobin) as blood returns to the pulmonary capillaries. This causes carbon dioxide buildup because deoxygenated hemoglobin normally transports considerable carbon dioxide as carbaminohemoglobin from the tissues (see Chapter 13). Treatment for oxygen poisoning consists of breathing air at sea-level pressure.

Carbon Monoxide Poisoning

Potentially lethal carbon monoxide gas combines about 200 times more readily with hemoglobin than does oxygen. Consequently, just a small quantity of carbon monoxide in the inspired mixture can induce tissue hypoxia. Carbon monoxide poisoning is of concern during deep dives because the partial pressures of all gases in the breathing mixture, including impurities, increase greatly.

The air in urban areas likely contains high levels of contaminants from automotive and industrial exhausts, including carbon monoxide and oxides of sulfur. One should never fill a scuba tank during air pollution or "unhealthy air" alerts. Aside from the contaminants present in ambient air, operating gasoline or diesel engine compressors contributes additional carbon monoxide and oil impurities. Placing the compressor's engine exhaust downstream from the air intake eliminates this potential source of contamination.

The antidote for carbon monoxide poisoning requires immediate breathing of hyperbaric oxygen. High pressures of inspired oxygen hasten dissociation of carbon monoxide from the hemoglobin molecule.

Women at No Greater Risk

Approximately 35% of recreational scuba divers in the United States are female. They do *not* experience a greater risk than males of equivalent physical fitness for decompression sickness, nitrogen narcosis, oxygen toxicity, air embolism, or diving accidents.

Little research has assessed the risks of open-circuit scuba diving to the fetus during pregnancy. Prudent guidelines recommend that pregnant women *refrain* from scuba diving during pregnancy to eliminate risk of fetal injury from maternal breathing of compressed air at elevated pressures.[35] However, firm data to support this recommendation remain lacking.[33]

DIVES TO EXCEPTIONAL DEPTHS: MIXED-GAS DIVING

Commercial, military, scientific, rescue, and technical divers often descend to depths in excess of 160 fsw. Recall that at depths greater than 60 fsw, diving with compressed air and saturation diving increase risk of oxygen toxicity. Diving lower than this depth requires breathing compressed mixed gases (nonair) with a lower Po_2. **FIGURE 26.10** lists the three main advantages of using nonair mixtures—specifically the reduced narcotic effects of nitrogen and reduced risk of oxygen toxicity—for dives to great depths. Oxygen always exists in the breathing mixture in mixed-gas diving, but it represents only a small fraction of the mix in dives to extreme depths. Precise management of oxygen concentrations becomes a primary consideration in **mixed-gas diving**. Three mixtures of oxygen, nitrogen, and helium are used today for deep and saturation diving:

1. *Nitrox* (nitrogen + oxygen)
2. *Heliox* (helium + oxygen)
3. *Trimix* (helium + nitrogen + oxygen)

Relatively shallow recreational dives employ nitrox, while heliox is used for deep diving, and trimix for dives to depths that may produce high-pressure nervous syndrome (see next section).[3]

Helium–Oxygen Mixtures

Helium, the second lightest known element, is the most common inert gas substituted for nitrogen in deep diving. Helium is colorless, odorless, tasteless, nonexplosive, and relatively nontoxic, and does not induce narcosis at any inspired pressure.[31]

Helium in the breathing mixture in diving came into its own during the 1939 rescue of remaining crew members and salvage of the submarine *Squalus* (see "Chronology of Selected Events in Diving History," earlier in the chapter). For these purposes, a compressor at the water's surface continually supplied the divers with a helium–oxygen (heliox) mixture. Because of helium's low density, breathing heliox mixtures reduces the typical increased breathing resistance imposed by nitrogen.

During rapid descent to depths in excess of 300 fsw up to 2280 fsw, divers breathing helium–oxygen mixtures can experience potentially incapacitating nausea, muscle tremors, and other central nervous effects. This phenomenon was first noted in the 1960s and termed ***high-pressure nervous syndrome*** (**HPNS**); initially, it was known as helium tremors. The condition probably results from the direct effects of extremes of hydrostatic pressure on excitable nerve cells. Slowing the rate of descent (compression) and adding a small amount of narcotic gas (e.g., 5% nitrogen) to the heliox breathing mixture relieves the tremor associated with HPNS.

Two other negative effects of breathing helium include:

1. Changes in voice characteristics (high-pitched, cartoon-like quality), which interfere with voice communication among divers. Electronic voice unscramblers remedy this effect.

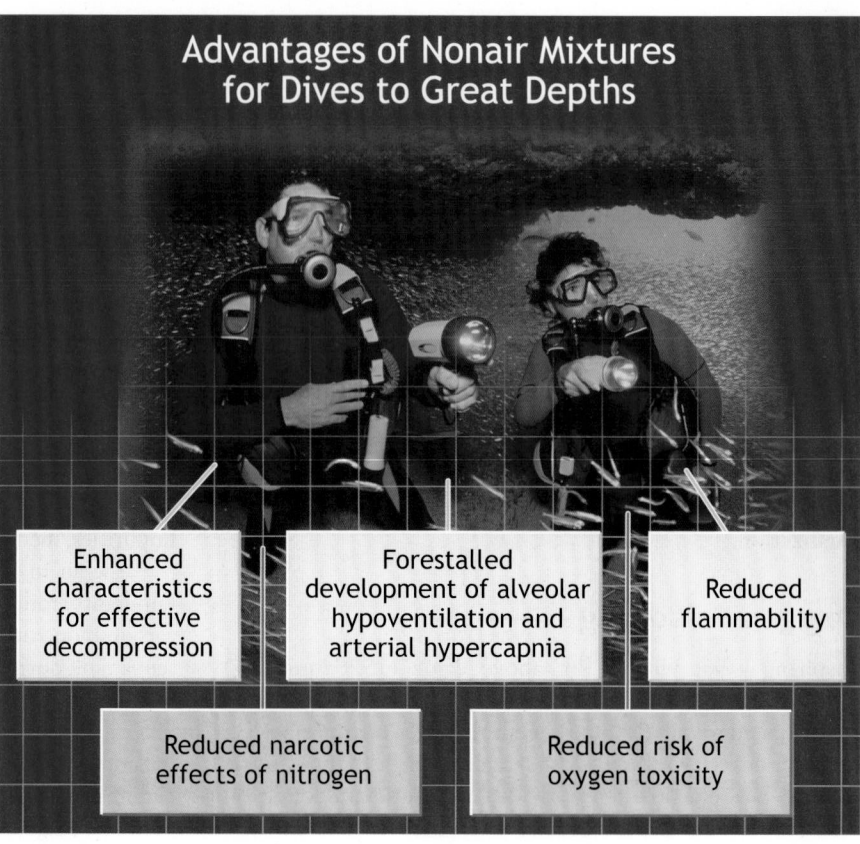

Advantages of Nonair Mixtures for Dives to Great Depths

Enhanced characteristics for effective decompression

Forestalled development of alveolar hypoventilation and arterial hypercapnia

Reduced flammability

Reduced narcotic effects of nitrogen

Reduced risk of oxygen toxicity

FIGURE 26.10 • Rationale for breathing gas mixtures other than compressed air when diving to great depths. Avoidance of nitrogen narcosis and oxygen poisoning are the overwhelming reasons for breathing nonair mixtures.

2. Considerable heat loss for divers living in a heliox environment, from helium's high thermal conductivity (six times that of air).[24] The thermal challenge contributes to weight loss, common among saturation divers.

Increased risk for central nervous system oxygen toxicity when breathing surface-supplied heliox gas makes it crucial that the diver not exceed the oxygen exposure limits put forth in **TABLE 26.5**.

 **Three Recommendations to Avoid High Pressure Nervous System (HPNS)**

1. Do not dive heliox (He+O_2) deeper than 400 fsw.

2. Do not dive trimix (He+N_2+O_2) deeper than 600 fsw. Adding 10% nitrogen to He+O_2 mix buffers mix so it can be used to 600 fsw without experiencing HPNS.

3. Use slow descent rates. Descending slower than one fsw per minute beyond 400 fsw on heliox and 600 fsw on trimix keeps HPNS at bay. Unfortunately, this slow rate of decent is only practical in commercial diving and is of no use in technical diving.

Source: National Oceanic and Atmospheric Administration (www.dive.noaa.gov).

TABLE 26.5	Representative Oxygen Partial Pressure Limits for Surface-Supplied Heliox Diving	
Exposure Time (min)	**Maximum Oxygen Partial Pressure (ata)**	
13	1.8	
20	1.7	
30	1.6	
40	1.5	
80	1.4	
Unlimited	**1.3**	

Adapted from U.S. Navy Diving Manual, Vol. 5, Superintendent of Documents, U.S. Government Printing Office, Washington, DC 20402, 2008.

Saturation Diving

Breathing a heliox mixture supports a safe dive to depths greater than 300 fsw, but the time the diver must remain "in-water" for decompression becomes prohibitive. Thus, dives below 300 fsw generally take place with **saturation diving** in a deep-diving system using a helium–oxygen–nitrogen (trimix) breathing mixture that maintains oxygen pressure between 0.4 and 0.6 ata (P_{O_2}, 300 to 450 mm Hg). In saturation diving, each inert gas in a mixture begins to concentrate in body tissues as depth and duration progress. Within 24 to 30 hr, the gases equilibrate and *saturate* body tissues to equal the pressures of the inspired gases. Once the tissues saturate, the decompression procedure remains identical regardless of the dive's duration.

The deep-diving system consists of a chamber where the divers live under pressure for up to 4 wk. The system also contains a deck decompression chamber and transfer capsule or diving bell for transport of personnel under pressure to and from the worksite. Once at the worksite, the divers exit, tethered to an umbilicus-supplied breathing apparatus. Saturation diving provides benefits in offshore oil-field work with dives up to 30 days at depths of 1500 fsw. Successful dives to depths of 2300 fsw in a dry chamber apply principles of saturation diving with a breathing mixture of hydrogen, helium, and oxygen. Decompression from a saturation dive takes 8 to 24 hr per 10-m ascent.

A critical consideration in saturation diving with heliox mixtures is to maintain normoxic P_{O_2}. Breathing the wrong mixture or the correct mixture at the wrong pressure creates the potential for a tragic fatality. Oxygen percentages must remain within ±0.10% of the desired value to avoid either hypoxia or oxygen toxicity. **Figure 26.11** shows the typical recommended percentage of oxygen in heliox for various diving depths. For example, the oxygen concentration to obtain a desired P_{O_2} of 0.35 ata (P_{O_2}, 270 mm Hg; green curve) at a depth of 1200 fsw requires a breathing mixture with approximately 0.7% oxygen.

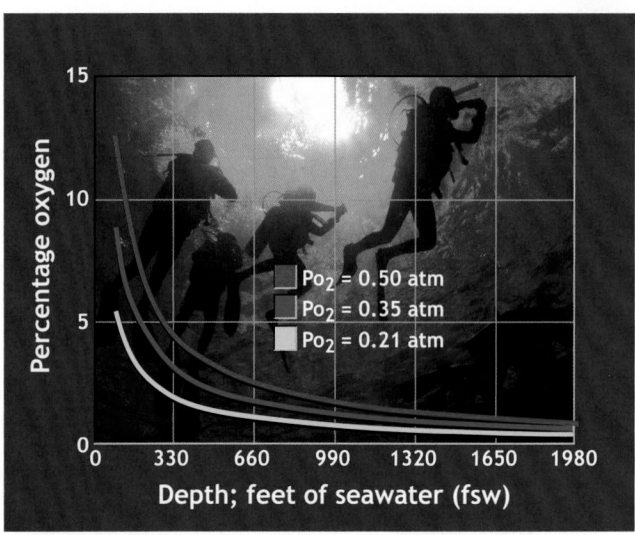

FIGURE 26.11 • Range of oxygen concentrations for saturation diving. The *green line* represents the oxygen concentration that maintains oxygen at 0.35 ata (P_{O_2} = 266 mm Hg), a common choice for P_{O_2}. The *yellow line* shows the oxygen needed to provide the normoxic level of 0.21 ata. The *red line* represents 0.5 ata (P_{O_2} = 380 mm Hg), the upper limit of continuous exposure to avoid whole-body oxygen toxicity. The low oxygen concentrations needed at great depths become difficult to mix and analyze within acceptable tolerance limits; thus, they are usually mixed as the diving chamber becomes pressurized. (Adapted with permission from Hamilton RW. Mixed-gas diving. In: Bove AA, Jefferson CD, eds. *Diving Medicine*. 4th Ed. Philadelphia: WB Saunders, 2004.)

Technical Diving

The term ***technical diving*** defines untethered dives (scuba or closed-circuit rebreathing) beyond the traditional compressed air range for military operations, science, salvage, and recreational pursuits. Many recreational scuba divers now consider the typical depth limit of 130 fsw imposed by diving with compressed air too restrictive. They wish to expand diving depths for personal achievement, recreation, and exploration (e.g., cave diving). Technical diving requires special equipment, expertise, and vigilant management of gas mixtures. Technical divers routinely use various mixtures of trimix compressed gas to dive below 300 fsw. Blending a depth-specific gas mixture allows the diver to control the risk of hyperoxia and the narcotic potential of nitrogen.

Closed-circuit nitrogen–oxygen and helium–oxygen scuba originally developed for military operations now appear in the recreational technical-diving community. These highly sophisticated systems maintain a constant partial pressure of oxygen in the inhaled mixture regardless of depth. **Figure 26.12** illustrates a closed-circuit mixed-gas system used by the U.S. Navy. An oxygen sensor (*19*) and microprocessor (*21*) in the breathing loop continually detect and regulate falling P_{O_2}. The sensors activate valves that add the precise quantity of 100% oxygen to regulate inspired P_{O_2} at 0.75 ata (427 mm Hg). One of two high-pressure gas bottles (*9* and *14*) supplies pure

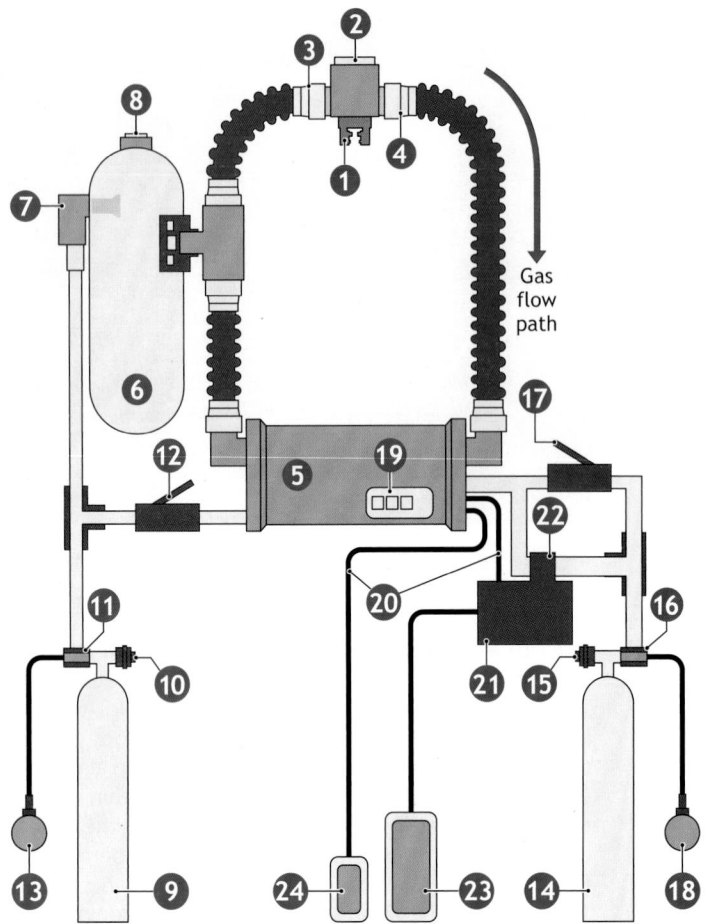

1. Mouthpiece
2. Mouthpiece shutoff
3. Upstream check-valve
4. Downstream check-valve
5. CO_2 absorbent canister
6. Counterlung
7. Diluent addition valve
8. Overpressure check-valve
9. Diluent supply cylinder
10. Diluent on-off valve
11. Diluent regulator
12. Manual diluent bypass
13. Diluent pressure gauge
14. Oxygen supply cylinder
15. Oxygen on/off valve
16. Oxygen regulator
17. Manual oxygen bypass
18. Oxygen pressure gauge
19. Oxygen sensor
20. Oxygen sensor cables
21. Main electronics
22. Oxygen solenoid valve
23. Primary display
24. Secondary display

FIGURE 26.12 • Closed-circuit mixed-gas system used by the U.S. Navy for diving to great depths. A microprocessor and oxygen sensors in the breathing loop continually detect falling Po_2 and activate valves that add the precise amount of 100% oxygen to regulate the partial pressure of inspired oxygen. A single high-pressure gas bottle supplies pure oxygen, and a second provides either air or a heliox mixture as a diluent. A chemical bed continually absorbs the carbon dioxide produced in metabolism.

oxygen, and the other provides either air or a heliox mixture as the diluent gas. As with the typical closed-circuit system, a chemical bed absorbs carbon dioxide produced by the body's metabolism. Monitors within the facemask provide continual feedback about Po_2 and diving depth. A fiberglass casing worn on the diver's back contains the microprocessor, gas bottles, breathing bag, and insulated carbon dioxide absorbent canister (cold decreases CO_2 absorbent life).

ENERGY COST OF UNDERWATER SWIMMING

As with surface swimming, drag forces impede the diver's forward movement and greatly increase the energy cost of swimming underwater. **FIGURE 26.13** shows the curvilinear relationship between oxygen consumption and underwater swimming speed. For example, a swimmer with a $\dot{V}O_{2max}$ of 35 mL · kg^{-1} · min^{-1} could swim underwater at a speed of 1.2 knots (1.4 mph) for only a few minutes. This speed creates minimal stress for a diver with a $\dot{V}O_{2max}$ of 65 mL · kg^{-1} · min^{-1}. The location and density of the gear can alter the diver's positioning in the water and increase the energy cost of swimming

by as much as 30% at slow speeds. The type of fin worn by the diver affects the depth and frequency of the kick, thus influencing drag and swimming economy.[29]

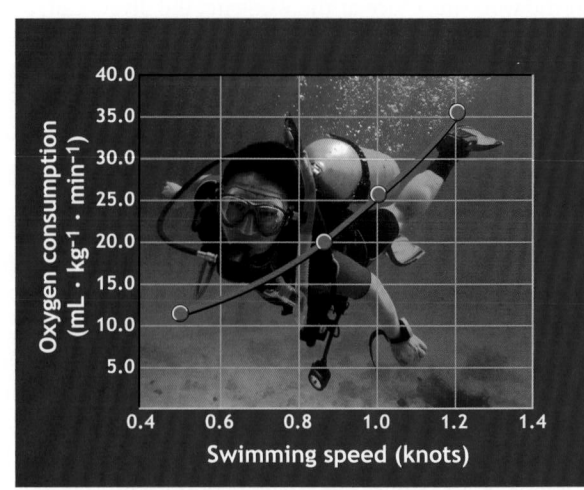

FIGURE 26.13 • Generalized curvilinear relationship between oxygen consumption (mL · kg^{-1} · min^{-1}) and underwater swimming speed (1.0 knot = 1.15 mph).

Summary

1. Breath-hold diving has been practiced for centuries. Deep-sea diving had its origins in the 14th century with the invention of diving bells supplied with surface air.

2. The underwater environment routinely exposes divers to high pressures (hyperbaria) and the possibility of rapidly changing pressures. Severe injury and even death ensue unless divers adjust to equalize pressures in the body's air-filled cavities.

3. Two factors limit snorkel size: increased hydrostatic pressure on the chest cavity during descent and increased pulmonary dead space from enlarging the snorkel's internal volume.

4. Duration of a breath-hold dive depends on time until arterial P_{CO_2} reaches the breath-holding breakpoint.

5. Hyperventilation considerably lowers arterial P_{CO_2} and increases breath-holding time; it also increases the likelihood of underwater blackout.

6. The point at which the diver's lung volume compresses to RLV generally determines maximum depth for breath-hold diving. Lung squeeze occurs below this critical depth when internal and external pressures cannot equalize.

7. Breath-hold diving by elite divers produces intense cardiovascular changes that resemble response patterns of diving mammals.

8. The sport of free diving has gained worldwide popularity, with many categories of dives where the object attempts to achieve maximum depth with a single breath of air before descending and returning to the surface.

9. Periodization training for free diving focuses on basic principles of training that then includes strength, cardiovascular, flexibility, and yoga regimens. It also includes specific dive training, with further specialized dive training to optimize a diver's ability to breath-hold for extended periods underwater by focusing on the ventilatory musculature to tolerate the highest levels of CO_2 possible.

10. Scuba supplies breathing mixtures at great depths and pressures.

11. Specific scuba hazards result from improper equalization of pressures in the lungs, sinus, and middle-ear spaces with the external water pressure. Important dangers include air embolism, pneumothorax, mask and middle-ear squeeze, and aerosinusitis.

12. Gases breathed at high pressures move across the alveolar membrane to dissolve and equilibrate in the fluids of all tissues.

13. High tissue oxygen and nitrogen pressures exert profound negative effects on physiologic function. The maximum recommended diving depth for breathing compressed air is about 30 m (98.4 ft).

14. Prolonged breathing of a gas with a P_{O_2} above 2 ata increases a diver's susceptibility to oxygen poisoning.

15. Closed-circuit scuba systems that use pure oxygen severely restrict dive depth and duration.

16. Nitrogen bubbles form in tissues when excess nitrogen fails to exit through the lungs if ascent progresses too rapidly. Decompression sickness, or bends, describes this painful condition.

17. Diving to depths below 60 fsw requires inhalation of compressed mixed gases. Precisely managing oxygen concentrations becomes a primary consideration.

18. Breathing mixtures of helium and oxygen (heliox) allows dives to depths of 2000 fsw. Heliox diving eliminates nitrogen narcosis risk and minimizes risk of oxygen poisoning.

19. Rapid descent to depths from 300 fsw to 2800 fsw breathing heliox mixtures produces nausea, muscle tremors, and other central nervous system effects termed *high-pressure nervous syndrome* (HPNS).

20. Drag forces that impede a diver's forward movement increase the energy cost of swimming underwater.

thePoint References are available online at **http://thepoint.lww.com/mkk8e.**

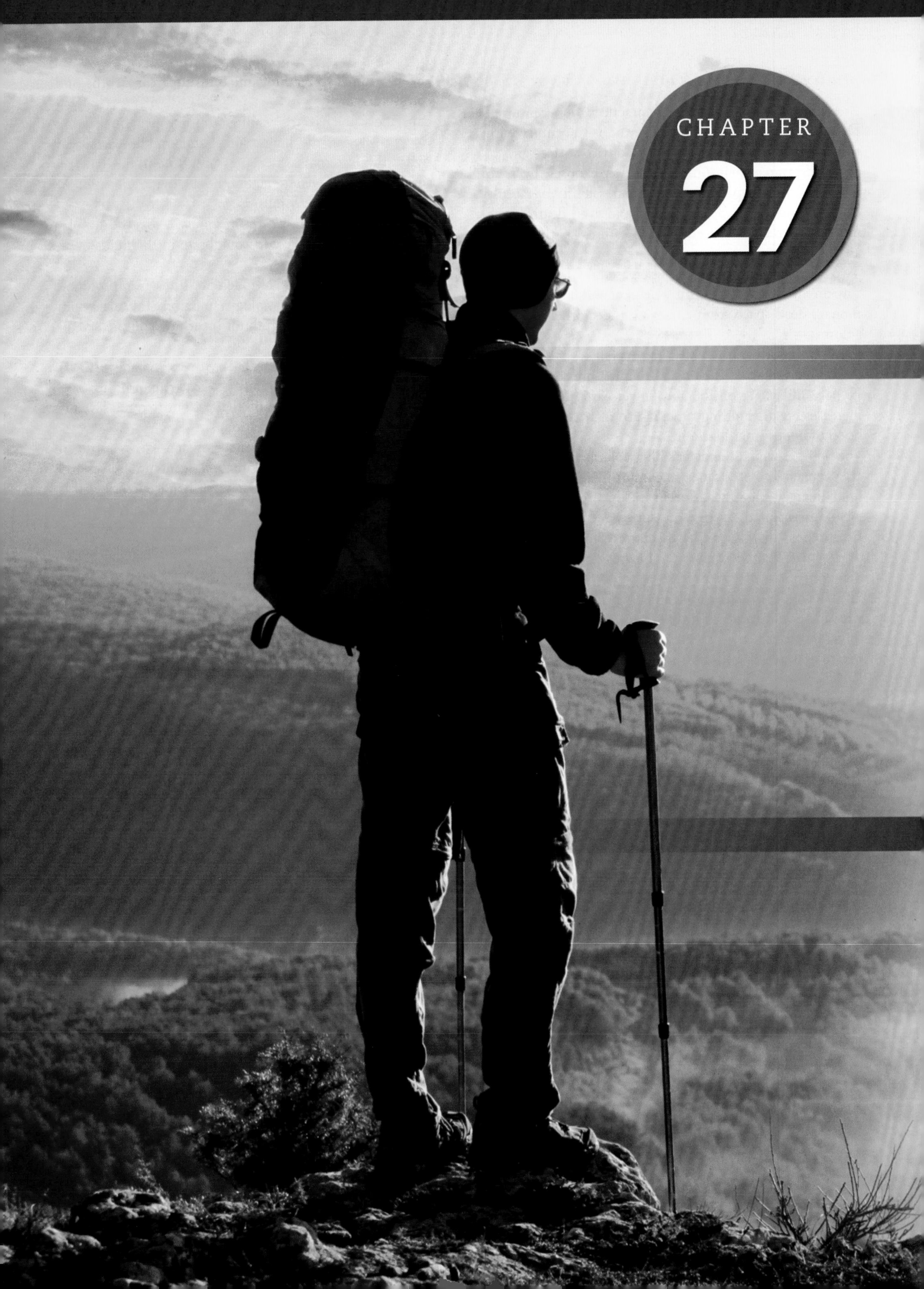

CHAPTER

27

Microgravity: The Last Frontier

- Define gravity and list three factors that affect the magnitude of gravitational force
- Differentiate between zero-g and weightlessness
- Outline two factors that contribute to a sense of "free fall" in a falling elevator
- Describe four strategies to simulate microgravity with inanimate objects and animals and humans
- Explain the importance of the "vomit comet" to train astronauts for space missions
- List five physiologic/anatomic responses to microgravity exposure; differentiate between short-term and long-term responses
- Give three reasons for denitrogenation prior to extravehicular activity in space and procedures to achieve this effect

- Outline four goals of exercise countermeasures to ensure astronaut health and safety during missions and return to Earth
- Describe the rationale for applying lower-body negative pressure and its role as a countermeasure during spaceflight
- Outline three interactions among energy balance, nutrition, and protein dynamics during space missions
- Describe the time course for postflight recovery for physiologic systems from 2-wk and 1-year space missions
- List 10 significant beneficial spin-off technologies from space biology research

Visit http://thePoint.lww.com/mkk8e to access the following resources.

- References: Chapter 27
- Appendix J: Accomplishments of the United States and Soviet Human Space Flight Programs
- Appendix K: Microgravity Web sites
- Interactive Question Bank
- Focus on Research: Microgravity's Effects on Muscle Fibers

THE WEIGHTLESS ENVIRONMENT

The pioneering efforts of mainly German, Russian, and American scientists and engineers advanced aerospace medicine from the early test flights of rocket-propelled jet aircraft to the technologic innovations of today's **International Space Station (ISS)** that orbits 220 nautical miles (1 nautical mile = 1852 m or 1.852 km; 1 nautical mile = 1.1508 miles or 6076 ft) above Earth (www.nasa.gov/mission_pages/station/main/index.html).

The remarkable successes of man's escape from Earth's atmosphere (at approximately 7 miles a second, 25,000 miles an hour, or 34 times the speed of sound) and subsequent return originated in antiquity, when prophets and philosophers could only dream of contacting celestial bodies. From flying machine designs of da Vinci's Renaissance drawings five centuries ago at the dawn of modern science to successful hot-air balloon ascents during the mid-1700s, the obsession to explore the universe has not waned. By 2011, the reliability of powerful rocketry and new aircraft design and composite materials made commercial, suborbital space adventure a reality (www.space.com/8325-space-tourism-firm-offer-suborbital-joy-rides-costs.html; www.faa.gov/about/office_org/headquarters_offices/ast/media/111460.pdf; www.faa.gov/about/office_org/headquarters_offices/ast/). Spectacular views of Earth can be seen from time-lapse still photos from the ISS as it circles Earth every 90 min (www.guardian.co.uk/science/video/2012/nov/29/earth-international-space-station-timelapse-video). Future research efforts will determine how best to tame the physiologic stressors imposed by yearlong flights to Mars—and eventually beyond.

The early jet flights could not test human responses to changing gravitational forces because that era's test aircraft could not accommodate specialized laboratory equipment. Nevertheless, knowing how to cope with the unique environmental stressors (and health challenges) of high-altitude exposure still required new understanding unavailable from conventional medicine. The field of **aerospace medicine** (www.asma.org) emerged from a need to deal with unconventional situations not encountered in normal gravity (g). Aerospace medical research progressed using the responses of mice, cats, dogs, monkeys, and eventually humans to spaceflight. Concurrently, research progressed by use of space cabin simulators on Earth. Scientists focused on human psychophysiologic responses to changing gravitational forces and prolonged isolation while performing complex motor and mental tasks. The experience from simulations and manned flights provided new understanding about spaceflights' impact on human structure, function, and adaptation.

The United States is not the only country committed to reinvigorating its efforts to future space exploration. The concept of an Advanced Crew Transportation System, or ACTS, also known as the "Euro-Soyuz" Crew Space Transportation System (CSTS; www.russianspaceweb.com/soyuz_acts.html), was developed by Russia during 2006 to replace the workhorse Soyuz spacecraft (www.astronautix.com/craftfam/soyuz.htm). Since then, the Russian Federal Space Agency

---

 Facts About the International Space Station (ISS)

- The ISS marked its 13th anniversary of continuous human occupation on November 2, 2013. Since Expedition 1, launched October 31, 2000, and docked November 2, 2000, the space station has been visited by 204 individuals.
- At the time of the 10th anniversary, the space station's odometer read more than 1.5 billion statute miles (the equivalent of eight round trips to the sun) spanning 57,361 orbits around Earth.

- As of June 2013, there have been:
  - 89 Russian launches
  - 37 Space Shuttle launches
  - 1 test flight and 2 operational flights.
- The final space shuttle mission Atlantis on July 8–21, 2011, delivered 4.5 tons of supplies in the Raffaello logistics module (www.nasa.gov/mission_pages/station/structure/elements/mplm.html).
  - A total of 162 spacewalks totaling about 1021 hr have been conducted in support of space station assembly.
  - The space station, including its large solar arrays, spans the area of a U.S. football field, including the end zones.
  - The station's complex now has more livable room than a conventional five-bedroom house with two bathrooms, a gymnasium, and a 360-degree bay window.
  - Approximately 2.3 million lines of computer code keep the station operational.
  - The station weighs 924,739 lb (419,455 kg).
  - Eight solar arrays generate 84 kilowatts of power.

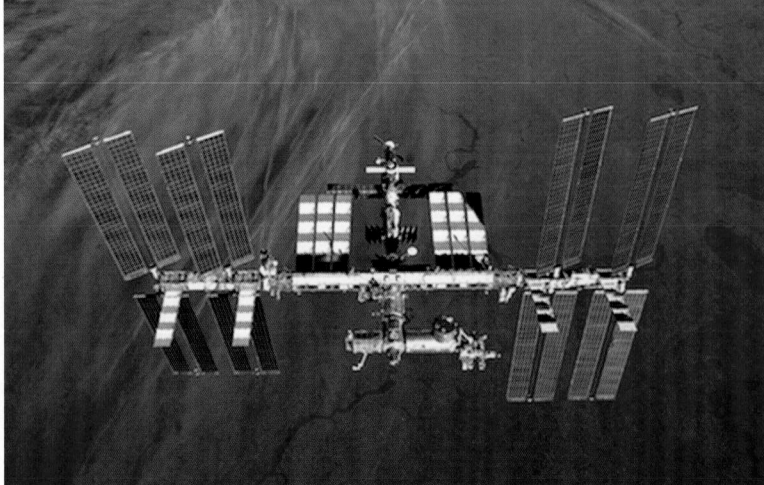

(www.roscosmos.ru/index.asp?Lang=ENG) has used considerable resources to develop the next generation manned transport, a modified Soyuz vehicle capable of achieving lunar orbit, including lunar vehicles designed to explore the terrain and obtain soil samples, perhaps in the 2016 to 2017 timeframe (www.russianspaceweb.com/luna_resurs.html).

Gravity

On Earth's surface, gravity provides an invisible attraction that makes any mass exert downward force or have weight. Gravity behaves in the same fundamental way between Earth and any object on it, between any of the planets that revolve about the sun in our solar system, or between a planet and its moons. The universality of the gravitational law, first proposed in 1687 by English physicist and mathematician **Sir Isaac Newton** (1642–1727), can be stated as follows and is depicted in the top of **FIGURE 27.1**.

> Every particle in matter in the universe attracts every other particle with a force directly proportional to the product of the masses of the particles and inversely proportional to the square of the distance separating them.

When a person sits in a chair on Earth, gravity's force pulls the person into the seat because the fixed chair provides an equal and opposite force (Newton's third law). Every mass (m) on Earth requires support from a force (F) equal to its weight (w, in Newtons), such that $F_w = mg$, where m is mass in kg and g is acceleration of gravity ($9.8 \ m \cdot s^{-2}$). Stated differently, the constant acceleration force per second (s) of descent on a freely falling body at or near Earth's surface has a value of 1g or the acceleration due to gravity, with an equivalent magnitude of 9.80665 or $9.80 \ m \cdot s^{-2}$, $980 \ cm \cdot s^{-2}$, or $32 \ ft \cdot s^{-2}$. On the moon's surface, in contrast, the attractive force of the moon and not Earth causes the acceleration of gravity, where $g = 1.6 \ m \cdot s^{-2}$. Someone on Earth who weighs 150 lb (68 kg) would weigh 354 lb (160.5 kg) on the planet Jupiter (about 5.2 times farther away from the sun than Earth). Near the sun's surface, with a much larger mass than the Earth or moon (or Jupiter), the g value increases tremendously by a factor of nearly 169 to $270 \ m \cdot s^{-2}$. In the near future when humans land on another planet or asteroid, a person's mass will remain the same, but weight will change depending on the force of gravity encountered.

When the first astronaut, Commander Neil Armstrong (1930–2012), stepped onto the moon on July 20, 1969, he weighed one-sixth his 165-lb Earth weight or 27.5 lb

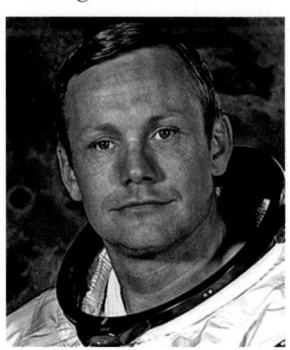

because the moon's gravity was one-sixth that of Earth. In essence, knowledge of an object's mass allows computation of its weight; conversely, knowing weight allows computation of mass. The general equation $F_w = mg$ allows for the easy conversion between mass and weight or weight and mass (and accounting for g).

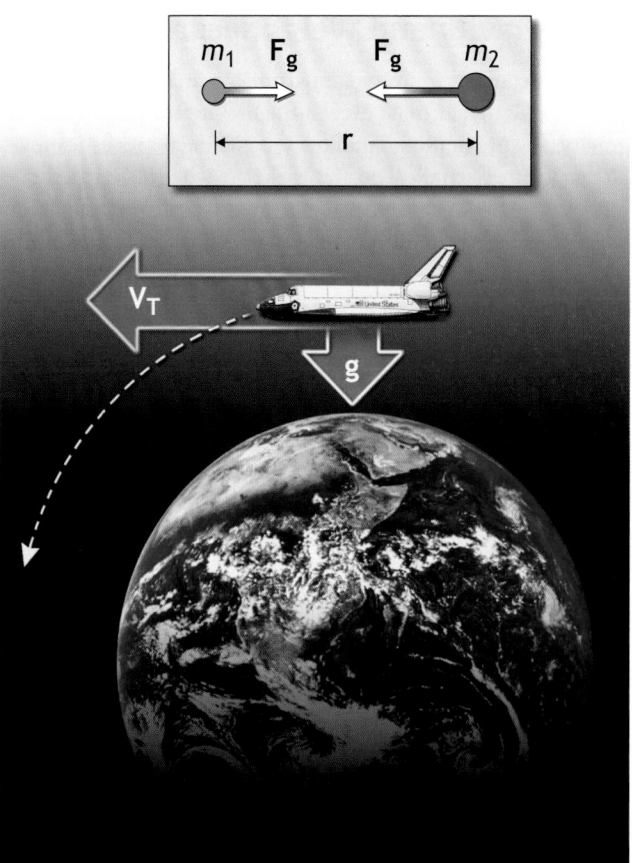

FIGURE 27.1 • (**Upper inset**) Two different size masses (m_1 and m_2), depicted as the green- and red-filled circles, and separated by a distance r exert attractive gravitational forces (F_g) on each other. The forces on each particle have equal magnitude even when their masses differ markedly. (**Lower inset**) Microgravity refers to the perceived "weightlessness" associated with free fall. The forces acting on an astronaut orbiting Earth in a spacecraft are not balanced—both astronaut and spacecraft accelerate toward Earth's center. They do not "fall" to the Earth because its surface is curved and they are moving at a tangential velocity (V_T) high enough to "balance" gravity's downward force on the spacecraft. No perceived force (i.e., weight) exists because nothing counteracts the force of gravity.

 ## Gravity on the Moon and Mars

Gravity's effect on celestial bodies always remains a positive number because it represents the magnitude of a vector quantity. The attractive force on the moon's surface experienced by the 12 astronauts who walked there from the Apollo 11 to 17 missions produces a g force of $1.6 \ m \cdot s^{-2}$, or approximately one-sixth that on Earth. When future astronauts eventually land on Mars, scheduled for mid-2030 (and landing on an asteroid in 2025 preceded in 2016 by the launch of OSIRIS-REx, a spacecraft that will travel to an asteroid and return soil samples to Earth), they will experience a g force of $3.7 \ m \cdot s^{-2}$, approximately 40% that on Earth's surface at sea level.

Microgravity and Weightlessness

To achieve an orbit around Earth or move away from it, the velocity of a rocket must exceed the downward pull of Earth's gravity. The gravitational pull on a rocket decreases as it moves farther from Earth. When the rocket reaches a specified distance from Earth sufficient for orbit, a traveler experiences a weightless feeling because *nearly* all of the forces acting on the body remain in balance. To reach a point in space where the gravitational pull from Earth equals one-millionth the force at Earth's surface requires traveling 6.37 million kilometers, or 16.6 times the distance from Earth to the moon, or 1400 times the highway distance between New York City and San Francisco. In a practical sense, a rock dropped from a window 5 m above the ground requires 1 s to touch ground. In an environment with only 1% of Earth's gravitational pull, the same drop takes 10 s. In a microgravity environment equal to one-millionth of the gravity on Earth, the same 5-m drop would take 1000 s, or approximately 17 min.

Spacecraft orbit Earth at a relatively close distance (typically 200 to 450 km [155 to 248 mi]), so astronauts experience only an *apparent* sense of weightlessness. In essence, the force of gravity never truly reaches an absolute value of zero (called **zero-g**) because some gravitational force still exists. Consequently, the term *microgravity*, not weightlessness (or zero-g), correctly describes what astronauts feel during spaceflight in Earth's orbit when the rocket's altitude exceeds approximately 160 km (100 mi) at a velocity of approximately 17,500 mph.

The 121-ft space shuttle orbiting laboratory can carry a payload of 29,479 kg into orbit, with each main engine producing a thrust of 170,068 kg at sea level while burning a mixture of liquid oxygen and hydrogen. After achieving orbital velocity, the astronaut and spacecraft continually accelerate toward a single point at Earth's center. They do not fall to Earth because of the planet's curved surface and because both craft and crew move at a high enough tangential velocity (V_T) to the Earth (V_T and g shown in green in Fig. 27.1). The spacecraft's speed creates an outward centrifugal force that "balances" the downward gravitational force on the spacecraft. When spacecraft velocity decreases (reduced V_T)—a planned maneuver during reentry—the craft "plunges" toward Earth under gravity's pull.

Passenger in a Falling Elevator

When an elevator descends quickly, one feels a lessening of weight because of reduced force between the feet and elevator floor. If the elevator cable suddenly snaps and the elevator plummets downward, the force against the feet equals zero until the elevator strikes bottom. Consider the example of a 60-kg (132-lb) woman riding in an elevator. If she could lift her feet off the floor before hitting the ground, she would float within the elevator compartment. No force pushes her up because she and the elevator fall together at the same speed and acceleration. This applies equally to any other objects in the elevator. If a scale were present in the elevator, the woman's weight would not register because the scale

Galileo's Famous Leaning Tower of Pisa "Falling" Experiment—Did It Happen?

The incomparable scientist Galileo Galilei (1564–1642), in his classic *Two New Sciences* published in 1638 (**www.juliantrubin.com/bigten/galileofallingbodies.html**), makes the case of a "thought-experiment" in which he, as legend has it, simultaneously dropped a cannonball and musket ball of different

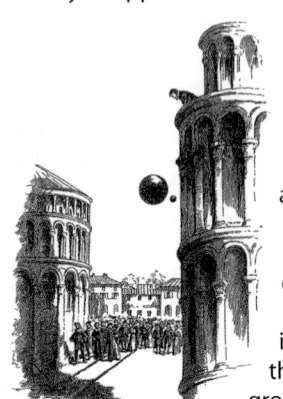

masses from the leaning Bell Tower of Pisa. The veracity of this occurrence was not put forth by Galileo, but later scientists and even his long-time secretary Vincenzio Viviani (1622–1703) claimed 15 years after the fact that Galileo observed that both objects fell downward at approximately the same rate and consequently touched the ground simultaneously. In reality, according to Galileo in *Two New Sciences*, the heavier ball actually struck the ground slightly ahead of the lighter object. In the centuries-old story about Galileo's demonstration of two falling masses (where *F* and *g* both must have equaled zero), it has become commonplace to restate that both objects reached the ground at the same time. What is remarkable about the retelling of this discovery over several centuries was the audacity of the experiment that shook up conventional wisdom about the important role of science and scientific experimentation. Galileo's scientific approach using an experimental paradigm overturned centuries of belief that adherence to religious dogma could adequately explain previously unexplainable phenomena. Galileo's famous undertaking may have been more myth than truth; it has been questioned by serious historians (and many social thinkers/academicians from the 1500s to the present) regarding the veracity of dropping differently weighted heavy and light objects from the Tower of Pisa (**www.uh.edu/engines/epi166.htm**; Martinez, A. *Science Secrets: the Truth About Darwin's Finches, Einstein's Wife, and Other Myths*. Pittsburgh, PA: University of Pittsburgh Press, 2011; Cooper, L. *Aristotle, Galileo, and the Tower of Pisa*. Ithaca, NY: Cornell University Press, 1935; Drake, S. *Galileo at Work: His Scientific Biography*. Chicago, IL: University of Chicago Press, 1979; Drake, S. *A History of Free Fall: Aristotle to Galileo, with an Epilogue on Pi in the Sky*. Toronto, ON: Wall & Emerson, 1989).

too would be falling. *During free-fall, everything in the elevator remains weightless because the person and elevator car (including a scale) accelerate downward at the same rate from gravity alone.*

Examples of Near–Zero-G During Spaceflight

Spaceflight provides the ubiquitous condition of near–zero-g. Liquids fail to remain in open cups or glasses, so drinks must be squeezed into the mouth from special containers. No "up" or "down" exists inside the space vehicle (**Fig. 27.2**); to keep from

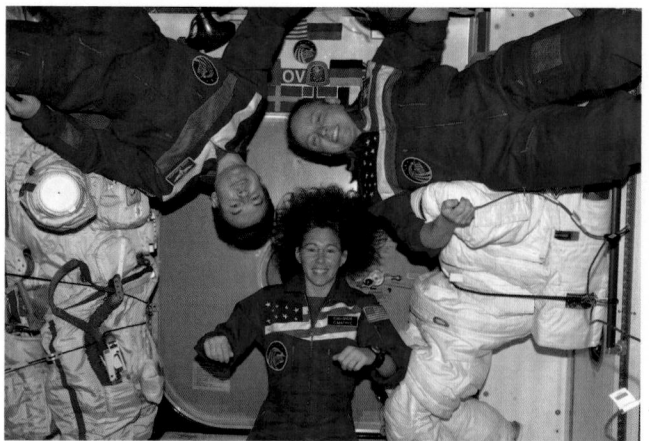

FIGURE 27.2 • Demonstration of microgravity aboard the International Space Station where no "up" or "down" exists. Astronaut Michael Fincke (right), Expedition 18 commander; astronaut Sandra Magnus, flight engineer; and cosmonaut Yury Lonchakov, flight engineer, pose between a Russian Orlan spacesuit and an extravehicular mobility unit (EMU) spacesuit in the Harmony node of the ISS. In a spacecraft, its crew and any objects aboard all fall toward but around Earth. Because they all fall together, the crew and objects appear to float compared with the spacecraft. (Photo courtesy of NASA, Lyndon B. Johnson Space Center, Houston, TX.)

floating freely, astronauts must anchor or tether themselves to a fixed object within the cabin (e.g., a wall or other attached object).

In microgravity, blood and fluid volumes shift upward and move into the thoracocephalic region. This causes a puffy-face appearance as fluid relocates from extracellular to intracellular spaces.[84] Correspondingly, a 2- to 5-cm decrease occurs in waist girth (a legitimate way in space to wear otherwise tight-fitting pants!). The initial net shift of fluid also produces eye redness, "bird-type" (skinny) legs, nasal congestion, headaches, and nausea. Concomitant reductions in blood volume affect cardiovascular function, manifested by decreased plasma and red blood cell volume,[35] increased venous pooling, blunted baroreceptor reflex, and **orthostatic intolerance**, defined as compromised venous return to the heart during upright posture in a gravity environment.

On Earth, the constant downward pressure of 1 g compresses intervertebral disks. In microgravity, removal of gravitational force causes disks to expand, making stature increase up to 5 cm (**Fig. 27.3A**). Figure 27.3B illustrates that posture also changes during microgravity exposure. Compared with preflight, joints move toward the midpoint in their range of motion so that hips and knees flex slightly, causing the body to crouch. Arms tend to float in front of the body unless consciously forced downward. Note the postural sway with the head protruding forward, with accompanying lordosis immediately upon return to Earth.

Strategies to Simulate Microgravity

Different strategies have simulated spaceflight's microgravity environment. This allows researchers to manipulate various experimental conditions before deciding on the best procedure(s) for a particular mission. One strategy uses sophisticated test equipment that creates zero-g conditions for relatively brief times with nonhuman objects dropped from towers and into tubes or within sounding rockets as they fall to Earth after achieving a maximum altitude. Another tactic uses parabolic airplane flights with living and nonliving objects, and a third strategy simulates microgravity conditions with animals and humans using head-down bed rest, confinement, water immersion, or immobilization.

Human Testing

Researchers have devised five basic strategies to simulate a microgravity environment and study its effects on humans:

1. Head-down bed rest
2. Wheelchair confinement of paraplegics
3. Water immersion
4. Immobilization and confinement
5. Parabolic flights

Head-Down Bed Rest. Head-down bed rest has yielded the most information about human physiologic dynamics in simulated microgravity (**Fig. 27.4A**). These studies confirmed experimental findings in space about physiologic responses and adaptations including psychologic stress, hormonal changes, and immune function[24,91]; this makes the head-down bed-rest strategy a useful spaceflight analogue. Subjects remain confined to bed for an extended time (weeks, months, or a year) in a horizontal or head-down tilt position (−3° to −12°), often followed by physiologic measurements to positive acceleration at forces up to 3g in a centrifuge.

Wheelchair Confinement of Paraplegics. Prolonged wheelchair confinement produces postural hypotension in paraplegics, who seldom experience full erect posture following their disability.[39] As in longer spaceflight missions (>21 days), years of sitting constrain fluctuations in hydrostatic gradients normally experienced by nonparaplegics during routine daily activities. Short-term exertion such as graded, arm-cranking to maximum[103] evaluates paraplegics' responses for heart rate, systolic and diastolic blood pressure, forearm vascular resistance (FVR), and vasoactive hormones. In general, exercise eliminated orthostatic hypotension and increased FVR and baroreflex sensitivity independent of blood volume changes. The positive cardiovascular adjustments in paraplegics to less frequent but relatively intense exercise have relevance as a postflight countermeasure to the potentially debilitating effects of prolonged missions on orthostatic stability and baroreflex functions on return to Earth's gravitational environment. The intriguing possibility of immediate benefit from short-term, intense postflight exercise would maximize overall mission efficiency by reducing time devoted to in-flight exercise and concomitant demands for additional food and water associated with daily exercise.[48]

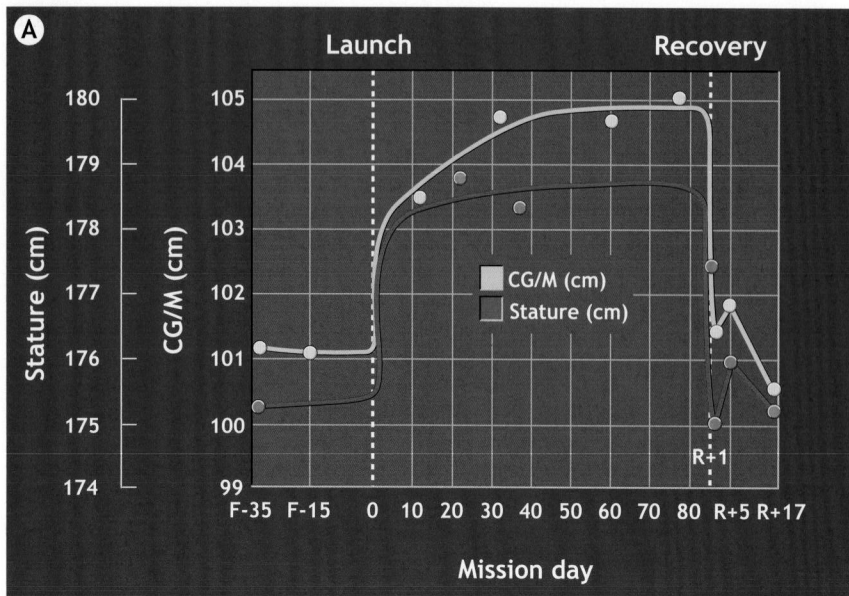

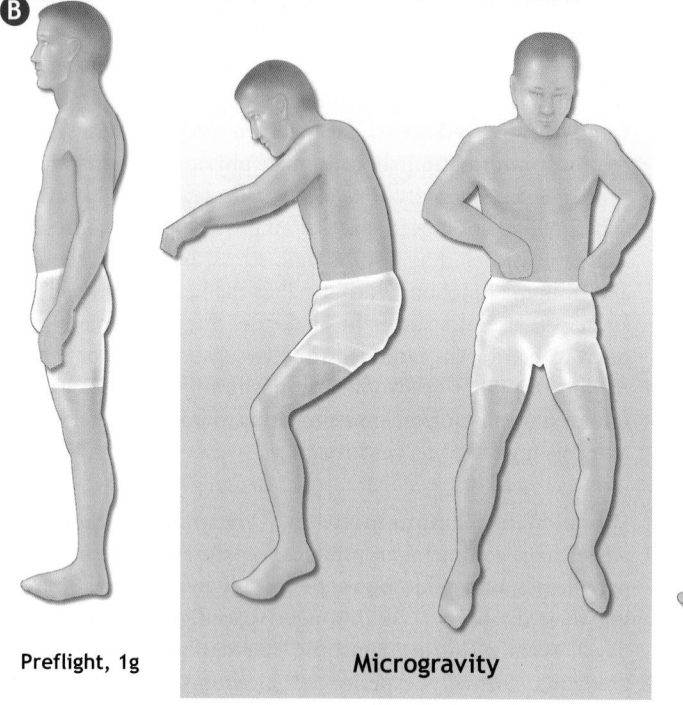

FIGURE 27.3 • **(A)** Change in the center of gravity/mass (CG ÷ M) and stature before (F), during an 84-day Skylab 4 mission, and 17 days postflight (R +17). **(B)** General changes in posture under conditions of Earth's gravity preflight (1g), microgravity, and postflight (1 g). (Reprinted from Thornton WE, et al. Anthropometric changes and fluid shifts. In: Johnson RS, Dietlein LF, eds. *Biomedical Results from Skylab*. NASA SP-377. Washington, DC: U.S. Government Printing Office, 1977.)

Water Immersion. Subjects lie supine in a water tank for up to 24 hr (wet immersion technique) or lie on a thin sheet to prevent the skin from touching the water (dry immersion technique). In NASA's Weightless Environment Training Facility (WETF; http://on.aol.com/video/learn-about-the-weightless-environment-training-facility-of-

nasa-304221617?icid=video_related_0), astronauts practice complex hand–eye coordination tasks to mimic skills required in extravehicular activities (EVA) during orbital missions (Fig. 27.4B).

Immobilization and Confinement.

1. Whole-body or segmental casts restrict limb and body movements in humans and animals. One approach immobilizes the nondominant arm in a sling, except during sleep and bathing, for 4 wk.[103] This procedure produces an effective analogue for simulating the effects of "weightlessness" on human skeletal muscle loading. Changes in muscle structure and function (e.g., torque production, cross-sectional area, histochemical muscle fiber analysis, and integrated electromyography [IEMG]) produce results similar in magnitude and direction to data obtained from humans following exposure to real and simulated microgravity environments.

2. Confining animals to a small cage severely restricts their movement.

3. A harness provides partial body support by suspending an animal in a head-down position with gravitational loading removed from the hind limbs.

Parabolic Flights. FIGURE 27.5A illustrates the strategy to evaluate physiologic responses to microgravity produced when NASA's KC-135 Stratotanker aircraft climbs rapidly at a 45° angle and then follows a path called a parabola (http://jsc-aircraft-ops.jsc.nasa.gov/Reduced_Gravity/KC_135_history.html). The four-engine turbojet aircraft produces a near–zero-g effect $(1 \times 10^{-3}g)$ for about 30 s (*center orange area* in the figure) just as the aircraft achieves 9500 m of the 10,000-m ascent (termed *pull-up*) before it slows. The plane then traces a parabola (pushover), descending rapidly at a 45° angle (termed *pull-out*) to 7300 m. The forces of acceleration and deceleration produce 2 to 2.5 times normal gravity during the pull-up and pull-out phases of the flight; the brief pushover at the apogee generates an environment with less than 1% of Earth's gravity. The nickname "vomit comet" aptly describes the gut-wrenching sensations produced during KC-135 training flights. The two insets show examples of practicing with tethered treadmill walking (left) and dynamic resistance training (right) during parabola practice. Online, videos from NASA show early reduced-gravity flights on the

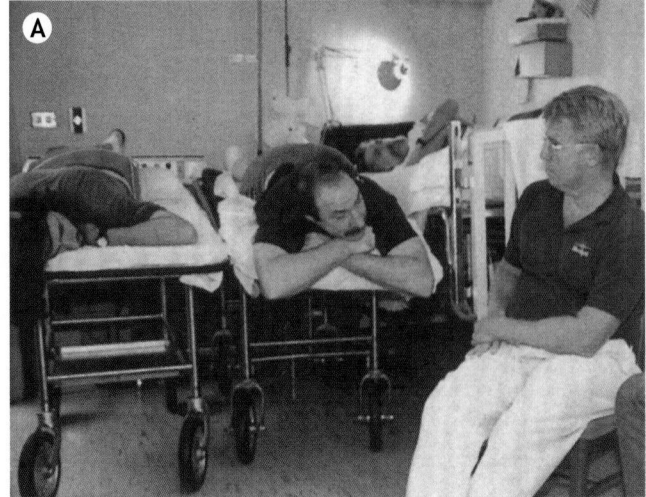

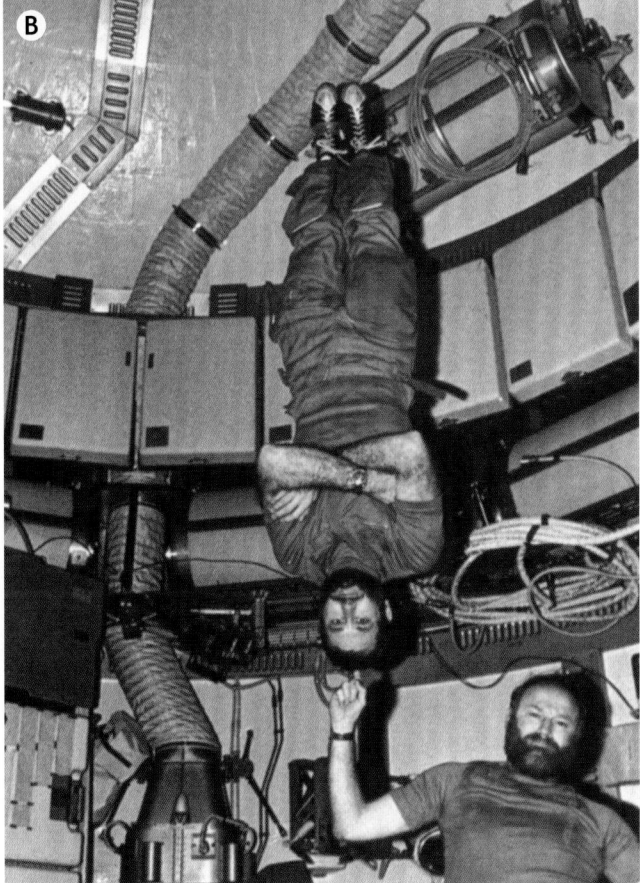

FIGURE 27.4 • **(A)** Bed-rest, head-down experimental strategy in the laboratory to simulate microgravity effects on postural hypotension and associated cardiovascular functions. **(B)** Demonstration of microgravity aboard spacelab where no "up" or "down" exists. (Photos courtesy of NASA, Lyndon B. Johnson Space Center, Houston, TX.)

KC-135 trainer with cats and birds (www.uh.edu/engines/epi166.htm), the physics of yo-yo training (www.youtube.com/watch?v=bpljytIwcaQ; with practical application for the tether assist) during microgravity on the ISS, and how

astronauts drink beverages from an open "space cup" during spaceflight.(http://io9.com/5893378/how-astronauts-use-space-cups-to-drink-in-low-gravity).

During repeated brief parabolic roller coaster–like maneuvers, scientists evaluate how humans and equipment function during intermittent forces that range from 1.8 g to near–zero-g, similar to those experienced during liftoff and reentry of space vehicles. Depending on the mission, astronaut training can include up to 60 **parabolic flights** daily for a week, providing about 3 hr of cumulative weightlessness. This specialized flight training prepares the space traveler for experiencing the initially high g-forces during lift-off in the time the spacecraft attains its escape velocity of 25,000 miles per hour (11,000 meters per second) to pull away from Earth's gravitational pull. The final flight of the KC-135 occurred on October 29, 2004; its replacement, a C-9 aircraft, is the military version of the DC-9 used by commercial airlines and military for medical evacuation, passenger transportation, and special missions.

The new field of bioastronautics focuses on biologic and medical effects of spaceflight on human systems. The National Space Biomedical Research Institute (NSBRI; www.nsbri.org) has developed long-range plans to implement research to reduce or prevent the known risks to astronaut health, safety, and mission performance.[36,41,128] In 2008, the NSBRI and NASA selected 33 research proposals to investigate questions of astronaut health and performance on future space exploration missions. The NSBRI supports research in many fields, particularly of importance to many aspects of exercise physiology. For example, the Human Factors and Performance Team studies ways to improve daily living and keep crewmembers and other personnel healthy, productive, and safe during exploration missions. The overall aims are to reduce performance errors and mitigate habitability, environmental, and behavioral factors that pose significant risks to mission success. The Team develops guidelines for human systems design and information tools to support crew performance. Team members examine ways to improve sleep and scheduling of work shifts,[102] including how specific types of lighting in the craft and habitat can improve alertness and performance. Other projects address improving the interactions between automated and manual control of a spacecraft and how environmental factors such as dust impact crew health.

Mathematical Modeling and Computer Simulations

Researchers generally consider an entire physiologic system (e.g., cardiovascular, thermoregulatory, hormonal, respiratory, muscular) or subdivide it into its component parts. For example, elements of the cardiovascular system include the heart, lungs, blood vessels, and blood. Each constituent can further subdivide into parts and factors such as vascular wall compliance, wall thickness, and blood flow within the heart's chambers or through its valves and specific vasculature. Researchers

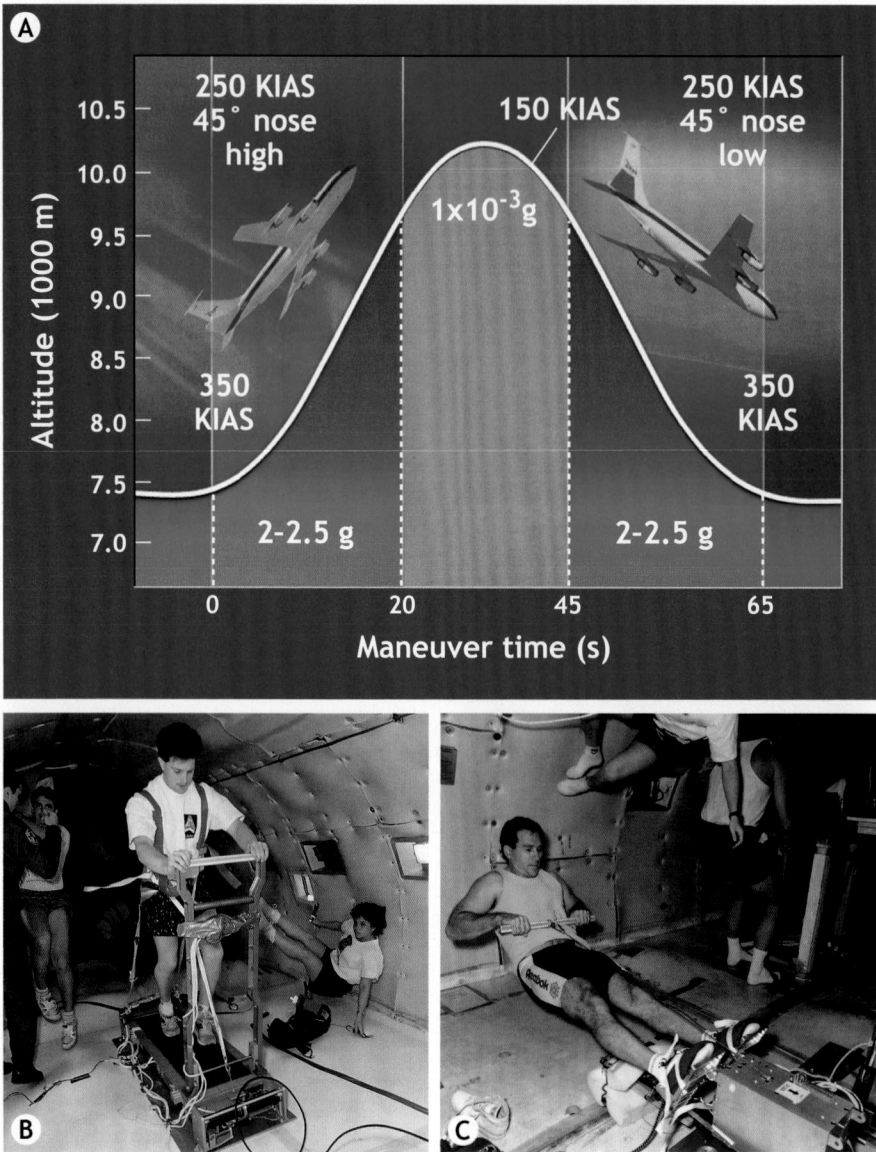

FIGURE 27.5 • **(A)** Parabolic (Keplerian trajectory) flight profile of NASA's KC-135 aircraft to achieve brief periods of weightlessness. KIAS refers to knots indicating air speed. (Reprinted from Nicogossian AE, et al. *Space Physiology and Medicine*. 3rd Ed. Philadelphia: Lea & Febiger, 1994.) From September 1995 to 2004, the KC-135 had flown 34,757 training, an equivalent of approximately 300 flight hours yearly. **(B)** Evaluating the shock absorption qualities caused by vibrations while running on a motorized treadmill during KC-135 flights. **(C)** Evaluating exercise equipment (aerobic and strength) during KC-135 flights. (Photos courtesy of NASA, Lyndon B. Johnson Space Center, Houston, TX.)

mathematically model each component on the basis of known values for a particular function (e.g., HR_{max} in young adults averages 200 b · min⁻¹).

Armed with facts about the entire physiologic system, a computer-based model recreates how the system would respond to weightlessness when changes affect single or multiple components. Researchers have applied mathematical models of the thermoregulatory and cardiovascular systems to establish design criteria for the astronaut's space suit. For example, the model predicts the range of energy expenditures an astronaut might encounter with

EVA (from 180 to 200 kcal · hr⁻¹) assessed during different space missions.[101]

HISTORICAL OVERVIEW OF AEROSPACE PHYSIOLOGY AND MEDICINE

Astronauts must overcome numerous challenges as they prepare to live in space for prolonged periods. Perhaps during the middle of this century, thousands of individuals will routinely travel into space, some establishing permanent space colonies relatively near Earth orbit, while others will participate in exploration-class Mars and asteroid missions.

The Early Balloonists

Almost 250 years ago, during the period in Europe when experimentation in science was thriving, a group of courageous explorers began to push the envelope for what could be considered "space travel." These pioneers, in essence the fathers of aerospace physiology and medicine, included Scottish meteorologists Alexander Wilson (1726–1753; first Regius Professor of Astronomy from the University of Glasgow) along with colleague Thomas Melville, in 1749 hoisted thermometers on six linked kites (balloons) with fuses attached to each to a height of 3000 feet so the thermometers could be dropped from different altitudes. These scientists were the first to record temperatures above Earth's surface. The Montgolfier brothers Joseph (1740–1810) and Etienne (1745–1799) in 1783 ascended over the Palace of Versailles, France, in a large-capacity hot-air balloon they designed. This early "space experiment" caused quite a stir, being observed by the King and Queen and their Court. Their balloon rose to 1000 to 1500 m and traveled about 2 km. The balloon, made of various fabrics (including silk) and lined with paper, was coated with alum as fireproofing, with about 2000 buttons holding its segments together. It stood 75 feet tall, 49 feet wide, and contained 77,000 cubic feet of hot air heated by burning straw and wool.

In 1783, French physicist and chemist Jac Alexander Cesar Charles (1746–1823) made one of the first free ascents with a passenger and gondola in a hydrogen-filled balloon. His contribution, which refined ballooning and allowed ascents to higher altitudes and longer distances, was to invent the valve at the balloon's apex to allow the release of hydrogen gas. An emerging cadre of science fiction writers began their descriptions of travel to "other worlds" (e.g., Jules Verne, *De la Terre a la Lune*, 1865; Edward Everett Hale, *Brick Moon*, serialized in *Atlantic Monthly* magazine in 1869–1870; Achille Eyraud, *Voyage a Venus*, 1875).

Balloons changed little over the next century, continuing to be filled with hot air, which rises because its density is lower than the colder air of the atmosphere. The balloons saw military action as "spies in the sky" during the American Civil War (almost exclusively by the North), and Napoleon used them to observe enemy troop positions during his many wars. World War I also saw the use of balloons for observations, including the extension of balloons into blimps and dirigibles. In 1931, Swiss physicist Auguste Piccard (1884–1963) and his colleague, Paul Kipfer (1884–1962), became the first humans to reach the stratosphere in Piccard's balloon, achieving an altitude of 51,762 feet (15,777 m). During this flight, in addition to making some scientific observations, Piccard and Kipfer demonstrated that Piccard's design worked. To allow people to survive in the stratosphere, Piccard designed the first pressurized gondola intended to keep air pressure within the gondola at a comfortable level even in the rarefied upper atmosphere. Piccard also designed a huge balloon that could lift the gondola while remaining partially inflated. This let the gas within the balloon expand as it ascended, giving steadily increasing lift. Piccard broke his record with an ascent to nearly 55,000 feet (16,764 m), and within a few years, others had risen to nearly 61,000 feet (18,593 m).[43] In his 2013 book, *Falling Upwards*, Richard Homes chronicles the rich history of early European and American aeronaut explorers, their balloons, and their adventures.

As humans venture into unexplored regions of space, new scientific knowledge about adaptations to microgravity affects exploration efforts. Research in exercise physiology and interrelated disciplines has considerably expanded knowledge about microgravity's effects on human structure and function, and adaptations and countermeasure strategies to minimize undesirable outcomes. Throughout the history of aerospace exploration, achieving each new milestone fostered new challenges to improve human safety and health while at the same time matching aircraft performance with the ambitious demands of flying faster and higher. A single historical event in 1957—the Russian **Sputnik 1** orbiting satellite (discussed below)—significantly impacted future research about physiologic function during high-altitude flights—thus accelerating man's quest to explore heavenly bodies beyond planet Earth.

Early Years

The first national civil aeronautics laboratory, now known as the National Aeronautics and Space Administration Langley Research Center, was established in 1917 in Hampton, Virginia. This research facility currently focuses on aeronautics, earth science, space technology and structures, and materials research (www.larc.nasa.gov). In 1951, the Aeromedical Association created a Space Medicine Branch for systematic evaluation of human function in a weightless environment (http://www.wpafb.af.mil/shared/media/document/AFD-081204-013.pdf). Two research laboratories, the U.S. Air Force School of Space Medicine and the Naval Aerospace Medical Institute (www.hq.nasa.gov/office/pao/History/SP-60/cover.html), also devoted time and resources to study space medicine. These military research facilities partnered with universities and private-sector laboratories to create a formidable team to study high-performance aircraft and unmanned guided missiles at high altitudes. Research eventually covered human adaptation to high-altitude exposure. This included development in the 1930s of pressurized suits to allow pilots to achieve higher altitudes than previously (50,000 ft), paving the way for the 1961–1963 Mercury series of suborbital flights and eventual lunar missions.[93] From 1951 to 1957, the two laboratories and auxiliary support facilities produced significant information, mostly about "hardware" aspects of spaceflight (www.hq.nasa.gov/office/pao/History/SP-60/cover.html) but also biomedical evaluations during suborbital flights with lower animal forms (bacteria, mice) and primates.

Wernher von Braun—The Father of Space Rocketry

Wernher von Braun (1912–1977), a German engineer strongly influenced in the early 1920s by Hermann Oberth, another German rocketry expert (see FYI on the Hubble Space Telescope, later in this chapter), played a prominent role in all aspects of rocketry and space exploration both in Germany and following World War II in the United States. Braun's PhD in physics from the University of Berlin contained theoretical insights and developmental experiments on 300- and 660-lb-thrust rocket engines. Braun became expert in liquid-fueled rocket aircraft and jet-assisted takeoffs, and played a prominent role in the Nazis' development of the feared V-2 rocket (meaning "Vengeance Weapon 2") that terrorized Europe with over 10,000 firings during WWII. After the war, Braun and his German rocket-development team surrendered

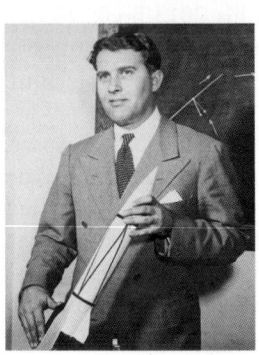

to U.S. troops. About 100 members of his group were sent to the U.S. Army Ordnance Corps test site at White Sands, New Mexico, where they assembled, tested, and supervised the launching of captured V-2s for high-altitude research purposes. Developmental studies were made of advanced ramjet and rocket missiles. At the end of the war, no doubt existed that the United States had definitively entered the field of guided missiles and advanced rocketry. Braun became technical director and later chief of the U.S. Army ballistic-weapon program. During the 1950s, he served as a national and international spokesperson for promoting space flight. In 1954, he developed a secret project to launch an Earth satellite Project Orbiter for military reconnaissance purposes. Before approval for its launch, the Soviets literally shocked the world by launching Sputnik 1 on October 4, 1957, followed by Sputnik 2 on November 3. A few months later on January 31, 1958, Braun and his army group were pressed to launch Explorer 1, the first U.S. satellite to go into orbit. And so the space race was "on" with the U.S. entry into orbital satellite deployment. As director of NASA's Marshall Space Flight Center in Huntsville, Alabama (**http://history.msfc.nasa.gov**), Braun led the development of the large space launch vehicles Saturn I, IB, and V. The engineering success of each rocket in the Saturn class of space boosters (the Saturn V eventually landed a man on the moon) contained millions of individual parts, and remains unparalleled in rocket history for its technical elegance and outstanding performance. Von Braun, a prolific writer, penned influential and authoritative books about rocketry and space travel. Examples include *Das Marsprojekt* (1952; *The Mars Project*); *Space Frontier*, rev. ed. (1971); *Across the Space Frontier* (1952); *Conquest of the Moon* (1953); *Exploration of Mars* (1956); *History of Rocketry and Space Travel*, rev. ed. (1969); and *Moon* (1970). Many excellent biographies chronicle the life and times of this influential space and rocket pioneer.

Suborbital Flights

In December 1946, experiments sponsored by the National Institutes of Health at Holloman's Aeromedical Field Laboratory (and later at Wright-Patterson Air Force Base and White Sands Air Force Base) studied cosmic radiation's effects on fungus spores (unsuccessful, as the cylinders carrying the microbes vanished on reentry) and how fruit flies survived without deleterious effects at an altitude of 171 km. The Albert Project (named for the monkey sealed in the nose cone of the V-2 rocket) attempted to record respiration during spaceflight, but the respiration apparatus failed just before launch and Albert perished. The mission was doomed anyway because the parachute recovery apparatus also failed on reentry.

A second launch (Albert II) occurred 1 year later on June 14, 1949, but the primate died on impact when the recovery chute again failed. Fortunately, respiratory and electrocardiographic instruments verified that the primate functioned well during the 83-mile ascent and return. Two additional V-2 rocket flights provided supportive evidence that a primate could successfully withstand reentry forces of 5.5g and exposure to cosmic radiation. A fifth V-2 launch substituted a mouse for the monkey, and an onboard camera photographed the mouse at fixed intervals. The mouse died on impact (once again the recovery system failed), but the mouse displayed normal muscular function and coordination during the subgravity flight. Additional flights in 1951 that monitored cardiovascular and respiratory dynamics of primates showed no negative responses during these relatively brief missions.

With subsequent travel, rocketry systems improved and the onboard monkey and mouse "animalnauts" survived intact during suborbital flights to altitudes of 36 miles. High-altitude balloon flights also proved successful. In September 1950, eight white mice withstood a 97,000-ft ascent without negative physiologic consequences. The balloon experiments continued with fruit flies, mice, hamsters, cats, and dogs for up to 24 hr. Most of these experiments ended in failure, mainly from equipment malfunction. Nonetheless, the invaluable experience gained from rocket and balloon launchings, instrumentation and recovery techniques, and the growing body of scientific data related to cosmic radiation and subgravity physiologic responses would greatly benefit subsequent human endeavors. The years 1946 through 1952 marked the practical beginning of Air Force research in space biology, setting the stage for the next round of experimentation with more powerful rockets.

High-Altitude Explorations

Between 1952 and 1957, research in high-altitude exploration matched the United States' enthusiasm for its embryonic space biology programs. Study areas included human reaction to subgravity or near–zero-g conditions, human reentry into Earth's atmosphere, effects of abrupt and sustained acceleration and deceleration on human response to rocket flight, and equipment design to better accommodate primate and human explorers as they pushed the envelope by ascending higher (120,000-ft balloon ascent) and for longer durations (up to 74 h). In 1952, the National Advisory Committee for Aeronautics (NACA; established in 1915 to foster aviation) proposed new research to extend airplane velocity to Mach 10 at altitudes from 12 to 50 miles, and identify problems with spaceflights at speeds that required a 25,039-mph (40,200 km $\cdot$ hr^{-1}, or 1.12×10^4 m $\cdot$ s^{-1}m) escape velocity from Earth's gravity.

Mach numbers were named to honor Austrian physicist Ernst Mach (1838–1916) who established basic principles of supersonics and ballistics. The Mach number represents the ratio of an object's velocity to the velocity of sound, which travels at 1089 ft $\cdot$ s^{-1} or 331.9 m $\cdot$ s^{-1} at 0°C. For example, Mach 10 refers to 10 times the speed of sound. Interestingly, Professor Mach rejected Newton's concepts of absolute time and space before Einstein, who cited Mach's inertial theories in the early 1900s in developing his relativity theory.

By 1954, characteristics for a new hypersonic research aircraft had been defined, and 1 year later, North American Aviation won the competition to build the X-15 airplane (http://history.nasa.gov/x15/cover.html). Construction began in September 1957, ushering in a new era that featured high-performance aircraft capable of hypersonic speeds (4250 mph) at altitudes close to the fringes of the atmosphere (67 mi, or 353,760 ft). Concurrently, the United States had committed to launch an Earth-orbiting satellite as part of the International Geophysical Year (July 1, 1957 to December 31, 1958) to gather scientific information about our planet. At the same time, the early phases of developing a potential space vehicle and sophisticated satellite program were about to change in sudden and dramatic fashion.

Sputnik: The Rocket Launch That Shocked the World

On October 4, 1957, the Russians shocked the world when their 83.6-kg, 58-cm diameter aluminum alloy Sputnik 1 became the first Earth-orbiting satellite (**Fig. 27.6**). One month later on November 3, a larger 508-kg Sputnik 2 remained in orbit for almost 200 days with a dog on board. These space milestones—achieved 4 mo before the Naval Research Laboratory launched its inaugural, tiny 1.6-kg Vanguard 1 orbiting, unmanned satellite—jolted the United States' scientific and government establishments into a sense of urgency to surpass Russia's apparent space technology supremacy. Two factors contributed to a "space race" to achieve dominance of this new frontier:

1. Fear of losing potential military superiority in space
2. Fear of losing the "education race" to an enlightened Russian youth who excelled in mathematics and science

MODERN ERA

In 1958, the newly formed NASA laid the groundwork for future discoveries that would affect almost every facet of our

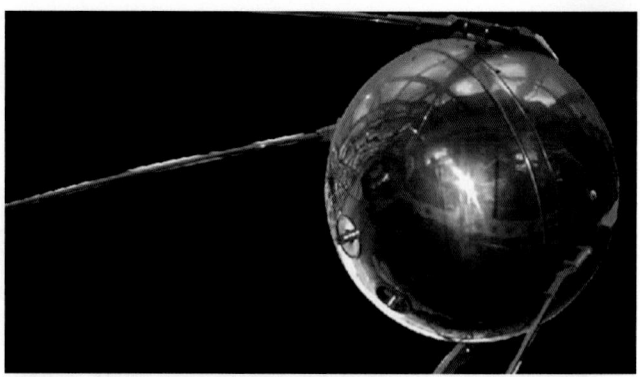

FIGURE 27.6 • Sputnik 1 satellite. This beach ball–sized sphere took just 98 min to orbit the Earth on its elliptical path—but its journey sent shockwaves around the globe. As a technical achievement (**www.nasa.gov/externalflash/SpaceAge/**), Sputnik caught the world's attention and the American public off-guard. The public feared that the Soviets' ability to launch satellites also translated into the capability to launch ballistic missiles that could carry nuclear weapons from Europe to the United States. Sputnik in Russian means "fellow traveler" or "traveling companion of the world." Sputnik 1 lofted into space by a powerful R7 Russian rocket. It carried a thermometer and two radio transmitters. Sputnik transmitted atmospheric information by radio (**www.astrosurf.com/luxorion/Documents/sat-sputnik.wav**), but its two transmitters only functioned for 21 days. After 57 days in orbit, it was destroyed while reentering the atmosphere.

lives. These included discoveries about rocketry and propulsion systems, physiologic requirements and adaptations to manned spaceflight, and more than 30,000 practical "technology-transfer" payoffs (see "Practical Benefits from Space Biology Research," later in this chapter) from interdisciplinary experiments in physical chemistry, microbiology, genetics, medicine, and exercise physiology.

NASA had two main goals: (1) launching a man into space and returning him safely to Earth and (2) developing the capability of humans to endure space missions.[97] Achieving this second goal had been a Herculean task because the current knowledge of microgravity's effects remained restricted to laboratory simulations. Scientists knew little about how humans would respond to the rigors of microgravity and what might happen during extended sojourns beyond Earth's gravitational field. Experts publicly expressed concern about possible deleterious effects of spaceflight on human function and overall health. In 1958, the National Academy of Sciences National Research Council Committee on Bioastronautics listed potential ill effects from human exposure to the space environment during launch and reentry (**Table 27.1**). Some concerns proved justified and are discussed in subsequent sections.

United States Races into Space

NASA's top priority besides initiating human spaceflight centered on a plan to allow humans to work for extended periods during prolonged space missions. NASA's two goals required

IN A PRACTICAL SENSE

Space Suits for Space Travel

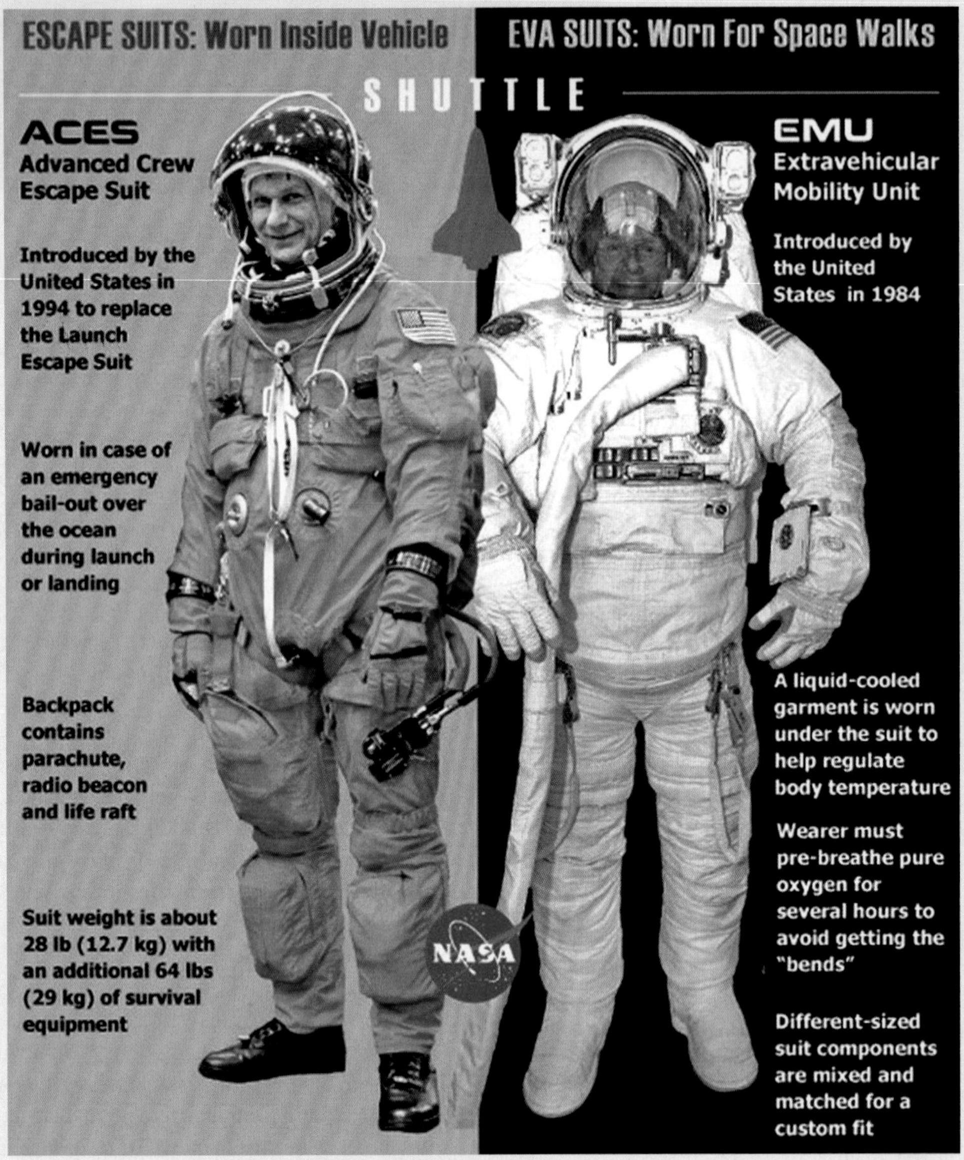

ESCAPE SUITS: Worn Inside Vehicle **EVA SUITS: Worn For Space Walks**

SHUTTLE

ACES
Advanced Crew
Escape Suit

Introduced by the
United States in
1994 to replace
the Launch
Escape Suit

Worn in case of
an emergency
bail-out over
the ocean
during launch
or landing

Backpack
contains
parachute,
radio beacon
and life raft

Suit weight is about
28 lb (12.7 kg) with
an additional 64 lbs
(29 kg) of survival
equipment

NASA

EMU
Extravehicular
Mobility Unit

Introduced by
the United
States in 1984

A liquid-cooled
garment is worn
under the suit to
help regulate
body temperature

Wearer must
pre-breathe pure
oxygen for
several hours to
avoid getting the
"bends"

Different-sized
suit components
are mixed and
matched for a
custom fit

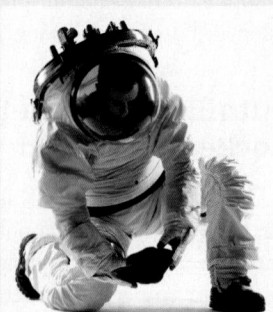

Modern space travel relies on two types of pressurized space suits, with a third suit in development for a future Mars mission:

1. *Advanced Crew Escape Suit* (ACES). This full-pressure suit, introduced in 1994, replaced the older Launch Escape Suit (LES; **www.nasa.gov/multimedia/3d_resources/ assets/aces.html**), first worn by U.S. Air Force pilots in the mid-1970s, replacing a similar suit worn by SR-71 and U-2 high-altitude reconnaissance pilots (**www.blackbirds. net/u2/u-2mission.html**). The LES was almost identical to the high-altitude suits worn by X-15 pilots and Gemini astronauts (**http://nssdc.gsfc.nasa.gov/planetary/ gemini.html**). Unlike the current full-pressure ACES, the high-altitude suits were partial pressure suits designed

to protect the crew in the event of loss of cabin pressure at altitudes up to 30 km. The suits also served to insulate the pilots from cold air or hostile water temperatures after a bailout in case of an accident. During reentry, an anti-G protection system consisted of pressure bladders in the legs and lower abdomen to attenuate blood pooling in the lower body. The current suit weighs 28 lb (12.7 kg) and can protect the crew from any contamination in the cabin atmosphere. An additional backpack weighing 64 lb (29 kg) contains a parachute, radio beacon, and life raft. The one-piece garment assembly incorporates integrated pressure bladders with a self-contained ventilation system. Oxygen, fed through a connector at the wearer's left thigh, travels to the helmet through a connector at the base of the neck ring. The helmet and gloves connect to the suit with locking rings. The international orange "pumpkin" color suit has a Dupont Nomex cover layer (flame-resistant meta-aramid material developed in the 1960s) that allows rescue units to easily spot the astronauts in case of an emergency ocean "ditching." Astronauts wear maximum-absorbency garment (MAG) urine-containment trunks underneath the suits that resemble "Depends" incontinence shorts and thermal underwear. Plastic tubing woven into the garments allows for liquid cooling and ventilation. A full pressure helmet with a locking clear visor and a black sunshade reduces any glare from reflected sunlight, especially during the approach and landing. Black leather "paratrooper-type" boots with zippers instead of laces help to prevent foot and ankle injuries and reduce foot swelling with suit pressurization. Each suit is sized individually for the astronaut. ACES have not failed during normal flight operations, although a report released by the Columbia Accident Investigation Board (www.nasa.gov/columbia/home/CAIB_Vol1.html) concluded that the suits would not have protected the astronauts at the altitude and velocity of the *Columbia* breakup in 2003.

2. *Extravehicular mobility unit (EMU) garment.* The EMU spacesuit serves many life-support functions; it provides for environmental protection outside of the spacecraft, mobility during extravehicular activities (EVA) in Earth orbit and during International Space Station (ISS) missions (see EVA example Fig. 27.4B), and intra-astronaut communications during spacewalks and constant communication with ISS and mission control on Earth. Introduced in 1982, the EMI consists of a two-piece semi-rigid suit, and was worn by NASA's astronauts prior to the termination of the Shuttle missions in 2011. The EMU consists of a hard upper torso (HUT) assembly, a primary life support system (PLSS), which incorporates the life support and electrical systems, arm sections, gloves, an Apollo-style "bubble" helmet, the extravehicular visor assembly (EVVA), and a soft lower torso assembly (LTA), incorporating the body seal closure (BSC), waist-bearing briefs, legs, and boots. The crew member wears a similar MAG to that worn in the ACES with thermal control

undergarment or "long johns." The liquid cooling and ventilation garment (LCVG) incorporates clear plastic tubing through which chilled liquid water flows to control body temperature. It also includes separate ventilation tubes for waste gas removal. The EMU provides support for 8.5 hr, with a 30-min reserve in case of primary life support failure. To perform an EVA from the space vehicle, the cabin pressure is reduced from 14.7 psi to 10.2 psi for 24 hr, after which the astronaut must prebreathe oxygen for 45 min. For ISS EVAs, the astronaut prebreathes for about 4 hr. The latest suits on ISS have increased battery capacity, improved cameras and radios, and a new caution and warning system. Another unique feature includes an additional battery to power heaters built into the gloves, allowing astronauts to keep their hands warm during nighttime passages on each 95-min orbit.

3. *Z-1 Prototype Spacesuit and Portable Life Support System (PLSS) 2.0.* Getting inspiration from the "Buzz Lightyear" character in the movie *Toy Story 3* (http://movies.yahoo.com/news/nasas-next-generation-spacesuit-looks-buzz-lightyear-050000433.html), the newly designed PLSS undergoing development and testing at the Lyndon B. Johnson Space Center (www.jsc.nasa.gov/roundup/online/2012/0312.pdf) will replace the 40-year-old EMU technology for use in future space explorations set to begin within two decades. The spacesuit will contain a large backpack with unique features, one of which doubles as a hatch that can latch onto another space vehicle so an astronaut can easily crawl through from the back without letting dust or foreign particles in or air out. The new backpack will sustain all of the astronaut's life-support needs including oxygen delivery, new technologies to provide more efficient cooling to better eliminate carbon dioxide and trace contaminants including temperature regulation for the crew member, continuous ventilation flow, and an electronics package that includes wireless communication among astronauts and the home base. Unique Z-1 features include new bearings on the legs, ankles, hips, and waist to help the wearer ambulate more naturally, including urethane-coated nylon and polyester layers for optimal control of the suit's internal pressure.

---

advanced technologies in rocket design and effective approaches to prepare test pilots for missions never attempted previously. To put a human into Earth orbit required new ways of looking at the man–machine interface. On the human side, engineers had to design a fail-safe life-support system, provide for food and water, integrate an efficient method to remove metabolic byproducts, and implement temperature control to ensure crew safety during liftoff, flight, and reentry. Research had to determine physiologic responses to extremes of acceleration and reduced gravity, including short- and long-term adjustments to prolonged weightlessness. Could a human function competently

during liftoff, propelled upward at thousands of miles per hour, and then perform flawlessly in maneuvering the space vehicle and returning it to Earth safely? Engineers needed to develop rocket engines with sufficient thrust to achieve escape velocity. The pilot's capsule required intricate communication and navigation controls. The capsule's weight and size had to dovetail with rocket design and launch requirements. In addition, a capsule recovery system required development for safe reentry. The human and engineering requirements facing NASA provided considerable challenges to say the least, but the race into space was on with no turning back.

TABLE 27.1	Potential Deleterious Effects of Weightlessness for Launch, Travel, and Reentry

- Anorexia
- Bone demineralization
- Cardiac arrhythmia
- Decreased g tolerance
- Decreased work capacity
- Dehydration
- Disorientation
- Diuresis
- Euphoria
- Fatigue
- Gastrointestinal disturbance
- Hallucinations
- Hypertension
- Hypotension
- Infectious illnesses
- Motion sickness
- Muscular incoordination
- Muscle atrophy
- Nausea
- Postflight syncope
- Pulmonary atelectasis
- Reduced blood volume
- Reduced plasma volume
- Renal calculi
- Restlessness
- Sleepiness
- Sleeplessness
- Tachycardia
- Urine retention
- Weight loss

Adapted from Dietlein LF. Skylab: a beginning. In: Johnston RS, Dietlein LF, eds. *Biomedical Results from Skylab* (NASA SP-377). Washington, DC: U.S. Government Printing Office, 1977.

thePoint   Appendix J, available online at **http://thepoint. lww.com/mkk8e**, chronicles the accomplishments of the United States and Soviet human space programs from Project Mercury to the International Space Station.

United States Human Space Program

The key achievements of the United States and Russian space programs relate to advances in space medicine and physiology. These superpowers played the dominant role in the space effort, but not without significant contributions from European, Japanese, and Canadian human space programs. Their remarkable successes culminated in the two 1998 launches of Russian and United States rockets to initiate assembly of the ISS.

Perhaps the most significant technologic achievement of the 20th century took place on July 20, 1969, when Apollo 11 astronauts Edwin "Buzz" Aldrin (1930–; **www.buzzaldrin. com**) and Neil Armstrong (1930–2012; **www.jsc.nasa.gov/ Bios/htmlbios/armstrong-na.html**) landed on the Moon's surface in the lunar module Eagle after it separated from the main spacecraft at 50,000 feet. With these words, "Houston, Tranquility Base here. The Eagle has landed," the world knew a momentous accomplishment had taken place. Seven hours later, Armstrong's hopeful words as he set foot on the lunar surface—"*One small step for man, one giant leap for mankind*"—resonated worldwide to demonstrate that humans could travel to the moon, explore its surface, and return safely to Earth. Aldrin joined him on the surface several minutes later, and for 2 hr they collected rocks, planted the American flag on lunar soil in the Sea of Tranquility, and took photographs. Thus, it had taken almost a decade and $25.4 billion to achieve the goal of putting a man on the moon that President

John F. Kennedy first stated to both houses of Congress on May 25, 1961:

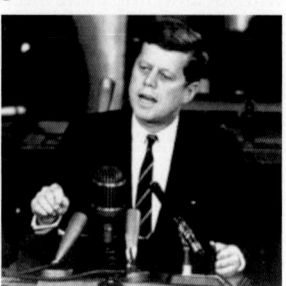

I believe that this nation should commit itself to achieving the goal, before this decade is out, of landing a man on the Moon and returning him safely to the Earth. No single space project in this period will be more impressive to mankind, or more important for the long-range exploration of space; and none will be so difficult or expensive to accomplish (**www.space. com/11775-president-kennedy-moonshot-moment.html**).

Indeed, the Apollo program achieved its three main objectives: (1) ensuring the safety and health of crew members, (2) preventing contamination of Earth by extraterrestrial organisms, and (3) studying specific effects of space exposure on the human body. During the pioneering and highly successful Apollo program, 12 astronauts walked on the moon during six lunar landings.

MEDICAL EVALUATION FOR ASTRONAUT SELECTION

Candidates for astronaut currently undergo extensive medical and psychologic evaluation[61,111]; the primary objective of U.S.–Russian cooperation in space medicine is to maintain the health and fitness of space crews aboard joint missions to the ISS.[55,95] Little factual information existed about what to expect during spaceflight or the personal characteristics necessary for mission success when NASA devised the first medical evaluation in 1959. Approximately 600 active military test pilots from the Navy, Air Force, Army, and Marine Corps served as the initial candidate pool. From this group, NASA invited 110 for further testing. Thirty-two pilot finalists qualified for the next phase of testing, which included the exhaustive 23-item test battery listed in **TABLE 27.2**.

First Astronauts

The test battery identified a final group of candidates believed best qualified to achieve the following five goals:

1. *Survive*—Demonstrate ability to fly in space and return safely.
2. *Perform*—Demonstrate ability to perform effectively under the conditions of spaceflight.
3. *Serve as a backup for automatic controls and instrumentation*—Increase the reliability of flight systems.
4. *Serve as a scientific observer*—Go beyond what the instruments and satellites can observe and report.
5. *Serve as an engineering observer and true test pilot*—Improve the flight system and its components.

In April 1959, NASA selected the final seven astronauts

TABLE 27.2	Physiologic and Psychologic Testing of the First American Project Mercury Astronauts

Physiologic Tests	Psychologic Tests
1. *Harvard step test:* Subject steps up 20 inches to platform and down once every 2 s for 5 min to measure physical fitness.	1. Extensive interviews (psychiatrists)
	2. Rorschach (ink blot)
2. *Treadmill maximum workload:* Subject walks at constant rate on moving platform elevated 1° each min; test continues until heart rate reaches 180 b·min^{-1}; test of physical fitness	3. Thematic apperception (stories suggested by pictures)
	4. Draw-a-person
	5. Sentence completion
	6. Self-inventory from 566-item questionnaire
3. *Cold pressor:* Subject plunges feet into tub of ice water; pulse and blood pressure measured before and during test.	7. Officer effectiveness inventory
	8. Personal-preference schedule from 225 pairs of self-descriptive statements
4. *Complex behavior simulator:* A panel with 12 signals, each requiring a different response, measures ability to react reliably in confusing situations.	9. Preference evaluation from 52 statements
	10. Determination of authoritarian attitudes
	11. Peer ratings
5. *Tilt table:* Subject lies on steeply inclined table for 25 min to measure heart's ability to compensate for unusual body position for extended duration.	12. Interpretation of the question "Who am I?"
	13. Wechsler Adult Scale
	14. Miller Analogies Test
6. *Partial pressure suit:* Subject is taken to simulated altitude of 65,000 ft for 1 hr in MC-1 partial pressure suit; measure of cardiovascular efficiency and breathing at low ambient pressures.	15. Raven Progressive Matrices
	16. Doppelt Mathematical Reasoning Scale
	17. Engineering analogies
	18. Mechanical comprehension
7. *Isolation:* Subject enters a dark, soundproof room for 3 hr to assess adaptation to unusual circumstances and coping without external stimuli.	19. Air Force Officer Qualification Test
	20. Aviation qualification test (United States Navy) space memory
8. *Acceleration:* Subject is placed in centrifuge with seat inclined at various angles; assesses near-multiple gravity forces.	21. Spatial orientation
	22. Gottschaldt Hidden Figures
9. *Heat:* Subject spends 2 hr in chamber at 130°F; measures reactions of heart and body functions to this stress.	23. Guilford-Zimmerman Spatial Visualization
10. *Equilibrium and vibration:* Subject seated on chair that rotates simultaneously on two axes; subject required to maintain chair on even keel using control stick with and without vibration; subject tested with and without blindfold.	
11. *Noise:* Subject exposed to different sound frequencies to determine susceptibility to high-frequency tones.	

An executive decision pronounced that the new astronauts would only be males with commissions in the armed services and with prior fighter pilot training and experience. This elite group, survivors of an extraordinarily elaborate search and selection process, would train to enter an unknown environment with a life-support system previously tested only during high-altitude balloon flights.

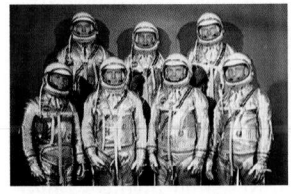

Project Mercury-7 astronauts. (Photo courtesy of NASA, Lyndon B. Johnson Space Center, Houston, TX.)

Although not made public at the time, a special flight-training program included a program for a final group of 13 highly qualified female aviators with extensive flight experience for future space missions. Shortly before the 13 finalists, known as the First Lady Astronaut Trainees (FLATS), were scheduled to report for testing at Pensacola, Florida, the Navy unceremoniously scuttled this effort, in part because of bureaucratic cronyism at the highest levels of the space agency.[2,161] Without official NASA support to conduct the tests, the Navy would not allow the use of their facilities. NASA's official position required that all astronauts be jet test pilots and have engineering degrees. Because no women could meet those requirements (although by every account they were as qualified for flight status as their male counterparts), no women could qualify to become an astronaut! Interestingly, test pilot Geraldine (Jerrie) Cobb was the first and only woman to undergo and successfully pass all three phases of Mercury astronaut testing (**Fig. 27.7**).[25] She passed the same medical tests at the same clinic that evaluated the final cadre of aspiring male test pilots who eventually were selected as the Mercury 7 crew (www.mercury13.com/). Cobb's autobiography and other books are highly recommended for insights into the male-dominated world of test pilots and into these women's zeal to become the first female NASA astronauts.[10,64,98]

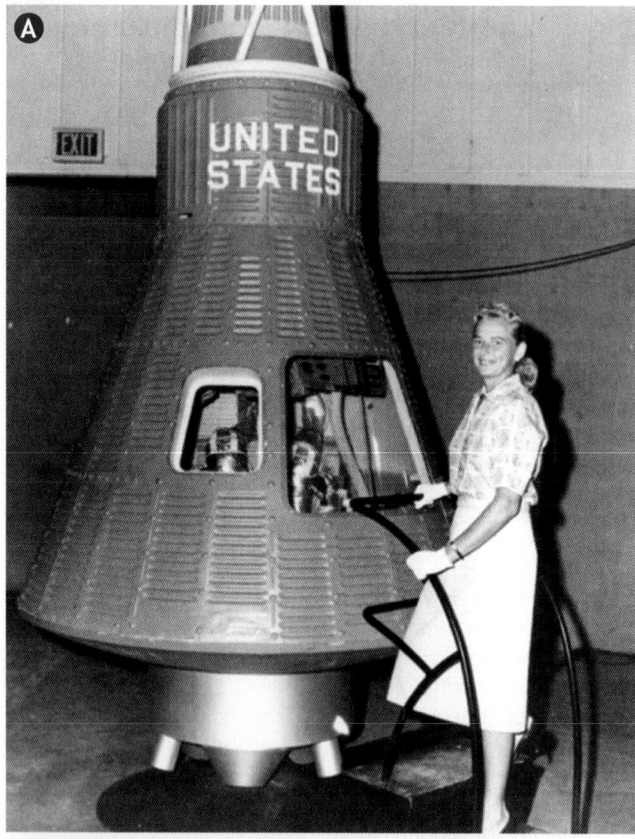

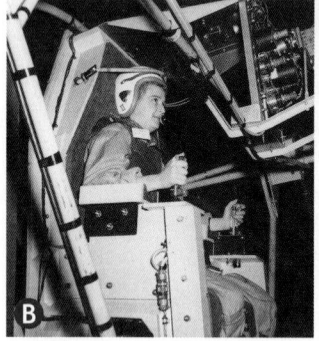
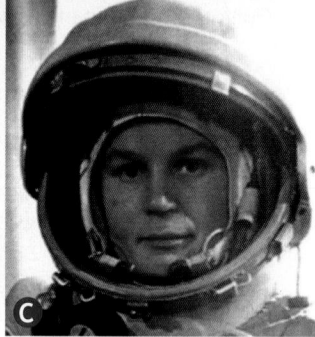

FIGURE 27.7 • **(A)** Test pilot Jerrie Cobb (1931–; www.jerrie-cobb.org) poses next to a Mercury spaceship capsule. She passed all of the training exercises and demanding medical tests, ranking in the top 2% of all astronaut candidates. **(B)** Cobb pilots the Gimbal Rig (formally called MASTIF, or Multiple Axis Space Test Inertia Facility) in the altitude wind tunnel at Lewis Research Center (now John H. Glenn Research Center; www.nasa.gov/centers/glenn/home/index.html) in April 1960. The Gimbal Rig trained astronauts to control the spin of a tumbling spacecraft. Dr. William Randolf "Randy" Lovelace II (1907–1965; www.nmspacemuseum.org/halloffame/detail.php?id=19), physician and NASA aerospace scientist who conducted the official Mercury program physical exams (without official NASA approval) at his private Lovelace Medical Foundation Clinic, now the Lovelace Respiratory Research Institute in Albuquerque, New Mexico. **(C)** Cosmonaut and engineer Valentina V. Tereshkova (1937–), the first female test pilot, flew into space aboard the Vostok 6 spacecraft (www.youtube.com/watch?v=GRBYDTlovjk) during 48 orbits and nearly 71 hr in space, 15 years before the first American woman achieved that goal. Her flight served as the first space mission where physiological measurements were collected about female response to microgravity.

In October 1962, in its annual report, the House Committee on Science and Astronautics issued these recommendations from the subcommittee on astronaut qualifications:

> After hearing witnesses, both Government and non-Government, including Astronauts Glenn and Carpenter, the subcommittee concluded that NASA's program of selection was basically sound and properly directed, that the highest possible standards should continue to be maintained, and that some time in the future, consideration should be given to inaugurating a program of research to determine the advantages to be gained by utilizing women as astronauts. (Report of the Special Subcommittee on the Selection of Astronauts: Qualifications for Astronauts. Committee on Science and Astronautics. U.S. House of Representatives. 87th Congress. Second Session. Serial S. Washington, DC: U.S. Government Printing Office, 1962.)

Ironically, it was Colonel John Glenn (who did not have an engineering degree before he became one of the Mercury astronauts and would have been eliminated from the program had NASA strictly enforced its regulations) who testified to the committee: "It is just a fact. The men go off and fight the wars and fly the airplanes and come back and help design and build and test them. The fact that women are not in this field is a fact of our social order. It may be undesirable."[114]

It was not until 1978 that NASA selected six women as astronaut candidates (http://womenshistory.about.com/od/aviationspace/a/timeline_space.htm), 15 years *after* cosmonaut Valentina Tereshkova from the USSR (Fig. 27.7C) became the first woman rocketed into space. She orbited Earth 48 times during a 3-day flight from June 17 to 19, 1963.

In addition to medical screening and testing, NASA conducts retrospective and longitudinal studies of astronauts matched against a large control group of Johnson Space Center employees. A behind-the-scenes view of astronaut training, written by the astronaut candidates in the form of journals, provides insights from the time they entered the program through spaceflight (www.nasa.gov/centers/johnson/astronauts/journals_astronauts.html).

Until about age 40, astronauts score better on health and fitness variables than non-astronaut controls. The comparative data provide an important baseline for future studies of the possible effects of short- and long-term microgravity exposure on parameters concerned with overall health and aging. NASA sponsors three types of studies:

1. *Data analysis from single flights.* Research involves ongoing data collection about space motion sickness symptoms experienced before, during, and after flights. Experiments aim to validate ground-based predictive tests of an individual's susceptibility to this malady and to define operationally acceptable countermeasures.[99,115]
2. *Longitudinal studies spanning several missions.* Such studies quantify the cumulative effects of repeated exposure to the space environment, particularly radiation effects on cancer risk and bone mineral loss.[13,60]

3. *Longitudinal studies throughout careers.* Long-term medical surveillance documents occupational injuries and maladies during or following space missions.[110] The longest-duration study of physiologic responses after microgravity exposure involves studies of astronaut John Glenn, Jr. (1921–), the first American to orbit Earth, who piloted the 1962 Friendship 7 Earth-orbital space mission.

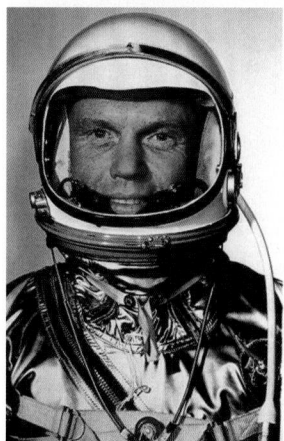

Thirty-six years later on October 29, 1998, at age 77, Glenn served as a Payload Specialist 2 on Shuttle Discovery STS-95 for an 8-day mission. The experiments involved studies of bone and muscle loss, balance, and sleep disorders (www.spaceflight.nasa.gov/shuttle/archives/sts-95/ index.html).

Occupational Health Program

In addition to NASA's exercise physiology laboratory, the Occupational Health Program (OHP; www.ohp.nasa.gov) consists of approximately 400 occupational medicine and environmental health professionals distributed across 10 primary NASA centers. This team provides comprehensive medical support to a diverse, highly technologic workforce of more than 60,000 civil servant and contractor employees involved in human exploration and development of space, aeronautics research, and Earth and space science activities. The traditional occupational health program elements include medical surveillance, industrial hygiene, health physics, emergency medical response, employee assistance programs, physical fitness programs, and overall health and wellness programs. Astronauts in training for a mission participate at the Johnson Space Center in developmental fitness regimens in modern facilities similar to most university and commercial gymnasia.

Radiation Effects. For astronauts living in low-Earth orbit for extended periods, including exploratory Mars missions and beyond, radiation exposure poses potentially serious health concerns.[134,166] Current preflight requirements include projecting a mission radiation dosage, assessing the probability of solar flares during the mission, and quantifying the radiation exposure history of flight crew members. Each crew member carries a passive dosimeter (radiation-measuring device), and highly sensitive dosimeters located throughout the spacecraft continually monitor radiation in case of solar flares or other radiation contingencies.[108] Different kinds of radiation during liftoff and aboard the spacecraft on short-duration missions at nominal orbit generally pose an "acceptable" level of hazard to astronaut health (e.g., blood-forming organs, lens of eyes, skin).[96,165]

BONE

Spaceflight has produced considerable biomedical information about human physiology in microgravity, beginning on May 5, 1961, with astronaut Alan Shepard's (1923–1998) solo flight aboard Freedom 7 (http://history.nasa.gov/40thmerc7/shepard.htm). This capstone event launched suborbitally to an altitude of 116 miles, 303 statute miles downrange from the Cape Canaveral launch complex. His 15-min, 28-s flight attained a final velocity of 5134 miles per hour and pulled a maximum of 11g's. From this point on, the race had begun for NASA and their astronaut heroes to explore uncharted paths outside of Earth's gravitational pull. In the ensuing 50 years, researchers have quantified physiologic adaptations to relatively brief space missions (1–14 d) and flights lasting longer than 2 wk, including postflight adaptations.

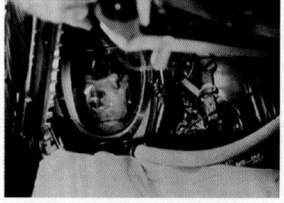

FIGURE 27.8 displays a generalized schema of the dynamics of physiologic functions during microgravity exposure. These include the effects of two major factors: reduced hydrostatic gradients (purple box left with white text) and reduced loading and disuse of weight-bearing tissues (purple box right with white text). The graphic reveals how these two factors impact the following six systems:

1. Cardiovascular and cardiopulmonary (orange)
2. Hematologic (dark blue)
3. Fluid, electrolyte, and hormonal (red)
4. Muscle (green)
5. Bone (light blue)
6. Neurosensory and vestibular (aqua)

Each system has been color coded as noted above, with arrows indicating how one system might influence another. For example, trace the pathways between a decrease in hydrostatic gradients and reduced total blood volume. How many different pathways interact to reduce total blood volume? Similarly, trace how altered sensory and balance information also affects blood volume and maximal exercise capacity. All of the different systems impact singularly yet often interact with each other, with all being impacted by the two main factors: reduced hydrostatic gradients and loading and disuse of weight-bearing tissues. Scientists who work in the field of aerospace medicine strive to unravel the separate yet compounding influences of the six main systems affected by space travel. Two of NASA's main research efforts focus on the impact of reduced bone density on risk of bone fractures and functional impact of skeletal muscle atrophy (reduced strength) on performing mission-related tasks.[87,118]

These physiologic responses to microgravity, in addition to the heart's reduced stroke volume related to orthostatic hypotension and possible syncope, have implications for developing and testing effective countermeasure strategies (see "Countermeasure Strategies," later in this chapter). Excellent summary resource materials exist about the body's cardiovascular, pulmonary, body fluid, sensory, bone loss, and musculoskeletal responses to microgravity.[18,29,44,45,47,52,56,77,131,148,162]

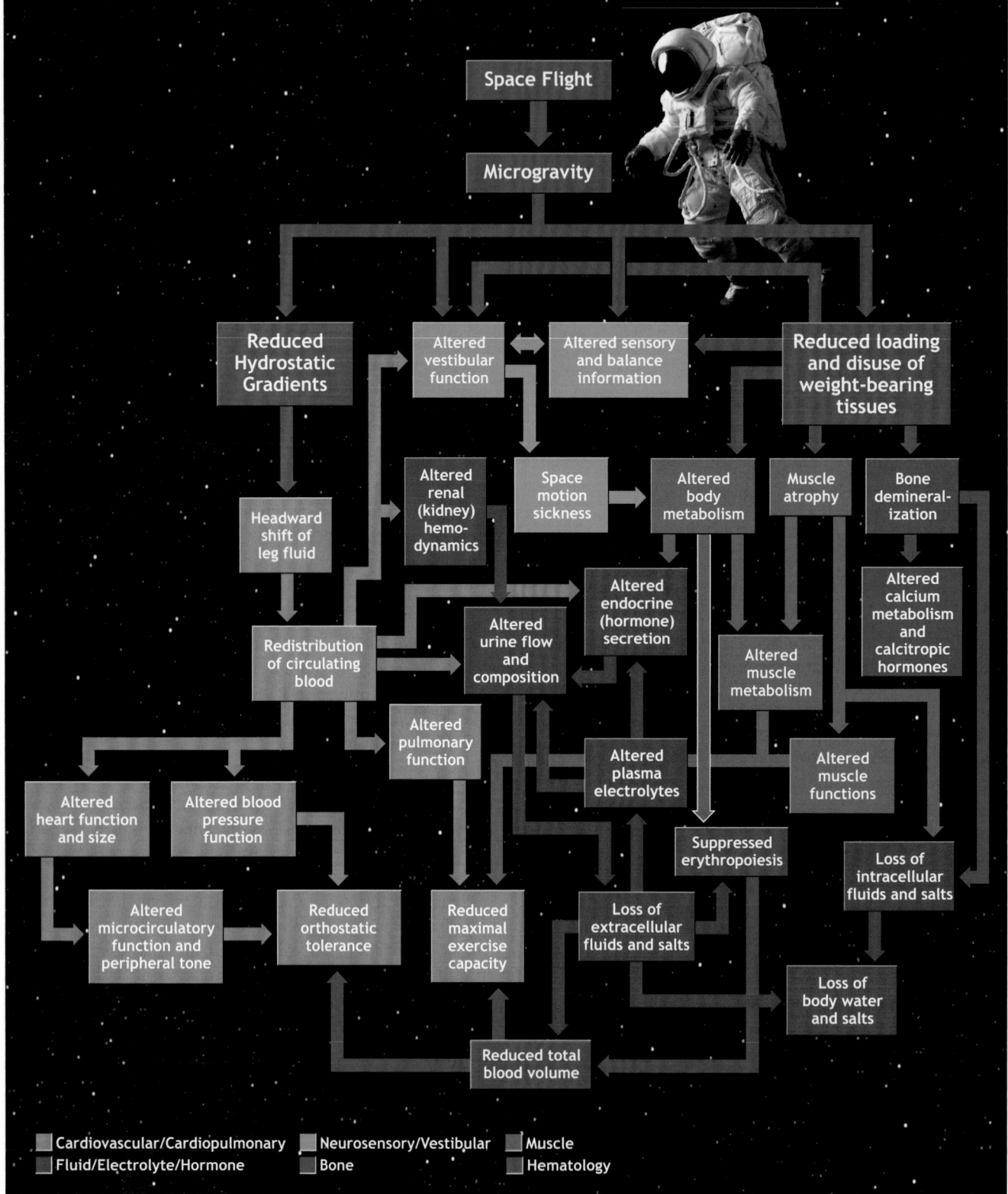

FIGURE 27.8 • General schema of microgravity's effects on physiologic alterations from (1) reduced hydrostatic gradients and (2) reduced loading and disuse of weight-bearing tissues. (Adapted from Lujan BF, White RJ. Human Physiology in Space; **www.nsbri.org/humanphysspace/**.)

thePoint Appendix K, available online at http://thePoint. lww.com/mkk8e, provides a list of popular websites related to microgravity.

Cardiovascular Adaptations

The decrease in total fluid volume during the first few days in microgravity reduces the heart's total work effort. With continued microgravity exposure, overall heart size decreases mainly from reduced left-ventricular end-diastolic volume. Such adaptations represent an appropriate response to microgravity without compromising "normal" cardiovascular function during a mission.[54]

TABLE 27.3 summarizes adaptations in 15 cardiovascular variables for space missions through 1992, while FIGURE 27.9A displays pre- to postflight changes in stroke volume during upright exercise expressed as a percentage of preflight baseline. Also shown in FIGURE 27.9B are changes in aerobic capacity ($\dot{V}O_{2max}$) not listed in Table 27.3) as a function of intensity and frequency of 20-min in-flight cycle ergometer exercise bouts during four different missions. The $\dot{V}O_{2max}$ declined regardless of training regimen, except for group 1, which maintained heart rate above 130 b·min^{-1} and exercised longer than 20 min more than three times weekly.

Experiments have measured changes in cardiac function (left- and right-ventricular mass and left-ventricular end-diastolic volume) assessed by magnetic resonance imaging to isolate whether microgravity per se or frank atrophy from physical inactivity produced changes in cardiac loading functions. In four astronauts on a 10-day mission and in controls on ground measured at 2, 6, and 12 wk of bed rest and 6 wk of routine daily activities, left-ventricular mass declined by 12% (67.9%). Cardiac atrophy occurs both during relatively long 6-wk periods of horizontal bed rest (inactivity) and after short-term spaceflight (microgravity). These findings suggest that physiologic adaptation to reduced myocardial load and work in real or simulated microgravity produces the cardiac atrophy, demonstrating the plasticity of cardiac muscle under different loading conditions.[105]

INTEGRATIVE QUESTION

Contrast the hemodynamic responses when a person moves from the upright to the upside-down position on Earth and in a microgravity environment.

Pulmonary Adaptations

Tight linkage exists between the cardiovascular, pulmonary, and metabolic systems. The cells' demand for oxygen during rest and physical activity remains invariant regardless of environment. Any change in external work above a resting baseline triggers immediate ventilatory responses that increase breathing rate and tidal volume. Augmented alveolar ventilation maintains an adequate pressure differential for oxygen

diffusion across lung tissues for delivery to the site of increased energy metabolism.

TABLE 27.4 summarizes changes in pulmonary variables during two Spacelab missions. FIGURE 27.10 depicts changes in pulmonary diffusing capacity for carbon monoxide measured preflight on days 2, 4, and 9 during the mission and within 6 hr before or after landing and then at days 1, 2, 4, and 6 postflight. Values are presented as a percentage of preflight standing. Note that diffusing capacity increases in the sitting and standing positions during 3 days in microgravity and then returns to preflight baseline values.

Denitrogenation and EVA

Before astronauts perform EVA maneuvers, they must "wash out" the nitrogen from their fluids and tissues to prevent decompression sickness (DCS or bends) from differentials in gas pressures within the cabin and EVA garment.[19,40,112] They do this by using a 10.2 lb per square inch atmosphere (psia) staged decompression of the shuttle for at least 12 hr. This also includes 100 min of **preoxygenation**, breathing 100% O_2 at 14.7 psia prior to decompression and before decompression to the suit pressure of 4.3 psia (equivalent to 9144-m altitude). Scientists have proposed several ways to induce **denitrogenation**. First, reduce the total pressure inside the spacecraft from 760 to 630 torr, the approximate barometric pressure of Denver, Colorado, to shorten overall time for denitrogenation prior to EVA. Second, have astronauts sleep in a special low-pressure compartment prior to EVA. One hour of preoxygenation with exercise improves resistance to DCS, illustrating the potentially positive exercise effect on ameliorating DCS during critical mission EVA maneuvers.

Body Fluid Adaptations

TABLE 27.5 summarizes preflight to postflight adaptations in 24 body fluid variables. FIGURE 27.11 reports data for three variables on early NASA and Salyut science missions:

1. Percentage change in plasma volume and red blood cell mass during Spacelab 1 and three Skylab missions (inset A)
2. Percentage change in total hemoglobin during four Salyut (Russian) missions (inset B)
3. Blood volume related to orthostatically stressed heart rate response during Apollo, SMEAT (Skylab Medical Experiments Altitude Tests), and Skylab missions (inset C).

Sensory System Adaptations

TABLE 27.6 summarizes spaceflight adaptations in the sensory system categories of audition, gustation and olfaction, somatosensory, and vision for relatively short (<14 d) and longer (>14 d) space missions. The bottom of the table lists general vestibular system changes. FIGURE 27.12A schematically shows an overview of multisensory interactions that readjust

TABLE 27.3   Changes in Cardiovascular Variables Associated with Microgravity

Physiologic Measure	Short Space Flights (1–14 d)	Long Space Flights (>2 wk)	
		Preflight vs. In-Flight	Preflight vs. Postflight
Heart rate (resting)	Variable in flight; increased after flight; peaks during launch and reentry; RPB up to 1 wk	Normal or slightly increased	Increased; RPB 3 w
Blood pressure (resting)	Normal; decreased after flight	Diastolic blood pressure reduced or unchanged	Decreased mean arterial pressure
Orthostatic tolerance	Decreased after flights longer than 5 hr; exaggerated cardiovascular responses to tilt test, stand test, and LBNP after flight; RPB 3–14 d	Exaggerated cardiovascular responses to in-flight LBNP (especially during first 2 wk); last in-flight test comparable to recovery-day test	Exaggerated cardiovascular responses to LBNP; RPB up to 3 wk
Total peripheral resistance	Decreased in flight; no increase at landing despite drop in stroke volume and increase in HR	Tendency toward decrease	Increased after landing
Cardiac size	Normal or slightly decreased C/T ratio after flight	C/T ratio decreased after flight	
Stroke volume	Increased in flight by as much as 60% (SLS-1); compensated by decreased HR	Increased early in flight then decreased	12% decrease on average
Left end-diastolic volume	Same as stroke volume	Same as in short-duration missions	16% decrease on average
Cardiac output	Elevated 30–40% in flight (SLS-1); reduced immediately after flight	Unchanged	Variable; RPB 3–4 wk
Central venous pressure	Elevated above resting supine level before launch; transient increase followed by levels below preflight upon attaining orbit	Not measured	Not measured
Left cardiac muscle mass thickness	Unchanged	Unchanged	11% decrease; return to normal after 3 wk
Cardiac electrical activity (ECG/VCG)	Moderate rightward shift in QRS and T waves after flight	Increased P-R interval, QT interval, and QRS vector magnitude	Slight increase in QRS duration and magnitude; increase in P-R interval duration
Arrhythmia	Usually PABs and PVBs; isolated cases of nodal tachycardia, ectopic beats, and supraventricular bigeminy in flights	PVBs and occasional PABs; sinus or nodal arrhythmia at release of LBNP in flight	Occasional unifocal PABs and PVBs
Systolic time intervals	Not measured	Not measured; PEP/ET ratio RPB 2 wk	Increase in resting and LBNP-stressed
Exercise capacity	No change or decreased <12% after flight; increased HR for same $\dot{V}O_2$; no change in efficiency; RPB 3–8 d	Submaximal exercise capacity unchanged	Decreased after flight; recovery time inversely related to amount of in-flight exercise rather than mission duration
Venous compliance in legs	Not measured	Increased: continues to increase for 10 d or more; slow decrease later in flight	Normal or slightly increased

RPB, return to preflight baseline; LBNP, lower-body negative pressure; C/T, cardiothoracic; ECG, electrocardiogram; VCG, vectorcardiogram; PAB, premature atrial beat; PVB, premature ventricular beat; HR, heart rate; SLS-1, Spacelab Life Sciences 1.
Data from Nicogossian AE, et al. *Space Physiology and Medicine*. 3rd Ed. Philadelphia: Lea & Febiger, 1994:216.

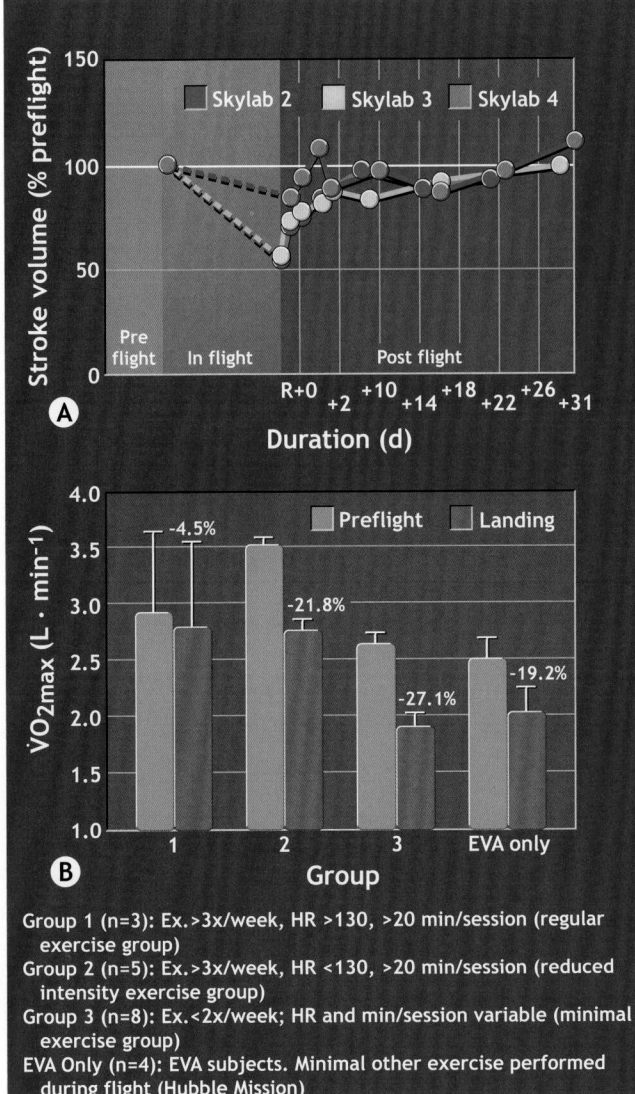

FIGURE 27.9 • Pre- to postflight changes in **(A)** stroke volume during upright exercise (Skylab 2–4). R, return to Earth, and **(B)** aerobic capacity related to intensity and frequency of 20-min in-flight cycle ergometry. (Data for A from Michel EL, et al. Results of Skylab medical experiment M171-metabolic activity. In: Johnson RS, Dietlein LF, eds. *Biomedical Results from Skylab*. NASA SP-377. Washington, DC: U.S. Government Printing Office, 1977. Data for B from Sawin CF. Biomedical investigations conducted in support of the extended duration orbiter medical project. *Aviat Space Environ Med* 1999;70:169.)

the sensory responses disturbed by microgravity. Sensorimotor integration plays a pivotal role in posture and movement control, ambulation, and manipulating objects at 1g, which necessitate proper adjustment in body orientation. In essence, the sensorimotor control system consists of a highly complex, tightly integrated neural complex that modulates vestibular, visual, somatosensory, tactile, and proprioceptive input within a central command-processing center. Disturbance in one part of the system usually initiates an override, readjustment, or temporary substitution by other system components to maintain the system's functional integrity.[50,81,106,156] Considerable

research has assessed how microgravity affects spatial orientation, postural control,[80] vestibuloocular reflexes, and vestibular processing.[57] Studies have also focused on mechanisms related to space motion sickness and perceptual motor performance.[100,101]

FIGURE 27.12B displays the immediate effects of spaceflight on postural reflexes in crew members from eight missions that lasted 4 to 10 days. Immediate postflight measurements were made within 1 to 5 hr in 10 of the 13 subjects. The greatest postural instability occurred in tests that required vestibular information. Note that few responses occurred below the established lower critical level of a normalized composite equilibrium score. In total, the experiments demonstrated a two-stage readaptation process that followed microgravity exposure. The first stage occurred quickly, within a few hours after landing; in a second, slower stage, stability returned to near normal in approximately 4 days. On longer Russian Mir missions (140 and 175 d), recovery of postural parameters to preflight levels required approximately 6 wk. Apparently, readaptation of postural control upon return from space coincides with mission duration, with a prominent role played by visual cues.

Musculoskeletal Adaptations

TABLE 27.7 examines musculoskeletal adaptations during exposure to microgravity. *NASA's greatest biomedical concern involves the 1% per month loss in weight-bearing bone mass during space missions.*[109]

Increased Calcium Loss

TABLE 27.8 summarizes data from 18 male crew members aboard Russian Mir station missions lasting between 4 and 14.4 mo. Bone mineral density (BMD) declined at all seven sites measured, with spine, neck of femur, trochanter, and pelvis decreasing more than 1% per month. On the shorter 4- to 14-day Gemini flights, BMD decreased 3 to 9% in the os calcis (heel bone).[158] Loss of BMD at the os calcis and radius occurred during Apollo Skylab missions and showed no recovery, even 97 days postflight.[147,157] During the Skylab 2 28-day orbital mission, crew members experienced a daily negative 50-mg calcium imbalance[163]; daily calcium loss averaged 140 mg on the 84-day mission. Increased bone calcium loss, if coupled with a high fluid and salt intake, could alter plasma filtrate composition and pH to favor supersaturation of kidney stone–forming salts.[164]

FIGURE 27.13 illustrates how reduced mechanical stress in microgravity affects calcium balance. Figure 27.13 (top) shows how three skeletal loading factors—reduced gravity (microgravity), normal gravity (1g), and above-normal gravity (2g)—adjust calcium distribution in the digestive (intestine), cardiovascular, renal (kidney), and skeletal (bone) systems. Under normal gravity conditions, the small intestine absorbs approximately 250 to 500 mg of calcium for every 1000 mg consumed, with the remainder excreted in feces (▼▼). In a microgravity environment, reduced

TABLE 27.4 Pulmonary System Changes Associated with Microgravity During Spacelab Life Sciences-1 (Flight STS-40, June 5, 1991) and German Spacelab Mission D-2 Aboard STS-55 (April 26, 1993)

Physiologic Response to Microgravity (1–14 d)	Reference Letter	Number of Subjects	Changes in Microgravity (In-Flight vs. Preflight Standing Measurements)
Pulmonary blood flow			
Total pulmonary blood flow (cardiac output)	A	4	18% increase
Cardiac stroke volume	A	4	4% increase
Diffusing capacity (carbon monoxide)	A	4	28% increase
Pulmonary capillary blood volume	A	4	28% increase
Diffusing capacity of alveolar membrane	A	4	27% increase
Pulmonary blood flow distribution	C	7	More uniform but some inequality remained
Pulmonary ventilation			
Respiration frequency	E	8	9% increase
Tidal volume	E	8	15% decrease
Alveolar ventilation	E	8	Unchanged
Total ventilation	E	8	Small decrease
Ventilatory distribution	B	7	More uniform but some inequality remained
Maximal peak expiratory flow rate	E	7	Decreased by ≤12.5% early in flight, then returned to normal
Pulmonary gas exchange			
O_2 uptake	E	8	Unchanged
CO_2 output	E	8	Unchanged
End-tidal Po_2	E	8	Unchanged
End-tidal Pco_2	E	8	Small increase when CO_2 concentration in spacecraft increased
Lung volumes			
Functional residual capacity	D	4	15% decrease
Residual lung volume	D	4	18% decrease
Closing volume	B	7	Unchanged as measured by argon bolus

Note: Pulmonary blood flow in normal subjects equals cardiac output. How well carbon monoxide diffuses into the blood is a standard clinical test of the integrity of the alveolar membrane and its surrounding capillary blood supply. The data indicate that more alveoli are expanded and ventilated in space than on Earth. Closing volume refers to the volume in the lung where the alveoli close in significant numbers.

A. Prisk OK, et al. Pulmonary diffusing capacity, capillary blood volume and cardiac output during sustained microgravity. *J Appl Physiol* 1993;75:15.

B. Guy HJB, et al. Inhomogeneity of pulmonary ventilation during sustained microgravity as determined by single-breath washouts. *J Appl Physiol* 1994;76:1719.

C. Prisk OK, et al. Inhomogeneity of pulmonary ventilation during sustained microgravity on Spacelab SLS-1. *J Appl Physiol* 1994;76:1730.

D. Elliott AR, et al. Lung volumes during sustained microgravity on Spacelab SLS-1. *J Appl Physiol* 1994;77:2005.

E. Prisk OK, et al. Pulmonary gas exchange and its determinants during sustained microgravity on Spacelab SLS-1. *J Appl Physiol* 1995;76:1290.

Adapted from West JB, et al. Pulmonary function in space. *JAMA* 1997;277:1957.

calcium intestinal absorption exacerbates calcium fecal loss (▼▼▼). Abnormal calcium excretion from bone resorption disrupts calcium homeostasis, which in turn decreases total body calcium and bone mass. With increased gravitational loading, calcium absorption by bone increases to spare overall calcium loss (▼). In Figure 27.13 (bottom), the flow diagram shows proposed parallel dynamics of the calcium–endocrine response and skeletal adaptation and altered bone composition and architecture to altered gravitational loading with adequate diet and endocrine balance.[65]

Without suitable countermeasures, progressive calcium losses during future missions of several years' duration will compromise astronaut well-being, increasing bone fracture risk upon return to Earth. Onboard, multimode exercise training and lower-limb exercise has not prevented BMD loss, despite United States and Soviet crewmembers' commitment to intense resistance-type daily workout regimens. Hopefully, future research using valid animal and bed-rest models will reveal the basic mechanism of bone remodeling during prolonged microgravity exposure.[129,149,169,171] Biochemical markers of bone turnover during 120 days of bed rest (skeletal unloading) showed the combined effects of accelerated bone resorption and retarded bone formation accounted for bone loss.[66] BMD measurements at the distal radius and tibia in 15

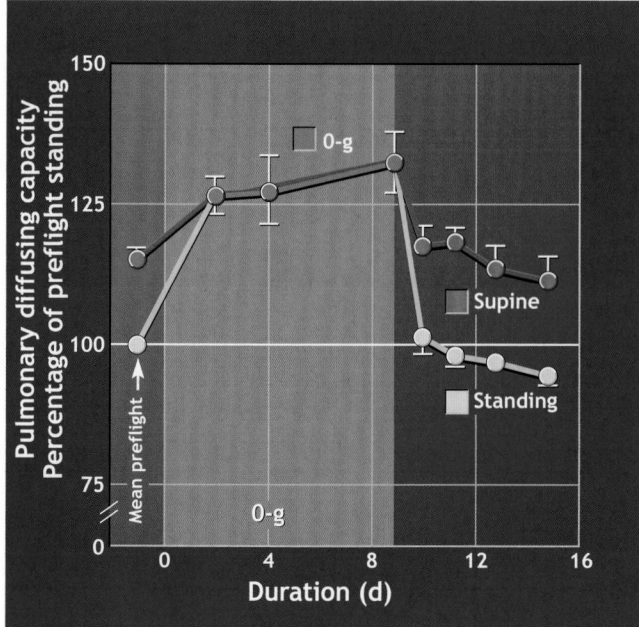

FIGURE 27.10 • Pulmonary diffusing capacity for carbon monoxide preflight on flight days 2, 4, and 9 and 6 hr following landing and on days 1, 2, 4, and 6 postflight. Data are referenced to the preflight standing value. (From Prisk GK, et al. Pulmonary diffusing capacity, capillary blood volume, and cardiac output during sustained microgravity. *J Appl Physiol* 1993;75:15.)

cosmonauts on the Mir space station on missions of 1, 2, and 6 mo revealed the following[154]:

1. Cancellous and cortical bone of the radius decreased progressively at each of the time points.
2. For the weight-bearing tibial site, cancellous BMD appeared normal after 1 mo and deteriorated thereafter. After 2 mo, bone loss became noticeable in the tibial cortices.
3. At 6 mo, cortical bone loss was less evident than cancellous bone loss; cumulative time in microgravity did not relate to BMD changes.
4. Tibial bone loss still persisted after return to Earth for durations similar to time in space (1 to 6 mo).

Alterations in circulation to bone during microgravity exposure can alter the balance between bone resorption and bone formation. Bone blood flow may play an important role in bone remodeling in microgravity.[22] Part of the solution to the problem of bone loss in prolonged microgravity lies in selecting crew members with the greatest resistance to bone loss, including applying targeted prevention and/or treatment strategies.[150] Carefully controlled, longitudinal studies in a microgravity environment (i.e., long-term studies on the ISS) become crucial to better understand skeletal biology. Altering the ratio of animal protein intake to potassium intake can affect bone metabolism in ambulatory and bed-rest subjects. Changing this ratio may help attenuate bone loss on Earth and during spaceflight.[170]

Skeletal Muscle Adaptations

Bone loss during prolonged microgravity exposure coincides with considerable decrements in muscle mass and strength.[167] Deterioration in muscle structure and function could compromise crew health and safety, including performance of critical EVA tasks, landing maneuvers, and procedures for leaving orbit on return to Earth. The absence of gravity virtually eliminates any load-bearing effects on antigravity muscles, rendering them susceptible to impaired performance in emergencies.

Concentric and Eccentric Strength

The important role of concentric and eccentric muscle actions during space missions has focused experiments on pre- and postflight assessment of submaximal and maximal muscle functions.[4,15,20,23,27,30,37,38,58] The preponderance of research in exercise countermeasures supports the use of resistance–exercise training on various modes of exercise equipment to increase "space-bound" muscle mass to improve its force-generating capacity and produce positive ultrastructural changes and complimentary neural components.[1,3,8,9,42,63,144] Standard concentric and eccentric methods, including isokinetic loading devices and newer onboard equipment,[5-7,124,127,143] produce such improvements. For example, concentric strength of Skylab crews tested isokinetically before and 5 days after the 28-day flight showed decrements of approximately 25% in leg extensor strength.[146] Greater losses would probably have occurred had testing been conducted immediately upon landing. Subsequently, longer Skylab missions (59, 84, and 59 d) provided preflight fitness and conditioning that emphasized strengthening exercises for the lower extremities. This emphasis on preflight fitness produced smaller strength decrements during flight than during Skylab 2. On longer (110–237 d) and short (7 d) Russian missions, isokinetic concentric strength declined up to 28%.[59] The 7-day Salyut 6 mission decreased torque–velocity relationships in the gastrocnemius/soleus, anterior tibialis, and ankle extensor musculature. On longer 110- to 237-day missions, cosmonauts' average triceps strength loss ranged between 20 and 50%. Considerable losses in peak torque occurred for isokinetic ankle flexion and extension at all measured angular velocities of movement (**FIG. 27.14**). Studies of cosmonauts investigated the use of functional electrostimulation (FES) to minimize atrophy, morphologic changes, and neuromuscular coordination patterns of skeletal muscles during prolonged space missions.[92] FES trains lower-extremity muscle groups using 1-s tetanic muscle actions followed by 2 s of relaxation continuously at 20 to 30% of maximum tetanic muscle force up to 6 hr daily.

Muscle Ultrastructural Changes

Permanent neuromuscular dysfunction has not yet been demonstrated during prolonged space missions.[21] Nevertheless, in-flight and postflight changes during missions of nearly 1 year reveal altered muscular coordination patterns, some

TABLE 27.5   Body Fluid Changes Associated with Microgravity

Physiologic Measure	Short Space Flights (1–14 d)[a]	Long Space Flights (>2 wk)[b]	
		Preflight vs. In-Flight	Preflight vs. Postflight
Total body water	3% decrease by flight day 4 or 5		Decreased after flight
Plasma volume	Decreased after flight (except Gemini 7 and 8); decreased in flight (SLS-1)		Markedly decreased after flight; RPB 2 w increased at R + 0; decreased R + 2 (hydration effect)
Hematocrit	Slightly increased after flight		Decreased after flight; RPB 2–4 wk after landing
Hemoglobin	Normal or slightly increased after flight	Increased in first in-flight sample; slowly declines later in flight	Decreased from near-preflight values on landing day; RPB 1–2 mo
Red blood cell (RBC) mass	Decreased after flight (approx. 9% on SLS-1); RPB at least 2 wk	Decreased ~15% during first 2–3 wk in flight; begins to recover after about 60 d; recovery of RBC mass independent of time spent in space	Decreased after flight; RPB 2 wk to 3 mo after landing
Red blood cell morphology	No significant changes after flight	Increased percentage of echinocytes; decrease in discocytes	Rapid reversal of in-flight changes in distribution of red blood cell shapes; increased potassium influx; RPB 3 d
Red blood cell half-life (^{51}Cr)	No change; verified on SLS-1		No change
Reticulocytes	Decreased after flight; RPB 1 wk		Decreases at landing, then shifts to increases over preflight values by 7 d after landing; greatest changes seen after longer flights
Iron turnover	No change		No change
Mean corpuscular volume	Increased after flight; RPB at least 2 wk		Variable, but within normal limits
White blood cells	Increased after flight, especially neutrophils; lymphocytes decreased; RPB 1–2 d; no significant change in T/B lymphocyte ratio		Increased, especially neutrophils; postflight reduction in number of T cells and T-cell function as measured by PHA responsiveness, RPB 3–7 d; transient postflight elevation in B cells, RPB 3 d
Plasma lipids	Decreased cholesterol and triacylglycerols in flight		
Plasma glucose	Decreased during and immediately after flight	Decreased for the first 2 mo, then leveled off	Postflight hyperglycemia with increased lactate and pyruvate
Plasma proteins	Occasional postflight elevations in α_2-globulin from increases of haptoglobin, ceruloplasmin, and α_2-macroglobulin; elevated IgA and C_3		No significant changes

TABLE 27.5	Body Fluid Changes Associated with Microgravity (Continued)		
	Short Space Flights (1–14 d)[a]	**Long Space Flights (>2 wk)**[b]	
Physiologic Measure		**Preflight vs. In-Flight**	**Preflight vs. Postflight**
Red blood cell enzymes	No consistent postflight changes	Decreased phosphofructokinase; no evidence of lipid peroxidation or red blood cell damage	No consistent postflight changes
Serum/plasma electrolytes	Increased K and Ca in flight (SLS-1); decreased Na in flight; decreased K and Mg after flight	Decreased Na, Cl, and osmolality; slight increase in K and PO_4	Postflight decreases in Na, K, Cl, Mg; increase in PO_4 and osmolality
Serum/plasma hormones	Decreased ANF, aldosterone, and ADH in flight (SLS-1); increased cortisol and angiotensin 1 in flight (SLS-1)	Increased cortisol; decreased ACTH, insulin	Postflight increases in angiotensin, aldosterone, thyroxine, TSH, and GH; decrease in ACTH
Insulin		Decreased during long missions	Decreased after flight
Serum/plasma metabolites and enzymes	Postflight increases in blood urea nitrogen, creatinine, and glucose; decreases in lactic acid dehydrogenase, creatinine phosphokinase, albumin, triacylglycerols, cholesterol, and uric acid		Postflight decrease in cholesterol, uric acid
Urine volume	Decreased after flight	Decreased early in flight	Decreased after flight
Urine electrolytes	Postflight increases in Ca, creatinine, PO_4, and osmolality; decreases in Na, K, Cl, Mg	Increased osmolality, Na, K, Cl, Mg, Ca, PO_4; decrease in uric acid excretion	Increased Ca excretion; initial postflight decreases in Na, K, Cl, Mg, PO4, uric acid; Na and Cl excretion increased in second and third week after flight
Urinary hormones	In-flight decreases in 17-OH-corticosteroids, increase in aldosterone; postflight increases in cortisol, aldosterone, ADH, and pregnanediol; decreases in epinephrine, 17-OH-corticosteroids, androsterone, and etiocholanolone	In-flight increases in cortisol, aldosterone, and total 17-ketosteroids; decrease in ADH	Increased cortisol, aldosterone, norepinephrine; decreases in total 17-OH-corticosteroids, ADH
Urinary amino acids	Postflight increases in taurine and β-alanine; decreases in glycine, alanine, and tyrosine	Increased in flight	Increased after flight

[a]Biomedical data from Mercury, Gemini, Apollo, ASTP, Vostok, Voskhod, Soyuz, Shuttle, Spacelab.
[b]Biomedical data from Skylab, Salyut, Mir missions.
SLS, Spacelab Life Sciences; RPB, return to preflight baseline; R, return to Earth.
Data from Nicogossian AE, et al. *Space Physiology and Medicine.* 3rd Ed. Philadelphia: Lea & Febiger, 1994:217.

delayed-onset muscle soreness (DOMS), and generalized muscular fatigue and weakness. Many unanswered questions remain about human muscle physiology and biochemical adaptations related to microgravity exposure in humans. Animal models using head-down, tail-suspended, non–weight-bearing rodents rely on reduced gravity's effects on skeletal muscle contractile morphology and physiology.

Placing rodents in a harness that elevates the hindquarters or tail (**Fig. 27.15A**), or using a partial weight-bearing apparatus (Fig. 27.15B), eliminates the normal loading of weight-bearing hind-limb muscles. The model mimics the fluid shifts of microgravity; it produces reduced sensory input to the motor centers and less mechanical stimulation of connective, muscular, and osseous tissues. Specifically, both spaceflight and non–weight-bearing confinement atrophies rat

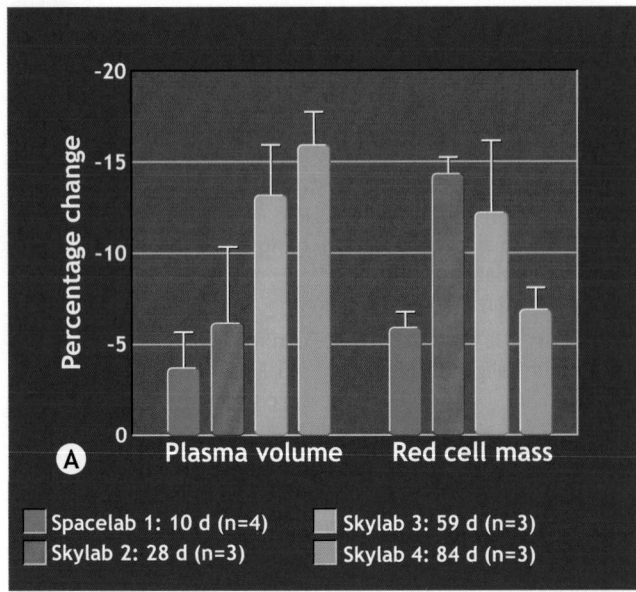

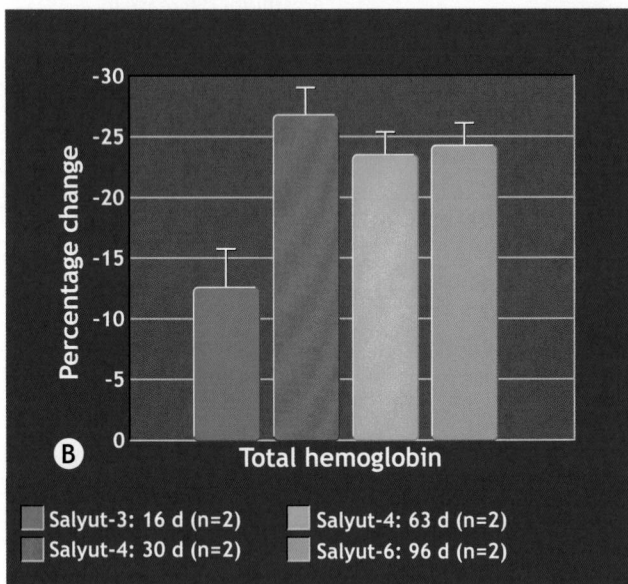

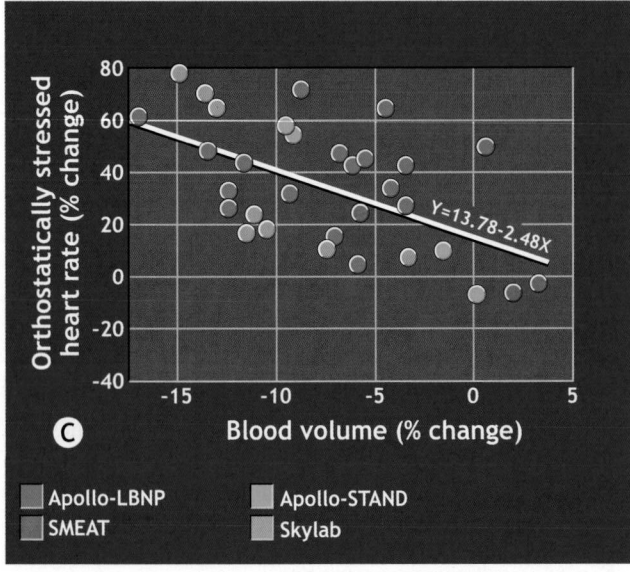

skeletal muscles, mainly the slow-twitch (type 1) leg-extensor fibers.[69,70,117,120,168] Also, non–weight bearing in microgravity reduces contractile activity assessed by EMG of male rat hindlimb soleus muscle by 75%.

Maximal Explosive Leg Power Before and After Space Missions

Figure 27.16 shows different duration spaceflight effects on maximal explosive power (MEP) and maximal cycling power (MCP) assessed preflight and 26 days postflight for astronauts exposed to microgravity for up to 180 days. *Inset A* shows the percentage of premission scores for MEP and MCP for four astronauts at four periods after mission completion. Astronaut 1, who spent 31 days in orbit, recovered nearly all MEP by 11 days postflight. For the other three astronauts, whose missions lasted 169 to 180 days, MEP recovery approached only 77% of the preflight value. For the two astronauts tested 26 days postflight, MEP for astronaut 3 was 80% of his premission score, while astronaut 4 achieved only 57%. In contrast, each astronaut's MCP, a measure of more sustained power output, recovered more rapidly throughout the postflight measurement period, with final scores within 10% of premission values. *Inset B* shows the ergometer–dynamometer to assess MEP, with *inset C* showing the relation between maximal cycling power and maximal explosive power, each expressed as a percentage of premission values. Subjects made six maximal pushes with both feet against the force platform for approximately 250 ms at a knee angle of 110° with a 2-min rest between pushes. MCP involved five to seven "all-out" pedal revolutions for 5 to 6 s on a bicycle ergometer following either 5 to 7 min of mild aerobic exercise or free-wheel pedaling.

On average, MCP deterioration exceeded MEP loss. The researchers attributed the differential deterioration in the two forms of maximal exercise to muscular and neurologic factors involved in each form of effort. In essence, the absence of gravity appears to rearrange postural muscle tone and locomotor coordination substantially. This adversely affects the motor control system; in one astronaut, it negatively affected the normal pattern of motor unit recruitment. Changes in neural drive during long-term missions of 90 to 180 days could impact the contractile and elastic characteristics of lower limb musculature.[71]

FIGURE 27.11 • Pre- to postflight changes in **(A)** plasma volume and red blood cell mass (Spacelab 1; Skylab 2–4), **(B)** total hemoglobin (Salyut 3–4, 6), and **(C)** blood volume in relation to orthostatically stressed heart rate (Apollo, Skylab, and SMEAT [Skylab Medical Experiments Altitude Tests]). Error bars in A and B represent standard errors of measurement. (Data for A and B redrawn from Convertino VA. Physiological adaptations to weightlessness: effects on exercise and work performance. *Exerc Sports Sci Rev* 1990;18:119.)

Microgravity's Effects on Muscle Fibers

From the beginning of manned spaceflight, researchers assumed that prolonged exposure to near–zero-g would negatively affect neuromuscular function. Soviet research showed that spaceflight impaired a number of neuromotor components. Some of these neural adaptations persisted for days and weeks after spaceflight. A principal issue not addressed by the Soviets was the degree to which neuromotor changes related to muscular components. UCLA researchers were first to objectify spaceflight's effects on human muscle fibers. They measured size and capillarization of single muscle fibers and enzyme activities of myofibrillar adenosine triphosphatase (ATPase), succinate dehydrogenase (SDH), and α-glycerophosphate dehydrogenase (GPD) of astronauts who flew either one 11-day or one of two 5-day missions. A 32% decrease in total SDH activity in type II fibers was the only significant difference in enzyme activity during spaceflight. SDH activity per unit mass of the fibers did not change for either type I or type II fibers, but SDH activity per fiber decreased from muscle atrophy. No loss of total activity occurred for ATPase or GPD because the increase in activity per unit mass countered any atrophy effect. Also, the absolute number of capillaries supplying each type of muscle fiber decreased significantly from spaceflight. Mean fiber size also decreased, so capillary number per unit muscle cross-sectional area (CSA) remained unchanged. The results confirmed that skeletal muscle adapts rapidly to microgravity exposure, with a significant loss in CSA, selected enzyme activity, and fiber capillarization. These highly variable responses partly related to physical fitness level before launch and the extent of in-flight exercise.

Source: Edgerton VR, et al. Human fiber size and enzymatic properties after 5 and 11 days of space flight. *J Appl Physiol* 1995;78:1733.

TABLE 27.6   Sensory System Changes Associated with Microgravity

Physiologic Measure	Short Space Flights (1–14 d)	Long Space Flights (>2 wk)	
		Preflight vs. In-Flight	Preflight vs. Postflight
Audition	No change in thresholds after flight	One report of lowered thresholds during a 1-yr flight	No change in thresholds after flight
Gustation and olfaction	Subjective and varied human experience; no impairments noted	Same as shorter missions	Same as shorter missions
Somatosensory	Subjective and varied human experience; no impairments noted	Subjective experiences (e.g., tingling in feet)	
Vision	Intraocular tension tends to increase during flight and decrease at landing; postflight decreases in visual field; retinal blood vessels constricted after flight; dark-adapted crews reported light flashes with eyes open or closed; decrease in visual motor task performance and contrast discrimination; no change in in-flight contrast discrimination or distant and near visual acuity	Light flashes reported by dark-adapted subjects; frequency related to latitude (highest in South Atlantic, lowest over poles)	No significant changes except transient decreases in intraocular pressure
Vestibular system	Forty to 70% of astronauts/cosmonauts exhibit in-flight neurovestibular effects including immediate reflex motor responses (postural illusions, sensations of tumbling or rotation, nystagmus, dizziness, vertigo) and space motion sickness (pallor, cold sweating, nausea, vomiting); motion sickness symptoms appear early in flight and subside or disappear in 2–7 d; postflight difficulties in postural equilibrium with eyes closed or other vestibular disturbances	In-flight vestibular disturbances are the same as for shorter missions; markedly decreased susceptibility to provocative motion stimuli (cross-coupled angular acceleration) after adaptation period of 2–7 days; cosmonauts reported occasional reappearance of illusions during long missions	Immunity to provocative motion continues for several days after flight; marked postflight disturbances in postural equilibrium with eyes closed; some cosmonauts exhibit additional vestibular disturbances after flight, including dizziness, nausea, and vomiting

Data used by permission from Nicogossian AE, et al. *Space Physiology and Medicine*. 3rd Ed. Philadelphia: Lea & Febiger, 1994:219.

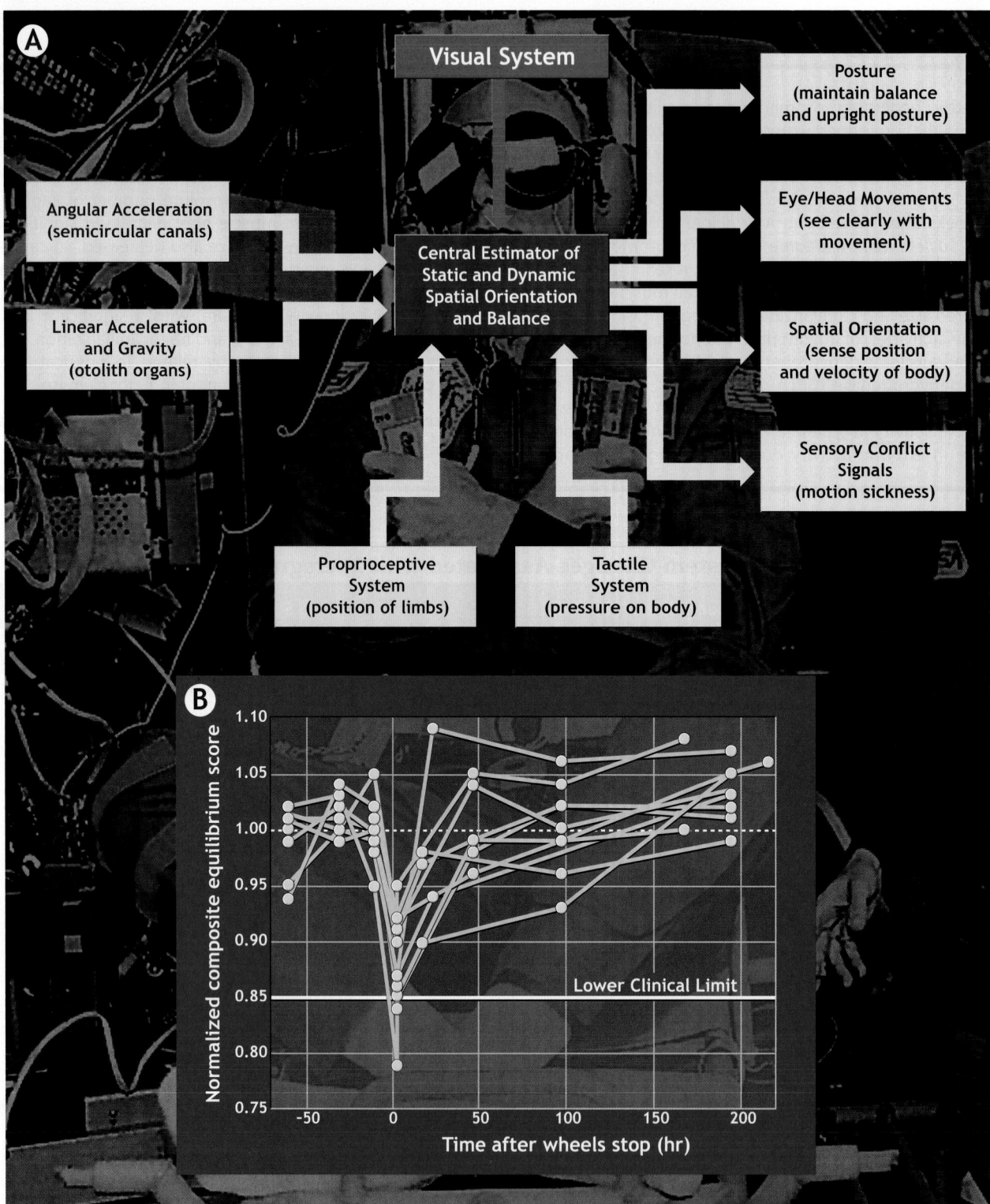

FIGURE 27.12 • **(A)** Schematic representation of sensory motor system that controls eye movements and posture and perception of orientation and motion. **(B)** Changes in anterior–posterior sway (composite equilibrium score) in 10 astronauts at various times after the space shuttle returned to Earth (wheels stop, 0 hr). The tests involved perturbation of a posture platform under different conditions of visual, vestibular, and proprioceptive input. Dashed horizontal line at 1.00 represents normal response. (Data reported in Daunton NG. Adaptation of the vestibular system to microgravity. In: Fregly MJ, Blatteis CM, eds. *Handbook of Physiology. Section 4, Environmental Physiology, Vol. 2.* American Physiological Society. New York: Oxford University Press, 1996:765. Data for A adapted from Young LR, et al. M.I.T./Canadian vestibular experiments on the Spacelab 1 mission: 2. Visual vestibular tilt interaction in weightlessness. *Exp Brain Res* 1986;64:299. Data for B adapted from Paloski WH, et al. Recovery of postural equilibrium control following spaceflight. *Ann NY Acad Sci* 1992;656:747; background photo of astronaut Dr. Martin Fettman provided by Dr. Fettman and used with his permission.)

TABLE 27.7   Musculoskeletal Changes Associated with Microgravity

Physiologic Measure	Short Space Flights (1–14 d)	Long Space Flights (>2 wk) Preflight vs. In-Flight	Long Space Flights (>2 wk) Preflight vs. Postflight
Stature	Slight increase during first week in flight (~1.3 cm); RPB 1 d	Increased during first 2 wk in flight (maximum 3–6 cm); stabilizes thereafter	Height returns to normal on R + 0
Body mass	Postflight weight losses average about 3.4%; about 2/3 of the loss from water loss, the remainder from loss of lean body mass and fat	In-flight weight losses average 3–4% during first 5 d; thereafter, weight either declines or increases for the remainder of mission; early in-flight losses probably from fluid loss; later losses are metabolic	Rapid weight gain during first 5 d after flight, mainly replenishment from fluid; slower weight gain from R + 5 days to R + 2 or 3 wk; amount of postflight weight loss inversely related to in-flight caloric intake
Protein synthesis	Elevated 40% on flight day 8 (SLS-1), suggesting a "stress response"		
Body composition		Fat is probably replacing muscle tissue; muscle mass is partially preserved depending on exercise regimen	
Total body volume	Decreased after flight	Center of mass shifts headward	Decreased after flight
Limb volume	In-flight leg volume decreases exponentially during the first flight day; thereafter, rate of decrease declines and plateaus within 3–5 d; postflight decrements in leg volume up to 3%; rapid increase immediately after flight, followed by slower RPB	Same as short missions early in flight; leg volume continues to decrease slightly throughout mission; arm volume decreases slightly	Rapid increase in leg volume immediately after flight followed by slow RPB
Muscle strength	Decreased during and after flight; RPB 1–2 wk		Postflight decrease in leg muscle strength, particularly extensors; increased use of in-flight exercise reduces postflight losses in strength regardless of mission duration; arm strength normal or slightly decreased after flight
EMG analysis	Postflight EMGs from gastrocnemius suggest increased susceptibility to fatigue and reduced muscular efficiency; EMGs from arm muscles show no change		Postflight EMGs from gastrocnemius show shift to higher frequencies, suggesting deterioration of muscle tissue; EMGs indicate increased susceptibility to fatigue; RPB in about 4 d
Reflexes (Achilles tendon)	Reflex duration decreased after flight		Reflex duration decreased after flight by 30% or more; reflex magnitude increased; compensatory increase in reflex duration about 2 wk after flight; RPB about 1 mo
Nitrogen and phosphorus balance		Negative balances early in flight shift to less negative or slightly positive balances later	Rapid return to markedly positive balances after flight

TABLE 27.7 **Musculoskeletal Changes Associated with Microgravity** *(Continued)*

	Short Space Flights (1–14 d)	Long Space Flights (>2 wk)	
Physiologic Measure		**Preflight vs. In-Flight**	**Preflight vs. Postflight**
Bone density	Os calcis density decreased after flight; radius and ulna show variable changes depending on measurement method		Os calcis density decreased after flight; amount of loss correlated with mission duration; little or no loss from non–weight-bearing bones; RPB is gradual; time course undetermined
Calcium balance	Progressive negative calcium balance in flight	Ca excretion in urine increases during first month in flight, then plateaus; fecal Ca excretion declines until day 10, then increases continually throughout flight; Ca balance becomes increasingly negative throughout flight	Urine Ca content drops below preflight baselines by day 10; fecal Ca content declines but does not reach preflight baseline by day 20; markedly negative Ca balance after flight, becomes less negative by day 10; Ca balance remains slightly negative on day 20; RPB at least several weeks

RPB, return to preflight baseline; SLS, Spacelab Life Sciences; R, return to Earth; EMG, electromyography.
Data used by permission from Nicogossian AE, et al. *Space Physiology and Medicine*. 3rd Ed. Philadelphia: Lea & Febiger, 1994:220.

COUNTERMEASURE STRATEGIES

Countermeasures systematically attempt to neutralize or minimize spaceflight's potentially harmful deconditioning effects on crew physiologic function, performance, and overall health during mission-critical maneuvers, particularly reentry and landing.[82] In the absence of gravity, no linear, downward head-to-foot acceleration forces (referred to as 1 Gz) act on the body. This makes normal biologic functions more susceptible to short- and longer-term maladaptations such as **space motion sickness** (SMS). This syndrome usually manifests within the first 72 hr of a mission and is often characterized by clumsiness, difficulty concentrating, disorientation, persisting sensation aftereffects, nausea, pallor, drowsiness, vomiting, vertigo while walking and standing, difficulty walking a straight line, blurred vision, and dry heaves. Some symptoms resemble those of terrestrial motion sickness. SMS symptoms often dissipate on their own or with medication during the first few days of spaceflight. On reentry after short-duration missions, SMS can manifest as a general reentry syndrome (GRS) that imposes potentially deleterious effects on astronaut performance. GRS symptoms include vertigo, nausea, instability, and fatigue induced by reimposition of increased +Gz during reentry and landing. In contrast to the relatively acute emergence of SMS, weeks and months of prolonged absence of normal gravitational loading adversely affect bone and muscular structure and function. Concurrently, fluid shifts within the vascular system produce considerable loss of electrolytes and bone minerals. Cumulative negative effects during sustained missions could trigger more severe medical complications that include increased risk for developing renal stones, orthostatic intolerance, neurosensory and motor dysfunctions, and musculoskeletal injuries (including bone fracture) in the weeks and months following return to Earth.

Without appropriate countermeasures, microgravity's deleterious effects mimic the adverse changes with prolonged bed rest. For example, 30 days of bed rest dramatically impairs skeletal muscle function; knee extensor strength declines nearly 23%, while knee flexor strength and leg volume decrease 10 to 12%. Reductions in limb volume result from decreased muscular cross-sectional area from muscle fiber protein loss. The 28-day Skylab 2 mission decreased muscular function and leg

TABLE 27.8 **Bone Loss on Mir Space Station Expressed as Percentage of Bone Mineral Density Lost Per Month**

Variable	Crew Members (*n*)	Mean Loss (%)	SD[a]
Spine	18	1.07[b]	0.63
Neck of femur	18	1.16[b]	0.85
Trochanter	18	1.58[b]	0.98
Total body	17	0.35[b]	0.25
Pelvis	17	1.35[b]	0.54
Arm	17	0.04[b]	0.88
Leg	16	0.34[b]	0.33

[a]Standard deviation.
[b]$p < 0.01$.
Reprinted from LeBlanc A, et al. Bone mineral and lean tissue loss after long duration space flight. *Am Soc Bone Miner Res* 1996;11:S323.

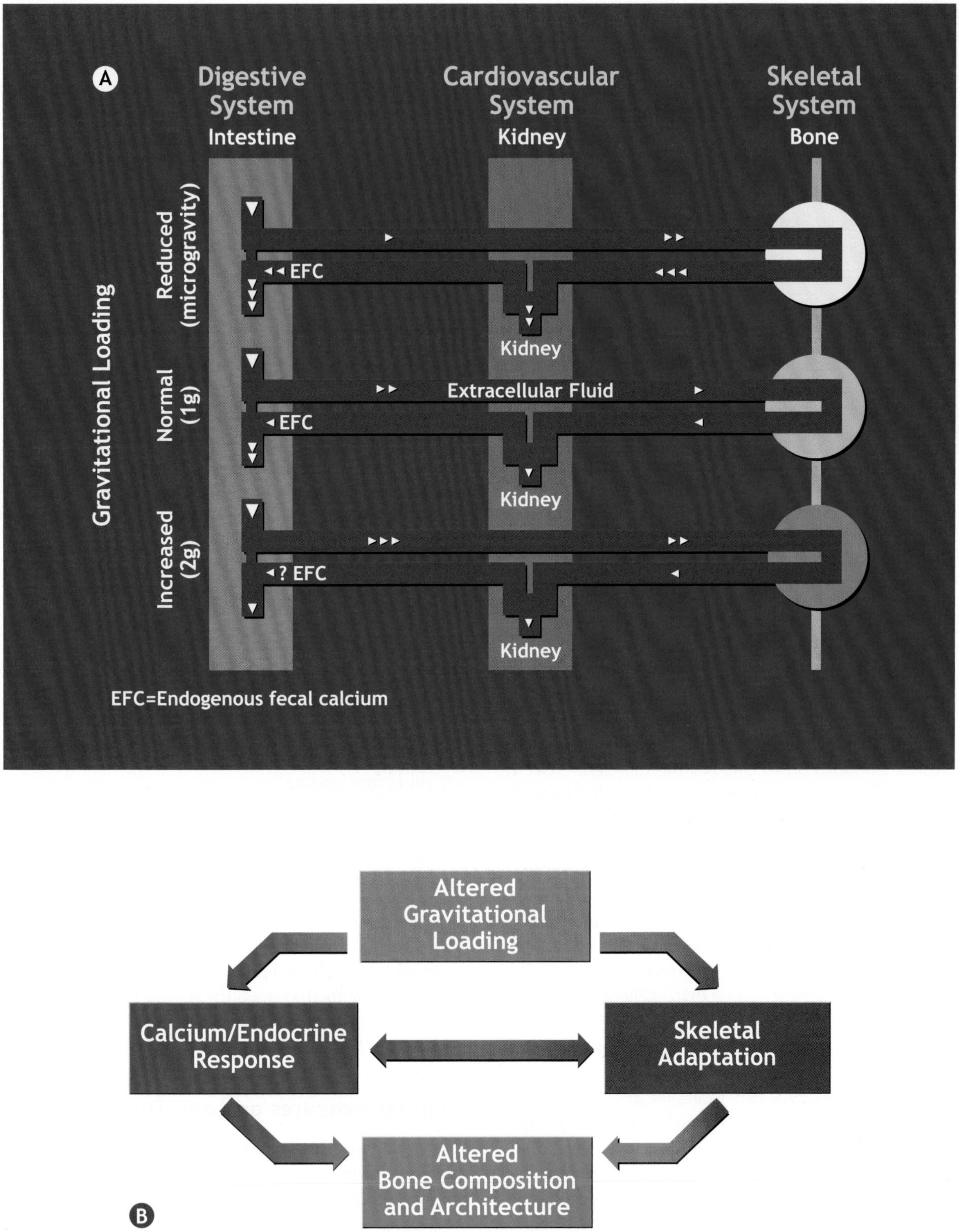

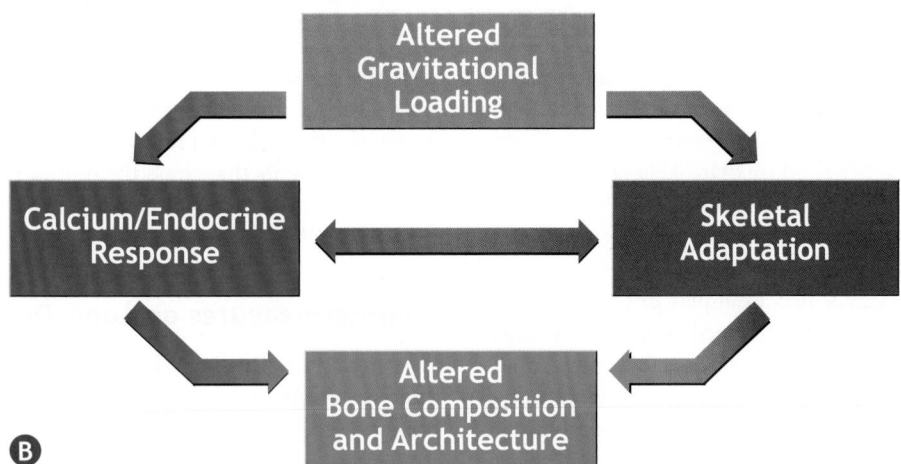

FIGURE 27.13 • Influence of gravitational loading (mechanical stress) on calcium balance. **(A)** How the digestive system (intestine), cardiovascular system (kidney), and skeletal system (bone) adjust calcium distribution in response to (1) reduced (microgravity), (2) normal (1g), and (3) increased (2g) gravitational skeletal loading. The degree of shading within the circles in the right panel represents the adaptation in whole-body bone mineral (darker shading, greater calcium accretion) to the different loading conditions. **(B)** Flow diagram proposing parallel calcium/endocrine and skeletal adaptive responses to changing gravitational loading, assuming adequate diet and endocrine balance. (Adapted from Morey-Holton ER, et al. The skeleton and its adaptation to gravity. In: Fregly MJ, Blatteis CM, eds. *Handbook of Physiology. Section 4, Environmental Physiology, Vol. 2.* American Physiological Society. New York: Oxford University Press, 1996.)

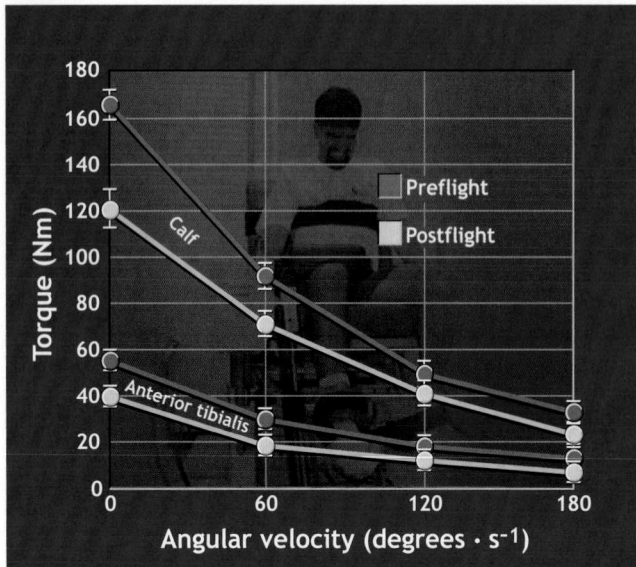

FIGURE 27.14 • Force–velocity relationship of ankle flexors (anterior tibialis) and extensor calf muscles measured by isokinetic dynamometry at four angular velocities in six cosmonauts before and after 110 to 237 days in microgravity on Salyut 7. (Data summarized from Convertino VA. Effects of microgravity on exercise performance. In: Garrett WE, Kirkendall DT, eds. *Exercise and Sport Science.* Philadelphia: Lippincott Williams & Wilkins, 2000.)

volume to an extent comparable with bed rest. The protein loss has been attributed in part to a normal adaptive response to decreased workload on weight-bearing muscles.[140] Decrements in cardiovascular function generally parallel losses in muscle strength and size,[142,145] including problems related to low back pain.[122] Projected travel time for an exploration-class mission to Mars requires approximately 6 mo of isolation in microgravity, more than a year of planetary habitation at 0.38g, followed by a 6-mo return trip to Earth in microgravity. Onboard countermeasures play a critical role in minimizing pathology or impaired motor task performance to preserve crew health and safety.[123,125,133] More than likely, gender-related factors affect these health and performance goals.[51] *In-flight resistance and endurance exercises show the greatest overall potential as exercise countermeasures to combat microgravity's sustained deleterious effects.* TABLE 27.9 lists examples of adverse effects and clinical consequences of prolonged microgravity exposure in four functional body areas and possible countermeasure strategies. The countermeasure strategies of fluid loading, G-suit inflation, pharmacologic agents, artificial gravity, and short-term physical exertion to elicit maximal effort help to minimize microgravity-induced orthostatic intolerance.[33] A compelling argument posits that combining multiple countermeasures could afford astronauts optimal protection against potential adverse effects of long-duration space missions.

On an ISS mission in September 2012, NASA astronaut Sunita "Suni" Williams completed the first simulated triathlon in space. Only the second female commander of the ISS, she also ran a simulated Boston Marathon during her last extended

ISS stay in 2007. Williams holds the female record for the longest continuous spaceflight of 195 consecutive days on ISS. She competed in the 2012 Malibu triathlon using equipment on board the ISS—the station's exercise bike, treadmill, and the iRED resistive exercise machine—to simulate the type of

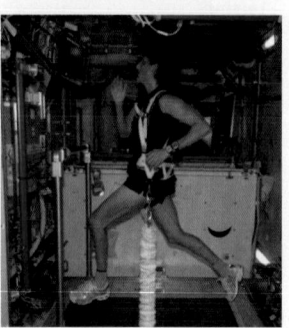

workout in a half-mile ocean swim. Williams, a committed fitness enthusiast, also holds the women's world records for six spacewalks, and the most spacewalking EVA time at 44 hr and 2 min. Watch this interesting and highly recommended video of Williams as she simulates the swim, bike, and treadmill portions of the marathon she completed (www.space.com/17641-astronaut-runs-triathlon-in-space-video.html). Note how she periodically takes air samples for analysis of expired air and energy expenditure calculations. Her workouts in the ISS "exercise physiology lab" illustrate the importance that NASA places on maintaining overall fitness during space missions.

In-Flight Exercise

Four predominant exercise modes have played important roles during in-flight workouts aboard space missions (**FIGURE 27.17 A-D**):

1. Treadmill walking and running
2. Cycle ergometry, including maximal effort performed 24 hr before landing[94]
3. Leg rowing
4. Upper- and lower-body multijoint dynamic resistance exercise

The interim Resistance Exercise Device (iRED; inset D), the resistance-exercise training equipment aboard the ISS, allows astronauts to exercise dynamically with increasing resistance throughout a full range of motion (ROM) for three basic movements that stress the hip, back, and spine. For each repetition, measurements includes peak force, average force, and ROM.[124]

Countermeasures on Long-Duration Missions

The prolonged Russian Mir missions made extensive use of exercise countermeasures based on considerable prior experience with extended space missions. Like their American counterparts, cosmonauts did not exercise during the flight's first 48 to 72 hr to provide sufficient recovery from SMS that affects nearly 70% of astronauts and cosmonauts on their first flight. On current space shuttle missions, an intramuscular injection of Phenergan relieved SMS, replacing Dexedrine and other drug combinations that evoke strong negative central nervous system responses.

Toward the end of the flight's first week and over the next 24 days, cosmonauts exercised twice daily, progressing to

Microgravity Compromises Immune System Function

Weightlessness negatively impacts human immune response during extended-duration missions.[a,b] A 5-mo experiment provided insights into immune cellular response. The studies involved two cultures of human cells: one free-floating in weightlessness without constraints, and the other in simulated gravity using an on-board centrifuge that generated a 1-g simultaneous control to isolate the effects of microgravity from the potential confounding variables of spaceflight. On return to Earth, the cells preserved in microgravity fared more favorably than the ones maintained in simulated gravity. The researchers hypothesized that the protein complex Rel/NF-κB, an important cellular signaling pathway active in human cells that controls DNA transcription and helps regulate immune response to infection, failed to function properly. The Rel/NF-κB complex supposedly serves as an important transcription factor in normal lymphatic β and T-cell functioning. When these cells receive the "correct" external stimulation, they activate a cascade of events that end with NF-κB entering the nucleus and turning on genes that control maturation, activation, and proliferation of the specialized immune cells. Without gravity, the Rel/NF-κB pathway becomes deactivated. In the absence of NF-κB regulation on genes, the body's immune cells remain at a disadvantage in the event of infection during a space mission. This is of great importance to space travel, particularly for future Mars missions, because such deregulation can lead to ineffective pro-inflammatory host defenses against infectious pathogens. Research continues to study means to productively combat this negative effect, particularly because of its additional deleterious effects on bone during prolonged microgravity missions.[b]

Sources:

[a]Chang TT, et al. The Rel/NF-κb pathway and transcription of immediate early genes in T cell activation are inhibited by microgravity. *J Leukoc Biol* 2012;92:1133.

[b]Sonnenfeld G. Editorial: Space flight modifies T cell activation—role of microgravity. *J Leukoc Biol* 2012;92:1125.

[c]Nakamura H, et al. Disruption of NF-κB1 prevents bone loss caused by mechanical unloading. *J Bone Miner Res* 2013;28:1457.

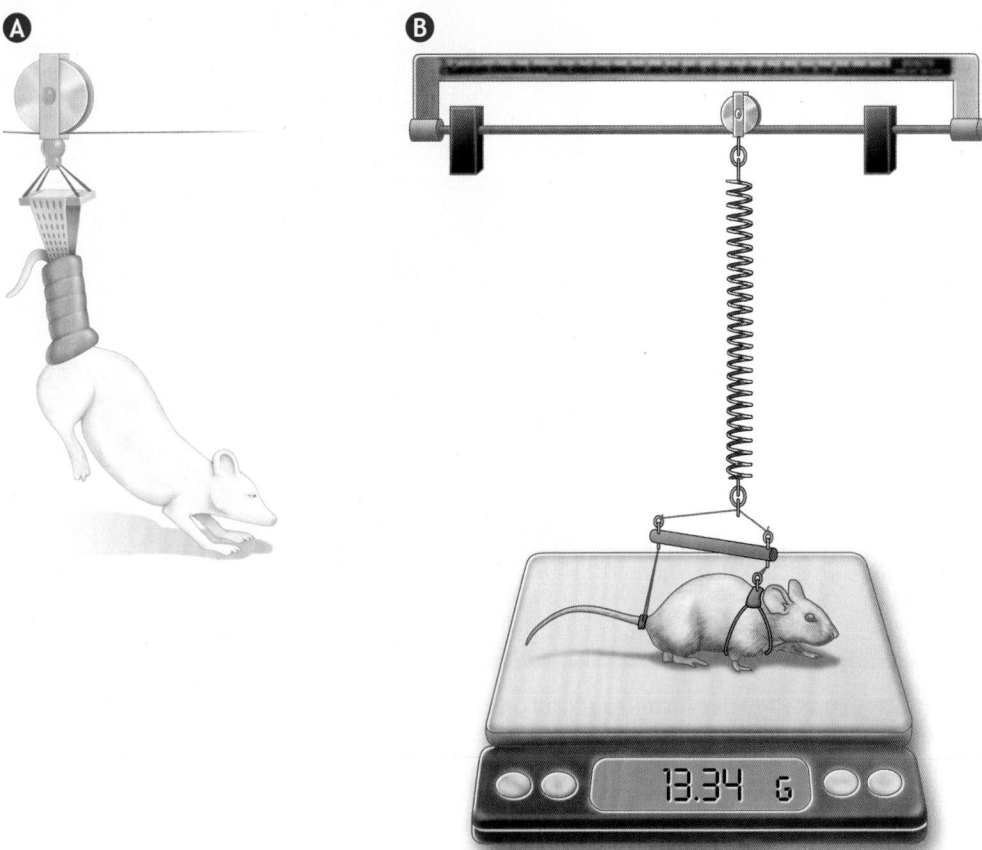

FIGURE 27.15 • **(A)** Hind-limb suspension. This uploading technique limits the activity or movement of the animal by immobilizing or restraining its hind limbs or tail to simulate the non–weight-bearing effects of microgravity. **(B)** Partial weight-bearing mouse model (referred to as hypodynamic or graded gravitational loading) can "unweight" the animal to a desired percentage of full body weight measured on the platform by adjusted movable rods at the top of the balance. Description of the method in Wagner ED, et al. Partial weight suspension: a novel murine model for investigating adaptation to reduced musculoskeletal loading. *J Appl Physiol* 2010;109:350; Swift JM, et al. β-1 Adrenergic agonist mitigates unloading-induced bone loss by maintaining formation. *Med Sci Sports Exerc* 2013;45:1665. Photographic images on which illustrations are based provided courtesy of Dr. Susan Bloomfield, Bone Biology Lab. Texas A&M University. College Station, TX.

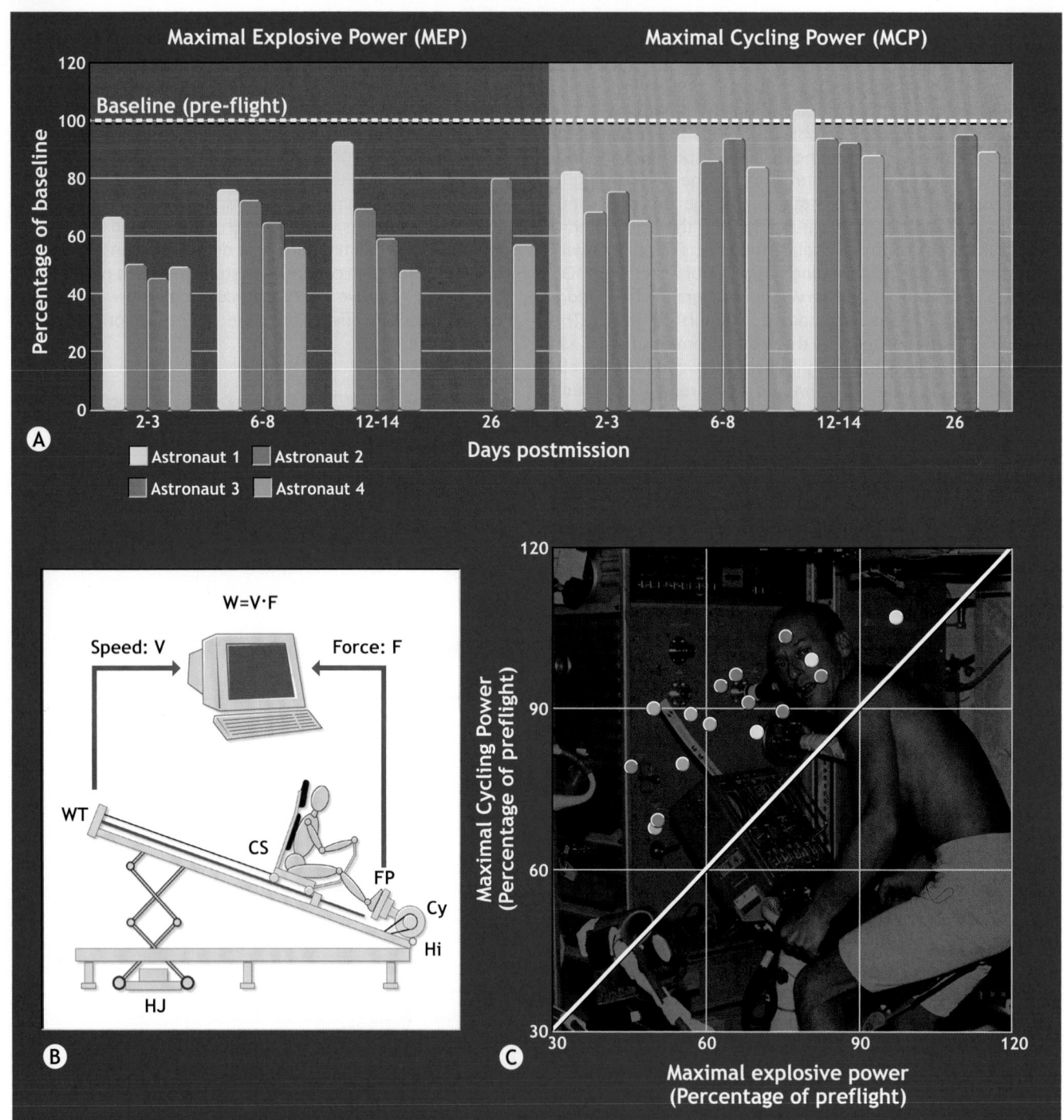

FIGURE 27.16 • **(A)** Effects of up to 180 days in microgravity on changes in maximal explosive power (MEP) and maximal cycling power (MCP). **(B)** The ergometer–dynamometer assessed MEP of the lower limbs by varying either force or velocity. HJ, hydraulic jack; WT, wire tachometer; CS, carriage seat; FP, force platform; Cy, isokinetic cycle ergometer; Hi, hinge. MEP was assessed within less than 0.3 s, and MCP was determined during all-out pedaling on a cycle ergometer for 5 to 6 s. **(C)**. Plot of MCP versus MEP scores expressed as a percentage of premission values. (Adapted with permission from Antonutto G, et al. Effects of microgravity on maximal power of lower limbs during very short efforts in humans. *J Appl Physiol* 1999;86:85.)

1 hr of continuous ergometer cycling at an initial workload of 900 kg-m · min⁻¹. Exercise intensity progressively increased to maintain heart rate between 80 and 90% of age-predicted maximum. They added 5 to 15 min of daily strengthening exercise (hamstrings, trunk extensors) using bungee-cord devices. On missions exceeding 1 mo, cosmonauts exercise twice daily

for 1 hr on a passive (subject-driven) treadmill with a restraint system similar to that used by space shuttle astronauts (see **FIG. 27.18** for a schematic of a U.S. Space Shuttle passive treadmill in which a rapid-onset centrifugal brake provided seven braking levels to control drag forces on the running track). To simulate gravitational forces, straps from their side—called

TABLE 27.9	Adverse Effects of Spaceflight and Proposed Countermeasures		
Area	**Major Findings**	**Clinical/Operational Consequences**	**Countermeasures under Evaluation**
Cardiovascular	Fluid loss Electrolyte changes Electrical activity disturbances Neuroreflex readjustments	Orthostatic intolerance	Fluid/electrolyte replenishment Exercise
Neurovestibular	Motion sickness Gait disturbances Motor performance degradation	Decreased productivity	Palliative treatments (intramuscular promethazine) Adaptation trainers
Musculoskeletal	Bone mass loss Muscle mass loss	Renal stone formation Muscle/joint injuries Bone fractures	Diet Exercise; lower-body negative pressure Drugs (biphosphonates, etc.)

Immunologic
  endocrinologic
	Changes in immune response *in vitro*
	Inappropriate hormonal secretion
	  or metabolism
		Susceptibility to infection (?)
		Synergistic radiation effects
		Allergic reactions and disorders
			Growth factors (?)

Note: Third column lists factors (renal stone formation, muscle/joint injuries, bone fractures) undocumented in NASA reports.
Reprinted from Nicogossian AE, et al. Countermeasures to space deconditioning. In: Nicogossian AE, et al., eds. *Space Physiology and Medicine*. 3rd ed. Philadelphia: Lea & Febiger, 1994:447.

subject load devices—secured the cosmonaut to the treadmill. Treadmill exercise, using a harness and bungee tether system, generated the effects of 0.5 to 0.7 g, while exercise on Salyut and Mir treadmills generated a "gravitational" pull of 0.62 g. The nonmotorized treadmill required astronauts to run at a positive percentage grade to overcome frictional resistance. At present, the treadmill provides the only mode of onboard exercise. Astronauts wore a monitor secured to the ear called an ear oximeter to record heart rate continuously by an infrared sensor that detects pulsating blood flow in the earlobe. A mechanical sensor wire on the side of the treadmill displaced distance run from the number of treadmill revolutions completed. Several of the exercise modes that served as a cornerstone for countermeasures strategies on shuttle missions now continue their important role on current ISS missions, and will remain a part of future travel to asteroids and Mars in the decades to come.

FIGURE 27.19 compares heart rate response during continuous (A) and intermittent (B) treadmill exercise during two shuttle missions. Astronauts did not attain assigned target heart rates (representing 60, 70, or 80% $\dot{V}O_{2max}$) when exercising continuously for 30 min during an 11-day mission. More than likely, altered running mechanics while wearing the bungee apparatus reduced ability to attain target heart rates.

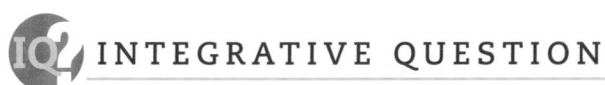

INTEGRATIVE QUESTION

What type of exercise training program would you advise an astronaut to undertake 6 mo prior to a Mars mission and during the mission?

Space Pharmacology

SMS remained the most persistent short-term problem during spaceflight missions, and future research with countermeasures will attempt to mitigate this problem, not only for ISS but future NASA missions. Approximately 50% of cosmonauts, 60% of Apollo astronauts, and 71% of first-time shuttle astronauts encountered mild-to-severe SMS. TABLE 27.10 lists the incidence and severity of SMS during 36 space shuttle flights through 1991. Note the decline in prevalence (mild, moderate, and severe) from 77 episodes to 34 episodes for crewmembers on their second shuttle flight. On the 1993 Space Shuttle Life Sciences mission (SLS-2), only one astronaut experienced nausea, but without sickness during the mission's first few days.[135]

SMS is not confined to orbital flight; nearly 10% of astronauts experience it during reentry or immediately upon landing, including training during parabolic flights. Ninety-two percent of cosmonauts report SMS upon return from missions that last several months or longer.[68] To date, no single pharmacologic treatment prevents or cures SMS. On shuttle missions, the disorder shows no preference for commanders, pilots, or mission specialists, gender or age, career versus noncareer astronauts, or first-time versus repeat flyers. Incomplete understanding of the cause(s) of SMS hampers its treatment, but pharmacologic treatment usually relieves most symptoms within the first 3 days in the space environment. Additional countermeasure strategies to minimize SMS effects include mechanical and electrical stimulation and biofeedback techniques. Despite these efforts, medication still provides the most effective pharmacologic therapy against SMS.

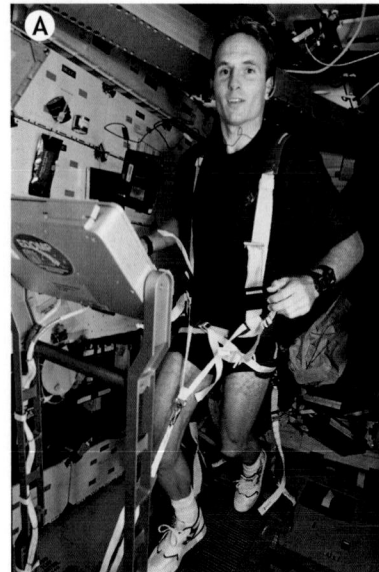
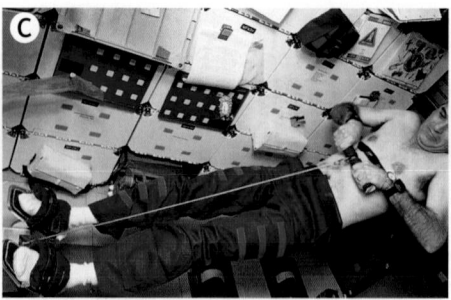
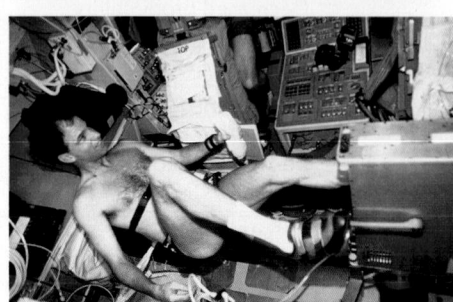
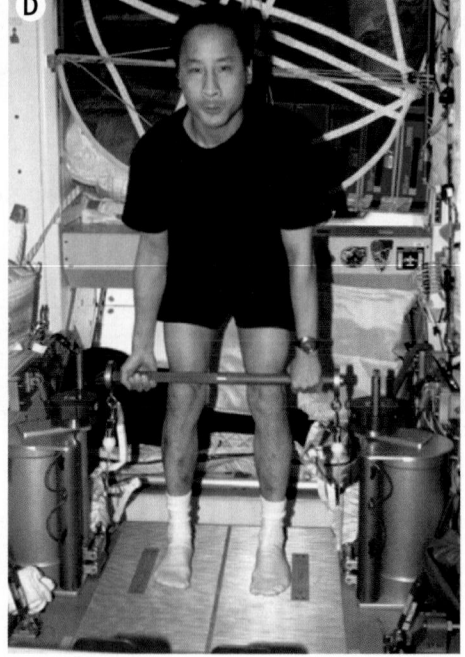
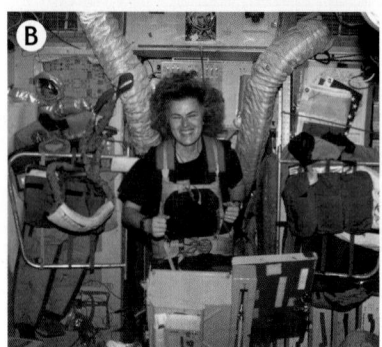
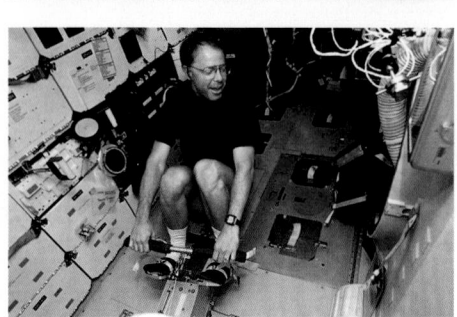

FIGURE 27.17 • Six examples of exercise training and measurement for different exercise modes during microgravity conditions. (**A** and **B**) Tethered treadmill exercise during a space shuttle mission. Note the strap arrangement around the upper body and straps anchored to the hips to keep the astronaut tethered to the treadmill. (**C**) Exercise training during different space shuttle missions showing back and arm, cycling, and rowing activity modes. (**D**) Astronaut using the short bar for the Interim Resistive Exercise Device (IRED) to perform upper-body strengthening exercise in the Unity node of the ISS. (Photos courtesy of NASA, Lyndon B. Johnson Space Center, Houston, TX.) (See also Alkner BA, et al. Effects of strength training using a gravity-independent exercise system, performed during 110 days of simulated space station confinement. *Eur J Appl Physiol* 2003;90:44; Convertino VA. Planning strategies for development of effective exercise and nutrition countermeasures for long-duration spaceflight. *Nutrition* 2002;18:880; Cowell SA, et al. The exercise and environmental physiology of extravehicular activity. *Aviat Space Environ Med* 2002;73:54; Lee SM, et al. Foot-ground reaction force during resistive exercise in parabolic flight. *Aviat Space Environ Med* 2004;75:405; and McCrory JL, et al. Locomotion in simulated zero gravity: ground reaction forces. *Aviat Space Environ Med* 2004;75:203.) A NASA sponsored YouTube video (**www.youtube.com/watch?v=doN4t5NKW-k**) provides an extensive tour of the ISS, including the exercise stations.

Lower-Body Negative Pressure

FIGURE 27.20 shows the in-flight lower-body negative pressure (LBNP) apparatus used aboard Skylab and Shuttle missions. This device serves two functions:

1. Assesses orthostatic deconditioning during spaceflight and postlanding
2. As a countermeasure against adverse orthostatic changes with short- and long-term missions

The LBNP device applies negative pressure to the lower limbs.[46,160] This forces fluid in the vascular system to migrate downward from the upper torso to the lower body—an effect that counters the in-flight response to microgravity. During three 6-mo Mir missions, cosmonauts wore thigh cuffs (rather than rely on an LBNP device) at 1, 3 to 4, and 5 to 5.5 mo and assessed cardiovascular parameters with echocardiography. Data were contrasted with control sessions 30 days preflight and 3 and 7 days postflight.[62] In all cosmonauts, a reduced vasoconstrictive response and a less efficient blood flow redistribution toward the brain coincided with orthostatic intolerance during postflight stand tests.[128] The vascular response to LBNP tests remained depressed during the flights. Thigh cuffs compensated partially for the cardiovascular changes induced by microgravity, but not for microgravity deconditioning. Upregulation of nitric oxide (NO; a potent vasodilator and natriuretic) may explain orthostatic intolerance in microgravity.[152] If this mechanism proves correct, administration of an inducible nitric oxide synthase (iNOS) inhibitor may attenuate orthostatic intolerance when astronauts return to Earth following a mission; it also may benefit patients following extended bed rest.

Assessing Orthostatic Deconditioning Effects

Disruptions in cardiovascular dynamics—heart rate, blood pressure, and leg volume changes—during space missions could compromise crew performance and mission success.[17,33] For example, orthostatic testing conducted after Gemini (14 days) and during Skylab (80 days) missions documented the degree of orthostatic deconditioning effects. The Gemini vehicles (including Mercury and Apollo) barely had enough room for the astronauts, so the mission could not accommodate an onboard LBNP chamber. Testing on Gemini took place only before and after flights. Also, Gemini flights used a tilt table rather than LBNP (Fig. 27.21A). A 15-min, 70° vertical LBNP tilt test produced dramatic changes in heart rate, systolic and diastolic blood pressure, and leg volume during the prolonged Skylab mission compared with the same variables assessed 3 wk prior to liftoff. Heart rate increased 100% from 70 b·min⁻¹ at rest at the start of the LBNP tilt test to 140 b·min⁻¹ at the end of the procedure. Systolic blood pressure declined more (30%) than diastolic blood pressure (<10%) during the tilt, whereas leg volume increased 10-fold during the test.

Figure 27.21B shows the pattern of resting heart rate in a 250-mm Hg LBNP test in one crew member during the 80-day Skylab 4 mission and 2 mo postflight. Although not as dramatic as the shorter-duration Gemini experiments, the resting heart rate increase in response to LBNP during Skylab confirmed the relative instability (and variability) of heart rate, particularly during the first month of spaceflight compared with the end of the mission. Heart rate with LBNP during preflight never exceeded 75 b·min⁻¹, but it always exceeded this value throughout the mission. On Skylab missions 2 and 3, resting heart rate averaged 109 b·min⁻¹, a 55% increase over preflight values.

LBNP Combined Countermeasures

A countermeasure combination of LBNP and increased fluid ingestion during spaceflight improves performance on an upright standing posture test postflight.[153] For example, two groups of 26 male astronauts consumed either no fluid or a loading volume of 32 oz of water or juice

plus eight salt tablets (to facilitate fluid retention) 1 hr before leaving Earth orbit during shuttle missions 1 through 8.[22] Crew members who used the liquid countermeasures did not experience syncope after landing mainly because about 40% of the ingested fluid increased plasma volume for nearly 4 hr. Astronauts who loaded fluid before reentry also had lower heart rates and maintained a more stable mean blood pressure. Overall, the hyperhydration countermeasures were more effective during short 3- to 7-day missions than during longer 10-day ones.

The protective benefits of *combined countermeasures* reduce the incidence of orthostatic intolerance assessed by postural tests postflight to only 5%.[121] In contrast, fluid loading alone prior to reentry loses its effectiveness after 7 days in microgravity[31] or during a 7-day, 6° head-down bed rest[28] because the vascular space cannot maintain enough fluid to restore plasma volume to a level that exerts benefits. Another countermeasure tactic reduces air temperature inside the space cabin the night before landing. Keeping the cabin "as cold as tolerable" helps to dissipate heat in the cabin, and ultimately in the space garments, during reentry and postlanding, when cabin air temperature can reach 26.7 to 32°C (80–90°F). The astronaut's liquid cooling garment uses a thermoelectric cooler to keep the precirculated water cool before it circulates through the full-torso garment. Reducing sweating response during reentry and landing minimizes fluid loss.

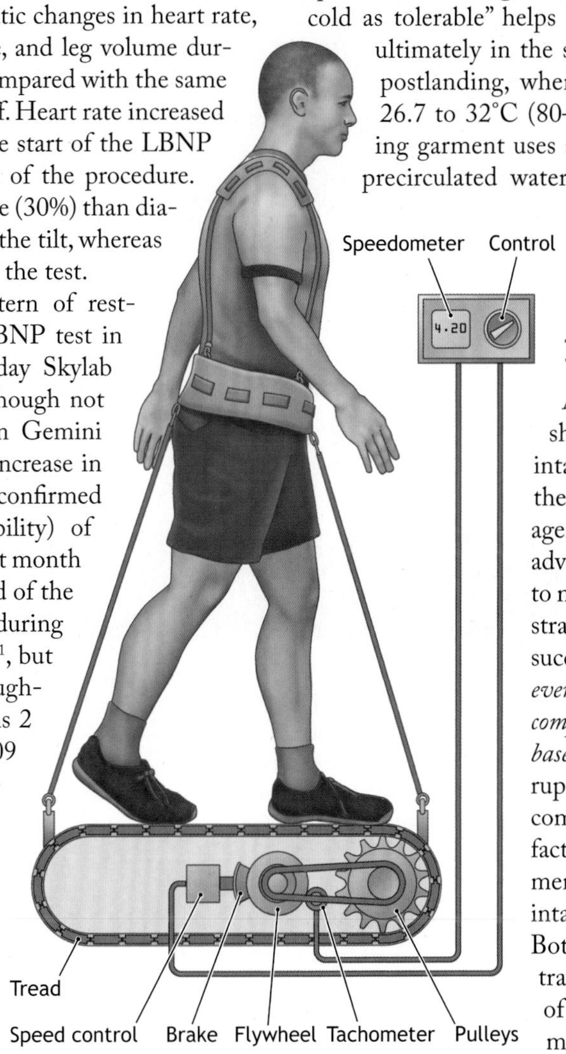

Nutrition

An optimal diet for spaceflight should theoretically provide energy intake equal to the energy required for the mission.[11,12,14,72–74,105] Dietary management also may counter the diverse, adverse effects of physiologic adaptation to microgravity.[48,148] This goal, seemingly straightforward, has not been reached successfully on most missions. *Almost every space journey produces weight loss compared with similar-duration ground-based activities on Earth.*[71,115,135,155] Disruption in energy balance results from combined effects of the two important factors: demands of the physical requirements of spaceflight and decreased food intake during microgravity exposure. Both factors negatively affect the space traveler's energy balance. The effects of a negative energy balance became manifested not only in weight loss but in impaired fluid, electrolyte, and mineral balance.[76,79] Each of these factors influences cardiovascular, musculoskeletal, immunologic, and endocrinologic functions. Cosmonauts

Speedometer   Control

Tread

Speed control   Brake   Flywheel   Tachometer   Pulleys

FIGURE 27.18 • Schematic details of subject-driven U.S. Space Shuttle treadmill. On each day in orbit on the ISS, each station crew member exercises for 1 hr of aerobic (treadmill or cycle ergometer) and 1 hr of dynamic resistance exercise (similar to lifting weights; www.nasa.gov/audience/foreducators/teachingfromspace/dayinthelife/exercise-adil-index.html).

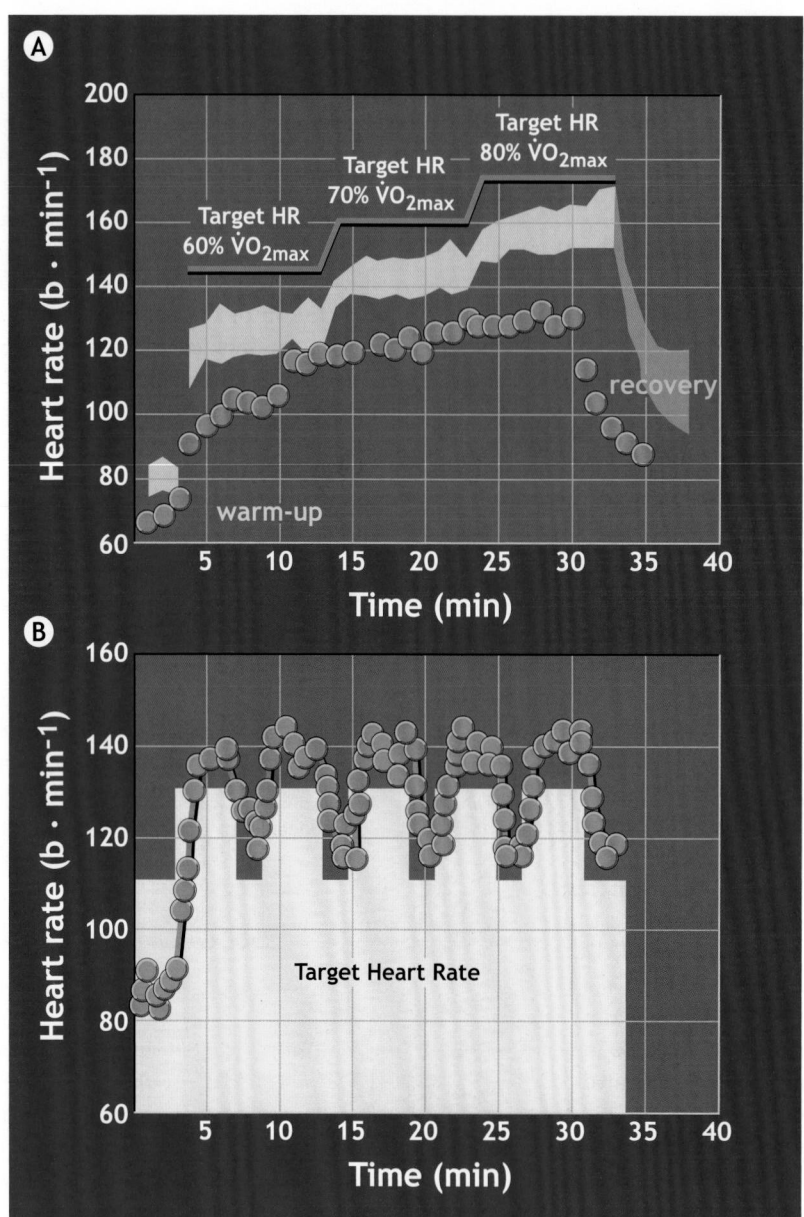

FIGURE 27.19 • **(A)** Heart rate during continuous treadmill exercise at 60, 70, and 80% of $\dot{V}O_{2max}$ on an 11-day shuttle mission. The *light-green shaded area* shows the exercise heart rate range during workout days 3 to 11. *Orange* circles represent heart rate during a familiarization run on flight day 2. The intense workouts helped to minimize orthostatic dysfunction upon landing. **(B)** Heart rate during five intervals of a treadmill exercise routine using the shuttle treadmill. (Adapted with permission from Lee SL, et al. Exercise Countermeasures Demonstration Project during the Lunar–Mars Life Support Test Project. Phase IIA. NASA. NASA/TP-98-206537. Lyndon B. Johnson Space Center, Houston, TX. 1998.)

in the Russian space program also have reported weight loss during extended missions.

Effects on Body Weight

Large individual variation in body weight occurred for crewmembers during three Skylab missions lasting 24, 56, and 84 days. On each mission, all crewmembers lost weight and did not regain it except for the commander whose weight returned to prelaunch values by mission's end. The most dramatic weight loss of 3 to 4% generally occurred over the first 10 days of each

mission, mainly from fluid loss. Weight loss reversed within 5 days after return to Earth. This same weight loss pattern during spaceflight and weight regain postflight occurred during the 1996 Life Sciences and Microgravity (LSM) mission.[136]

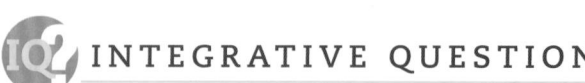 **INTEGRATIVE QUESTION**

How would you measure an astronaut's body weight in microgravity? (Hint: Refer to these citations for insights.)[53,121]

TABLE 27.10	**Incidence and Severity of Space Motion Sickness During 36 Space Shuttle Flights**			
	Number of Crew Members			
Motion Sickness Rating	**First Shuttle Flight**	**Later Shuttle Flight**	**Totals**	
None	32 (29%)	28 (45%)	60 (35%)	
Mild	36 (33%)	24 (39%)	60 (35%)	
Moderate	29 (27%)	10 (16%)	39 (23%)	
Severe	12 (11%)	0 (0%)	12 (7%)	
Total	**109 (64%)**	**62 (36%)**	**171 (100%)**	

Reprinted from Nicogossian AE, et al. Countermeasures to space deconditioning. In: Nicogossian AE, et al., eds. *Space Physiology and Medicine*. 3rd Ed. Philadelphia: Lea & Febiger, 1994:230.

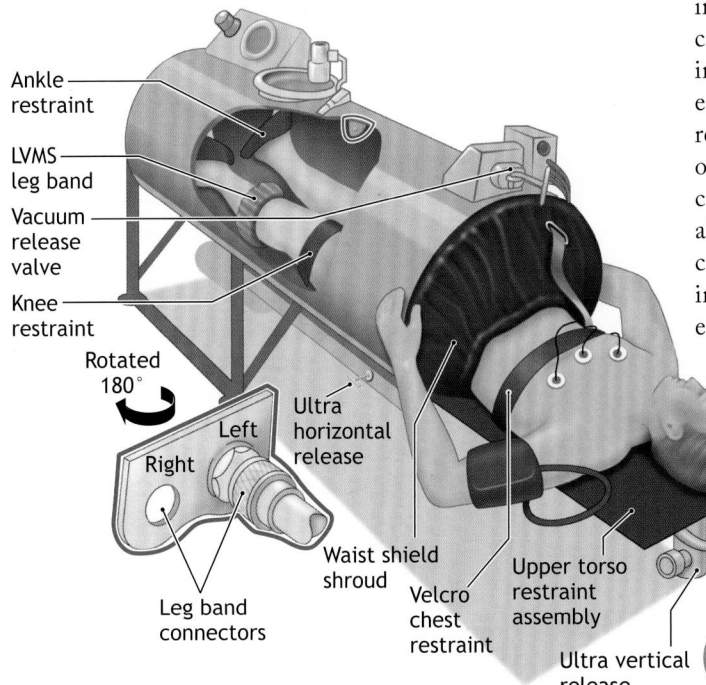

FIGURE 27.20 • Schematic diagram of the lower-body negative pressure (LBNP) apparatus used aboard Skylab illustrating the upper- and lower-body restraint assembly, including the leg volume measuring system (LVMS) leg band. The waist seal shroud maintains controlled and regulated negative pressure from 0 to 50 mm Hg below ambient pressure. During ground tests, a vacuum provides negative pressure; during flight, negative pressure occurs from the space vacuum. (Reprinted with permission from Nicogossian AE, et al., eds. *Space Physiology and Medicine*. 3rd Ed. Philadelphia: Lea & Febiger, 1994.)

Altered Protein Dynamics. *Atrophy of skeletal muscles that support posture and locomotion represents a characteristic maladaptation to microgravity during short- and long-duration exposures.*[49] Decreases in lean body mass, muscle volume, and muscle strength and changes in muscle fiber micro-architecture[168] accompany space-induced muscle atrophy. Such changes suggest poor adaptation in whole-body protein (nitrogen) balance.[88,135,137,] Isotopic methods that assess tissue protein turnover show that astronauts increase protein breakdown rate by approximately 30% on mission days 2 to 8, thereby producing negative nitrogen balance. In addition, increases occur in urinary cortisol, fibrinogen, and interleukin-2 (IL-2). These changes suggest that space-flight triggers a stress response similar to response patterns from physical injury. In both of these stressful situations, tissue protein serves as a substrate for energy metabolism that fosters a negative nitrogen balance (protein catabolism). This supports the recommendation of a daily protein intake of 1.5 g per kilogram, of body mass during space travel.[78] In addition, long space missions (4 to 9 mo on the Russian Mir Space Station) and shorter-duration space shuttle flights (up to 15 d) were associated with decreased oxidative damage owing to reduced oxygen radical production (in the electron transport chain) from reduced energy intake. Increased oxidative damage occurs postflight from combined increases in metabolic rate and possible loss of in-flight host antioxidant defenses.[139] The potential beneficial effects of postflight antioxidant supplementation remain unknown. On the two shuttle missions, daily calorie intake and nitrogen balance were affected negatively compared with preflight values. Based on Russian data aboard the Salyut-7 space mission, the estimated energy cost of twice-daily in-flight exercise sessions was approximately 20 kcal per kilogram of body mass. Adding this energy requirement to an already inadequate daily energy intake would provoke further protein loss to absorb the energy deficit.[67] Research must determine effective combinations of exercise and nutritional supplementation to stabilize energy and protein balance during space missions, including development of renal stones that can seriously impact the health of the crew member and mission.[107]

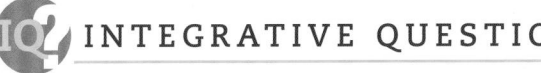

INTEGRATIVE QUESTION

Explain whether consuming additional protein during a space mission would help to restore fat-free body mass.

Energy Expenditure and Energy Balance Dynamics on the Space Shuttle

The 1996 LMS shuttle mission measured energy expenditure and energy balance in four crew members for 12 days before liftoff, during the 17-day flight, and 15 days postflight.[136]

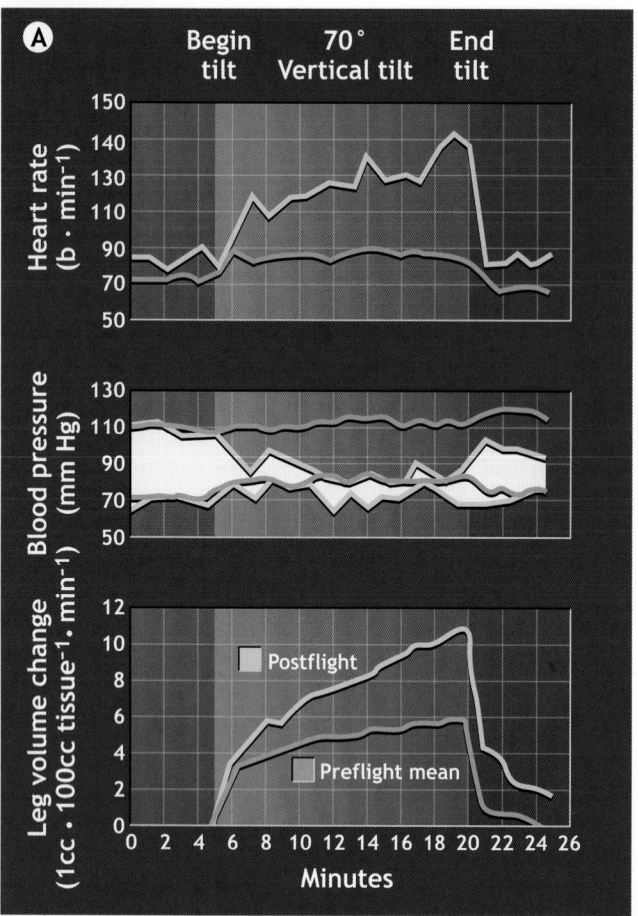

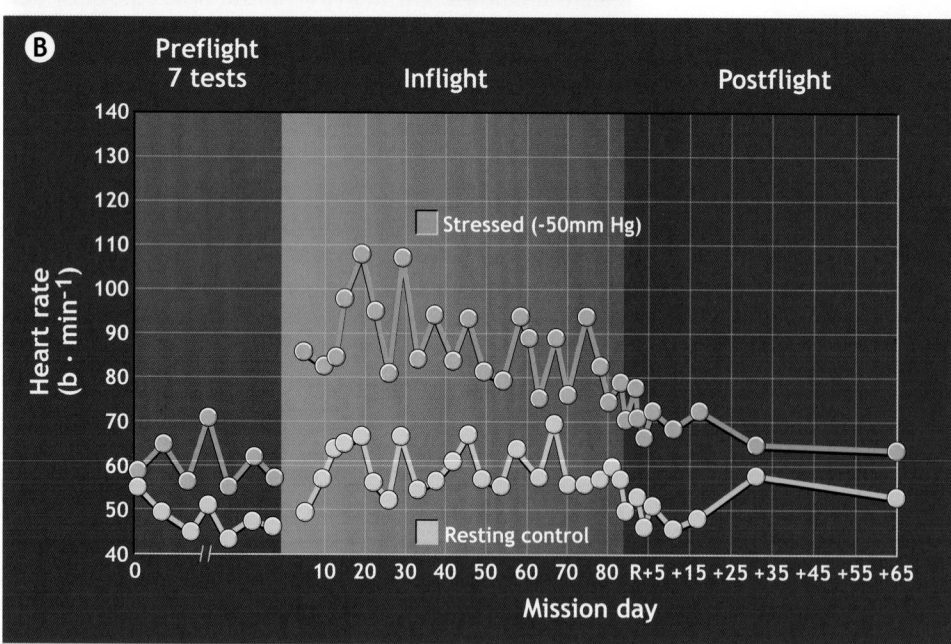

FIGURE 27.21 • LBNP evaluation of cardiovascular dynamics during space missions: **(A)** Gemini 14-day pre- to postflight changes in heart rate, blood pressure, and leg volume. **(B)** Resting heart rate in a 250-mm Hg LBNP test in one crew member during an 80-day Skylab mission. (Reprinted with permission from Charles JB, et al. Cardiopulmonary function. In: Nicogossian AE, et al., eds. *Space Physiology and Medicine*. 3rd Ed. Philadelphia: Lea & Febiger, 1994.)

In addition, a complementary bed-rest study with a 6° head-down tilt to simulate microgravity evaluated energy expenditure and energy balance in eight subjects. The bed-rest study had three phases: (1) 15-day pre–bed-rest ambulatory period, (2) 17 days of bed rest (except when subjects exercised to match the in-flight exercise routines), and (3) a 15-day recovery period. Subjects in both experiments performed submaximal and maximal bicycle ergometer exercise tests on days 13 and 8 before launch and on days 4 and 8 postflight. During spaceflight days 2, 8, and 13, crewmembers performed an additional ergometer test to assess cardiorespiratory responses to exercise at 85% $\dot{V}O_{2max}$.

Measurements included doubly labeled water (DLW; $^2H_2^{18}O$) and body composition by dual-energy x-ray absorptiometry (DXA) before and after spaceflight/bed rest to quantify positive energy balance (fat stored) or negative energy balance (fat catabolized). Subjects quantified each food item consumed and not consumed with a bar code reader and verbal description (using a cassette recorder) to estimate the contents remaining in the individual food package. During pre- and postflight periods, subjects consumed prepared meals of known nutrient content. The Spacelab contained a system to collect, measure, and save a 20-mL daily urine sample to estimate nitrogen balance from nitrogen and creatinine excretion.

FIGURE 27.22 A displays three energy intake periods expressed as kcal·kg^{-1}·d^{-1} during preflight, flight, and postflight. Note that within each period, a relative stabilization or adaptation took place for energy intake. This probably occurred from resetting of setpoint mechanisms that regulate energy balance. The *histogram inset* at the lower right expresses average energy intake in kcal daily to highlight the dramatic 45% lower in-flight energy intake (1708 kcal·d^{-1}) compared with the remarkably similar values preflight (3025 kcal·d^{-1}) and postflight (3151 kcal·d^{-1}) intakes.

FIGURE 27.22B compares the energy intake during the first 2 wk of spaceflight for Skylab missions 2, 3, and 4 and the two shuttle LMS missions. Astronauts on the shuttle LMS (*bottom red curve*) remained in substantial negative energy balance throughout the flight. Astronauts on the previous three Skylab missions participated in a metabolic balance study, so daily energy intakes remained fairly stable during the different-duration missions. In contrast, astronauts on shuttle LMS consumed food ad libitum. At the same time, they performed vigorous

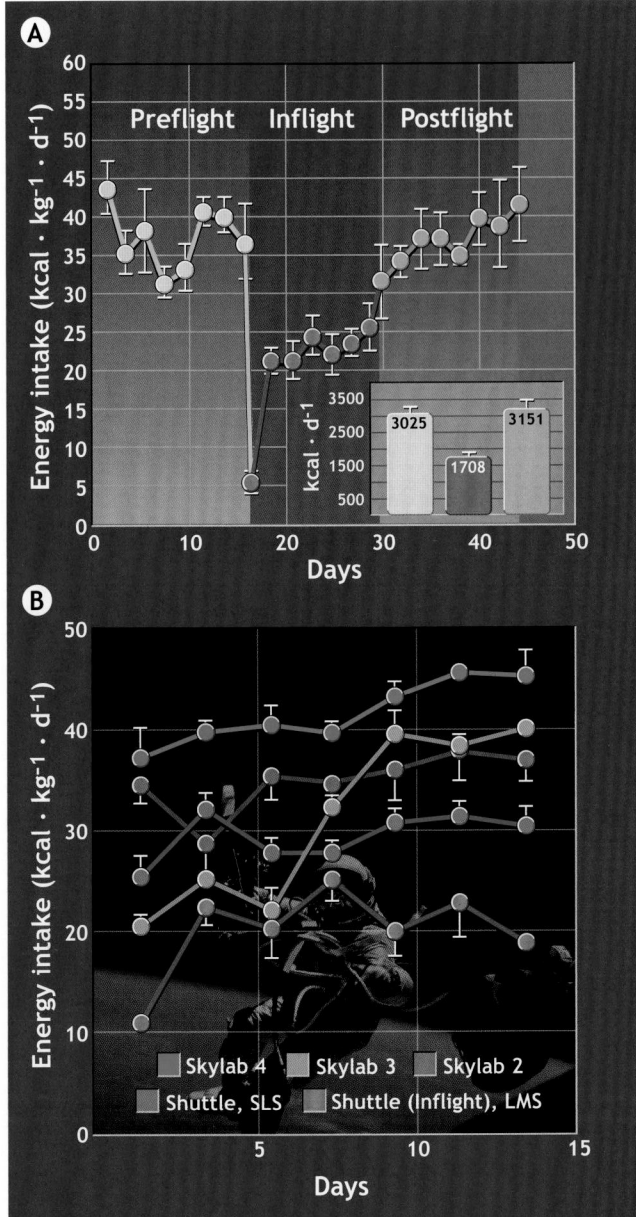

FIGURE 27.22 • **(A)** Daily energy intake before, during, and after spaceflight on shuttle LMS. The histogram inset expresses the data as average kcal·d⁻¹ during each mission phase. **(B)** Daily energy intake during the first 2 wk of spaceflight for Skylab missions 2 (28 d), 3 (56 d), and 4 (84 d); two shuttle missions (SLS-1 and SLS-2 combined); and shuttle LMS. (Data adapted with permission from Stein TP, et al. Energy expenditure and balance during spaceflight on the space shuttle. *Am J Physiol* 1999;45:R1739.)

daily exercise that contributed to their relatively high average total daily energy expenditure of 40.8 kcal·kg⁻¹·d⁻¹ (3238 kcal). No differences occurred among the three methods of estimating energy balance. This result supported the validity of the methodology and main two research conclusions:

1. Severe negative energy balance and corresponding loss of body mass, body fat, and protein could compromise

a mission and adversely affect an astronaut's health in a manner resembling prolonged malnutrition.
2. High levels of physical activity during spaceflight may disrupt mechanisms that maintain energy balance.

International Space Station (ISS) Experiments on Nutrition and Body Composition

One of the difficulties facing space medicine scientists is how to plan for optimal nutrient requirements during long-duration space exploration missions.[75] The ISS provides a unique vehicle to assess nutritional changes during long-duration spaceflights of 128 to 195 days. An interesting series of experiments aboard the ISS has examined body composition, bone metabolism, hematology, general blood chemistry, and blood levels of selected vitamins and minerals in 11 astronauts before and after such long-duration missions. Crewmembers consumed an average of 80% of their recommended energy intake, and on landing day their body weight registered significantly lower than before flight. Hematocrit, serum iron, ferritin saturation, and transferrin were decreased and serum ferritin significantly increased after flight. The finding that other acute-phase proteins were unchanged after flight suggests that the changes in iron metabolism were not solely responsible for an inflammatory response. Urinary 8-hydroxy-29-deoxyguanosine concentration was greater and red blood cell superoxide dismutase was depressed after flight, indicating increased oxidative damage. The astronauts consumed vitamin D supplements during flight, yet serum 25-hydroxycholecalciferol decreased after flight. Bone resorption was increased after flight, but bone formation did not consistently rise 1 day after landing. Bone loss, compromised vitamin D status, and oxidative damage are among critical nutritional concerns that require resolution for long-duration space travelers.[132]

Nutritionally Related Effects of Spaceflight on Physiologic Functions

Since the first space missions, researchers have tracked adaptations in physiologic function during microgravity exposure. A prevailing theory about such changes concerns the interactions among nutritional variables and endocrine functions and their combined effects on cardiopulmonary, hormonal, skeletal, and body fluid functions, and body mass and composition.[34,99,130,141] FIGURE 27.23 shows the triad of nutritionally related effects of spaceflight on different physiologic systems. The interrelated triad components—fluid shifts, physical unloading of weight-bearing structures, and metabolic changes—in many ways link to shifts in endocrine function. The inset table shows endocrine changes during stress, simulated microgravity (bed rest), and spaceflight. Note the responses to bed rest do not generally mirror endocrine changes in spaceflight, but instead mimic stress-mediated responses. An attractive hypothesis posits that endocrine effects of spaceflight relate more to nutritional changes characterized by stress-related models, not a model that includes bed rest. The similarity between the catabolic effects of increased demands on energy metabolism (and negative energy balance) and catabolic effects of spaceflight "stress" help to explain space-induced decreases in body mass, lean body mass, and bone density. This includes shifts in extracellular and intracellular water compartments.

Body Composition Changes. FIGURE 27.24 shows percentage changes in body composition variables of 10 astronauts assessed by densitometry and bioelectrical impedance analysis before and 2 days following 7- to 16-day missions. No changes occurred in body fat or extracellular water, with the 2.3% decline in body mass attributable to a loss in fat-free body mass (FFM). Note that all three components of FFM (water, protein, and mineral) declined from 3 to 4% in post-flight measures. The 3% loss of intracellular water—attributable to decreased protein and mineral levels within other tissues including muscle—explains the decrease in total-body water. An integrative approach assesses regional body composition (calf muscle volume)[159] and MRI-derived characteristics of muscle (transverse relaxation of calf muscles) following multiple shuttle/Mir missions lasting 16 to 28 wk.[86]

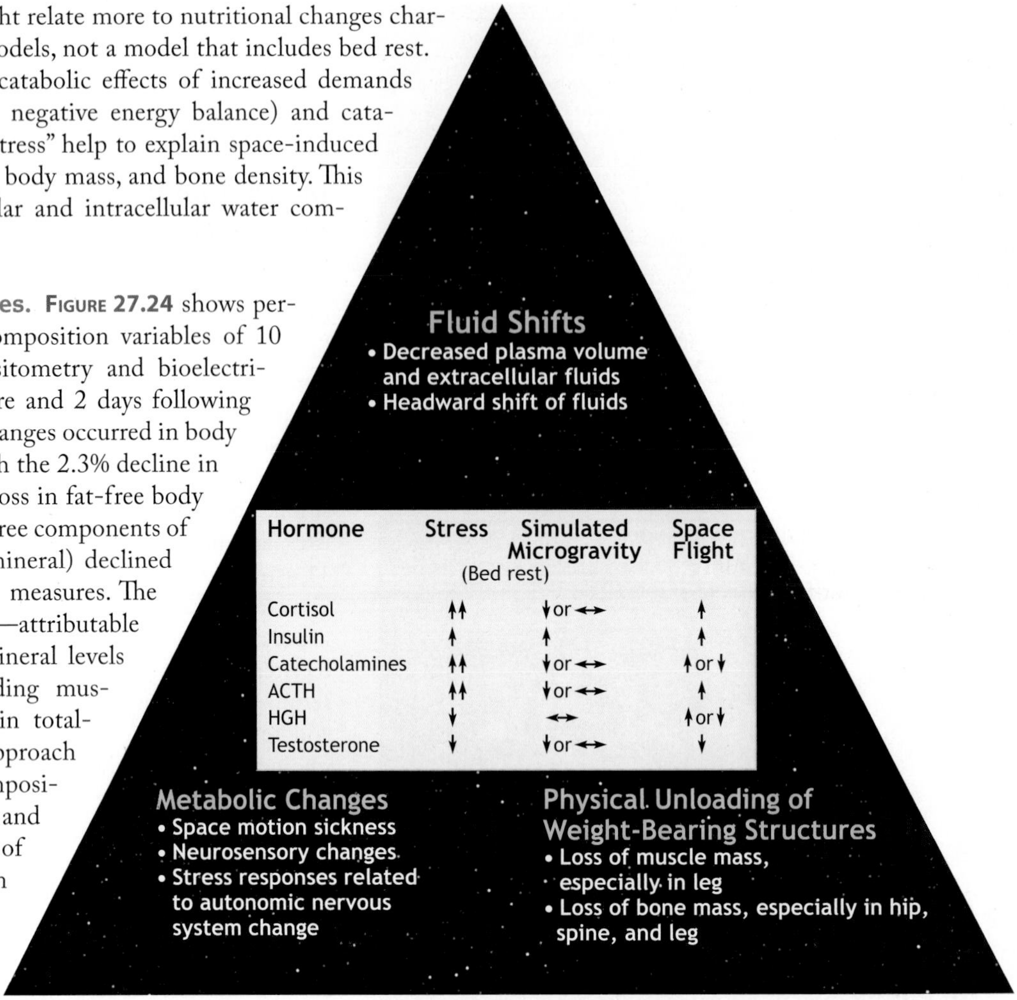

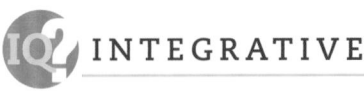 INTEGRATIVE QUESTION

Explain what role diet and exercise should play in prolonged-duration space missions.

OVERVIEW OF PHYSIOLOGIC RESPONSES TO SPACEFLIGHT

Numerous research reports discuss short- and long-term consequences of spaceflight on human physiology.[16,83,113] From the first single-pilot flights of Project Mercury in the early 1960s to the extended Soviet Soyuz missions of the 1990s and latest manned Chinese space missions, scientists have pondered how best to minimize deleterious effects of microgravity during flight and upon return to Earth. FIGURE 27.25 diagrams two main physical stressors from space travel:

1. Decreased hydrostatic pressure gradients within the cardiovascular system (displayed on right)
2. Decreased weight loading on muscles (displayed on left)

Fluid Shifts
- Decreased plasma volume and extracellular fluids
- Headward shift of fluids

Hormone	Stress	Simulated Microgravity (Bed rest)	Space Flight
Cortisol	↑↑	↓ or ↔	↑
Insulin	↑	↑	↑
Catecholamines	↑↑	↓ or ↔	↑ or ↓
ACTH	↑↑	↓ or ↔	↑
HGH	↓	↔	↑ or ↓
Testosterone	↓	↓ or ↔	↓

Metabolic Changes
- Space motion sickness
- Neurosensory changes
- Stress responses related to autonomic nervous system change

Physical Unloading of Weight-Bearing Structures
- Loss of muscle mass, especially in leg
- Loss of bone mass, especially in hip, spine, and leg

FIGURE 27.23 • Triad of nutritionally related effects of spaceflight on physiologic systems. The inset shows endocrine changes during stress, simulated microgravity (bed-rest studies), and spaceflight. ↑, increase; ↑↑, large increase; ↓, decrease; ↔, no change. (Adapted with permission from Lane HW, Gretebeck RJ. Nutrition, endocrinology, and body composition during space flight. *Nutr Res* 1998;18:1923.)

Both factors ultimately increase physiologic strain (*blue box at the bottom*) and negatively affect an astronaut's physical performance (*red box at the bottom*).

Note that the three effects (decreased $\dot{V}O_{2max}$ and muscular strength and increased fatigability), combined with an increased thermal load, add substantially to the total physiologic strain. Exercise countermeasures (specifically site-specific lower-body eccentric and concentric resistance exercise) coupled with relatively intense cardiovascular workouts on a cycle ergometer and treadmill can mitigate deleterious effects from prolonged microgravity sojourns. This is particularly important when astronauts return to a 1g Earth environment.

Short- and Long-Term Responses

Two categories, short and long term, describe the time course of physiologic response and adaptation in transition from

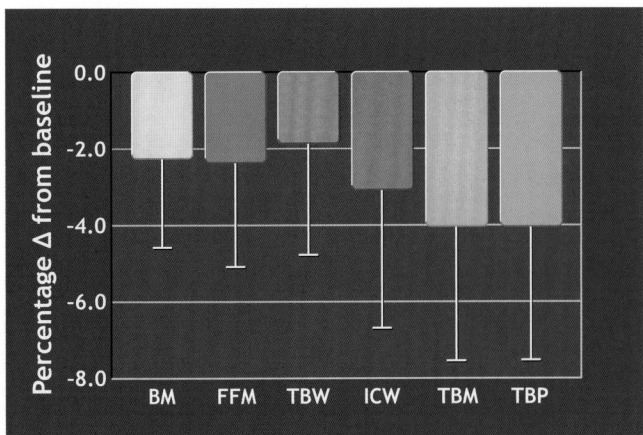

FIGURE 27.24 • Percentage changes (Δ) in body composition variables of 10 astronauts assessed by densitometry and multifrequency bioelectrical impedance analysis before and 2 days after 7- to 16-day missions. BM, body mass; FFM, fat-free body mass; TBW, total body water; ICW, intracellular water; TBM, total body mineral; TBP, total body protein. (Data used with permission from Greenisen MC, et al. Functional performance evaluation. In: Extended Duration Orbiter Medical Project. NASA Johnson Space Center final report. 1989–1995. [NASA/SP-1999-534] NASA. Lyndon B. Johnson Space Center, Houston, TX, 1999.)

Earth's 1g environment to microgravity in low-Earth orbit and then return to 1g following a mission. Short-term responses occur within 24 hr or the first few days of a mission. The second category describes longer-term changes following a mission. **FIGURE 27.26** presents a generalized flow diagram of the immediate or short-term (<24 hr) and delayed or long-term (>24 hr) responses. Both immediate and delayed responses eventually contribute to orthostatic hypotension (*bottom red box*), the most common malady following spaceflight.

In space, body fluids no longer move "downward" from gravity's pull, so fluids redistribute toward the chest and upper body (note facial puffiness from cranial edema in the two inset photos on the left). Lower-body fluid loss gives the legs a birdlike appearance. Excess fluid buildup in the torso triggers fluid elimination by the kidneys. Mean arterial pressure increases in the cranial region from a preflight normal of 70 mm Hg to 100 mm Hg in space (Fig. 27.26 Top), while mean pressure at the feet declines 50% from its normal 200 mm Hg; heart volume also decreases slightly in microgravity. The immediate change in body fluid distribution activates a plethora of additional responses and lower sympathetic nervous system activity. Restricted stimulation environments such as spaceflight and other stress-inducing situations from prolonged confinement and isolation share many of the same responses and adaptations.[90]

Time Course of In-Flight Adaptations

FIGURE 27.27 depicts the time course for shifts in four main categories of physiologic function during 1 year of sustained microgravity. The *green horizontal line* represents baseline function on Earth (denoted as 0% change). Within the first 3 wk, up to a 10% change in cardiovascular function reflects a deconditioning response; within 14 days, a 10% change occurs in body fluid redistribution; and within 3 mo, bone mass declines by 5%. Bone mass declines further, to 15%, between months 5 and 6, when it stabilizes for several months before decreasing farther to 17% after 1 year. Like bone mass, muscle structure and function deteriorate at a slower rate than do cardiac deconditioning and fluid redistribution, but the magnitude of the decrement reaches higher values that approach 20% from baseline values. Note the similar, parallel decline in bone mass and muscle mass as a function of deconditioning throughout a year.

Time Course of Postflight Readaptations

FIGURE 27.28 shows how 3 mo of recovery (readaptation) affects neurovestibular and cardiovascular functions, fluid and electrolyte balance, red blood cell mass, and lean body mass. For reference, the *lower horizontal line*, indicated by the *arrow at bottom left* (*1g set point*), represents baseline measures expected under normal 1g conditions. The *colored lines* for each variable indicate average trends, but with considerable inter- and intraindividual differences exist in the basic response variables.

Analysis of the recovery curves reveals two characteristics:

1. The response rate is nonlinear, with some processes appearing bimodal with relatively high rate constants.
2. Recovery time varies depending on the variable evaluated.

For example, the rapid change in fluid distribution during the first few weeks of microgravity exposure shown previously in Figure.28 recovers to baseline within the first week of return to 1g (*yellow curve*). In contrast, the *aqua curve* for lean body mass and *magenta curve* for cardiovascular deconditioning require approximately 6 wk to approach baseline.

NASA'S NEW VISION FOR THE FUTURE OF SPACE EXPLORATION

A June 2012 report articulates NASA's multi-destination human space exploration strategy using a capability-driven approach (www.nasa.gov/pdf/657307main_Exploration%20Report_508_6-4-12.pdf). NASA posits that the United States should foster a safe, robust, affordable, sustainable, and flexible space program by developing a set of core evolving capabilities instead of specialized, destination-specific hardware. These core capabilities will allow NASA the flexibility to conduct increasingly complex missions to a range of destinations over time. NASA believes that expanding such an approach will increase scientific knowledge, enable technological and economic growth, and inspire global collaboration and achievement.

One of NASA's ambitious goals over the next two decades hopefully will succeed in sending humans to a range of destinations beyond low Earth orbit (LEO), including cis-lunar space (visualized as a sphere with a circumference slightly larger than the orbit of the Moon, within which are thousands of artificial satellites, countless pieces of space debris, and micro asteroids), near-Earth asteroids (NEAs), the Moon, and Mars

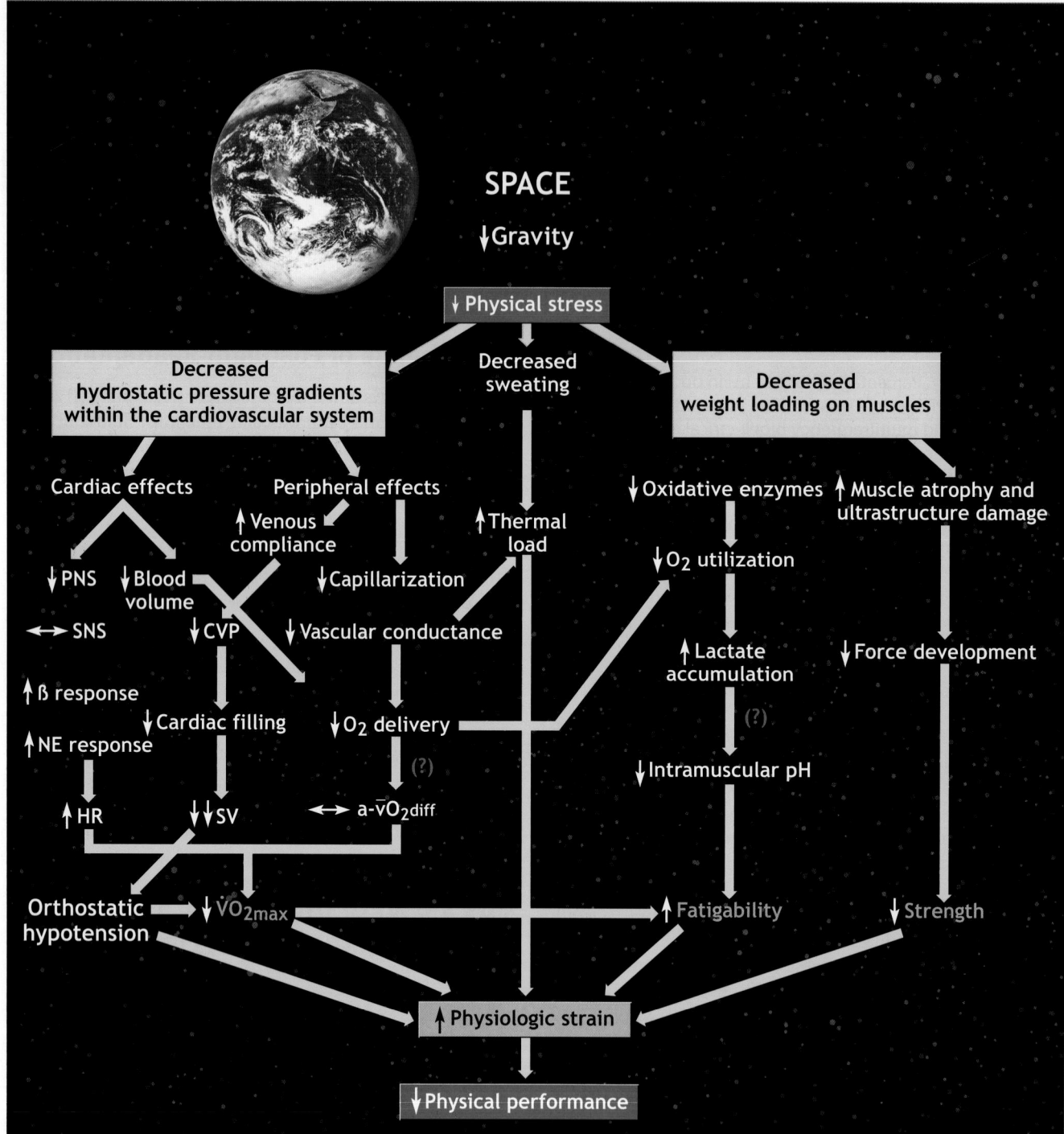

FIGURE 27.25 • Model of the relationship between physical stress of the space environment and adaptation of cardiovascular and muscular systems, with resulting increased physiologic strain and decreased physical performance. SNS, sympathetic nervous system; CVP, central venous pressure; β, beta-adrenergic; NE, norepinephrine; HR, heart rate; SV, stroke volume; a–$\bar{v}O_2$diff, arteriovenous oxygen difference; ↑, increase; ↓, decrease; ↓↓, large decrease; ↔, no change. (Reprinted with permission from Convertino VA. Effects of microgravity on exercise performance. In: Garrett WE, Kirkendall DT, eds. *Exercise and Sport Science*. Philadelphia: Lippincott Williams & Wilkins, 2000.)

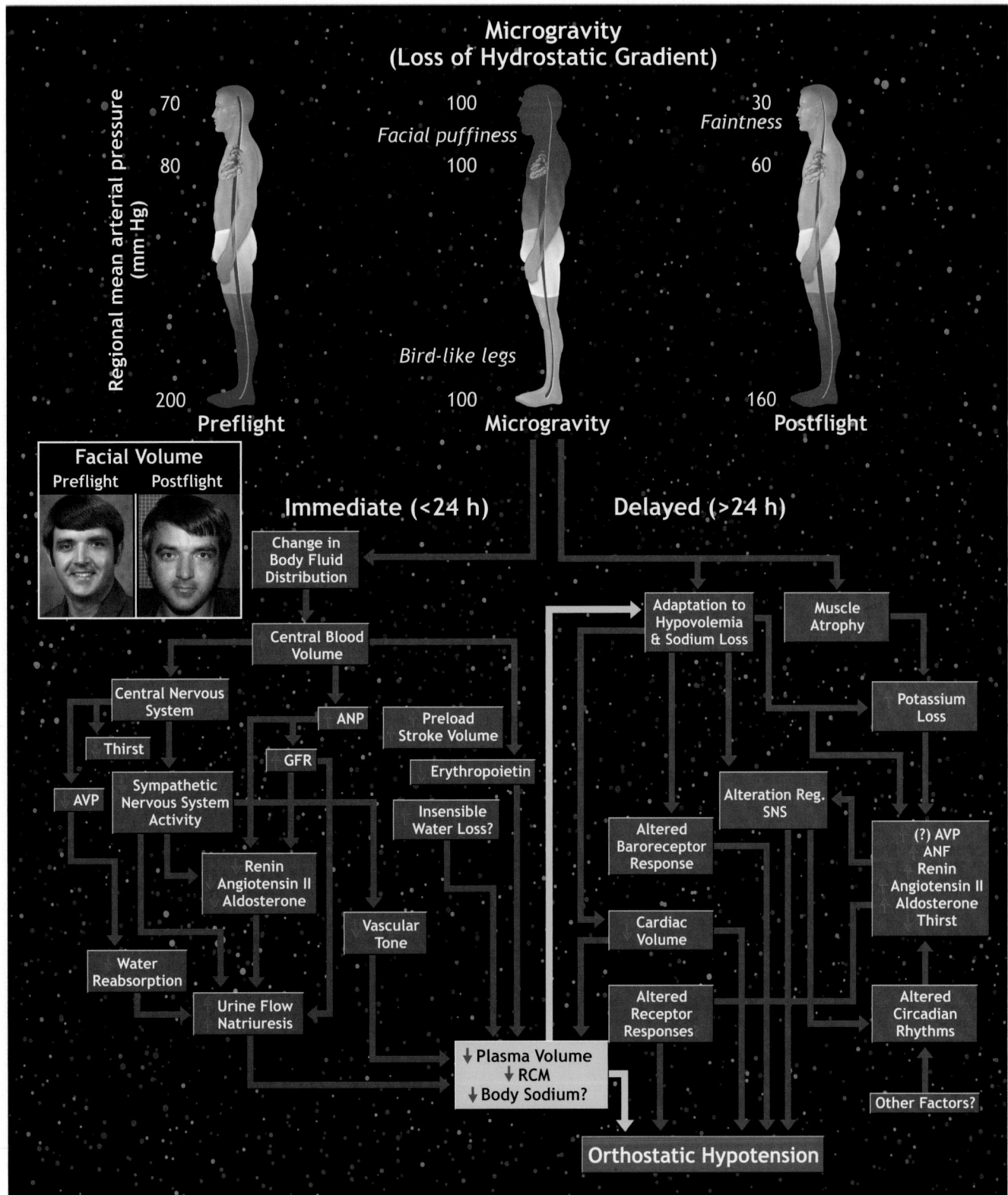

FIGURE 27.26 • Proposed immediate (<24 hr) and delayed (>24 hr) responses to microgravity compared with those under preflight (1g) and postflight (1g) conditions. AVP, arginine vasopressin; ANP, atrial natriuretic peptide; GFR, glomerular filtration rate; RCM, red cell mass; SNS, sympathetic nervous system; ↑, increase; ↓, decrease, ?, possible. (Photos courtesy of NASA, Lyndon B. Johnson Space Center, Houston, TX. Figures denoting changes in mean arterial pressure were adapted with permission from Hargens AR, et al. Control of circulatory function in altered gravitational fields. *Physiologist* 1992;35:S80. Additional graphic information adapted from Maillet A, et al. Cardiovascular and hormonal changes induced by isolation and confinement. *Med Sci Sports Exerc* 1996;28:S53.)

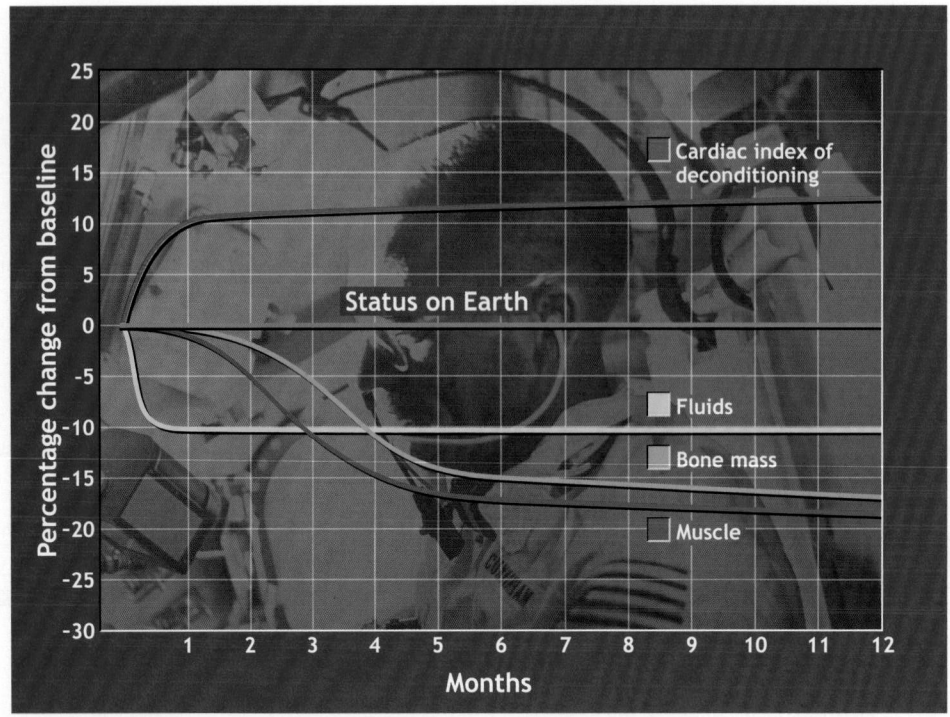

FIGURE 27.27 • Time course of four main shifts in physiologic function during 1 year in microgravity. The horizontal green line represents baseline function on Earth at 1g (denoted as zero percent change). The cardiac index of deconditioning (*red line*) reflects severity of orthostatic intolerance to gravitational stress. (Adapted with permission from: Nicogossian A, et al. Overall physiologic response to space flight. In: Nicogossian AE, et al., eds. *Space Physiology and Medicine*. 3rd Ed. Philadelphia: Lea & Febiger, 1994.)

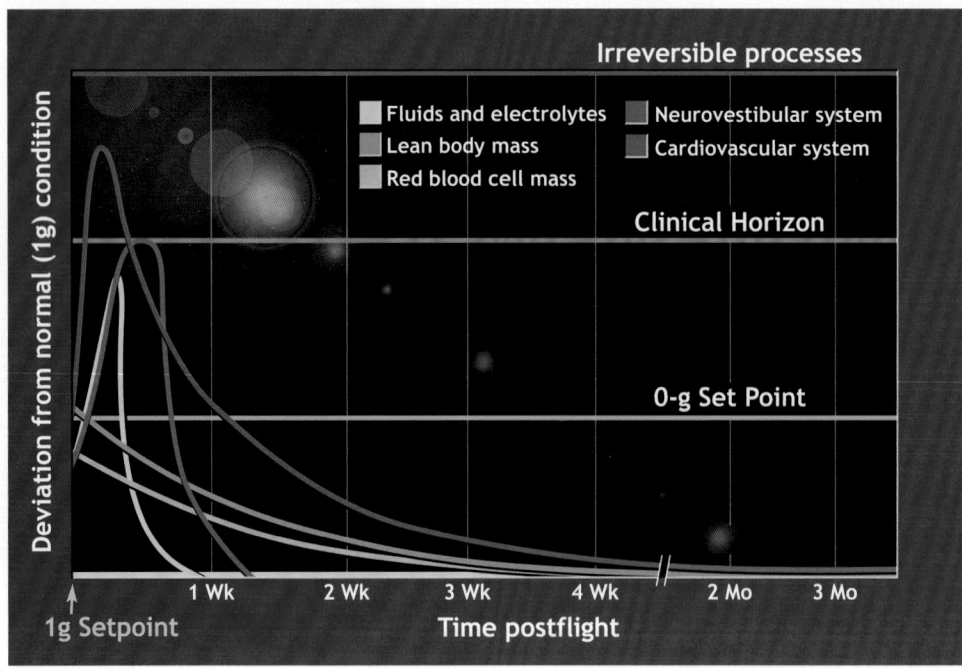

FIGURE 27.28 • Time course of physiologic shifts during 3 mo of readaptation to 1g, in which flight duration only minimally affects the readaptations. (Adapted with permission from Nicogossian AE, et al., eds. *Space Physiology and Medicine*. 3rd Ed. Philadelphia: Lea & Febiger, 1994.)

Hubble Space Telescope

Ever since the invention of early telescopes over 410 years ago, the biggest obstacle for obtaining clear images of distant objects was overcoming distortions caused by the atmosphere. It was obvious that to obtain a clear image, a major requirement was to place the telescope on a mountaintop or, even more audacious, launched into space. This is exactly what accomplished German physicist and engineer Hermann Oberth (1894–1989) first suggested in a 1923 book he authored about rocket travel into outer space (*Die Rakete zu den Planetenräumen* [The Rocket into Interplanetary Space]). As rocket launchings became more commonplace with larger engines with greater thrust and range, the idea of launching a telescope into space became feasible. In 1969, preparations were being made to launch a Large Space Telescope (LST), but it took another 6 years before the European Space Agency (http://sci.esa.int/science-e/www/area/index.cfm?fareaid=31) began work with NASA on a plan that would eventually become Hubble. Congress approved funding for such a telescope in 1977, with the reusable Space Shuttle providing a new mechanism for delivering it into space. The Large Space Telescope was renamed the Hubble Space Telescope (HST) in honor of Edwin P. Hubble (www.biography.com/people/edwin-hubble-9345936), an American astronomer who made the momentous discovery, while working diligently at the Mount Wilson Observatory's 100-inch Telescope in Southern California, that some of the numerous distant, faint clouds of light in the universe were actually entire galaxies—similar to the Milky Way. A cogent timeline about the early development

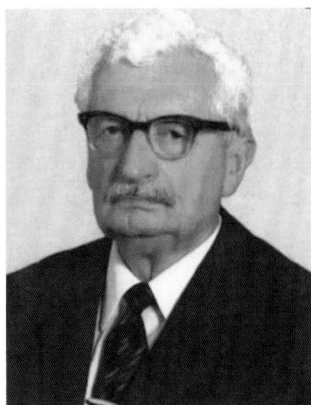

Hermann Oberth

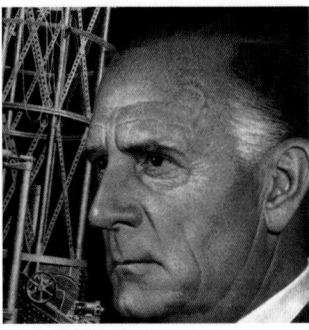

Edwin P. Hubble

and current use of the Hubble Space Telescope can be found at www.chara.gsu.edu/CHARA/MWI-Video-640-web.mov. Hubble's original notion of an "expanding" universe formed the basis of the Big Bang theory, which states that the universe began with an intense burst of energy at a single moment in time. After continuous years of flawless service, NASA had periodically conducted astronaut missions to service and upgrade Hubble's gyroscopes, electronic boxes, batteries, and state-of-the-art scientific instrumentation to make the Hubble a more capable orbiting observatory. In an ambitious undertaking, the Space Shuttle Endeavor ferried a crew of seven to fix Hubble during 5 days of spacewalks. Two new cameras were installed during the fix (http://hubblesite.org/gallery/album/), which subsequently took many of Hubble's most famous photos from deep space that included distant stars, galaxies, nebulae, and celestial bodies (e.g., Mars, Saturn, Jupiter). In December 1993, the first new images from Hubble reached Earth. Hubble has been serviced five times, the final time in 2009 with five back-to-back spacewalks during an 11-day mission (http://hubblesite.org/the_telescope/team_hubble/servicing_missions.php). NASA plans to replace Hubble with the new James Webb Space Telescope (JWST), scheduled to launch in 2018. This Earth-orbiting astronomical observatory will be three times the size of Hubble, and was designed to work best at infrared wavelengths to study the distant universe, looking for the first stars and galaxies that ever emerged (www.jwst.nasa.gov). The JWST will have a large mirror, 6.5 m (21.3 ft) in diameter and a sunshield the size of a tennis court. JWST will reside in an orbit about 1.5 million km (1 million miles) from the Earth. The telescope was named after James Webb (1906–1992), who crafted the Apollo program and was a staunch supporter of space science and an effective NASA administrator.

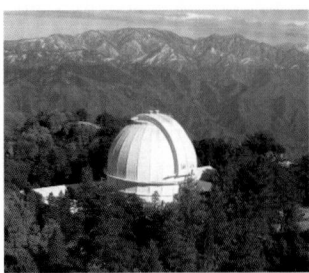

Mount Wilson Observatory

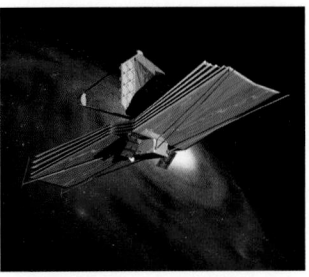

James Webb Space Telescope

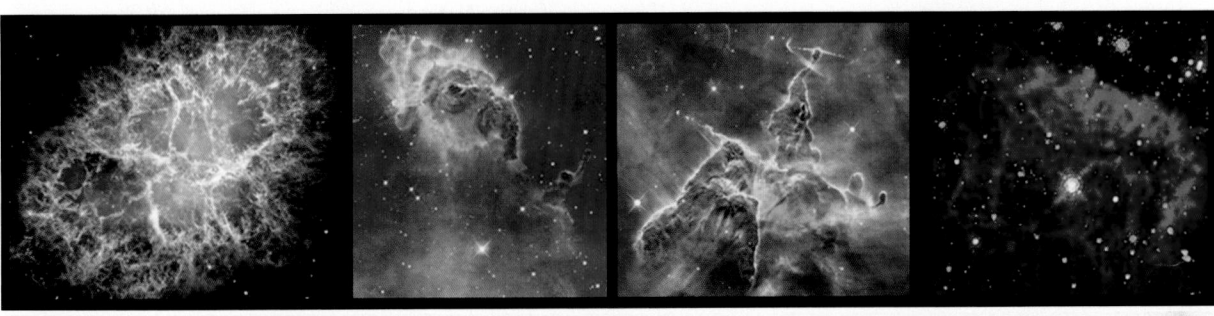

and its moons. Initially, exploring the vast expanse of space surrounding Earth and Moon, including the Lagrange points—locations in space where gravitational forces and the orbital motion of a body balance each other—will establish a human presence outside of LEO in preparing for more complex missions beyond the Earth's gravitational influence. Human exploration missions in this area, called *cis-lunar space*, will provide new knowledge about how humans live and work in space, and building capabilities for future in-space activities and deep-space missions. Robotic missions have paved the way for human exploration of NEAs. Exploring a NEA could reveal information about how the solar system formed, how life began on Earth, how to predict and mitigate the threat of asteroid impacts, and if there is a way to harness the resources found in asteroids for future space exploration. Prior human and robotic missions to the Moon produced a wealth of scientific information about Earth's satellite, illuminating the vast potential of the Moon. An extended human mission would lead to new discoveries about the Moon, the Earth, our solar system, and the universe. NASA's plan for landing a human on the surface of Mars would enable incredible scientific discoveries. Exploring Mars represents the first step to long-term, human space exploration beyond the inner solar system by driving technology innovation necessary to sustain humans on another planet.

PRACTICAL BENEFITS FROM SPACE BIOLOGY RESEARCH

Of a $3 trillion budget, less than 1% is spent on the entire United States space program. That amounts to less than one penny for every dollar the government spends on different programs. The average American spends more of their budget on a monthly cable bill or eating out at fast-food restaurants. For every dollar the United States spends on research and development in the space program, seven dollars come back as corporate and personal income taxes from increased jobs and economic growth (http://spinoff.nasa.gov/).

Hundreds of companies that apply NASA technology in non–space-related areas create hundreds of thousands of jobs that ultimately affect citizens worldwide. Technologies developed over the past 50 years to meet the challenges of space exploration have produced more than 30,000 secondary commercial applications in seven categories dating back to 1976.

1. Computer Technology
2. Consumer/Home/Recreation
3. Environmental and Resource Management
4. Health and Medicine
5. Industrial Productivity/Manufacturing
6. Public Safety
7. Transportation

Details about the seven categories through 2011 can be found at http://spinoff.nasa.gov/Spinoff2011/pdf/Spinoff2011.pdf:

NASA maintains an active database of all its programs and technologies with commercial potential and benefits (www.sti.nasa.gov/tto/spinoff2001/cbs_div.html). TABLE 27.11 lists examples of spin-off technologies from the Apollo Space Program, and TABLE 27.12 lists spin-off contributions from the Space Shuttle Program.

 ## Newly Won Knowledge Pays Huge and Unexpected Dividends

According to Professor Werner von Braun (www.nmspacemuseum.org/halloffame/detail.php?id=29; see the FYI earlier in this chapter): "The greatest gain from space travel consists in the extension of our knowledge. In a hundred years this newly won knowledge will pay huge and unexpected dividends." Little did von Braun know how prescient his prediction would become. The following web sites provide details about the many spin-offs from space exploration:

Web site	Content
http://spaceflight.nasa.gov/shuttle/benefits/	Space Shuttle Benefits from NASA Spinoff Magazine
www.spacefoundation.org/programs/space-technology-hall-fame	Space Technology Hall of Fame
http://spinoff.nasa.gov/spinoff/database	Office of the Chief Technologist, Value for NASA, Benefits for the Nation
http://spinoff.nasa.gov/	NASA spin-off technologies
www.forbes.com/.../10-nasa-spinoff-technology-products-and-the-op; http://ipp.gsfc.nasa.gov/optimus/	Ten NASA Spinoff Technology Products and the Optimus Prime Contest
http://science.howstuffworks.com/innovation/nasa-inventions/nasa-high-tech-products1.htm	What High-Tech Products Came from NASA Technology?
www.neurope.eu/article/nasa-spinoff-technology-continues-benefit-society	NASA Spinoff Technology Continues to Benefit Society

TABLE 27.11   Examples of Spin-off Technologies from the Apollo Space Program

Spin-Off Device
• Digital signal-processing techniques, originally developed to computer-enhance pictures of the moon for the Apollo program, are an indispensable part of computer-aided tomography (CAT) scan and magnetic resonance imaging (MRI) technologies in hospitals worldwide.
• As a medical CAT scanner searches the human body for tumors or other abnormalities, the industrial version or advanced computed tomography inspection system finds imperfections in aerospace castings, rocket motors, and nozzles.
• Cool suits, which kept Apollo astronauts comfortable during moon walks, are worn by race car drivers, nuclear reactor technicians, shipyard workers, persons with multiple sclerosis, and children with a congenital disorder known as hypohidrotic ectodermal dysplasia.
• Kidney dialysis machines were developed from a NASA-developed chemical process that removed toxic waste from used dialysis fluid.
• A cardiovascular conditioner developed for astronauts in space led to the development of a physical therapy and athletic development machine used by football teams, sports clinics, and medical rehabilitation centers.
• Cordless power tools and appliances.
• Athletic shoe design and manufacture incorporated technology from NASA spacesuits into a shoe's external shell. A stress-free "blow molding" process is used in the shoe's manufacture.
• Insulation barriers made of aluminum foil laid over a core of propylene or Mylar, which protected astronauts and their spacecraft's delicate instruments from radiation, protects cars and trucks, and dampens engine and exhaust noise.

TABLE 27.12   Examples of Spin-off Technologies from the Space Shuttle Program

Spin-off Device	Description
Artificial heart	Technology used in space shuttle fuel pumps led to the development of a miniaturized ventricular assist pump.
Automotive insulation	NASCAR racing cars use materials from the space shuttle thermal protection system to protect drivers from extreme engine heat.
Balance evaluation systems	Medical centers use balance systems to measure the equilibrium of space shuttle astronauts upon return from space; the balance systems diagnose and treat patients that suffer from head injury, stroke, chronic dizziness, and central nervous system disorders.
Bioreactor	A rotating cell culture apparatus simulates some aspects of the space environment or microgravity on the ground. Tissue samples grown in the bioreactor help to design therapeutic drugs and antibodies.
Diagnostic instrument	NASA technology created a compact laboratory instrument for hospitals and doctors' offices that analyzes blood in 30 s, which once required 20 min.
Gas detector	Ford Motor Company uses a gas-leak detection system, originally developed to monitor the shuttle's hydrogen propulsion system, to produce a natural gas-powered car.
Infrared camera	A sensitive infrared handheld camera that observes the blazing plumes from the shuttle can scan for fires. The camera localizes hot spots for firefighters.
Infrared thermometer	Infrared sensors developed to remotely measure distant star and planet temperatures led to the development of the handheld optical sensor thermometer. Placed inside the ear canal, the thermometer provides an accurate reading in 2 s or less.
Land mine removal device	The same rocket fuel that helps launch the space shuttle destroys land mines. A flare device, using leftover fuel donated by NASA, is placed next to the uncovered land mine and ignited from a safe distance with a battery-triggered electric match. The explosive burns away, neutering the mine and rendering it harmless.
Lifesaving light	Special lighting technology developed for plant growth experiments on space shuttle missions treats brain tumors in children. Physicians use light-emitting diodes to eradicate cancerous tumors.
Prosthesis material	The foam insulation to protect the shuttle's external tank replaced the heavy, fragile plaster to produce light, virtually indestructible master molds for prosthetics.
Video stabilization software	Image-processing technology that analyzes space shuttle launch video and studies meteorologic images helps law enforcement agencies improve crime-solving video. The technology removes defects from image jitter, image rotation, and image zoom-in video sequences.

FINAL WORDS

As we close this chapter, NASA's Curiosity Mars Rover, launched November, 26, 2011, from Cape Canaveral, Florida, successfully landed on the Martian surface 9 mo later following a perfect 350 million mile flight that will undertake initial surface operations lasting two Earth years. You can read about Curiosity online, for instance at **http://mars.nasa.gov/msl/**. Curiosity, depicted in **FIGURE 27.29** and in a self-portrait in **FIGURE 27.30**, includes the equipment listed in the legend to carry out its eight main objectives: determining the nature/amount of organic compounds, identifying the building blocks of life, looking for traces of past life, investigating Martian geology (**FIG. 27.31**), discovering how rocks/soils were formed, assessing atmospheric evolution, trying to understand the current water cycle, and identifying the surface radiation from the sun.

Building on its success with the ongoing rover expedition, particularly the landing on the planet that required failsafe technologies (www.youtube.com/watch?v=ISmWAyQxqqs), NASA has announced plans for additional Mars missions (www.nasa.org/mars). In 2016, the InSight lander (**I**nterior **E**xploration using **S**eismic **I**nvestigations, **G**eodesy and **H**eat **T**ransport) will return to Mars for additional geologic evolution studies (**http://insight.jpl.nasa.gov/home.cfm**). In addition, the Mars Atmosphere and Volatile EvolutioN (MAVEN) mission, part of NASA's Mars Scout program, will launch in late 2013 as the first mission devoted to understanding the Martian upper atmosphere (www.nasa.gov/mission_pages/maven/main/index.html). The MAVEN orbiter shown in the artist rendering will explore the Red Planet's upper atmosphere, ionosphere, and interactions with the sun and solar wind.

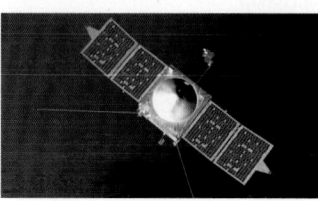

The data from the MAVEN orbiting laboratory will determine the role that loss of volatile compounds—carbon dioxide, nitrogen dioxide, and water—from the Mars atmosphere to space has played through time, giving insight into the history of Mars' atmosphere and climate, liquid water, and planetary

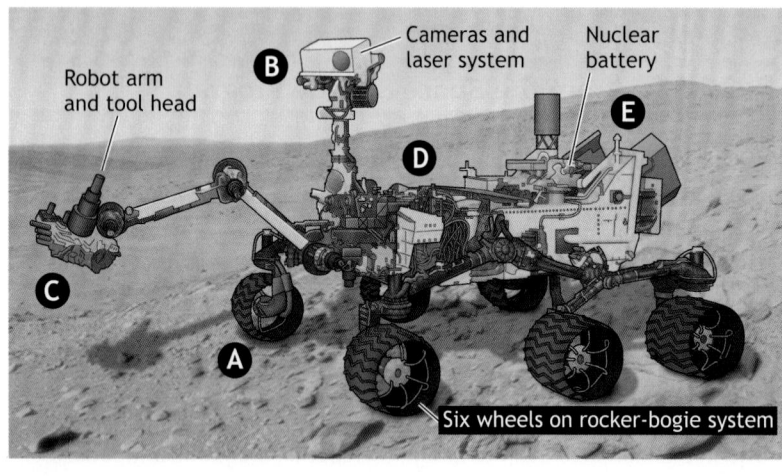

Robot arm and tool head

B Cameras and laser system

Nuclear battery

E

D

C

A

Six wheels on rocker-bogie system

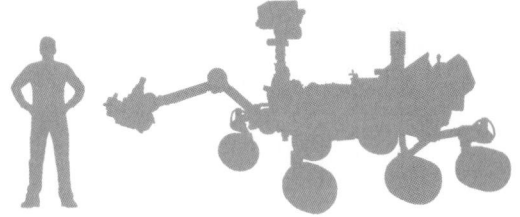

Length: 3 m/10 ft

Weight: 900 kg

Width: 2.8 m

Mast height: 2.1 m

Robot arm reach: 2.2 m

A Curiosity can trundle around its landing site looking for interesting rock features to study at a top speed of about 4 cm/s.

B Curiosity has 17 cameras to identify particular targets, and a laser will zap rocks to probe their chemistry. The 2 cameras on the mast provide multiple spectra and true-color imaging at 1600 X 1200 pixels. The cameras operate up to 10 frames a second hardware-compressed, with video at 720p (1280 X 720).

C If Curiosity detects a significant signal, it positions specialized instruments (including a microscope) on its arm for close-up investigation.

D Two hi-tech analysis labs inside the rover body can analyze samples drilled from rock or scooped from soil.

E Antennas on the rover deck can transmit the results to Earth, with return commands telling the rover where to drive next.

FIGURE 27.29 • Mars Curiosity rover landed on the red planet on August 16, 2012. The rover weighed 1980 lb, including 180 lb of scientific equipment. The rover, 9.5 ft long, 8.9 ft wide, and 7.2 ft tall, has onboard plutonium generators to deliver heat and electricity for at least 14 years. The primary goal is to determine whether Mars has ever had the conditions to support life. In addition, Curiosity is equipped with tools to brush and drill into rocks, to scoop up, and to sort and sieve samples. The Curiosity carries a special laser to zap rocks and its beam will identify atomic elements in them. Curiosity also includes a variety of analytical techniques to discern chemistry in rocks, soil, and the atmosphere, and try to make the first definitive identification of organic, carbon-rich compounds. (Curiosity image courtesy of NASA/JPL-Caltech/Malin Space Science Systems).

Apollo Space Mission's 41-Year Anniversary

The Apollo program was designed to land humans on the Moon and return them safely to Earth. Six of the missions, Apollos 11, 12, 14, 15, 16, and 17, achieved this goal. Apollos 7 and 9 were Earth-orbiting missions to test the Command and Lunar Modules, and did not return lunar data. Apollos 8 and 10 tested various components while orbiting the Moon, and returned photography of the lunar surface. Apollo 13 did not land on the Moon due to a malfunction, but also returned photographs. The six missions that landed on the Moon returned a wealth of scientific data and almost 400 kilograms of lunar samples. Experiments included soil mechanics, meteoroids, seismic, heat flow, lunar ranging, magnetic fields, and solar wind studies. The Apollo missions provided a wealth of new "spin-off" technologies with real-world current applications (i.e., cell phones, lasers, MRI technology, built-in HR monitoring on exercise equipment).

This photo shows the 363-foot tall Apollo 17 spacecraft launching from the Kennedy Space Center in Florida on December 7, 1972. Apollo 17, the final lunar landing mission in NASA's Apollo program, was the first nighttime liftoff of the Saturn V launch vehicle (**http://nssdc.gsfc.nasa.gov/planetary/lunar/apollo.html**). Aboard were astronaut Eugene A. Cernan, commander; astronaut Ronald E. Evans, command module pilot; and scientist-astronaut Harrison H. Schmitt, lunar module pilot. (Photo courtesy of NASA, Lyndon B. Johnson Space Center, Houston, TX.)

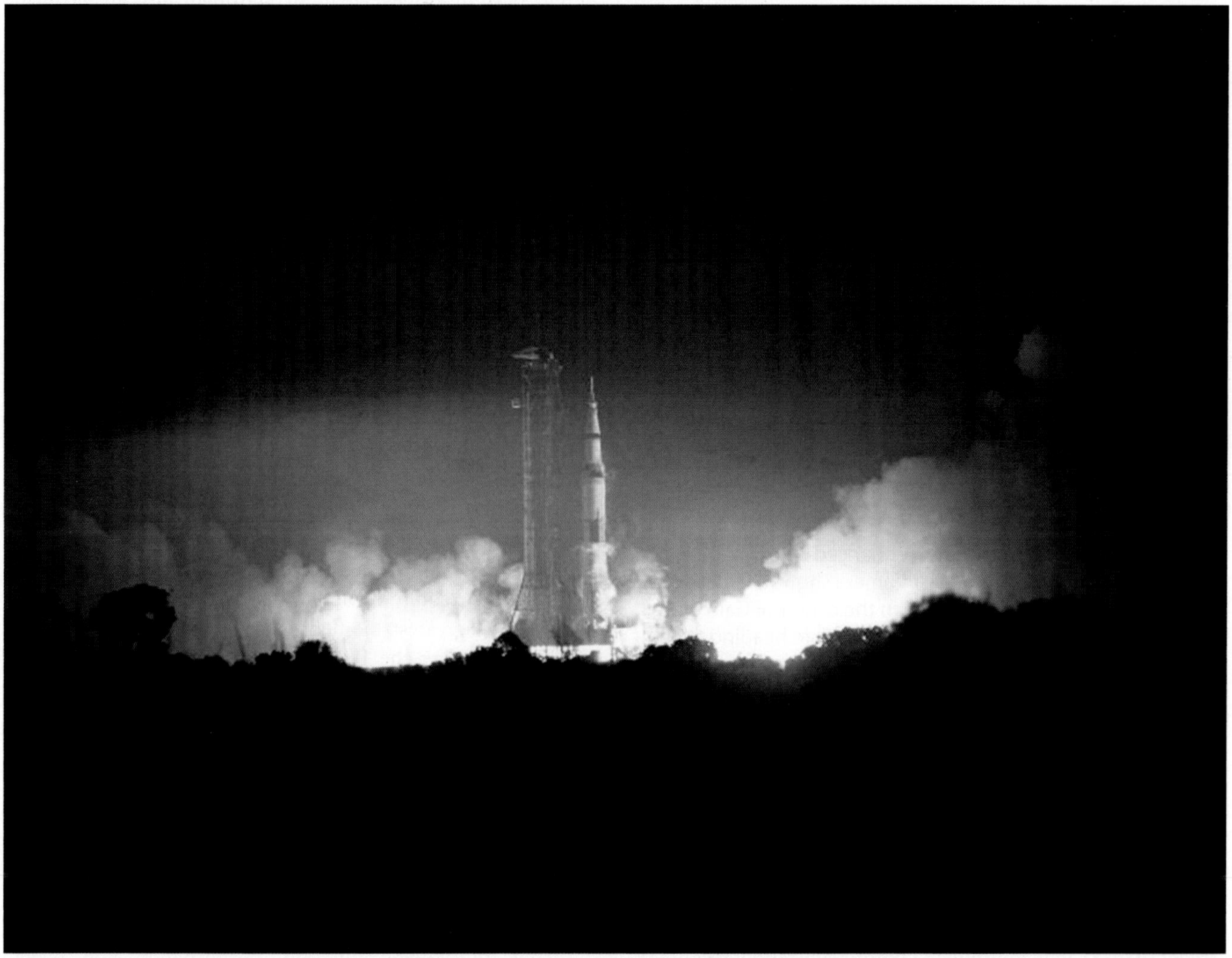

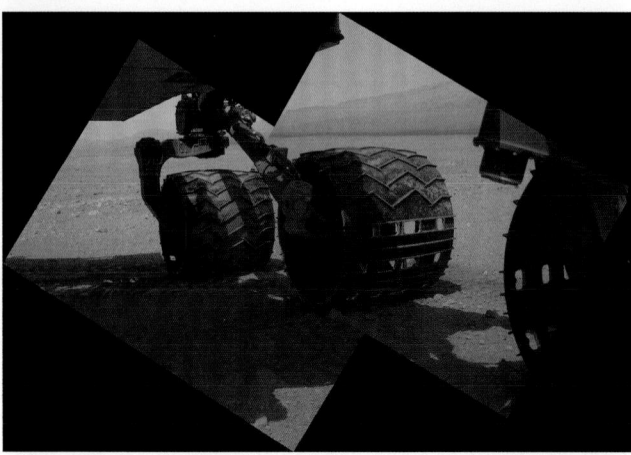

FIGURE 27.30 • Color self-portrait images of the rover captured by the Mars Hand Lens Imager (MAHLI) on November 1, 2012. (Photo courtesy of NASA/JPL-Caltech/MSSS.)

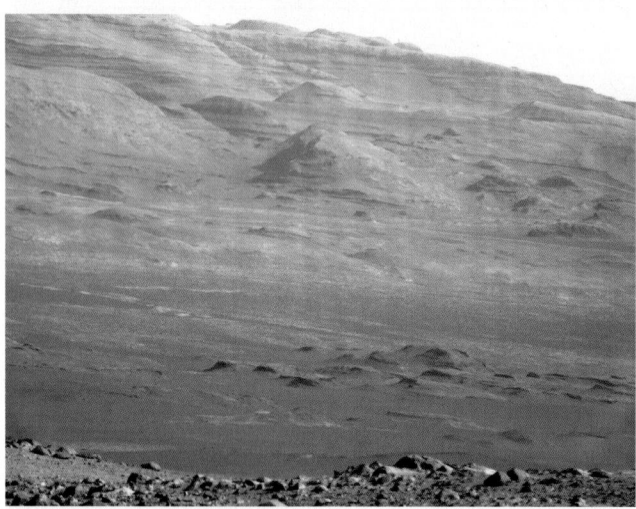

FIGURE 27.31 • High-resolution enhanced color image taken by Curiosity's 100-mm Mast Camera shows the base of Mount Sharp, the 3-mile high peak in the center of Gale Crater where the rover landed in August 2012. Before heading to the mountain, Curiosity bored into a Martian rock to determine its chemical makeup. (Photo courtesy of NASA/JPL-Caltech/MSSS.)

habitability. Such projects are part of NASA's larger plan leading to future human explorations.

We are hopeful that the United States, along with its dedicated international space partners (www.nasa.gov/mission_pages/station/research/partners.html) including private-sector entrepreneurs (www.thespacereview.com/article/1916/1), will continue to commit substantial resources to space exploration so the next generation of space explorers (maybe one of you reading this text) will develop better ways to understand the impact of the last frontier on humankind. In fact, one private space travel venture (www.goldenspikecompany.com) believes human lunar expeditions can be launched using existing rocketry and commercial crew spacecraft. The company estimates the cost for a two-person lunar surface

mission will start at $1.4 billion, and their ambitious plan calls for a lunar landing by 2020. This indeed ushers in a new era and exciting time ahead for private lunar missions and NASA's planned schedule of interplanetary travel explorations.

Summary

1. On Earth's surface, gravity provides an invisible attraction force that makes any mass exert downward force or have weight. Sir Isaac Newton (1642–1727) discovered the universality of the gravitational law.

2. The escape velocity of an object or celestial body depends on the mass and radius of that body. Escape velocity from Earth equals 25,039 mi·hr⁻¹.

3. The force of gravity never reaches an absolute zero value (called zero-g) because a gravitational force still exists. The term *microgravity*, not weightlessness or zero-g, best describes what an astronaut perceives during spaceflight.

4. When an elevator descends quickly, one perceives a lessening of weight from the reduced force between the feet and elevator floor.

5. On October 4, 1957, the Russians' Sputnik 1 became the first Earth-orbiting satellite. One month later, Sputnik 2 remained in orbit for almost 200 days with a dog on board.

6. NASA established two main early goals: first, launch a man into space and return him safely to Earth and, second, develop human capability to endure space missions.

7. The most significant technological achievement of the 20th century took place when Apollo 11 astronauts first landed on the moon's surface on July 20, 1969.

8. During the first few days in microgravity, fluid shifts from the lower body to the upper body. Total fluid volume also decreases to reduce the heart's work effort.

9. The greatest postural instability in microgravity occurs in tests that require vestibular information.

10. NASA's greatest biomedical concern during space missions involves the 1% per month loss in weight-bearing bone mass.

11. Permanent neuromuscular dysfunction has not occurred during prolonged space missions.

12. In-flight and postflight changes during missions of nearly 1 year reveal altered muscular coordination patterns, delayed-onset muscle soreness, and generalized muscular fatigue and weakness.

13. Countermeasure strategies attempt to minimize spaceflight's potentially harmful deconditioning effects on crew physiologic function, performance, and overall health during mission-critical maneuvers with reentry and landing.

14. Without gravity, normal biologic functions become more susceptible to short- and longer-term maladaptations such as space motion sickness (SMS).

15. The energy balance equation has not been satisfied successfully on most space missions because of the

increased energy demands of spaceflight and decreased food intake.

16. Maladaptations to microgravity include decreases in lean body mass, muscle volume, and muscle strength, altered muscle fiber microarchitecture, and atrophy of skeletal muscles that support posture and locomotion.

17. New technologies developed by NASA over the past 50 years have produced more than 30,000 secondary commercial spin-off applications, many of the advances providing life-altering breakthroughs in computer technology, consumer/home/recreation, transportation, environmental and resource management, industrial productivity/manufacturing, health and medicine, and public safety.

thePoint References are available online at
http://thepoint.lww.com/mkk8e.

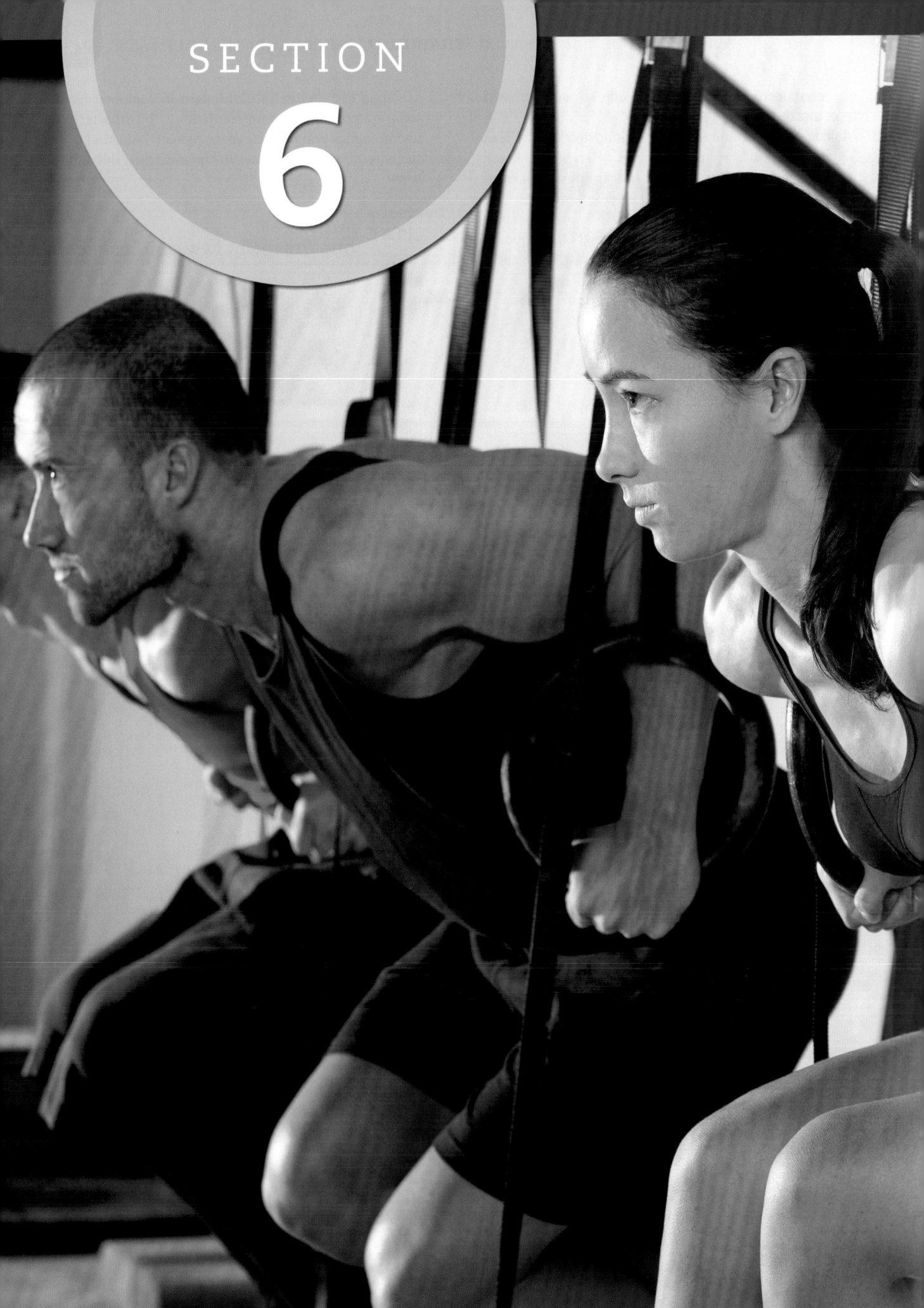

Body Composition, Energy Balance, and Weight Control

Six major reasons justify an accurate appraisal of body composition in a comprehensive program of total physical fitness:

1. Provides a starting point to base current and future decisions about weight loss and weight gain.

2. Provides realistic goals about how to best achieve an "ideal" balance between the body's fat and nonfat compartments.

3. Relates to general health status and plays an important role in the health and fitness goals of *all* individuals.

4. Monitors *changes* in the fat and lean components during physical activity regimens of different durations and intensities.

5. Allows allied health practitioners (sports nutritionist, dietician, personal trainer, chiropractor, coach, athletic trainer, physical therapist, physician, health coach, exercise leader) to interact with the individuals they deal with to provide quality information related to exercise training, nutrition, weight control, exercise, and rehabilitation.

6. Provides objective information relating body composition assessment to sports performance, and the changes in body composition from varied training and physical activity regimens.

Many diverse methods, both complex and simple, assess human body composition. Of the simpler methods, the popular height–weight tables continue as a frequently used standard in the medical community and elsewhere to assess overweight and obesity status.[37,99,173] This approach is of limited value because "overweight" and excess body fat do not necessarily coincide. For example, many large-sized athletes typically exceed the average weight for height by gender but otherwise possess relatively low levels of body fat. Most of these individuals obviously do not require weight loss, which might adversely affect their sports performance. In contrast, a prudent weight loss program would surely benefit the extreme number of overweight men and women not only in the United States but worldwide. This group spends nearly $60 billion each year to purchase diet books, products, and services at more than 1500 weight-control clinics in the United States in the hope of permanently reducing excess fat. Medicaid and Medicare finance almost half of the more than $190 billion spent annually in 2012 on the nation's obesity-related medical costs. Since 1980, obesity rates have risen threefold in some areas of North America, the United Kingdom, Eastern Europe, the Middle East, the Pacific Islands, Australasia, and China. Worldwide, more than 1 billion people now are defined as overweight, with 300 million classified as clinically obese (www.worldometers.info)! And the number continues to increase annually.

From antiquity to the present, regular physical activity and dietary restraint have played an important role to combat the overweight and obese conditions. In Galen's treatise *De Sanitate Tuenda* [*On Hygiene*], penned five centuries after Hippocrates communicated about overweight and obesity in his many writings (refer to p. xxiii in the Introduction), he describes the treatment for an obese patient using a combination of physical activity and food restriction as follows[144]:

> *Now, I have made any sufficiently stout patient moderately thin in a short time by compelling him to do rapid running, then wiping off his perspiration with very soft or very rough muslin, and then massaging him maximally with diaphoretic inunctions, which the younger doctors customarily call restoratives, and after such massage leading him to the bath, after which I did not give him nourishment immediately, but bade him rest for a while or do something to which he was accustomed, then led him to the second bath and then gave him abundant food of little nourishment, so as to fill him up but distribute little of it to the entire body.*

This section discusses body composition, its components and assessment, and differences in body size and composition between sedentary and physically active men and women. We also consider topics relevant to obesity and discuss the use of diet and physical activity for weight management, as Hippocrates, Galen, and others considered over 3000 years ago.

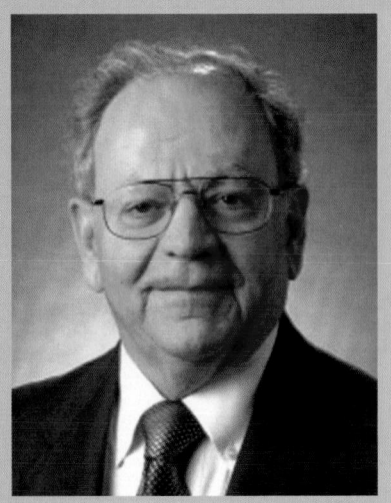

INTERVIEW WITH
Dr. Claude Bouchard

Education: BPed (Laval University, Quebec City, Canada); MSc (University of Oregon, Eugene); PhD (population genetics, University of Texas, Austin); postgraduate training (Deutsche Sporthochschule, Institute for Research on Circulation and Sport Medicine, Cologne; Growth Research Center, Université de Montreal)

Current Affiliation: Professor and John W. Barton, Sr. Endowed Chair in Genetics and Nutrition Professor, Louisiana State University System, Pennington Biomedical Research Center, Baton Rouge, LA

Honors, Awards, and ACSM Honor Award Statement of Contributions: See Appendix C, available online at http://thepoint.lww.com/mkk8e

Research Focus: Genetics of adaptation to exercise and nutritional interventions, and genetics of obesity and its comorbidities

Memorable Publication: Bouchard C, et al. Genomic scan for maximal oxygen uptake and its response to training in the HERITAGE Family Study. *J Appl Physiol* 2000;88:551.

What first inspired you to enter the exercise science field? What made you decide to pursue your advanced degree and/or line of research?

➤ As a student in what was known as College Classic (the equivalent of high school, but it takes 9 years and emphasizes the humanities), I became fascinated with human movement and performance. At that time, it was a very diffuse interest—that is, I was curious about the biomechanics, the exertion and the physiology, or the medical aspect, and the aesthetic of human movement. I had several career options but came rapidly to the conclusion that I would move on to the local university, Université Laval, to learn about exercise and sports with the goal of approaching them from a scientific point of view. As you can see, even before I became a student in physical education, I was fascinated by science and human movement.

During my undergraduate studies, I was very frustrated by the poor science to which I was exposed, so I decided to go on to graduate studies. For 2 years during the summer, I traveled with friends on the East Coast of the United States and in the Midwest for the purpose of visiting universities and meeting faculty to select one for a master's degree program. I visited at least 15 such institutions and finally ended up at the University of Oregon, an institution that had been highly recommended to me. There, I was exposed to the teachings of Sigerseth, Clarke, Brumbach, Poley, and others.

After earning my master's degree in Oregon, I felt that I was not quite ready to benefit from a PhD program. Following the advice of a few of my friends, I decided to go to the Sporthochschule in Cologne to work with Professor Wildor Hollmann. He was the Director of the Institute für Kreislaufforschung und Sportmedizin, or the Institute for Research on Circulation and Sport Medicine. I knew that I could not obtain a degree there but wanted to get more hands-on research experience. By then, my interests included not only performance but also the health implications of exercise. I stayed there for 18 months and learned much.

Then I was offered a position at my alma mater, Laval University in Quebec. I decided to accept the position with the expectation to leave after 3 years or so to obtain my PhD.

If I had done so immediately, I would have entered an endocrinology PhD program, as I had made contact to be admitted in the lab of Professor Hans Selye at the Université de Montreal. But I became so involved in the development of the programs and the facilities at Laval University that it was 8 years before I left for my doctoral studies. By then, I had decided that genetics and biological individuality would be the focus of my research for the last decades of my career.

I opted to work with Professor Robert Malina, a colleague who had training in both physical education and biological anthropology, at the University of Texas. I spent 3 productive years there, which I completed with 10 months of postgraduate work at the Université de Montreal in the Human Growth and Development Center.

Obviously, mine has not been a linear career path. But I always felt that I was sharpening the focus of my research interest all along. Every phase in my career has been a useful one in the sense that it took me closer to what I am doing today—investigating the genetic and molecular basis of the response to exercise and of obesity and its comorbidities. It would have been impossible to select this line of research 35 years ago, since the field did not exist. The study of individual differences could not even be contemplated at the molecular level then.

Who were the most influential people in your career, and why?

➤ Three scientists have played key roles at different times of my career. The first was Professor Fernand Landry. He was a faculty member at the University of Ottawa, but he was from the same city where I was born and went to the same colleges and community organizations that I later attended. He stimulated my interest in the biological sciences in general and the marvels of the human body's adaptation to exercise and training. He had a lasting impact on my career choices.

The second was Professor Wildor Hollmann. I got to know him very well during my stay in Cologne at his Institute. He stimulated my interest in the general topic of physical activity and health, particularly cardiovascular health. He was a very kind and patient mentor.

The last one was Professor Robert Malina. We became good friends during my doctoral studies at the University of Texas. Bob is a scholar with a strong interest in human diversity. We shared this research focus and many of the small pleasures of life.

What advice would you give to students who express an interest in pursuing a career in exercise science research?

➤ You will eventually need to become highly specialized in your own research pursuit, but try to acquire a broad-based understanding of the parent discipline. If you elect to become an exercise molecular biologist, you will find it useful to become an excellent biologist first. Maintaining a reasonable understanding of the changes occurring in biology in general will be a strong asset throughout your career. First, you will derive more satisfaction from your own research because you will be able to see the general implications of your work. Second, you are likely to find that a career in exercise science is more interesting if you understand what is going on in the broader field of science to which you are related.

What interests have you pursued outside of your professional career?

➤ At age 20, I learned to ski and enjoyed it tremendously for many years. I shifted progressively from downhill to cross-country skiing, which I still like to do. At present, my preferred activities are hiking, fly fishing for trout and salmon, working out at the gym, reading, classical music, and wine tasting. I also enjoy traveling, but these days most of my travel is for business purposes.

Where do you see the exercise science field (particularly your area of greatest interest) heading in the next 20 years?

➤ In the next 20 years, the field of exercise science will incorporate the advances in molecular biology and genetics, something that it has failed to do in the past 10 years. The techniques of genomics and proteomics will become common technologies in our field. The benefits should be enormous, as exercise science can offer a wealth of opportunities to verify the functional consequences of DNA sequence variations in people who are not symptomatic for any disease. Such advances in the field of exercise science should make it possible for the exercise science discipline to become a significant player in preventative medicine and public health, as it will be able to develop the probes to identify those who are likely to benefit most from a physically active lifestyle. It will also change the way exercise science contributes to sports performance, as it will have the tools to identify the talented individuals at an early age.

You have the opportunity to give a "last lecture." Describe its primary focus.

➤ It would be on the extent and the causes of biological individuality and its implications for human health in a Darwinian evolutionary perspective.

What has been the most interesting/enjoyable aspect of your involvement in science? What was the least interesting/enjoyable aspect?

➤ The most enjoyable aspect is that you always think out of the commonly accepted paradigm and look toward the future.

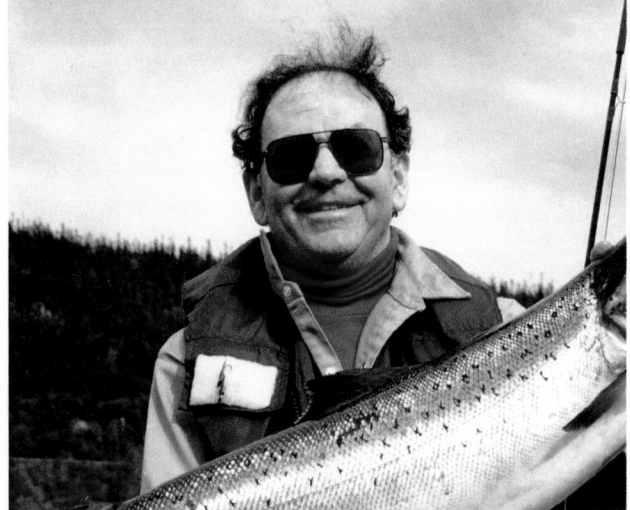

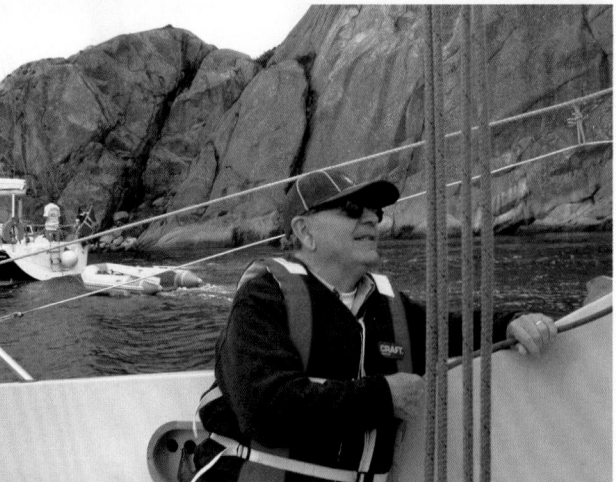

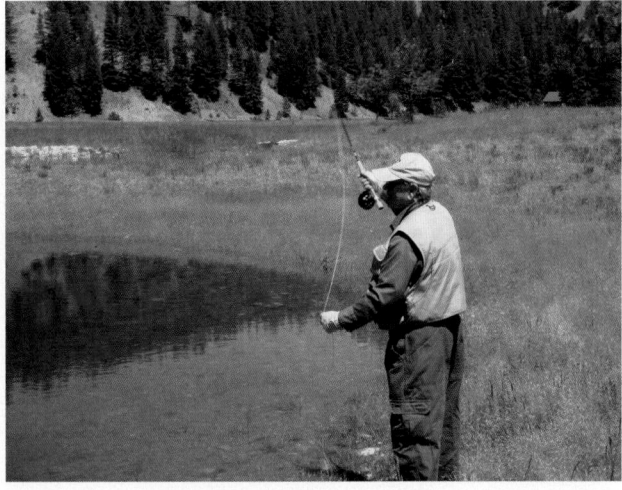

You verify one fact only to refocus on the new questions generated by the previous experience. You also constantly meet people who are of the same mind, colleagues who are always trying to be innovative and creative in the presence of the same set of facts as you. The life of a scientist is never dull if you have the chance to interact with the best in your field.

The least enjoyable aspect is the fact that you have to hunt for research funds all the time, particularly if you run a large laboratory operation. At one point, there were 55 people working on my research projects, and I was spending at least a third of my time writing grant applications or renewals to maintain all of these positions.

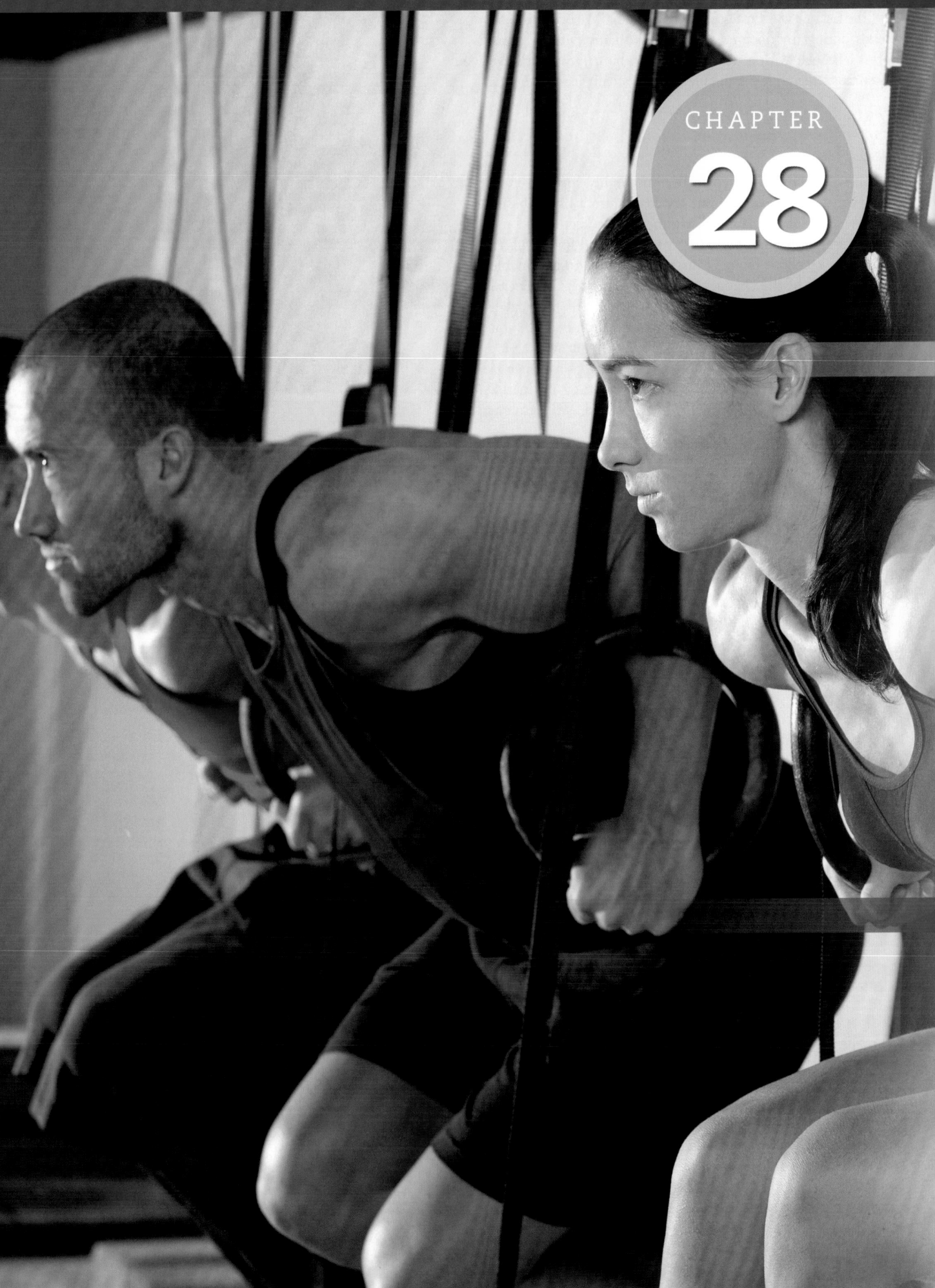

Body Composition Assessment

- Summarize the early research on inadequacies of height–weight tables

- Distinguish among the terms *overweight*, *overfat*, and *obesity*

- Outline current systems to classify overweight and obese conditions

- Delineate characteristics of the "reference man" and "reference woman," including values for storage fat, essential fat, and sex-specific essential fat

- Discuss the prevalence of menstrual irregularities within the general population and specific athletic groups, and factors associated with their occurrence

- Describe Archimedes' principle applied to human body volume measurement

- Discuss limitations in assumptions for computing percentage body fat from whole-body density

- Summarize the rationale, strengths, and weaknesses of air-displacement plethysmography for assessing body composition

- Give the anatomic locations for six frequently measured skinfolds and girths

- Describe how skinfolds and girths provide meaningful information about body fat and its distribution

- Discuss the rationale for bioelectrical impedance analysis and factors that affect body composition estimates with this technique

- Summarize the rationale, strengths, and weaknesses of near-infrared interactance, ultrasound, computed tomography, magnetic resonance imaging, and dual-energy x-ray absorptiometry to assess body composition

- Give representative average values with variation limits for percentage body fat of typical young and older adult men and women

ANCILLARIES at-a-Glance

Visit http://thePoint.lww.com/mkk8e to access the following resources.

- References: Chapter 28
- Appendix D: The Metric System and Conversion Constants in Exercise Physiology
- Appendix H: Supplemental Animations and Videos
- Appendix L: Evaluation of Body Composition—Girth Method
- Interactive Question Bank
- Focus on Research: Overweight But Not Overfat

The life insurance actuary-based **height–weight tables** (weight measured with normal indoor clothing and height measured with 1-inch heels) provide a popular means to assess the extent of "overweightness" on the basis of gender and body frame size (see the upcoming "In a Practical Sense"). These tables give unreliable information about an individual's relative body composition (muscle, bone, and fat). Rather, they provide statistical landmarks based on the average ranges of body mass related to stature associated with the lowest mortality rate for persons' ages 25 to 59 years. They do not consider specific causes of death or quality of health (morbidity) before death.

A person may weigh considerably more than the average weight-for-height standard yet still rate "underfat" for body composition; "extra" weight for this person exists as muscle mass. According to the tables, the desirable body weight (assuming a large frame size) for a professional American football player 188-cm (74 in.) tall and weighing 116 kg (255 lb) ranges between 78 (172 lb) and 88 kg (194 lb). Similarly, body weight without regard for frame size for young adult men 188-cm (74 in.) tall averages 85 kg (187 lb). Using either criterion, conventional standards would classify this player as overweight, implying that he should lose at least 28 kg (62 lb) just to achieve the upper limit of the desirable body weight range. He must lose an additional 3 kg (6.6 lb) to match his "average" American male counterpart. If the player followed these guidelines, he most likely would no longer play football and could jeopardize overall health. Body fat for the football player (even though he weighed 31 kg (68 lb) more than the average) was only 12.7% of body mass, compared with about 15.0% body fat for untrained young men of "normal" weight.

Four Limitations of Height–Weight Tables

1. Uses unvalidated estimates of body frame size
2. Developed from data derived primarily from white populations
3. Specific focus on mortality data that may not reflect obesity-related comorbidities
4. Provides no assessment of body composition

Navy physician and research scientist Albert Behnke (1898–1993; see a brief profile in the preface to this text) first observed body composition variations between elite athletes and untrained individuals in studies of football players in the early 1940s. Careful evaluation of each player's body composition revealed that extreme muscular development primarily contributed to excess weight. These observations point out that the term **overweight** refers only to a body mass in excess of some standard, usually the average for a given stature. Being above an average, ideal, or desirable body mass based on height–weight tables should not necessarily dictate whether someone begins a reducing regimen, particularly among physically active individuals. A better alternative determines body composition by one of the laboratory or field techniques reviewed in this chapter. TABLE 28.1 lists terms and definitions common to the area of body composition evaluation.

OVERWEIGHT, OVERFATNESS, AND OBESITY: NO UNANIMITY FOR TERMINOLOGY

Confusion surrounds the precise meaning of the terms *overweight*, *overfat*, and *obesity* applied to body weight and body composition. Each term often takes on a different meaning depending on the situation and context of use. The medical literature infers the term *overweight* to an overfat condition despite the absence of accompanying body fat measures while **obesity** refers to individuals at the extreme of the overweight (overfat) continuum.

Research and contemporary discussion among diverse disciplines reinforces the need to distinguish between overweight, overfat, and obesity to ensure consistency in use and interpretation. In proper context, the overweight condition refers to a body weight that exceeds some average weight for stature, and perhaps age, usually by some standard deviation unit or percentage. The overweight condition frequently accompanies an increase in body fat, but not always (e.g., male power athletes), and may or may not coincide with the comorbidities glucose intolerance, insulin resistance, dyslipidemia, and hypertension.

With objective measures of body fat, one can more accurately place body fat level on a continuum from low to high, independent of body weight. Overfatness then would refer to a condition where body fat exceeds an age- and/or gender-appropriate average by a predetermined amount. In most situations, "overfatness" represents the correct term when assessing individual and group body fat levels.

The term *obesity* refers to the overfat condition that accompanies a constellation of comorbidities that include one or all of the following nine components of the "**obese syndrome**":

1. Glucose intolerance
2. Insulin resistance
3. Dyslipidemia
4. Type 2 diabetes
5. Hypertension
6. Elevated plasma leptin concentrations
7. Visceral adipose tissue accumulation
8. Increased coronary heart disease risk
9. Increased cancer risk

In all likelihood, excess body fat, not excess body weight per se, explains the relationship between above average body weight and disease risk. Such findings emphasize the importance of distinguishing the composition of excess body weight to determine an overweight person's disease risk.

Individuals may be overweight or overfat yet not exhibit components of the obese syndrome. For these individuals, we urge caution in using the term *obesity* (the correct term would be *overfatness*) in all cases of excessive body weight. We acknowledge that these terms are often used interchangeably (as we at times do in this text) to designate the same condition.

THE BODY MASS INDEX: A POPULAR CLINICAL STANDARD

Clinicians and researchers use the **body mass index** (**BMI**), derived from body mass and stature, to assess "normalcy" for body weight. This measure exhibits a somewhat higher yet still moderate association with body fat and disease risk than other estimates based simply on stature and body mass. A new body shape index incorporating waist girth adjusted for body mass and stature provides another way to identify risk factors for premature mortality across the range of age, sex, BMI, and for white and black ethnicities (but not Mexican ethnicity).[95] Adding abdominal girth to the BMI assessment also has been successfully tested among Canadians.[168]

BMI Computation

BMI computes as follows:

$$\text{BMI} = \text{Body mass (kg)} \div \text{Stature (m}^2)$$

Example

Male—stature: 175.3 cm, 1.753 m (69 in.); body mass: 97.1 kg (214.1 lb)

$$\text{BMI} = 97.1 \div (1.753)^2$$
$$= 31.6 \text{ kg} \cdot \text{m}^{-2}, \text{ or simply } 31.6$$

TABLE 28.1	Terms Frequently Used in Describing and Measuring Body Composition
Term	**Definition**
Abdominal fat	Subcutaneous and visceral fat in the abdominal region
Adipose tissue mass (ATM)	Fat (about 83%) plus its supporting structures (about 2% protein and 15% water); consists predominantly of white adipocytes (cells with a single fat droplet, mainly as triacylglycerol)
Anthropometry	Standardized techniques (e.g., calipers, tapes) to quantify (or predict) body size, proportion, and shape (*anthropo*, human; *metry*, measure)
Body density (Db)	Body mass (BM) expressed per unit body volume (body mass ÷ body volume)
Body mass index (BMI, kg · m²)	Ratio of BM to stature squared (body mass, kg ÷ stature, m²)
Densitometry	Archimedes' principle of water displacement to estimate whole-body density; other terms include *hydrostatic weighting, hydrodensitometry, underwater weighing*
Essential lipids	Compound lipids (phospholipids) needed for cell membrane formation—about 10% of total body fat
Fat mass (FM)	All extractable lipids from adipose and other body tissues
Fat-free body mass (FFM)	All residual lipid-free chemicals and tissues, including water, muscle, bone, connective tissue, and internal organs
Intra-abdominal fat	Visceral fat in the abdominal cavity
Lean body mass (LBM)	FFM plus essential body fat
Minimal body mass	BM plus essential fat (includes sex-specific essential fat); 48.5 kg for the reference woman; computed from bone diameters, stature, and constants
Non-essential lipids	Triacylglycerols found mainly in adipose tissue—about 90% of total body fat
Reference man and reference woman	Behnke's reference standards for men and women that partition body mass into lean body mass, muscle, and bone, with fat subdivided into storage and essential fat; standards for body dimensions developed from military and anthropometric surveys
Relative body fat (%BF)	FM expressed as a percentage of total body mass
Residual lung volume	Volume of air remaining in the lungs after a forced maximal exhalation
Specific gravity	Body mass in air divided by loss of weight in water (body mass ÷ [body mass − body weight in water])
Stature	Height expressed in metric units; for example, 72 in. = 182.88 cm = 1.829 m
Subcutaneous fat	Adipose tissue located beneath the skin
Visceral adipose tissue (VAT)	Adipose tissue within and surrounding thoracic (e.g., heart, liver, lungs) and abdominal (e.g., liver, kidneys, intestines) cavities

IN A PRACTICAL SENSE

Determining Body Frame Size from Stature and Two Bone Diameters

Body frame size (BFS) becomes a useful measure to evaluate "normalcy" of body weight with standardized charts that categorize weight by frame size (bony structure). A combination of stature and bony widths (bone diameter measurements) adequately defines BFS because BFS relates to the fat-free body mass (bone and muscle) and not body fat.

MEASUREMENTS

1. Stature (height [Ht]) measured in cm

2. Biacromial diameter (cm) measured as the distance between the most lateral projections of the acromial processes (see figure)

3. Bitrochanteric diameter (cm) measured as the distance between the most lateral projection of the greater trochanters (see figure)

CALCULATIONS

Regression analyses determine BFS values for women and men from Ht and sum of the biacromial and bitrochanteric bone diameters (ΣBia + Bitroc) with the following equations:

Female: BFS = Ht + 10.357 + (ΣBia + Bitroc)

Male: BFS = Ht + 8.239 + (ΣBia + Bitroc)

STEPS

1. Measure stature and biacromial and bitrochanteric diameters; use the average of two measurements.

2. Sum the average biacromial and bitrochanteric diameter measurements (ΣBia + Bitroc).

3. Compute BFS by substituting in the appropriate gender-specific formulas (example illustrated in TABLE 1).

4. Determine frame-size category by referring to TABLE 2.

EXAMPLE

Table 1 shows calculations of BFS for a male and a female of different heights and bony diameters. The male's height corresponds to a value below the 10th percentile for height-by-age

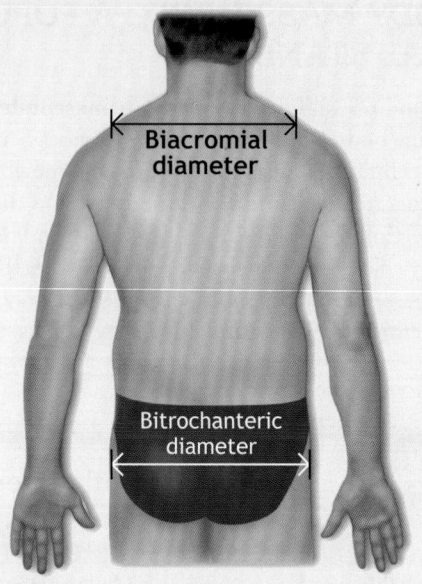

Biacromial diameter

Bitrochanteric diameter

for men in the U.S. population. This height, combined with large breadth measurements, results in a medium frame-sized ranking (Table 2). In contrast, the female's height of 173.4 cm (68.3 in.) ranks above the 90th percentile for the U.S. population. Her small breadth measurements also resulted in a medium frame-sized ranking (Table 2).

TABLE 2   **BFS Categories**

Sex	Frame-Size Category		
	Small	Medium	Large
Male	<1459.3	1459.4–1591.9	<1592.0
Female	>1661.9	1662.0–1850.7	>1850.08

Reprinted from Katch VL, Freedson PS. Body size and shape: derivation of the "HAT" frame-size model. *Am J Clin Nutr* 1982;36:669.

TABLE 1   **Example of BFS Calculations for a Male and Female of Different Heights and Bone Measurements**

Variable	Subject A (Male)	Subject B (Female)
Ht	167.3 cm	173.4 cm
Biacromial diameter	48.0 cm	29.8 cm
Bitrochanteric diameter	35.0 cm	22.2 cm
ΣBia + Bitroc	83.0 cm	52.0 cm
BFS value	1461.4 cm [BFS = Ht × 8.239 + ΣBia + Bitroc] [BSF = 167.3 × 8.239 + 83.0] [BSF = 1461.4]	1847.9 cm [BFS = Ht × 10.357 + ΣBia + Bitroc] [BSF = 173.4 × 10.357 + 52.0] [BSF = 1847.9]
Frame-size category (from Table 2)	Medium	Medium

Reprinted from Katch VL, Freedson PS. Body size and shape: derivation of the "HAT" frame-size model. *Am J Clin Nutr* 1982;36:669.

The importance of this easily obtained index is its curvilinear relationship with all-cause mortality. As BMI increases throughout the range of moderate and severe overweight, so also does risk increase for cardiovascular complications (including hypertension and stroke), certain cancers, diabetes, Alzheimer's disease, gallstones, sleep apnea, osteoarthritis, rheumatoid arthritis, and renal disease.[89,126,134,156]

A large prospective study of more than 1 million United States adults during 14 years of follow-up revealed the relationships between BMI and mortality risk.[25a] Smoking status and presence or absence of disease at time of enrollment in the study substantially modified the association between BMI and risk of premature death from all causes. Men and women who never smoked and remained disease free at the study's start experienced the greatest health risk from excess weight. Excessive leanness related to increased death risk among current and former smokers with a history of disease. In healthy people, lowest relationship between BMI and mortality occurred between a BMI of 23.5 and 24.9 for men (e.g., 5'10" at 174 lb) and 22.0 and 23.4 for women (e.g., 5'5" at 150 lb), with a gradient of increasing risk associated with moderate overweight. Among white men and women with the highest BMI, relative death risk equaled 2.58 (men) and 2.00 (women) compared with counterparts with a BMI of 23.5 to 24.9 (relative risk of 1.00).

New Standards for Overweight and Obesity

In 1998, the expert panel of the National Heart, Lung and Blood Institute lowered the BMI demarcation point for "overweight" from 27 to 25. Based on the association between excess body weight and disease, individuals with a BMI of 30 or more were categorized as obese. Persons with a BMI of 30 average 30 lb overweight. For example, a 6'0" man weighing 221 lb and a woman weighing 186 lb at 5'6" each have a BMI of 30, and each is approximately 30 lb overweight. These revised standards place nearly 130 million, or 62%, of Americans in the overweight and obese categories—up from 72 million under the previous standard. Of this total, 30.5% (59 million people) classify as obese. For the first time, overweight persons with a BMI above 25 outnumber persons of desirable weight! More black, Mexican, Cuban, and Puerto Rican males and females classify as overweight than their white counterparts. FIGURE 28.1 shows the computed BMI and accompanying weight classifications with associated health risks. Note the accelerated risk of diabetes and gallstones (purple bars) in persons moderately to morbidly obese.

FIGURE 28.2 presents the revised (2000) growth charts for boys and girls ages 2 to 20 years in the United States. No absolute BMI standard exists to classify children and adolescents as overweight and obese. Expert panels recommend BMI-for-age to identify the increasing number of children and adolescents at the upper end of the distribution who are either overweight (≥95th percentile) or at risk for overweight (≥85th percentile and ≤95th percentile; see Chapter 30). Less specific recommendations exist for the lower end of the distributions,

but BMIs in this lower range may indicate underweight or at risk for underweight.[50,189]

One in Five American Children are Obese

Research on a representative sample of American preschoolers born in 2001 indicates that nearly one in five (more than half a million) 4-year-old children are overfat, with an alarmingly high one in three rate among American Indian children. Obesity is also more prevalent among Hispanic and black children but the disparity becomes most startling among American Indians whose obesity rate doubles whites. The alarming statistics are that 13% of Asian children, 16% of whites, 21% of blacks, 22% of Hispanics, and 31% of American Indians are obese.

BMI Limitations

Current classification for overweight (and obesity) assumes that the relationship between BMI and percentage body fat (and disease risk) remains independent of age, gender, ethnicity, fitness status, and race, but this is not the case.[38,53,77] For example, Asians have a higher body fat content at a given BMI than Caucasians and thus show greater risk for obesity-related illness. A higher body fat percentage for a given BMI also exists among Hispanic American women compared with European American and African American women.[45] Failure to consider these sources of bias alters the proportion of individuals defined as obese by measured percentage body fat.[77,124] The accuracy of BMI in diagnosing obesity is limited for individuals in the intermediate BMI ranges, particularly in men and in older adults.[152]

The BMI, like the height–weight tables, fails to consider the body's proportional composition or the all-important component of body fat distribution, referred to as **fat patterning**. In addition, factors other than excess body fat—bone, muscle mass, and even increased plasma volume induced by exercise training—affect the BMI equation's numerator. A high BMI could lead to an incorrect interpretation of overfatness in lean individuals with excessive muscle mass because of genetic makeup or exercise training.[141]

The possibility of misclassifying someone as overweight (or obese) by applying BMI standards pertains particularly to large-size field athletes, bodybuilders, weightlifters, heavier wrestlers, and most professional American football players. FIGURE 28.3 plots the average BMI for all National Football League (NFL) roster players at each 5-year interval between 1920 and 1996 based on 53,333 players. Average body fat content of players measured during the late 1970s through the 1990s fell below the range typically associated with population data for men. Those with body fat evaluated by densitometry during this era included all roster players of the New York Jets, Washington Redskins, New Orleans Saints, and Dallas Cowboys. Almost all players from 1960 onward classify as overweight based on BMI measures. For the BMI data up to 1989, values for linebackers, skill players, and defensive backs represent the low category for disease risk, while the BMIs for offensive and defensive linemen place them at "moderate" risk. After 1989, risk for linebackers increased from the low to moderate category. The BMIs for offensive and defensive linemen through 2013 (data not shown), the largest NFL players, quickly approached a high risk and remained in that category. This does not bode well from a health perspective for these large-size players, at least based on BMI risk predictions for the general population.

In contrast to professional football players, the BMI for the National Basketball Association (NBA) players for the 1993–1994 season averaged only 24.5. This relatively low BMI places them in the very low risk category, yet height–weight standards would classify them as overweight.

Another category of world-class athletes—racing cyclists who participated in the Tour de France—had remarkably low BMIs. In the 1997 race, the BMI for 170 competitors averaged 21.5 (1.79 m stature (70.5 in.), 68.7 kg (151.1 lb) body mass). Three years later in the 2000 race, the BMI for 162 competitors remained essentially unchanged (21.5; 1.79 m [70.5 in.] stature, 69.1 kg [152.0 lb] body mass). The results were almost identical in 2005 for the 189 riders; their stature remained the same (1.79 m, 70.5 in.), with weight increasing slightly to 71 kg (156.2 lb). The 2012 Tour de France winner, celebrated British Olympic cycling champion Bradley Wiggins, was taller than most Tour riders (1.90 m; 75.2 in.) but weighed just about the same as Tour counterparts (69.0 kg; 151.8 lb). On average, the variation in stature and body weight among cycling teams remains remarkably small. The homogeneity in body size variables among these top-level performers makes it unlikely that body composition variables per se determine individual differences in cycling performance.

Miss America and BMI: Underweight Role Models?

Many consider Miss America beauty pageant contestants to possess the ideal combination of beauty, grace, and talent. Each competitor survives the rigors of local and state contests, satisfying judges that finalists have "ideal qualities" worthy of role-model status. The consummate image of the Miss America physique to some extent shapes society's generalized "ideal" for female size and shape. An important question concerns whether such images, televised worldwide to millions

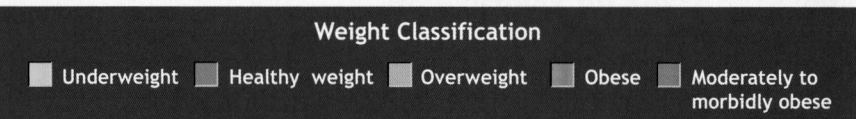

Weight in pounds

Height	120	130	140	150	160	170	180	190	200	210	220	230	240	250
4'6"	29	31	34	36	39	41	43	46	48	51	53	56	58	60
4'8"	27	29	31	34	36	38	40	43	45	47	49	52	54	56
4'10"	25	27	29	31	34	36	38	40	42	44	46	48	50	52
5'0"	23	25	27	29	31	33	35	37	39	41	43	45	47	49
5'2"	22	24	26	27	29	31	33	35	37	38	40	42	44	46
5'4"	21	22	24	26	28	29	31	33	34	36	38	40	41	43
5'6"	19	21	23	24	26	27	29	31	32	34	36	37	39	40
5'8"	18	20	21	23	24	26	27	29	30	32	34	35	37	38
5'10"	17	19	20	22	23	24	26	27	29	30	32	33	35	36
6'0"	16	18	19	20	22	23	24	26	27	28	30	31	33	34
6'2"	15	17	18	19	21	22	23	24	26	27	28	30	31	32
6'4"	15	16	17	18	20	21	22	23	24	26	27	28	29	30
6'6"	14	15	16	17	19	20	21	22	23	24	25	27	28	29
6'8"	13	14	15	17	18	19	20	21	22	23	24	25	26	28

Height in feet and inches

Weight Classification

■ Underweight   ■ Healthy weight   ■ Overweight   ■ Obese   ■ Moderately to morbidly obese

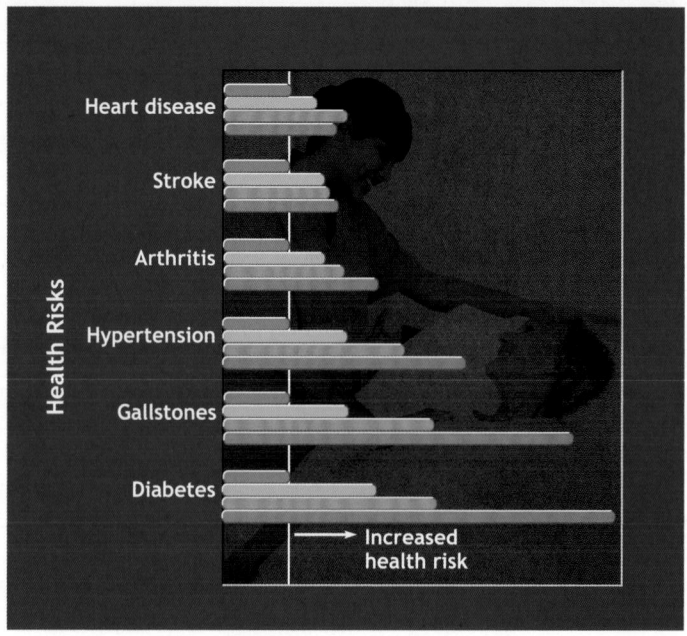

Heart disease
Stroke
Arthritis
Hypertension
Gallstones
Diabetes

Health Risks

→ Increased health risk

FIGURE 28.1 • Body mass index (BMI), weight classifications, and associated health risks.

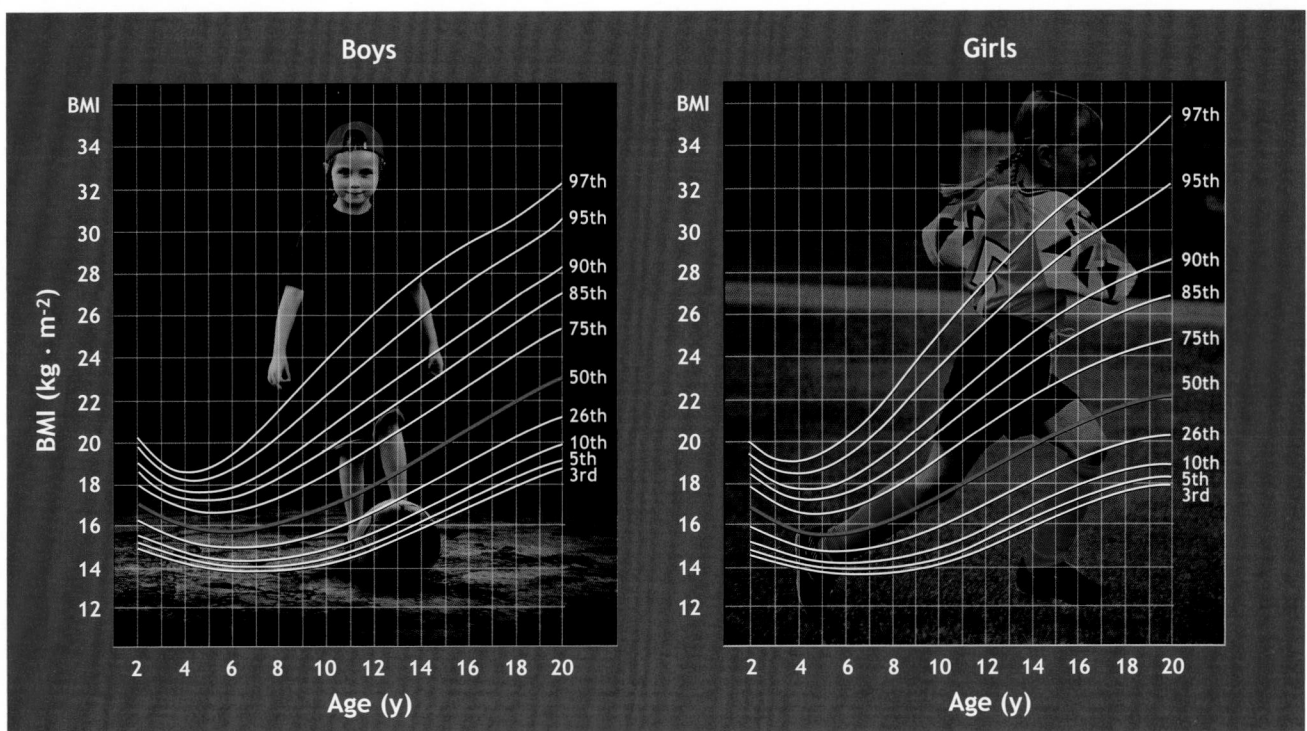

FIGURE 28.2 • Body mass index-for-age percentiles for boys and girls ages 2 to 20 years. Developed by the National Center for Health Statistics in collaboration with the National Center for Chronic Disease Prevention and Health Promotion (2000). (Reprinted with permission from Kuczmarski RJ, et al. CDC growth charts: United States. Advance Data 2000;314. From Vital and Health Statistics of the Centers for Disease Control and Prevention/National Center for Health Statistics.)

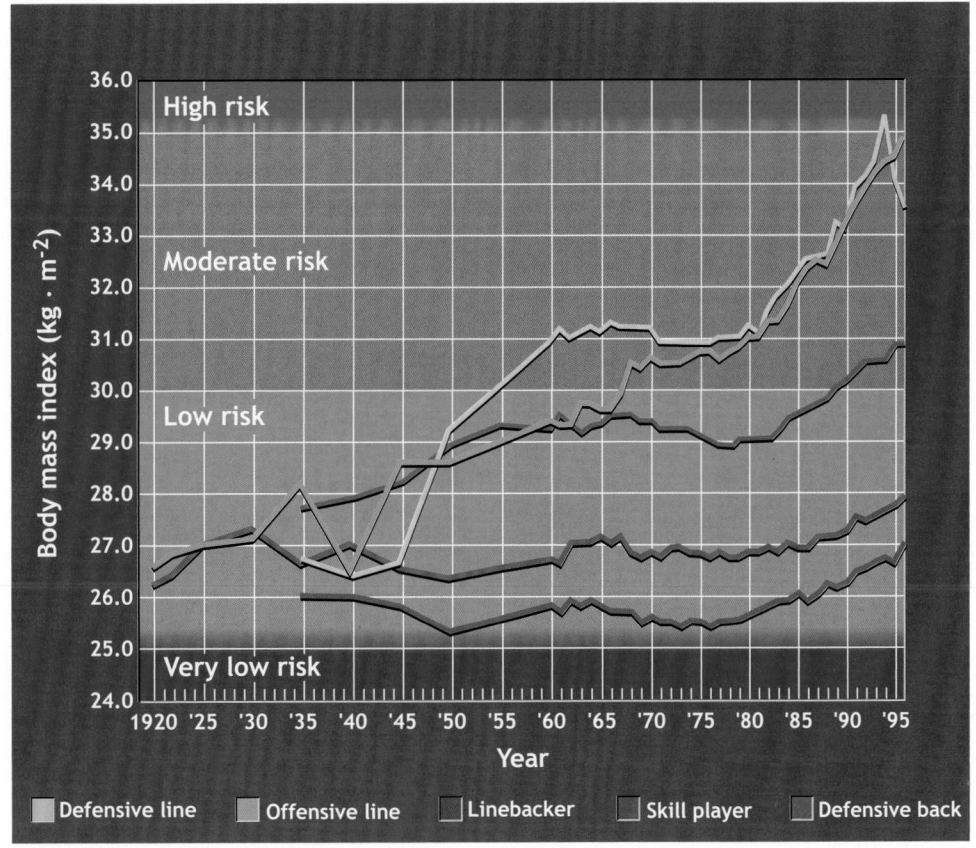

FIGURE 28.3 • BMIs for all players in the National Football League between 1920 and 1996 (n = 53,333). Categories include offensive and defensive linemen, linebackers, skill players (quarterbacks, receivers, backfield), and defensive backs. (Data compiled by Monahan K and Katch F, Exercise Science Department, University of Massachusetts, Amherst, 1996.)

When a Model is Not Ideal

In 1967, only an 8% difference existed in body weight between professional fashion models and the average American woman. Today, a model's body weight averages about 23% lower than the national average. Twenty years ago, gymnasts weighed about 20 lb more than their present-day counterparts. It should come as little surprise that disordered eating patterns and unrealistic weight goals (and general dissatisfaction with one's body) remain so common among girls and women of *all* ages.

of viewers, reinforce an unhealthful message to young women who attempt to emulate such ideal physiques.

FIGURE 28.4 shows the BMIs and accompanying anthropometric data of Miss America contestants from available data between 1922 and 1999 (excluding 1927–1933, when the pageant was not held, and from 2000 on, when data no longer were readily available to the general public). Behnke's standard for the reference woman in Figure 28.5C is also included for comparison of body size. The *bottom horizontal white dashed line* in Figure 28.4A designates the World Health Organization (WHO) cutoff for undernutrition established at a BMI of 18.5.[205] The *top horizontal white dashed line* represents the BMI for the reference woman (see Fig. 28.5; stature: 1.638 m [64.5 in.]; body mass: 56.7 kg [126.7 lb]; BMI: 21.1). The downward slope of the regression line from 1922 to 1999 shows a clear tendency for relative undernutrition from the mid-1960s to approximately 1990. Using the WHO cutoff, the BMIs of 30% ($n = 14$) of the 47 Miss America winners fell below 18.5. Raising the BMI cutoff to 19.0 adds another 18 women, or a total of 48% of the winners with undesirable values. Approximately 24% of contest winners had BMIs between 20.0 and 21.0, and no winner after 1924 had a BMI equaling that of the reference woman!

Interestingly, 1965 was the last year we could locate girth measurements from official press releases or newspaper coverage of the contest. We compared the percentage difference between the Miss America girth averages with the corresponding measurements for the reference woman (*bottom yellow row* of Fig. 28.4C). For the average bust, waist, and hip values (35.1, 24.0, 35.4 in., respectively), Miss America's measurement exceeded the reference woman's bust measurement by 2.6 inches (8%) but fell 7% below for the waist value (21.8 in.) and 5% (21.7 in.) for the hips. Unfortunately, no contemporary data exist from 1966 through 2013 to compare the current Miss America's physique with historical data.

COMPOSITION OF THE HUMAN BODY

In 1921, Czech anthropologist J. Matiega described a four-component model consisting of the weight of the skeleton (S), skin plus subcutaneous tissue (Sk + St), skeletal muscle (M), and a remainder (R).[118] The sum of the four components equaled the body mass.

Over the past 90 years, researchers have focused on body composition and how best to measure the various components. One methodology partitions the body into two distinct compartments:

1. Fat-free body mass
2. Fat mass

The density of homogenized samples of fat-free body tissues in small mammals equals $1.100 \text{ g} \cdot \text{cm}^{-3}$ at 37°C (98.6°F).[151] Fat-free tissue maintains a water content of 73.2%,[133] with potassium at 60 to 70 $\text{mmol} \cdot \text{kg}^{-1}$ in men and 50 to 60 $\text{mmol} \cdot \text{kg}^{-1}$ in women.[20] Fat stored in adipose tissue has a density of $0.900 \text{ g} \cdot \text{cm}^{-3}$ at 37°C.[125] Subsequent body composition studies expanded the two-component model to account for biologic variability in three (water, protein, fat) or four (water, protein, bone mineral, fat) distinct components.[201,203] Women and men differ in relative quantities of specific body composition components. Consequently, gender-specific reference standards provide a framework to evaluate on a relative basis what constitutes "normal" body composition. Behnke's model for the reference man and reference woman (Fig. 28.5) proves useful for such purposes.[16]

Reference Man and Reference Woman

FIGURE 28.5 shows the body composition compartments for the reference man and reference woman. This different color schema partitions body mass into lean body mass, muscle, and bone, with total body fat subdivided into storage and essential fat components. This model integrates the average physical dimensions from thousands of individuals measured in large-scale civilian and military anthropometric surveys with data from laboratory studies of tissue composition and structure.

The reference man is taller and heavier, his skeleton weighs more, and he possesses a larger muscle mass and lower body fat content than the reference woman. These differences exist even when expressing fat, muscle, and bone as a percentage of body mass. Just how much of the gender difference in body fat relates to biologic and behavioral factors, perhaps from lifestyle differences, remains unclear. Undoubtedly, hormonal differences play an important role. The concept of reference standards does not mean that men and women should strive to achieve this body composition or that the reference man and woman reflect some healthful standard. Instead, the reference model proves useful for statistical comparisons and interpretations of data from other studies of elite athletes, individuals involved in exercise training, different racial and ethnic groups, and the underweight and the obese.

Essential and Storage Fat

In the reference model, total body fat exists in two storage sites or depots: essential fat and storage fat. **Essential fat** consists of the fat in the heart, lungs, liver, spleen, kidneys, intestines, muscles, and lipid-rich tissues of the central nervous system and bone marrow. *Normal physiologic functioning requires this fat.* In the heart, for example, dissectible fat from cadavers represents approximately 18.4 g, or 5.3%, of an average heart weighing 349 g in males and 22.7 g, or 8.6%, of a heart weighing 256 g in females.[204] Importantly, essential fat in the female includes additional **sex-specific essential fat**. Whether this fat provides reserve storage for metabolic fuel is unclear.

The **storage fat** depot includes fat primarily in adipose tissue. The adipose tissue energy reserve contains approximately 83% pure fat, 2% protein, and 15% water within its supporting structures. Storage fat includes the visceral fatty tissues that protect the organs within the thoracic and abdominal cavities from trauma, and the larger adipose tissue volume deposited beneath the skin's surface. A similar proportional distribution of storage fat exists in men and women (12% of body mass in men, 15% in women), but the total percentage of essential fat in women that includes the sex-specific fat averages four times the value in men. *The additional essential fat most likely serves biologically important functions for childbearing and other hormone-related functions.* Considering the reference body's total quantity of storage fat (approximately 8.5 kg; 18.7 lb), this depot theoretically represents 63,500 kcal of available energy, or the energy equivalent of playing pickup basketball nonstop for 107 hr, golfing without a cart or walking at a normal pace on a track for 176–180 continuous hours, or treading water in a swimming pool without a break for 10 days straight!

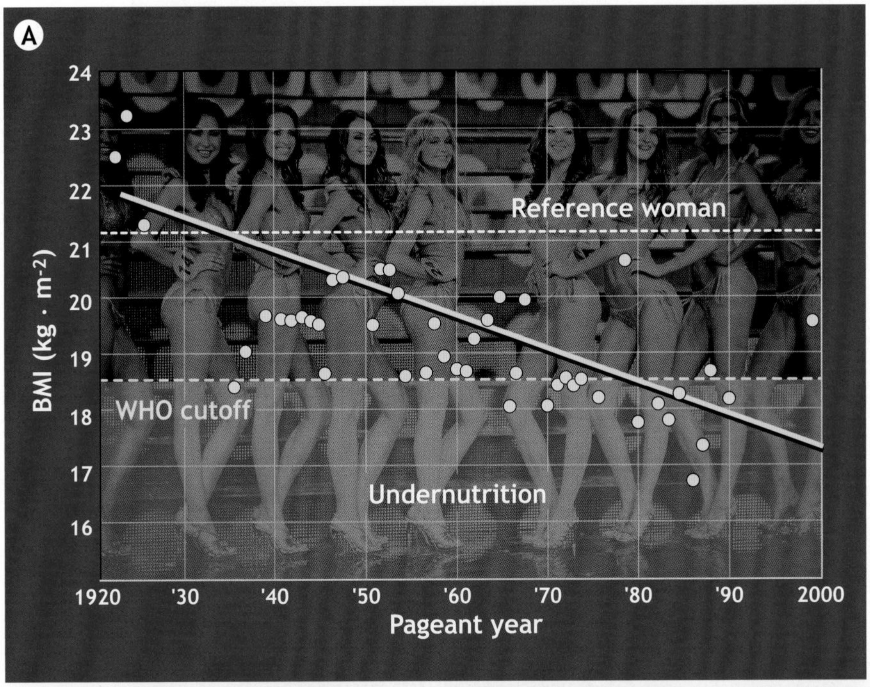

FIGURE 28.6 partitions the distribution of body fat for the idealized reference woman. As part of the 5 to 9% sex-specific fat reserves, breast fat probably contributes no more than 4% of body mass for women whose total fat content ranges between 14 and 35%.[88] We interpret this to mean that other substantial sex-specific fat depots exist (e.g., pelvic, buttock, and thigh regions) that contribute to the female's body fat stores.

Fat-Free Body Mass Versus Lean Body Mass. The terms *fat-free body mass (FFM)* and *lean body mass* refer to

FIGURE 28.4 • (A) Body mass index (BMI) of 47 Miss America pageant contestants from 1922 to 1999. The *top* horizontal *white dashed line* represents the BMI for Behnke's reference woman (21.1 kg·m⁻²). The bottom horizontal *white dashed line* designates the World Health Organization's (WHO's) BMI demarcation for undernutrition (18.5 kg·m⁻²). **(B)** Available data for age, height (in.), and weight (lb) for the contest winners. **(C)** Selected girths for 24 Miss America winners from 1926 to 1965. Despite our best efforts, we were unable to locate height or weight data for Miss America winners from 2000 on.

(B)

1922–1948				1951–1968				1970–1999			
	Age	Ht	Wt		Age	Ht	Wt		Age	Ht	Wt
1922	18	65	135	1951	20	65.5	119	1970	21	65.5	110
1923	19	65	140	1952	25	70	143	1971	21	68	121
1924	18	66	132	1953	19	66.5	128	1972	22	67	118
1926	18	52.5	118	1954	20	68	132	1973	23	68	120
1936	22	66	114	1955	19	68.5	124	1974	23	69	125
1937	17	66.5	120	1957	19	67	120	1976	18	70.5	128
1939	19	67	126	1958	20	68.5	130	1979	22	64	121
1941	19	65.5	120	1959	21	65	114	1980	22	67	114
1942	21	65	118	1960	21	67	120	1983	25	67	115
1943	21	68	130	1961	18	66	116	1984	20	66	110
1944	21	67	125	1962	19	65.5	118	1985	20	68	120
1945	18	70	136	1964	21	66.5	124	1986	21	69	114
1946	21	68	123	1965	22	124	124	1987	21	68.5	116
1947	21	67	130	1966	19	115	115	1988	24	70	131
1948	18	69	138	1967	19	116	116	1990	24	67.5	118
				1968	19	135	135	1999	24	69	133

(C)

				Girths (in)				
	Bust	Waist	Hips	Calf	Thigh	Ankle	Biceps	Wrist
1926	33	24.5	33.5	12.5	19.5	7	—	—
1935	33	23	35.5	—	—	—	—	—
1926	34	23.5	34.5	13	19	8.5	9.5	5.5
1941	34	24	36	14	23	8	11	6
1942	34	24	34.5	—	—	—	—	—
1943	36	23	35	—	—	—	—	—
1944	36.5	25	37.5	13	19.5	8	—	—
1945	35.5	25	35	14.5	20	8.5	—	—
1946	35.5	25.5	36	13.5	22	8.5	—	—
1947	35	35	—	—	—	—	—	—
1948	37	37	—	—	—	—	—	—
1951	35	35	—	—	—	—	—	—
1952	36	24	36	—	—	—	—	—
1953	35	23	35	—	—	—	—	—
1954	37	24	36	—	—	—	—	—
1955	34.5	22	35	—	—	—	—	—
1957	35	23	35	—	—	—	—	—
1958	35	25	36	—	—	—	—	—
1959	34	22	35	—	—	—	—	—
1960	36	24	36	—	—	—	—	—
1961	35	22	35	—	—	—	—	—
1962	35	24	35	—	—	—	—	—
1964	35	23	35	—	—	—	—	—
1965	36	24	36	—	—	—	—	—
Ref W*	36.1	30.3	36.8	14.1	21.6	8.9	12.5	6.8

Ref W* = Behnke's reference woman; stature = 163.8 cm, body mass = 56.7 kg

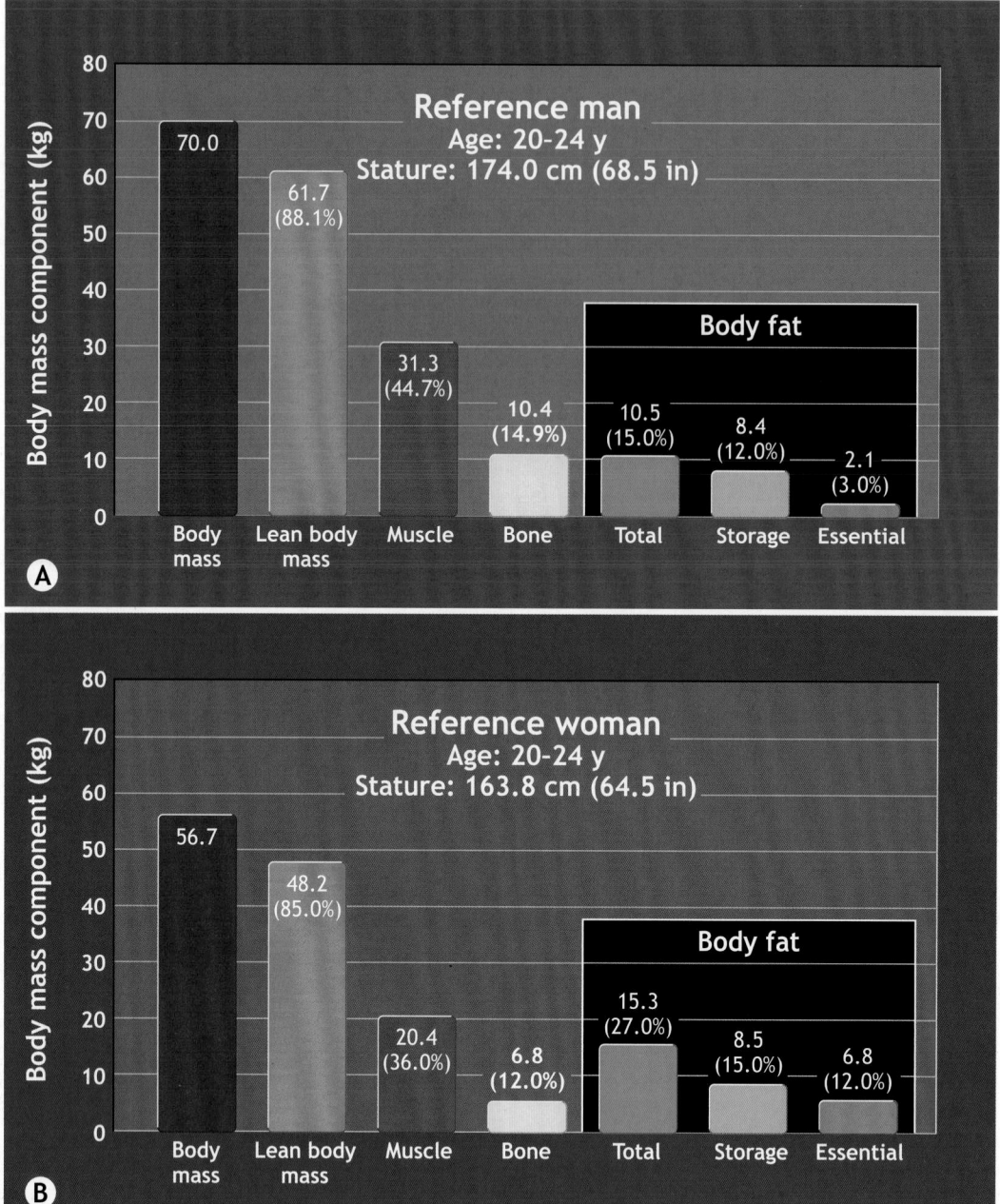

FIGURE 28.5 • Behnke's theoretical model for the body composition of the reference man **(A)** and reference woman **(B)**. Values in parentheses indicate percentage of total body mass.

specific entities. Lean body mass contains the small percentage of non–sex-specific essential fat equivalent to approximately 3% of body mass. In contrast, FFM represents the body mass devoid of *all* extractable fat (FFM = body mass – fat mass). Behnke emphasizes that FFM refers to an *in vitro* entity appropriate to carcass analysis. He considered lean body mass as an *in vivo* entity relatively constant in water, organic matter, and mineral content throughout the active adult's life span. *In normally hydrated, healthy adults, the FFM and lean body mass differ only in the essential fat component.*

Figure 28.5 showed that lean body mass in men and **minimal body mass** in women consist chiefly of essential fat (plus sex-specific essential fat for women), muscle, water, and

bone. The whole-body density of the reference man with 12% storage fat and 3% essential fat is 1.070 g·cm⁻³; the density of his FFM is 1.094 g·cm⁻³. If the reference man's total body fat percentage equals 15.0% (storage fat plus essential fat), the density of a hypothetical fat-free body attains the upper limit of 1.100 g·cm⁻³.

In the reference woman, the average whole-body density of 1.040 g·cm⁻³ represents a body fat percentage of 27%; of this, approximately 12% consists of essential body fat. A density of 1.072 g·cm⁻³ represents the minimal body mass of 48.5 kg (106.7 lb). In actual practice, density values that exceed 1.068 for women (14.8% body fat) and 1.088 g·cm⁻³ for men (5% body fat) rarely occur except in young, lean athletes.

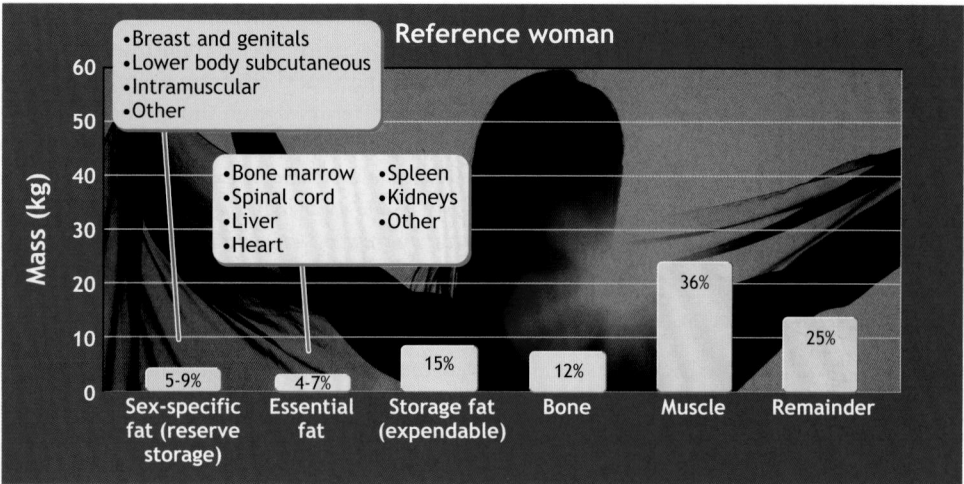

FIGURE 28.6 • Theoretical model for body fat distribution for the reference woman with body mass of 56.7 kg (124.7 lb), stature of 163.8 cm (64.5 in.), and 27% body fat. (Reprinted with permission from Katch VL, et al. Contribution of breast volume and weight to body fat distribution in females. *Am J Phys Anthropol* 1980;53:93.)

Minimal Leanness Standards

A biologic lower limit exists beyond which a person's body mass cannot decrease without impairing health status or altering normal physiologic functions.

Men

To estimate the lower body fat limit in men (i.e., lean body mass), subtract storage fat from body mass. For the reference man, the lean body mass (61.7 kg) includes approximately 3% (2.1 kg) essential body fat. Encroachment into this reserve may impair optimal health and capacity for vigorous physical activity.

Low body fat values exist for male world-class endurance athletes and some conscientious objectors to military service who voluntarily reduced body fat stores during a prolonged experiment with semistarvation. The low fat levels of marathon runners, which ranges from 1 to 8% of body mass, probably reflect adaptation to severe training for distance running.[104] A low body fat level reduces the energy cost of weight-bearing physical activity; it also provides a more effective gradient to dissipate metabolic heat generated during prolonged, intense activity.

Considerable variation exists in the FFM of different athletes, with values ranging from a low of 48.1 kg in some jockeys to over 100 kg in football linemen and field-event athletes. Seven elite sumo wrestlers (*sekitori*, ranked in one of the top two professional sumo divisions) possessed an average FFM of 109 kg.[94]

Women

In comparison to the lower limit of body mass for the reference man (with 3% essential fat), the lower limit for the reference woman includes approximately 12% essential fat. This theoretical lower limit developed by Dr. Behnke, termed *minimal body mass*, is 48.5 kg for the reference woman. Generally, the leanest women in the population do not possess less than 10 to 12% body fat, a narrow range at the lower limit for most women in good health. *Behnke's theoretical concept of minimal body mass in women that incorporates 12% essential fat corresponds to the lean body mass in men that includes 3% essential fat.*

Leanness, Regular Physical Activity, and Menstrual Irregularity

Physically active women, mainly participants in the "low weight" or "appearance" sports (e.g., distance running, bodybuilding, figure skating, diving, ballet, and gymnastics), increase their likelihood for one of three maladies:

1. Delayed onset of menstruation
2. Irregular menstrual cycle (**oligomenorrhea**)
3. Complete cessation of menses (**amenorrhea**)

Menstrual and ovarian dysfunction results largely from changes in the pituitary gland's normal pulsatile secretion of luteinizing hormone regulated by gonadotropin-releasing hormone from the hypothalamus.

Amenorrhea occurs in 2 to 5% of women of reproductive age in the general population, but it can reach 40% in some athletic groups.[153,177] As a group, ballet dancers remain lean, with a greater incidence of menstrual dysfunction and eating disorders and a higher mean age at menarche than age-matched, nondance counterparts.[51] One third to one half of female endurance athletes exhibit some menstrual irregularity. In premenopausal women, irregularity or absence of menstrual function accelerates bone loss and increases risk of musculoskeletal injury during exercise and causes a longer interruption of training (see Chapter 2).[15,136]

A prolonged level of physical stress may disrupt the hypothalamic–pituitary–adrenal axis and modify the output of gonadotropin-releasing hormone, which results in irregular menstruation (**exercise stress hypothesis**). A concurrent hypothesis maintains that energy (fat) reserves inadequate to sustain pregnancy induce cessation of ovulation (**energy availability hypothesis**).

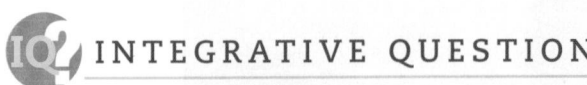

INTEGRATIVE QUESTION

Explain if gender-related patterns of regular physical activity and caloric intake account for the true sex differences in body fat level.

Lean-to-Fat Ratio

An optimal **lean-to-fat ratio** is important to normal menstrual function, perhaps through peripheral fat's role that converts androgens to estrogens or through adipose tissue's production of leptin, a hormone intimately linked to body fat levels and appetite control (see Chapter 30) and initiation of puberty.[174] A linkage exists between hormonal regulation of sexual maturity onset and level of stored energy from accumulated body fat.

Some researchers assert that 17% body fat represents a lower-end critical level for the onset of menstruation, with 22% fat needed to sustain a normal menstrual cycle.[51,52] They reason that lower body fat levels trigger hormonal and metabolic disturbances that affect menses. *Objective data indicate that many physically active females who are below the supposedly critical 17% body fat level have normal menstrual cycles with high levels of physiologic and exercise capacity.* Conversely, some amenorrheic athletes maintain body fat levels considered average for the population. One of our laboratories compared 30 athletes and 30 nonathletes, all with less than 20% body fat, for menstrual cycle regularity.[86] Four athletes and three nonathletes, ranging from 11 to 15% body fat, maintained regular cycles, whereas seven athletes and two nonathletes had irregular cycles or were amenorrheic. For the total sample, 14 athletes and 21 nonathletes maintained regular menstrual cycles. These data indicate that normal menstrual function *does not require* a critical body fat level of 17 to 22%.

Potential causes of menstrual dysfunction include the complex interplay of seven factors[93]:

1. Physical
2. Nutritional
3. Genetic
4. Hormonal
5. Regional fat distribution
6. Psychological
7. Environmental

An intense bout of physical activity triggers the release of an array of hormones, some of which disrupt normal reproductive function.[60,198] Intense and/or prolonged exertion that releases cortisol and other stress-related hormones also can alter ovarian function via the hypothalamic–pituitary–adrenal axis.[35,114]

Consuming well-balanced, nutritious meals on a regular basis helps to prevent or reverse athletic amenorrhea without requiring the athlete to reduce training volume or intensity.[113] The approach may take up to 1 year of nonpharmacologic

intervention that includes weight gain with continuation in physical activity.[7] When injuries to young amenorrheic ballet dancers prevent them from exercising regularly, normal menstruation resumes even though body weight remains low.[80,208] *Proponents of this "energy deficit" explanation maintain that physical exertion per se exerts no deleterious effect on the reproductive system other than the potential impact of its additional energy cost on creating a negative energy balance.*[6,111,112,115]

The effects and risks of sustained amenorrhea on the reproductive system remain unknown. A gynecologist/endocrinologist should evaluate failure to menstruate or cessation of the normal cycle because it may reflect pituitary or thyroid gland malfunction or premature menopause,[14,110] perhaps from ovarian failure related to a genetic aberration in the X chromosome.[12] As we point out in Chapter 2, prolonged menstrual dysfunction affects bone mass profoundly and negatively.

Delayed Onset of Menstruation and Cancer Risk

The delayed onset of menarche in chronically active young females may offer positive health benefits. Female athletes who start training in high school or earlier show a lower lifetime occurrence of cancers of the breast and reproductive organs, and non–reproductive-system cancers than less-active counterparts.[52] Even among older women, regular activity protects against reproductive cancers. Swedish researchers studied the country's entire female population ages 50 to 74 years in 1994–1995.[132] Higher levels of occupational and leisure-time physical activity in normal-weight nonsmokers during ages 18 to 30 years related to lower postmenopausal endometrial cancer risk. Women who exercise an average of 4 hr a week after menarche reduce breast cancer risk by 50% compared with age-matched inactive women.[18] One proposed mechanism for reduced cancer risk links lower total estrogen production or a less potent estrogen form over the athlete's lifetime with fewer ovulatory cycles from delayed menstruation onset.[105,194] Lower body fat levels in physically active individuals also may contribute to lowered cancer risk because peripheral fatty tissues convert androgens to estrogen.

COMMON TECHNIQUES TO ASSESS BODY COMPOSITION

Two procedures evaluate body composition:

1. Direct measurement by chemical analysis of the animal carcass or human cadaver
2. Indirect estimation by hydrostatic weighing, simple anthropometric measurements, and other clinical and laboratory procedures

Direct Assessment

Two approaches directly assess body composition. One technique dissolves a cadaver in a chemical solution to determine its mixture of fat and fat-free components. The other approach involves physically dissecting the fat mass, muscle, bone, and other cadaver organ tissues to determine body composition. Considerable research has chemically assessed body composition in various animal species, but few studies with humans have been conducted.[29,30,31] These labor-intensive and tedious analyses require specialized laboratory equipment and involve ethical questions and legal hurdles in obtaining cadavers for research purposes.

Direct body composition assessment suggests that while considerable individual differences exist in total body fatness, the compositions of skeletal mass and the fat-free and fat tissues remain relatively stable. The assumed constancy of these tissues allows researchers to develop mathematical equations to indirectly predict the body's fat percentage.

Indirect Assessment

Diverse indirect procedures assess body composition. One involves Archimedes' principle applied to hydrostatic weighing (also referred to as *hydrodensitometry* or *underwater weighing*). This method computes percentage body fat from body density (ratio of body mass to body volume). Other procedures predict body fat from skinfold thickness and girth measurements (anthropometry), x-ray, total body electrical conductivity or bioimpedance (including segmental impedance), near-infrared interactance, ultrasound, computed tomography, air plethysmography, and magnetic resonance imaging.

Hydrostatic Weighing: Archimedes' Principle

The Greek mathematician, engineer, researcher, and inventor Archimedes (287–212 BC) discovered a fundamental principle currently applied to evaluate human body composition. Legend has it that an itinerant scholar of that time described the circumstances surrounding the event (http://ed.ted.com/lessons/mark-salata-how-taking-a-bath-led-to-archimedes-principle):

> King Hieron of Syracuse suspected that his pure gold crown had been altered by substitution of silver for gold. The King directed Archimedes to devise a method for testing the crown for its gold content without dismantling it. Archimedes pondered over this problem for many weeks without succeeding, until one day, he stepped into a bath filled to the top with water and observed the overflow. He thought about this for a moment, and then, wild with joy, jumped from the bath and ran naked through the streets of Syracuse shouting, "Eureka, Eureka! I have discovered a way to solve the mystery of the King's crown."

Archimedes reasoned that a substance such as gold must have a volume proportional to its mass; measuring the volume of an irregularly shaped object would require submersion in water with collection of the overflow. To apply his reasoning, Archimedes took lumps of gold and silver of the same mass as the crown and submerged each in a water-filled container. He discovered the crown displaced more water than the lump of gold and less than the lump of silver. This could only mean that the crown consisted of *both* silver and gold as the king suspected.

Essentially, Archimedes compared the **specific gravity** of the crown with the specific gravities for gold and silver. He also reasoned that an object submerged or floating in water becomes buoyed up by a counterforce that equals the weight of the volume of water it displaces. This buoyant force supports an immersed object against gravity's downward pull so an object loses weight in water. *The object's loss of weight in water equals the weight of the volume of water it displaces, so its specific gravity refers to the mass of an object in air divided by its loss of weight in water.* The loss equals the weight in air minus the weight in water.

Specific gravity = Weight in air ÷ Loss of weight in water

In practical terms, suppose a crown weighs 2.27 kg in air and 0.13 kg less, or 2.14 kg, when weighed underwater (**Fig. 28.7**). Dividing the crown's mass (2.27 kg) by its weight loss in water (0.13 kg) yields a specific gravity of 17.5. This ratio differs considerably from gold's specific gravity

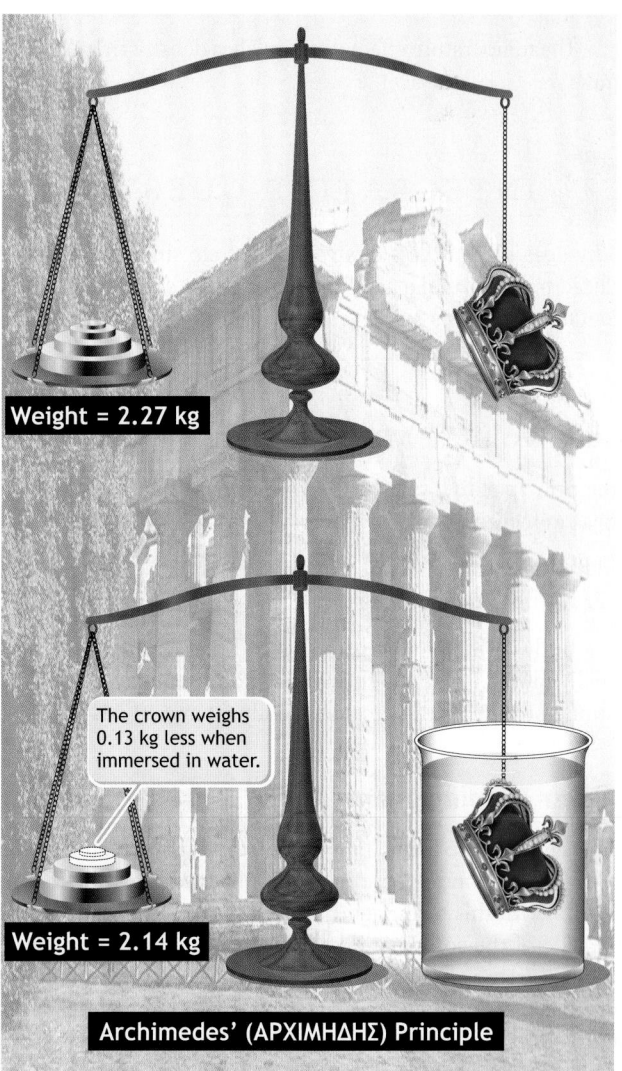

Weight = 2.27 kg

The crown weighs 0.13 kg less when immersed in water.

Weight = 2.14 kg

Archimedes' (ΑΡΧΙΜΗΔΗΣ) Principle

FIGURE 28.7 • Archimedes' principle of buoyant force to determine the volume and, subsequently, specific gravity of the king's crown.

of 19.3, so we too can conclude as Archimedes supposedly did: "Eureka, the crown is a fraud!" The physical principle of hydrostatic water displacement Archimedes discovered allows us to use water submersion to determine the body's volume. Dividing body mass by its volume yields body density (**density = mass ÷ volume**), and from this, an estimate of percentage body fat.

One can think of specific gravity as an object's "heaviness" related to its volume. Objects of the same volume may vary considerably in density defined as mass per unit volume. One gram of water occupies exactly 1 cm^3 at a temperature of 4°C (39.2°F); the density equals 1 g·cm^{-3}. Water achieves its greatest density at 4°C; increasing water temperature increases the volume of 1 g of water and decreases its density. One must correct the volume of an object weighed in water for water density at the weighing temperature.

thePoint Appendix D, available online at http://thepoint. lww.com/mkk8e, shows metric system conversion constants in exercise physiology.

The temperature effect distinguishes density from specific gravity.

INTEGRATIVE QUESTION

Why does a solid piece of steel or concrete sink rapidly when placed in water while a ship made of either substance readily floats?

Body Volume Measurement

The principle discovered by Archimedes applies body volume measurement in one of two ways:

1. Water displacement
2. Hydrostatic weighing

Body volume requires accurate measurement because small volume variations substantially affect the density calculation and computed percentage body fat and FFM.

Water Displacement

One can measure the volume of an object submerged in water by the corresponding rise in the level of water within a container. With this technique, a finely calibrated tube secured to the side of the container that measures the rise of water permits accurate volume measurements. One also can submerge an object in a container filled with water to a preset mark and collect the overflow. The amount of the overflow, when weighed accurately, corresponds to the volume of the submerged object because 1 g or mass is equivalent to 1 mL volume. With this method when weighing a submerged human, one must account for the volume of air remaining in the lungs

during full head submersion. The usual protocol assesses this lung volume before the subject enters the tank and subtracts it from the total body volume determined by **water displacement**. Water displacement has proved effective in assessing arm and leg volumes and their corresponding changes with exercise training, tissue changes with weight gain or loss, or changes in body dimensions from physical inactivity.

Hydrostatic Weighing

Hydrostatic weighing provides the most common application of Archimedes' principle to determine body volume. It computes body volume as the difference between body mass measured in air (M_a) and body weight measured during water submersion (W_w; the correct term because body mass remains unchanged under water). *Body volume equals loss of weight in water with the appropriate temperature correction for water's density.*

FIGURE **28.8** illustrates measurement of body volume by hydrostatic weighing using four different methodologies. The first step in each method accurately assesses the subject's body mass in air, usually within ±50 g. The subject, who wears a thin nylon swimsuit, sits in a lightweight, plastic tubular chair suspended from the scale and submerged beneath the water's surface. A swimming pool serves the same purpose as the tank, with the scale and chair assembly suspended from a support at the side of the pool or diving board. The tank maintains a comfortable water temperature near 95°F (35°C), similar to skin temperature. Water temperature provides the correction factor to determine water density at the weighing temperature. A diver's belt secured around the waist (or placed across the lap) stabilizes the subject from floating toward the surface during submersion. The underwater weight of this belt and chair (tare weight) is subtracted from the subject's total weight underwater.

Seated with the head above water, the subject makes a forced maximal exhalation while slowly lowering the head under the water. The breath is held for 5 to 8 s to allow the scale pointer to stabilize at the midpoint of the oscillations or rely on an electronic readout with appropriate instrumentation. The subject repeats the procedure 8 to 12 times to obtain a dependable underwater weight score. Even when achieving a full exhalation, a small volume of air, the residual lung volume, remains in the lungs. Body volume calculation requires subtracting the buoyant effect of the residual lung volume measured immediately before, during, or following the underwater weighing. Failure to account for residual lung volume *underestimates* whole-body density because the lungs' air volume contributes to buoyancy. This omission creates a "fatter" person when converting body density to percentage body fat. Even under field conditions (i.e., sports training site; Figure 28.8B and C), assessment of residual volume cannot be neglected.

Variations with Menstruation. Normal fluctuations in body mass (chiefly body water) related to the menstrual cycle generally do not affect body density and body fat assessed by hydrostatic weighing. Some females experience noticeable increases in body water (>1.0 kg) during menstruation. Water retention of this magnitude affects body density and introduces a small error in computing percentage body fat.[25]

Calculating Body Composition from Body Mass, Body Volume, and Residual Lung Volume. Data for two professional football players, an offensive guard and a quarterback, illustrate the sequence of steps in computing body density, percentage fat, fat mass, and FFM (Table 28.2). Mass ÷ volume is the conventional formula for computing density, with density expressed in grams per cubic centimeter ($g \cdot cm^{-3}$), mass in kilograms, and volume in liters. The difference between M_a and W_w equals body volume after applying the appropriate water temperature correction (D_w). Air remaining in the lungs and other body "spaces" (abdominal viscera, sinuses) contributes some buoyancy at the time of underwater weighing. In the extreme, consuming 800 mL of a carbonated beverage increases gastric gas volume by approximately 600 mL. This *underestimates* body density by hydrostatic weighing by 0.7% and *overestimates* percentage body fat by 11% compared with measures made before drinking the beverage.[135] In most subjects, abdominal gas and sinus air volume remain small (<100 mL) and inconsequential. *This contrasts with the relatively large and variable residual lung volume, which requires measurement and subsequent subtraction from total body volume.*

Whereas the residual lung volume decreases slightly in a person immersed in water compared with residual volume in air (from water's compressive force against the thoracic cavity), the difference exerts only a small effect on computed percentage body fat.[70] Consequently, most laboratories measure residual lung volume in air just prior to underwater weighing.

The following formula computes body density (D_b) from underwater weighing variables:

$$D_b = Mass \div Volume$$
$$= M_a \div [(M_a - W_w) \div D_w] - RLV$$

For ease in computation, the following formula can be used to compute body density:

$$D_b = M_a \times D_w/(M_a - W_w - RLV \times D_w)$$

The lower part of Table 28.2 presents body composition results for the two football players based on body density.

Validity of Hydrostatic Weighing to Estimate Body Fat. Experimental evidence supports the validity of hydrostatic weighing to estimate the body's fat content. Behnke's early studies of Navy divers placed 64 subjects into two groups based on their measured body density assessed by hydrostatic weighing. The mean difference between the groups in body mass (12.4 kg) and body volume (13.3 L) allowed Behnke to easily

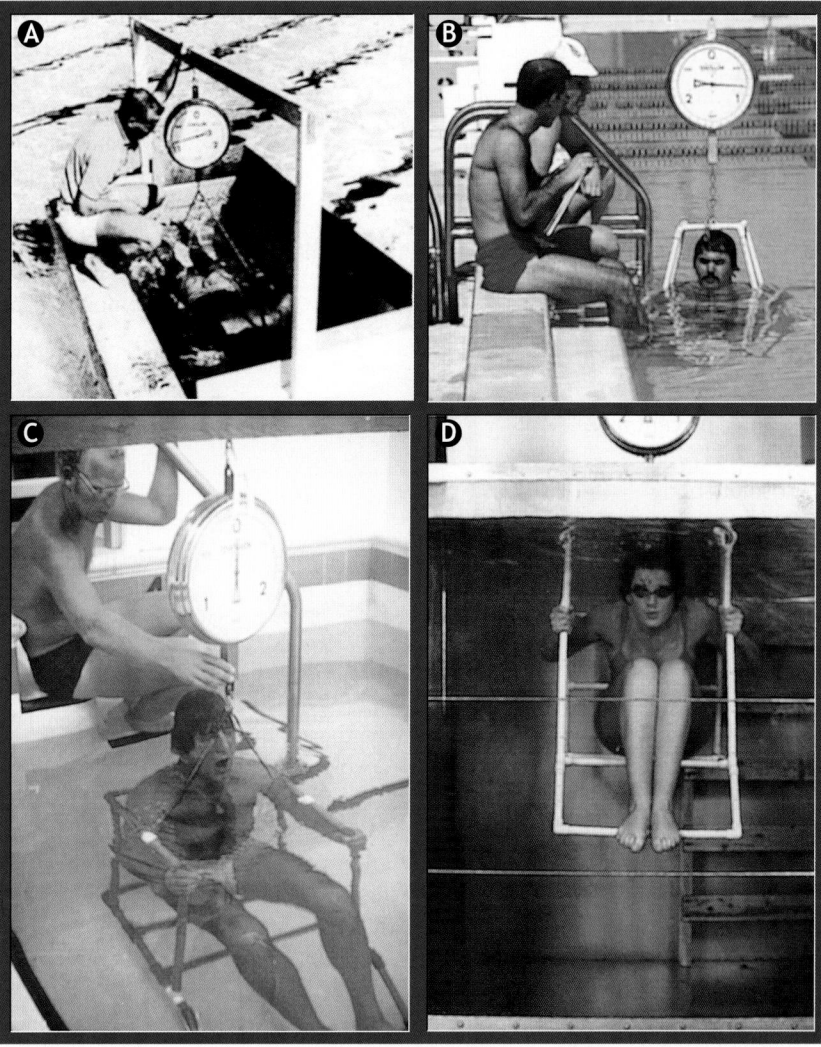

FIGURE 28.8 • Measuring body volume by underwater weighing. Prone and supine underwater weighing methods provide the same values with residual lung volume measured before, during, or after the underwater weighing. Measurements taken **(A)** prone in a swimming pool (constructed by textbook author F. Katch for his master's degree project at the University of California at Santa Barbara); **(B)** seated in a swimming pool (body volume measured during spring training of the Boston Red Sox baseball team by textbook authors VK and FK); **(C)** seated on a PVC piping chair in a therapy pool (New York Jets football team training camp by textbook authors VK and FK); and **(D)** seated in a stainless steel tank with Plexiglas front in the laboratory (textbook author FK laboratory, Exercise Science Department, University of Massachusetts, Amherst, MA). An autopsy scale recorded underwater weight during water submersion. For any of the methods, subjects can use a snorkel with nose clip if they express apprehension about submersion. The final calculation of underwater weight must account for these added objects.

TABLE 28.2 Measurements of Two Professional Football Players from Underwater Weighing

Variable	Symbol	Defensive Lineman	Running Back
Body mass (kg)	M_a	121.73	97.37
Net underwater weight (kg)	W_w	7.30	6.52
Water temperature correction	D_w	0.99336	0.99336
Residual lung volume (L)	RLV	1.213	1.374
Total body volume (L)	TBV	113.89	90.08
Body density ($g \cdot cm^{-3}$)	D_b	1.0688	1.0809
Body Composition			
Relative percentage body fat (%)[a]	%Fat	13.1	8.0
Absolute body fat (kg)	FM	15.9	7.2
Fat-free body mass (kg)	FFM	105.8	90.2

[a]Siri equation, %fat = (495/density) − 450.

discern body composition differences between the groups. The ratio of the average differences (Δ mass ÷ Δ volume) equaled 0.933 $g \cdot cm^{-3}$, a value within the density range of 0.92 to 0.96 $g \cdot cm^{-3}$ for human adipose tissue. The difference in body mass between the high- and low-density groups represented the density of adipose tissue. Body density for a group of heavy but lean professional football players, with lean body mass 20 kg higher than the Navy divers, averaged 1.080 $g \cdot cm^{-3}$. Behnke stated, "Here indeed was a presumptive demonstration that fat could be 'separated' from bone and muscle *in vivo* or 'the silver from the gold' by application of a principle renowned in antiquity."[16]

The lower and upper limits of body density among humans range from 0.93 $g \cdot cm^{-3}$ in the massively obese to nearly 1.10 $g \cdot cm^{-3}$ in the leanest males. This coincides nicely with the 1.10 density of fat-free tissue and 0.90 for homogenized samples of fat tissue from small mammals at 37°C.

Computing Body Density. For illustrative purposes, suppose a 50-kg person weighs 2 kg submerged in water. According to Archimedes' principle, loss of weight in water of 48 kg equals the weight of the displaced water. One can easily compute the volume of water displaced by correcting for the density of water at the weighing temperature. In this example, 48 kg of water equals 48 L, or 48,000 cm^3 (1 g of water = 1 cm^3 by volume at 39.2°F [4°C]). Measuring the person at a water temperature of 39.2°F (4°C) requires no density correction for water temperature. In practice, researchers use warmer water

and apply the appropriate density value for water at the weighing temperature.

The density of this person, computed as mass divided by volume, equals 50,000 g (50 kg) ÷ 48,000 cm^3, or 1.0417 $g \cdot cm^{-3}$. The total volume of any body segment can be determined using densitometry, for example, the volume of the hands.[72] The next step estimates percentage body fat and mass of the fat and fat-free tissues.

Computing Percentage Body Fat. An equation that incorporates whole-body density estimates the body's fat percentage. The simplified equation, derived by UC Berkeley biophysicist William Siri (1919–1998), substitutes 0.90 $g \cdot cm^{-3}$ for the density of fat and 1.10 $g \cdot cm^{-3}$ for the density of the fat-free tissues.[163] The final derivation, referred to as the **Siri equation**, computes percentage body fat as:

Percentage body fat = (495 ÷ body density) − 450

This equation assumes the two-component model of body composition; the density of fat extracted from adipose tissue equals 0.90 $g \cdot cm^{-3}$ and 1.10 $g \cdot cm^{-3}$ for fat-free tissue at 37°C. The pioneer researchers in this area maintained that each of these densities remains relatively constant among individuals despite large individual variations in total fat and FFM. They also assumed that the densities of the lean tissue components of bone and muscle remained the same among individuals.

In the previous example (body mass: 50 kg; body volume: 48 L), the whole-body density of 1.0417 $g \cdot cm^{-3}$ converted to percentage fat by the Siri equation equaled 25.2%.

$$\text{Percentage body fat} = (495 \div 1.0417) - 450$$
$$= 25.2\%$$

Several formulas other than Siri's equation also estimate percentage body fat from body density.[24,91] The basic difference among the formulas in calculating body fat generally averages less than 1% body fat units for body fat levels between 4 and 30%.

Limitations of Density Assumptions. The generalized density values for the fat-free (1.10 $g \cdot cm^{-3}$) and fat (0.90 $g \cdot cm^{-3}$) tissue compartments represent averages for young and middle-age adults. These "constants" vary among individuals and groups, particularly the density and chemical composition of the FFM. Such variation places some limitation in partitioning body mass into fat and fat-free components and predicting percentage body fat from whole-body density.[54] More specifically, average density of the FFM is higher for blacks and Hispanics than for whites (1.113 $g \cdot cm^{-3}$ blacks, 1.105 $g \cdot cm^{-3}$ Hispanics, and 1.100 $g \cdot cm^{-3}$ whites).[142,158,169] Racial differences also exist among adolescents.[176] Consequently, existing equations formulated from assumptions for whites to calculate body composition from body density in blacks or Hispanics *overestimates* FFM and *underestimates* percentage body fat. The following modification of the Siri equation computes percentage body fat from body density for blacks:

Percentage body fat = (437.4 ÷ body density) − 392.8

Applying constant density values for the different tissues in growing children or aging adults also introduces errors in predicting body composition. For example, the water and mineral contents of the FFM continually change during the growth period, including the demineralization of osteoporosis with aging. Reduced bone density makes the density of the fat-free tissue of young children and older adults lower than the assumed 1.10 g·cm^{-3} constant. This invalidates assumptions of constant densities of fat and fat-free masses in the two-compartment model and *overestimates* relative body fat calculated from densitometry. For this reason, many researchers do not convert body density to percentage body fat in children and aging adults. Others apply a **multicompartment model** to adjust for such factors to compute percentage body fat from body density in prepubertal children.[164,196] **TABLE 28.3** provides equations adjusted to maturation level to predict percentage body fat from whole-body density of boys and girls ages 7 to 17.

Adjust for Large Musculoskeletal Development. Chronic resistance training affects the density of the FFM, altering body fat estimation from whole-body density determinations. White male weightlifters with considerable muscular development and nontrained controls were assessed for body density, total body water, and bone mineral content.[130] Comparisons included estimations of percentage body fat with both the two-compartment model and a four-compartment model using the body's fat, water, mineral, and protein content and corresponding densities. Percentage body fat estimated from body density (two-compartment Siri equation) produced higher values than percentage body fat from the four-compartment model for the weight trainers but not for untrained controls. A *lower* FFM density in weight trainers than in controls, 1.089 versus 1.099 g·cm^{-3}, explained this discrepancy; it resulted from larger water and smaller mineral and protein fractions of the FFM in the resistance-trained men. For them, incorrect assumptions underlying the Siri equation *overestimated* percentage body fat.

For the weightlifters, muscularity increased disproportionately to changes in bone mass. A lower FFM density

occurred because the density of their fat-free muscle (1.066 g·cm^{-3} at 37°C) fell below the 1.1 g·cm^{-3} value assumed in the Siri equation. Disproportionate increases in muscle mass relative to increases in bone mass accounted for the reduced density of the FFM below 1.1 g·cm^{-3}, *overpredicting* percentage body fat from the two-compartment model. If resistance training does indeed progressively lower FFM density, then applying the Siri equation fails to accurately reflect true body composition changes from this training mode.

Based on revised densities of the FFM (1.089 g·cm^{-3}) and fat mass (0.9007 g·cm^{-3}), a modified equation more accurately appraises resistance-trained white males[130]:

Percentage body fat = (521 ÷ body density) − 478

Computing Fat Mass. Using data from the previous example, fat mass computes by multiplying body mass by percentage body fat as follows:

$$\text{Fat mass} = \text{Body mass} \times (\% \text{ fat}/100)$$
$$= 50 \text{ kg} \times 0.252$$
$$= 12.5 \text{ kg}$$

Further computations subdivide this person's fat mass into essential and storage fat. A female with 25.2% body fat has approximately 12% essential fat, or 6.0 kg (0.12 × 50 kg); the remaining 13.2% (6.6 kg) exists as storage fat (0.132 × 50 kg). For a male with 3% essential fat and 22.2% storage fat (based on 25.2% body fat), the corresponding values equal 1.5 kg for essential fat and 11.1 kg for storage fat. Clearly, for a man and woman with identical percentage body fat, the man rates "fatter" because storage fat represents a larger percentage of total body fat. Each gram of body fat (83% pure fat) contains approximately 7.5 kcal (7500 kcal per kg). One can compute the approximate potential energy stored in each fat depot. For storage fat in this example, the values are 49,500 kcal for the woman and 83,260 kcal for the man; for essential fat, including a female's sex-specific fat, the values are 45,000 kcal for the woman and 11,250 kcal for the man.

	Body Fat Estimates Using Age- and Gender-Specific Conversions to Account for Age-Related Changes in the	
TABLE 28.3	**Density of the Fat-Free Body Mass**	

Age (y)	Boys	Girls
7–9	% Fat = (5.38/BD − 4.97) × 100	% Fat = (5.43/BD − 5.03) × 100
9–11	% Fat = (5.30/BD − 4.89) × 100	% Fat = (5.35/BD − 4.95) × 100
11–13	% Fat = (5.23/BD − 4.81) × 100	% Fat = (5.25/BD − 4.84) × 100
13–15	% Fat = (5.08/BD − 4.64) × 100	% Fat = (5.12/BD − 4.69) × 100
15–17	% Fat = (5.03/BD − 4.59) × 100	% Fat = (5.07/BD − 4.64) × 100

Reprinted from Lohman T. Applicability of body composition techniques and constants for children and youth. *Exerc Sports Sci Rev* 1986;14:325.

Computing Fat-Free Body Mass. Compute FFM by subtracting fat mass from body mass.

$$\textbf{Fat-free body mass} = \textbf{Body mass} - \textbf{Fat mass}$$
$$= 50 \text{ kg} - 12.5 \text{ kg}$$
$$= 37.5 \text{ kg}$$

BOD POD Measurement of Body Volume

A relatively new procedure assesses body volume and its changes for groups that range from infants to older adults, to collegiate wrestlers and exceptionally large athletes like American professional football and basketball players.[49,181,207] The method has adapted helium-displacement plethysmography first reported in the late 1800s. The subject sits inside a small chamber marketed commercially as **BOD POD** (Fig. 28.9A). Measurement requires only 3 to 5 min, with high reproducibility of test scores ($r > 0.90$) within and across days. After being weighed to the nearest ±5 g on an electronic scale (*bottom left* of BOD POD illustration), the subject sits comfortably in the 750-L volume, dual-chamber fiberglass shell. The molded front seat separates the unit into front and rear chambers. The electronics, housed in the rear chamber, contain the pressure transducers, breathing circuit, and air circulation system.

The BOD POD determines body volume by measuring the initial volume of the empty chamber and then the volume with the person inside. To ensure measurement reliability and accuracy, the person wears a tight-fitting swimsuit.[187] Body volume represents the initial volume minus the reduced chamber volume with the subject inside. The subject breathes several breaths into an air circuit to assess pulmonary gas volume, which when subtracted from measured body volume yields body volume. Body density computes as body mass (measured in air) divided by body volume (measured in BOD POD, including a correction for a small negative volume caused by isothermal effects related to skin surface area). The Siri equation converts body density to percentage body fat.

Some Discrepancies in the Literature

Figure 28.9B shows the regression of percentage body fat assessed by hydrostatic weighing (HW) versus percentage body fat assessed by BOD POD (BP) in an ethnically diverse group of adult women and men. A difference of only 0.3% (0.2% fat units) occurred between body fat determined by the two methods, with a validity coefficient of $r = 0.96$. In contrast to these rather impressive findings, BOD POD assessments of collegiate football players, while producing reliable scores, underpredicted percentage body fat compared with hydrostatic weighing and DXA.[33] Underprediction of body fat also occurred in a heterogeneous sample of black men who varied considerably in age, stature, body mass, percentage body fat, and self-reported physical activity level and socioeconomic status.[193] The method underpredicted percentage body fat compared with densitometry (−1.9% fat units) and DXA (−1.6% fat units). Similar underpredictions compared with DXA-derived body fat (−2.9% fat units)

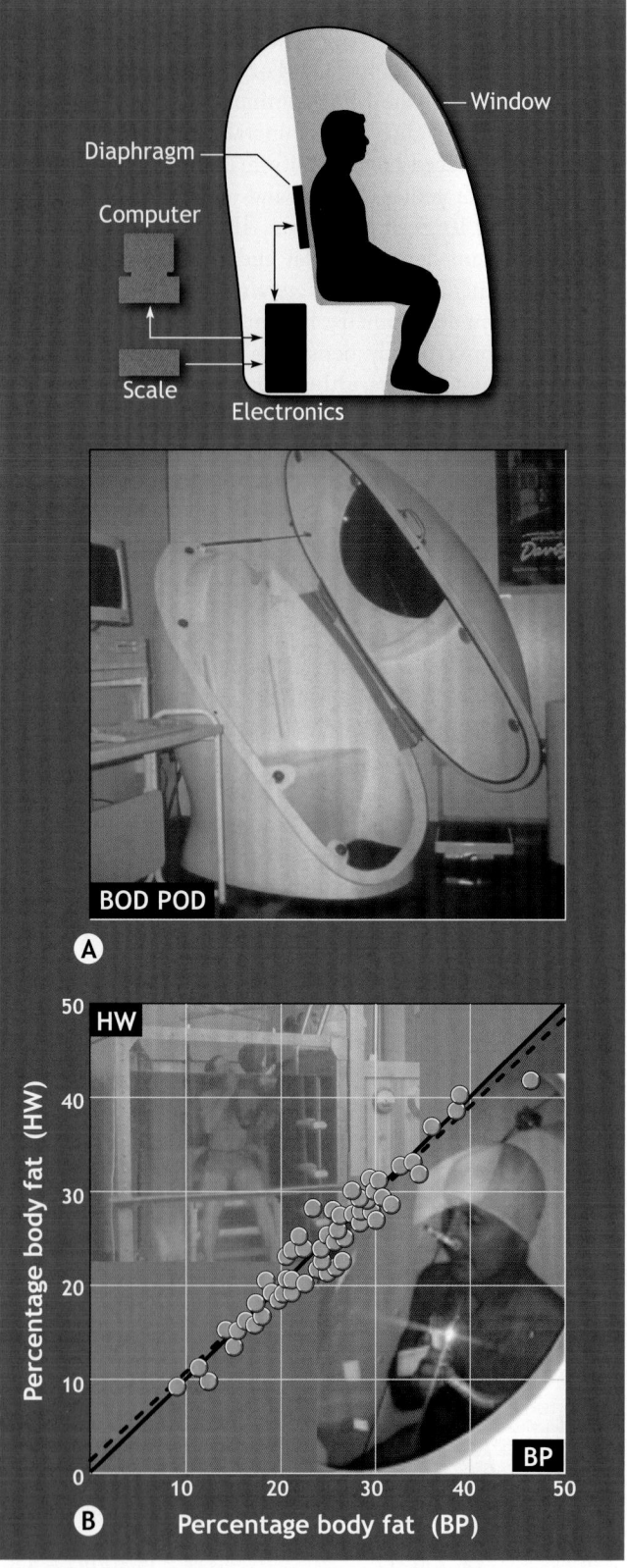

FIGURE 28.9 • **(A)** BOD POD for measuring human volume. (Photo courtesy of Dr. Megan McCrory, Purdue University, West Lafayette, IN.) **(B)** Regression of percentage body fat by hydrostatic weighing (HW) versus percentage body fat by BOD POD (BP). (Data from McCrory MA, et al. Evaluation of a new air displacement plethysmograph for measuring human body composition. *Med Sci Sports Exerc* 1995;27:1686.)

occurred in 54 boys and girls 10 to 18 years of age.[108] BOD POD also underestimated body fat of young adults compared with body fat predictions from a four-component model.[48,128] The method overestimated percentage body fat among lean individuals in a heterogeneous group of adults.[186] A BOD POD validation study in children ages 9 to 14 concluded that compared with DXA, total body water, and densitometry, BOD POD precisely and accurately estimated fat mass without introducing bias estimates.[46] The method has also been shown to accurately detect body composition changes from a small-to-moderate weight loss in overweight women and men.[197] Numerous studies have assessed the efficacy of BOD POD compared with other body composition methods in children; young, middle-age, and older adults; obese persons; and athletes.[5,8,11,17,32,47,147,188]

Skinfold and Girth Measurements

In field situations, two relatively simple anthropometric procedures that measure either subcutaneous fat (skinfolds) or circumferences (girths) predict body fatness with reasonable accuracy.

Subcutaneous Fat Measurement with Skinfolds

The rationale for using skinfolds to estimate body fat comes from the interrelationships among three factors:

1. Adipose tissue directly beneath the skin (subcutaneous fat)
2. Internal fat
3. Whole-body density

The Caliper. By 1930, a pincer-type caliper accurately measured subcutaneous fat at selected anatomic sites. The three calipers shown in FIGURE 28.10 operate on a principle similar to a micrometer that measures distance between two points. Measuring skinfold thickness requires firmly grasping a fold of skin and subcutaneous fat with the thumb and forefingers, pulling it away from the underlying muscle tissue following the natural contour of the skinfold. When calibrated, the pincer jaws exert a relatively constant tension of $10 \text{ g} \cdot \text{mm}^{-2}$ at the point of contact with the double layer of skin plus subcutaneous adipose tissue. The caliper dial indicates skinfold thickness in mm recorded within 2 s after applying the full force of the caliper. This time limitation avoids skinfold compression when taking the measurement. For research purposes, the investigator has considerable experience in taking measurements and demonstrates consistency in duplicating values for the same subjects on the same day, consecutive days, or weeks apart. A rule of thumb to achieve consistency requires duplicate or triplicate practice measurements on approximately 50 individuals who vary in body fat. Careful attention to detail usually ensures high measurement reproducibility.

Measurement Sites. Common anatomic sites for skinfold measurements include triceps, subscapular, suprailiac, abdominal, and upper thigh sites. The investigator should take a minimum

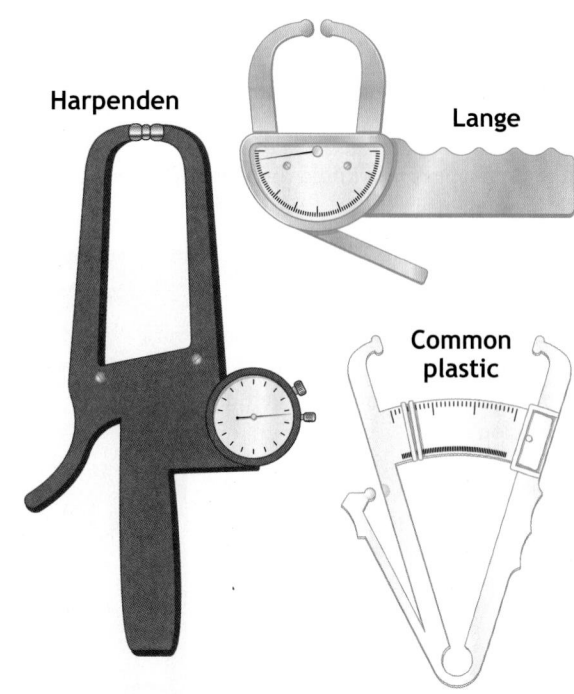

FIGURE 28.10 • Common calipers for skinfold measurements. The Harpenden and Lange calipers but not the plastic calipers provide constant tension at all jaw openings.

of two or three measurements in rotational order at each site on the right side of the body with the subject standing. The average value represents the skinfold score. FIGURE 28.11 shows the anatomic location of five of the more frequently measured sites:

1. *Triceps*: Vertical fold at the posterior midline of the right upper arm, halfway between the tip of the shoulder and tip of the elbow; elbow remains in an extended, relaxed position
2. *Subscapular*: Oblique fold, just below the bottom tip of the right scapula
3. *Iliac* (iliac crest): Slightly oblique fold, just above the right hipbone (crest of ileum); the fold follows the natural diagonal line
4. *Abdominal*: Vertical fold 1 in. to the right of the umbilicus
5. *Thigh*: Vertical fold at the midline of the right thigh, two thirds the distance from the middle of the patella (kneecap) to the hip

Other measurement sites include the *chest* (diagonal fold with long axis directed toward the right nipple; on the anterior axillary fold as high as possible) and the *biceps* (vertical fold at the posterior midline of the right upper arm).

Usefulness of Skinfold Scores

Skinfold measurements provide meaningful information about body fat and its distribution. We recommend two ways to use skinfolds. The first sums the skinfold scores to indicate relative fatness among individuals. The sum-of-skinfolds and individual values reflect either absolute or percentage skinfold changes before and after an intervention program.

One can draw the following conclusions from the skinfold data in Table 28.4 obtained from a 19-year-old female college student before and after a 16-wk aerobic conditioning program:

1. Largest changes in skinfold thickness occurred at the iliac and abdomen sites
2. Triceps showed the largest percentage decrease and the subscapular the smallest percentage decrease
3. Total reduction in subcutaneous skinfolds at the five sites was 16.6 mm, or 12.6% below the "before" condition

A second use of skinfolds incorporates population-specific mathematical equations to predict body density or percentage body fat. The equations prove accurate for subjects similar in age, gender, training status, fatness, and race to the group from which they were derived.[22,43,66,135,138,146] *When meeting these criteria, predicted body fat for an individual usually ranges between 3 and 5% body fat units computed from body density with hydrostatic weighing.*

Our laboratories developed the following equations to predict percentage body fat from triceps and subscapular skinfolds in young women and men[83–85]:

Young women, ages 17 to 26 years

% Body fat = 0.55A + 0.31B + 6.13

Young men, ages 17 to 26 years

% Body fat = 0.43A + 0.58B + 1.47

In both equations, A is triceps skinfold (mm) and B is subscapular skinfold (mm).

We computed the "before" and "after" percentage body fat of the woman who participated in the 16-wk physical conditioning program (Table 28.4). Percentage body fat equals 24.4% by substituting the pretraining values for triceps (22.5 mm) and subscapular (19.0 mm) skinfolds into the equation.

$$\% \text{ Body fat} = 0.55A + 0.31B + 6.13$$
$$= 0.55\,(22.5) + 0.31(19.0) + 6.13$$
$$= 12.38 + 5.89 + 6.13$$
$$= 24.4\%$$

Substituting posttraining values for triceps (19.4 mm) and subscapular (17.0 mm) skinfolds produced a body fat value of 22.1%.

$$\% \text{ Body fat} = 0.55(19.4) + 0.31(17.0) + 6.13$$
$$= 10.67 + 5.27 + 6.13$$
$$= 22.1\%$$

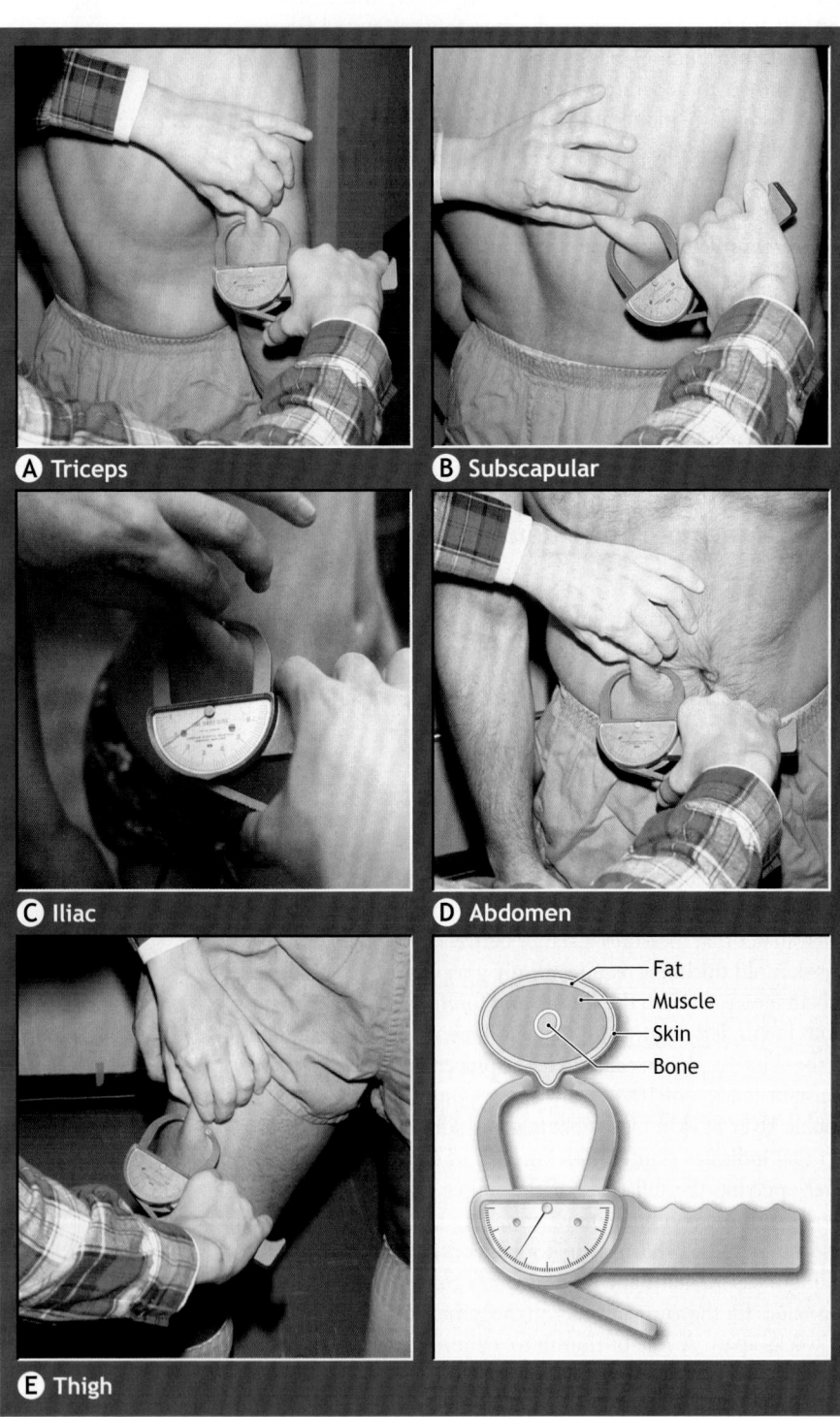

FIGURE 28.11 • Anatomic location of five common skinfold sites: **(A)** Triceps. **(B)** Subscapular. **(C)** Iliac. **(D)** Abdomen. **(E)** Thigh. Measurements taken on the right side of the body in the vertical plane except diagonally at subscapular and iliac sites.

TABLE 28.4 — Changes in Selected Skinfolds of a Young Woman During a 16-Week Exercise Program

Skinfolds (mm)	Before	After	Absolute Change	Percentage Change
Triceps	22.5	19.4	−3.1	−13.8
Subscapular	19.0	17.0	−2.0	−10.5
Suprailiac	34.5	30.2	−4.3	−12.8
Abdomen	33.7	29.4	−4.3	−12.8
Thigh	21.6	18.7	−2.9	−13.4
Sum	**131.3**	**114.7**	**−16.6**	**−12.6**

Percentage body fat determined before and after a physical conditioning or weight-loss program provides a convenient way to evaluate alterations in body composition, independent of body weight changes.

Skinfold Prediction for Athletes

Predict body fat in athletes from an equation validated against a four-component model (total body water, bone mineral by DXA, and body density by underwater weighing).

$$\% \text{ Body fat} = 8.997 + 0.24658\ (3\ \text{SKF}) - 6.343\ (\text{gender}) - 1.998\ (\text{race})$$

where 3 SKF = sum of skinfolds in mm at abdomen, thigh, and triceps; gender = 0 for female, 1 for male; race = 0 for white, 1 for black.

Source: Evans EM, et al. Skinfold prediction equation for athletes developed using a four-component model. *Med Sci Sports Exerc* 2005;37:2006.

Skinfolds and Age

In young adults, approximately one half of total fat consists of subcutaneous fat, with the remainder visceral and organ fat. With advancing age, proportionately more fat deposits internally than subcutaneously. The same skinfold score reflects a greater total percentage of body fat as one ages. *For this reason, use age-adjusted* **generalized equations** *to predict body fat from skinfolds or girths in older men and women.*[75,76,150,174] Researchers also have cautioned that acceleration of the "obesity epidemic" may require adjustment of generalized equations to predict body fat in subjects whose sum of seven skinfolds (chest, axilla, triceps, subscapular, abdominal, iliac, thigh) exceeds 120 mm.[137]

User Beware

Assessing skinfolds requires expertise with the proper measurement techniques. The particular caliper style, whether metal, spring-loaded, plastic, electronic, or wide and thin pincer pads, may contribute to errors of measurement.[57] Another

source of error occurs when trying to assess skinfold thickness in extremely obese people; in such individuals, skinfold thickness often exceeds the width of the caliper's jaws. For these reasons, we advocate that girth measurements be used as the assessment technique of choice (see next section).

 INTEGRATIVE QUESTION

A friend complains that three different fitness centers determined her percentage body fat from skinfolds as follows: 25%, 29%, and 21%. How can you reconcile the differences in these values?

Measurement of Girths

A linen or plastic measuring tape (not a metal tape) applied lightly to the skin surface allows the tape to remain taut but not tight. This avoids skin compression, which produces below-normal scores. We advocate taking a minimum of two duplicate measurements at each site and averaging the scores. FIGURE 28.12 shows six common anatomic landmarks for anthropometric measurement:

1. **Right upper arm (biceps):** arm straight and extended in front of the body; measurement taken at midpoint between the shoulder and the elbow
2. **Right forearm:** maximum girth with arm extended in front of the body
3. **Abdomen:** 1 inch above the umbilicus
4. **Buttocks:** maximum protrusion with heels together
5. **Right thigh:** upper thigh, just below the buttocks
6. **Right calf:** widest girth midway between ankle and knee

Equations to predict body fat based on girths exist for each gender and different age groups.[83,127,180] The equations for these subgroups show considerable population specificity, not general applicability. This means that a particular equation applies to the particular group upon which the equations were developed. For example, equations developed on younger subjects should never be used to predict body fat in older age groups, but unanimity is not universal on this point.[101] We believe that this same specificity approach should apply to males and females and particular athletic groups. The equations do not apply to the following categories of individuals:

1. Overly thin or excessively fat
2. Regularly train in strenuous endurance sports or activities with substantial resistance-training, and subsequent muscular-enlargement component
3. Differ in race from the specific group used to derive the original equations

Usefulness of Girth Scores

Girths prove most useful in ranking individuals within a group according to relative fatness. As with skinfolds, girth-based equations predict body density and/or percentage body fat with a certain degree of error, albeit relatively small.

thePoint Appendix L, available online at http://thepoint. lww.com/mkk8e, presents equations and constants for young and older men and women to predict body fat within ±2.5 to 4.0% body fat units of the actual value.

This means that on average for about 70 of every 100 people measured, the equations will predict body fat within the 2.5 to 4.0% body fat compared to the person's body fat had it been assessed by a valid criterion such as hydrostatic weighing, DXA, or BOD POD (see "Hydrostatic Weighing and BOD POD Measurement of Body Volume," earlier in this chapter, and "Dual-Energy X-Ray Absorptiometry," later in this chapter). The prediction error depends on whether the individual portrays physical characteristics similar to the original validation group. Such relatively small errors make girth predictions particularly useful in nonlaboratory settings. Specific equations based on girths also estimate body composition of obese adult men and women.[21,179,195]

Along with predicting percentage body fat, girth scores can analyze patterns of body fat distribution, including changes in fat patterning during weight loss.[62,191] *Fat patterning* refers to the distribution of body fat on the trunk and extremities. Not surprisingly, those equations that use the more labile sites of fat deposition (e.g., waist and hips instead of upper arm or thigh in females and abdomen in males) provide the greatest accuracy to predict changes in body composition.[50]

Body Fat Predictions from Girths

From the appropriate tables in Appendix L, on http://thepoint.lww.com/mkk8e, substitute the corresponding constants A, B, and C in the formula shown at the bottom of each table. This requires one addition and two subtraction steps. The following five-step example shows how to compute percentage fat, fat mass, and FFM for a 21-year-old man who weighs 79.1 kg:

Step 1. Measure upper arm, abdomen, and right forearm girths with a cloth tape to the nearest 0.25 in. (0.6 cm): upper arm = 11.5 in. (29.21 cm); abdomen = 31.0 in. (78.74 cm); right forearm = 10.75 in. (27.30 cm)

Step 2. Determine the three constants *A*, *B*, and *C* corresponding to the three girths from the table: *A*, corresponding to 11.5 in. = 42.56;

B, corresponding to 31.0 in. = 40.68; and *C*, corresponding to 10.75 in. = 58.37.

Step 3. Compute percentage body fat by substituting the constants from step 2 in the formula for young men as follows:

$$\text{Percentage fat} = A + B - C - 10.2$$
$$= 42.56 + 40.68 - 58.37 - 10.2$$
$$= 83.24 - 58.37 - 10.2$$
$$= 24.87 - 10.2$$
$$= 14.7\%$$

Step 4. Determine fat mass

$$\text{Fat mass} = \text{Body mass} \times (\% \text{ fat} \div 100)$$
$$= 79.1 \text{ kg} \times (14.7 \div 100)$$
$$= 79.1 \text{ kg} \times 0.147$$
$$= 11.6 \text{ kg}$$

Step 5. Determine FFM

$$\text{FFM} = \text{Body mass} - \text{Fat mass}$$
$$= 79.1 \text{ kg} - 11.6 \text{ kg}$$
$$= 67.5 \text{ kg}$$

Bioelectrical Impedance Analysis

In the single mode of low-frequency **bioelectrical impedance analysis (BIA)**, a small alternating current flowing between two electrodes passes more rapidly through hydrated fat-free body tissues and extracellular water than through fat or bone tissues because of the greater electrolyte content (lower electrical resistance) of the fat-free component. In essence, the body's water content conducts the flow of electrical charges, so when current flows through the fluid, sensitive instrumentation can detect the water's impedance. Impedance to electric current flow, calculated by measuring current and voltage, is based on Ohm's law (R = V/I, where R = resistance, V = voltage, and I = current). These relationships can quantify the volume of water within the body, and from this, percentage body fat and FFM.

FIGURE 28.13A and B show an example for single-frequency BIA. A person lies on a flat, nonconducting surface with injector (source) electrodes attached on the dorsal surfaces of the foot and wrist and detector (sink) electrodes attached between the radius and ulna (styloid process)

1. **Abdomen:** 1 in. above the umbilicus
2. **Buttocks:** Maximum protrusion of buttocks with the heels together
3. **Right thigh:** Upper thigh, just below the buttocks
4. **Right upper arm (biceps):** Palm up, arm straight and extended in front of the body; taken at the midpoint between the shoulder and the elbow
5. **Right forearm:** Maximum girth with the arm extended in front of the body
6. **Right calf:** Widest girth midway between the ankle and knee

FIGURE 28.12 • Landmarks for measuring various girths at six common anatomic sites.

IN A PRACTICAL SENSE

How to Predict Percentage Body Fat from Girths for Overly Fat Men and Women

Estimating percentage body fat (%BF) in the overly fat by skinfold prediction becomes problematic from difficulty securing accurate and repeatable measurements owing to an extensive mass of subcutaneous fat. In addition, with increasing levels of body fatness, the proportion of subcutaneous fat to total body fat changes, thereby affecting the relationship between skinfolds and body density (Db). The following four factors limit skinfold use with the overly fat population:

1. Difficulty of site selection and palpation of body landmarks
2. Skinfold thickness may exceed caliper jaw aperture
3. Variability in adipose tissue composition affects skinfold compressibility
4. Poorer objectivity in skinfold measures as body fat increases

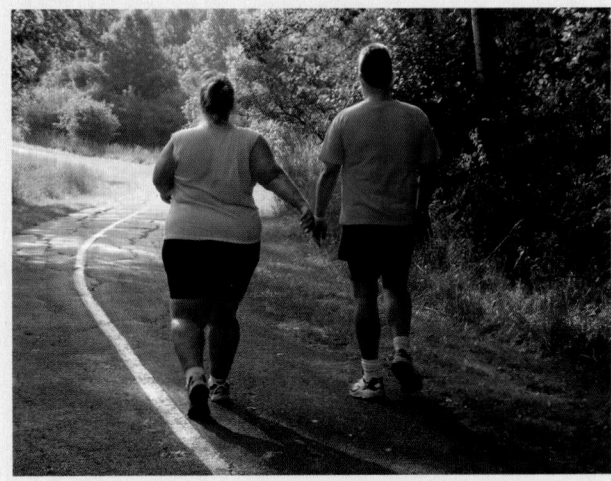

PREDICTING PERCENTAGE BODY FAT

Use the following equations to predict %BF in obese (>30%BF) women (age 20–60 years) and obese (>20%BF) men (age 24–68 years).

Women

$$\%BF = 0.11077\ (ABDO) - 0.17666\ (HT) + 0.14354\ (BW) + 51.03301$$

Men

$$\%BF = 0.31457\ (ABDO) - 0.10969\ (BW) + 10.8336$$

where ABDO = the average of (1) waist girth (taken horizontally at the level of the natural waist—narrowest part of the torso, as seen from the anterior) and (2) abdomen girth (taken horizontally at the level of the greatest anterior extension of the abdomen, usually, but not always, at the level of the umbilicus). Duplicate measurements are taken and averaged. BW = body weight in kilograms; HT = stature in centimeters.

EXAMPLES

1. Overly Fat Woman

Waist girth = 115 cm;
Abdomen girth = 121 cm; HT = 165.1 cm; BW = 97.5 kg

$$\%BF = 0.11077\ (ABDO) - 0.17666\ (HT) + 0.14354\ (BW) + 51.03301$$

$$= 0.11077\ [(115 + 121)/2] - 0.17666\ (165.1) + 0.14354\ (97.5) + 51.03301$$

$$= 13.07 - 29.17 + 13.995 + 51.03301$$

$$= 48.9$$

2. Overly Fat Man

Waist girth = 131 cm;
Abdomen girth = 136 cm; BW = 135.6 kg

$$\%BF = 0.31457\ (ABDO) - 0.10969\ (BW) + 10.8336$$

$$= 0.31457\ [(131.0 + 136.0)/2] - 0.10969\ (135.6) + 10.8336$$

$$= 41.995 - 14.873 + 10.8336$$

$$= 37.9$$

Sources:
Tran ZV, Weltman A. Predicting body composition of men from girth measurements. *Hum Biol* 1988;60:167.
Weltman, A, et al. Accurate assessment of body composition in obese females. *Am J Clin Nutr* 1988;48:1178.

and at the ankle between the medial and lateral malleoli. A painless, localized electrical current (approximately 800 µA at a frequency of 50 kHz) is introduced, and the impedance (resistance) to current flow between the source and detector electrodes determined. Conversion of the impedance value to body density—adding body mass and stature; gender, age, and sometimes race; level of fatness; and several girths to the

equation—computes percentage body fat from the Siri equation or other density conversion equations. Body composition prediction with such a system depends on the additional input data as part of the BIA equation. Any unreliability of data input produces different prediction results. This becomes more pronounced for individuals at the extremes of body composition. For example, a difference of only 5 mm in a girth measurement or a difference of 1.5 cm in "true" stature from measurement to measurement can produce up to a 2% change in an output variable—unrelated to any real change in a computed body composition variable such as fat mass or FFM. Figure 28.13C illustrates the segmental measurement approach including electrode configuration and how electric current (I) and voltage (V) are assessed for the right arm, trunk, and right leg.

Influence of Hydration Level and Ambient Temperature

Hydration level affects the accuracy of BIA to incorrectly determine an individual's body fat content.[96,140] Hypohydration and hyperhydration alter the body's normal electrolyte concentrations; this in turn affects current flow independent of real body composition changes. For example, voluntary fluid restriction decreases the impedance measure. This lowers the percentage body fat estimate; hyperhydration produces the opposite effect (higher body fat estimate). Skin temperature, influenced by ambient conditions, also affects whole-body resistance and BIA prediction of body fat. Predicted body fat is lower in a warm environment because moist skin produces less impedance to electrical flow than in a cold one.

Even with normal hydration and environmental temperature, body fat predictions with BIA prove less valid than with hydrostatic weighing as the criterion. BIA tends to overpredict body fat in lean and athletic subjects and underpredict body fat in obese subjects.[116,159] BIA often predicts body fat less accurately than do girths and skinfolds.[23,41,87,170] Whether BIA detects small changes in body composition during weight loss remains unclear.[98,148] Conventional BIA technology cannot determine regional fat distribution.

At best, BIA represents a noninvasive, safe, relatively easy, and generally reliable means to assess total body water. The technique requires that experienced personnel make measurements under standardized conditions. Particularly important factors include electrode placement and the subject's body position, hydration status, plasma osmolality and sodium concentration, skin temperature, recent physical activity, and previous food and beverage intake.[19,97,98,193] For example, eating several successive meals within a short time interval progressively decreases bioelectrical impedance, possibly from the combined effect of increased electrolytes and a redistribution of extracellular fluid, which decreases computed percentage body fat.[165] Body fatness and racial characteristics also influence BIA's predictive accuracy.[4,143,171] The tendency to overestimate percentage body fat increases among black athletes[67,159] and lean subjects.[172] Fatness-specific BIA equations exist that predict body fat for obese and nonobese American Indian, Hispanic, white men and women,[191] and diverse population groups.[42,161,157,206] With proper measurement standardization, the menstrual cycle does not affect body composition assessment by BIA.[121]

Applicability of BIA in Sports and Exercise Training

Coaches and athletes require a safe, easily administered, and valid tool to assess body composition and detect changes with caloric restriction or physical conditioning. A major limitation in achieving these goals concerns BIA's lack of sensitivity to detect small body-compositional changes, particularly without appropriate control over factors that affect measurement accuracy and reliability. For example, sweat-loss dehydration from prior physical activity or reduced glycogen reserves (and associated loss of glycogen-bound water) from an intense training session reduces body resistance (impedance) to electrical current flow. This overestimates FFM and underestimates percentage body fat.

Chapter 29's "In a Practical Sense" includes BIA equations, in addition to equations using skinfolds and girths, to estimate body density and percentage body fat for athletes in general and athletes in specific sports. Without sport-specific equations, population-based generalized equations that account for age and gender usually provide an acceptable alternative to estimate body fat.[76,162,175]

Near-Infrared Interactance

Near-infrared interactance (**NIR**) applies technology developed by the U.S. Department of Agriculture to assess body composition of livestock and the lipid content of various grains. The commercial versions to assess human body composition use principles of light absorption and reflection. A fiber optic probe or light wand emits a low-energy beam of near-infrared light into the single measuring site at the anterior midline surface of the dominant biceps. A detector within the same probe measures the intensity of the reemitted light, expressed as optical density. Shifts in wavelength of the reflected beam as it interacts with organic material in the arm interfaces with a manufacturer's prediction equation that includes adjustments for subject's body mass and stature, estimated frame size, gender, and physical activity level to compute percentage body fat and FFM. The safe, portable, lightweight equipment requires minimal training to use and necessitates little physical contact with the subject during measurement. These test administration aspects make NIR popular for body composition assessment in health clubs, hospitals, and weight-loss centers. The important question about the usefulness of NIR concerns its validity.

Questionable Validity of NIR

Early research indicated a relationship between spectrophotometric measures of light interactance at various body sites and body composition assessed by total body water.[36] Subsequent studies with humans have not confirmed NIR's validity versus hydrostatic weighing or skinfold measurements. NIR does not accurately predict body fat across a broad range of body fat levels; it often provides less accuracy than skinfolds,[23,65,185] but has proved more useful in young females using rapid Fourier transform NIR, a laboratory instrument that uses infrared spectroscopic techniques.[79] In general, it overestimates body fat in lean men and women and underestimates it in fatter subjects.[122] The data in **FIGURE 28.14** show the inadequacy of NIR compared with skinfold measurements to predict body fat compared to hydrostatic weighing. In more than 47% of

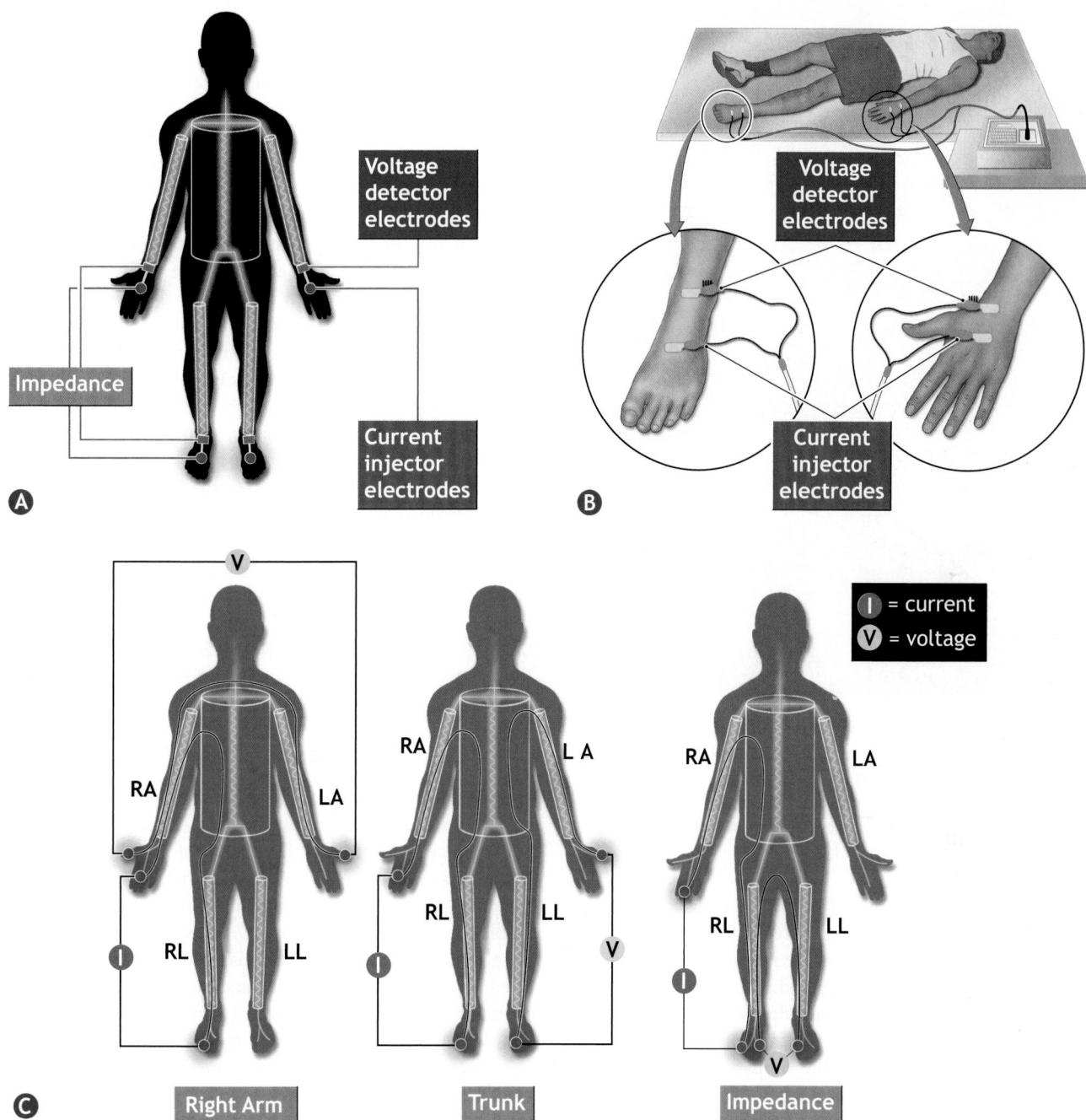

FIGURE 28.13 • Method to assess body composition by bioelectrical impedance analysis. **(A)** Four-surface electrode technique (whole-body impedance) applies current via one pair of distal (injector) electrodes, while the proximal (detector) electrode pair measures electrical potential across the conducting segment. **(B)** Standard placement of electrodes and body position during whole-body impedance measurement. **(C)** Segmental measurement illustrating assessment of current (*I*) and voltage (*V*) for the right arm, trunk, and right leg.

the subjects, an error greater than 4% body fat units occurred with NIR, with the largest errors at the extremes of body fatness. NIR produced large errors when estimating body fat for children[27] and youth wrestlers,[69] and underestimated body fat in collegiate football players.[68] NIR did not accurately assess body composition changes from resistance training.[23] *In general, research does not support NIR as a robust, valid method to* *assess human body composition across a broad range of ages, sexes, and racial and athletic categories.*

Ultrasound Assessment of Fat

Ultrasound technology can assess the thickness of different tissues (fat and muscle) and image the deeper tissues such as

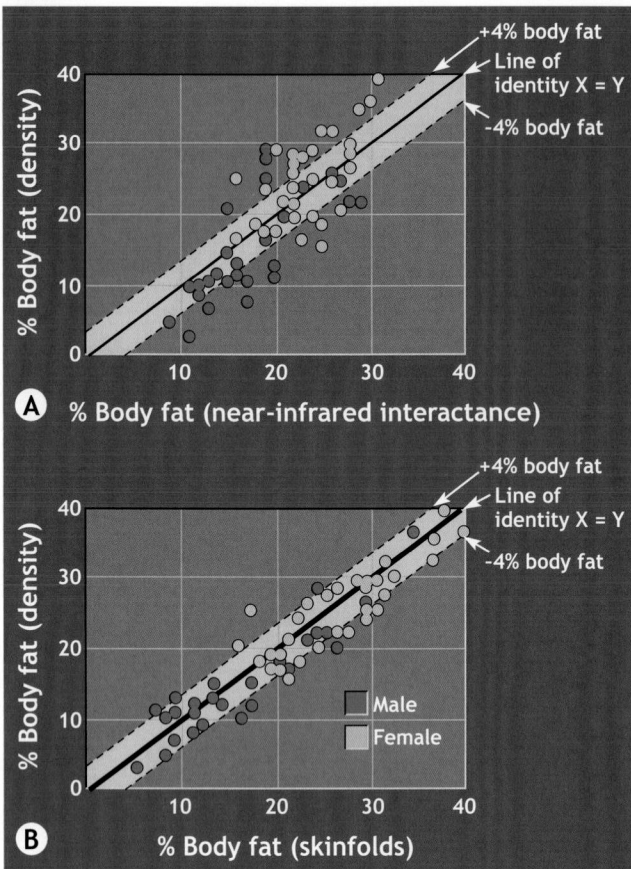

FIGURE 28.14 • Comparison of near-infrared interactance (Futrex-5000) **(A)** and skinfolds **(B)** for assessing percentage body fat. Shaded area around line incorporates 64% body fat units. (Adapted with permission from McLean K, Skinner JS. Validity of Futrex-5000 for body composition determination. *Med Sci Sports Exerc* 1992;24:253.)

a muscle's cross-sectional area. The method converts electrical energy through a probe into high-frequency (pulsed) sound waves that penetrate the skin surface into the underlying tissues. The sound waves pass through adipose tissue to penetrate the muscle layer. The waves then reflect against the bone to the fat–muscle interface to produce an echo, which returns to a receiver within the probe. The simplest A-mode type of ultrasound does not produce an image of the underlying tissues. Rather, the time required for sound wave transmission through the tissues and back to the transducer converts to a distance score that indicates fat or muscle thickness. With the more expensive and technically demanding B-mode ultrasound, a two-dimensional image provides considerable detail and tissue differentiation.

Ultrasound exhibits high reliability for repeat measurements of subcutaneous fat thickness at multiple sites in the lying and standing positions on the same day and different days.[74,82] The technique can determine total and segmental subcutaneous adipose tissue volume.[2] It has also shown validity for assessing FFM of high school wrestlers, which may prove useful as a field-based body composition assessment method,[182] and other athletic groups as part of a

multicomponent model that considers variability in the density of the body's fat mass.[3] Ultrasound proves particularly useful with obese persons who show considerable variation and compression of subcutaneous body fat with skinfold measures. When used to map muscle and fat thickness at different body regions and quantify changes in topographic fat patterns, ultrasound serves as a valuable adjunct to body composition assessment. In hospitalized patients, ultrasonic fat and muscle thickness determinations aid in nutritional assessment during weight loss and weight gain. Ultrasonic imaging also serves a clinical role in assessing tissue growth and development, including fetal development and structure and function of the heart and other organs. With imaging devices, reflected sound waves from the soft tissues convert to a real-time image for convenient visualization or for computer digitization of area, volume, and diameter directly from the image. Color and multiple-frequency imaging allows clinicians to trace blood flow through organs and tissues or, with the use of miniaturized probes, identify internal tissues, vessels, and organs. In consumer-oriented research, ultrasonic imaging of thigh fat depth provided evidence that treatments using two topical cream applications to the thighs and buttocks to reduce "cellulite" (so-called dimpled fat) failed to reduce local fat thickness compared with control conditions.[34]

Computed Tomography, Magnetic Resonance Imaging, and Dual-Energy X-Ray Absorptiometry

Computed Tomography

Computed tomography (**CT**) scanning revolutionized medicine when first introduced in the mid-1970s as organs and bones became visible with the clarity of anatomy textbooks. By use of an array of x-ray emitters and detectors, the CT scan generates detailed cross-sectional, two-dimensional radiographic images of body segments when an x-ray beam (ionizing radiation) passes through tissues of different densities. The CT scan produces pictorial and quantitative information about total tissue area, total fat and muscle area, and thickness and volume of tissues within an organ.[56,129,190]

Figure **28.15A–C** shows CT scans of the upper legs and a cross section at the midthigh of a professional walker who covered 11,200 miles walking through the 50 states in 50 wk. Total cross section and muscle cross section increased and subcutaneous fat decreased correspondingly in the midthigh region in the "after" scans (not shown). Studies have demonstrated the efficacy of CT scans to establish the relationship between simple skinfold and girth anthropometric measures at the abdomen and total abdominal fat volume measured from single or multiple pictorial "slices" through this region.[160] The single cut through the L4 to L5 region minimizes radiation dose and provides the best view of visceral and subcutaneous fat. Figure **28.16** illustrates the high association ($r = 0.82$) between waist circumference and deep **visceral adipose tissue** (**VAT**) area; men with larger waist girth also possessed greater VAT. The relationship exceeded the association between

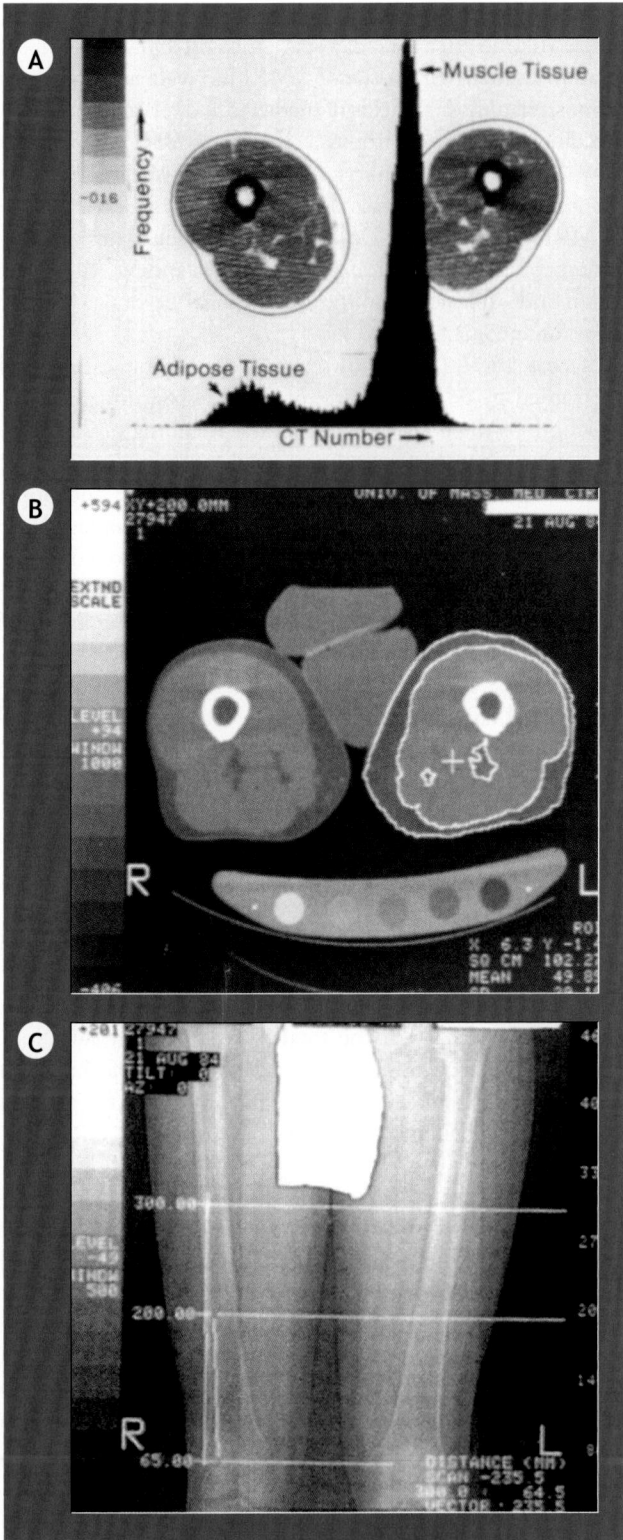

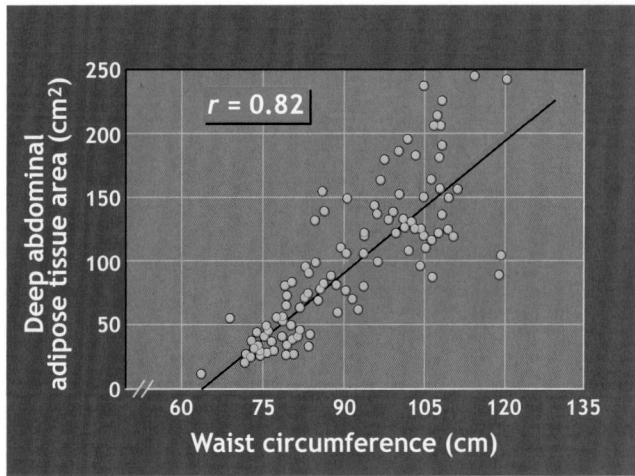

FIGURE 28.16 • Relationship between deep visceral adipose tissue (VAT) determined by CT scanning and waist girth in 110 men, ages 18 to 42 years, who varied considerably in percentage body fat by densitometry. The best predictors of VAT included (a) abdominal skinfold thickness in mm, (b) waist girth in cm, and (c) waist–hip ratio. VAT (cm²) = −363.12 + (−1.113a) + 3.478b + 186.7c. For example, if abdominal skinfold is 23.0 mm, waist girth is 92.0 cm, and waist–hip ratio is 0.929, then by substitution in the equation, VAT + 104.7 cm². (Adapted with permission from Dépres J-P, et al. Estimation of deep abdominal adipose-tissue accumulation from simple anthropometric measurements in men. *Am J Clin Nutr* 1991;54:471.)

subcutaneous fat thickness (skinfolds) and VAT. An increased amount of deep abdominal adipose tissue relates to increased risk for type 2 diabetes, blood lipid profile disorders, lung disease, and hypertension, including cardiometabolic factors and cardiovascular disease.[28,61,73,107] Chapter 30 discusses health risks from the deep type of abdominal obesity.

Magnetic Resonance Imaging

Physician and research scientist Raymond Vahan Damadian (1936–) first proposed the idea for **magnetic resonance imaging** (**MRI**) in a grant application in 1969 dealing with soft tissue imaging of cancers. The first published article on the topic of his novel idea appeared in 1971. MRI, patented in 1974 and first constructed at the Downstate Medical Center in Brooklyn, New York, in 1976, provided a noninvasive assessment of detailed, high-resolution contrasts of the body's tissue compartments without the potential risks of damaging ionizing radiation common with x-ray and CT scanning.[1,81,103] The schematic drawing in Figure **28.17A** shows the arrangement of the different muscular structures. The yellow areas that surround the thigh correspond to both subcutaneous and internal fat, with minimal fat intrusion located among and within the different muscles. The femur bone appears at the center of the cross-section. Figure **28.17B** shows an MRI transaxial image of the midthigh of a 30-year-old male middle-distance runner. Computer software subtracts fat and bony tissues (*white areas*) to compute thigh muscle cross-sectional area With MRI, electromagnetic radiation (not ionizing radiation as in CT scans) in a strong magnetic

FIGURE 28.15 • CT scans. **(A)** Plot of pixel elements (CT scan) illustrating the extent of adipose and muscle tissue in a cross section of the thigh. The two other views show **(B)** a cross section of the midthigh and **(C)** an anterior view of the upper legs prior to a 1-year walk across the United States by a champion walker. (CT scans courtesy of Dr. Steven Heymsfeld, George A. Bray, Jr., endowed Chair in Nutrition, Pennington Biomedical Research Center, Louisiana State University, Baton Rouge, LA.)

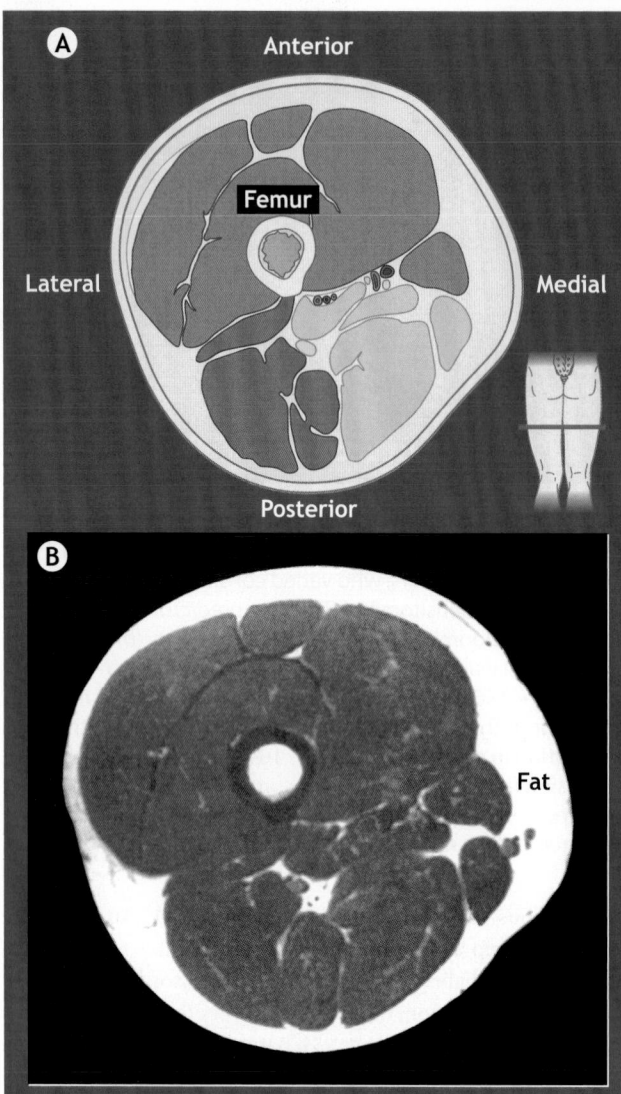

FIGURE 28.17 • (A) Arrangement of muscular structures at the midthigh region as shown at the top of the cross-sectional drawing. The yellow areas that surround the thigh correspond to subcutaneous and internal fat, with minimal fat located among the different muscles. The femur bone appears at the center of the cross-section. **(B)** Transverse MRI scan of the right thigh that corresponds to the structures in A. (Adapted with permission from Moore KL, Dalley AF, Agur AMR. *Clinically Oriented Anatomy.* 7th Ed. Baltimore: Wolters Kluwer Health, 2013.)

field excites the hydrogen nuclei of the body's water and lipid molecules, which vary in concentration depending on the tissue source; it is more concentrated in fat, less so in water and blood, and least in bone. The nuclei then project a detectable signal that rearranges under computer software to visually represent various body tissues. MRI can quantify total and subcutaneous adipose tissue in individuals of varying body fatness. Combined with muscle mass analysis, MRI assesses changes in a muscle's lean and fat components following resistance training, changes in muscle volume in and out of training, as a diagnostic tool for various pathologies (e.g., ligamentous knee damage or femoral condyle necrosis), or during different stages of growth

and aging.[78,178] MRI analysis has assessed postflight changes in muscle volume after a 17-day space mission and 16- to 28-wk duration shuttle/*Mir* missions.[102] MRI has wide acceptance for diagnosis in almost all fields of medicine and related disciplines, including muscular dystrophy.[55] The latest MRI technologies allow imaging of pacemakers with fiber optic leads rather than wire leads, MRI compatible defibrillators, and FONAR stand-up MRI developed by Dr. Damadian, which scans patients in numerous weight-bearing positions—standing, sitting, in flexion and extension, and the conventional lie-down position (www.fonar.com).

FIGURE **28.18** (**top**) shows a plot of percentage body fat determined by MRI scanning of 30 transaxial images along the length of the body and underwater weighing of 20 Swedish women, ages 23 to 40 years. Total fat from scans of the calves, thighs, lower and upper trunk, and lower and upper arms provided the basis for computing MRI percentage body fat. Good agreement emerged between the two body fat estimates ($r = 0.84$). Similar validity emerged between MRI-determined total body fat and hydrostatic weighing and total body water estimates of body fat.[123]

Figure 28.18 (**bottom three graphs**) shows the distribution of total adipose tissue, subcutaneous adipose tissue, and nonsubcutaneous adipose tissue measures from different body regions. The *bar graphs* show the smallest to the largest adipose tissue depots. Of all body regions, adipose tissue in the lower trunk (both subcutaneous and nonsubcutaneous) contained the greatest percentage of total body fat (38.5%); the lower arm region included 2.7%, the smallest amount. The *pie chart* at the lower right of the figure shows the relative amounts of adipose tissue in each body compartment in relation to the MRI-determined total volume of body fat. Subcutaneous fat accounted for 75.2% of the total 21.8 L of body fat. Non-subcutaneous fat accounts for the remaining 24.8%, making it reasonable to conclude that "excess" fat deposits to the greatest extent in the subcutaneous tissues.

MRI Comparison of Lean and Obese. Seventeen MRI-derived tissue slices from groups of lean and obese females provided comparative data for total fat and VAT volume at four anatomic sites between the top of the patella and sternal notch. Body fat determined by densitometry for the lean women (BMI: 20.6) averaged 25.4%; the obese women's BMI averaged 42.4, with about 42% body fat. The three graphs in FIGURE **28.19** display differences between the relatively lean (*orange* data points) and obese (*blue* data points) groups in total body tissue expressed as the sum of fat and nonfat tissues, total adipose tissue, and subcutaneous adipose tissue at the 17 sites. The results show a fairly consistent pattern in MRI-derived adipose tissue volumes. The overfat subjects possessed 165% more subcutaneous adipose tissue and 155% more total adipose tissue. Abdominal and upper-thigh regions showed the largest fat accretion. Interestingly, the lean women had a greater amount of nonfat tissue (not shown) at the upper-thorax and lower-thigh regions. The inset graph shows the strong relationship between MRI-determined percentage of body adipose tissue (four instead of 17 sites) and percentage

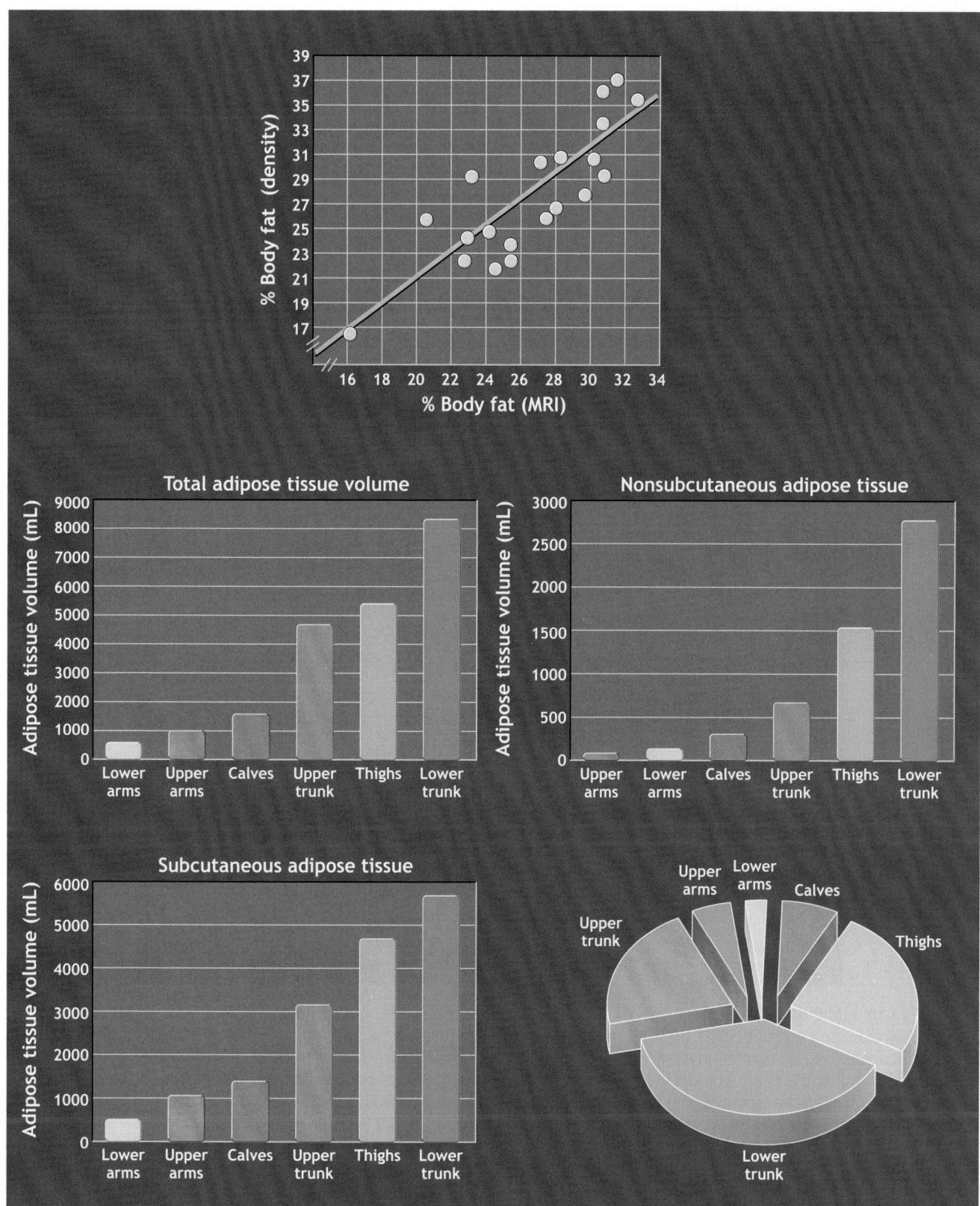

FIGURE 28.18 • **(Top)** Percentage body fat determined by hydrostatic weighing (density) and MRI scanning (graph created from individual data points presented in the original article). **(Bottom three graphs)** Distribution of adipose tissue (total, subcutaneous, and nonsubcutaneous) within the various body compartments; arrangement progresses from smallest to largest. The *right pie chart* displays the relative distribution of adipose tissue in different body regions. (Adapted with permission from Sohlstrom A, et al. Adipose tissue distribution as assessed by magnetic resonance imaging and total body fat by magnetic resonance imaging, underwater weighing, and body-water dilution in healthy women. *Am J Clin Nutr* 1993;58:830.)

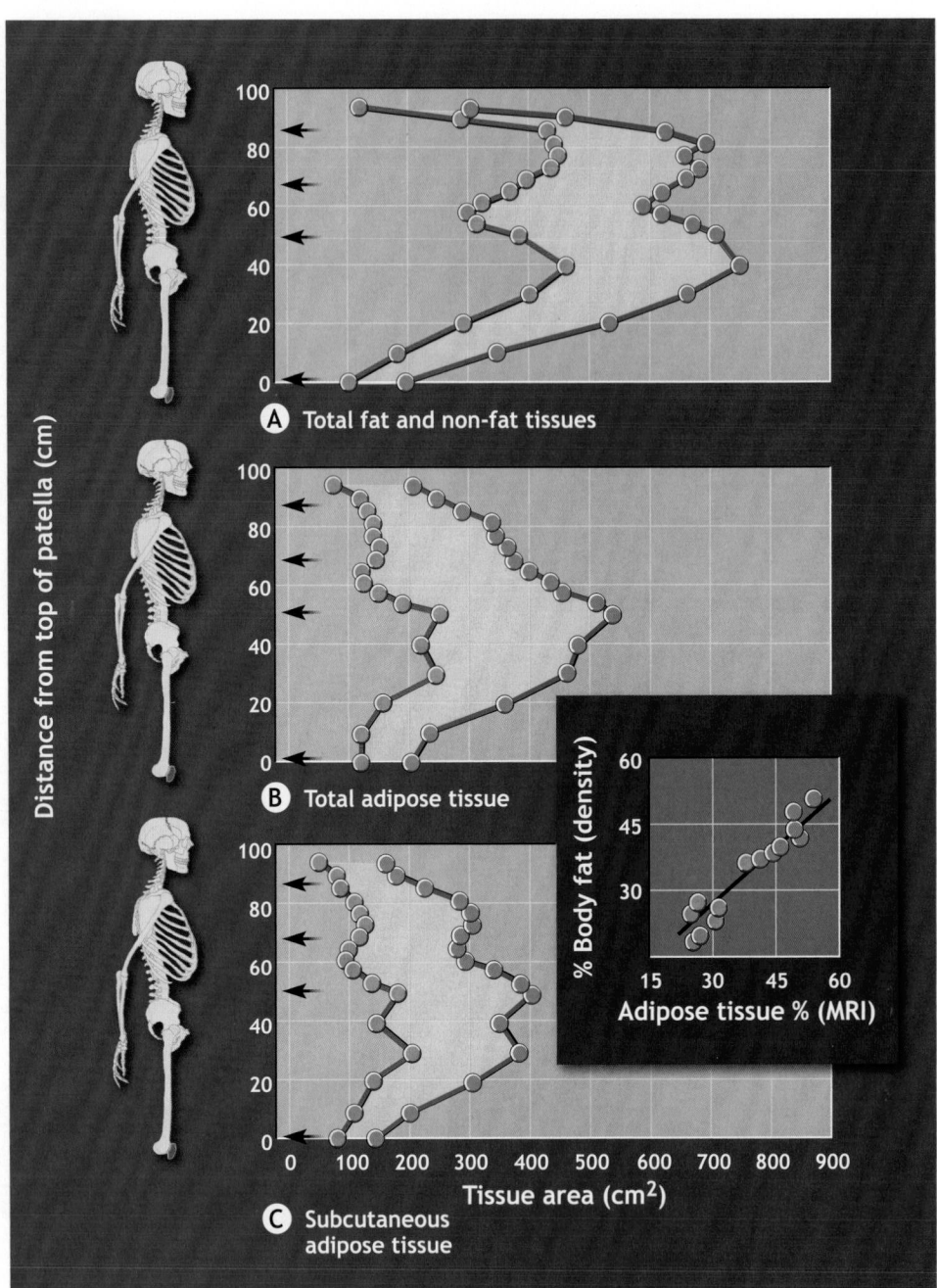

FIGURE 28.19 • MRI-determined distribution of body tissues in seven lean (*red*) and seven obese (*blue*) females. **(A)** Total body tissues (sum of fat and nonfat tissues). **(B)** Total adipose tissue. **(C)** Subcutaneous adipose tissue. *Arrows* to the right of the *y*-axis indicate the four anatomic markers in relation to position on the skeleton. The *inset graph* displays the relationship between percentage body adipose tissue (using four instead of 17 MRI sites) and percentage body fat determined by hydrostatic weighing in obese and lean subjects. (Adapted with permission from Fowler PA, et al. Total and subcutaneous adipose tissue in women: the measurement of distribution and accurate prediction of quantity by using magnetic resonance imaging. *Am J Clin Nutr* 1991;54:18.)

body fat determined by densitometry. MRI yields a wealth of useful information for accurately assessing total and regional body composition.

Exercise Training. MRI and dual-energy x-ray absorptiometry (discussed next) assessed changes in regional trunk and extremities and whole-body fat mass, lean body mass, and bone mineral content at 3 and 6 mo of resistance training

in 31 women.[139] MRI measured changes in thigh muscle morphology in a subset of 11 women exercisers. The women decreased fat mass by 10% and body mass and soft tissue lean mass by 2.2%, but bone mineral content did not change compared with nontraining groups of men and women. Soft tissue lean mass was distributed less in women's arms than in men's both before and after training. The most striking training-induced differences occurred in the tissue composition of the women's arms (31% loss in fat mass without change in lean mass) compared with the legs (5.5% gain in lean mass without change in fat mass). Fat decreased in the trunk by 12% without change in soft tissue lean mass. The changes for fat mass by MRI and DXA showed close relationships (range between $r = 0.72$ and $r = 0.92$). Both techniques also similarly assessed increases in lean leg tissue mass. This experiment reinforced the importance of appraising changes in regional tissue morphology (including total body changes) with an experimental treatment—in this case, the effects of resistance training.

Dual-Energy X-Ray Absorptiometry

Dual-energy x-ray absorptiometry (DXA) reliably and accurately quantifies fat and nonbone regional lean body mass, including the mineral content of the body's deeper bony structures.[90,93,109,145,154] It has become the accepted clinical tool to assess spinal osteoporosis and related bone disorders.[44,100] When used for body composition assessment, DXA does not require assumptions concerning the biologic constancy of the fat and fat-free components inherent with hydrostatic weighing.[13]

With DXA, two distinct low-energy x-ray beams with short exposure with low radiation dosage penetrate bone and soft tissue areas to a depth of approximately 30 cm. The subject lies supine on a table so the source and detector probes slowly pass across the body over a 12-min period. Computer software reconstructs the attenuated x-ray beams to produce an image of the underlying tissues and quantify bone mineral content, total fat mass, and FFM. Analysis can include selected trunk and limb regions for detailed study of tissue composition and its relation to disease risk and the effects of exercise training and detraining.[106,117,202]

DXA shows excellent agreement with other independent estimates of bone mineral content. Strong relationships also exist between DXA-determined total body fat and body fat by either densitometry,[63,119] segmental body composition (upper- and lower-extremity mass), total body potassium, or total body nitrogen[120] and abdominal adiposity.[54] Studies have focused on body fat estimation by DXA with other methods in young children,[40] prepubertal children,[26,71,167] younger and older men[10] and women,[9,131] older adults,[58,166] and changes during intense resistance training.[155,184] **Figure 28.20** shows the strong association between percentage body fat estimates by DXA and hydrostatic weighing over a broad age range in men and women. The strength of the prediction decreases for older and fatter subjects but remains within the typical range for comparisons among discrete methodologies. Using a more robust model of body composition assessment, the error is less than 2% body fat units between DXA and densitometry in the heterogeneous age group of adults shown in the figure.[64]

 INTEGRATIVE QUESTION

Outline your response to a friend who asks: "Why am I considered 'overfat' by some criteria for obesity while my body fat assessment with other methods falls within normal limits?"

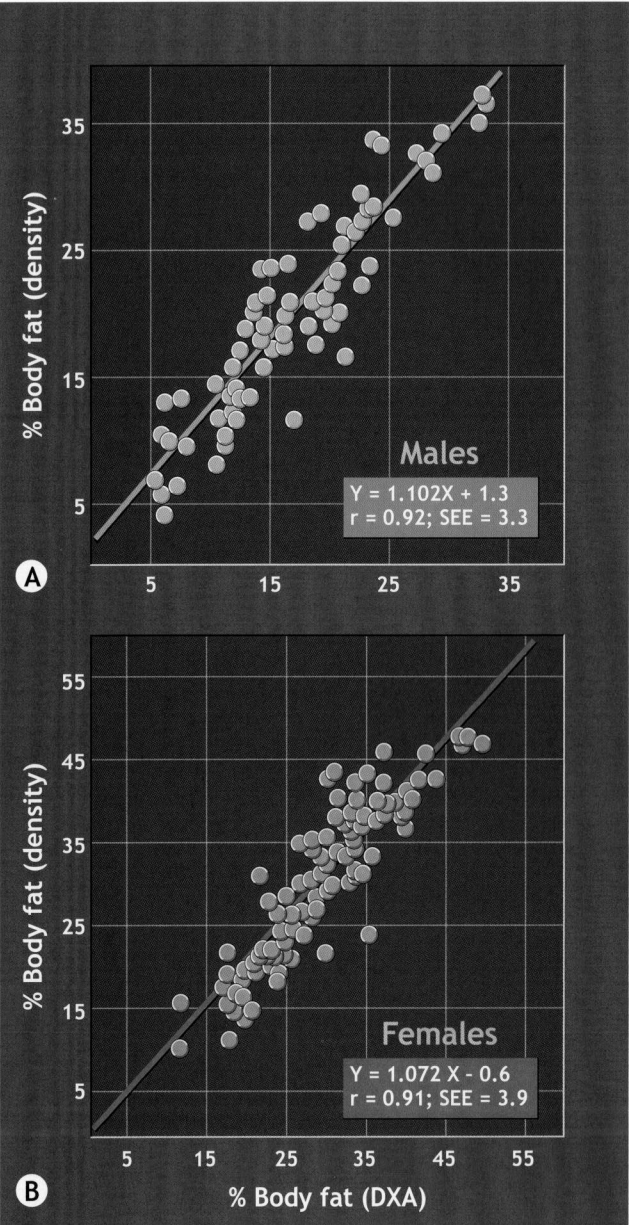

FIGURE 28.20 • Comparison of total body fat determined by hydrostatic weighing and DXA in men **(A)** and women **(B)**. (Adapted with permission from Snead DB, et al. Age-related differences in body composition by hydrodensitometry and dual-energy absorptiometry. *J Appl Physiol* 1993;74:770.)

AVERAGE PERCENTAGE BODY FAT

Table 28.5 lists average values for percentage body fat in samples of men and women throughout the United States. The column headed "68% Variation Limits" indicates the range of percentage body fat that includes approximately 68 of every 100 persons measured. As an example, the average percentage body fat of 15.0% for young men from the New York sample includes the 68% variation limits from 8.9 to 21.1% body fat. This means that for every 68 of 100 young men measured, percentage fat ranges between 8.9 and 21.1%. Of the remaining 32 young men, 16 possess more than 21.1% body fat, while 16 other men have a body fat percentage below 8.9. *In general, percentage body fat for young adult men averages between 12 and 15%; the average value for women falls between 25 and 28%.*

The general trend of available body composition data of men and women of different ages indicates a distinct tendency for percentage body fat to steadily increase with advancing age. The mechanisms that lead to increased body fat with age are not clearly understood. The trend does not necessarily imply a desirable or normal aging process because participation in vigorous physical activity throughout life frequently blunts body fat accretion with age.[183,199,200] Regular physical activity maintains or increases bone mass while preserving muscle mass. A sedentary lifestyle, in contrast, increases storage fat, particularly in the abdominal region, and reduces muscle mass. This occurs even if daily caloric intake remains unchanged.

DETERMINING GOAL BODY WEIGHT

Average values for percentage body fat approximate 15% for young men and 25% for young women. In contact sports and activities that require a high level of muscular power (e.g., football, sprint swimming and running), successful performance typically requires a large fat-free body mass with average or below-average body fat. Successful athletes in weight-bearing endurance activities generally possess a relatively light body mass with low body fat. *Proper assessment of body composition, not body weight, determines a person's ideal body weight. For athletes,* **goal body weight** *must coincide with optimizing sport-specific measures of physiologic functional capacity and exercise performance.* The following equation computes a goal body weight based on a desired percentage body fat level:

$$\text{Goal body weight} = \text{Fat-free body mass} \div (1.00 - \text{desired \%fat})$$

TABLE 28.5 Average Values of Body Fat for Younger and Older Women and Men from Selected Studies

Study	Age Range	Stature (cm)	Mass (kg)	% Fat	68% Variation Limits
Younger women					
North Carolina, 1962	17–25	165.0	55.5	22.9	17.5–28.5
New York, 1962	16–30	167.5	59.0	28.7	24.6–32.9
California, 1968	19–23	165.9	58.4	21.9	17.0–26.9
California, 1970	17–29	164.9	58.6	25.5	21.0–30.1
Air Force, 1972	17–22	164.1	55.8	28.7	22.3–35.3
New York, 1973	17–26	160.4	59.0	26.2	23.4–33.3
North Carolina, 1975	—	166.1	57.5	24.6	—
Army Recruits, 1986	17–25	162.0	58.6	28.4	23.9–32.9
Massachusetts, 1998	17–31	165.2	57.8	21.8	16.7–27.9
Older women					
Minnesota, 1953	31–45	163.3	60.7	28.9	25.1–32.8
	43–68	160.0	60.9	34.2	28.0–40.5
New York, 1963	30–40	164.9	59.6	28.6	22.1–35.3
	40–50	163.1	56.4	34.4	29.5–39.5
North Carolina, 1975	33–50	—	—	29.7	23.1–36.5
Massachusetts, 1993	31–50	165.2	58.9	25.2	19.2–31.2
Younger men					
Minnesota, 1951	17–26	177.8	69.1	11.8	5.9–11.8
Colorado, 1956	17–25	172.4	68.3	13.5	8.3–18.8
Indiana, 1966	18–23	180.1	75.5	12.6	8.7–16.5
California, 1968	16–31	175.7	74.1	15.2	6.3–24.2
New York, 1973	17–26	176.4	71.4	15.0	8.9–21.1
Texas, 1977	18–24	179.9	74.6	13.4	7.4–19.4
Army Recruits, 1986	17–25	174.7	70.5	15.6	10.0–21.2
Massachusetts, 1998	17–31	178.1	76.4	12.9	7.8–19.0
Older men					
Indiana, 1966	24–38	179.0	76.6	17.8	11.3–24.3
	40–48	177.0	80.5	22.3	16.3–28.3
North Carolina, 1976	27–50	—	—	23.7	17.9–30.1
Texas, 1977	27–59	180.0	85.3	27.1	23.7–30.5
Massachusetts, 1993	31–50	177.1	77.5	19.9	13.2–26.5

Suppose a 91-kg (200-lb) man, currently with 20% body fat, wants to know how much fat weight to lose to attain a body fat composition of 10%. The computations progress as follows:

$$\text{Fat mass} = 91 \text{ kg} \times 0.20$$
$$= 18.2 \text{ kg}$$
$$\text{Fat-free body mass} = 91 \text{ kg} - 18.2 \text{ kg}$$
$$= 72.8 \text{ kg}$$
$$\text{Goal body weight} = 72.8 \text{ kg} \div (1.00 - 0.10)$$
$$= 72.8 \text{ kg} \div 0.90$$
$$= 80.9 \text{ kg} (178 \text{ lb})$$
$$\text{Goal fat loss} = \text{Current body weight} - \text{Goal body weight}$$
$$= 91 \text{ kg} - 80.9 \text{ kg}$$
$$= 10.1 \text{ kg} (22.2 \text{ lb})$$

If this athlete lost 10.1 kg (22.2 lb) of body fat, his new body weight of 80.9 kg (178.0 lb) would contain fat equal to 10% of body mass. These calculations assume no change in FFM during weight loss. Moderate caloric restriction plus increased daily energy expenditure through exercise induce fat loss and conserve the FFM. Chapter 30 discusses prudent yet effective approaches to reduce body fat.

Summary

1. Standard height–weight tables reveal little about the body's composition. Studies of athletes show clearly that overweight does not necessarily coincide with excessive body fat.
2. BMI relates more closely to body fat and health risk than simply body mass and stature. BMI still fails to consider the body's proportional composition.
3. Total body fat consists of essential fat and storage fat. Essential fat contains fat present in bone marrow, nerve tissue, and organs; storage fat represents the energy reserve that accumulates as adipose tissue beneath the skin and visceral depots.
4. Essential fat averages 3% of body mass for men and 12% for women. Storage fat averages 12% of body mass for men and 15% for women.
5. An individual probably cannot reduce body fat below the essential fat level and still maintain optimal health.
6. Menstrual dysfunction in athletes who train hard and maintain low body fat levels relates to the interaction between the physiologic and psychologic stress of regular training, hormonal balance, energy and nutrient intake, and body fat.
7. Delayed onset of menarche in chronically active young females may confer health benefits because they show a lower lifetime occurrence of reproductive organ and other cancers.
8. Popular indirect methods of body composition assessment include hydrostatic weighing and anthropometric prediction methods that incorporate skinfold and girth measurements.
9. Hydrostatic weighing determines body density with subsequent estimation of percentage body fat. The computation assumes a constant density for the body's fat and fat-free tissue compartments.
10. The air displacement BOD POD method provides a reasonable alternative to hydrostatic weighing for body volume determination and subsequent body composition assessment.
11. The error inherent in predicting body fat from whole-body density lies in assumptions concerning the densities of the fat and fat-free components.
12. Body composition assessments that use skinfolds and girths exhibit population specificity; they are most valid with subjects similar to those who participated in the equations' original derivation.
13. Hydrated fat-free body tissues and extracellular water facilitate electrical flow compared with fat tissue from the greater electrolyte content of the fat-free component.
14. Impedance to electric current flow in BIA analysis relates to the body's fat quantity.
15. Near-infrared interactance should be used with caution to assess body composition in the exercise sciences; this methodology currently lacks verification with adequate validity.
16. Ultrasound, CT, MRI, and DXA indirectly assess body composition, with each having a unique application for expanding knowledge of the compositional components of the live human body.
17. Average young adult males possess a body fat content of approximately 15% and women 25%.
18. Goal body weight computes as fat-free body mass: 1.00 − desired %fat.

the Point References are available online at **http://thepoint.lww.com/mkk8e.**

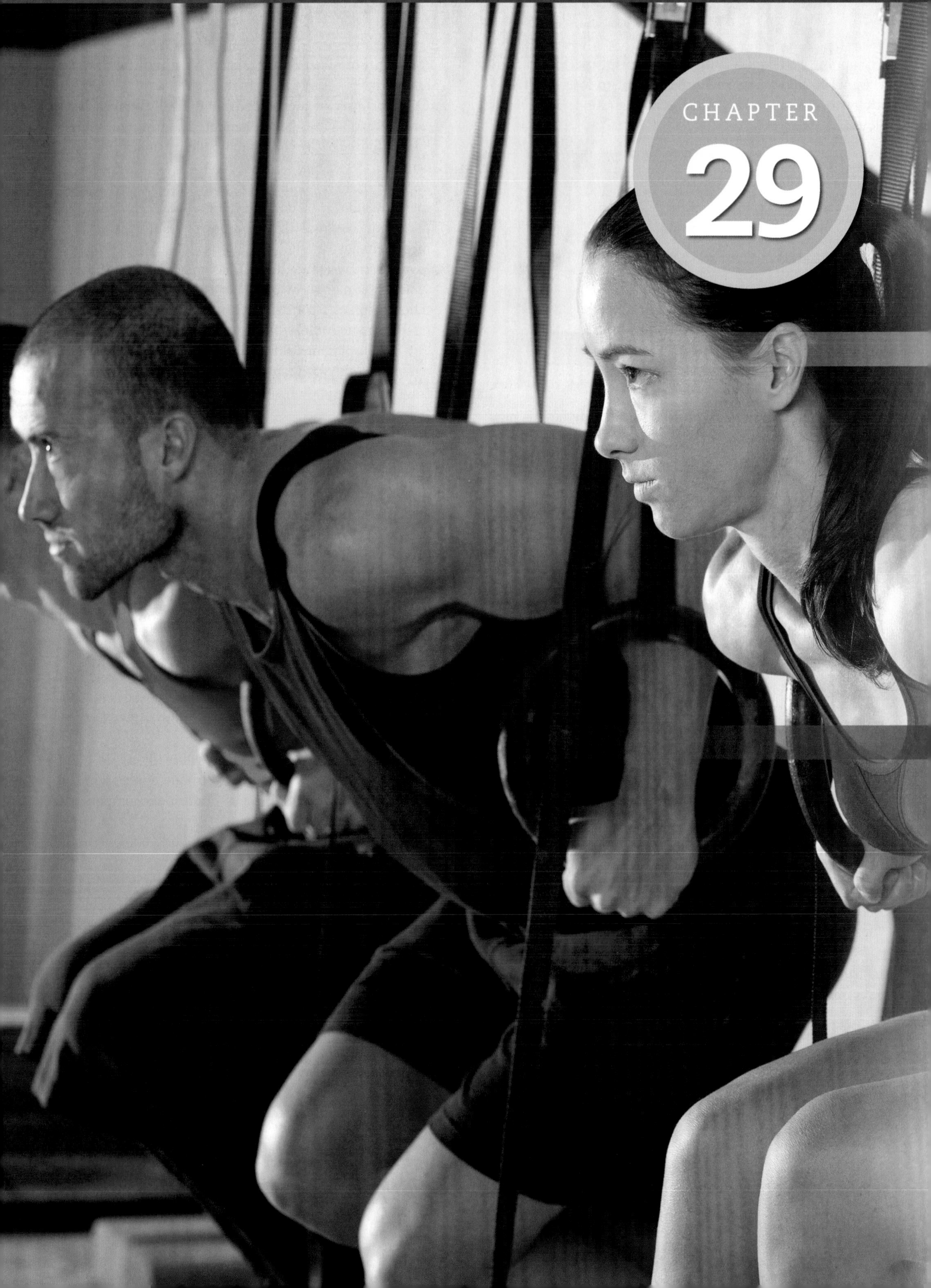
CHAPTER
29

Physique, Performance, and Physical Activity

CHAPTER OBJECTIVES

- Compare body composition characteristics of average young men and women with elite competitors in endurance running, wrestling, triathlon, professional golf, and weightlifting and bodybuilding

- Contrast body fat values for male and female competitive swimmers with runners and give possible reasons for the differences

- Summarize body composition characteristics, including body mass index, of early American professional football players and modern-day counterparts; compare modern professionals with current collegiate players

- Contrast body composition characteristics of elite high school wrestlers and less successful counterparts

- Contrast body composition, girths, and excess muscle mass of male and female bodybuilders

- Compare ratios of fat-free body mass (FFM) to fat mass of female bodybuilders with other elite female athletes

- Discuss the upper limit of FFM in "large-sized" athletes

ANCILLARIES ◉ at-a-Glance

Visit http://thepoint.lww.com/mkk8e to access the following resources.

- References: Chapter 29
- Appendix H: Supplemental Animations and Videos
- Interactive Question Bank
- Focus on Research: Body Composition Analysis by Dissection

Body composition evaluation partitions gross body mass into two major structural components—body fat and fat-free body mass (FFM). In Chapter 28, we characterized the major physique differences between men and women of different ages. Pronounced physique differences also exist among participants of the same gender in most high skill sports.

Different anthropometric methodologies have quantified physique status. Visual appraisal often describes individuals as small, medium, and large or as thin (**ectomorphic**), muscular (**mesomorphic**), or fat (**endomorphic**). This older approach, termed *somatotyping* and proposed by psychologist/physician William H. Sheldon (1898–1977), describes body shape by placing a person into categories such as thin or muscular, and grading them on a 1-to-7 scale for ectomorphy, mesomorphy, and endomorphy. He based his somatotypology work on measurements from nude posture photographs taken of undergraduates enrolled in physical education classes (Harvard University, Mt. Holyoke College, Princeton University, Radcliffe College, Smith College, Swarthmore College, Vassar College, Wellesley College, and Yale University) (you can read about this work at www.nytimes.com/1995/01/15/magazine/the-great-ivy-league-nude-posture-photo-scandal.html?pagewanted=all&src=pm). Sheldon's work was turned over to the Smithsonian Institution, which has sealed all public access to the photos (http://www.nytimes.com/1995/01/21/us/nude-photos-are-sealed-at-smithsonian.html). His detractors contend that Sheldon's visual appraisal method attempted to correlate body type differences with social hierarchy (and even intelligence; www.ncbi.nlm.nih.gov/pubmed/18447308). Nonetheless, somatotyping quantifies neither body dimensions (e.g., size of the abdomen in relation to the hips) nor how biceps development compares with thigh or calf development. Somatotyping served previously as a simple but ineffective methodology to analyze meaningful differences in physique status of world-class athletes[5–9,13] and familial heritabilities,[39,58] but in this chapter we focus on the objectively determined body fat and FFM components of body composition.

This chapter examines the physiques of champion athletes in different sport and competition categories. Our review quantifies aspects of physique for Olympic competitors, endurance runners, collegiate and professional American football players, triathletes, high school wrestlers, champion male and female bodybuilders, collegiate gymnasts, PGA golfers, and NBA basketball players. It remains instructive to cite earlier published studies on body composition of top athletes to illustrate basic differences in physique status among highly skilled male and female competitors in different sport categories and changes in this status over time.

PHYSIQUES OF CHAMPION ATHLETES

Early studies of 1964 Tokyo and 1968 Mexico City summer Olympic competitors linked physique to a high level of sports achievement.[13,14,27,43] For swimmers, for example, the best male swimmers were heavier and taller and had larger chest, upper-arm, and thigh girths and upper- and lower-limb lengths than counterparts not ranking in performance among the top 12 athletes. The best female breaststroke swimmers, also taller and heavier, possessed larger arm span, foot and arm lengths, and hand and wrist breadths than less successful competitors. Governing bodies of the different sports should encourage scientific cooperation among exercise physiology and sports medicine researchers to assess body composition. The measurement process should begin early in the development of the most promising young athletes and systematically follow them as they train for higher-level competition. This would provide longitudinal data as the athlete progresses in skill level throughout their competitive endeavors. Subtle differences in physique characteristics among athletes in the same sport may help to unravel an age-old question: "What physique characteristics (and other performance variables) about an athlete make them achieve truly outstanding performances compared to less successful peers in the same sport?"

Michael Phelps—World Champion Swimmer Anomaly?

An anomaly in body proportions seems apparent in world and Olympic champion swimmer Michael Phelps, winner of 18 gold medals and 22 overall medals since the 2004 Athens Olympic Games. Of the 48 men's swimming events in the three Olympics (Athens 2004, Beijing 2008, London 2012), Phelps has amassed 46% of the awarded medals. This equates to more medals won by any of the previous outstanding athletes who participated in multiple Games and won medals in different Games (Carl Lewis, track; Mark Spitz, swimming; Paavo Nurmi, running; and Larisa Latyina, gymnastics). The question arises: What makes Michael Phelps so good?

Limited body composition data are available to shed light on this question. Phelps' arm span measures 203 cm, 10 cm more than his stature. This exceeds the nearly perfect arm to leg to torso ratios of Leonardo da Vinci's Vitruvian Man (see "Notable Achievements by European Scientists," in the Introduction to this text). This, coupled with his foot size of 14 that reportedly bends 15 degrees farther at the ankle than other swimmers,

Michael Phelps, winner of 18 gold medals and 22 overall medals since his first 2004 Athens Olympic games. Image © Mitch Gunn.

TABLE 29.1	Comparison of Swimming Speed in Goldfish and Michael Phelps (100-m butterfly time of 51.25 s)		
		Goldfish	Phelps
Absolute speed, mph		0.85	4.4
Absolute speed, km · hr^{-1}		1.37	7.1
Relative speed, body lengths · s^{-1}		4.5	1.0

turn his feet into virtual "dolphin-like flippers." The added flexibility apparently applies to his knees and elbows, which should theoretically increase the efficiency of the propulsive characteristics of each stroke. Phelps' larger upper body compared to his relatively smaller-proportioned lower body helps to explain his superior thrust through the water at about 4.7 mph, the speed of a brisk walk but not nearly as fast as a small goldfish when adjusted for body length (TABLE 29.1).

Even if one accounts for the Beijing Games Water Cube as one of the world's fastest pools (the 3-m depth is the deepest allowed, and the 10 lanes apparently reduce speed-robbing turbulence), it is difficult to argue that pool characteristics explain how Phelps so convincingly demolished existing world records. A counterargument that the swimsuit Phelps wore during the Games provided the "edge" in these records is that Phelps wore the full-length LZR suit in only three of his eight races—the 200-m freestyle, the 4 × 100-m, and 4 × 200-m freestyle relays. He swam without this suit in his five butterfly and individual medley contests. Phelps and his counterparts did not wear the LZR suit in the 2012 London Games because that equipment was banned from competition by the Fédération Internationale de Natation (FINA; www.fina.org/H2O/), but instead wore redesigned suits to comply with new Olympic suit rules. Phelps's unique physical dimensions coupled with incomparable stroke mechanics honed after thousands of hours and 16 years of carefully supervised workouts obviously played a key role in his extraordinary achievements.

As noted in Chapter 10, a swimmer's morphology alters the horizontal components of lift and drag. Selected anthropometric variables influence the magnitude of propulsive and resistive forces that affect the swimmer's forward movement.[10,11] In well-trained freestyle swimmers, arm length, leg length, and hand and foot size—factors governed largely by genetics—influence stroke length and stroke frequency.[23]

Fat–Free-to-Fat Ratio

FIGURE 29.1 compares the ratio of fat-free body mass (FFM) to fat mass (FM) derived from the world literature for the specific sport among male and female competitors. The *inset tables* present data for average body mass, percentage body fat, and FFM. Male marathon runners and gymnasts have the

largest FFM:FM; American football offensive and defensive linemen and shot putters show the smallest ratios. Among females, bodybuilders have the largest FFM:FM values (equal of males), while the smallest FFM:FMs emerge for field-event participants. Surprisingly, female gymnasts and ballet dancers rank intermediate compared with other female sport participants.

Racial Differences

Racial differences in physique may affect athletic performance.[65,72] Black sprinters and high jumpers, for example, have longer limbs and narrower hips than white counterparts. From a mechanical perspective, a black sprinter with leg and arm size identical to a white sprinter has a lighter, shorter, and slimmer body to propel. This might confer a more favorable power–body mass ratio at any given body size. Greater power output relative to body mass gives an advantage in jumping and sprint-running events where success depends on generating rapid energy for short durations. The advantage diminishes in the throwing events that require propulsion of an absolute mass. Compared with whites and blacks, Asian athletes have short legs relative to upper torso components, a dimensional characteristic beneficial in short- and longer-distance races and in weightlifting. Successful weightlifters of all races compared with other athletic groups have relatively short arms and legs for their stature.

The 1988 Seoul Olympics were a focal point for the start of serious discussions about racial differences in performance, specifically endurance running events because Kenya's top male runners won gold in the 800-m, 1500-m, and 5000-m runs and the 3000-m steeplechase races.[54,75] These East African athletes, from a population of about 500,000 people located in a highland region above the Great Rift Valley (the continuous geographic trench, approximately 6000 km (3700 mi) in length, that runs from northern Syria to central Mozambique in South East Africa), won about 40% of top international distance running competitions—with three times more top finishes than any other country worldwide. The Kenyans won 14 medals in the 2008 Beijing Olympic Games; in 2011, the Kenyans achieved the 20 fastest marathon times. Ironically, Patrick Makau set a new world record of 2:03:38 at the Berlin Marathon in September 2011 but did not make the 2012 London Olympic Games team of runners! From that initial "awakening" in Seoul, considerable research has focused on individual differences in physiological factors (muscle fiber type, $\dot{V}O_{2max}$, fractional $\dot{V}O_{2max}$ utilization, and running economy; see Chapter 14),[3,24,46,51,63,76] including genetic factors[12,15,34,68,69,80] to explain superior athletic accomplishments among some African and non-African groups.

Percentage Body Fat of Elite Athletes

Considerable literature describes body fat levels of male and female competitive athletes in diverse sports.

Body Dimensions Relate to Superior Performance

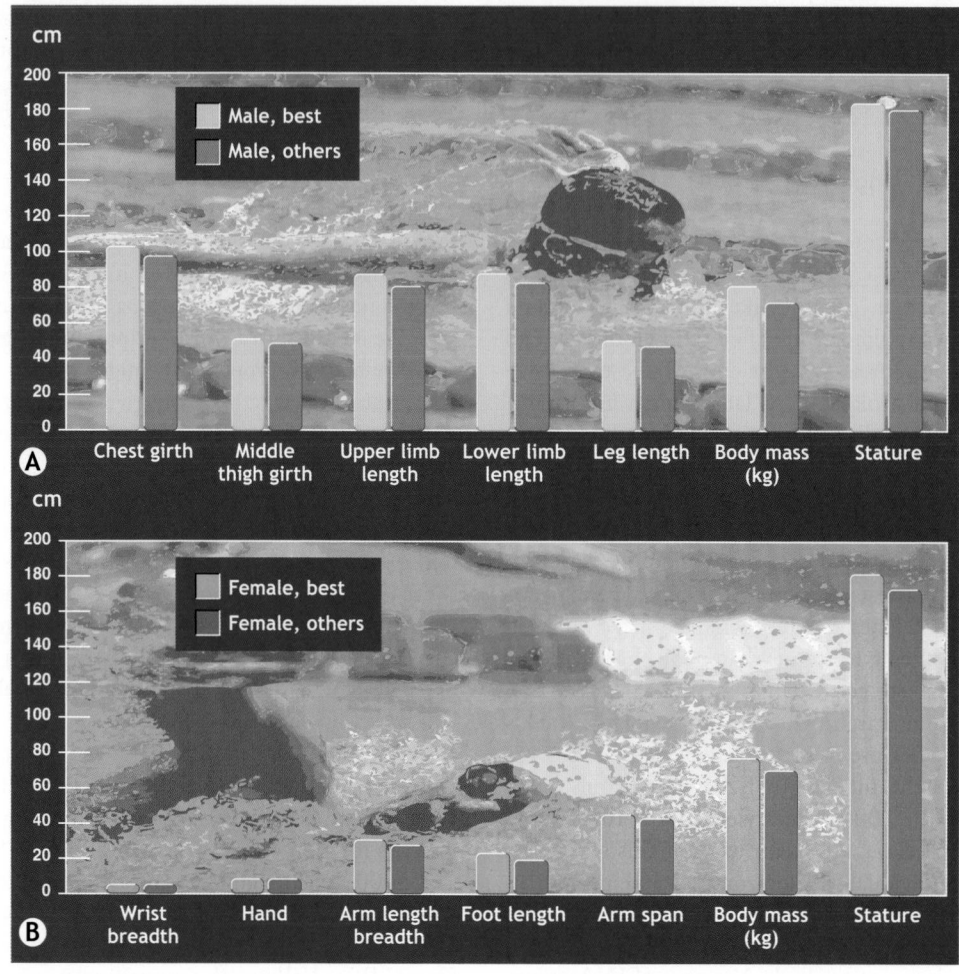

The **(A)** figure compares the body mass, stature, chest girth, upper- and lower-limb girths, and leg length for 12 male swimmers rated "best" in the 200- and 400-m freestyle with less successful counterparts. The **(B)** compares selected body size variables between the 12 "best" 50-, 100-, and 200-m female breaststroke swimmers with other competitors. It is evident that the best male swimmers are heavier and taller and have larger chest, upper-arm, and thigh girths and upper- and lower-limb lengths than counterparts not ranking among the top 12. The best female breaststroke swimmers, also taller and heavier, possess larger arm span, foot and arm lengths, and hand and wrist breadths than less successful competitors. The y-axis (cm) applies to all variables except body mass (kg).

Image reprinted with permission from McArdle WD, Katch FI, Katch VL. *Sports and Exercise Nutrition*. 4th Ed. Philadelphia: Wolters Kluwer Health, 2013, as adapted with permission from Mazza JC, et al. Absolute body size. In: Carter JE, Ackland TR, eds. *Kinanthropometry in Aquatic Sports. A Study of World-Class Athletes*. Champaign, IL: Human Kinetics, 1994.

By Category

FIGURE 29.2 presents six classifications of sports activities based on common characteristics and performance requirements, with percentage body fat rankings within each category for male and female competitors. This compendium provides an overview of percentage body fat of athletes within a broad grouping of relatively similar sports.

Field Event Athletes

FIGURE 29.3 shows body composition obtained by hydrostatic weighing and anthropometry—percentage body fat, fat weight, FFM, and lean-to-fat ratio—for the 10 top American athletes in the discus, shot-put, javelin, and hammer throw 2 years before the 1980 Moscow Olympics. Comparative data describe international elite middle- and long-distance runners

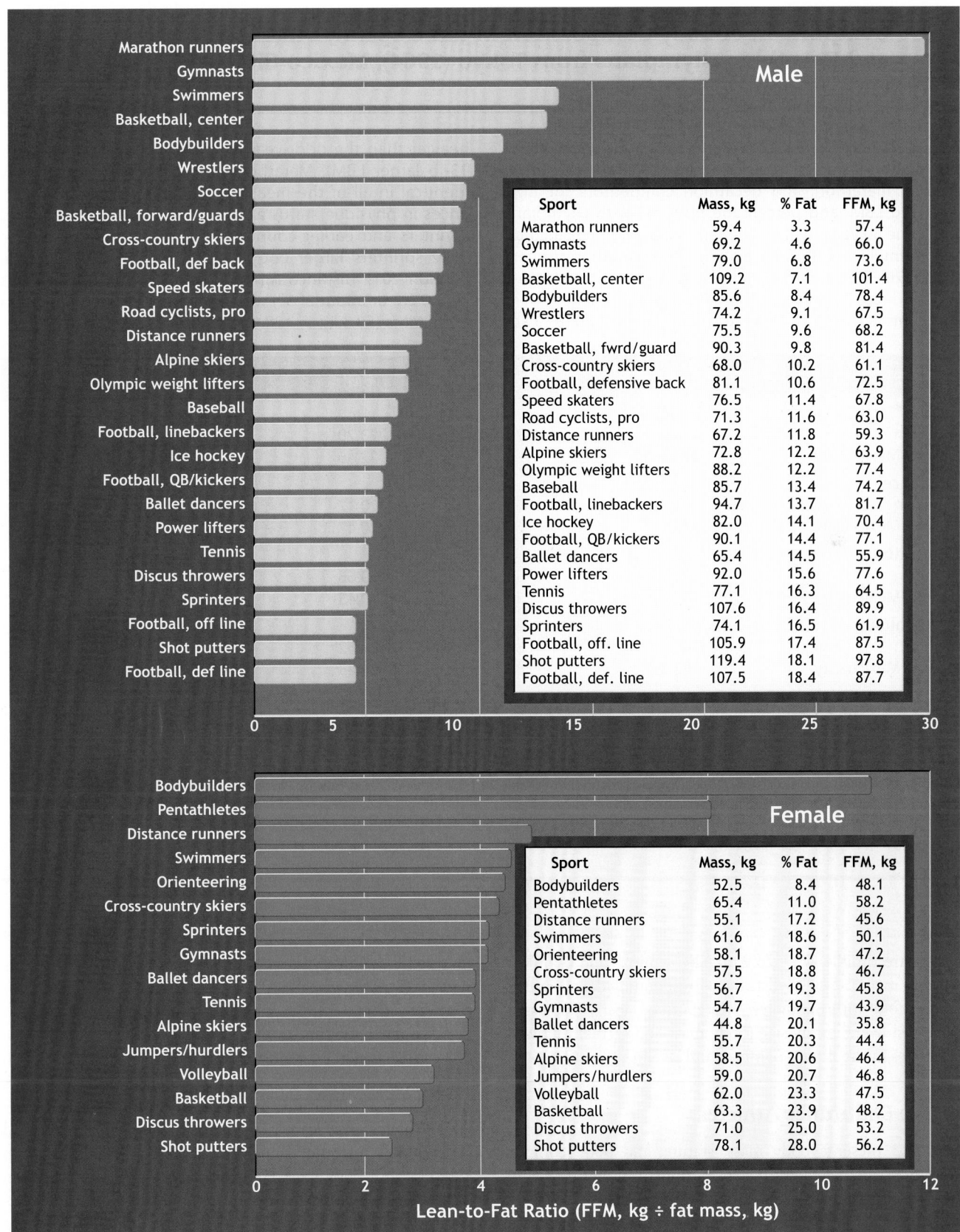

FIGURE 29.1 • Comparison of the lean–fat ratio among male and female competitors in diverse sports. Values are based on the average body mass and percentage body fat for each sport from various studies in the literature. The lean–fat ratio is FFM (kg) ÷ fat mass (kg). Values in the *inset tables* represent averages for body composition if the literature contained two or more citations about a specific sport. The equation of Siri (Chapter 28) converted body density to percentage body fat.

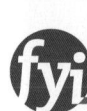

Comparison of Body Composition in Male Sprint, Distance, Marathon, and Decathlon Olympians from Tokyo (1964), Mexico City (1968), and London (2012)

The 2012 London Olympics presented a unique opportunity to compare the current physique status of elite male sprint, distance, marathon, and decathlon competitors for BMI, calculated LBM, and percentage body fat with Olympians from some 50 years earlier. The remarkable findings include the extremely low BMIs for distance and marathon runners (19.7 to 20.2), and the similarity in BMI among the 1964—1968 and 2012 athletes. The 2012 sprint athletes were slightly more than 3 in. taller (8 cm) and almost 20 lb (9 kg) heavier than the prior-year Olympians (and had 5.9-kg or 13-lb larger LBM). Marathoners in both eras were nearly identical in all of the measures; the most apparent differences in physique status among the 2012 decathletes and sprinters and earlier counterparts are highlighted by the 2012 sprinters' larger body weight, height, and LBM. The London 2012 distance runners were the shortest athletes (171.9 cm or about 5' 5") while marathoners were lowest in body mass (58.3 kg or 128.6 lb).

EVENT[a]	Height, cm	Weight, kg	BMI	LBM,[b] kg	Body Fat[c]
Sprint[d]					
London	184.9	79.3	23.20	69.7	12.1
Tokyo, Mexico City[e]	176.9	70.3	22.46	63.8	9.2
Distance[f]					
London	171.9	62.8	20.17	60.3	4.0
Tokyo, Mexico City	172.8	61.1	20.47	60.9	3.3
Marathon					
London	172.2	58.3	19.66	60.5	NA[g]
Tokyo, Mexico City	169.5	58.7	20.43	58.6	1.7
Decathlon					
London	188.0	87.0	24.62	72.1	7.5
Tokyo, Mexico City	182.3	80.5	24.23	67.8	15.8

[a]Top 8 finishers, 2012 London Olympics.
[b]Calculated by Behnke's method: LBM (lean body mass) = h² × 0.204, where h = stature, dm (from reference 2).
[c]Body fat (%) = (Body mass − LBM)/Body mass × 100.
[d]Sprint athletes included 100 m, 200 m, 4 × 100 m, 110-m hurdles.
[e]Data for Tokyo (1964) and Mexico City (1968) Olympics adapted from Table 29.1, McArdle, WD et al. *Exercise Physiology. Energy, Nutrition, and Human Performance*. 7th Ed. Baltimore: Lippincott Williams & Wilkins, 2010.
[f]Distance athletes included 3000 steeplechase, 5000 m, 10,000 m.
[g]Could not compute because average body mass lower than calculated LBM.

(average treadmill $\dot{V}O_{2max}$ 76.9 mL·kg⁻¹·min⁻¹) and Behnke's reference man. TABLE 29.2 lists the corresponding data for girth and skinfold anthropometry. Shot putters clearly possessed the largest overall body size (body mass and girths) followed by athletes in the discus, hammer, and javelin throw.

Female Endurance Athletes

TABLE 29.3 presents body mass, stature, and body composition of 11 female long-distance runners of national and international caliber.[78] The runners averaged 15.2% body fat (hydrostatic weighing), similar to reported data for high school cross-country runners but considerably lower than the 26% body fat for sedentary females of the same age, stature, and body mass.[2,35] Compared with other athletic groups, the runners have relatively less fat than collegiate basketball players (20.9%),[61] gymnasts (15.5%),[62] younger distance runners (18%),[43] swimmers (20.1%),[37] tennis players (22.8%),[37] or triathletes.[28]

Interestingly, the runners' average body fat equaled the 15% value generally reported for nonathletic males. The 6 to 9% body fat levels of several apparently healthy runners in Table 29.3 fall within the range for topflight male endurance athletes. The leanest women in the population, based on Behnke's reference standards, have essential fat equal to 12 to 14% of body mass. This apparent discrepancy between estimated fat content of distance runners and the theoretical lower limit for body fat in women requires further study. Note the relatively high body fat (35.4%) for one of the best runners, suggesting that, at least for this runner, other factors override the "dead weight" and the regulatory limitations to distance running imposed by excess fat.

Male Endurance Athletes

TABLE 29.4 presents body composition data for 10 male elite middle- and long-distance runners and eight elite marathoners. The group included Steve Prefontaine, former American record holder in the 800- and 1500-m runs, and Frank Shorter, the 1976 Olympic gold medalist in the marathon. A representative sample of 95 untrained college-age men provides comparison data. Both groups of runners have extremely low body fat values considering that essential fat theoretically constitutes about 3% of body mass. Clearly, these competitors represent the lower end of the lean-to-fat continuum for top-flight endurance athletes.

For body dimensions and structure, male distance runners generally have smaller girths and bone diameters than untrained males.[13] Structural differences, particularly bone diameters, reflect a genetic influence similar to the distinct anthropometric characteristics typical of world-class aquatic athletes.[5] The best long-distance runners inherit a slight build with well-proportioned skeletal dimensions. *The prime ingredients for a champion include a genetically optimal physique profile blended with a lean body composition, highly developed aerobic system, optimal distribution of muscle fiber architecture, and proper psychologic mindset for protracted intense training.* Interestingly, the body size and composition (length of lower limbs, skinfold thicknesses, circumference of extremities, skeletal muscle mass, BMI, and percentage body fat) and training volume (weekly training hours, running years, the number of finished marathons) of male Caucasian ultraendurance runners is not as important as their personal best marathon time in predicting performance in a 24-hr endurance race.[40]

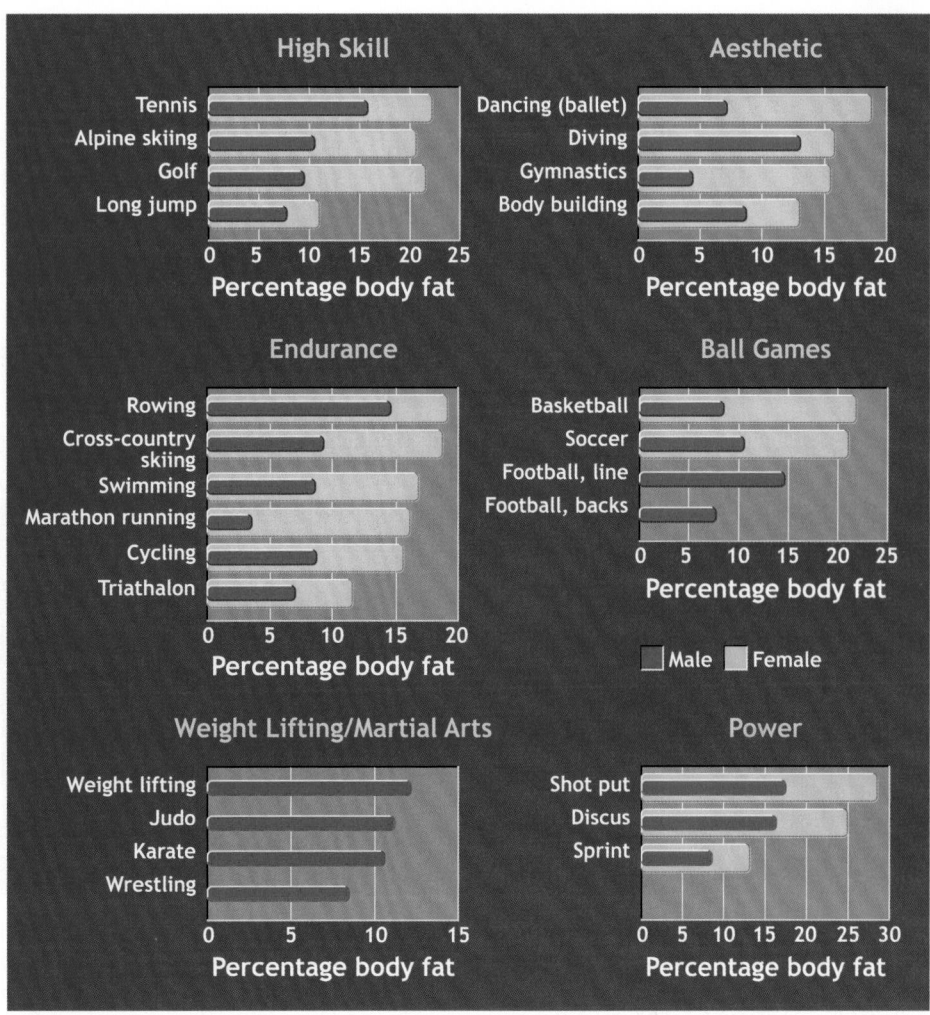

FIGURE 29.2 • Percentage body fat in athletes grouped by sport category. The value for males is displayed within the bar (in *red*) when a corresponding value exists for females (in *yellow*). The values for percentage body fat (from body density by the Siri equation) represent averages from the literature.

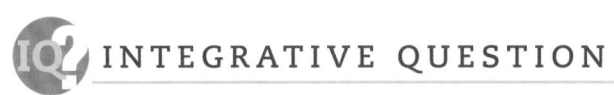

INTEGRATIVE QUESTION

Discuss the physiologic and anthropometric characteristics necessary for successful endurance running performance.

Swimmer Sets Swim Record from Cuba to Florida and Expends 29,000 Calories

On September 3, 2013, Diana Nyad, a 64-year-old endurance swimmer, made a record-setting 110 mile, non-stop swim without a shark cage, from Havana, Cuba to Key West, Florida. She completed the swim in about 54 hours, treading water at intervals to consume food and drink, and averaged 1.6 mph. We have estimated her total caloric expenditure during the swim as roughly 29,000 kcal, based on an average swim velocity of 0.715 m.s^{-1} (1 mph = 0.447 m.s^{-1}). Figure 10.13 shows the oxygen consumption for front crawl swimming for elite swimmers, and using her swim velocity of 0.715 m.s^{-1} translates to about 1.8 L.min^{-1} or 9 kcal per min, or in 54 hours (3240 min), roughly 29,000 kcal. In 1975, Nyad completed a swim around Manhattan, NY, in slightly less than 8 hours, and four years later, swam 102 miles from North Bimini, Bahamas to Juno Beach, FL in about 28 hours.

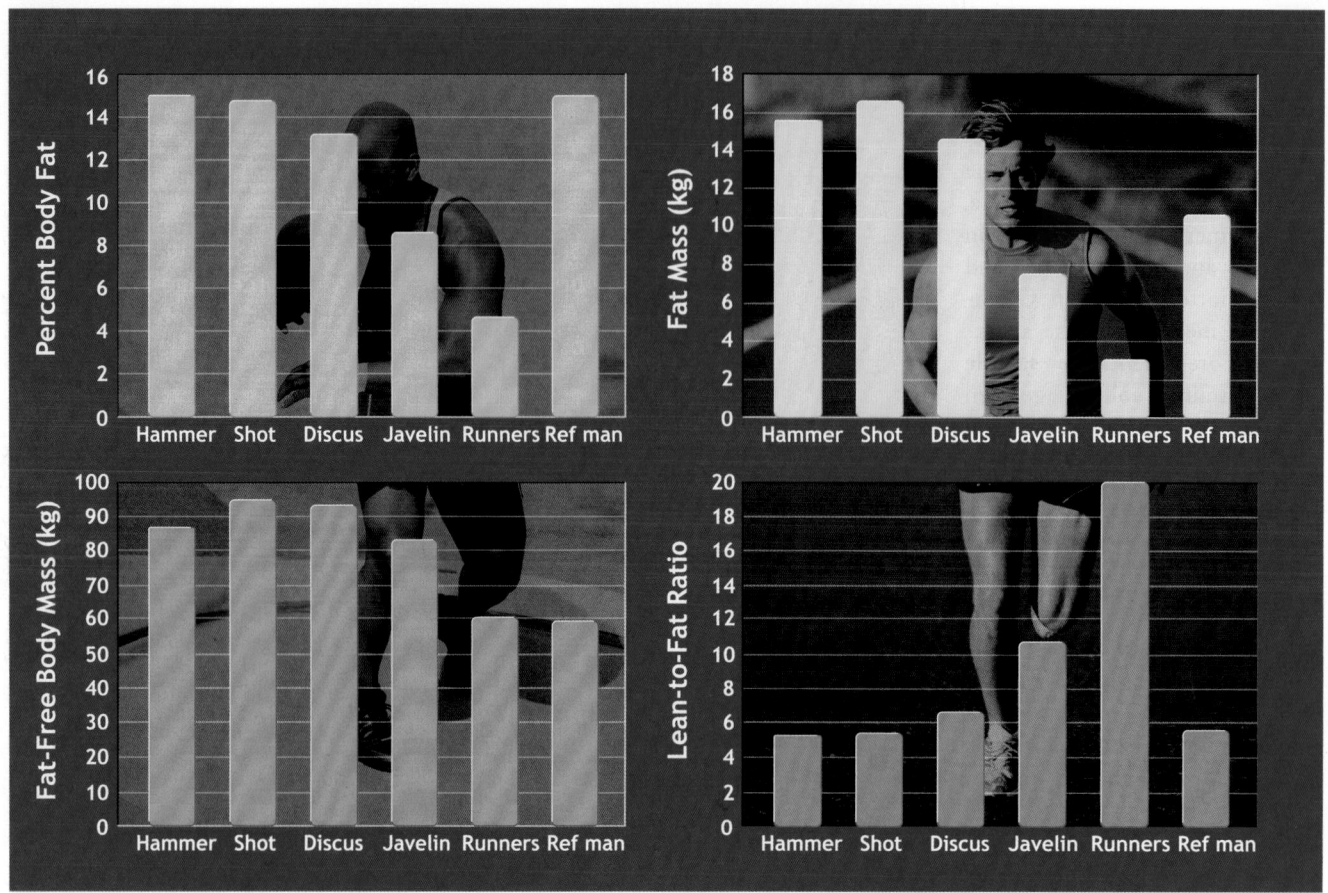

FIGURE 29.3 • Body composition determined by hydrostatic weighing of the top 10 American male athletes in the discus, shot-put, javelin, and hammer throw. Data collected by textbook authors (FK and VK) at a 1978 U.S. Olympic minicamp at the University of Houston, Houston, TX. Athletes include former gold medalist Wilkins (discus) and world record holder Powell (discus). (Data for the international elite middle- and long-distance runners from Pollock ML, et al. Body composition of elite class distance runners. *Ann NY Acad Sci* 1977;301:361. Reference man [*Ref man*] data from Behnke's model in Chapter 28.)

Triathletes. The triathlon combines continuous endurance performance in swimming, bicycling, and running. The extreme triathlon, the ultraendurance Ironman competition, requires competitors to first swim 3.9 km (2.4 mi), then bicycle 180.2 km (112 mi), and finish with a standard marathon run of 42.2 km (26.2 mi). The course records for the Ironman triathlon in Kailua-Kona, Hawaii, stand at 8:03:56 for men, set in 2011 by Australian Craig Alexander, and for women in 2009 by Britain's Chrissie Wellington with a winning time of 8:54:02. The serious triathlete's training averages nearly 4 hr daily, covering a total of 280 miles a week by swimming 7.2 miles (30:00 min per mi pace), bicycling 227 miles (18.6 mph), and running 45 miles (7:42 min per mi pace).[55] Percentage body fat of six male and three female participants in the 1982 Ironman triathlon ranged between 5.0 and 11.3% for men and 7.4 and 17.2% for women. Body fat averaged 7.1% for the top 15 male finishers, with corresponding $\dot{V}O_{2max}$ of 72.0 mL · kg^{-1} · min^{-1}. In subsequent research, body fat was unrelated to training volume for both men (14.4%) and

women (22.8%).[41] The authors concluded that body fat correlated weakly to total race time in male and female triathletes. A follow-up study showed that low levels of body fat and a high training volume benefited ultraendurance triathletes in cycling and running, whereas cycling speed in training benefited total race time.[42] Triathletes' body fat content and aerobic capacity are comparable to those of other athletes in single endurance sports,[57] with an overall physique most closely resembling that of elite cyclists[56] or swimmers[47] rather than runners. Aerobic capacity of these athletes during swimming consistently averages below values during treadmill running or stationary cycling.[44] Significant reductions occurred in percentage body fat and skeletal muscle mass following one ultraendurance event in which athletes swam 11.6 km, cycled 540 km, and ran 126.6 km within 58 hr.[1]

A longitudinal study evaluated the effects of a triathlon season on bone dynamics and hormonal status in seven male competitive triathletes at the beginning of training and 32 wk later.[50] Total and regional bone mineral density (BMD) was

TABLE 29.2	Skinfold and Girth Anthropometry of the Top 10 American Athletes in the Discus, Shot-Put, Javelin, and Hammer Throw					
Measurement[a]	Discus	Shot-Put	Javelin	Hammer	Runners	Ref Man
Body mass, kg	108.2	112.3	90.6	104.2	63.1	70.0
Stature, cm	191.7	187.0	186.0	187.3	177.0	174.0
Skinfolds, mm						
Triceps	13.0	15.0	11.9	12.7	5.0	—
Scapular	18.0	23.8	12.5	21.5	6.4	—
Iliac	24.5	29.6	17.0	27.4	4.6	—
Abdomen	25.6	31.4	18.4	29.1	7.1	—
Thigh	16.4	15.7	13.3	17.3	6.1	—
Girths, cm						
Shoulders	129.8	133.3	121.5	127.4	106.1	110.8
Chest	113.5	118.5	104.6	111.3	91.1	91.8
Waist	94.1	99.1	86.6	94.8	74.6	77.0
Abdomen	97.5	101.5	87.8	98.0	74.2	79.8
Hips	110.4	112.3	102.0	108.7	87.8	93.4
Thighs	66.3	69.4	61.5	67.3	51.9	54.8
Knees	41.5	42.9	40.0	41.0	36.2[b]	36.6
Calves	42.6	43.6	39.5	41.5	35.4	35.8
Ankles	25.4	24.9	24.1	24.3	21.0	22.5
Biceps	41.8	42.2	37.7	39.9	28.2	31.7
Forearms	33.1	33.7	30.8	32.4	26.4	26.4
Wrists	18.7	18.9	18.2	18.4	16.0	17.3
Diameters, cm						
Biacromial	44.5	43.8	43.2	44.8	39.5	40.6
Chest	33.1	33.7	30.8	32.6	31.3	30.0
Bi-iliac	31.3	31.2	29.6	30.4	28.0	28.6
Bitrochanter	35.5	34.9	33.7	34.8	32.2	32.8
Knee	10.2	10.5	10.0	10.2	9.5	9.3
Wrist	6.3	6.2	6.0	6.2	5.6	5.6
Ankle	7.6	7.6	7.5	7.4	—	7.0
Elbow	7.6	7.6	7.6	7.2	—	7.0

[a]Details about measurement procedures from Katch FI, Katch VL. The body composition profile: techniques of measurement and applications. *Clin Sports Med* 1984;3:31. Data correspond to the athletic groups presented in Figure 29.3.
[b]Not measured; value computed from the ratio for the reference man calf to knee.

determined by dual-energy x-ray absorptiometry, and specific biochemical markers assessed bone turnover. The triathlon season had a small but favorable effect on BMD at the lumbar spine and skull, but no effect on total body or proximal femur BMD. No changes occurred in hormonal levels. For nine professional cyclists who participated in the Giro d'Italia 3-wk stage race in Italy, markers of bone activity measured 1 day prerace, and 12 and 22 days during the race indicated resorption of bone brought on by the race.[48]

Swimmers versus Runners

Male and female competitive swimmers generally have higher body fat levels than distance runners, despite swim training's considerable energy requirement. The cool water of the training environment generally produces lower core temperatures than equivalent land exercise. Speculation exists that a lower core temperature in swim training may prevent the depressed appetite that often accompanies intense training on land.

Limited evidence indicates similar daily energy intake for male collegiate swimmers (3380 kcal) and distance runners (3460 kcal), which balances training energy expenditure. In contrast, female swimmers averaged a higher daily energy intake of 2490 kcal compared with 2040 kcal for running counterparts.[33] Swimmers had higher estimated daily energy expenditure than runners. The swimmers' energy expenditure surpassed energy intake, placing them in a slightly *negative* energy balance. A *positive* energy balance with intake greater than output cannot explain typically higher body fat levels in male (12%) and female (20%) swimmers than in male (7%) and female (15%) runners.

TABLE 29.3		Body Composition of Female Endurance Runners				
Subject	Age (y)	Stature (cm)	Mass (kg)	FFM (kg)	Body Fat (kg)	(%)
1[a]	24	172.7	52.6	49.5	3.1	5.9
2[b]	26	159.8	71.5	46.2	25.3	35.4
3[c]	28	162.6	50.7	47.6	3.1	6.1
4	31	171.5	52.0	47.3	4.7	9.0
5	33	176.5	61.2	50.8	10.4	17.0
6	34	166.4	52.9	44.8	8.1	15.2
7	35	168.4	55.0	48.7	6.3	11.6
8	36	164.5	53.1	44.3	8.8	16.6
9	36	182.9	61.5	50.4	11.1	18.1
10	36	182.9	65.4	55.7	9.7	14.8
11	37	154.9	53.6	44.0	9.6	18.0
Average	32.4	169.4	57.2	48.1	9.1	15.2

[a]World's best time in marathon (2:49:40) as of 1974.
[b]World's best time in 50-mile run (7:04:31); established 18 mo after the body composition evaluation.
[c]Noted U.S. distance runner. Five consecutive national and international cross-country championships.
Reprinted from Wilmore JH, Brown CH. Physiological profiles of women distance runners. *Med Sci Sports* 1974;6:178.

TABLE 29.4		Body Composition Characteristics of Elite Male Middle- and Long-Distance Runners and Elite Marathoners					
Group	Stature (cm)	Mass (kg)	Density (g·cm^{-3})	Body Fat (%)	FFM (kg)	Fat Mass (kg)	Sum 7 Skinfolds (mm)
Distance runners							
Brown	187.3	72.10	1.07428	10.8	64.31	7.79	53.0
Castaneda	178.6	63.34	1.09102	3.7	61.00	2.34	32.5
Crawford	171.8	58.01	1.09702	1.2	57.31	0.70	32.5
Geis	179.1	66.28	1.07551	10.2	59.52	6.76	49.0
Johnson	174.6	61.79	1.08963	4.3	59.13	2.66	35.5
Manley	177.8	69.10	1.09642	1.5	68.06	1.04	32.0
Ndoo	169.3	53.97	1.08379	6.7	50.35	3.62	33.5
Prefontaine	174.2	68.00	1.08842	4.8	64.74	3.26	38.0
Rose	175.6	59.15	1.08248	7.3	54.83	4.32	31.5
Tuttle	176.8	61.44	1.09960	0.2	61.32	0.12	31.5
Mean	170.5	60.92	1.08916	4.5	58.18	2.74	34.5
Marathon runners							
Cusack	174.6	64.19	1.08096	7.9	59.12	5.07	45.5
Galloway	180.9	65.76	1.08419	6.6	61.42	4.34	43.0
Kennedy	167.0	56.52	1.09348	2.7	54.99	1.53	37.0
Moore	184.1	64.24	1.09193	3.3	62.12	2.12	37.0
Pate	179.6	57.28	1.09676	1.3	56.54	0.74	32.5
Shorter	178.4	61.17	1.09475	2.2	59.82	1.35	45.0
Wayne	172.1	61.61	1.07859	8.9	56.13	5.48	42.5
Williams	177.2	66.07	1.09569	1.8	64.88	1.19	41.5
Mean	176.8	62.11	1.08954	4.3	59.38	2.73	40.5

Data from Pollock ML, et al. Body composition of elite class distance runners. *Ann NYAcad Sci* 1977;301:361.

Subsequent research from the same laboratory evaluated energy expenditure and fuel use for swimmers and runners during each form of training (45 min at 75 to 80% $\dot{V}O_{2max}$) and 2 hr recovery.[19] The hypothesis assumed that differences in hormonal response and substrate catabolism between the two activity modes accounted for body fat differences between groups. The small between-group differences in energy expenditure, substrate use, and hormone levels could not account for body fat differences.

American Football Players

The first detailed body composition analyses of American professional football players in the early 1940s demonstrated the inadequacy of determining a person's optimal body mass from height–weight standards.[74] The body fat content of the players averaged only 10.4% of body mass, while FFM averaged 81.3 kg. Certainly these men were heavy but not "fat." The heaviest lineman weighed 118 kg (260 lb) (17.4% body fat; 97.7 kg FFM), whereas the lineman with the most body fat (23.2%) weighed 115.4 kg (254 lb). Body mass of a defensive back with the least fat (3.3%) was 82.3 kg (181 lb) with an FFM of 79.6 kg.

TABLE 29.5 presents a clearer picture of average values for body mass, stature, percentage body fat, and FFM of college and professional football players grouped by position.[77,79] The *Pro, older* group consists of 25 players from the 1942 Washington Redskins, the first professional players measured for body composition by hydrostatic weighing. The *Pro, modern* group consists of 164 players from 14 teams in the National Football League (NFL; 69% veterans, 31% rookies). One hundred seven members of the 1976–1978 Dallas Cowboys and New York Jets make up the third group. Four groups of collegiate players include candidates for spring practice at St. Cloud State College in Minnesota, the University of Massachusetts (U Mass), and Division III Gettysburg College, and teams from 1973–1977 University of Southern California (USC) national champions and participants in two Rose Bowls. Body composition measurements for this data set featured the criterion hydrostatic weighing with correction for measured residual lung volume.

One would generally expect modern-day professional players to have a larger body size at each position than a representative collegiate group. This occurred for comparisons with St. Cloud and U Mass players, but the USC players generally maintained a physique similar to that of modern professionals. With the exception of defensive linemen, the USC players at each position showed nearly the same body fat content as current professionals but they weighed less. For FFM, the USC players weighed no more than 4.4 kg less than professionals at each position. The average defensive lineman in the NFL outweighed his USC counterpart in FFM by only 1.8 kg. Total body mass of the professional linemen exceeded USC counterparts, primarily because the professionals possessed 18.2% body fat versus the collegians'

14.7%. These data suggest that in general, elite college and professional players maintain similar body size and body composition.

As a group, professional players of almost 75 years ago were lower in body fat (10.4%), shorter, and had lower total body mass and FFM than professionals of 30 years ago. The exceptions, defensive and offensive backs and receivers, were almost identical to current players in body size and composition. The biggest differences in physique emerged for the defensive linemen; modern players were 6.7 cm taller, 20 kg heavier, fatter by 4.2 percentage points of body fat, and had 12.3 kg more FFM. Obviously, "bigness" was not an important factor in line play during the 1940s. To illustrate this point, FIGURE 29.4A shows the average body weights for all roster players in the NFL ($n = 51,333$) over a 76-year period.[36] From 1920 to 1985, offensive linemen were the heaviest players; this changed beginning with the 1990 season, when defensive linemen achieved the same body mass as offensive linemen and then surpassed them. The body weight for offensive linemen appeared to have leveled off at nearly 280 lb (127 kg), but the weigh of defensive linemen continued to increase, particularly from 1990 to 1996, when they averaged 16 lb more (double the weight gain for offensive linemen for the comparable period). On average, offensive linemen were 1.3 lb per year heavier from 1920 to 1995. At this rate of increase, they should have attained 300-plus lb by the year 2007 (with an average height of 6' 8")! At this size, BMI would be 35.2, classifying them as high for disease risk. Not surprisingly, the data for the height–weight statistics for the 2007 (and 2008) Super Bowl offensive and defensive lines exceeded these predictions, where average body mass exceeded 300 lb (136 kg). This comparison clearly placed the team BMI values of 37.0 and 37.5 in the "obese" category (TABLE 29.6). Data for the 2012 and 2013 Super Bowl teams revealed similar findings for BMI excess for the 2009 data, the number of 300-pounders per team averaged 12 players at this weight. If we assume that the 2013 player rosters carry the average number of 300-pounders as the 2012 Super Bowl teams (15 for Patriots and 13 for Giants), then 14 players per team would predict that 448 players on the 32 NFL teams would exceed 330 lb (150 kg). At this rate of increase, the 2015 season will see a record of more than 500 players with a body weight in excess of 330 lb and projected to 1000 players in 2020!

The BMI data for 2168 NFL players based on 2004 team rosters were consistent with the data presented in Figure 29.4 and Table 29.6—almost all of the players had a BMI that exceeded 25 (97%), 56% had BMIs greater than 30, 26% had BMIs greater than 35, and 3% had BMIs greater than 40.[25] Compared to 20- to 39-year-old men in a 1999–2002 national survey, the percentage of NFL players within the same age range with a BMI of 30 or greater was twice that of the national sample (56% vs. 23%). The percentage of players with a BMI of 40 or greater was similar to that among

TABLE 29.5 **Body Composition of Collegiate and Professional Football Players Grouped by Position**

Position[a]	Level	nF	Stature (cm)	Mass (kg)	Body Fat (%)	FFM (kg)
Defensive backs	St. Cloud[b]	15	178.3	77.3	11.5	68.4
	U Mass[c]	12	179.9	83.1	8.8	76.8
	USC[d]	15	183.0	83.7	9.6	75.7
	Gettysburg[e]	16	175.9	79.8	13.6	68.9
	Pro, modern[f]	26	182.5	84.8	9.6	76.7
	Pro, older[g]	25	183.0	91.2	10.7	81.4
Offensive backs and receivers	St. Cloud	15	179.7	79.8	12.4	69.6
	U Mass	29	181.8	84.1	9.5	76.4
	USC	18	185.6	86.1	9.9	77.6
	Gettysburg	18	176.0	78.3	12.9	68.2
	Pro, modern	40	183.8	90.7	9.4	81.9
	Pro, older	25	183.0	91.7	10.0	87.5
Linebackers	St. Cloud	7	180.1	87.2	13.4	75.4
	U Mass	17	186.1	97.1	13.1	84.2
	USC	17	185.6	98.8	13.2	85.8
	Gettysburg	—	—	—	—	—
	Pro, modern	28	188.6	102.2	14.0	87.6
Offensive linemen and tight ends	St. Cloud	13	186.0	99.2	19.1	79.8
	U Mass	23	187.5	107.6	19.5	86.6
	Gettysburg	15	182.6	110.4	26.2	81.0
	USC	25	191.1	106.5	15.3	90.3
	Pro, modern	38	193.0	112.6	15.6	94.7
Defensive linemen	St. Cloud	15	186.6	97.8	18.5	79.3
	U Mass	8	188.8	114.3	19.5	91.9
	USC	13	191.1	109.3	14.7	93.2
	Gettysburg	11	178.0	99.4	21.9	77.6
	Pro, modern	32	192.4	117.1	18.2	95.8
	Pro, older	25	185.7	97.1	14.0	83.5
All positions	St. Cloud	65	182.5	88.0	15.0	74.2
	U Mass	91	184.9	97.3	13.9	83.2
	USC	88	186.6	96.6	11.4	84.6
	Gettysburg	60	178.0	90.6	18.1	73.3
	Pro, modern	164	188.1	101.5	13.4	87.3
	Pro, older	25	183.1	91.2	10.4	81.3
	Dallas-Jets[h]	107	188.2	100.4	12.6	87.7

[a]Grouping according to Wilmore JH, Haskel WL. Body composition and endurance capacity of professional football players. *J Appl Physiol* 1972;33:564.
[b]Data from Wickkiser JD, Kelly JM. The body composition of a college football team. *Med Sci Sports* 1975;7:199.
[c]UMass data from Coach Robert Stull and F Katch, University of Massachusetts. Data collected during spring practice, 1985; %fat by densitometry.
[d]USC data from Dr. Robert Girandola, University of Southern California, Los Angeles, 1978, 1993.
[e]Data courtesy of Dr. Kristin Steumple, Department of Exercise and Sport Science, Gettysburg College, Gettysburg, PA, 2000.
[f]Data from Wilmore JH, et al. Football pros' strengths—and CV weakness—charted. *Phys Sportsmed* 1976;4:45.
[g]Data from Dr. A. R. Behnke.
[h]Data from Katch FI, Katch, VL. Body composition of the Dallas Cowboys and New York Jets football teams, unpublished, 1978.

20- to 39-year-old men in a 1999–2002 survey (3.0% vs. 3.7%). Compared to the National Institutes of Health classification categories of obesity (Chapter 30), 564 players (36% of the sample) qualified as obesity class 2, with 65 players in obesity class 3. The authors concluded, as have we, based on the most recent BMI data for NFL players, that the high prevalence of obesity (overweight based on BMI) in this group of large men warrants further investigation to determine the long-term health consequences of excessive weight compared to stature. The roster data for each of the 2007 and 2008 NFL teams (including 2010 to 2013 rosters) make this very point—large-sized athletes, in the short term, are at higher-than-normal risk for a variety of diseases based on their body size. It also may be of interest to note that the top

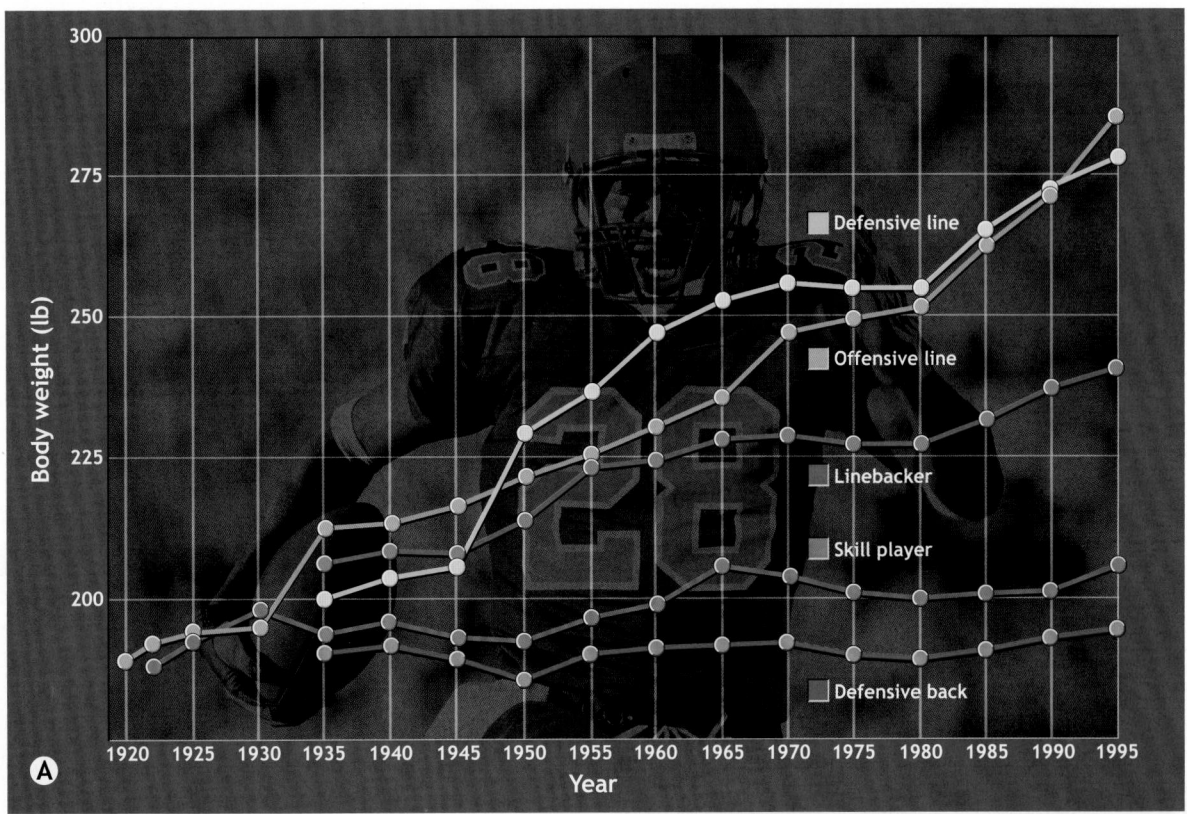

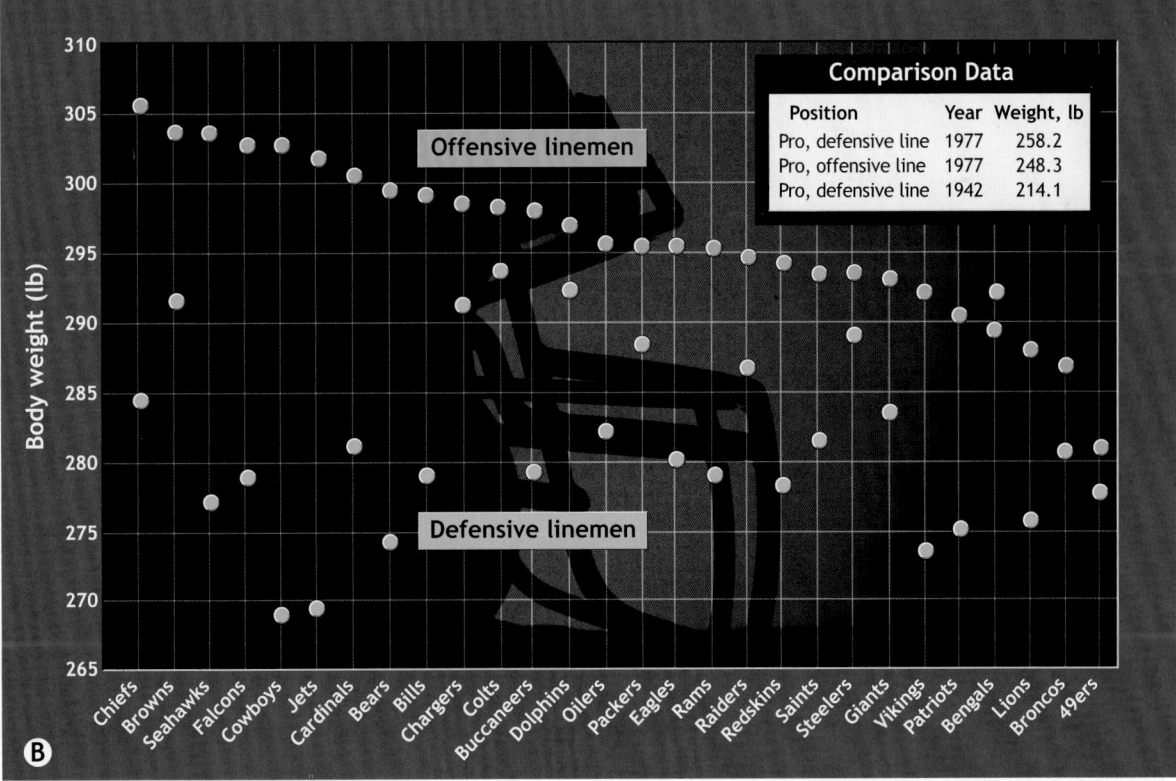

FIGURE 29.4 • **(A)** Average body weight by position for all roster players in the NFL between 1920 and 1995. **(B)** Average body weight of all roster offensive and defensive linemen in the NFL in 1994. Team rankings progress from the heaviest to lightest body weight for the team's offensive linemen. (From active team rosters for 28 NFL teams as of the first regular-season weekend, September 4–5, 1994.) The comparison body weight data for the pro offensive and defensive line (1977) shown in the *inset box* are combined data for the New York Jets and Dallas Cowboys football teams (collected by textbook authors FK and VK). The 1942 data were provided by Dr. Albert Behnke from his studies of the Washington Redskins. (Data courtesy of the National Football League public relations department.)

IN A PRACTICAL SENSE

Predicting Body Fat from Skinfolds, Girths, and BIA Measurements for Different Athletic Groups

Appropriate assessment of body composition allows determination of optimal body weight for competition, comparisons between athletes within the same sport, and monitoring changes in the body's lean and fat components resulting from dietary modification and/or exercise training. A valid appraisal of body composition also provides an important first step in identifying potential eating disorders and formulating nutritional counseling. In the absence of body fat appraisal by hydrostatic weighing, predictions using skinfolds and/or girth measurements and bioelectric impedance analysis (BIA) have been used for diverse athletic groups.

The body's fat-free component can vary, making multicomponent models most effective to convert whole-body density to percentage body fat. The accompanying table presents population-specific skinfold, anthropometric (girth), and BIA equations for body composition assessment of athletes in general and in specific sport categories.

Method	Sport	Gender	Equation	Reference
Skinfolds	All	Women (18-29 yr)	Db (g · cm^{-3})^a = 1.096095 - 0.0006952 (Σ4SKF)^b + 0.0000011 (Σ4SKF)^2 - 0.0000714 (age)	32
	All	Boys (14-19 yr)	Db (g · cm^{-3})^a = 1.10647 - 0.00162 (subscapular SKF) - 0.00144 (abdomen SKF) - 0.00077 (triceps SKF) + 0.00071 (midaxillary SKF)	20
	All	Men (18-29 yr)	Db (g · cm^{-3})^a = 1.112 - 0.00043499 (Σ7SKF)^c + 0.00000055 (Σ7SKF) - 0.00028826 (age)	31
	All	Men and Women	%BF = 10.566 + 0.12077 (7SKF)^d - 8.057 (gender) - 2.545 (race)	16
	Wrestling	Boys (HS)	Db (g · cm^{-3})^a = 1.0982 - 0.000815 (Σ3SKF)^e - 0.00000084 (Σ3SKF)^2	67
BIA	All	Women (NR)	FFM (kg) = 0.73 (HT^2/R) + 0.23 (X$_c$) + 0.16 (BW) + 2.0	30
	All	Women (college)	FFM (kg) = 0.73 (HT^2/R) + 0.116 (BW) + 0.096 (X$_c$) - 4.03	49
	All	Men (college)	FFM (kg) = 0.734 (HT^2/R) + 0.116 (BW) + 0.096 (X$_c$) - 3.152	49
	All	Men (19-40 yr)	FFM (kg) = 1.949 + 0.701 (BW) + 0.186 (HT^2/R)	55
Anthropometry (girths)	All	Women (18-23 yr)	FFM (kg) = 0.757 (BW) + 0.981 (neck C) - 0.516 (thigh C) + 0.79	53
	Ballet	Females (11-25 yr)	FFM (kg) = 0.73 (BW) + 3.0	26
	Wrestling	Boys (13-18 yr)	Db (g · cm^{-3})^a = 1.12691 - 0.00357 (arm C) - 0.00127 (AB C) + 0.00524 (forearm C)	35
	Football	White men (18-23 yr)	%BF = 55.2 + 0.481 (BW) - 0.468 (HT)	29

Modified from Heyward VH, Stolarczyk LM. Applied body composition assessment. Champaign, IL: Human Kinetics, 1996.

^{a}Use the following formulas to convert body density (Db) to % body fat (BF): Men %BF = [(4.95/Db) - 4.50] X 100; Women %BF = [(5.01/Db) - 4.57] X 100; Boys (7-12yr) %BF = [(5.30/Db) - 4.89] X 100; Boys (13-16yr) %BF = [(5.07/Db) - 4.64] X 100; Boys (17-19yr) %BF = [(4.99/Db) - 4.55] X 100. ^{b}4SKF (mm) = sum of four skinfolds: triceps + anterior suprailiac + abdomen + thigh. ^{c}7SKF (mm) = sum of seven skinfolds: chest + midaxillary + triceps + subscapular + abdomen + anterior suprailiac + thigh. ^{d}7SKF(mm) = subscapular + triceps + chest + midaxillary + suprailiac + abdominal + thigh; gender = 0 for female, 1 for male; race = 0 for white, 1 for black. ^{e}HT = height (cm); R = resistance (Ω); Xc = reactance (Ω); BW = body weight (kg); C= circumference (cm); thigh (cm) at the gluteal fold; AB (cm): average abdominal circumference = [(AB$_1$ + AB$_2$)/2], where AB$_1$ (cm) = abdominal circumference anteriorly midway between the xyphoid process of the sternum and umbilicus, and laterally between the lower end of the rib cage and iliac crests, and AB$_2$ (cm) = abdominal circumference at the umbilicus level; NR = age not reported; HS = high school.

50 NFL running backs of all time from 1970 to 2007 (based on total yards rushed) had an average BMI of 29.6 (range 35.1–25.8); it was only slightly higher at 29.7 for the top 10 rushers (www.pro-football-reference.com/blog/?p=489; www.dailyiowan.com). The relationship between total yards rushed and BMI for these 50 exceptional running backs was $r = 0.14$, indicating that for this select group a player's BMI does not relate to on-field achievements. This low correlation is due in part to the relatively low variance in BMI among these athletes.

IN A PRACTICAL SENSE *(continued)*

CALCULATION EXAMPLES

Boy Athlete (18 yr)

Data: Subscapular (SS) skinfold: 10 mm; abdominal (AB) skinfold: 18 mm; triceps (TRI) skinfold: 10 mm; midaxillary (MA) skinfold: 8 mm

$Db = 1.10647 - (0.00162 \times SS_{SKF}) - (0.00144 \times AB_{SKF}) - (0.00077 \times TRI_{SKF}) + (0.00071 \times MA_{SKF})$

$\quad = 1.10647 - (0.00162 \times 10) - (0.00144 \times 18) - (0.00077 \times 10) + (0.00071 \times 8)$

$\quad = 1.10647 - 0.0162 - 0.02592 - 0.0077 + 0.00568$

$\quad = 1.06233$

$\%BF = \left[(499 \div Db) - 455\right]$

$\quad = \left[(499 \div 1.06233) - 455\right]$

$\quad = 14.7\%$

Female Ballet Dancer (20 yr)

Data: Body weight: 55.0 kg

$FFM(kg) = (0.73 \times BW) + 3.0$

$\quad = 43.15\,kg$

$\%BF = \left[(BW - FFM) \div BW\right] \times 100$

$\quad = \left[(55 - 43.15) \div 55\right] \times 100$

$\quad = 21.5\%$

Male Football Player (20 yr)

Data: Body weight: 105.0 kg; stature: 188 cm

$\%BF = 55.2 + (0.481 \times BW) - (0.468 \times HT)$

$\quad = 55.2 + (0.481 \times 105) - (0.468 \times 188)$

$\quad = 55.2 + 50.51 - 87.98$

$\quad = 17.7\%$

A Worrisome Trend Even Among Less Skilled and Younger Players. Exceptionally high BMIs also occur at less elite levels of collegiate competition. The average BMI of 33.1 for the Division III 1999 Gettysburg offensive line ($n = 15$) (29.9 for 2000 offensive line, $n = 13$),[64] and the BMI of 31.7 for other NCAA Division III American football linemen ($n = 26$; 1994–1995) raises similar concern about potential health risks (e.g., high blood pressure, insulin resistance, and type 2 diabetes) for such large young men (stature: 1.84 m [72.4 in.] ; body mass: 107.2 kg [236 lb]) and long-term outlooks remain undetermined but certainly are not encouraging.[59] At the high school level, the BMI of *Parade* magazine's All-American football teams increased dramatically beginning in the early 1970s through 1989 and then further increased in rate of gain to the year 2004.[73] The plot in FIGURE 29.5 shows a clear shift at 1972 in the slope of the regression line (*yellow line*) relating BMI to year of competition compared with age-matched individuals from large-scale epidemiologic normative data (*red line*). This shift toward a higher BMI coincided with either improved nutrition and training and/or the emerging prevalence among high school athletes of performance-enhancing drugs (chiefly anabolic steroids).[4] Particularly disturbing are the most recent 2013 data for high school offensive and defensive linemen, for which the BMI averaged 34.8, slightly greater than the average 2008 BMI value. For the 2013 linemen data (value not shown) with the last data point for the *Parade* magazine 2008 high school football players, the BMI has in just 13 years increased dramatically now comparable to the average BMI values for the 2012 Bowl Championship Series (BCS) National Champion collegiate linemen and both 2012 NFL Super Bowl teams!

2004–2005 Division I Big Ten Collegiate Football Players

A unique data set exists for Division I Big Ten collegiate football players from 2004–2005. Forty-three percent of 1124 football players had BMIs that exceeded 30. An additional 14% had BMIs above 35. The study pointed out that bigger size did not correlate with more victories. The Iowa team was the lightest team in the Big Ten, with an average BMI of 28.5, but won a share of the conference championship. In contrast, Indiana had the highest average team BMI with 30.9, followed by Penn State (30.3) and Michigan (30.2). Wisconsin's offensive line's BMI averaged 38.3, and the Badgers boasted a conference-high 11 linemen who exceeded 300 lb. Unfortunately, the same analysis is unavailable for 2010–2012 roster players at these same institutions. TABLE 29.7 lists the team rank for BMI from high to low. This surely represents a situation where achieving the lowest rank of 10 is cherished instead of the "We're Number 1!" ranking.

The implications of such huge body mass for these and other large athletes in terms of health risk and long-term outlook remain undetermined but certainly are worrisome.

Average Body Mass and Stature for the 2007 NFL Super Bowl Offensive and Defensive Linemen

TABLE 29.6

Variable	Colts	Bears
Body mass	301.3 lbs (136.6 kg)	302.2 lbs (137.5 kg)
Stature	75.1 in (190.8 cm)	75.9 in (192.8 cm)
BMI, kg · m⁻²	37.5	37.0
BMI classification	Obese	Obese

2006 team rosters; obese = BMI >30.0; normal weight = BMI 22.0–25.9

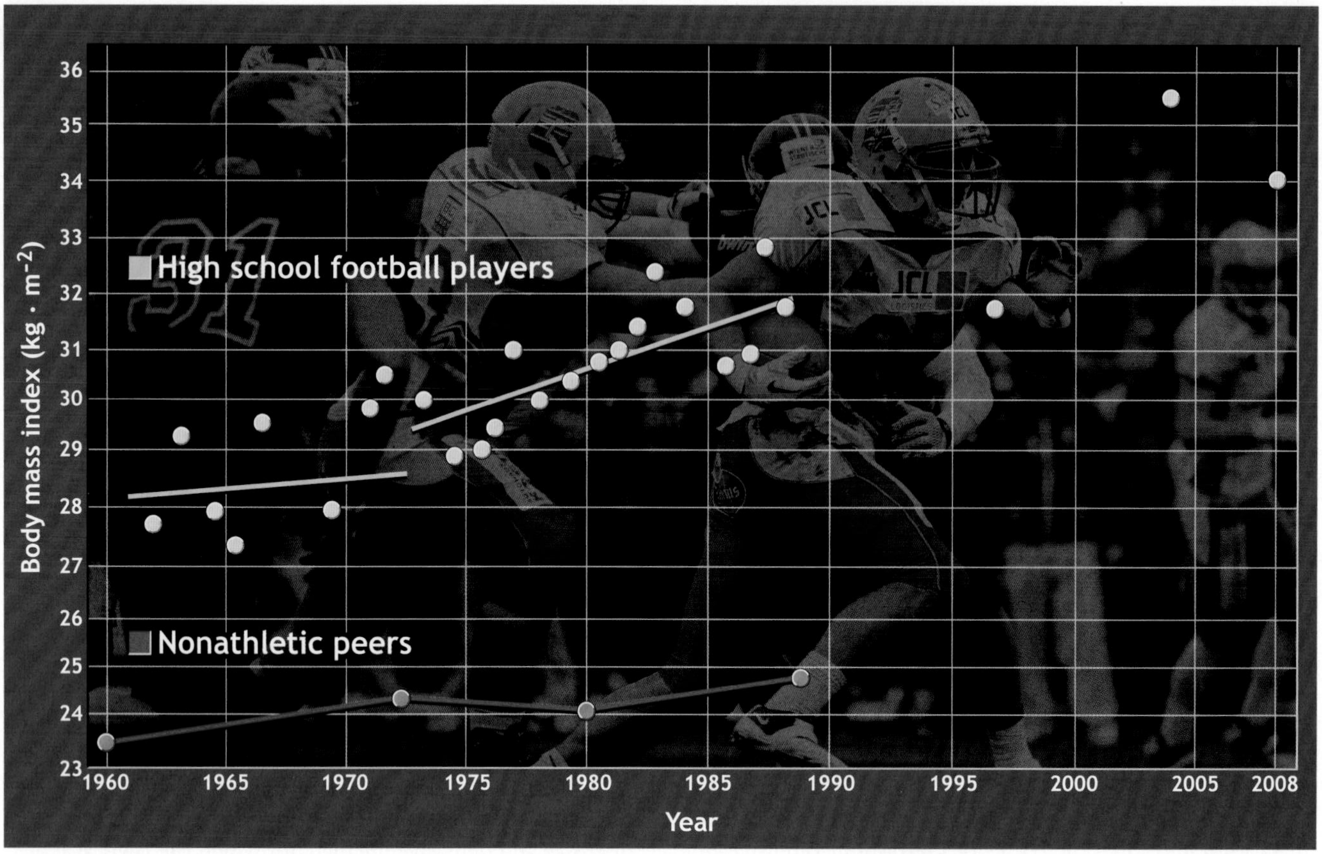

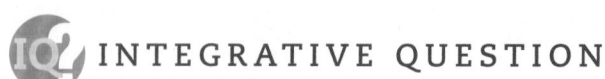

FIGURE 29.5 • BMIs of elite Parade All-American high school football offensive and defensive linemen over time compared with nonathlete counterparts (http://www.parade.com/9489/katemeyers/meet-the-2013-parade-all-america-football-team/).

One of the underreported but important health risks concerns disordered breathing problems during sleep prevalent among large-sized Canadian professional football players.[22] The average neck girth (45.2 cm; 17.7 in.) and elevated BMI (31.5) predicted risk for sleep-disordered breathing and apnea (and accompanying snoring). Certainly the large-sized elite high school players (and large top collegiate and NFL players) are likely to exhibit sleep-associated disorders that could affect field performance and future health. As we emphasize in Chapter 28, use of BMI to classify individuals as overfat can mislead, as confirmed in a study of 85 collegiate American football players.[52] The BMI overestimated the prevalence of overweight and obesity in 51% of the players, with only 14 players qualified as obese using bioelectrical impedance techniques to assess body composition. Nonetheless, the offensive linemen exceeded the at-risk criteria for BMI (>30), waist girth (>102 cm; 40.2 in.), and percentage body fat (>25%). It probably is fair to state that large high school players about to enter college and collegiate football players will still exhibit multiple criteria for obesity, a worrisome finding indeed, in addition to their large BMI.

Average BMI of Division I Big Ten Collegiate American Football Offensive and Defensive Linemen

TABLE 29.7

Team Rank	Average BMI of Linemen (kg · m⁻²)
1. Indiana	30.9
2. Penn State	30.3
3. Michigan	30.2
4. Michigan State	30.1
5. Ohio State	30.0
6. Illinois	29.8
7. Northwestern	29.6
8. Wisconsin	29.5
9. Minnesota	29.4
10. Iowa	28.5
11. Purdue	28.5

Data for 2004–2005 reported from the *Daily Iowan*, 2007, www.dailyiowan.com.

INTEGRATIVE QUESTION

A football coach wishes to field a team whose players are not overly fat. He selects the frequently used BMI to screen out players with excessive body fat. What are the possible outcomes of his decision for football performance?

Other Longitudinal Trends in Body Size for Professional Basketball and Baseball Players. To expand upon longitudinal trends for body size among elite athletes, we determined stature and body mass for two groups of professional athletes: (1) all NBA players from 1970 to 1993 (*n* ranged from 156 to 400 yearly) and (2) Major League Baseball players from 28 teams during the 1986, 1988, 1990, 1992, and 1995 seasons (*n* = 5031 roster players). The BMI for the champion 2013 World Series Boston Red Sox starting lineup, designated hitter, and 4 rotation pitchers averaged 27.2 (stature 186.8 cm; body mass 94.9 kg), and for the St. Louis Cardinals (stature 189.1 cm; body mass 99.1 kg), a comparable value of 27.7.

For the NBA players (Fig. 29.6A), average body mass increased by 3.8 lb (1.7 kg) or 1.8% during the 23-year interval. Stature increased more slowly; it changed by only 1 inch or less than 1% over the same interval. The NBA players' BMI during this time remained within a narrow range of 0.8 BMI units, from 23.6 to 24.4. Major League Baseball players (shown in *red*) show slightly higher mean BMI values than do the basketball players. Compared with American professional and collegiate football players, baseball and basketball athletes have maintained BMIs within guidelines considered relatively healthful for minimizing mortality and disease risk.

Increasing Trend for NFL Players to Exceed 300 Pounds

The accompanying figure illustrates the number of NFL players exceeding 300 lb (136 kg) in 10-year intervals from 1970 to 2010, including a projected value of about 1000 players for the year 2020! The projected value is approximately 500 players in the 2015 season. The inset figures show the number of 2013 Super Bowl offensive and defensive linemen that exceeded 300 lb, including averages for body weight, stature, and BMI.

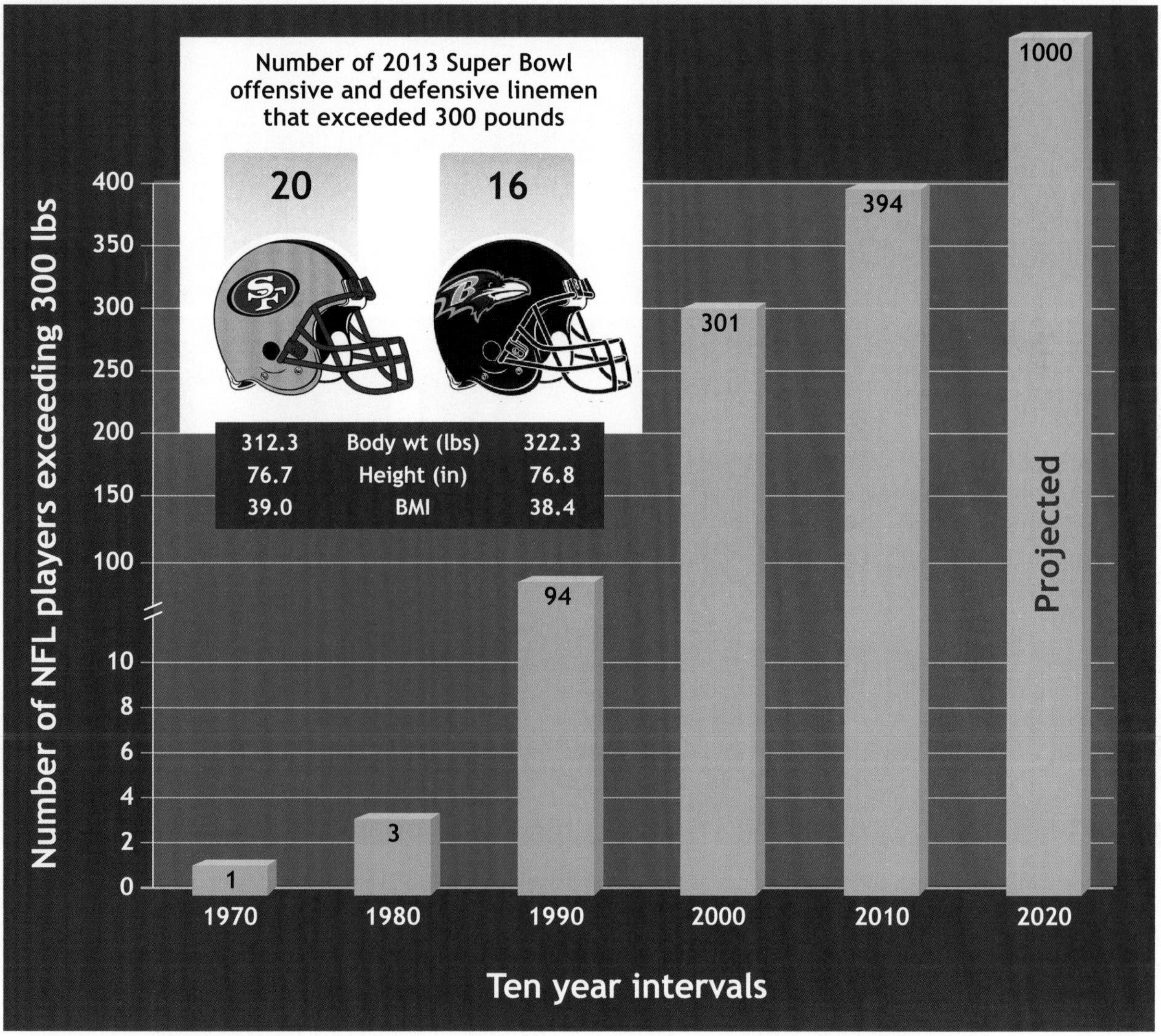

Number of NFL players exceeding 300 lbs vs **Ten year intervals**

Inset: **Number of 2013 Super Bowl offensive and defensive linemen that exceeded 300 pounds**

20		16
312.3	Body wt (lbs)	322.3
76.7	Height (in)	76.8
39.0	BMI	38.4

Bar values: 1970 = 1; 1980 = 3; 1990 = 94; 2000 = 301; 2010 = 394; 2020 = 1000 (Projected)

(Image adapted with permission from McArdle WD, Katch FI, Katch VL. *Sports and Exercise Nutrition*. 4th Ed. Philadelphia: Wolters Kluwer Health, 2013.)

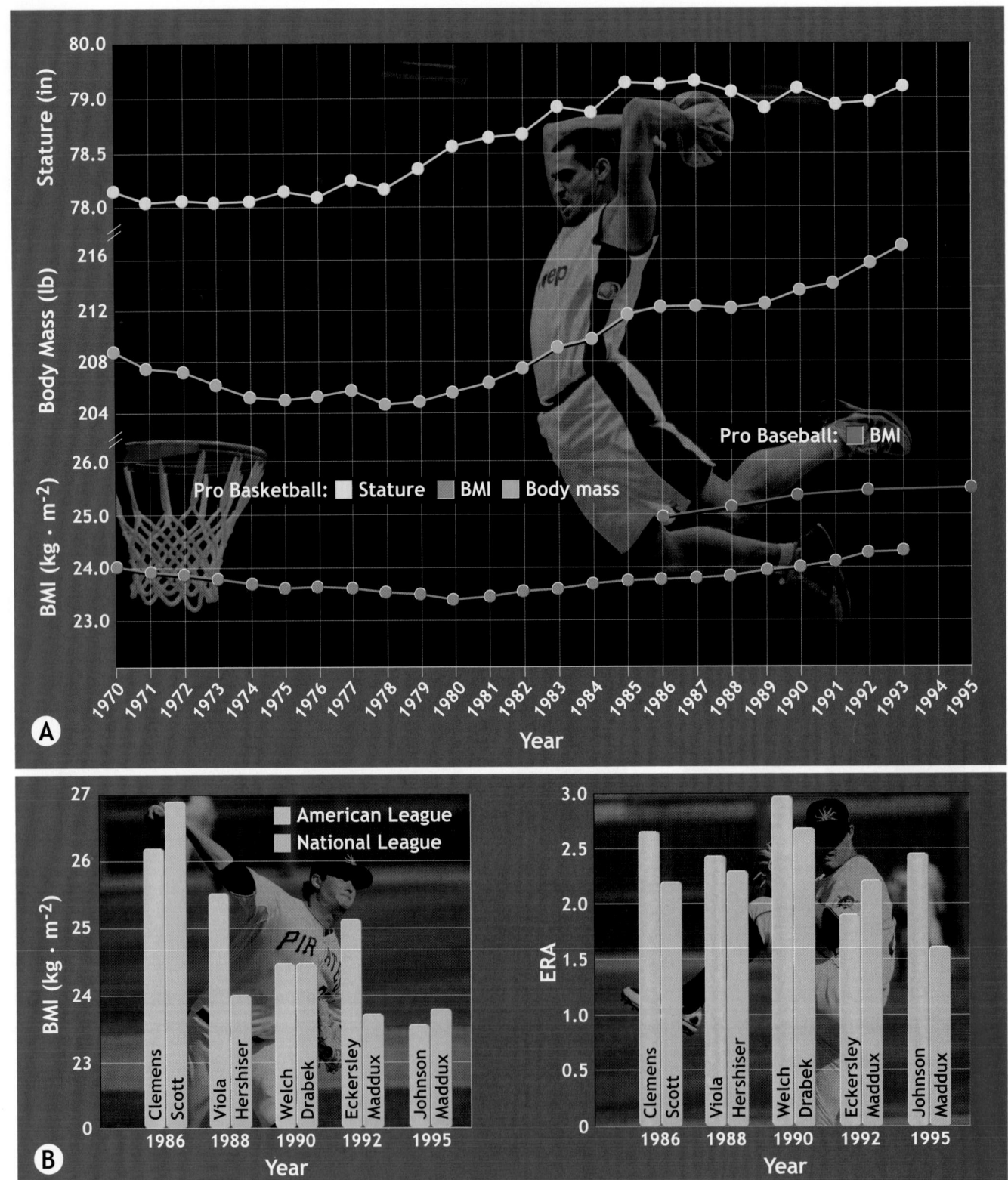

FIGURE 29.6 • BMI, body mass, and stature of professional NBA players (1970–1993) and BMI of Major League Baseball players (1986–1995). (Adapted with permission from McArdle WD, Katch FI, Katch VL. *Sports and Exercise Nutrition*. 4th Ed. Philadelphia: Wolters Kluwer Health, 2013. Data for NBA players from team rosters compiled by F. Katch; Major League Baseball data from team rosters courtesy of Major League Baseball.)

INTEGRATIVE QUESTION

Explain if a singular prototype for body composition (%fat, FFM) consistently emerges when one analyzes the body composition of elite athletes in different sports.

Professional Golfers. Limited data exist on the body composition of professional male and female golfers, although height and weight for current male tour PGA players are available from popular golf magazines and online (http://columbusdispatch.sportsdirectinc.com/golf/pgplayers.aspx?page=/data/pga/players/A_players.html; http://chicagosports.sportsdirectinc.com/golf/pga-players.aspx?page=/data/pga/players/P_players.html)

TABLE 29.8 lists the height, weight, and BMI for 2005 PGA Champion Tour players, PGA tour champions, and the 2011 top 20 PGA players (n = 18) and 257 golfers stratified by proficiency levels. Data for Behnke's reference man (refer to Chapter 28) are included for comparison. Interestingly, little difference if any exists in the height, weight, and BMI for the two groups of professional players with other tour golfers. The mortality ratio for these highly skilled golf athletes based on BMI would rate as very low (refer to Fig. 28.1). The most recent study of the Swedish Golf Federation's membership registry and the nationwide Mortality Registry corroborates this classification for health status based on standardized mortality ratios for 300,818 Swedish golfers (203,778 males and 97,040 females) with stratification for age, sex, and socioeconomic status.[18] Swedish golfers had mortality rates about 60% of those in the general population for both sexes and in all age groups after adjustment for socioeconomic status. In a comparison study of 257 golfers stratified by proficiency levels based on handicap index, their average BMI index was only marginally higher than the two pro groups. All three golf groups were still taller, heavier, and had a larger BMI compared to Behnke's reference man. This contrasts to the high school and professional football players who classify as obese and fall in the high range for mortality risk. For the obese NFL players, one half fall in the severely obese range with BMI that reaches 35, and those with a BMI above 40 classify as morbidly obese.

Weightlifters and Bodybuilders

Men. Resistance-trained bodybuilders, Olympic weightlifters, and power weightlifters exhibit remarkable muscular development and FFM combined with a relatively lean physique.[38] Percentage body fat computed from body density by underwater weighing averaged 9.3% in bodybuilders, 9.1% in power weightlifters, and 10.8% in Olympic weightlifters. Considerable leanness exists for each group

of athletes, even though height–weight tables classify up to 19% of these men as overweight. The groups did not differ in skeletal frame size, FFM, skinfolds, and bone diameters. The only differences occurred for shoulders, chest, biceps, and forearm girths; bodybuilders were larger at each site. The bodybuilders exhibited nearly 16 kg more muscle than predicted for their size; power weightlifters, 15 kg; and Olympic weightlifters, 13 kg. The three- or four-compartment model for body composition prediction is useful for assessing body composition changes in male bodybuilders during training.[70]

Women. Bodybuilding gained widespread popularity among women in the United States during the late 1970s. As women aggressively undertook the vigorous demands of resistance training, competition became more intense and achievement level increased. Bodybuilding success depends on a lean appearance complemented by a well-defined yet enlarged musculature, raising interesting questions about the women's body composition. How lean do the competitors become, and does a relatively large muscle mass accompany low body fat levels?

Body composition assessment of 10 competitive female bodybuilders averaged 13.2% body fat (range, 8.0 to 18.3%) and 46.6 kg (103 lb) FFM.[21] Except for champion gymnasts, who also average about 13% body fat, bodybuilders were 3 to 4% shorter, 4 to 5% lighter, and had 7 to 10% lower total body fat mass than other top female athletes. The bodybuilders' most striking compositional characteristic, a dramatically large FFM:FM ratio of 7:1, nearly doubles the 4.3:1 ratio for other female athletic groups. This difference presumably occurred without steroid use. Interestingly, 8 of the 10 bodybuilders reported normal menstrual function with concurrent relatively low body fat. When female bodybuilders trained for competition during a 12-wk preparation period, the major portion of the total weight lost (−5.8 kg; from 18.3% to 12.7% body fat) occurred primarily from reduced fat mass and not fat-free mass (−1.4 kg decline).[71] A 25.5-mm decline in the sum of eight skinfolds accompanied the body composition changes. This experiment reveals that healthy females at the lower end of the body fat continuum can still reduce fat mass over a 3-mo training duration to a level that approaches the theoretical boundary for storage fat without apparent deleterious, acute health effects.

Men versus Women. TABLE 29.9 compares body composition, girths, and excess body mass of male and female bodybuilders. Excess mass represents the difference between actual body mass and body mass-for-stature from the Metropolitan Life Insurance tables. Overweight for the men corresponded to a 14.8-kg (32.6 lb; 18%) excess; and for the women, a 1.2-kg (2.6 lb; 12%) excess. Obviously, excess body mass in these lean athletes primarily reflected FFM as increased skeletal muscle mass.

TABLE 29.8 Comparison of Height, Body Weight, and BMI for 2005 Champions Tour and PGA Golf Tour Champions and 2011 Top 20 PGA Players

Group[a]	Height (cm)	Weight (kg)	BMI
PGA Tour (n = 33)	182.0	84.1	25.4
Champions Tour (n = 18)	181.0	85.8	26.2
PGA Tour 2011[b] (n = 19)	184.0	81.2	24.0
Behnke reference man	174.0	70.0	23.1

[a]PGA TOUR Annual 2006, published by Boston Hannah International, www.bostonhannah.com
[b]2011 players: Casey, Donald, Els, Fowler, Furyk, D. Johnson, Kuchar, McDonwell, Michelson, Oglivy, Poulter, Rose, Schwartzel, Scott, Stricker, Watney, Watson, Wilson, Woods.

Contrasts of the girth data allow comparison of individuals (or groups) who differ in body size. The analysis shows that gender differences in girths when scaled to body size (referred to as "adjusted" in the table) do not differ as much compared to the uncorrected absolute girth values. Relative to body size, females exceed the male bodybuilders in 7 of 12 body areas. Women probably can alter muscle size to almost the same relative extent as men, at least when scaled to body size. The larger hip size in women probably reflects greater fat stores in this location.

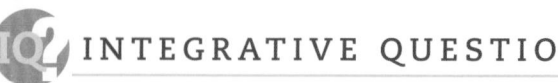

INTEGRATIVE QUESTION

Do established gender differences in body composition justify sex-specific normative standards to evaluate different components of physical fitness and motor performance?

UPPER LIMIT FOR FAT-FREE BODY MASS

The FFM for Japanese elite sumo wrestlers (*seki-tori*—top-ranked, salaried sumo wrestler who performs in the highest divisions of sumo http://www.youtube.com/watch?v=gGJe42jSTYc) averages 109 kg (240 lb).[45] These athletes share the distinction of being among the world's largest, along with some American professional football players who weigh 159 kg (350 lb).

TABLE 29.9 Body Composition and Anthropometric Girths of Male and Female Bodybuilders

Sex	Age (y)	Mass (kg)	Stature (cm)	Fat (%)	FFM (kg)	Excess Mass[a] (kg)
Male[b] (n = 18)	27.0	82.4	177.1	9.3	74.6	14.8
Female[c] (n = 10)	27.0	53.8	160.8	13.2	46.6	1.2

Body Part (cm)	Males Raw	Males Adjusted[d]	Females Raw	Females Adjusted[d]	% Difference (Males vs. Females) Raw	% Difference (Males vs. Females) Adjusted[d]
Shoulders	123.1	37.1	101.7	36.7	17.4	1.1
Chest	106.4	32.1	90.6	32.7	14.9	−1.9
Waist	82.0	24.7	64.5	23.3	21.3	5.7
Abdomen	82.3	24.8	67.7	25.1	15.3	−1.2
Hips	95.6	28.8	87.0	31.4	9.0	−9.0
Biceps relaxed	35.9	10.8	25.8	9.3	28.1	13.9
Biceps flexed	40.4	12.2	28.9	10.4	28.5	14.8
Forearm	30.7	9.2	24.0	8.7	21.8	5.4
Wrist	17.4	5.2	15.1	5.4	13.2	−3.8
Thigh	59.6	17.9	53.0	19.1	11.1	−6.7
Calf	37.3	11.2	32.4	11.7	13.1	−4.5
Ankle	22.8	6.9	26.3	7.3	11.0	−5.8

[a]Body mass minus body mass estimated from height–weight tables.
[b]Katch VL, et al. Muscular development and lean body weight in bodybuilders and weightlifters. *Med Sci Sports* 1980;12:340.
[c]Freedson PS, et al. Physique, body composition, and psychological characteristics of competitive female bodybuilders. *Phys Sportsmed* 1983;11:85.
[d]Calculated as $Gi/\sqrt{mass\,(kg)/stature\,(dm)^{0.7}}$, where Gi equals any one of the girths. The term $(mass/stature^{0.7})$ is a frame structure estimate of perimetric (girth) size. The adjusted values are the perimetric equivalent adjusted girths due to sex differences because they are corrected for whatever differences may exist from differences in body size.

thePoint Appendix H, available online at http://the point.lww.com/mkk8e, provides a list of supplemental animations and videos, including a video of sumo wrestling.

It seems unlikely that athletes in this weight range would possess less than 15% body fat; the FFMs of the largest football play-ers at 15% body fat theoretically correspond to 135 kg (298 lb). In reality, a football player with a body mass of 159 kg (351 lb) would more likely have 20 to 25% body fat. At 20% body fat, the FFM would be about 127 kg (280 lb), certainly the highest value ever measured hydrostatically. But this value remains hypothetical in the absence of reliable data. Even for an exceptionally large professional basketball player (body mass, 138.3 kg [305 lb]; stature, 210.8 cm [83 in.]), percentage body fat is unlikely to be less than 10% of body mass. Thus, fat mass equals 13.8 kg and FFM equals 114.2 kg—perhaps an upper limit FFM value for an athlete of such dimensions.

To gain additional insight into the question of an upper limit in FFM among athletes, we reviewed more than 35 years of body composition data from our laboratories to determine the largest FFM values calculated densitometrically. Thirty-five athletes exceeded an FFM of 100 kg; the top five values were 114.3, 109.7, 108.4, 107.6, and 105.6. The three top values were larger than the two values of 106.5 kg reported for defensive football linemen from 1969–1971 data[3] and for other resistance-trained athletes.[17]

The body composition of an exceptionally large professional football player (NFL Oakland Raiders; unpublished data, Dr. Robert Girandola, Department of Kinesiology, University of Southern California) determined by repeated trials of underwater weighing exceeds values for FFM presented in the research literature. The former defensive player (deceased, 2005 car accident), with a body fat content of 11.3% (body mass: 141.4 kg; stature: 193 cm; BMI: 38.4), had a FFM of 125.4 kg, the uppermost value we are aware of. With the continuing increase in the body size of professional football offensive and defensive players, this player's large FFM, determined in 1997 before he turned professional, will probably not remain the peak value for FFM, as body composition data on other large athletes become available. In the absence of additional data using criterion body composition assessment techniques, we assume that 125.4 kg (276 lb) represents the current upper limit for this component of body composition in elite "power" athletes.

Summary

1. Athletes generally have physique characteristics unique to their specific sport. Field-event athletes have a relatively large FFM and a high percentage of body fat; distance runners possess the least amount of lean tissue and fat mass.
2. Champion performance blends unique physique characteristics and highly developed physiologic support systems.
3. Male and female triathletes possess a body composition and aerobic capacity most similar to elite competitive bicyclists.
4. Body composition analyses of American football players reveal they are among the heaviest of all athletes, yet maintain a relatively lean body composition. At the highest levels of competition, Division I collegiate and professional football players show remarkable similarity in body size and composition.
5. Top-rated high school football linemen in 2013 are comparable to the stature and body mass (and BMI) of 2007–2013 NFL Super Bowl participants and 2012 NCAA Division I champion offensive and defensive collegiate football linemen.
6. Professional male golfers and those of high skill level have normal BMI ratios compared to other groups of athletes.
7. Competitive male and female swimmers generally have higher body fat levels than distance runners. The difference probably results from self-selection related to economically exercising in the different environments rather than real metabolic effects caused by the environments.
8. Female bodybuilders alter muscle size to the same relative extent as male bodybuilders.
9. The FFM–FM ratio of competitive female bodybuilders exceeds the FFM–FM ratio of other elite female athletes.
10. A value of 125.4 kg (276.5 lb) represents the current upper limit of FFM of elite power athletes.

thePoint References are available online at http://thepoint.lww.com/mkk8e.

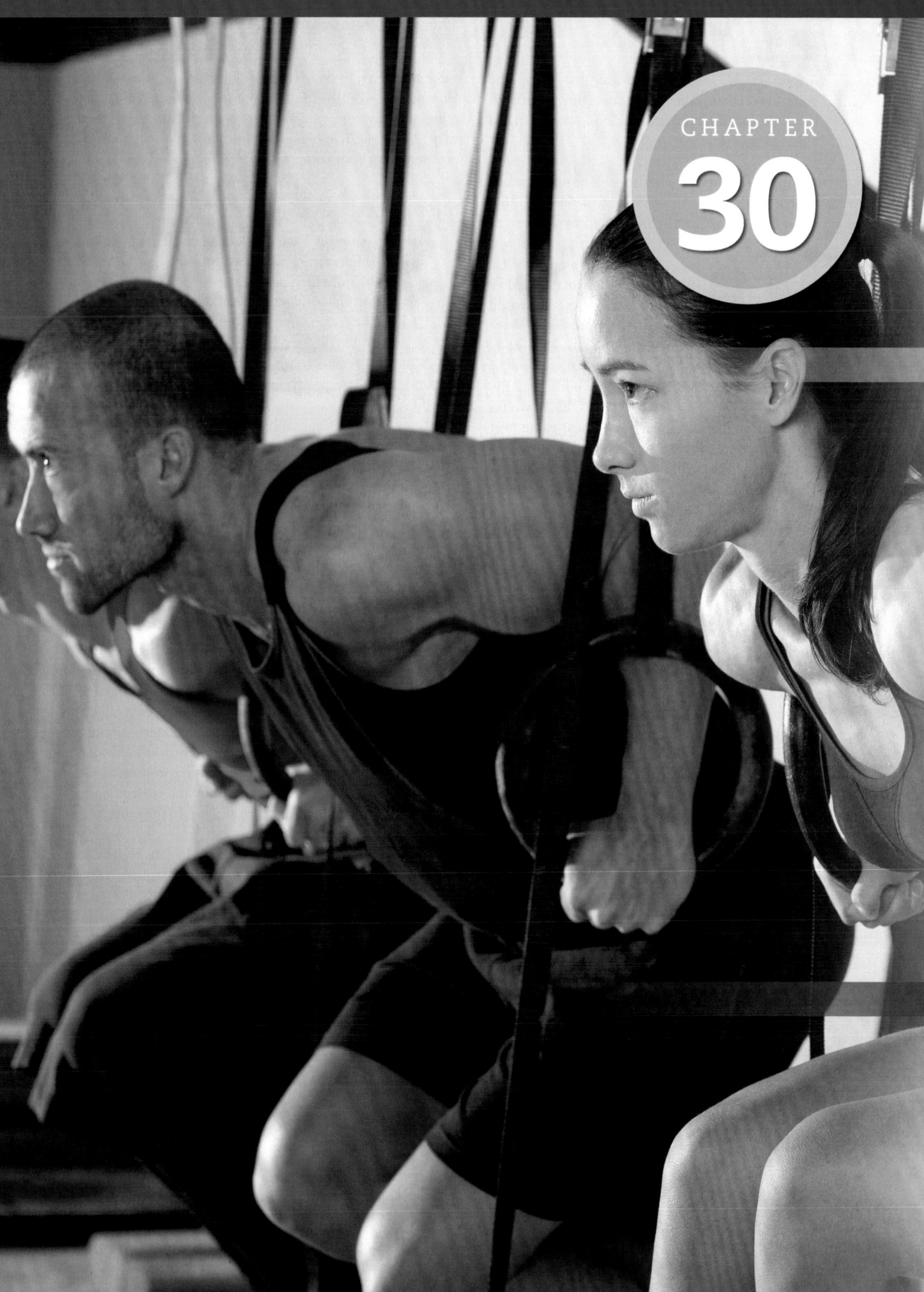

Overweight, Overfatness (Obesity), and Weight Control

CHAPTER OBJECTIVES

- Discuss the worldwide impact of being overweight, overfat, and obese in the United States and worldwide

- Evaluate the contribution of inherited factors to the development of excess body fat

- List 10 key health risks of excessive body weight and fat

- Describe how excess body weight in childhood and adolescence relates to adult risk for overfatness and poor health

- Discuss each of the following three criteria to assess excessive body fat: percentage body fat, regional fat distribution, and fat cell size and number

- Compare fat cell size and number in individuals with average body fat and the massively obese

- Discuss how genetic factors create white and brown fat cells and the impact this has on the tendency for fat gain.

- Describe two general effects of weight gain and loss on adult fat cell size and number

- Outline three approaches to "unbalance" the energy balance equation to trigger weight loss

- Describe four characteristics of individuals who successfully maintain prolonged weight loss

- Summarize two proposed advantages and disadvantages of ketogenic diets, high-protein diets, and very low-calorie diets (VLCD)

- Present the most salient rationale for including regular physical activity in a weight-loss program

- Review how moderate increases in physical activity for a previously sedentary, overly fat person affect daily food intake and energy expenditure on a short- and long-term basis

- Explain why combining regular physical activity with moderate food restriction may provide the most effective option for successful weight loss

- Summarize how different modes of physical activity affect body composition during weight loss

- Explain whether specific target exercises in one part of the body induce localized fat loss in that region

- Give specific diet and increased physical activity advice to gain body weight to improve appearance or enhance sports performance

ANCILLARIES ◉ at-a-Glance

Visit http://thepoint.lww.com/mkk8e to access the following resources.

- References: Chapter 30
- Appendix F: Energy Expenditure in Household, Occupational, Recreational, and Sports Activities
- Interactive Question Bank
- Focus on Research: Genetic Tendency to Gain Weight

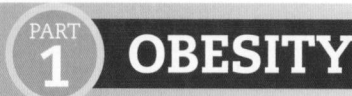

OBESITY

HISTORICAL PERSPECTIVE

Biblical scholars throughout history have preached against the ills of excessive food intake and sedentary living. The 12th-century Jewish sage Rabbi Moses ben Maimon (also known as Maimonides; 1138–1204) quotes the incomparable Greek physician Galen (AD 129–201; refer to the section titled "In the Beginning: Origins of Exercise Physiology from Ancient Greece to America in the Early 1800s," in "Roots and Historical Perspectives," before Chapter 1) in one of his many essays on health, that excess fat is harmful to the body and makes it sluggish, disturbs its functions, and hinders its movements. Maimonides also taught that everyone who practices a sedentary lifestyle and does not exercise will live a painful life. He posited that excessive eating mimics a deadly poison in the body that precipitates all illnesses.

Hippocrates (b. 460–377 BC), the ancient Greek physician regarded as the "Father of Medicine," opined that obesity represented a major health risk that led to death from many diseases. The Hippocratic texts conveyed the overarching belief that obesity deviated from the norm or ideal so essential for maintaining a healthy balance to all aspects of life. Galen and other physicians of that era wrote essays that extolled the virtues of walking, running, wrestling, rope climbing, and vigorous, physically active pursuits in addition to baths, massage, rest, and an "appropriate" lifestyle as antidotes to rebalance one's health. Interestingly, Hippocrates believed that obese individuals should undertake physical activity before eating and to eat while still breathing hard as a viable strategy to reduce excess weight. The practice of modulating food intake for dietary control of disease conditions was promoted in the first half of the 9th century by an ancient Assyrian physician, Yuhanna ibn Masawayh (known in the Western world as Jean Mesue; CE 777–857 http://journals.cambridge.org/action/displayAbstract;jsessionid=FDE876854DE3306E6355D6522B2D7A00.journals?fromPage=online&aid=5703544). This prolific medical writer practiced medicine in Baghdad and served as personal physician to four caliphs. Known for his medical aphorisms, Mesue produced the first known treatise concerning dietetics, incorporating ideas from the earlier writings of Galen. He was one of the first ancient "medical nutritionists" to describe the properties of 140 foodstuffs from plants and animals and their effects on the human body. He also performed anatomical dissections on apes, exploring how to better understand bodily functions.

For the past 20 centuries, medical practitioners, writers, philosophers, scientists, and theologians throughout the world have advocated a sensible approach to healthy living, but apparently without much lasting impact. The following quote provides a succinct summary of the historical development of scientific and cultural ideas about obesity gleaned from the ancients to the present[15]:

> Scholarly theses on this subject began to appear in the late 16th century, with the first monographs published in the 18th century. The values of dietary restriction, increasing exercise, and reducing the amount of sleep were identified early in medical history dating at least from the time of Hippocrates. These concepts were often framed in a manner that implied a "moral" weakness on the part of the overweight individual. Cases of massive obesity were identified in stone-age carvings and have been described frequently since the time of Galen and the Roman Empire. More specific types of obesity began to be identified in the 19th century. Following the identification of the cell as the basic building block of animals and plants, fat cells were described and the possibility that obesity was due to too many fat cells was suggested. After the introduction of the calorimeter by Lavoisier, the suggestion that obesity might represent a metabolic derangement has been suggested and tested. Standards for measuring body weight appeared in the 19th century. The possibility that familial factors might also be involved was clearly identified in the 18th and 19th centuries. Most of the concepts that are currently the basis for research in the field of obesity had their origin in the 19th century and often earlier.

OBESITY REMAINS A WORLDWIDE EPIDEMIC

In our modern scientific era, no clear answer exists to a seemingly simple question: Why have so many people gained so much weight and fat, and what can be done to reduce the problem? An excessive gain in body fat results from a complex interaction of genetic, environmental, metabolic, physiologic, behavioral, social, and perhaps racial influences (see the section Overweight, Overfatness, and Obesity: No Unanimity for Terminology, in Chapter 28).[22,68] Individual differences in specific factors that predispose humans to gain fat include at least the following 10 factors:

1. Disordered eating patterns and eating environment
2. Food packaging that promotes spontaneous food purchases
3. Distorted body image
4. Reduced resting metabolic rate
5. Lowered diet-induced thermogenesis
6. Reduced levels of spontaneous nonexercise activity thermogenesis (NEAT)
7. Lowered basal body temperature
8. Susceptibility to viral infections
9. Diminished cellular adenosine triphosphatase, lipoprotein lipase, and other enzymes
10. Reduced levels of metabolically active brown adipose tissue

Large numbers of individuals struggle to lose weight or just maintain body weight. Only one-fifth of Americans attempting to lose weight use the recommended combination of eating fewer calories and engaging in increased amounts of physical activity. Those attempting weight loss often rely on potentially harmful dietary practices and drugs while ignoring sensible weight-loss programs. Notwithstanding the upswing in attempts to lose weight, people throughout the industrialized nations are considerably more overweight than people of a generation ago. Obesity, unfortunately, remains an equal-opportunity affliction; this epidemic now afflicts all regions of the United States.[140]

Four Reasons for Classifying Overweight and Obesity

1. Provides meaningful comparisons of body weight status within and among populations
2. Identifies individuals and groups at increased risk of morbidity and mortality
3. Identifies priorities for intervention at individual and community levels
4. Establishes a firm basis to evaluate diverse intervention strategies

Source: World Health Organization

FIGURE 30.1 compares data from the National Health and Nutrition Examination Survey (NHANES; www.cdc.gov/nchs/products/pubs/pubd/hestats/overweight/overwght_adult_03.htm) of obesity prevalence (percent) among adults (Fig. 30.1A) and children (Fig. 30.1B) as well as the total number of obese children, adolescents, and adults in the Unites States who classify as obese (Fig. 30.1C). Current estimates place the combined number of both overweight and obese Americans at nearly 140 million (69% of the population, including 35% of college students[130]), an unprecedented increase from "only" 56% in 1982. If current trends continue, more than half of adult Americans in most states will be obese by 2030. This expansion of the obesity epidemic has strained the nation's medical burden, with an estimated 6 to 10 million additional cases of diabetes and up to 12 million additional heart disease and stroke patients. The situation would become so out of control that the obesity rate in Colorado, the current state with the *lowest* obesity rate in 2012 at 20.7%, would more than double to 44.8%, outpacing Mississippi in 2012 at 34.9%! Overweight occurrence is particularly high among women and Hispanic, African American, and Pacific Islander minority groups.

Similar increases in obesity have occurred worldwide,[59,219] contributing to the rising onslaught of diabetes and cardiovascular disease—prompting the World Health Organization (www.who.int/en/) and the International Obesity Task Force (www.iotf.org) to declare a **global obesity epidemic**. For example, FIGURE 30.2 shows estimates for women and men obesity assessed by BMI for 2009 from selected European countries. Yugoslavia and Greece have the largest percentage of obese women and men, defined as BMI that exceeds 30 kg·m⁻², while Switzerland has the lowest

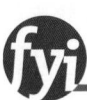

Perspective About the Size of the Obesity Epidemic

An October 2013 report from the National Center for Health Statistics, part of the Centers for Disease Control and Prevention (www.cdc.gov/nchs/), suggests a leveling off in the rate of increase in obesity among U.S. adults. In 2012, 34.9% of adult were obese, roughly 35 pounds in excess of a healthy body weight and not significantly different for the 35.7% value in 2010. Despite such encouraging data, and to give perspective about the sheer magnitude of the obesity epidemic, 70 to 80 million obese people equals the entire current population of either France, the United Kingdom, or Italy, or the combined 2012 populations of Belgium, Portugal, Sweden, Switzerland, Denmark, Finland, Norway, and Israel. In the United States for the year 2013, the total number of obese individuals equals the combined number of men, women, and children living in Michigan, New York, Florida, and Ohio (or Alabama, California, Kentucky, Massachusetts, Oregon, and Tennessee). If these millions of overfat people carried "only" an excess 20 lb of fat, it would approximate 4.2 trillion "extra kcal," the equivalent stored energy to power a walk around the Earth's 25,000 mile equator approximately 2.3 million times!

---

percentage of obese adults. Worldwide, about 310 million people are obese and nearly 790 million more are overweight. Obesity now ranks as the second leading cause of preventable deaths in the United States (about 330,000 deaths yearly; deaths from tobacco use ranks first—exceeding all deaths from HIV, illegal drug and alcohol use, motor vehicle injuries, suicides, and murders combined). The total annual cost of about $140 billion related to obesity (www.cdc.gov/obesity/index.html) accounts for approximately 10% of the U.S. health care expenditures.[2]

FIGURE 30.3 depicts the powerful effect of excess body weight in predicting survival at an older age. Overweight, but not obese, nonsmoking men and women in their mid-30s to mid-40s die at least 3 years sooner than normal-weight counterparts, a risk just as damaging to life expectancy as chronic cigarette smoking. Obese individuals with a BMI 30 or larger (*red lines*) can expect about a 7-year decrease in longevity. Survival rates progressively increase as BMI decreases. Correctly, contemporary physicians (and those from antiquity) tell us to eat less and increase the time spent in more vigorous physical activity. In industrialized nations, economic factors operate to counter this advice: Food continues to become cheaper, readily available, and more fat laden, while most occupations have not changed or have decreased their exertional demands.

A milestone in American governmental action regarding obesity took place on December 1, 2003. The United States Preventive Services Task Force (www.ahrq.gov/clinic/uspstfix.htm), a government advisory group composed of medical

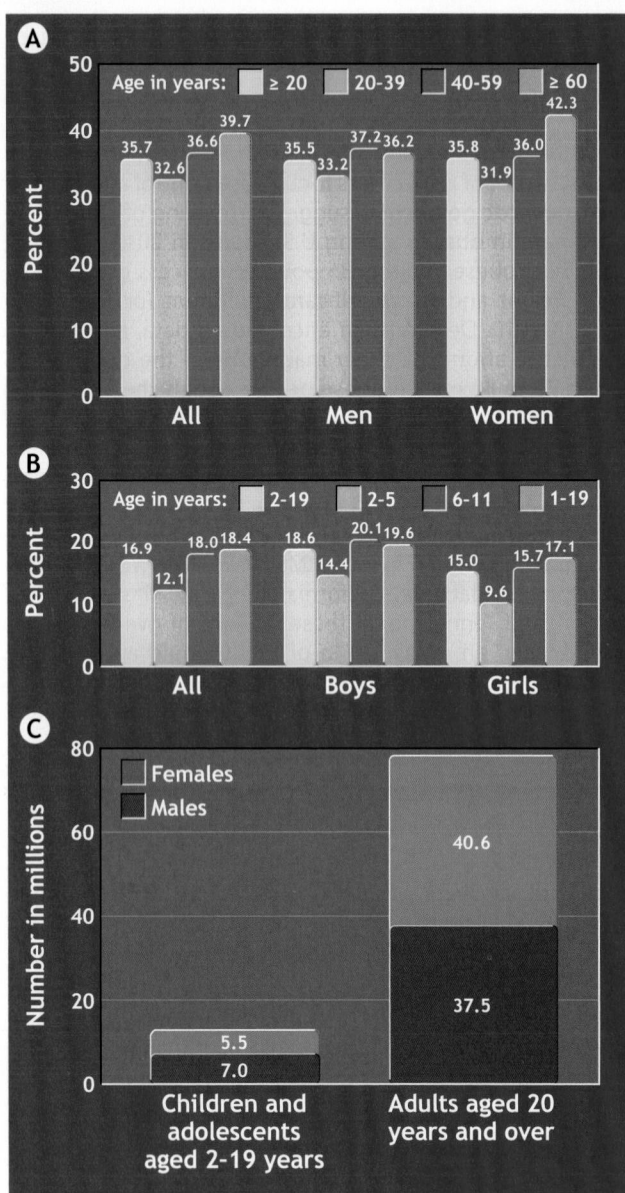

FIGURE 30.1 • **(A)** Prevalence of obesity among adults aged 20 and above by sex and age in the United States, 2009–2010. **(B)** Prevalence of obesity among children and adolescents ages 2 to 19 by sex and age in the United States, 2009–2010. **(C)** Number of obese children, adolescents, and adults in the United States, 2009–2010. Data from CDC NCHS Health E-Stat. *Prevalence of Overweight, Obesity, and Extreme Obesity Among Adults: United States, Trends 1960–1962 Through 2009–2010* (**www.cdc.gov/nchs/data/databriefs/db82.htm**).

experts, urged physicians to weigh and measure all patients and recommend counseling and behavior therapy strategies for those who classify as obese using BMI. Specifically, the group recommended that doctors prescribe intensive behavior therapy at least twice monthly (in individual or group sessions) for up to 3 mo under the supervision of a health-professional team of psychologists, registered dietitians, and

exercise specialists. These guidelines represent a major shift in how the health care system treats obesity, hopefully prompting health plans and insurers to pay for obesity treatment. Apparently, this plea had some effect. After a quarter century of increases, obesity prevalence has not measurably increased from 2005 to 2009, even though levels still remain far too high—approximately 39% of U.S. adults ages 20 and older through 2013.

fyi One Third of Americans Now Classified as Ill by AMA

At its annual 2013 meeting, the American Medical Association (**www.ama-assn.org**) formally recognized obesity as a disease, a decision that will now make physicians pay more attention to this condition that affects one in three Americans and causes insurance companies to cover prevention and treatment strategies that include drugs, surgery, and counseling. Those opposing this decision argue that the means for classification, the body mass index, is simplistic and flawed. For example, some individuals classified as obese are healthy with no specific disease symptoms (or treatment requirements) whereas others below this classification have excess body fat and accompanying comorbidities. Others argue that obesity is more of a risk factor for disease than a disease itself. The opposing AMA point of view argues that obesity is a "multimetabolic and hormonal disease state" leading to diverse medical outcomes like type 2 diabetes and cardiovascular disease.

Children experience an equally depressing situation because the prevalence of overweight in children (BMI ≥95th percentile for age and sex) has attained grim proportions, with the total reaching almost 13 million or 17% of American youth ages 2 to 19 classified as obese according to the Centers for Disease Control and Prevention.[26,149,198] A comprehensive report released by the National Academies of the Institute of Medicine (**www.iom.edu**) on the causes and solutions for childhood obesity in the United States indicates that in the last 30 years obesity has tripled among children ages 6 to 11, particularly in rural America, to nearly 15%. The rates have doubled for those ages 2 to 5 (>10%) and from age 12 to 19 to more than 15%. Pediatric obesity represents childhood's most common chronic disorder, particularly prevalent among poor and minority children.[54,211] About 70% of obese youth possess multiple risk factors for diabetes, elevated cholesterol, hypertension, risk for bone and joint disorders, and social and psychological problems including stigmatization and poor self-esteem. Part of this rise in body weight relates to the nearly 300% increase between 1977 and 1996 in the foods that children consume from restaurants and fast-food outlets.[197] Soft drink consumption in young consumers accounts

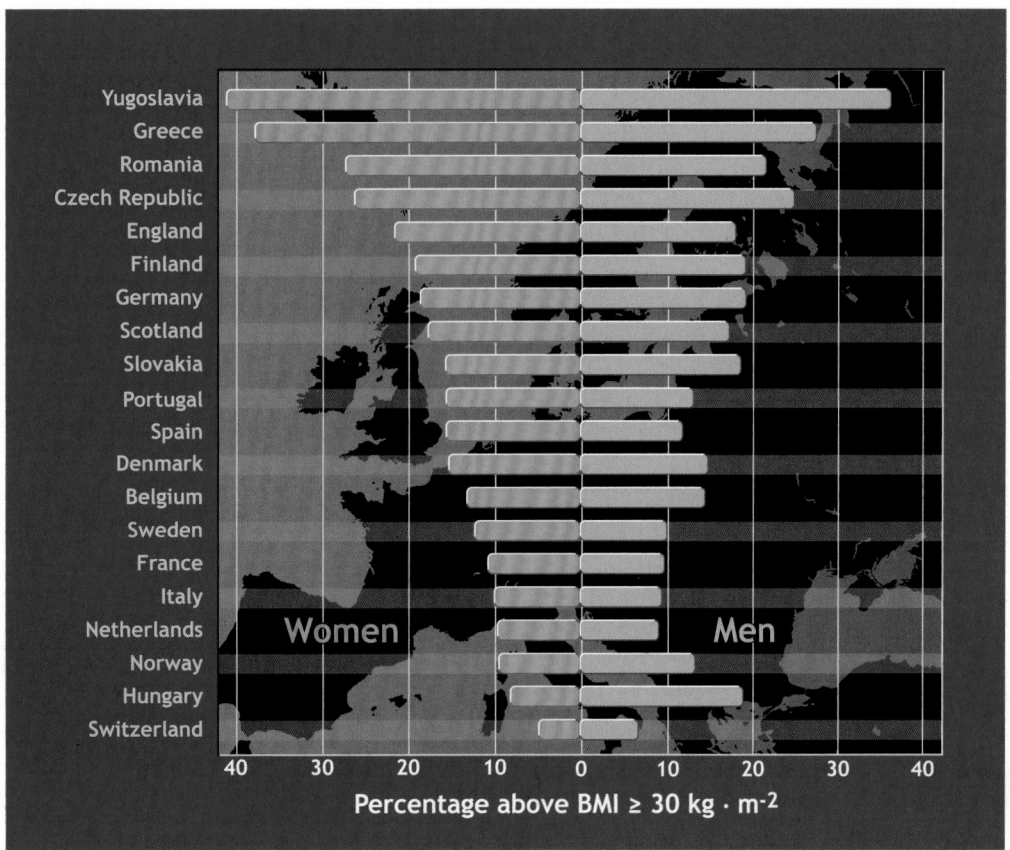

FIGURE 30.2 • The obese condition expands across Europe. Adult levels of obesity (BMI above 30 kg · m⁻²) in 20 European countries during 2007–2009. Data from the International Obesity Taskforce (www.iotf.org), a global network of expertise and research-led think tank and advocacy arm of the International Association for the Study of Obesity (www.iaso.org).

for an additional 188 kcal each day above energy intakes of children who do not consume these beverages. Excessive fatness in youth represents an even greater adult health risk than obesity begun in adulthood. Overweight children and adolescents, regardless of final body weight in adulthood, exhibit higher risk of a broad range of illnesses than adolescents of normal weight.

The New York City Board of Health's Sugary Drinks Portion Cap Rule took a proactive stance to combat the increasing weight of its citizens by banning the sale of "oversized"

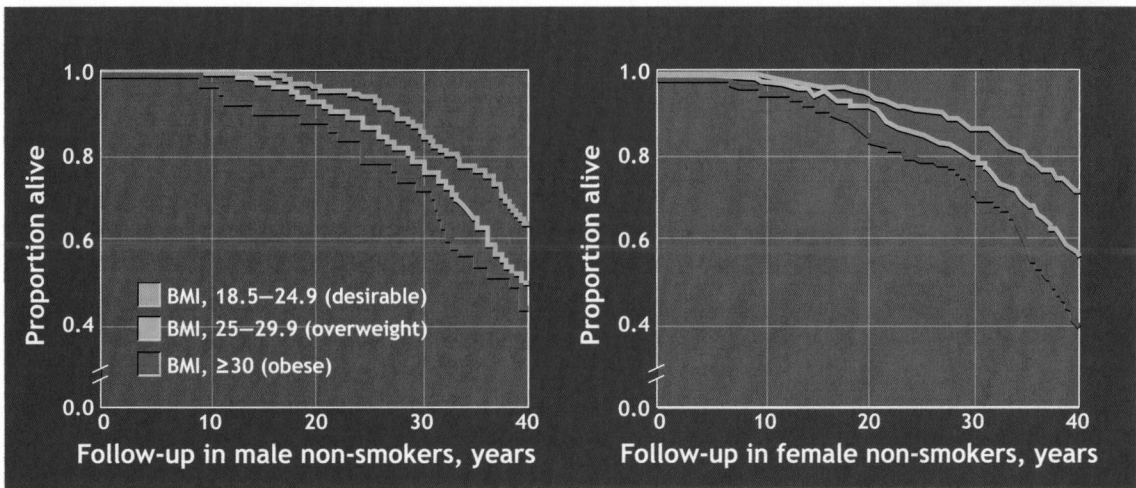

FIGURE 30.3 • Survival estimates for women and men categorized by body mass index (BMI). (Adapted with permission from Peeters A, et al. Obesity in adulthood and its consequences for life expectancy. *Ann Intern Med* 2003;138:24.)

soft drinks at restaurants, fast-food chains, theaters, delis, office cafeterias, and most other eateries. People who buy sugary drinks at such establishments still have the option to purchase an additional 16-oz beverage. The ban, begun in March 2013 exempts sugary drinks sold at supermarkets or most convenience stores and alcoholic and dairy-based beverages sold at New York City establishments. However, as of July 30, 2013 a New York appeals court upheld a ruling striking down as unconstitutional the City's ban on large sugary drinks. Turning back the ban by the court temporarily halted the groundbreaking legislation, pending an appeal for future adjudication.

 ## Sugary Drinks: Difficult to Dethrone

Nearly half of the U.S. population over age 2 drinks at least one sugary beverage every day, and 70% of boys ages 2 to 19 drink sugary beverages daily. One fourth of Americans consume 200 or more calories daily from sugary soft drinks, and 5% slurp at least 567 liquid calories—the equivalent of four 12-oz regular sodas. In only one year, the latter total of 1460 12-oz cans of soda would theoretically be the equivalent of 60 lb of body fat from the added 207,000 calories! For caffeine junkies, 1460 cans of Pepsi or Coke would contribute about the same amount of caffeine (about 55,000 mg) in 367 Tall, 12-oz cups of Starbucks Caffe Americano.

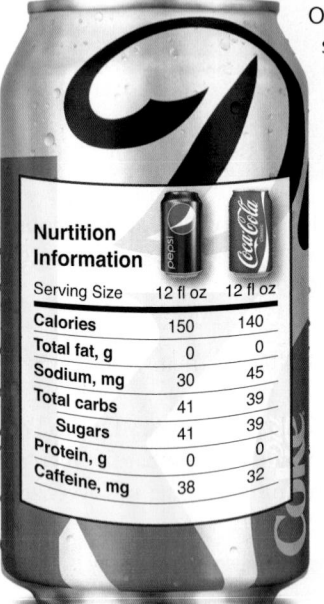

Nurtition Information		
Serving Size	12 fl oz	12 fl oz
Calories	150	140
Total fat, g	0	0
Sodium, mg	30	45
Total carbs	41	39
Sugars	41	39
Protein, g	0	0
Caffeine, mg	38	32

INCREASED BODY FAT: A PROGRESSIVE LONG-TERM PROCESS

Excess accumulation of body fat or overfatness represents a heterogeneous disorder in which energy intake chronically exceeds energy expenditure. The disruption in energy balance that often begins in childhood profoundly affects the likelihood for achieving adult obesity. For example, obese children at ages 6 to 9 have a 55% chance of becoming obese as adults—a risk 10 times that of children of normal weight. Simply stated, a child generally does not "outgrow" an overly fat condition.

 ## Childhood Obesity Rates

The stunning four-decade rise in childhood obesity that began in the 1970s has appeared to have plateaued, at least temporarily. An analysis of height and weight of more than 8000 children shows that the percentage of obese youngsters has somewhat stabilized since 1999 in every age and racial group surveyed (although childhood overweight and obesity continues to increase as documented by BMI and overall body size as shown in the inset figure[1,2]). Researchers from the Centers for Disease Control and Prevention[1] suggest that educational and regulatory campaigns to get children to increase their levels of daily physical activity and to consume healthier foods remain a top priority.

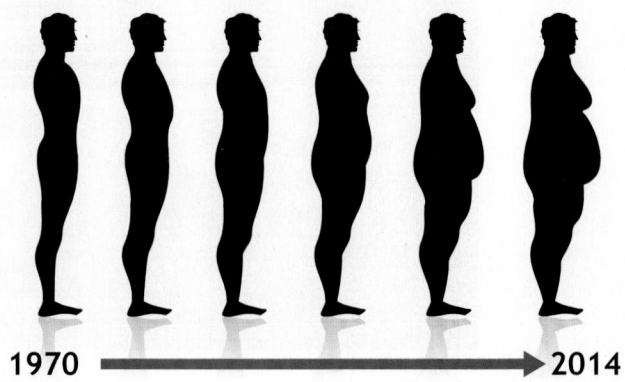

1970 ➝ **2014**

Sources:
1. www.cdc.gov/healthyyouth/obesity/facts.htm.
2. Moreno G, et al. Prevalence and prediction of overweight and obesity among elementary school students. *J Sch Health* 2013;83:157.

Ages 25 to 44 are the "danger" years when adults develop excessive fatness.[31] Middle-age men and women invariably weigh more than college-age counterparts of the same stature. Between ages 20 and 40, Americans gain about 2 lb yearly for a 40-lb gain in body weight. Women tend to gain the most weight; about 14% add more than 30 lb between ages 25 and 34. The degree to which this "creeping overfatness" in adulthood reflects a normal biologic pattern remains unclear.

Generally an Overfed Nation

A general increase in energy intake has occurred over a 30-year period among adult Americans. Every man and woman now consumes an average of 445 more calories daily than in 1970. This translates to 162,790 additional calories per person yearly! Of this 445 daily calorie increase, grains (mainly refined) accounted for 188 calories; added fats and oils, 188 calories; caloric sweeteners, 42 calories; dairy fats, 16 calories; fruits and vegetables, 15 calories; and meats, 8 calories. Only dairy products declined by 12 calories.

The most disturbing dramatic increase occurred in consumption of added sugars. In 1970, the average daily per capita calorie intake from added sugars (adjusted for spoilage and other waste) amounted to 332 calories. In 2010, the amount jumped 10% to 367 calories per day per person. Most of this increase came from high-fructose corn syrup (HFCS), glucose, and other corn sweeteners. Figure 30.4A shows the most current 2010 data for food consumption from the different food sources, expressed as calories a day, for the average American. Flour and cereal products provided more calories daily than any other food group. Figure 30.4B reveals how the typical American diet does not dovetail with the most recent MyPlate dietary recommendations (www.choosemyplate.gov/dietary-guidelines.html). As a percentage of total food intake, Americans overconsume meats by about 17% and grains by about 22%, while substantially underconsuming fruits by about 60%, vegetables by about 40%, and dairy products by about 50%. Such mismatches in food consumption patterns would seem to be particularly troublesome for overweight and obese individuals who need to dramatically upgrade their daily dietary and physical activity patterns.

GENETICS INFLUENCES BODY FAT ACCUMULATION

The notable interaction between genetics and environment makes it difficult to quantify the role of each in obesity development. Research with twins, adopted children, and specific segments of the population attributes up to 80% of the risk of becoming obese to genetic factors. For example, heavier than normal newborns become fat adolescents only when the father or particularly the mother is overweight.[61] Little risk exists for an overweight toddler to grow into an obese adult if both parents are of normal weight. But if a child under age 10, regardless of current weight, has one or both obese parents, the child has more than twice the normal risk of becoming an obese adult.[209,227] Even for normal-weight prepubertal girls, body composition and regional fat distribution relate to the body composition characteristics of both parents.[208]

One's genetic makeup does not necessarily cause obesity, but instead lowers the *threshold* for its development because of the impact of susceptibility genes.[160] Researchers have identified key genes and specific DNA sequence variants that relate to the molecular causes of appetite and satiety that predispose a person to gain excessive body fat. A more complete understanding of the genetic role in body fat accretion requires identification of the key genes and their mutations (including the relevant proteins) that contribute to chronic energy imbalance. Dr. Claude Bouchard, the John W. Barton, Dr. Endowed Chair in Genetics and Nutrition at the Pennington Biomedical Research Center (www.pbrc.edu) and one of the individuals we profile in the introduction to Section 6, continues to play a key role in the search for and identification of obesity genes.

Inherited factors contribute to variability in weight gain among individuals fed an identical daily caloric excess and can contribute to the tendency to regain lost weight. Studies of individuals who represent nine different kinds of relatives indicate that genetic factors that affect metabolism and appetite determine about 25% of the total transmissible variation among persons in percentage body fat and total fat mass (Fig. 30.5). A larger percentage variation in body fat status relates to a 30% transmissible cultural effect—an unhealthy expression of patterns of preexisting genes. The remaining 45% nontransmissible effect may change as new research frontiers explore the multi-dimensional aspect of the obese condition. *In an obesity-producing environment—sedentary and stressful, with ready access to inexpensive, large-portion, high-calorie, good-tasting food—the genetically susceptible obesity-prone individual gains weight and possibly lots of it.* Athletes in weight-related sports with a genetic propensity for obesity must constantly battle to maintain optimal body weight and composition for competitive performance.

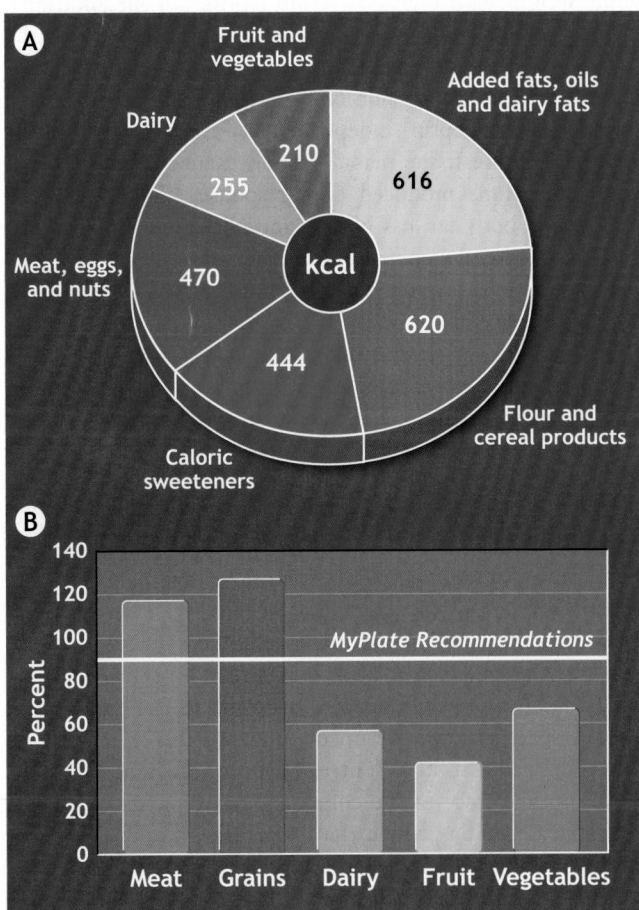

FIGURE 30.4 • **(A)** The circle represents the total number of calories consumed daily (2615 kcal) by the typical adult American; the individual circle segments refer to the daily caloric contribution of the six food categories. **(B)** How the typical American adult fails to meet or exceed the MyPlate recommendations. (Source: USDA Economic Research Service; www.ers.usda.gov.)

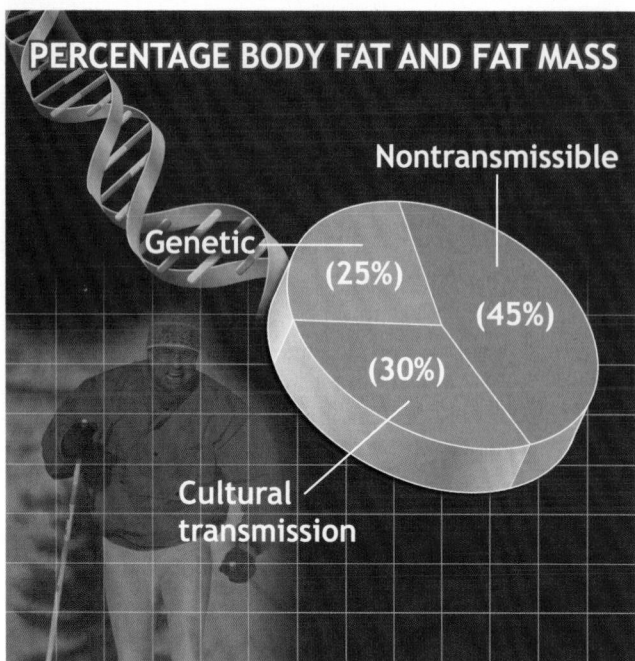

PERCENTAGE BODY FAT AND FAT MASS

Nontransmissible

Genetic

(25%)

(45%)

(30%)

Cultural transmission

FIGURE 30.5 • Total transmissible variance for body fat. Total body fat and percentage body fat were determined by hydrostatic weighing. (Adapted with permission from Bouchard C, et al. Inheritance of the amount and distribution of human body fat. *Int J Obes* 1988;12:205.)

A Mutant Gene and Leptin

Human obesity links to a mutant gene that synthesizes leptin (derived from the Greek root *leptos*, meaning "thin"). This crucial body weight–regulating hormonal substance, produced by fat and released into the bloodstream, acts on the hypothalamus to affect how much one eats, how much energy one expends, and ultimately how much one weighs.

The genetic model in FIGURE 30.6 proposes that the *ob* gene normally becomes activated in adipose tissue and perhaps muscle tissue, where it encodes and stimulates production of a body fat–signaling, hormone-like protein (*ob* **protein** or **leptin**), which then enters the bloodstream. This satiety signal molecule travels to the arcuate nucleus, a collection of specialized neurons in the mediobasal hypothalamus that controls appetite and metabolism and develops soon after birth. Normally, leptin blunts the urge to eat when caloric intake maintains ideal fat stores. Leptin may affect certain neurons in the hypothalamic region that stimulate the production of chemicals that suppress appetite and/or reduce the levels of neurochemicals that stimulate appetite.[76,119,142] Such mechanisms would explain how body fat remains intimately "connected" via a physiologic pathway to the brain to regulate energy balance. In a way, the adipocyte serves an endocrine-like function. With a gene defective for either adipocyte leptin production and/or hypothalamic leptin sensitivity, as probably exists in humans, the brain inadequately assesses the body's

adipose tissue status. This would enable the continuation for the urge to eat. In essence, leptin availability or its lack affects the neurochemistry of appetite and brain's dynamic "wiring" to dysregulate appetite and possibly cause obesity in adulthood.

The hormone–hypothalamic biologic control mechanism helps to explain the extreme difficulty overfat persons have in sustaining fat loss. In children and adults, when energy balance remains in steady state, plasma leptin circulates in direct proportion to adipose tissue mass, with four times more leptin in obese compared to lean individuals. Consequently, human obesity may resemble a relative state of leptin resistance similar to obesity-related insulin resistance.[70] High blood leptin concentrations associate strongly with the combination of four core metabolic disturbances in the insulin-resistant metabolic syndrome—upper-body obesity, glucose intolerance, hypertriglyceridemia, and hypertension (see Chapter 20). These unique metabolic disturbances ultimately act as a conduit to trigger higher incidence for heart disease, stroke, and type 2 diabetes.[199] Weight loss reduces serum leptin concentration, while weight gain increases serum leptin.[113] Four additional factors—gender, hormones, pharmacologic agents, and the body's current energy requirements—also affect leptin production. Neither short- nor long-term physical activity meaningfully affects leptin, independent of the activity's effects on total adipose tissue mass.[42,150] Subcutaneous recombinant leptin injections produced dose–response effect with body weight and body fat loss in lean and obese men and women with elevated endogenous serum leptin concentrations.[80] This suggests a potential role for leptin and related hormones in treating obesity.[163]

The linkage of genetic and molecular abnormalities to obesity allows researchers to view overfatness as a disease rather than a psychologic flaw. Early identification of one's genetic predisposition toward obesity makes it possible to begin diet and physical activity interventions before obesity sets in and fat loss becomes exceedingly difficult if not highly improbable.

Leptin alone does not determine body fatness nor explain why some people eat whatever they want and gain little weight, while others become overfat with the same caloric intake. Besides *defective leptin production*, defective receptor action increases resistance to endogenous satiety chemicals. A specific gene, the uncoupling protein-2 gene *UCP2* (www.ncbi.nlm.nih.gov/entrez/dispomim.cgi?id5601693), adds another piece to the complex obesity puzzle. The gene activates a specific protein that burns excess calories as heat energy without coupling to other energy-consuming processes. This **futile metabolism** blunts excess fat storage. Individual differences in gene activation and alterations in metabolic activity lend credence to the common claim "Every little bit of excess I eat turns to fat." A drug that turns on the *UCP2* gene to synthesize more of the heat-generating protein could provide a pharmacologic windfall to shed excess body fat. Other newly discovered molecules that control eating include AGRP (agouti-related protein), a protein controlled by leptin that may affect hypothalamic cells to increase caloric intake. The brain also synthesizes melanin-concentrating hormone when leptin levels increase.[134] An excess of this protein molecule increases an animal's appetite, causing it to eat and gain weight. Future drugs that inhibit or "destabilize" brain chemicals may ultimately provide the long-term "solution" to control eating and subsequent overfat condition.

Influence of Racial Factors

Racial differences in food consumption and physical activity patterns, and cultural attitudes toward body weight, help to

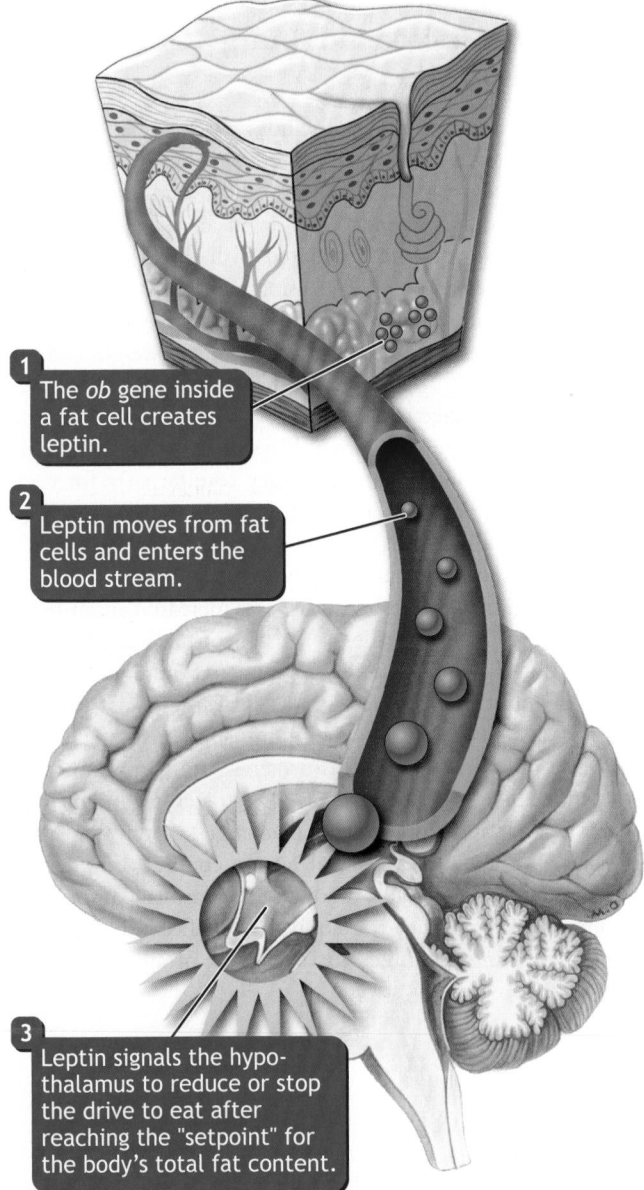

1 The *ob* gene inside a fat cell creates leptin.

2 Leptin moves from fat cells and enters the blood stream.

3 Leptin signals the hypothalamus to reduce or stop the drive to eat after reaching the "setpoint" for the body's total fat content.

FIGURE 30.6 • A genetic model for obesity. A malfunction of the satiety gene markedly affects production of the satiety hormone leptin. This disrupts events that occur in the hypothalamus, the center responsible for adjusting the body's fat level.

explain the greater prevalence of nearly 50% obesity among black women than the 33% of white women. Small differences in resting energy expenditure (REE), related to racial differences in lean body mass,[18] contribute to the racial differences in obesity.[81,93] This "racial" effect, which also exists among children and adolescents,[201,207] predisposes a black female to gain weight and regain it after weight loss. On average, black women burn nearly 100 fewer kcal daily during rest than white counterparts. The slower rate of caloric expenditure persists even after adjusting for differences in body mass and body composition. A 100-kcal reduction in daily metabolism translates to nearly 1 lb of fat gained each month. Total daily energy expenditure of black women averages 10% lower than whites, owing to a 5% lower REE and 19% lower physical activity energy expenditure.[22] Additionally, obese black women showed greater decreases in REE than white women following energy restriction and weight loss.[66] The combination of a lower initial REE and more profound depression of REE with weight loss suggests that overweight black women, including athletes, experience greater difficulty achieving and maintaining goal body weight than overweight white women.

Obesity in African Americans and Mexican Americans

Vast income, racial, and regional disparities exist among those classified overweight or obese.

RACIAL DISPARITIES

1. Mexican American and African American children ages 6 to 11 are more likely to be overweight or obese than white children.

2. Almost 43% of Mexican American children and 37% of African American children classify as obese or overweight, compared with 32% of white children. African American obese children are more likely to develop diabetes than obese white children.

CONSEQUENCES

1. An obese child costs the health care system about three times more than a child of normal weight.

2. Childhood obesity costs $14 billion annually in direct health costs (www.healthycommunitieshealthyfuture.org/learn-the-facts/economic-costs-of-obesity/). Average total health expenses of the obese child under Medicaid averages $3743 annually versus $1138 for all children covered by private insurance.

A Word of Caution

One must carefully evaluate methods to explore purported racial differences in body composition characteristics and their implications on health and physical performance.[32,218]

For example, interethnic and interracial differences in body size, structure, and body fat distribution often mask true differences in body fat at a given BMI. A single generalized BMI–health risk model that combines all ethnic and racial groups obscures the potential to document chronic disease risks among different ethnically and racially diverse population groups.[63,188] As discussed in Chapter 28, the nature and magnitude of the relationship between body mass or BMI and health risk may vary among racial and ethnic groups.

PHYSICAL INACTIVITY: A CRUCIAL COMPONENT IN EXCESSIVE FAT ACCUMULATION

Regular physical activity, through either recreation or occupation, can help to minimize weight and fat gain. This effect thwarts the tendency to regain lost weight and counters a common genetic variation that makes people more likely to gain excess weight.[84,91,92,160,194] Maintaining a physically active lifestyle contributes positively to the prevention and treatment of obesity-related health outcomes, independent of its effect on weight loss.[75]

Individuals who maintain weight loss show greater muscle strength and engage in more physical activity than counterparts who regained lost weight.[221] Variations in physical activity alone accounted for more than 75% of regained body weight. Such findings highlight the need to identify and promote strategies that increase regular physical activity. Current national guidelines by the Surgeon General and Institute of Medicine recommend a minimum of 30 to 60 min of moderate physical activity daily. *We endorse an increase to 80 to 90 min of physical activity, six to seven days a week (preferably seven) over and above regular routines, to combat the obesity epidemic in the U.S. population.* We also affirm that individuals modify their daily routines to encourage more whole body movement while minimizing the most common relatively nonactive sedentary behaviors.

Physical Activity and Body Fat Accumulation Throughout Life

From age 3 mo to 1 year, the total energy expenditure of infants who later became overweight averaged 21% lower than infants with normal weight gain.[166] For children ages 6 to 9 years, percentage body fat inversely related to physical activity level in boys but not girls.[8] Obese preadolescent and adolescent children generally spend less time in physical activity or engage in less intense physical activity than normal-weight peers.[35,125,216] By the time young girls attain adolescence, many do not engage in any leisure-time physical activity. For girls, the decline in time spent in physical activity averaged nearly 100% among blacks and 64% among whites between ages 9

and 10 and 15 and 16.[109] By age 16, 56% of the black girls and 31% of the white girls reported no leisure-time physical activity.

Physically active lifestyles lessen the "normal" pattern of fat gain in adulthood. For young and middle-age men who engage in regular physical activity, time spent active relates inversely to body fat level.[136] Not surprisingly, middle-age long-distance runners remain leaner than sedentary counterparts. No relationship emerges between the runners' body fat level and caloric intake. Perhaps the relatively greater body fat among middle-age runners results from less-vigorous training, not greater food intake.[112]

Benefits of Increased Energy Output with Aging

Maintaining a lifestyle that includes a regular and consistent level of endurance activity attenuates but does not fully forestall the tendency to add weight through middle age. Sedentary men and women who begin an exercise regimen lose weight and body fat compared with those who remain sedentary; those who stop exercising gain body weight relative to those who remain more physically active. Moreover, a proportionality exists between the amounts of weight change and activity dose.[229,230] **FIGURE 30.7** displays the inverse association among distance run and BMI and waist circumference for males in all age categories. Physically active men typically remained leaner than sedentary counterparts for each age group; men who ran longer distance each week weighed less than those who ran shorter distance. The typical male who maintained a constant weekly running distance through middle age gained 3.3 lb, and waist size increased about three quarters of an inch regardless of distance run. Such findings suggest that by age 50, a physically active man can expect to weigh about 10 lb more with a 2-in. larger waist than he weighed at age 20 despite maintaining a constant level of increased physical activity. This proclivity to gain weight and girth may relate to reduced levels of testosterone and growth hormone that induce age-related changes in physique and increase abdominal and visceral fat. To counter weight gain in middle age, one should gradually increase the amount of weekly physical activity the equivalent of fast walking, jogging, or running 1.4 miles for each year of age starting at about age 30.

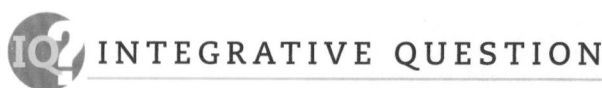

INTEGRATIVE QUESTION

What evidence documents that body fat accumulation among children and adults does not necessarily result from excessive food intake?

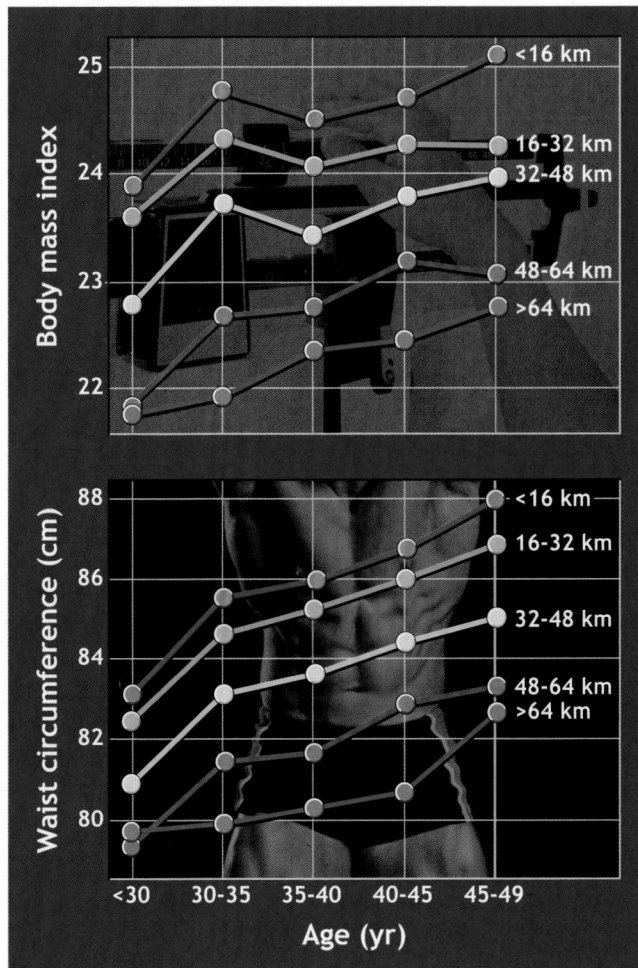

FIGURE 30.7 • Relationship among average body mass index (top) and waist circumference (bottom) and age for men who maintained constant weekly running for varying distances (<16 to >64 km · wk⁻¹). Men who annually increase their running distance by 1.39 miles (2.24 km) per week compensate for the anticipated weight gain during middle age. (Adapted with permission from Williams PT. Evidence for the incompatibility of age-neutral overweight and age-neutral physical activity standards from runners. *Am J Clin Nutr* 1997;65:1391.)

HEALTH RISKS OF EXCESSIVE BODY FAT

Obesity represents an unfortunate *cause* of preventable death in America. The combined effects of poor diet and physical inactivity caused approximately 330,000 deaths in the year 2000, a 33% jump over 1990. If the body weight of Americans continues to increase at its current rate, by 2020 one in five health care dollars spent on middle-age Americans will result from excessive body fat. Impaired glucose tolerance and overall diminished quality of life emerge even among obese children and adolescents.[24,175,183] Hypertension, elevated blood sugar, postmenopausal breast cancer, and elevated total cholesterol and low high-density

lipoprotein-cholesterol heighten an overweight individual's risk of poor health at any given level of excess weight. Increased loads on the major joints can lead to pain and discomfort, complications from osteoarthritis, inefficient body mechanics, and reduced mobility.[82]

Extra Pounds Weigh Heavily on Lifespan Quality and Life

Extra Pounds Can Shorten Life

The body mass index (BMI) classification of *obesity* alone does raise premature death risk but merely being *overweight* also carries significant health risks. Individuals who classify as overweight by BMI were 13% more likely to die during a 5- to 28-year follow-up period than counterparts with weight in an ideal range. For those classified as obese, the increased risk ranges from 44 to 88% of dying prematurely.

Factors That Inhibit Life Extension

The rising trend in obesity may underlie the slight dip in life expectancy in the United States to 77.8 years. Heart disease and cancer continue to rank as the two top killers, accounting for about 50% of all deaths. Stroke declined from its number three position for the first time in five decades, replaced by chronic lower respiratory diseases, which include asthma, emphysema, and chronic bronchitis (**www.cdc.gov/nchs/fastats/lcod.htm**).

Physical Fitness Makes Good Medicine

Enhancing physical fitness interacts with the overfat condition to lower disease risk.[173] Men ages 30 to 83 years who are overweight but physically fit suffered fewer deaths from all causes than unfit but normal-weight men.[126] Unfit, lean men have a higher risk of all-cause mortality than overfat, fit men. Such findings support the theory that general fitness status plays a more important role than fatness status in mitigating all-cause mortality; thus, the preferred strategy emphasizes increased physical activity for overweight men and women to improve cardiovascular fitness rather than relying on diet and weight loss alone to improve the individual's health risk profile.

Staying healthy and maintaining a normal body weight also may reduce the risk of mental decline and impaired cognitive function as one ages.[182] The prevalence of obesity has counteracted the decline over previous years in coronary disease among middle-age women.[87] Obese and overweight individuals with two or more heart disease risk factors should reduce weight, while overweight persons without any other risk factors should at least maintain current body weight. Even a modest weight reduction improves insulin sensitivity and blood lipid profile, and prevents or delays diabetes onset in high-risk individuals.[39,66]

Obesity and Cancer Risk

The American Cancer Society's *Guidelines on Nutrition and Physical Activity for Cancer Prevention* states: "Be as lean as possible throughout life without being underweight" to reduce cancer risk. Clear evidence links obesity to breast cancer in postmenopausal women and adenocarcinoma of the lower esophagus, and cancers of the colon, rectum, uterus, kidney, and pancreas. Supportive evidence indicates that obesity relates positively to cancers of the liver, cervix, gallbladder, and ovaries including non-Hodgkin lymphoma, multiple myeloma, and aggressive prostate cancer. Up to one third of common cancers in industrialized nations link to excess weight and diminished physical activity. Excess weight also can decrease the chance of cancer survival. According to statistics released by the American Institute of Cancer Research (www.aicr.org), excessive body fat causes nearly one half of endometrial cancers and one third of esophageal cancers. If Americans maintained normal body weights at a BMI ≤25.0, endometrial cancer would decrease by 49%, esophageal cancer by 35%, pancreatic cancer by 28%, kidney cancer by 24%, gallbladder cancer by 21%, breast cancer by 17%, and colon cancer by 9%.

The bottom line: regular physical activity, a healthful diet, and losing excess weight provides a potent way to reduce cancer risk and improve its outcome once detected.

Excessive Fatness in Childhood and Adolescence Predicts Adverse Health Effects in Adulthood

The origin of adult obesity and its adverse health consequences often begins in childhood. Children who gain more weight than peers tend to become overweight adults with increased risk for hypertension, elevated insulin, hypercholesterolemia, and heart disease.[40] Being overweight during adolescence links to adverse health effects 55 years later. The Harvard Growth Study from 1922 to 1935 evaluated 3000 schoolchildren annually on a variety of health variables, including triplicate measures of body mass and stature, at the same time each year until they left or graduated high school.[34] Of the initial group, the researchers studied 1857 subjects for an additional 8 years. Subjects were designated as either lean, corresponding to the 25th to 50th percentile for BMI, or overweight, which exceeds the 75th percentile for BMI. Compared with leaner subjects, overweight children as adults showed a greater risk of mortality from all causes and a twofold higher coronary heart disease risk. Women overweight during adolescence were eight times more likely to report problems with personal care and routine living tasks such as walking, stair climbing, and lifting, and a 1.6-fold increase in arthritis than women rated lean in adolescence.

The alarming rise in obesity during childhood and adolescence requires immediate interventions to prevent subsequent risk for disease as these children grow into adulthood. FIGURE 30.8 shows the percentile cutoffs for a two-level procedure recommended by the American Academy of Pediatrics to identify either overweight children (BMI >95th percentile requiring in-depth medical assessment) and those at risk of becoming overweight (BMI 85th–95th percentile, requiring second-level screening including family history and risk factor assessment).

Defined Health Risks

Considerable information exists regarding increasing levels of body fat and defined health risks in children, adolescents, and adults. Excessive body fat relates closely to the alarming increase in type 2 diabetes among children. For adults with diabetes, 70% classify as overweight and nearly 35% as obese.

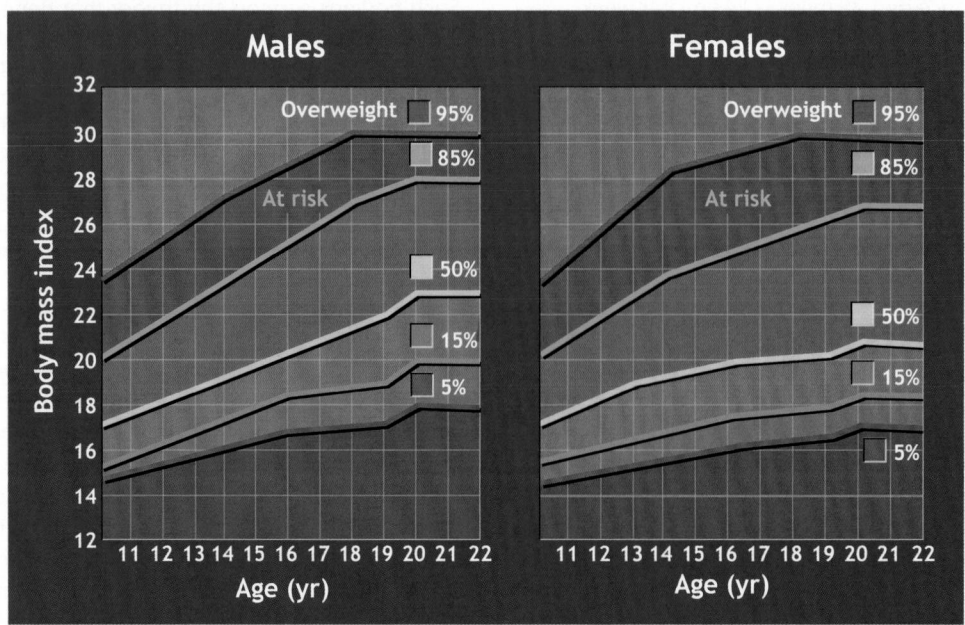

FIGURE 30.8 • Two-level procedure using BMI to identify overweight adolescents and adolescents at risk of becoming overweight. (Adapted with permission from Green M, ed. *Bright Futures: Guidelines for Health Supervision of Infants, Children And Adolescents.* Arlington, VA: National Center for Education in Maternal and Child Health, 1994; www.mchlibrary.info/pubs/default.html.)

Five Potential Serious Medical Complications of Diabetes

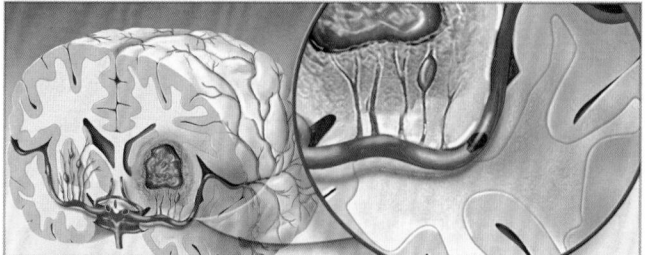

Stroke: Impairs neurologic function, leading to numbness, weakness, difficulty with speech, coordination, or walking.

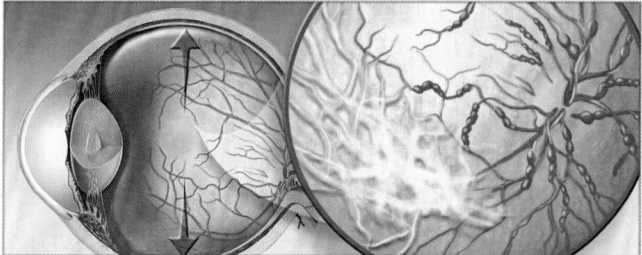

Eye disease: Causes blind spots or, in the extreme, blindness.

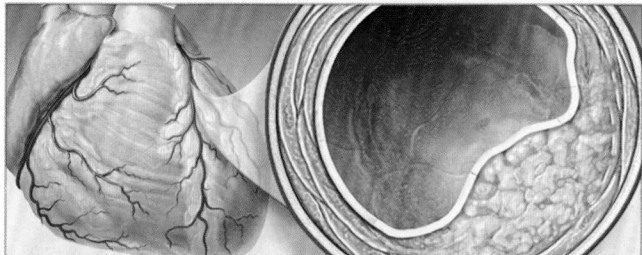

Heart disease: Causes heart attacks and congestive heart failure.

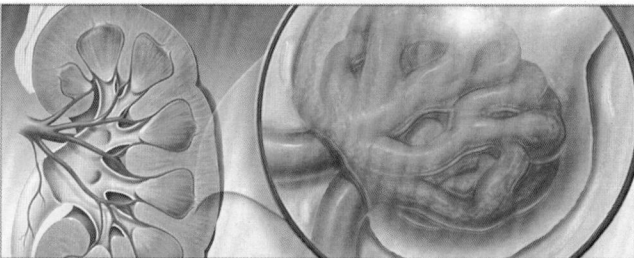

Kidney disease: Causes kidney failure.

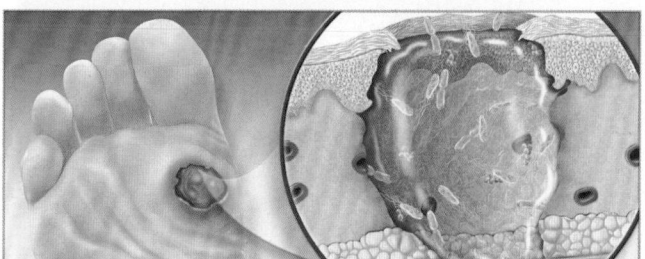

Circulatory problems: Causes sores that heal poorly. In extreme situations, gangrene develops and can lead to amputations.

A moderate 4 to 10% increase in body weight after age 20 associates with 1.5 times greater risk of death from coronary artery disease and nonfatal myocardial infarction.[168] Even maintaining body weight at the high end of the normal range increases heart disease risk. An 8-year study of nearly 116,000 female nurses observed that all but the thinnest women showed increased risk for heart attack and chest pains.[131] Nurses of average body weight experienced 30% more heart attacks than thinner counterparts, while the risk for a moderately overweight nurse averaged 80% higher. This means that a woman who gains 9 kg (19.8 lb) from her late teens to middle age doubles her heart attack risk. Epidemiologic evidence indicates excess body weight as an independent and powerful risk for congestive heart failure.[107]

Weight gain also increases risk for cancers of the breast, colon, esophagus, prostate, kidney, and uterus.[19,200,234] Maintaining a BMI below 25 could prevent one of every six cancer deaths in the United States or about 90,000 deaths yearly.[19] One half of cardiovascular deaths and one third of colon, endometrial, and breast cancer deaths linked to the overweight condition.

Researchers followed a cohort of 82,000 female nurses ages 30 to 55 years every 2 years from 1976 to determine whether initial BMI modifies the relation between long-term weight gain or weight loss and hypertension risk. FIGURE 30.9 depicts the relative risk for hypertension adjusted for multiple factors linked to hypertension in three groups stratified for BMI at age 18. For women in the first and second BMI tertiles at age 18 (BMI ≥22.0), weight loss in later years did not reduce

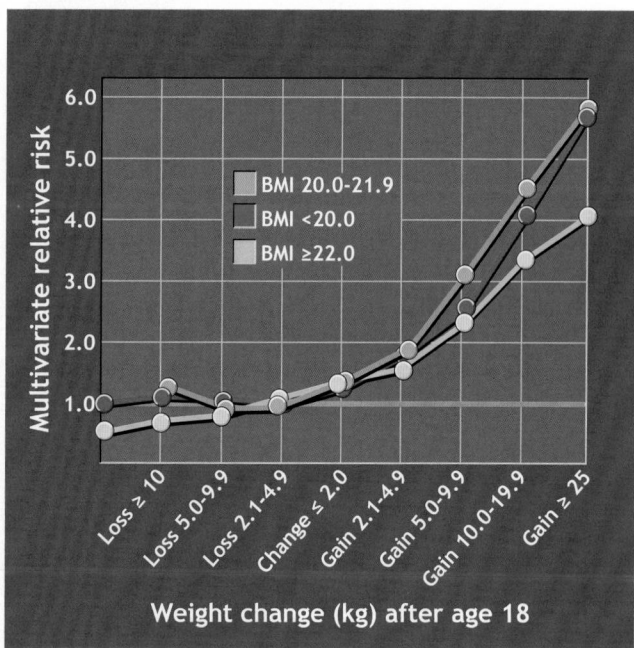

FIGURE 30.9 • Multivariate relative risk for hypertension according to weight change after age 18 years within strata of BMI at age 18. Risk adjusted for age, BMI at age 18, stature, family history of myocardial infarction, parity, oral contraceptive use, menopausal status, postmenopausal use of hormones, and smoking status. Horizontal pink line indicates normal risk. (Adapted with permission from Huang Z, et al. Body weight, weight change, and risk for hypertension in women. *Ann Intern Med* 1998;128:81.)

Specific Health Risks of Excessive Body Fat

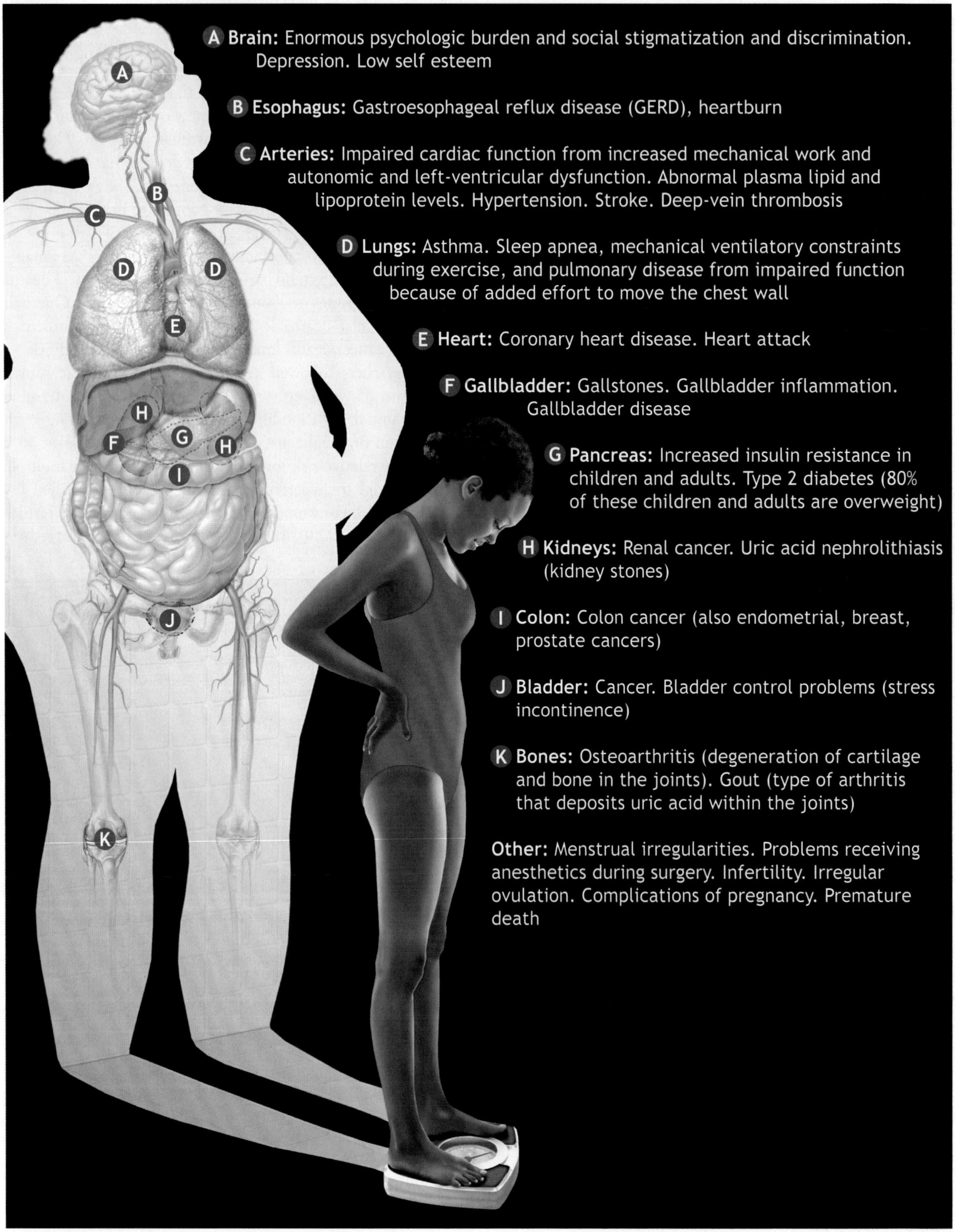

A **Brain:** Enormous psychologic burden and social stigmatization and discrimination. Depression. Low self esteem

B **Esophagus:** Gastroesophageal reflux disease (GERD), heartburn

C **Arteries:** Impaired cardiac function from increased mechanical work and autonomic and left-ventricular dysfunction. Abnormal plasma lipid and lipoprotein levels. Hypertension. Stroke. Deep-vein thrombosis

D **Lungs:** Asthma. Sleep apnea, mechanical ventilatory constraints during exercise, and pulmonary disease from impaired function because of added effort to move the chest wall

E **Heart:** Coronary heart disease. Heart attack

F **Gallbladder:** Gallstones. Gallbladder inflammation. Gallbladder disease

G **Pancreas:** Increased insulin resistance in children and adults. Type 2 diabetes (80% of these children and adults are overweight)

H **Kidneys:** Renal cancer. Uric acid nephrolithiasis (kidney stones)

I **Colon:** Colon cancer (also endometrial, breast, prostate cancers)

J **Bladder:** Cancer. Bladder control problems (stress incontinence)

K **Bones:** Osteoarthritis (degeneration of cartilage and bone in the joints). Gout (type of arthritis that deposits uric acid within the joints)

Other: Menstrual irregularities. Problems receiving anesthetics during surgery. Infertility. Irregular ovulation. Complications of pregnancy. Premature death

hypertension risk. Weight gain after age 18 markedly increased hypertension risk compared to women who maintained a stable body weight. For women with BMIs exceeding 22.0, subsequent weight loss dramatically decreased hypertension risk. Weight gain increased hypertension risk similarly to that of the lighter group of women. Obesity now ranks with the four other major heart attack risk factors—high cholesterol, hypertension, cigarette smoking, and sedentary lifestyle—in contrast to its former status formally listed only as a *contributing* risk factor.

CRITERIA FOR EXCESSIVE BODY FAT: HOW FAT IS TOO FAT?

In Chapter 28, we discussed limitations of the height–weight tables and BMI to assess body composition. Three approaches more appropriate for measuring a person's fat content include:

1. Percentage of body mass composed of fat
2. Distribution or patterning of fat at different anatomic regions
3. Size and number of individual fat cells

Percentage of Body Fat

What determines the demarcation between a normal level of body fat and an excess? In Chapter 28, we suggested the following serve as the "normal" body fat range for adult men and women—the "average" percentage body fat value ±1 standard deviation. For men and women ages 17 to 50 years, this variation equals 5% body fat units. Using this statistical boundary, overfatness then corresponds to a body fat level that exceeds the average value +5% body fat. For example, in young men whose body fat averages 15% of body mass, the borderline for excessive fatness becomes 20% body fat. For older men whose fat averages 25%, overfatness would include body fat in excess of 30%. For young women, overfatness corresponds to body fat content above 30%; for older women, borderline obesity corresponds to about 37% body fat. We emphasize that just because the average value for percentage body fat increases with age, this does not dictate that people should become fatter as they age. In our opinion, one criterion for determining "too fat" emerges from data for younger men and women—above 20% for men and above 30% for women. With this single gender-specific standard, average age-related population values do not become the reference standard and thus the acceptable criterion. We also recognize that this classification standard based on an average for young adults becomes overly rigorous when applied to an older population. It probably places more than 50% of adults in the overly fat category, a value below the 69% value for overweight and obese Americans using BMI as the standard. It also closely corresponds to proposed gender-based body fat standards computed for young adults from the relationship between BMI and four component estimates of percentage body fat for African Americans and whites.[62]

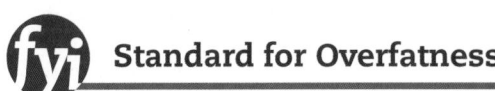

Standard for Overfatness

Men: above 20%; **Women**: above 30%

We consider that the overfatness exists along a continuum from the upper limit of normal (20% body fat for men and 30% for women) to as high as 50% and a theoretical maximum of nearly 70% of body mass in the massively obese. This latter group's weight ranges from 170 to 250 kg (374 to 550 lb) or higher. This can create a life-threatening situation in such extreme cases as the body's total fat content exceeds lean body mass!

Distribution or Patterning of Fat at Different Anatomic Regions

The patterning of the body's adipose tissue, independent of total body fat, alters health risks in children, adolescents, and adults.[33,60,210,235,237] FIGURE 30.10 shows two types of regional fat distribution. Increased health risk from fat deposition in the

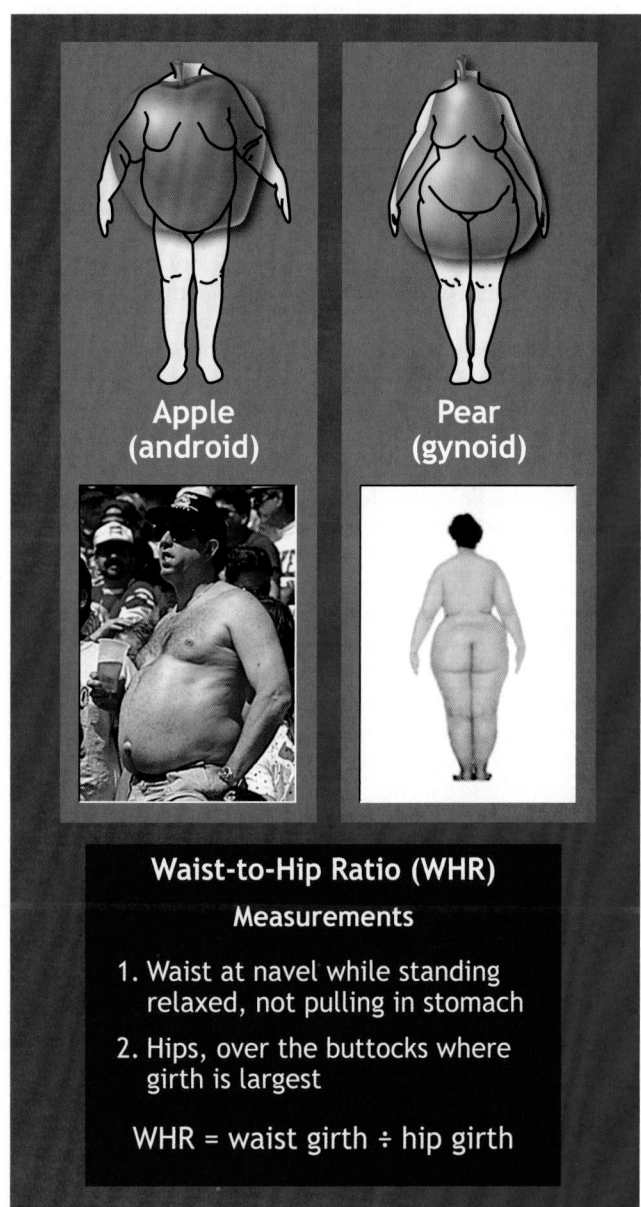

Waist-to-Hip Ratio (WHR)

Measurements

1. Waist at navel while standing relaxed, not pulling in stomach
2. Hips, over the buttocks where girth is largest

WHR = waist girth ÷ hip girth

FIGURE 30.10 • Male (android pattern) and female (gynoid pattern) fat patterning, including waist-to-hip girth ratio.

abdominal area (**central** or **android-type obesity**), particularly internal visceral deposits, may result from this tissue's active lipolysis with catecholamine stimulation. Fat stored in this region shows greater metabolic responsiveness than fat in the gluteal and femoral regions known as **peripheral** or **gynoid-type obesity**. Increases in central fat more readily support processes that cause heart disease[186] and metabolic syndrome.[165]

In men, the amount of fat located inside the abdominal cavity (intraabdominal, or *visceral adipose tissue*) is twice as large compared to that of women.[12] For men, visceral fat percentage increases progressively with age, whereas this fat deposition in women begins to increase at menopause onset.[115] Central fat deposition particularly in the abdominal region with increasing levels of fatness shown in the figure, independent of fat storage in other anatomic areas, reflects an altered metabolic profile that increases health risk.

As a general guideline, waist-to-hip girth ratios that exceed 0.80 for women and 0.95 for men increase death risk even after adjusting for BMI.[37,164] One limitation of the ratio is it poorly captures the specific effects of each girth measure. Waist and hip circumferences reflect different aspects of body composition and fat distribution. Each has an independent and often opposite effect on cardiovascular disease risk. An increased waist girth represents the so-called malignant form of obesity characterized by central fat deposition that may cripple the body's ability to mobilize and/or utilize insulin, setting the stage for type 2 diabetes and heart disease. This region of fat deposition provides a reasonable indication of the accumulation of intra-abdominal (visceral) adipose tissue. This makes abdominal girth the trunk measure of clinical choice as a practical measure to evaluate the metabolic and health risks and accelerated mortality with obesity.[101,144,178,196] *Over a broad range of BMI values, men and women with high abdominal girth values possess greater relative risk for cardiovascular disease, type 2 diabetes, cancer, dementia, and cataracts (the leading cause of blindness worldwide) than individuals with small waist circumference or peripheral obesity.*[96,214,228]

Excess weight distribution in the abdominal area (and correspondingly high blood insulin levels) also increases colorectal cancer risk.[83,103] A waist girth that exceeds 91 cm (36 in.) in men and 82 cm (32 in.) in women nearly doubles the risk of this cancer.[174] The unnumbered figure in the following FYI shows how to apply three BMI categories and waist girth measurements (above and below 40 inches for men and 34.6 inches for women) to assess a person's risk of health problems ranked from least risk to very high risk.

Waist Girth and Health Risk With Normal Body Mass Index

Researchers at the American Cancer Society examined the association between waist circumference and overall mortality among 48,000 men and 56,343 women age 50 and older in the Cancer Prevention Study II Nutrition Cohort (**www.cancer.org/research/researchprogramsfunding/cancer-prevention-study-overviews**). Waist girths exceeding 47 inches in men and 43 inches in women associated with approximately twice the likelihood of dying during the study period. Surprisingly, a larger waistline linked to greater mortality for men and women regardless of normal BMI levels.

For men not overweight, an average excess at the abdominal waist of 3.9 inches increased death risk by 16% compared to counterparts with the same BMI but a slimmer waist girth. For normal-weight women, an extra 3.9 inches at the abdominal waist increased risk by 25%.

More than half of U.S. men ages 50 to 79 have a waist girth considered "abdominally obese" (≥40.1 inches), whereas 70% of women in this age category have an "abdominally obese" waist girth of ≥34.6 inches. The researchers concluded the following: "Regardless of body weight, avoiding gains in waist circumference may reduce risk of premature mortality. Even if you have not had a noticeable weight gain, if you notice your waist size increasing, that's an important sign it's time to eat better and start exercising more."

Source: Jacobs EJ, et al. Waist circumference and all-cause mortality in a large US cohort. *Arch Intern Med* 2010;170:1293.

Related References

Kanhai DA, et al. The risk of general and abdominal adiposity in the occurrence of new vascular events and mortality in patients with various manifestations of vascular disease. *Int J Obes (Lond)* 2012;36:695.

Lee JS, et al. Survival benefit of abdominal adiposity: a 6-year follow-up study with dual x-ray absorptiometry in 3,978 older adults. *Age (Dordr)* 2012;34:597.

Adipocyte Size and Number: Hypertrophy versus Hyperplasia

Adipocyte size and number provide another way to assess and classify obesity. Adipose tissue mass increases in two ways:

1. **Fat cell hypertrophy**: Existing adipocytes enlarge or fill with fat
2. **Fat cell hyperplasia**: Total adipocyte number increases

One technique for studying adipose cellularity involves sucking small fragments of subcutaneous tissue usually from the triceps, subscapular, buttocks, and/or lower abdomen into a syringe through a needle inserted directly into the fat depot. Chemical treatment of the tissue sample isolates the individual adipocytes for accurate sizing and counting. Dividing fat mass in the tissue sample by adipocyte number determines the average quantity of fat in each cell. One can estimate total adipocyte number by determining total body fat by a criterion method such as hydrostatic weighing or DXA. For example, an individual who weighs 88 kg (194 lb) with 13% body fat has a total fat mass of 11.4 kg (0.13 × 88 kg). Dividing 11.4 kg by the average fat content per cell estimates total adipocyte number. If the average adipocyte contains 0.60 μg of fat, then this person's body contains 19 billion adipocytes (11.4 kg ÷ 0.60 μg).

$$\text{Total adipocyte number} = \text{Mass of body fat} \div \text{Fat content per cell}$$

Abdominal Obesity Associated with Death Risk

Researchers have examined the association of BMI (measured without wearing shoes), waist girth (narrowest torso girth), and waist-to-hip ratio with the risk of death among 359,387 participants without prior history of cancer, heart disease, or stroke at baseline from nine countries in the European Prospective Investigation into Cancer and Nutrition (EPIC; **http://epic.iarc.fr/**). The mean age at baseline was 51.5 ± 10.4 years; 65.4% of the participants were women. After 9.7 years, 4% or 14,723 participants had died. The lowest risks of death related to BMI occurred at a BMI of 25.3 for men and 24.3 for women. By definition, BMI <18.5 refers to underweight, 18.5 to <25.0 refers to normal weight, 25.0 to <30.0 refers to overweight, and ≥30.0 refers to obesity. After adjustment for BMI, waist girth and waist-to-hip ratio strongly associated with death risk. The correlations for BMI with waist girth and waist-to-hip ratio were $r = 0.85$ and 0.55 (men) and $r = 0.84$ and 0.38 (women). BMI remained significantly associated with death risk when the statistical analysis included either waist circumference or waist-to-hip ratio. The authors advocate the use of waist girth or waist-to-hip ratio including BMI to assess death risk, particularly among persons with a relatively low BMI.

Waist girth	BMI category		
	Normal 18.5 - 24.9 kg · m⁻²	Overweight 25 - 29.9 kg · m⁻²	Obese class I 30 - 34.9 kg · m⁻²
Men: < 102 cm Women: < 88 cm	Least risk	Increased risk	High risk
Men: ≥ 102 cm Women: ≥ 88 cm	Increased risk	High risk	Very high risk

Applying BMI and waist girth measurements in adult men and women from least risk to very high risk for health and medical problems. For men, 102 cm = 40 inches; for women, 88 cm = 34.6 inches. (Data from the world literature, including Douketis, JD. Body weight classification. *CMAJ* 2005;172:995.)

In one of our laboratories, needle biopsy and photomicrographic techniques extracted fat and measured the average fat content of adipocytes at three anatomic sites. **FIGURE 30.11** shows adipocytes from the upper buttocks of one of this textbook's authors whose total fat mass at the time equaled 17.02 kg (body mass: 89.1 kg; 19.1% body fat) with 0.73 μg of fat per cell; the estimated total adipocyte number was 23.3 billion (17.02 kg ÷ 0.73 μg). Over the next 28 years, a weight gain of 3.2 kg presumably was accounted for by an increase in total fat mass (without increasing FFM; more than likely it related to a decline in FFM with aging). The additional fat accretion can probably be explained by increases in the size of individual fat cells without fat cell proliferation.

Fat Cell Development and Adipocytes

Pioneering research in the early 1980s began to search for a molecular trigger to explain the link between newly developing fat cells called preadipocytes, the precursors to fat cells, and subsequent obesity. Researchers studied cellular differentiation to determine why some fat cells became excessively large and abundant and others remained normal in size without increasing their number. It had been determined that either the conservation of energy or the expenditure of energy differed in the development of adult white adipose tissue and infant brown adipose tissue. Specific genes were identified that first were expressed in preadipocytes compared to mature fat cells. Once identified, attention focused on what transcription factors and enhancers "turned on" those genes. From hundreds of turned-on genes during fat cell differentiation, the *aP2* gene became a good candidate as an appropriate model to study differentiation between brown fat cell versus white fat cell growth and development.[67] Research in the 1990s originally identified the peroxisome proliferation-activated receptor gamma (PPARγ) as the "master gene" of white fat cell development. Subsequent research has demonstrated that this human gene also serves the following three functions[53,179,206]:

1. Serves as a receptor for antidiabetic drugs (TZD drug class or thiazolidinediones)
2. Triggers cellular metabolic effects to decrease adiposity
3. Functions in the control of cell proliferation, atherosclerosis, macrophage function, and immunity

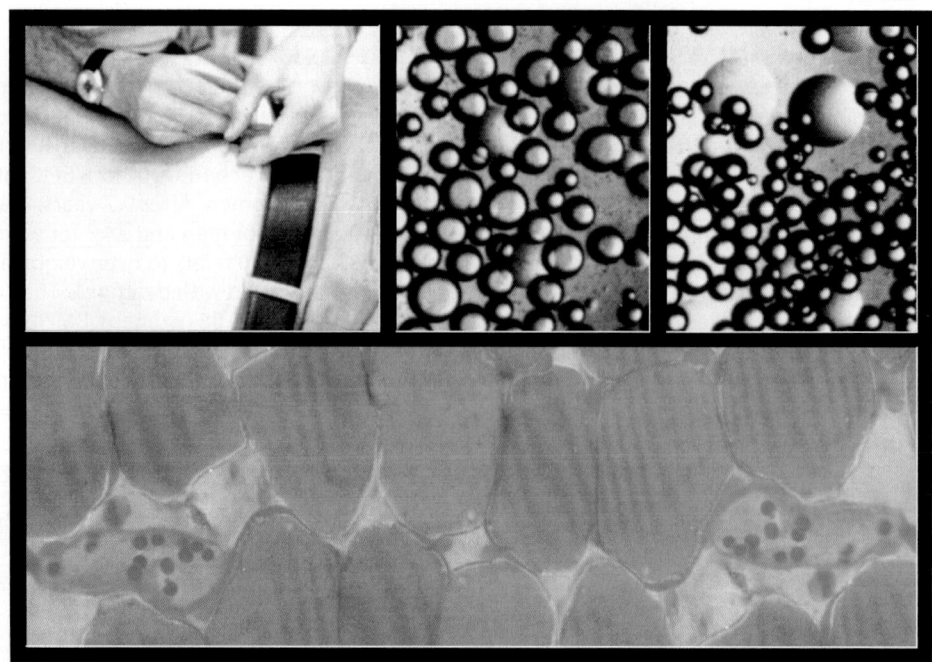

FIGURE 30.11 • *(Upper panel)* Needle biopsy to extract adipocytes from the upper buttocks region. A small area is sterilized and anesthetized, and the biopsy needle placed beneath the skin surface to extract minute samples of fluid and tissue that is further analyzed to isolate a representative sample of fat cells. Photomicrographs of the adipocytes from the buttocks of a physically active professor before *(center)* and after *(right)* 6 months of marathon training. Adipocyte diameter averaged 8.6% smaller after training. The average volume of fat in each cell decreased by 18.2%. The large spherical structures in the background are lipid droplets. Bottom panel. Cross section of human adipocytes × 440. (From Geneser F. Color atlas of histology. Philadelphia: Lea & Febiger, 1985. Top panel two photomicrographs courtesy of P. M. Clarkson, Muscle Biochemistry Laboratory, Department of Kinesiology, University of Massachusetts, Amherst, MA.)

The brown fat present in infants, but presumably not in adults, has one main function: to serve as a heat source for the baby's survival. Heat production occurs metabolically by leaking hydrogen ions across the mitochondrion's inner membrane, generating heat called futile metabolism instead of converting it into ATP for other metabolic processes in white lipid droplets. **Figure 30.12** shows a schematic diagram of these basic metabolic differences between how brown fat uses its mitochondria to convert food into the end product *heat* rather than what occurs in white fat to produce the end product *ATP* to power cellular functions.

Cellularity Differences Between Nonobese and Obese Persons

Figure 30.13 compares body mass, total fat, and adipose tissue cellularity in 25 subjects, 20 of whom classified as clinically obese (BMI ~40.0). The body mass of the obese averaged more than twice that of the nonobese, and they had nearly three times more body fat. In cellularity, adipocytes in the obese averaged 50% larger with nearly three times more cells (75 vs. 27 billion). *Cell number represents the major structural difference in adipose tissue mass between the severely obese and nonobese persons.*

Relating total body fat content to cell size and cell number further demonstrates the contribution of adipocyte

 Molecular Biology to the Rescue

In 2004, researchers discovered the protein molecule PGC-1α that binds to the important PPARγ molecule and activates genes important to brown fat–specific differentiation.[51,177,189] The gene for PGC-1α expressed in white fat cells impacted an uncoupling protein (UCP1) that caused mitochondria to produce heat (thermogenesis or uncoupled mitochondrial respiration). Interestingly, this same gene also causes muscles with aerobic exercise training to switch their fiber type to more oxidative fibers (type II to type I).[73] The gene PRDM16 serves as one of the master "regulators" of brown fat differentiation. It stimulates brown adipogenesis by binding to PPARγ and activating its transcriptional function. This gene activates the PGC-1α gene and accelerates the expression of nine other brown fat–specific genes, and with some molecular tinkering, makes the energy-wasting brown fat cells behave more like the energy-conserving white fat cells. The bottom line of research with preadipocyte cells and PRDM16 and PGC-1α relates to their possible roles in regulating mitochondrial function. This approach in fat cell and obesity research shifts focus to the molecular basis of energy expenditure. Researchers hope that discovery of a new drug or combination of drugs, even if they have only a 1 to 2% internal metabolic effect for augmenting caloric expenditure in obese individuals, could over time with other management methods positively impact the obese condition.[30,224]

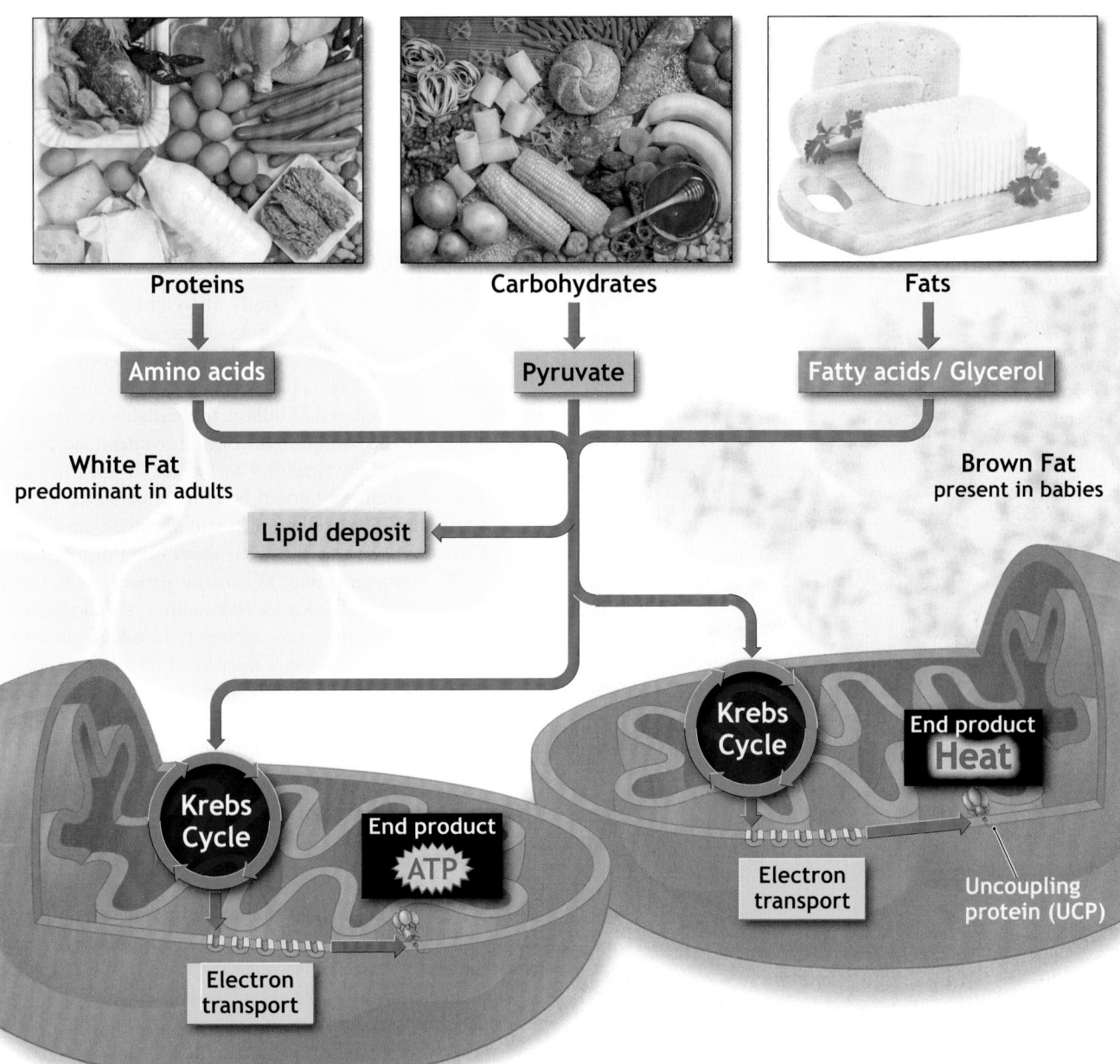

FIGURE 30.12 • A unique set of molecular switches governs fat cell differentiation. Two master regulator genes, PPARgamma with RXR (a cofactor retinoic acid receptor) initiates white fat development; when PRDM16 switches on, the preadipocyte activates PGC-1 (plays a central role in regulating cellular energy metabolism) along with other genes, which define the brown fat phenotype. The evidence is now abundantly clear that fat cells are not simply inert globs of lipid. Instead, they are dynamic and influential in exchanging chemical signals with the brain and reproductive and immune systems. Existing fat cells grow and shrink, and absorb and release energy-rich lipids as needed depending on substrate availability and utilization. When overloaded with surplus calories, fat cells can initiate cell division to absorb the oversupply; once they hypertrophy as they fill with excess fat, they remain in a state of flux until a shift occurs in the energy balance equation. Molecular remodeling of fat cells has the potential to shift the balance in favor of expenditure rather than storage. If the mechanism for brown fat production could be determined and "turned on" in obese adults (as both cell types originate from the same precursor cells), and if metabolic pathways in obese individuals could utilize the heat-producing mechanisms from brown fat, the extra heat energy from these cells might compete with the energy storage function of white fat cells and shift the energy balance equation in the direction of fat loss.

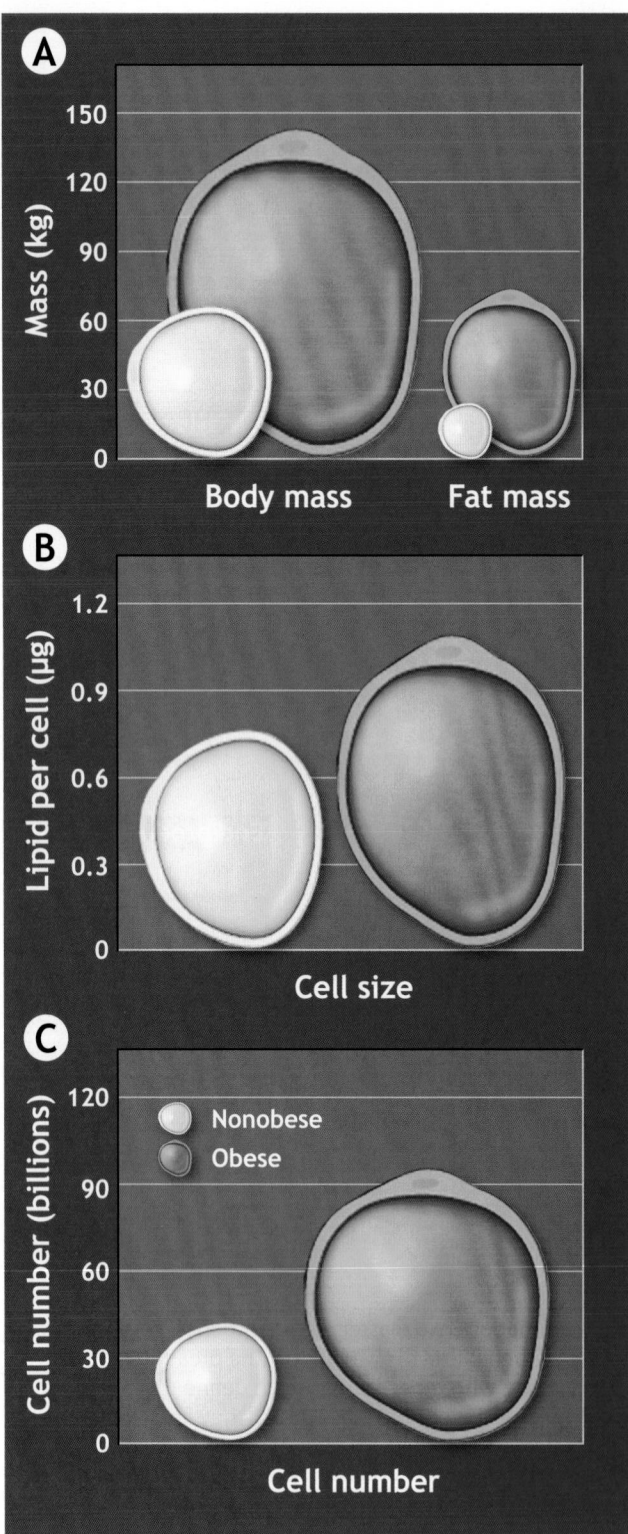

FIGURE 30.13 • Comparison of body mass, total fat, and adipose tissue cellularity in 25 subjects, 20 of whom classified as clinically obese.

For comparison, an average-size person has between 25 and 30 billion adipocytes, whereas the clinically severe obese may have more than three to five times this number, particularly when excessive fatness occurs in childhood or adolescence. Differences also exist in the composition of the fatty acid structures in perivisceral, omental, and subcutaneous adipose tissue regions among overweight/obese males and females.[64]

Effects of Weight Loss

FIGURE 30.14 shows a classic study of weight loss effects on adipose tissue characteristics of 19 obese adults during two stages of weight loss. During the first stage, subjects reduced body mass by 46 kg (149 to 103 kg). Adipocyte number before weight reduction averaged 75 billion; this remained unchanged even after the 46-kg weight reduction. In contrast, adipocyte size decreased by 33% from 0.9 to 0.6 μg of lipid per cell. When subjects attained normal body mass of 75 kg by losing an additional 28 kg, cell number still remained unchanged but cell size continued to shrink to about one third that in a nonobese comparison group. When the patients achieved a "normal" body mass and body fat level, adipocytes had become considerably smaller than the nonobese. *In adults, the major change in adipose cellularity in weight loss is shrinkage of adipocytes with no change in cell number.* These findings suggest that weight loss in obese persons does not really "cure" their obesity, at least for total adipocyte number.

Effects of Weight Gain

An interesting series of studies in the late 1960s and early 1970s evaluated the dynamics of weight gain on adipose tissue cellularity. In one study, adult male volunteers with an initial average body fat content of 15% deliberately increased daily caloric intake by three times normal to about 7000 kcal for 40 wk.[184] For a typical subject, body mass increased 25% and percentage body fat nearly doubled from 14.6 to 28.2%. Fat deposition represented 10.5 kg of the 12.7 kg of weight gained during the overfeeding period. In a similar experiment with subjects with no personal or family history of obesity, voluntary overeating increased body mass by 16.4 kg.[171] In both experiments, adipocytes increased substantially in size with *no change* in cell number. When caloric intake decreased and subjects attained normal weight, total body fat declined and the adipocytes reverted to their original size. *In general, moderate weight gain from overeating in adults enlarges existing adipocytes rather than stimulating new adipocyte development.*

Possibility of New Adipocyte Formation

Extreme accumulation of body fat in adults stimulates increased adipose cellularity because adipocyte size reaches an upper limit of about 1.0 μg fat, beyond which no further hypertrophy occurs. At extremes of obesity, almost all adipocytes attain their hypertrophic limit. In this situation, the preadipocyte pool provides additional adipocytes to increase cell number, with a concomitant increase in the quantity

number to obesity. As body fat increases, adipocytes eventually reach a biologic upper size limit. Once this occurs, cell number becomes the key factor determining any further fat accretion. Even doubling adipocyte size does not explain the large difference in total fat mass between obese and average persons.

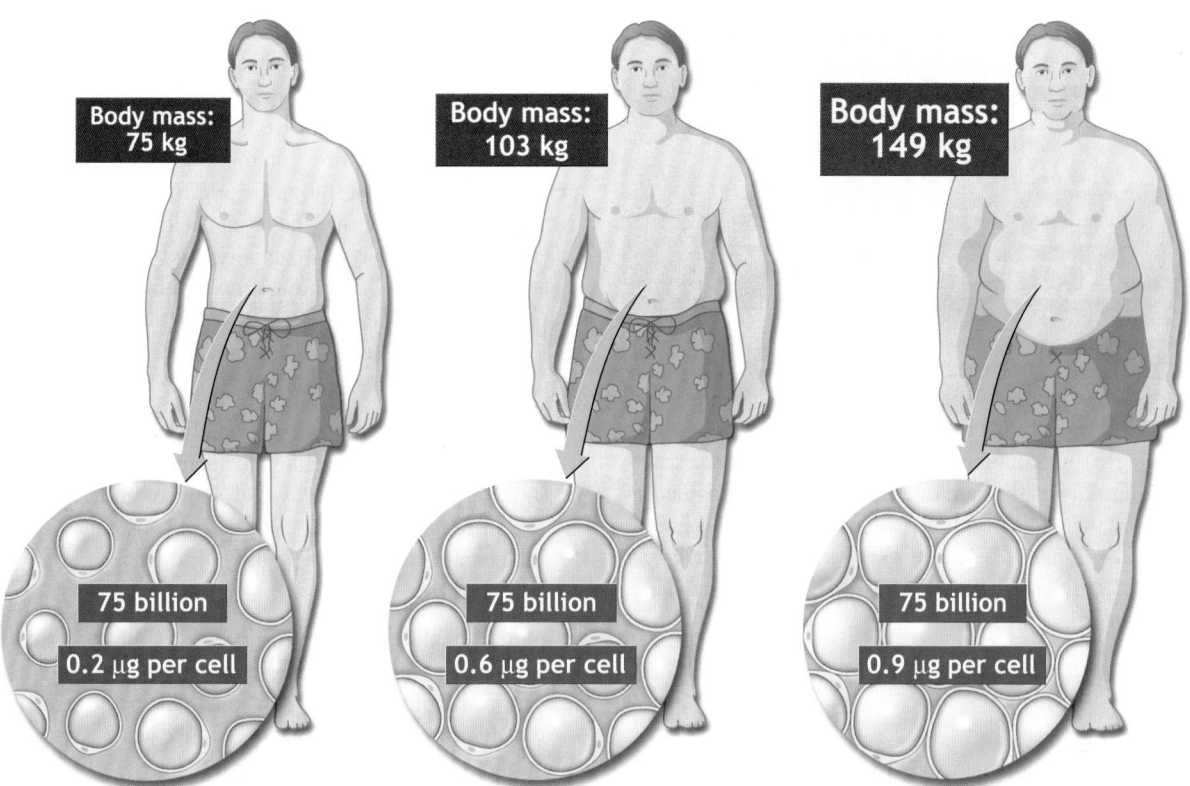

FIGURE 30.14 • Changes in adipose cellularity with weight reduction in obese subjects. (Data from Hirsch J. Adipose cellularity in relation to human obesity. In: Stollerman GH, ed. *Advances in Internal Medicine*, Vol. 17. Chicago, IL: Year-Book, 1971.)

of fat stored within the liver and between muscle fibers. *In maturity-onset severe obesity, in which the already obese adult gains even more body fat, hypercellularity may accompany the increasing size of existing adipocytes.* The increased number of cells at this point constitutes a failure of adipocyte regulation that unfortunately leads to further fat accumulation.

Summary

1. Obesity or excess accumulation of body fat represents a heterogeneous disorder with a final common pathway where energy intake chronically exceeds energy expenditure.

2. Over the past 35 years, the average body weight of adult Americans has increased considerably. Currently, nearly 140 million American (69% of the population) classify as either overweight (BMI 25 to <30) or obese (BMI ≥30), with 39% of adults classified as obese. Worldwide, about 310 million people are obese and nearly 790 million more are overweight.

3. Fifteen to 20% of American children and 12% of adolescents (up from 7.6% in 1976 to 1980) classify as overweight. Excessive body fatness, childhood's most common chronic disorder, is most prevalent among poor and minority children.

4. Genetic factors account for 25 to 30% of excessive body fat accumulation. Genetic predisposition does not necessarily cause excessive fatness, but in the right environment, the genetically susceptible individual gains body fat.

5. A defective gene for adipocyte leptin production and/or hypothalamic leptin insensitivity causes the brain to assess adipose tissue status improperly. Excessive food intake creates a chronic positive energy balance.

6. Excessive body fat is a leading cause of preventable death in the United States.

7. Comorbid hypertension, elevated blood sugar level, postmenopausal breast cancer, and elevated total cholesterol and low HDL cholesterol levels increase an overweight person's risk of poor health at any level of excess weight.

8. The overfatness threshold for adult men and women should more closely reflect percentage body fat levels of younger adults—men above 20%, women above 30%.

9. Body fat patterning affects health risks independent of total body fat. Fat distributed in the abdominal region (central, or android-type, obesity) poses a greater risk than fat deposited at the thighs and buttocks (peripheral, or gynoid-type, obesity).

10. Body fat increases in two ways before adulthood: enlargement of individual adipocytes (*fat cell hypertrophy*) and increase in total cell number (*fat cell hyperplasia*).

11. Modest adult weight gain and loss changes adipocyte size with little change in cell number. In extreme weight gain, adipocyte number increases once cell size reaches a hypertrophic limit.

PRINCIPLES OF WEIGHT CONTROL: DIET AND PHYSICAL ACTIVITY

PART 2

For many adults, body weight fluctuates only slightly during the year, even though annual food intake averages more than 830 kg (1826 lb). This represents an impressive constancy considering that slight increases in daily food intake translate to substantial weight gain over time if unaccompanied by compensatory increases in energy expenditure. *The human body functions in accord with the laws of thermodynamics. If total food calories exceed daily energy expenditure, excess calories accumulate and store as fat in adipose tissue.*

ENERGY BALANCE: INPUT VERSUS OUTPUT

The first law of thermodynamics, often called the law of conservation of energy, discovered by German physician Julius

Robert Mayer (1814–1878; www.ghtc.usp.br/server/HFIS/Mayer-Joule-Carnot-Isis-1929.pdf) posits that energy can be transferred from one system to another in many forms but cannot be created or destroyed. In human terms, this means that the energy balance equation dictates that body mass remains constant when total caloric intake from food equals total caloric expenditure The latter includes the thermic effect of food (TEF), physical activity, and resting metabolism. **FIGURE 30.15** shows that any chronic imbalance on the energy output or input side of the equation changes body weight.

There are three ways to unbalance the energy balance equation to produce weight loss:

1. Reduce caloric intake below daily energy requirements
2. Maintain caloric intake and increase energy expenditure through additional physical activity above daily energy requirements
3. Decrease daily caloric intake and increase daily energy expenditure

When considering the sensitivity of the energy balance equation, if caloric intake exceeds output by only 100 kcal daily, the surplus calories consumed in a year equal 36,500 kcal (365 days × 100 kcal). Because 0.45 kg (1.0 lb) of body fat contains about 3500 kcal (each 1 lb [454 g] of adipose tissue contains about 86% fat, or 390.4 g; therefore,

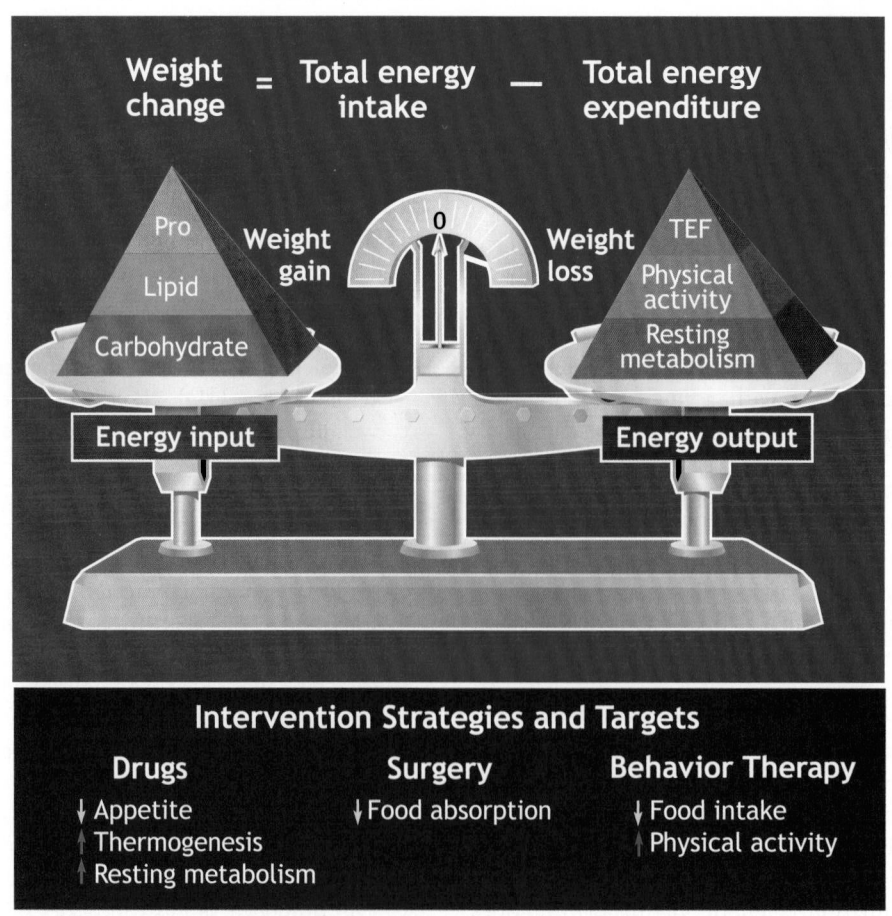

FIGURE 30.15 • The energy balance equation plus intervention strategies and specific targets to alter energy balance in the direction of weight loss. *Pro*, protein; *TEF*, thermic effect of food.

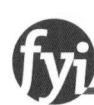

Consuming Excess Calories Produces Fat Gain Regardless of Nutrient Source

The quantity of food consumed, not the food's composition, determines fat gain. A recent study challenges the claim that altering the mixture of macronutrient components in the diet—protein, fats, carbohydrates—profoundly affects fat gain.[1] Twenty-five young, healthy men (*n* = 16) and women (*n* = 9) with BMIs between 19 and 30 were deliberately fed 1000 excess calories a day for 56 days. Carbohydrate intake for both groups remained steady at about 42% of total calories consumed. Those on the low-protein diet (about 5% of total calories) gained less weight (largely attributed to a reduction in lean body mass) than those on a normal- or high-protein regimen (largely attributed to an increase in lean body mass). The body fat of all participants increased by about the same amount, a surprising finding suggesting that it is not the diet's macronutrient composition but rather the excess of calories consumed in terms of body fat accretion. These findings also cast doubt on the validity of BMI measures as a proper means to assess an individual's body fat level. On the opposite side of the energy balance debate,[2] study participants lost total, abdominal, and hepatic fat with consumption of all low-calorie diets regardless of whether they emphasized a lower percentage of fat, protein, or carbohydrate. No differences in fat loss were attributable to the diet's macronutrient composition.

Sources:

[1]Bray G, et al. Effect of dietary protein content on weight gain, energy expenditure, and body composition during overeating: a randomized controlled trial. *JAMA* 2012;307:47.

[2]deSouza RJ, et al. Effects of 4 weight-loss diets differing in fat, protein, and carbohydrate on fat mass, lean mass, visceral adipose tissue, and hepatic fat: results from the POUNDS LOST trial. *Am J Clin Nutr* 2012;95:614.

390.4 g × 9 kcal·g^{-1} = 3514 kcal per lb), this caloric excess causes a yearly gain of about 4.7 kg (10.3 lb) of body fat. In contrast, if daily food intake decreases by just 100 kcal and energy expenditure increases by 100 kcal (e.g., by walking or jogging one extra mile daily), then the yearly deficit equals the energy in 9.5 kg (21 lb) of body fat.

A Prudent Recommendation

The objective of weight-loss programs has changed dramatically over past decades. The previous approach assigned a **goal body weight** that coincided with an "ideal" weight based on body mass and stature. Achievement of goal body weight heralded the weight-loss program's success. Currently, the World Health Organization (www.who.int/en), the Institute of Medicine of the National Academy of Sciences (www.iom.edu), and the National Heart, Lung and Blood Institute (www.nhlbi.nih.gov) recommend that an overweight/obese person reduce initial body weight by 5 to 15%. Setting the initial weight loss goal beyond the 5 to 15% recommendation

often gives patients an unrealistic and potentially unattainable target in light of current treatment methods.

DIETING FOR WEIGHT CONTROL

The first law of thermodynamics affirms that weight loss occurs whenever energy output exceeds energy intake, regardless of the diet's macronutrient mixture. Advantages of relatively high percentages of unrefined complex carbohydrates in a reduced-calorie diet include their moderate-to-low glycemic index; high vitamin, mineral, and phytochemical content; low energy density; and low saturated fatty acid levels. A prudent dietary approach to weight loss unbalances the energy balance equation by reducing energy intake by 300 to 1000 kcal below daily energy expenditure. Moderately reduced energy intake (300 to 500 kcal daily) produces greater fat loss relative to the energy deficit than more severe energy restriction. Individuals who create larger daily deficits to lose weight more rapidly tend to regain weight compared to those who lose weight at a slower rate.

New Controversy: Can You Really Reduce One Pound a Week with a 3500-kcal Deficit?

The 3500-kcal rule posits that 3500 kcal are "used up" for each one pound of weight loss, a model advocated in this text, on respected government-and health-related web sites, and scientific research publications. Nonetheless, new research suggests that this rule grossly overestimates actual weight loss. The authors demonstrate this overestimation and risk of applying the 3500-kcal rule even as a convenient weight-loss estimate by comparing predicted against actual weight loss in seven experiments conducted in confinement under total supervision or objectively measured energy intake. The researchers have made downloadable applications housed in Microsoft Excel and Java, which simulate a rigorously validated, dynamic model of expected weight change. The first two tools, available at **http://www.pbrc.edu/sswcp**, offer a convenient alternative method to provide individuals with projected weight loss and weight gain estimates in response to changes in dietary energy intake. A second tool, which can be downloaded at **http://www.pbrc.edu/mswcp**, projects estimated weight loss simultaneously for multiple subjects, a useful adjunct to inform weight change in varied experimental designs and statistical analysis. The new tools offer a convenient and potentially more accurate alternative to the 3500-kcal rule than incorporated in most smartphone apps and commercial weight-loss reducing regimens.

Source: Thomas DM, et al. Can a weight loss of one pound a week be achieved with a 3500-kcal deficit? Commentary on a commonly accepted rule. *Int J Obes (Lond)* 2013. Apr 8. doi: 10.1038/ijo.2013.51. [Epub ahead of print].

Suppose an overfat woman who normally consumes 2800 kcal daily and maintains a body mass of 79.4 kg wishes to reduce weight only by caloric restriction (dieting). She maintains regular daily energy expenditure but reduces food intake to 1800 kcal to create a 1000-kcal daily deficit. In 7 days, the accumulated deficit equals 7000 kcal, or the energy equivalent of 0.9 kg (2.0 lb) of body fat. Actually, considerably more than 0.9 kg would be lost during the first week because initially the body's glycogen stores make up a large portion of the energy deficit. Stored glycogen compared to stored fat contains fewer calories per gram and considerably more water. For this reason, short periods of caloric restriction often encourage the dieter but produce a large percentage of water and carbohydrate loss per unit weight loss with only a small decrease in body fat. As weight loss continues, a larger proportion of body fat supports the energy deficit created by food restriction (see Fig. 30.21 later in this chapter). To reduce body fat by an additional 1.4 kg, the dieter must maintain the reduced caloric intake of 1800 kcal for another 10.5 days; at this point, body fat theoretically decreases at a rate of 0.45 kg every 3.5 days.

Long-Term Success

The potential for successful long-term weight loss maintenance generally varies inversely with the initial degree of fatness (FIG. 30.16). Note that as the degree of obesity increases from overweight to obese to severe to morbidly obese, the chances for success markedly diminish. For most individuals, unfortunately, initial success in weight loss relates poorly to long-term success. Participants in supervised weight-loss programs that include pharmacologic or behavioral interventions generally lose about 8 to 12% of their original body mass. Unfortunately, typically one to two thirds of the lost weight returns within a year, and almost all of it within 5 years.[108,138,146] FIGURE 30.17 illustrates clearly that over a 7.3-year follow-up of 121 patients, return to original weight occurred in 50% of the individuals within 2 to 3 years, and only seven people remained at their reduced body weights. These discouraging but typical statistics highlight the extreme difficulty of long-term maintenance of a low-calorie diet; it becomes particularly difficult in the relaxed

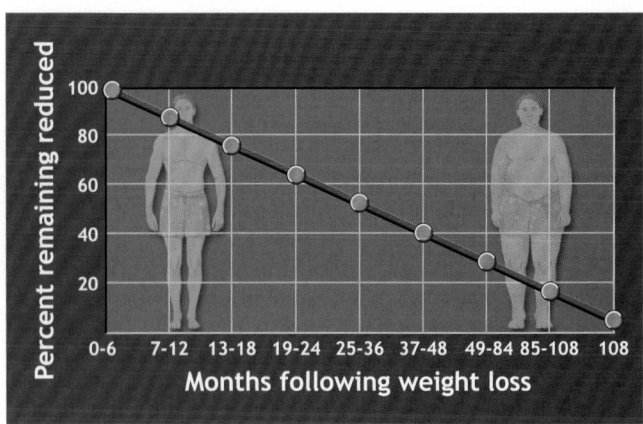

FIGURE 30.17 • General trend for percentage of patients remaining at reduced weights at various time intervals following accomplished weight loss.

atmosphere of one's home with ready access to food and often little emotional support.

(fyi) More Fat and Less Muscle With Regained Weight

Typically, weight regained after weight loss represents more fat and less muscle compared to the composition of weight lost. An experiment determined if the composition of body weight regained after intentional weight loss corresponded to the composition of body weight lost. Seventy-eight obese, sedentary, postmenopausal women reduced weight an average of 26 lb over 5 mo by reducing daily energy intake by 400 kcal 3 days a week. On average, 67% of the weight lost was fat and 33% lean body tissue. One year after the program ended, 54 women regained at least 2.0 kg. For them, 81% of regained weight was fat and 19% lean tissue. Specifically, for every 1 kg fat lost during weight-loss intervention, 0.26 kg lean tissue was lost; for every 1 kg fat regained over the following year, only 0.12 kg lean tissue was regained.

Source: Beavers KM, et al. Is lost lean mass from intentional weight loss recovered during weight regain in postmenopausal women? *Am J Clin Nutr* 2011;94:767.

National Weight Control Registry: Clues to Long-Term Success

Among lifetime members of a commercial weight-loss organization that promotes prudent caloric restriction, behavior modification, group support, and moderate physical activity, more than half maintained their original weight loss goal after 2 years, and more than a third after 5 years.[79,139] Behavior modification, a common intervention in weight loss programs, provides a set of principles and techniques to alter physical activity and eating habits. The therapy increases skills for replacing existing habits with new more-healthful habits. Behavior therapy characteristics include eating well-balanced meals with reduced portion size, restricting daily caloric intake by 500 to 700 kcal,

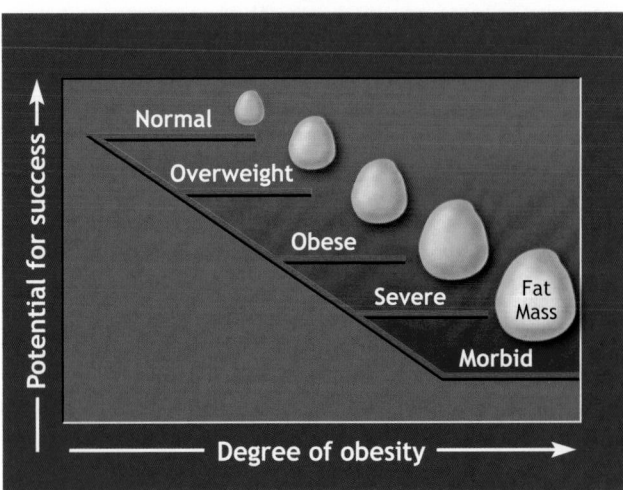

FIGURE 30.16 • Likelihood of success in long-term maintenance of weight loss inversely relates to the level of obesity at the start of intervention.

keeping meticulous records of food intake and physical activity, and increasing daily physical activity by at least 200 to 300 kcal.

A project recruited 784 individuals (629 women, 155 men) in the 10,000-member National Weight Control Registry (NWCR; www.nwcr.ws/), the largest database of individuals who successfully achieved prolonged weight loss. Criteria for NWCR membership included being 18 years or older and maintaining weight loss of at least 30 lb (13.6 kg) for 1 year or longer. Participants fill out a lifestyle questionnaire every year. Participants averaged 66 lb (30 kg) of weight loss, while 14% lost more than 100 lb (45.4 kg). Members maintained the required minimum 30-lb weight loss for a 5.5-year average, and 16% maintained the lost weight for 10 years or longer. Most participants had been overweight since childhood; nearly half had one overweight parent, and more than 25% had both parents overweight. *Genetic background may have predisposed these persons to obesity, but an impressive weight loss and its maintenance proves that heredity alone need not predestine a person to excessive fatness.*

Can Intestinal Bacteria Cause and/or Cure Obesity?

The human large intestine contains tens of trillions of bacteria and viruses. In fact, the total number of microbes that exist and colonize inside and outside of the body surfaces exceeds the total number of human cells by 10-fold. Thus, one can view humans as a composite of both human and microbial cells. Researchers worldwide are devising experiments to tease out the separate influence of how human and microbial genetics impact future human characteristics. When the microbial colonies multiply after one's birth, can their presence "signal" or "trigger" changes in physiologic and metabolic functions, as for example, the development of obesity and other health-related aspects? Based on rodent models, the answer seems to be yes for gut "microbiota" playing a predisposing role in obesity development. In a novel set of experiments involving humans and mice, researchers at the Center for Genome Science and Systems Biology at Washington University in St. Louis, MO demonstrated that when gut bacteria from four obese (Ob) and lean (Ln) human twin pairs were transplanted into "normal" germfree mice, the mice with the injected bacteria from the Ob twins became fat, and the mice injected with bacteria from the Ln twins remained unaffected. The researchers also demonstrated that different proportions of high fat and low fat mouse chow changed the structural composition of short-chain fatty acid fermentation (increased in Ln) and metabolism of branched-chain amino acids (increased in Ob) following the bacterial transport. The next step on the road to practical application in humans is to determine which bacteria cause the effect, so that pure bacteria extracts can serve as the agent for inducing possible changes in obesity status. The researchers hope that insights gleaned from mouse models can frame the design of human studies to better understand the pathogenesis of complex diseases, and to develop new gut microbiome-directed therapeutics that improve health.

Source: Ridaura V, et al. Gut microbiota from twins discordant for obesity modulate metabolism in mice. *Science* 2013;341:1241212.

About 55% of the NWCR members used either a formal program or professional assistance to lose weight; the rest succeeded on their own. Regarding weight-loss methods, 89% modified food intake and maintained relatively high levels of physical activity that equated to 2800 kcal weekly on average to achieve goal weight loss. Only 10% relied solely on diet, and 1% used physical activity exclusively. The diet strategy of nearly 90% of participants restricted their intake of certain types and/or amounts of foods—44% counted calories, 33% limited general lipid intake, and 25% restricted actual grams of lipid consumed. Forty-four percent ate the same foods they normally ate but in reduced amounts (TABLE 30.1).

The registry members' belief in the importance of increased physical activity for weight maintenance represents a significant finding; nearly all of them exercised as part of their strategy. Many walked briskly for at least 1 hr daily. About 92% exercised at home, and one third exercised regularly with friends. Women primarily walked and did aerobic dancing, while men chose competitive sports and resistance training. The data in Table 30.1 also show that successful weight loss had far-reaching, positive effects on their lives. At least 85% improved general quality of life, level of energy, physical mobility, general mood, self-confidence, and physical health. Only 1.6% ($n = 13$) worsened in any of these areas. Such observations reaffirm that weight loss strategies that include moderately reducing energy intake and increasing energy expenditure can effectively thwart a genetic predisposition to obesity. Small weight regains were common despite the success of these individuals in maintaining a large percentage of their weight losses. Very few of these individuals were able to lose the weight again after any regain.[152]

A follow-up study in 2008 extended the results presented above, providing more details about the weekly energy expenditure patterns among the 887 men and 2796 women who enrolled in the NWCR between 1993 and 2004.[25] Interestingly, NWCR participants expended an average of 2621 kcal·wk^{-1} in physical activity, but the range of expenditure (2252 kcal·wk^{-1}) was almost as large as the average. Approximately 25.3% reported >1000 kcal·wk^{-1} and 34.9% reported >3000 kcal·wk^{-1}. The amount of activity reported by men has decreased over time, while no significant change occurred for women. The large amount of individual variability in energy expenditure makes it extremely difficult to pinpoint what amount of activity would constitute as optimum to maintain weight loss.

Structured Assistance May Prove Useful for Successful Weight Loss

Effective approaches for weight loss are required to combat the increased prevalence of overweight and obesity in primary medical care and community settings. The usefulness of commercial providers of weight loss services (e.g., Weight Watchers; www.weightwatchers.com) versus the

TABLE 30.1 (Top) Dietary Strategies to Achieve Weight Loss of Participants of the NWCR. (Bottom) Effects of Weight Loss on Various Dimensions of Life Reported by Participants

	Percentage		
Strategy	**Women**	**Men**	**Total**
Restricted intake of certain types or classes of food	87.8	86.7	87.6
Ate all foods but limited the quantity	47.2	32.0	44.2
Counted calories	44.8	39.3	43.7
Limited % lipid intake	31.1	36.7	33.1
Counted lipid grams	25.7	21.3	25.2
Followed exchange diet	25.2	11.3	22.5
Used liquid formula	19.1	26.0	20.4
Ate only one or two food types	5.1	6.7	5.5

	Percentage		
Area of Life	**Improved**	**No Difference**	**Worsened**
Quality of life	95.3	4.3	0.4
Level of energy	92.4	6.7	0.9
Mobility	92.3	7.1	0.6
General mood	91.4	6.9	1.6
Self-confidence	90.9	9.0	0.1
Physical health	85.8	12.9	1.3
Interactions with:			
Opposite sex	65.2	32.9	0.9
Same sex	5.0	46.8	0.4
Strangers	69.5	30.4	0.1
Job performance	54.5	45.0	0.6
Hobbies	49.1	36.7	0.4
Spouse interactions	56.3	37.3	5.9

Reprinted from Klem MI, et al. A descriptive study of individuals successful at long-term maintenance of substantial weight loss. *Am J Clin Nutr* 1997;66:239.

standard treatment in primary care practices in Australia, Germany, and the United Kingdom was evaluated in 772 overweight and obese adults in a randomized controlled trial.[97] Participants received either 12 mo of standard care defined by national treatment guidelines or 12 mo of free membership to the commercial program. Two hundred and thirty (61%) of the participants completed the commercial program and 214 (54%) participants completed standard care. Weight loss after 12 mo was 5.1 kg for the commercial program participants versus 2.3 kg for the standard care. The researchers concluded: "Referral by a primary health-care professional to a commercial weight loss program that provides regular weighing, advice about diet and physical activity, motivation, and group support can offer a clinically useful early intervention for weight management in over-weight and obese people that can be delivered on a large scale."

Weight Loss Improves Disease-Risk Biomarkers

Weight loss by obese individuals often exerts a pro-found effect on biologic factors related to disease risk.[43,137] FIGURE 30.18 shows the percentage changes from initial body weight and change in biomarkers of disease risk in obese patients over a 27-mo period using two energy-restricting meal plans. In phase 1 during the first 3 mo, group A (n = 50) attempted to consume an energy-restricted diet of 1200 to 1500 kcal daily composed of conventional, self-selected meals prepared by the subjects; group B (n = 50), assigned the same caloric intake, substituted two meals and two snack-replacement shakes, soups, hot chocolate, and snack bars (Slim-Fast; www.slim-fast.com) for self-selected foods. In phase 2 (months 4 to 27), all subjects consumed self-selected diets of equal caloric value with one meal and one

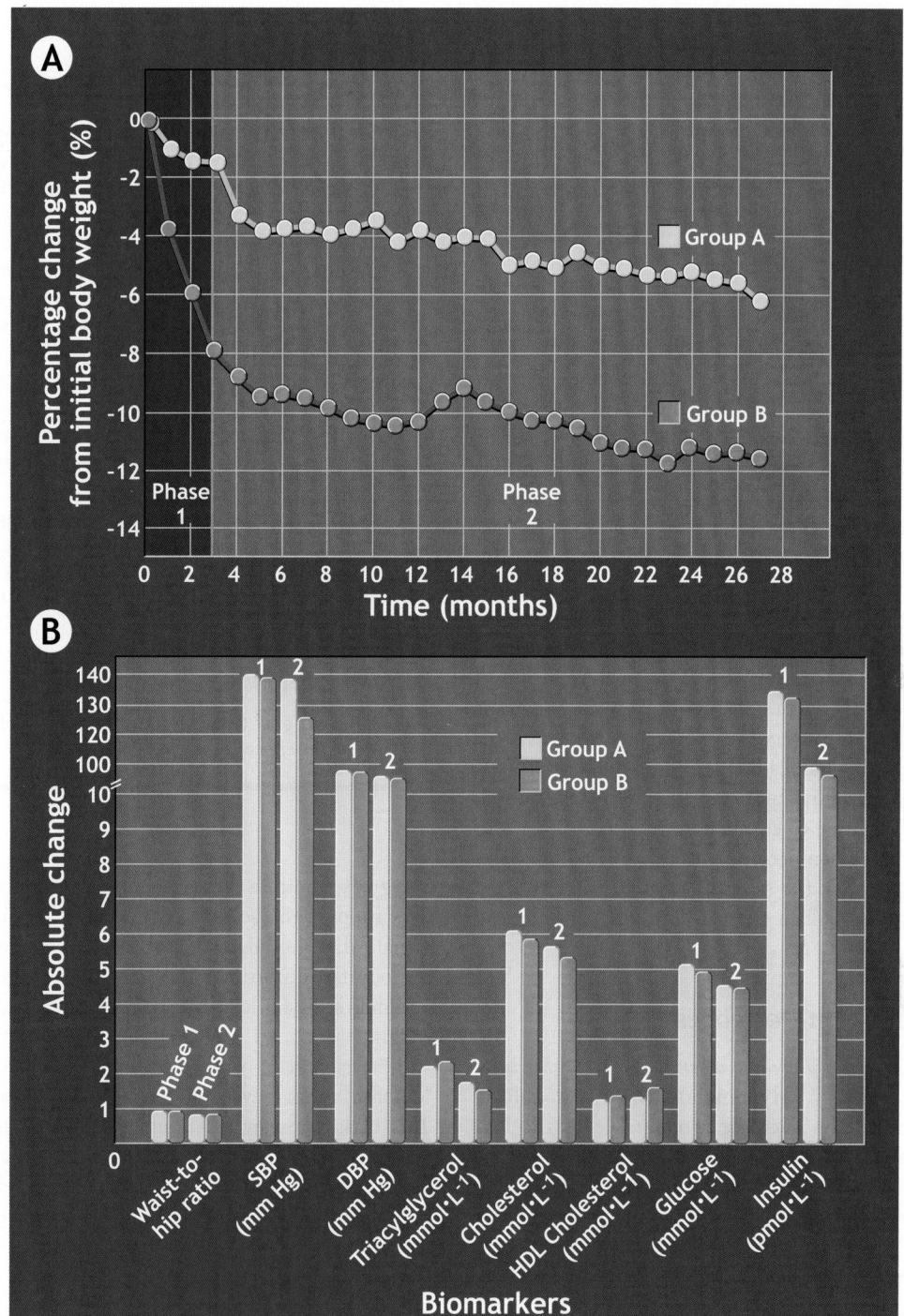

FIGURE 30.18 • **(A)** Average percentage change from initial body weight of obese patients during 27 mo of treatment with an energy-restricted diet containing 1200 to 1500 kcal. **(B)** Absolute changes in biomarkers for groups A (energy-restricted, self-selected, self-prepared meals) and B (Slim-Fast replacement meals) from baseline (Phase 1) to 27 mo of energy restriction (Phase 2). SBP, systolic blood pressure; DBP, diastolic blood pressure. (Adapted with permission from Detschuneit HH, et al. Metabolic and weight-loss effects of a long-term dietary intervention in obese patients. *Am J Clin Nutr* 1999;69:198.)

shake replacement. Unequivocal results emerged from both study phases. Group B's greater weight loss during the 3-mo phase 1 period was attributed to a larger caloric deficit created with the eating plan. Thereafter, both groups reduced on average an additional 0.1% of initial body weight each month (4.2 kg for group A and 3.0 kg for group B). The bottom figure shows absolute changes in eight disease biomarkers during phases 1 and 2. Both groups reduced systolic blood pressure and plasma insulin, glucose, and triacylglycerol concentrations over the 27-mo weight-loss period.

A modest but sustained weight loss produced long-term health benefits reflected by improvement in documented risk factors.

Setpoint Theory: A Case Against Dieting

One can lose large amounts of weight in a relatively short time period by simply not eating. Unfortunately, success is short-lived, and eventually the urge to eat wins out and the lost weight returns. Some argue that this failure to maintain weight loss represents a genetically determined "setpoint" for body weight or body fat that differs from what the person would like. Proponents of a **setpoint theory** maintain that all persons fat or thin have a well-regulated internal control mechanism located deep within the lateral hypothalamus that maintains with relative ease a preset level of body weight and/or body fat within a limited range.

In a practical sense, the setpoint ensures that a person's body weight remains relatively constant when not counting intake calories. Physical activity may lower a person's setpoint, whereas dieting exerts no effect. Each time body weight decreases below one's preestablished setpoint, internal adjustments that affect food intake and regulatory thermogenesis resist the change and conserve and/or replenish body fat. For example, resting metabolism slows, thus conserving total energy output and the individual becomes obsessed with food, unable to control the urge to eat. In contrast, on the opposite end of the spectrum, when persons overeat and gain body fat above their normal level, the setpoint resists this change by increasing resting metabolism and causing the person to lose interest in food.

Resting Metabolism Decreases

Resting metabolism often decreases when dieting progressively produces weight loss.[141,226] Hypometabolism with caloric deficit often exceeds the decrease attributable to the loss of body mass or FFM independent of the person's weight status or prior dieting history. A depressed metabolism conserves energy, causing the diet to become progressively less effective despite restricted caloric intake. This produces a weight-loss plateau. Further weight loss occurs at a slower pace than predicted from the mathematics of restricted energy intake.

A close coupling exists between daily total energy expenditure or TEE required to maintain a constant FFM in obese and nonobese subjects at their usual body weights.[127a] When body weight decreased by 10% below the usual weight, TEE declined more than could be explained by the normal relation between energy expenditure and FFM. Both obese and normal-weight subjects became more energy efficient, requiring disproportionately lower energy intake to maintain the lower body weight. Conversely, increasing body weight by 10% above usual weight produced a 15 to 20% unanticipated *increase* in

A Challenge to the Weight-Loss Equation

A new weight loss model considers the immediate and continuous slowing of the metabolic rate as weight loss progresses, limiting anticipated weight loss. This weight loss model relies on controlled feeding studies that show a "metabolic slowdown" and loss of weight directly contribute to reduced energy expended in physical activity. For example, every reduction in food intake of 10 kcal a day for a typical overweight adult would lead to a weight loss of only *one-half pound* yearly, not the *one pound* a year loss predicted in the classic weight loss model, with the next half pound taking about 2 more years to lose. Cutting 250 kcal daily produces a weight loss of about 25 lb in 3 years. These observations cast further doubt on the sole reliance on dietary restriction to achieve weight loss, often touted by many physicians, as the most effective weight loss method. The online simulator accessed at the National Institute of Diabetes and Digestive and Kidney Diseases (www.niddk.nih.gov; http://bwsimulator.niddk.nih.gov) provides a Web-based tool for people of varying body weights, diets, and physical activity habits to tailor a desired rate of weight loss based on short- and long-term physical activity habits.

Source: Hall KD, et al. Quantification of the effect of energy imbalance on bodyweight. *Lancet* 2011;378:826.

energy expenditure that countered the gain in body fat. These data support the setpoint concept, or "high-level command signal," that modulates metabolism to defend a specific level of body fat; unfortunately in the obese, regulation occurs at a higher body fat level, which makes it more difficult to lose weight.

Figure 30.19 shows further evidence of the body's "defense" against even moderate fluctuations in body weight. This classic research carefully monitored body mass, resting oxygen consumption or minimal energy requirement, and caloric intake of six obese men for 31 days. During the prediet period (*red*), body weight and resting oxygen consumption stabilized with a daily food intake of 3500 kcal. Thereafter, daily caloric intake decreased to 450 kcal shown in the bottom inset in yellow. When the subjects switched to the low-calorie diet, body weight and resting metabolism decreased, but the percentage decline in metabolism exceeded the body weight decrease. The dashed line in the upper figure represents the expected weight loss for the 450-kcal diet. The decline in resting metabolism (*middle figure*) conserved energy to make the diet progressively less effective. More than half of the total weight loss occurred over the first 8 days of dieting; the remaining weight loss occurred during the final 16 days. A plateau in the theoretical weight-loss curve often frustrates and discourages dieters, causing them to abandon attempts at weight loss.

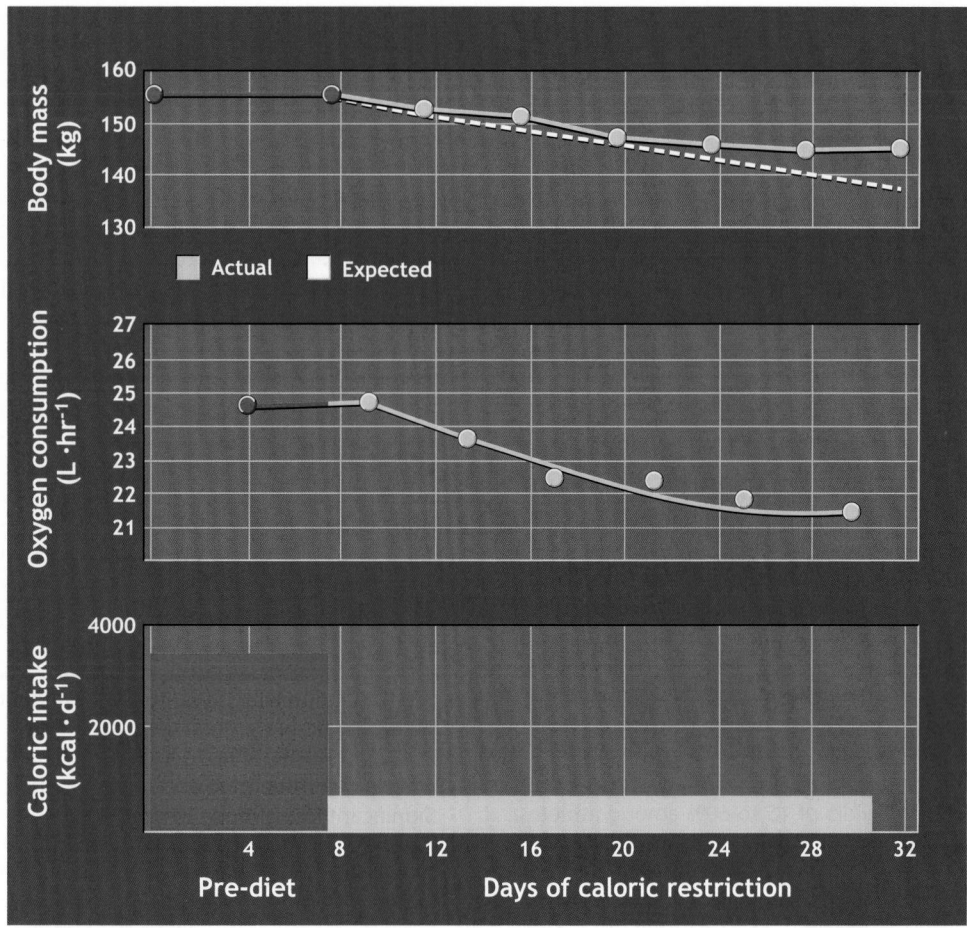

FIGURE 30.19 • Results of a classic study of the effects of two levels of caloric intake on body mass and resting oxygen consumption. Failure of the actual weight loss to keep pace with that predicted on the basis of food restriction (*dashed line*) often leaves the dieter frustrated and discouraged. (Adapted with permission from Bray G. Effect of caloric restriction on energy expenditure in obese subjects. *Lancet* 1969;2:397.)

Biologic Feedback Mechanism

Further disconcerting news awaits those who anticipate permanent fat loss. When overfat people lose weight, adipocytes increase their level of the fat-storing enzyme lipoprotein lipase (LPL).[108] This adaptation facilitates body fat synthesis, and the fatter the person before weight loss, the greater the LPL production with weight loss. In essence, the fatter one is at the start, the more vigorously the body attempts to regain the lost weight. This observation supports the existence of a dedicated biologic feedback mechanism between the brain and the body's fat levels and helps to explain the difficulty overfat individuals have maintaining weight loss.

The setpoint theory delivers unwelcome news for those with a setpoint "tuned" too high; encouragingly, regular moderate-level intensity physical activity may lower the setpoint level. Concurrently, regular physical activity conserves and even increases FFM, raises resting metabolism if FFM increases, and induces metabolic changes that facilitate fat catabolism. Each of these healthful adaptations augments

the weight-loss effort., In the section "Misconception 1: Increased Physical Activity Increases Food Intake," we discuss how food intake tends to decline initially, despite the increase in energy output, for overly fat men and women who begin to exercise regularly. As a physically active lifestyle continues and body fat decreases, caloric intake balances daily energy requirements to stabilize body mass at a new, lower level.

Challenge to the Setpoint Proponents. Some research challenges the argument that individuals who lose weight necessarily *maintain* the initial depressed metabolism that predisposes them to weight regain.[220] Undoubtedly, energy restriction produces a *transient state* of hypometabolism if the dieter maintains the state of negative energy intake. This adaptive downregulation in resting metabolism does not persist when individuals lose weight but then reestablish balance where energy intake equals energy expenditure at their lower body weight. Consequently, research that fails to establish energy balance following weight loss gives the inaccurate

IN A PRACTICAL SENSE

Recognizing Warning Signs of Disordered Eating

Disordered eating refers to a broad spectrum of complex behaviors, core attitudes, coping strategies, and conditions that share an emotionally based, inordinate, and often pathologic focus on body shape and weight.

ANOREXIA ATHLETICA

A cluster of personality traits exists among some athletes that often shares a commonality with patients with clinical eating disorders. The same traits that help an athlete excel in sports—compulsive, driven, dichotomous thinker, perfectionist, competitive, compliant and eager to please ("coachable"), and self-motivated—increase the risks for developing disordered eating patterns. This risk grows for individuals whose normal, genetically determined body size and shape deviate from the "ideal" imposed by the sport. The term *anorexia athletica* describes the continuum of subclinical eating behaviors of athletes who fail to meet the criteria for a true eating disorder but who exhibit at least one unhealthy method of weight control, including fasting, vomiting, or use of diet pills, laxatives, or diuretics ("water pills"). Clinical observations indicate a prevalence of disordered eating behaviors of 15 to 60% among athletes, depending on the sport.

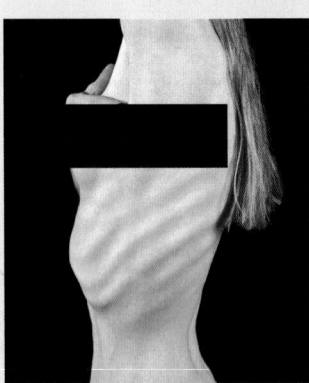

Typical "thin and underweight" physique with anorexia nervosa. In the 1930s, three basic methods were available to manage anorexia nervosa; change of environment, forced feeding, and psychotherapy. The first published photo of an anorectic in an American medical journal appeared in the *N Engl J Med* 207(5): Oct, 1932.

For many athletes, patterns of disordered eating coincide with the competitive season and abate when the season ends. For them, the preoccupation with body weight may not reflect a true underlying pathology but a desire to achieve optimum physiologic function and competitive performance. For a small number of athletes, the season never ends and they develop a full-blown eating disorder. Anorexia nervosa and bulimia nervosa are the two most common eating disorders. A third category, binge-eating disorder, does not include purging behavior.

ANOREXIA NERVOSA

Originally described in ancient writings, *anorexia nervosa* is an unhealthy physical and mental state characterized by a crippling obsession with body size. A "nervous loss of appetite" reflects preoccupation with dieting and thinness and refusal to eat enough food to maintain normal body weight. The relentless pursuit of thinness (present in about 1 to 2% of the general population) includes an intense fear of weight gain and fatness (despite a low body weight) and failure to menstruate regularly (amenorrhea). Anorectic persons have a distorted body image; they actually perceive themselves as fat despite their emaciation.

Anorexia nervosa usually begins with a normal attempt to lose weight through dieting (TABLE 1). With prolonged dieting, the individual continues to eat less until practically no food is consumed. Eventually, food restriction becomes an obsession, and the anorectic person achieves no sense of satisfaction despite continued weight loss.

TABLE 1	Warning Signs of Anorexia Nervosa

- Preoccupation with being too fat despite maintenance of normal body weight
- Loss of menstrual cycle (amenorrhea)
- Frequent commenting about body weight or shape
- Significant loss of body weight
- Weight too low for athletic performance
- Ritualistic concern and preoccupation with dieting, counting calories, cooking, and eating meals
- Excessive concern about body weight, size, and shape, even after weight loss
- Feeling of helplessness in the presence of food
- Severe shifts in mood
- Guilt about eating
- Compulsive need for continuous, vigorous physical activity that exceeds training requirements for a specific sport
- Maintenance of a skinny look (body weight less than 85% of expected weight)
- Prefers to eat in isolation
- Wears baggy clothes to disguise thin-looking appearance
- Episodes of bingeing and purging

BULIMIA NERVOSA

The term *bulimia*, literally meaning "ox hunger," refers to "gorging" or "insatiable appetite." In bulimia nervosa, far more common than anorexia nervosa, purging and intense feelings of guilt and shame almost always follow the episodes of binge eating (TABLE 2). Approximately 2 to 4% of all adolescents and adults in the general population (almost exclusively female, including 5% of college women) have bulimia nervosa. Unlike the continual semistarvation of anorexia nervosa, binge eating characterizes bulimia nervosa. The bulimic person consumes calorically dense food within several hours (often at night and out of sight), usually containing between 1000 and 10,000 calories. This is

IN A PRACTICAL SENSE *(continued)*

TABLE 2	Warning Signs of Bulimia Nervosa

- Excessive concern about body weight, body size, and body composition
- Frequent gains and losses in body weight
- Visits to the bathroom following meals
- Fear of not being able to stop eating
- Eating when depressed
- Compulsive dieting after binge-eating episodes
- Severe shifts in mood (depression, loneliness)
- Secretive binge eating but never overeating in front of others
- More frequent criticism of own body size and shape
- Personal or family problems with alcohol or drugs
- Irregular menstrual cycle (oligomenorrhea)

followed by fasting, self-induced vomiting, taking laxatives or diuretics, or compulsive exercising solely to avoid gaining weight.

BINGE-EATING DISORDER

Episodes of bingeing, often without the subsequent purging behavior common to bulimia, characterize binge-eating disorder. Individuals eat more rapidly than normal until they can consume no additional food. Food intake greatly exceeds that determined by the physiologic hunger drive. Binge eating, often in private, occurs with feelings of guilt, depression, or self-disgust. These individuals suffer greater self-anger, shame, lack of control, and frustration than nonbingeing overfat individuals. The diagnosis of binge-eating disorder requires that the individual experiences a lack of control over eating and marked psychologic distress when it occurs. The person must binge at least an average of 2 days a week for 6 mo. Binge eating differs from the overfat condition because the same level of self-anger, shame, lack of control, and frustration about binge eating does not necessarily accompany obesity. Little factual information exists about the prevalence of binge-eating disorder; it may occur in approximately 2% of the U.S. population.

References

Agras WS, et al. Report of the National Institutes of Health workshop on overcoming barriers to treatment research in anorexia nervosa. *Int J Eat Disord* 2004;35:509.

Field AE, Colditz GA. Exposure to the mass media, body shape concerns, and use of supplements to improve weight and shape among male and female adolescents. *Pediatrics* 2005;116:214.

Hay P, Bacaltchuk J. Bulimia nervosa. *Clin Evid* 2004;12:1326.

Klump KL, Gobrogge KL. A review and primer of molecular genetic studies of anorexia nervosa. *Int J Eat Disord* 2005;37:S43.

Silber TJ. Anorexia nervosa among children and adolescents. *Adv Pediatr* 2005;52:49.

Striegel-Moore RH, et al. Eating disorders in white and black women. *Am J Psychiatry* 2003;160:1326.

Striegel-Moore RH, Franko DL. Epidemiology of binge eating disorder. *Int J Eat Disord* 2003;34:S19.

impression that individuals who lose weight necessarily battle a prolonged overcompensating reduction in resting energy expenditure until they return to their original body weight.

Dieting Extremes

Professional organizations have voiced strong opposition to some dietary practices, particularly extremes of fasting and low-carbohydrate, high-fat, and high-protein diets. Dietary extremes raise concern about athletes and other adolescents and young adults who routinely engage in bizarre and often pathogenic weight-control behaviors (see "In a Practical Sense: Recognizing Warning Signs of Disordered Eating"). Researchers currently are studying a subgroup of bulimia that occurs without the binging.[105,106] These individuals do not binge-eat and generally maintain a normal body weight, yet feel compelled to purge usually by vomiting, even after eating only a small or normal food amount. Dangers of this subset of eating disorder are similar to bulimia—dehydration; electrolyte imbalance; potential dental problems from self-induced vomiting; and emotional and psychological problems, including body image problems, anxiety, and depression.

Low Carbohydrate–Ketogenic Diets

Ketogenic diets emphasize carbohydrate restriction while generally ignoring total calories and the diet's cholesterol and saturated fat content.

Billed as a "diet revolution" and championed by the late Robert C. Atkins, MD (1930–2003),[7] a version of the diet was first promoted in the late 1800s and has appeared in various forms since then. Long disparaged by the medical establishment, advocates maintain that restricting daily carbohydrate intake to 20 g or less for the initial 2 wk, with some liberalization afterward, causes the body to mobilize considerable fat for energy. This generates excess plasma ketone bodies—byproducts of incomplete fat breakdown from inadequate carbohydrate catabolism; ketones supposedly suppress appetite. Theoretically, the ketones lost in the urine represent unused energy that should further facilitate weight loss. Some advocates claim that urinary energy loss becomes so large that dieters can eat all they want if they just restrict carbohydrates.

The singular focus of the low-carbohydrate diet craze may eventually reduce caloric intake, despite claims that dieters need not consider calorie intake as long as lipid represents the excess. Initial weight loss also may result largely from dehydration caused by an extra solute load on the kidneys that increases water excretion. Water loss does not reduce body fat. Low-carbohydrate intake also sets the stage for lean tissue loss because the body recruits amino acids from muscle to maintain blood glucose via gluconeogenesis—an undesirable side effect for a diet designed to induce body fat loss.

Three clinical trials compared the Atkins-type, low-carbohydrate diet with traditional low-fat diets for weight loss.[58,172,236] The low-carbohydrate diet was more effective in achieving a modest weight loss for severely overweight persons. Some measures of heart health also improved as reflected by a more favorable lipid profile and glycemic control in those who followed the low-carbohydrate diet for up to 1 year.[193] Such findings add a measure of credibility to low-carbohydrate diets and challenge conventional wisdom concerning the potential dangers from consuming a high-fat diet.

Importantly, Atkins-type, high-fat, low-carbohydrate diets require systematic long-term evaluation up to 5 years for safety and effectiveness, particularly related to the blood lipid profile. The diet, which places no limit on the amount of meat, fat, eggs, and cheese a person consumes, poses nine potential health hazards:

1. Raises serum uric acid levels
2. Potentiates development of kidney stones
3. Alters electrolyte concentrations to initiate cardiac arrhythmias
4. Causes acidosis
5. Aggravates existing kidney problems from the extra solute burden in the renal filtrate
6. Depletes glycogen reserves contributing to a fatigued state
7. Decreases calcium balance and increases risk for bone loss
8. Causes dehydration
9. Retards fetal development during pregnancy from inadequate carbohydrate intake

For high-performance endurance athletes who train at or above 70% of maximum effort, switching to a high-fat diet is ill advised because the body needs to maintain adequate blood glucose and glycogen packed in the active muscles and liver storage depots. Fatigue during intense physical activity for more than 60 min duration occurs more rapidly when athletes consume high-fat meals than with carbohydrate-rich meals.

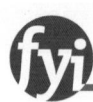

Confirming Evidence to Reduce Dietary Animal Fat

The long-anticipated results of a 25-year epidemiological Swedish study concluded that over time, reducing dietary animal fat decreased blood cholesterol levels. In contrast, a high-fat, low-carbohydrate diet increased these levels. On average, individuals who switched from a lower fat diet to one higher in fat and lower in carbohydrate saw blood cholesterol levels increase—despite increased use of cholesterol-lowering medication. While low-carbohydrate/high-fat diets may help short-term weight loss, these results demonstrate that long-term weight loss is not maintained, and this diet increases blood cholesterol with a potential, major impact on cardiovascular disease risk.

Source: Johansson I, et al. Associations among 25-year trends in diet, cholesterol and BMI from 140,000 observations in men and women in Northern Sweden. *Nutr J* 2012;11:40.

High-Protein Diets

Low-carbohydrate, high-protein diets may shed pounds in the near term, but their long-term success remains questionable and may even pose health risks.[50] These diets have been promoted to the overly fat as "last-chance diets." Earlier versions consisted of protein in liquid form advertised as "miracle liquid." Unknown to the consumer, the liquid protein mixture often contained a blend of ground-up animal hooves and horns, with pigskin mixed in a broth with enzymes and tenderizers to "predigest" it. Collagen-based blends produced from gelatin hydrolysis supplemented with small amounts of essential amino acids did not contain the highest-quality amino acid mixture and lacked required vitamins and minerals, particularly copper. A negative copper balance coincides with electrocardiographic abnormalities and rapid heart rate.[52] Protein-rich foods often contain high levels of saturated fat, which increase the risk for heart disease and type 2 diabetes. Diets excessively high in animal protein increase urinary excretion of oxalate, a compound that combines primarily with calcium to form kidney stones.[161] The diet's safety improves if it contains high-quality protein with ample carbohydrate, essential fatty acids, and micronutrients.[157]

Some argue that an extremely high protein intake suppresses appetite through reliance on fat mobilization and subsequent excess ketone formation. The elevated thermic effect of dietary protein, with its relatively low coefficient of digestibility (particularly for plant protein), reduces the net calories available from ingested protein compared with a well-balanced meal of equivalent caloric value. This point has some validity, but one must consider additional factors when formulating a sound weight-loss program, particularly for physically active individuals. A high-protein diet has the potential for these four deleterious outcomes:

1. Strain on liver and kidney function and accompanying dehydration
2. Electrolyte imbalance

3. Glycogen depletion
4. Lean-tissue loss

Semistarvation Diets

Therapeutic fasting or **very low-calorie diets** (**VLCD**) may benefit severe clinical obesity where body fat exceeds 40 to 50% of body mass. The diet provides between 400 and 1000 kcal daily as high-quality protein foods or liquid meal replacements. Dietary prescriptions usually last up to 3 mo but only as a "last resort" before undertaking more-extreme medical approaches for morbid obesity that include various surgical treatments (collectively called *bariatric surgery*; http://asmbs. org). Surgical treatments that considerably reduce stomach size and reconfigure the small intestine induce a sustained weight loss, but are only prescribed for patients with a BMI of at least 40, or a BMI of 35 when accompanied by other comorbidities.

Dieting with VLCD requires close supervision, usually in a hospital setting. Proponents maintain that severe food restriction breaks established dietary habits, which in turn improves long-term prospects for success. These diets also may depress appetite to help compliance. Daily medications that accompany a VLCD include calcium carbonate for nausea, bicarbonate of soda and potassium chloride to maintain consistency of body fluids, mouthwash and sugar-free chewing gum for bad breath from a high level of ketones from fatty acid catabolism, and bath oils for dry skin. *For most individuals, semistarvation does not compose an "ultimate diet" or proper approach to weight control.* A VLCD provides inadequate carbohydrate, with the glycogen-storage depots in the liver and muscles depleting rapidly. This impairs physical tasks that require either intense aerobic effort or shorter-duration anaerobic power output. The continuous nitrogen loss with fasting and weight loss reflects an exacerbated lean tissue loss, which may occur disproportionately from critical organs like the heart. The success rate remains poor for prolonged fasting.[145]

Most diets produce weight loss during the first several weeks, although body water makes up much of this initial lost weight. In addition, lean tissue loss occurs with dieting alone, particularly in the early phase of a VLCD. An individual can certainly reduce weight through dieting alone, but few persons achieve long-term success in favorably altering body size and composition.

FACTORS THAT AFFECT WEIGHT LOSS

Hydration level and duration of the energy deficit affect the amount and composition of weight lost.

Early Weight Loss Largely Water

FIGURE 30.20 presents the general trend for the percentage composition of daily weight loss during 4 wk of dieting. Approximately 70% of weight lost over the first week of energy deficit consists of water. Thereafter, water loss progressively lessens, representing only about 20% of the weight lost in the second and third weeks; concurrently, body fat loss accelerates from 25 to 70%. During the fourth week of dieting, reductions in body fat produce about 85% of the weight loss without further increase in water loss. Protein's contribution to weight loss increases from 5% initially to about 15% after the fourth week. In practical terms, counseling efforts should emphasize that the weight lost during the initial attempts to reduce weight, when successful, consists chiefly of water and not fat; it takes approximately 4 wk to establish the desired pattern of fat loss for each pound of weight loss.

Hydration Level

Restricting water during the first several days of a caloric deficit increases the proportion of body water lost and decreases the *proportion* of fat lost. More total weight loss occurs with restricted daily water intake, but the additional weight lost comes solely from water as dehydration progresses. *Dieters lose the same quantity of body fat regardless of fluid intake level.*

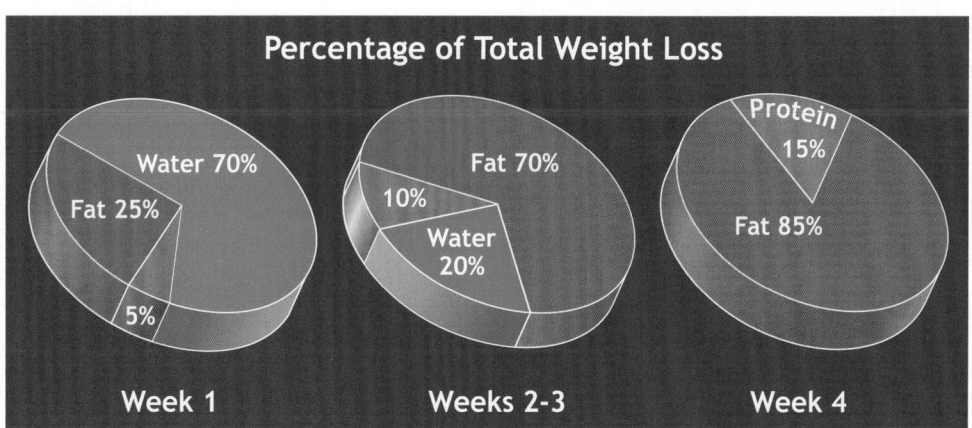

FIGURE 30.20 • General trend for the percentage composition of the weight lost during 4 wk of caloric restriction.

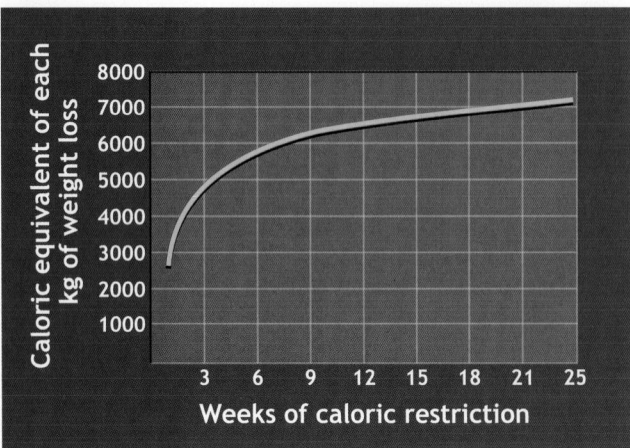

FIGURE 30.21 • General trend for the energy (caloric) equivalent of the weight lost in relation to the duration of caloric restriction. As caloric restriction progresses, the energy equivalent per unit of weight lost increases to about 7000 kcal per kilogram after 20 wk. This occurs because of the large initial body water loss (no calorie value) early in weight loss.

Longer-Term Deficit Promotes Fat Loss

FIGURE **30.21** reinforces the important concept that the caloric equivalent of the weight lost increases as duration of caloric restriction progresses. After about 8 wk on a diet, the caloric equivalent of weight loss exceeds twice that in the first week and continues to increase throughout a 25-wk period. *This points out the importance of maintaining a caloric deficit for extended durations.* Shorter periods of caloric restriction produce larger percentages of water and carbohydrate loss per unit weight reduction with only a minimal decrease in body fat.

INCREASED PHYSICAL ACTIVITY FOR WEIGHT CONTROL

Conventional wisdom views excessive food intake as the prime cause of the overfat condition. Many believe the only way to reduce unwanted body fat requires caloric restriction by dieting. This overly simplistic strategy partly accounts for the dismal success in maintaining weight loss over the long term, refocusing debate on the contribution of food intake to obesity.[75,180] A sedentary lifestyle consistently emerges as an important factor in weight gain in children, adolescents, and adults.[17,169,204]

Not Simply Gluttony

Excess weight gain often parallels reduced physical activity rather than increased caloric intake. Physically active individuals who eat the most often weigh the least and maintain the highest levels of physiologic fitness.

Fat Loss Best with Aerobic Activity

General guidelines for an optimal, well-balanced physical activity program recommend a blend of aerobic activity, resistance exercise, and joint flexibility movements. Resistance training helps to prevent muscle loss (sarcopenia) with aging. Aerobic activity excels for its calorie burning effects in combating excess body fat; it most likely curbs insulin resistance that increases diabetes and heart disease risk. Aerobic activity also reduces deep abdominal (visceral) fat. Middle-age men and women with elevated LDL or low HDL cholesterol were assigned to aerobic training, resistance training, or both. Aerobic training consisted of the equivalent of 12 miles a week at a vigorous intensity on a treadmill, elliptical trainer, or stationary cycle. Resistance training consisted of three sets of eight exercises with eight to 12 repetitions per set, three times weekly. Following 8 mo of training, the resistance-trained group lost only subcutaneous abdominal fat, while the aerobically trained group lost both visceral fat and subcutaneous fat, including fat from around the liver. Aerobic training also decreased the tendency for insulin resistance. The take-away message—combine regular aerobic physical activity for fat loss and to curb insulin resistance with resistance training to counter the tendency to lose muscle that occurs with aging.

Source: Slentz CA, et al. Effects of aerobic vs. resistance training on visceral and liver fat stores, liver enzymes, and insulin resistance by HOMA in overweight adults from STRRIDE AT/RT. *Am J Physiol Endocrinol Metab* 2011;301:E1033.

Obese infants do not characteristically ingest more calories than recommended dietary standards. For children ages 4 to 6 years, daily energy expenditure averaged 25% below the current recommendation for energy intake at this age. A low level of daily physical activity primarily produced the depressed energy output.[21] More specifically, 50% of boys and 75% of girls in the United States fail to engage in even moderate physical activity three or more times weekly.[1] Physically active children tend to be leaner than less active counterparts. For preschool children, no relationship emerged between total energy intake, or the fat, carbohydrate, and protein composition of the diet and percentage body fat.[8] Excessive fatness relates directly to the number of hours spent watching television (a consistent marker of inactivity) among children, adolescents, and adults.[5,65,89] For example, 3 hr of television viewing a day led to a twofold increase in obesity and a 50% increase in diabetes.[88] Each 2-hr-per-day increment of TV watching coincides with a 23% increase in obesity and a 14% rise in diabetes risk. Excessive television watching, playing video games, and otherwise remaining inactive characterizes overweight minority teens. Estimates indicate that reducing the amount of time spent watching television, playing video games, or using a computer would substantially reduce the incidence of metabolic syndrome.[69]

Minimizing time devoted to such behaviors can help combat childhood fat gain.[167]

The observation that overfat children often eat the same or even less than peers of average body weight also pertains to less physically active adults as they slowly, progressively gain weight. *Overweight individuals often do not eat more on average than persons of normal weight.* Consequently, it remains neither prudent nor justifiable to emphasize dieting alone to effectively induce long-term weight loss.

When Reality Meets the Road

The inset photo illustrates the reality faced daily by millions of Americans when they go out to eat and reinforces the extreme difficulty in combating overeating and the obesity epidemic—the portion sizes are huge!

This hit home when two of the textbook authors stopped for breakfast at a roadside eatery (Tony's I-75 Restaurant, exit 136, Birch Run, Michigan; **http://www.youtube.com/ watch?v=oswFTZPBZl8**) while traveling to the 2013 American College of Sports Medicine National Convention. What a surprise when the order arrived of scrambled eggs, toast, hash browns, and a side of bacon. When asked if a mistake had been made in the bacon side-order, the waiter confirmed that all bacon sides weigh in at 1 lb (58 pieces, about 2418 kcal with 184 g or 6.5 oz of fat–more than seven times the recommended daily intake)! A colleague could not finish his vegetarian omelet due to its sheer size. He was told the standard omelet contained 12 eggs (888 kcal and about 2200 mg of cholesterol just for the eggs)! The restaurant proudly advertises its specialty—the United States of Bacon.

The Most Desirable Solution—Increase Energy Output

Physically active men and women usually maintain a desirable body composition. An increased level of regular physical activity combined with dietary restraint maintains weight loss more effectively than long-term caloric restriction alone.[3,213] A negative energy balance induced by increased caloric expenditure, through either lifestyle activities or formal conditioning programs, unbalances the energy balance equation for weight loss, improves physical fitness and the health risk profile, and favorably alters body composition and body

fat distribution for children and adults.[49,151,169,185,218] Regular physical activity produces less accumulation of central adipose tissue associated with aging.[100,170,212] Overweight women show a dose–response relationship between amount of physical activity and long-term weight loss.[94] Obese adolescents and adults improve body composition and visceral fat distribution from both moderate physical activity and more vigorous activity that improves cardiovascular fitness, with more intense physical activity being most effective.[90] For obese boys and girls, the most favorable body composition changes occur with long-duration aerobic exercise and high-repetition resistance training, combined with a behavior-modification component.[71,129,135] Additional spin-off from regular physical activity includes slowing of the age-related loss in muscle mass, possible prevention of adult-onset fatness, improvement in obesity-related comorbidities, decreased mortality, and beneficial effects on existing chronic diseases.[14,74,127,132,195]

Two Misconceptions About Physical Activity

Two arguments attempt to counter the increased physical activity approach to weight loss. One maintains that physical activity inevitably increases appetite to produce a proportionate increase in food intake that negates the caloric deficit that increased physical activity produces. The second argument claims that the relatively small calorie-burning effect of a normal exercise workout does not "dent" the body's fat reserves as effectively as food restriction.

Misconception 1: Increased Physical Activity Increases Food Intake

Sedentary persons often do not balance energy intake with energy expenditure. Failure to accurately regulate energy balance at the lower end of the physical activity spectrum contributes to the "creeping obesity" observed in highly mechanized and technically advanced societies. In contrast, regular participation in physical activity maintains appetite control within a reactive zone where food intake more readily matches daily energy expenditure.

In considering the effects of physical activity on appetite and food intake, one must distinguish the activity type and duration and the participant's body fat status. Lumberjacks, farm laborers, and endurance athletes consume about twice as many daily calories as sedentary individuals. And marathon runners, cross-country skiers, and cyclists consume about 4000 to 5000 kcal daily, yet they are the leanest people in the population. Obviously, their large caloric intake meets the energy requirements of training while maintaining a relatively lean body composition.

For the overweight or obese person, the extra energy required for increased physical activity more than offsets moderate physical activity's small compensatory appetite-stimulating effect. To some extent, the large energy reserve of the over-fat person makes it easier to tolerate weight loss and physical activity without the obligatory increase in caloric intake typically observed for leaner counterparts.[110,175] No difference emerged in fat, carbohydrate, or protein intake or total calories consumed for overweight men and women during 16 mo of supervised, moderate-intensity exercise training compared with a sedentary control group.[46] *In essence, a weak coupling exists between the short-term energy deficit induced by physical activity and energy intake. Increased physical activity by overweight, sedentary individuals does not necessarily alter physiologic needs and automatically produce compensatory increases in food intake to balance additional energy expenditure.*

INTEGRATIVE QUESTION

Respond to the person who claims: "The only way to lose weight is to stop eating. It's that simple!"

Misconception 2: Physical Activity Does Not Burn Many Calories

A common misconception concerns the supposed negligible contribution to weight loss of the calories burned in typical physical activity. Some argue correctly that it requires an inordinate amount of short-term activity to lose just 0.45 kg of body fat: for example, chopping wood for 10 hr, playing golf for 20 hr, performing mild calisthenics for 22 hr, or playing ping-pong for 28 hr or volleyball for 32 hr. Consequently, a 2- or 3-mo physical activity regimen can produce only a small fat loss in an overfat person. From a different perspective, if one played golf (no cart) for 2 hr daily (350 kcal) 2 days per week (700 kcal), it would take about 5 wk to lose 0.45 kg of body fat. Assuming the person plays year-round, golfing 2 days a week produces a 4.5-kg yearly fat loss, provided food intake remains constant. Even an activity as innocuous as chewing gum burns an extra 11 kcal each hour, a 20% increase over normal resting metabolism. Stepping in place while watching television commercials during a 1-hr show produces an average of 25.2 min of increased energy expenditure and 4.3 kcal liberated during each minute of stepping.[191] *Simply stated, the calorie-expending effects of increased physical activity add up over time. A caloric deficit of 3500 kcal equals a 0.45-kg body fat loss, whether the deficit occurs rapidly or systematically over time.*

When estimating the energy cost of performing various physical activities, one assumes that exercise energy expenditure remains constant among persons of a particular body size. In Chapter 8, we noted that energy cost data for most physical activities represent averages, often based on only a few observations of a few subjects. A wide range of values exists because of individual differences in performance style and technique; terrain, temperature, and wind

Calories In versus Calories Out: The Amount of Physical Activity Required for a 150-lb Person to Burn Off the Calories in Some Popular Foods

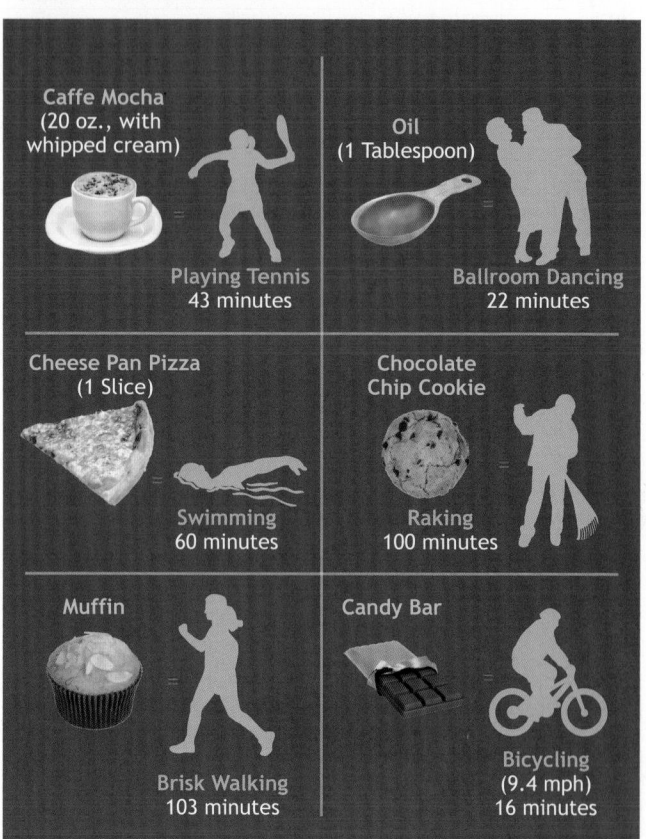

resistance (environmental factors); and intensity of participation. Consequently, energy expenditure values for the physical activities presented in Appendix F (available online at http://thepoint.lww.com/mkk8e) do not represent constants. Rather, they reflect "average" values applicable under "average" conditions when applied to the "average" person of a given body weight. However, the data do provide useful approximations to establish the energy cost of diverse physical activities.

thePoint Appendix F, available online at http://thepoint.lww.com/mkk8e, shows energy expenditure values for household, occupational, recreational, and sports activities.

The Recovery "Afterglow." Controversy exists about the quantitative contribution of excess postexercise oxygen consumption to the total energy expended.[111] With low-to-moderate exercise, as performed by most persons who exercise for weight control, the contribution of recovery metabolism—the so-called **recovery afterglow**—to total energy expenditure remains small relative to exercise energy expenditure, ranging up to 75 kcal for exercise durations of 80 min.[159] In addition, exercise training induces faster adjustments in postexercise energetics that reduce the magnitude of the total recovery oxygen consumption. *Calories burned during physical activity represent the most important factor in total exercise energy expenditure, not calories expended during recovery.*

fyi Vigorous Physical Activity May Boost Recovery Metabolism

A bout of vigorous physical activity may increase recovery oxygen consumption for up to 14 hr. Ten young adult men bicycled for 45 min at a vigorous pace equivalent to 73% $\dot{V}O_{2max}$. Energy expenditure was then measured for 24 hr while the men recovered in a metabolic chamber. In the 14-hr period following cycling, the men burned 190 more calories than on a day when they remained sedentary. This 37% recovery calorie-burning bonus occurred in addition to the 520 calories burned during cycling.

Source: Knab AM, et al. A 45-minute vigorous exercise bout increases metabolic rate for 14 hours. *Med Sci Sports Exerc* 2011;43:1643.

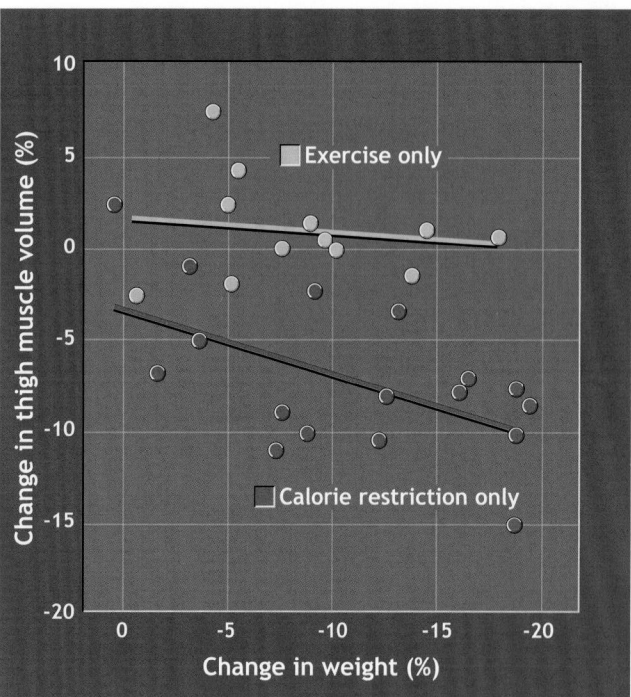

FIGURE 30.22 • Conserve the lean and lose the fat. Relationship between the magnitude of weight loss and the magnitude of change in thigh muscle volume (sum of right and left thighs) in a group losing weight by only caloric restriction and a group losing weight by only exercise. (Adapted with permission from Weiss EP, et al. Lower extremity muscle size and strength and aerobic capacity decrease with caloric restriction but not with exercise-induced weight loss. *J Appl Physiol* 2007;102:634.)

EFFECTIVENESS OF REGULAR PHYSICAL ACTIVITY

Adding physical activity to a weight-loss program favorably modifies the composition of the weight lost in the direction of greater fat loss, less lean tissue loss, and the maintenance or even enhancement of physical capacity.[9,222] This muscle-sparing effect of regular physical activity is clearly illustrated in **FIGURE 30.22**, which compares the effect of about 10 lb of weight loss over 12 mo induced by either *only* caloric restriction (*red data points*) or *only* physical activity (*yellow data points*) on MRI-assessed thigh muscle volume of 50- to 60-year-old men and women. Decreases in thigh muscle volume of 6.8% and composite knee flexion strength (27%), and $\dot{V}O_{2max}$ (27%) occurred only in the caloric restriction group, whereas $\dot{V}O_{2max}$ increased 15.5% in the group losing weight via exercise. Clearly, muscle mass, muscle strength, and aerobic capacity decreased in response to 12 mo of weight loss by caloric restriction, but not in response to similar exercise-induced weight loss.

The effectiveness of regular physical activity for weight loss relates closely to the degree of excess body fat. Obese persons generally lose weight and fat more readily with increased physical activity than normal-weight persons.[169] Aerobic physical activity and resistance training, even without dietary restriction, provide positive spin-off to the weight loss effort. They alter body composition favorably (reduced

body fat with a small increase in FFM) for the otherwise healthy overweight person, postmenopausal woman, cardiac patient, and physically challenged individual.[116,181,203] Adolescent males who engaged regularly in vigorous activities showed less abdominal fat than sedentary counterparts.[41] This indicates that regular physical activity and improved aerobic fitness may target excess fat accumulation in the abdominal–visceral area to a greater extent than peripheral fat deposits. Even when an activity program produces no weight loss, substantial reductions occur in abdominal subcutaneous and visceral fat.[170] This response certainly diminishes the tendency toward insulin resistance and resulting predisposition to type 2 diabetes. **TABLE 30.2** shows the effects of regular physical activity for weight loss by six sedentary, overfat young men who exercised 5 days a week for 16 wk by walking 90 min each session. The men lost nearly 6 kg (13 lb) of body fat, a decrease in percentage body fat from 23.5 to 18.6%. Exercise capacity also improved as did HDL cholesterol (↑15.6%) and the HDL-to-LDL cholesterol ratio (↑26%).

Most of the health-related metabolic improvements in the obese with regular physical activity relate to total activity volume and quantity of fat loss rather than enhanced

TABLE 30.2	Effectiveness of a 16-Week Walking Program on Body Composition and Blood Lipid Changes in Six Overfat, Young Men		
Variable	**Pre-Training**[a]	**Post-Training**[a]	**Difference**
Body mass (kg)	99.1	93.4	−5.7[b]
Body density, $g \cdot mL^{-1}$	1.044	1.056	+0.012[b]
Body fat (%)	23.5	18.6	−4.9[b]
Fat mass (kg)	23.3	17.4	−5.9[b]
Fat-free body mass (kg)	75.8	76.0	+0.2
Sum of skinfolds (mm)	142.9	104.8	−38.1[b]
HDL cholesterol, $mg \cdot dL^{-1}$	32	37	5.0[b]
HDL/LDL cholesterol	0.27	0.34	+ 0.07[b]

[a]Values are means.
[b]Statistically significant.
Reprinted from Leon AS, et al. Effects of a vigorous walking program on body composition, and carbohydrate and lipid metabolism of obese young men. *Am J Clin Nutr* 1979;33:1776.

cardiorespiratory fitness.[37,38] Ideal physical activity consists of continuous, large-muscle activities with moderate-to-high caloric cost such as circuit-resistance training, walking, running, rope skipping, stair stepping, cycling, and swimming. Many recreational sports and games also are effective in promoting weight control, but precise quantification and regulation of energy expenditure becomes difficult. Aerobic physical activity stimulates fat catabolism, establishes favorable blood pressure responses, and generally promotes cardiovascular fitness. Interestingly, aerobic exercise training may elevate resting metabolism independent of any FFM change.[233] No selective effect exists for running, walking, or bicycling; each promotes fat loss with equal effectiveness.[154] Expenditure of an extra 300 kcal daily (e.g., jogging for 30 min) should produce a 0.45-kg fat loss in about 12 days. This represents a yearly caloric deficit equivalent to the energy in 13.6 kg (29.9 lb) of body fat.

Resistance Training

Resistance training provides an important adjunct to aerobic training for weight loss and weight maintenance, and overall decreases in cardiovascular disease risk. The energy expended in circuit-resistance training—continuous exercise using low resistance and high repetitions—averages about 9 kcal a minute. This activity mode yields substantial calories during a typical 30- to 60-min workout. Even conventional resistance training that involves less total energy expenditure positively affects muscular strength and FFM during weight loss compared with programs that rely solely on food restriction.[10,215] Individuals who maintain high muscular strength levels tend to gain less weight than weaker counterparts.[124] Standard resistance training performed regularly reduces coronary heart disease risk, improves glycemic control, favorably modifies the lipoprotein profile, and increases resting metabolic rate (when FFM increases).[85,157,202]

 Use It or Lose It

A meta-analysis that examined the overall value of progressive resistance exercise among healthy aging adults showed that this exercise form helps older adults build muscle mass and increase strength to function better in activities of daily living. Sedentary adults, with an average age of 50, added 2.4 lb of lean muscle and increased overall strength by up to 30% after 18 to 20 wk of resistance training. The amount of weight lifted and frequency and duration of the training sessions interact in a dose–response manner to facilitate improvement. Sedentary adults above age 50 typically lose up to 0.4 lb of muscle yearly.

Source: Peterson MD, Gordon PM. Resistance exercise for the aging adult: clinical implications and prescription guidelines. *Am J Med* 2011;124:194.

Comparisons of conventional resistance training with endurance training indicate unique resistance-training benefits on body composition.[16,215] **TABLE 30.3** summarizes the effects of 12 wk of either endurance exercise or resistance training on nondieting, untrained young men. Endurance training reduced percentage body fat (hydrostatic weighing) from reduced fat mass (1.6 kg; no change in FFM), while resistance training decreased body fat mass by 2.4 kg and increased the FFM by 2.4 kg. Because FFM remains metabolically more active than body fat, conserving or increasing this tissue depot with exercise training maintains a higher level of resting metabolism, average daily metabolic rate, and possibly fat oxidation during rest, all factors that counteract the age-related increase in adiposity.[20,44,187]

FIGURE 30.23 shows body composition changes for 40 obese women placed into one of four groups: (1) control, no exercise and no diet; (2) diet only, no exercise (DO); (3) diet

TABLE 30.3	Changes in Body Composition After 12 Weeks of Either Resistance Training or Endurance Training					
	Controls		**Resistance Trained**		**Endurance Trained**	
Variable	**Pretreatment**	**Posttreatment**	**Pretreatment**	**Posttreatment**	**Pretreatment**	**Posttreatment**
Relative body fat (%)	20.1 ± 8.5	20.2 ± 8.5	21.8 ± 6.2	18.7 ± 6.6[a]	18.4 ± 7.9	16.5 ± 6.4[a]
Fat mass (kg)	16.2 ± 10.8	16.3 ± 10.5	17.2 ± 7.6	14.8 ± 6.2[a]	14.4 ± 7.9	12.8 ± 7.1[a]
Fat-free body mass (kg)	64.3 ± 5.4	64.4 ± 6.6	61.9 ± 8.3	64.4 ± 9.0[a]	64.1 ± 8.2	64.7 ± 8.6
Total body mass (kg)	80.5 ± 8.1	80.7 ± 8.5	79.4 ± 8.3	79.2 ± 7.6	78.5 ± 8.2	77.5 ± 7.9

All values means ± SD.
[a]Significant difference between pre- and posttest measurements ($p < 0.05$).
Reprinted from Broeder CE, et al. Assessing body composition before and after resistance or endurance training. *Med Sci Sports Exerc* 1997;29:705.

plus resistance exercise (D + E), and (4) resistance exercise only, no diet (EO). The women trained 3 days a week for 8 wk. They performed 10 repetitions each of three sets of eight strength exercises. Body mass decreased for DO (4.5 kg) and D + E (3.9 kg), compared with EO (+0.5 kg) and controls (+0.4 kg). Importantly, FFM increased for EO (+1.1 kg), whereas the DO group lost 0.9 kg of FFM. The authors concluded that augmenting a calorie-restriction program with resistance-exercise training preserves FFM better than dietary restriction alone.

Dose–Response Relationship for Energy Expended and Weight Lost

The total energy expended in physical activity relates in a dose–response manner to the effectiveness of physical activity for weight loss.[9,95] *A reasonable goal progressively increases moderate activity to between 60 and 90 min daily or a level that burns 2100 to 2800 kcal weekly.*[55,98] To combat the worldwide obesity epidemic, the public health perspective must promote a population's need to increase *total* daily energy expenditure substantially and regularly rather than increase effort intensity solely to induce a training response. An overly fat person who starts out with light physical activity such as slow walking accrues a considerable caloric expenditure simply by extending exercise duration. The focus on duration offsets the inadvisability of having a sedentary, obese individual begin a program with more strenuous physical activity. Also, the energy cost of weight-bearing physical activity relates directly to body weight; the overweight person expends considerably more calories in such activity than someone of average weight.

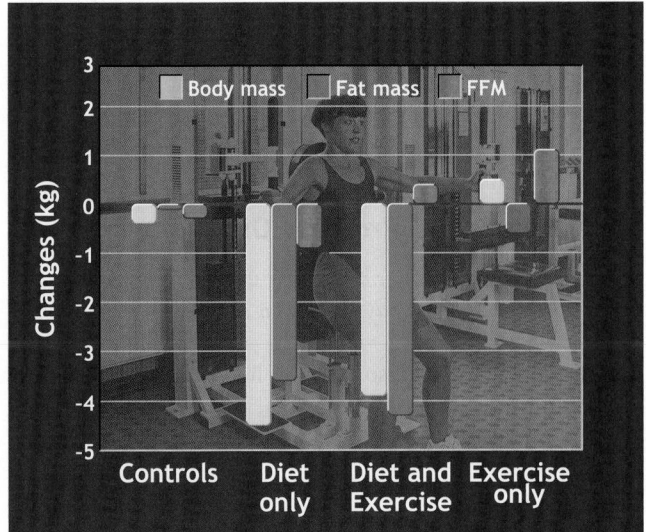

FIGURE 30.23 • Changes in body composition with combinations of resistance exercise and/or diet in obese females. (Adapted with permission from Ballor DL, et al. Resistance weight training during caloric restriction enhances lean body weight maintenance. *Am J Clin Nutr* 1988;47:19.)

 INTEGRATIVE QUESTION

Among physically active men and women, how can individuals who consume the most calories weigh less than those who consume fewer calories?

Walking–Running for Different Durations

The duration of physical activity affects fat loss. **TABLE 30.4** lists changes in body fat for three groups of men who exercised for 20 wk by walking and running for either 15, 30, or 45 min per workout. Data also include distance covered and total duration of weekly workouts, training heart rate, body mass, sum of six skinfolds, and waist girth.

The three exercise groups decreased body fat, skinfolds, and waist girth compared with sedentary controls. Body weight also decreased with exercise, except for the 15-min group, whose weight remained stable. Comparing the three groups, the 45-min group lost more body fat than either the 30- or 15-min groups. This difference was closely linked to the

TABLE 30.4 **Effects of Three Training Durations of Walking and Running on Body Composition Changes**

	Control (n = 16)		15 Minute (n = 14)		30 Minute (n = 17)		45 Minute (n = 12)	
	Training Group							
Variable	**Pre**	**Post**	**Pre**	**Post**	**Pre**	**Post**	**Pre**	**Post**
Body mass (kg)	72.1	73.2	76.9	76.3	80.6	78.9	70.9	69.9
Body fat (%)	12.5	13.0	13.7	13.2	14.2	13.6	13.2	12.0
Sum skinfolds (mm)	73.8	79.6	83.0	77.0	90.0	83.8	77.5	67.0
Waist girth (cm)	82.7	84.9	84.3	82.8	88.2	86.1	83.6	81.8
Distance covered per workout (mi)	Week 4		1.56		2.89		4.13	
	8		1.54		2.95		4.46	
	13		1.79		3.19		4.82	
	17		1.75		3.24		5.06	
Total time of exercise (min:s)	Week 4		14:58		30:25		41:18	
	8		14:11		28:40		42:48	
	13		15:51		29:43		43:19	
	17		14:53		30:12		42:27	
Training heart rate (b · min⁻¹)	Week 4		179		175		174	
	8		179		174		169	
	13		182		175		177	
	17		180		175		175	
Intensity (%max HR)	Week 4		89.4		83.8		84.5	
	8		89.8		73.4		81.0	
	13		94.0		90.1		89.5	
	17		92.5		90.2		88.1	

Reprinted from Milesis CA, et al. Effects of different durations of physical training on cardiorespiratory function, body composition, and serum lipids. *Res Q* 1976;47:716.

greater caloric expenditure with longer activity (i.e., a dose–response relationship).

Exercise Frequency

To determine the optimal exercise frequency for weight loss, subjects exercised for 30 to 47 min for 20 wk by either running or walking, with activity intensity maintained between 80 and 95% of maximum heart rate.[155] Training twice weekly produced no changes in body weight, skinfolds, or percentage body fat, but training 3 and 4 days weekly did. Subjects who trained 4 days a week reduced body weight and skinfolds more than subjects who trained 3 days a week. Percentage body fat decreased similarly in both groups. Individuals should participate in physical activity a *minimum* of 3 days a week to favorably alter body composition; the additional caloric expenditure with more frequent activity produces even greater results. The threshold energy expenditure for weight loss probably remains highly individualized. The calorie-burning effect of each activity session should eventually reach *at least* 300 kcal whenever possible. This generally occurs with 30 min of moderate-to-vigorous running, swimming, bicycling, or circuit-resistance training or 60 min of brisk walking.

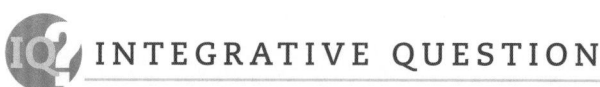

INTEGRATIVE QUESTION

Why should individuals limit weight loss to no more than 2 lb of body weight weekly?

Start Slowly and Progress Gradually

The initial stage of a physical activity–weight-loss program for a previously sedentary, overly fat person should be developmental with moderate intensity demands. The individual should adopt long-term goals and personal discipline and restructure eating and physical activity behaviors. Unduly rapid training progressions prove counterproductive because most overfat individuals initially resist increasing their physical activity. During the first few months, intervals of faster-paced walking can replace slow walking. Meaningful changes in body weight and body composition require a minimum of 12 wk. Most overfat persons can realistically expect to reduce body weight by 5 to 15% with programs that focus on modifying eating and exercise behaviors. Behavioral approaches should foster lifestyle changes in daily physical activity.[205]

For example, walking or bicycling can replace the auto, stair climbing can replace the elevator, and manual tools can replace power tools.[4,47] Eating less and moving more proves more effective in a group situation than going it alone. Persons who joined a weight-loss program with several friends or family members lost more weight than individuals who participated alone.[232] This also holds true for individuals who receive face-to-face behavioral support or participation in Web technologies that offer virtual-world weight loss engagement.[99]

Self-Selected Energy Expenditures: Mode of Physical Activity

No selective effect exists among diverse modes of big-muscle aerobic activity with equivalent energy expenditures to favorably reduce body weight, body fat, skinfold thickness, and girths, yet other differences may emerge. For example, Figure 30.24A shows that men and women generally self-select a higher energy expenditure level (with accompanying higher heart rates) at similar ratings of perceived exertion when running for 20 min on a treadmill than when performing simulated cross-country skiing (NordicTrack; www.nordictrack.com), cycle ergometry, or aerobic riding (HealthRider; www.healthrider.com).[117] Men selected a higher absolute level of exercise intensity and oxygen consumption than women in each exercise mode (Fig. 30.24B); treadmill running generated the greatest total oxygen consumed (energy expended) for both groups. For individuals without physical activity limitations, running usually provides the most suitable activity mode for maximizing energy expenditure during self-selected intensities of continuous physical activity.

Caloric Restraint Plus Physical Activity: The Ideal Combination

Combinations of increased physical activity and caloric restraint offer considerably more flexibility for achieving a negative caloric imbalance than either exercise alone or diet alone.[48,123,231] Dietary restraint plus increased physical activity through lifestyle changes offer health and weight-loss benefits similar to those from combining dietary restraint and a vigorous program of structured physical activity.[4] Adding physical activity to a weight-control program facilitates longer-term maintenance of fat loss than total reliance on either food restriction alone or increased activity alone.[95,158] Table 30.5 summarizes the benefits of physical activity to a weight-loss program.

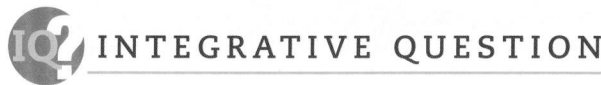

INTEGRATIVE QUESTION

Why might large-scale studies that compare diet only and physical activity plus diet often show only a small, added weight loss benefit for the activity-plus-diet group?

How can an overfat person using increased physical activity and dietary restraint maintain a weight loss of about 1 lb (0.45 kg) a week to reduce body weight by 20 lb (9.1 kg)? A prudent 1-lb per week fat loss requires 20 wk. The weekly energy deficit to achieve this goal must average 3500 kcal with a daily deficit of 500 kcal. One half-hour of moderate physical activity (about 350 "extra" kcal) performed 3 days a week adds 1050 kcal to the weekly deficit. Consequently, the weekly caloric intake need only decrease by 2400 kcal or about 350 kcal daily instead of 3500 kcal to lose the desired pound of body fat each week. If the number of activity days increases from 3 to 5, daily food intake requires only a 250-kcal decrease. Extending the duration of the 5-day-per-week workouts from 30 min to 1 hr produces the desired weight loss without reducing food intake. In this case, extra physical activity creates the entire 3500 kcal deficit. If the intensity of the 1-hr session performed 5 days a week increases by only 10% (cycling at 22 mph instead of 20 mph; running at 6.6 mph instead of 6.0 mph), the number of calories expended each week with physical activity increases by an additional 350 kcal (3500 kcal × 0.10). This new weekly deficit of 3850 kcal (550 kcal per day) allows the dieter to *increase* daily food intake by 50 kcal and still maintain a 1-lb weekly fat loss.

Clearly, physical activity combined with mild dietary restriction effectively *unbalances* the energy balance equation for weight loss. This approach produces less-intense feelings of hunger and less psychologic stress than one that relies exclusively on caloric restriction. Furthermore, both aerobic and resistance activities protect against FFM loss that occurs with weight loss by diet alone. This occurs partly from the favorable effect of regular exercise on mobilization and use of fatty acids from adipose tissue depots.[133] Combining physical activity with weight loss produces desirable reductions in blood pressure at rest and in situations that typically elevate blood pressure such as intense physical activity and emotional distress.[192] Physical activity also facilitates protein retention in skeletal muscle and retards its rate of breakdown. *The fat-burning, protein-sparing benefits of regular activity contribute to facilitated fat loss in a weight-loss program.*

Reality Check. Regardless of the approach to weight loss, a statement from the National Task Force on the Prevention and Treatment of Obesity (www.ncbi.nih.gov) best sums up the difficulty in solving the overly fat condition on a long-term basis: "Obese individuals who undertake weight loss efforts should be ready to commit to lifelong changes in their behavioral patterns, diet, and physical activity."[147] Unfortunately, despite the importance of regular physical activity, fewer than one-half the people (about 40%) trying to lose or maintain weight were regularly active during leisure-time in a nationally representative sample.[121,122]

The benefits of regular physical activity for weight loss and weight maintenance outlined in Table 30.5 come primarily from highly structured experimental research on relatively small numbers of subjects who significantly increased physical activity with high compliance. On the other hand,

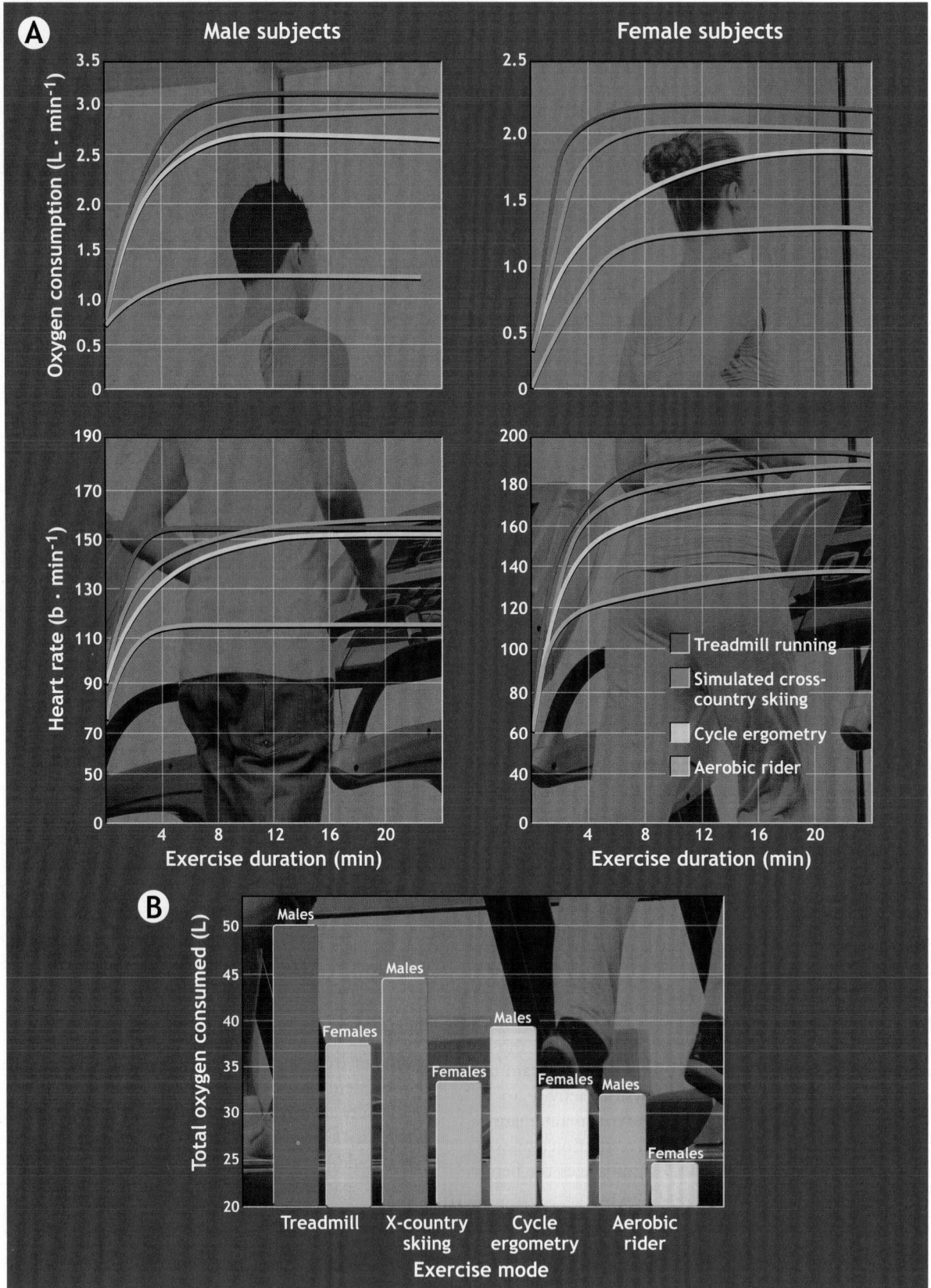

FIGURE 30.24 • **(A)** Oxygen consumption and heart rate for a representative male and female subject during 20 min of self-selected exercise consisting of treadmill running, leg-cycle ergometry, simulated cross-country skiing, or aerobic riding. **(B)** Total oxygen consumed by males and females during 20 min of each form of exercise at the same rating of perceived exertion. (Adapted with permission from Kravitz L, et al. Exercise mode and gender comparisons of energy expenditure at self-selected intensities. *Med Sci Sports Exerc* 1997;29:1028.)

TABLE 30.5	Benefits of Adding Exercise to Dietary Restriction for Weight Loss

- Increases overall size of the energy deficit
- Facilitates lipid mobilization and oxidation, especially from visceral adipose tissue depots
- Increases relative body fat loss by preserving fat-free body mass
- Bunts the drop in resting metabolism that accompanies weight loss by conserving and even increasing fat-free body mass
- Requires less reliance on caloric restriction to create an energy deficit
- Contributes to long-term success of the weight-loss effort
- Provides significant health-related benefits
- Offsets the deterioration in immune system function that often accompanies weight loss

large-scale intervention studies (randomized clinical trials) that compare diet only with a combination of diet and regular physical activity produce generally less remarkable results. In some cases, adding physical activity did not augment weight loss; when a benefit occur, the extra weight loss remained small. Clearly, the relatively modest amount of extra physical activity in the exercise group combined with high noncompliance to the exercise regimen in large-scale studies accounts for some blunting of an exercise effect. *The key to unlocking the benefits of regular physical activity for weight control in the general population lies in effective implementation of psychologic–behavioral factors that favor increased regular physical activity and reducing the amount of time spent sedentary.*

 INTEGRATIVE QUESTION

Outline a prudent, effective plan for a middle-age woman who wants to shed 10 kg of excess weight. Provide the rationale for each recommendation.

Spot Reduction Does Not Work to Selectively Reduce Local Fat Deposits

The notion of spot reduction emanates from the belief that an increase in a muscle's metabolic activity stimulates relatively greater fat mobilization from the adipose tissue in proximity to the active muscle. As such, moving a specific body area region to "sculpt" should selectively reduce more fat from that area than moving a different muscle group at the same metabolic intensity. Advocates of spot reduction recommend performing large numbers of sit-ups or side-bends to reduce excessive abdominal and hip fat. The promise of spot reduction with physical activity seems attractive from an aesthetic and health risk standpoint—unfortunately, critical evaluation of the research evidence does not support its use.[114,120,148]

 Physical Activity Prevents Fat Infiltration into Muscle

Considerable evidence suggests that loss of strength and muscle mass appear to be inevitable consequences of aging, and that body fat increases with aging. Eleven men and 31 women completed a randomized trial consisting of either a physical activity group (PA; *n* = 22) or successful aging health educational control group (SA; *n* = 20). Isokinetic knee extensor strength and computed tomography–derived mid-thigh skeletal muscle and adipose tissue cross-sectional areas (CSA) were assessed at baseline and at 12 mo following randomization. Total body weight and muscle CSA decreased in both groups, but these losses were not different between groups. Strength adjusted for muscle mass decreased (−20.1 ± 9.3%) in SA. The loss of strength was essentially prevented in PA (−2.5 ± 8.3%). In addition, a significant increase (18.4 ± 6.0%) in muscle fat infiltration occurred in SA, but this gain was nearly completely prevented in PA (2.3 ± 5.7%). These results show that regular physical activity prevents both the age-associated loss of muscle strength and increase in muscle fat infiltration in older adults.

Source: Goodpaster BH et al. Effects of physical activity on strength and skeletal muscle fat infiltration in older adults: a randomized controlled trial. *J Appl Physiol* 2008;105:1498.

 INTEGRATIVE QUESTION

Give specific examples of how small adjustments in daily energy expenditure and daily food intake can alter body fat content over time.

To examine claims for spot reduction, researchers compared the girths and subcutaneous fat stores of the right and left forearms of high-caliber tennis players.[72] As expected, the girth of the dominant or playing arm exceeded the nondominant arm because of a modest muscular hypertrophy from the activity overload of tennis. Measurements of skinfold thickness, however, clearly showed that regular and prolonged tennis training did not reduce subcutaneous fat in the playing arm. Another study evaluated fat biopsy specimens from abdominal, subscapular, and buttock sites before and after 27 days of sit-up exercise training.[104] The number of sit-ups increased from 140 at the end of the first week to 336 on day 27. Despite the considerable amount of localized physical activity, adipocytes in the abdominal region were no smaller than adipocytes in the unexercised buttocks or subscapular control regions.

The negative energy balance created through regular physical activity contributes to reducing total body fat. Physical activity stimulates the mobilization of fatty acids via hormones and enzymes that act on fat depots throughout the body. Body areas of greatest fat concentration and/or lipid-mobilizing enzyme activity supply the greatest amount of this energy. *Physical activity does not cause greater fatty acid release from the fat pads directly over the active muscle.*

Possible Gender Difference in Responsiveness to Physical Activity

An interesting question concerns the possibility of a gender difference in the responsiveness of weight loss to regular physical activity. A meta-analysis of 53 research studies on this topic concluded that men generally respond more favorably than women to the effects of physical activity on weight loss.[9] One possible explanation involves the gender difference in body fat distribution. As discussed previously, fat distributed in the upper body and abdominal regions (central fat) shows active lipolysis to sympathetic nervous system stimulation and becomes preferentially mobilized for energy during physical activity.[6,217] Consequently, the greater upper-body fat distribution in men may contribute to a greater sensitivity to lose fat in the abdominal region with regular physical activity. Women also may more effectively preserve energy balance with increased physical activity.[45,47,225] Men often reduce energy intake with training, whereas the depression of food intake with exercise may be less for women.

WEIGHT LOSS RECOMMENDATIONS FOR WRESTLERS AND OTHER POWER ATHLETES

Weightlifters, gymnasts, and other athletes in sports that require a high level of muscular strength and power per unit of body mass often must reduce body fat without compromising athletic performance. Any increase in relative muscular strength and short-term power output capacity should improve competitive performance. The following discussion focuses on wrestlers, but applies to all physically active individuals who desire to reduce body fat without negatively affecting health, safety, and physical capacity.

To reduce injury and medical complications from short- and longer-term periods of weight loss and dehydration, the ACSM, NCAA, and AMA recommend assessing each wrestler's body composition. The National Federation of State High School Associations required the adoption of weight certification beginning with the 2005 season. This assessment takes place several weeks prior to the competitive season to determine a **minimal wrestling weight** based on percentage body fat. *Five percent body fat (determined using hydrostatic weighing or population-specific skinfold equations) represents the lowest acceptable level for safe wrestling competition.* The hydrostatic weighing or skinfold assessment of body fat recommended by the NCAA has been cross-validated by the more rigorous four-component body composition assessment and found to be acceptable for accuracy and precision.[27,28] For wrestlers under age 16, 7% body fat represents the recommended lower limit. Importantly, percentage body fat must be determined in the euhydrated state because dehydration of between 2 and 5% body weight through fluid restriction and exercise in a hot environment (techniques commonly used by wrestlers) violates the assumptions necessary for accurate and precise prediction of minimal wrestling weight.[11] TABLE 30.6 outlines a practical application to determine minimal wrestling weight and an appropriate competitive weight class. The ACSM also recommends that weight loss should progress gradually and not exceed a 1- to 2-lb reduction per week. At the same time, the athlete should continue to consume a well-balanced, nutritious diet.

Prudent Recommendations for Wrestlers

The Gatorade Sports Science Institute (**www.gssiweb.com**) presents nutrition guidelines for wrestlers, with downloads available in PDF format. This includes general body composition and nutritional recommendations for wrestlers once their appropriate wrestling weight has been established and achieved. Coaches should regularly assess their wrestlers' body composition and hydration and nutrition status. In response to the deaths of three collegiate wrestlers in 1997 from excessive weight loss largely from dehydration, the NCAA introduced rule changes for the 1998–99 season to discourage dangerous weight-cutting practices and increase safe participation.[29] In addition to establishing a minimal wrestling weight, another rule change measures urine-specific gravity (density of urine to the density of water). This assessment of hydration status ensures euhydration of wrestlers at weight certification. Athletes with a urine-specific gravity of 1.020 or less are considered euhydrated, while those with specific gravity in excess of 1.020 cannot have body fat measured to determine minimum competitive wrestling weight for the season. Urine-specific gravity reflects hydration status, but it lags behind true hydration status during rapid body fluid turnover with acute dehydration as used by wrestlers to make weight. Such a scenario would fail to detect a large number of dehydrated wrestlers.[156]

GAINING WEIGHT: THE COMPETITIVE ATHLETE'S DILEMMA

Gaining weight to enhance body composition and physical performance in activities that require muscular strength and power or aesthetic appearance poses a unique problem not easily resolved. Most persons focus on weight loss to reduce excess

TABLE 30.6	**Using Anthropometric Equations to Predict a Minimal Wrestling Weight and to Select a Competitive Weight Class**

A. To predict body density (BD), use one of the following equations. (For each skinfold, record the average of at least three trials in mm.)

1. Lohman equation[a]
    BD = 1.0982 − (0.00815 × [triceps + subscapular + abdominal skinfolds])
         + (0.00000084 × [triceps + subscapular + abdominal skinfolds]^2)
2. Katch and McArdle equation[b]
    BD = 1.09448 − (0.00103 × triceps skinfold) − (0.00056 × subscapular skinfold) − (0.00054 × abdominal skinfold)
3. Behnke and Wilmore equation[c]
    BD = 1.05721 − (0.00052 × abdominal skinfold) + (0.00168 × iliac diameter) + (0.00114 × neck circumference)
         + (0.00048 × chest circumference) + (0.00145 × abdominal circumference)
4. Thorland equation[d]
    BD = 1.0982 − (0.000815 × [triceps + abdominal skinfolds])^2 + (0.00000084 × [triceps + abdominal skinfolds])

B. To determine fat percentage, use the Brožek equation:
   % Fat = [4.570 + BD − 4.142] × 100

C. To determine fat-free weight and to identify a minimum weight class, follow the examples below:

1. Fifteen-year-old wrestler who weighs 132 lb has a body density of 1.075 g · cc^{-1} and hopes to compete in the 119-lb weight class.
2. Percentage fat is (4.570 + 1.075 − 4.142) × 100 = 10.9%
3. Fat weight and fat-free weight are:
    a. 132.0 lb × 0.109 = 14.4 lb fat
    b. 132.0 lb − 14.4 lb fat = 117.6 lb fat-free weight

D. To calculate a minimal wrestling weight:

1. Realize that the recommended minimum body weight for those 15 years and younger contains 93% (0.93) fat-free weight and 7% fat (0.07)
2. Divide the wrestler's calculated fat-free weight by the greatest allowable fraction of fat-free weight to estimate minimal wrestling weight: 117.6 ÷ (93/100) = 117.6 ÷ 0.93 = 126.5 lb

E. To allow for a 2% error, perform the following calculations:

1. 126.5 minimal weight × 0.02 = 2.5 lb error allowance
2. 126.5 lb − 2.5 lb = 124.0 lb minimum wrestling weight

F. Conclusion: This boy cannot wrestle in the 119-lb weight class; rather, he must compete in the 125-lb class.

[a]Lohman TG. Skinfolds and body density and their relationship to body frames: a review. *Hum Biol* 1981;53:181.
[b]Katch FI, McArdle WD. Prediction of body density from simple anthropometric measurements in college-age men and women. *Hum Biol* 1973;l45:445.
[c]Behnke AR, Wilmore JH. *Evaluation and Regulation of Body Build and Composition.* Englewood Cliffs, NJ: Prentice Hall, 1974.
[d]Thorland W, et al. New equations for prediction of a minimal weight in high school wrestlers. *Med Sci Sports Exerc* 1989;21:S72.
Reprinted from Tipton CM. Making and maintaining weight for interscholastic wrestling. *Gatorade Sports Science Exchange* 1990;2(22).

body fat and improve overall health and appearance. Body weight and fat gain per se occurs all too readily by tilting the body's energy balance to favor greater caloric intake. Weight gain for athletes should represent increases in muscle mass and accompanying connective tissue. Generally, this form of weight gain occurs if increased caloric intake—carbohydrate for adequate energy and protein sparing, plus the amino acid building blocks of protein for tissue synthesis—accompanies a balanced, progressive resistance-exercise regimen.

Unsupported Hype

Athletes attempting to increase muscle mass often fall easy prey to health food and diet supplement manufacturers who market "high-potency, tissue-building" substances—chromium, boron, vanadyl sulfate, β-hydroxy-methyl butyrate, and various protein and amino acid mixtures—none of which reliably increases muscle mass. Concerning protein supplementation, no evidence indicates that commercially prepared mixtures of powdered protein, predigested amino acids, or special high-protein "cocktails" promote muscle growth any more effectively than protein consumed in a well-balanced diet (see Chapter 23).[118]

Increase the Lean, Not the Fat

Endurance training usually increases FFM only slightly, but the overall effect reduces body weight because of fat loss from the calorie-burning and possible appetite-depressing effects of this activity. In contrast, muscular overload through resistance training, supported by adequate energy and protein intake with sufficient recovery, increases muscle mass and strength. Adequate energy intake ensures that no catabolism of protein available for muscle growth occurs from an energy deficit. *Thus, intense aerobic training should not coincide with resistance training to increase muscle mass.*[77] More than likely, the added energy and perhaps protein demands of concurrent resistance and aerobic exercise training impose a limit on muscle growth and responsiveness to resistance training. In addition, on the molecular level, aerobic training may inhibit signaling to the protein synthesis machinery of skeletal muscle to negatively impact the muscle's adaptive response to resistance training.[13,143] A prudent recommendation increases daily protein intake to about 1.6 to 2.0 g per kilogram of body mass during the resistance-training period.[128] The individual should consume a variety of plant and animal proteins; relying solely on animal protein (high in saturated fatty acids and cholesterol) potentially increases heart disease risk.

If all calories consumed in excess of the energy requirement during resistance training sustained muscle growth, then 2000 to 2500 extra kcal could supply each 0.5-kg increase in lean tissue. In practical terms, 700 to 1000 kcal added to the well-balanced daily meal plan supports a weekly 0.5- to 1.0-kg gain in lean tissue and additional energy needs for training. This ideal situation presupposes that all extra calories synthesize lean tissue. Chapter 23 provided specific recommendations for nutrient timing to optimize muscle responsiveness to resistance training.

How Much Gain to Expect

A 1-year program of heavy-resistance training for young, athletic men increases body mass by about 20%, mostly from lean tissue accrual. The rate of lean tissue gain rapidly plateaus as training progresses beyond the first year. For athletic women, first-year gains in lean tissue mass average 50 to 75% of the absolute values for men, probably from the women's smaller initial lean body mass. Individual differences in the daily quantity of nitrogen incorporated into body protein (and protein incorporated into muscle) also limit and explain differences among persons in muscle mass increases with resistance training. FIGURE 30.25 lists eight specific factors that affect the responsiveness of lean tissue synthesis to resistance training.

Individuals with relatively high androgen–estrogen ratios and greater percentages of fast-twitch muscle fibers probably increase lean tissue to the greatest extent. Muscle mass increases most at the start of training in individuals with the largest relative FFM (FFM corrected for stature and body fat).[215] Regularly monitoring body mass and body fat verifies whether the combination of training and additional food intake increases lean tissue and not body fat. This requires an accurate (valid) appraisal of body composition at regular intervals throughout the training period.

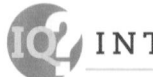 **INTEGRATIVE QUESTION**

Outline recommendations to a high school student who wishes to increase body weight to improve physical appearance and sports performance.

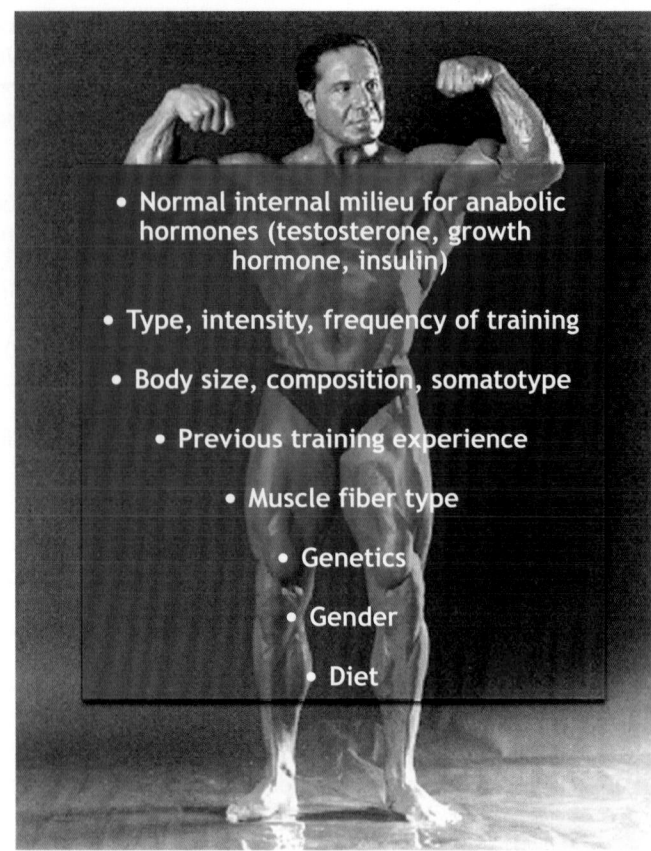

FIGURE 30.25 • Specific factors affecting the magnitude of lean tissue synthesis with resistance training. (Photo of Bill Pearl, courtesy of Bill Pearl.)

Summary

1. Three ways to unbalance the energy-balance equation to produce weight loss: reduce energy intake below energy expenditure, maintain normal energy intake and increase energy expenditure, and decrease energy intake and increasing energy expenditure.
2. Long-term maintenance of weight loss through dietary restriction has a success rate less than 20%. Typically, one to two thirds of the lost weight returns within a year and almost all of it within 5 years.
3. A caloric deficit of 3500 kcal, created through either diet or physical activity, represents the equivalent of the calories in 0.45 kg of adipose tissue.
4. Prudent dieting effectively promotes weight loss. Disadvantages of extremes of caloric restriction include loss of FFM, lethargy, malnutrition, and depressed resting metabolism.
5. Reduced resting metabolism represents a well-documented response to weight loss through dieting.
6. Rapid weight loss during the first few days of caloric deficit mainly reflects loss of body water and stored glycogen; greater fat loss occurs per unit of weight lost as caloric restriction continues.
7. The calories burned in physical activity accumulate. Over time, regular extra physical activity creates a considerable energy deficit.

8. The precise role of physical activity in appetite suppression or stimulation remains unclear, but moderate increases in physical activity may depress appetite and energy intake of a previously sedentary, overweight person.

9. Physical activity combined with caloric restriction offers a flexible and effective way to achieve weight loss.

10. Physical activity enhances fat mobilization and catabolism to accelerate body fat loss.

11. Regular aerobic activity retards lean tissue loss while resistance training increases FFM.

12. Selective activation of specific body regions by "spot exercise" proves no more effective for localized fat loss than more general physical activity of equivalent caloric expenditure.

13. Differences in body fat distribution partially explain gender difference in responsiveness to physical activity–induced weight loss.

14. Athletes should gain weight as lean body tissue. Modest increases in caloric intake with systematic resistance training effectively produce this effect.

15. Ideally, 700 to 1000 extra kcal per day supports a weekly 0.5- to 1.0-kg gain in lean tissue and resistance training energy requirements.

the**Point**   References are available online at **http://thepoint.lww.com/mkk8e.**

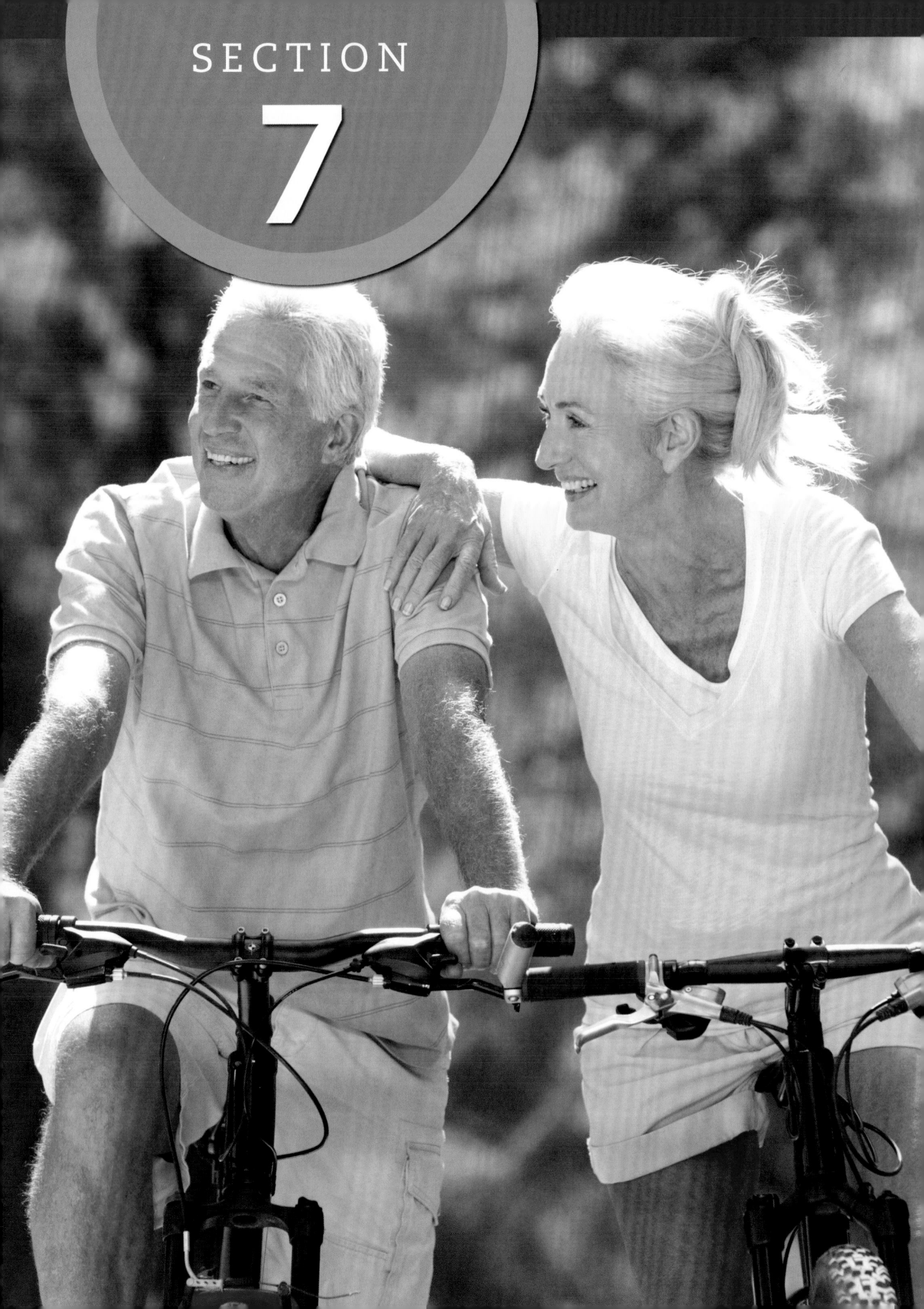

Exercise, Successful Aging, and Disease Prevention

OVERVIEW

The physiologic and exercise capacities of older persons usually rate below those of younger peers. It remains uncertain how these differences reflect true biologic aging or the effect of disuse from alterations in lifestyle and reduced physical activity. Recent research reveals that older men and women no longer conform to a sedentary stereotype with little or no initiative for active pursuits. Seniors now routinely participate in a broad range of physical activities and exercise programs. Maintenance of an active lifestyle into later years helps older adults retain a high level of functional capacity. In addition, regular physical activity offers considerable protection against and rehabilitation from a variety of disabilities, diseases, and risk factors, particularly those related to cardiovascular health. Within this framework, the exercise physiologist provides skills and contributions to encourage regular exercise in the clinical setting.

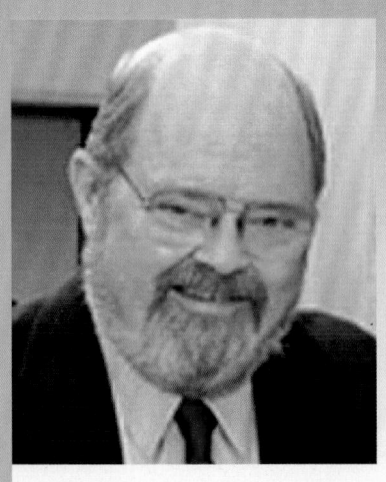

INTERVIEW WITH
Dr. Steven N. Blair

Education: BA (Kansas Wesleyan University, Salina, KS); MS and PED (Indiana University, Bloomington, IN); postgraduate training (Scholar in Preventive Cardiology, Stanford University School of Medicine, Palo Alto, CA)

Current Affiliation: Professor and Faculty Affiliate, Prevention Research Center, Department of Exercise Science, University of South Carolina, Columbia, SC

Honors, Awards, and ACSM Citation Award Statement of Contributions: See Appendix C, available online at http://thepoint.lww.com/mkk8e

Research Focus: My research has two major foci: (1) The Aerobics Center Longitudinal Study, an investigation of the relation of physical activity, cardiorespiratory fitness, and health outcomes and (2) randomized clinical trials of physical activity interventions and their health-related outcomes.

Memorable Publication: Blair SN, et al. Physical fitness and all-cause mortality: a prospective study of healthy men and women. *JAMA* 1989;262:2395.

What first inspired you to enter the exercise science field? What made you decide to pursue your advanced degree and/or line of research?

➤ I participated in sports in high school and college, and decided during my college career that I wanted to be a physical education teacher and athletic coach.

What influence did your undergraduate education have on your final career choice?

➤ My physical education teachers and coaches encouraged and influenced me to continue my education with graduate school. I had conducted a small, independent research project as an undergraduate and found that I liked defining a problem, collecting data, and trying to make sense of the results. In graduate school, I developed an interest in an academic research career, but I think it was the solid foundation in the liberal arts and specific areas of physical education that influenced my career direction.

Who were the most influential people in your career, and why?

➤ Gene Bissell was a strong early mentor. He is a man of uncompromising principles, dedication, and genuine concern for his students. He once forfeited a win in football when, after the game was over, he realized that an official had missed a call. When Coach Bissell pointed out the infraction, the league office replied that sometimes calls are missed and that is just one of the breaks of the game. Coach Bissell refused to accept that ruling and insisted that his team be declared the loser.

I had several influential mentors at Indiana University. Karl and Carolyn Bookwalter gave me a research assistantship, helped me with my first publication, and generally introduced me to the world of scientific writing. Arthur Slater-Hammel introduced me to the scientific process, taught me about

experimental design, and was the director of my doctoral dissertation. George Cousins was inquisitive and skeptical—two traits I consider essential for a scientist.

My first academic job was at the University of South Carolina. My interests soon turned to preventive cardiology, with a specific interest in exercise as a preventive and therapeutic modality. In the early 1970s I wrote an application for the Multiple Risk Factor Intervention Trial (MRFIT), and we received a grant to serve as one of 20 MRFIT clinical centers. I learned much from leaders of the MRFIT, including Professors Jerry Stamler, Henry Taylor, Paul Ogelsby, Henry Blackburn, Steve Hulley, Mark Kjelsburg, Lew Kuller, and many others.

In 1978, I had an opportunity to work with Bill Haskell and Peter Wood at the Stanford University Heart Disease Prevention Program. I have had literally hundreds of hours of discussion with them over the years about various issues in exercise science and public health, and I continue to learn from their work and examples.

I also had the great opportunity to develop a relationship with Dr. Ralph S. Paffenbarger, who has considerably influenced my research over the past 20 years. "Paff" has made enormous contributions to the epidemiology of physical activity and health. His work is a model of rigorous methodology, clear thinking, poetic writing, and carefully drawn conclusions. He continues to be a good friend, research collaborator, mentor, and inspiration.

Last, I will mention colleagues at the Cooper Institute. I feel very fortunate that Dr. Cooper had the vision to establish the database for the Aerobics Center Longitudinal Study. My many colleagues at the Cooper Institute have been instrumental in our work over the past 20 years. I have learned much from them, and any success we have had is due in large part to their hard work, dedication, and scientific expertise.

What has been the most interesting/enjoyable aspect of your involvement in science? What was the least interesting/enjoyable aspect?

➤ The most interesting/enjoyable aspect of science for me is the discovery that accompanies research. Nothing is more exciting than seeing the results of an analysis that yield something new and perhaps unexpected.

The least desirable aspects of my scientific life are the constant scrambling for funds to support our research activities and the routine administrative tasks that are inherent in managing an enterprise of 25 to 30 people.

What is your most meaningful contribution to the field of exercise science, and why is it so important?

➤ I think that our work on low cardiorespiratory fitness as a predictor of morbidity and mortality in middle-age and older women and men is a meaningful contribution to exercise science. Our report on fitness and mortality that was published in the *Journal of the American Medical Association* in 1989 seemed to come at the right time and struck a responsive chord in both the scientific and lay communities. This research helped influence several statements on the significance of physical inactivity on public health, which have had a substantial effect on exercise science, public health, and clinical medicine.

I am also proud of our research on lifestyle physical activity interventions. Our epidemiological studies revealed a curvilinear, dose–response relation between cardiorespiratory fitness and mortality, with the steepest part of the curve at the low end of the fitness continuum. Moderate levels of fitness are associated with reduced risk, and moderate amounts and intensities of physical activity can produce these moderate levels of fitness. We designed a randomized clinical trial to test the hypothesis that behaviorally based lifestyle physical activity intervention would be as effective as a traditional, structured exercise program in increasing physical activity, improving cardiorespiratory fitness, and improving other health parameters. I am pleased that this work is leading to greater flexibility and more options for exercise programming to achieve health benefits.

What advice would you give to students who express an interest in pursuing a career in exercise science research?

➤ Obtain a strong foundation in science as an undergraduate. Read widely in your area of interest and become familiar with the leading researchers in this area of investigation. Talk to your professors about your plans and seek their advice. Do not be afraid to approach well-known researchers and ask for their advice in making your career choices. Most of them are very nice people and will be flattered if you come well prepared with good questions. As you begin to narrow your choice of institutions for graduate school, make up a visitation schedule and try to visit at least three or four programs that you think match your needs. Go to the very best program that will accept you.

What interests have you pursued outside your professional career?

➤ I like to garden, and my wife and I are proud of our landscaping and flowers. We have season tickets to the symphony, opera, summer musicals, and one of the Dallas theaters. We both use running as our main form of exercise, and we run nearly every day and have over the past 30 years. We like to travel and feel fortunate that my work has afforded us many opportunities to travel in the United States and abroad.

Where do you see the exercise science field (particularly your area of greatest interest) heading in the next 30 years?

➤ Genetic epidemiology will make important contributions to our understanding of which individuals are at greatest risk of a sedentary way of life. We will work out in much greater detail the specific types, amounts, and intensities of activity that prevent or delay specific diseases or conditions. We will finally establish appropriate public health surveillance systems to monitor accurately patterns and trends of physical activity and physical fitness in people of all ages. Physical inactivity will be recognized as the major and most expensive public health problem in the United States.

We will learn much more about how to help sedentary individuals adopt and maintain physical activity. These advances, however, may not be sufficient to overcome the ever more toxic environment in which we live, as indicated by our continuing to engineer physical activity out of daily life. The threat posed to our public health and well-being by an increase in the prevalence of sedentary habits may finally cause us to seriously consider, develop, and implement policy and legislative solutions to encourage more physical activity.

You have the opportunity to give a "last lecture." Describe its primary focus.

➤ I would describe the joys of scientific discovery and the pleasure of collaborating with colleagues to address important public health issues. I would illustrate how hazardous it is to be sedentary and unfit, and how a fit and active way of life can bring benefits to virtually all demographic groups. I would outline the seriousness of the public health problem of inactivity and try to issue a rousing call to action to encourage all to help address this problem. After accepting sustained applause, and even standing ovations and shouts of "Bravo," I would exit the stage and leave the work to the younger generation.

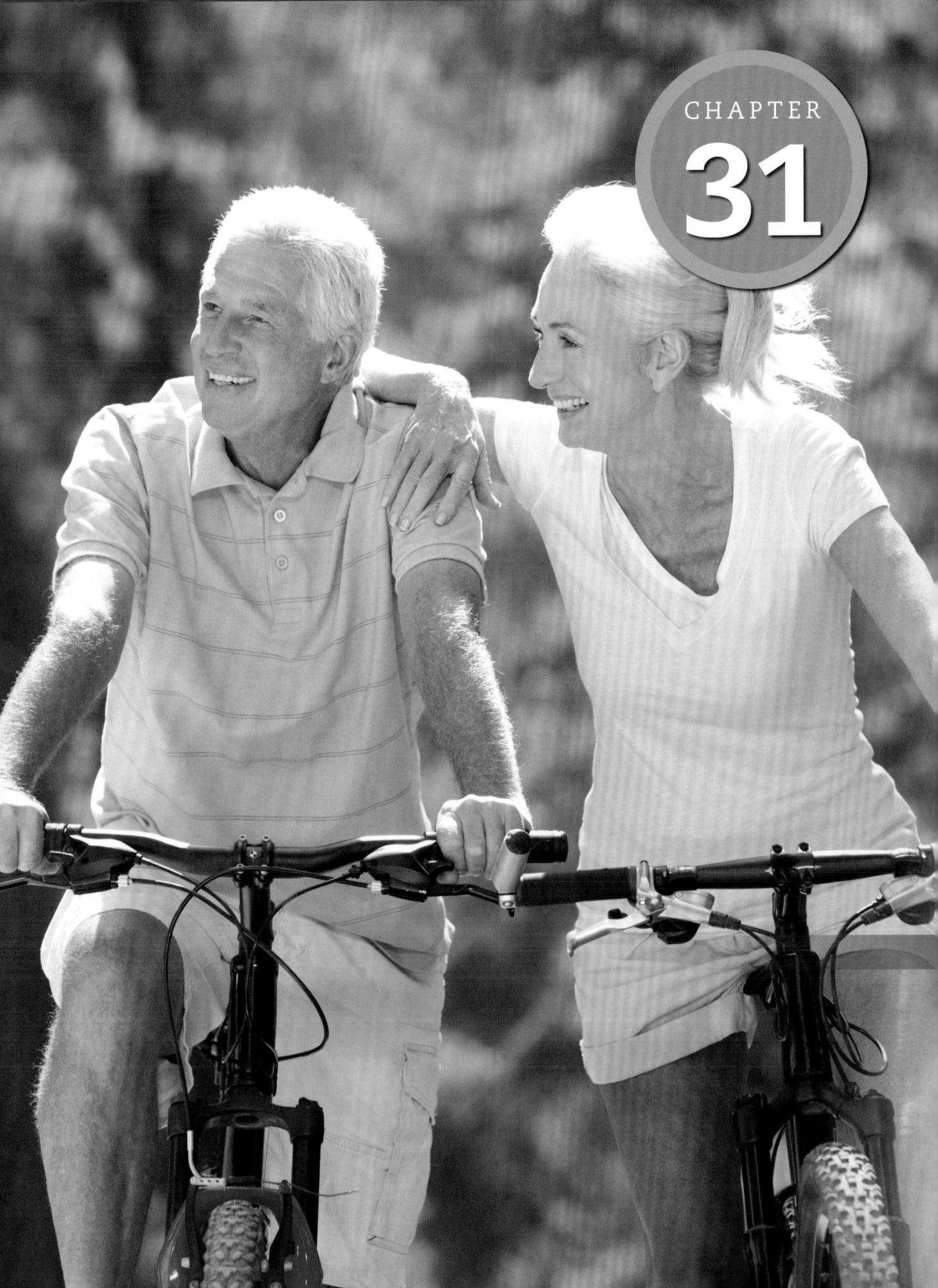

Physical Activity, Health, and Aging

CHAPTER OBJECTIVES

- Summarize aging trends in the American population

- Describe the physical activity level of typical adult American men and women

- Outline the major findings of the Surgeon General's report on the population's physical activity participation

- Answer the question: How safe is exercise?

- List factors that increase the likelihood of experiencing an exercise catastrophe

- Contrast physiologic responses to physical activity of children and adults and their implications for evaluating physiologic function and exercise performance

- List important age-related changes in muscular function, nervous system function, cardiovascular function, pulmonary function, and body composition components

- Summarize the potential benefits of moderate resistance training for older adults

- Discuss the following statement: A sedentary lifestyle causes losses in functional capacity at least as great as the effects of aging itself

- Describe research about the role of regular physical activity in coronary heart disease prevention and life extension

- Indicate the types and levels of physical activity that induce the greatest improvement in risk-factor profile and overall health

- Describe vulnerable plaque and its proposed role in sudden death

- List the major modifiable heart disease risk factors and how regular physical activity affects each

- Outline the normal dynamics of homocysteine, its proposed role in coronary heart disease, and factors that affect plasma levels

- Discuss the prevalence of heart disease risk factors in children

ANCILLARIES ◉ at-a-Glance

Visit http://thepoint.lww.com/mkk8e to access the following resources.

- References: Chapter 31
- Interactive Question Bank
- Animation: Acute Inflammation
- Focus on Research: Physical Inactivity: A Significant Coronary Heart Disease Risk

THE GRAYING OF AMERICA

Older adults—those age 85 and older—make up the fastest growing segment of American society. Thirty years ago, age 65 represented the onset of old age. Gerontologists now consider 85 the demarcation of "**oldest-old**" and age 75, "**young-old**." According to the 2010 U.S. census (2010; www.census.gov/prod/cen2010/briefs/c2010br-09.pdf), nearly 13% of the country's population (a 15.1% increase from 2000), or 40 million U.S. citizens, exceed age 65. Between 2000 and 2010 the rate of increase in the population 65 years and over increased almost twice as fast that the total U.S. population. Males show more rapid growth in the older population than females. By the year 2030, 20% of the population, or about 72 million, will exceed age 85. No longer viewed as a quirk of nature, 2 in 10,000 Americans now live to age 100. Demographers project that by the middle of this century, more than 800,000 Americans will exceed age 100, with many maintaining relatively good health. Life-expectancy calculators can be found online and include that of the National Center for Health Statistics (www.cdc.gov/nchs/fastats/lifexpec.htm).

Some demographers project that half of the girls and a third of the boys born in developed countries near the end of the 20th century will live in three centuries. In the short term, disease prevention, water purification and better sanitation, improved nutrition and health care, and more effective treatment of age-related heart disease and osteoporosis help people to live longer. Far fewer persons now die from infectious childhood diseases, so those with the genetic potential actualize their proclivity for longevity. On a different but parallel front, anticipated breakthroughs in genetic therapies may slow the aging of individual cells. Gene therapies and rapid progress in stem cell research could boost human life spans to a much greater extent than improved medical treatment or even eradication of some diseases. The goal of current research seeks to increase the quality of life in older age, not simply to extend life. One focus concerns the development of new ways to replace worn-out organs and tissues including liver, bone, and heart or help the body to regenerate them.

Physical inactivity relates causally to nearly 30% of all deaths from heart disease, colon cancer, and diabetes. Lifestyle changes could reduce mortality from these ailments and greatly improve cardiovascular and functional capacities, quality of life, and independent living.[32,82,169] Accumulating evidence indicates that both aerobic and resistance training are important for maintaining cognitive and brain health in old age, an effect produced, in part, by vascular-mediated mechanisms such as increases in brain perfusion and the ability of cerebral blood vessels to respond to blood flow demands[47,125,139,228] The equivalent of a daily brisk 30-min walk associates with a lower risk of cognitive impairment. As physical activity levels increased, the rate of cognitive decline decreased.[223] The greatest health benefits would come from strategies that promote regular physical activity throughout one's lifetime.[2,3,74,144]

At any age, behavioral changes—becoming more physically active, quitting cigarette smoking, and controlling body weight and blood pressure—act independently to delay all-cause mortality and aging effects caused by diseases and environmental factors.[29,188] Persons with more healthful lifestyles survive longer, and the risk of disability and the necessity to seek home health care is postponed and compressed into fewer years at the end of life.[225,226]

 Older Yet Still Competing

The increased number of 65-and-over participants in marathons and ultramarathons aptly illustrates the exercise capacities of active older individuals. More than 240 individuals in the 70-90 year age group finished the 2011 New York City Marathon, the largest number of "aged" participants in the event's history.

Runners by Age Group Completing 2011 New York City Marathon

Age Group	Men	Women	Total
18-19	96	47	143
20-24	718	642	1360
25-29	2597	2861	5458
30-34	3950	3122	7072
35-39	4889	2878	7767
40-44	5910	3070	8980
45-49	4577	2131	6708
50-54	3762	1469	5231
55-59	1782	610	2392
60-64	1106	291	1397
65-69	363	87	450
70-74	158	28	186
75-79	35	6	41
80-89	9	4	13

THE NEW GERONTOLOGY

Gerontologists maintain that research on the elderly should focus on improving "**healthspan**," or the total number of years a person remains in excellent health, not simply to increase life span. Healthspan addresses areas beyond age-related diseases and prevention to recognize that *successful aging* requires maintenance of enhanced physiologic function and physical fitness. *Vitality, not longevity per se, remains the primary goal.*

Researchers now view much of the physiologic deterioration previously considered "normal aging" as dependent on lifestyle and environmental influences subject to considerable modification with proper diet and physical activity.[33,59] For those who achieve older age, low muscular strength, diminished cardiovascular function, and poor joint range of motion, as well as sleep disturbances, relate directly to functional limitations regardless of disease status.[91,140,184] Successful aging includes four main components:

1. Physical health
2. Spirituality
3. Emotional and educational health
4. Social satisfaction

Maintaining and even enhancing physical and cognitive functions, fully engaging in life, and participating in productive activities and interpersonal relations contribute to achieving these goals.

Healthy Life Expectancy: A New Concept

The Centers for Disease Control and Prevention (CDC; www.cdc.gov) report that about one-third of people age 65 or older report functional limitations of one kind or another; among people age 85 or older, about two-thirds report functional limitations. Current estimates indicate that more than two-thirds of 65-year-olds will need assistance to deal with a loss in functioning at some point during their remaining years of life (www.cbo.gov/publication/44363)

To estimate healthful longevity, the World Health Organization (WHO) has introduced the concept of **healthy life expectancy**—the expected number of years a person might live in the equivalent with full health. This involves **disability-adjusted life expectancy (DALE)**, which considers the years of ill health, weighted according to severity and subtracted from expected overall life expectancy to compute the equivalent years of healthy life. While WHO is still in the process of updating their DALE database for 2014, previous rankings by country remain pertinent today and show substantially more years lost to disability in poorer countries from the impact of injury, blindness, and paralysis, and from the debilitating effects of malaria, a tropical disease that most frequently strikes children and young adults. **FIGURE 31.1** shows the DALE for a sample of 14 countries. Of the 191 countries evaluated, DALE estimates of healthy life expectancy reached 70 years in 24 countries and 60 years in more than half. Thirty-two countries fell at the lower extreme, where DALE estimates were less than 40 years.

Japanese citizens experience the longest healthy life expectancy of 74.5 years. Surprisingly, the United States ranks 24th, with 70.0 years of healthy life for babies born in 1999 (72.6 years for females and 67.5 years for males). Native Americans, rural African Americans, and inner-city poor experience health characteristics similar to those living in underdeveloped countries. The HIV/AIDS epidemic, tobacco-related diseases, violent deaths, and prevalence of coronary heart disease all contribute to the United States' lower ranking among industrialized nations.

 New Advice for Osteoarthritis: Keep Moving and Lose Weight

Osteoarthritis, a degenerative joint disease once considered an ailment of older adults, occurs with increased frequency in younger individuals due to obesity and sports injuries. This disease, which occurs when the cartilage that cushions the spaces between the joints wears away, as in the knee joint shown in the inset, afflicts some 12.1% of the U.S. population (nearly 21 million individuals) age 25 and older and leads to more than 1 million joint replacements each year.

Traditional medical treatment advised individuals with this condition to go easy to reduce the stress on their joints. Current medical advice now recommends that arthritic patients combine regular low-impact activity such as aquatic exercise, cycling, swimming, and walking with weight loss and the strengthening of muscles that support joints to improve health and quality of life compared to medication alone. Even a small weight loss of 10 lb can reduce knee osteoarthritis risk (and reduce pain if the condition exists).

Acknowledgment: Dr. Grahm Hurvitz, MD, Ryu-Hurvitz Orthopedic Clinic, Santa Barbara, California (**http://santabarbaraorthopedicsurgery.com/physician-Graham_Hurvitz_MD.html**) assisted with anatomical structure identification.

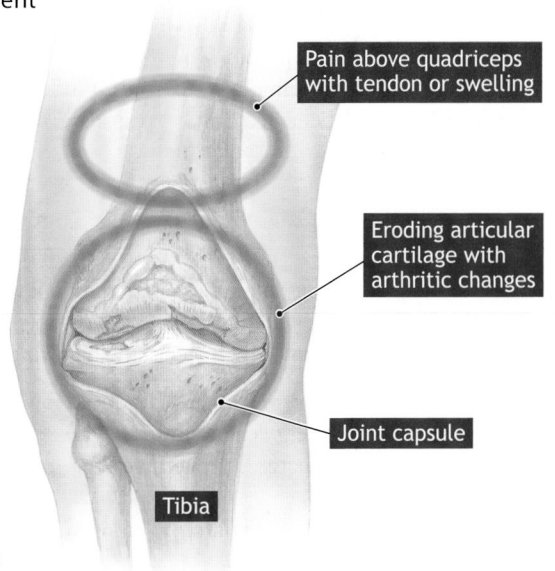

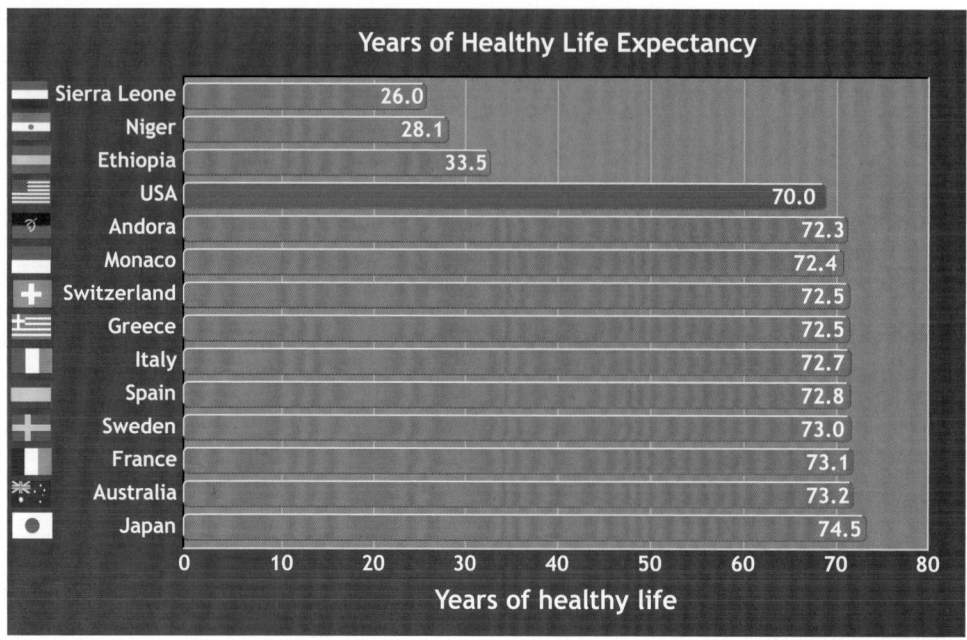

FIGURE 31.1 • Disability-adjusted life expectancy rankings (DALE; an estimate of healthy life expectancy) of populations of selected countries as assessed by the World Health Organization. Of all countries surveyed, the United States ranked 24th, with Japan ranked at the top.

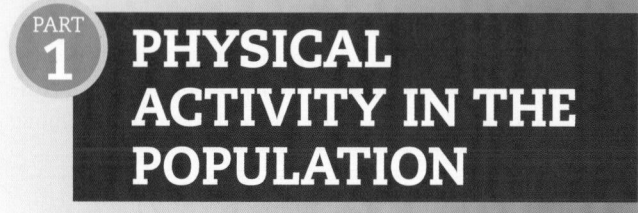

PART 1 PHYSICAL ACTIVITY IN THE POPULATION

PHYSICAL ACTIVITY EPIDEMIOLOGY

Epidemiology involves quantifying factors that influence the occurrence of illness to better understand, modify, and/or control a disease pattern in the general population. The specific field of **physical activity epidemiology** applies the general research strategies of epidemiology to study physical activity as a health-related behavior linked to disease and other outcomes.

Terminology

Physical activity epidemiology applies specific definitions to characterize behavioral patterns and outcomes of the group(s) under investigation. Relevant terminology includes the following:

- **Physical activity**: Body movement produced by muscle action that increases energy expenditure
- **Exercise**: Planned, structured, repetitive, and purposeful physical activity
- **Physical fitness**: Attributes related to how well one performs physical activity
- **Health**: Physical, mental, and social well-being, not simply absence of disease

- **Health-related physical fitness**: Components of physical fitness associated with some aspect of good health and/or disease prevention
- **Longevity**: Length of life

Within this framework, *physical activity* becomes a generic term, with *exercise* its major component. Similarly, the definition of *health* focuses on the broad spectrum of well-being that ranges from complete absence of health (near death) to the highest levels of physiologic function. Such definitions often challenge how we measure and quantify health and physical activity objectively. They provide a broad perspective to study the role of physical activity in health and disease.

The trend in physical fitness assessment during the past 40 years deemphasizes tests that stress motor performance and athletic fitness (i.e., speed, power, balance, and agility). Instead, current assessment focuses on functional capacities related to overall health and disease prevention. The four most common components of **health-related physical fitness** are aerobic and/or cardiovascular fitness, body composition, abdominal muscular strength and endurance, and lower back and hamstring flexibility (see **FIG. 31.2** and "In a Practical Sense," in this chapter).

Physical Activity Participation

More than 30 different methods assess diverse aspects of physical activity. They include direct and indirect calorimetry, self-reports and questionnaires, job classifications, physiologic markers, behavioral observations, mechanical or electronic monitors, and activity surveys. Each approach offers unique advantages but also has disadvantages depending on the situation and population studied. Obtaining valid estimates of physical activity of large groups is difficult because such studies, by necessity, apply self-reports of daily activity and exercise participation rather than direct monitoring or objective measurement.

A discouraging picture of physical activity participation worldwide, both of work/occupational and of leisure-time activity, emerges consistently as emphasized in the Surgeon General's report on United States citizens' physical activity and data provided by others:[138,159,208,215]

U.S. Adult Population

- Only about 15% engage in vigorous physical activity during leisure time, three times a week for at least 30 min.
- More than 60% do not engage in physical activity regularly.
- Twenty-five percent lead sedentary lives (i.e., do not exercise at all).
- Walking, gardening, and yard work are the most popular leisure-time activities.
- Twenty-two percent engage in light-to-moderate physical activity regularly during leisure time (five times a week for at least 30 min).
- Physical inactivity occurs among women more than men, blacks and Hispanics more than whites, older more than younger adults, and less-affluent more than wealthier persons.
- Participation in fitness activities declines with age; a large number of older citizens have such poor functional capacity they cannot rise from a chair or bed, walk to the bathroom, or climb a single stair without assistance.
- At best, no more than 20% and possibly less than 10% of adults in the United States, Australia, Canada, and England obtain sufficient regular physical activity at an intensity that imparts discernible health and fitness benefits.

U.S. Children and Teenagers

Physical activity data from a longitudinal study of boys and girls between ages 9 and 15 indicate that moderate-to-vigorous physical activity declined with age over the study period.[142] By age 15, daily physical activity decreased to just 49 min on weekdays and about 30 min per weekend day, well below the government's recommended 60-min duration. Overall, boys were only slightly more active than girls, moving an average of 18 more min daily. The percentage of children who met the government's 1-hr recommendation of moderate daily

Activities of Those Americans Who Report Regular Physical Activity

fyi

Activity	Percentage	
	Male	Female
Walking	39	48
Resistance training	20	9
Cycling	16	15
Running	12	6
Stair climbing	10	12
Aerobics	3	10

activity shifted markedly over time. Between ages 9 and 11, almost every child in the study was moving at least an hour a day. But by age 15, only 31% met the guideline during the week, and just 17% on the weekend.

Other data on the physical activity patterns of children, adolescents, and teenagers indicate the following:

- Nearly one half of those between ages 12 and 21 do not exercise vigorously on a regular basis; a sharp decline in physical activity occurs during adolescence regardless of gender.
- Fourteen percent report no recent physical activity; this lack of activity occurs more frequently among females, particularly black females.
- Twenty-five percent engage in light-to-moderate physical activity (e.g., walk or bicycle) nearly every day.
- Participation in all types of physical activity declines strikingly with increasing age and school grade.
- More males than females participate in vigorous physical activity, strengthening activities, and walking or bicycling.
- Daily attendance in school physical education programs declined from 42% in early 1990 to less than 25% in 2005.

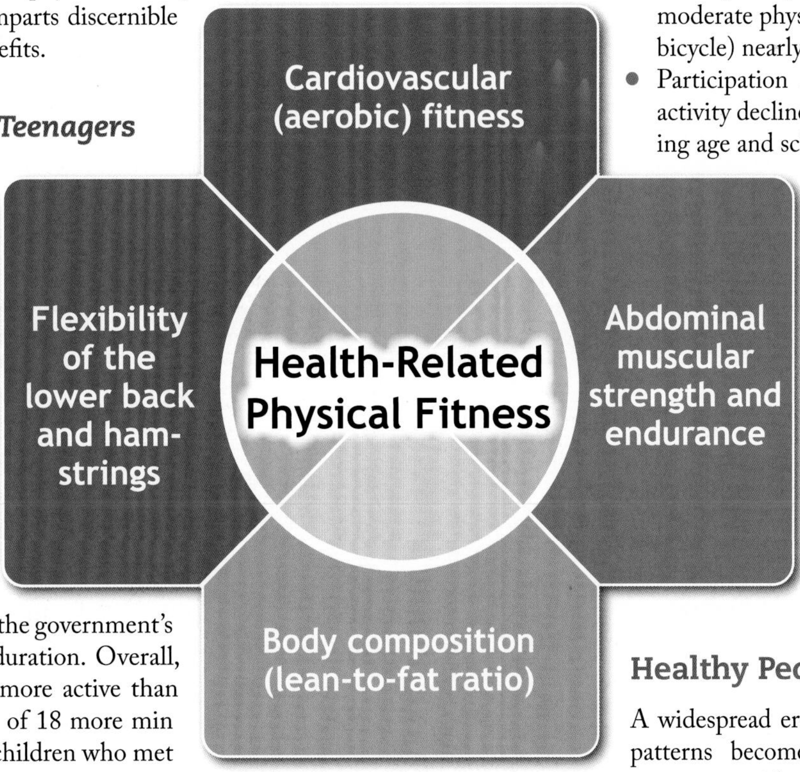

Healthy People 2020

A widespread erosion of physical activity patterns becomes particularly apparent with increasing age among American adolescents and

FIGURE 31.2 • Health-related physical fitness components.

IN A PRACTICAL SENSE

Assessing Hip-and-Trunk and Shoulder–Wrist Flexibility

Two types of flexibility include (1) static flexibility, full range of motion (ROM) of a specific joint and (2) dynamic flexibility, torque or resistance encountered as the joint moves through its ROM. Field tests commonly assess static flexibility indirectly through linear measurement of ROM.

FIELD TESTS OF HIP-AND-TRUNK AND SHOULDER–WRIST STATIC FLEXIBILITY

Administer a minimum of three trials following a standardized warm-up.

TEST 1: HIP-AND-TRUNK FLEXIBILITY (MODIFIED SIT-AND-REACH TEST)

Starting Position

Sit on the floor with the back and head against a wall, legs fully extended, with the bottoms of the feet against the sit-and-reach box. Place hands on top of each other, stretching the arms forward while keeping the head and back against the wall. Measure the distance from the fingertips to the box edge with a yardstick. This represents the zero, or starting, point (FIG. A).

Movement

Slowly bend and reach forward as far as possible (move head and back away from the wall), sliding the fingers along the yardstick; hold the final position for 2 s (FIG. B).

Score

Total distance reached to the nearest 1/4 inch represents the final score.

Modified Sit-and-Reach Ratings: Men (Score in Inches)

Rating	Age Range (yr)					
	18–25	26–35	36–45	46–55	56–65	65+
Excellent	>20	>20	>19	>19	>17	>17
Good	18–20	18–19	17–19	16–17	14–17	13–16
Above Average	17–18	16–17	15–17	14–15	12–14	11–13
Average	15–16	15–16	13–15	12–13	10–12	9–11
Below Average	13–14	12–14	11–13	10–11	8–10	8–9
Poor	10–12	10–12	9–11	7–9	5–8	5–7
Very Poor	<10	<10	<8	<7	<5	<5

Source: YMCA Sit-and-Reach Test; Shape Up America.
www.shapeup.org/fitness/assess/flex2.html

Modified Sit-and-Reach Ratings: Women (Score in Inches)

Rating	Age Range (yr)					
	18–25	26–35	36–45	46–55	56–65	65+
Excellent	>24	>25	>22	>21	>20	>1720
Good	21–23	20–22	19–21	18–20	18–19	18–19
Above Average	20–21	19–20	17–19	17–18	16–17	16–17
Average	18–19	18	16–17	15–16	15	14–15
Below Average	17–18	16–17	14–15	14–15	13–14	12–13
Poor	14–16	14–15	11–13	11–13	10–12	9–11
Very Poor	<13	<13	<10	<10	<9	<8

Source: YMCA Sit-and-Reach Test; Shape Up America.
www.shapeup.org/fitness/assess/flex2.html

Test 1: Hip-and-trunk flexibility (modified sit-and-reach test)

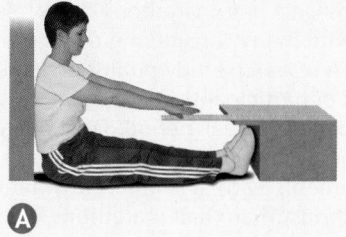

Test 2: Shoulder-wrist flexibility (shoulder-and-wrist elevation test)

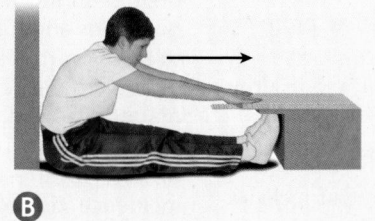

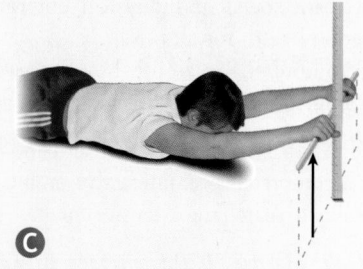

TEST 2: SHOULDER–WRIST FLEXIBILITY (SHOULDER-AND-WRIST ELEVATION TEST)

Starting Position

Lie prone on the floor with the arms fully extended over-head; grasp a yardstick with the hands shoulder-width apart.

Movement

Raise the stick as high as possible (FIG. C).

- Measure the vertical distance (nearest 0.5 in.) the yard-stick rises from the floor.
- Measure arm length from the acromial process to the tip of the longest finger.
- Subtract the average vertical score from arm length.

Score

Arm length 2 average vertical score (nearest 0.25 in.)

SHOULDER-AND-WRIST ELEVATION RATINGS BASED ON COLEGE-AGE MEN AND WOMEN (SCORE IN INCHES)

Rating	Men	Women
Excellent	6.00 or less	5.50 or less
Good	8.25–6.25	7.50–5.75
Average	11.50–8.50	10.75–7.75
Fair	12.50–11.75	11.75–11.00
Poor	12.75 or more	12.00 or more

Source: Adapted from Johnson BL, Nelson JK. *Practical Measurements for Evaluation in Physical Education.* 4th Ed. New York: Macmillan, 1986.

adults; the decline is greater for adolescent and adult females than for males.[36] Regardless of the cause for progressive inactivity as adults age, *increased* levels of physical activity predict *decreased* levels of all-cause morbidity and mortality and the relationship appears to be graded.[28,92]

The "*Physical Activity Pyramid*" illustrated in **FIGURE 31.3** summarizes major goals for increasing the level of regular physical activity in the general population and emphasizes diverse forms of behavioral and lifestyle options.

Healthy People 2020, launched on December 2, 2010, represents a set of goals and objectives with 10-year targets designed to guide national health promotion and disease prevention efforts to improve the health of all people in the United States.

Released by the U.S. Department of Health and Human Services each decade, the Healthy People initiative reflects the idea that setting objectives and providing science-based benchmarks to track and monitor progress can motivate and focus action. Healthy People 2020 represents the fourth generation of this initiative, building on a foundation of the previous three decades of work.

These goals and objectives are used as a tool for strategic management by the federal government, states, communities, and other public- and private-sector partners. The comprehensive set of objectives and targets are used to measure progress for health issues in specific populations and serves to meet the following objectives:

1. A foundation for disease prevention and wellness activities across various state and local sectors and within the federal government
2. A model for measurement at the state and local levels

What is new in Healthy People 2020? *Healthy People 2020 commits to the vision of a society in which all people live long, healthy lives* (www.healthypeople.gov/). New features aim to make this vision a reality:

1. Emphasizing ideas of health equity that address social determinants of health and promote health across all stages of life
2. Replacing the traditional print publication with an interactive website as the main vehicle for dissemination
3. Maintaining a website that allows users to tailor information to their needs and explore evidence-based resources for implementation

Healthy People 2020 is designed to achieve four primary goals:

1. Attain high-quality, longer lives free of preventable disease, disability, injury, and premature death
2. Achieve health equity, eliminate disparities, and improve the health of all groups
3. Create social and physical environments that promote good health for all
4. Promote quality of life, healthy development, and healthy behaviors across all life stages

The U.S. Department of Health and Human Services maintains a comprehensive, interactive online presence that includes the ability to search the extensive database of the U.S. government.

- *Healthy People 2020 Homepage*: http://www.healthypeople.gov/2020/default.aspx
- *Data 2020 Search*: http://www.healthypeople.gov/2020/data/searchData.aspx
- *Healthy People 2020 Topics and Objectives*: http://www.healthypeople.gov/2020/topicsobjectives2020/default.aspx

Safety of Exercising

Several well-publicized reports of sudden cardiac death during physical activity have raised the question of exercise safety.[111,187] Despite an overall increase in exercise participation, the death rate during exercise has declined over the past 30 years. In one report of cardiovascular episodes over a 65-mo period, 2935 exercisers recorded 374,798 hr of activity that included 2,726,272 km of running and walking. No deaths occurred during this time, with only two nonfatal cardiovascular complications. This amounted to two complications per 100,000 hr of physical activity for women and three complications for men. For individuals involved in marathon running, recent estimates place the occurrence of sudden cardiac arrest at approximately 1 in 57,000 runners, with the event most common among older runners and occurring over the last 4 miles of the race-course.[231]

Intense physical exertion raises a small risk of

An Overblown Risk for Marathoners

About 2 million people in the Unites States annually participate in long-distance running races. Several reports of deaths during marathons and half-marathons have raised questions about safety, with many considering these events to be "high-risk" activity. A research study published in 2012 quantified the actual risk of participants in all organized U.S. marathons over more than a 10-year period. Data analysis compiled from 10.9 million participants identified 59 cases of cardiac arrest (86% men), with a significantly higher incidence during marathons than half-marathons. Death occurred in 71% of the cases. This translated into only a small risk of 1 in 184,000 of cardiac arrest during or immediately after a race.

Source: Kim JH, et al. Cardiac arrest during long-distance running races. *N Engl J Med* 2012;366:130.

sudden death (e.g., one sudden death per 1.51 million episodes of exertion) during the activity compared with resting an equivalent time, particularly for sedentary persons, as shown in FIGURE 31.4. Nonetheless, the longer-term reduction in overall death risk from regular physical activity outweighs any small potential for acute cardiovascular complications.

Regular exercisers have considerably less risk of death during physical activity.[6] A 12-year follow-up of more than 21,000 male physicians showed that men who exercised at least five times a week had a much lower sudden death risk during vigorous exertion—about sevenfold less—than those who exercised only once weekly.[9] The likelihood of an exercise catastrophe—cerebrovascular accident, aortic dissection and rupture, lethal arrhythmias, myocardial infarction—increases under the following eight conditions:

1. Genetic predisposition (family history of sudden death at a relatively young age)
2. History of fainting or chest pain with physical activity
3. Unaccustomed vigorous activity
4. Exercise performed with accompanying psychologic stress

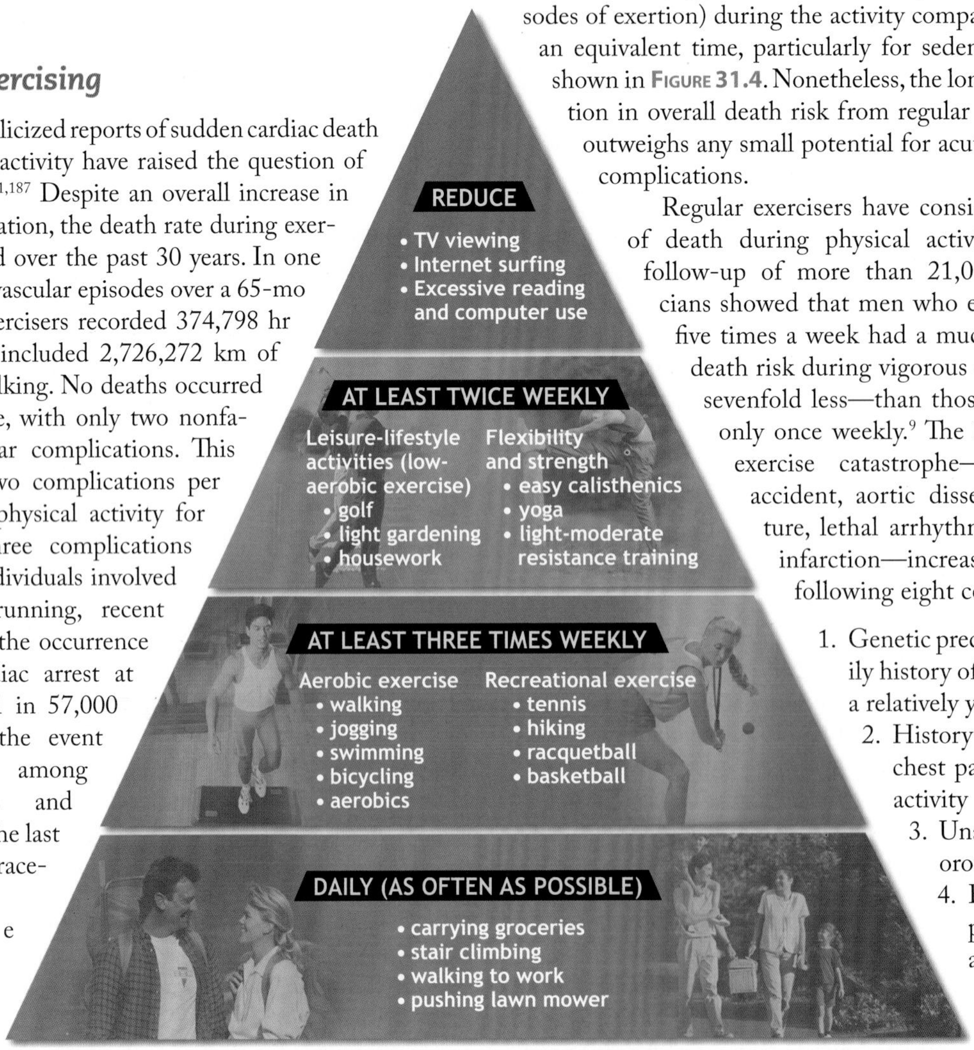

Physical Activity Pyramid

REDUCE
- TV viewing
- Internet surfing
- Excessive reading and computer use

AT LEAST TWICE WEEKLY

Leisure-lifestyle activities (low-aerobic exercise)
- golf
- light gardening
- housework

Flexibility and strength
- easy calisthenics
- yoga
- light-moderate resistance training

AT LEAST THREE TIMES WEEKLY

Aerobic exercise
- walking
- jogging
- swimming
- bicycling
- aerobics

Recreational exercise
- tennis
- hiking
- racquetball
- basketball

DAILY (AS OFTEN AS POSSIBLE)
- carrying groceries
- stair climbing
- walking to work
- pushing lawn mower

FIGURE 31.3 • The Physical Activity Pyramid: Prudent goals for increasing daily physical activity.

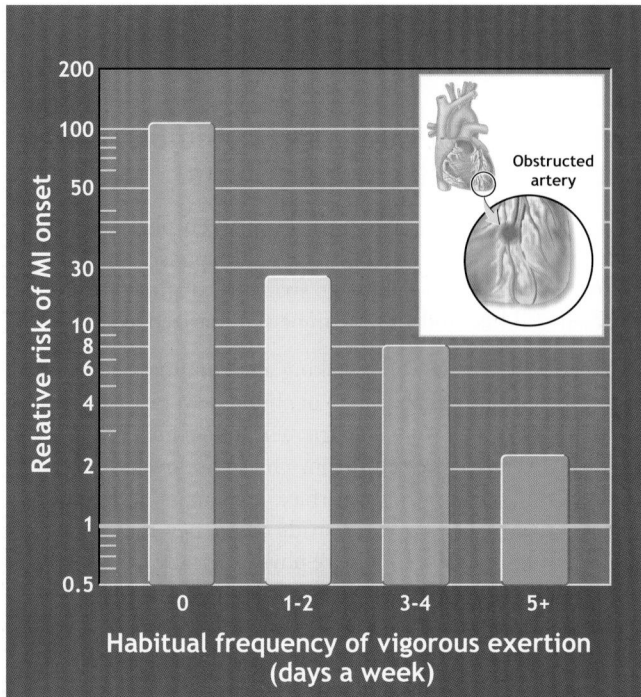

FIGURE 31.4 • Triggering acute cardiac events. Relative risk of myocardial infarction associated with vigorous exertion (≥6 METs) according to habitual frequency of vigorous physical activity. The horizontal solid line indicates risk of myocardial infarction with no exertion. (From Mittleman MA. Trigger of acute cardiac events: new insights. *Am J Med Sports* 2005;4:99.)

5. Extremes of environmental temperature
6. Straining-type activities that requires a considerable static muscle-action component (e.g., shoveling wet snow)
7. Exercise during viral infection or when feeling ill
8. Co-mingling of prescription drugs or dietary supplements (e.g., ephedra)

Musculoskeletal injuries represent the most prevalent exercise complications. A longitudinal study of aerobic dance injuries in 351 participants and 60 instructors during nearly 30,000 hr of activity reported 327 medical complaints.[66] Just 84 of the injuries caused disability (2.8 per 1000 person-hours of participation) and only 2.1% required medical attention. National estimates from self-reported frequency and severity of injuries in five common physical activities—walking, gardening, weightlifting, outdoor bicycling, and aerobics—report relatively low injury rates.[120,163] Most injuries required no treatment or reduction in physical activity. Age does not affect incidence of orthopedic problems for activities of moderate intensity and duration. For activities that involve running, the greatest orthopedic injury risk occurs in those who run for prolonged durations.[11]

Prospective epidemiologic research evaluated clinically significant medical incidents and emergencies for 7725 low-risk, apparently healthy corporate fitness enrollees in a supervised facility at a major medical center.[141] Almost 3 years of surveillance reported 15 medically significant events (0.048 per 1000 participant-hours) and two medical emergencies (both recovered), which equaled a rate of 0.0063 per 1000 participant-hours. Such a low rate of medical incidents in a supervised health-fitness facility illustrates convincingly that the health-related fitness benefits outweigh any small risk of participation.

Prehabilitation Reduces Sports and Recreational Injuries

For most individuals, participation in sports/athletic/recreational activities poses little risk, particularly in younger individuals. For individuals older than 40 years, and particularly those 60 years and older, a carefully planned and systematic **prehabilitation program** to ensure readiness for participation reduces exercise-induced disability further. Prehabilitation conditioning emphasizes joint stretching, muscle activation, core stability and strength, balance, and muscle coordination. Such an approach ensures maximum motor unit recruitment and joint stability.

Sedentary Environmental Death Syndrome

A review of the world literature over the last 50 years concludes that inactivity alone results in a constellation of problems and conditions eventually leading to premature death.

The term *sedentary environmental death syndrome* (SeDS), coined by Professor Frank Booth (see Interview in final Chapter), aptly identifies this deteriorating condition.[28] Research evidence reveals the following:

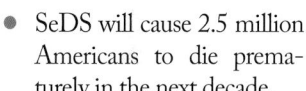

- SeDS will cause 2.5 million Americans to die prematurely in the next decade.
- SeDS will cost $2 to 3 trillion in healthcare expenses in the United States in the next decade.
- Chronic diseases have increased because of physical inactivity. In the United States, type 2 diabetes has increased ninefold since 1958, obesity has doubled since 1980, and heart disease remains the number one cause of death.
- U.S. children are now getting SeDS-related diseases—they are increasingly overweight, showing fatty streaks in their arteries, and developing type 2 diabetes (a disease formerly restricted to adults).
- SeDS relates to the following conditions: high blood triacylglycerol, high blood cholesterol, high blood glucose, type 2 diabetes, hypertension, myocardial ischemia, arrhythmias, congestive heart failure, obesity, breast cancer, depression, chronic back pain, spinal cord injury, stroke, disease cachexia, debilitating illnesses, fall resulting in broken hips, vertebral/femoral fractures.
- Efforts to lessen time watching television or videos or using a computer, if coupled with increases in physical

activity above daily routines, could substantially decrease the prevalence of metabolic syndrome. Individuals who do not engage in any moderate or vigorous physical activity during leisure time have about twice the odds of having metabolic syndrome as those who exercise up to 150 min a week or more.

Summary

1. Physical activity epidemiology evaluates the nature, extent, and demographics of exercise participation in a large population. Such data often reflect disease occurrence and other health-related outcomes.

2. A discouraging picture exists about physical activity participation by adult Americans. Only 10 to 15% of adults in the United States obtain enough regular physical activity of adequate intensity to impart health and fitness benefits.

3. Health benefits accrue from including a moderate amount of physical activity on most if not all days of the week.

4. Intense physical effort raises a small risk of sudden death during the activity compared with resting for an equivalent time, particularly for sedentary people. The longer-term health benefits of regular physical activity far outweigh the risk of acute cardiovascular complications.

5. The Healthy People 2020 initiative attempts to achieve four primary goals: first, attain high-quality, longer lives free of preventable disease, disability, injury, and premature death; second, achieve health equity, eliminate disparities, and improve the health of all groups; third, create social and physical environments that promote good health for all; and fourth, promote quality of life, healthy development, and healthy behaviors across all life stages.

6. For activities that involve running, the greatest orthopedic injury potential exists among individuals who run for extended durations.

7. Prehabilitation, particularly among older individuals, that utilizes core strengthening training can reduce injury potential in exercising.

8. Physical inactivity promotes unhealthy gene expression; increasing regular physical activity in the population must become a top public health priority.

PART 2 AGING AND PHYSIOLOGIC FUNCTION

AGE TRENDS

Physiologic and performance measures improve rapidly during childhood and achieve a maximum between late adolescence and approximately age 30. Functional capacity declines thereafter, with deterioration varying at any age depending on lifestyle and genetic characteristics.

Differences in Exercise Physiology Between Children and Adults

One must consider the interaction between physical activity and aging when evaluating physiologic responses and exercise performance across a broad age span. The distinct differences between children and adults can be summarized as follows:

- During weight-bearing walking and running, oxygen consumption ($mL \cdot kg^{-1} \cdot min^{-1}$) of children averages 10 to 30% higher than adults at a designated submaximal pace.[230] The lower exercise economy from children's lower ventilatory efficiency, greater body surface area–mass ratio, shorter stride length, and greater stride frequency makes a standard walking or running pace physiologically more stressful and performance scores poorer.

- Performance disadvantages exist even though children typically maintain equal or somewhat higher aerobic powers than adults. Also, walking and running economy and percentage $\dot{V}O_{2max}$ sustainable during activity at the lactate threshold continually improve as children age, independent of aerobic power changes. This limits the usefulness of a single walking or running performance test to predict $\dot{V}O_{2max}$ throughout childhood and adolescence.[45]

- Children exhibit lower absolute aerobic power values ($L \cdot min^{-1}$) than adults from a smaller fat-free body mass (FFM; see Fig. 11.11 in Chapter 11). Consequently, children are disadvantaged when exercising against a standard external resistance (unadjusted for body size) in stationary cycling and arm cranking. The fixed oxygen cost ($L \cdot min^{-1}$) of this activity represents a greater percentage of children's smaller absolute aerobic power. During weight-bearing activity, energy expenditure relates directly to body mass, so children are not disadvantaged by a smaller body size.

- Children score lower than adults on tests of anaerobic power because they cannot generate a high level of blood lactate during maximal effort. Lower intramuscular levels of the glycolytic enzyme phosphofructokinase may contribute to children's poorer anaerobic performance.

- Children breathe larger air volumes (greater ventilatory equivalent) than adults at any level of submaximal oxygen consumption.

- Adults score higher than children on perception of effort (rating of perceived exertion, or RPE) when both exercise at equivalent percentages of aerobic power. Greater pulmonary discomfort owing to the higher respiratory rate and ventilatory equivalent of children may produce this effect.[210]

- Children and adults increase muscle strength with resistance training. Prepubescent children, unlike pubescent children and adults, have limited ability to increase muscle mass, presumably because of their relatively low androgen levels.

INTEGRATIVE QUESTION

What factors would explain the relatively poor performances of children in a 10-km run compared with adults of equal aerobic power?

Muscular Strength

Age and gender affect muscular strength and muscular power, with the magnitude of each effect influenced by the muscle group studied and the type of muscle action. The following summarizes general trends in muscular strength and power of adults with increasing age:

- Men and women attain their highest strength levels between ages 20 and 40, the time when muscle cross-sectional area is largest. Thereafter, concentric strength of most muscle groups declines, slowly at first and then more rapidly after middle age.
- Accelerated strength loss in middle age coincides with weight loss and increase in chronic diseases such as stroke, diabetes, arthritis, and coronary heart disease.
- Muscles of older adults act with less force, have slower relaxation rates, and show a downward shift in their force–velocity relationship.[34]
- The capacity for power generation declines faster than that for maximal strength.[88]
- Declines in eccentric strength begin at a later age and progress more slowly than for concentric strength. Strength loss begins at a later age for women than for men.[123]
- Arm strength for men and women deteriorates more slowly than leg strength.[129]
- Rate of decline in muscular power with aging is similar among male and female weightlifters including world record holders, elite master athletes, and healthy, untrained individuals.[205]
- Strength loss among older adults directly relates to limited mobility and fitness status and potential for increased incidence of accidents from muscle weakness, fatigue, and poor balance.[96,204]

Age Trends Among Elite Weightlifters and Powerlifters

Master athletes more accurately reflect the effects of physiologic aging because such healthy, motivated athletes maintain a rigorous training schedule to compete at the highest level. **Figure 31.5** illustrates age trends for weightlifting and powerlifting records of the U.S. weightlifting and U.S. powerlifting organizations (www.usawa.com; www.usapowerlifting.com). These four findings indicate the following:

1. Peak lifting performance declines for men and women with aging. Weightlifting performance follows a curvilinear trend, while powerlifting performance declines linearly with age.

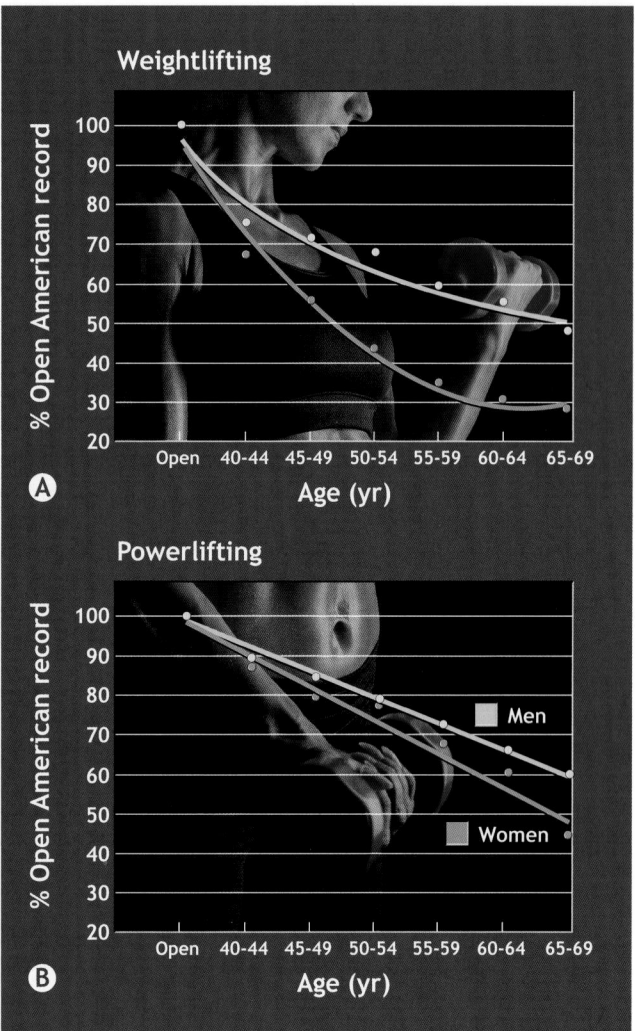

FIGURE 31.5 • Age-related sex differences in **(A)** weightlifting (average snatch and clean and jerk scores) and **(B)** powerlifting (average deadlift, squat, and bench press scores) based on analysis of top age-group records of the U.S. Weightlifting and U.S. Powerlifting Organizations. (From Anton MA, et al. Age-related declines in anaerobic muscular performance: weightlifting and powerlifting. *Med Sci Sports Exerc* 2004;36:143.)

2. The rate and overall magnitude of decline in performance with age are markedly greater in weightlifting than powerlifting.
3. The magnitude of decline in peak muscular power is greater in lifting tasks that require more complex and explosive power movements (weightlifting).
4. Sex differences in age-related performance decrements emerge only in events that require more complex and explosive power movements, with performance declining in women to a greater extent than in men.

The above list indicates a gender- and task-specific influence of age on muscular performance among elite resistance-trained athletes. More powerful and complex tasks undergo greater decline with age than tasks that require simpler movement patterns; women experience greater age-related declines in such tasks.

Muscle Mass Decrease

Motor unit remodeling represents a normal, continuous process that involves motor endplate repair and reconstruction. Remodeling progresses by selective denervation of muscle fibers, followed by terminal sprouting of axons from adjacent motor units. Motor unit remodeling gradually deteriorates in old age. This leads to **denervation muscle atrophy**, an irreversible degeneration of muscle fibers, particularly type II fibers; the condition associates with chronic inflammation and reduction in circulating growth hormone (GH), insulin-like growth factor-1 (IGF-1), muscle-specific isoforms of IGF, mitochondria number and capacity, cell nuclei, and endplate structures.[12,41,71,72]

Age-associated muscle wasting, termed *sarcopenia*, is magnified by reduced physical activity and progressively reduces muscle cross section, mass, and function, even after adjusting for changes in body mass and stature.[26,30,93] Muscle fibers tend to "*type group*" because fast- and slow-twitch fibers lose their typical chessboard distribution and cluster within groups of similar type—perhaps from denervation and subsequent fiber necrosis. Older adults have more than twice the noncontractile content in locomotor muscles as younger adults.[100] Impaired neural drive does not explain the decline in muscle strength with age because older adults achieve full muscle activation during a maximal voluntary muscle action.[48]

The primary cause of reduced strength between ages 25 and 80 relates to a 40 to 50% reduction in muscle mass from muscle fiber atrophy and loss of motor units, even among healthy, physically active adults. **FIGURE 31.6A** shows that muscle-fiber loss begins near ages 50 to 60. Reduction in total muscle area (Fig. 31.6B)

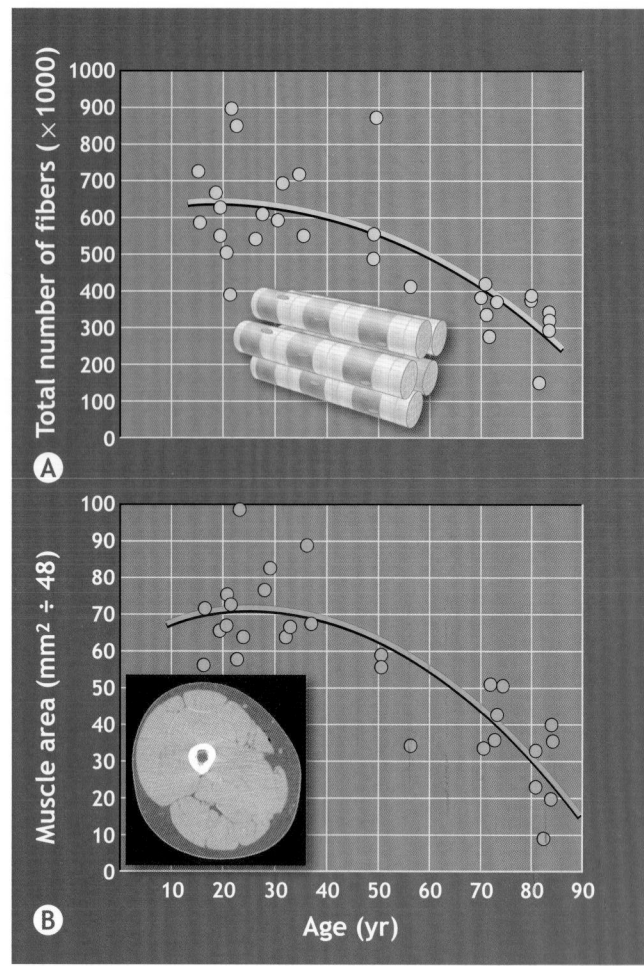

FIGURE 31.6 • Relationship between age and **(A)** total number of muscle fibers and **(B)** muscle cross-sectional area. Muscle size begins to decrease at approximately age 30, decreasing 10% by age 50. Thereafter, muscle area declines more precipitously, largely from decreased total number of muscle fibers. (From Lexell J, et al. What is the cause of the ageing atrophy? Total number, size, and proportion of different fiber types studied in whole vastus lateralis muscle from 15- to 83-year-old men. *J Neurol Sci* 1988;84:275; CT scan © LifeART Imaging Collection.)

 ### Potassium-Rich Foods May Blunt Muscle Loss with Aging

A mild but slowly increasing metabolic acidosis develops with aging, which may trigger a muscle-wasting response that contributes to the incidence of slips, falls, and fractures in this population. Consuming alkaline-producing plant foods high in potassium may neutralize this response.

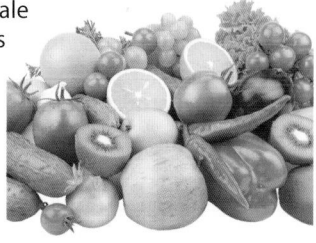

Researchers evaluated 384 male and female volunteers ages 65 or older to determine the association of 24-hr urinary potassium and an index of fruit and vegetable content of the diet and percentage of lean body mass at the start of the study and 3 years later.

Subjects whose diets were potassium rich averaged 3.6 lb of lean tissue mass more than those with only half that potassium intake. This conservation of lean tissue mass almost offsets the 4.4 lb of lean tissue typically lost in a decade in this age group.

Source: Dawson-Hughes B, et al. Alkaline diets favor lean tissue mass in older adults. *Am J Clin Nutr* 2008;87:662.

usually parallels reduced fiber size, particularly fast-twitch fibers in the lower extremities. This proportionately increases the area occupied by slow-twitch (type I) muscle fibers.

In a longitudinal study of age-related declines in muscular strength, nine men initially evaluated for muscular strength and muscle fiber composition 12 years earlier were remeasured.[65] Knee and elbow extensor and flexor strengths tested at slow and fast angular velocities decreased by 20 to 30%. Muscle cross-sectional area for the same muscle groups evaluated by CT scans decreased between 13 and 16%. Muscle biopsies from the vastus lateralis muscle showed a 42% reduction in type I fibers without changes in mean fiber type area. Capillary-to-fiber ratio decreased with aging by 0.31 units lower after 12 years. The researchers concluded that changes in muscle cross-sectional area largely contributed to the strength decline from ages 65 to 77.

Resistance Training for Older Adults

Moderate resistance training provides a remarkably safe way to stimulate protein synthesis and retention while slowing the "normal" and somewhat inevitable loss of muscle mass and strength with aging.[3,64,87,130] Muscle fiber size and mechanical performance, particularly rate of force development, were consistently elevated in older adults exposed to lifelong resistance training.[1] Older men who resistance-train demonstrate greater absolute gains in muscle size and strength than women, but the percentage improvement is similar between genders, yet gains are somewhat less than those of younger counterparts.[106,213]

Healthy men between ages 60 and 72 years who trained for 12 wk with standard-resistance exercise at loads equivalent to 80% of 1-RM demonstrate how well older adults respond to resistance training. Figure 31.7 shows that muscle strength increased progressively throughout training. At week 12, knee-extension strength increased by 107% and knee-flexion strength by 227%. Improvement rate of 5% per training session matched similar increases reported for young adults. Fast- and slow-twitch muscle fiber hypertrophy accompanied dramatic strength improvements. In other research, muscle cross-sectional area and strength in 70-year-olds who had resistance-trained since age 50 equaled values for a group of 28-year-old university students.[103] *Older individuals possess impressive plasticity in physiologic, structural, and performance characteristics despite the fact that the capacity to respond to muscle growth cues—mechanical load, nutrition, neural activity, hormones, and growth factors—declines with age.*[170]

Muscle responds to vigorous training with rapid improvement into the ninth decade of life (Figure 31.8). Improved muscle strength, bone density, dynamic balance, and overall functional status with regular physical activity can minimize or reverse the syndrome of physical frailty. For men and women ages 70 to 89, a regular program of aerobic, strength, flexibility, and balance training prevented both loss of muscle strength and increase in muscle fat infiltration associated with advancing age.[67] Regular strengthening and balance movements provide the most effective way to reduce orthopedic injury from high prevalence of falls in older men and women.[167]

Even for older persons disabled with knee osteoarthritis, regular aerobic or resistance exercises induce beneficial effects on measures of disability, pain, and physical performance.[55] For disabled older female cardiac patients, a 6-mo program of resistance training improved muscular strength and physical capacity in a wide range of household physical activities and also improved endurance, balance, coordination, and flexibility.[7] This relative preservation in muscle structure and function may provide an important physical reserve capacity to retain muscle mass and function above the critical threshold for independent living at old age.

Mechanisms that explain how middle-age and older adults respond to resistance training include enhanced motor unit recruitment and innervation patterns and muscular hypertrophy (see Chapter 22). The magnitude of strength adaptations depends on the number of sets and repetitions and intensity, duration, and frequency of training, just as it does in younger counterparts.

Neural Function

A nearly 40% decline in the number of spinal cord axons and a 10% decline in nerve conduction velocity reflect the cumulative effects of aging on central nervous system function. These changes likely contribute to the age-related decrement in neuromuscular performance assessed by simple and complex reaction and movement times. Partitioning reaction time into central processing time and muscle action time, aging most

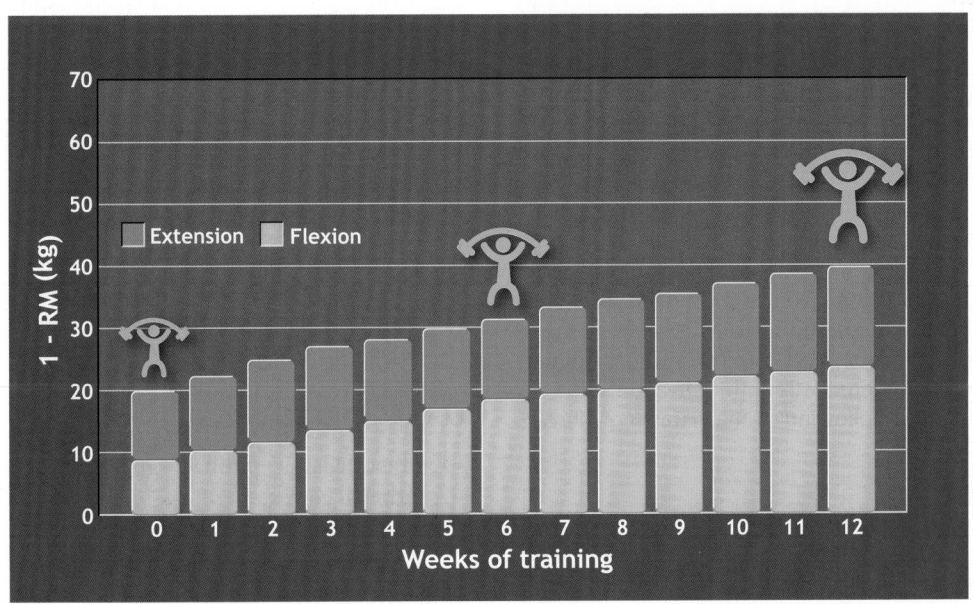

FIGURE 31.7 • Weekly measurements of dynamic muscle strength (1-RM) in left knee extension (*green*) and flexion (*orange*) during resistance training in older men. (From Frontera WR, et al. Strength conditioning in older men: skeletal muscle hypertrophy and improved function. *J Appl Physiol* 1988;64:1038.)

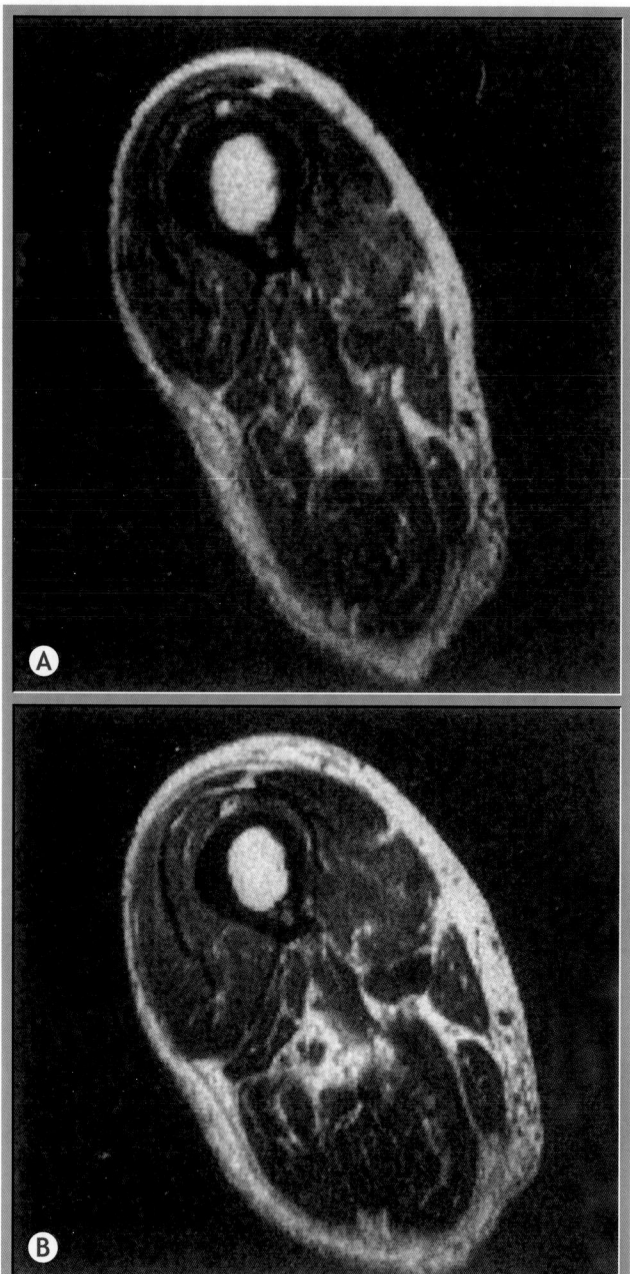

FIGURE 31.8 • Plasticity in physiologic response to resistance training among older adults. Magnetic resonance images taken at the mid-thigh region of a male subject 92 years of age before **(A)** and after **(B)** 112 wk of resistance training of the knee extensor and flexor muscles. Quadriceps lean cross-sectional area increased by 44% in this individual. (From Harridge SD, et al. Knee extensor strength, activation, and size in very elderly people following strength training. *Muscle Nerve* 1999;22:831.)

adversely affects the time to detect a stimulus and process the information to produce the response. Knee-jerk reflexes do not involve neural processing in the brain, so aging affects them less than voluntary responses that involve reaction and movement. Physical inactivity may also be responsible for a large portion of the loss of neuromuscular function seen in

older adults. Highly active versus low-active older women achieve greater peak torque, faster rate of torque development, shorter motor time, faster rate of EMG rise, and greater onset of EMG magnitude.[114] **Figure 31.9** shows slower movement times for simple and complex tasks by older subjects than by younger subjects with similar physical activity levels. In all instances, the young or old active groups moved considerably faster than the less-active age group. *A physically active lifestyle and specific training (combined aerobic, balance, coordination, and strength) affects neuromuscular functions positively at any age to slow the age-related decline in cognitive performance associated with speed of information processing.*[220]

Physically active older adults who have relatively high cardiorespiratory fitness are less likely to experience cognitive decline and dementia with a lower risk of mortality from dementia.[47,124] Biologic mechanisms for such protection include reduced vascular risk, body fat, and levels of inflammatory markers and enhanced neuronal health and function (**Fig. 31.10**). Regular physical activity also increases mitochondrial biogenesis in the brain, which may have important implications for age-related dementia (often characterized by mitochondrial dysfunction).[197] Exercise interventions associate with short-term improvements in cognitive function in sedentary elders.[17,21,37] Older individuals who remain physically active for 20 years or longer show reaction speeds that equal or exceed inactive younger adults. These findings support the value of regular physical activity for slowing biologic aging of select neuromuscular functions. The potential magnitude of these changes and amount of physical activity required to induce meaningful responses remain controversial.[186]

Endocrine Changes

Endocrine function changes with age. Approximately 40% of individuals ages 65 and 75 years and 50% of those older than age 80 have impaired glucose tolerance that leads to type 2 diabetes (see Chapter 20). Increased disease prevalence among older adults largely relates to the controllable factors of poor diet quality, inadequate physical activity, and increased body fat, particularly in the visceral–abdominal region.[4]

Advancing age lowers pituitary gland release of the thyroid-stimulating hormone thyrotropin, including reduced thyroxine output. Thyroid dysfunction directly impacts metabolic function, with resultant decreases in metabolic rate, glucose metabolism, and protein synthesis.

Figure 31.11 depicts changes in three hormonal systems associated with aging:

1. Hypothalamic–pituitary–gonadal axis
2. Adrenal cortex
3. GH/IGF axis

Hypothalamic–Pituitary–Gonadal Axis

In females, alteration in the interaction between stimulating hormones from the hypothalamus and anterior pituitary gland

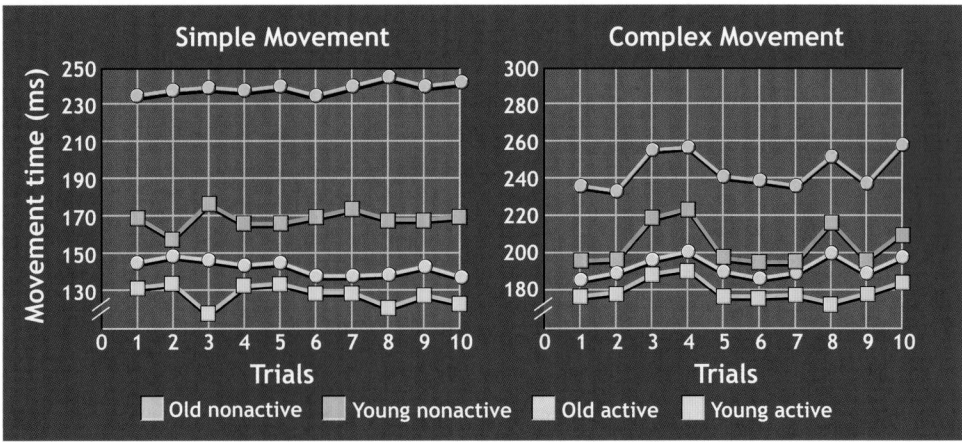

FIGURE 31.9 • Simple and complex movement time in subjects classified as young active, old active, young nonactive, and old nonactive. Note the slower movement times (higher scores) in simple and complex tasks by the old and young nonactive subjects than by their active counterparts. (From Spirduso WW. Reaction and movement time as a function of age and physical activity level. *J Gerontol* 1975;30:435.)

and gonads decreases ovarian estradiol output. This effect probably initiates permanent cessation of menses (**meno-pause**). Changes in hypothalamic–pituitary–gonadal axis activity in males occur more slowly than in females. Serum total and free testosterone, for example, gradually decline with aging in males. Decreased gonadotropic secretions from the anterior pituitary gland characterize male **andropause**.

Adrenal Cortex

Adrenopause refers to reduced adrenal cortex output of dehydroepiandrosterone (DHEA) and its sulfated ester DHEAS. DHEA exhibits a long, progressive decline after age 30, in contrast to glucocorticoid and mineralocorticoid adrenal steroids whose plasma levels remain relatively high with aging.

By age 75, DHEA plasma levels achieve only 20 to 30% of the value in young adults. This has evoked speculation that plasma DHEA levels might serve as a biochemical marker of biologic aging and disease susceptibility. Animal research suggests that exogenous DHEA protects against cancer, atherosclerosis, viral infections, obesity, and diabetes; enhances immune function; and even extends life. Despite its quantitative significance as a hormone in humans, researchers know little about DHEA's role in the following four areas of concern:

1. Health and aging
2. Cellular or molecular mechanism(s) of action
3. Possible receptor sites
4. Potential for adverse effects from supplemental use among young adults with normal DHEA levels

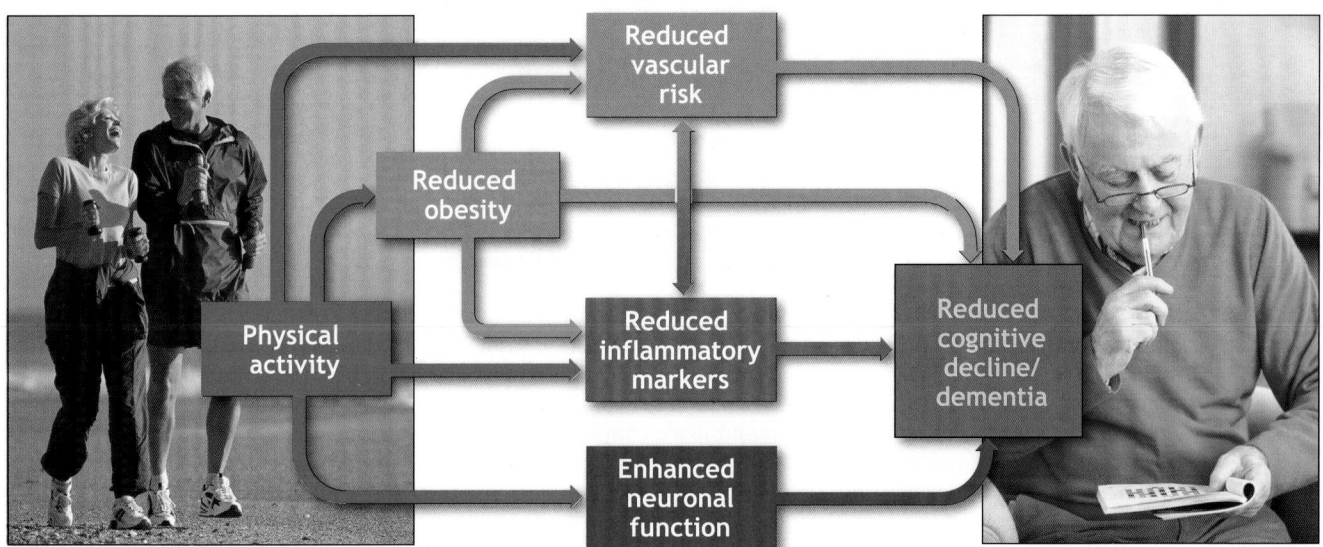

FIGURE 31.10 • Potential mechanisms that may underlie the association between physical activity and reduced risk of cognitive decline and dementia in older adults.

Chapter 23 discusses the case for ergogenic effects of DHEA supplements (and potential risks) on adult men and women.

Growth Hormone/Insulin-Like Growth Factor Axis

Mean pulse amplitude, duration, and fraction of secreted GH gradually decrease with aging, a condition termed *somatopause*. A parallel decrease also occurs in circulating levels of IGF-1, which stimulates tissue growth and protein synthesis. The interaction between the hypothalamus and anterior pituitary gland probably triggers the age-related GH decrease.

The extent to which changes in gonadal function (menopause and andropause) contribute to adrenopause and somatopause (present in both sexes) remains uncertain. Evidence indicates that muscle size and strength, body composition and bone mass alterations, and progression of atherosclerosis relate directly to hormonal changes with aging. Hormone replacement therapy, nutritional supplementation, and regular physical activity can delay or even prevent aspects of immune function deterioration and hormone-related aging dysfunction.[158]

Pulmonary Function

Mechanical constraints on the pulmonary system progress with age to cause deterioration in static and dynamic lung function. Pulmonary ventilation and gas exchange kinetics during the transition from rest to submaximal exercise also slow substantially.[44] In older men, aerobic training increases gas exchange kinetics to levels that approach values for fit young adults.[16] Likewise, older endurance-trained athletes demonstrate greater pulmonary functional capacity than their sedentary peers. Values for vital capacity, total lung capacity, residual lung volume, maximum voluntary ventilation, $FEV_{1.0}$, and $FEV_{1.0}/FVC$ in athletes above age 60 remain higher than predicted from body size and higher than values for sedentary, healthy individuals.[68] Such findings indicate that regular physical activity retards pulmonary function decline with aging.

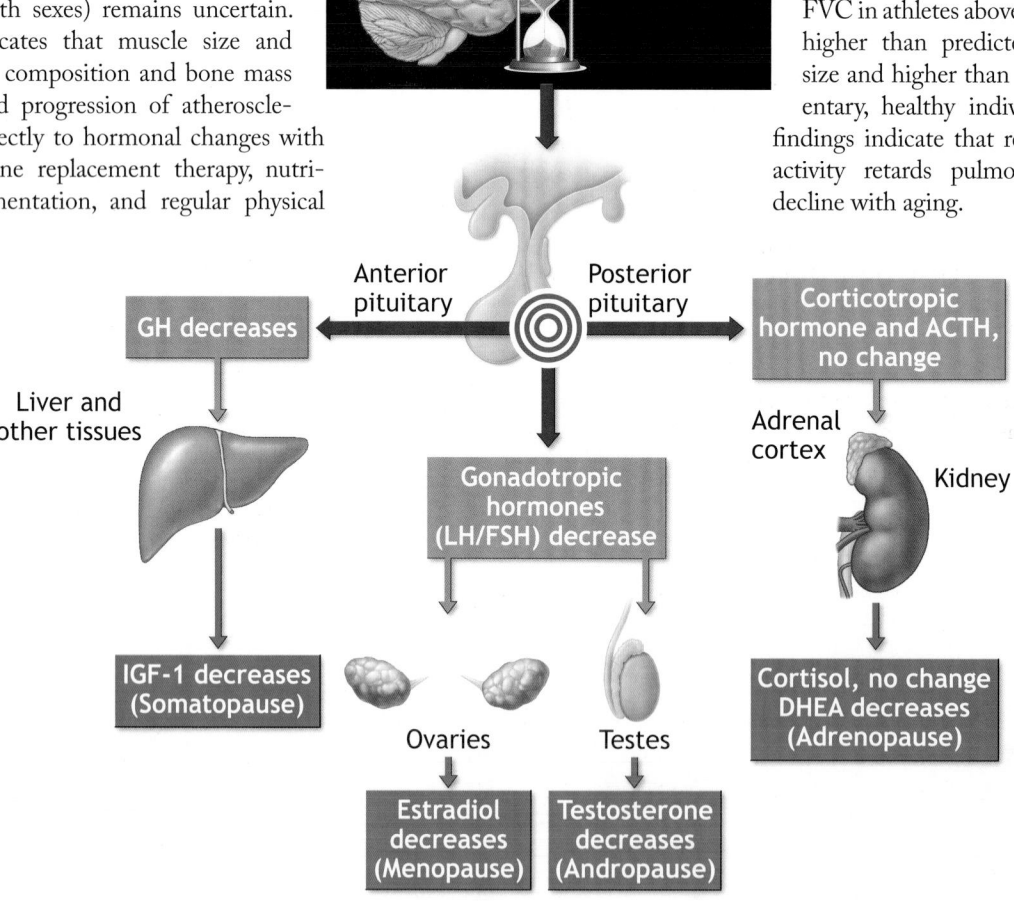

FIGURE 31.11 • Age-related decline in three hormone systems that affect the rate of biologic aging. **(Left)** Decreased growth hormone (GH) release by the anterior pituitary depresses production of IGF-1 by the liver and other tissues, which inhibits cellular growth (a condition of aging termed *somatopause*). **(Center)** Decreased output of gonadotropic luteinizing hormone (LH) and follicle-stimulating hormone (FSH) by the anterior pituitary, coupled with reduced estradiol secretion from the ovaries and testosterone from the testes, causes menopause (females) and andropause (males). **(Right)** Adrenocortical cells responsible for DHEA production decrease their activity (termed *adrenopause*) without clinically evident changes in this gland's corticotropin (ACTH) and cortisol secretion. A central pacemaker in the hypothalamus and/or higher brain areas mediates these processes to produce aging-related changes in peripheral organs (ovaries, testicles, and adrenal cortex). (Brain, liver, and ovary images used with permission from Moore KL, Dalley AF, Agur AMR. *Clinically Oriented Anatomy.* 7th Ed. Baltimore: Wolters Kluwer Health, 2013.)

Cardiovascular Function

Cardiovascular function and aerobic power do not escape age-related decrements.

Aerobic Power

The precise effect of regular aerobic training on the age-related decline in aerobic power remains unresolved. Cross-sectional data reveal that $\dot{V}O_{2max}$ declines between 0.4 and 0.5 mL·kg^{-1} each year (approximately 1% per year) in adult men and women, although the rate of decline accelerates somewhat in advancing age, particularly for men.[62,90,234] Extrapolating this average rate of decline reduces aerobic power by age 100 to a level that equals the resting oxygen consumption. This represents a somewhat severe and unrealistic estimate because differences exist in the age-related rate of decline in $\dot{V}O_{2max}$ in sedentary and active individuals.[175] The decline in $\dot{V}O_{2max}$ with advancing age occurs nearly twice as fast in sedentary compared to physically active men and women. Studies of men who varied considerably in age, aerobic power, body composition, and lifestyle revealed that maintaining relatively stable physical activity and body composition levels over time produced an average yearly decline in $\dot{V}O_{2max}$ of 0.25 mL·kg^{-1}·min^{-1}. No decline in aerobic power occurred in individuals who maintained constant training during a 10-year period.[99,160]

For most individuals, regular aerobic exercise cannot fully prevent the age-related decline in aerobic power with aging.[60,201,214] For example, the aerobic power of 50-year-old endurance athletes decreased between 8 and 15% per decade despite continued exercise over a 20-year period.[161] *Even with this decline, research consistently shows that physically active older men and women maintain a 10 to 50% higher aerobic power than sedentary counterparts.*

Factors other than physical activity level influence the age-related decline in $\dot{V}O_{2max}$. Heredity undoubtedly plays a crucial role, as does increased body fat and decreased skeletal muscle mass.[175] In the later decades of life, declines in maximal cardiac output and a-$\bar{v}O_2$ difference contribute equally to the age-related decrease in $\dot{V}O_{2max}$.[232] Aging also relates to a decline in a muscle's oxidative function from reduced synthesis of mitochondrial and other proteins.[185] An analysis of aerobic power of young and older endurance-trained men and women (**Fig. 31.12**) indicates an average 0.5 L·min^{-1} lower $\dot{V}O_{2max}$ per kilogram of limb (appendicular) muscle mass for older athletes, independent of age-associated decreases in muscle and increases in fat. No clear answer exists as to how much the lower aerobic power per kilogram of limb muscle mass in the older subjects reflects reduced oxygen extraction by active muscles and/or reduced oxygen delivery via decreased cardiac output and/or active muscle blood flow. Leg blood flow and vascular conductance during cycle ergometer exercise averaged 20 to 30% lower in older endurance-trained men than in younger peers at similar submaximal oxygen consumptions.[164] Consequently, older athletes achieve an equivalent submaximal oxygen consumption at reduced leg blood flows by increased local oxygen extraction (a-$\bar{v}O_2$ difference) from the available blood supply. For a group of older untrained women, a diminished leg

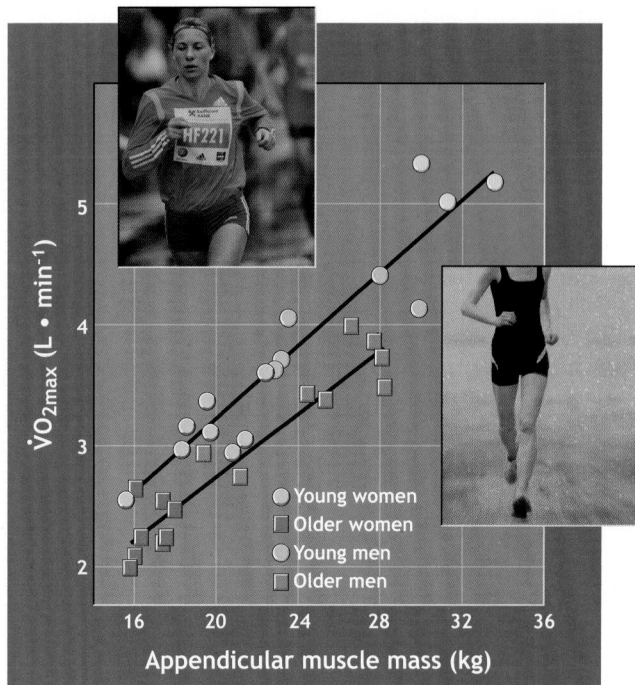

FIGURE 31.12 • Individual maximal oxygen consumption values ($\dot{V}O_{2max}$) related to appendicular muscle mass in young (*top line*) and older (*bottom line*) endurance-trained women and men. For an equivalent appendicular muscle mass, $\dot{V}O_{2max}$ averaged 0.5 L·min^{-1} less for older subjects. These data suggest that aerobic power per kilogram of appendicular muscle mass decreases with age in highly trained men and women. (From Procter DN, Joyner MJ. Skeletal muscle mass and the reduction of $\dot{V}O_{2max}$ in trained older subjects. *J Appl Physiol* 1997;82:1411.)

blood flow during peak exercise contributed considerably to their lower $\dot{V}O_{2peak}$ than untrained younger counterparts. The diminished leg blood flow occurred from both central (cardiac output) and peripheral (reduced vascular conductance) limitations.[165]

Central and Peripheral Cardiovascular Functions

Decrements in central and peripheral functions linked to oxygen transport and use influence the age-related decline in aerobic power.

Heart Rate. *A decline in maximum exercise heart rate represents a well-documented change with age.* This age effect reflects reduced medullary outflow of sympathetic activity (depressed β-adrenergic stimulation) that occurs similarly in men and women. Several longitudinal studies of elite athletes reveal that decreases in maximum heart rate from ages 50 to 70 years are smaller than typically predicted and indicative of a training response.[161,203]

Cardiac Output. *Maximum cardiac output decreases with age in trained and untrained men and women because of a lower maximum heart rate and stroke volume.* The stroke volume decline reflects the combined effects of reduced left-ventricular systolic and diastolic myocardial performance. Healthy older adults often compensate for a diminished maximum heart rate with increased cardiac filling (end-diastolic volume preload), which subsequently increases stroke volume by the Frank-Starling mechanism.[61,234]

Large Artery Compliance. *Compliance of large arteries in the cardiothoracic circulation declines with age due to changes in the arterial wall's structural and nonstructural properties.*[157,181] The inability of the internal diameter of an artery to expand and recoil in response to fluctuations in intravascular pressure during the cardiac cycle associates with impaired cardiovascular function and elevated heart disease risk factors—hypertension, stroke, atherosclerosis, thrombosis, myocardial infarction, and congestive heart failure. Regular endurance activities slow or prevent the "stiffening" of the large arteries with advancing age and slow the decline in limb vasodilator capacity with healthy aging.[166,198,202]

Peripheral Factors. *Reduced peripheral blood flow capacity accompanies age-related decreases in muscle mass.* Decreased capillary-to-muscle fiber ratio and reduced arterial cross-sectional area produced lower blood flow to active muscle.[192]

Physiologic Loss with Aging: Lifestyle or Chronologic Age?

Sedentary living and unhealthy behaviors produce losses in functional capacity at least as great as the effects of aging. A high degree of trainability exists among older men and women and may not only slow but even reverse the decline in functional capacity with aging.[183] Positive training-induced adaptations in skeletal muscle structure and function, substrate metabolism, and cardiovascular function often equal those for younger individuals. Both low- and higher-intensity physical activity enable older individuals to retain cardiovascular functions at a higher level than age-paired sedentary subjects. Active middle-aged men who endurance-trained over a 10-year period forestalled the usual 9 to 15% decline in aerobic power.[98] At age 55, the men maintained the same values for blood pressure, body mass, and $\dot{V}O_{2max}$ as 10 years earlier.

Endurance Performance

Comparing endurance performance of athletes of different ages provides further evidence for the impressive effects of regular exercise on preservation of cardiovascular function throughout life. Age-group, world-record times for 50-, 100-, and 200-km runs for men and women are always recorded by the youngest athletes. For longer runs, however, older runners often excel. For example, data for the 70- to 74-year-old group marathon record is 2:59:10 (6:40 per mile pace), set in 2003 by 73-year-old Canadian marathon and international track and field superstar athlete Ed Whitlock. This was the first time anyone above age 70 ran a sub-3-hr marathon (http://www.runnersworld.com/runners-stories/ed-whitlock-runs-330-marathon-age-81).

This time would have placed him 608th in the 2008 New York City Marathon, or in the top 1.6% of the 38,111 finishers; 994 runners bettered 3 hr in that marathon. In February 2013, at age 81, Whitlock, smashed the age-group world record at the Toronto Marathon with a time of 3:30:28.4. This was nearly 15 min faster than the previous world record for that age, and roughly 45 min faster than that day's average marathon finisher—regardless of age. He also crushed the world record in the half-marathon, despite coming back from serious injuries. He now holds just about every record in the 70-plus age group, including records in the mile, half-marathon, and marathon distances. Whitlock spoke about his accomplishments at a conference on exercise, lifestyle, and aging well at Concordia University in May, 2013 (http://performcentre.concordia.ca/en/about-perform/videos/). That individuals in their eighth and ninth decades of life successfully run for 12 to 14 hr affirms the tremendous cardiovascular potential of older men and women who continue vigorous training as they age.

Oldest Marathoner

In 2011 Fauja Singh became the oldest and fastest 100-year-old marathoner, completing the Toronto Waterfront Marathon in 8:25:15. The run marked the eighth marathon for Singh; in 2003 in the same marathon, he set a world record in the 90-plus category of 5:40:1.

Sprint Performance

FIGURE 31.13 illustrates the relationship between age and 100-m sprint performance in male and female master sprinters ages

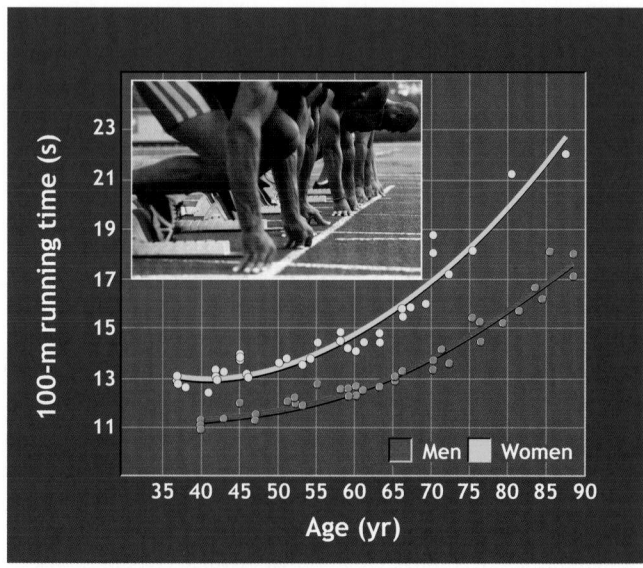

FIGURE 31.13 • Individual values of 100-m running time as a function of age in male and female sprinters. (From Korhonen MT, et al. Age-related differences in 100-m sprint performance in male and female master runners. *Med Sci Sports Exerc* 2003;35:1419.)

35 to 88 years. Performance declined in both groups of athletes with age, the decreases becoming more evident after age 60. Remarkable similarities exist for age-related decrements in running velocity between sexes. Running velocity during the different phases of the run declined from 5 to 6% per decade in men and 5 to 7% per decade in women. Reduced stride length and increase in contact time of the foot with the ground primarily accounted for the overall performance deterioration with age.

Body Composition

Cross-sectional studies indicate that after age 18, men and women progressively gain body weight and fat until the fifth or sixth decade of life, at which time total body mass decreases despite increasing body fat. This results partly from a disproportionately greater death rate among the obese in the upper age group, leaving fewer of these individuals to measure.

Most age-trend studies do not track the same subjects over time; instead, they evaluate different subjects in different age categories at the same time. From such **cross-sectional data**, one attempts to generalize about an individual's expected age-related changes, but sometimes this creates misleading generalizations. For example, today's 70- and 80-year-olds typically are shorter than 20-year-old college students. This observation does not necessarily mean that individuals become shorter with age (although this does happen to some extent). Instead, the young adults of the current generation receive better nourishment than 80-year-olds received at age 20.

The limited **longitudinal data** collected on the same subjects over time show trends in body fat changes similar to data from cross-sectional studies. It is not known whether body fat increases during adulthood represent a normal biologic pattern or simply reflect sedentary lifestyle choices.

Longitudinal observations of individuals who maintain a physically active lifestyle support a biologic tendency to gain fat with age. FIGURE 31.14 shows body composition changes for 21 endurance athletes who continued to train over a 20-year period starting at age 50. Despite maintaining a relatively constant body mass during the prolonged period of training, gains occurred in body fat and abdominal obesity while FFM declined. The roughly 3% body fat unit increase per decade paralleled increases in waist girth. The magnitude of increase in body fat and decrease in FFM, while discouraging to some, averages at least 20% less than reported for nonathletes. Habitual endurance exercise confers at least some "protection" from the effects of aging on body composition.

Bone Mass

Osteoporosis poses a major problem with aging, particularly among postmenopausal women. This condition produces loss of bone mass as the aging skeleton demineralizes and becomes porous. Bone mass can decrease by 30 to 50% in persons above age 60. As emphasized in Chapter 2, regimens of

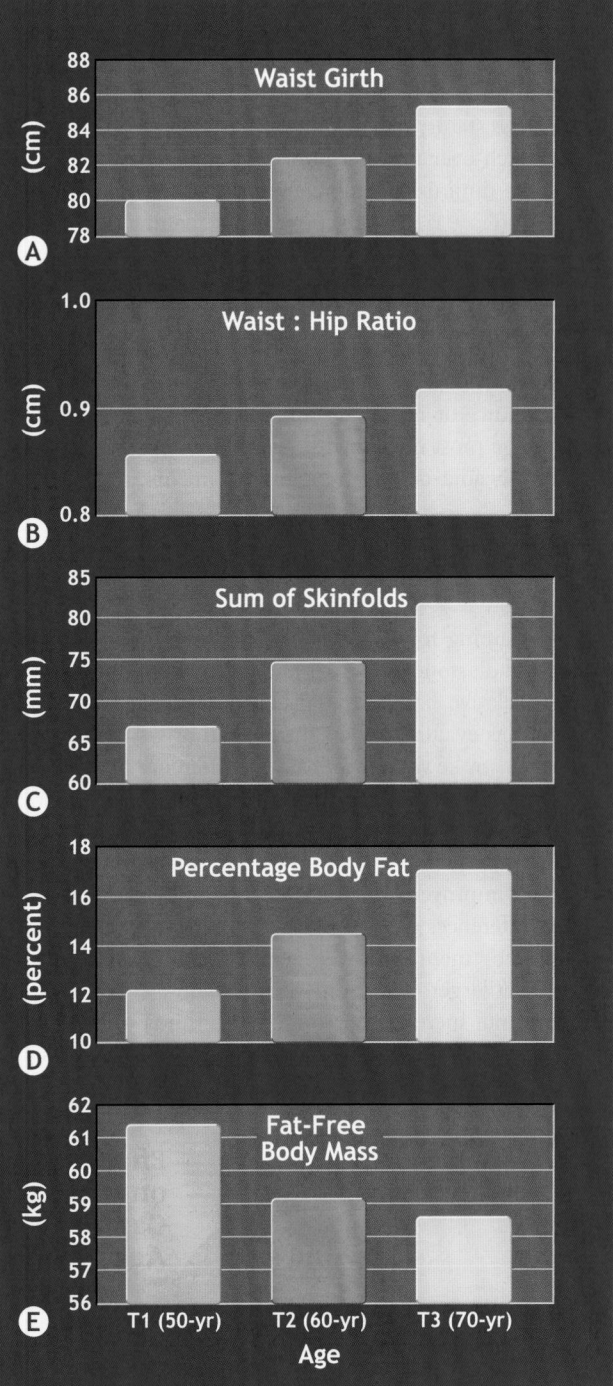

FIGURE 31.14 • Changes in **(A)** waist girth, **(B)** waist–hip girth ratio, **(C)** sum of skinfolds, **(D)** percentage body fat, and **(E)** FFM for 21 endurance athletes who continued to train over a 20-year period, starting at age 50. (From Pollock ML, et al. Twenty-year follow-up of aerobic power and body composition of older track athletes. *J Appl Physiol* 1997;82:1508.)

weight-bearing activity and resistance exercise not only retard bone loss but also often increase bone mass in older men and women.[5] In postmenopausal women, regular physical activity augments hormone replacement therapy to increase total bone mineral density and preserve these gains.[69,105]

TRAINABILITY AND AGE

Exercise training improves physiologic responses at any age. Several factors affect the magnitude of the training response, including initial fitness status, genetics, and specific type of training.

Research over the past 50 years has modified the classic view of the diminished improvements from physical activity with aging (**FIG. 31.15**). The current view maintains that over a broad age range, improvements in physiologic function result from an appropriate training stimulus, often at a rate and magnitude independent of age. Older men and women and younger adults show similar adaptations of muscle fiber size, capillarization, and glycolytic and respiratory enzymes to specific endurance or resistance-training exercise. These adaptations emerge most readily with relatively intense exercise that continuously adjusts to training improvements.

Aerobic Trainability Among Older Adults: Perhaps a Gender Difference

Exercise training for healthy older men enhances the heart's systolic and diastolic properties and increases aerobic power to the same relative extent (15–30%) as in younger adults.[31,53,180] Research has evaluated the contribution of training-induced increases in stroke volume and a-$\bar{v}O_2$ difference to aerobic fitness improvements in healthy older men and women. Nine to 12 mo of endurance training increased $\dot{V}O_{2max}$ by 19% in men and 22% in women (**TABLE 31.1**). These values represent the high end of improvement typically observed for younger adults. Gender differences emerged in certain aspects of the training response. For men, improved aerobic power was associated with a 15% larger maximum stroke volume (corresponding cardiac output increase represented two thirds of the $\dot{V}O_{2max}$ increase) and 7% greater maximum a-$\bar{v}O_2$ difference (representing one third of the $\dot{V}O_{2max}$ increase).

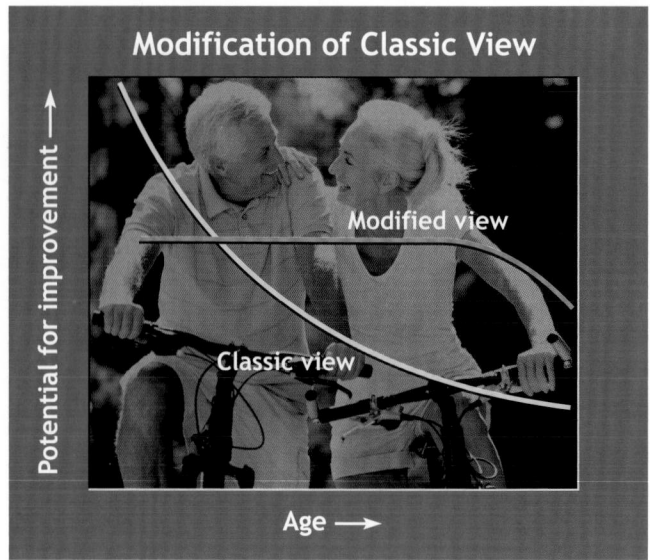

FIGURE 31.15 • New view of old beliefs. Traditional (classic) versus the more current view of the expected improvements from physical training with aging.

For the women, the a-$\bar{v}O_2$ difference explained the total $\dot{V}O_{2max}$ increase, with no change in left-ventricular performance at maximal exercise. This indicates that training-induced increases in aerobic power for older women depend on peripheral adaptations in trained muscle and suggests that sex hormones influence gender-related adaptations to endurance training.[102] The lack of a stroke volume increase among older women with training may result from three factors:[192–194]

1. Blunting of the normal increase in plasma volume
2. Depression of cardiopulmonary baroreflex sensitivity
3. Estrogen deficiency–related decrease in vascular compliance (i.e., increased vascular stiffness)

TABLE 31.1	**Effects of 9 Months of Endurance Training on Maximal Oxygen Consumption and Cardiovascular Function in 15 Men Age 63 ± 3 yr, and 16 Women Age 64 ± 3 yr**				
	$\dot{V}O_{2max}$ L·Min^{-1}	$\dot{Q}_{max}$ L·Min^{-1}	HR$_{max}$ B·Min^{-1}	SV$_{max}$ mL	a-$\bar{v}O_{2diff}$ mL·dL^{-1}
Men					
Before	2.35	17	170	101	13.8
After	2.8[a]	19[a]	164[a]	116[a]	14.8[a]
Women					
Before	1.36	11.2	161	70	12.2
After	1.66[a]	11.5	164	70	14.4[a]

Values are means; $\dot{V}O_{2max}$, maximal O_2 consumption; $\dot{Q}_{max}$, maximal cardiac output; HR$_{max}$, maximal heart rate; SV$_{max}$, stroke volume at maximal exercise; a-$\bar{v}O_{2diff}$, arteriovenous O_2 content difference at maximal exercise.
[a]p ± 0.01 vs. before training.
Reprinted from Spina RJ, et al. Differences in cardiovascular adaptations to endurance-exercise training between older men and women. *J Appl Physiol* 1993;75:849.

These apparent gender differences in physiology do not impair endurance performance in older women, as reflected by male–female similarities in ultradistance running performance.

Summary

1. Physiologic and performance capabilities usually decline after age 30. Many factors, including diminished physical activity level, affect the rate of decline.
2. Regular physical activity and training enable older persons to retain higher levels of functional capacity, notably cardiovascular and muscular function.
3. Biologic aging relates to changes in three hormonal systems: hypothalamic–pituitary–gonadal axis, adrenal cortex, and growth hormone–insulin-like growth factor axis.
4. Four factors are important when evaluating physiologic and performance differences between children and adults: exercise economy, FFM, anaerobic power, and anabolic hormone levels.
5. The primary cause of age-associated reduction in muscle strength between ages 25 and 80 is a 40 to 50% reduction in muscle mass from a loss of motor units and muscle fiber atrophy.
6. Considerable plasticity exists in physiologic, structural, and performance characteristics among older individuals; this plasticity enables marked and rapid strength improvement with training into the ninth decade of life.
7. A physically active lifestyle affects neuromuscular functions positively at any age and possibly slows the age-related decline in cognitive performance associated with speed of information processing.
8. VO_{2max} declines approximately 1% each year in adult men and women.
9. Physically active older men and women maintain a higher aerobic power than their sedentary peers at any age.
10. Sedentary living causes losses in functional capacity at least as great as aging itself.
11. Regular exercise improves physiologic function at any age; initial fitness, genetics, and type and amount of training control the magnitude of change.
10. Active older athletes average at least 20% less body fat and 20% more FFM than their nonathletic peers; this suggests that habitual physical activity confers some protection from the negative effects of aging on body composition.

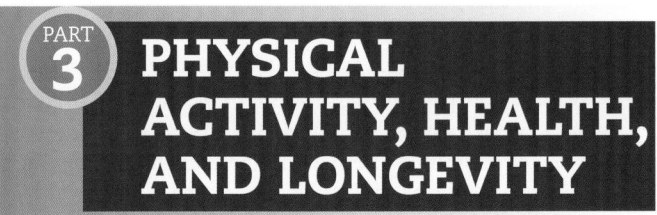

PHYSICAL ACTIVITY, HEALTH, AND LONGEVITY

Physical activity may not necessarily represent a "fountain of youth," yet the preponderance of evidence shows that regular

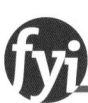

The Federal Government Takes a Stand

In 2012, many federal government agencies joined together to craft an update of the *Physical Activity Guidelines for Americans*. The major findings identified "strategies to increase physical activity among youth" and can be read online at **www.health.gov/paguidelines/midcourse/pag-mid-course-report-final.pdf**.

physical activity retards the decline in functional capacity associated with typical aging and disuse.

PHYSICAL ACTIVITY, HEALTH, AND LONGEVITY

In one of the first studies of the possibility that sport and regular physical activity prolongs life, former Harvard University oarsmen exceeded their predicted longevity by 5.1 years per man.[74] Other early studies showed similar but more modest life-span extensions.[13] Methodologic problems in this research included inadequate record keeping, small sample size, improper statistical procedures to estimate expected longevity, and no accounting for socioeconomic status, body type, tobacco use, and family background.

Subsequent research contradicted these findings and showed that participation in athletics as a young adult did *not* ensure good health and longevity later in life.[168] *Maintaining increased physical activity and fitness throughout life provided significant health and longevity benefits.*[24,178,209,238] A continuing longitudinal study of the health consequences of different fitness levels in 25,341 men and 7080 women revealed that low aerobic fitness was a more important precursor of all-cause mortality than any of the other risk factors.[24a] In addition, inverse risk gradients emerged across categories of low, moderate, and high fitness, with a lower death rate among moderately fit individuals compared to the low-fitness group. The least fit men and women were nearly twice as likely to die from all causes as the most fit counterparts during an 8-year follow-up. *Low physical fitness emerged as a more powerful risk factor for death than high blood pressure, high cholesterol, obesity, and family history.*

Enhanced Quality to a Longer Life: The Harvard Alumni Study

The lifestyles and exercise habits of 17,000 Harvard alumni who entered college between 1916 and 1950 provide evidence that *moderate* aerobic exercise equivalent to jogging 3 miles daily at a pace slightly faster than fast walking promotes good health and adds several years to life. The results of long-term studies show four direct benefits from regular physical activity:

1. Counters the life-shortening effects of cigarette smoking and excess body weight

2. Reduces death rate by one half in individuals with hypertension who exercise regularly
3. Counters genetic tendencies toward early death with a lifestyle of regular physical activity; reduces death risk by 25% for individuals with one or both parents who died before age 65 (a significant health risk)
4. Decreases mortality rate by 50% for physically active men whose parents live beyond age 65

Persons who do more physical activity further reduce their risk of dying from any cause.[153a] Men who walked nine or more miles each week, for example, had a 21% lower mortality rate than men who walked three miles or less. Life expectancy was higher for men who exercised at the equivalent of light sport activity than sedentary men. Life expectancy of Harvard alumni increased steadily from a weekly activity energy expenditure of 500 kcal up to 3500 kcal, a value equivalent to 6 to 8 hr of strenuous physical effort. The active men lived an average of 1 to 2 years longer than their sedentary classmates. Weekly activity beyond 3500 kcal conferred no additional health or longevity benefits.

Vigorous Exercise and Longevity

The Harvard alumni study examined only the total amount of weekly physical activity, not its intensity, in relation to heart disease and mortality. Further research from the same population revealed that vigorous regular activity exerts the greatest effect on extending life,[117] and reducing major chronic disease risk including cardiovascular disease.[39] Men who expended at least 1500 kcal weekly in vigorous activity during the 20-year study—equivalent to 6 METs or more (e.g., jogging or walking briskly, lap swimming, singles tennis, fast cycling, or heavy yard chores for 1 hr, performed three or four times weekly)—had a 25% lower death rate than the most sedentary men. The most active men showed the greatest life expectancies, largely from reduced deaths from cardiovascular disease. The benefits of vigorous activity also extended to overweight smokers. Risk associated with a sedentary lifestyle equaled the risk of smoking one pack of cigarettes daily or being 20% overweight. Subsequent research by these men and others[8] showed that the activity equivalent of a 1-hr brisk walk 5 days weekly or a vigorous workout at least once weekly cut stroke risk almost in half; brisk walking for 30 min 5 days weekly reduced stroke risk by 24%.[118,119] Other stroke-protective activities included stair climbing or participating in moderate activities such as gardening, dancing, and bicycling. An intensive post-stroke conditioning program also facilitates the stroke survivor's recovery of motor skills.

Epidemiologic Evidence

A critique of 43 studies of the relationship between physical inactivity and coronary heart disease concluded that lack of regular physical activity contributes to heart disease in a cause-and-effect manner; the sedentary person has about twice the risk of developing heart disease as the most active

individual.[162] The strength of the association between lack of exercise and heart disease risk equals that for hypertension, cigarette smoking, and high serum cholesterol. This makes physical inactivity the greater heart disease risk because more people lead sedentary lifestyles than possess one or more of the other primary risk factors. The life-protecting benefits of regular physical activity link more with preventing early mortality than extending life span. Surprisingly, only light-to-moderate regular walking, gardening, stair climbing, and household chores produce health benefits for previously sedentary middle-age and older men and women.[22,104,120,174] These sedentary individuals represent the largest percentage of the population at greatest risk for chronic disease.

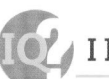 **INTEGRATIVE QUESTION**

Discuss whether physical activity benefits a person's health profile even if the intensity does not produce a training effect.

REGULAR MODERATE PHYSICAL ACTIVITY PROVIDES SIGNIFICANT BENEFITS

A sedentary lifestyle represents an independent and powerful predictor of coronary heart disease risk and mortality, so encouraging the most sedentary 25% of the American adult population to become only moderately active would yield substantial public health benefits.[23,35,112,171] Even moderate activity such as walking reduces the level of diabetic, hypertensive, and cholesterol medication required by patients.[237] For postmenopausal women, walking briskly for 2.5 hr weekly (about 30 min a day 5 days a week) reduced heart disease risk by 30%—a reduction comparable to that achieved with cholesterol-lowering drugs—regardless of race, age, or how much the women weighed.[134] Women who did the most activity reduced risk by 63%. To further assess the health-related benefits of regular physical activity, research assessed the effect of miles walked each day on overall mortality rate in 707 nonsmoking men ages 61 to 81 years.[70a] An inverse relationship between distance walked and mortality emerged after adjusting for overall physical activity and other risk factors. Men who walked less than 1 mile daily had a cumulative death incidence in 7 years that required 12 years for the most active men who walked at least 2 miles daily. Over 7 years, 43.1% of the less active men died compared with 21.5% of the most active walkers.

Corroborative research compared the leisure-time physical activity of 333 patients ages 25 to 74 years who suffered a first heart attack and 503 control subjects without a heart attack selected randomly and matched for age and gender.[121a] After adjustments for heart disease risks of age, smoking, diabetes, and hypertension, regular walkers reduced cardiac arrest risk by 73%. Those who gardened regularly reduced risk by 66% compared with sedentary peers (risk ratio set at 1.00).

Walking or gardening for more than 60 min a week reduced risk similarly to high-intensity leisure-time physical activity. The benefits of walking also applied to women who regularly walked 3 mph or faster for at least 3 hr weekly; cardiac arrest risk decreased up to 40% below the risk for sedentary women. Risk was reduced by one half for women who walked briskly (≥3.0 mph) for 5 hr a week.[133] These findings complement and further support physical activity recommendations from the CDC (www.cdc.gov/physicalactivity/) and ACSM (greatist.com/fitness/acsm-releases-new-exercise-guidelines) to accumulate 30 min or more of moderate-intensity activity on most days of the week.

Influence of Physiologic Factors

In addition to simple physical activity data, physiologic measures like a low level of cardiorespiratory fitness (including low exercise capacity, low $\dot{V}O_{2max}$, low heart rate recovery, and failure to achieve target heart rate) provide a strong independent predictor of increased risk for cardiovascular disease and all-cause mortality.[38,56,236]

One study directly examined aerobic fitness, rather than verbal or written reports of physical activity habits, and heart disease risk in more than 13,000 men and women observed over an average of 8 years.[23a] To isolate the effect of physical fitness, the study accounted for cigarette smoking, high cholesterol and blood sugar levels, hypertension, and family history of heart disease. Based on age-adjusted death rates per 10,000 person-years, the least-fit group averaged more than three times the death rate of the most-fit individuals. The greatest health benefits emerged for the group rated just above the most sedentary category. For men, the decrease in death rate from the least-fit category to the next category exceeded 38 (64.0 vs. 25.5 deaths per 10,000 person-years). Enhanced aerobic fitness benefits women to a similar if not greater extent.[149] For every increased score of 1 MET in exercise capacity, the risk of death from all causes decreased by 17%.[134] To move from the most sedentary category to the next highest group—the change that produced the greatest health benefits—requires only such moderate-intensity effort as walking briskly for 30 min twice weekly.

Studies of Finnish men complement the above findings.[97] Aerobic power and leisure-time physical activity showed an inverse, graded, independent association with risk for acute myocardial infarction. After adjusting for genetic effects and other familial factors that predict mortality, current aerobic fitness and physical activity level still conferred significant protection from death.[110] Physical fitness also counters the negative impact of existing disease. For example, an inverse and independent relationship emerges between aerobic power and incidence of fatal and nonfatal cardiovascular events and all-cause mortality in male and female hypertensives followed over 16.5 years.[155]

TABLE 31.2 summarizes 30 years of research relating physical activity level or physical fitness to chronic disease or medical conditions. Clearly, a strong inverse association exists between regular physical activity and level of aerobic fitness

General Trend for Effects of Regular Physical Activity and/or Increased Physical Fitness and Risk for Chronic Disease Conditions

TABLE 31.2

Disease or Condition	Trends Across Activity or Fitness Categories and Strength of Evidence[a]
All-cause mortality	↑↑↑
Coronary artery disease	↑↑↑
Hypertension	↑↑
Obesity	↑↑↑
Stroke	↑
Peripheral vascular disease	→
Cancer	
Colon	↑↑
Rectum	→
Stomach	→
Breast	↑
Prostate	↑
Lung	↑
Pancreas	→
Type 2 diabetes	↑↑↑
Osteoarthritis	→
Osteoporosis	↑↑

[a]→, *No apparent difference* in disease rates across activity or fitness categories; ↑, *some* evidence of reduced disease rates across activity or fitness categories; ↑↑, *good* evidence of reduced disease rates across activity or fitness categories, control of potential confounders, good methods, some evidence of biologic mechanisms; ↑↑↑, *excellent* evidence of reduced disease rates across activity or fitness categories, good control of potential confounders, excellent methods, extensive evidence of biologic mechanisms, relationship is considered causal.

and all causes of death. *Moderate-intensity regular activity substantially reduces the risk of dying from heart disease, cancer, and other causes.*

Structured Physical Activity Not Necessary

Researchers monitored two groups of 116 sedentary men and 119 women ages 35 to 60 years during a 2-year randomized clinical trial.[52] One group spent 20 to 60 min vigorously swimming, stair stepping, walking, or biking at a fitness center up to 5 days a week. The other group incorporated 30 min a day of "lifestyle" activities such as extra walking, raking leaves, stair climbing, walking around the airport while waiting for a plane, and participating in a walking club most days of the week. The lifestyle participants also learned cognitive and behavioral strategies to increase daily physical activity. For each of the programs, the intervention consisted of 6 mo of intensive activity followed by 18 mo of maintenance. At the end of 24 mo, *both* groups showed similar improvements in physical activity level, cardiorespiratory fitness, systolic and diastolic blood pressure, and body fat percentage. These findings reinforce the conclusion that the health-derived benefits from regular physical activity do not require highly structured or vigorous exercise.

Can Increasing Physical Activity Levels Improve Health and Extend Life?

Current level of physical activity and physical fitness relates to health risk, but an important question concerns whether a sustained *increase* in regular activity can further reduce disease risk. To answer this question, previously sedentary, apparently healthy male Harvard alumni reported whether they changed their typical physical activity and other lifestyle habits over an 11- to 15-year period. Regardless of age, sedentary men who adopted a more moderate to vigorous level of regular activity had a 51% lower risk of dying than men who remained sedentary. For lifestyle change and heart disease mortality risk, becoming more physically active on a regular basis provided risk reduction benefits equivalent to quitting cigarette smoking, reducing body weight, or controlling blood pressure.

Source: Paffenbarger RS Jr, et al. Physical activity, all-cause mortality, and longevity of college alumni. *N Engl J Med* 1993;328:538.

INTEGRATIVE QUESTION

Respond to the statement: The fact that overwhelming epidemiologic evidence links on-the-job or leisure-time physical activity to reduced coronary heart disease risk does not necessarily prove that exercise causes improved cardiovascular health.

Summary

1. Vigorous physical activity early in life contributes little to increased longevity or health in later life. A physically active lifestyle throughout life confers significant health benefits.

2. Regular, moderate physical activity counters the life-shortening effects of coronary heart disease risks that include cigarette smoking and excess body weight. A sedentary person runs almost twice the risk of developing heart disease as the most active individuals.

3. The risk of coronary heart disease from sedentary living equals that for hypertension, cigarette smoking, and high serum cholesterol. The life-protecting benefits of physical activity relate more to preventing early mortality than to extending overall life span.

4. A moderate amount of regular physical activity substantially reduces risk of dying from heart disease, cancer, and other medically related maladies.

5. The greatest health benefits emerge when a person alters a sedentary lifestyle and becomes just moderately physically active.

6. Strategies that modify lifestyle toward increased daily physical activity beneficially alter factors associated with coronary heart disease risk.

PART 4 CORONARY HEART DISEASE

Coronary heart disease (CHD) involves degenerative changes in the intima, or inner lining, of the larger arteries that supply the myocardium.

CHANGES ON THE CELLULAR LEVEL

Damage to arterial walls begins as a multifactorial, largely immunologically mediated, inflammatory response to injury, perhaps from hypertension, cigarette smoking, infection, homocysteine, elevated cholesterol, or free radicals. One response triggers the chemical modification of various compounds, which includes oxidation of low-density lipoprotein cholesterol (LDL-C). This initiates a complex series of changes that produce lesions that sometimes bulge into the vessel lumen or protrude outward into the arterial wall. Lesions initially take the form of fatty streaks, the first signs of atherosclerosis. With further inflammatory damage from continued lipid deposition and proliferation of smooth muscle cells and connective tissue, the vessel congests with lipid-filled plaques, fibrous scar tissue, or both. Progressive occlusion gradually reduces blood flow capacity, with ensuing myocardial ischemia (reduced supply of oxygen).

C-Reactive Protein: An Indication of Arterial Inflammation

About half of persons with heart disease have normal or just moderately elevated cholesterol levels, which has led researchers to consider other factors in the heart disease process. Guidelines from major health agencies (www.nlm.nih.gov/medlineplus/ency/article/003356.htm) propose an important role for inflammation testing to judge whether persons need aggressive treatment to protect their hearts and vascular system. Mounting evidence indicates that painless chronic low-grade arterial inflammation, including that of the coronary arteries, is central to every stage of atherosclerotic disease and a major trigger for heart attack—more substantial even than high cholesterol. The inflammation produces heart attacks by weakening blood vessel walls, making plaque burst, and interfering with substances that increase myocardial circulation. C-reactive protein (CRP), a plasma protein discovered in 1930 by American internist and microbiologist William Smith Tillett (1892–1974) and American virologist and epidemiologist Thomas Francis (1900–1969) (http://www.clinchem.org/content/55/2/209.long), is produced by the liver and adipocytes to help fight injury, inflammation, and infection. Levels of this protein rise dramatically during acute and more chronic inflammatory reactions in the body. This compound may be just as important an independent coronary artery disease risk factor as elevated LDL cholesterol.

 See the animation "Acute Inflammation" on http://thePoint.lww.com/mkk8e for a demonstration of this process.

Not Just For the Blood Lipid Profile: New Recommendations

CRP reduction with statin drugs (and associated reduction in plaque size) may be as crucial as cholesterol reduction in preventing heart attacks.[148,172] In 2010, the U.S. Food and Drug Administration approved a new indication for the use of statin drugs (primarily used for lowering LDL cholesterol) to treat men age 50 and older (women 60 and older) who present with elevated C-reactive protein (CRP; >2.0 mg·L⁻¹) and at least one other cardiac risk factors even without high LDL levels (www.theheart.org/article/1046095.do). The American Heart Association and the American College of Cardiology recommend CRP testing for intermediate-risk patients with a 10 to 20% risk of cardiovascular events over 10 years based on traditional risk factors.

CRP frequently rises when arteries begin to accumulate plaque. High CRP levels also associate with the development of hypertension,[182] a finding that suggests that hypertension is part of an inflammatory disorder. Normal CRP levels average 1.5 mg·dL⁻¹ of blood. Individuals with abnormally high CRP levels (>3.0 to 4.0 mg·dL⁻¹) are four times more likely to experience impaired blood flow to the heart. They also are twice as likely to die from heart attacks and strokes as individuals with high cholesterol—a finding that explains why some persons with low cholesterol develop heart disease or why lowering cholesterol sometimes fails to prevent serious heart problems. Strategies to lower CRP include weight loss, abstinence from cigarette smoking, consuming a healthful diet, and regular physical activity (e.g., combined aerobics with resistance training).[199]

Vulnerable Plaque: Difficult to Detect Yet Lethal

Vulnerable plaque, a soft type of metabolically active, unstable plaque, does not necessarily produce coronary artery narrowing but tends to fissure and burst. The rupture of unstable plaque—the sudden breakdown of fatty plaques in the lining of coronary arteries—exposes the blood to thrombogenic compounds. This triggers a cascade of chemical events that can produce clot formation or **thrombus** and subsequent myocardial infarction and possible death. The sudden, complete obstruction of a coronary artery frequently occurs in blood vessels with only mild-to-moderate obstructions (<70% blockage). Arterial blockage often occurs before a coronary vessel has narrowed enough to produce angina symptoms or electrocardiographic (ECG) abnormalities or to indicate the need for revascularization procedures (e.g., coronary bypass surgery or balloon angioplasty). Acute disruption and rupture of arterial plaque and subsequent clot formation provides a plausible explanation for sudden death from acute physical and emotional exertion in middle-age men with coronary artery disease compared with sudden death under resting conditions. The beneficial effects of cholesterol-lowering strategies on heart disease risk do not always improve coronary blood flow. Stability of vulnerable plaque may improve with reduction in overall blood cholesterol.[122] This stabilizing effect would reduce the likelihood of rupture of existing coronary artery plaque.

Vascular Degeneration Begins Early in Life

Landmark studies of atherosclerosis in young American soldiers killed in Korea in the 1950s showed advanced lesions in men whose ages averaged 22 years.[54] These surprising findings focused attention on the possible childhood origins of atherosclerosis. Researchers now know that fatty streaks and clinically significant fibrous plaques develop rapidly during adolescence through the third decade of life. In children and adolescents with metabolic syndrome, CRP levels are also elevated.[63] Autopsies of 93 young persons ages 2 to 39 years, most of whom died from trauma, revealed that fatty streaks and fibrous plaques in the aorta and coronary arteries appear early and progress in severity with aging.[19] Body mass index, systolic and diastolic blood pressure, and total serum cholesterol, triacylglycerols, and LDL-C were strongly and positively related to the extent of vascular lesions in the deceased young people (high-density lipoprotein cholesterol [HDL-C] related negatively). History of cigarette smoking magnified the vascular damage.[173] As the number of risk factors increased, so did the severity of atherosclerosis in these asymptomatic individuals. Analyses of microscopic qualities of coronary atherosclerosis in 760 teenagers and young adults who died from accidents, suicide, and murder indicated that many had arteries so clogged that they could suffer a myocardial infarction.[137] Two percent of those ages 15 to 19 and 20% of those 30 to 34 had advanced plaque formation, the blockages considered most likely to break off and precipitate a heart attack or stroke. Collectively, the autopsy findings support the wisdom of primary prevention of atherosclerosis through risk factor identification and intervention early in childhood or adolescence.

Risks Develop at an Early Age

A dismal picture emerges for selected markers of cardiovascular health for American adolescents, suggesting that the current generation of teenagers may increase their risk for heart

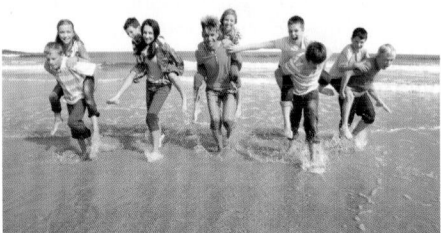

disease later in life. An analysis of data from the Centers for Disease Control and Prevention found that 5450 adolescents between 12 and 19 years of age performed poorly overall on the criteria set by the American Heart Association for ideal cardiovascular health. Particularly noteworthy was the poor quality of their diet. Not one adolescent reported meeting recommended targets on five different nutrition categories, including consuming at least 4.5 servings of fruits and vegetables per day, 3 whole-grain servings daily, 2 or more servings of fish a week, consuming less than 1500 mg of sodium daily, and drinking less than 3 oz of sugar-sweetened drinks a week. Just 16.4% of boys and 11.3% of girls rated ideal on all of the other six criteria. For the physical activity category, 50% of boys and 60% of girls failed to meet the optimal goal of exercising 60 min a day; worse yet, between 10% and 20% reported getting no exercise at all!

FIGURE 31.16 shows the progressive occlusion of an artery from a buildup of calcified fatty substances in atherosclerosis. The first overt sign of atherosclerotic change occurs when lipid-laden macrophage cells cluster under the endothelial lining in the artery to form a bulge or fatty streak. Over time, proliferating smooth muscle cells migrate to the inner endothelial layer and accumulate to narrow the lumen (center) of the artery. A thrombus forms and plugs the artery, depriving the myocardium of normal blood flow and oxygen supply. When the thrombus blocks one of the smaller coronary vessels, a portion of the heart muscle dies (necrosis) and the person suffers a heart attack or **myocardial infarction (MI)**. MIs are caused by blockage in one or more arteries that supply the heart, cutting off myocardial blood supply or sudden spasms (constrictions) of a coronary vessel that causes tissue necrosis from oxygen deprivation. MI contrasts with **cardiac arrest** from irregular neural–electrical transmission within the myocardium. The latter results from chaotic, unregulated beating of the heart's upper chambers (atrial fibrillation) or lower chambers (ventricular fibrillation).

If coronary artery narrowing progresses to produce brief periods of inadequate myocardial perfusion, the person may experience temporary chest pains, termed *angina pectoris* (see Chapter 32). These pains usually appear during exertion because physical activity increases myocardial blood flow demand. Anginal attacks provide painful, dramatic evidence of the importance of adequate myocardial oxygen supply.

 INTEGRATIVE QUESTION

Design an experiment to evaluate the effects of (1) aerobic training and (2) standard resistance training on cardiovascular risk factors in middle-age women. Indicate controls, measurement variables, and tests to show a training effect.

Cardiovascular Disease Epidemic

Cardiovascular disease (CVD) currently ranks as the leading health problem and primary cause of death among Americans younger than age 85 (http://www.cdc.gov/heartdisease/facts.htm). Heart disease is a resource-intensive chronic condition that is expensive to treat.

Prevalence and Control of Cardiovascular Disease and Risk Factors: An Issue for Many Americans

According to the Centers for Disease Control and Prevention (www.nhlbi.nih.gov/resources/docs/2012_ChartBook_508.pdf) estimates for cardiovascular disease are alarming. Over 82,600,000 individuals currently suffer from CVD in the U.S. Overwhelmingly, the greatest prevalence occurs for hypertension and coronary heart disease. There are over 1,255,000 heart attacks per year and more than 470,000 recurrent yearly heart attack events.

- An estimated 31.9 million U.S. adults ≥20 years of age have total serum cholesterol levels ≥240 mg·dL^{-1}, with a prevalence of 13.8%. Based on 2007 to 2010 data, 33.0% of adults ≥20 years of age have hypertension. This represents 78 million adults with hypertension. The prevalence of hypertension is nearly equal between men and women. African American adults have the highest prevalence of hypertension in the world (44%).
- Among hypertensive adults, ≈82% are aware of their condition and 75% use antihypertensive medication, but only 53% of those with documented hypertension control their condition to target levels.
- In 2010, an estimated 19.7 million Americans had diagnosed type 2 diabetes mellitus, representing 8.3% of the adult population. An additional 8.2 million had undiagnosed diabetes mellitus, and 38.2% had prediabetes, with abnormal fasting glucose levels. African Americans, Mexican Americans, Hispanic/Latino individuals, and other ethnic minorities bear a strikingly disproportionate incidence of diabetes mellitus in the United States.
- The prevalence of diabetes mellitus continues to increase dramatically over time, in parallel with the increases in overweight and obesity prevalence.

CORONARY HEART DISEASE RISK FACTORS

Research over the past 50 to 60 years has identified various personal characteristics, behaviors, and environmental factors linked to increased CHD susceptibility. Many of these

Stages of coronary artery deterioration

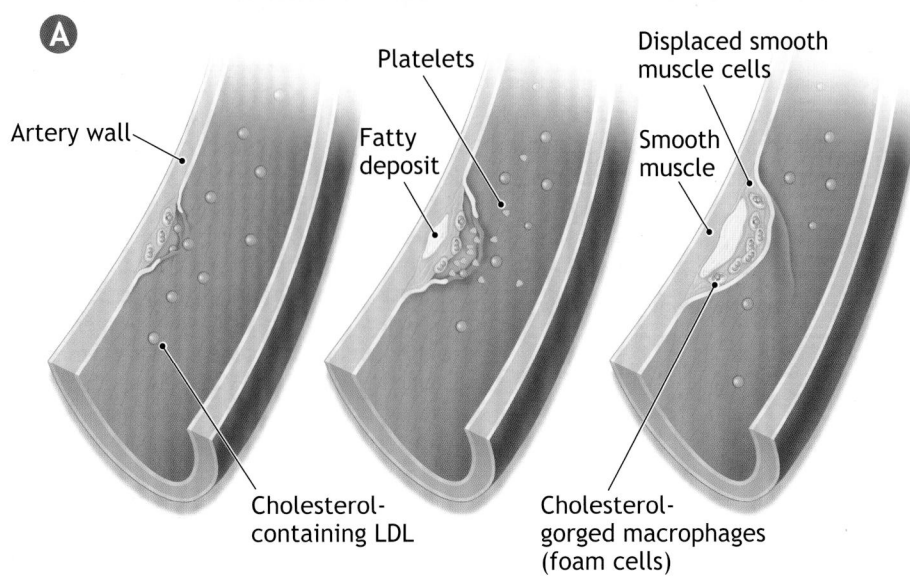

A

Artery wall

Platelets

Fatty deposit

Displaced smooth muscle cells

Smooth muscle

Cholesterol-containing LDL

Cholesterol-gorged macrophages (foam cells)

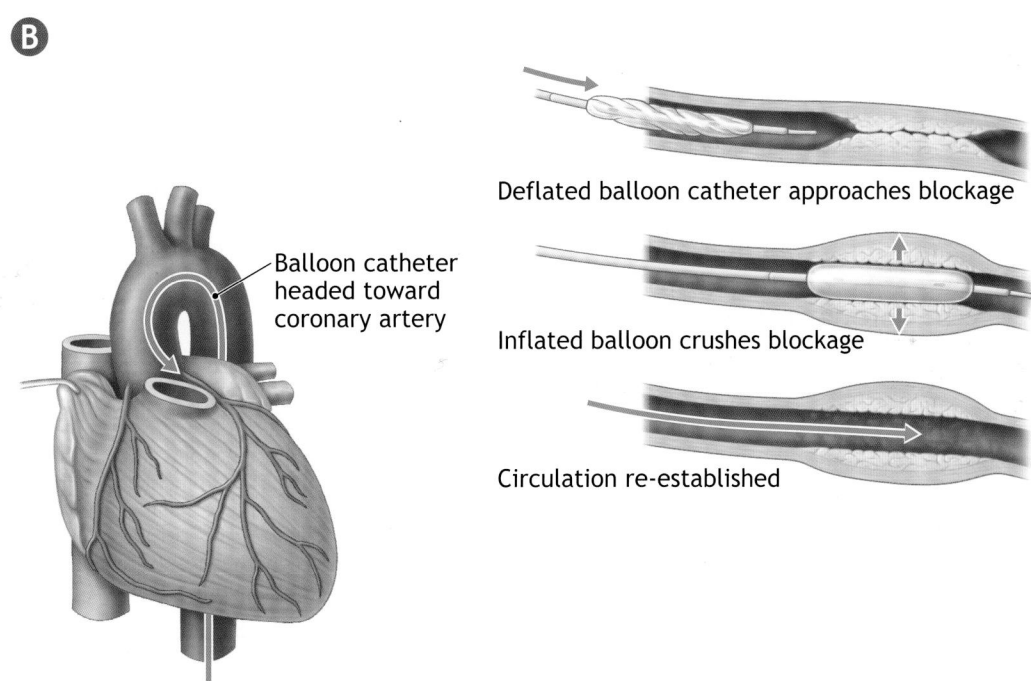

B

Balloon catheter headed toward coronary artery

Deflated balloon catheter approaches blockage

Inflated balloon crushes blockage

Circulation re-established

FIGURE 31.16 • (A) Deterioration of a coronary artery from deposits of fatty substances that roughen the vessel's center. When a thrombus (blood clot) forms above the plaque, complete blockage of the artery produces a myocardial infarction or heart attack. A coronary artery bypass graft (CABG) creates a new "transportation route" around the blocked region to allow the required blood flow to deliver oxygen and nutrients to the previously "starved" surrounding heart muscle. The saphenous vein from the leg is the most commonly used bypass vessel. CABG involves sewing the graft vessels to the coronary arteries beyond the narrowing or blockage, with the other end of the vein attached to the aorta. Medications (statins) lower total and LDL cholesterol, and daily low-dose aspirin (81 mg) reduces post-CABG artery narrowing beyond the insertion site of the graft. Repeat CABG surgical mortality averages 5 to 10%. **(B)** Angioplasty procedure to fix a blocked coronary artery. (Adapted with permission from Moore KL, Dalley AF, Agur AMR. *Clinically Oriented Anatomy*, 7th Ed., as used with permission from *Stedman's Medical Dictionary*. 27th Ed. Baltimore: Wolters Kluwer Health, 2013.)

factors relate strongly to CHD risk, but the associations do not necessarily imply a causal relationship (e.g., male-pattern baldness).[127] In some instances, it remains unclear whether risk-factor modification offers effective disease protection.

Until definite proof emerges, it seems prudent to assume that either elimination or reduction of one or more of the modifiable risk factors will reduce the likelihood of CHD and cumulative disability in later years. For example, a radical heart risk–reduction program that includes a vegetarian diet limiting fat intake to no more than 10% of total calories and including regular physical activity, stress-management training, and support meetings substantially reduces subsequent heart attack rate and other adverse heart events such as bypass operations and angioplasty procedures.[152] In contrast, patients in conventional care steadily worsened over the same 5-year period. TABLE 31.3 lists modifiable and unmodifiable risk factors most frequently implicated in CHD.

Determining the quantitative importance of any single CHD risk factor remains difficult because of the interrelationships among blood lipid abnormalities, type 2 diabetes, heredity (gene polymorphism), and obesity.[27,225]

Age, Gender, and Heredity

Age represents a CHD risk factor largely from its association with hypertension, elevated blood lipid levels, and glucose intolerance. After age 35 in men and age 45 in women, the chances of dying from CHD increase progressively and dramatically.

TABLE 31.3 Modifiable and Unmodifiable Risk Factors Most Frequently Implicated in Coronary Heart Disease

Modifiable Factors	Unmodifiable Factors
Diet	Age
Elevated blood lipids	Gender
Hypertension	Ethnic background
Personality and behavior patterns	Male-pattern baldness, particularly lack of hair on the crown of the head; possibly from raised androgen levels
Cigarette smoking	Family history
High serum uric acid	
Sedentary lifestyle	
Pulmonary function abnormalities	
Excessive body fat	
Diabetes mellitus	
ECG abnormalities	
Tension and stress	
Poor education	
Elevated homocysteine	
Sleep apnea	

Sleep Disorders: An Underdiagnosed and Undertreated CHD Risk Factor

The prevalence of sleep disorders, primarily obstructive sleep apnea (OSA), continues to increase worldwide. Adult prevalence rates of OSA from different countries vary, with an overall estimation of approximately 3 to 7% for adult men and 2 to 5% for adult women. OSA is higher in the subgroups of overweight or obese subjects, older adults, and those of different ethnic origins. African American ethnicity also may be a significant OSA risk factor. The increased prevalence of OSA among American Indian and Hispanic adults and increased severity among Pacific Islanders and Maoris is explained mainly by their high obesity indices.

In the United States, approximately one in six individuals, or 43 million, suffer from sleep loss and an additional 20 to 30 million experience intermittent sleep-related problems that directly or indirectly impacts CHD via insulin resistance and hypertension, obesity and diabetes, increased carotid wall thickness, and nocturnal myocardial ischemia from apnea-associated oxygen desaturation. The National Commission on Sleep Disorders Research (**www.nhlbi.nih.gov/health/prof/sleep/reschpln.htm**) attributes $15.9 billion as the direct cost of disordered sleep, with an estimated $50 to $100 billion in indirect and related costs. The NIH's National Institute of Neurological Disorders and Stroke (**www.ninds.nih.gov**), National Heart, Lung and Blood Institute (**www.nhlbi.nih.gov/health/prof/sleep/**), National Center on Sleep Disorders Research (**www.nhlbi.nih.gov/about/ncsdr/index.htm**), National Sleep Foundation (**www.sleepfoundation.org**), and Patient Education Institute (**www.nlm.nih.gov/medlineplus/sleepdisorders.html**) provide excellent resources about sleep disorders.

Sources:
Altin R, et al. Evaluation of carotid artery wall thickness with high-resolution sonography in obstructive sleep apnea syndrome. *J Clin Ultrasound* 2005;33:80.
Harsch IA, et al. Insulin resistance and other metabolic aspects of the Obstructive sleep apnea syndrome. *Med Sci Monit* 2005;11:RA70.
Lam JC. Obstructive sleep apnea: Definitions, epidemiology and natural history. *Indian J Med Res* 2010;131:165.
Wieber SJ. The cardiac consequences of the obstructive sleep apnea-hypopnea syndrome. *Mt. Sinai J Med* 2005;72:10.

In contrast to the beliefs of many physicians who still adhere to the antiquated notion that cardiovascular disease is primarily a man's illness, current facts indicate otherwise (www.cdc.gov/dhdsp/data_statistics/fact_sheets/fs_women_heart.htm):[80,135,218]

- Heart disease is the leading cause of death for women in the United States, killing 292,188 women in 2009—that's 1 in every 4 female deaths.
- Although heart disease is sometimes thought of as a "man's disease," around the same number of women and men die each year of heart disease in the United States. Despite increases in awareness over the past decade, only 54% of women recognize that heart disease is their number 1 killer.

- Heart disease is the leading cause of death for African American and white women in the United States. Among Hispanic women, heart disease and cancer cause roughly the same number of deaths each year. For American Indian or Alaska Native and Asian or Pacific Islander women, heart disease is second only to cancer.
- About 5.8% of all white women, 7.6% of black women, and 5.6% of Mexican American women have coronary heart disease.
- Almost two-thirds (64%) of women who die suddenly of coronary heart disease have no previous symptoms.

A troubling and enduring gap still remains in the diagnosis and treatment for women with heart disease. Women often have different heart attack symptoms than men. One such difference, more common in women, is something called *coronary microvascular disease*. In this malady, the small blood vessels that feed the heart become damaged, causing them to spasm or squeeze shut. Plaque does not necessarily create blockages in these vessels as it does in the heart's large arteries. Disease genesis appears related to a drop in estrogen levels during menopause combined with traditional heart disease risk factors. Little is known about the most effective means to diagnose and treat this disorder.

In addition, women account for about half of the coronary artery disease deaths in the United States, yet they receive only about one-third of the nearly 1 million annual intervention procedures. To close this gap, the American Heart Association (AHA) recommends gender-specific guidelines that encourage doctors to make greater use of cardiac imaging tests in women, which includes single photon emission computed tomography and stress echocardiography (see Chapter 32).[89] The AHA also recommends an increase in the application of life-saving procedures such as balloon angioplasty and drug-coated stents to open previously blocked arteries. Special attention should be paid to women with diabetes, who have a particularly high heart disease risk, as do women with metabolic syndrome and polycystic ovary syndrome (a hormonal disorder among women of reproductive age). The pattern of coronary artery blockage may also differ between sexes. Men exhibit discrete blockages at distinct focal points, making them more amenable to stenting, while women show a more diffuse blockage that occupies a longer segment of the vessel. The good news is that current trends in smoking cessation, diet improvement, and increase in postmenopausal hormone prescriptions largely account for the current decline in coronary artery disease in middle-age women.[81]

Heart attacks that strike at an early age tend to run in families. Familial predisposition relates to a genetic role in determining risk of heart disease. The following sections examine blood lipid abnormalities, obesity, cigarette smoking, and physical inactivity related to CHD (Chapters 15 and 32 discuss hypertension). These modifiable factors represent the "big five" heart disease risks proposed by the AHA. Each exists as a potent, independent CHD risk that can change considerably with lifestyle modification.

 INTEGRATIVE QUESTION

Explain how risk factor modification can affect change in disease risk.

Blood Lipid Abnormalities

Serum cholesterol levels in adults have declined substantially in the United States over the past 40 years, a decline that coincides with a decreased national incidence of CHD. Despite this support for the effectiveness of public health programs geared to lowering heart disease risks, nearly 30% of adults still require intervention for high cholesterol levels.[95] Unfortunately, data from the CDC indicate that approximately 60% of persons with high cholesterol levels did not know those levels were high. Of those who knew, only 14% were taking a cholesterol-lowering drug. An abnormal blood lipid level, or **hyperlipidemia**, plays an important role in atherosclerosis genesis.

AHA Recommendations for Cholesterol and Triacylglycerol

FIGURE 31.17 shows the rate of increase in death risk from CHD related to total serum cholesterol. The inset table presents the American Heart Association (www.heart.org/HEARTORG/) serum cholesterol and lipoprotein and triacylglycerol level classifications for adults (www.heart.org/idc/groups/heart-public/@wcm/@hcm/documents/downloadable/ucm_300301.pdf). Recommendations also include that individuals above age 20 have a fasting "lipoprotein profile" every 5 years (9 to 12 hr following the last meal and without liquids or pills).

Cholesterol guidelines focus both on total cholesterol and its lipoprotein components based on findings concerning effects of the powerful cholesterol-lowering statin drugs on heart health (i.e., reduced risk of heart attack, bypass surgery, plaque growth in coronary vessels, angioplasty).[25,115,147,179]

Early treatment becomes crucial because of a strong association between high serum cholesterol as a young adult and cardiovascular disease in middle age. A cholesterol level of 200 mg·dL^{-1} or lower is usually deemed desirable, although risk for a fatal heart attack begins to rise at 150 mg·dL^{-1}. A cholesterol level of 230 mg·dL^{-1} increases heart attack risk to about twice that of 180 mg·dL^{-1}, and 300 mg·dL^{-1} increases the risk fourfold. For triacylglycerol, 150 to 199 mg·dL^{-1} is considered as an upper-limit normal level, with 200 to 499 considered high. The latter requires modifications in physical activity, diet, and possibly drug intervention if accompanied by other CHD risk factors.

Lipids do not circulate freely in blood plasma; they combine with a carrier protein to form lipoproteins. Lipoproteins are composed of a hydrophobic cholesterol core and a coat of free cholesterol, phospholipid, and regulatory protein (**apolipoprotein [Apo]**). **TABLE 31.4** lists the four different

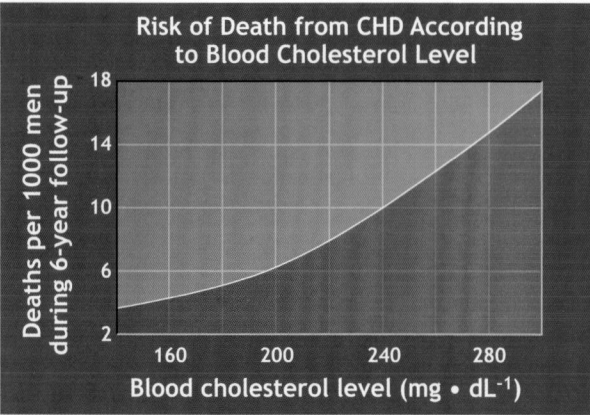

Risk of Death from CHD According to Blood Cholesterol Level

American Heart Association Recommendations and Classifications for Total Cholesterol and HDL and LDL cholesterol and Triacylglycerol

Total cholesterol*	Category
≥ 240	High blood cholesterol. A person with this level has more than twice the risk of heart disease as someone with cholesterol below 200.
200 to 239	Borderline high
≤ 200	Desirable level that puts you at a lower risk for heart disease. Cholesterol level of 200 or higher raises risk.

HDL cholesterol	Category
< 40	Low HDL cholesterol. A major risk factor for heart disease.
40 to 59	Higher HDL levels are better.
≥ 60	High HDL cholesterol. An HDL of 60 mg • dL⁻¹ and above is considered protective against heart disease.

LDL cholesterol	Category
> 190	Very high; cholesterol-lowering drug therapies even without heart disease or risk factors.**
160-189	High; cholesterol-lowering drug therapies even if there is no heart disease but 2 or more risk factors present.
130-159	Borderline high; cholesterol-lowering drug therapies if heart disease is present.
100-129	Near optimal; doctor may consider cholesterol-lowering drug therapies plus dietary modification if heart disease is present.
< 100	Optimal; no therapy needed.

Triacylglycerol	Category
< 150	Normal
150-199	Borderline high
200-499	High
≥ 500	Very high

* All levels in mg • dL⁻¹.

** In men under age 35 and premenopausal women with LDL cholesterol levels of 190 to 219 mg • dL⁻¹, delay drug therapy except in high-risk patients with diabetes.

FIGURE 31.17 • Death risk from coronary heart disease (CHD) in relation to total serum cholesterol level in middle-aged men. *Inset.* The American Heart Association recommendations and classifications for serum cholesterol, lipoproteins, and triacylglycerol levels for adults.

lipoproteins, their approximate gravitational densities, and their percentage composition in the blood. *Serum cholesterol consists of a composite of the total cholesterol contained in each of the different lipoproteins.* Discussions commonly refer to hyperlipidemia, but the more meaningful focus addresses the different types of **hyperlipoproteinemia**.

Cholesterol distribution among the various lipoproteins provides a more powerful predictor of heart disease risk than total blood cholesterol. Specifically, elevated HDL-C levels relate causally with a lower heart disease risk even among individuals with total cholesterol below 200 mg • dL⁻¹. Overwhelming evidence links high LDL-C and apolipoprotein (B) levels with increased CHD risk.[113] A more effective evaluation of heart disease risk than either total cholesterol or LDL-C levels divides total cholesterol by HDL-C. *A ratio greater than 4.5 indicates high heart disease risk; a ratio of 3.5 or lower represents a more desirable risk level.*

LDL-C, synthesized in the liver, and very low-density lipoprotein cholesterol (VLDL-C) transport fats to cells, including the smooth muscle walls of arteries. Upon oxidation, LDL-C participates in artery-clogging, plaque-forming atherosclerosis by stimulating monocyte–macrophage infiltration and lipoprotein deposition.[189] LDL-C's surface coat contains the specific apolipoprotein (Apo B) that facilitates cholesterol removal from the LDL-C molecule by binding to LDL-C receptors of specific cells. Prevention of LDL-C oxidation, in contrast, slows CHD progression. In this case, any potential benefit of dietary antioxidants such as vitamins C and E and β-carotene, within a food matrix and not as isolated dietary supplements, on heart disease risk may lie in their ability to blunt LDL-C oxidation (see Chapter 2).[49,73,109]

LDL-C targets peripheral tissue and contributes to arterial damage. HDL-C is also produced in the liver. Its levels relate to genetic factors.[90] HDL-C facilitates reverse cholesterol transport: it promotes surplus cholesterol removal from peripheral tissues, including arterial walls, for transport to the liver for bile synthesis and subsequent excretion. The apolipoprotein A-1 (Apo A-1) in HDL-C activates **lecithin acetyl transferase (LCAT)**. This enzyme converts free cholesterol into cholesterol esters, facilitating cholesterol removal from lipoproteins.[153]

LDL Particle Size Assessment Also Important

In addition to routine cholesterol screening, clinicians employ a variety of other tests to assess heart disease risk, in particular LDL particle size. A blood sample containing a larger proportion of small LDL particles with high density is more atherogenic (up to 300% greater heart disease risk) than larger particles that appear less dense or "fluffy" for any given level of LDL. This risk may relate to increased deposition in the plaque-forming subendothelial arterial space, an increased uptake by macrophages, and increased susceptibility to oxidation, both early steps in plaque formation, or may be the result of a decreased clearance from reduced affinity for the LDL receptor. Small dense LDL particles associate with high triacylglycerol levels, so the assessment of this blood lipid

TABLE 31.4	Approximate Composition of Serum Lipoproteins			
	Chylomicrons	Very Low-Density Lipoproteins (VLDL:Prebeta)	Low-Density Lipoproteins (LDL:Beta)	High-Density Lipoproteins (HDL:Alpha)
Density (g·cm^{-3})	0.95	0.95–1.006	1.006–1.019	1.063–1.210
Protein (%)	05–1.0	5–15	25	45–55
Lipid (%)	99	95	75	50
Cholesterol (%)	2–5	10–20	40–45	18
Triacylglycerol (%)	85	50–70	5–10	2
Phospholipid (%)	3–6	10–20	20–25	30

(value >140 mg·dL^{-1} represents increased risk) may prove useful in targeting individuals with small, dense LDL particles. Effective treatments include physical activity, weight loss, niacin supplements, and fibrates.

Factors That Affect Blood Lipids

Six behaviors that favorably affect cholesterol and lipoprotein levels include:

1. Weight loss
2. Regular aerobic physical activity (independent of weight loss)
3. Increased dietary intake of water-soluble fibers (fibers in beans, legumes, and oat bran)
4. Increased dietary intake of polyunsaturated-to-saturated fatty acid ratio and of monounsaturated fatty acids
5. Increased dietary intake of unique polyunsaturated fatty acids in fish oils (omega-3 fatty acids) and elimination of trans-fatty acids
6. Moderate alcohol consumption

Four variables that adversely affect cholesterol and lipoprotein levels include:

1. Cigarette smoking
2. Diet high in saturated fatty acids and preformed cholesterol and trans-fatty acids
3. Emotionally stressful situations
4. Oral contraceptives

Specific Effects of Physical Activity

Short-Term Effects. Reaching the threshold that changes blood lipid and lipoprotein levels in a single exercise session requires considerable physical activity. For example, healthy trained men needed to expend 1100 kcal in one exercise bout to elevate HDL-C, 1300 kcal of exercise to lower LDL-C, and 800 kcal of exercise to decrease triacylglycerol levels.[57]

Long-Term Effects. A single exercise session produces only transient favorable changes in lipid and apolipoprotein concentrations, yet the change persists with exercising at least every other day.[43]

LDL-C. Exercising regularly usually produces only small reductions in LDL-C level when controlling for serum cholesterol-related factors of body fat and dietary lipid and cholesterol intake. Regular physical activity may improve the quality of this circulating lipoprotein by promoting a less oxidized form of LDL-C to reduce atherosclerosis risk.[213] In addition, regular aerobic activity increases the success of dietary efforts to favorably alter high-risk lipoprotein profiles.[195]

HDL-C. Endurance athletes usually maintain relatively high HDL-C levels, while favorable alterations occur for sedentary men and women of all ages who engage in regular moderate-to-vigorous aerobic activity.[50] To some extent, exercise intensity and duration exert independent effects in modifying specific CHD risk factors. In general, duration exerts the greatest effect on HDL-C, while intensity most favorably modifies blood pressure and waist girth.[235] A favorable change in lipoprotein profile does not necessarily require that intensity of effort reach a level to improve cardiovascular fitness. With the exception of triacylglycerols, exercise-induced lipid alterations usually progress independent of body weight changes.[116] For overweight individuals, the typical increase in HDL-C with training diminishes without concomitant weight loss.[145,207] Favorable activity-related lipoprotein changes probably result from enhanced triacylglycerol clearance from plasma in response to physical activity.

Protection from Gallstones. The benefits of regular aerobic activity on modifying cholesterol and lipoprotein profiles extend to protection against painful gallstones and accompanying gallbladder removal (the usual treatment for 500,000 Americans yearly, two thirds of whom are female). The National Institutes of Health (NIH) reports that gallstone formation and its consequences are the most common and costly digestive disease, costing $5 billion yearly and requiring hospitalization and surgery. Increased physical activity protects against the development of gall bladder disease.[108] Overall, women who exercised 30 min daily reduced their need for gallbladder surgery by 31%.[121] Physical activity increases the movement of the large intestine and improves blood glucose and insulin regulation; both factors reduce gallstone risk.

Regular physical activity also may reduce the cholesterol content of bile, the digestive juice stored in the gallbladder. Eight percent of gallstones are solid cholesterol.

Other Influences

Even trained endurance athletes exhibit considerable variability in HDL-C levels, with some elite runners' values approaching the median value for the general population. No single factor—nutrition, body composition, or training status—distinguishes runners with high HDL-C values from runners with lower values. This suggests that genetic factors exert a strong influence on the blood lipid profile. In fact, a specific gene produces endothelial lipase (EL), an enzyme that may affect HDL-C production.[94] Turning on this gene increases EL synthesis, which may lower HDL-C and subsequently increase cardiovascular risk.

Standard resistance training exerts little or no effect on serum levels of triacylglycerol, cholesterol, or lipoproteins. From a dietary perspective, substituting soy-derived protein for protein from animal sources improves the cholesterol and lipoprotein profile, particularly in persons with high blood cholesterol.[14] A moderate daily alcohol intake—2 oz (30 mL) of 90-proof alcohol, three 6-oz glasses of wine, or slightly less than three 12-oz beers—reduces an otherwise healthy person's risk of heart attack and stroke independent of their physical activity level.[40,177] The heart-protective benefit of alcohol consumption also applies to individuals with type 2 diabetes.[219] The mechanism for the benefit remains elusive, yet a moderate alcohol intake increases HDL-C and its subfractions HDL_2 and HDL_3. The polyphenols in red wine may inhibit LDL-C oxidation, thus blunting a critical step in plaque formation.[146] Moderate wine intake also tends to associate with more heart-healthy dietary choices, with a positive impact on plasma lipids. Excessive alcohol consumption offers no lipoprotein benefit and increases liver disease and cancer risk.

Lipoprotein(a). **Lipoprotein(a) [Lp(a)]** represents a diverse class of protein particles formed in the liver when two distinct apolipoproteins unite. Lp(a) structurally resembles LDL-C but contains an additional unique apolipoprotein(a) coat. Heredity determines elevated Lp(a) levels, which occur in approximately 20% of the population. The independent risk for atherosclerosis, thrombosis, and acute MI increases when Lp(a) levels exceed 25 to 30 mg·dL^{-1} with raised LDL-C levels.[20] Dietary changes and either short- or long-term physical activity exert little or no effect on serum Lp(a) concentrations.[79,84,85,131]

Dietary Fiber, Insulin, and CHD Risk. Insulin resistance and associated hyperinsulinemia relate to CHD risk factors of age, obesity, central body fat distribution, smoking, physical inactivity, hypertension, dyslipidemia, and abnormalities in blood-clotting factors. *Insulin resistance and consequent hyperinsulinemia act as independent CHD risk factors.*[176]

The combined effects of established CHD risk factors account for approximately 50% of the observed variability in insulin resistance and hyperinsulinemia within the population. The question then is what other factors might contribute to excessive insulin output and, by implication, increased CHD risk. Perhaps total lipid or saturated fatty acid intake and dietary carbohydrates are possible causal factors. Dietary fiber also may play a key role in optimizing insulin response.[128] For example, dietary fiber reduces insulin secretion by slowing the rate of nutrient digestion and glucose absorption following a meal. A low-fiber meal with its inherently high glycemic index stimulates more insulin secretion than a high-fiber meal of equivalent carbohydrate content. Dietary fiber can serve a dual role in heart-disease prevention by attenuating the insulin response to a carbohydrate-containing meal and reducing the tendency to accumulate body fat from insulin's facilitatory role in fat synthesis. Excessive body fat increases insulin resistance, which ultimately leads to hyperinsulinemia.

Immunologic Factors. An immune response likely triggers plaque development within arterial walls. During this process, mononuclear immune cells produce proteins called *cytokines*, some of which stimulate plaque buildup whereas others inhibit plaque formation. Regular physical activity can stimulate the immune system to inhibit agents that facilitate arterial disease. For example, 2.5 hr of weekly exercise for 6 mo decreased cytokine production that aids in plaque development by 58%, while cytokines that inhibit plaque formation increased by nearly 36%.[190]

Beyond Cholesterol: Homocysteine and Coronary Heart Disease

Homocysteine, a highly reactive, sulfur-containing amino acid, forms as a byproduct of methionine metabolism. Researchers in the 1960s and 1970s described three different inborn errors of homocysteine metabolism that involved B-vitamin enzymes. High levels of homocysteine in the blood and urine were common to all three disorders of the afflicted individuals, and half of these persons developed arterial or venous thrombosis by age 30. Researchers postulated that moderate elevation of homocysteine in the general population predisposes individuals to atherosclerosis in a manner similar to elevated cholesterol concentration. A nearly lockstep association occurs between plasma homocysteine levels and heart attack and mortality in men and women.[70,126,229,233]

FIGURE 31.18A proposes a mechanism for homocysteine's negative impact on cardiovascular health. The homocysteine model helps explain why some persons with low-to-normal cholesterol levels contract heart disease. In the presence of other conventional CHD risks such as smoking and hypertension, synergistic effects magnify the negative impact of homocysteine.[132,216,240] This metabolic abnormality occurs in nearly 30% of CHD patients and 40% of patients with cerebrovascular disease. Excessive homocysteine causes blood platelets to clump, fostering blood clots and deterioration of smooth muscle cells that line the arterial wall. Chronic homocysteine exposure eventually scars and thickens arteries and provides a fertile medium for circulating LDL-C to initiate damage.

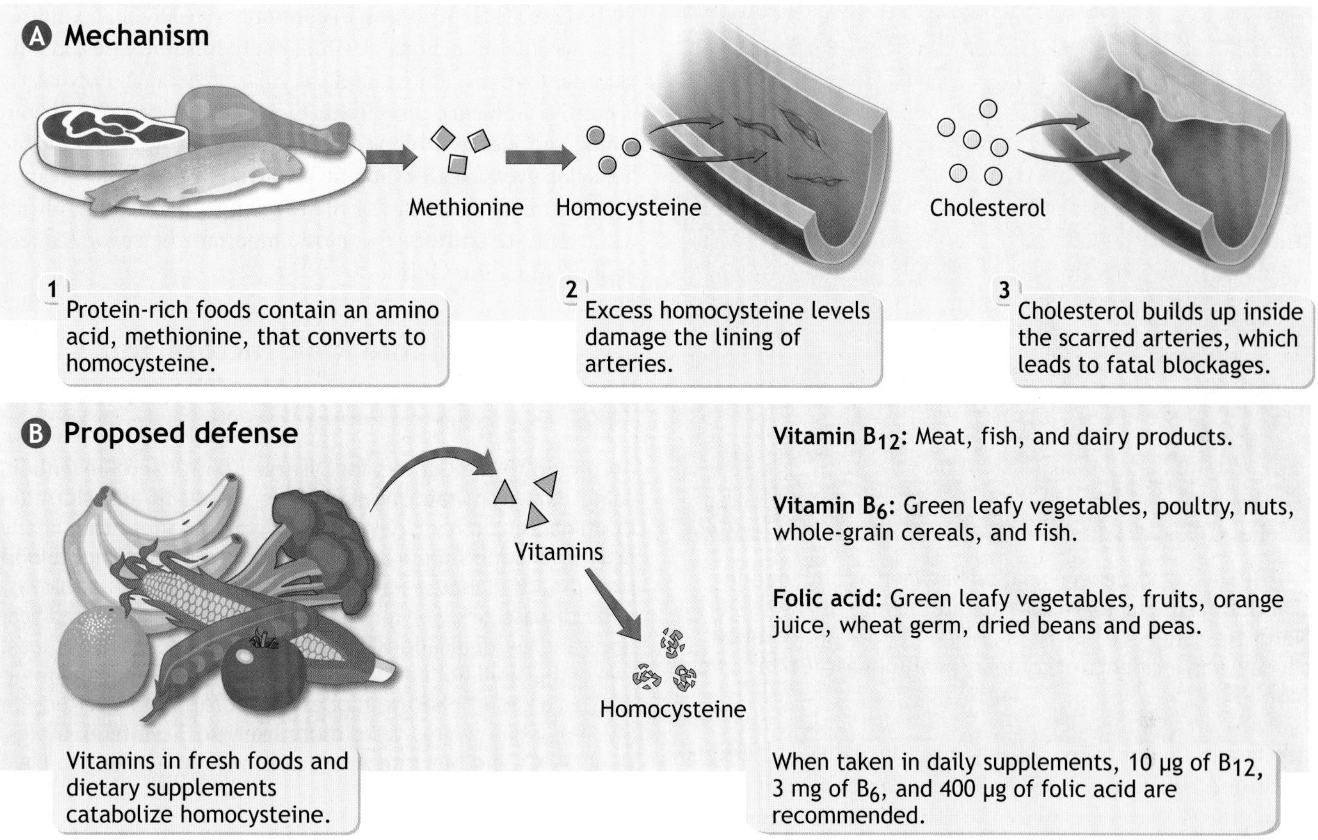

A Mechanism

Methionine   Homocysteine

Cholesterol

1 Protein-rich foods contain an amino acid, methionine, that converts to homocysteine.

2 Excess homocysteine levels damage the lining of arteries.

3 Cholesterol builds up inside the scarred arteries, which leads to fatal blockages.

B Proposed defense

Vitamins

Homocysteine

Vitamin B$_{12}$: Meat, fish, and dairy products.

Vitamin B$_6$: Green leafy vegetables, poultry, nuts, whole-grain cereals, and fish.

Folic acid: Green leafy vegetables, fruits, orange juice, wheat germ, dried beans and peas.

Vitamins in fresh foods and dietary supplements catabolize homocysteine.

When taken in daily supplements, 10 µg of B$_{12}$, 3 mg of B$_6$, and 400 µg of folic acid are recommended.

FIGURE 31.18 • **(A)** Mechanism for how the amino acid homocysteine damages the lining of arteries and sets the stage for cholesterol infiltration into a vessel. **(B)** Proposed defense against the possible harmful effects of elevated homocysteine levels.

Resting homocysteine levels exerted an independent increased risk on a continuum for vascular disease similar to that of smoking and hyperlipidemia. A powerful multiplicative interaction effect also emerges in the presence of other risks, particularly cigarette smoking and hypertension. Persons in the highest quartile for homocysteine levels experience nearly twice the risk of heart attack or stroke of those in the lowest quartile. Why some persons accumulate homocysteine remains uncertain, but evidence points to a deficiency of B vitamins (B$_6$, B$_{12}$, and particularly folic acid; Fig. 31.18B); lifestyle factors of cigarette smoking and coffee and high meat intake also associate with elevated homocysteine concentrations.[143,151,189,200]

No clear standard currently exists for normal or desirable homocysteine levels. Most evidence indicates that the current "normal range" of 8 to 20 mmol per liter of plasma is too high. Evidence suggests as little as 12 mmol can double heart disease risk. Until recently, debate has focused on whether normalizing homocysteine reduces risk of arterial occlusive disease that precipitates heart attack and stroke. Consequently, little is known regarding whether an elevated homocysteine level is simply a CHD risk factor or an actual CHD cause (not an effect).[136,150] A double-blind, randomized, controlled trial published in 2004 determined whether once-daily high doses of folic acid (2.5 mg), vitamin B$_6$ (25 mg), and vitamin B$_{12}$ (0.4 mg) over a 2-year period lowered homocysteine levels and reduced recurrent stroke risk in patients with ischemic stroke.[212] Reduction of total homocysteine averaged 2.0 mmol · L^{-1} greater in the group that received the high-dose supplement than in the group receiving lower doses. The moderate homocysteine reduction produced no effect on vascular outcomes during a 2-year follow-up.

Research on the effects of physical activity on homocysteine levels remains inconclusive. Intense training may increase homocysteine levels accompanied by changes in vitamin B$_{12}$ and folate status.[51,76,77] Other data indicate that individuals who engage in long-term activity, and who exhibit higher plasma folate levels, show reduced homocysteine levels.[75,107,154] Also, resistance training reduced homocysteine in older adults.[224] The American Heart Association does not recommend taking folic acid or other B vitamins to lower CHD risk.

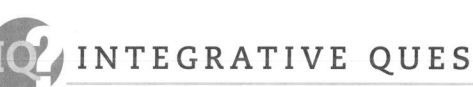

INTEGRATIVE QUESTION

In addition to extending life span, what other reasons would make sense for maintaining a physically active lifestyle throughout middle and older age?

CHD Risk Factor Interactions

Many risk factors interact with each other and with CHD. FIGURE 31.19 shows that the presence of three primary CHD

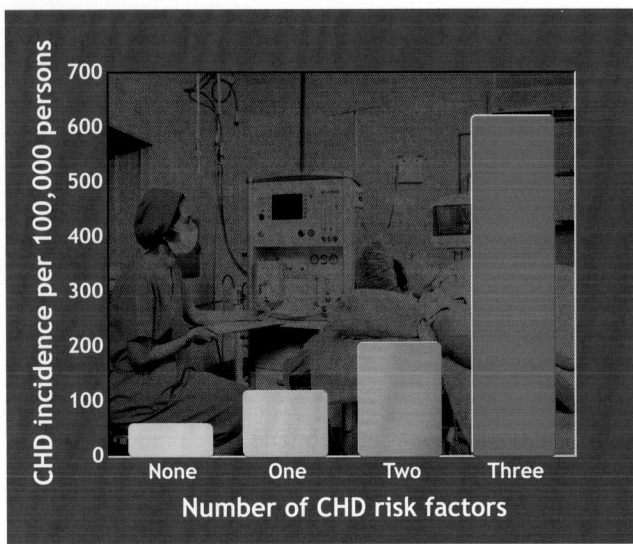

FIGURE 31.19 • General relation between a combination of abnormal risk factors (cholesterol ≥250 mg · dL⁻¹; systolic blood pressure ≥160 mm Hg; smoking ≥1 pack of cigarettes per day) and incidence of coronary heart disease (CHD).

risk factors in the same person magnify individual effects. With one risk factor, a 45-year-old man's chance of CHD during the year averages twice the risk for a man without risk factors. With three risk factors, this man's chance for angina, heart attack, or sudden death increases to nearly 10 times the level for those without risk factors.

Some researchers posit that the five major modifiable cardiovascular risk factors—cigarette smoking, physical inactivity, diabetes mellitus, hypertension, and hypercholesterolemia—account for only about 50% of individuals who subsequently develop CHD. Other novel markers and nontraditional risk factor candidates have been investigated to increase cardiovascular risk predictability.[27,225] TABLE 31.5 presents different novel risk factors that independently associate with atherosclerotic vascular disease.

Several reports directly challenge this "only 50%" claim for the aforementioned five risk factors. Analysis of data from 14 randomized clinical trials (N = 122,458) and three observational studies (N = 386,915) showed that in contrast to previous belief, 80 to 90% of patients who developed clinically significant CHD and more than 95% of patients who experienced a fatal CHD event had at least one of the five traditional major risk factors, including overweight/obesity. Remarkably, these findings may even underestimate the true extent of the relationship, given the self-report design of the observational studies and number of patients unaware or not diagnosed as having risk factors at the time of evaluation.

These findings have enormous public health implications for targeting a large segment of the population at risk of developing CHD. Smoking is arguably the single most important modifiable and preventable cardiovascular disease risk factor and one of the strongest predictors of premature CHD. Equally important CHD predictors include obesity and physical inactivity.

Many CHD risks link in common to behavioral patterns; they become influenced by similar and, in some cases, identical interventions. For example, regular physical activity exerts a positive influence on obesity, hypertension, type 2 diabetes, stress, and elevated blood lipid profile. No other modifiable behavior exerts such a potent positive effect for the greatest number of persons, causing many to argue that regular physical activity constitutes the most important behavioral intervention to reduce CHD.

Modifiable Risk Factors and Cardiovascular Health

According to the Centers for Disease Control and Prevention, using data from the ongoing National Health and Nutrition Examination Survey (**www.cdc.gov/nchs/nhanes.htm**), nearly 50% of all adult Americans have high cholesterol, high blood pressure, or diabetes—all conditions that increase cardiovascular disease risk, yet remain treatable by lifestyle modifications and/or medications. One in eight Americans has at least two of the conditions and one in 33 has all three. African Americans as a group had the highest proportion of hypertension (42.5%), while whites were more likely to have high cholesterol (29%), and Mexican Americans were more likely to have diabetes (26%).

Risk Factors in Children

The frequent occurrence of multiple CHD risk factors in young children emphasizes the need for early CHD initiatives to reduce atherosclerosis risk later in life.[211,236] Risk factors assessed in childhood and adolescence associate with the thickness of the carotid artery later in life. As with adults, the association between body fat and serum lipid levels becomes readily apparent in overfat children; the fattest children usually have higher levels of serum cholesterol and triacylglycerols. General adiposity and visceral adipose tissue also relate to unfavorable hemostatic factors that increase CHD morbidity and mortality in adulthood.[58] Of 62 overfat children ages 10 to 15 years, only one child had just one CHD risk factor.[18] Of the remaining children, 14% had two risk factors, 30% three, 29% four, 18% had five, and the remaining five children, or 8%, had six. A subsample then enrolled in a 20-wk program to evaluate the effects on the risk profile of either diet plus behavior therapy or regular exercise plus diet plus behavior therapy. No changes resulted in multiple-risk reduction in either the control group or those receiving diet plus behavior treatment. In contrast, children undergoing exercise plus diet plus behavior therapy dramatically reduced multiple risks (FIG. 31.20). These encouraging findings demonstrate that a supervised program of moderate food restriction and physical activity with behavior modification reduces CHD risk factors in obese adolescents. Adding regular physical activity augmented the effectiveness of risk-factor intervention.

TABLE 31.5   Novel Risk Factors for Atherosclerotic Vascular Disease

Inflammatory Markers	Hemostatic/ Thrombosis Markers	Platelet-Related Factors	Lipid-Related Factors	Other Factors
• C-reactive protein	• Fibrinogen	• Platelet aggregation	• Low-density lipoprotein (LDL)	• Homocysteine
• Interleukins (e.g., IL-6)	• von Willebrand factor antigen	• Platelet activity	• Lipoprotein (a)	• Lipoprotein-associated phospolipase A(2)
• Serum amyloid A	• Plasminogen activator inhibitor 1 (PAI-1)	• Platelet size and volume	• Remnant lipoproteins	• Microalbuminuria
• Vascular and cellular adhesion molecules	• Tissue-plasminogen activator		• Apolipoproteins A1 and B	• Insulin resistance
• Soluble CD40 ligand	• Factors V, VII, VIII		• High-density lipoprotein subtypes	• PAT-1 genotype
• Leukocyte count	• D-dimer • Fibrinopeptide A • Prothrombin fragment 1+2		• Oxidized LDL	• Angiotensin-converting enzyme genotype • ApoE genotype • Infectious agents: cytomegalovirus, *Chlamydia pneumonia, Helicobacter pylori,* herpes simplex virus • Psychosocial factors

Autopsy evidence and prevalence of CHD risk factors among preadolescents and adolescents indicate that heart disease begins in childhood. Usually, the most sedentary children who watch the most TV have more body fat and a higher BMI than more physically active peers.[15] School-based programs that increase the level of daily physical activity, reduce risk factors, and increase students' knowledge about risk factors and benefits of physical activity can produce a long-term positive effect on activity habits and overall health.[101,217] Because regular physical activity upgrades or stabilizes a poor risk factor profile, school curricula at all grade levels, especially kindergarten and the elementary grades, should strongly encourage more physically active lifestyles. Not implementing required daily physical education in the school curriculum at all grade levels, especially in elementary school, seems counterproductive from a public health policy standpoint.

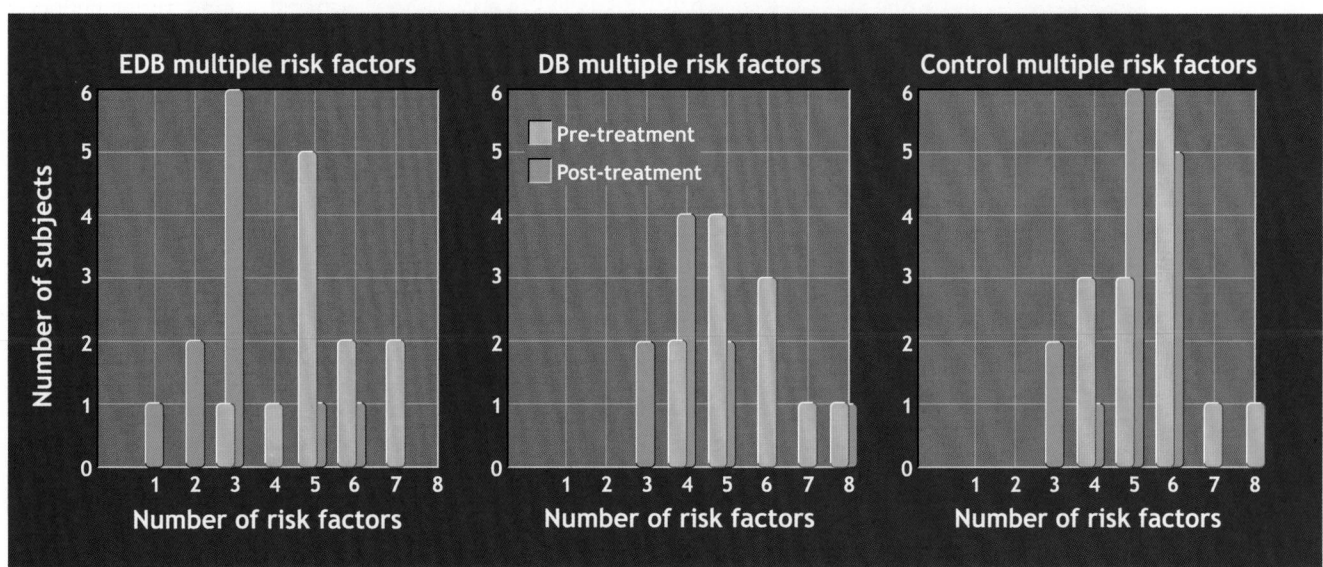

FIGURE 31.20 • Multiple coronary heart disease risk factors for obese adolescents before and after treatment. *DB*, diet + behavior change group; *EDB*, exercise + diet + behavior change group. (From Becque DB, et al. Coronary risk incidence of obese adolescents: reduction by exercise plus diet intervention. *Pediatrics* 1988;81:605.)

Calculate Your CHD Risk

Risk inventories assess an individual's susceptibility to CHD. Several different quantitative methods estimate CHD risk. **The Framingham Risk Score** (updated 2010; http://cvdrisk.nhlbi.nih.gov/calculator.asp), derived from the Framingham Heart Study Cohort, predicts 10-year risk of mortality from CHD and nonfatal myocardial infarction.[46,206] The Framingham Risk Score considers age, gender, smoking status, total cholesterol, high-density lipoprotein cholesterol, systolic blood pressure, and diabetes.

An alternative risk scoring method, the **European SCORE**, was developed in 2003 by the European Society of Cardiology (www.escardio.org) to estimate 10-year risk of fatal cardiovascular disease in European nations in primary prevention.[42] SCORE estimates total cardiovascular risk rather than risk of CHD alone by totaling calculated coronary and noncoronary components. The variables used for SCORE include age, gender, total cholesterol, systolic blood pressure, and smoking status.

Figure 31.21 presents the AHA risk inventory. To assess risk profile, determine the numerical value that best describes a person's status. Find the applicable box and circle the number in it. For example, a 19-year-old person circles the number 1 in the box labeled "10 to 20 years." After checking all the rows, the circled numbers are totaled. The total number of points represents the risk score; see the table in the footnote for relative risk category.

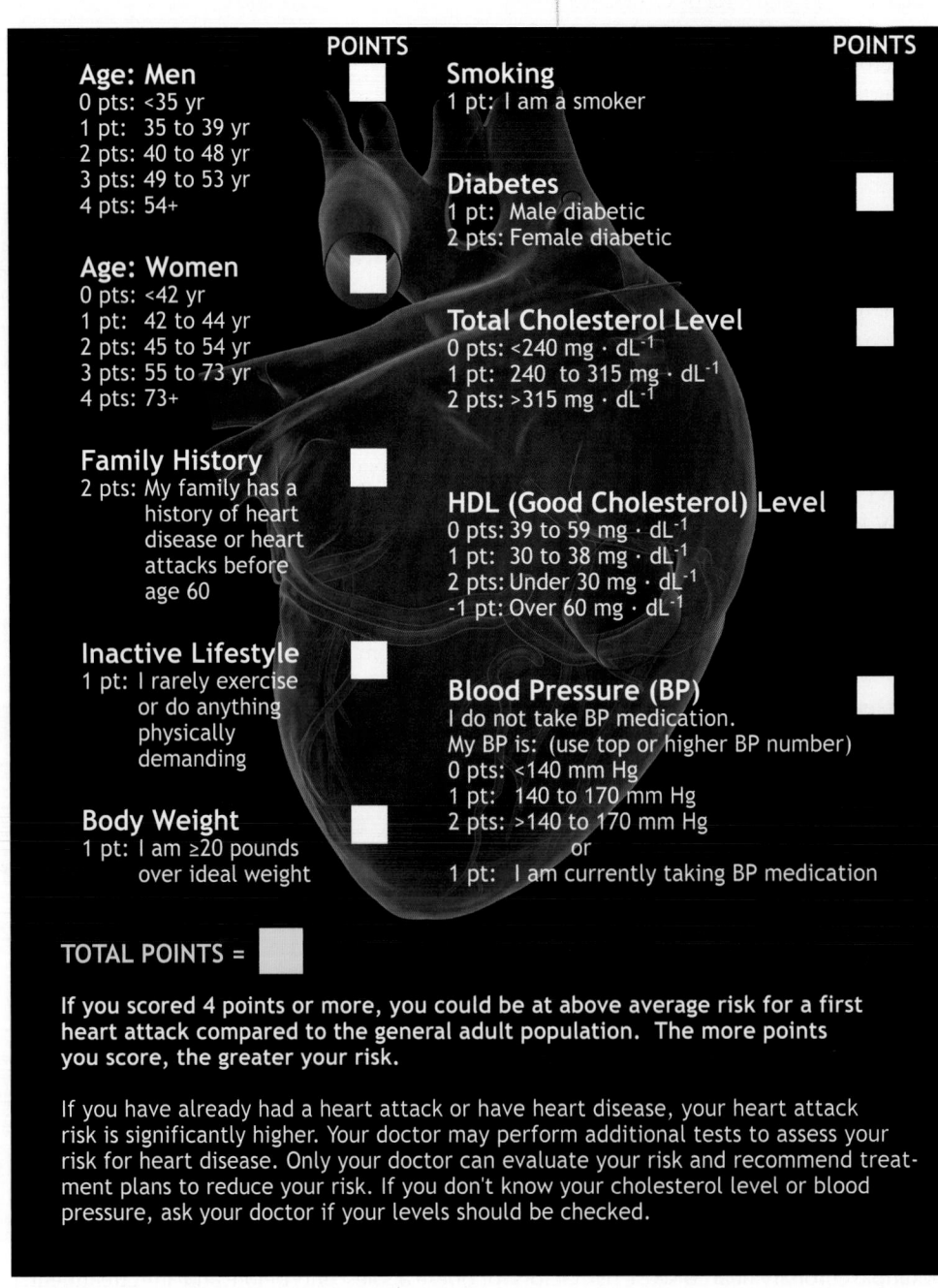

FIGURE 31.21 • American Heart Association's checklist to evaluate coronary heart disease risk.

Summary

1. CHD represents the most prevalent cause of death in the Western world. Its pathogenesis involves degenerative changes in the inner lining of the arterial wall that progressively occlude blood vessels.

2. Major CHD risk factors include age and gender, blood lipid abnormalities, hypertension, cigarette smoking, obesity, physical inactivity, diet, family history, and ECG abnormalities during rest and exercise. Prudent treatment attempts to eliminate or reduce "modifiable" CHD risk factors.

3. Painless chronic low-grade arterial inflammation is central to every stage of atherosclerotic disease and a major trigger for heart attack. High levels of C-reactive protein reflect the inflammatory process.

4. A serum cholesterol level of 200 mg·dL^{-1} or lower is desirable, but experts recommend lower values to achieve the lowest CHD risk.

5. Treatment of elevated cholesterol should begin early in life because of a strong association between serum cholesterol level as a young adult and cardiovascular disease in middle age.

6. The distribution of HDL-C and LDL-C provides a more powerful predictor of heart disease risk than total serum cholesterol concentration alone.

7. LDL-C upon oxidation participates in atherosclerosis by stimulating monocyte–macrophage infiltration and lipoprotein deposition.

8. HDL-C facilitates reverse cholesterol transport by removing surplus cholesterol from peripheral tissues (including arterial walls) for transport to the liver for bile synthesis and excretion via the small intestine.

9. Favorable alterations in HDL-C occur in sedentary men and women of all ages who regularly participate in moderate to intense aerobic exercise.

10. A high level of homocysteine exerts a powerful independent risk for vascular disease.

11. Dietary fiber exerts a dual role to prevent hyperinsulinemia by decreasing circulating insulin levels directly and thwarting obesity with its associated insulin resistance.

12. Cigarette smokers experience almost twice the risk of death from heart disease as nonsmokers. One mechanism for risk involves the adverse effects of smoking on lipoprotein levels.

13. Sedentary men and women face approximately twice the risk of a fatal heart attack than more physically active counterparts. Maintenance of a physically active lifestyle throughout life lowers CHD risk factors and disease occurrence.

14. The interaction of CHD risk factors magnifies their individual effects on overall disease risk.

15. Nutrition, physical activity, and weight control programs favorably alter CHD risk factors and usually improve an individual's health profile.

the**Point** References are available online at **http://thepoint.lww.com/mkk8e.**

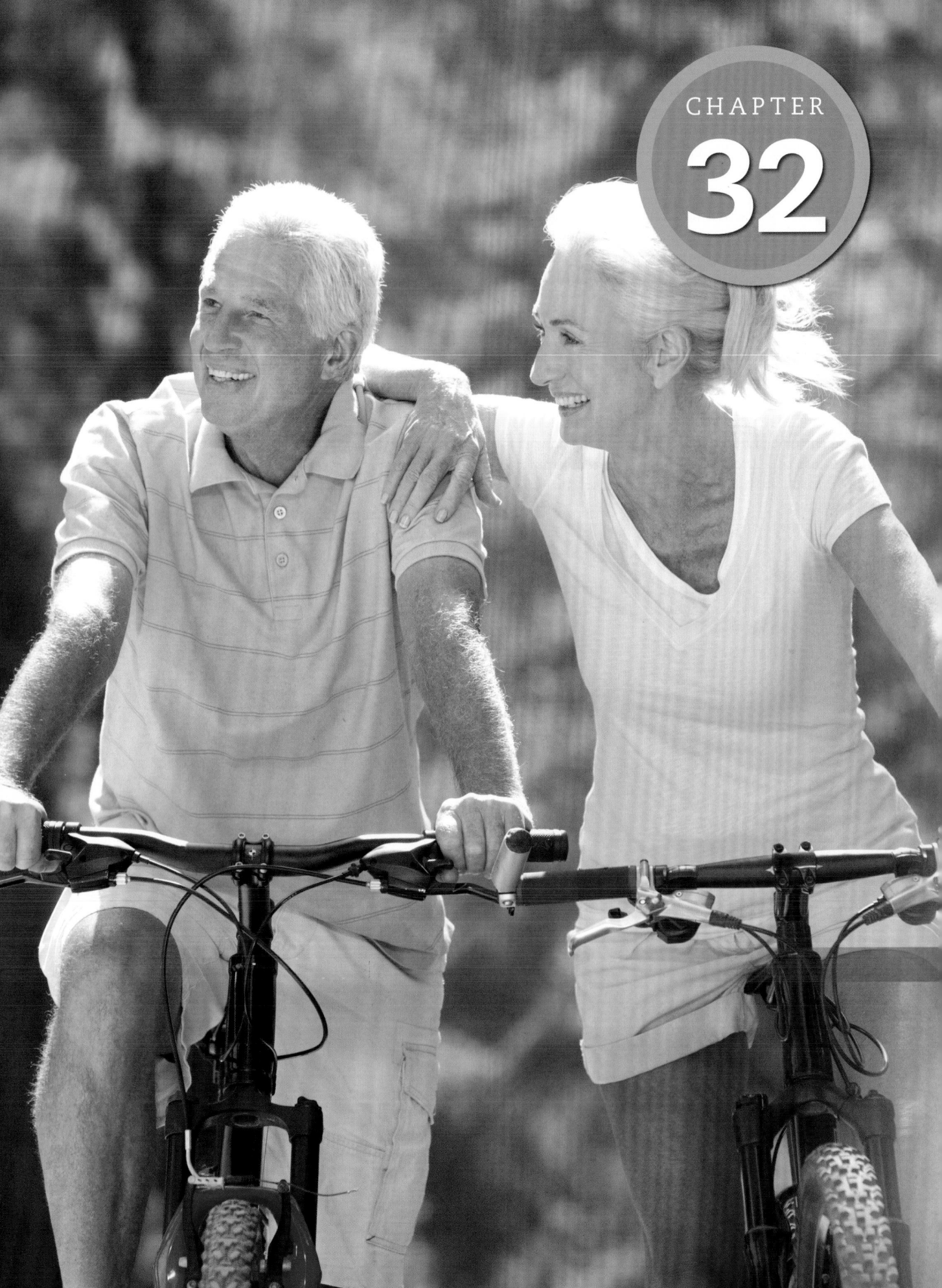

Clinical Exercise Physiology for Cancer, Cardiovascular, and Pulmonary Rehabilitation

CHAPTER OBJECTIVES

- Discuss the role of the exercise physiologist and health and fitness professional in the clinical setting

- Summarize the benefits of physical activity for cancer prevention and rehabilitation and make activity recommendations for persons with cancer

- Review the potential benefits of aerobic physical activity for moderate hypertension

- Discuss the role of regular physical activity in congestive heart failure

- Discuss the general components in the clinical assessment for cardiac disease

- Summarize noninvasive and invasive procedures to identify specific cardiac dysfunctions

- Describe three phases of cardiac rehabilitation, including objectives, required levels of supervision, and prudent physical activities

- Give three reasons to include graded exercise stress testing for coronary heart disease screening

- Describe five objective indicators of coronary heart disease during an exercise stress test

- List 10 reasons to discontinue a stress test

- Define the following terms for stress test results: *true positive*, *false positive*, *true negative*, and *false negative*

- Outline one approach to individualize an exercise prescription

- Discuss the heart transplant patient's responses and adaptations to regular aerobic activity and resistance training

- Categorize and describe five diseases that affect the pulmonary system

- Outline two proposed mechanisms for exercise-induced bronchospasm and factors that modify its severity

- Describe three neuromuscular diseases and the role that physical activity plays in their rehabilitation

- Describe the major classifications of cognitive/emotional diseases and the potential for physical activity as adjunctive therapy

ANCILLARIES 👁 at-a-Glance

Visit http://thePoint.lww.com/mkk8e to access the following resources.

- References: Chapter 32
- Appendix H: Supplemental Animations and Videos
- Interactive Question Bank
- Animation: Asthma
- Animation: Congestive Heart Failure
- Animation: Coronary Angiography: Left Coronary System—Part A
- Animation: Coronary Angiobraphy: Left Coronary System—Part B
- Animation: Edema
- Animation: Stroke
- Focus on Research: Physical Fitness Protects Against Death

THE EXERCISE PHYSIOLOGIST IN THE CLINICAL SETTING

Regular physical activity plays an increasingly important role in the global prevention of disease, in rehabilitation from injury, and as adjunctive therapy for medically related disorders. Attention now focuses on understanding the mechanisms by which physical activity improves health, physical fitness, and rehabilitation potential of patients challenged by chronic disease and disability. TABLE 32.1 lists clinical areas for of physical activity interventions for major diseases and disorders.

The clinical exercise physiologist has become an integral component in the team approach to health and total patient care (FIG. 32.1). In the clinical setting, the exercise physiologist focuses primarily on restoring patient mobility and functional capacity while working closely with physical therapists, occupational therapists, and physicians. The exercise physiologist has an expanded role in clinical practice because of fundamental relationships among measures of functional capacity, physical fitness, and overall good health. *The World Health Organization (WHO; www.who.int) defines health as "a state of complete physical, mental and social well-being, not merely the absence of disease and infirmity."* This definition considers good health an ability to complete physical tasks successfully and maintain functional independence.

Vital Link Between Sports Medicine and Exercise Physiology

One traditional view of **sports medicine** concerns rehabilitating athletes from sports-related injuries. In its broader context, sports medicine relates to scientific and medical aspects of physical activity, physical fitness, health, and sports performance. The WHO defines physical fitness as ability to perform muscular work satisfactorily. This definition encompasses one's capacity to perform physical activity

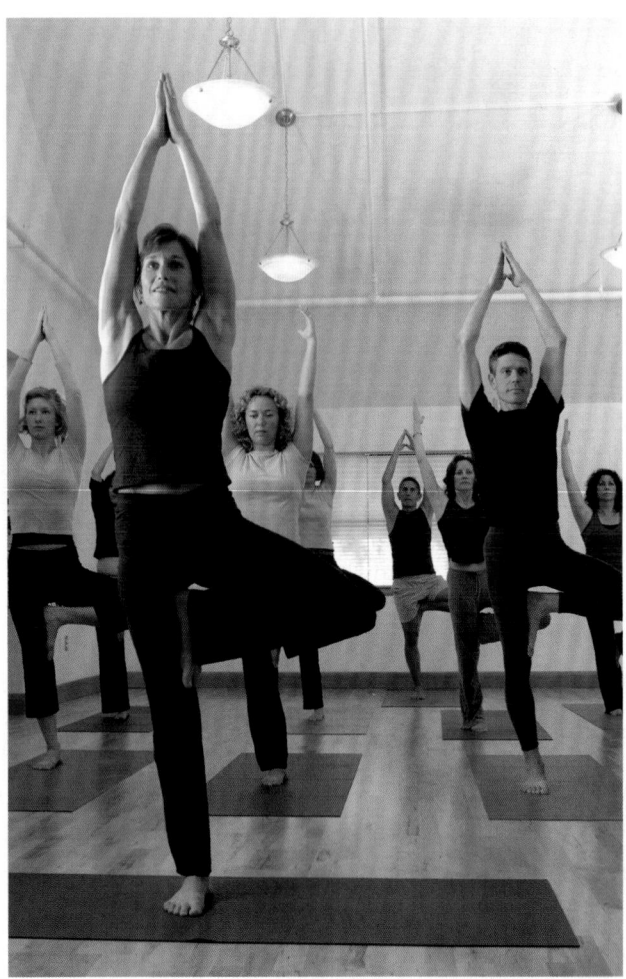

FIGURE 32.1 • Exercise physiologists work in cooperation with local community groups to help supervise diverse activity programs to improve overall health and fitness. This includes games and individual and organized sports, recreational activities from archery to Zumba dance, and popular classes that emphasize balance training, posture, movement control, strength, flexibility, and aerobic and strength conditioning.

TABLE 32.1	Clinical Areas and Corresponding Diseases and Disorders Where Regular Physical Activity Applies
Clinical Areas	**Diseases and Disorders**
Cardiovascular Diseases and Disorders	Ischemia; Chronic heart failure; Dyslipidemia; Cardiomyopathies; Cardiac valvular disease; Heart transplantation; Congenital heart deformations
Pulmonary Diseases and Disorders	Chronic obstructive pulmonary disease; Cystic fibrosis; Asthma and exercise-induced asthma
Neuromuscular Diseases and Disorders	Stroke; Multiple sclerosis; Parkinson's disease; Alzheimer's disease; Polio; Cerebral palsy
Metabolic Diseases and Disorders Immunologic and Hematologic Diseases and Disorders	Obesity (adult and pediatric); Diabetes; Renal disease; Menstrual dysfunction Cancer; Breast cancer; Immune deficiency; Allergies; Sickle cell disease; HIV and AIDS
Orthopedic Diseases and Disorders	Osteoporosis; Osteoarthritis and rheumatoid arthritis; Back pain; Sports injuries
Aging	Sarcopenia
Cognitive and Emotional Disorders	Anxiety and stress disorders; Mental retardation; Depression

at work, at home, or on the athletic field. Sports medicine closely links to clinical exercise physiology because the sports medicine profession treats a broad spectrum of individuals. Individuals with low functional capacity recovering from injury, disease, and medical interventions comprise one end of the continuum; the other extreme encompasses healthy, able-bodied, and disabled athletes with well-developed levels of total body fitness. Carefully prescribed physical activity contributes to overall good health and quality of life (TABLE 32.2).

TABLE 32.2 Health Benefits of Regular Physical Activity[a]

Physical Activity Benefit	Surety Rating	Physical Activity Benefit	Surety Rating
Fitness of Body		**Cigarette Smoking**	
Improves heart and lung function	****	Improves success in quitting	**
Improves muscular strength/size	****	**Diabetes**	
Cardiovascular Disease		Prevention of type 2	****
Coronary heart disease prevention	****	Treatment of type 2	***
Regression of atherosclerosis	**	Treatment of type 1	*
Treatment of heart disease	***	Improvement in diabetic's life quality	***
Prevention of stroke	**	**Infection and Immunity**	
Cancer		Prevention of the common cold	**
Prevention of colon cancer	****	Improves overall immunity	**
Prevention of breast cancer	**	Slows progression of HIV to AIDS	*
Prevention of uterine cancer	**	Improves life quality of HIV-infected	****
Prevention of prostate cancer	**	persons	
Prevention of other cancer	*	**Arthritis**	
Treatment of cancer	*	Prevention of arthritis	*
Osteoporosis		Treatment/cure of arthritis	*
Helps increase bone mass and density	****	Improvement life quality/fitness	****
Prevention of osteoporosis	***	**High Blood Pressure**	
Treatment of osteoporosis	**	Prevention of high blood pressure	****
Blood Cholesterol/Lipoproteins		Treatment of high blood pressure	****
Lowers blood total cholesterol	*	**Asthma**	
Lowers LDL cholesterol	*	Prevention/treatment of asthma	*
Lowers triacylglycerols	***	Improvement in asthmatic's life quality	***
Raises HDL cholesterol	***	**Sleep**	
Low Back Pain		Improvement in sleep quality	***
Prevention of low back pain	**	**Psychologic Well-Being**	
Treatment of low back pain	**	Elevation in mood	****
Nutrition and Diet Quality		Buffers effects of mental stress	***
Improvement in diet quality	**	Alleviates/prevents depression	****
Increase in total energy intake	***	Anxiety reduction	****
Weight Management		Improves self-esteem	****
Prevention of weight gain	****	**Special Issues for Women**	
Treatment of obesity	**	Improves total body fitness	****
Helps maintain weight loss	***	Improves fitness while pregnant	****
Children and Youth		Improves birthing experience	**
Prevention of obesity	***	Improves health of fetus	**
Controls disease risk factors	***	Improves health during menopause	***
Reduction of unhealthy habits	**		
Improves odds of adult activity	**		
Older Adults and the Aging Process			
Improvement in physical fitness	****		
Counters loss in heart/lung fitness	**		
Counters loss of muscle	***		
Counters gain in fat	***		
Improvement in life expectancy	****		
Improvement in life quality	****		

****	Strong consensus with little or no conflicting data
***	Most data supportive, but more research required for clarification
**	Some supportive data, but much more research needed
*	Little or no data to support

[a]Based on a total physical fitness program that includes physical activity to improve aerobic and musculoskeletal fitness.
From Newman CC. The human body. *ACSM's Health Fitness J* 1998;2(3):30.

TRAINING AND CERTIFICATION PROGRAMS FOR PROFESSIONAL EXERCISE PHYSIOLOGISTS

During the past half-century, regular physical activity continues to gain widespread acceptance as an integral part of rehabilitative programs of care and health maintenance for a growing list of chronic diseases and disabling conditions. Likewise, expanding public interest in physical activity for health promotion has stimulated a parallel need to certify qualified professionals to provide sound advice and supervision regarding physical activities for preventative and rehabilitative purposes. In 1975, the **American College of Sports Medicine** (ACSM; www.acsm.org) initiated the first ACSM Clinical and Health/Fitness Certification program. The ACSM continues to be the preeminent organization to offer certification programs, newsletters, and continuing education credits (CEUs, or CECs) to support the professional growth of health and fitness professionals.

The ACSM certifications consist of two different tracks:

1. *Health/Fitness Track* for those who want to provide leadership in fitness assessment and exercise programming of a preventative nature for apparently healthy individuals and for controlling diseases in corporate, commercial, and community settings. This track includes three levels of certification: Health/Fitness Director (HFD), Health/Fitness Instructor (HFI), and Exercise Leader (EL).
2. *Clinical Track* for professionals who work with groups at high risk or with existing disease in addition to apparently healthy individuals. This track includes two levels of certification: Program Director (PD) and Exercise Specialist (ES).

Competency-based certification at a given level requires a knowledge and skills base commensurate with that specific certification. Additionally, each level has a minimum experience requirement, level of education, or other ACSM certifications. Certification programs continually undergo review and revision to ensure the highest level of professionalism. Numerous groups and organizations offer different types of "certifications," some without undergraduate degree requirements and some requiring a short examination or "experience" to replace core content. These so-called *"certifications,"* without approved standards and exclusions, confuse the public about the level of competence or care provided by a "certified" exercise professional.

CLINICAL APPLICATIONS OF EXERCISE PHYSIOLOGY TO DIVERSE DISEASES AND DISORDERS

The following sections present clinical applications of exercise physiology for the major areas of oncology, cardiovascular diseases, pulmonary system disabilities, neuromuscular diseases and disorders, renal disease, and psychologic disorders. We focus on these disabilities because the clinical exercise physiologist mostly deals with these conditions.

ONCOLOGY

Cancer represents a group of diseases collectively characterized by uncontrolled growth of abnormal cells. More than 100 different types of cancers exist, mostly in adults. **Carcinomas** develop from epithelial cells that line the surface of the body, glands, and internal organs. They account for 80 to 90% of all cancers that include prostate, colon, lung, cervical, and breast cancer. Cancers also can arise from cells of the blood (**leukemias**), the immune system (**lymphomas**), and connective tissues such as bones, tendons, cartilage, fat, and muscle (**sarcomas**).

The current population of more than 13.7 million cancer survivors (projected to rise to 18 million by 2022; www.cancer.org/acs/groups/content/@epidemiologysurveilance/documents/document/acspc-033876.pdf) illustrates the ongoing need for rehabilitative and maintenance options for health professionals in this expanding area. The most serious outcomes for current cancer patients and survivors include loss of body mass and functional status. Depressed functional status includes difficulty walking even short distances and serious fatigue that limits completion of simple household chores. Approximately 75% of cancer survivors report extreme fatigue during and following radiotherapy or chemotherapy treatment. Weight loss, decreased muscular strength, and suboptimal cardiovascular endurance accompany these decrements. Maintaining and restoring functional capacity challenges the cancer survivor, even those considered "cured." Sufficient rationale now justifies physical activity intervention for cancer patients during and following different treatment modalities to not only facilitate the recovery process but to prevent the disease from coming back. Guidelines by the American Cancer Society urge doctors to talk to their cancer patients about eating healthfully, exercising, and reducing body weight if they are above norms for desirable weight for age and gender.

Recent Cancer Statistics

Cancer has currently replaced heart disease as the top killer of Americans younger than age 85, and approximately one third of the population have some form of cancer (www.cancer.gov/cancerinformation). New methodologies and increased surveillance and reporting techniques now allow the American Cancer Society to update cancer statistics yearly. Figure 32.2 represents the most recent statistics for cancer deaths for the U.S. population for 2013 (www.cancer.org/research/cancerfactsfigures/cancerfactsfigures/cancer-facts-figures-2013).

Clinical Features

Clinical features of cancer relate to the effects of three primary cancer treatment modalities: *surgery*, *radiation*, and *systemic (pharmacologic) therapy*, which includes application of proteonomics that use proteins as biomarkers for clinical diagnosis.

1. **Surgeries** include operations to remove high-risk tissues to prevent cancer development, biopsies of abnormal tissue to diagnose cancer, excision of tumors with curative intent, insertion of central venous catheters to support

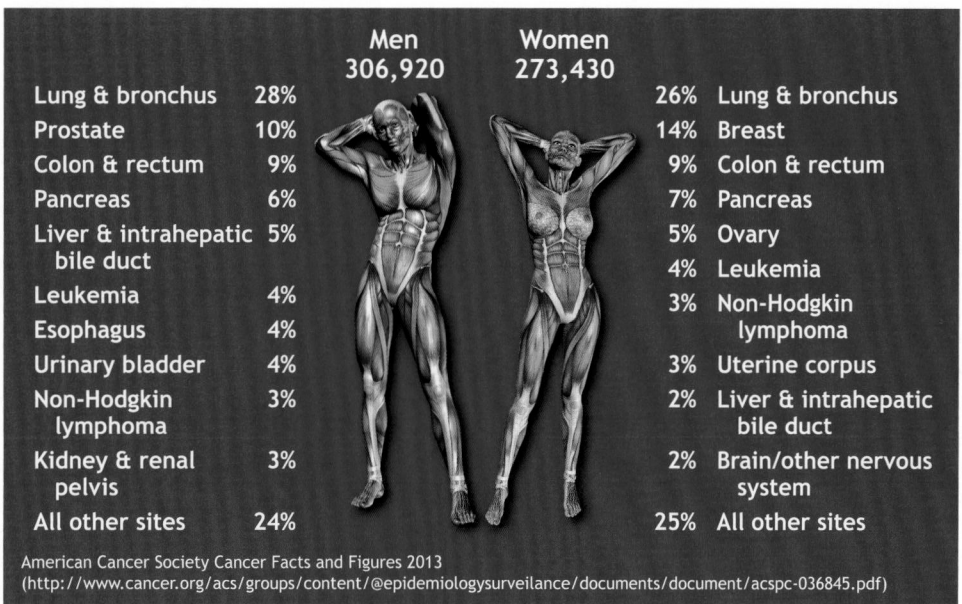

FIGURE 32.2 • Estimated cancer deaths in United States, 2013. Modified and reprinted by the permission of the American Cancer Society. *Cancer Facts and Figures 2013*. Atlanta: American Cancer Society, Inc.

chemotherapy infusions, reconstruction after definitive surgery, and palliative or symptom relief for incurable disease such as partial bowel removal or resection.

2. **Radiation** involves photon penetration into a specific tissue to produce an ionized (electrically charged) particle that damages DNA to inhibit cell replication and produce cell death. Daily radiation treatment typically lasts between 5 and 8 wk. Pharmacologic therapy is prescribed for many advanced solid tumors if cancer cells metastasize beyond the primary site and regional lymph nodes.

3. **Chemotherapy**, endocrine therapy, and biologic therapy represent the three major types of systemic therapy.

TABLE 32.3 presents common clinical symptoms, effects, and outcome from surgery, radiation therapy, and systemic therapy interventions.

TABLE 32.3 Cancer Therapies and Their Complications

Type of Treatment	Description and Effects/Outcome
Surgery	**Lung:** reduced lung capacity, dyspnea, deconditioning **Neck:** reduced range of motion, muscle weakness, occasional cranial nerve palsy **Pelvic region:** urinary incontinence, erectile dysfunction, deconditioning **Abdomen:** deconditioning, diarrhea **Limb amputation:** chronic pain, deconditioning
Radiation Therapy	**Skin:** redness, pain, dryness, peeling, sloughing, reduced elasticity **Brain:** nausea, vomiting, fatigue, memory loss **Thorax:** some degree of irreversible lung fibrosis, heart may receive radiation causing pericardial inflammation or fibrosis, premature atherosclerosis, cardiomyopathy **Abdomen:** vomiting, diarrhea **Pelvis:** diarrhea, pelvic pain, bladder scarring, occasional incontinence, sexual dysfunction **Joints:** connective tissue and joint capsule fibrosis; possible decreased range of motion
Systemic Therapy	**Chemotherapies** [depending on type and amount]: extreme fatigue, anorexia, nausea, anemia, neutropenia, muscle pain, sensory and motor peripheral neuropathy, ataxia, anemia, vomiting, loss of muscle mass, deconditioning, infection **Endocrine Therapies** [depending on type and amount]: fat redistribution (truncal and facial obesity), proximal muscle weakness, osteoporosis, edema, infection, weight gain, extreme fatigue, hot flashes, loss of muscle mass **Biologic Therapies** [depending on type and amount]: fevers or allergic reactions, chills, fever, headache, extreme fatigue, low blood pressure, skin rash, anemia

Reprinted from Courneya KS, et al. In Myers J, ed. *ACSM's Resources for Clinical Exercise Physiology for Special Populations*. 2nd Ed. Baltimore: Lippincott Williams & Wilkins, 2009.

Cancer Rehabilitation and Physical Activity

Regular physical activity helps cancer patients recuperate and return to a normal lifestyle with greater independence and functional capacity.[21,62,81] The most serious health outcomes for most cancer survivors include loss of body mass and decreased energy level and functional status. This occurs predominantly following surgery and during chemotherapy and radiation therapy.[29,31,52] Loss of functional status includes difficulty walking more than one block and chronic fatigue that limits completion of routine household chores. As mentioned above, approximately 75% of cancer survivors report extreme fatigue during radiation therapy or chemotherapy, probably from weight loss and muscle atrophy and loss of cardiovascular endurance. Home-based activity regimens reduce feelings of fatigue and enhance life quality and other biosocial outcomes following cancer diagnosis.[26,150] Maintaining and restoring function present distinct challenges to the cancer survivor. Evidence justifies exercise intervention for breast cancer survivors,[69,87,137,151] and nutrition intervention plus regular physical activity reduces risk of contracting additional cancers.[144,165,168]

Listed below are 10 general preventative and intervention goals for patients who face sustained periods of inactivity, disuse, and bed rest:

1. Improve overall functional status.
2. Improve active motion for nonrestrictive segments and joints.
3. Prevent loss of flexibility by active motion and passive movements.
4. Stimulate peripheral and central circulation through active motion exercise based on current functional level.
5. Increase ventilatory function with systematic breathing exercises.
6. Prevent thrombosis through physical activities.
7. Prevent loss of motor control and muscle strength and endurance with resistance exercises.
8. Reduce rate of bone loss through weight-bearing aerobic and muscle-strengthening exercises.
9. Through active aerobic and resistance exercise, slow the loss of fat-free body mass and subsequent reduction of BMR that accompanies deconditioning.
10. Monitor signs of increased fatigue or weakness, lethargy, dyspnea, pallor, dizziness, claudication, or cramping during or following exercise.

The overall goal of the health-care team is to attempt to rehabilitate the patient to a level of function that allows return to work and pursuit of normal recreational activities. **FIGURE 32.3** shows the effects of a 6-wk physical activity rehabilitation program of treadmill walking weekdays at 80% of peak heart rate during a stress test for five cancer patients suffering severe fatigue. During the first 3 wk, each patient walked five intervals of 3 min with 3 min of active recovery. Walkng duration increased weekly, with the number of exercise intervals reduced until the patient could complete one continuous 30- to 35-min bout during week 6. Submaximal heart rate and blood lactate

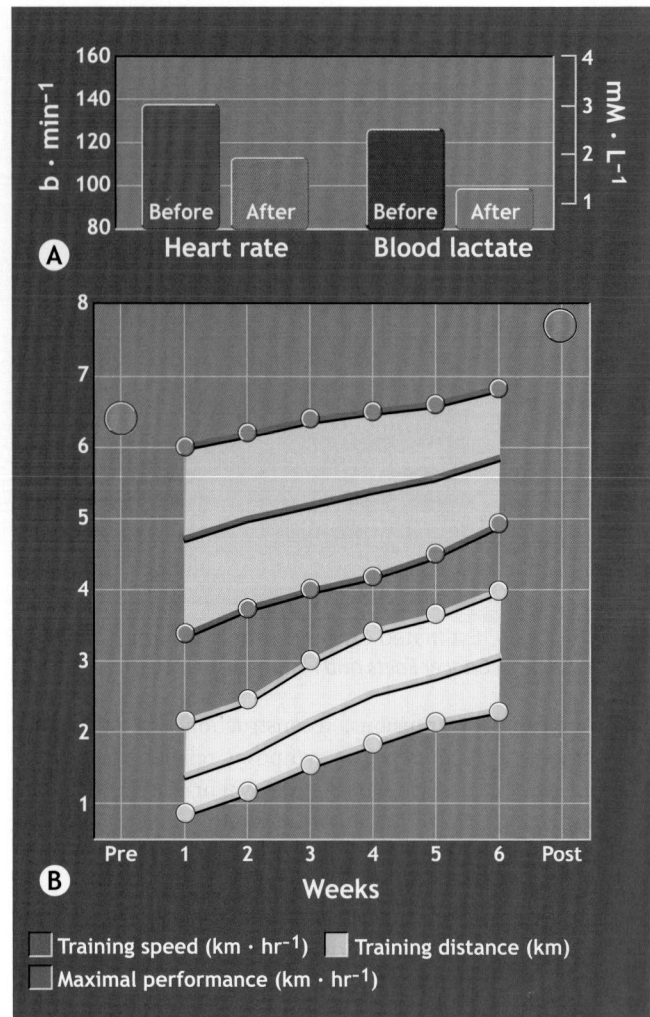

FIGURE 32.3 • (A) Reduction in heart rate and blood lactate concentration during submaximal walking at 5 km · hr⁻¹ following 6 wk of exercise rehabilitation in five cancer patients suffering from severe fatigue. **(B)** Weekly changes in training speed (km · hr⁻¹) and daily distance walked (km) and pre- and posttraining maximal exercise performance. (Reprinted with permission from Dimeo F, et al. Aerobic exercise as therapy for cancer fatigue. *Med Sci Sports Exerc* 1998;30:475.)

concentration decreased during exercise (Fig. 32.3A), while walking speed and distance and maximal performance on the stress test increased (Fig. 32.3B). All subjects increased daily physical activity level without substantial limitations, and each reported increased daily vigor. This clinical investigation did not meet the rigors of experimental research design (e.g., no nonexercise control patients); nevertheless, the results highlight the positive potential of regular physical activity for cancer patient rehabilitation.

Physical Activity: Protective Effects on Cancer Occurrence

Firm epidemiologic evidence confirms an inverse relation between amount of occupational or leisure-time physical activity and reduction in *all-cause* cancer risk. For example, one review concludes "the magnitude of the protective effect of physical activity on estrogen-dependent cancer warrants including low-to-moderate activity as a prudent preventive strategy."[93] Other large-scale, community-based studies of colorectal, breast, and prostatic hyperplasia indicate that increased physical activity reduces cancer risk and mortality.[34,75,104,134] A study of nearly 122,000 women found that exercising at least 1 hr daily reduced breast cancer risk by 20%.[144] The benefits may differ depending on menopausal status, with a greater risk reduction for post-menopausal women.[50] The proportion of men at high risk for colon cancer would decrease considerably if men eliminated the modifiable risk factors of physical inactivity and excessive red meat consumption, obesity, alcohol consumption, cigarette smoking, and low folic acid intake.[135]

Regular physical activity exerts at least the following nine effects to thwart cancerous tumor formation:

1. Lowers circulating levels of blood glucose and insulin
2. Increases corticosteroid hormones
3. Increases antiinflammatory cytokines
4. Augments insulin-receptor expression in cancer-fighting T cells
5. Promotes interferon production
6. Stimulates glycogen synthetase
7. Enhances leukocyte function
8. Improves ascorbic acid metabolism
9. Exerts beneficial effects on provirus or oncogene activation

 **Physical Activity and Cancer Risk**

The evidence of a causal link for physical activity and reduced cancer risk is strong for colon cancer; weaker for postmenopausal breast and endometrium cancers; and limited (suggestive) for lung, prostate, ovary, gastric, and pancreatic cancers. Average risk reductions range between 20 and 30%. The protective effects of physical activity on cancer risk are hypothesized to act through multiple interrelated pathways including decreased adiposity, decreased sexual and metabolic hormones, changes in biomarkers and insulin resistance, improved immune function, and reduced levels of inflammation.

Source: Kruk J, Czerniak U. Physical activity and its relation to cancer risk: updating the evidence. *Asian Pac J Cancer Prev* 2013;14:3993.

Physical Activity Prescription and Cancer

Limited research exists regarding the proper physical activity prescription for cancer patients, including the proper timing of activity relative to the various phases of cancer treatment. Determining the best time to initiate physical activity intervention in the recovery process remains problematic, but not without encouraging results. Thirty-five stomach cancer patients were placed in a physical activity or control group immediately following curative surgery.[116] From postoperative day 2, patients performed arm and leg ergometer exercise twice daily, 5 days weekly for 14 days at 60% of maximal heart rate. The early physical

activity intervention increased natural killer cell cytotoxic activity in the exercise group compared with the control group.

In light of limited information, exercise prescription recommendations for cancer rehabilitation generally include symptom-limited, progressive, and individualized physical activities.[88,176] Ambulation of any kind as soon as practical becomes important for the most sedentary and deconditioned patients. Emphasis should focus on intervals of low-to-moderate aerobic activity performed several times daily rather than one relatively strenuous bout of continuous exercise. A dose–response relationship seems to emerge between increased physical activity and improved health and functional capacity.[69] Most sedentary patients derive clinically significant benefits by accumulating up to 30 min of daily walking or equivalent energy expenditure in other activities. Health benefits accrue whether activity takes the form of structured exercise, home-based programs, or sport, household, occupational, or recreational activities.

Cancer patients initially receive a symptom-limited, graded exercise stress test (GXT) on a treadmill or cycle ergometer to form their exercise prescription. Testing procedures remain the same as for healthy individuals except the patient receives greater attention about sensations of fatigue. Generally, patients should not exercise to maximum. The exercise prescription initially aims to produce ambulation if no specific contraindications exist. The prescription also provides for range-of-motion movements and other activities to improve muscular strength, augment fat-free body mass (FFM), and improve overall mobility (e.g., submaximal static exercises of the antigravity muscles, deep breathing exercises, and dynamic trunk rotation movements). Progression and intensity of activity are individualized, with initial work–rest ratios of 1:1 increasing to 2:1. Eventually, continuous activity for up to 15 min replaces the intermittent bouts.

Based on a review of 25 or more studies involving exercise interventions in post-diagnosis cancer patients in 2010 the American Cancer Society and the American College of Sports Medicine jointly released the following consensus recommendations for physical activity for cancer survivors (www.cancer.org/acs/groups/content/@behavioralresearchcenter/documents/document/acspc-027699.pdf):

- Recommended the same age-appropriate guidelines from the United States Department of Health and Human Services *Physical Activity Guidelines for Americans*
  — 150 minutes per week of moderate intense aerobic physical activity or 75 minutes per week of vigorous activity
  — Strength training 2 to 3 times per week, 8 to 10 exercises of 10 to 15 repetitions per set, with at least one set per session
- Avoid inactivity
- Return to normal daily activities as quickly as possible
- Continue normal daily activities and exercise as much as possible during and after non-surgical treatments.

More detailed exercise guidelines for *early stage* cancer patients and survivors need to be modified as needed for specific patients. Concerning exercise mode, walking and cycling are recommended as safe and generally well tolerated that involve large muscle groups, with a recommended frequency of 3 to 5 times a week. More deconditioned patients need to begin with daily sessions of shorter duration and lower intensity. In general, moderate intensity exercise sessions (50-75% HR reserve, RPE 11-14) of between 20 and 30 minutes duration are recommended, with modifications as needed, including short exercise bouts (3–5 minutes) followed by rest periods.

Breast Cancer Rehabilitation and Physical Activity

Carcinoma of the breast, the most common form of cancer in white females ages 40 years and older, causes the greatest number of deaths in women between 40 and 55 years of age. In 2001, 192,200 new invasive breast cancer cases were diagnosed and almost 22% of those women died. By age 30, the chance of being diagnosed with breast cancer remains just 1 in 2000; by age 40, the chances increase considerably to 1 in 233, and by age 60, 1 in 22. Ten risk factors for breast cancer follow:

1. Family history: especially a mother, sister, or daughter who had breast or ovarian cancer
2. Age: above age 60
3. Personal history of cancer
4. First menstrual period started before age 12
5. Menopause started after age 55
6. Hormones: prior history of estrogen plus progestin following menopause
7. Breast density: you have dense breast tissue verified by mammogram
8. Abnormal breast cells: atypical hyperplasia or carcinoma in situ
9. First child born after age 30 or no childbirth
10. High-fat diet and excess body weight

Most studies of physical activity for cancer patients have demonstrated physiologic and psychologic benefits of regular activity.[36,78,80,157,171] Unfortunately, most of this research remains limited because it did not involve randomized controlled trials and/or it used small sample sizes. Research with breast cancer patients has mainly incorporated aerobic training rather than resistance exercise as the exercise modality. High levels of estrogens have been implicated in the development and growth of breast cancer. One postulated mechanism for the beneficial effects of aerobic activity for women at high risk for breast cancer relates to the estrogen-lowering effects of this form of exercise and the concurrent reduction in breast cancer recurrence and new diagnosis.[91] Following menopause, fat cells, not the ovaries, are the main source of estrogen, and regular aerobic activity provides a potent means to control body weight. Breast cancer patients who are physically active and less overweight have a greater chance of surviving the disease.[62,80,168]

Resistance exercise during cancer management can effectively counteract disease and treatment side effects and contribute to the maintenance of a positive body image.[113,158] In a study from one of our laboratories, 28 patients recovering from breast cancer surgery enrolled in a 10-wk program of circuit-resistance training to evaluate the effects of exercise on depression, self-esteem, and anxiety.[152] Patients performed hydraulic

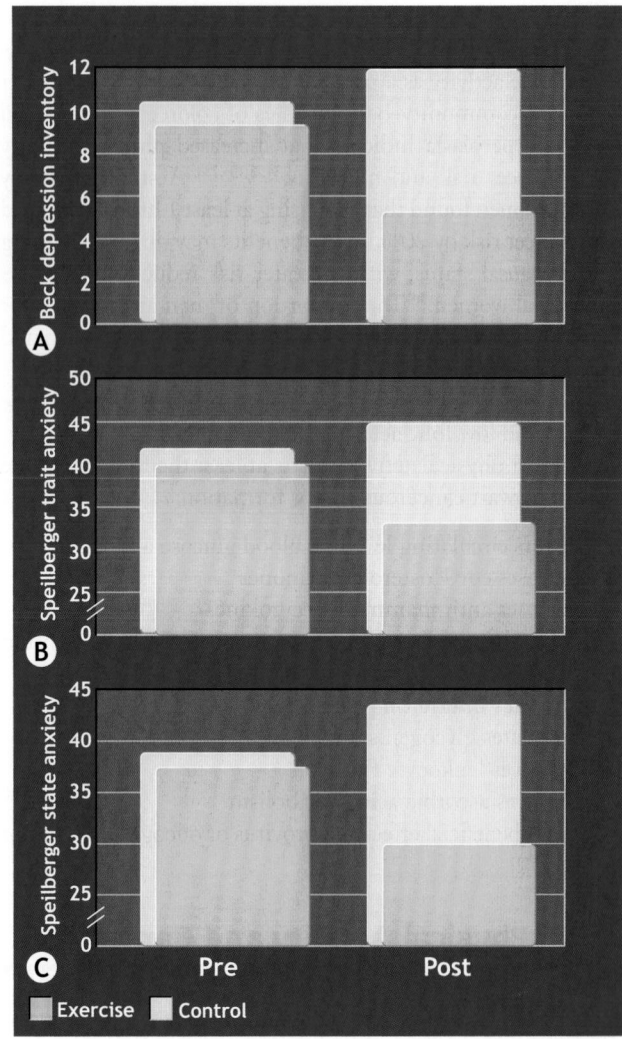

FIGURE 32.4 • Effects of 10 wk of moderate aerobic exercise on depression **(A)**, trait **(B)**, and state **(C)** anxiety in 28 women recovering from breast cancer surgery. (Reprinted with permission from Segar ML, et al. The effect of aerobic exercise on self-esteem and depressive and anxiety symptoms among breast cancer survivors. *Oncol Nurs Forum* 1998;25:107.)

resistance exercises in a 14-station aerobic exercise circuit 4 days a week with a self-paced, individualized program adjusted to their needs and fitness levels. **FIGURE 32.4** shows that exercisers decreased depression by 38% compared with a 13% increase for nonexercising counterparts recovering from breast cancer surgery. The exercisers also decreased trait anxiety by 16% and state anxiety by 20%, whereas nonexercising patients increased in both variables. These potent exercise effects on psychosocial variables during breast cancer rehabilitation bode well for advocating structured, comprehensive activity programs.

CARDIOVASCULAR DISEASE

This section examines the prevalence of different diseases of the cardiovascular system, possible causes and diagnosis of the disease, and specific applications of physical activity for cardiovascular disease rehabilitation.

TABLE 32.4	Cardiac Diseases That Cause Functional Impairment		
	Diseases Affecting the Heart Muscle	Diseases Affecting the Heart Valves	Diseases Affecting the Cardiac Nervous System
	CHD	Rheumatic fever	Arrhythmias
	Angina	Endocarditis	Tachycardia
	Myocardial infarction	Mitral valve prolapse	Bradycardia
	Pericarditis	Congenital deformations	
	Congestive heart failure		
	Aneurysms		

Cardiovascular Disease and Exercise Capacity

When designing aerobic activity programs for cardiac patients, three factors should be considered:

1. Specific pathophysiology of the disease
2. Mechanisms that may limit exercise performance
3. Individual differences in functional capacity

TABLE 32.4 lists three general categories of heart disease that cause functional impairment. Diseases of the myocardium predominate, particularly with advancing age. *Any one of the following terms indicates myocardial disease: degenerative heart disease (DHD), atherosclerotic cardiovascular disease, arterio- sclerotic cardiovascular disease, coronary artery disease (CAD), or* **coronary heart disease (CHD)**.

Hypertension represents a primary risk for CHD, so we first discuss blood pressure stratification and subsequent treat- ment recommendations. We then review the role of regular physical activity in preventing and treating hypertension.

Blood Pressure: Classification and Risk Stratification

Hypertension (www.ash-us.org) afflicts between 38 and 64% of men and 37 and 74% of women between ages 45 and 74 (see Fig. 15.9 in Chapter 15). Prevalence increases sharply with age, particularly for blacks than whites. FIGURE 32.5 pres- ents the prevalence of hypertension in black and white males and females. Note that total prevalence is only slightly higher in blacks than in whites (28.1% vs. 23.2%), yet in young adults, hypertension occurs more frequently in blacks, particularly black women. In the 35 to 44 age range, hypertension occurs in one third as many white women (8.5%) as black women (22.9%).

TABLE 32.5 presents the standard classification of blood pressure for adults ages 18 years and older. TABLE 32.6 provides recommendations for initial screening and subsequent risk stratification and treatment for hypertensive patients. Chronic hypertension damages arterial vessels; it serves as a primary risk for arteriosclerosis, heart disease, stroke, and kidney fail- ure. In many instances, regular exercise provides a prudent first

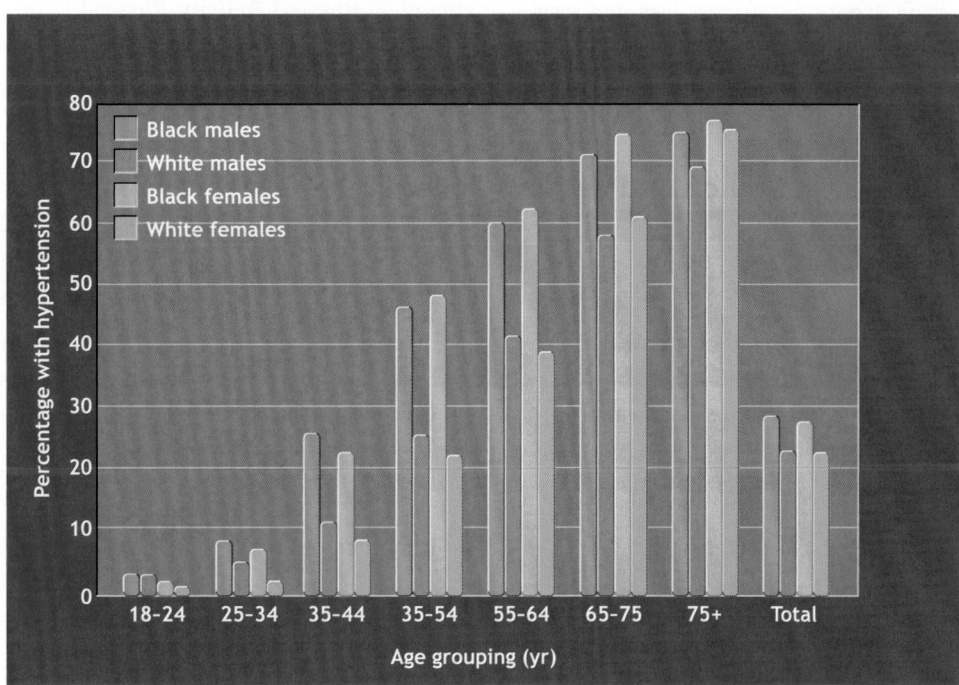

FIGURE 32.5 • Prevalence of hypertension for blacks versus whites for both males and females or different age groupings. (Reprinted with permission from Wolz M, et al. Statement from the National High Blood Pressure Education Program: prevalence of hypertension. *Am J Hypertens* 2000;13:103.)

TABLE 32.5 Classification of Blood Pressure for Adults Age 18 Years and Older

Category[a]	Systolic (MM Hg)	and/or	Diastolic (MM Hg)
Optimal	<120	and	<80
Normal	120–129	and	80–84
High normal	130–139	or	85–89
Hypertension			
Stage 1	140–159	or	90–99
Stage 2	160–179	or	100–109
Stage 3	>180	or	>110

[a]This classification system should be used with individuals not taking anti-hypertensive medication and not acutely ill. When systolic and diastolic blood pressures fall into different categories, the higher category should be used to classify status. For example, 160/92 mm Hg would be stage 2 and 174/120 mm Hg, stage 3.

From the sixth report of the Joint Committee on Prevention, Detection, Evaluation, and Treatment of High Blood Pressure (JNVI), Public Health Service, National Institutes of Health, National Heart, Lung and Blood Institute, NIH Publication No. 98-4080, November 1997.

line of defense to treat mild hypertension (140–159 mm Hg systolic; 90–99 mm Hg diastolic) and moderate hypertension (160–179 mm Hg systolic; 100–109 mm Hg diastolic).

Regular Physical Activity and Hypertension

Systolic and diastolic blood pressures decrease by 6 to 10 mm Hg with aerobic training in previously sedentary men and women regardless of age. Beneficial results occur with normotensive and hypertensive subjects during rest and physical activity.[30,47,57,92,174] Regular physical activity as preventative therapy also controls the tendency for blood pressure to increase over time in individuals at risk for hypertension.[130]

Patients with mild hypertension respond favorably to exercise training, a response also noted among children and adolescents (in the pediatric population).[4,90,103,119] In fact, hypertension medication may be reduced by progressively increasing effort intensity by walking faster each week.[175]

TABLE 32.7 shows that average resting systolic blood pressure decreased from 139 to 133 mm Hg in seven middle-age male patients following 4 to 6 wk of interval training. During submaximal exertion, systolic pressure decreased from 173 to 155 mm Hg, while diastolic pressure decreased from 92 to 79 mm Hg. Training produced approximately a 14% decrease in mean arterial exercise blood pressure. Similar results occurred for an apparently healthy yet borderline hypertensive group of 37 middle-age men following 6 mo of regular aerobic training.[20] For hypertensive older men and women, 9 mo of low-intensity, aerobic activity lowered systolic blood pressure by 20 mm Hg and diastolic pressure by 12 mm Hg.[59] FIGURE 32.6 shows changes in resting blood pressure with aerobic training and 1 mo of detraining in hypertensive older adults who trained at the lactate threshold three to six times a week for 36 wk. Baseline values 3 mo prior to training indicate subjects' blood pressures with normal antihypertensive drug therapy. Regular exercise with continued medication produced decreases of 15 mm Hg in systolic blood pressure, 11 mm Hg in mean arterial pressure, and 9 mm Hg in diastolic blood pressure. Blood pressure returned to pretraining levels within 1 mo for the five subjects who discontinued training. The ACSM's "Position Stand on Physical Activity, Physical Fitness, and Hypertension" can be accessed at www.acsm-msse.org.

TABLE 32.6 Risk Stratification and Recommended Treatment for Hypertension

Blood Pressure Stages (MM Hg)	Risk Group A (No Risk Factors; No TOD[a] or CCD[b])	Risk Group B (One Risk Factor Not Including Diabetes; No TOD or CCD)	Risk Group C (TOD and/or CCD and/or Diabetes, with or Without Other Risk Factors)
High-normal 130–139/85–89	Lifestyle modification	Lifestyle modification	Drug therapy
Stage 1 140–159/90–99	Lifestyle modification	Lifestyle modification	Drug therapy
Stages 2 and 3 >160/>100	Drug therapy	Drug therapy	Drug therapy

A person with diabetes, blood pressure of 142/94 mm Hg, and left-ventricular hypertrophy classifies as having stage 1 hypertension with target organ disease (left-ventricular hypertrophy) and another major risk factor (diabetes). This patient would be classified as stage 1, risk group C, and recommended for immediate drug therapy.

[a]TOD, target organ disease.

[b]CCD, clinical cardiovascular disease.

From the sixth report of the Joint Committee on Prevention, Detection, Evaluation, and Treatment of High Blood Pressure (JNVI), Public Health Service, National Institutes of Health, National Heart, Lung and Blood Institute, NIH Publication No. 98-4080, November 1997.

| TABLE 32.7 | Blood Pressure During Rest and Submaximal Exercise Before and After 4 to 6 Weeks of Training in Seven Middle-Age CHD Patients | | | | | |

| Measure[a] | Rest | | | Submaximal Exercise | | |
| | Average Value | | Difference (%) | Average Value | | Difference (%) |
	Before	After		Before	After	
Systolic blood pressure (mm Hg)	139	133	−4.3	173	155	−10.4
Diastolic blood pressure (mm Hg)	78	73	−6.4	92	79	−14.1
Mean blood pressure (mm Hg)	97	92	−5.2	127	109	−14.3

[a]Intra-arterial catheter.

Adapted from Clausen JP, et al. Physical training in the management of coronary artery disease. *Circulation* 1969;40:143.

The precise mechanism(s) for how regular physical activity lowers blood pressure remains unclear but two contributing factors include the following:

1. Reduced sympathetic nervous system activity with training and possible normalization of arteriole morphology decrease peripheral resistance to blood flow, which lowers blood pressure.[3,128]
2. Altered renal function facilitates the kidneys' elimination of sodium, which subsequently reduces fluid volume and hence blood pressure.

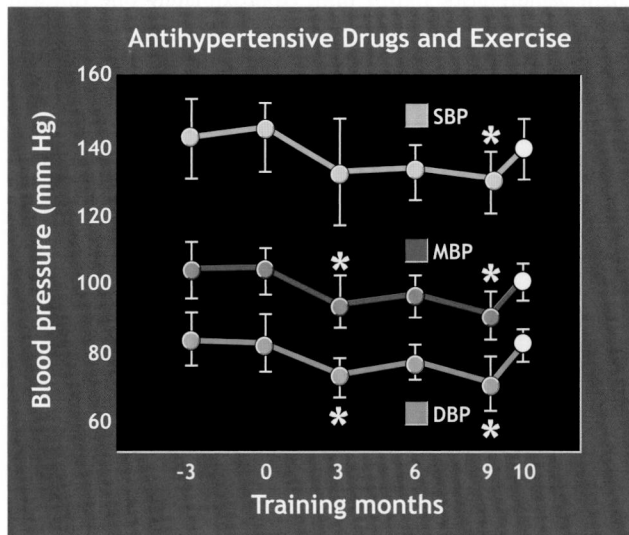

FIGURE 32.6 • Blood pressure changes in older subjects who received hypertensive medication following 9 mo of exercise training at the lactate threshold and after 1 mo of detraining (five subjects). Baseline values 3 mo before training (−3) indicate subjects' blood pressures with their normal antihypertensive drug therapy only. *SBP*, systolic blood pressure; *MBP*, mean blood pressure; *DBP*, diastolic blood pressure; * statistically significant from baseline value. (Reprinted with permission from Motoyama M, et al. Blood pressure lowering effect of low intensity aerobic training in elderly hypertensive patients. *Med Sci Sports Exerc* 1998;30:818.)

Not all research supports physical activity as a strategy to treat hypertension.[25,49] Even when research shows that regular physical activity lowers blood pressure, the studies often have methodologic shortcomings and inadequate design, particularly a lack of appropriate control subjects who have their blood pressure measured but do not exercise. *Despite these limitations, it remains prudent to recommend regular aerobic activity (and proper diet to induce weight loss when necessary) as a first-line strategy to manage borderline hypertension.*[4,84,159]

Improved fitness often neutralizes increased mortality associated with elevated blood pressure. Even if regular physical activity does not return elevated blood pressure to a normal level, aerobic training confers important independent health benefits. Aerobically fit individuals with hypertension achieved a 60% lower mortality rate than unfit normotensive peers.[13] More severe elevations in blood pressure require pharmacologic intervention (over 60 drugs and 30 pill combinations are available for treatment; refer to Fig. 15.10 in Chapter 15).

Chronic Resistance Training Effects on Blood Pressure

Despite the relatively large rise in blood pressure during resistance exercise, long-term resistance training does not elevate resting blood pressure.[24,40,60] Resistance training reduces the typical short-term blood pressure increases during this exercise mode. Trained bodybuilders, for example, show smaller increases in systolic and diastolic blood pressures with resistance exercise than novice bodybuilders and untrained individuals.[40,147] The diminished blood pressure response posttraining becomes most evident when a person exercises at the same absolute load during pretraining and posttraining.[106] Some resistance training protocols lower resting blood pressure,[58,173] but aerobic exercise training (not standard resistance training) confers the greater blood pressure–lowering benefits for hypertensives.[84,85,127] *As a general guideline, resistance training should not serve as the sole activity mode to lower blood pressure in hypertensive individuals.*

Diseases of the Myocardium

Recent advances in molecular biology have isolated a possible genetic link to CHD. The gene, termed the *atherosclerosis susceptibility (ATHS) gene*, appears on chromosome 19 close to the gene that regulates the receptor that removes low-density lipoprotein cholesterol (LDL-C) from the blood. The ATHS gene accounts for nearly 50% of all cases of CHD in the United States.[122] It apparently expresses a set of characteristics—abdominal obesity, low levels of high-density lipoprotein cholesterol (HDL-C), and high levels of LDL-C—that triple a person's risk of myocardial infarction (MI), or heart attack.

thePoint Appendix H, available online at http://the point.lww.com/mkk8e, provides a list of supplemental animations and videos on this subject.

Symptoms rarely present in the early stages of CHD. As the disease progresses and coronary arteries narrow, clinical symptoms become evident and advance with increasing severity. The first sign of CHD is often slight angina pain accompanied by decreased functional capacity. This eventually leads to ischemia (reduced blood flow) and possible myocardial tissue necrosis. In severe cases, the person experiences persistent chest pain, anxiety, nausea, vomiting, and dyspnea. Chronic, untreated angina weakens the myocardium and eventually produces heart failure as cardiac output fails to meet metabolic demands. Pulmonary congestion with a persistent cough often accompanies heart failure. At this stage, the patient becomes dyspneic even when sitting at rest and can suffer a sudden MI.

CHD pathogenesis progresses in five stages:

1. Injury to the endothelial cell wall of the coronary artery
2. Fibroblastic proliferation of the inner lining (intima) of the artery
3. Further obstruction of blood flow as fat accumulates at the junction of the arterial intima and middle lining
4. Cellular degeneration and subsequent formation of hyalin (a translucent, homogeneous substance produced in degeneration) within the arterial intima
5. Calcium deposition at the edges of hyalinated area

The major disorders caused by reduced myocardial blood supply in CHD include angina pectoris, MI, and congestive heart failure.

Angina Pectoris

Chest-related pain, called **angina pectoris**, occurs in approximately 30% of initial

TABLE 32.8	Comparison of Symptoms of Angina Pectoris and Heartburn
Angina Pectoris	**Heartburn**
• Gripping, viselike feelings of pain or pressure behind the breast bone	• Frequent feeling of heartburn
• Pain that radiates to the neck, jaw, back, shoulders, or arms (usually left)	• Frequent use of antacids to relieve pain
• Toothache	• Heartburn that wakes person up at night
• Burning indigestion	• Acid or bitter taste in mouth
• Shortness of breath	• Burning chest sensation
• Nausea	• Discomfort after eating spicy food
• Frequent belching	• Difficulty swallowing

manifestations of CHD. This temporary but painful condition indicates that coronary blood flow and oxygen supply momentarily reach inadequate levels. Current theory suggests that metabolites within an ischemic segment of the heart muscle stimulate myocardial pain receptors. The sensation of angina pectoris includes squeezing, burning, and pressing or choking in the chest region, sensations that often mimic the discomforts of benign heartburn (TABLE 32.8). Anginal pain usually lasts 1 to 3 min. Approximately one third of individuals who experience recurring anginal episodes die suddenly from an MI. Chronic stable angina (often called *walk-through angina*) occurs at a predictable level of physical exertion. Drugs that promote coronary artery vasodilation and reduce systemic peripheral vascular resistance (e.g., nitroglycerin) commonly treat this condition. FIGURE 32.7 illustrates the usual pain pattern with an acute episode of angina pectoris. Pain generally appears in the left shoulder along the arm to the elbow or occasionally in the midback region near the left scapula along the spinal cord.

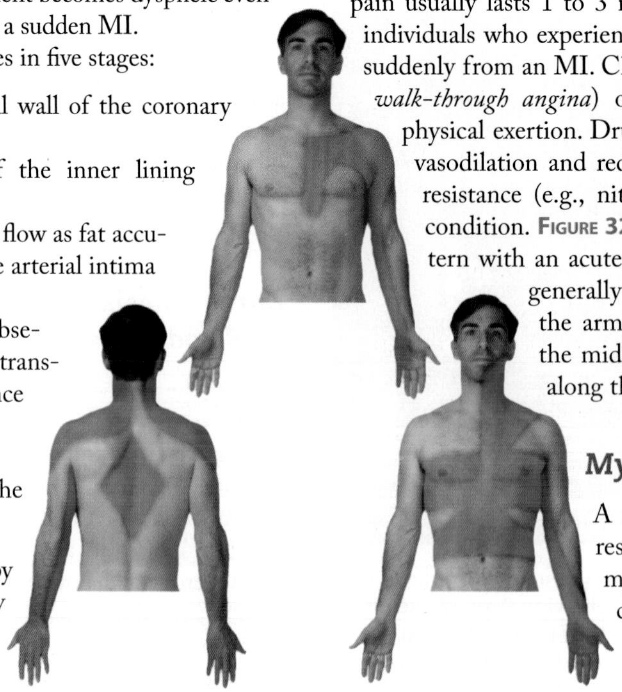

Myocardial Infarction

A **myocardial infarction (MI)** can result from sudden insufficiency in myocardial blood flow, usually from coronary artery occlusion. A prior clot or thrombus formed from plaque accumulation in one or more coronary vessels (see Chapter 31) can trigger sudden occlusion. Severe fatigue for several days without specific pain frequently precedes the onset of MI. FIGURE 32.8

FIGURE 32.7 • Locations for pain generally associated with angina pectoris. Pain of cardiac origin, although usually referred to the left side, may be referred to the right side, both sides, or midback. (Reprinted with permission from Moore KL, Dalley AF, Agur AMR. *Clinically Oriented Anatomy*. 7th Ed. Baltimore: Wolters Kluwer Health, 2014.)

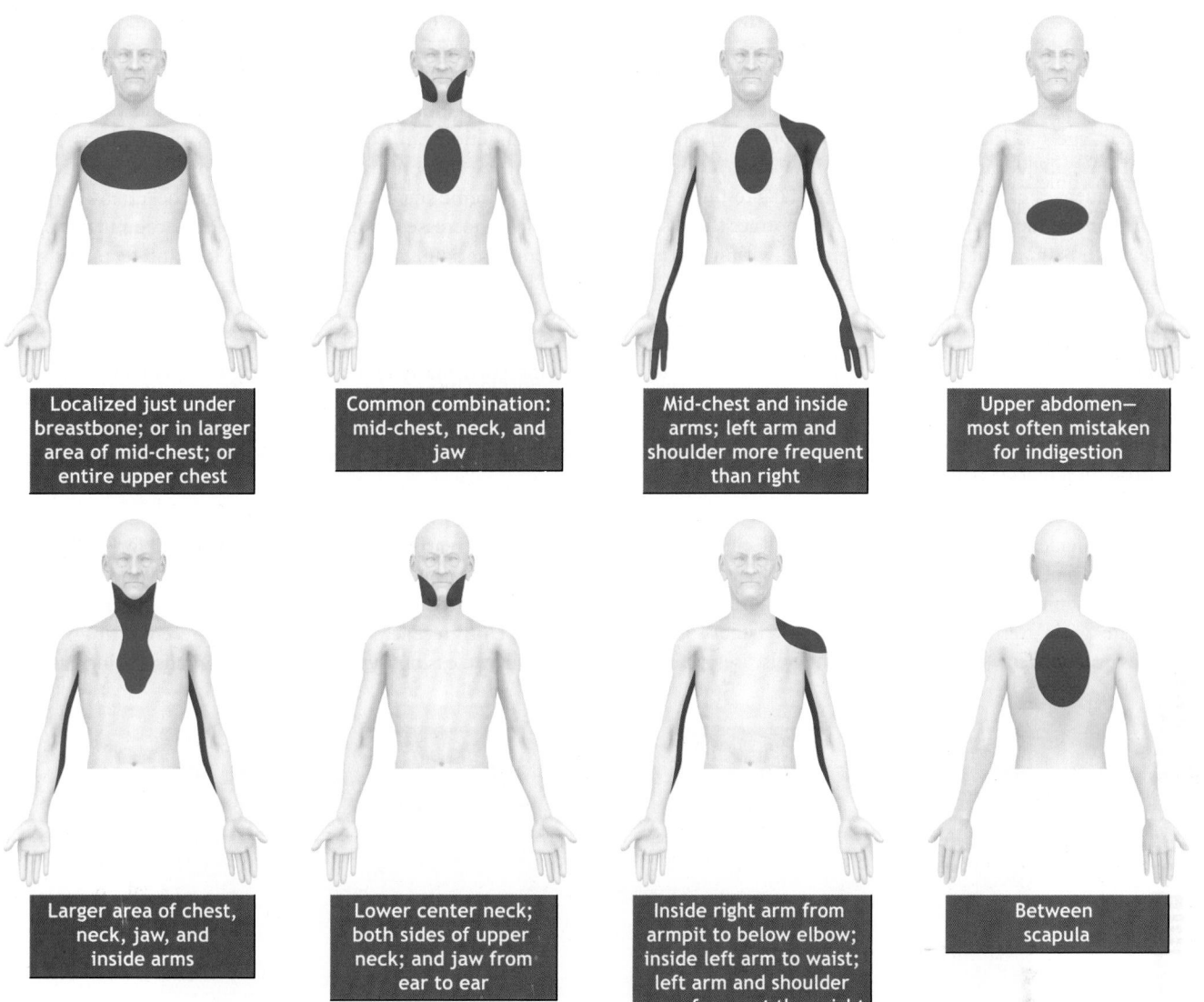

FIGURE 32.8 • Anatomic locations for early warning signs of myocardial infarction. Note the diverse locations for pain.

shows the varied locations for pain and discomfort that represent early warning of an MI. During the infarction, severe, unrelenting chest pain can persist for more than 1 hr.

Congestive Heart Failure

More than 5 million Americans and 22 million people globally have **congestive heart failure**. In congestive heart failure (CHF; chronic decompensation or heart failure), the heart fails to pump adequately to meet other organ needs. This causes fluid to back up into the lungs, which can leave the patient struggling to breathe. CHF results from one or all of the following seven factors:

1. Narrowed arteries from CHD that limit myocardial blood supply
2. Past MI with accompanying scar tissue (necrosis) that diminishes myocardial pumping efficiency

3. Chronic hypertension
4. Heart valve disease from past rheumatic fever or other pathology
5. Primary disease of the myocardium, called *cardiomyopathy*
6. Defects present in the heart at birth (*congenital heart disease*)
7. Infection of heart valves and/or myocardium (*endocarditis or myocarditis*)

A "failing" heart keeps pumping, but inefficiently. Heart failure produces shortness of breath and fatigue upon minimal exertion. As blood flowing from the heart slows, blood returning to the heart through the veins backs up, causing fluid to accumulate in the lungs and edema in legs and ankles. When fluid collects in the lungs, it interferes with breathing and causes shortness of breath, especially when lying supine. CHF also affects the kidneys' disposal of sodium and water, further accentuating edema.

See the animation "Edema" on http://thePoint.lww. com/mkk8e for a demonstration of this process.

CHF is the leading cause for hospitalization of persons older than age 65. It is responsible for more than 800,000 hospital stays, including many repeat visits. FIGURE 32.9 shows the consequences of CHF when the heart fails to pump adequately. For the most part, CHF patients contract the disease before age 60 and about 20% of patients die within 1 year of diagnosis. Nearly half die within 5 years.

CHF usually develops slowly as the heart gradually weakens and performs less effectively. Three primary causes of CHF include:

1. Chronic hypertension
2. Intrinsic myocardial disease
3. Structural defects (e.g., diseased heart valves)

These three conditions produce an oversized, misshapen heart with inadequate pump performance reflected by a low resting left-ventricular ejection fraction (LVEF)—a marker of life-threatening heart dysfunction—and failure to increase heart rate with exercise.[43,82] Associated risk factors include diabetes, alcoholism, and chronic lung diseases such as emphysema. CHF symptoms produce extreme disability, but symptom intensity frequently bears little relation to disease severity.[5,129] Patients with a low LVEF may not exhibit symptoms, while individuals whose hearts demonstrate normal pump function can experience severe disability. Heart disease and chronic hypertension contribute to disease progression. At the extreme stage, cardiac output from the left and/or right ventricles decreases to an extent that blood accumulates in the abdomen and lungs and sometimes in legs and feet. This stage of CHF produces fatigue, shortness of breath, and eventual flooding of the alveoli with blood, a condition termed *pulmonary congestion*. Impaired blood flow may also damage other organs, particularly kidneys, resulting in renal failure.

 See the animation "Congestive Heart Failure" on http://thePoint.lww.com/mkk8e for a demonstration of this process.

CHF Treatment and Rehabilitation. Before the 1980s, rest was advocated for all stages of CHF as the immediate treatment to reduce stress on the compromised cardiovascular system. Until recently, patients routinely received drugs aimed primarily at easing symptoms (e.g., digitalis to increase the

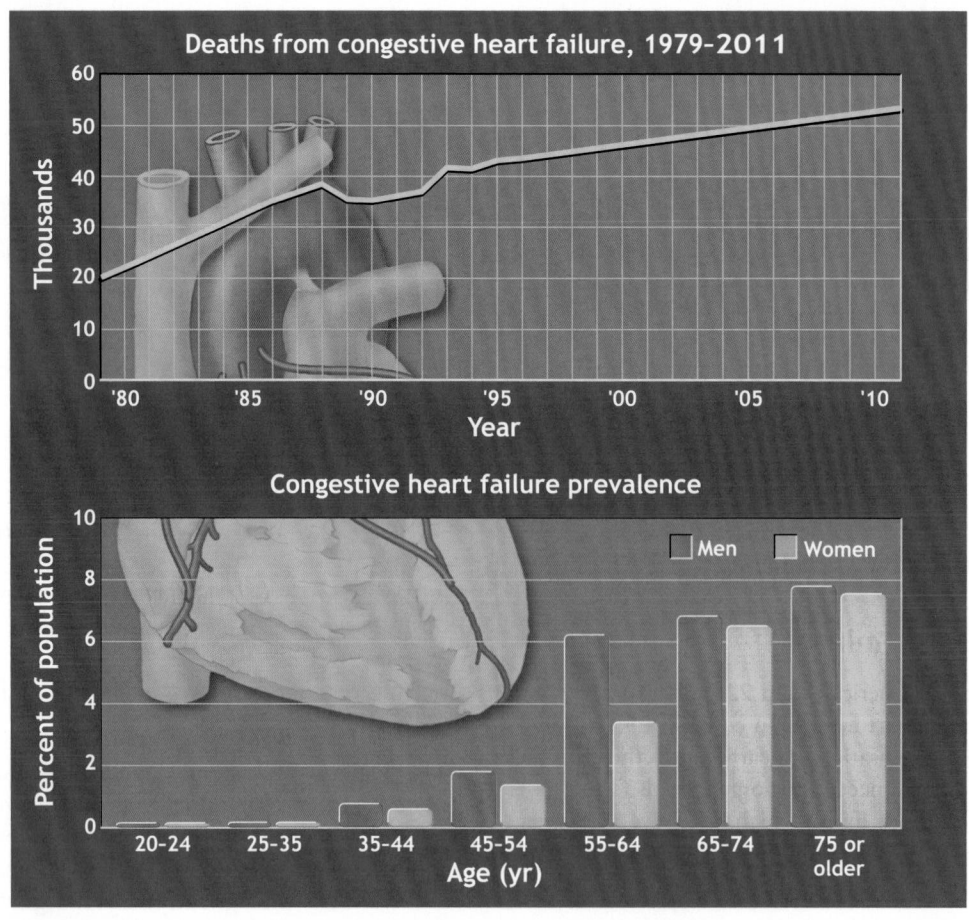

FIGURE 32.9 • Consequences of congestive heart failure (CHF) from impaired pumping ability of either the right or left heart or both. The prevalence of and deaths from CHF increase with age; nearly one third (1.4 million) contract the disease before age 60 years. (Data from National Center for Health Statistics and American Heart Association, 2000; heart image adapted with permission from Moore KL, Dalley AF, Agur AMR. *Clinically Oriented Anatomy*. 7th Ed. Baltimore: Wolters Kluwer Health, 2014.)

heart's pumping function, called the inotropic effect). Current recommendations promote a four-drug regimen with two traditional drugs, digitalis and a diuretic to increase fluid excretion by kidneys, with newer angiotensin-converting enzyme (ACE) inhibitors and β-blockers. Fifty years ago, Sir James Whyte Black (1924–2010), Scottish physician and pharmacologist who established the physiology department at the University of Glasgow, reported the first clinically significant β-blockers—propranolol and pronethalol—for medical management of angina pectoris. Read about β-blockers online at http://www.healthline.com/health/heart-disease/beta-blockers.

Surgical treatment replaces damaged heart valves or repairs myocardial aneurysms—bulging areas that form on the myocardial wall. Cardiac transplantation represents the extreme treatment of progressive disability from CHF, yet the shortage of donor organs persists. For patients awaiting a transplant, electrically powered pump implants placed in the abdomen below the heart mechanically assist ventricular function.

CHF and Regular Physical Activity. Clinicians have reevaluated the role of regular physical activity because many of the functional deteriorations in CHF duplicate those that accompany extreme physical deconditioning. Reduced physical fitness and intrinsic changes in skeletal muscle exacerbate the patient's physical incapacity.[55] Current therapy advocates regular activity as an effective adjunct in CHF rehabilitation.[61,101,120]

Clinical practice indicates that regular, moderate physical activity formulated from a symptom-limited GXT with medications benefits relatively low-risk, stable, compensated patients.[33,112,142,163,177] Even intense endurance and resistance-exercise training increases cardiac function, physical capacity, and peripheral muscle function and quality of life in CHF patients.[38] Physical activity benefits often accrue independent of the degree of baseline left-ventricular dysfunction.[2] These benefits include improvements in functional capacity, exercise tolerance, muscle metabolism, level for dyspnea and ventilatory response to exertion, risk for arrhythmias, left-ventricular function, quality of life, and shift toward greater dominance of vagal (parasympathetic) tone.

It remains controversial whether the benefits of exercise rehabilitation for CHF link directly to enhanced central circulatory function—either improved myocardial performance per se or disease reversal reflected by reduced heart size.[10,43,61] To a large extent, peripheral adaptations with regular activity enhance function and foster symptomatic improvements.

The clinician supervises an physical activity program for compensated patients with controlled fluid volume status and absence of unstable or exercise-induced ventricular arrhythmias. The GXT provides the basis for the exercise prescription. For patients with marked exercise intolerance, relatively brief intervals of 2 to 5 min of light activity with 1 to 3 min of recovery afford benefits. The prescription also includes multiple exercise sessions interspersed throughout the day. Because of the usually abnormal heart-rate response in CHF patients, exercising at between 40 and 60% $\dot{V}O_{2peak}$ provides a more objective standard to establish initial intensity

of effort. Alternatively, a rating of perceived exertion (RPE) on the Borg scale of "light" to "somewhat hard" (see Fig. 21.19 in Chapter 21) and/or 2 on the dyspnea scale ("mild, some difficulty"; see Fig. 32.18) generally proves effective. Supervisory personnel should recognize the six warning symptoms of cardiac decompensation:

1. Dyspnea
2. Hypotension
3. Cough
4. Angina
5. Lightheadedness
6. Arrhythmias

After the patient begins to increase physical activity, exercise duration can increase to 20 to 40 min at least three times weekly. Following 6 to 12 wk of supervised activity, patients usually can undertake an unsupervised home exercise program.

Aneurysm

Aneurysm describes an abnormal dilation in the wall of an artery, vein, or cardiac chamber. Vascular aneurysms develop when a vessel wall weakens from trauma, congenital vascular disease, infection, or atherosclerosis. Aneurysms are either arterial or venous according to their specific regions of origin (e.g., thoracic aneurysm). Most aneurysms develop without symptoms and often are discovered during a routine x-ray. The most common symptoms include chest pain with a specific palpable, pulsating mass in the chest, abdomen, or lower back.

Heart Valve Diseases

Three medical conditions relate to heart valve abnormalities:

1. **Stenosis**: Narrowing or constriction that prevents heart valves from opening fully; may result from growths, scars, or abnormal calcified deposits
2. **Insufficiency** (also called regurgitation): Occurs when a heart valve closes improperly and blood moves back into a heart chamber
3. **Prolapse**: Occurs when enlarged valve leaflets in the mitral valve bulge backward into the left atrium during ventricular systole

Valvular abnormalities increase the heart's workload, causing it to pump harder to propel blood through a stenosed valve or to maintain cardiac output if blood seeps backward into one of its chambers during diastole. Rheumatic fever, a serious group A streptococcal bacterial infection, scars and deforms heart valves. The most common symptoms include fever and joint pain. Penicillin and other antibiotics treat this inflammatory condition, which typically occurs in children 5 to 15 years old.

Cardiac Nervous System Diseases

Cardiac diseases that affect the heart's electrical conduction system include the following: dysrhythmias (arrhythmias) that cause the heart to beat too rapidly (**tachycardia**), too slowly (**bradycardia**), or with extra contractions (**ectopic**, **extrasystole**, or **premature ventricular contractions** or PVCs) that possibly lead to fibrillation. Dysrhythmias can produce changes in circulatory dynamics that cause hypotension (extremely low blood pressure), heart failure, and shock. They often occur after a stroke induced by increased physical exertion or other stressful conditions.

Sinus tachycardia describes a resting heart rate *above* 100 b·min⁻¹; *bradycardia* describes a resting heart rate *below* 60 b·min⁻¹. Sinus bradycardia occurs frequently in endurance athletes and young adults and generally represents a benign dysrhythmia; it may benefit cardiac function by producing a longer ventricular filling time during the cardiac cycle.

ASSESSING CARDIAC DISEASE

Before initiating an intervention program of physical activity, the healthcare team decides on the health screening necessary. This always includes a medical history, physical examination, and various laboratory assessments, and pertinent physiologic testing.

Purpose of Health Screening and Risk Stratification

Assessment of specific risk factors and/or symptoms for chronic cardiovascular, pulmonary, and metabolic diseases optimizes safety during exercise testing and program participation. Proper preparticipation screening accomplishes the following three goals:

1. Identifies and excludes persons with medical contraindications to physical activity
2. Identifies persons who require in-depth medical evaluation because of age, symptoms, and/or risk factors
3. Identifies persons with clinically significant disease who require medical supervision when exercising

Before beginning a physical conditioning program, the ACSM recommends that age, health status, symptoms, and risk factor information classify individuals into one of three risk strata to ensure their safety (see ACSM Risk Stratification inset, below).[5] Proper risk stratification provides a basis to recommend further testing, medical assessment, or diagnostic interventions before exercise participation. "In a Practical Sense: Par-Q to Assess Readiness for Physical Activity,"

IN A PRACTICAL SENSE

Par-Q to Assess Readiness for Physical Activity

ORIGINAL PAR-Q

Common sense is your best guide in answering these questions. Please read each question carefully and check yes or no if it applies to you.

The Physical Activity Readiness Questionnaire (Par-Q) has been recommended as minimal screening for entry into moderate-intensity exercise programs. Par-Q was designed to identify the small number of adults for whom physical activity might be inappropriate or those who should receive medical advice concerning the most suitable type of activity.

YES ___ NO ___ 1. Has your doctor ever said that you have heart trouble?

YES ___ NO ___ 2. Do you frequently have pains in your heart and chest?

YES ___ NO ___ 3. Do you often feel faint or have spells of severe dizziness?

YES ___ NO ___ 4. Has a doctor ever said your blood pressure was too high?

YES ___ NO ___ 5. Has your doctor told you that you have a bone or joint problem that has been aggravated by exercise or might be made worse with exercise?

YES ___ NO ___ 6. Is there a good physical reason not mentioned here why you should not follow an activity program even if you wanted to?

YES ___ NO ___ 7. Are you over age 65 and not accustomed to vigorous exercise?

IF YOU ANSWERED YES TO ONE OR MORE QUESTIONS:

If you have not recently done so, consult with your personal physician by telephone or in person BEFORE increasing your physical activity and/or taking a fitness test. Show your doctor a copy of this quiz. After medical evaluation, seek advice from your physician as to your suitability for:

- Unrestricted physical activity, probably on a gradually increasing basis
- Restricted or supervised activity to meet your specific needs, at least on an initial basis; check in your community for special programs or services

IF YOU ANSWERED NO TO ALL QUESTIONS:

If you answered no honestly to all Par-Q questions, you have reasonable assurance of your present suitability for:

- A graduated exercise program—a gradual increase in proper exercise promotes good fitness development while minimizing or eliminating discomfort
- An exercise test—simple tests of fitness (such as the Canadian Home Fitness Test) or more complex types may be undertaken if you so desire
- Postpone exercising—if you have a temporary minor illness, such as a common cold, postpone any exercise program

IN A PRACTICAL SENSE *(continued)*

PAR-Q (REVISED 1994)

One limitation of the original Par-Q was that about 20% of potential exercisers failed the test—many of these exclusions were unnecessary because subsequent evaluations showed that the individuals were apparently healthy. The revised Par-Q (rPar-Q) was developed to reduce the number of unnecessary exclusions (false positives). The revision can determine the exercise readiness of apparently healthy middle-age adults with no more than one major risk factor for coronary heart disease.

YES ___ NO ___ 1. Has your doctor ever said that you have a heart condition and recommended only medically supervised activity?

YES ___ NO ___ 2. Do you have chest pain brought on by physical activity?

YES ___ NO ___ 3. Have you developed chest pain in the past month?

YES ___ NO ___ 4. Do you lose your balance because of dizziness, or do you ever lose consciousness?

YES ___ NO ___ 5. Do you have a bone or joint problem that could be worsened by a change in your physical activity?

YES ___ NO ___ 6. Is your doctor currently prescribing drugs (for example, water pills) for high blood pressure or a heart condition?

YES ___ NO ___ 7. Do you know of any other reason why you should not do physical activity?

Note: Postpone testing if you have a temporary illness such as a common cold or are not feeling well.

IF YOU ANSWERED YES TO ONE OR MORE QUESTIONS:

Talk with your doctor by phone or in person before you start becoming much more physically active or before you have a fitness appraisal. Tell your doctor about the rPar-Q and which questions you answered with yes.

- You may be able to do any activity you want—as long as you start slowly and build up gradually. Or, you may need to restrict your activities to those that are safe for you. Talk with your doctor about the kinds of activities you wish to participate in and follow his or her advice.
- Find out which community programs are safe and helpful for you.

IF YOU ANSWERED NO TO ALL QUESTIONS:

If you answered no honestly to all rPar-Q questions, you can be reasonably sure that you can:

- Start becoming much more physically active—begin slowly and build up gradually; this is the safest and easiest way to go
- Take part in a fitness appraisal—this is an excellent way to determine your basic fitness so that you can plan the best way for you to live actively.

Delay becoming much more active:

- If you are not feeling well because of a temporary cold or fever—wait until you feel better, or
- If you are or may be pregnant—talk to your doctor before you start becoming more active.

Please note: If your health changes so that you then answer yes to any of the above questions, tell your fitness or health professional. Ask whether you should change your physical activity plan.

Source: *Par-Q and You.* Gloucester, Ontario: Canadian Society for Exercise Physiology, 1994.

 ## ACSM Risk Stratification for Beginning an Exercise Program

Low risk	Men <45 years Women <55 years Asymptomatic with ≤1 risk factor[a,b]
Moderate risk	Men ≥45 years Women ≥55 years Or with ≥2 risk factors[a,b]
High risk	Individuals with ≥1 sign/symptom of cardiovascular or pulmonary disease[c] or known cardiovascular (cardiac, peripheral vascular, or cerebrovascular), pulmonary (obstructive pulmonary disease, asthma, cystic fibrosis), or metabolic (diabetes, thyroid disorder, renal, or liver) disease

[a]Risk factors: family history of heart disease, cigarette smoking, hypertension, hypercholesterolemia, impaired fasting glucose, obesity, sedentary lifestyle.
[b]HDL ≥60 mg · dL^{-1} (subtract one risk factor from the sum of other risk factors because high HDL decreases CHD risk).
[c]Signs/symptoms of cardiovascular and pulmonary disease: pain, discomfort in chest, neck, jaw, left arm; shortness of breath at rest or with mild exertion; dizziness or syncope; orthopnea or paroxysmal nocturnal dyspnea; ankle edema; tachycardia; intermittent claudication; heart murmur; unusual fatigue or shortness of breath with mild activity.
Source: *ACSM's Guidelines for Exercise Testing and Prescription.* 9th Ed. Baltimore, Lippincott Williams & Wilkins, 2013.

TABLE 32.9   Diagnosis of Chest Pain

Pain/Complaint/Findings	Possible Causes	Stimuli	Possible Pathology
Pressure, ache, tightness or burning in midsternum, left shoulder, arm; sweating; nausea; vomiting; S–T segment changes	MI	Exertion; cold; smoking; heavy meal; fluid overload	CHD
Sharp pain worsens with inspiration, improves with sitting	Inflammation	Acute MI	Pericarditis
Chest tightness with breathlessness; low-grade fever	Infection	IV drug use; microbes	Myocarditis; endocarditis
Sharp, stabbing pain; breathlessness; cough; loss of consciousness	Pulmonary	Recent surgery	Pulmonary embolism
Burning pain; indigestion relieved by antacids	Referred pain	Heavy meal, spicy food	Esophageal reflux
Angina pain; breathlessness; wide pulse pressure; ventricular hypertrophy on ECG	Ventricular outflow tract obstruction	Exertion; CHD	Aortic stenosis; mitral valve prolapse

in this chapter provides the Physical Activity Readiness Questionnaire (Par-Q), commonly used as a minimal first-pass, preparticipation screening tool.

Patient History

A thorough patient history, including past and current medical problems, documents the most common patient complaints and establishes the CHD risk profile. Most CHD symptoms include chest pain, so the differential diagnosis of this pain is a primary focus. TABLE 32.9 lists symptoms, possible causes, and related pathology of chest pain. A patient history typically includes the following nine entries:

1. Medical diagnosis of diseases
2. Previous physical examination findings to uncover abnormalities
3. Recent illnesses, hospitalizations, or surgical procedures
4. History of significant symptoms
5. Orthopedic concerns
6. Medications
7. Work record
8. Family background
9. Psychologic record

Physical Examination

The physical examination includes vital signs (body temperature, heart rate, breathing rate, and blood pressure) and possible indications of problems. Assessments encompass auscultation of lungs; palpation and inspection of lower extremities for edema; tests of neurologic function (reflexes and cognition); and inspection of the skin, especially of the lower extremities in diabetics. Resting cardiorespiratory variables sometimes provide indirect, noninvasive clues to cardiovascular dysfunction. For example, sinus tachycardia or abnormal bradycardia and increased breathing rate and systolic blood pressure can contraindicate exercise without further evaluation.

The clinical exercise physiologist assesses the patient's heart rate and blood pressure response to graded exercise in order to prescribe physical activity and identify potential warning signs. For example, a systolic blood pressure increase of 20 mm Hg or more with low-intensity exercise of 2 to 4 METs often reflects abnormal myocardial oxygen demand that signals some form of cardiovascular impairment. Similarly, failure of systolic blood pressure to increase (hypotensive response) can indicate blunted ventricular function; a depressed response intense activity (e.g., failure to achieve systolic blood pressures above 140 mm Hg) frequently indicates the presence of dormant cardiac disease.

Heart Auscultation

Listening to heart sounds (auscultation) during the cardiac cycle can assess cardiac performance. The exercise physiologist should become familiar with the different abnormal heart sounds and learn to identify associated murmurs (www.wilkes.med.ucla.edu/intro.html). Auscultation can uncover valvular conditions (e.g., MVP, diagnosed by click-murmur sounds) and congenital heart abnormalities (regurgitation sounds in ventricular septal defects; http://filer.case.edu/dck3/heart/listen.html).

Laboratory Tests

Laboratory studies with chest x-ray, electrocardiogram (ECG), blood lipid and lipoprotein analyses, and serum enzyme testing help to assess the extent of CHD.

The chest x-ray reveals the size and shape of the heart and lungs, whereas resting and exercise ECGs assess myocardial electrical conductivity and degree of oxygenation. Clinical exercise physiologists require considerable experience reading and interpreting ECGs. Chapter 31 discusses various ECG abnormalities and atypical physiologic responses to exercise. Careful ECG monitoring during a

TABLE 32.10   Normal and Abnormal ECG Changes During Exercise

Normal ECG Response in Healthy Individuals	Abnormal ECG Response with CHD
1. Slight increase in P wave amplitude	1. Appearance of bundle branch block at a critical HR
2. Shortening of P–R interval	2. Recurrent or multifocal PVCs during exercise and recovery
3. Shift to the right of QRS axis	3. Ventricular tachycardia
4. S–T segment depression <1.0 mm	4. Appearance of bradyarrhythmias, tachyarrhythmias
5. Decreased T-wave amplitude	5. S–T segment depression/elevation of >1.0 mm 0.08 s after J point
6. Single or rare PVCs during exercise and recovery	6. Exercise bradycardia
7. Single or rare PVCs or PACs	7. Submaximal exercise tachycardia
	8. Increase in frequency or severity of any known arrhythmia

PVC, premature ventricular contraction; PAC, premature atrial contraction.

GXT provides more extensive evaluation to target individuals with possible CHD. Table 32.10 presents common ECG changes during exercise in healthy persons and anomalies associated with abnormal ECG responses with CHD.

Alterations in serum enzymes often confirm the existence of an acute MI. With myocardial cell death (necrosis) or prolonged ischemia, the following three cardiac muscle enzymes leak into the blood from increased plasma membrane permeability:

1. Creatine phosphokinase (CPK)
2. Lactate dehydrogenase (LDH)
3. Serum glutamic oxaloacetic transaminase (SGOT)

Elevated CPK levels reflect either skeletal or cardiac muscle fiber damage. To pinpoint the source of the enzyme leak, electrophoresis or radioimmunoassay analysis separates CPK into three different isoenzymes: MM-isoenzyme, unique to skeletal muscle; BB-isoenzyme, specific to brain tissue; and MB-isoenzyme, specific for cardiac muscle necrosis. LDH fractionates into different isoenzymes (as does CPK), one of which increases during an MI. An acute MI also raises SGOT. Additional blood tests for CHD diagnosis include serum homocysteine (see Chapter 31), lipoprotein (a), fibrinogen, tissue-type plasminogen activator (tPA), and C-reactive protein (CRP).

Invasive Physiologic Tests

Invasive cardiovascular testing provides information unattainable through noninvasive procedures. This includes the extent, severity, and location of coronary atherosclerosis, degree of ventricular dysfunction, and specific cardiac abnormalities.

Radionuclide Studies. Radionuclide studies require injecting a radioactive isotope (e.g., mostly technetium-99) into the circulation during rest and exercise (http://my.clevelandclinic.org/services/radionuclide_scanning/hic_radionuclide_scanning_nuclear_medicine_scanning.aspx). Two examples include:

1. **Thallium imaging**: Evaluates areas of myocardial blood flow and tissue perfusion to differentiate between a true-positive and false-positive S–T segment depression obtained by ECG evaluation during a GXT

2. **Nuclear ventriculography**: Radiographic imaging procedure that analyzes regional left-ventricular contractility following injection of radioactive isotope contrast material

Pharmacologic Stress Testing. A pharmacologic stress test benefits individuals unable to undergo routine exercise stress testing because of extreme deconditioning, peripheral vascular disease, orthopedic disabilities, neurologic disease, or other health problems. This test involves systematic intravenous drug infusion (e.g., dobutamine, dipyridamole, or adenosine) every 3 min until the patient receives the appropriate dosage. Echocardiography and/or thallium scanning then monitor for changes in wall motion abnormalities or coronary perfusion limitations, respectively. Heart rate response, arrhythmias, angina symptoms, S–T segment depression, and blood pressure dynamics also reflect myocardial viability during a pharmacologic stress test.

Cardiac Catheterization. A fine tube or catheter inserted into a vein or artery passes into the heart's right or left side. The intracardiac catheter can sample blood, assess pressure differentials within the heart's chambers or vessels, and add contrast media to evaluate cardiac function.

Coronary Angiography. Radiography images the coronary circulation by injecting a contrast medium, essentially a dye, that flows into the coronary vasculature. The technique, highly effective to evaluate the extent of coronary atherosclerosis, serves as the gold standard to assess coronary blood flow and provides the baseline for other test comparisons. Unlike thallium imaging, angiography cannot determine how easily blood flows within portions of the myocardium and cannot be applied during exercise. The angiogram shown in Figure 32.10 pinpoints impaired blood flow (see circle drawn around occluded part of the vessel) in the carotid artery (shown in red). Resectioning a vessel or removing its atherosclerotic plaques improves blood flow to reduce stroke occurrence.

 See the animations "Coronary Angiography: Left Coronary System-Part A" and "Coronary Angiography: Left Coronary System-Part B" on http://thePoint.lww.com/mkk8e for a demonstration of this process.

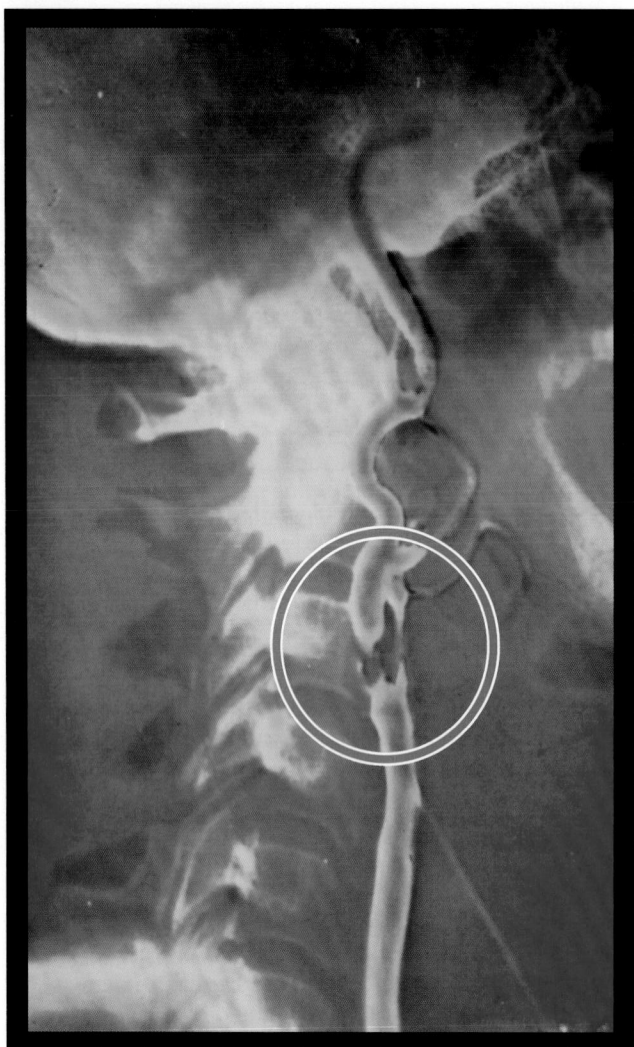

FIGURE 32.10 • Angiogram showing constriction and absence of blood flow through the right carotid artery (*in red*). (Courtesy of Dr. Barry Franklin, Beaumont Hospital, Birmingham, MI.)

thePoint Appendix H, available online at http://thepoint.lww.com/mkk8e, provides a list of supplemental animations and videos on this subject, including an animation of angiography.

Noninvasive Physiologic Tests

Echocardiography. Pulses of reflected ultrasound (echo) assess the functional and structural characteristics of the myocardium. Ultrasound (high-frequency sound waves) identifies the heart's anatomic components during a cardiac cycle and measures their distances from the echo transducers to accurately estimate heart chamber and vessel size and myocardial wall thickness. Echocardiograms diagnose heart murmurs, evaluate valvular lesions, and quantify congenital defects and myopathies. The echocardiogram is preferred to the ECG for recognizing chamber enlargement, inefficient ventricular contractility, myocardial hypertrophy, and other structural abnormalities.

Ultrafast CT Scan. This 10-min, noninvasive test uses an ultrafast electron beam computed tomographic (EBCT) scan to assess calcium deposition within plaque in coronary artery linings (www.hopkinsmedicine.org/healthlibrary/test_procedures/cardiovascular/ultrafast_computed_tomography_ultrafast_ct_scan_92,P07987/). Test results determine how aggressively to treat blood lipid abnormalities (e.g., diet and physical activity vs. drug therapy) and other CHD risk factors. Testing to detect coronary calcium deposition with EBCT is highly sensitive in men and women with coronary disease validated by coronary angiography.[56] Exclusion of coronary calcium buildup helps to characterize individuals with a low probability of significant stenosis.

Graded Exercise Stress Testing. *The graded exercise stress test (GXT) evaluates the cardiac function under conditions that exceed resting requirements in defined, progressive increments to increase myocardial workload.* The GXT also objectifies the functional capacity of patients with known disease and evaluates progress following surgery or other therapeutic interventions.

TABLE 32.11 presents subjective and objective information obtained during a GXT for designing an exercise prescription.

TABLE 32.11	**Data from an Exercise Stress Test to Diagnose and Formulate an Exercise Prescription**

Subjective data
- Angina pain
- Dyspnea ratings
- Fatigue and weakness
- Leg discomfort
- Dizziness
- Rating of perceived exertion (RPE)

Objective data
- **Physical examination data**
  - Breathing sounds
  - Murmurs and gallops
  - Blood pressure
  - Pulmonary function tests (before or after exercise)
  - Heart rate response
  - Blood gas parameters
  - Rate-pressure product (RPP = HR X systolic blood pressure)
- **Physical performance data**
  - Time on treadmill/cycle ergometer
  - Maximum work or power output
- **Electrocardiogram data**
  - S–T segment changes
  - Rate responses
  - Dysrhythmias
  - Conduction abnormalities
- **Cardiorespiratory data**
  - Lactate threshold
  - Carbon dioxide output
  - Minute ventilation
  - Oxygen consumption
  - Respiratory exchange ratio (R)

The cardiologist and exercise physiologist supervise the exercise test, interpret the data, and prescribe the appropriate exercise intervention.

Prudent Pre-exercise Evaluation

For a sedentary person with undetected CHD, a sudden burst of strenuous physical activity can inordinately strain cardiovascular function. Medical evaluation before initiating an activity program reduces this risk considerably. A GXT provides a crucial component of the medical evaluation.

The term *GXT* generally describes the systematic use of exercise for the following four purposes:

1. ECG observations
2. Evaluating patients with exertional discomfort
3. Determining pharmacologic and therapeutic treatment strategies
4. Evaluating physiologic adjustments to increasing metabolic demands to objectify physical activity recommendations

Multistage bicycle and treadmill tests represent the most common stress testing modes. These tests, graded for intensity, usually include several levels of 3 to 5 min of submaximal effort that bring the person to a self-imposed fatigue level or end point. The graded nature of testing allows intensity to increase in small increments to pinpoint ischemic manifestations and rhythm disorders such as anginal pain or ECG abnormalities. With heart disease, exercise testing provides a reliable, quantitative index of the person's functional impairment; this objectifies the diagnosis and subsequent exercise prescription.[45] Testing generally does not require maximal effort, but the person should attain at least 85% of age-predicted maximum heart rate.

Exercise stress testing cannot show the extent of CHD or its specific location. Twenty-five to 40% of people with relatively advanced CHD with significant blockage in one or more coronary arteries achieve a normal GXT evaluation. Interestingly, an abnormal heart rate recovery (i.e., failure of heart rate to decrease by more than 12 b · min^{-1} in the first minute after peak exercise) predicts, independent of ECG assessment, subsequent mortality in patients referred specifically for exercise electrocardiography.[121] This indicates that recovery heart rate provides additional prognostic information to complement interpretation of the exercise stress test.

Reasons for Stress Testing

Stress testing serves the following six functions in a CHD evaluation:

1. *Diagnoses overt heart disease and screens for "silent" coronary disease in seemingly healthy adults.* Approximately 30% of persons with confirmed CHD have a normal resting ECG. Graded exercise testing generally uncovers 70% of the abnormalities.
2. *Assesses exercise-related chest symptoms.* For individuals older than age 40 who suffer chest or related pain in the left shoulder or arm during physical exertion, ECG analysis identifies myocardial abnormalities and more precisely diagnoses exercise-induced pain.
3. *Screens candidates for entry into preventative and cardiac rehabilitative exercise programs.* Test results provide an objective framework to design a program based on current functional capacity and health status. Repeat testing assesses progress and adaptations to regular exercise and provides for program modification.
4. *Uncovers abnormal blood pressure responses.* Individuals with normal resting blood pressure sometimes show greater than normal increases in systolic blood pressure during mild-to-moderate activity, which may signify developing cardiovascular complications.
5. *Monitors effectiveness of therapeutic interventions (drug, surgical, dietary) to improve heart disease status and cardiovascular function.* A patient's capacity to achieve a target heart rate without complications often confirms success of coronary bypass surgery.
6. *Quantifies functional aerobic capacity ($\dot{V}O_{2peak}$) to evaluate its deviation from normal standards.*

 INTEGRATIVE QUESTION

Give recommendations for a middle-age man who experiences breathlessness and chest discomfort while walking the golf course yet wants to begin an aerobic activity program.

Who Requires Stress Testing?

TABLE 32.12 outlines screening and supervisory procedures for exercise testing that conform to policies and practices of the ACSM and the AMA.

Informed Consent

All testing and exercise training must be performed on "informed" volunteers. **Informed consent** should raise the subject's awareness about all potential participation risks. It must include a written statement that the person had an opportunity to ask questions about the procedures, with sufficient information clearly stated so that consent occurs from a knowledgeable (informed) perspective. A legal guardian or parent must sign the consent form for minors. Individuals need assurance that test results remain confidential and that they can terminate testing or training at any time and for any reason. A sample informed consent for exercise stress testing can be found at http://circ.ahajournals.org/content/91/3/912.full.[133]

Stress Testing Contraindications

Absolute contraindications

A stress test should not take place without direct medical supervision if the following contraindications exist:

- Resting ECG suggesting acute cardiac disease
- Recent complicated MI
- Unstable angina pectoris

TABLE 32.12

ACSM Recommendations for Current Medical Examination and Exercise Stress Testing (GXT) and Physician Supervision of GXT Prior to Participation in Exercise Program

Risk Category	Medical Examination and GXT	MD Supervision
Low risk Men <45 years Women <55 years; asymptomatic with <1 risk factor[a,b]	Moderate exercise; not necessary Vigorous exercise; not necessary	Moderate exercise; not necessary Vigorous exercise; not necessary
Moderate risk Men HDL-C <45 mg · dL^{-1} Women HDL-C <55 mg · dL^{-1}; recommended with >2 risk factors[a,b]	Moderate exercise; not necessary, Vigorous exercise; recommended	Moderate exercise; not necessary Vigorous exercise; recommended

High risk
Individuals with >1 sign/symptom of
  cardiovascular or pulmonary disease[c] or
  known cardiovascular (cardiac, peripheral
  vascular, or cerebrovascular), pulmonary
  (obstructive pulmonary disease, asthma,
  cystic fibrosis), or metabolic (diabetes,
  thyroid disorder, renal or liver) disease
	Moderate exercise; recommended
	Vigorous exercise; recommended
		Moderate exercise; recommended
		Vigorous exercise; recommended

[a]Risk factors: family history of heart disease; cigarette smoking; hypertension; hypercholesterolemia; impaired fasting glucose; obesity; sedentary lifestyle.
[b]HDL >60 mg · dL^{-1} (subtract one risk factor from the sum of other risk factors because high HDL decreases CHD risk).
[c]Signs and symptoms of cardiovascular and pulmonary disease: pain, discomfort in chest, neck, jaw, left arm; shortness of breath at rest or with mild exertion; dizziness or syncope; orthopnea or paroxysmal nocturnal dyspnea; ankle edema; tachycardia; intermittent claudication; heart murmur; unusual fatigue or shortness of breath with mild activity.
Adapted from Franklin BA, et al. *ACSM's Guidelines for Exercise Testing and Prescription*. 9th Ed. Baltimore: Lippincott Williams & Wilkins, 2009.

- Uncontrolled ventricular arrhythmias
- Uncontrolled atrial arrhythmias that compromise cardiac function
- Third-degree AV heart block without pacemaker
- Acute CHF
- Severe aortic stenosis
- Active or suspected myocarditis or pericarditis
- Recent systemic or pulmonary embolism
- Acute infections
- Acute emotional distress

Relative contraindications

A GXT can be administered with caution and with medical personnel in the test area under the following conditions:

- Resting diastolic blood pressure ≤115 mm Hg or systolic blood pressure ≤200 mm Hg
- Moderate valvular disease
- Electrolyte abnormalities
- Frequent or complex ventricular ectopy
- Ventricular aneurysm
- Uncontrolled metabolic disease (diabetes, thyrotoxicosis)
- Chronic infectious disease (hepatitis, mononucleosis, AIDS)
- Neuromuscular or musculoskeletal disorders
- Pregnancy (complicated or in the last trimester)
- Psychologic distress and/or apprehension about participating in the test

GXT Termination

Graded exercise testing is generally safe when following recognized guidelines and taking proper precautions. TABLE 32.13 lists reasons why test termination may be required before the person attains maximum volitional fatigue.

TABLE 32.13

Criteria for Terminating a Graded Exercise Test by Apparently Healthy Adults

- Onset of angina or angina-like symptoms
- Significant drop of 20 mm Hg in systolic blood pressure or failure of systolic blood pressure to rise with an increase in exercise intensity
- Excessive rise in blood pressure: systolic pressure >260 mm Hg or diastolic pressure >115 mm Hg
- Signs of poor perfusion: light-headedness, confusion, ataxia, pallor, cyanosis, nausea, or cold and clammy skin
- Failure of heart rate to increase with increasing exercise intensity
- Noticeable change in heart rhythm
- Subject requests to stop
- Physical or verbal manifestations of severe fatigue
- Failure of testing equipment
- Early-onset horizontal or downsloping S–T segment depression or elevation (>4 mm)
- Increasing ventricular ectopy; multiform PVCs
- Sustained supraventricular tachycardia

Stress Test Outcomes

The clinical success of the GXT depends on its predictive outcome; this means how effectively the test correctly diagnoses a person with heart disease.

Four possible GXT outcomes include:

1. **True positive** (successful test): The GXT correctly identifies a person with heart disease.
2. **True negative** (successful test): The GXT correctly identifies a person without heart disease.
3. **False positive** (unsuccessful test): The GXT incorrectly identifies a normal person as having heart disease.
4. **False negative** (unsuccessful test): The GXT incorrectly identifies a person with heart disease as normal.

A test's **sensitivity** refers to the percentage of persons for whom the test detects an abnormal (positive) response. This represents a true-positive condition that only subsequent follow-up can verify. False-negative results (unsuccessful test) occur 25% of the time, and false-positive (unsuccessful test) results approximately 15%. Factors that contribute to false-negative results include the patient's failure to reach an ischemic threshold, failure to recognize non-ECG signs and symptoms associated with underlying CHD, and technical or observer errors. Various drugs and conditions also increase the probability of false-negative results, particularly if the person takes β-blockers, nitrates, or calcium channel blocking agents.

A test's **specificity** refers to the number of true-negative test results—correctly identifying someone without CHD. More false-positive results occur under the influence of the drug digitalis and hypokalemia (low blood potassium levels), mitral valve prolapse, pericardial disorders, and anemia.

Stress Testing the "Oldest-Old"

The stress testing guidelines in Table 32.12 do not apply to individuals 75 years and older, those considered among the "oldest-old."[59] Only a small, highly select subgroup of these individuals participates in vigorous physical activity or can successfully complete a stress test. For example, approximately 30% of persons ages 75 to 79 years can achieve a maximal physical effort, 25% of those ages 80 to 84 years, and only 9% of those 85 years or older.[75] The oldest-old differ markedly from younger (<70 yr) persons in two key areas relative to stress testing:

1. High prevalence of asymptomatic CHD
2. Coexistence of other chronic conditions and physical limitations

Older, asymptomatic men and women exhibit increased ECG abnormalities, many of which diminish the diagnostic accuracy of the GXT. The prevalence of asymptomatic ischemic episodes uncovered by the exercise ECG increases dramatically among older adults with no history of MI or ECG abnormalities. Given the large reservoir of asymptomatic CHD among older persons, routine exercise stress testing would likely initiate a cascade of requirements for follow-up invasive cardiac procedures.[170] In the absence of strong evidence to support aggressive evaluation in older adults, this practice places many at unnecessary risk for complications from invasive assessment. For this reason, empirical screening for older adults prescribes physical activity based on the person's previous activity experiences and overall sense of well-being. This approach to exercise testing, training, and safety monitoring observes the widely accepted geriatric dictum *"start low and go slow."*

Exercise-Induced Indicators of CHD

Physical activity creates the greatest demand for coronary blood flow, making exercise testing an effective means of probing for CHD.

Angina Pectoris

Myocardial ischemia—usually from restricted coronary circulation induced by atherosclerosis—stimulates sensory nerves in the walls of the coronary arteries and myocardium. Pain or discomfort generally manifests in the upper chest region, yet frequently presents as increased pressure or constriction in the left shoulder or arm, neck, or jaw (see Figs. 32.7 and 32.8). Impaired cardiac performance—reduced stroke volume and cardiac output and generally diminished left-ventricular contractility—also accompanies angina. The pain usually subsides after a few minutes of inactivity, without permanent myocardial damage. Physical activity frequently precipitates an angina episode, yet angina also can occur at rest, called *Prinzmetal's angina* or *variant angina*, with attacks usually occurring in the late evening or nighttime through early morning. Approximately two thirds of people who have variant angina, caused by a coronary artery spasm, have severe blockage in at least one major coronary vessel. *Stable angina indicates predictable chest pain on exertion or under mental or emotional stress.*

Electrocardiographic Abnormalities

Alterations in the heart's normal pattern of electrical activity often indicate insufficient myocardial oxygen supply. Such electrical "clues" rarely emerge unless myocardial metabolic and blood flow requirements exceed resting conditions.

Figure 32.11A shows a tracing of the dynamic electrical activity of the myocardium throughout the cardiac cycle. Standard ECG paper contains 1-mm and 5-mm squares. Horizontally, each small square represents 0.04 s (with normal paper speed of 25 mm·s^{-1}); each large square represents 0.2 s. On the vertical axis, a small square indicates a 0.1-mV deflection with a calibration of 10 mm·mV^{-1}. One normal heartbeat (cardiac cycle) consists of five major electrical waves labeled P, Q, R, S, and T. The P wave indicates the electrical impulse (wave of depolarization) before atrial contraction. The Q, R, and S waves, collectively known as the **QRS complex**, represent depolarization of the ventricles immediately before their contraction. Ventricular repolarization generates the T wave. The cause of **S–T segment depression** (Fig. 32.11B) remains unknown, yet this abnormal deviation correlates with other CHD indicators that include coronary artery narrowing. *Individuals with significant S–T segment depression usually have severe, extensive obstruction in one or more coronary arteries.* The amount of S–T segment depression relates directly to the chances of dying from CHD. Generally, persons with 1- to 2-mm S–T segment depression during exercise exhibit a nearly fivefold increase in CHD mortality. The death risk increases approximately 20-fold for those with more than

2-mm depression. Current opinion advocates including nonspecific ECG findings in the overall heart disease risk assessment.[27] Even nonspecific minor S–T segment or T-wave abnormalities or both (termed ST–T abnormalities) provide a disquieting hint of increased long-term risk of mortality from cardiovascular disease.

During a standard ECG-monitored treadmill test, special electrodes can identify extremely subtle electrical patterns to predict a patient's risk for ventricular fibrillation. The test, termed the *alternans test*, identifies electrical alternation of the heart. Specifically, it uses a device to analyze T-wave alternans, which represent beat-to-beat electrical fluctuations of just one-millionth of a volt. T-wave alternans reflect abnormalities in the way myocardial cells recover after transmitting the heart's electrical impulse. Oscillation of the cells' impulse can initiate a chain reaction that produces arrhythmias, fibrillation, and subsequent sudden cardiac arrest in some 350,000 individuals in the United States. Predicting

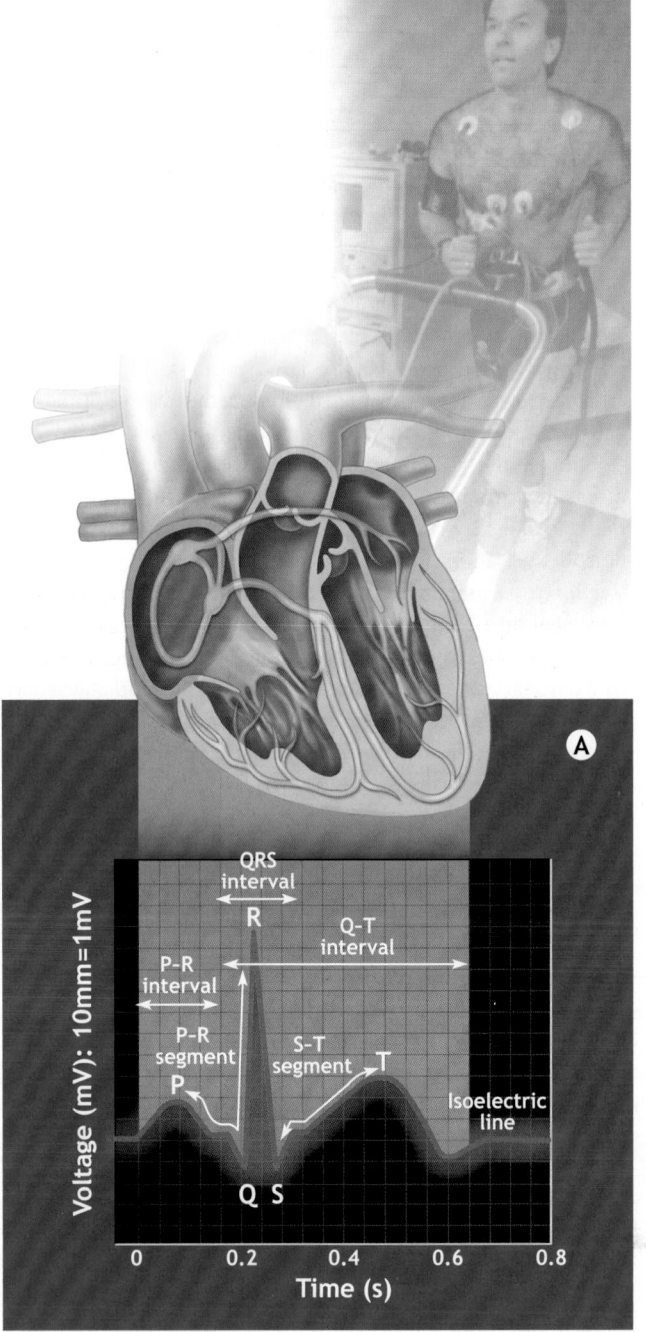

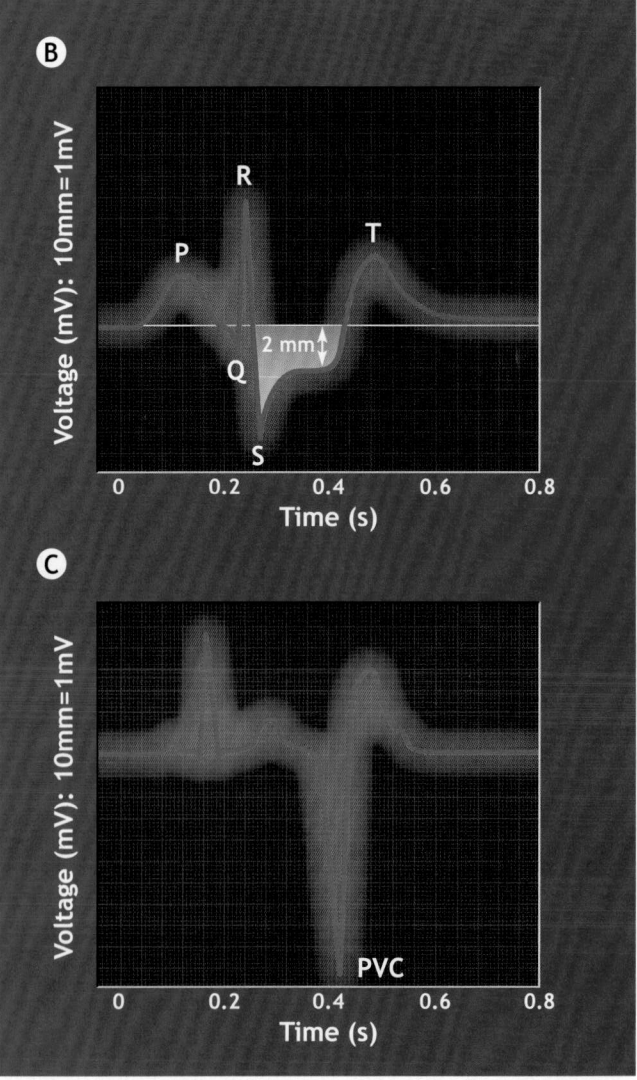

FIGURE 32.11 • **(A)** Normal ECG tracing with an upward-sloping S–T segment. **(B)** ECG tracing showing an abnormal horizontal S–T segment depression (*shaded area*) of 2 mm, measured from a stable baseline. **(C)** ECG tracing illustrating a premature ventricular contraction (*PVC*).

risk for sudden death via T-wave alternans gives high-risk patients medical protection that might include an implanted defibrillator (placed beneath the skin of the chest) to automatically correct abnormal cardiac electrical activity. The defibrillator activates a built-in pacemaker to restabilize the heart's rhythm if it detects minor arrhythmias. If that fails, the pacemaker delivers a small defibrillating electrical jolt that resets the rhythm.

Cardiac Rhythm Abnormalities

Graded exercise testing uncovers abnormalities in the pattern of the heart's electrical activity. A preventricular contraction (PVC; Fig. 32.11C) during exercise often reflects abnormal alteration in cardiac rhythm or **arrhythmia**. In this case, the normal depolarization wave through the atrioventricular node does not stimulate the ventricles. Instead, portions of the ventricle spontaneously depolarize. This disorganized electrical activity produces an "extra" ventricular beat (*QRS complex*) without the P wave (atrial depolarization) that normally precedes it.

PVCs in exercise generally herald the presence of severe ischemic atherosclerotic heart disease that often involves two or more major coronary vessels. This specific myocardial electrical instability with exercise has greater predictive value than S–T segment depression for CHD diagnosis. Patients with exercise-induced PVCs have a 6 to 10 times greater risk of sudden death from abnormal course or fine rapid movements of the ventricles (**ventricular fibrillation**) than patients without this instability. Fibrillation risk becomes more prevalent for individuals with family history of this occurrence. With fibrillation, the ventricles do not contract in a unified manner, and cardiac output falls dramatically. Sudden death ensues unless normal ventricular rhythm returns. Mitigating this risk requires implanting an electrical stimulator to correct the abnormal myocardial electrical conductance pattern.

Other Exercise-Induced CHD Indicators

Blood pressure and heart rate responses to physical activity provide three useful non-ECG indices of possible CHD:

1. **Hypertensive exercise response**: Normally, systolic blood pressure progressively increases during graded exercise from approximately 120 mm Hg at rest to 160 to 190 mm Hg during peak-intensity of effort. The change in diastolic pressure is generally less than 10 mm Hg. In exercise, systolic blood pressure can rise to well above 200 mm Hg, whereas the diastolic pressure can approach 150 mm Hg. This abnormal hypertensive response provides a significant clue to the presence of cardiovascular disease.

2. **Hypotensive exercise response**: Inability for blood pressure to increase during graded exercise reflects cardiovascular malfunction. For example, failure of systolic blood pressure to increase by at least 20 or 30 mm Hg often results from diminished cardiac reserve.

3. **Heart rate response**: A rapid, large increase in heart rate (tachycardia) early in graded exercise often indicates cardiac dysfunction. Likewise, abnormally low exercise heart rates (bradycardia) in non–endurance-trained individuals may reflect unhealthy function of the heart's SA node. Inability of heart rate to increase during graded exercise (**chronotropic incompetence**), particularly when accompanied by extreme fatigue, indicates cardiac strain and CHD. An attenuated maximal exercise heart rate in apparently healthy men and women raises cardiovascular disease mortality risk.[89,97] Specifically, failure to achieve at least 85% of age-predicted maximum heart rate during exercise predicts eventual all-cause mortality, independent of any exercise-induced myocardial perfusion defects.[98]

STRESS TEST PROTOCOLS

A survey conducted in 2000, based on 75,828 exercise tests performed at Veterans Affairs Medical Centers with cardiology divisions, reported that 78% used the treadmill, with 82% preferring the Bruce or Modified Bruce protocol. Four major cardiac events occurred (3 MIs and one sustained ventricular tachycardia), representing an event rate of 1.2 per 10,000 exercise tests.[115]

Bruce and Balke Treadmill Tests

Chapter 11 outlines protocols for the Bruce and Balke GXTs. Each test has distinct advantages and disadvantages. For example, the Bruce test provides more abrupt increases in exercise intensity between stages. This may improve sensitivity to detect ischemic ECG responses, but the patient must possess adequate fitness to tolerate increased exercise levels. Both protocols begin at relatively high levels of exercise for cardiac patients and older individuals and often require modification. The Bruce protocol incorporates lower initial exercise levels, whereas the Balke test includes a preliminary 2- to 3-min initial stage at 2 mph and 0% grade.

Choice of a specific exercise test considers overall health, age, and the person's fitness status. A stress test generally begins at a low level, with increments in intensity every several minutes. A warm-up, either separately or incorporated within the test protocol, eases the patient into exercise. Total exercise duration should average at least 8 min. A test much longer than 15 min adds little additional information because the most meaningful cardiac and physiologic data emerge within this time interval.

Bicycle Ergometer Tests

Bicycle ergometers have distinct advantages for exercise stress testing. In contrast to the treadmill, power output on the ergometer is readily computed and remains independent of the person's body mass. Most bicycle ergometers are portable, safe, and relatively inexpensive. Generally, two types of ergometers have application for graded exercise testing:

1. Electrically braked ergometers
2. Weight-loaded, friction-type ergometers

With electrically braked ergometers, the preselected power output remains fixed within a range of pedaling frequencies. With weight-loaded ergometers, power output, usually expressed in kg-m $\cdot$ min^{-1} or watts (1 W = 6.12 kg-m $\cdot$ min^{-1}), relates directly to frictional resistance and pedaling rate.

The general guidelines for treadmill testing also apply to testing with the bicycle ergometer. Test protocols provide 2- to 4-min stages of graded exercise with an initial resistance between 0 and 15 or 30 watts; power output generally increases in 15- to 30-watt increments per stage. The subject usually pedals the weight-loaded ergometer at either 50 or 60 revolutions per minute.

Arm-Crank Ergometer Tests

Arm cranking has application for graded exercise testing in special situations (e.g., cardiac assessment during upper-body effort) and for disabled individuals. Chapters 15 and 17 point out that arm exercise lowers $\dot{V}O_{2peak}$ up to 30%, and maximum heart rate generally averages 10 to 15 b $\cdot$ min^{-1} lower than with treadmill or bicycle exercise. Blood pressure is also difficult to measure during arm-crank exercise. Furthermore, submaximal arm cranking produces higher blood pressure, heart rate, and oxygen consumption values than the same power output with leg exercise. Nevertheless, graded exercise protocols similar to those developed for leg cycling tests apply to evaluating a patient's response to upper-body exercise. The initial frictional resistance remains lower in arm exercise, with smaller increments in power output adjusted accordingly.

 INTEGRATIVE QUESTION

What type of exercise prescription most benefits a patient with CHD who experiences angina during upper-body work in his job as a plasterer or paperhanger?

Stress Testing Safety

*The safety of stress testing largely depends on knowing who **not** to test (prescreening health histories reveal noncandidates for testing), knowing when to terminate a test, and preparing for emergencies.* TABLE 32.14 summarizes the results of 12 reports about exercise stress testing complications (morbidity and mortality during and after the test) involving 2 million exercise tests with different supervision levels.[18,46,82,161]

Only 16 high-risk but apparently healthy patients suffered coronary episodes in approximately 170,000 submaximal and maximal stress tests. This represents about one person per 10,000, or approximately 0.01% of the total group. For more

than 9000 stress tests, no cardiovascular episodes occurred for subjects with increased heart disease risk. In other reports, risk of coronary episodes for healthy, middle-age adults during a maximum stress test equaled about 1 in 3000.[47] Test risk in most middle-age men and women generally increases to about 6 to 12 times more than for young adults. For patients with documented CHD (including previous myocardial infarction or episodes of angina), risk of cardiovascular incident in stress testing increases 30 to 60 times above normal. Based on total risk analyses, many experts believe that a *lower* "overall risk" exists for those who take a GXT and then initiate a regular physical activity program than for those who take no GXT and remain sedentary.

Despite differences in testing techniques, purposes, safety precautions, type, and mode of testing, three conclusions about risk during or immediately following a GXT appear warranted:

1. Low risk of death (≤0.01%)
2. Low risk of an acute MI (≤0.04%)
3. Low risk of complications that require hospitalization, including acute MI or serious arrhythmias (≤0.2%)

Clearly, the risk–benefit ratio favors GXT testing as part of the medical evaluation process.

PRESCRIBING PHYSICAL ACTIVITY AND EXERCISE

An exercise prescription should improve fitness, promote overall health by reducing risk factors, and ensure a safe and enjoyable activity experience. *Prescribing physical activity involves successful integration of exercise science with behavioral objectives to enhance patient compliance and goal attainment.*

Heart rate and oxygen consumption (or exercise intensity) measured during the stress test provide the basis for the exercise prescription. The prescription individualizes exercise based on current fitness and health status, with emphasis on intensity, frequency, duration, and exercise type.

Initiating a physical activity program at the proper level takes on added importance for CHD patients because beginners do not often recognize their limitations.

Practical Illustration

FIGURE 32.12 illustrates a practical approach that permits functional translation of treadmill or bicycle exercise test responses to the exercise prescription. The figure depicts data for a male cardiac patient generated from an algorithm of responses from the Bruce treadmill protocol for level-ground ambulation. Heart rate (*A*) was plotted as a function of time, with a mathematical line of best fit (*B*) applied to the data points. A target zone for heart rate (*shaded portion, C*) represented approximately 75 to 85% of the maximum heart rate of 170 b $\cdot$ min^{-1}. The individualized prescription is then detailed for pace (13.8 to 15.4 mi $\cdot$ min^{-1}, *D*) and/or METs (4.1 to 5.9, *E*). The acceptable intensity range in area C, based on heart rate response during the exercise test,

TABLE 32.14 **Summary Reports of Incidence of Morbidity and/or Mortality During or Following a Graded Exercise Test (1969–1995)**

Study	GXT Tests	Type of Subject	Morbidity Rate (per 10,000)	Mortality Rate (per 10,000)	Total Complications[b] (per 10,000)
1	50,000[a]	Variety	5.2	0.4	5.6
2	18,707	Variety	3.8	0.9	4.7
3	>12,000	Variety	—	2.5	—
4	58,047	Variety	2.1	0.3	2.4
5	71,914[a]	Variety	0.7	0.1	0.8
6	28,133	Variety	3.2	0	3.2
7	4,050	Variety	0.3	0	0.3
8	170,000[a]	Variety	2.4	1.0	3.4
9	353,638[a]	Athlete	0	0	0
10	712,285[a]	CHD patients	1.4	0.2	1.6
11	518,448[a]	Variety	8.4	0.5	8.9
12	1377[a]	Severe CHD	232	0	232

[a]Direct physician supervision of GXT.

[b]Complications defined as the occurrence of serious arrhythmias during exercise testing (i.e., ventricular fibrillation, ventricular tachycardia, or bradycardia) that mandated immediate medical treatment (cardioversion, use of intravenous drugs, or closed-chest compression).

1. Atterhog JH, et al. *Am Heart J* 1979;98:572.
2. Cahalin LP, et al. *J Cardiopulm Rehabil* 1987;7:269.
3. Blessey RL. *Exercise Standards and Malpractice Reporter* 1989;3:69.
4. DeBrusk RF. *Exercise Standards and Malpractice Reporter* 1988;2:65.
5. Franklin BA, et al. *Chest* 1997;111:262.
6. Gibbons L, et al. *Circulation* 1989;80:846.
7. Knight JA, et al. *Am J Cardiol* 1995;75:390.
8. Lem V, et al. *Heart Lung* 1985;14:280.
9. Rochmis P, Blackburn H. *JAMA* 217:1971;1061.
10. Scherer D, Kaltenbach M. *Dtsch Med Wochenschr* 1979;33:1161.
11. Stuart RJ Jr, Ellestad MH. *Chest* 1980;77:94.
12. Young, et al. *Circulation* 1984;70:184.

Reprinted from Franklin BA, et al. *ACSM's Guidelines for Exercise Testing and Prescription*. 9th Ed. Baltimore: Lippincott Williams & Wilkins, 2009.

includes the following recreational activities: aerobics, bicycling, canoeing, light-to-moderate volleyball, skating, skiing, tennis and badminton, swimming, skating, touch football, and waterskiing. This practical approach to prescribing physical activity may improve the prescription's effectiveness and adherence for healthy, previously sedentary individuals and CHD patients.

Improvements in CHD Patients

A properly prescribed and monitored physical activity program safely improves a cardiac patient's functional capacity. Exercise training post-MI may also favorably modulate some of the deleterious changes in the myocardium's connective tissue metabolism seen in response to the MI, which may negate the deleterious effects of increased cardiac stiffness characteristics and associated diastolic function abnormalities seen after a heart attack.[178] Clinical symptoms (e.g., ECG abnormalities) often improve or disappear. This occurs partly from structural and functional changes in the myocardium. Cardiac patients and healthy individuals respond to exercise training with physiologic adjustments that reduce cardiac work at any given external exercise load. For example, reduced exercise heart rate and blood pressure (two major determinants of myocardial workload and oxygen consumption) reduce myocardial effort. The reduced rate–pressure product (HR × SBP) delays the onset of anginal pain and allows effort of greater intensity and duration. For individuals whose occupations predominantly require arm activities, training (and testing) should emphasize this musculature because physical conditioning benefits are highly specific and generally not transferable among muscle groups.

The Program

Joint recommendations of the ACSM and AHA for cardiovascular screening of 18- to 65-year-olds before enrollment or participation in activities at health/fitness facilities can be accessed online at http://circ.ahajournals.org/cgi/reprint/CIRCU-LATIONAHA.107.185649 (*Circulation* 2007;116:1081). The recommendations also discuss staff qualifications and emergency policies related to cardiovascular safety.

The most effective preventive and rehabilitative physical activity programs focus on individual needs. Low- to moderate-intensity regimens evoke greater adherence than

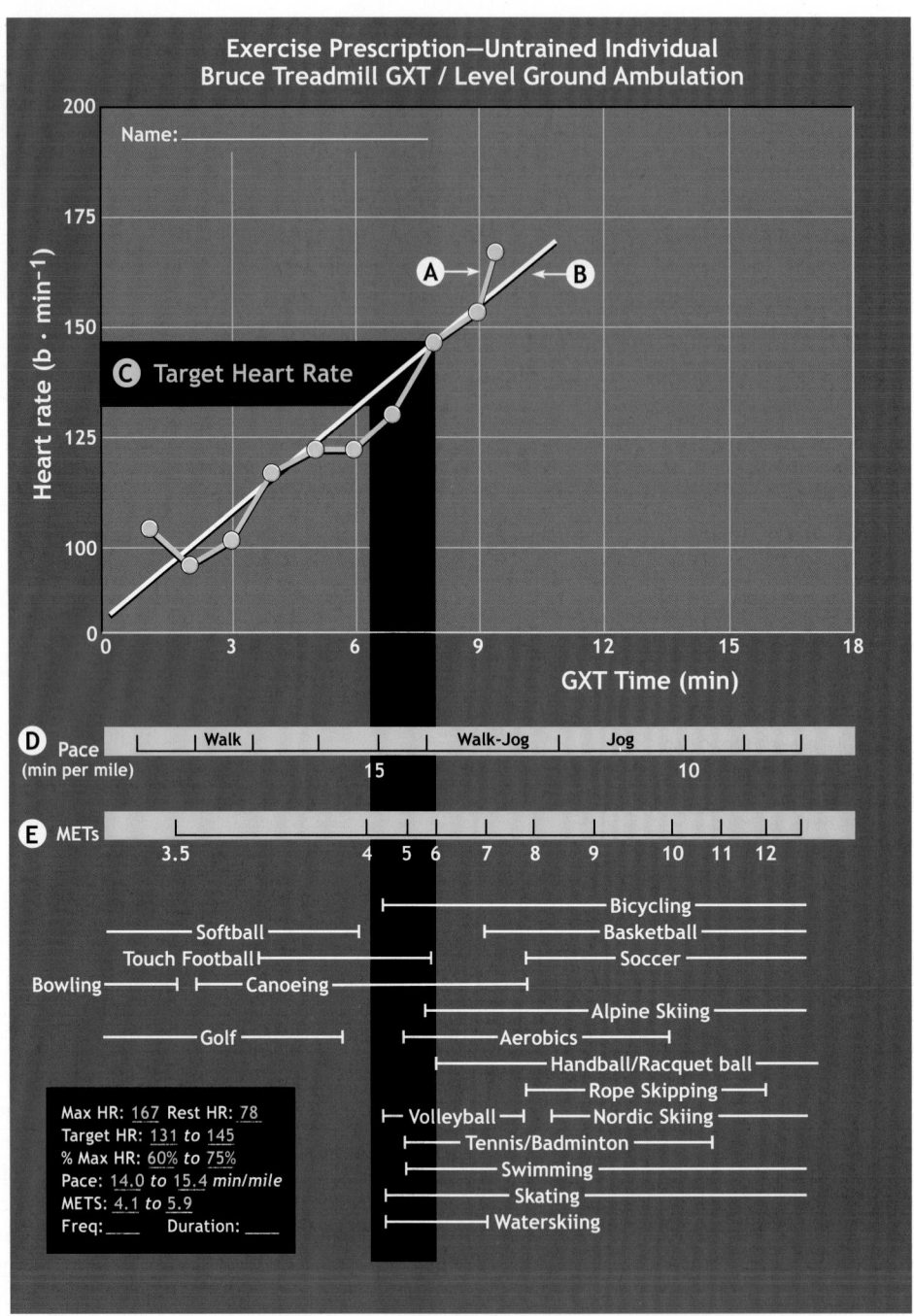

FIGURE 32.12 • Exercise prescription based on functional translation algorithm for level-ground ambulation. Letters in figure identified in text. (Reprinted with permission of Dr. Carl Foster, University of Wisconsin–LaCrosse.)

intense physical activity. Prescribed activities usually include rhythmic big-muscle movements that stimulate cardiovascular improvement; examples include walking, jogging, cycling, rope skipping, swimming, stair-climbing and cross-country ski simulation, dynamic calisthenics, and higher-intensity interval training, even among older adults and patients with congestive heart failure.[1,109,110] On an outpatient basis, less restricted activities such as mountain biking serve as a recreational adjunct to rehabilitate regularly active MI patients with stable CHD.[77]

Chapter 21 discusses guidelines for decision making concerning training frequency, duration, and intensity. Ideally, the personalized exercise prescription should include a recommendation for weight loss and dietary modification (if necessary), warm-up and cool-down exercises, and a developmental flexibility and strength program. Some heart disease patients exhibit a reduced exercise heart rate response with correspondingly reduced maximum heart rate. In such cases, target heart rates based on age-predicted maximum for the general, healthy population grossly overestimate the appropriate training intensity. *This supports the wisdom of exercise stress testing each patient to symptom-limited maximum and then formulating the exercise prescription from the test's heart rate data.*

TABLE 32.15	ACSM Categories for Exercise Programs Related to Patient Symptoms		
Type	**Participants**	**Entry MET Level**	**Supervision**
A. Unsupervised	Asymptomatic	8+	None
B. Supervised			
1. Inpatient	All symptomatics—post-myocardial infarction, postoperative, pulmonary disease	3	Supervised ambulatory therapy
2. Outpatient	All symptomatics—post-myocardial infarction, postoperative, pulmonary disease	3+	Exercise specialist, physician on call
3. In home	Symptomatic + asymptomatic	>3–5	Unsupervised; periodic hospital reevaluation
4. Community	Symptomatic + asymptomatic, 6–8 wk postinfarct, 4–8 wk postoperative	>5	Exercise program director + exercise specialist

Adapted with permission from Franklin BA, et al. *ACSM's Guidelines for Exercise Testing and Prescription*. 9th Ed. Baltimore: Lippincott Williams & Wilkins, 2009.

Supervision Level

The ACSM has categorized several types of exercise programs with specific criteria for entry and supervision (TABLE 32.15). These programs are either unsupervised or supervised, with four subdivisions in the supervised category. Unsupervised programs meet the needs of asymptomatic participants of any age with functional capacities of at least 8 METs and without known major risk factors. The supervised programs focus on patients with specific needs. These include asymptomatic physically active or inactive persons of any age with CHD risk factors but no known disease (B4) and symptomatic individuals, including individuals with recent onset of CHD and those with a changed disease status (B1 to B3).

Resistance Exercise Provides Benefits

Resistance exercises added to a cardiac rehabilitation program restore muscular strength, promote preservation of FFM, improve psychologic status and quality of life, and increase glucose tolerance and insulin sensitivity.[48,106,107] Combining resistance training and aerobic training yields more pronounced physiologic adaptations (improved aerobic capacity, muscle strength, and lean body mass) in patients with coronary artery disease than aerobic training alone.[105] For patients with advanced heart disease, no adverse effects occur while performing weightlifting arm exercise at 50, 65, and 85% of 1-RM.[86] In comparisons of resting and exercise responses, no changes occurred in pulmonary wedge pressures, S–T segment of the ECG, or incidence of dysrhythmias. Contraindications to resistance training for cardiac patients parallel those for aerobic training.[136] The following six conditions preclude cardiac patients from participating in resistance training:

1. Unstable angina
2. Uncontrolled arrhythmias
3. Left-ventricular outflow obstruction (e.g., hypertrophic cardiomyopathy with obstruction)
4. Recent history of CHF without follow-up and treatment

5. Severe valvular disease, hypertension (systolic blood pressure >160 mm Hg and/or diastolic blood pressure >105 mm Hg)
6. Poor left-ventricular function and exercise capacity below 5 METs with anginal symptoms or ischemic S–T segment depression

Resistance Training Prescription. Cardiac patients should exercise with light resistance in the range of 30 to 50% of 1-RM because of exaggerated blood pressure responses with straining-type exercise. In the absence of contraindications, elastic bands, light (1–5 lb) cuff and hand weights, light free weights, and wall pulleys can be applied at entrance to an outpatient program. Do not initiate low-level resistance training until 2 to 3 wk post-MI. Introduce barbells and/or weight machines after 4 to 6 wk of convalescence.

Most cardiac patients begin range-of-motion movements using relatively light weights for the lower and upper extremities. In accordance with AHA recommendations, they should perform one set of 10 to 15 repetitions to moderate fatigue, using 8 to 10 different exercises such as chest press, shoulder press, triceps extension, biceps curl, lat pull-down, lower back extension, abdominal crunch/curl-up, quadriceps extension or leg press, leg curl, and calf raise. Exercises performed 2 to 3 days a week produce favorable adaptations.[136] The RPE should range from 11 to 14 on the Borg scale ("fairly light" to "somewhat hard"). *To minimize dramatic blood pressure fluctuations during lifting, patients should be warned to avoid straining, performing the Valsalva maneuver, and gripping weight handles or bars tightly.*

Cardiac Medications and Exercise Response

Knowledge of the physiologic effects of drug intervention allows the clinical exercise physiologist to properly assess patient response during physical activity. TABLE 32.16 presents six classifications of common cardiac drugs along with trade names, side effects, and possible effects on exercise responses.

TABLE 32.16   Cardiac Medications: Their Use, Side Effects, and Effects on Exercise Response

Type/Trade Name	Use	Side Effects	Effects on Exercise Response
I. Antianginal agents			
A. Nitroglycerin compounds [*Amyl nitrate; Isordil; Nitrostat*]	Smooth muscle relaxation; decrease cardiac output	Headache, dizziness, hypotension	Hypotension; increase exercise capacity
B. β-Blockers [*Inderal; propranolol; Lopressor; Corgard; Biocadren*]	Block β receptors; decrease sympathetic tone; decrease HR, myocardial contractility, BP	Bradycardia, heart block, insomnia, weakness, nausea, fatigue, increased cholesterol and blood sugar	Decrease HR; hypotension; decrease cardiac contractility
C. Calcium antagonists [*Verapamil; nifedipine; Procardia*]	Block influx of calcium; dilate coronary arteries; suppress dysrhythmias	Dizziness, syncope, flushing, hypotension, headache, fluid retention	Hypotension
II. Antihypertensive agents			
A. Diuretics [*Thiazides, Lasix, Aldactone*]	Inhibit Na^+ and Cl^- in kidney; increase excretion of sodium and water, and control high BP and fluid retention	Drowsiness, dehydration, electrolyte imbalance; gout, nausea, pain, hearing loss, elevated cholesterol and lipoproteins	Hypotension
B. Vasodilators [*Hydralazine, Captopril, Apresoline, Loniten, Minoxidil*]	Dilate peripheral blood vessels; used in conjunction with diuretics; decrease BP	Increase HR and contractility; headache, drowsiness, nausea, vomiting, diarrhea	
C. Drugs interfering with sympathetic nervous system [*Reserpine, Propranolol, Aldomet, Catapres, Minipress*]	Decrease BP, HR, and cardiac output by dilating blood vessels	Drowsiness, depression, sexual dysfunction, fatigue, dry mouth, stuffy nose, fever, upset stomach, fluid retention, weight gain	Hypotension
III. Digitalis glycosides, derivatives [*Digoxin Lonoxin digitoxin*]	Strengthen heart's pumping force and decrease electrical conduction	Arrhythmias, heart block, altered ECG, fatigue, weakness, headache, nausea, vomiting	Increase exercise capacity; increase myocardial contractility
IV. Anticoagulant agents [*Coumadin, sodium heparin, aspirin, Persantine*]	Prevent blood clot formation	Easy bruising, stomach irritation, joint or abdominal pain, difficulty swallowing, unexplained swelling, uncontrolled bleeding	
V. Antilipidemic agents [*Cholestyramine, Lopid, Niacin, Atromid-S, Mevacor, Questran, Zocor, Lipitor*]	Interfere with lipid metabolism and lower cholesterol and low-density lipoproteins	Nausea, vomiting, diarrhea, constipation, flatulence, abdominal discomfort, glucose intolerance, myalgia, liver dysfunction, muscle fatigue	
VI. Antiarrhythmic agents [*Cardioquin, procaine, quinidine, lidocaine, Dilantin, propranolol, bretylium tosylate, verapamil*]	Alter conduction patterns throughout the myocardium	Nausea, palpitations, vomiting, rash, insomnia, dizziness, shortness of breath, swollen ankles, coughing up blood, fever, psychosis, impotence	Hypotension; decrease HR; decrease cardiac contractility

INTEGRATIVE QUESTION

Why would participating in a weightlifting competition pose a risk to a person with advanced CHD?

CARDIAC REHABILITATION

A comprehensive **cardiac rehabilitation program** focuses on improving longevity and quality of life, in addition to risk factor modification.[35,126] After diagnosis and intervention (e.g., aggressive risk factor reduction, bypass surgery, angioplasty), the exercise physiologist evaluates the cardiac patient for functional capacity and ensuing classification and rehabilitation.[37] TABLE 32.17 outlines functional and therapeutic classifications of heart disease from the New York Heart Association while TABLE 32.18 presents guidelines for risk stratification from the AHA (www.american-heart.org) to categorize patients for subsequent rehabilitation. Patients differ greatly in symptoms, functional capacities, and rehabilitation strategies. The rehabilitation program incorporates stringent guidelines to promote low-risk treatment.[41,64,166] CHD patients with mild ischemia tolerate steady-rate exercise at intensities consistent for aerobic training, without progressive deterioration in left-ventricular function. For patients without ischemia, left ventricular function in prolonged physical effort remains similar to healthy controls.[42] Five important aspects of a successful cardiac rehabilitation program include:

1. Appropriate patient selection
2. Concurrent medical, surgical, and pharmacologic therapies
3. Comprehensive patient education
4. Appropriate exercise prescription
5. Careful patient monitoring during rehabilitation

Traditional cardiac rehabilitation programs consist of three distinct phases with different objectives, physical activities, and required supervision. More contemporary programs have changed on the basis of new theories of risk stratification, exercise safety data, and changes in the healthcare industry. Current programs recognize individual differences in rehabilitation when determining program length, degree of supervision, and required ECG monitoring.

Contemporary cardiac rehabilitation includes inpatient and outpatient programs and services, with emphasis on outcome measures. Almost all postsurgery patients benefit from inpatient activity intervention, risk factor assessment, lifestyle activity and dietary counseling, and patient and family education. Patients stay at the hospital an average of 3 to 5 days postsurgery before release.

Inpatient Programs

Inpatient cardiac rehabilitation focuses on the following four objectives:

1. Medical surveillance
2. Identification of patients with significant impairments before discharge
3. Rapid patient return to daily activities
4. Preparation of patient and family to optimize recovery upon discharge

In-hospital physical activity during the first 48 hr following an MI and/or cardiac surgery is restricted to self-care movements, including arm and leg range of motion and intermittent sitting and standing to maintain cardiovascular reflexes. After several days, patients usually sit and stand without assistance, perform self-care activities, and walk independently up to six times daily, provided none of the following contraindications exist:

- Unstable angina
- Elevated resting blood pressure

	Functional and Therapeutic Classifications of Heart Disease from the New York Heart Association.
TABLE 32.17	

Functional Capacity Classification		Therapeutic Classification	
Class I:	No limitation of physical activity. Ordinary physical activity does not cause undue fatigue, palpitation, dyspnea, or anginal pain	Class A:	Physical activity need not be restricted
Class II:	Slight limitation of physical activity. Comfortable at rest, but ordinary physical activity results in fatigue, palpitation, dyspnea, or anginal pain	Class B:	Ordinary physical activity need not be restricted, but unusually severe or competitive efforts should be avoided
Class III:	Marked limitation of physical activity. Comfortable at rest, but less than ordinary activity causes fatigue, palpitation, dyspnea, or anginal pain	Class C:	Ordinary physical activity should be moderately restricted, and more strenuous efforts should be discontinued
Class IV:	Unable to carry on any physical activity without discomfort. Symptoms of cardiac insufficiency or of the anginal syndrome may be present even at rest; any physical activity increases discomfort	Class D:	Ordinary physical activity should be markedly restricted
		Class E:	Patient should be at complete rest and confined to bed or chair

Adapted with permission from Franklin BA, et al. *ACSM's Guidelines for Exercise Testing and Prescription.* 9th Ed. Baltimore: Lippincott Williams & Wilkins, 2009.

TABLE 32.18	**Guidelines for Risk Stratification from the AHA When Considering an Exercise Program**				
AHA Classification	**NYHA[a] Class**	**Exercise Capacity**	**Angina/Ischemia and Clinical Characteristics**	**ECG Monitoring**	
A. Apparently healthy			Less than 40 years of age; without symptoms, no major risk factors, and normal GXT	No supervision or monitoring required	
B. Known stable CHD, low risk for vigorous exercise	I or II	5–6 METs	Free of ischemia or angina at rest or on the GXT; EF = 40 to 60%	Monitored and supervised only during prescribed sessions (6–12 sessions); light resistance training may be included in comprehensive rehabilitation programs	
C. Stable CHD with low risk for vigorous exercise but unable to self-regulate activity	I or II	5–6 METs	Same disease states and clinical characteristics as class B but without the ability to self-monitor exercise	Medical supervision and ECG monitoring during prescribed sessions; nonmedical supervision of other exercise sessions	
D. Moderate-to-high risk for cardiac complications during exercise	≥III	<6 METs	Ischemia (≥4.0 mm S–T depression) or angina during exercise; two or more previous MIs; EF <30%	Continuous ECG monitoring during rehabilitation until safety established; medical supervision during all exercise sessions until safety established	
E. Unstable disease with activity restriction	≥III	<6 METs	Unstable angina; uncompensated heart failure; uncomfortable arrhythmias	No activity recommended for conditioning purposes; attention directed to restoring patient to class D or higher	

[a]NYHA, New York Heart Association; EF, ejection fraction; CHD, coronary heart disease; GXT, graded exercise test.
Adapted with permission from Franklin BA, et al. *ACSM's Guidelines for Exercise Testing and Prescription*. 9th Ed. Baltimore: Lippincott Williams & Wilkins, 2009.

- Orthostatic systolic blood pressure above 200 mm Hg with symptoms
- Critical aortic stenosis
- Acute systemic illness or fever
- Uncontrolled atrial or ventricular arrhythmias
- Uncontrolled sinus tachycardia above 120 b·min⁻¹
- Uncompensated CHF
- Active pericarditis or myocarditis
- Recent embolism or thrombophlebitis
- Resting S–T segment displacement of 2 mm or more
- Severe orthopedic conditions

Outpatient Programs

Upon discharge, the patient should know appropriate and inappropriate physical activities and dietary guidelines and have a prudent and progressive plan of risk reduction with specific exercise prescription. Enrollment in an outpatient activity program is the ideal. Four goals for **outpatient cardiac rehabilitation** include:

1. Monitoring and supervising patient to detect changes in clinical status
2. Returning patient to premorbid/vocational/recreational activities

3. Assisting patient to implement at-home, unsupervised activity program
4. Providing family support and education

Most outpatient program sites encourage multiple physical activities that include resistance exercise and walking, cycling, and swimming. Supervision should include personnel trained in CPR and advanced life support, and in some cases, a home defibrillator known as an automated external defibrillator (AED; www.heartstarthome.com/content/heartstart_featured.asp).

PULMONARY DISEASES

The clinical exercise physiologist's involvement in treating patients with pulmonary disease focuses on improving ventilatory capacity, decreasing the energy cost of breathing, and increasing overall level of physiologic function. The personal history, physical examination, pertinent laboratory data, and imaging studies provide important background information. Cardiovascular system disorders almost always affect pulmonary function, which eventually leads to varying degrees of pulmonary disability. Conversely, pulmonary disease intimately relates to cardiovascular complications. Patients with pulmonary disease and disabilities often benefit from exercise rehabilitation. Pulmonary abnormalities classify as either obstructive (normal airflow impeded) or restrictive (lung volume dimensions reduced). Despite the convenience of this classification system, pulmonary disorders often reflect both restrictive and obstructive impairment.

Restrictive Lung Dysfunction

Abnormal reduction in pulmonary ventilation, along with diminished lung expansion, decreased tidal volume, and loss of functioning alveolar–capillary units, characterize a large and diverse group of pulmonary disorders collectively termed *restrictive lung disease (RLD)*.

The genesis of RLD involves pathophysiology of three aspects of pulmonary ventilation:

1. Lung compliance
2. Lung volumes and capacities
3. Physiologic work of breathing

In RLD, the chest and lung tissues stiffen and resist expansion under the normal pressure differentials of breathing. The additional resistance to lung expansion requires greater pulmonary force to maintain adequate alveolar ventilation. This increases the energy cost of normal ventilation and accounts for up to 50% of the total oxygen requirement during physical activity.[74] Eventually, the progression of RLD negatively affects all lung volumes and capacities. Diminished inspiratory and expiratory reserve volumes occur consistently under all conditions.

TABLE 32.19 lists major RLD conditions, along with their causes, signs and symptoms, and suggested treatments. Known causes of RLD include rheumatoid arthritis, immunologic pathology, massive obesity, diabetes mellitus, trauma from injury, penetrating wounds, radiation, burns, other inhalation injuries, poisoning, and complications from drug therapy, including reactions to antibiotics and antiinflammatory drugs.

Chronic Obstructive Pulmonary Disease

Chronic obstructive pulmonary disease (COPD), also termed *chronic airflow limitations (CAL)*, comprises several respiratory tract diseases that obstruct airflow (e.g., emphysema, asthma, and chronic bronchitis). The disease destroys lung parenchyma, causing a mismatch between regional alveolar air and blood flow. This ultimately affects the lung's mechanical function to compromise gas exchange (ventilation–perfusion ratio) at the alveolar level. *A dramatic decrease in exercise tolerance almost always accompanies COPD*. The natural history of COPD spans 20 to 50 years and closely parallels a history of chronic cigarette smoking. The National Heart, Lung, and Blood Institute (NHLBI; www.nhlbi.nih.gov) projects that COPD will be the third leading cause of death by 2020.

Changes in pulmonary function measures, most notably decreased expiratory flow rate and increased residual lung volume, usually form the diagnosis of COPD. The classic disease symptoms include spontaneous spasms of bronchial smooth muscle that produce chronic cough, increased mucus production, inflammation and thickening of the mucosal lining of the bronchi and bronchioles, wheezing, and dyspnea upon exertion. The FYI "Differences Among Major COPD Diseases" distinguishes conditions by anatomic location and pathology.

Factors predisposing to COPD include chronic cigarette smoking (greater effect in women than men; particularly on the increase among college students),[143] air pollution, occupational exposure to irritating dusts or gases, heredity, infection, allergies, aging, and drugs. *COPD rarely occurs in nonsmokers*. The airways narrow to obstruct pulmonary airflow in all forms of COPD. Airway narrowing hinders ventilation by trapping air in the bronchioles and alveoli; in essence, the disease increases pulmonary physiologic dead space. The obstruction also increases resistance to airflow (chiefly in expiration), hinders normal gas exchange, and

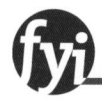 **Differences Among Major COPD Diseases**

Name	Area Affected	Result
Bronchitis	Membrane lining bronchial tubes	Inflammation of bronchial lining
Bronchiectasis	Bronchial tubes (bronchi or air passages)	Breakdown of alveolar walls; air spaces enlarged
Emphysema	Air spaces beyond terminal bronchioles (alveoli)	Bronchial dilation with inflammation
Asthma	Bronchioles (small airways)	Bronchioles obstructed by muscle spasm; swelling of mucosa; thick secretions
Cystic fibrosis	Bronchioles	Bronchioles become obstructed and obliterated; plugs of mucus cling to airway walls, leading to bronchitis, atelectasis, pneumonia, or pulmonary abscess

reduces exercise performance by increasing the energy cost of breathing. The latter reduces ventilatory capacity to hinder full arterial oxygen saturation and carbon dioxide elimination. Patients with severe COPD exhibit decreased whole-body mechanical efficiency during physical activity.[141] This suggests that factors associated with the respiratory effort also magnify the energy requirements of whole-body activity to further negatively impact physical capacity. Exercise intervention can sometimes reverse peripheral abnormalities associated with COPD.[172]

The following sections focus on four major COPD diseases:

1. Chronic bronchitis
2. Emphysema
3. Cystic fibrosis
4. Asthma and exercise-induced bronchospasm

TABLE 32.19 Restrictive Lung Diseases[a]

Causes/Type	Etiology	Signs and Symptoms	Treatment
I. Maturational			
a. Abnormal fetal lung development	Premature birth (hypoplasia-reduced lung tissue)	Asymptomatic; pulmonary insufficiency	No specific treatment
b. Respiratory distress syndrome (hyaline membrane disease)	Insufficient maturation of lungs due to premature birth	↑ Respiration rate; ↓ lung volumes; ↓ P_{AO_2}; acidemia; rapid and labored respiration pressure	Treat mother prior to birth (corticosteroids); hyperalimentation; continuous positive airway
c. Aging	Aging and cumulative effects of pollution, noxious gas, inhaled drug use, and cigarette smoking	↑ Residual volume; ↓ vital capacity; repetitive periodic apnea	No specific treatment; increase physical activity
II. Pulmonary			
a. Idiopathic pulmonary fibrosis	Unknown origin (perhaps viral or genetic)	↓ Lung volumes; pulmonary hypertension; dyspnea; cough; weight loss, fatigue	Corticosteroids; maintain adequate nutrition and ventilation
b. Coal workers' pneumoconiosis	Repeated inhalation of coal dust over 10–12 years	↓ TLC, VC, FRC; ↓ lung compliance; dyspnea; ↓ P_{AO_2}; pulmonary hypertension; cough	Nonreversible, no known cure
c. Asbestosis	Long-term exposure to asbestos	↓ Lung volumes; abnormal x-ray; ↓ P_{AO_2}; dyspnea on exertion, shortness of breath	Nonreversible, no known cure
d. Pneumonia	Inflammatory process caused by various bacteria microbes, viruses	↓ Lung volumes; abnormal x-ray; tachypneic dyspnea; high fever, chills, cough; pleuritic pain	Drug therapy (antibiotic)
e. Adult respiratory distress syndrome	Acute lung injury (fat emboli, drowning, drug-induced, shock, blood transfusion, pneumonia)	Abnormal lung function tests; P_{AO_2} <60 mm Hg; extreme dyspnea; cyanotic; headache; anxiety	Intubation and mechanical ventilation
f. Bronchogenic carcinoma	Tobacco use	Variable, depending on type and location of growth	Surgery, radiation, chemotherapy; specific drainage
g. Pleural effusions	Accumulation of fluid within pleural space; heart failure; cirrhosis	Shortness of breath; pleuritic chest pain; ↓ P_{AO_2}	
III. Cardiovascular			
a. Pulmonary edema	↑ Pulmonary capillary hydrostatic pressure secondary to left ventricular failure	↑ Respiration rate; ↓ lung volumes; ↓ P_{AO_2}; arrhythmias; report feelings of suffocation, shortness of breath, cyanotic, cough	Drug therapy, diuretics; supplemental oxygen
b. Pulmonary emboli	Complications of venous thrombosis	↓ Lung volumes; ↓ P_{AO_2}; tachycardia; acute dyspnea, shortness of breath; syncope	Heparin therapy; mechanical ventilation

TABLE 32.19	Restrictive Lung Diseases^a (Continued)		
Causes/Type	**Etiology**	**Signs and Symptoms**	**Treatment**
IV. Neuromuscular			
a. *Spinal cord injury*	Trauma paralysis of respiratory muscle	↓ Lung volumes; hypoxemia; fatigue; shortness of breath; inability to cough; ↓ voice volume	Active and passive chest wall stretching
b. *Amyotrophic lateral sclerosis*	Degenerative disease of nervous system	↓ Lung volumes; ↓ maximum voluntary volume	No treatment except supportive therapy
c. *Poliomyelitis*	Viral infectious disease that attacks motor nerves	Paralysis of diaphragm; shortness of breath	No treatment except supportive therapy
d. *Guillain-Barré syndrome*	Demyelinating disease of motor neurons	Profound muscular weakness; ↓ lung volumes	Passive range-of-motion exercises; active exercise
e. *Neuromuscular diseases (myasthenia gravis, tetanus, muscular dystrophy)*	Diseases of neuromuscular system, genetic or other cause resulting in chronic muscular weakness and wasting	Weakness, fatigue, loss of muscle function and strength, paralysis affects pulmonary system with eventual loss of function	Drugs; passive and active exercise; supportive therapy
V. Musculoskeletal			
a. *Diaphragmatic paralysis*	Loss or impairment of motor function of diaphragm muscle due to specific lesion	↓ Lung volumes; dyspnea, shortness of breath	Not needed
b. *Kyphoscoliosis*	Excessive anteroposterior and lateral curvature of thoracic spine (cause unknown)	↓ Lung volumes; exertional dyspnea	Use of orthotic devices; active exercise
c. *Ankylosing spondylitis*	Chronic inflammatory disease of spine (inherited)	Exertional dyspnea	No treatment

^awww.nlm.nih.gov/medlineplus/; www.cvm.msu.edu/RESEARCH/PULMON/site/respiratory_diseases/diseases/Heaves/mainFrame.html

Chronic Bronchitis

Acute bronchitis, an inflammation of the trachea and bronchi, usually is self-limiting and of short duration. In contrast, prolonged exposure to nonspecific irritants produces **chronic bronchitis**. Over time, the swollen mucous membranes and increased mucus production obstruct airways, causing wheezing and chronic coughing. Partial or complete airway blockage from mucus secretion produces inadequate arterial oxygen saturation, diminished carbon dioxide elimination, and pulmonary edema. Eventually, the patient develops the characteristic look of a "blue bloater" (FIG. 32.13). Chronic bronchitis develops slowly and worsens over time. Patients usually have a history of cigarette smoking for decades. Functional capacity decreases considerably, and fatigue occurs readily with mild exertion. If left untreated, this disease leads to premature death.

Emphysema

An abnormal, permanent enlargement of air spaces distal to the terminal bronchioles characterizes **emphysema**. The disease occurs most frequently among chronic cigarette smokers. It develops as a consequence of chronic bronchitis; its symptoms include dyspnea, hypercapnea, persistent cough, cyanosis, and digital clubbing (evidence of chronic hypoxemia; FIG. 32.14). Emphysemic patients consistently demonstrate low physical capacity and extreme dyspnea with exertion; patients appear thin and often lean forward with arms braced on the knees to support the shoulders and chest to ease breathing. The chronic effects of trapped air and alveolar distension change the size and shape of the chest, causing the characteristic emphysemic "barrel chest" appearance (FIG. 32.15). Regular physical activity does not improve pulmonary function of individuals with emphysema, but it enhances cardiovascular fitness, strengthens both respiratory and nonrespiratory musculature, and improves psychologic status.[11] In selected patients with severe emphysema, lung-volume reduction surgery has improved pulmonary function, physical capacity, and quality of life. Its effects on longevity remain uncertain.[53]

Cystic Fibrosis

The term *cystic fibrosis* (CF; www.cff.org) originates from the diagnosis of cysts and scar tissue observed on the pancreas during autopsy. Pancreatic cysts and scar tissue often exist

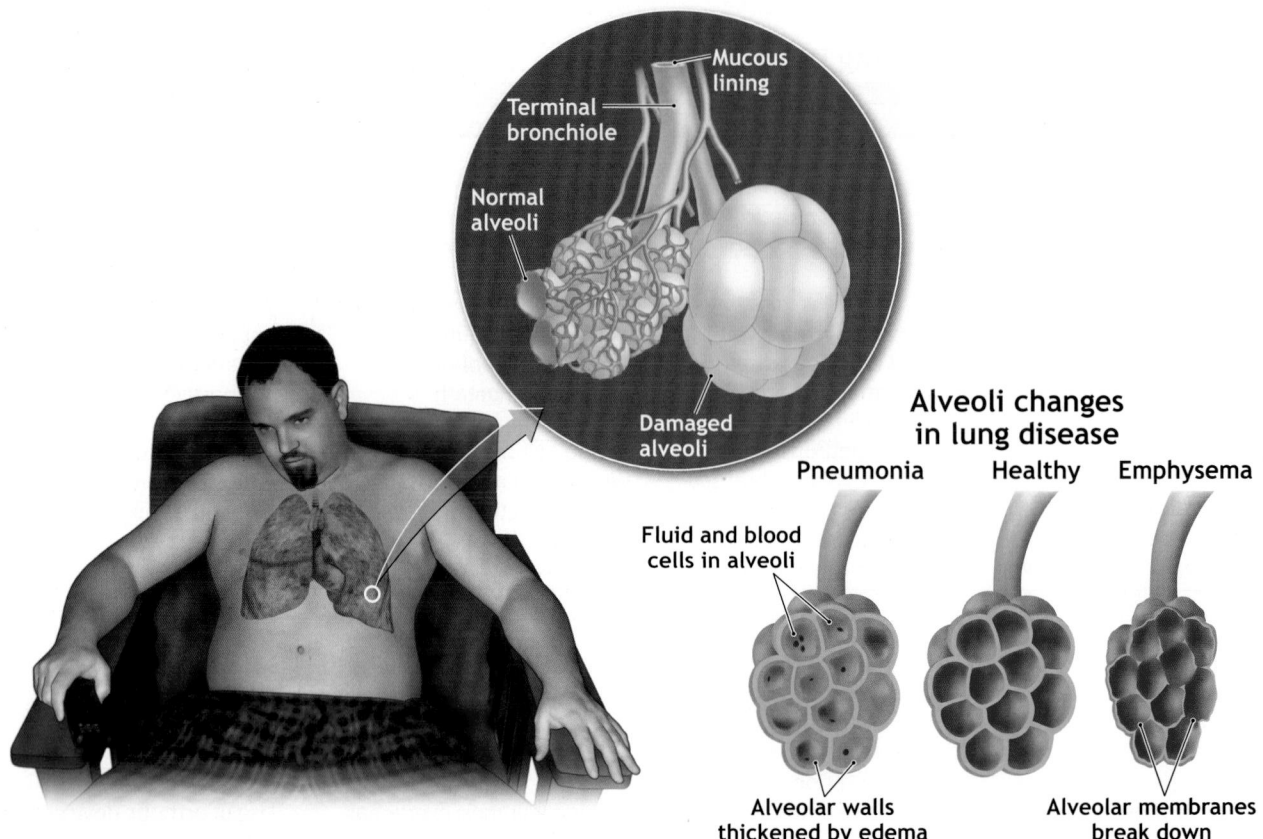

FIGURE 32.13 • A person with chronic bronchitis usually develops cyanosis and pulmonary edema with the characteristic appearance known as the "blue bloater." (*Insert*) Effects of chronic bronchitis: misshapen or large alveolar sacs with reduced surface for oxygen and carbon dioxide exchange.

but do not reflect the primary characteristics of the disease. TABLE 32.20 lists clinical signs and symptoms of this inherited debilitating, life-threatening disease characterized by thickening secretions of all exocrine glands (e.g., pancreatic, pulmonic, gastrointestinal). Glandular secretions plug the lung bronchioles and ultimately lead to chronic cough, difficulty breathing, and obstruction in lung tissue. CF, the most common inherited disease (both parents must carry the recessive trait) in whites, afflicts approximately 1 in 2000 infants in the United States.

Approximately 5% (12 million) of Americans carry the gene for CF located on chromosome 7, first identified in 1985 by research scientists John R. Riordan at Mayo Clinic Scottsdale, in Arizona, and Lap-Chee Tsui at the Research Institute of The Hospital for Sick Children, in Toronto. This produces defective or missing cystic fibrosis transmembrane conductor regulator (CFTR) proteins, which results in poor ion flow across cell membranes, including the lung. FIGURE 32.16 shows the approximate gene location on the chromosome 7 map.

A positive sweat electrolyte (chloride) test result diagnoses CF. Patients possess a faulty copy of the gene that allows cells to construct a channel for the passage of chloride ions. Consequently, the resulting poor ion flow across

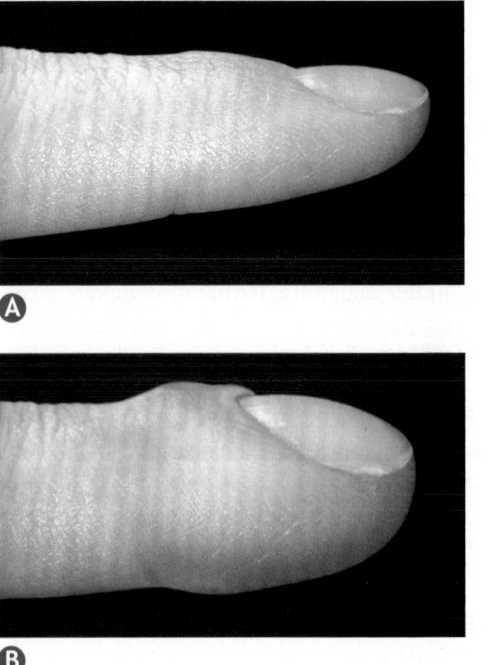

FIGURE 32.14 • Normal digit configuration (A) and digital clubbing (B). Club fingers and toes indicate chronic tissue hypoxia, a common diagnosis in emphysema.

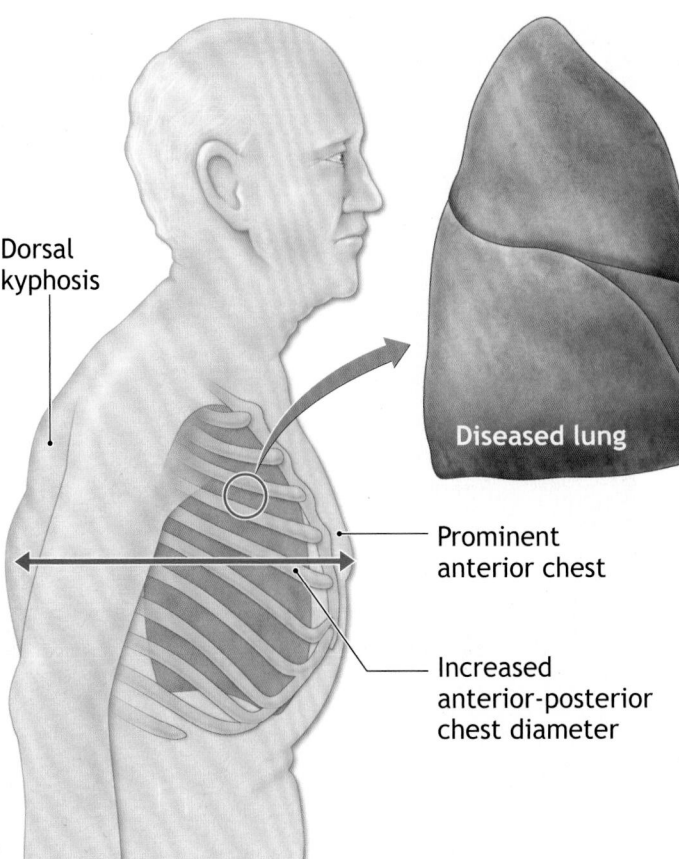

cell membranes causes salt to accumulate in the cells that line the lungs and digestive tissues, making the surrounding mucus thicker and salty. These mucous secretions, the critical feature of CF, obstruct ducts and passages in the pancreas, liver, and lungs.

Pulmonary impairment represents the most common and severe manifestation of CF. Airway obstruction leads to chronic lung hyperinflation. Over time, RLD superimposes on the obstructive disease that leads to chronic hypoxia, hypercapnea, and acidosis. These three maladies increase the risk of arterial desaturation during exercise. The disease progresses to pneumothorax and pulmonary hypertension and eventually death.

Treatment of CF includes antibiotics, the FDA-approved mucus-thinning drug Pulmozyme, TOBI (tobramycin) solution for inhalation, high dosages of ibuprofen, enzyme supplements, nutritional intervention, and frequent mucous secretion removal. In most instances regular exercise is recommended as part of the physiotherapy for cystic fibrosis as it delays the development of pulmonary disease in patients via mechanisms that improve airway hydration and mucociliary clearance and reduce markers of inflammation.[19] Assessments of physical capacity of children with CF suggest a positive role for regular physical activity. For example, aerobic fitness correlates inversely with 8-year mortality.[123] The anaerobic power of children with CF is lower than healthy counterparts, although CF patients rely more on anaerobic pathways during strenuous activity.[14,15] The kinetics of oxygen uptake slow in cystic fibrosis patients.[66]

Increased minute ventilation with aerobic activity helps to clear airways of excessive secretions.[148,179] For example, 20 to 30 min of aerobic exercise replaces one session of secretion removal for some children. Thus, increasing physical fitness can delay CF's crippling effects. An abnormally high NaCl loss in the sweat increases the likelihood of plasma hypoosmolality with a concomitant reduction in thirst drive. A flavored drink with relatively high salt content (e.g., 50 mmol · L^{-1}) enhances drinking and reduces exercise dehydration risk in CF patients.[94]

Pulmonary Assessments

Exercise physiologists do not diagnose pulmonary disease, but understanding the different tests and their results assists in planning and implementing exercise interventions. *Pulmonary*

FIGURE 32.15 • Emphysema traps air in the lungs, making exhalation difficult. With time, changes occur in the physical features of the patient, hence the name "pink puffer."

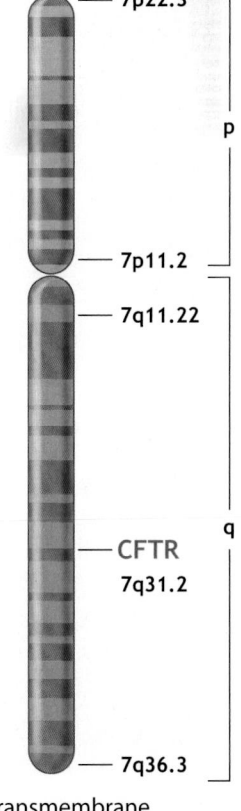

FIGURE 32.16 • CFTR, cystic fibrosis transmembrane conductance regulator. (Photo courtesy of NCBI Entrez.)

Clinical Signs and Symptoms of Cystic Fibrosis and Related Pulmonary Involvement

TABLE 32.20

Early-stage clinical signs and symptoms of cystic fibrosis
- Persistent cough and wheezing
- Recurrent pneumonia
- Excessive appetite but poor weight gain
- Salty skin or sweat
- Bulky, foul-smelling stools (undigested lipids)

Late-stage clinical signs and symptoms of cystic fibrosis with pulmonary involvement
- Tachypnea (rapid breathing)
- Sustained chronic cough with mucus production on vomiting
- Barrel chest
- Cyanosis and digital clubbing
- Exertional dyspnea with decreased exercise capacity
- Pneumothorax
- Right heart failure secondary to pulmonary hypertension

disease diagnosis involves several different objective measures that include chest imaging, flow and volume tests, blood gas analyses, and cytologic and hematologic evaluations.

thePoint Appendix H, available online at http://the point.lww.com/mkk8e, provides a list of supplemental animations and videos on this subject, including a discussion of working with dyspnea.

X-Ray

Chest and lung imaging continue as the most popular pulmonary assessment techniques. These include the conventional medical x-ray in which roentgen rays, named in honor of 1901 Physics Nobel Laureate Wilhelm Konrad Röntgen (1845–1923, who took the first x-ray of his wife's hand [see image below]), penetrate human tissues to provide an image (known as a radiograph or roentgenogram) of the chest's anatomy on film. This standard diagnostic tool screens for abnormalities, provides a baseline for subsequent assessments, and monitors disease progression. A chest radiograph shows body fat, water, tissue, bone, and air space. The low density of air in the lungs allows greater roentgen ray penetration, which produces a dark image. Relatively dense bone represents the other extreme; it allows fewer roentgen rays to penetrate its tissue, thus producing a white image. FIGURE 32.17A illustrates a normal chest radiograph taken in the posteroanterior (PA) position. FIGURE 32.17B shows the same radiograph with the normal anatomic structures labeled. Abnormal radiographic densities identify specific lung lesions.

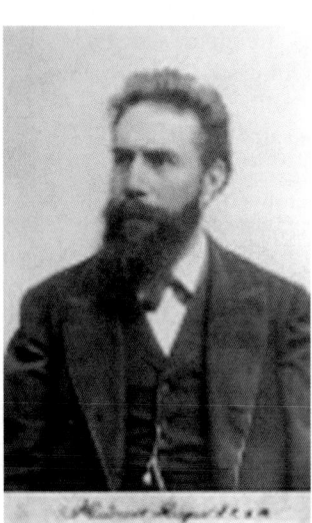

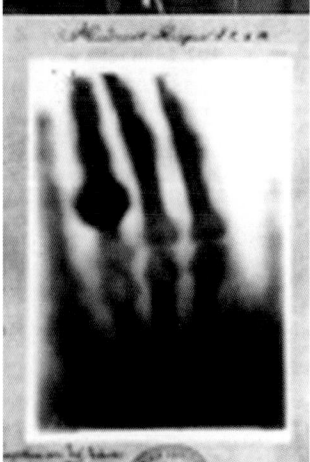

Computed Tomography

Most clinical radiologists consider computed tomography (CT) scanning, invented in 1972, the single greatest advance in radiography of anatomic structures since the 1895 discovery of roentgen rays. This coveted discovery earned the 1979 Nobel Prize in Physiology or Medicine to Godfrey N. Hounsfield (1919–2004) and Allan M. Cormack (1924–1998) http://www.nobelprize.org/ nobel_prizes/medicine/

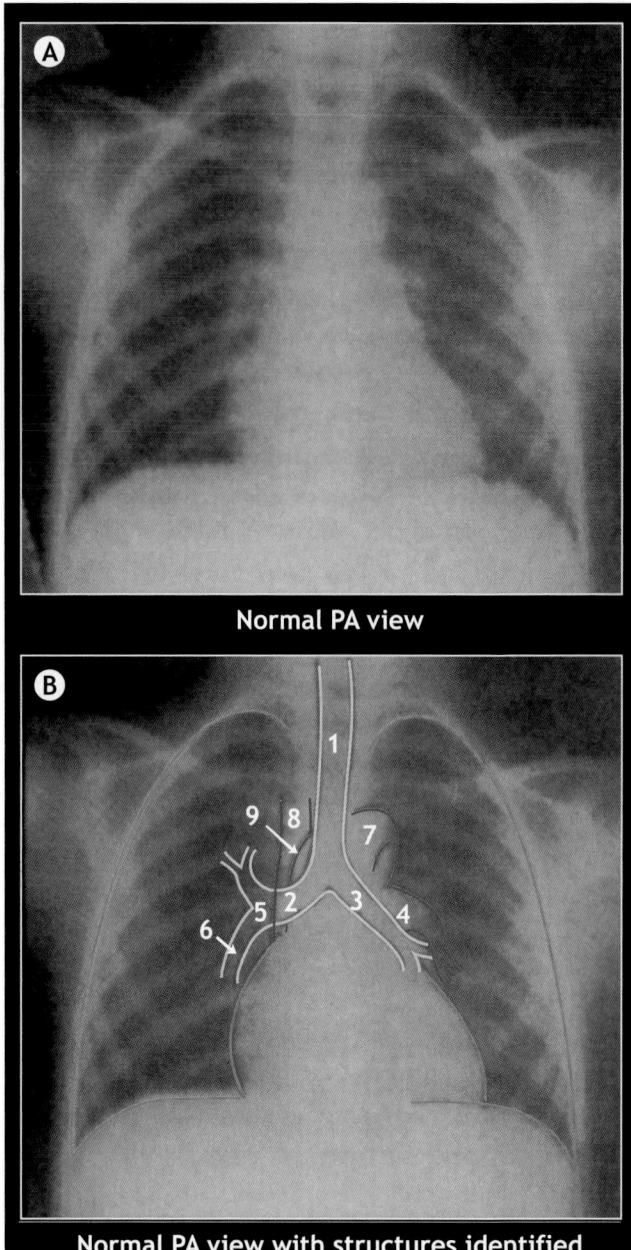

Normal PA view

Normal PA view with structures identified

FIGURE 32.17 • Chest x-ray. **(A)** Radiograph showing a normal chest x-ray in the posteroanterior (PA) view. **(B)** Radiograph showing labeling of the normal anatomic structures. 1, trachea; 2, right mainstem bronchus; 3, left mainstem bronchus; 4, left pulmonary artery; 5, pulmonary vein to the right upper lobe; 6, right interlobular artery; 7, aortic knob; 8, superior vena cava; 9, ascending aorta.

laureates/1979/). CT uses a narrow x-ray beam that moves across the body to define adjacent cross-sectional columns of tissue known as a translation. Another pass of the beam progresses at a different angle or rotation. Repeated translations and rotations in different directions in a given plane with subsequent digitization produce a clear computer-summated image of x-ray transmission data for diagnostic interpretation.

Other Measures

Chapter 12 discussed static and dynamic lung function tests with simple spirometry. Carefully collected spirometric forced vital capacity (FVC), forced expiratory volume in 1 s ($FEV_{1.0}$), maximum voluntary ventilation (MVV), peak expiratory flow (PEF), and lung compliance provide crucial diagnostic information. To measure compliance, the patient swallows a balloon catheter. The technician positions the catheter in the lower third of the esophagus and connects it to a manometer to measure esophageal pressure. The relation of lung volume change to any change in pressure within the catheter then establishes the curve for lung compliance.

Other useful functional tests include pulmonary diffusing capacity (DL or DLCO, expressed in $mL \cdot min^{-1} \cdot mm\ Hg^{-1}$), which measures how much gas enters pulmonary blood per unit time per unit pressure differential across the alveolar–capillary membrane. Flow-volume loops provide graphic representations of events occurring during forced inspiration and expiration. Recording the flow versus volume in an X–Y presentation diagnoses central or peripheral airway obstructions.

Blood gas analyses provide important information to assess problems related to acid–base balance, alveolar ventilation, and level of arterial oxygen saturation and carbon dioxide elimination. Cytologic and hematologic tests identify microorganisms that cause pulmonary disease.

Pulmonary Rehabilitation and Physical Activity Prescription

Pulmonary rehabilitation programs receive considerably less attention than programs for cardiovascular and musculoskeletal diseases. The lack of emphasis on pulmonary rehabilitation stems from a failure of rehabilitation to improve pulmonary function significantly or "cure" these potentially deadly diseases.

thePoint   Appendix H, available online at http://thepoint.lww.com/mkk8e, provides a list of supplemental animations and videos on this subject, including a discussion of ongoing research about dyspnea.

Nevertheless, successful pulmonary rehabilitation places central focus on increased physical activity because of its positive impact on exercise capacity, respiratory and nonrespiratory muscle functions, ventilatory equivalents for oxygen, psychologic status, quality-of-life variables (e.g., self-esteem and self-efficacy), frequency of hospitalization, and disease progression.[11,23,125] The spiral of progressive physical deconditioning from a sedentary lifestyle (as patients attempt to avoid dyspnea) is not just the direct effect of COPD.[138,154] Peripheral and respiratory muscle weakness frequently contribute to the COPD patients' poor exercise performance and

physiologic incapacity.[65,153] Within this framework, the eight major goals for pulmonary rehabilitation include:

1. Improving health status
2. Improving respiratory symptoms (shortness of breath and cough)
3. Recognizing early signs that require medical intervention
4. Decreasing frequency and severity of respiratory problems
5. Maximizing arterial oxygen saturation and carbon dioxide elimination
6. Enhancing daily functional capacity through improved muscular strength, joint flexibility, and cardiorespiratory endurance
7. Modifying body composition to enhance functional capacity
8. Optimizing nutritional status

The overall pulmonary rehabilitation program emphasizes general patient care, pulmonary respiratory care, exercise and functional training, education about the disease, and psychosocial management.

Since breathlessness is the primary determinant of exertional tolerance for the individual with COPD, *ratings of shortness of breath* can be used to monitor exercise intensity. Intensity should not be limited by shortness of breath before patients experience moderate exertion. Intermittent exercise comprised of short intervals of activity alternating with regular rest periods usually allows for higher intensities of effort. After accommodating to a regular physical activity schedule the individual may be able to sustain a higher percentage of peak capacity for 30 to 40 minutes per training session. Regular physical activity benefits typically increase as the training load gradually progresses. For most COPD patients, 15 minutes of moderate physical activity, 3 days per week is probably the minimum amount to ensure the appropriate benefits.

Physiologic monitoring during exercise rehabilitation typically includes measurement of heart rate, blood pressure, respiratory rate, arterial oxygen saturation by pulse oximetry, and dyspnea. Dyspnea monitoring as a target for physical training involves a perceived **dyspnea scale** (FIG. 32.18) similar to the ratings of perceived exertion scale.[44,73] The dyspnea scale emphasizes symptoms of breathing difficulty rather than perceptions of whole-body physical distress, which the RPE measures. Self-monitoring effort intensity in this manner has two inherent advantages:

1. Respiratory disease usually impairs pulmonary function rather than cardiovascular response
2. Target heart rate for training healthy individuals usually exceeds the peak heart rate achieved when stress testing pulmonary patients.

The most common reasons for stopping activity include extreme shortness of breath, fatigue, palpitations, chest discomfort, and a 3 to 5% decrease in pulse oximetry.

The pretraining GXT and spirometric analyses form the basis for the exercise prescription.[28] Interpretation of the exercise stress test includes examining three factors:

1. Whether the test terminated because of cardiovascular or ventilatory end points
2. The difference between pre- and postexercise pulmonary function (e.g., a decrease of 10% in $FEV_{1.0}$ indicates the need for bronchodilator therapy before exercise)
3. Need for supplemental oxygen during exercise (e.g., a pre- to posttest decrease in Pao_2 of more than 20 mm Hg or a Pao_2 below 55 mm Hg)

Exercise prescriptions based on cycling, walking, treadmill exercise, and stair climbing for patients with **mild lung disease**—shortness of breath with intense exercise—remains similar to requirements for healthy subjects. Exercise for patients with **moderate lung disease**—shortness of breath with normal daily activities or clinical symptoms of RLD or COPD—typically achieves an intensity no greater than 75% of the ventilatory reserve, or the point where the patient becomes noticeably dyspneic. For most patients, this exercise intensity usually falls in the middle of the calculated training heart rate range—50 to 70% of age-predicted maximum with a goal of 60 to 80% of maximum—and corresponds to 40 to 85% of maximum MET level on the GXT. In this case, exercise duration averages 20 min, three times weekly. If the patient can exercise only for a shorter duration (e.g., 5 to 15 min per session), exercise frequency can increase to 5 to 7 days weekly.

Patients with **severe lung disease**—shortness of breath during most daily activities and FVC and $FEV_{1.0}$ below 55% of predicted values—require a modified approach to exercise testing and prescription. Low-level, discontinuous testing usually begins at 2 to 3 METs with increments every 2 to 3 min. Exercise prescription relies on symptom-limited walking speeds and distances. Brief bouts of interval exercise also provide an option. The low level of the initial training prescription means that patients should exercise a minimum of once daily. Even small gains in physical tolerance add to improving daily function and quality of life.

General activities and specific expiratory muscle training effectively improve respiratory muscle function and reduce sensations of respiratory effort during physical activity in nearly all patients with pulmonary disease.[22,96,162] Two approaches achieve this goal:

1. Resistance training of the ventilatory musculature with a continuous positive airway pressure (CPAP) device; this specifically overloads the respiratory muscles similarly to progressive resistance exercise for nonrespiratory skeletal muscles
2. Increasing respiratory muscle force and endurance capacity through regular aerobic training

 INTEGRATIVE QUESTION

Why might regular physical activity prove more effective for coronary heart disease patients than patients with pulmonary disease?

Pulmonary Medications

Pulmonary medications include bronchodilators, antiinflammatory agents, decongestants, antihistamines, mucokinetic agents, respiratory stimulants, depressants, and paralyzing and antimicrobial agents. The drugs promote bronchodilation, facilitate removal of lung secretions, improve alveolar ventilation and arterial oxygenation, and optimize breathing patterns. TABLE 32.21 lists the most commonly administered pulmonary drugs.

PHYSICAL ACTIVITY AND ASTHMA

Asthma Statistics

The latest available statistics indicate that asthma has increased in severity and scope (www.aaaai.org/media/resources/media_kit/asthma_statistics.stm). Hyperirritability of the pulmonary airways followed by bronchial spasm, edema, and mucus secretion characterize this obstructive pulmonary disease (FIG 32.19) Common asthma symptoms include chest tightness, coughing, wheezing, and/or shortness of breath.

 See the animation "Asthma" on **http://thePoint. lww.com/mkk8e** for a description and explanation of this condition.

A high level of physical fitness does not confer immunity from asthma.[39,100,124,131,167] The recreational road runner is more likely to report symptoms of allergy and/or asthma but

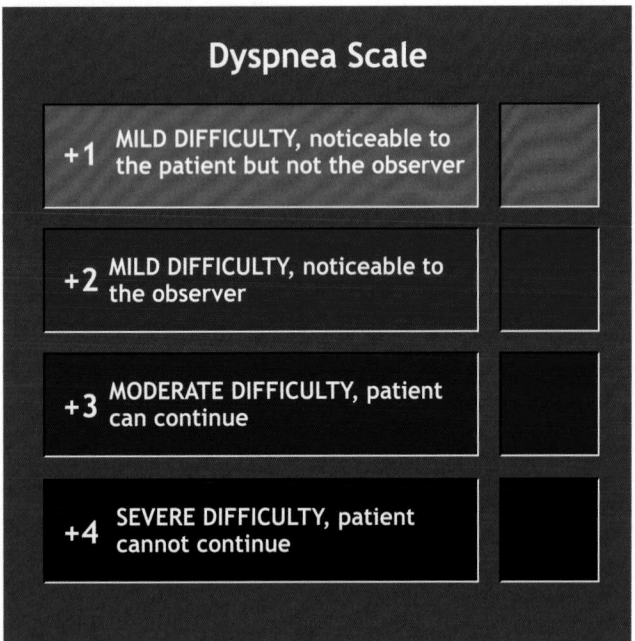

FIGURE 32.18 • Dyspnea scale. Subjective ratings of dyspnea on a scale of 1 to 4 during graded exercise testing. Dyspnea usually accompanies poor exercise capacity and an impaired systolic blood pressure response.

TABLE 32.21   Major Pulmonary Bronchodilator Drugs: Their Uses and Side Effects

Drug/Name	Action and Clinical Uses	Side Effects
Sympathomimetics Isoproterenol, ephedrine, Bronkosol, Alupent, Brethine, Proventil, Ventolin (Albuterol inhaler)	Decrease intracellular calcium; smooth muscle relaxation; bronchodilation	Tachycardia, palpitations, GI distress, nervousness, headache, dizziness
Methylxanthines Amnodur, Elixophyllin, Theo-dur, Choladril	Increase cAMP; block cAMP decrease	Agitation, hypotension, chest pain, nausea, tachycardia, palpitations, GI distress, nervousness, headache, dizziness
α-Sympatholytics	Block cAMP decrease; bronchodilation	Agitation, hypotension, chest pain, nausea, tachycardia, palpitations, GI distress, nervousness, headache, dizziness
Parasympatholytics Atrovent, atropine sulfate	Block parasympathetic stimulation and prevents increases in cGMP; prevents bronchoconstriction	Central nervous system stimulation with low doses and depression with high doses; delirium, hallucinations, decreased GI activity
Glucocorticoids Prednisone, Cortisol, Azmacort, Vanceril	Decrease inflammatory response; bronchodilation	Obesity, growth suppression, hyperglycemia and diabetes, mood changes, irritability or depression, thinning of skin, muscle wasting
Cromolyn sodium Intal, Fivent	Prevents influx of calcium ions, thus blocking mast cell release of mediators responsible for bronchoconstriction; bronchodilation	Throat irritation, hoarseness, dry mouth, cough, chest tightness, bronchospasm

less likely to have prescription medication than the Olympic athlete.[111,139] Based on data from the last five Olympic games, a study by the University of Western Australia has identified those athletes with asthma and airway hyperresponsiveness. With a prevalence of around 8%, these are the most common chronic conditions among Olympic athletes, and could be related to the nature of their intense training.[39] Studies of Finnish elite track and field athletes report physician-diagnosed asthma in 17% of long-distance runners, 8% of power athletes, and 3% of nonathletic controls, while 35% of figure skaters showed a significant increase in airway resistance following skating routines.[68,102]

For nearly 90% of persons with asthma and 30 to 50% of those suffering from allergic rhinitis and hay fever, physical activity provides a potent stimulus for bronchoconstriction, termed ***exercise-induced bronchospasm***. Reduced vagal tone and increased catecholamine release from the sympathetic nervous system during exertion *normally* relax pulmonary airway smooth muscle.[9] Initial bronchodilation with activity occurs in healthy persons and asthmatics. For the asthmatic, bronchospasm accompanied by excessive mucus secretion follow initial bronchodilation. An acute episode of airway obstruction often occurs within 5 to 15 min postexercise; recovery usually occurs spontaneously within 30 to 90 min. One useful technique to detect an exercise-induced asthmatic response applies progressive exercise increments. A spirometric evaluation of FVC and $FEV_{1.0}$ takes place after each exercise period and during 10 to 20 min of recovery. *A 10 to*

15% reduction in pre-exercise $FEV_{1.0}$/FVC confirms the diagnosis of exercise-induced bronchospasm.[71,95,108] For elite athletes who perform in cold-weather sports (e.g., biathlon, canoeing/kayaking, cross-country skiing, ice hockey, Nordic combined, and speed skating), combining pulmonary function testing with near-maximal sport-specific exercise testing, preferably in a cold, dry environment, provides greater sensitivity for screening than laboratory-based warm air environmental challenges or self-reported symptoms.[74,145,146]

Sensitivity to Thermal Gradients and Fluid Loss

Several mechanisms help to explain bronchospastic responses to exercise. An attractive theory relates to how ventilation in exercise and recovery alters the rate and magnitude of heat and water exchange in the tracheobronchial tree. As the incoming breath of air moves down the respiratory tract, heat and water move away from the airway lining as the air warms and humidifies. The conditioning of inspired air ultimately cools and dries the respiratory mucosa. Drying increases mucosal lining osmolality, with accompanying mast cell degranulation. This in turn releases powerful proinflammatory mediators that trigger bronchoconstriction (e.g., leukotrienes, histamine, and prostaglandins). Rewarming the airways following physical activity dilates the bronchial microcirculation to increase blood flow. Bronchial vasculature engorgement precipitates edema that constricts the airway, independent of any constrictive

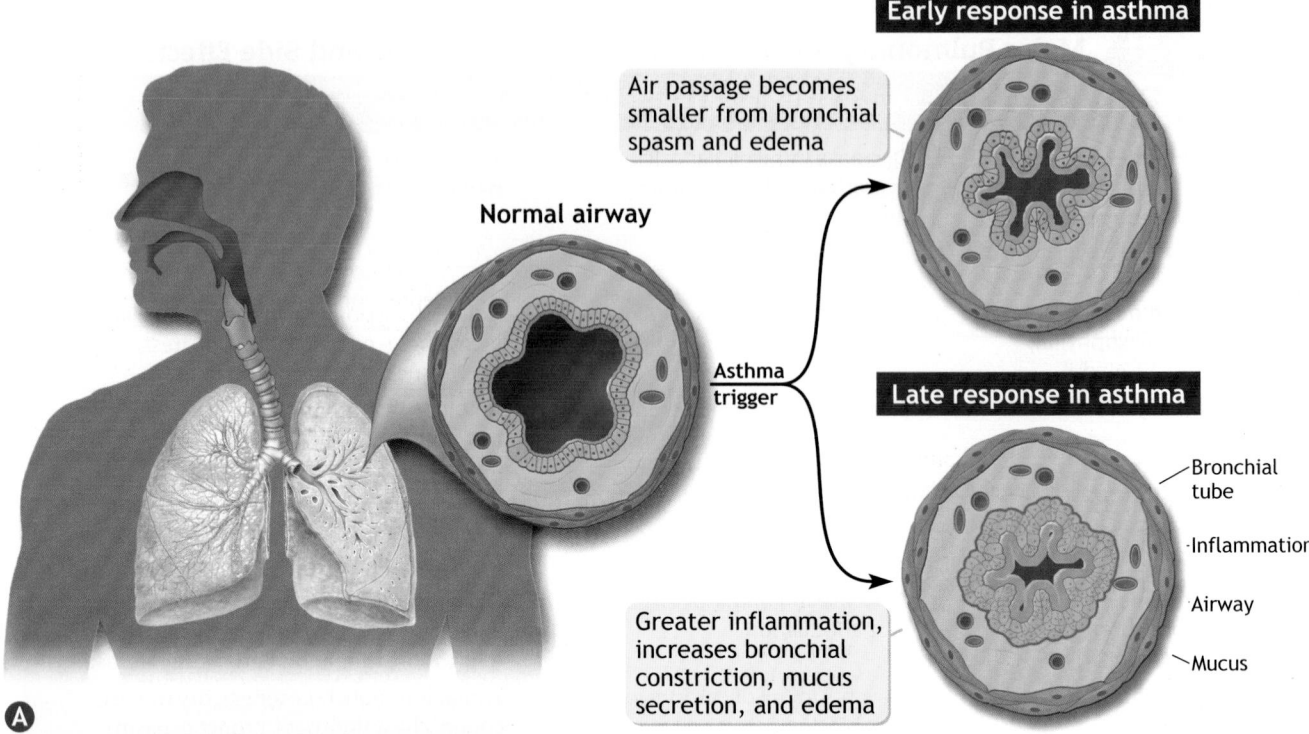

Early response in asthma

Air passage becomes smaller from bronchial spasm and edema

Normal airway

Asthma trigger

Late response in asthma

Bronchial tube

Inflammation

Airway

Mucus

Greater inflammation, increases bronchial constriction, mucus secretion, and edema

A

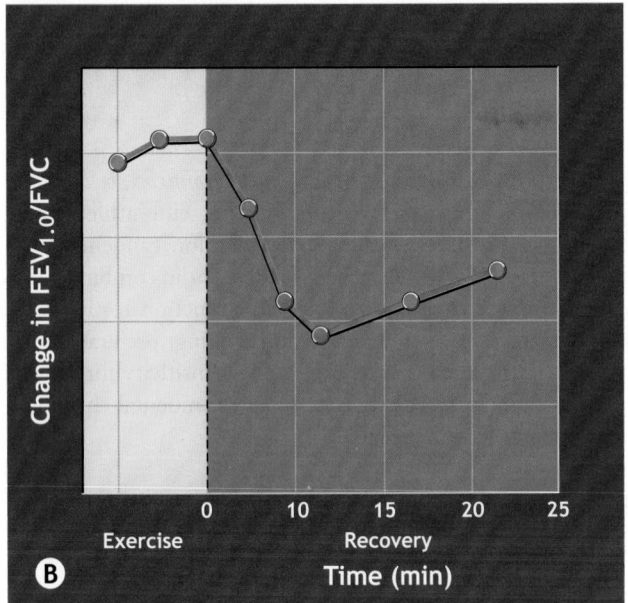

B

FIGURE 32.19 • **(A)** Typical response to an asthma attack. **(B)** Pattern of dynamic lung function ($FEV_{1.0}/FVC$) during an episode of exercise-induced bronchospasm.

action of bronchial smooth muscle. Bronchial cooling during activity and rewarming in recovery also stimulate chemical mediator release that induces bronchoconstriction.

Regardless of the precise mechanism, the large volume of incompletely conditioned inspired air taxes the tracheobronchial tree's smaller airways, causing mucosal temperature to decrease. Heat loss from the airways during physical activity relates directly to the degree of bronchoconstriction. In susceptible individuals, the thermal gradient generated by the combination of airway cooling during exercise and subsequent rewarming in recovery intensifies bronchospastic processes.

Environmental Impact

A warm–humid (summer) environment suppresses the magnitude of exercise-induced bronchospasm regardless of air temperature. Inhaling ambient air fully saturated with water vapor limits airway epithelial cell disruption and injury and often abolishes an asthmatic's bronchospastic exercise response.[16] This explains why persons with asthma tolerate walking or jogging on a warm, humid day or swimming in an indoor pool, in contrast to outdoor winter sports that typically trigger an asthmatic attack.[79,149]

Benefits of Warm-Up and Medication

Fifteen to 30 min of a light-to-moderate, continuous warm-up or a strategy that includes at least some repeat high-intensity warm-up intervals initiate a **refractory period** where subsequent intense activity does not trigger as severe a bronchoconstrictive response.[9,12,140,160] The warm-up benefit continues for up to 2 hr, perhaps from prostaglandin release. Prolonging the cooldown period also reduces the severity of postexercise bronchoconstriction; this could occur by slowing airway rewarming and subsequent bronchiole vascular dilation and edema.

Effective pre-exercise medications limit bronchoconstriction for those desiring to exercise regularly without adversely affecting exercise performance. Medications include bronchodilators such as theophylline or the leukotriene-receptor antagonist montelukast or β_2-agonists (salmeterol) and inhaled heparin therapy or anti-inflammatory corticosteroids or cromolyn sodium.[17,32,118]

Exercise training does not eliminate or cure an asthmatic condition; instead, it increases pulmonary airflow reserve and reduces ventilatory work by potentiating exercise bronchodilation. This lets asthmatics maintain higher airflow and sustain relatively intense effort despite impaired pulmonary function. For asthmatic children, aerobic training, primarily swimming and cycle ergometry, improves $\dot{V}O_{2max}$ and suppresses asthmatic symptoms.

NEUROMUSCULAR DISEASES, DISABILITIES, AND DISORDERS

Neuromuscular diseases and disabilities affect the brain in specific ways. Progressive degeneration or trauma to specific brain neurons induces distinct impairment that ranges from simple to complex.

Stroke

Stroke refers to a potentially fatal reduction in the brain's blood flow from ischemia (restricted blood flow) or hemorrhage (bleeding). The resulting brain injury affects multiple systems depending on injury site and amount of damage sustained. Effects include motor and sensory impairment and language, perception, and affective and cognitive dysfunction. Strokes cause severe limitations in mobility and cognition or can be less severe with short-term, nonpermanent consequences (www.strokeassociation.org/STROKEORG/AboutStroke/About-Stroke_UCM_308529_SubHomePage.jsp).

 See the animation "Stroke" on http://thePoint.lww.com/mkk8e to learn more about the different types of strokes.

Clinical Features

Clinical features of stroke depend on location and severity of injury. Signs of a hemorrhagic stroke include altered levels of consciousness, severe headache, and elevated blood pressure. Cerebellar hemorrhage usually occurs unilaterally and associates with disequilibrium, nausea, and vomiting. TABLE 32.22 presents the typical physical and psychologic conditions and comorbidities associated with a stroke.

Cerebral blood flow (CBF) represents the primary marker to assess ischemic strokes. When CBF drops below $10\ mL \cdot 100\ g \cdot min^{-1}$ of brain tissue (normal CBF = 50–55 $mL \cdot 100\ g \cdot min^{-1}$), synaptic transmission failure occurs; cell death results at a CBF of $\leq 8\ mL \cdot 100\ g \cdot min^{-1}$.

Stroke produces physical and cognitive damage. Left-hemisphere lesions typically associate with expressive and receptive language deficits compared with right-hemisphere lesions. Motor impairment from a stroke usually triggers hemiplegia (paralysis) or hemiparesis (weakness). Damage to descending neural pathways produces abnormal regulation of spinal motor neurons. This adversely changes

postural and stretch reflexes and produces difficulty with voluntary movement. Deficits in motor control involve muscle weakness, abnormal synergistic organization of movement, impaired regulation of force, decreased reaction times, abnormal muscle tone, and loss of active range of joint motion.

Exercise Prescription

The emphasis for stroke survivors centers on rehabilitation of movement (passive and active-assisted flexibility and muscle strength) during the first 6 mo of recovery. The few exercise-training studies with stroke patients support physical activity to improve mobility and functional independence and prevent or reduce further disease and functional impairment.[8,99,169]

Stroke survivors vary widely in age, degree of disability, motivational level, and number and severity of comorbidities, secondary conditions, and associated circumstances. The specific exercise prescription focuses on reducing these conditions and improving functional capacity.

Multiple Sclerosis

Multiple sclerosis (MS) represents a chronic, often disabling disease characterized by destruction of the myelin sheath or demyelination that surrounds CNS nerve fibers (www.nationalmssociety.org/index.aspx). Lesions of inflammatory demyelination can be present in any part of the brain and spinal cord.

Clinical Features

Two or more areas of demyelination confirm the diagnosis of MS. This disease usually develops between ages 20 and 40. Frequently a history emerges of transient neurologic deficits that include extremity numbness, weakness,

TABLE 32.22	Physical and Psychologic Conditions and Comorbidities in Stroke Patients	
Physical Conditions	**Psychologic Conditions**	**Comorbidities**
Aphasia	Cognitive impairment	Coronary heart disease
Balance problems	Emotional instability	Diabetes mellitus
Falls	Cognitive impairment	Hypertension
Fatigue	Depression	Hyperlipidemia
Muscle weakness	Memory loss	Obesity
Obesity	Low self-esteem	Peripheral vascular disease
Paralysis	Social isolation	
Paresis		
Spasticity		
Visual impairment		

blurred vision, and diplopia (double vision) in childhood or adolescence prior to more persistent neurologic deficits that lead to the definitive diagnosis. Fatigue is the most common symptom of MS. MS occurs worldwide at a higher frequency in latitudes farther from the equator (40°). For as yet unknown reasons, MS prevalence in the United States below the 37th parallel is 57 to 78 cases per 100,000, whereas the prevalence rate above the 37th parallel averages 140 cases per 100,000. Patients with a definite MS diagnosis often have a variety of other autoimmune illnesses such as systemic lupus erythematosus, rheumatoid arthritis, polymyositis, and myasthenia gravis. A person who has a first-degree relative with MS has a 12- to 20-fold increased chance of developing MS.

Exercise Prescription

MS patients benefit from a comprehensive health prescription that involves aerobic, strength, balance, coordination, and flexibility exercises. About 80% of MS patients report adverse effects to heat exposure. This occurs whether generated environmentally by outside climatic changes or internally via fever or exercise-induced thermogenesis. This effect makes continuous exercise training difficult and not well tolerated. Nevertheless, MS patients still can improve cardiovascular function. Stationary cycling, walking, and low-impact chair or water aerobics provide excellent training choices depending on personal interest and level and nature of physical impairment. Ideal activity consists of walking in a climate-controlled area that provides stable temperatures, a level surface, and opportunity to rest frequently. Controlling body temperature is a primary consideration in the exercise prescription. A realistic and achievable goal for structured activity provides training three times a week for a minimum of 30 min each session divided into three 10-min periods.

Parkinson's Disease

Parkinson's disease (**PD**) belongs to a group of conditions called motor system disorders, which are the result of the loss of dopamine-producing brain cells (www.parkinson.org).

Clinical Features

Four clinical symptoms of PD include:

1. Varying degrees of tremor
2. Decrease in spontaneity and movement (bradykinesia)
3. Rigidity
4. Impaired postural reflexes

These conditions produce extreme gait and postural instability that increases falling episodes and difficulty walking. Some patients exhibit a complete lack of movement (akinesia). Functional problems hinder getting out of bed or a car and rising from a chair. Other problems include difficulties dressing, writing, talking, and swallowing. A person with PD

generally experiences difficulty with more than one task at a time. As the disease progresses, these problems become more pronounced, and the person eventually loses ability to perform activities of daily living. In the last stage of the disease, the person becomes wheelchair and/or bed bound.

Exercise Prescription

Most exercise prescriptions for PD patients are individualized and directed toward interventions that affect associated motor control problems. They emphasize slow, controlled movements for specific tasks through various ranges of motion while lying, sitting, standing, and walking. Treatment protocols include range-of-motion activities that emphasize slow static stretches for all major muscle–joint areas, balance and gait training, mobility, and/or coordination exercises.

RENAL DISEASE

Treatment modalities for the major metabolic diseases of diabetes (see Chapter 20), obesity (see Chapter 30), and renal dysfunction use regular exercise as adjunctive therapy. This section reviews aspects of renal disease related to exercise physiology.

Chronic renal disease occurs when kidneys no longer adequately carry out their filtering functions. Acute renal failure occurs from a toxin (e.g., drug allergy or poison) or severe blood loss or trauma. Diabetes is the primary cause of kidney disease, responsible for about 40% of all kidney failures; hypertension is the second cause, responsible for about 25%. Genetic diseases, autoimmune diseases, and birth defects most commonly cause kidney ailments.

Clinical Features

Common symptoms of chronic kidney disease, sometimes referred to as uremia (retention in the blood of waste products normally excreted in urine), include the following ten characteristics:

1. *Changes in urination*: These include making more or less urine than usual, feeling pressure when urinating, changes in the color of urine, foamy or bubbly urine, or having to get up frequently at night to urinate.
2. *Swelling of the feet, ankles, hands, or face*: Fluid the kidneys are unable to remove stays in the tissues.
3. *Fatigue or weakness*: Buildup of wastes or a shortage of red blood cells (anemia) causes these problems as the kidneys begin to fail.
4. *Shortness of breath*: Kidney failure is sometimes confused with asthma or heart failure because fluid builds up in the lungs.
5. *Ammonia breath or an ammonia or metal taste in the mouth*: Waste build-up causes bad breath, changes in taste, or an aversion to protein foods such as meat.
6. *Back or flank pain*: The kidneys are located on either side of the spine in the back.

7. *Itching*: Waste accumulation causes severe itching, especially of the legs.
8. *Loss of appetite*
9. *Nausea and vomiting*
10. *Increased hypoglycemic episodes, if diabetic*

Chronic uremia eventually progresses to **end-stage renal disease** (**ESRD**) that requires life-long dialysis or kidney transplant. The number of renal transplants has increased steadily worldwide in the last decade and generally offers a more normal lifestyle and full rehabilitation. Nearly 80% of transplant patients function at near normal levels compared with 40 to 60% of those treated with dialysis. Almost 75% of transplant patients resume work compared with 50 to 60% of patients who receive dialysis.

Exercise Prescription

Regular physical activity is important in rehabilitating dialysis and transplant patients to better adapt to their illness. The rehabilitation program should begin prior to the start of dialysis to optimize beneficial effects. Normal low-level endurance training (following ACSM guidelines) reduces muscle protein degradation in moderate renal insufficiency, reduces resting blood pressure in some hemodialysis patients, and modestly improves aerobic capacity in patients who undergo hemodialysis.

No longitudinal data exist about aerobic training effects or a more physically active lifestyle on patient survival with chronic uremia or kidney transplants. Uremic patients who maintain diverse physical activity report enhanced quality of life, increased physical capacity, improved muscle strength and function, decreased blood pressure, and improved inflammation and oxidative stress biomarkers.[67,72]

COGNITIVE/EMOTIONAL DISEASES AND DISORDERS

The National Institute of Mental Health (www.nimh.nih.gov) estimates that about 26% of Americans ages 18 and older—about 1 in 4 adults—suffer from a diagnosable mental disorder in a given year. In addition, 4 of the 10 leading causes of disability in the United States and other developed countries are mental disorders—major depression, bipolar disorder, schizophrenia, and obsessive–compulsive disorder. Suicide, closely linked to depression, represents the third leading cause of death among 10- to 24-year-olds. Also, 6 to 8% of all outpatients in primary care settings suffer major depression. Despite the large numbers of depressed patients, mental disorders remain underdiagnosed; only about one third of those diagnosed receive treatment.

The five major classifications of cognitive/emotional diseases include:

1. **Major depressive disorder**—commonly referred to as "depression"
2. **Dysthymia**—mildly depressed on most days over a period of at least 2 years

3. **Seasonal affective disorder**—recurrence of the depressive symptoms during certain seasons (e.g., winter)
4. **Postpartum depression**—in women who have recently given birth; typically occurs in the first few months after delivery, but can happen within the first year after giving birth
5. **Bipolar disorder** (previously known as manic-depressive illness)—characterized by extremes in mood and behavior that last for at least 2 wk

 Use It or Lose It

Regular physical activity during adolescence may protect against dementia in old age. Researchers already know that physically active older people are less likely to suffer cognitive impairment than sedentary counterparts, and some research indicates that physical activity during middle age also confers a protective effect. A study from the *Journal of the American Geriatrics Society* evaluated exercise effects at age 50, age 30, and down through the teenage years. Those who were physically active at each point in life got higher cognition test scores than those who were inactive, with exercise in the teenage years having the most powerful effect. One possible explanation for this effect is that physical activity in the teen years helps to stave off conditions like obesity, type 2 diabetes, and hypertension that also carry greater risk for cognitive decline.

Source: Middleton LE, et al. Physical activity over the life course and its association with cognitive performance and impairment in old age. *J Am Geriatr Soc* 2010;58:1322.

Clinical Features

Depression has no single cause but often results from a combination of factors or events. Whatever its cause, depression is not just a "state of mind." Depression relates to physical changes in the brain and a chemical imbalance of neurotransmitters.

Women are almost twice as likely to suffer from depression as men, partly because of hormonal changes from puberty, menstruation, menopause, and pregnancy. Men are more likely go undiagnosed and less likely to seek help. Men may show the typical symptoms of depression but tend to be angry and hostile or mask their condition with alcohol or drug abuse. Suicide remains a serious risk for depressed men, who are four times more likely than women to kill themselves. Depression among older adults poses a unique situation. Older persons often lose loved ones and have to adjust to living alone. Physical illness depresses normal levels of physical activity, further contributing to depression. Loved ones may attribute signs of depression to normal aging, and many older persons are reluctant to talk about their symptoms. Consequently, older persons may not receive proper treatment for depression. TABLE 32.23 presents common signs and symptoms of depression.

TABLE 32.23	Twelve Common Signs and Symptoms of Depression

1. Loss of enjoyment from things that were once pleasurable
2. Loss of energy
3. Feelings of hopelessness or worthlessness
4. Difficulty concentrating
5. Difficulty making decisions
6. Insomnia or excessive sleep
7. Stomachache and digestive problems
8. Decreased sex drive
9. Aches and pains (e.g., recurrent headaches)
10. Change in appetite causing weight loss or gain
11. Thoughts of death or suicide
12. Attempting suicide

Four common factors in depression include:

1. **Family situation**—trauma and stress from financial problems, breakup of a relationship, death of a loved one, other major life changes
2. **Pessimistic personality**—higher risk for individuals who have low self-esteem and a negative outlook
3. **Health status**—medical conditions such as heart disease, cancer, and HIV that contribute to depression
4. **Other psychologic disorders**—anxiety disorders, eating disorders, schizophrenia, and substance abuse that often appear with depression

Exercise Prescription

Exercise studies in clinically depressed populations include both hospitalized and ambulatory patients. Overall, the data support the positive effects of regular physical activity including resistance training on depressive symptoms.[7,117,156] In most cases, physically active patients had significantly decreased depression scores.

No one kind of exercise has the greatest impact on depression, yet most studies have used running or other aerobic-type activities. Interestingly, positive psychologic outcomes do not depend on achieving physical fitness. Such fitness-related indicators as lower blood pressure and increased aerobic capacity frequently do improve.

The exercise prescription for patients with depression considers the following eight factors:

1. **Anticipate barriers**. Common symptoms of depression—fatigue, lack of energy, and psychomotor retardation—pose formidable barriers to physical activity. Feelings of hopelessness and worthlessness also interfere with motivation to exercise.
2. **Keep expectations realistic**. Make physical activity recommendations with caution. Depressed patients often self-blame and may view exercise as another occasion for failure. Do not raise false expectations that can arouse anxiety and guilt. Explain that physical activity provides an adjunct but not a substitute for primary treatment.
3. **Design a feasible plan**. Make the exercise prescription realistic and practical, not an additional burden to compound the patient's sense of futility. Consider the individual's background and history. For severely depressed patients, postpone exercise until medication and psychotherapy alleviate symptoms. Previously sedentary patients should start with a light activity schedule; for example, just a few minutes of walking each day.
4. **Accentuate pleasurable aspects**. Guide the choice of physical activity by the patient's preferences and circumstances. Use pleasurable activities that are easily added to the patient's schedule.
5. **Include group activities**. Depressed, isolated, and withdrawn patients are most likely to benefit from increased social involvement. The stimulation of being outdoors in a pleasant setting may enhance mood; exposure to light exerts therapeutic effects for seasonal depression.
6. **State specifics**. Walking is almost universally acceptable, carries minimal risk of injury, and benefits mood enhancement. In keeping with recent ACSM recommendations for healthy adults, a goal of 20 to 60 min of walking or other aerobic activity, three to five times a week, remains reasonable. The ACSM also recommends resistance and flexibility training 2 to 3 days weekly.
7. **Encourage compliance**. Improved fitness may be a valuable consequence of exercise participation but is not necessary to produce an antidepressant effect. Compliance increases with less physically demanding programs.
8. **Integrate physical activity with other treatments**. The primary treatments for depression should not present obstacles to increasing physical activity. Antidepressant medication can improve a patient's well being when depression impairs their ability to function.

Summary

1. In the clinical setting, the exercise physiologist focuses on total patient care and restoring patient mobility and functional capacity.
2. Disability refers to diminished functional capacity compounded by an inactive lifestyle. Handicapped denotes a physical performance frame of reference defined by society.
3. Exercise plays an important role in cancer risk reduction, perhaps by increasing levels of anti-inflammatory cytokines.
4. The exercise prescription for cancer patients is symptom-limited, progressive, and individualized, with improved ambulation the primary goal.
5. A carefully planned, circuit–resistance-exercise program decreases depression and state and trait anxieties for women recovering from breast cancer surgery.
6. Cardiovascular disease affects the heart muscle directly, the heart valves, or neural regulation of cardiac function each with a specific pathogenesis and intervention strategy.
7. Myocardial pathologies include angina pectoris, myocardial infarction, pericarditis, congestive heart failure

(CHF), and aneurysm. Moderate-intensity physical activity and prescribed medications provide benefits with relatively low risk for stable, compensated CHF patients.

8. Heart valve diseases include stenosis, insufficiency (regurgitation), prolapse, and endocarditis. Congenital malformations include ventricular or atrial septal defects and patent ductus arteriosus. Dysrhythmias (bradycardia, tachycardia, and premature ventricular contractions) are diseases of the heart's nervous system.

9. Cardiac patient assessment includes medical history, physical examination, heart auscultation to uncover murmurs and valvular problems, and laboratory tests (chest x-ray, ECG, blood lipid analyses, serum enzyme testing).

10. Physiologic assessments for CHD include noninvasive tests (echocardiography, exercise stress testing, and ECG analysis). Invasive testing includes radionuclide thallium imaging, cardiac catheterization, and coronary angiography.

11. Resistance exercise in cardiac rehabilitation restores and maintains muscular strength, promotes preservation of FFM, improves psychologic status and quality of life, and increases glucose tolerance and insulin sensitivity.

12. Graded exercise stress testing provides low-risk screening for CHD preventative and rehabilitative physical activity programs.

13. Multistage bicycle and treadmill tests usually include several levels of 3 to 5 min of submaximal exercise to a self-imposed fatigue level.

14. Alterations in the heart's normal electrical activity pattern often indicate insufficient myocardial oxygen supply.

15. Significant S–T segment depression heralds severe, extensive obstruction in one or more coronary arteries.

16. PVCs in exercise generally indicate severe atherosclerotic heart disease, often involving two or more major coronary vessels.

17. Sudden death from ventricular fibrillation averages 6 to 10 times higher in patients with frequent PVCs.

18. Significant deviations from normal blood pressure and heart rate responses during graded exercise testing often indicate underlying cardiovascular pathology.

19. Stress tests have four possible outcomes: true positive (test successful); false negative (person with CHD misdiagnosed); true negative (test successful); false positive (healthy person misdiagnosed).

20. Cardiac patients improve functional capacity to the same extent as healthy counterparts with a properly prescribed and monitored exercise program.

21. RLD and COPD represent the two major categories of pulmonary disease. RLD increases chest–lung resistance to inflation. COPD disrupts expiratory flow capacity and ultimately impedes aeration of alveolar blood.

22. Regular physical activity effectively manages pulmonary disease by providing guidelines for exercise intensity, patient monitoring, and exercise progression

23. Exercise-induced bronchospasm associates with ambient temperature and humidity and their drying effects on the respiratory mucosa.

24. Drying increases mucosal lining osmolality, which stimulates release of powerful mediators that trigger bronchoconstriction.

25. Physical training does not "cure" asthma; instead, it increases airflow reserve and reduces breathing work during physical activity.

26. The few exercise-training studies with stroke patients supports physical activity as a strategy to improve mobility and functional independence and reduce further disease and functional impairment.

27. Fatigue represents the most common MS symptom; other symptoms include muscle weakness in the extremities, clumsiness, and numbness and tingling. Patients benefit from a comprehensive health prescription that involves aerobic, strength, balance, and flexibility activities.

28. Clinical symptoms of Parkinson's disease (PD) include varying degrees of tremor, decreased spontaneity and movement (bradykinesia), rigidity, and impaired postural reflexes.

29. Individualized exercise prescriptions for PD attempt interventions that affect associated motor control problems. They emphasize slow, controlled movements for specific tasks through various ranges of motion while lying, sitting, standing, and walking.

30. Overall, research supports the positive effects on depressive symptoms of regular physical activity, including resistance training.

the**Point** References are available online at **http://thepoint.lww.com/mkk8e.**

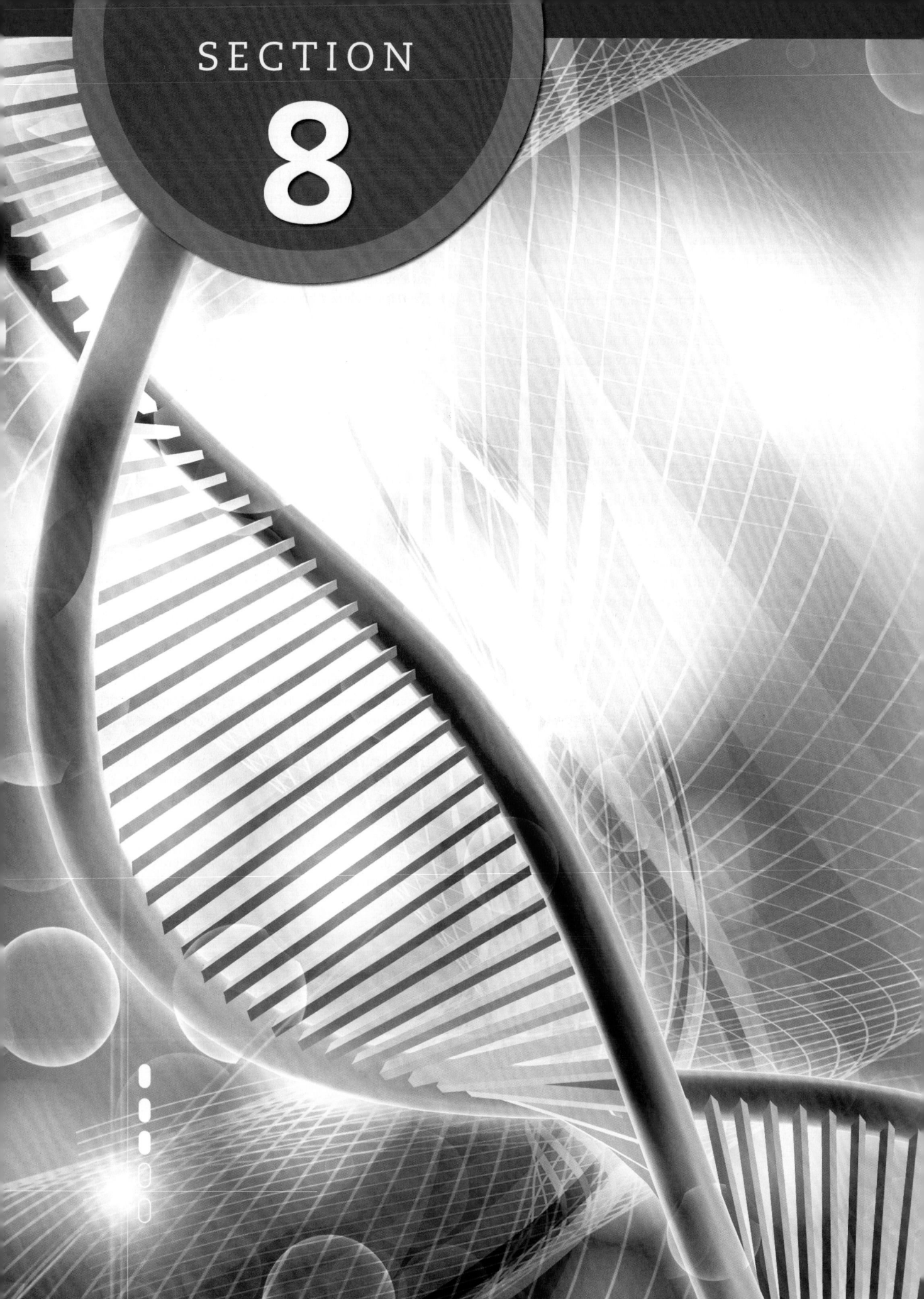

SECTION

8

On the Horizon

The most sensible way to prepare for the challenges and opportunities arising from progress in the identification of the genetic and molecular basis of health and disease is to become familiar with this field and to learn its tools.

Bouchard C, Malina R, Pérusse L. *Genetics of Fitness and Physical Performance*. Champaign, IL: Human Kinetics, 1997.

OVERVIEW

The early 1950s ushered in the dawn of the modern age of molecular biology, and the past 15 years of exercise physiology research has, fortunately, embraced this opportune field. Techniques now available to study how genetic characteristics shape human behavior are revolutionizing almost every facet of human physical activity and sports medicine. The new generation of exercise physiologists has a fantastic opportunity to study the molecular world of genes and their role in human exercise performance and health and disease. This section traces the early historical origins of how the pioneers in the emerging field of basic biology, heredity, and genetics developed their views that eventually led to the modern study in their quest to understand the molecular basis of life.

INTERVIEW WITH
Dr. Frank W. Booth

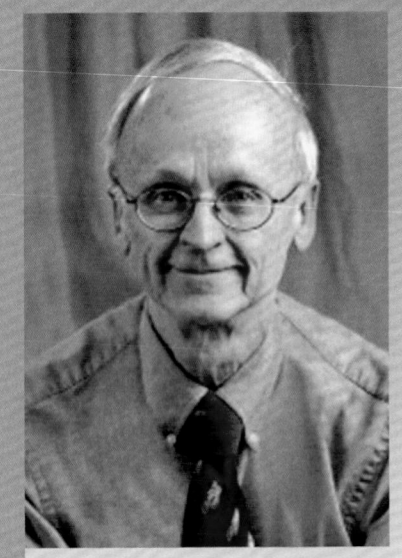

Education: BS (Denison University, Granville, OH); PhD (Exercise Physiology, University of Iowa, Ames); postgraduate studies (School of Aerospace Medicine, Brooks Air Force Base, San Antonio, TX); Department of Preventive Medicine, Washington University School of Medicine, St. Louis, MO.

Current Affiliation: Professor, Department of Veterinary Biomedical Sciences, College of Veterinary Medicine; Department of Physiology and Dalton Cardiovascular Research Institute, University of Missouri, Columbia.

Honors, Awards, and ACSM Citation Award Statement of Contributions: See Appendix C, available online at http://thepoint.lww.com/mkk8e

Research Focus: Molecular basis of how physical inactivity increases the risk of unhealthy syndromes and diseases in humans and companion animals.

Memorable Publication: Booth FW. Perspectives on molecular and cellular exercise physiology. *J Appl Physiol* 1988;65:1461.

What influence did your undergraduate education have on your final career choice?

➤ The courses I took as part of my biology program, along with Dr. Haubrich's encouragement, were the primary influences. I loved my comparative anatomy class, where we did animal dissections. This caused me to think about how things worked in humans. My favorite course was philosophy of religion, a course that really made me think.

Who were the most influential people in your career, and why?

➤ Four individuals exerted a profound effect on my thinking about my career. First, Dr. Haubrich made me think critically about the science of exercise, although I didn't think of it as a "real" science back then. On team bus trips, or when I would speak with him in his office, we would discuss science in general. I always wondered what was happening to my body during all those hours in the pool. I recall writing a paper for one of my classes about "metabolic pathways" that really turned me on about the topic.

What first inspired you to enter the exercise science field? What made you decide to pursue your advanced degree and/or line of research?

➤ My biology advisor at Denison University, Dr. Robert Haubrich, also was the assistant swim coach. Because I was on the swim team, he and I had many talks together, not only about swimming but science in general, including discussions about exercise and training methods. Dr. Haubrich knew of my interest in biology and sports, and one day after practice gave me a flyer advertising a new graduate program in exercise physiology at the University of Iowa. As soon as I finished reading it, I knew graduate school was what I wanted to pursue, so I applied to the program.

Second, Dr. Charles Tipton (see "Interview" in the front matter) at the University of Iowa taught me to explore mechanisms of exercise adaptations. He stressed honesty, as he was a real "straight shooter." Dr. Tipton encouraged me to convey what was on my mind and not simply to tell people what they wanted to hear. He was instrumental in getting me to communicate precisely what I thought and to be human yet honest in doing so. From a physiological–metabolic perspective, Dr. Tipton consistently tried to uncover why something occurred. I've never lost that burning desire to seek out basic explanations.

The third person was Dr. James Barnard, a fellow graduate student and now a professor at UCLA. Jim was an exemplary student (perhaps the smartest I've met), always getting A's in the hardest courses. His ability and enthusiasm for knowledge motivated me to push myself intellectually, both in coursework and in the laboratory. Jim was a great role model for me.

The fourth person, Dr. John Holloszy (see "Interview" in Section 2), mentored my postdoctoral work and taught me to think more critically. As I was continually around other "postdocs" and scientists who were trying to devise creative ways to explain biologic phenomena, there was no way to "hide" from contributing. More than any person I know, Dr. Holloszy possessed the most amazing intuitive "feel" for which experimental procedures would work and which would not. He taught me the basic tenets about how to do science. My interactions with Dr. Holloszy and the other postdoctoral students in conducting various experiments and writing up the results of our work were invaluable in shaping my career in science.

What has been the most interesting/enjoyable aspect of your involvement in science? What was the least interesting/enjoyable aspect?

➤ I cherish the camaraderie of exercise science colleagues, particularly those with whom I have in-depth discussions about various science topics. The individuals who open up and share the truth about their research are the ones I truly enjoy knowing and relating to. The ideal and most enjoyable environment enables one to speak freely, to really express truthful opinions about a topic. I do not enjoy people who tell you what they want you to hear or know for purposes of personal gain (i.e., to build their own ego or self-promote) instead of communicating with respect for the purity of scientific discovery.

What is your most meaningful contribution to the field of exercise science, and why is it so important?

➤ This is a very difficult question for which I have no answer. I suspect that the answer will emanate from the judgments of others. However, I do love applying cutting-edge technology to try to answer mechanistic questions concerning exercise. It is important to try to get to the bottom of things, and using new techniques often provides the key to unlocking the required information. Sometimes, it takes months to perfect the procedure you need for an experiment, and then months more to finally get it to work properly.

What advice would you give to students who express an interest in pursuing a career in exercise science research?

➤ It is important for the student to be excited by a course or topic. Sometimes, undergraduate students have difficulty making a decision about their future. I encourage students with an interest in discovering new insights about any exercise-related topic to become involved with a professor's research projects. Even in graduate school, there is a wide range of "true" desire to continue to pursue research interests. However, those students who experience joyous feelings when searching for the unknown will know deep down they have found a suitable path to follow. If a student can find a mentor, then by all means take advantage of the situation, and do whatever it takes to become deeply involved in the intellectual pursuit.

What interests have you pursued outside your professional career?

➤ I am basically a big-time workaholic. Except for evening runs with my dog Swim, I pretty much start in the lab early and end late. I love vigorous exercise and try to do as much as I can when time permits.

Where do you see the exercise science field (particularly your area of greatest interest) heading in the next 20 years?

➤ Our field needs to produce the very best science to counter the cultural trends that have created a sedentary society with all of its ailments and diseases. Discovering the benefits of exercise and conveying those benefits to the public, from the broadest possible topic areas to the molecular basis of disease, remains our best chance to prevent many diseases and upgrade the nation's health. The field needs to cooperate with multiple partners in a major public health effort to convince the world about the long-term health benefits of regular exercise. We as scientists must systematically provide the medical evidence and cross-disciplinary connections to show that exercise, not drugs, exerts the greatest impact on disease to improve health. All of us must become strong advocates, using education and laboratory-based research to convince people everywhere to pursue a healthy lifestyle.

You have the opportunity to give a "last lecture." Describe its primary focus.

➤ The basis of my talk would involve how regular exercise affects daily living. I would focus not just on the physiologic function and performance aspects, but also on exercise's effects on chronic ills like diabetes, pulmonary and kidney diseases, heart disease, and cancer. For the ever-increasing number of American citizens living in nursing homes, I would discuss the profound effect of sedentary living on muscular atrophy and reduced strength, two factors that limit these individuals' ability to carry out even the simplest tasks of daily living. I would emphasize that relying on pills to tackle disease contributes relatively little to a happy and healthy life. I would also hope to convince the audience that the exercise biologist's role is not simply to study the effects of physical activity or enhance sport performance. The "new" exercise physiologist must reintroduce regular physical activity into an unhealthy, overweight, and sedentary population that is genetically programmed to expect physical activity. I refer to this unhealthy state as SeDS, an abbreviation for sedentary death syndrome.

Achievement of a future, healthy world must involve cooperative effort among diverse public and private organizations that invest enough money in fundamental research to make a real difference. Talking a good game simply will not do it; putting sufficient resources to work will create newer and better opportunities for success through proper research.

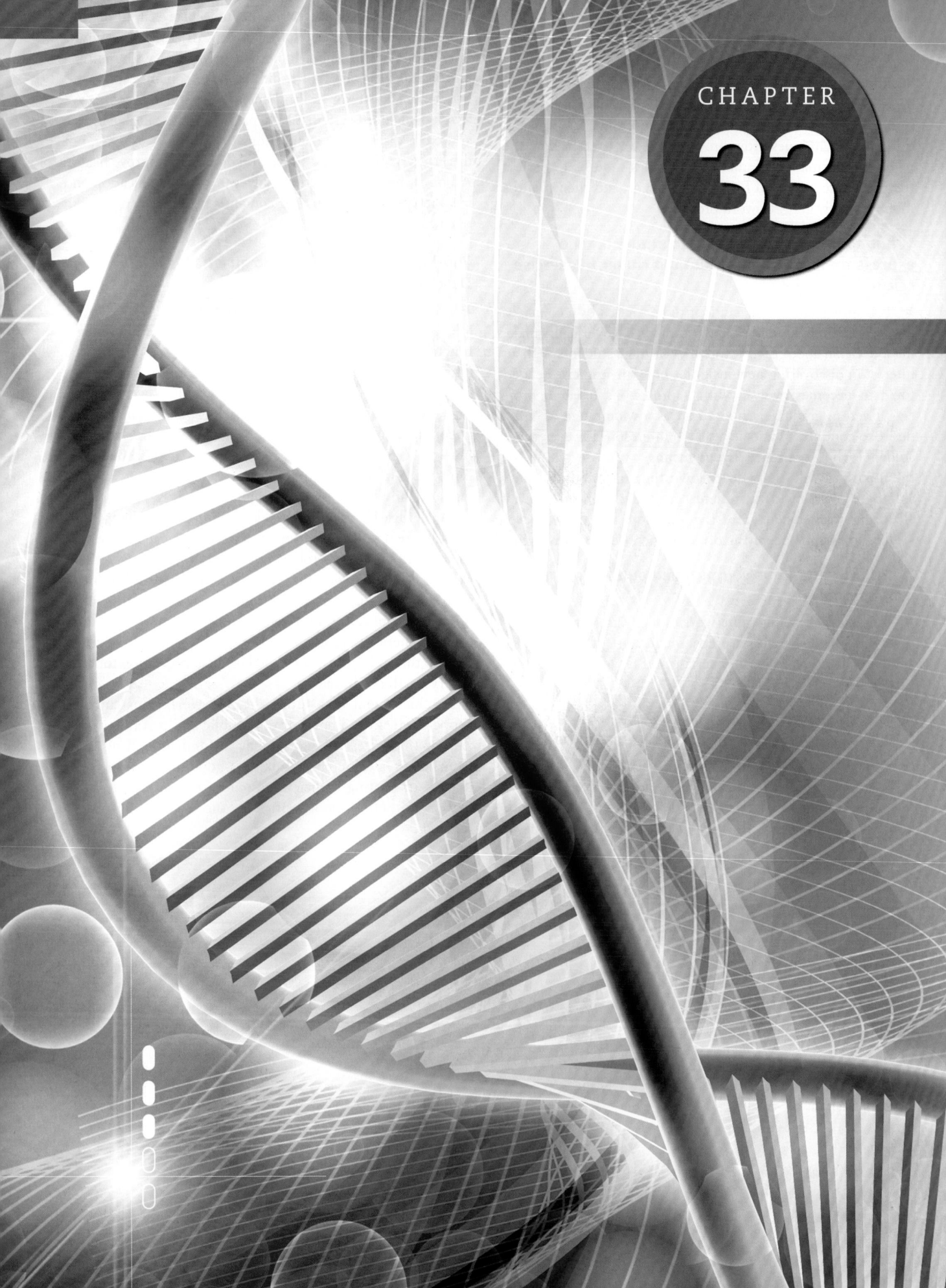

Molecular Biology: A New Vista for Exercise Physiology

Today's exercise physiology faculty and students are cooperating in research projects with basic science, clinical and environmental medicine, chemistry, **molecular biology** and **molecular genetics, pharmacogenetics** (www.ncbi.nlm.nih.gov/About/primer/pharm.html), **epigenetics** (www.nature.com/nature/supplements/insights/epigenetics/), **pharmacogenomics** (www. ornl.gov/sci/techresources/Human_Genome/medicine/pharma.shtml),**bioinformatics** (www. ncbi.nlm.nih.gov/About/primer/bioinformatics.html), **metagenomics** (www.ploscompbiol. org/article/info%3Adoi%2F10.1371%2Fjournal.pcbi.1000667), and other emerging disciplines, many with their own specialty journals, in the physical and life sciences.

Exercise physiology/kinesiology scientists now probe for answers about the molecular basis of physical activity and inactivity as it relates to diseases and dysfunctions (e.g., http://hlknweb.tamu.edu/articles/phd_exercise_physiology; www.kin.hs.iastate.edu/research/immunology/; http://catalog.utk.edu/preview_program.php?catoid=5&poid=1613&returnto=398; www.mcgill.ca/study/2012-2013/faculties/education/undergraduate/programs/bachelor-science-kinesiology-bsckinesiology-kinesiology). Topics run the gamut from the

Gene: segment of DNA with an ordered nucleotide sequence for encoding a specific functional substance (i.e., a protein or RNA molecule)

Molecular biology: study of the molecular basis of life

Molecular genetics: study of the structure and sequence of the molecules that carry genetic information

Genetics: branch of science that studies patterns of inheritance of specific traits in successive generations

Pharmacogenetics: genetic engineering to design specific drugs to target specific disease conditions of an individual's genetic code; this field investigates how genetic diversity affects the efficacy and side effects of targeted drugs

Epigenetics: study of heritable changes in gene function that occur without a change in DNA sequence

Pharmacogenomics: application of genomic methods and perspectives to study drug-responsive genes

Bioinformatics: understanding the underlying chemical codes of organisms by interpreting gene sequences, converting primary linear code into complex three-dimensional structures, managing automated screens, and running combinatorial chemistry syntheses

Metagenomics: the study of a mixture of genetic material from different organisms contained in an environmental sample

Protein: relatively large molecule composed of one or more chains of amino acids in a specific order (determined by the base sequence of nucleotides in the gene coding for the protein); proteins (perhaps up to 140,000 different structures in the body) provide for unique structure, function, and regulation of cells, tissues, and organs; examples include hormones, enzymes, and antibodies

Proteomics: systematic analysis of the protein expression of healthy and unhealthy genomes at the molecular level by identifying, characterizing, and quantifying proteins

Genome: an organism's complete genetic information (DNA and RNA)

Gene expression: converting a gene's coded information by transcription and translation into cellular structures; expressed genes include those transcribed (copied) from DNA nucleotide sequences into mRNA and then translated by ribosomes into specific nucleotide sequences to form protein

role of **genetics** in training and exercise performance to skeletal muscle and neurovestibular adaptations to microgravity. Occupational, physical, and rehabilitation medicine can apply the new strategies of gene therapy to transfer genetic material to enhance a patient's production of specific growth factors (e.g., www.ncmrr.org/Sites/ChildrensNationalMedicalCenter/tabid/182/Default.aspx). These small **protein** molecules stimulate cell proliferation, migration, and differentiation; and they promote matrix synthesis to facilitate healing of injured or surgically repaired tissues with limited blood supply and slowed cell growth that impair normal processes of tissue repair.[99]

In addition to delivering therapeutic proteins to injured tissues, molecular biology provides a way to engineer new tissues (https://biology.mit.edu/research/molecular_medicine_human_disease). Such biologic substitutes—exogenous structures and/or tissue scaffolding—can link gene therapy procedures to support tissue regeneration and healing from athletic trauma. Molecular biology also focuses on how short-term and ongoing physical activity interact to foster structural and functional adaptations that enhance exercise performance and desirable health outcomes.

Booth and colleagues[15,16,17,18] assert that future exercise physiology research should emphasize primary disease prevention, with a focus on uncovering the environmental roots of modern chronic diseases notably type 2 diabetes, almost entirely preventable with increased physical activity.[88] Such maladies annually cause in excess of 350,000 premature deaths and play a role in $4 to 7 trillion in healthcare costs for conditions associated with sedentary living, not to mention the toll on human suffering. Booth, whose contributions are chronicled just prior to this chapter, coined the term *SeDS* (**sedentary environmental death syndrome**) to characterize the effects of a sedentary lifestyle on unhealthy outcomes.[17,19,20,21,150]

Studying the basic biology of organisms at the molecular level offers novel ways to illuminate disease mechanisms and strategies that best combat them. Research challenges also emerge in the exercise biology sciences. More than two decades ago, Baldwin made a compelling case that the membership of the American College of Sports Medicine should exploit new fields and technologies involved with "molecular exercise sciences.[8] Booth and Baldwin (and the authors of this text) maintain that exercise physiology and sports medicine have progressed over the past decades from an exercise biochemistry focus at the organ level to an emphasis on molecular biology at the cellular level. We posit that our field has already shifted to the molecular age, as evidenced by research emphasis in integrative biology and **proteomics** (http://panomics.pnnl.gov). A literature search on PubMed (www.ncbi.nlm.nih.gov:80/entrez) reinforces the point. A tremendous proliferation has occurred in molecular biology interdisciplinary research through 2013 related to the exercise sciences (**Figure 33.1**). As of October 10, 2013, the word **genome** generated 873,331 articles (a 1260% increase from 2001!). Citations with the terms *gene* and *muscle* also increased tremendously, from 502 citations in 2001 to 16,184 in 2005 and to 82,930 on October 10, 2013. Not unexpectedly, the number of citations for "gene" on this same date exceeded 1.82 million, an increase of 250% or 521,203 articles in just 8 years! Other combinations of terms are included to provide a frame of comparison for the future. A clear but recent trend has emerged—inclusion of the term *health* to both gene and **gene expression** has far outpaced, on a percentage basis, the total number of new citations compared to the other terms. This indicates a bountiful and unprecedented explosion of new multidisciplinary research in specific exercise- and health-related areas in molecular biology investigation.

Although funding for genomics, at its peak in 2003–2004, totaled $437 million (from the U.S. Department of Energy [DOE] and the National Institutes of Health), the DOE no longer funds research in this area.

the**Point** Appendix M, available online at http://thepoint.lww.com/mkk8e, contains citations and links to considerable supplemental information related to topics of interest in molecular biology, including a timeline of events about genetics before Mendel, salient events in genetics and molecular biology to 2005, and a link to Watson and Crick's one-page classic 1953 paper in *Nature* about their deduction of DNA's structure, which nearly six decades later unraveled the pieces to the primordial jigsaw puzzle of the **Human Genome Project**.

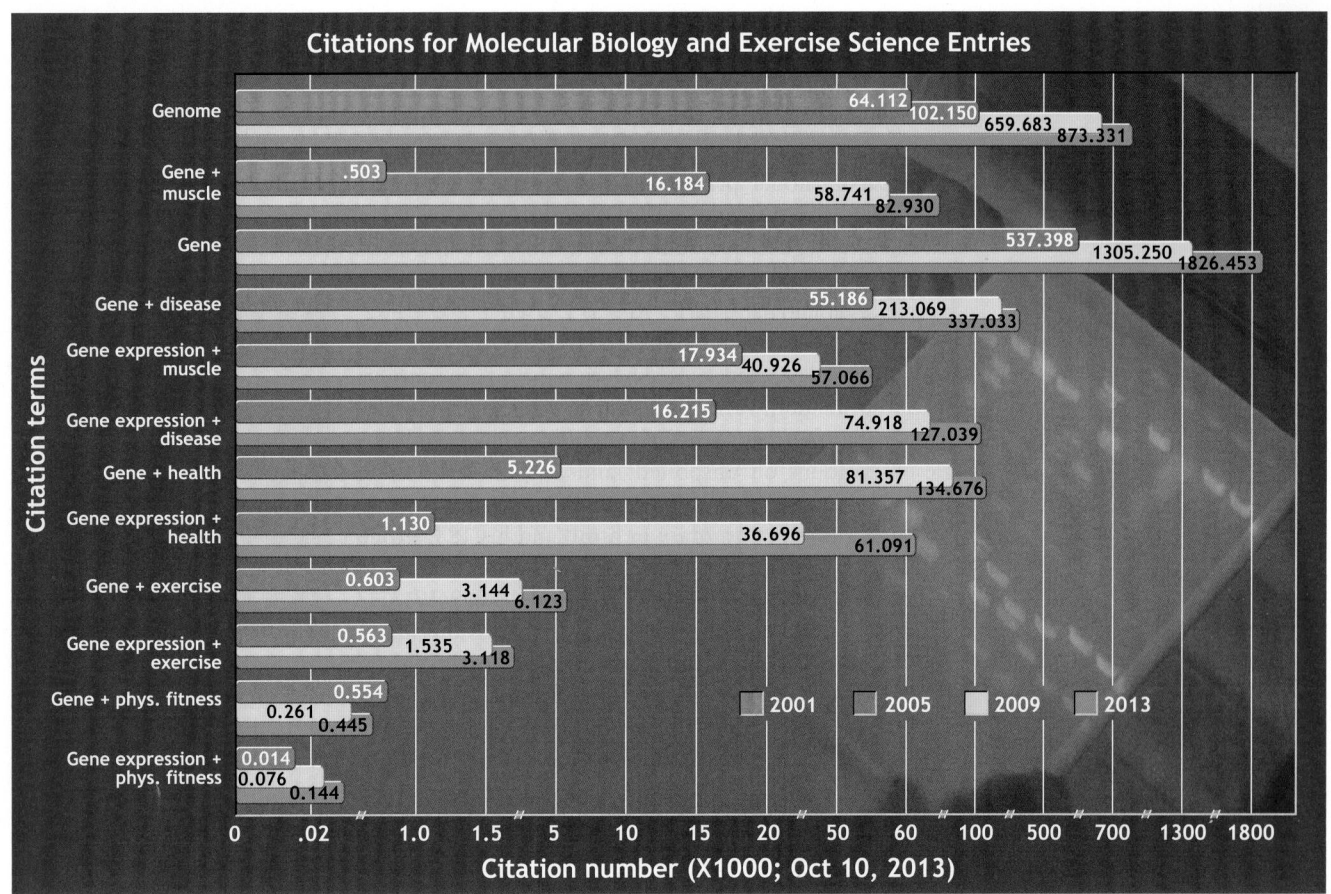

Citations for Molecular Biology and Exercise Science Entries

FIGURE 33.1 • Comparison of citations from 2001 to 2013 (as of October 10, 2013) for molecular biology terms with exercise science entries

In all likelihood, future limits to athletic performance will be determined less by an athlete's innate physiology and anatomy (and commitment to training) and more by surgical enhancement (e.g., more flexible tendons) and genetic interventions engineered for faster-acting, more powerful muscles, greater oxygen transport, and more rapid circulation. The continuing use by athletes of banned substances, uncovered at every international Olympiad since 2000 (and the Tour de France for many years before that), highlights the challenges facing the World Anti-Doping Association (WADA; www.wada-ama.org), the independent drug-testing agency charged with curbing continuing illegal drug use in future Olympic Games. Breakthroughs in gene therapy techniques in the coming years will likely infiltrate the athlete's arsenal of "tricks" in time for a future Olympiad or other world-class competitions. As increasing numbers of amateur and professional athletes in many sport disciplines cheat with advanced molecular techniques to gain a competitive edge, both students and an educated general public will confront specialists in exercise physiology concerning the implications of the molecular biology of gene therapy and "genetic ergogenics."

HISTORICAL TOUR OF MOLECULAR BIOLOGY

The road to uncovering DNA's three-dimensional structure began with an innocent discovery by Swiss physiologist Friedrich Miescher (1844–1895), professor of physiology at the University of Basel, Switzerland, and a charter member of the 1889 First International Congress of Physiologists. In 1869, Miescher identified what he considered a new biologic substance. Cells obtained from fish sperm and human tissue cells obtained from pus in discarded surgical bandages contained unusual proportions of nitrogen and phosphorus in their **nucleus**. Miescher called the substance *nuclein*, which one of his students, Richard Altman (1852–1900), later termed *nucleic acid* because of its slightly acidic properties. Altman, also remembered for

Human Genome Project: government-sponsored project (Department of Energy and National Institutes of Health) to (1) create an ordered set of DNA segments from known chromosomal locations, (2) develop new computational methods to analyze genetic maps and DNA sequence data, and (3) develop new techniques and instruments for detecting and analyzing DNA (i.e., deciphering the complete sequence of genetic instructions in humans). Hundreds of robotic sequencing machines work around the clock to analyze nucleotide sequences using the Sanger-Coulson dideoxy DNA sequencing method to map different genomes

Nucleus: structure that contains the cell's genetic material (chromosomal DNA)

creating an anilin-acid fuchsin histological pigment, stained mitochondria crimson against a yellow background (www.chemistryexplained.com/Ne-Nu/Nucleic-Acids.html#b). Ten years after Altman's primary experiments, Ludwig Albrecht Kossel 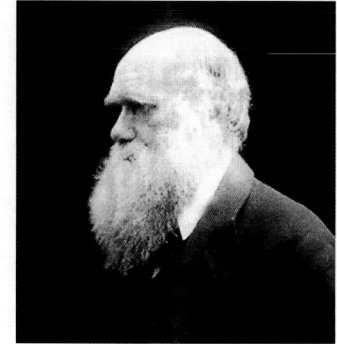 (1853–1927), a German physiological chemist, won the 1910 Nobel Prize in Physiology or Medicine for his pioneering work on proteins and the nucleic substances and their cleavage products (www.nobelprize.org/nobel_prizes/medicine/laureates/1910/kossel-bio.html).

As late as the second half of the 19th century, chemists and biologists did not know what role, if any, genes played in transmitting hereditary information in plants or animals. This changed when English naturalist, geologist, avid anti-slavery advocate, and biologist Charles Robert Darwin (1809–1882) (www.public.coe.edu/departments/Biology/darwin_bio.html) proposed a theory of evolution based on **natural selection** of random variation.[40] Darwin developed his theory gradually after many years of insightful geologic and biologic observations on unspoiled lands, particularly along the western coast of South America, including the Galapagos Islands (www.gct.org/darwin.html) and his 1835–1836 recording of his shore observations in New Zealand and Australia (https://www.mja.com.au/journal/2009/191/11/charles-darwin-s-impressions-new-zealand-and-australia-and-insights-his-illness). His ideas about evolution

Natural selection: Darwin's basic idea that species survive because more favorable phenotypic traits pass down through successive generations

Charles Darwin

emerged mainly from observations of subtle differences among plant and animal species during his 57-mo, 2-day voyage around the world (www.aboutdarwin.com/voyage/voyage03.html), begun in 1831 aboard the British survey ship HMS *Beagle* (**FIG. 33.2**).[38] Darwin's careful observations about the distribution and continuation of animal and plant phenotypic traits were first published on November 26, 1859, 10 years before Miescher discovered nuclein.

English naturalist and explorer, evolutionist, anthropologist, and prolific writer and essayist Alfred Russel Wallace (1823–1913; www.wku.edu/~smithch/index1.htm) had independently formed his own views regarding natural selection at about the same time Darwin completed his work dealing with evolution theory. Except for sharing his thoughts with selected colleagues in various disciplines, Darwin had not yet made them widely known in formal publications. Darwin's reading of Wallace's 1855 paper about natural selection, *On the Tendency of Varieties to Depart Indefinitely From the Original Type* (reprinted in *Contributions of the theory of natural selection*[160]) no doubt accelerated his pace to publish his single-volume discourse on evolutionary theory. It was Wallace who encouraged Darwin to use the phrase "survival of the fittest" (coined by

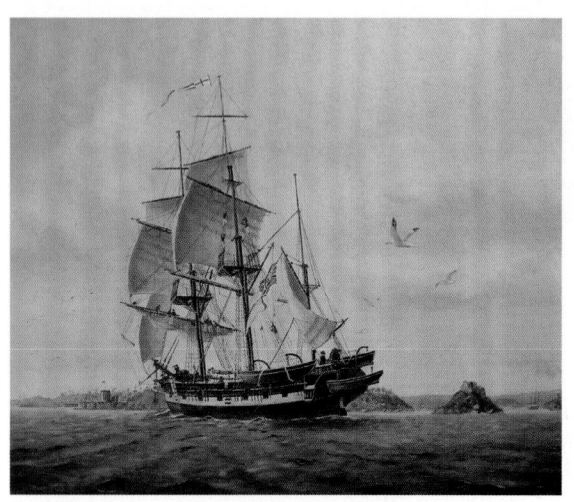

FIGURE 33.2 • The HMS *Beagle* (235 tons, 27 m length, 7 m breadth, 6 canons) engaged in three survey missions from 1826 to 1843, with Charles Darwin the naturalist on the second survey. "On the morning of 27 December 1831, HMS Beagle, with a crew of seventy-three men, sailed out of Plymouth harbor under a calm easterly wind and drizzly rain. Darwin became seasick almost immediately and started to have second thoughts about the voyage." (www.aboutdarwin.com/voyage/voyage03.html). HMS *Beagle* courtesy of marine artist Ron Scobie, ASMA (www.ronscobie-marineartist.com). Further details about Darwin's travels are summarized at www.aboutdarwin.com/index.html, and every letter written by and to Darwin between 1837 and 1859 are chronicled in the "Darwin Correspondence Project" (www.aboutdarwin.com/links/links_070.html and http://darwin-online.org.uk). The original *Beagle Diary* (also available in mp3 format for online download at the Darwin Online Website above, is housed in a museum at Darwin's home, Down House, Kent, England (www.english-heritage.org.uk/daysout/properties/home-of-charles-darwin-down-house/).

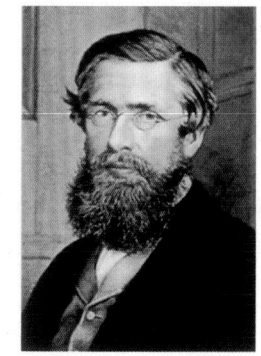

Alfred Russel Wallace

British sociologist and philosopher Herbert Spencer [1820–1903]) to convey the basic idea about natural selection to the general public.

Darwin's carefully crafted, thought-provoking treatise *On the Origin of the Species, by Means of Natural Selection, or the Preservation of Favoured Races in the Struggle for Life*[39] indirectly provided empirical "data" on how environmental pressures selected for the survival of a species' observable characteristics (traits) from one generation to the next. Darwin's theory explained how adaptive modifications to environmental stressors impacted the common descent of current animal and plant species and how natural selection preserved a species' survival.

Interestingly, Miescher's discovery of nuclein came 4 years after Austrian monk Gregor Johann Mendel's (1822–1884) elegant 25-year breeding experiments with 10,000 varieties of edible pea plants, *Pisum sativum*. Mendel vigilantly tracked the peas' inherited characteristics and in 1865 submitted his findings, "Versuche über Pflanzen-Hybriden," to an obscure natural history society journal. The work appeared in 1866 and about 1902 was translated into English by William Bateson (1861–1926; http://www.dnalc.org/view/16206-Biography-5-William-Bateson-1861-1926-.html).[11] Darwin's unifying evolution theory and Mendel's experiments on heredity formed "scientific pillars" of insights embraced by a relatively new field of study—molecular biology—that would subsequently dominate fundamental discoveries in biology, chemistry, genetics, nutrition, and medicine to this date and surely beyond.

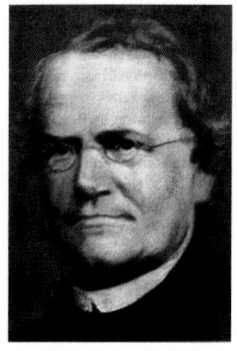

Gregor Johann Mendel

 ## Discovery of Darwin's Inherited Medical Malady

Using molecular biology methods, British scientists in 2005 unraveled the cause of Darwin's 40 years of suffering from long bouts of vomiting, gut pain, headaches, severe fatigue, skin problems, and depression.[28] Darwin's family history revealed a major inherited component of predisposed hypolactasia (aversion to milk and cream). The authors concluded that Darwin's multifold symptoms (including long periods of isolation from friends and colleagues) and illness highlights a missed observation—the importance of lactose in mammalian and human evolution.

Mendel's meticulous scientific insights remained relatively obscure for nearly three decades until three scientists—German botanist Carl Correns (1864–1933; www.dnalc.org/view/16223-Biography-6-Carl-Correns-1864-1933-.html; using maize and peas), Dutch botanist Hugo De Vries (1848–1935; www.britannica.com/EBchecked/topic/633337/Hugo-de-Vries; working with flowering plants), and Austrian agronomist Erich van Tschermak-Seysenegg (1871–1962; www.eucarpia.org/secretariate/honorary/tschermak.html; using peas)—rediscovered his research in about 1900. It would take nearly 65 years after Mendel's initial publication and enormous progress in biochemical techniques to unravel further secrets highlighting the mysteries of hereditary transmission in human cells.

In 1929, Phoebus A. T. Levene (1869–1940; www.jbc.org/content/277/22/e11) discovered that the essential components of the nucleic acids DNA and **ribonucleic acid (RNA)** were long chains of repeating **nucleotides**. However, it remained unclear to Levene and others how these molecules assembled. If the genes indeed contained the hereditary information, scientists needed to know the process involved. Twenty-five years later, a major breakthrough—Watson and Crick's discovery of DNA's structure (see below)—delivered the biggest biologic thunderbolt since Darwin. The significance of this breakthrough had its impact on at least nine other crucial scientific milestones as of 2013:

1. 1966—cracking the DNA genetic code
2. 1972 to 1973—splicing pieces of DNA together to form genes (called *recombinant molecules*) and then inserted into bacteria to produce human proteins
3. 1977—elucidating the complete genetic information of a microorganism, paving the way for the Human Genome Project
4. 1981—creating the first **transgenic** animal by inserting a viral gene into the DNA of a mouse, permitting such animals to serve as models for the study of human diseases
5. 1984—devising the **polymerase chain reaction (PCR)**, an ingenious method of sequencing DNA from minute samples of DNA

Deoxyribonucleic acid (DNA): double-helix molecule (two complementary chains of nucleotides) containing an organism's total hereditary information

Ribonucleic acid (RNA): nucleic acid that contains the sugar ribose; usually single stranded

Nucleotide: segment of a nucleic acid containing a 5-carbon sugar, phosphate group, and nitrogen-containing base

Transgenic: transforming genes from one species into another

Polymerase chain reaction (PCR): technique for artificially amplifying the number of copies of a target DNA sequence, usually by 106- to 109-fold, during repeated cycles of denaturation, annealing with primer, and extension with DNA polymerase

See the animation "Polymerase Chain Reaction (PCR)" on **http://thePoint.lww. com/mkk8e** for a demonstration of this process.

6. 1997—cloning the first mammal, the lamb Dolly, from an adult sheep cell
7. 2000 to 2004—deciphering the human genome; sequencing the genome of the fruit fly *Drosophila melanogaster*; sequencing the DNA of rice (first decoding of a crop); initial sequencing and comparative analysis of the mouse and brown Norway rat genomes; producing a single embryonic stem cell line from a human blastocyst through somatic cell nuclear transfer (SCNT) technology, (representing the first published report of cloned human stem cells)
8. 2005 to 2009—creating human stem cell lines from human embryos by cloning, then extracting patient-specific, immune-matched human embryonic stem cells to create genetic matches in patients with disease or injury
9. 2009 to 2014—controversies continue over human and animal cloning; research on human stem cells advances understanding of debilitating genetic malfunctions (e.g., amyotrophic lateral sclerosis [ALS; Lou Gehrig's disease]), Alzheimer's disease, blindness, blood disorders, malfunctions in blood supply, cancers, cartilage damage, rheumatoid arthritis, diabetes, hearing loss, heart and circulatory disease, infertility, lung damage, memory loss due to brain tumor treatment, multiple sclerosis, muscular dystrophy, organ replacement, platelet transfusions, spinal cord injury; genetic modification of crops; gene analysis companies compete for cloud-based solutions for gene mapping

REVOLUTION IN THE BIOLOGIC SCIENCES

In 1953, James Dewey Watson (1928– ; **www.nobelprize.org/nobel_prizes/medicine/ laureates/1962/watson-bio.html**), an American postdoctoral student who earned a PhD in genetics from Indiana University at age 22, teamed with English physicist Francis Harry Compton Crick (1916–2004; **www.nobelprize.org/nobel_prizes/medicine/laureates/ 1962/crick-bio.html**), who was pursuing a PhD in x-ray studies of protein in the influential Cavendish Laboratory, Cambridge, England (**www.phy.cam.ac.uk/history/**). At Cavendish, Professor Sir Lawrence Bragg (1890–1971; British physicist and X-ray crystallographer and 1915 Nobel Prize winner in Physics; **www.nobelprize.org/nobel_prizes/physics/laure-**

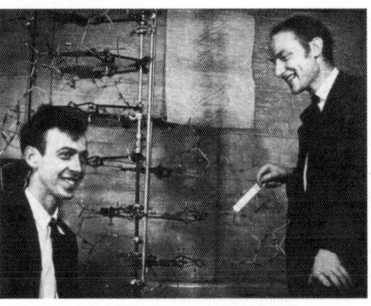

Watson (left) and Crick (right) at the Cavendish Laboratory next to their DNA ball and wire model, May 1953.

ates/1915/wl-bragg-bio.html) developed the use of X-ray crystallography as a powerful tool to understand the structure of biological molecules. Bragg was instrumental in allowing Watson and Crick to pursue their model-building work at his laboratory (**http://pauling blog.wordpress.com/2009/04/30/the-watson-and-crick-structure-of-dna/**).

Watson and Crick's breakthrough, deduced from other scientists' published and unpublished research, posited that the DNA molecule consisted of two poly-nucleotide linear strands coiled around each other to form a **double helix**.[161]

The young researchers constructed a ball-and-wire model of DNA, proposing that the two helical strands connected like spiral staircase steps by nucleotide **base pairs** held together by **hydrogen bonds**. Their eventual 1962 Nobel Prize rewarded their contribution about DNA's architecture and the three-dimensional fit of its molecular components. We now know that this discovery was fueled in part by substantial theoretical contributions previously gleaned about DNA's helical structure from rival Kings College, London, colleague Rosalind Elsie Franklin (1920–1957; **www.sdsc.edu/ScienceWomen/ franklin.html**).

In their 1953 landmark publication in *Nature* describing DNA's molecular structure, Watson and Crick state that their research efforts were stimulated by "a knowledge of the general nature of the unpublished experimental results and ideas of Drs. M. H. F.

Double helix: two DNA strands twisted in a spiral around each other

Base pairs: two complementary nucleotide bases (G-C or A-T) in a double-stranded DNA molecule held together by hydrogen bonds

Hydrogen bonds: weak, interactive bonding from simultaneous attraction of a positive hydrogen atom to other atoms with negative charges

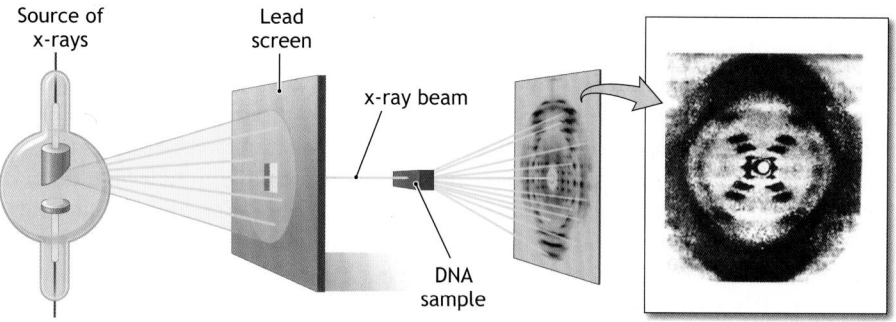

FIGURE 33.3 • The technique of X-ray crystallography bombards crystals with thin x-ray beams of single (monochromatic) wavelength to determine a substance's three-dimensional crystal structure. The right photo shows Franklin's x-ray photograph of DNA; she focused the x-ray beam on extra-wet DNAB fibers for a longer-than-usual time, with a 62-hr exposure to obtain the vivid photo of DNA's cruciform pattern. Without her knowledge or permission, this x-ray was shown to Watson and Crick, who put it together with their knowledge about base pairing and correctly deduced that DNA must have originated from a helix-shaped molecule.

Wilkins (1926–2004; www.nobelprize.org/nobel_prizes/medicine/laureates/1962/wilkins-bio.html) and R. E. Franklin and coworkers at King's College, London." This statement, interpreted with the hindsight of many years of investigative follow-up by historians and researchers, paints quite a different picture of Franklin's prior crucial discoveries about DNA's structure, which eventually led Watson and Crick to deduce DNA's final configuration correctly. Franklin's sophisticated x-ray diffraction photo reflecting her expertise with x-ray crystallography (shown to Watson and Crick surreptitiously without Franklin's knowledge) provided the missing piece about DNA's double helix that empowered Watson and Crick to quickly decipher the puzzle after viewing the photo (**Fig. 33.3**). Interestingly, unlike many biologists, Watson and Crick did not conduct experiments. Their technique involved thinking, arguing, and rethinking ideas and concepts about how to put together pieces of a complicated puzzle with many interconnected components.

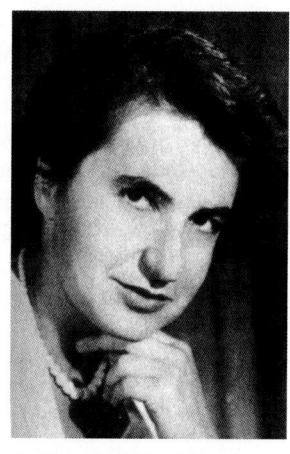

Dr. Rosalind Franklin

(fyi) Rosalind Franklin: An Unsung Hero in the Discovery of the Double Helix

For a historic perspective, we recommend two books with different views about how the DNA puzzle was solved. Watson's[163] colorful personal interpretation details one of the most important discoveries in all of science by one of the scientists who made the discovery. Sayre[138] provides a compelling and insightful first full account of Rosalind Franklin's previously unacknowledged major contribution to discovering DNA's structure. From our viewpoint, these revelations reveal a seldom seen but ugly side of some in the basic sciences—cutthroat ways and blind ambition run roughshod over other researchers' contributions without proper attribution.

From Watson's and Crick's decisive "discovery," we know definitively that DNA's helical structure carries the biologic blueprint for specifying the *order* in which the body's 20 amino acids assemble to create a protein. Each protein has its own unique amino acid sequence; this sequence ultimately dictates the protein molecule's final shape and distinctive chemical and functional characteristics. We also know that each double-helix strand provides a **template** for synthesizing a new strand, something Watson and Crick

Template: copy, replica, or pattern; sequence of nucleotides from which a complementary DNA or RNA strand forms

had hinted at in their seminal 1953 paper published in the prestigious scientific journal *Nature*. A **template strand** represents an original DNA strand. Once faithfully copied, each newly created double-helix strand represents a duplicate of its predecessor, with its genetic code sequence perfectly preserved. This mechanism of self-replication preserves the genetic flow of information to ensure that successive generations receive the same coded DNA "messages." In fact, all living things on Earth share a common molecular plan. Each of a human's 100 trillion cells relies on four basic molecular building blocks—nucleic acid, protein, lipid, and polysaccharide—along with other nano-sized biomolecules—to perform their functions efficiently. In addition, all living cells shuttle the flow of information from DNA to RNA to protein. The full impact of what Watson and Crick deduced about DNA's structural configuration cannot be overstated: their contribution and subsequent years of investigation have impacted every facet of biomedical science, from how primordial DNA formed and survived to the nature of deadly diseases and the all-out search for their eventual cure. Their unraveling of DNA's structure has profoundly impacted all of science, particularly subsequent discoveries about human, viral, plant, and animal genomes (see next section).

The fields of molecular biology have shown explosive growth during the past five decades. Discoveries have been so startling that almost every year since 1958 a Nobel Prize has been awarded for research related to molecular biology. Since its 1901 inception, four of the only 10 women awarded a Nobel Prize in science won for molecular biology–related research.[106]

THE HUMAN GENOME

The **human genome** represents the full complement of genetic material in a human cell. The December 1999 issue of *Nature* featured a milestone scientific achievement—the sequence or "genetic map" for 12 contiguous segments of human chromosome 22, the second smallest of the 23 chromosomes (chromosome 22 contains about 1.6 to 1.8% of the total genomic DNA).[44] On June 26, 2000, a private company, Celera Genomics (www.celera.com), and the publicly funded National Human Genome Research Institute (www.genome.gov) announced completion of the first assembly draft of the human genome. By November 2000, more than half the genome had been identified, sequenced, and recorded in public databases (e.g., www.acedb.org). The Human Genome Project (www.ornl.gov/sci/TechResources/Human_Genome/home.html) achieved its major objective of producing a high-quality version of the human genome sequence, freely available in April 2003 in public databases.

To unravel the submicroscopic secrets of genetic material, sophisticated detection techniques help scientists "decode" the human genome. Most of the decoded DNA sequences never become part of the final transcript that ultimately directs **protein synthesis**.

The total number of base pairs determines genome size. The human genome, distributed among 23 pairs of **chromosomes** that each repeat over and over like a genetic stutter without interruption, imparts our individual uniqueness. At conception, one complete chromosome set from the father (22 plus an **X** or **Y sex chromosome**) joins with one complete set from the mother (22 plus an X sex chromosome) to give each human offspring 46 chromosomes. The helical DNA structures (**genotype**) contain the genetic blueprint or "roadmap" of instructions for almost every aspect of our being (**phenotype**). The phenotype reflects the expression of our gene pool from the physical dimensions, texture, color, composition, and shape of every internal and external body part to our personalities with all their idiosyncrasies. The size of the human genome greatly exceeds that of other organisms. For example, the bacterium *Escherichia coli* shown in Figure 33.4A (*E. coli*; primary member of the large bacterial family *Enterobacteriaceae*) contains 4.6 million base pairs, while yeast contains 15 million base pairs. In contrast, the smallest human chromosome (the male or Y chromosome; Fig. 33.4B) consists of 58 million base pairs (http://ghr.nlm.nih.gov/chromosome=Y) and occupies an estimated 20,000 to 25,000 total genes in the human genome. The largest human chromosome contains 250 million base pairs. For some idea of the enormity of the genetic structures, consider the following analogies:

A double-spaced 8.5 × 11–inch page of text using normal margins contains about 3000 letters, or roughly 250 words. Porting the human genome to pages would equal the number of letters in 1000

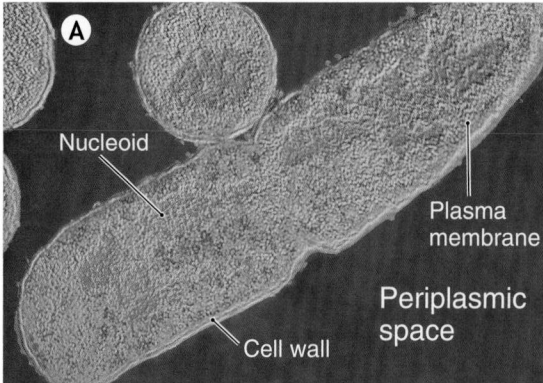
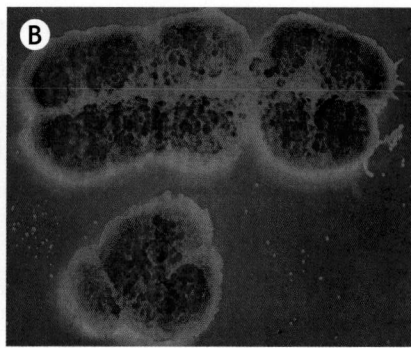

FIGURE 33.4 • (A) The bacterium *Escherichia coli* (*E. coli*). **(B)** The smallest human chromosome. Human males have X (larger; top) and Y (smaller; bottom) chromosomes.

copies of the Sunday *New York Times* or about 1200 copies of this text. Stated another way, reading one letter of code every second would require about 100 years without a break to peruse the entire genome! A single DNA strand in one **diploid** human cell with 23 pairs of chromosomes, if unwound and stacked end to end, would stretch to the height of a person 60 inches tall, yet it occupies a width of only 50-trillionths of an inch.

The human DNA sequence includes the longest continuous stretch of DNA ever deciphered and assembled, with over 23 million letters. The sequencing of chromosome 22 allowed scientists for the first time to view the entire DNA of a chromosome. At least 27 human disorders link to chromosome 22 genes, including ovarian, colon, and breast cancers; cataracts; congenital heart disease; schizophrenia; **neurofibromatosis**; mental retardation; and disorders of the nervous system and fetal development (www.ornl.gov/sci/techresources/Human_Genome/launchpad/chrom22.shtml).

Scientists view sequencing of the human genome as somewhat analogous to completing an intricately detailed inaugural chapter in the human genetic instruction book, which in turn comprises many complex chapters. An international collaboration from eight laboratories in the United Kingdom, Japan, the United States, Canada, and Sweden helped to complete the analysis of the body's 23 chromosomes through 2006, and through June, 2013, over 70 leading healthcare, research, and disease advocacy organizations from more than 40 countries initiated a global alliance for genetic health dedicated to enabling the secure sharing of genomic and clinical data in a technical and regulatory effective and responsible manner (www.ornl.gov/sci/techresources/Human_Genome/project/timeline.shtml; www.broadinstitute.org/news/globalalliance). Knowing the identity and order of the chemical components of the DNA of the 23 pairs of human chromosomes has provided an important tool to determine the basis of health and disease.

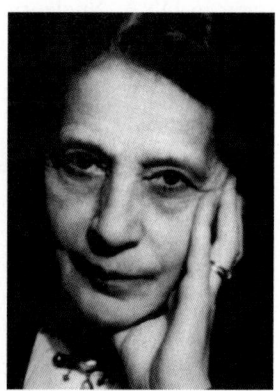

Dr. Lise Meitner

In a material sense, a relatively few discrete genetic instructions ultimately determine all of the subtlety of the human species, including the thousands of years of accomplishment in fields of study from architecture to poetry and medicine to computer science and zoology. Anatomic and psychological differences between any two unrelated individuals really reflect relatively few differences in their genomic blueprint—perhaps one or two gene sequences out of thousands. For example, NBA basketball champions Kobe Bryant, Lebron James, and brilliant Austrian physicist Lise Meitner (1878–1968[142], www.atomicarchive.com/Bios/Meitner.shtml; deprived of a Nobel Prize for contributing to the discovery of nuclear fission because of her religion and professional animosities) are far more alike than they are different. The variety among individuals approaches infinity!

Template: copy, replica, or pattern; sequence of nucleotides from which a complementary DNA or RNA strand forms

Template strand: original DNA strand that guides the synthesis of a new DNA strand by complementary base pairing

Diploid: having two representatives of every chromosome (i.e., two copies of each gene)

Neurofibromatosis: hereditary disorder characterized clinically by the combination of patches of hyperpigmentation in both cutaneous and subcutaneous tumors over the entire body

NUCLEIC ACIDS

Figure 33.5 shows the central configuration differences between the two nucleic acids, DNA and RNA; the three *yellow text boxes* highlight the important differences. When cells divide, both DNA and RNA carry and then transmit the hereditary information, ensuring, for example, that liver cells produce liver cells, and from generation to generation through reproductive cells. Within all living cells, genes encode the hereditary set of instructions that determine an organism's unique characteristics, from a simple bacterium such as *Streptococcus pneumoniae* to the tremendously complex multicellular human species, *Homo sapiens*. As organisms within a species increase in complexity, the total information stored within the genome also increases. In subsequent sections, we describe just how much encoded information must be transcribed and translated to ultimately create the proteins that characterize the thousands of unique cells, tissues, and organs that define the organism. Think of DNA as the raw material or building blocks of genes, and RNA as the link or intermediary to protein synthesis. Three Internet sites provide a starting point for the study of DNA and the revolution it spawned (www.dnai.org/index.htm; www.dnaftb.org/dnaftb/) including animations for discrete molecular biology processes (www.dnalc.org/resources/animations/; www.learnerstv.com/animation/animation.php?ani=%20169&cat=biology)

DNA and RNA

Nucleic acid: large molecule containing nucleotide subunits

Polymer: high-molecular-weight substance linked together by repeating similar or identical subunits (e.g., glucose polymer starch); long-chain molecule linkage forms two- and three-dimensional networks

Polynucleotide: two or more nucleotides joined together; the phosphate at carbon 59 of one sugar combines at the 39 position of another sugar

Deoxyribose: sugar with five carbon atoms

The **nucleic acids** DNA and RNA consist of polarized **polymers** of repeating subunits, or nucleotides. A nucleotide consists of a nitrogen-containing organic base having six carbon atoms, a 5-carbon sugar, and a phosphate molecule (**Fig. 33.6**). A nucleotide's main support structure or "backbone" consists of the sugar and phosphate molecules. The sugar–phosphate backbone lies on the outside of the helix, with the amine bases on the inside. In this configuration, a base on one strand points at a base on the second strand. When nucleotides join to form **polynucleotides**, they link at specific carbon locations on the sugar molecule. These locations, numbered in the *red circles* from 1′ to 5′, begin with 1′ to the right of the oxygen (O) atom in the ring. The "prime" symbol (′) distinguishes the carbons in the sugar from carbons in the base. Note from Figure 33.5 that RNA has one additional O atom in its sugar. Thus, the ribose sugar in RNA differs from the **deoxyribose** sugar in DNA. Nucleotides link when the phosphate at carbon 5′ of one sugar combines at the carbon 3′ position of another sugar. The phosphate group attaches to the 5′ carbon;

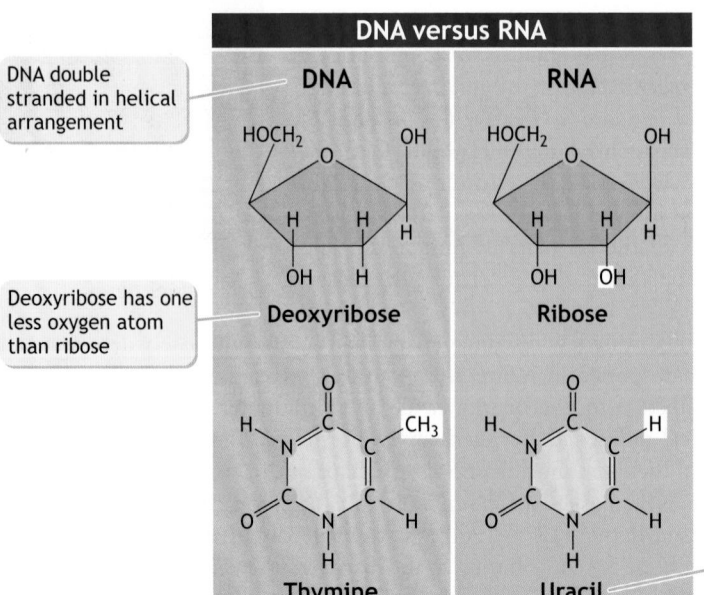

FIGURE 33.5 • Differences in molecular configuration between DNA and RNA.

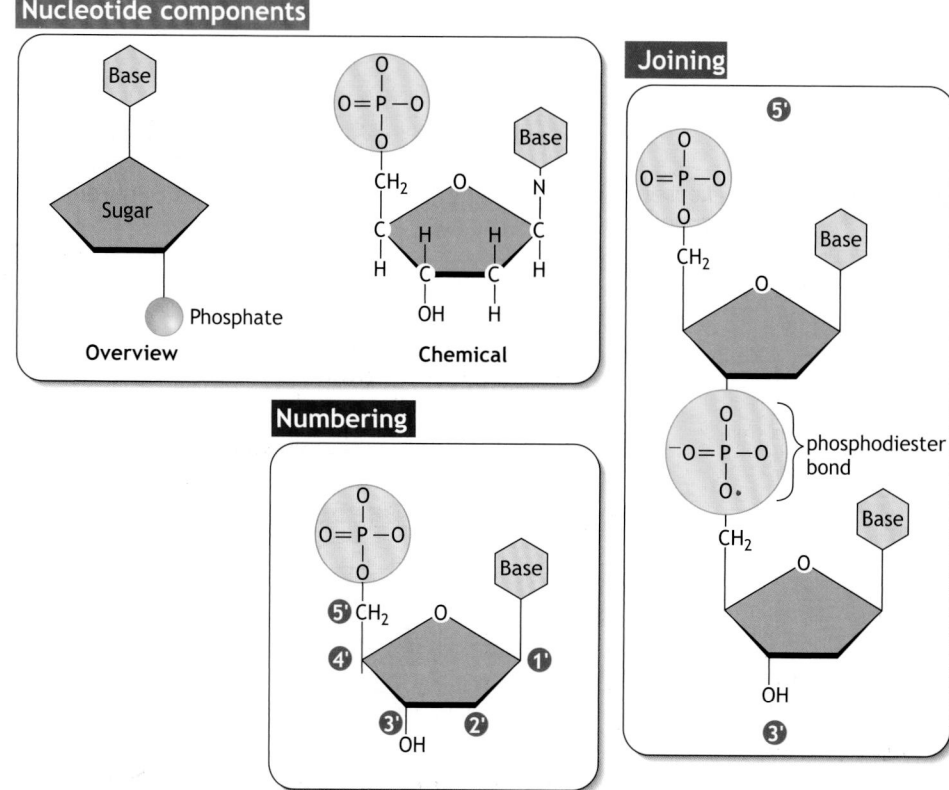

FIGURE 33.6 • The components of a nucleotide, nucleotide-numbering nomenclature, and how nucleotides join together by phosphodiester bonding.

Metaphase: step in mitosis (or meiosis) in which microtubules organize into a spindle and chromosomes move to the cell's equator to align in pairs but have not yet migrated to the poles

Histone: positively charged small nuclear protein molecule cluster that binds to DNA (DNA winds around it) before it uncoils at the replication site; histones neutralize negatively charged DNA

Nucleosome: DNA coiled around a cluster of histone proteins; linked nucleosomes form chromatin

Electron microscope: electron beams with wavelengths thousands of times shorter than visible light replace light, allowing significantly higher resolution and magnification; the electrons pass through an ultrathin, specially prepared stained section of an embedded and dehydrated specimen maintained in a vacuum

Chromatid: one of the two double-stranded DNA daughter molecules of a duplicated, mitotic chromosome joined by a centromere

Mitosis: separation of duplicated chromosomes to create identical daughter cells with mirror-image (genetically identical) chromosomes; prophase, metaphase, anaphase, and telophase are the four phases of mitosis

Centromere: region of a mitotic chromosome (indentation) before replication where two daughter chromatids join

Daughter chromosome: descendent chromosome following replication of the original (mother) chromosome

the base attaches to the 1′ carbon. DNA and RNA synthesis always proceeds in the 5′ to 3′ direction.

The top of **FIGURE 33.7** shows the successive levels or stages of DNA packaging in a chromosome, proceeding from condensed **metaphase** (*upper left*) to supercoiled (*middle right*), loosely condensed, and uncondensed chromatin fiber stages. The negatively charged DNA molecule encircles and binds to a cluster of eight positively charged **histone** proteins (http://genome.nhgri.nih.gov/histones/). The histone purple ball-like structure clamps the DNA to the core of the molecule. The term *nucleosome* describes DNA wrapped around the puck-shaped histone proteins. Examining this region by **electron microscopy** reveals that one beadlike nucleosome contains 146 nucleotide base pairs wound twice like a rope around one cluster of the eight histones. The cluster contains two each of four different protein subunits (H2A, H2B, H3, H4), with each specific subunit having a different molecular mass. A DNA strand with about 60 base pairs and a ninth histone molecule links each cluster to the next one. During replication, the DNA uncoils from the histone core. The DNA molecule shown at the *bottom* of the figure eventually packs into the single metaphase chromosome displayed at the *top left* of the figure. The *inset table* of Figure 33.7 provides relevant information about chromosome folding in the DNA double helix, nucleosomes, 30-nm fiber, loops, minibands, and **chromatids**.

The packaging of DNA within cells reflects a remarkable architectural accomplishment. The *inset table* summarizes DNA folding and how compacting the molecule enhances the efficiency of replication. In the compacted configuration as chromosomes, no transcription takes place, to ensure that DNA remains intact to survive **mitosis**. The chromatids listed in the *last line of the table* with 1 million minibands represent duplicate strands of DNA held together by a **centromere** just before the DNA separates into two **daughter chromosomes**. **FIGURE 33.8** shows the details for chromosome 2 and the general nomenclature for identifying specific genes on the short p and long q arms of a chromosome. Figure 33.8B reveals the architectural details of a condensed metaphase chromosome with its kinetochore microtubules.

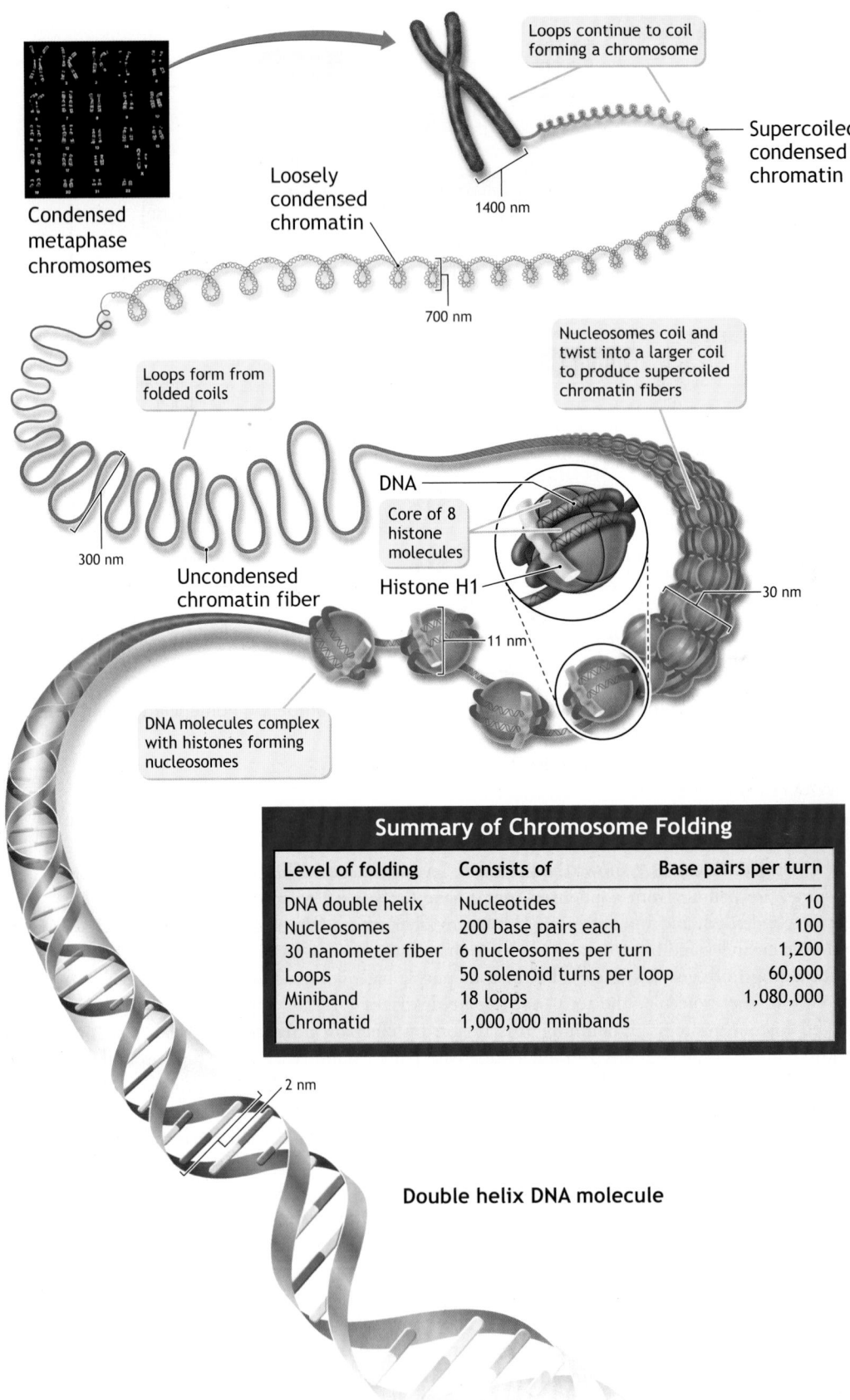

Loops continue to coil forming a chromosome

Supercoiled condensed chromatin

1400 nm

Loosely condensed chromatin

Condensed metaphase chromosomes

700 nm

Nucleosomes coil and twist into a larger coil to produce supercoiled chromatin fibers

Loops form from folded coils

DNA

Core of 8 histone molecules

Histone H1

30 nm

11 nm

300 nm

Uncondensed chromatin fiber

DNA molecules complex with histones forming nucleosomes

Summary of Chromosome Folding		
Level of folding	**Consists of**	**Base pairs per turn**
DNA double helix	Nucleotides	10
Nucleosomes	200 base pairs each	100
30 nanometer fiber	6 nucleosomes per turn	1,200
Loops	50 solenoid turns per loop	60,000
Miniband	18 loops	1,080,000
Chromatid	1,000,000 minibands	

2 nm

Double helix DNA molecule

FIGURE 33.7 • Double-helix DNA molecule packaged in a chromosome from the condensed metaphase stage, to supercoiled stage, to loosely condensed stage, and uncondensed chromatin fiber stage. The inset table provides summary details about chromosome folding from the DNA double helix to the chromatid. nm (nanometer), one-millionth mm.

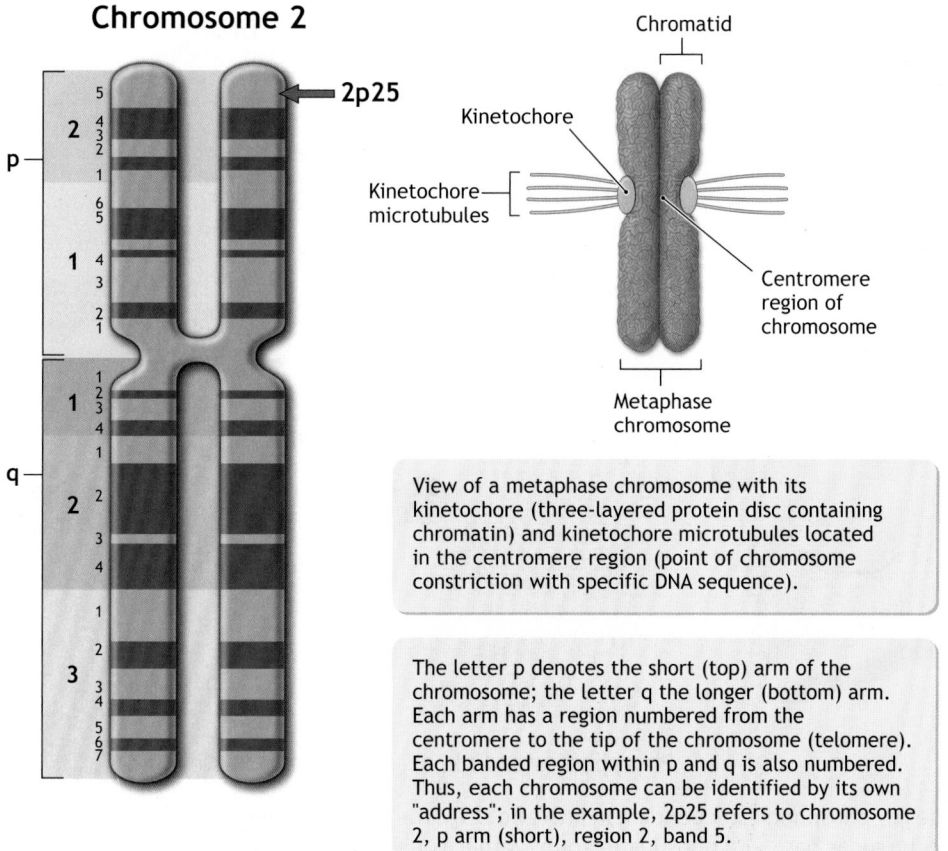

Chromosome 2

View of a metaphase chromosome with its kinetochore (three-layered protein disc containing chromatin) and kinetochore microtubules located in the centromere region (point of chromosome constriction with specific DNA sequence).

The letter p denotes the short (top) arm of the chromosome; the letter q the longer (bottom) arm. Each arm has a region numbered from the centromere to the tip of the chromosome (telomere). Each banded region within p and q is also numbered. Thus, each chromosome can be identified by its own "address"; in the example, 2p25 refers to chromosome 2, p arm (short), region 2, band 5.

FIGURE 33.8 • Chromosome 2. (*Left*) Identification of gene 2p25 on chromosome 2. (*Right*) Metaphase chromosome.

Linking Nucleotides: Phosphodiester Bonding

The chemical reaction when two nucleotides link together eliminates a water molecule, a process termed **dehydration synthesis**; it involves the phosphate molecule from one nucleotide and the hydroxyl (OH) molecule of another nucleotide. The resultant **phosphodiester bond** shown for RNA and DNA (**FIG. 33.9**) represents a relatively strong **covalent bond**. The new polymer, now two units long, still has free phosphate and OH groups for linking to other nucleotides. This linkage forms an incredibly long chain with thousands of nucleotides, although the example shows only a few. In DNA measurement, the term *kilobase* (**kb**) represents a unit of DNA fragment length equal to 1000 nucleotides. Another nucleic acid, adenosine triphosphate (ATP), contains a 5-carbon sugar base (**adenine**) and three phosphate groups. Unlike DNA and RNA, which transfer genetic information, ATP continually transfers chemical energy to power the body's cells throughout life.

Structure of DNA

FIGURE 33.10 shows a DNA molecule composed of a sequence of sugar phosphate chains with hydrogen bonding between the nitrogenous bases. In the double-stranded DNA molecule, the strands are not identical. They lie parallel but line up in opposite directions. One strand runs in the 5′ to 3′ direction, and its **complementary strand** runs from 3′ to 5′. The top left of the figure illustrates the **antiparallel** arrangement of the double stranded DNA strands, including a close-up view of the hydrogen bonding (shown as red dots) between the base pairs that holds the parallel spiral ribbons together. The deduction by Watson and Crick of the antiparallel nature of the DNA strands resolved one of the remaining mysteries about DNA's structure and ultimately how replication proceeds.

Dehydration synthesis: removal of the equivalent of a water molecule from two subunit molecules that form a new, larger molecule

Phosphodiester bond: strong covalent bond formed when two nucleotides link together, eliminating a water molecule; bonding involves the phosphate molecule from one nucleotide and the hydroxyl (OH) molecule of another nucleotide

Covalent bond: sharing one or more pairs of electrons between two atoms

Kilobase (kb): a unit of length for DNA fragments equal to 1000 nucleotides

Adenine: one of the four bases in DNA; always pairs with thymine adenosine triphosphate (ATP), contains a 5-carbon sugar base (adenine) and three phosphate groups. Unlike DNA and RNA that transfer genetic information, ATP continually transfers chemical energy to power the body's cells throughout life

Complementary strand: when one DNA strand runs in the 5′ to 3′ direction, the complementary strand runs oppositely from 3′ to 5′.

Antiparallel: arranged in parallel but with opposite orientation as in DNA

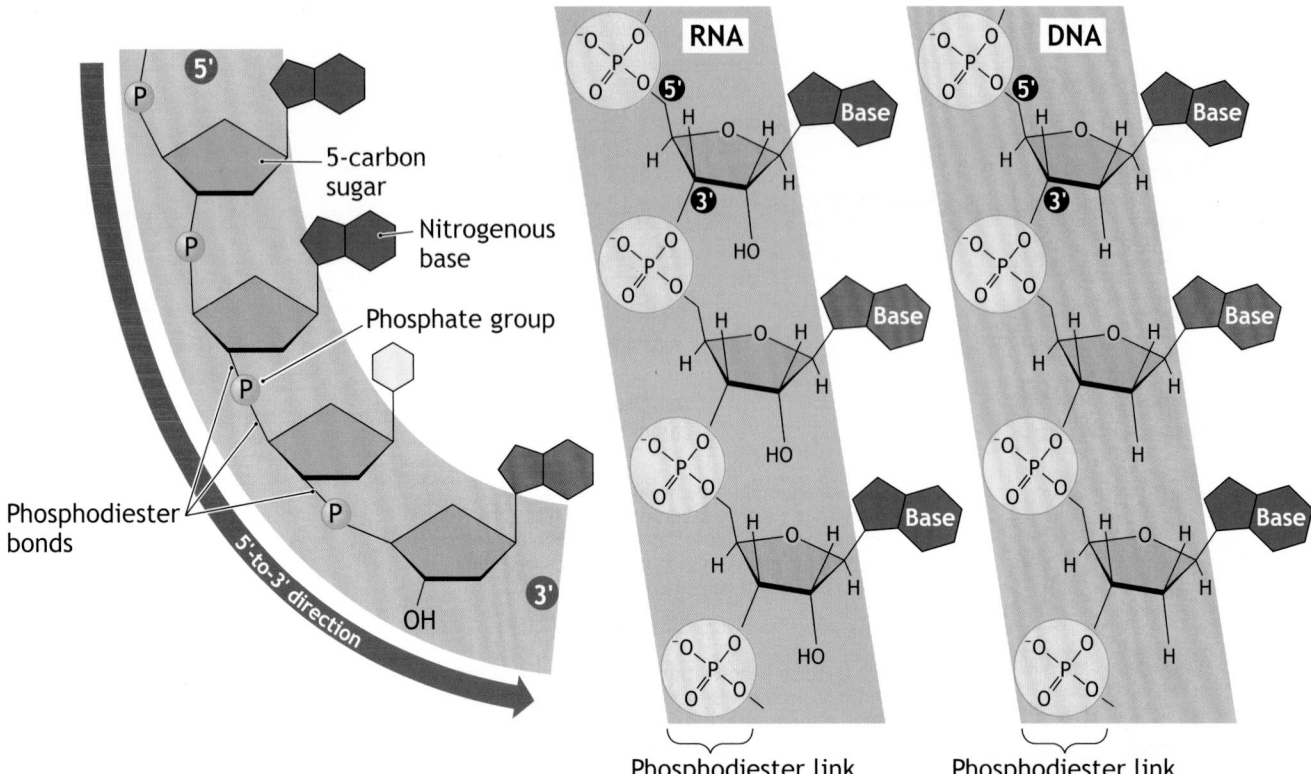

FIGURE 33.9 • Linking of nucleotides by phosphodiester bonding in RNA and DNA. The general schema shown at the bottom left illustrates the relative position of the sugar, base, and phosphate groups within a nucleotide along the 5′ to 3′ direction, including phosphodiester bonding.

Base Pairing

Guanine: one of the four bases in DNA; always pairs with cytosine

Cytosine: one of the four bases in DNA; always pairs with guanine

Thymine: one of the four bases in DNA; always pairs with adenine

Chargaff's rule: pyrimidine content (T C) equals purine content (A G), where ([T] [A]; [G] [C]); (A T)/(G C) varies between different organisms but is constant within an organism

Complementary bases: pairing in DNA between bases A–T or T–A, and C–G or G–C

Purine: nitrogen-containing, double-ring basic compound in nucleic acids; purines in DNA and RNA include adenine and guanine

Pyrimidine: nitrogen-containing, single-ring basic compound in nucleic acids; pyrimidines include cytosine and thymine in DNA and cytosine and uracil in RNA

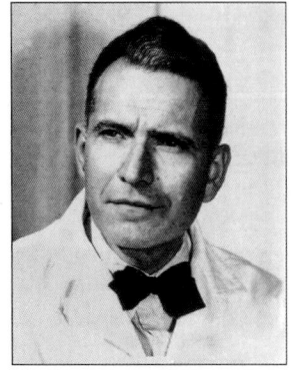

Erwin Chargaff

One of the "golden rules" of DNA's molecular arrangement, displayed in **FIGURE 33.11**, relates to the pairing of the four bases, the letters of the DNA alphabet. **Guanine** (**G**; shown in purple) always links with **cytosine** (**C**; shown in light blue) and **adenine** (**A**; shown in pink) always links with **thymine** (**T**; shown in gold) in the same proportions within all DNA molecules. Stated somewhat differently, whenever a G base occurs in one of the strands, a C base occurs opposite it in the opposing strand. Likewise, when an A base occurs in one strand, a T base occurs in the other strand. In 1950, Erwin Chargaff (1905–2002; www.jbc.org/content/280/24/e21) of Columbia University confirmed the proportionality of the four bases and determined the relative amounts of each base in DNA. In essence, Chargaff discovered key "facts" required to determine DNA's basic chemical structure. **Chargaff's rule** determined regularities among the four chemical bases of DNA (www.nytimes.com/2002/06/30/nyregion/erwin-chargaff-96-pioneer-in-dna-chemical-research.html). The molar amount of thymine always equaled the molar amount of adenine, and similarly, molar amounts of guanine always equaled cytosine on one DNA strand ([T] = [A]; [G] = [C]).

Watson and Crick relied on this information to piece together DNA's structure. In their model, each rung of the DNA ladder consists of a purine connected to a pyrimidine. The term *base pairing* refers to the joining of **complementary bases** (G with C, or A with T). The G and A nitrogenous bases consist of two rings (called a **purine**), while the two other bases, C and T, have a single ring (called a **pyrimidine**). Thus, each base pair consists of one larger purine base mated to a smaller pyrimidine base (http://library.med.utah.edu/NetBiochem/pupyr/pp.htm). Adenine and thymine form two strong hydrogen

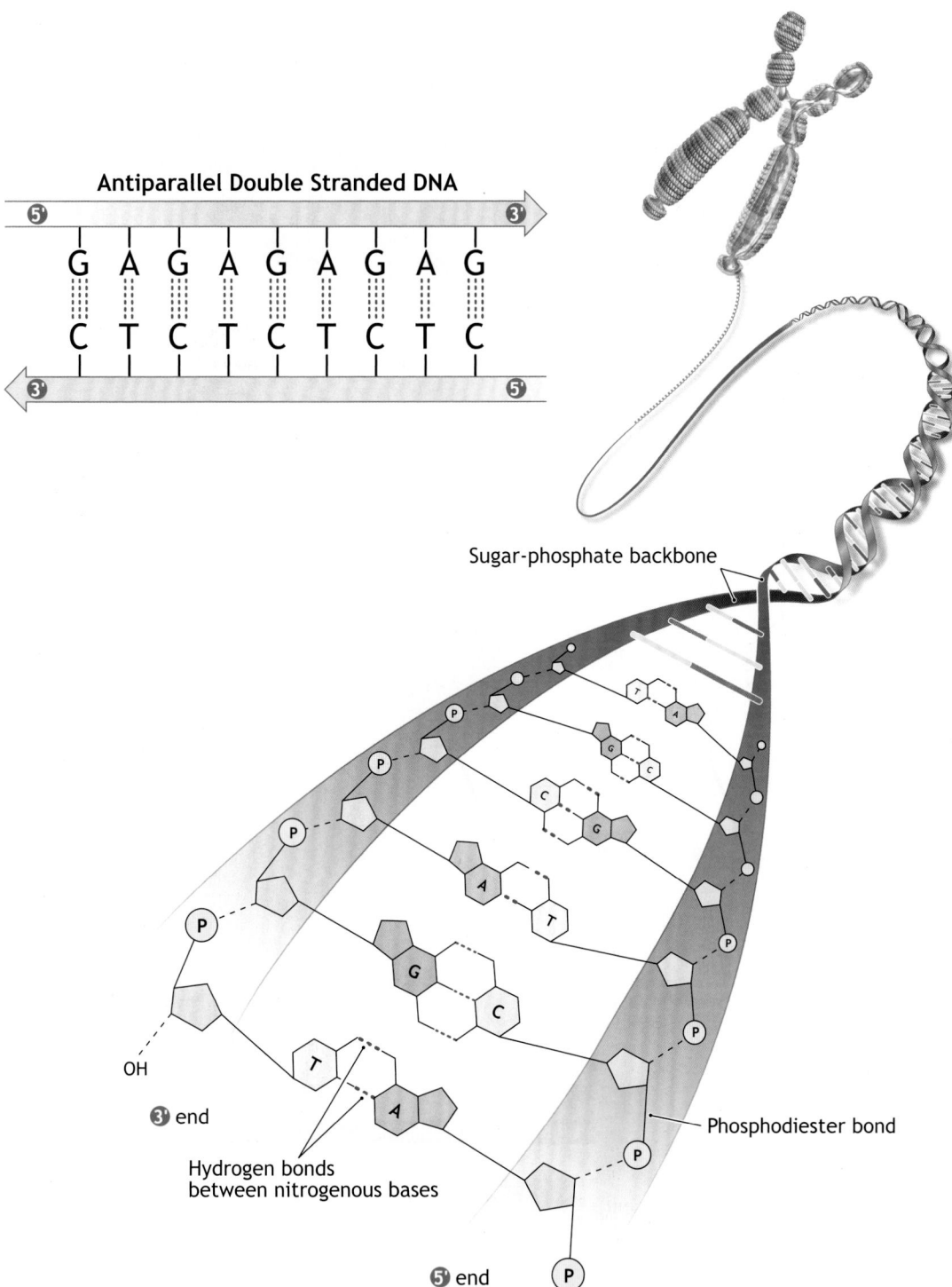

Antiparallel Double Stranded DNA

5' → 3'
G A G A G A G A G
C T C T C T C T C
3' ← 5'

Sugar-phosphate backbone

OH

3' end

Hydrogen bonds
between nitrogenous bases

5' end

Phosphodiester bond

FIGURE 33.10 • DNA molecule. Top: Antiparallel arrangement of a DNA double strand from the 5' to 3' and 3' to 5' directions. Note the hydrogen bonding between G and C and A and T. Bottom: DNA molecule with its sequence of sugar–phosphate chains and hydrogen bonding between nitrogenous bases. The specific sequence of base pairs ultimately determines every protein's specific characteristics. Adenine always binds with thymine.

bonds between the base pairs, but not with G or C. Similarly, G and C form three strong hydrogen bonds to keep the C–G base pair intact, but not with A or T. The additive effect of millions of relatively weak hydrogen bonds within the DNA molecule keeps the helix from separating. Applying Chargaff's rule within an organism, the pyrimidine content (TC) equals

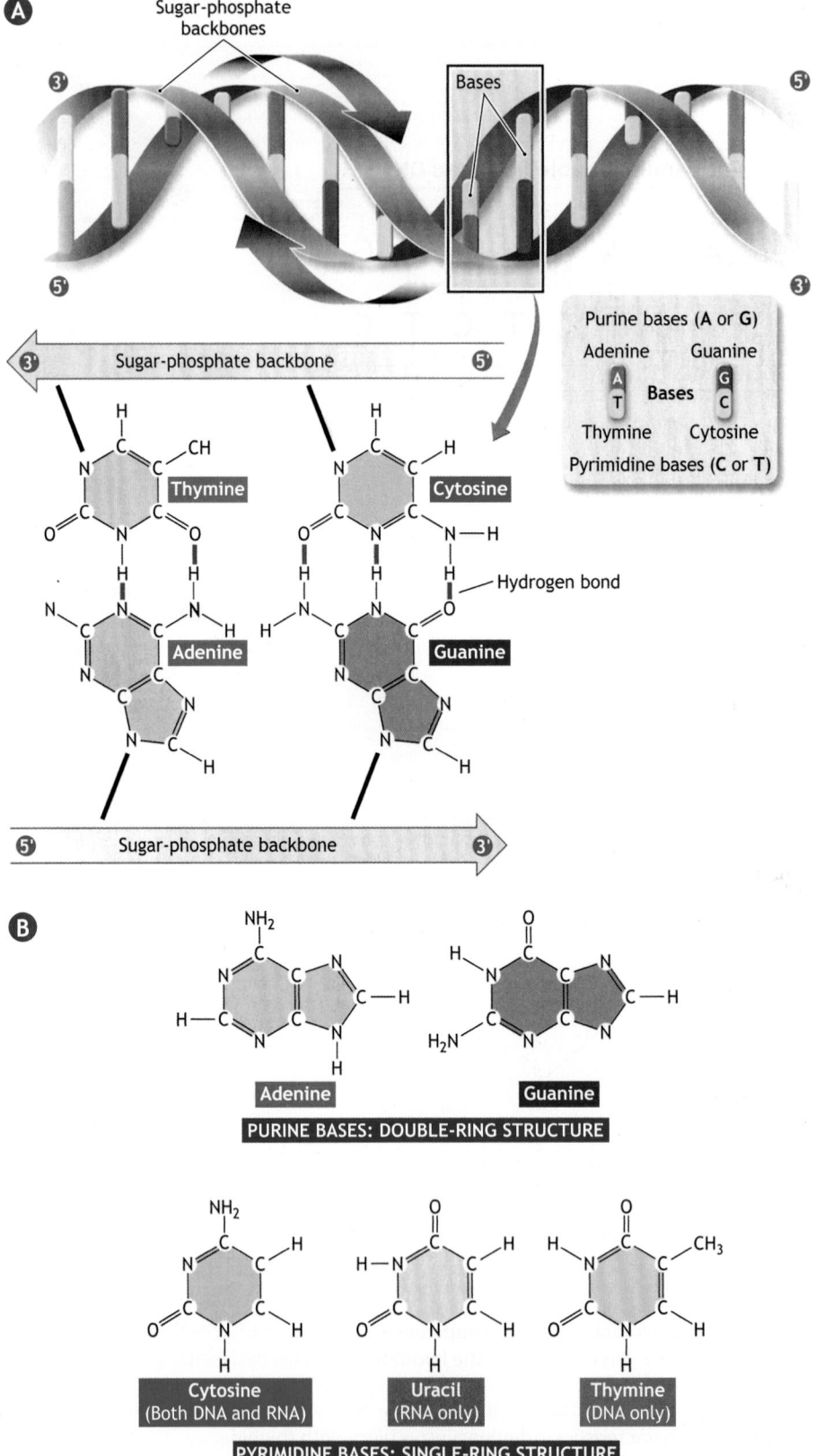

FIGURE 33.11 • Base pairing. **(A)** Configuration details of the DNA double-helix molecule with base pairing and hydrogen bonding for adenine (A)–thymine (T) and guanine (G)–cytosine (C). The two spiral ribbons represent the sugar (deoxyribose)–phosphate backbone of DNA. Note that two hydrogen bonds shown in dark red form between A and T and three form between G and C. This happens because the two polynucleotide chains that contain them lie antiparallel to each other. **(B)** The five bases are classified as purines (A and G) or pyrimidines (C, uracil, T).

the purine content (AG); however, the relative amounts of pyrimidines and purines differ among organisms.

Figure 33.11A illustrates the DNA double-helix molecule, with the base pairing and hydrogen bonding for A–T and G–C. Precise x-ray measurements have determined that the DNA double helix has a width of 2.0 nm (nanometers; 10^{-9} m [or 10 Å] one-millionth millimeter, or 1000 nm = 1 mm), with exactly 10 base pairs in each full turn, with the height of each turn equal to 3.4 nm. Figure 33.11B shows the five bases classified as either purine or pyrimidine bases. Note the pyrimidine base **uracil** (shown in grey). In RNA (next section), uracil replaces thymine, so that adenine pairs with uracil as A–U. The inclusion of uracil helps to distinguish RNA from DNA—besides RNA's extra oxygen atom in the ribose sugar and usually single-strand configuration. The simple mnemonic "cut the pie" helps to associate the pyrimidine or purine bases: CUT represents cytosine, uracil, and thymine, with the pyrimidines represented by pie.

The heat required to dissociate the H bonds between DNA's two strands determines the DNA molecule's **melting point**. Proportionality exists between the number of bonds in the base pair and the energy required to break the bonds. Thus, the three hydrogen bonds that hold C and G together require more heat to break (higher melting point) than the two hydrogen bonds between A and T.

Forms of RNA

The three forms of RNA include:

1. **Messenger RNA (mRNA)** molecules, which serve as a template for protein synthesis, based on the molecular sequence from a small section of the DNA molecule

 See the animations "Protein Synthesis Overview" and "Protein Synthesis" on http://thePoint.lww.com/mkk8e for a demonstration of this process.

2. **Transfer RNA (tRNA)** molecules, which, as the name implies, transfer amino acids to the growing peptide chain on the ribosome
3. **Ribosomal RNA (rRNA)** molecules, which account for about 50% of the mass of ribosomes and whose structures aid in assembling amino acids into polypeptides

Each of the three RNA forms has its own **polymerase**, or complex enzyme: polymerase I is associated with rRNA, polymerase II with mRNA, and polymerase III with tRNA. RNA polymerases, unlike their DNA counterparts, do not require a **primer** to initiate RNA chain synthesis. The term *primase* refers to the RNA polymerase that produces the primer for DNA synthesis. The three RNA polymerases have between 6 and 10 protein subunits that differ in molecular structure and regulatory function. About 97% of cellular RNA exists as rRNA; mRNA accounts for about 2%; and tRNA less than 1%. Compared with the DNA in a single chromosome that contains up to 250 million base pairs, RNA contains no more than a few thousand, which makes an RNA molecule considerably shorter. This makes sense because RNA carries only part of the information from one segment of the DNA molecule that it copied. Later in this chapter we discuss how mRNA duplicates DNA's genetic information and the roles of rRNA and tRNA in protein synthesis.

 See the animation "DNA Synthesis" on http://thePoint.lww.com/mkk8e for a demonstration of this process.

Codons and Nature's Genetic Code

First presented by Marshall Nirenberg 🔲 (1927–2010; 1968 Nobel Prize in Physiology or Medicine; interpretation of the genetic code and its function in protein synthesis; www.nobelprize.org/nobel_prizes/medicine/laureates/1968/nirenberg-bio.html) and Johann Matthaei (1927-; www.genomenewsnetwork.org/resources/timeline/1961_Nirenberg.php) best known for discovering that the RNA sequence "UUU" directs the addition of phenylalanine to any growing protein chain) of the National Institutes of Health in 1961 at the International Congress of Biochemistry in Moscow (and 3 years later by

Uracil: base that replaces thymine in RNA that pairs with the adenine base

Melting point: The temperature range or a solid where it changes state from solid to liquid, and the solid and liquid phases exist in equilibrium

Messenger RNA (mRNA): molecule that carries genetic information (complementary copy of one of the two DNA strands) between a gene and the ribosomes that translate the genetic information into proteins

Transfer RNA (tRNA): RNA molecules that transport a specific amino acid to ribosomes; translating information in the mRNA nucleotide into the amino acid sequence of a polypeptide

Transfer RNA (tRNA): molecules, which, as the name implies, transfer amino acids to the growing peptide chain on the ribosome

Ribosomal RNA (rRNA): structural part of a ribosome that contains RNA molecules and whose structures aid in assembling amino acids into polypeptides.

Polymerase (DNA or RNA): enzyme that catalyzes nucleic acid synthesis on preexisting nucleic acid templates; assembles RNA from ribonucleotides or DNA from deoxyribonucleotides

Primer: a short nucleotide segment that pairs with a single DNA strand at a free 3-OH end (template strand) so DNA polymerase can synthesize a DNA chain; cells use RNA primers, while the PCR method uses DNA primers

Primase: enzyme that synthesizes the RNA primer to initiate DNA synthesis

Codon: sequence of three DNA or RNA bases (nucleotides) that encode (specify) a single amino acid

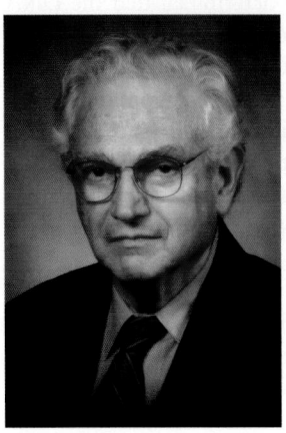

Marshall Nirenberg

Methionine: nutritionally essential amino acid; most natural source of active methyl groups in the body; the triplet sequence A-U-G on mRNA codes this amino acid

Philip Leder (1934-) and Marshall Nirenberg; 1927–2010), the coded message carried by the mRNA molecule exists as a series of three bases, or **codons** (http://users.rcn.com/ jkimball.ma.ultranet/BiologyPages/C/Codons.html). Each DNA and RNA three-letter codon block of information corresponds to one of the body's 20 amino acids. A codon codes for one amino acid, but most amino acids are represented by more than one codon. If only one base coded for an amino acid, only four amino acids could be coded instead of 20. Even if two adjacent bases coded for an amino acid, there would still not be enough combinations to make 20 amino acids. Fortunately, scientists deduced that three bases coding for an amino acid (4^3 = 64 combinations) met the requirement to include all the amino acids. For example, the triplet sequence A-U-G on mRNA displayed in **FIGURE 33.12** (*green box within left yellow panel*) refers to a specific code for the sulfur-containing essential amino acid **methionine**. The A (adenine) is called the first letter; U (uracil), the second letter; and G (guanine), the third letter. With only 20 amino acids and 64 codons, several codons code for more than one amino acid. In fact, most amino acids have more than one codon or sequence of letters, with no intervening code disrupting the sequence.

Sequencing of Codons

The amino acid serine exemplifies a four-codon sequence that differs only in the base occupying the third nucleotide or letter. The sequence is U-C-U, U-C-C, U-C-A, and U-C-G, with identical first two letters. The first two bases are the defining letters of the codon sequence.

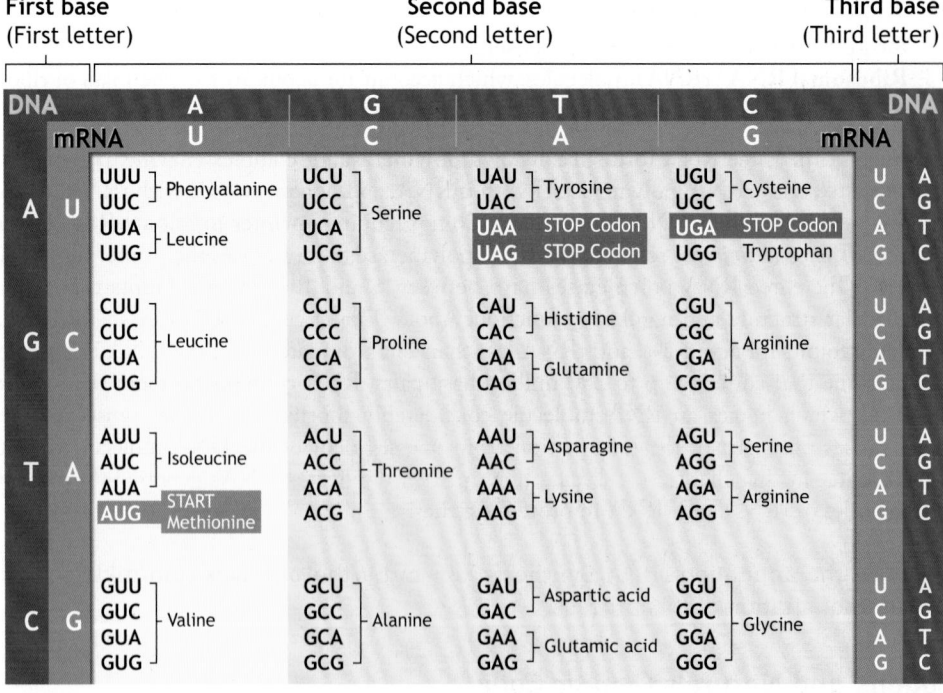

FIGURE 33.12 • The codon table—the alphabet of the universal genetic code. From the time that Watson and Crick correctly deduced DNA's helical structure in 1953, different coding schemes attempted to explain DNA's alphabetic configuration (including imaginative proposals by physicists George Gamow, Richard Feynman, and Edward Teller); in 1964, Paul Leder and Marshall Nirenberg established the final code-breaking sequences for RNA synthesis.[79] The three-letter codon "word" in mRNA is complementary to the corresponding three-letter codon within DNA from which it was transcribed. An alternative codon "wheel" has been developed (www.dna20.com/resources/bioinformatics-tools/codons-and-amino-acids).

Reading from the 5′ end of each codon, the first and second letters remain generally constant for each amino acid, while the base in the third position "wobbles." Thus, for example, the codon for phenylalanine contains a U or C as the third letter. Because both U-U-U and U-U-C code for phenylalanine, phenylalanine is inserted into a newly synthesized polypeptide if U-U-U or U-U-C is "read" during **translation** or protein synthesis.

Similar to the English alphabet with its 26 letters, the *codon table* in Figure 33.12 provides the genetic code "alphabet," but with only four distinct letters—the code words in the analogy. When we exclude the three **stop codons** (*red boxes*) that signal termination of linkages in polypeptide chains, the remaining 61 codons represent the useful information for protein synthesis. The stop codons, U-A-A, U-A-G, and U-G-A, signal the end of a genetic message (i.e., termination of protein synthesis), like periods at the end of a sentence. When the translation machinery encounters one of these chain terminators, translation halts, releasing the polypeptide from the translation complex. Recall that the start codon for methionine (A-U-G) initiates polypeptide formation; it also can code for methionine within peptide chains. A Codon Wheel Table provides a relatively simple alternative compared to the codon table in Figure 33.12 to view the first, second, and third nucleotides in the codon (**www.dna20.com/resources/bioinformatics-tools/codons-and-amino-acids**).

HOW DNA REPLICATES

A **DNA replication fork** refers to the Y-shaped region of replicating DNA molecules. As the double helix unwinds, nucleotide duplication occurs on both strands at a rate of about 50 nucleotide additions per second. Each strand serves as a template to create two new daughter strands by complementary base pairing. This mechanism provides each daughter helix with one intact strand from the parent (original strand) and one newly synthesized strand. Each strand, a complementary mirror image of the other, can serve as a template to reconstruct the other strand. **Figure 33.13** presents a schematic overview of DNA replication. Replication begins with the untwisted, unzipped appearance of two DNA strands (the **helicase** unwinds a segment of the DNA) on the *top*, where replication starts at specific zones called **origins of replication** and ends where **RNA primers** (*green*) start new DNA chains on the leading strand. Unwinding a segment of DNA breaks the hydrogen bonds between the two complementary strands of DNA. Several origins of replication exist along a chromosome, replicating simultaneously in *opposite* directions. Multiple replications reduce the time to propagate DNA by an order of magnitude because complete duplication of one strand of human DNA takes approximately 6 hr. The number of base pairs along the chromosome's replication region ranges from 10,000 up to 1 million, with an average of about 100,000 base pairs.

 See the animation "DNA Synthesis/Replication" on **http://thePoint.lww.com/mkk8e** for a demonstration of this process.

Three Stages of DNA Replication

Figure 33.14 amplifies the three stages of DNA replication illustrated in Figure 33.13. In **Stage 1**, helicase enzymes (*orange*) unwind the molecule's double helix. This stabilizes the strands, while **single-strand binding protein (SSB)** maintains separation between the two DNA strands. In **Stage 2**, **DNA polymerase** (*purple sphere*) immediately acts on DNA's **leading strand** to add nucleotides *toward* the strand's 3′ end (*red*). The process of creating the strand, called **continuous synthesis**, proceeds uninterrupted. The other DNA strand, known as a **lagging strand**, is created in shorter segments with gaps in its structure *away* from the replication fork, compared with the leading strand. In **Stage 3**, **discontinuous synthesis**, a 10-nucleotide RNA primer under the influence of **DNA polymerase I**, adds 1000 nucleotides ahead of the lagging strand's 5′ end until its gap fills. Thus, new DNA nucleotides replace the existing RNA nucleotides. **DNA ligase** then affixes the newly created, smaller **Okazaki fragments**, 100 to 200 nucleotides long, to the lagging strand in the 5′ to 3′ direction to make a complete DNA strand.

Translation: polypeptide formation (protein synthesis) on a ribosome using the amino acid sequence specified by an mRNA nucleotide sequence

Stop codon: three of the 64 codon combinations that terminate a polypeptide assembly

DNA replication fork: Y-shaped region of replicating DNA molecules where the enzymes replicating a DNA molecule bind to an untwisted, single DNA strand

Helicase: enzymes that catalyze (use the energy of nucleotide hydrolysis) to unwind and separate double-stranded DNA or RNA during its replication

Origins of replication: sites on DNA where replication begins

RNA primer: small segment of 10 RNA nucleotides complementary to the parent DNA template that adds DNA nucleotides to it to synthesize a new DNA strand

Single-strand binding protein (SSB): protein that keeps separated strands of DNA from rejoining

DNA polymerase: enzyme responsible for creating new DNA strands during replication or repair

Leading strand: new DNA daughter strand formed during continuous synthesis of DNA

Continuous synthesis: process of creating a DNA strand

Lagging strand: new shorter DNA strand formed during discontinuous synthesis; joined end to end by DNA ligase away from the replication fork

Discontinuous synthesis: RNA primer 10 nucleotides long under the influence of DNA polymerase I that adds 1000 nucleotides ahead of the lagging strand's 59 end until its gap fills

DNA polymerase I: enzyme that makes small bits of DNA to fill in gaps between Okazaki fragments during stage 3 discontinuous synthesis

DNA ligase: enzyme that binds short Okazaki fragments of the lagging strand into a continuous strand in DNA replication during stage 3 discontinuous synthesis

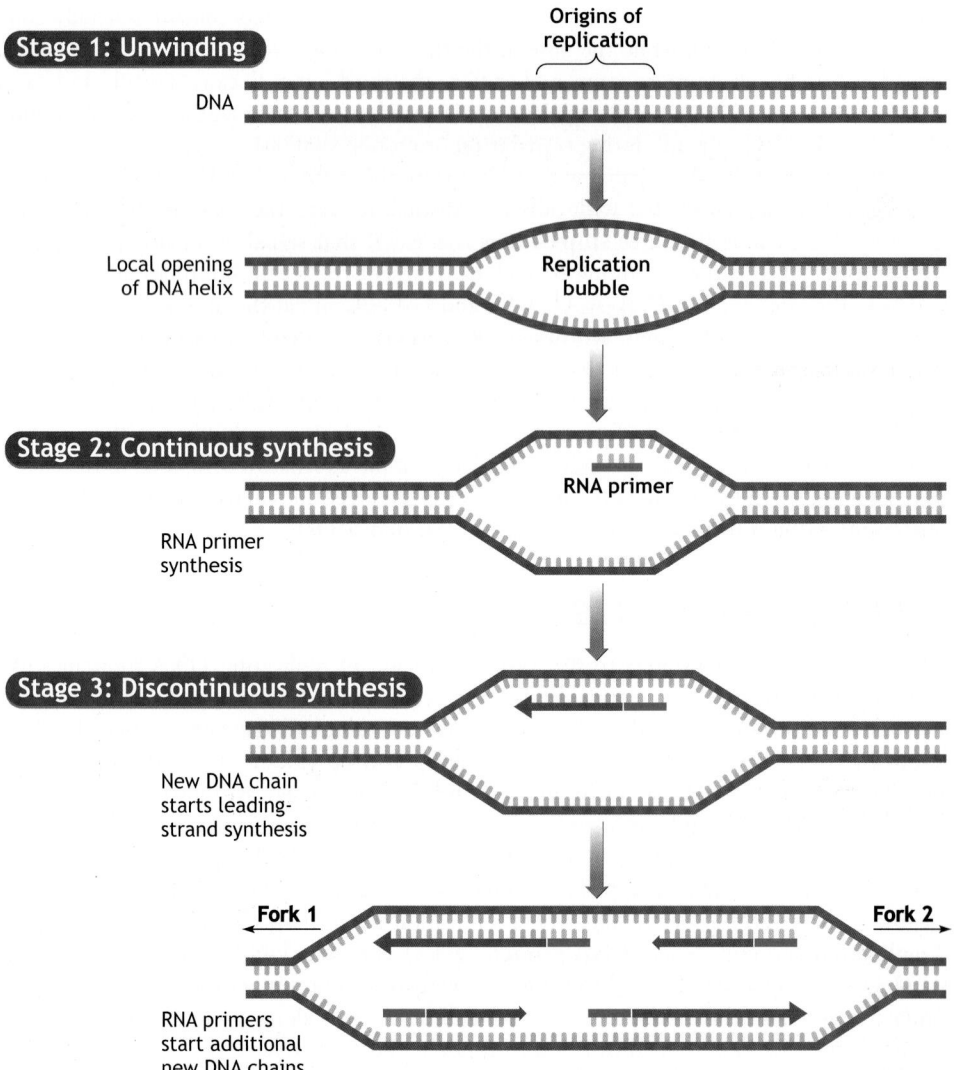

FIGURE 33.13 • Replication bubble and DNA replication. Note the straight (not helical) double strands of DNA in stage 1 after untwisting by DNA gyrase and unwinding by helicase. The DNA represents an elongated bubble as the double strand opens and DNA begins to divide (stage 2, continuous synthesis). In stage 3 (discontinuous synthesis), replication proceeds in opposite directions along each end of the Y-shaped replication forks.

Okazaki fragments: short DNA segments 100–200 nucleotides long assembled by discontinuous replication in the 5′ to 3′ direction away from the replication fork; forms the lagging strand

Pivotal Role for DNA Polymerase

DNA polymerase plays the central role in life's processes because this enzyme consistently duplicates the genetic information from generation to generation. The rich instructional bank of DNA information, modified and improved over more than 3 billion years, builds proteins and other molecules atom by atom according to selective molecular directions. For every cell that divides, DNA polymerase duplicates its entire DNA, so that cells transfer one copy to each daughter cell. DNA polymerase can be considered the most accurate of the thousands of enzymes because it creates an exact DNA copy, transmitting less than one "error" in a billion bases. Stated another way, one might find only one grammatical mistake in a thousand novels! The excellent match of C to G and A to T provides much of the specificity needed for this high accuracy, but DNA polymerase adds an extra step. After it copies each base, it "proofreads" it and deletes any wrong base sequence from its grasp. Polymerases can vary in structure from relatively "simple" to complex. In humans, polymerases are complex structures that unwind the helix, build an RNA primer, and construct a new strand. Some even have a ring-shaped structure that clamps the polymerase to the DNA strand. Polymerase function varies from day-to-day DNA repair and maintenance to the complex task of DNA replication

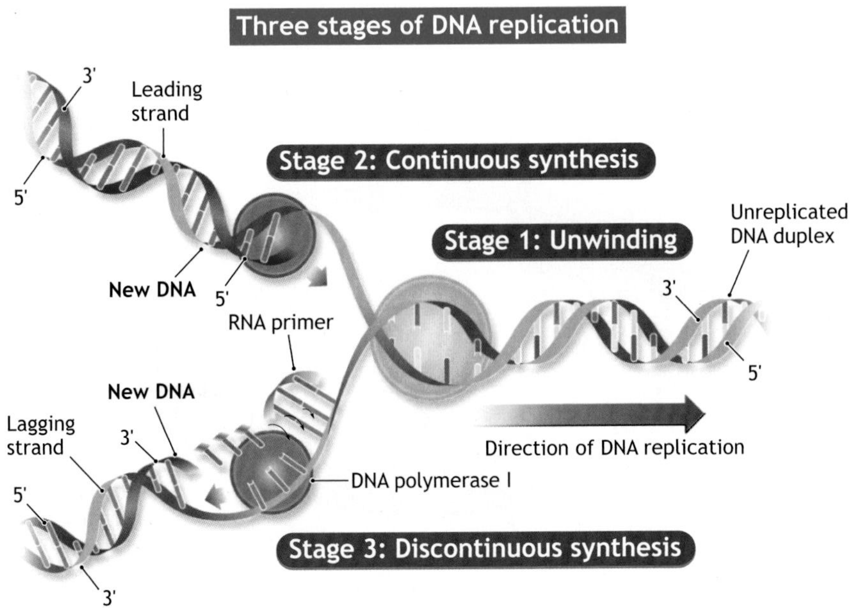

Three stages of DNA replication

FIGURE 33.14 • Three stages of DNA replication. Stage 1, unwinding; Stage 2, continuous synthesis; Stage 3, discontinuous synthesis.

when the cell divides. Here, we discuss the important role of DNA polymerase in forensic medicine in building a large quantity of identical DNA strands from a miniscule amount of DNA from a crime scene or paternity case.

See the animation "DNA Repair" on **http://thePoint.lww.com/mkk8e** for a demonstration of this process.

What Controls DNA Synthesis?

Several molecular control mechanisms trigger DNA synthesis in cells. The **cell cycle** illustrated in **FIGURE 33.15** depicts the four phases of a cell's life and accompanying three important checkpoints. Similar to a clock or thermostat, each phase has defined "on" and "off" periods regulated by enzymes that start and terminate a particular stage. DNA replication (synthesis) occurs in the S phase (*yellow* arrow), which lasts approximately 6 hr. The three checkpoints serve as the thermostat's sensors, each with specific regulator enzymes called **cyclins** governing a specific function. Toward the end of the **G1** (growth) stage (*orange* stage), cyclin enzymes achieve a critical activity level that triggers a response when the cell achieves adequate size within a favorable environment. If cell size and environment prove satisfactory, the cell proceeds to S phase for DNA synthesis. Following DNA synthesis, the G1 cyclins degrade as the cell prepares to enter **mitosis** (M phase). The next checkpoint occurs between the **G2** and M phases (*purple* arrow), a crucial time in the cell cycle. When the DNA has been replicated without error, the cell enters mitosis and then progresses to complete **telophase**. Mitosis produces two cells genetically identical to the original parent cell.

Cell Life Cycle Controllers

Figure 33.15 also provides insights about the workings of cell life cycle controllers. Cyclin-dependent **kinases** (cdk1 and cdk2) activate specific cyclins. Once this occurs, the complex of the two **protein kinases** regulates how the cell proceeds through its cycle. After each stage, cyclin degradation temporarily halts cdk activity. With mitosis complete, the process begins again, accumulating cyclins for the next initial G1 growth stage.

The cdk2 protein "turns on" in the transition between the G1 and S stages; cdk1 drives the cell cycle from stage G2 to M stage. In other words, the cyclin-dependent protein kinases phosphorylate their target cyclin proteins through the different stages of the cell cycle. Signaling proteins called growth factors operate in concert during the cycle. For example, mitosis-promoting

Cell cycle: four stages of a cell's life cycle

Cyclins: specific cell-regulator enzymes that activate and deactivate protein kinases in the cell cycle and help to control progression from one stage in the cycle to the next; they are destroyed after their function by a ubiquitin-signaled process

G1: period within the cell cycle preceding DNA synthesis

Mitosis: nuclear division that produces two daughter nuclei identical to the original nucleus

G2: period within the cell cycle from the end of DNA synthesis and start of the M phase

Telophase: final stage in mitosis (or meiosis); the spindle disappears and daughter sets of separated chromosomes decondense, the cytoplasm splits, a nuclear envelope resurrounds the chromosomes, and nucleoli appear

Kinase: enzyme that shuttles a phosphate group (PO4) from ATP or another nucleoside triphosphate to a different molecule

Protein kinase: enzyme that transfers phosphate groups to other proteins, changing their activity

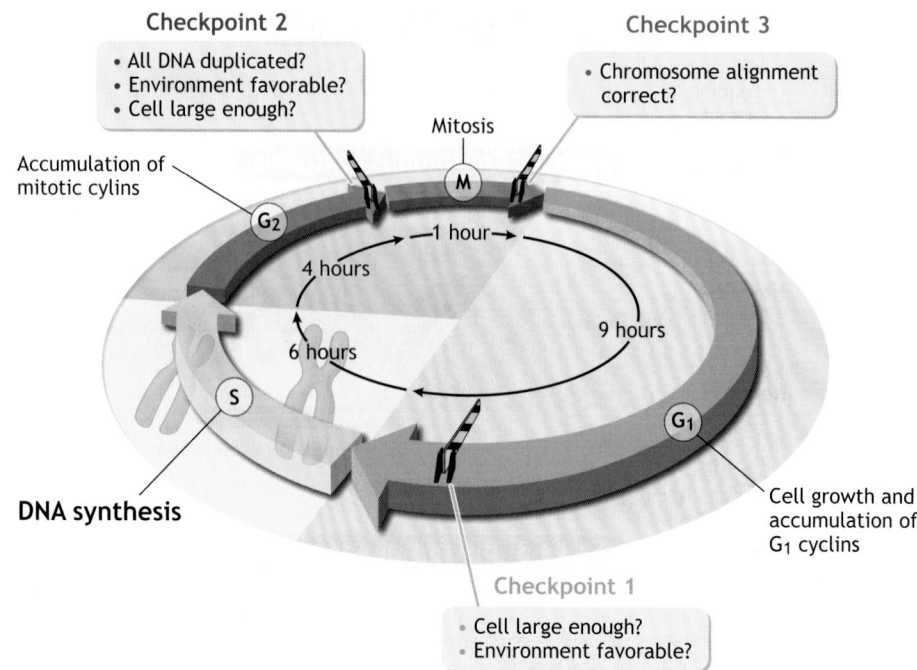

FIGURE 33.15 • Four stages of the cell cycle and its molecular control mechanisms. Note the three checkpoints and the question(s) posed prior to DNA synthesis during the S phase.

Erythropoietin: hormone produced by the kidneys that initiates red blood cell precursors and their maturation to erythrocytes

Insulin-like growth factor (IGF): small protein hormone with the potent effect of increasing aspects of cellular growth and development; IGF-1 (also known as somatomedin C) controls the general effects of growth hormone on growth

Cancer: accelerated, unplanned growth and division of mutant cells that form larger than normal cell clusters that become tumors

Transcription: RNA polymerase assembles an mRNA molecule complementary to the gene's nucleotide (making an RNA copy of a gene)

factor (MPF) governs the sequence of events between the G1 and M phases of the cell cycle. Other growth factors also exert their effect. The hormone **erythropoietin**, produced by the kidneys (see Chapters 20, 23, and 24), initiates proliferation of red blood cell precursors and their maturation to erythrocytes; nerve growth factor (NGF) modulates neuronal cell growth during development of the nervous system; interleukin-2 participates in immune cell proliferation; and **insulin-like growth factor** (**IGF**) facilitates many metabolic events related to muscle cellular growth and development,[54,135] including a role in the brain's center for smell,[139] a role in muscle strength and aerobic training in older adults,[153] and a role in increased breast cancer risk and/or death.[71]

A unique feature of growth factors relates to how they control the transition stages during cellular growth and differentiation. Failure to work in concert with cyclins and kinases during cellular proliferation terminates control of cellular proliferation, causing cells to continue to divide unchecked, which may serve both positive and negative functions. Unchecked cell division can precipitate lethal effects because DNA synthesis may progress to the M stage by successfully reproducing a mutant **cancer** gene. If highly specialized genes called tumor suppressors (e.g., the *p53* gene) cannot halt the cell cycle long enough for DNA repair enzymes to function, then cell growth proceeds rapidly and unchecked to produce tumors. Deleterious mutations also can pass to progeny cells; the successive buildup of mutations in all likelihood ultimately develops into cancer.

PROTEIN SYNTHESIS: TRANSCRIPTION AND TRANSLATION

Protein synthesis involves two prominent events:

1. **Transcription** in the cell nucleus that creates a single-stranded RNA copy of the genetic information stored in the double-stranded DNA molecule
2. RNA translation in the cell cytoplasm to form proteins

In essence, the DNA molecule's nucleotide base sequence defines the protein's ultimate three-dimensional shape.

Our tour of protein synthesis begins by considering a "roadmap" of the prominent events in assembling proteins from precursor biomolecules (i.e., lipids, carbohydrates, proteins, and nucleic acids). The tour originates in the cell's ribosomes and ends with creation of a fully **functional protein**—a unique molecule whose structure dictates its operation and specific mode of action.

Functional protein: protein with its own set of genetically determined information to carry out specific function(s)

Generalized Overview of Protein Synthesis

FIGURE 33.16 provides a generalized overview of six important stages in protein synthesis. Prior to stage 1, DNA, under enzyme control, "untwists" to expose its code. Before DNA's hydrogen bonds break, DNA topoisomerase enzymes (e.g., **DNA gyrase**) "relax" the **supercoiled DNA** by literally cutting the DNA to create a double-stranded break, but maintain a hold on both ends of the DNA. The two halves of the molecule then rotate relative to each other (untwist) before rejoining. Once the strand untwists, **DNA helicase** unwinds the helical DNA molecule by separating the hydrogen bonds between the base pairs. The single-strand binding protein (SSB) binds to one of the unpaired DNA strands to inhibit its reemerging with its neighbor (complementary) strand. This prevents the strands from recoiling and re-forming the double helix. **DNA polymerase III (Pol III)** serves as a "verifier" to ensure that the bases pair correctly. If they do, the enzyme joins the nucleotides together. If not, the mismatched base pair is rejected. "How DNA Replicates," earlier n this chapter, provides further details about the DNA **replication bubble** and DNA's three stages of replication.

DNA gyrase: enzyme that relaxes supercoiled DNA

Supercoiled DNA: configuration of twisted DNA packed into a cell prior to replication

DNA helicase: enzyme that catalyzes the unwinding of double-helical DNA by using energy released from ATP hydrolysis

DNA polymerase III (Pol III): enzyme involved in making DNA when chromosomes replicate

Replication bubble: site where DNA divides

See the animation "ATPase" on **http://thePoint.lww.com/mkk8e** for a demonstration of this process.

Stage 1 signifies the start of transcription. This involves copying a discrete section of the genetic sequence directly from the DNA template to the growing RNA strand. The enzyme **RNA polymerase I** (depicted in gold in Figure 33.16 and referred to as "I" because it was discovered before the other polymerases), binds to the specific **promoter** (initiator) region at the beginning of a gene. Roger David Kornberg 🌐 (1947-) American biochemist from Stanford University, Palo Alto, CA, won the 2006 Nobel Prize in Chemistry for creating detailed molecular images of RNA polymerase during various stages of the eukaryotic transcription process (**www.nobelprize.org/nobel_prizes/chemistry/laureates/2006/press.html**). Linking to a specific nitrogenous base sequence, it "alerts" transcription to initiate formation of the complementary RNA strand. When RNA polymerase arrives at the end of the gene, it receives a "stop" signal from one of three nucleotide sequences (U-A-A, U-A-G, U-G-A; see Fig. 33.12) and disengages from the DNA. The newly assembled RNA strand, called the **primary RNA transcript** of the gene (stage 2), is processed and eventually exits the nucleus to the cytoplasm through the octagon disk-shaped **nuclear pore complex**. This complex selectively transports proteins across the nuclear envelope after specific protein receptors dock with the protein, allowing it to enter its channel and pass to the cytoplasm. Note that once mRNA leaves the nucleus in stage 2, it links to the ribosome's poly A site and waits to bind to the appropriately coded amino acid floating freely in the cytoplasm. A specific orientation of mRNA on the ribosome exposes only one codon at a time to match and bind with its anticodon contained on a tRNA.

RNA polymerase I: enzyme that synthesizes RNA from a DNA template

Promoter: site on DNA where RNA polymerase binds and initiates transcription (promotes gene expression); required for expression and regulation of gene transcription

Primary RNA transcript: mRNA molecule transcribed as an exact complement to a gene

Nuclear pore complex: octagonal, disk-shaped structure that allows proteins to cross the nuclear envelope into the cytoplasm after protein receptors dock with the protein

Within the cytoplasm, translation proceeds through stage 3 (tRNA binds amino acids), stage 4 (tRNA binds to a ribosome, signifying the start of amino acid assembly), and stage 5 (the growing peptide chain increases in length), until stage 6, when a fully functional protein forms. The *red bar at the bottom* of Figure 33.16 summarizes the two crucial aspects of protein synthesis following DNA molecule **replication**:

Replication: duplication of DNA prior to cell division

1. Transcription of information in the genetic code from DNA molecules to RNA molecules in the nucleus (RNA synthesis) for decoding
2. Translation of genetic information in the cytoplasm to synthesize proteins

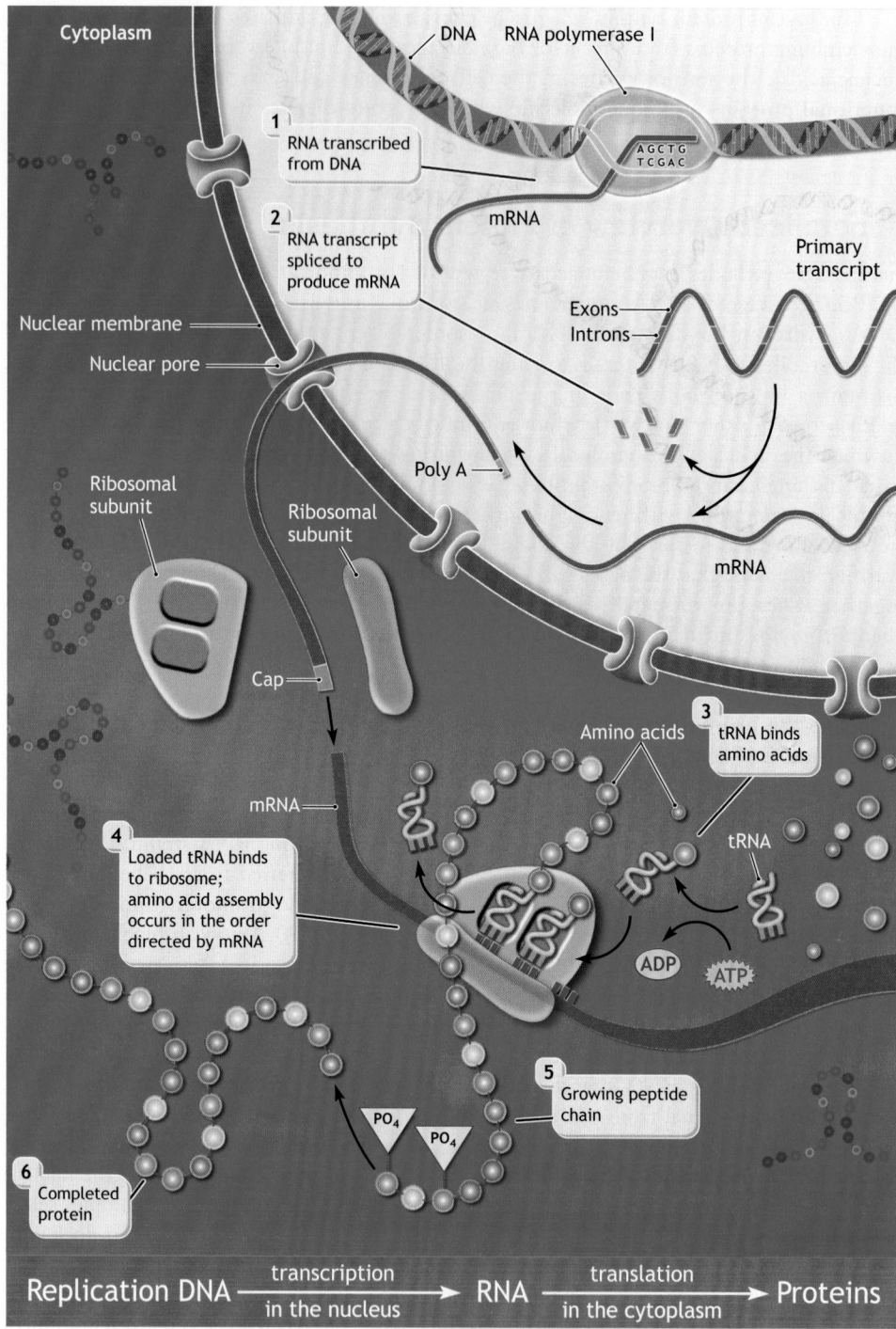

FIGURE 33.16 • Generalized overview of six stages (*numbered yellow boxes*) in protein synthesis. Notable features include the schematic depiction of events during transcription (stages labeled 1 and 2 within the cell's nucleus) and translation (stages labeled 3 to 6 in the cell's cytoplasm). The *bottom inset box* summarizes the two principle aspects of protein synthesis (transcription and translation) following replication of the DNA molecule.

Transcription of the Genetic Code: RNA Synthesis and Gene Expression

A gene, located along a specific chromosome at a specific site, contains the sequence code or "plan" for protein synthesis. The gene within the DNA molecule ranges from several thousand to millions of bases. Unlocking the regulation of a particular gene provides the driving force for many molecular biologists' passion for the field.

The *left side* of Figure 33.17 highlights the five stages of gene expression in human cells. The same two basic sequences of molecular events occur whether in the simplest **bacteria** or **prokaryotes** (organisms without membrane-bound structures including a nucleus) that dominated Earth during its first 2 billion or so years of evolution or in **eukaryotes** that evolved about 1.5 billion years ago. The eukaryotes include thousands of uni- and multicellular organisms, including humans, with membrane-bound **organelles**. The cells of these organisms include a true nucleus with chromosomes. The DNA in prokaryotes remains single stranded and the main events—transcription and translation—occur coupled, not separately in the nucleus and cytoplasm, respectively. In eukaryotes, in contrast, translating the code

Bacteria: primitive, single-celled organisms used to study genetic characteristics and to clone mammalian genes

Prokaryote: cell or organism lacking a structurally discrete nucleus or nuclear membrane; contains a single circular chromosome

Eukaryotes: multicellular organisms with membrane-bound organelles and a true nucleus containing multiple linear chromosomes (Greek; from eu-karyon, or "true nucleus")

Organelle: intracellular structure within a cell that carries out specialized functions (e.g., mitochondrion)

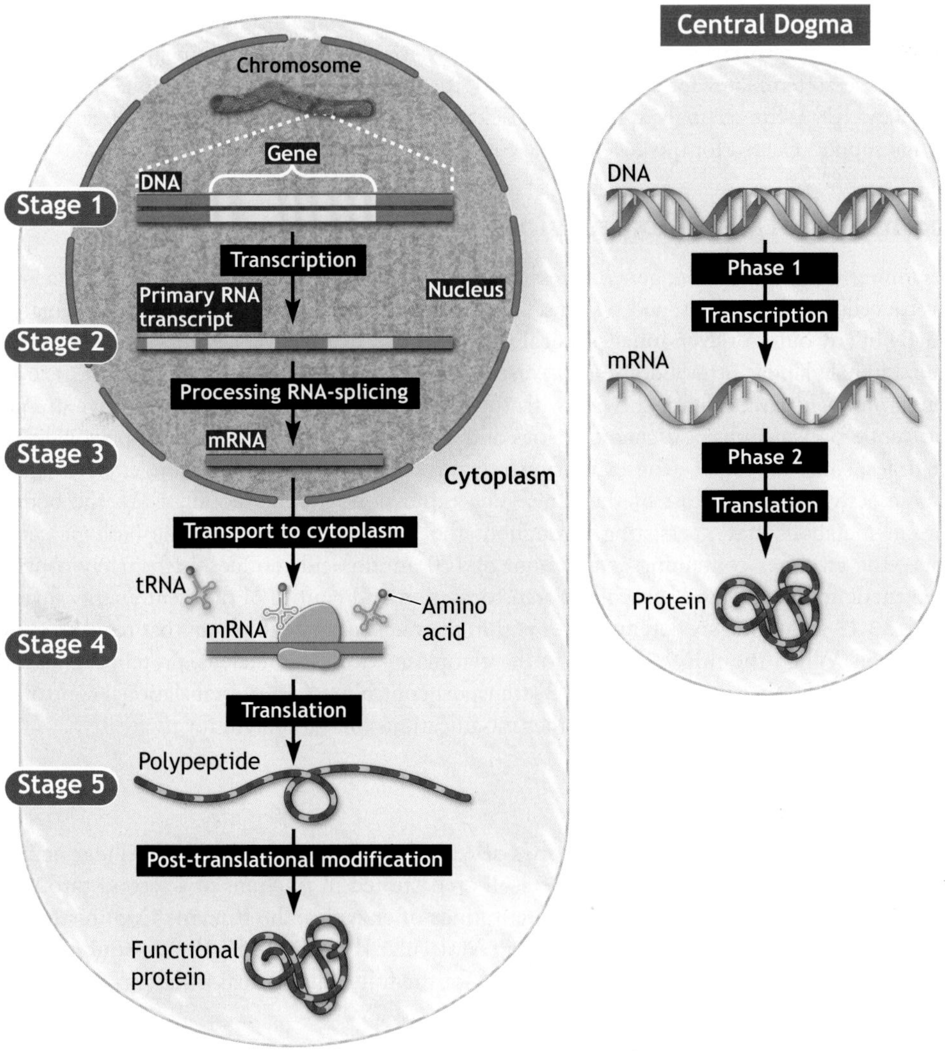

FIGURE 33.17 • Gene expression and translation. (*Left*) Five stages of gene expression in eukaryotes. Transcription (stage 1) produces an mRNA copy of the gene. In translation (stage 4), the information in mRNA molecules "directs" which amino acid to produce and where to position the amino acids when the ribosomes synthesize polypeptides. Translation refers to the creation (assembly) of a protein on the ribosome; mRNA copies the specific coded information from the DNA strand. Posttranslational modifications can alter polypeptides in their transition to a functional protein (stage 5). (*Right*) Crick's 1956 working hypothesis (central dogma) posits that two distinct phases play the defining role in expressing the genetic information encoded in DNA molecules. In phase 1 (transcription), RNA polymerase enzyme assembles an mRNA molecule with its nucleotide sequence complementary to the gene's nucleotide sequence. In phase 2 (translation), a ribosome assembles a polypeptide (protein) in which mRNA's nucleotide sequence specifies the final amino acid configuration.

for protein synthesis does not occur until the RNA strand exits the nucleus. The *right* figure illustrates the proposed flow of genetic information that Francis Crick in 1956 termed the **central dogma**.

The Watson and Crick hypothesis posited that chromosomal DNA functions as the template for RNA molecules. These molecules then move to the cytoplasm to dictate a protein's amino acid arrangement. The *down arrow at the top of* Fig. 33.17 (left) from DNA emphasizes the proposition that DNA provides the template for self-replication. The next phase emphasizes that all cellular RNA molecules were made on (transcribed from) DNA templates. Concomitantly, RNA templates determined (translated) the proteins. The unidirectionality of the two arrows between stages 3 (transport to cytoplasm) and 4 (translation) and 4 (translation) and 5 (post-translational modification) indicates that protein templates would never determine RNA sequences, nor would RNA templates create DNA. With few exceptions, the central dogma has stood the test of time and remains essentially valid. Except in some instances in which the reproductive cycle of **retroviruses** adds a step using a reverse transcriptase enzyme, proteins almost never serve as templates for RNA. If they did, the arrows would go bidirectionally between DNA and RNA. Interestingly, at the time Crick proposed the central dogma, little direct experimental support existed for this mechanistic concept that RNA serves as DNA's template.

Examples of Gene Expression

Beginning with conception, gene expression lays the eventual groundwork for each person's diverse cells, tissues, organs, and systems. Gene expression explains why no two people match exactly in any outer or even inner physical traits. No two hearts, livers, kidneys, brains, vertebrae, adrenal glands, intra-abdominal fat distributions, teeth, nostrils, ears, or fingerprints ever match precisely. Even identical twins with the same starting genetic machinery have unique and subtle outward physical characteristics and often not-so-subtle distinctive personalities. At times, some aspect of gene expression remains repressed or "off," no longer needing to remain active or "on." Most of the time, gene expression "fits" or modulates to the body's current metabolic state, persisting throughout the individual's life span. The biologic catalysts—the enzymes containing a minimum of 100 amino acid residues—effectively control the genetic machinery and subsequent transformation and control of different energy forms. FIGURE **33.18** shows the six potential sites within the nucleus and cytoplasm that regulate gene expression. When the mRNA travels to the cytoplasm from the nucleus, protein regulation via translation in the cytoplasm at sites 3 (transport control) to 6 (post-translational control of protein function) can begin, as can further modifications once a protein forms at site 6.

Protein Enzymes

Acting as biomolecular switches, enzymes selectively regulate thousands of cellular activities, coupling some and uncoupling others, all orchestrated in fractions of a second throughout an organism's life. To categorize different kinds of enzymes, the Enzyme Commission of the International Union of Biochemistry and Molecular Biology (IUBMB; **www.iubmb.org**) devised a nomenclature and numbering system for the following six major classes of enzymes, each with subgroups and sub-subgroups:

1. *Oxidoreductases*: catalyze oxidation–reduction reactions
2. *Transferases*: catalyze transfer of functional groups between molecules
3. *Hydrolases*: catalyze hydrolytic cleavage
4. *Lyases*: catalyze removal of a group from or addition of a group to a double bond, or other changes involving electron rearrangement
5. *Isomerases*: catalyze intramolecular rearrangement
6. *Ligases*: catalyze reactions that join two molecules

Transcription Control

Diverse "switches" or regulator enzyme **activator proteins** and **repressor proteins** affect gene expression during transcription. These switches operate at the site of the active gene and also at

Central dogma: Crick's belief that the genetic information flow creates proteins from DNA (transcription in the nucleus) and RNA (translation in the cytoplasm) to protein

Retrovirus: RNA virus that can enter a cell using reverse transcriptase to reproduce a copy of itself into the genome; a retrovirus carrying an oncogene can transform a host cell into a cancerous cell

Activator protein: binds to DNA at enhancer sites to position RNA polymerase correctly on the gene

Repressor protein: blocks action of RNA polymerase on DNA that turns genes "off"

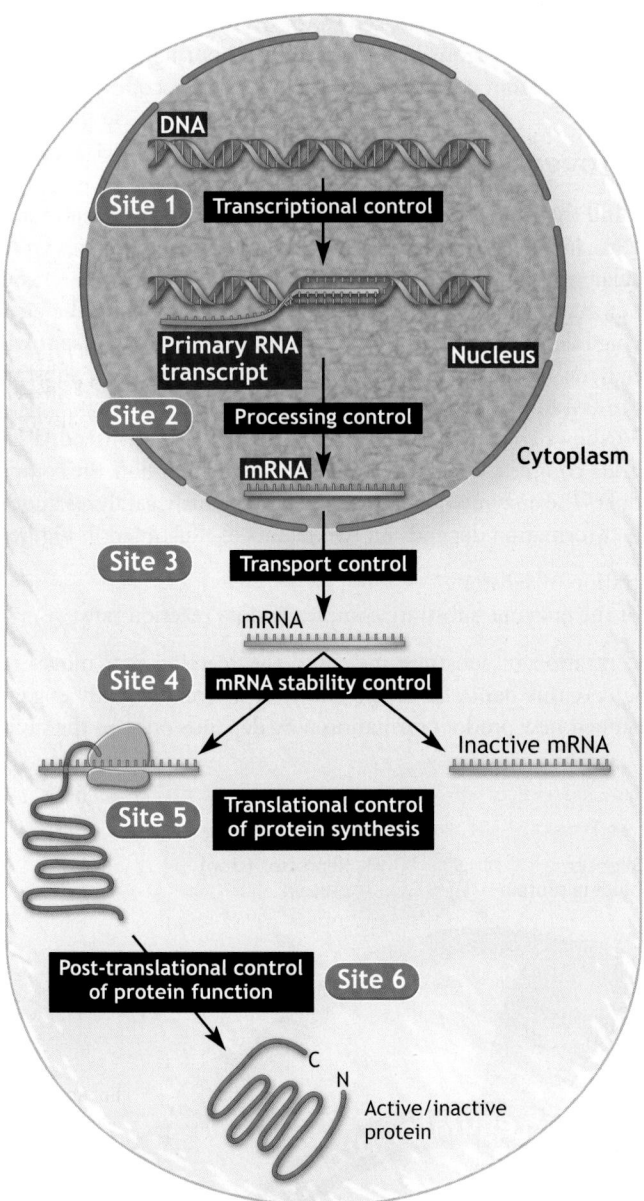

FIGURE 33.18 • Six potential sites regulate gene expression.

sites thousands of nucleotides away from the starting site. This geography of operation provides great regulatory freedom in how genes initially switch on and off prior to and during transcription. For example, some enzymes accelerate the capture of RNA polymerase to enhance transcription, while others repress transcription by delaying different sequences of events. In essence, activator and repressor proteins control transcription rate in the following two ways:

1. Activator proteins bind to DNA at sites called *enhancer sites*. FIGURE 33.19 shows the transcription complex (proteins involved in transcription) correctly positioning RNA polymerase at the proper gene location. The folding of the DNA strand brings the enhancer site into close proximity to the transcription complex. This increases communication between the activator proteins and the transcription complex. Another group of proteins, termed *coactivator proteins*, transmits signals from activator proteins to other factors (called *basal factors*) close to the DNA strand, helping to position RNA polymerase correctly at the precise location in DNA's **coding region**.

2. Repressor proteins bind to "silencer" protein binding sites along the DNA strand (the darker blue protein region at the top of the strand under the larger repressor or stop

Enhancer site: where gene expression increases from contact with the transcription complex

Coactivator protein: transmits signals from activator proteins to basal factors

Coding region: location on the DNA strand where transcription occurs

protein). The silencer sequence, adjacent to or overlapping the enhancer region, can prevent an activator protein from binding to a neighboring enhancer site. This delays or cancels transcription from initiating at a discrete mRNA coding sequence.

Enzyme Turnover Number

Some enzymes fulfill their functions more quickly than others. An important way to measure an enzyme's performance relates to how quickly it binds to and releases from its substrate(s) during biomolecular reactions; that is, its turnover rate or number. To encourage a reaction, an enzyme must correctly position or orient itself with its substrate. The electrical properties of a substrate change depending in part on its correct spatial arrangement with the substrate. In essence, the enzyme's positive and negative charges align with the substrate's positive and negative charges to favorably continue a chemical reaction.

FIGURE **33.20A** shows an enzyme arranging to link up with its intended substrate to create an enzyme–substrate complex. Once the enzyme fulfills its function, the complex breaks down, releasing its product. The enzyme then almost instantaneously catalyzes another reaction. The rate of end-product formation depends on two factors as illustrated in Figure 33.20B:

1. The concentration of substrate
2. The nature of the enzyme–substrate complex and its reaction rate

As the concentration of substrate increases, the reaction rate moves toward its maximum (*yellow* line). At this point, all of the enzymes' active sites fully engage the substrate's active sites. Continued new product formation now depends only on the rapidity of substrate

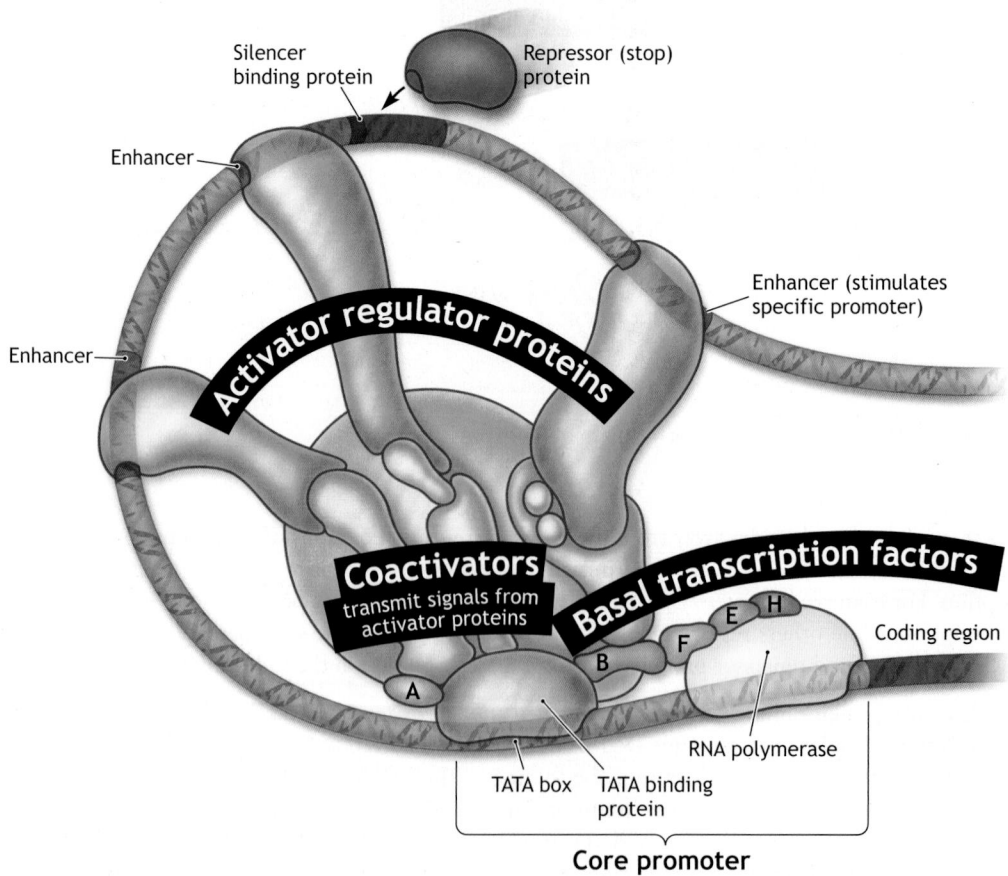

FIGURE 33.19 • Structure of transcription complex involved in transcriptional control. At the start of the coding sequence along DNA's double helix (*purple* ropelike structure), the basal (transcription) factors labeled (*from left to right*) A, TATA binding protein, B, F, E, and H correctly position RNA polymerase and then release it to transcribe mRNA.

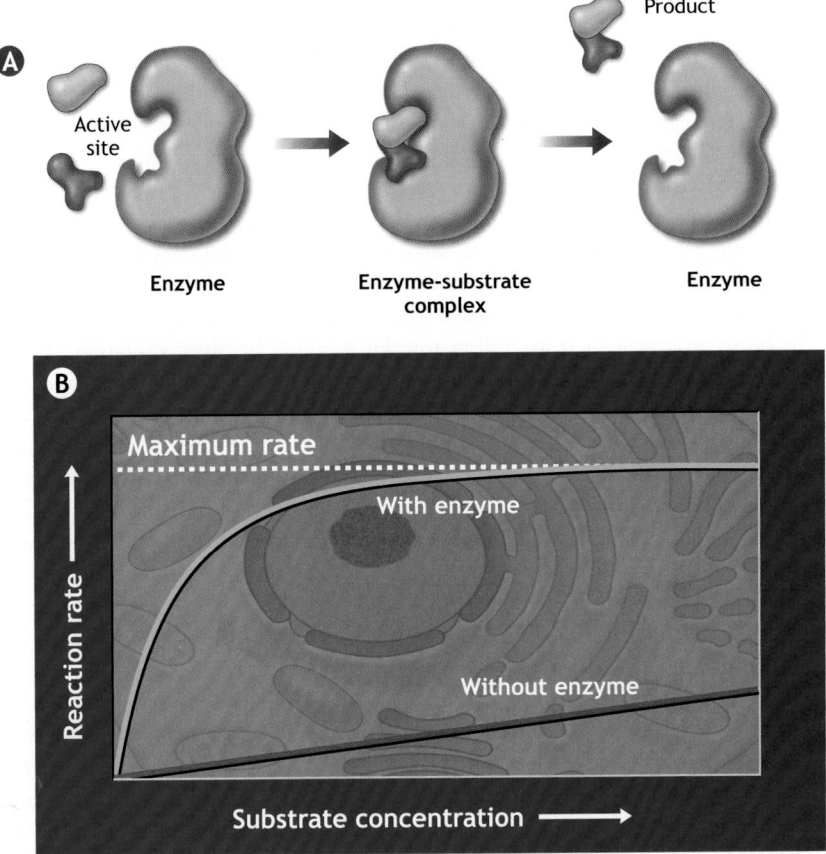

FIGURE 33.20 • **(A)** Enzyme–substrate interaction. **(B)** Reaction rate versus substrate concentration with and without enzyme action.

processing, referred to as **turnover number**. This can vary tremendously, from 1 to 10,000 molecules per second, but a turnover number of 1000 substrate molecules per second characterizes many enzymes. A high turnover ensures that enzymes remain "turned on" at their optimal concentration during gene expression. The enzyme's binding sites, while they remain in the "on" position with their substrate for extremely brief periods, may do so more dynamically than previously believed. Instead of remaining coupled for the entire period, other similar binding sites may switch places with the originally bound site (analogous to "hit-join-and-run"), suggesting that enzyme molecules maintain more mobility than previously believed. The bottom red line shows a typical reaction rate without an enzyme present despite increasing substrate availability.

> **Turnover number:** maximum number of molecules of substrate that an enzyme can convert to a product per unit of time; for example, catalase (5×10^4) is about 2500 times more active than amylase (1.9×10^4)

Gene Expression and Human Exercise Performance

The current and future exercise physiology research will continue to build upon the rapidly developing knowledge base about gene expression and the human gene map for exercise performance and health-related phenotypes (see *Med Sci Sports Exerc* 2001;33:885, with annual updates through 2012, and the obesity gene map database, http://obesitygene.pbrc.edu, with access to recent publications from the HERITAGE Family study, Québec Family Study, Cardia Fitness Study, Swedish Obese Subjects Study, Genathlete, and Hypgene).[130]

In the not too distant future, exercise scientists will routinely incorporate simplified molecular biologic techniques to assess an individual's potential for strength, speed, endurance, and other traits that can be "turned on" to selectively enhance exercise performance. It might seem far-fetched now, but choosing astronauts for extended-duration missions to other planets may rely on analyzing molecular biology to "select" candidates who possess genes more resistant to bone loss or spatial disorientation with prolonged microgravity exposure.

Coaches and trainers will undoubtedly apply technologies from molecular medicine to genetically screen young children for gene clusters that indicate potential for desirable athletic traits (and traits related to training responsiveness), such as predominance of a specific muscle fiber type, abundance of targeted aerobic enzymes, muscle capillaries, or left-ventricular cavity size.

Today, sports scientists use laboratory and field testing to screen athletes for performance and physiologic capacities, including the application of molecular genetics with the ACTN3 gene that encodes the protein actinin in skeletal muscle to assess potential for sports and athletic performance.[2,103,115,120,125,128] Gene expression is tightly controlled. When muscle tissue rebuilds, gene expression for actin and myosin protein filament enlargement remains "on," while gene expression for generating new muscle cells remains "off" because cellular hypertrophy, not hyperplasia, usually prevails. These "on–off" genes are referred to as "**housekeeping genes.**" In body processes such as coding for the proteins involved in aerobic metabolism, gene expression does not shut down but remains continually on until death. The same applies to all cell and tissue metabolic activities controlled by enzymes that dominate cellular and subcellular events. Organisms from bacteria to humans use the same two basic principles of gene expression. First, an RNA duplicate is made of a particular gene with its unique coding sequence on a DNA template that represents some combination in succession of G, C, T, A. Second, the RNA copy containing the sequence of the **genetic code** on the **ribosome** (located outside the nucleus) orchestrates the sequential construction of amino acids into a protein possessing unique biomolecular characteristics.

Exons and Introns

The primary RNA transcript molecule contains all of the information needed from the gene to create a protein. This molecule's structure discovered by Crick,[162] called a coding region or **exon**, shown in the green primary transcript within the nucleus in **FIGURE 33.21**, also contains additional, unwanted stretches of nucleotide "spacers," or noncoding regions termed *introns* (introns shown within the primary RNA transcript of Fig. 33.21). The 1993 Nobel Prize in Physiology or Medicine was awarded to British molecular biologist Sir Richard John Roberts (1943–) and American geneticist and microbiologist Phillip Allen Sharp (1944–) for their discovery of "split genes" or introns (**http://nobelprize.org/nobel_prizes/medicine/laureates/1993/press.html**). Approximately 97% of DNA consists of introns. An example of just three exons and two introns shows the individual numbering for the base pair sequences within each exon and intron. For example, the numbers 1–30 designate the base pairs for the first exon along the RNA strand, while 105–146 signify the base pairs for the last exon. The two introns with their base pairs have the numbers 30–31 and 104–105. During transcription, note the removal of intron links 30–31 and 104–105, leaving the remaining three exons that splice together (their base pairs now numbered 1–146) to create the final mRNA transcript. This must occur before the mRNA strand leaves the nucleus and enters the cytoplasmic space (cytosol).

The cytoplasm cannot receive partially processed transcripts. Intron removal likely occurs because these structures provide no known usable code for any part of the polypeptide initially specified by the gene. These clusters of repeated, apparently nonfunctional and random DNA sequences scattered throughout the genome exist as either short interspersed elements of 500 or fewer base pairs (called SINEs) or long interspersed elements of more than 1000 base pairs (LINEs) in length. The mature mRNA transcript displayed at the bottom of Figure 33.21 contains the correct sequence of codes to create proteins. The example shows the specified order for seven amino acids inserted into the elongating polypeptide chain, determined originally during translation based on codon sequence.

RNA Splicing

RNA splicing removes unwanted intron sequences from the primary transcript before it is translated, allowing translation to avoid those sequences. Introns usually occupy an area 10 to 30 times greater than exons. Small nuclear RNA (snRNA; composed of proteins and a special type of RNA) play a contributing role in RNA splicing. Another protein (small nuclear ribonucleoprotein, or snRNP) contains snRNA. This structure can bind to the 5′ end of an intron, while a different snRNP binds to the intron's 3′ end. Introns interact to form a loop that joins

Housekeeping genes: genes automatically switched "on" all the time to maintain essential cell functions

Genetic code: sequence of nucleotides, coded in triplets (codons) along the mRNA that determine the amino acid sequence in protein synthesis; the gene's DNA sequence can predict the mRNA sequence; the genetic code in turn predicts the amino acid sequence

Ribosome: small cellular component (organelle) composed of specialized ribosomal RNA; site of polypeptide (protein)

Exon: protein-coding DNA sequence of a gene

Intron: DNA base noncoding sequence that interrupts a gene's protein-coding sequence; the sequence transcribes into RNA but gets excised from the "message" before it translates into protein

RNA splicing: excision of unwanted sequence of introns from the primary transcript so the exons fuse together

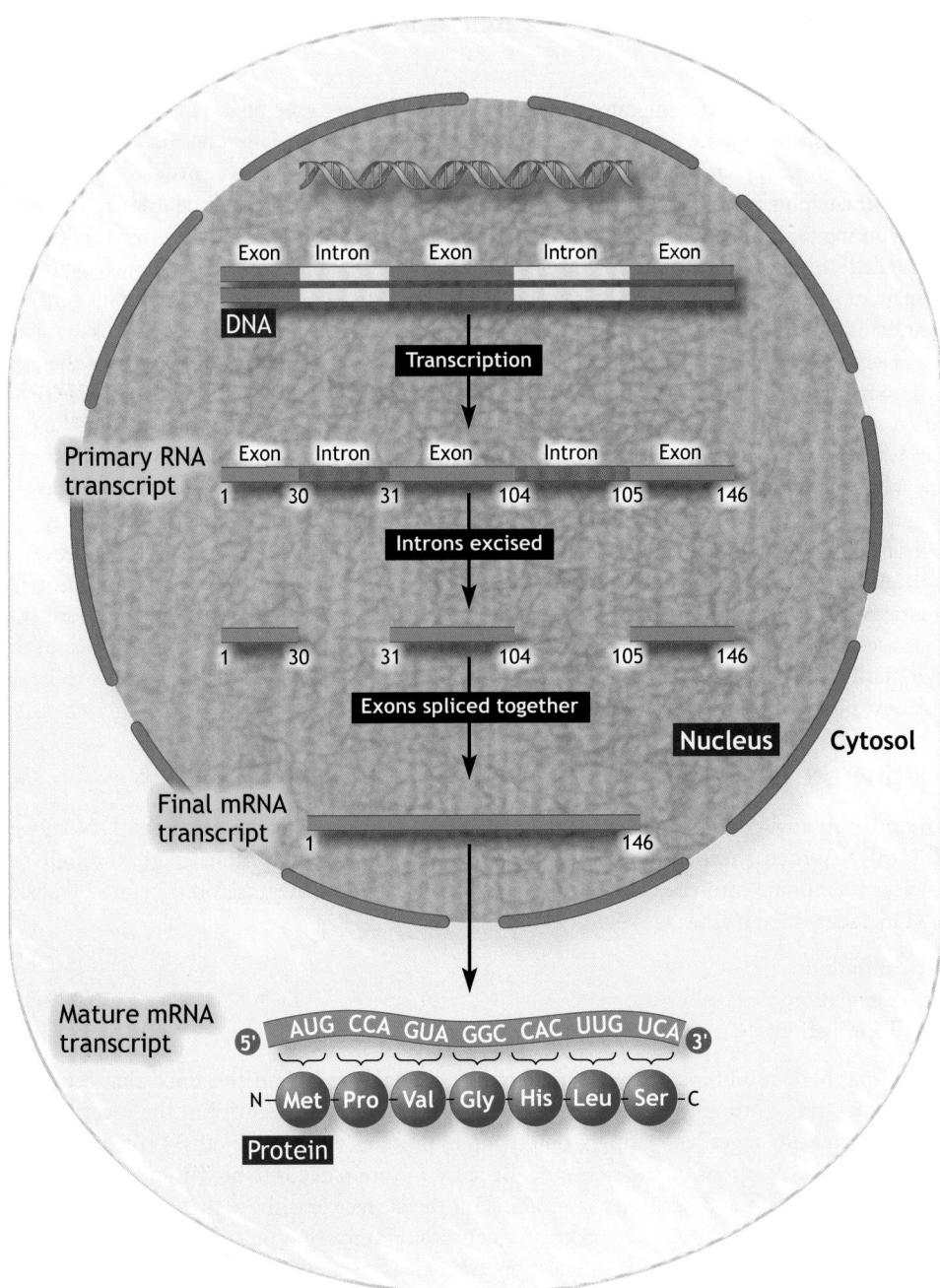

FIGURE 33.21 • Example of exons and introns, individual numbering for the base pair sequences, and intron excision and exon splicing to form the final (mature) mRNA transcript. For this structure, note the three-letter codons shown in *white* lettering along the *green* mRNA, and the corresponding amino acids listed in the *blue* circles below. The codon table in Figure 33.12 lists the full names of these amino acids.

the free ends of the intron. A collection of snRNPs is known as a *spliceosome*. Its function is to excise the intron, allowing the entron to join it but without the snRNPs. The final, mature mRNA strand is shorter than the primary transcript, owing to the excision of about 90% of the introns in the primary transcript prior to translation. Consider exon splicing a unique phase of protein construction at the start of protein assembly. Splicing manipulates intron sequencing in many ways to form **polypeptides**. The hemoglobin (Hb) molecule, for example, requires 432 nucleotides to encode its 144 amino acids, yet before intron excision, 1356 nucleotides exist in the primary mRNA transcript of the *Hb* gene. Regulation of gene expression occurs by changes in how splicing takes place during different stages of a cell's development and type.

Spliceosome: found within the nucleus of eukaryotes and composed of about 300 distinct proteins and a group of five RNAs in non-coding intervening sequences

Polypeptide: unbranched string of amino acids linked by peptide bonds formed during gene translation

mRNA Packaging: Polyadenylic Acid and Guanosine Triphosphate—Tails and Caps

Polyadenylic acid [poly(A)] tail: chain 100–200 adenine nucleotides long; joins one end at the 39 region of the final transcribed mRNA before the RNA transcript migrates through the nuclear pore

Guanosine triphosphate (GTP): initiates translation when it binds mRNA at the 5′ end of the molecule to the smaller of the ribosome's two subunits; referred to as the "cap" on the final transcribed mRNA

Before the RNA transcript migrates through the nuclear pore as the final transcribed mRNA, a **polyadenylic acid (poly[A]) tail**, 100–200 adenine nucleotides long, joins one end at the 3′ region via the action of the enzyme poly(A) polymerase, and a terminal portion or "cap" (methylated **guanosine triphosphate [GTP]**) joins near the 5′ end. Much as a college student wears a cap and gown during the graduation ceremony before entering the "real" world, so mRNA must be "capped and tailed" to prepare the transcribed molecule for translation before it exits the nucleus to participate in subsequent protein synthesis. The newly formed cap performs the important function of initiating translation when it binds the mRNA to the smaller of the ribosome's two subunits.

FIGURE 33.22 A shows how the GTP cap and poly(A) tail join to RNA. Note that the capping enzyme (symbolized by the *shorter curved purple arrow*) cleaves two phosphates (*circles enclosed in red*) from GTP and one phosphate from the mRNA strand. In forming the cap, the GTP now attaches near the end of the first base of the mRNA. Figure 33.22B illustrates the addition of the poly(A) tail when a specific endonuclease enzyme (*orange*) recognizes the sequence A-A-U-A-A-A on the mRNA and snips the strand near that point. This permits a tail of 100–200 adenine residues to affix to the 3′ end of the mRNA strand. The addition of poly(A) promotes mRNA stability. It permits the mRNA molecule to maintain translation for up to several weeks, sometimes producing 100,000 protein molecules. Recall that transcription that uses DNA occurs inside the cell's nucleus, whereas ribosomal assembly takes place in the cytoplasm. The capping and tailing function enables the mRNA to exit the nucleus to begin the next phase of protein synthesis.

Exiting the Nucleus

The mRNA now contains a copy of the specific nucleotide sequence from the DNA gene. The mRNA then shuttles the "coded message," after the transcription stage, through the nuclear membrane into the cytoplasm where protein synthesis (translation) begins. Translation includes three main stages:

1. Initiation
2. Elongation
3. Termination

Using high-resolution x-ray crystallography, researchers have determined that a tunnel-like groove runs through the middle of the larger 50S subunit, providing the location that links amino acids together.[118] Thirty-one separate proteins affix to the outside of the subunit where they also reach inside the ribosome. Because a protein needs to be within a 3 Å distance to induce any effect and because the proteins on the surface and those that reach around the surface remain within 18 Å, the source of any protein interaction must be RNA. In this case, adenosine 2486 is the nucleotide in question, with an associated nitrogen atom. Therefore, the RNA gives the catalytic power to protein synthesis—in essence, ribosomes serve as ribozymes. This finding helps to explain why some bacteria remain resistant to antibiotics. A mutation on one of the ribosomal proteins within the ribosomal groove locks up with part of the antibiotic molecule, preventing the peptide from exiting the region and thus stopping further antibiotic binding and subsequent damage to the bacterium.

Translation of the Genetic Code: Ribosomal Assembly of Polypeptides

Translation initiates protein construction. Once the mRNA enters the cytoplasm through the nuclear pore, it seeks out a ribosome with which to bind. The nucleus is the original source of the millions of ribosomes in the cell's cytoplasm. A ribosome consists of a large and a small subunit, the latter fitting into a depression on the ribosome's larger surface. A ribosome has three sites that associate with mRNA:

1. A-site (A for attachment)
2. P-site (P for polypeptide)
3. E-site (E for exit)

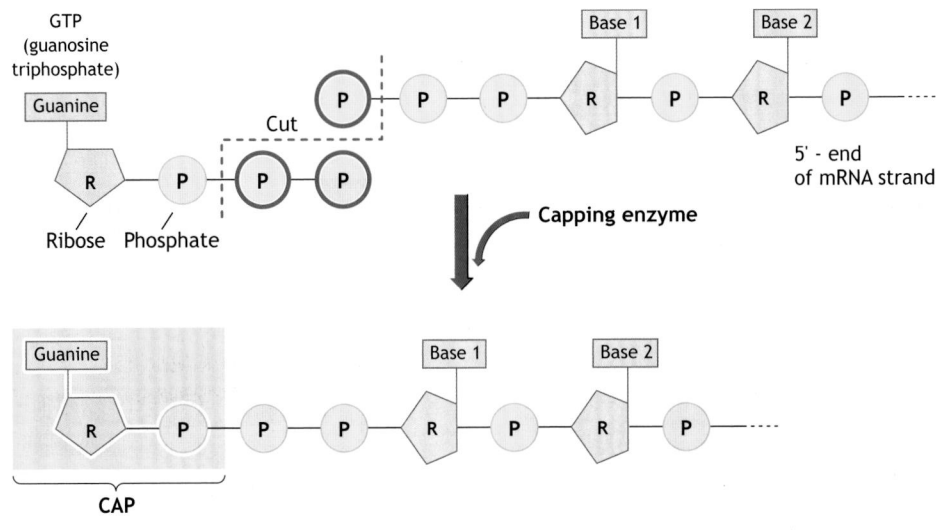

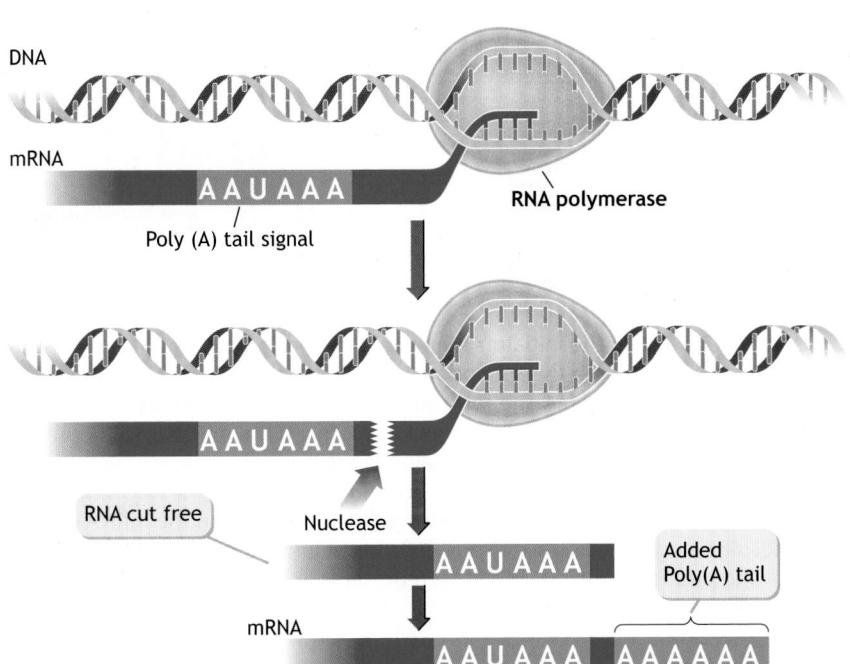

FIGURE 33.22 • Caps and tails. **(A)** Addition of a guanosine triphosphate (GTP) cap to mRNA. The red dashes indicate where the "cut" occurs by the action of the capping enzyme. **(B)** Addition of a poly(A) tail to mRNA. The mRNA molecule exits the nucleus once capping and tailing occurs, carrying the "coded message" for the upcoming translation phase in protein synthesis.

Ribosomes and Polypeptide Synthesis: Initiation of Protein Construction

The cell's ribosomes provide the catalysts for initiating protein synthesis and serve as submicroscopic factories to produce polypeptides. **FIGURE 33.23** illustrates a four-step sequence of a ribosome binding to one end of an mRNA molecule (Step 1) and the subsequent three-nucleotide increments down the mRNA molecule. Decoding of genetic information occurs when the ribosomes bound to mRNA translate a genetic code sequence. The tRNA then interacts with a specific amino acid, adding one at a time to the end of the progressively elongating **polypeptide chain**. Sequential linking of amino acids by **peptide bonding** ultimately forms the specific protein with its unique genetically determined information to achieve its specific function(s).

Polypeptide chain: repeated polypeptide units

Peptide bonding: chemical linking that binds amino acids in a protein; formed when the carboxyl group of one amino acid reacts with a second amino acid's amino group

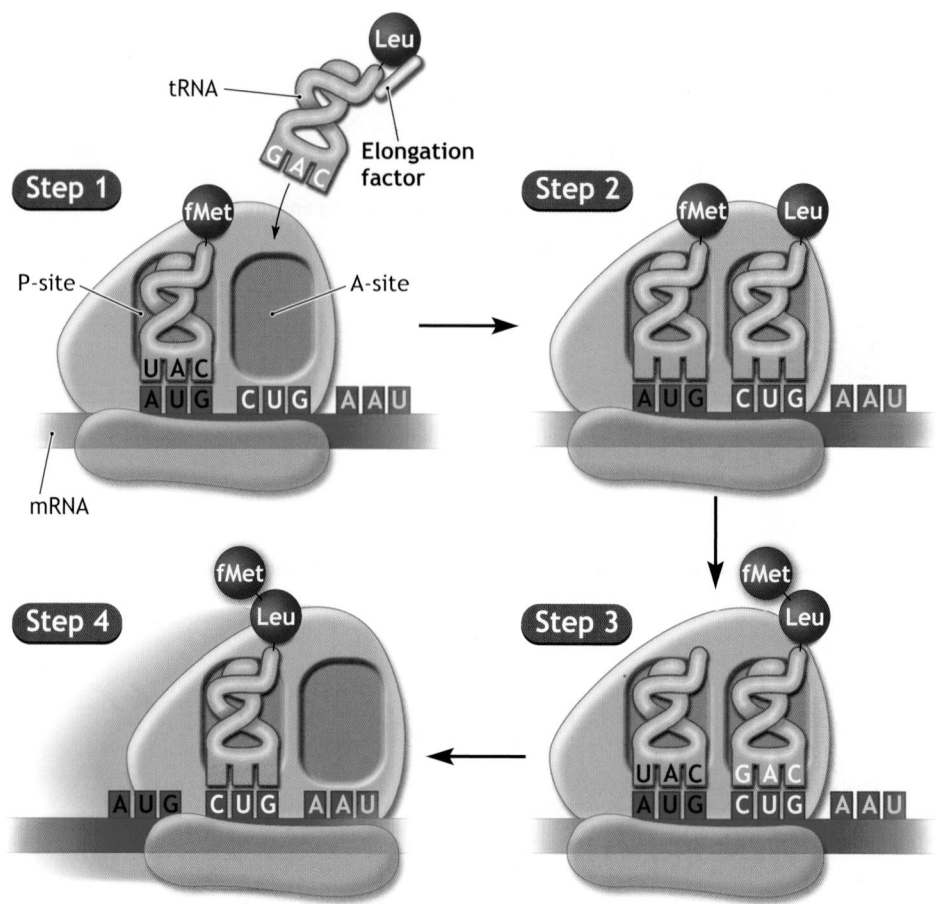

FIGURE 33.23 • Ribosomes, the initiators for protein synthesis. Polypeptide synthesis proceeds from the top in Step 1 with the anticodon of tRNA complementary to the mRNA codon. The tRNA occupies the ribosome's A-site, with an anticodon complementary to the mRNA's codon at the opposite A-site. The ribosome translocates down the mRNA one codon at a time. In Step 2 the lengthening polypeptide chain fMet (f, formyl-methionyl; Met, amino acid methionine) is transferred to Leu (leucine), the incoming amino acid. The ribosome ejects the original tRNA (Step 3) with its amino acid, exposing the next codon on the mRNA chain. When the tRNA molecule recognizes the next exposed codon, it binds to that codon, thus lengthening the growing peptide chain (Step 4). fMet represents an addition to the lengthening polypeptide chain already occupied by Leu.

Role of tRNA

The computer-generated tRNA molecule shown at the top left in **FIGURE 33.24** has a three-dimensional structure resembling a cloverleaf, with an amino acid at one end and three nitrogenous bases that match the mRNA's codon, called an **anticodon**, at the other end. The tRNA with matching codon serves as a relay or go-between in protein synthesis. In effect, the tRNA acts as a "personal shuttle" to deliver a specific free-floating amino acid to the ribosome's A-site. For example, the triplet U-A-C represents the codon for the amino acid methionine. When the tRNA with the matching U-A-C anticodon (it carries no other amino acid) interacts with the free-floating U-A-C amino acid, it binds to it by action of the activating enzyme **aminoacyl-tRNA synthetase**. Each amino acid's specific activating enzyme serves two purposes:

1. It deciphers and then binds (couples) to a specific amino acid.
2. It identifies the anticodon on the tRNA molecule.

Some activating enzymes decipher the sequence of one anticodon and thus only one tRNA, while others recognize multiple tRNA molecules. Thus, the activating enzyme "reads" the genetic code on both the particular amino acid, such as the essential amino acid tryptophan

Anticodon: three complementary bases at the end of a tRNA molecule that recognize and bind to an mRNA codon

Aminoacyl-tRNA synthetase: activating enzyme that covalently links amino acids to the 39 ends of their cognate tRNA

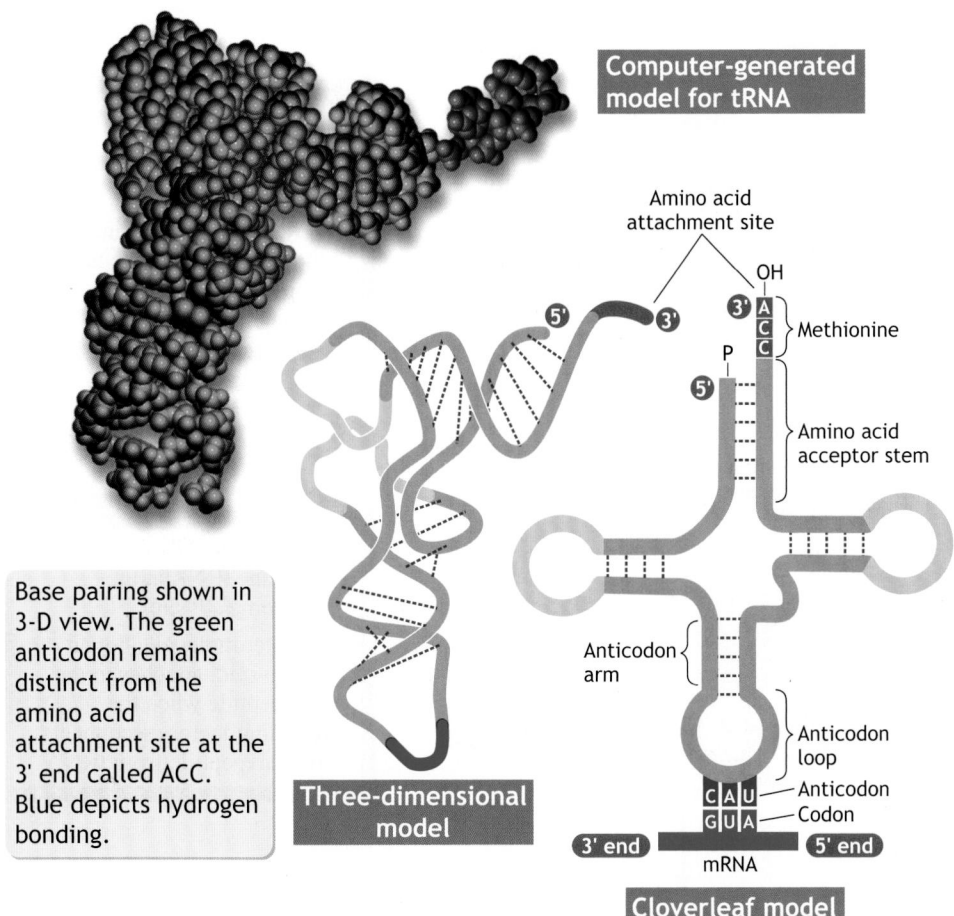

FIGURE 33.24 • Three views of tRNA: computer-generated model, three-dimensional model, and cloverleaf model. Note that the anticodon displayed in the cloverleaf model (complementary three-nucleotide sequence) matches up with the mRNA codon using complementary (antiparallel) binding between the anticodon (*blue*) and codon (*green*).

and its tRNA tryptophan anticodon sequence A-C-C. Figure 33.24 shows three views of tRNA:

1. Computer-generated model
2. Three-dimensional representation that highlights internal base pairing with hydrogen bonding
3. Two-dimensional cloverleaf model with the tRNA anticodon shown in *blue*

This example represents the complementary three-nucleotide sequence C-A-U matching mRNA's codon G-U-A.

Polypeptide Elongation and Termination

The polypeptide chain increases in length when an amino acid from tRNA **translocates** to it. The A-U-G codon shown in Figure 33.23 within the mRNA message initiates the "start" signal for peptide elongation. The same A-U-G sequence that encodes tryptophan also encodes methionine. The first A-U-G message "sensed" in the mRNA molecule initiates translation. The ribosome translocates down the mRNA a distance of three nucleotide blocks (one codon) at a time. After each third nucleotide, the ribosome ejects the original tRNA with its amino acid, exposing the next codon on the mRNA chain. When the tRNA molecule recognizes the next exposed codon, it binds to it, thus lengthening the growing peptide chain. The elongation procedure for building the polypeptide continues repeatedly until a stop codon terminates the process.

Translocation: describes movement along the ribosome by an mRNA molecule a distance of three nucleotide blocks (one codon) at a time

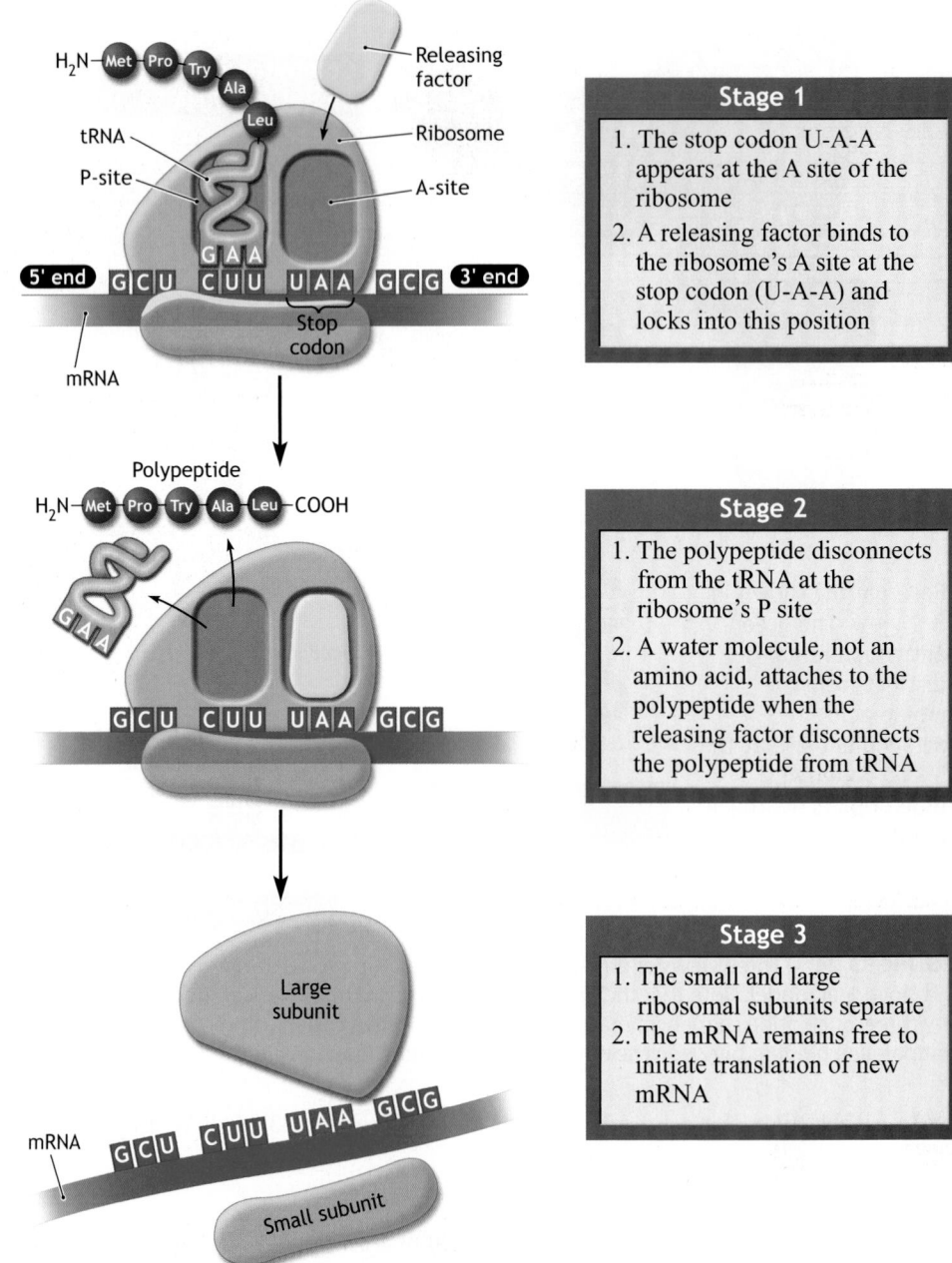

FIGURE 33.25 • Three stages in polypeptide termination.

In the three stages in polypeptide termination, the three "stop" codons or base sequences include U-A-A, U-A-G, and U-G-A (FIGURE 33.25). These codons "turn off" the signal in the mRNA message, preventing addition of another amino acid sequence to the chain. Stage 1 shows the stop codon U-A-A on the mRNA strand within the A-site of the ribosome, where one of three kinds of releasing factors—eRF1, eRF2, or eRF3—locks into position to split apart the linking covalent bond. In stage 2, the polypeptide chain releases from tRNA at the ribosome's P-site, to effectively end protein synthesis. Once the polypeptide and tRNA uncouple from the termination complex, the small and large ribosomal units recycle along with mRNA in stage 3 for further mRNA translation.

Protein Delivery System: The Golgi Complex

Once the ribosome produces its polypeptide, newly formed strands can exit a cell through its outer membrane into the external interstitial fluid environment. The highly membranous

Golgi complex structures within the cell provide the transfer mechanism for moving materials from the cell to its external environment. Italian physiologist and microscopist Camillo Golgi 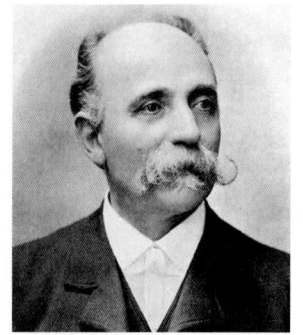 (1843–1926), who shared the 1906 Nobel Prize in Physiology or Medicine with Spanish researcher Santiago Ramon y Cajal (1852–1934) for their work on the structure of nervous system anatomy (http://nobelprize.org/nobel_prizes/medicine/articles/golgi/). These scientists first called attention in 1898 to these minute intracellular structures using the light microscope (www.nature.com/milestones/milelight/timeline.html). Many biologists of his time doubted the existence of such structures; 60 years later, the electron microscope confirmed their existence in exquisite detail.

The Golgi complex receives a polypeptide from the cell's **endoplasmic reticulum**. FIGURE 33.26 shows polypeptide transport into the Golgi complex, where this molecule shown as blue dots may become a **glycoprotein** (technically, a protein having a carbohydrate as the nonprotein component). When a polysaccharide binds to a lipid, it forms a **glycolipid**. Glycoproteins or glycolipids then collect within the flattened, membranous sacs called the *cisternae region of the Golgi complex*, where specialized enzymes modify the protein component. The transport vesicles that hold proteins that pass from the endoplasmic reticulum pinch off and break away from the roughened endoplasmic surfaces. The tiny vesicles attached to the cell's outer membrane expel their contents to the extracellular spaces via secretory vesicles. In essence, but not always, the Golgi complex takes up the polypeptide on one of its surfaces and then modifies and repackages it into molecules that leave the Golgi complex via a transport vesicle at its other membrane.

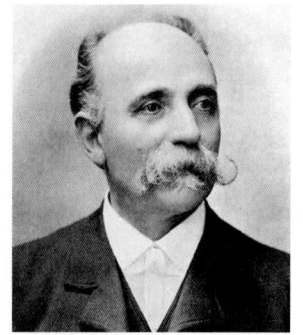
Camillo Golgi

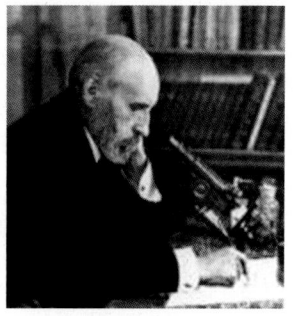
Santiago Ramon y Cajal

Golgi complex: stack of membrane-bound vesicles between the endoplasmic reticulum and plasma membrane; involved in posttranslational modification of proteins, and sorting and delivering them to different intracellular compartments

Endoplasmic reticulum: tubules, vesicles, and flattened sac structures of the cell's endomembrane system; ribosomes cover its outer rough, granular surface

Glycoprotein: protein complexed with a polysaccharide

Glycolipid: polysaccharide bound to a lipid

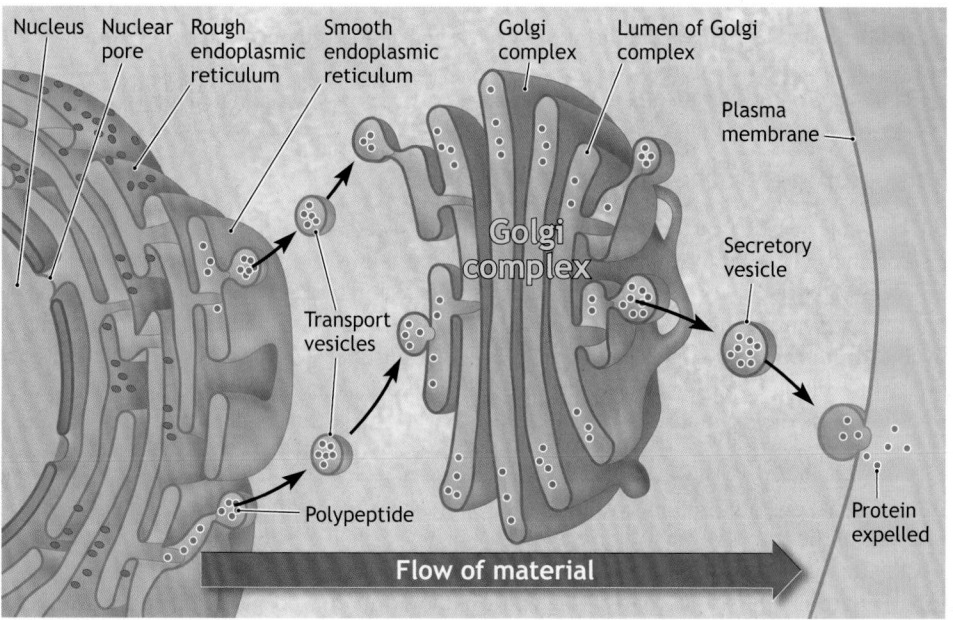

FIGURE 33.26 • Polypeptide transport into the Golgi complex. The Golgi complex accepts polypeptides on one of its surfaces after the ribosomes release them, repackaging them as glycoproteins, and expels them contained in secretory vesicles for final expulsion through the plasma membrane or delivery to another cell area. The Golgi structures modify proteins within their lumen for use within cells or outside of cells once they pass through the plasma membrane.

TABLE 33.1   **Eight Categories of Proteins and Their Biologic Functions**

Protein Category	Function	Example
1. Contractile	Form muscles	Actin, myosin
2. Enzyme	Catalyze biological processes	Protease
3. Hormone	Regulate body functions	Cortisol
4. Protective	Fight infection	Antibodies
5. Storage	Store nutrients	Calcium within bone
6. Structural	Form structures	Endoplasmic reticulum
7. Transport	Deliver substances among cells, tissues, and organs	Hemoglobin
8. Toxic	Defense mechanism	Snake venom (disintegrins)

Termination of Protein Synthesis

The end-point of protein synthesis creates one of thousands of completed or functional proteins, each with a specific function and mode of action depending in part on its structure. Table 33.1 shows eight categories of proteins and their biologic functions.

It usually takes between 20 s and 2 min to synthesize most proteins, depending on the protein's complexity. The Hb molecule and its amino acid sequence serves as an excellent example of the four levels of protein structure highlighted in black (Fig. 33.27). This generalized example begins with the linear sequence of amino acids from the amino acid at the amino-terminal end through to the carboxyl-terminal residue. The polypeptide strand formed when peptide linkages join amino acid monomers represents protein's **primary structure**. In a **secondary structure**, the protein can twist into a three-dimensional form known as an α **helix**. It can also fold back onto itself to give a flat look (β-pleated sheets), with regular repeating interactions using hydrogen bonding among closely linked residues in the primary sequence. Interactions among residues farther apart in the primary structure determine a **tertiary structure**, such as disulfide bond formation between two cysteine residues. In this conformation, the protein literally folds up on itself, much like a roll of pretzel dough twisting into a pretzel. The topology of the α helices and β-pleated sheets play important roles in determining the final shape assumed by a protein.[34] The complex Hb molecule consists of two α subunits and two β subunits (tetramer). The term *quaternary structure* refers to protein's subunit structure; Hb contains multiple subunits.

Hemoglobin and the Evolutionary Tree

The Hb molecule illustrated in Figure 33.27 contains two α and two β chains; the heme group is associated with each chain. The central iron atom (shown in *red*) binds with one oxygen molecule and acts as a magnet to attract and hold it. Interestingly, our closest genetic relative, the chimpanzee, has an identical α chain. The Hb amino acid sequence in cows and pigs diverges from that of humans by about 12%, while for chickens the divergence increases to 25%. Molecular biologists have constructed an evolutionary tree for many proteins (e.g., the iron-containing mitochondrial cytochromes) as a way of tracking evolution.

Primary structure: specific linear sequence of amino acids determined by the nucleotide sequence of the gene that encodes the protein

Secondary structure: coiled protein similar to the pairing of strands in DNA or folded back onto itself to give a flat look; formed from regular repeating interactions among closely linked residues in the primary sequence using hydrogen bonding

Helix: one possible secondary structure of polypeptides; right-handed peptide chain maintained by hydrogen (H) bonds between carbon (C) and oxygen (O) atoms of every fifth amino acid along the chain. The degree of rotation remains regular for bonds on either side of the carbon (with nitrogen, C, H, and amino side chain attached to it) along the polypeptide chain

Tertiary structure: final three-dimensional folding of a polymer chain; interactions between residues remain farther apart

Quaternary structure: highly complex, three-dimensional structure or functional protein formed by joining two or more polypeptides

FIGURE 33.27 • Four protein structures (primary, secondary, tertiary, quaternary) in the synthesis of the complex hemoglobin molecule first deciphered by British molecular biologist Max Perutz (1914–2002; shared 1962 Nobel Prize for Chemistry; www.nobelprize.org/nobel_prizes/chemistry/laureates/1962/perutz-bio.html) in 1960 and published in *Nature* (1960;185:416). The purified molecule's precise arrangement was calculated from the way its crystals diffracted a beam of x-rays. Hemoglobin's tertiary structure contains eight helical regions; the quaternary structure contains four polypeptide chains (two and two). Knowledge of the configuration of new protein structures has increased exponentially since Perutz first worked out the details of hemoglobin's structure; as of July 9, 2001, the Protein Data Bank (www.rcsb.org/pdb/) contained 15,531 unique structures into which proteins can fold. Of these, x-ray diffraction identified 12,817 unique structures and Alpha polypeptide NMR identified 2384 chains.

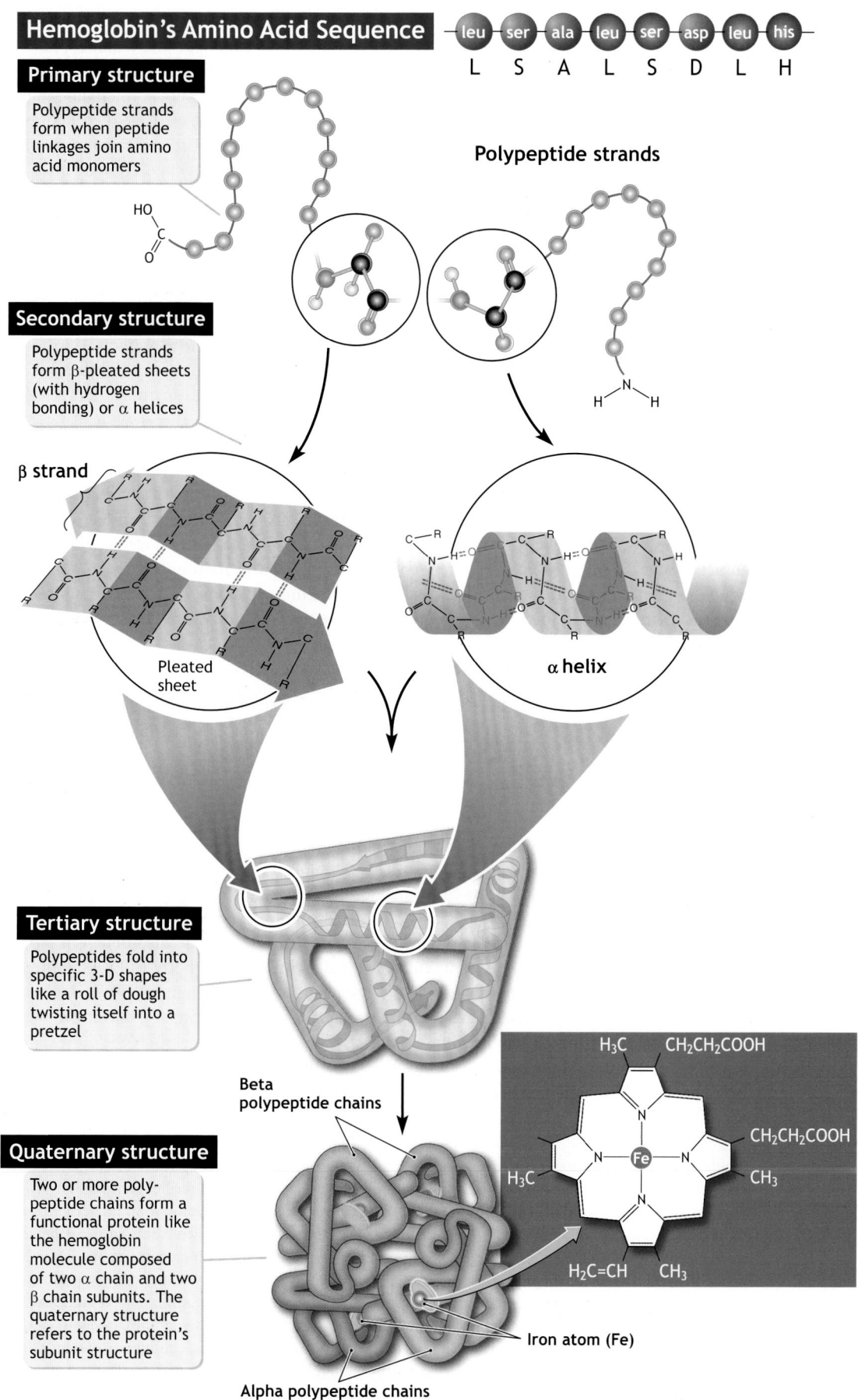

Hemoglobin's Amino Acid Sequence

leu – ser – ala – leu – ser – asp – leu – his

L S A L S D L H

Primary structure

Polypeptide strands form when peptide linkages join amino acid monomers

HO
C
O

Polypeptide strands

H – N – H

Secondary structure

Polypeptide strands form β-pleated sheets (with hydrogen bonding) or α helices

β strand

Pleated sheet

α helix

Tertiary structure

Polypeptides fold into specific 3-D shapes like a roll of dough twisting itself into a pretzel

Beta polypeptide chains

H_3C CH_2CH_2COOH

CH_2CH_2COOH

H_3C Fe CH_3

$H_2C=CH$ CH_3

Quaternary structure

Two or more polypeptide chains form a functional protein like the hemoglobin molecule composed of two α chain and two β chain subunits. The quaternary structure refers to the protein's subunit structure

Iron atom (Fe)

Alpha polypeptide chains

Some proteins change relatively slowly, taking hundreds of millions of years to evolve. Histones change at a rate of 0.25 mutations per 100 amino acids per 100 million years. In contrast, other proteins such as neurotoxins and immunoglobulins mutate more rapidly (rates of 110 to 140 mutations per 100 million years). Variation in the resistance to change makes "sense" because crucial cellular functions like energy generation in the citric acid cycle or correct folding of DNA requires that gene sequences remain almost invariant. Proteins sensitive to relatively large variations in their operational properties sustain faster evolutionary changes.

Proteolysis: The Ultimate Fate of Proteins

Proteolysis: protein degradation

Protein synthesis from amino acids and degradation into amino acid constituents progresses unabated throughout life. The rates of protein synthesis and degradation, a process called **proteolysis**, regulate the organism's total protein content at any given time independent of the proteins' structural configurations (bone or muscle) or functions (metabolic and intracellular enzymes). For example, the structural proteins[a] in bone may not decay significantly for months or years, while enzyme proteins in intermediary metabolism or those that regulate cell growth may survive for only minutes or fractions of a second. The enzymes that control proteolysis, called *proteases*, hydrolyze the amino acids' peptide bonds, splitting them into the constituent molecules. **Figure 33.28** illustrates how a relatively large rounded trash can–shaped **proteasome** formed from protease enzymes degrades the unwanted proteins in the cell's cytoplasm. These cylindrical structures capture proteins destined for destruction by recognizing a small marker or tag protein (**ubiquitin**) that attaches by covalent bonding to an active site on the protein. Once tagged, the ubiquinated protein enters the proteasome, which degrades it to small peptide units before expelling it along with the ubiquitin tag. Proteasomes degrade many types of proteins, from denatured or misfolded ones to misformed or oxidized amino acids.

Proteasome: proteolytic enzyme that degrades unwanted proteins in the cytoplasm of eukaryotic cells

Ubiquitin: small protein that attaches by covalent bonding to a protein "marked" for destruction by proteosomes

Summary of Main Sequence of Events in Protein Synthesis

Table 33.2 charts the sequence of key events in the flow of genetic information in living cells from DNA → RNA → protein.

MUTATIONS

Mutation: gene with permanently altered or defective genetic information that causes heritable changes

The slightest aberration in the sequence of the 3 billion letters of the genome can produce catastrophic and irreversible effects on health and well-being. Fortunately, an exquisite array of internal repair mechanisms or specialized protein complexes correct mismatches along the double helix, thus avoiding a phalanx of dreadful, life-altering genetic disorders. On a daily basis, factors in the external environment continually threaten the body's DNA from cosmic and ultraviolet radiation bombardment, to radioactive decay and gamma waves, including dangerously reactive free radical species, discussed later in this chapter. A **mutation** results from a minor alteration or "misspelling" in the DNA sequence that cripples the corresponding RNA or protein. Many human diseases generally form from protein abnormalities caused by a change in the sequence of only one of the 3×10^9 or more DNA nucleotide pairs in the

---

[a]Collagen, the most plentiful structural protein, accounts for about one-fourth of the body's protein. In essence, it forms molecular cables that strengthen the tendons and plentiful, resilient sheets that support the skin and internal organs. This simple protein, composed of three chains wound together in a tight triple helix, contains more than 1400 amino acids in each chain. Collagen forms from a repeated sequence of three amino acids; every third amino acid is glycine, a small amino acid that fits perfectly inside the helix. Many of the remaining positions in the chain are filled by two amino acids, proline and hydroxyproline, the latter a modified version of proline. Hydroxyproline formation involves modifying normal proline amino acids after building the collagen. The reaction requires vitamin C to assist in the addition of oxygen. Unfortunately, vitamin C deficiency slows hydroxyproline production and stops new collagen construction, ultimately causing scurvy. When heated, collagen's triple helix unwinds and the chains separate. When the denatured mass of tangled chains cools down, it soaks up the surrounding water like a sponge to form gelatin commonly used in cooking.

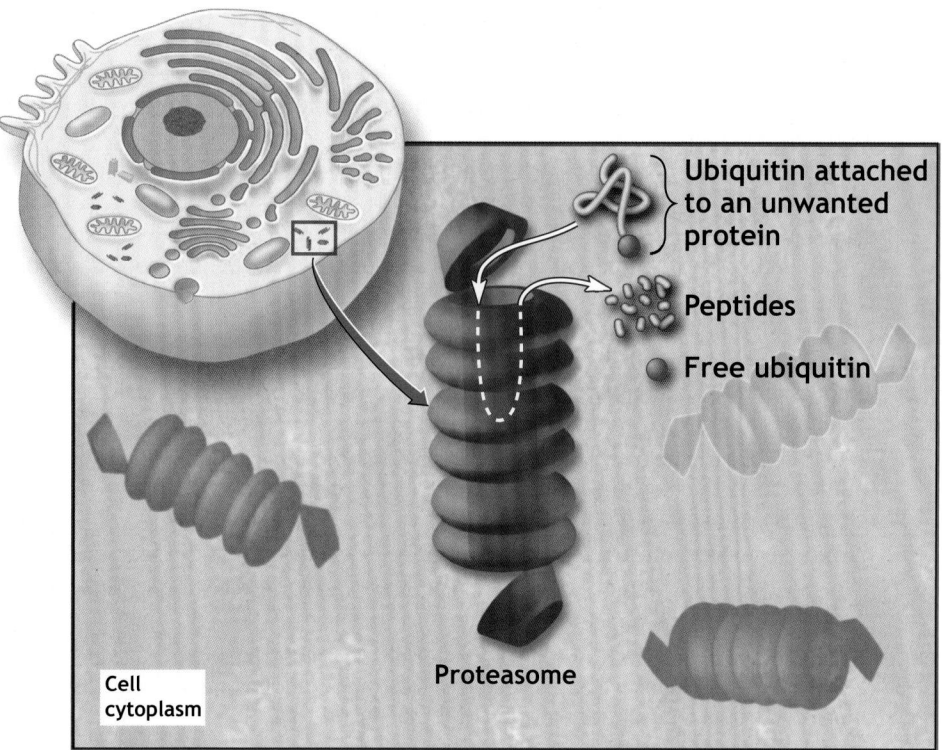

FIGURE 33.28 • Proteasomes in the cell cytoplasm maintain a balance between protein synthesis and protein degradation. The free ubiquitin tag (*displayed in red*) attaches to an active site on the designated protein, identifying it for degradation to its peptide components within the proteasome's cylindrical structure. Once ejected, the ubiquitin recycles to another unwanted protein.

human genome. Not all of the coding sequences in amino acids make "sense." The term *junk DNA* (also called *noncoding DNA*) used to describe such DNA sequences. So-called junk DNA replicates inside a cell the same way any other DNA molecules replicate but without gene expression.

 Inherited Blood Disorder Can Be Deadly

Sickle cell anemia, a form of sickle cell disease (**http://www.nhlbi.nih.gov/health/health-topics/topics/sca/**), provides a salient example when an abnormality occurs in the hemoglobin molecule illustrated in the second row of the table below:

Normal hemoglobin β-chain amino acids						
Valine	Histidine	Leucine	Threonine	Proline	Glutamic acid	Glutamic acid
Sickle cell anemia hemoglobin β-chain amino acids				↓		
Valine	Histidine	Leucine	Threonine	Proline	Valine	Glutamic acid

In the sickle cell condition, the amino acid valine shown in red substitutes for glutamic acid and alters hemoglobin's β chain because of a codon change from G-A-A to G-U-A.

Sickle cell anemia: usually fatal hereditary disease affecting hemoglobin; develops when the amino acid valine substitutes for glutamic acid because of a change in its codon nucleotide sequence from G-A-A to G-U-A; the disease afflicts two of every 1000 African Americans; the erythrocyte becomes irregular, thin, elongated, and crescent-shaped, severely affecting oxygen-transport capacity

Scientists used to believe that these inherited sequences perform no currently known "genetically useful" purpose,[12,156] yet recent data show just the opposite (www.medicalnewstoday.com/articles/250006.php).

TABLE 33.2	**Essential Concepts and Sequence of Events in Protein Synthesis**
1.	A nucleotide sequence from DNA provides the genetic information required to begin transcription into RNA.
2.	The enzyme RNA polymerase binds to the specific promoter region of a gene; nucleotide sequences in the DNA indicate where to begin and end transcription.
3.	RNA polymerase manufactures messenger RNA (mRNA) molecules to mirror the base sequence of DNA; transcription copies a sequence of the genetic code direction from DNA to an mRNA strand; this includes both coding and noncoding segments of genetic information.
4.	The RNA transcript contains the information it needs to create a protein; RNA splicing removes random, intervening sequences of unwanted "junk" nucleotides (introns) from mRNA.
5.	The mRNA strand (linked entrons) carrying a duplicate copy of the genetic code shuttles the "coded message" (sequence of codons), exiting the nucleus and entering the cytoplasm to begin protein synthesis.
6.	Translation initiates protein construction; the A-U-G codon acts as the "start" signal.
7.	In the cytoplasm, the mRNA molecule searches to bind with a ribosome (ribonucleoprotein, a "protein-manufacturing machine").
8.	The anticodon of transfer RNA (tRNA) positions itself to match up with a three-nucleotide sequence of codons, each codon corresponding to one amino acid; the codon contains a copy or transcription of the DNA code.
9.	With the four RNA nucleotides, 64 different codons in the genetic code exist, with each amino acid having at least one (and usually more than one) codon.
10.	Binding takes place at the ribosome's attachment site between the tRNA molecule (carrying the same genetic sequence on its anticodon) and the complementary base sequence of the mRNA codon (e.g., G-A-C with C-U-G).
11.	The ribosome, coupled to one end of the mRNA molecule, shifts (translocates) over one codon (three nucleotide blocks) to the polypeptide site, allowing exposure of a new codon; a new incoming tRNA (with its amino acid) links to the ribosome's attachment site; the amino acid at the ribosome's polypeptide region releases and binds to a new amino acid on tRNA at the ribosome's attachment site; thus, the tRNA with one amino acid now gains another amino acid, then another one, and so on; successive addition of new amino acids elongates the peptide chain.
12.	Protein synthesis terminates when a chain-terminating nonsense "stop" codon (UAA, UAG, UGA) turns off the signal for adding more amino acids to the peptide chain.
13.	A complete (fully assembled) protein exists in one of four geometric configurations (primary, secondary, tertiary, quaternary), shown in Figure 33.26.

Junk DNA: DNA sequences that perform no currently known useful purpose but still remain part of chromosomes

Junk DNA Not "Junk." Over 30 papers published in prestigious journals in 2012 rejected the notion that most DNA was "junk," simply being accumulated over time during routine evolutionary development.[81,104,119] Project ENCODE (Encyclopedia of DNA Elements; www.genome.gov/10005107; www.genome.gov/27549810; www.nature.com/encode/#/threads) developed based on the accumulated work of diverse groups of researchers across the United States, United Kingdom, Spain, Singapore, and Japan. The database relied on more than 1600 sets of experiments on 147 types of tissue with technologies standardized across the consortium. O ENCODE found that 80% of the human genome serves a purpose and is biochemically active. The scale of the international effort has been remarkable. The experiments relied on innovative uses of next-generation DNA sequencing technologies, due mainly to advances enabled by NHGRI's DNA sequencing technology development program

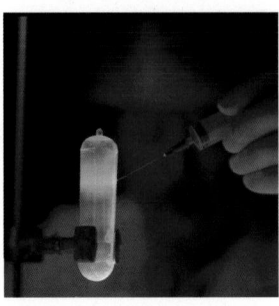

Purified DNA (Image courtesy www.genome.gov)

(www.capconcorp.com/meeting/2012/STM/purpose.asp). A multiyear concerted effort by over 40 researchers in 32 laboratories worldwide produced the first holistic view of how the human genome actually functions. ENCODE researchers use many of the latest techniques to assess DNA and its variations among different population groups. The inset photo shows purified DNA, fluorescing orange under UV light. In total, ENCODE generated more than 15 trillion bytes of raw data, consuming the equivalent of more than 300 years of computer time to analyze.

Varieties of Mutations

The guiding principle of the central dogma discussed earlier implicitly states that any change in the inherited genetic material produces a ripple effect on replication, transcription, and translation. This ultimately means that a mutation in the original daughter chromosomes passes on sets of characteristics to the next generation so the offspring inherits the mutation. One can accomplish little short of a temporary, stop-gap measure using **genetic engineering** to replace the defective sequences or arrest their development a distance far removed from the gene. For example, small deletions hundreds of thousands of bases away from a particular gene (*PAX6*) can alter the gene's expression and cause a mutation in which a typical characteristic (e.g., iris in the eye) fails to develop, producing a developmental syndrome called aniridia (**www.aniridia.org**). Poorly understood processes can *silence* genes up to 90 million bases down the chromosome. Once transcription uses the DNA template to make an RNA copy of the inherited mutated sequences, the altered RNA translates the defective code during protein synthesis. All of the body's vital processes depend on proteins for their intended functions; unfortunately, mutated genes pose a serious health hazard.

The doggerel in Table 33.3 provides eight examples of different types of mutations and what can happen to disrupt the orderly sequence in the genetic code.

A graphic example points out the probability for "errors" to creep into a DNA sequence. If the total DNA compacted in the body's 10 trillion cells was laid end to end like a long link of sausages, it would stretch from Earth to the sun 667 times—not a trivial length 93 million miles one-way to the sun! Consequently, a single genetic code mismatch can wreak havoc on the "normal" sequence of DNA nucleotides and hence genes. A defect in code sequence often remains quiescent for nearly a lifetime before it emerges. For example, it may take 60 years before a seemingly minor misalignment in a receptor gene devastates heart function, causing congestive heart failure within a few months. When researchers can identify this human gene variant years before its expression, as discussed below, newly developed, highly specific drugs hopefully will eradicate the defect. Within the next decade, new classes of drugs will target specific mutated cells instead of the current "shotgun" approach that attempts to cripple just about all cells with a massive pharmacologic overdose.

Genetic engineering: laboratory-altered DNA that changes its characteristics, usually in four stages that involve: (1) cleaving the source DNA, (2) creating recombinants, (3) cloning copies of recombinants, and (4) locating cloned copies for the desired gene; screening makes the desired clones resistant to antibiotics and gives them different properties for easy identification

TABLE 33.3 Types and Examples of Genetic Mutations

Mutation Type	Example of Disruption in the Coding Sequence
Wild type	The cat sat on the mat
Substitution	The rat sat on the mat
Insertion (single)	The cat spat on the mat
Insertion (multiple)	The cattle sat on the mat
Deletion (single)	The c-t sat on the mat
Deletion (multiple)	The cat——the mat
Inversion (small)	The tac sat on the mat
Inversion (large)	Tam echt no tas tac echt

 **The Fight Against Chromosome 21 Mutations**

Mutations along a stretch of genes on chromosome 21 give rise to Alzheimer's disease, amyotrophic lateral sclerosis (**www.alsa.org**), epilepsy, deafness, autoimmune disease, birth defects, and manic depression. For Down syndrome (named after English physician John Langdon Down [1828–1896] who observed individuals in a British asylum in 1866 and published *Observations on an Ethnic Classification of Idiots*; **www.ndss.org**), researchers have been on a quest to develop animal models of this genetic form of mental insufficiency and other genetic abnormalities in hopes of developing genetically engineered strategies to eradicate them. Gene testing may also prove useful for patients who often respond differently to warfarin (Coumadin; **www.drugs.com/coumadin.html**), a widely prescribed anti–blood-clotting drug because of newly identified genetic variations.[74,80]

Misjudgments in drug doses can critically affect the clotting mechanism to potentially cause fatal bleeding. One gene, known as vitamin K epoxide reductase gene (*VKORC1*), makes the enzyme that destroys warfarin in the body. DNA variations responsible for changing the gene's activity and the amount of protein it makes account for 25% of the overall variation in warfarin dosage; patients with a particular variation of the gene usually took similar doses of warfarin.

Single Nucleotide Polymorphisms

Single-nucleotide polymorphism (SNP): polymorphism due to variation at a single nucleotide

Pharmaceutical and computer chip manufacturers have partnered to develop techniques to identify specific molecular markers called **single nucleotide polymorphisms**, or **SNPs** (pronounced *snips*), thousands of which reside within each person's genetic code (**www.ncbi.nlm.nih.gov/snp**). Most of these tiny nucleotide genetic code "snippets" normally configure with no deviant code. Some, however, have a single "mismatch" in the nucleotide sequence that predisposes an individual to a particular disease or injury (e.g., knee ligament tear in football or gymnastics), which may be identified in the future with genetic probing to identify the risk[26]) or renders the immune system resistant to drug treatment.

Identifying a specific gene variant will allow appropriate lifestyle changes in nutrition, weight loss, exercise training, or introduction of a particular class of drugs to prevent emergence of the disease or disability, or delay its onset. Thirteen major multinational companies have formed a nonprofit alliance (**www.hapmap.org**) to identify 300,000 variants on human chromosomes and develop drugs that target diseases by their genetic profile. A new Entrez database, dbSNP (**www.ncbi.nlm.nih.gov/sites/entrez?db=snp**), similar in operation to the Entrez nucleotide database collection (**www.ncbi.nlm.nih.gov/sites/entrez?db=nucleotide**) that includes GenBank (**www.ncbi.nlm.nih.gov/Genbank/**) and BLAST (**http://blast.ncbi.nlm.nih.gov/Blast.cgi**), also has been created. These NCBI genome resource guides include detailed information about mammals, birds, amphibians, echinoderms, fish, insects, worms, plants, fungi, and protozoa.

SNP assessment (**Fig. 33.29**) uses microarrays of biochips or a "library" of artificial DNA to compare the individual's DNA sample with the chips' existing gene sequences. SNP identification (explained in the yellow text boxes) has current application in the identification and differentiation of different ancestral lines.[124]

A microarray DNA chip represents a spatial array of oligonucleotide probes arranged on a tiny supporting surface. The probe, representing sequences of nucleotides in known genes, is synthesized on the support surface, allowing the researcher to know each probe's position and sequence. With this information, the DNA chip can identify organisms and select genes by hybridization of the source DNA to the chips' oligonucleotide probes. One of the hallmarks of this process is to achieve 100% accuracy because even a small error or incorrect identification could prove disastrous from a worldwide health standpoint.[30] For example, 99.9% accuracy in matching the 300,000 biochip SNPs for only 1000 people would create 300,000 errors!

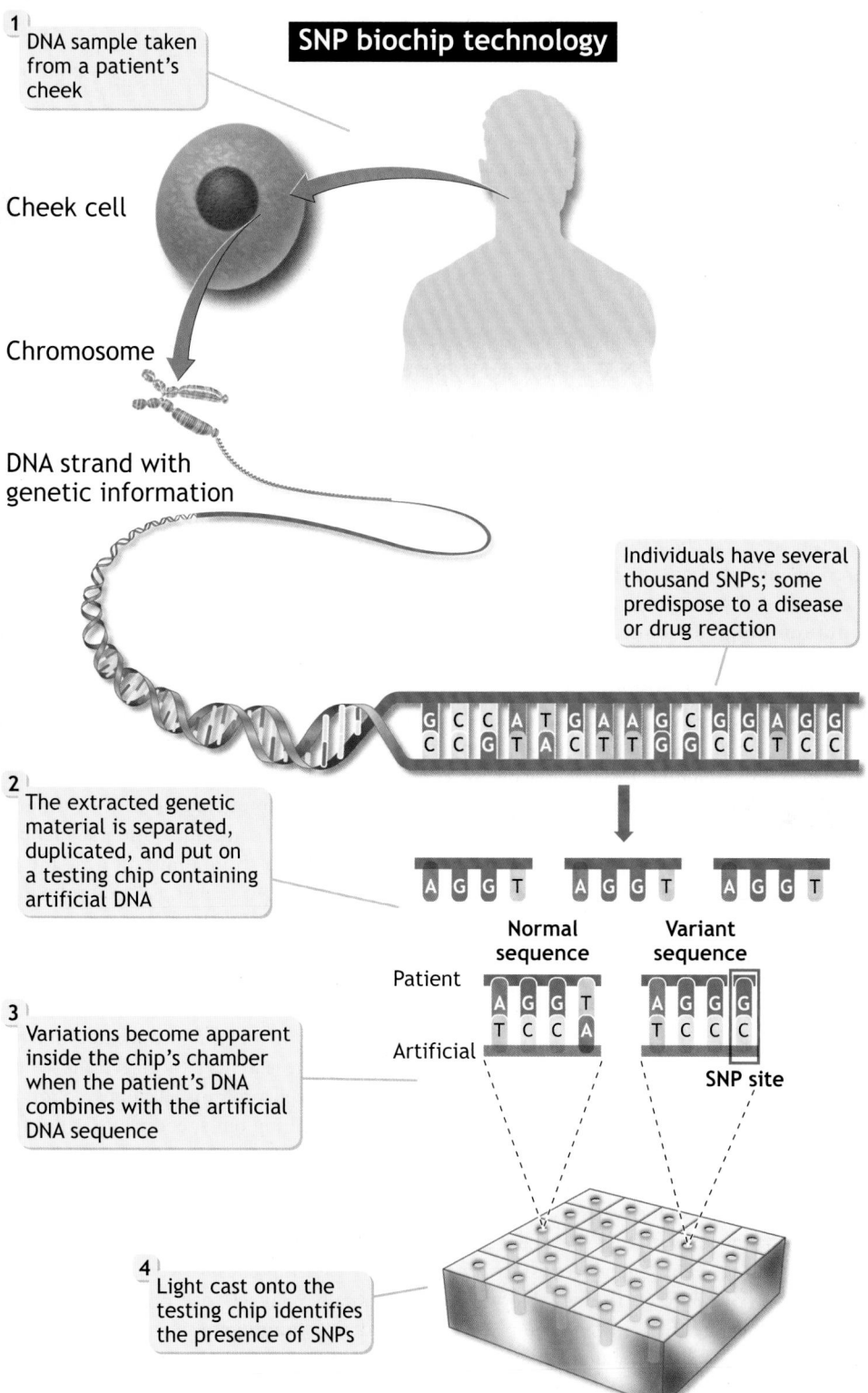

FIGURE 33.29 • Four main stages in SNP biochip technology that looks at many genes at once to determine which are expressed in a particular cell type. Thousands of individual genes can be spotted on a single square-inch slide. Note the relative size of the SNP biochip, made possible by barcode-scanning the microarrays on the biochip. Rapidly identifying the microarrays allows them to link to genes, probe samples, reagents, and experimental protocols. Consult **www.lab-on-a-chip.com** for research links about microarray technology, and Agilent Technologies for new products and specifications (**www.agilent.com**).

Photolithography: optimal technology for etching (transferring) electrical circuits on suitable media (silicon wafer with silicon dioxide)

Mutagen: ionizing radiation, ultraviolet radiation, or a chemical agent that disrupts the genetic machinery (sequence of DNA code) and causes mutations

Teratogen: agent that causes extreme mutations

Carcinogen: any agent that causes cancer; for example, smoke from cigarettes contains known carcinogenic agents (e.g., carbon monoxide, formaldehyde, and the metals aluminum, copper, lead, mercury, and zinc)

Benign tumor: tumor that remains in one location; it no longer responds to normal growth control and lacks the capacity to invade distant sites

Malignant tumor: tumor that invades other tissues and forms secondary or tertiary cancers

Sarcoma: cancers forming from connective, muscle, or bone tissue

Carcinoma: cancers formed from epithelial tissue

Metastasize: spread of cancerous cells from the original tumor mass to form secondary cancers (metastases) elsewhere in the body

Oncogene: mutant gene that promotes the loss of cellular growth control, transforming a cell to a malignant state; many oncogenes directly or indirectly control a cell's growth rate

Vasculogenesis: *in vivo* formation of blood vessels by differentiation of vascular precursor cells; in implanted bioartificial organs, molecular biology techniques can stimulate the growth of new blood vessels or treat peripheral vascular diseases, wounds, and ulcers from compromised microvasculature

Angiogenesis: new blood vessel formation, usually during embryo development but can also occur abnormally around malignant tumors

The technique of **photolithography** involves a combination of etching, chemical deposition, and chemical treatments in repeated steps on an initially flat substrate or wafer (**www.youtube.com/watch?v=9x3Lh1ZfggM**). Etching microcircuits on a silicon chip could also encode a single biochip containing the entire human genome. Figure 33.29 illustrates the four main stages to identify SNPs and their specific genetic sequences or anomalies. The challenge to molecular biologists is to map as many SNP genotypes as possible for purposes of analyzing an individual's genome with the hope of discovering any predisposition or susceptibility to disease.[91,98,107,154]

Cancer

The body's defense mechanisms include "error-correcting" proteins that literally "erase" an apparent aberration in DNA sequencing. Unfortunately, the external effects of ionizing and ultraviolet radiation and chemical and pharmacologic **mutagens** exert catastrophic effects on genetic machinery, specifically the code sequence in DNA. In extreme cases of mutations, structural defects in embryos produce gross deformities such as missing limbs and multiple organs. In these cases, the extreme form of chemical mutagen known as a **teratogen** (*teras* in Greek means "monster") produces the effect.

The term *carcinogen* refers to any agent that causes cancer (**www.osha.gov/SLTC/carcinogens/**). In cancer, cell growth proceeds unchecked, forming larger than normal cell clusters that become tumors. A **benign tumor** remains in one location; cells from a **malignant tumor** migrate to invade other tissues and form secondary cancers. Cancers that form from connective tissue, muscle, or bone are called **sarcomas**; the most prevalent breast and lung cancers, called **carcinomas**, originate from epithelial tissue. Malignant tumors tend to **metastasize** or spawn cells that invade healthy tissue when they travel via the lymphatic or vascular circulation to form new secondary cancers termed *metastases*. Mutation of a gene into an **oncogene** or cancer-causing gene often produces numerous cancers, many of which cannot be eradicated by surgery and/or drugs that target specific cells or tissues. Cancer occurs from a failure to "turn on" specific genes that code nucleotide sequences to repress uncontrolled cell division. A tumor cell can develop from a mutation in any of the stages that regulate cell growth and differentiation. In colon cancer, for example, loss of the *APC* gene (adenomatous polyposis coli) on chromosome 5q alters the gut's normal epithelial tissue lining. Abnormal alterations in DNA can induce malignant colon carcinoma and metastasis. Cell-imaging technology (**www.nature.com/nature/supplements/tech/7310/;**) can pinpoint the exact location in tissues that produce high levels of the protein thymosin β-4 believed to trigger tumor growth.[144,169] Digital computer images that identify the location of specific tissue proteins allow researchers to determine when new proteins invade tumor cells or when normally produced proteins disappear. Protein imaging has opened new vistas in cancer screening for searching out specific molecules for comparison between normal and disease states, and developing strategies to arrest existing cancers (**http://webinar.sciencemag.org/webinar/archive/protein-tagging-technologies-cell-imaging-and-analysis**).

Researchers know that as some cancerous cells become more lethal, they form into primitive channels to create blood vessels, a process called **vasculogenesis** (**www.ncbi.nlm.nih.gov/books/NBK53252/**). The new blood vessels eventually connect with preexisting vessels at the tumor's edge. This process, completely independent of **angiogenesis**, may explain why therapies that attack angiogenesis may not treat some cancers effectively. **Figure 33.30** shows angiogenesis and subsequent tumor vascularization. First, the tumor proliferates as it forms a small mass of cells (note the lack of blood vessels in Figure 33.30A). Without blood vessels the tumor remains small. Second, protein factors stimulate the endothelial cells of nearby blood vessels to grow toward the tumor cells (Fig. 33.30B). Third, blood vessels proliferate, creating almost unlimited tumor growth. Note the approximate quadrupling of tumor cells (Fig. 33.30C).

Researchers have developed gene therapy strategies to attack tumor growth (e.g., angiogenesis inhibitors) in clinical trials (**www.cancer.gov/CLINICALTRIALS**). For example, in 2003, a pharmaceutical company in cooperation with the National Cancer Institute received FDA approval to market Velcade (bortezomib; **www.fda.gov/CDER/**

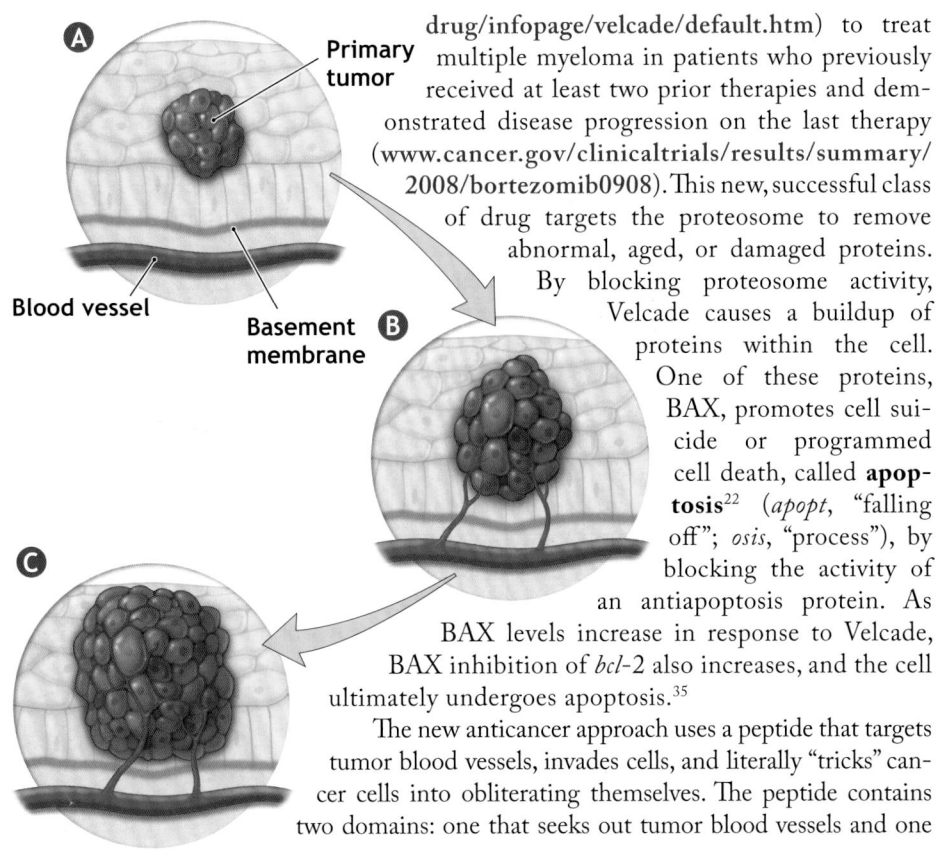

Primary tumor

Blood vessel

Basement membrane

A

B

C

drug/infopage/velcade/default.htm) to treat multiple myeloma in patients who previously received at least two prior therapies and demonstrated disease progression on the last therapy (www.cancer.gov/clinicaltrials/results/summary/2008/bortezomib0908). This new, successful class of drug targets the proteosome to remove abnormal, aged, or damaged proteins. By blocking proteosome activity, Velcade causes a buildup of proteins within the cell. One of these proteins, BAX, promotes cell suicide or programmed cell death, called **apoptosis**[22] (*apopt*, "falling off"; *osis*, "process"), by blocking the activity of an antiapoptosis protein. As BAX levels increase in response to Velcade, BAX inhibition of *bcl*-2 also increases, and the cell ultimately undergoes apoptosis.[35]

The new anticancer approach uses a peptide that targets tumor blood vessels, invades cells, and literally "tricks" cancer cells into obliterating themselves. The peptide contains two domains: one that seeks out tumor blood vessels and one

Gene therapy: introducing genes into cells (genetic surgery) to alter phenotype (i.e., cure diseases like cystic fibrosis using engineered adenovirus carrying a "good" gene to replace the crippled cystic fibrosis gene); gene therapy cures symptoms but cannot correct the genetic defect in next-generation germ cells

Apoptosis: death of a cell following preprogrammed "instructions"; the dead cell is eventually removed by phagocytosis; a small family of proteases called caspases transmit the apoptotic death signal

FIGURE 33.30 • Angiogenesis and subsequent tumor vascularization.

that triggers apoptosis. This normally occurring process in invertebrate and vertebrate biology represents one of nature's numerous defensive mechanisms to purge the organism of cells damaged by mutation, viral invasion, external radiation, malignancy, and other deleterious cellular events (not always abnormalities).

Researchers study four main areas of apoptosis:[1,121,123]

1. Molecular mechanisms involved in apoptosis induction
2. Control of intracellular protease pathways responsible for induction
3. Biochemical events during apoptosis, particularly events that mediate cell death
4. Role of mechanisms in normal development and disease

Anticancer drugs foster eradication of specific cancers once SNPs or related technology identifies them. A subsequent section discusses the fight against mutation-caused diseases with a new generation of genetically engineered vaccines.

Mitochondrial DNA Mutations and Diseases

Scientists normally view the chromosomes as the sole repository for DNA. DNA, however, also exists in mitochondria. The Mitomap database (www.mitomap.org) reports published and unpublished data on human mitochondrial DNA variation. The complete human mitochondrial genome, including the human mitochondrial sequence published in 2008, consists of 16,569 base pairs, with the genetic blueprint for 37 molecules that produce about 90% of the body's energy needs.

Chapters 5 and 6 described energy release during cellular respiration, when electron transfer ultimately produces water by uniting oxygen and hydrogen in the synthesis of significant quantities of energy-rich ATP. Researchers have determined the mitochondrial DNA (mtDNA) codes for 13 proteins that regulate respiratory chain oxidation and for 24 RNA molecules (2 tRNAs, 22 rRNAs) that manufacture subunits of respiratory chain proteins. Thus, a defect or mutation in mtDNA can induce devastating and unpredictable effects on basic cellular metabolic processes that can devastate neural, muscular, renal, and endocrine tissues. FIGURE 33.31 lists 12 diseases associated with mtDNA mutations. The ring of DNA displayed in the schematic view shows different base pairs of mtDNA, numbered counterclockwise from the top center position labeled O_H in *white*. Mitochondrial DNA mutations also may be implicated in aging, affecting the impact of **free radicals** on tissues of the cardiovascular system. In addition to the study of serious human diseases caused by deleterious mutations, other uses of mtDNA fall into two additional categories: **forensic medicine** and molecular anthropology. In forensic medicine, mtDNA analysis proves particularly useful because the high number of nucleotide polymorphisms called *sequence variants* allow discrimination among individuals and/or biologic samples. Even when degraded by environmental insult or time, minute samples of body fluids or fragments of hair, skin, muscle, bone, and blood may yield enough material for typing the mtDNA locus.[7,73,93,145] The likelihood of recovering mtDNA in small or degraded biologic samples exceeds that for nuclear DNA. Mitochondrial DNA molecules exist in hundreds to thousands of copies per cell compared with only two nuclear copies per cell. Also, because mtDNA is inherited only from the mother, any maternally related individual can provide a reference sample in situations where an individual's DNA cannot be directly compared with a biologic sample. In **molecular anthropology**, mtDNA analysis examines the extent of genetic variation in humans and the relatedness of world populations, including other mammals.[27,62,78,110,112,127,133,134]

Free radical: highly reactive ionized atom or molecule with a single unpaired electron in the outer orbit; can cause a mutation by reacting violently with DNA

Forensic medicine: branch of medicine concerned with the uses of medical knowledge applied to the law

Locus: location of a specific gene on a chromosome

Molecular anthropology: application of molecular biology and genetics to contemporary populations and origins of ancient specimens

 Mitochondrial DNA and the Evolutionary Tree

Mitochondrial DNA (mtDNA), because of its unique mode of maternal inheritance, can reveal ancient population histories and delineate migration patterns, expansion dates, and geographic homelands (**www.talkorigins.org/faqs/homs/mtDNA.html**). mtDNA has been extracted and sequenced from Neanderthal skeletons, providing evidence that modern humans do not share a close relationship with Neanderthals in the human evolutionary tree. The Neanderthal mtDNA studies strengthen the arguments that Neanderthals should be considered a separate species that did not contribute significantly to the modern gene pool.[57,122,129]

The mitochondrial DNA Analysis Unit of the FBI laboratory (**www.fbi.gov/about-us/lab/biometric-analysis/mtdna**) began conducting mtDNA analysis in 2001, and its various laboratories currently conduct more than a million examinations annually from skin, fabric, hair, bones, and teeth. The unit also maintains the National Missing Person DNA Database (NMPDD) to identify missing and unidentified persons, and the Scientific Working Group DNA Analysis Methods (SWGDAM) mtDNA Population Database, an integrated software and database resource for forensic comparisons. In addition, the Nuclear DNA Unit (NDNAU) provides forensic biologic services to the FBI and other duly constituted law enforcement agencies to support the investigative and intelligence priorities through evidence testing using forensic, serological, and nuclear DNA methodologies.

As Richard Dawkins, author and winner at the British Broadcast Awards 2009 of the three part Best Documentary Series, "The Genius of Charles Darwin," said, "DNA neither cares nor knows. DNA just is. And we dance to its music."

the**Point**   Appendix H, available online at http://thepoint.lww.com/mkk8e, provides a list of supplemental animations and videos on this subject.

Disease	Features
Alzheimer's disease	Progressive loss of cognitive capacity
CPEO (chronic progressive external ophthalmoplegia)	Paralysis of eye muscles and mitochondrial myopathy
Diabetes mellitus	High blood glucose levels; numerous complications
Dystonia	Abnormal movements involving muscular rigidity; degeneration of brain's basal ganglia
KSS (Kearns-Sayre syndrome)	CPEO combined with retinal degeneration, heart disease, hearing loss, diabetes, kidney failure
Leigh's syndrome	Progressive motor and verbal skill loss and degeneration of basal ganglia (potentially lethal childhood disease)
LHON (Leber's hereditary optic neuropathy)	Permanent or temporary blindness stemming from optic nerve damage

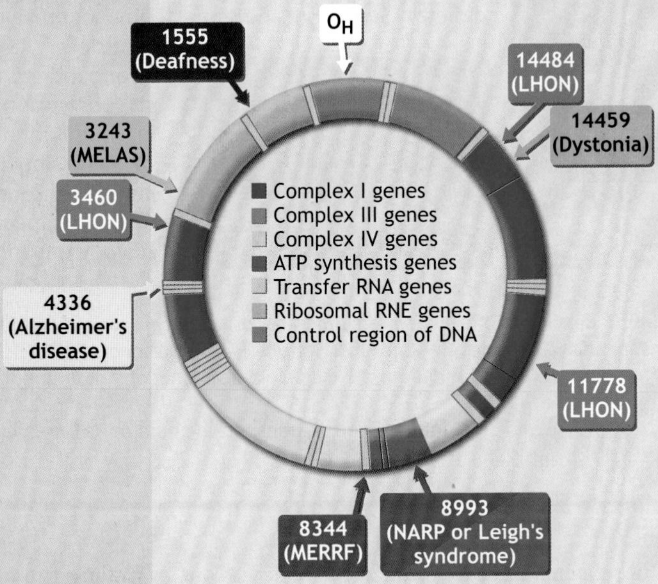

1555 (Deafness)

3243 (MELAS)

3460 (LHON)

4336 (Alzheimer's disease)

O$_H$

14484 (LHON)

14459 (Dystonia)

11778 (LHON)

8344 (MERRF)

8993 (NARP or Leigh's syndrome)

- Complex I genes
- Complex III genes
- Complex IV genes
- ATP synthesis genes
- Transfer RNA genes
- Ribosomal RNE genes
- Control region of DNA

FIGURE 33.31 • Mitochondrial DNA diseases. The ring of DNA displayed in the central schematic view shows the genes associated with a particular disorder. Many of the mitochondrial DNA diseases are inherited, but they also can occur spontaneously in the developing embryo and become widespread during fetal development. The mutations also can form in different tissues (at different times during the life span), often taking years to become fully expressed and often potentially lethal or severely debilitating. Adapted from Wallace, D. C., M. T. Lott, and M. D. Brown. "Report of the Committee on Human Mitochondrial DNA." *Human Gene Mapping, 1995: A Compendium.* Ed. A. Jamie Cuticchia, Michael A. Chipperfield, and Patricia A. Foster. pp. 1284, Figure 1. © 1996 The Johns Hopkins University Press. Reprinted with permission of Johns Hopkins University Press. Also available at **www.mitomap.org**.

Disease	Features
MELAS (mitochondrial encephalomyopathy, lactic acidosis and strokelike episodes)	Dysfunction of brain tissue (often causing seizures, transient regional paralysis and dementia) with mitochondrial myopathy and toxic blood acidity
MERRF (myoclonic epilepsy and ragged red fibers)	Seizures combined with mitochondrial myopathy, hearing loss, and dementia
Mitochondrial myopathy	Deterioration of muscle; poor exercise tolerance; muscle often displays ragged red fibers filled with abnormal mitochondria
NARP (neurogenic muscle weakness, ataxia and retinitis pigmentosa)	Muscle strength and coordination loss; regional brain degeneration and retinal deterioration
Pearson's syndrome	Childhood bone marrow dysfunction (leading to loss of blood cells) and pancreatic failure; survivors often progress to KSS

NEW HORIZONS IN MOLECULAR BIOLOGY

Watson and Crick's pioneering achievements in deciphering the molecular structure of DNA ushered in a new era. Advanced genetic engineering techniques affect not only medically related research [31,82,141] but also strategies involving improvements in food's nutrient content and in human exercise performance.[14,69,149]

 Supercharged Carrots and Lettuce

Researchers have uncovered a way to tweak a gene that increases the transport of calcium— a nutrient relatively low in foods from the plant kingdom—across carrot and lettuce leaf cell membranes into vacuoles. The scientists loaded their super-vegetables with a modified calcium–proton antiporter (known as short cation exchanger 1, or sCAX1), which pumps calcium into plant cells. For carrots, volunteers absorbed 41% more calcium compared to a group that consumed the "typical" carrot. The supercharged lettuce contained 25 to 32% more calcium than controls. The relevance of this tinkering and nutrient-boosting enhancement of a dietary staple is its potential to impact prevalent nutritional disorders (e.g., building strong bones in osteoporosis prevention). Such studies highlight the possibility of increasing plant nutrient content through expression of high-capacity molecular biology transporters.

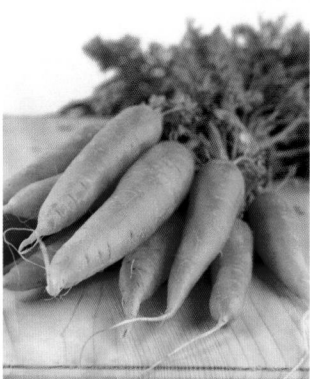
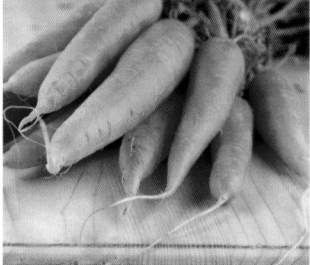

Sources:
1. Morris J, et al. Nutritional impact of elevated calcium transport activity in carrots. *PNAS* 2008;105:1431.
2. Park S, et al. Sensory analysis of calcium-biofortified lettuce. *Plant Biotechnol J* 2009;7:106.
3. Manohar, M., et al. Plant cation/H+ exchangers (CAXs); biological functions and genetic manipulations. *Plant Biol* (Stufttg) 2011;13:561.
4. Cho, D., et al. Vacuolar CAX1 and CAX2 influence auxin transport in guard cells via regulation of apoplastic pH. *Plant Physiol* 2012;160:1293.

The successful sequencing of the human genome was one of the most remarkable scientific feats in the history of medical science. Understanding the genetic blueprint of human life has transformed the discovery of innovative new drugs to battle existing medically related diseases.

Medically Related Research

Almost every aspect of the allied medical professions now benefit from molecular biology/molecular genetics research.[89,95,108] Within the past 30 years, researchers in many fields have created new strategies to fight many diseases, including cancer, AIDS, asthma, diabetes, influenza, heart and vascular disease, rheumatic fever, and malaria. The new disease fighters use genetic engineering to improve the immunologic antigen defense machinery against viral, bacterial, fungal, or parasitic **pathogens**. All pathogens contain antigens in their structure, so the new generation of genetically engineered vaccines severely blunt their destructive effects. FIGURE 33.32 provides a capsule view of four disease-fighting approaches with vaccine techniques that manipulate the genetic code.

1. *Live **vector** vaccines* (www.niaid.nih.gov/daids/vaccine/live.htm). Genes from a dangerous **virus** such as HIV are inserted into a harmless human virus. When injected, the altered virus prompts a strong **immune response** to combat the pathogen.

Pathogen: any virus, microorganism, or other substance that causes disease; *Streptococcus* bacteria cause scarlet fever, rheumatic fever, and pneumonia in humans; in plants, destructive diseases caused by bacteria (mostly pseudomonads) include blights, soft rots, and wilts. Viruses cannot replicate independently; they exist only within the cells of other organisms. Viruses usually contain a protein coating (capsid) and a lipid-rich protein envelope around the capsid ("a piece of bad news wrapped up in a protein") and reproduce using the metabolic apparatus of their host

Vector: plasmid, retrovirus, or bacterial or yeast artificial chromosome used to transfer a segment of foreign DNA among cells or species to produce more end product; the vector represents the genome that transports alien DNA into a host cell

Virus: small structure that grows by infecting other cells; adenovirus, retrovirus, and adeno-associated viruses are the most commonly used viral gene vectors

Immune response: immediate defensive reaction of the immune system upon encountering an invasion by a foreign substance such as a pathogen

Live vector vaccines

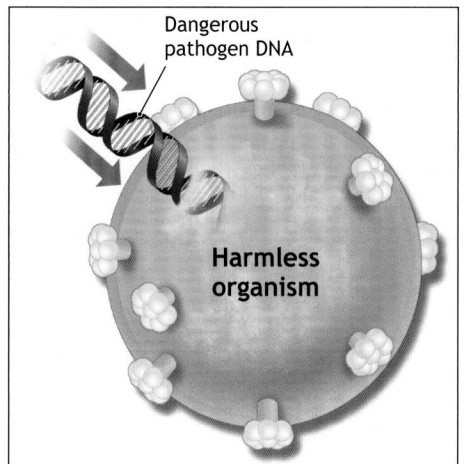

Reassortment vaccines

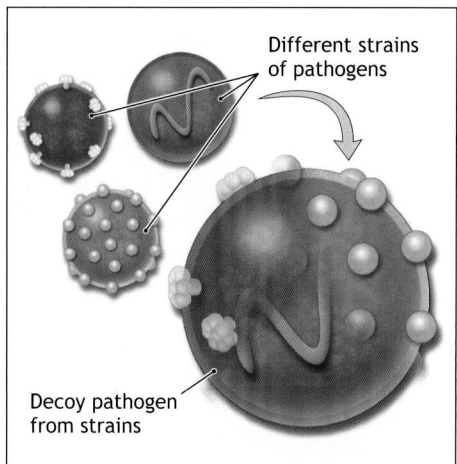

Naked vaccines

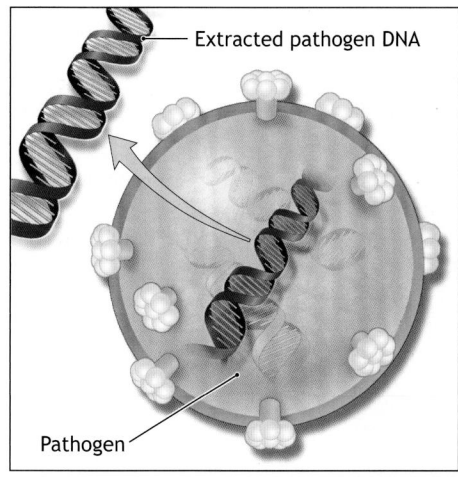

Recombinant subunit vaccines

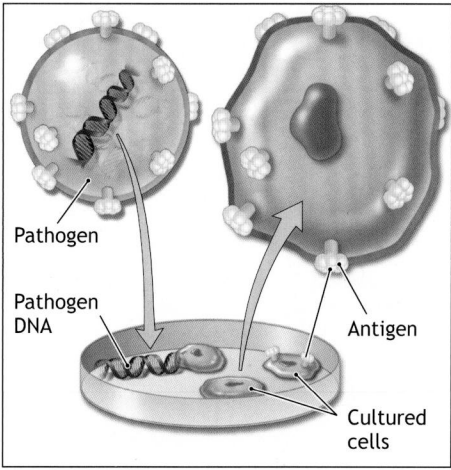

FIGURE 33.32 • Genetic-engineering a new generation of four vaccine types to fight human diseases.

2. *Reassortment virus vaccines* (**http://virology-online.com/viruses/Influenza.htm**). Combining genes from different pathogenic strains creates a decoy virus that looks dangerous to the pathogen but remains harmless while triggering an appropriate immune response.

3. *Naked DNA vaccines* (**www.niaid.nih.gov/daids/vaccine/dna.htm**). A pathogen's DNA is injected directly into the body. The cells incorporate the DNA, using the preprogrammed specific genetic "instructions" to create antigens to fight offending pathogens or existing tumors.

4. *Recombinant subunit vaccines* (**www.niaid.nih.gov/daids/vaccine/recombinant.htm**). Culturing a pathogen's genetic code or genes produces massive quantities of a specific antigen. The disease-fighting vaccine is made from the cultured antigens rather than from the whole pathogen.

Some genetically engineered vaccines trick the immune system into creating antibodies to seek out and destroy undesirable molecules before they cross the blood–brain barrier. For example, small cocaine molecules escape the body's protein antibody defenses without mechanisms to stop them. Engineered vaccines can create a larger cocaine derivative, which the immune system can then recognize and disarm. This aspect of genetic design offers innovative strategies to battle addictive diseases.

FIGURE **33.33** lists the body's 22 numbered chromosomes, including X and Y chromosomes, and specific genes on each chromosome linked to many cancers and metabolic–endocrine,

Chromosome 1
- Malignant melanoma
- Prostate cancer
- Deafness

Chromosome 2
- Congenital hypothyroidism
- Colorectal cancer

Chromosome 3
- Susceptibility to HIV infection
- Small-cell lung cancer
- Dementia

Chromosome 4
- Huntington's disease
- Polycystic kidney disease

Chromosome 5
- Spinal muscular atrophy
- Endometrial carcinoma

Chromosome 6
- Hemochromatosis
- Dyslexia
- Schizophrenia
- Myoclonus epilepsy

Chromosome 7
- Growth hormone deficient dwarfism
- Pregnancy-induced hypertension
- Cystic fibrosis
- Severe obesity

Chromosome 8
- Hemolytic anemia
- Burkitt's lymphoma

Chromosome 9
- Dilated cardiomyopathy
- Fructose intolerance

Chromosome 10
- Congenital cataracts
- Late onset cocayne syndrome

Chromosome 11
- Sickle-cell anemia
- Albinism

Chromosome 12
- Inflammatory bowel disease
- Rickets

Chromosome 13
- Breast cancer, early onset
- Retinoblastoma
- Pancreatic cancer

Chromosome 14
- Lukemia/T-cell lymphoma
- Goiter

Chromosome 15
- Marfan's syndrome
- Juvenile epilepsy

Chromosome 16
- Polycystic kidney disease
- Familial gastric cancer
- Tuberous sclerosis-2

Chromosome 17
(shown at right)

Chromosome 18
- Diabetes mellitus
- Familial carpal tunnel syndrome

Chromosome 19
- Myotonic dystrophy
- Malignant hyperthermia

Chromosome 20
- Isolated growth hormone deficiency
- Fatal familial insomnia

Chromosome 21
- Autoimmune polyglandular disease
- Amyotrophic lateral sclerosis

Chromosome 22
- Ewing's sarcoma
- Giant-cell fibroblastoma

X chromosome
- Colorblindness
- Mental retardation
- Gout
- Hemophilia
- Male pseudo-hermaphroditism

Y chromosome
- Gonadal dysgenesis

Mitochondrial DNA
- Leber's hereditary optic neuropathy
- Diabetes and deafness
- Myopathy and cardiomyopathy
- Dystonia

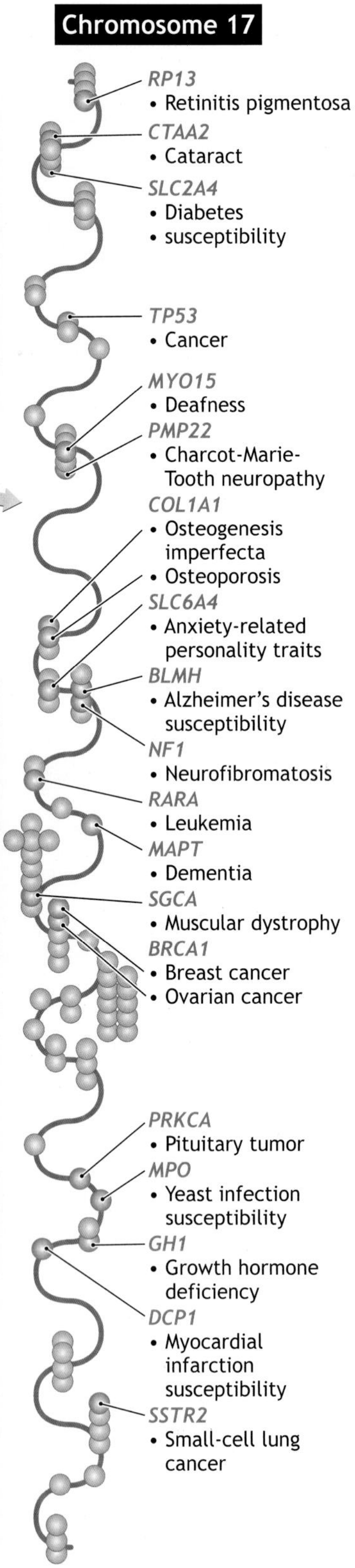

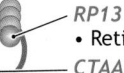

RP13
- Retinitis pigmentosa

CTAA2
- Cataract

SLC2A4
- Diabetes
- susceptibility

TP53
- Cancer

MYO15
- Deafness

PMP22
- Charcot-Marie-Tooth neuropathy

COL1A1
- Osteogenesis imperfecta
- Osteoporosis

SLC6A4
- Anxiety-related personality traits

BLMH
- Alzheimer's disease susceptibility

NF1
- Neurofibromatosis

RARA
- Leukemia

MAPT
- Dementia

SGCA
- Muscular dystrophy

BRCA1
- Breast cancer
- Ovarian cancer

PRKCA
- Pituitary tumor

MPO
- Yeast infection susceptibility

GH1
- Growth hormone deficiency

DCP1
- Myocardial infarction susceptibility

SSTR2
- Small-cell lung cancer

FIGURE 33.33 • Links on the body's chromosomes to specific cancer, metabolic–endocrine, neurologic–psychiatric, and cardiovascular disorders. **(A)** Close-up of disorders found on chromosome 17. On this chromosome, *red* designates the specific gene name and its location.

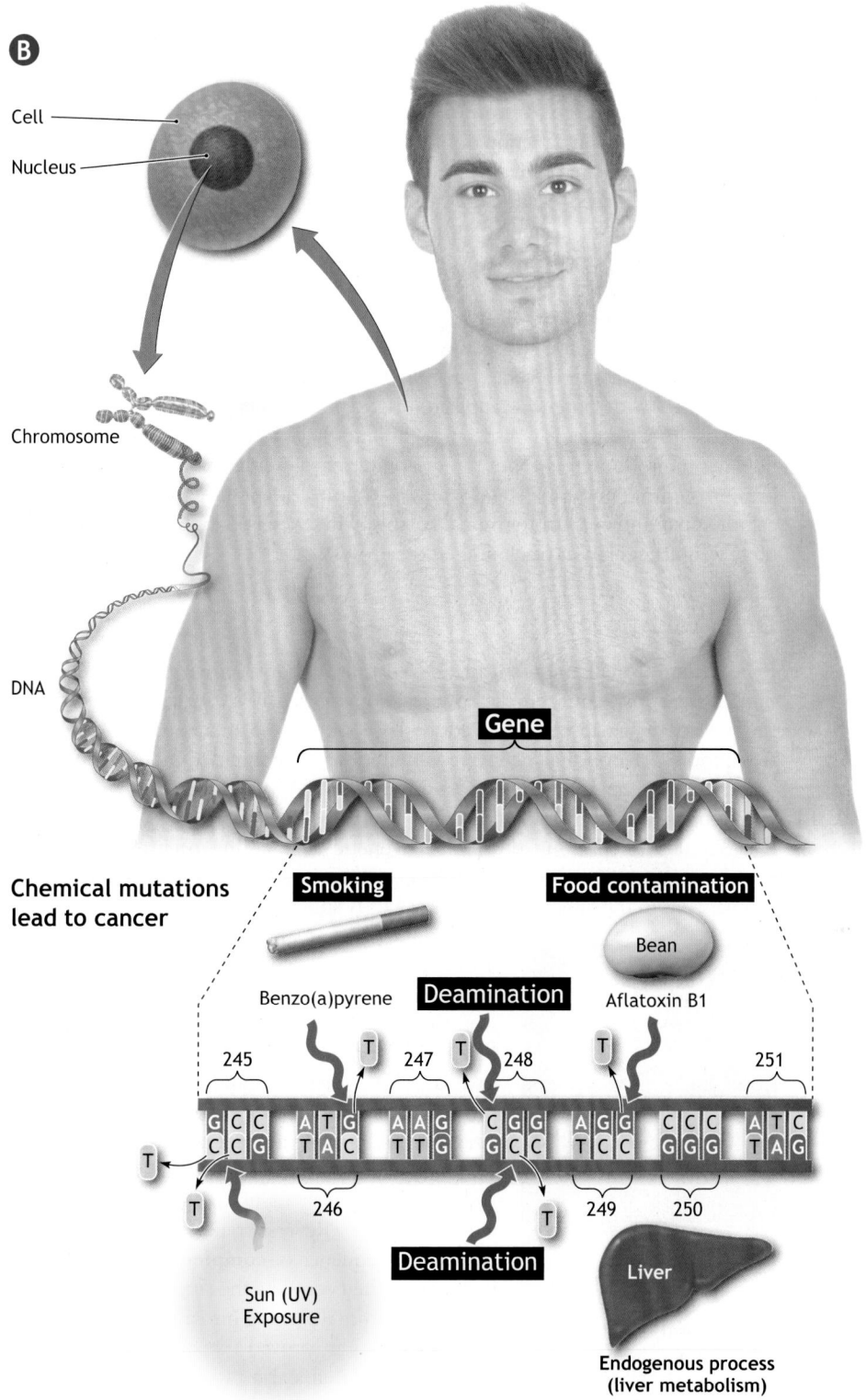

FIGURE 33.33 • **(B)** Graphic illustrating how different carcinogens (chemical and other) affect the nucleotide sequence of the *p53* gene responsible for about 50% of human cancers. The *p53* gene's name comes from the product it encodes, a polypeptide with a molecular mass of 53,000 daltons (1 dalton equals 1/12th the mass of carbon 12; for comparison, a water molecule weighs 18 daltons, and hemoglobin weighs 64,500 daltons).

neurologic–psychiatric, and cardiovascular disorders. Figure 33.33A profiles chromosome 17 on which seven deadly cancers have already been identified. Researchers estimate that chromosome 17 contains from 1200 to 1300 genes (depending on the technique of assessment), and includes about 81 million DNA building blocks—about 2.5 to 3.0% of the body's total DNA (http://ghr.nlm.nih.gov/chromosome/17; www.genome.gov/11508982). Figure 33.33B shows the mechanism of action of two different chemical carcinogens (smoking and food contamination) on this particular nucleotide sequence of the tumor suppressor gene *p53*. About 50% of human cancers occur from inactivating this gene. Each carcinogen produces a distinctive nucleotide substitution. Note the C or G substitution that displaces six T nucleotides.

Many areas of medicine other than cancer benefit from new findings in molecular biology.[157] Individuals with advanced sleep-phase syndrome (ASPS) cannot resist the urge either to sleep or to wake up early.[45] Research indicates that ASPS does not reflect a learned behavior or some other factor but follows a specific inherited pattern. Eventually, researchers may tie disorders to a single gene, opening new vistas to the genetics of the biologic clock in humans,[47,64,77] with potential applications to many aspects of human exercise performance. Some of the same medical research techniques have found their way into the arsenal of technologies to probe secrets about topics of interest to exercise physiologists. These include blood pressure control; endurance and strength-training adaptations; maturational shifts related to caloric input and output; hormonal balance with exercise; and pulmonary, cardiovascular, and body weight regulation (including anorexia nervosa).[56,113]

DNA Technologies

By isolating a small fragment of DNA from a chromosome in an animal species including humans, scientists can "remake" an exact copy of the DNA segment in a test tube to preserve the precise sequence of its nucleotide base pairs. Researchers use several terms to describe this process of eventual gene reconfiguration or manipulation on chromosomes—genetic engineering, **gene splicing**, or **recombinant DNA** (www.rpi.edu/dept/chem-eng/Biotech-Environ/Projects00/rdna/rdna.html).

A crucial step along the path to genetic engineering occurred in 1967 when Arthur Kornberg (1918–2007; 1959 Nobel Prize in Physiology or Medicine; discovered the mechanisms in the biologic synthesis of DNA and RNA) synthesized biologically active DNA (www.nobelprize.org/nobel_prizes/medicine/laureates/1959/).

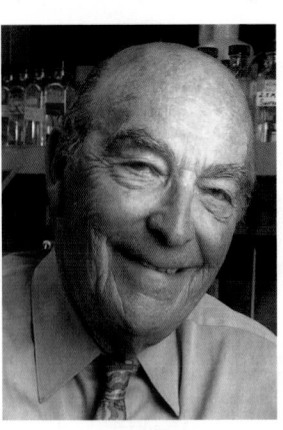

Arthur Kornberg

Three years later in 1970, David Baltimore (1938–), Renato Dulbecco (1914–2012), and Howard Temin (1934–1994) won the 1975 Nobel Prize in Physiology or Medicine for their discoveries concerning the interaction between tumor viruses and a cell's genetic material (www.nobelprize.org/nobel_prizes/medicine/laureates/1975/). They discovered that a specific enzyme tumor virus called **reverse transcriptase** made a DNA copy from RNA. The researchers used purified mRNA from muscle or liver tissue to show that this enzyme interacts with the mRNA. Reverse transcriptase duplicates the mRNA to the specific sequence of **complementary DNA (cDNA)**. DNA polymerase then converts the single-stranded DNA to a double strand for eventual cloning into a **bacteriophage** or other vector. These experiments proved transfer of the content stored in the genetic material to DNA; subsequent experiments also proved that purified DNA from one cell introduced into other cells produce new particles of RNA tumor virus.

In 1973, two American researchers, Stanford University, Palo Alto, CA Stanley Cohen (1922–), cofounder of Genentech (www.gene.com), one of the first biotechnology corporations, and Herbert Boyer (1936–), 1986 Nobel Prize in Physiology or Medicine with Rita Levi-Montalcini (1909–2012; for discovering cell growth factors) at the University of California, San Francisco, built upon the research described above (www.nobelprize.org/nobel_prizes/medicine/laureates/1986/). They introduced the recombinant DNA technique shown schematically in **FIGURE 33.34**. They successfully cut DNA from an amphibian gene (primitive frog *Xenopus*) into segments, using a **restriction endonuclease** enzyme (EcoRI) to

---

Gene splicing: attaching a fragment of DNA from one species (e.g., mammal) to another species (e.g., bacterium) to clone mammalian DNA

Recombinant DNA: forming a hybrid DNA molecule by fusing DNA fragments from different species; attaching a segment of DNA from one species to a second species, followed by inserting the hybrid molecule into a host organism such as a bacterium

Reverse transcriptase: enzyme that allows a single-stranded RNA template to synthesize a double-stranded DNA copy for insertion elsewhere in the genome

cDNA: single-stranded DNA complementary to an RNA and synthesized from it using reverse transcriptase; this kind of DNA only codes exons

Bacteriophage: any virus that infects bacteria

Restriction endonuclease: enzyme that cleaves a specific short DNA nucleotide sequence whenever it occurs at a target site

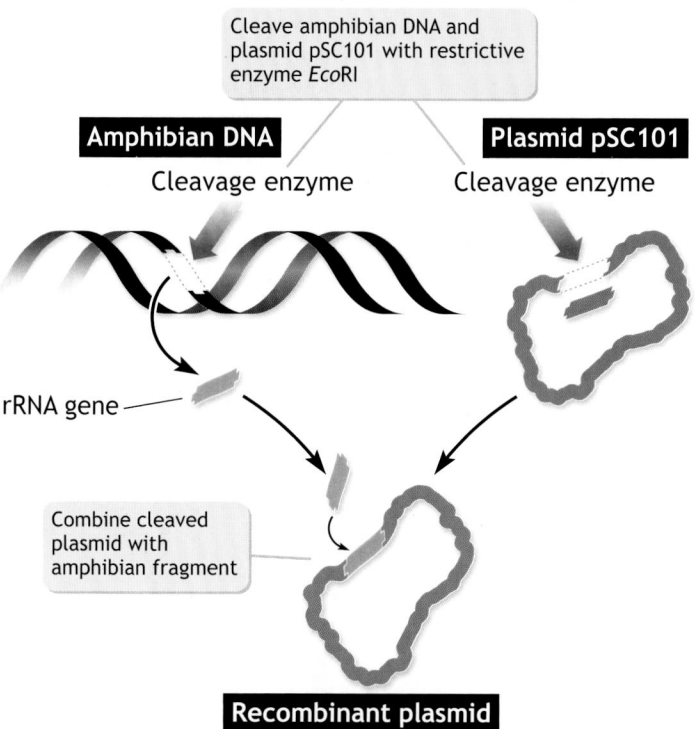

FIGURE 33.34 • Drs. Stanley Cohen and Herbert Boyer produced the first recombinant DNA organism in 1973. Their pioneering experiment combined the cleaved plasmid vector (pSC101 shown at the *right*) with a fragment of amphibian DNA (shown at the top *left*) using restriction endonuclease enzyme (EcoR1) to produce the recombinant plasmid shown at the bottom. The cells that contained the plasmid that carried the tetracycline gene grew and formed a cell colony (containing the frog ribosomal RNA gene).

cut the plasmid. They then rejoined the 9000-nucleotide segment to form a circular plasmid called pSC101, so named by Cohen because it was the 101st plasmid he isolated.

Their experimental procedure, explained further in the section on RNA cloning, produced the first plasmid to clone a vertebrate gene. In essence, the frog–bacterial molecule represented recombinant DNA using gene splicing to rejoin the two ends of the pSC101 plasmid. This technique can be likened to "cutting" and "pasting" text or images from one section of a document to another in a computer software program. The endonuclease first cleaves the amphibian DNA, setting it free. The two ends of the rRNA gene now join the pSC101 plasmid cleaved by *EcoR1*. Fundamentally, gene splicing creates a new genetic blueprint in a test tube that leapfrogs nature's own genetic engineering methods based on natural selection, a process that has commingled genes within Earth's plant and animal species over tens of millions of years of evolution. What took nature millions of years to accomplish scientists can now duplicate in a day and produce thousands of copies of DNA's exact nucleotide sequence from a particular gene in a given genome. By manipulating DNA's configuration, a newly created gene can be inserted into cells of plants and animals to create new cells or species with unique characteristics expressed by the new genetic instructions.

DNA Cloning Isolates Human Genes

DNA **cloning** progresses in several stages. The first involves mechanically breaking the genetic material within a DNA sample or, alternatively, using restriction endonucleases that precisely cut the nucleotide sequence along DNA's double helix into smaller segments to facilitate manipulation. The collection of DNA pieces formed by endonuclease cleavage

Cloning: creating a cell(s) or molecule(s) from a single ancestral cell or molecule

Genomic library: collection of DNA fragments from an organism's genome; a library includes noncoding DNA and cDNA

represents single, random segments of the organism's entire DNA, which includes all of the genetic material. The term *genomic library* describes the collection of cloned fragments. Many genomic libraries exist in the public domain (e.g., **www.musagenomics.org/genomics_tools/ genome_resources.html**), so researchers can use them without having to reduplicate the particular DNA sequences of interest. **FIGURE 33.35** shows formation of a genomic library from a strand of human DNA. This basic strategy led to tremendous advances in the role such techniques play related to almost all aspects of the medical sciences.[10,68,165]

A restriction endonuclease cleaves a short strand of human double helix chromosomal DNA, usually four to six base pairs in length, into millions of fragments. Restriction endonucleases have become a fundamental tool in molecular biology research because treatment of DNA with the same restriction endonuclease allows any two DNA fragments to join

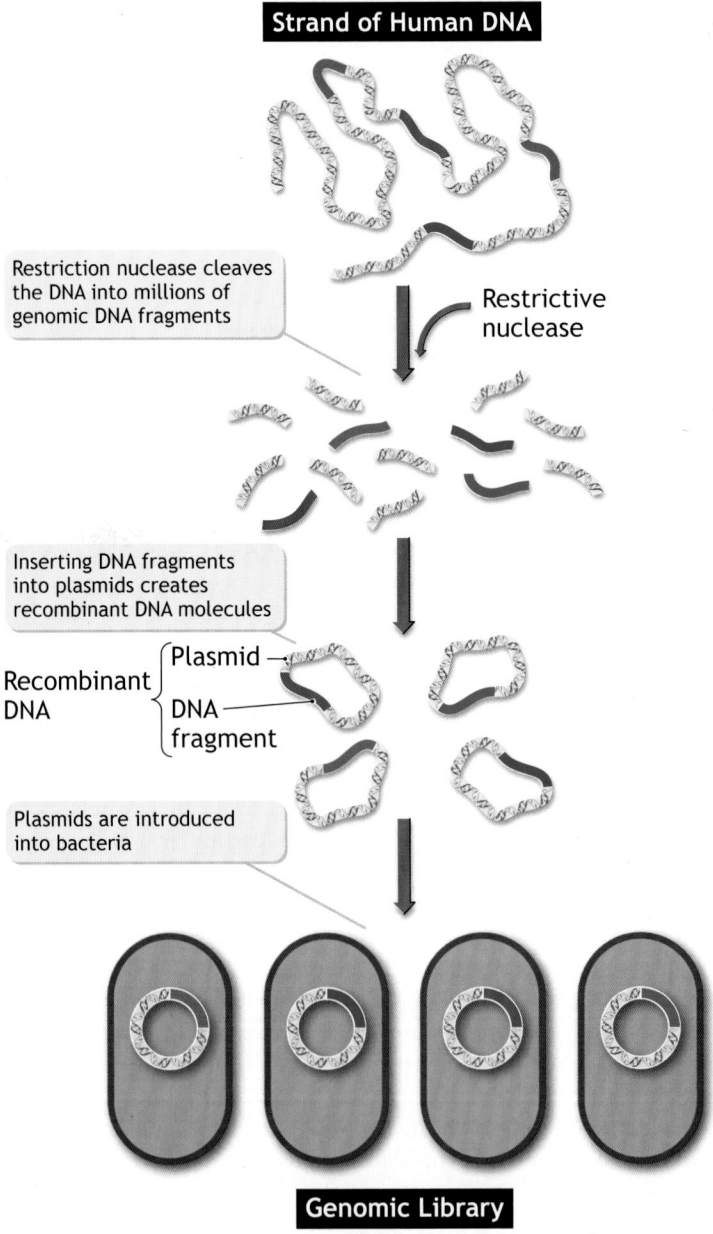

Strand of Human DNA

Restriction nuclease cleaves the DNA into millions of genomic DNA fragments

Restrictive nuclease

Inserting DNA fragments into plasmids creates recombinant DNA molecules

Recombinant DNA { Plasmid — DNA fragment

Plasmids are introduced into bacteria

Genomic Library

FIGURE 33.35 • Creating a genomic library from human DNA. The library consists of bacteria with specific DNA fragments contained in carrier substances such as plasmids. Note in the example how four different-colored DNA segments (*red, blue, purple, green*) from the original human DNA shown at the top end up within the bacterial host. The rest of the DNA fragments can also make clones.

together—providing for an essentially endless supply of DNA for further experimentation. One of the most widely used chemical techniques, **gel electrophoresis** (Greek *phoresis*, "to be carried"), perfected by 1948 Chemistry Nobel Laureate Arne Wilhelm Tiselius 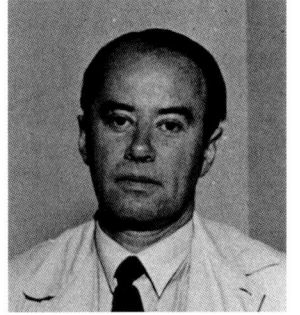 (1902–1971; for research on electrophoresis and adsorption analysis, and discoveries concerning the complex nature of the serum proteins), separates DNA fragments within an electric field (www.nobelprize.org/nobel_prizes/chemistry/laureates/1948/tiselius-bio.html). The DNA strands inserted into a circular plasmid carrier molecule recombine the DNA (hence the term *recombinant DNA*). This occurs when the enzyme DNA ligase, with addition of ATP, covalently links the DNA fragment to the previously opened **plasmid** composed of several thousand nucleotide pairs. Once inserted, the ligase rejoins the ends of the plasmid to produce the new recombinant plasmid molecule known as a vector. Recombinant plasmids are then inserted into

Arne Wilhelm Tiselius

bacteria (e.g., *E. coli*) to ensure that only one bacterium receives one plasmid. At this stage, the total culture of bacteria represents the genomic library illustrated in Figure 33.35.

The next stage of DNA cloning grows the bacterium in a nutrient-rich broth that sustains cell multiplication that doubles its number every hour. This doubles the number of recombinant DNA copies. By simple multiplication, doubling the number of DNA copies each hour over 24 hr produces almost 17 million new copies from a single bacterium! The bacteria are then broken apart or lysed, and the millions of DNA copies culled from the larger bacterial chromosome and other cellular contents to provide pure replicas of the original DNA segment. Recovering this segment occurs after the specific **restriction enzyme** isolates the segment from plasma DNA for separation by gel electrophoresis (see Fig. 33.38).

Practical Application in Bioremediation

Implementation of bacterial cloning has practical applications in the field of bioremediation, which uses bacteria to degrade dangerous compounds.[96,170] For example, the pink-colored bacteria that smell like rotten cabbage, *Deinococcus radiodurans* (*D. radi*), shown in **FIGURE 33.36**, have been genetically cloned from strains of *E. coli* previously made resistant to toxic wastes (www.genomenewsnetwork.org/articles/07_02/deinococcus.shtml). *D. radi* was isolated in 1956 from a can of ground beef that had been "sterilized" by gamma radiation but still spoiled. Researchers determined that *D. radi* survived approximately 17 kGy (1.7 million rads), a value equal to 3000 times the lethal human radiation dose. The economic value of *D. radi* is straightforward; easily producing trillions of copies of the new bacterium can save hundreds of billions of dollars in biohazard cleanup. For example, *D. radi* consumes heavy metals and radioactive waste, thus it can scavenge toxic wastes buried at 1000 sites throughout the United States and other sites worldwide, a legacy from nuclear weapons production between 1945 and 1986. Researchers have also fused a gene that encodes toluene dioxygenase (the enzyme that decomposes toluene) to a

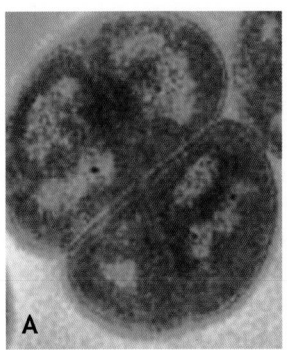 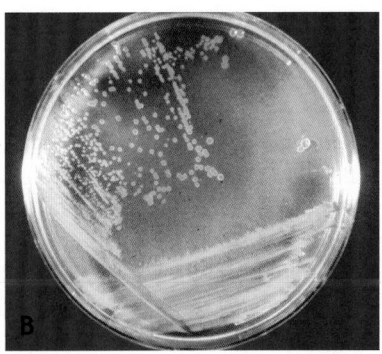

FIGURE 33.36 • Bioremediation. **(A)** Electron photomicrograph of *D. radi* (sequenced in the DOE Microbial Genome Program as a cluster of four cells or tetrad). *D. radi* and related species have been identified worldwide,[77] including in Antarctic granite and in tanks of powerful cobalt-60 irradiators in Denmark. **(B)** *D. radi* growing on a nutrient agar plate; the orange color is from carotenoid pigment. (Images from the Uniformed Services University of the Health Sciences, Bethesda, MD; www.usuhs.mil).

Gel electrophoresis: separation of electrically charged substances (e.g., proteins) through a gel mesh according to size; smaller substances migrate faster than larger substances when they pass through the electric field from the top (negative) to bottom (positive) electrode through a slab of agarose gel, a polysaccharide extracted from seaweed

Plasmid: small circular molecule in bacteria without chromosomal DNA; serves as a vector for transferring genes among cells

Restriction enzyme: cuts DNA at precise locations and, with DNA ligase, reassembles the pieces into a desired order; cutting between G and A leaves overhanging "sticky end" chains because base pairs formed between the two overhanging portions "glue" the two strands together where the sticky ends match, assembling them into customized genomes (e.g., designer bacteria that make insulin or growth hormone, or genes for disease resistance added to agricultural plants)

D. radi promoter (site that activates the gene) and then inserted it into one of the bacterium's chromosomes. The resulting recombinant bacterium "upgraded" *D. radi* for degrading toluene and other organic compounds at levels exceeding those at radioactive waste sites. *D. radi* not only survives high radiation doses, but also long periods of dehydration and ultraviolet irradiation. *D. radi* apparently repairs its radiation-damaged DNA base pairs by use of redundant genetic "signals." The 2-billion-year-old microbe has from 4 to 10 DNA molecules. The protein, RecA, matches the damaged DNA base pairs and splices them together. During the repair process, cell-building activities shut down and the broken DNA pieces stay in place. The complete genome of *D. radi* has been decoded and can be accessed from the J. Craig Venter Institute Web site, (www.jcvi.org). The DNA of *D. radi* consists of 3.3 million chemical base units. The genome contains two circular chromosomes, one of about 2.6 million and the other 400,000 base pairs, and two smaller circular molecules (megaplasmid of 177,000 base pairs and plasmid of 45,000 base pairs). Despite its high tolerance for radioactivity, *D. radi* decomposes at 45°C (113°F).

In addition to unraveling the secrets of *D. radi*, the Institute published the first diploid human genome (Levy S, et al. The diploid genome sequence of an individual human. *PLoS Biol* 2007;5:e254; www.plosbiology.org/article/info:doi/10.1371/journal.pbio.0050254) and ongoing Global Ocean Sampling Expedition (www.jcvi.org/cms/research/projects/gos/overview/), The quest was to unlock the secrets of the oceans by sampling, sequencing, and analyzing the DNA of the ocean's microorganisms. Thus far, scientists have uncovered more than 60 million genes and thousands of novel protein families from the seawater organisms during global circumnavigation experiments, ongoing sampling in waters off the California and western coast of the United States, and sampling with other collaborators in Antarctica and deep-sea ocean vents. In addition, researchers sequenced the microbial flora found in human environments (www.jcvi.org/cms/publications/listing/; oral cavity, vagina, digestive tract).

Locating Specific Genes with Plasmids

Creating cloned DNA involves locating a specific gene within the plasmid or viral culture. Consider the analogy of entering a five-story department store that lacks signs or a computer database to search for a single unmarked item. One could begin searching on the first floor, proceeding to every shelf and cupboard of every floor until finding the item, but the inefficiency of this strategy seems obvious. To facilitate locating a specific gene, a specific **DNA probe** of known nucleotide sequence, labeled with colored fluorescent markers or radioisotopes, searches the pool of millions of copies of DNA fragments. The probes used in **hybridization** reactions capture a single DNA or RNA strand to form another nucleic acid with a complementary nucleotide sequence. The probe searches the genomic library until it locates a matching code on a specific chromosomal gene or a specific RNA sequence in cells or tissues.

Searching for a single gene remains complicated because the gene can contain both coding exons and noncoding introns. If the clone with its isolated sequences contains only exons (i.e., only the uninterrupted coding sequences), then the new genomic library is called a **cDNA library** (the *c* refers to a copy or complementary DNA). Different cDNA libraries reflect different tissues because the libraries contain the specifically transcribed mRNA from the original source tissue. A cDNA library contains the gene's coding regions, often including the leading and trailing sequences of the mRNA. The absence of chromosomal DNA serves as a cDNA clone's most distinguishing feature. The enzyme reverse transcriptase uses the source cell or tissue mRNA to construct DNA. Cloning cDNA molecules is similar to cloning genomic DNA fragments. Each different type of tissue (e.g., heart, liver, kidney) has a different cDNA library associated with it. Cloned DNA makes it possible to manufacture exact copies of "pure" genetic material relatively quickly from among millions of nucleotide sequences. The uninterrupted coding sequence for a particular gene gives the cDNA clone a clear advantage for duplicating the gene in bulk or deducing a protein's amino acid sequence. Like genomic libraries, cDNA libraries exist in the public domain for sharing among researchers; commercial vendors also make them available for purchase. Many Internet sites provide valuable links to databases for

DNA probe: radioactive or fluorescent-labeled nucleotide that identifies, isolates (targets), or binds to a gene or gene product

Hybridization: selective binding of two complementary nucleic acid strands (DNA or RNA) to detect specific nucleotide sequences

cDNA library: contains the genes' coding regions, including leading and trailing mRNA sequences

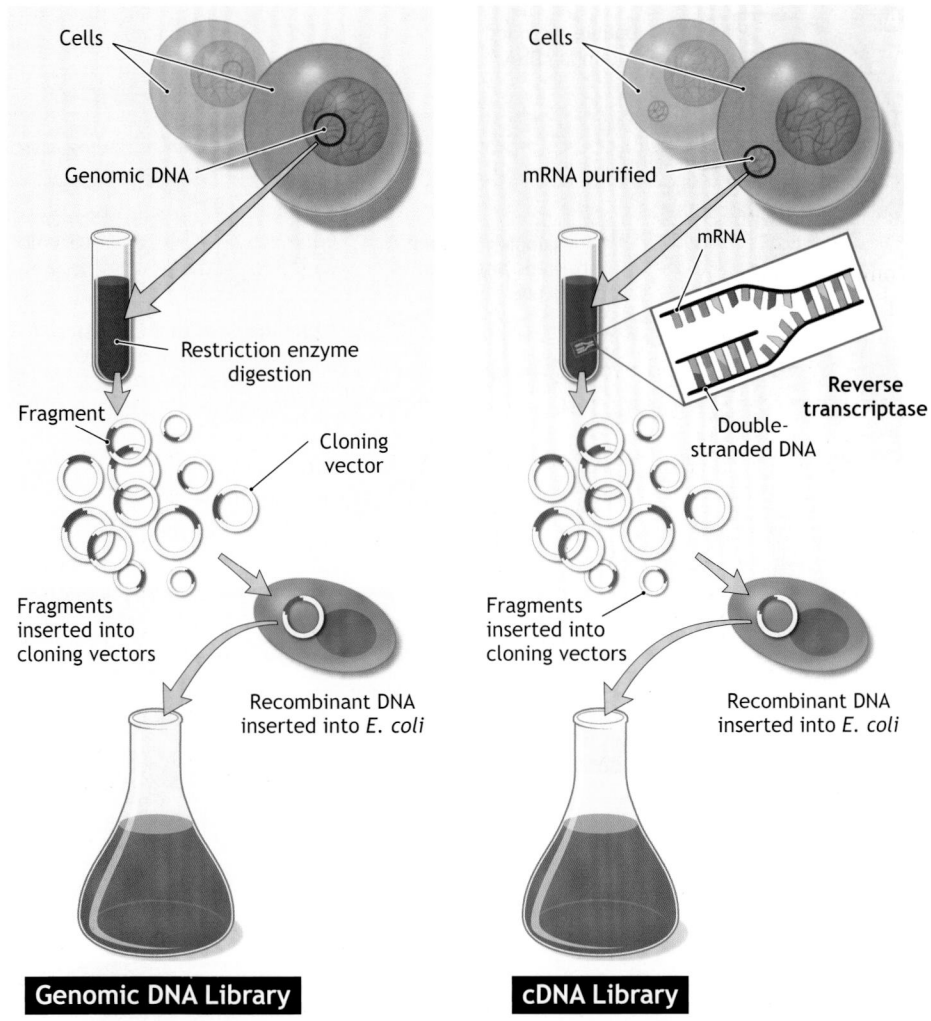

FIGURE 33.37 • Basic differences in creating genomic DNA and cDNA libraries.

mammals and other vertebrates, fungi, plants, eukaryotes, prokaryotes, viruses, specific gene groups, and large-scale genome sequencing centers (e.g., www.ddbj.nig.ac.jp). **FIGURE 33.37** illustrates the basic difference in creating genomic DNA and cDNA libraries. In both cases, fragments of digested DNA (shown as *purple* fragments) are inserted into cloning vectors such as a bacteriophage or phage (from the Greek "to devour"), a virus that invades and then replicates within bacteria. These structures populate the biosphere, and are omnipresent in sea water, soils, and animal intestinal flora (McGrath S, van Sinderen D (eds). *Bacteriophage: Genetics and Molecular Biology* Caister Academic Press. Norfolk, England, 2007).

Electrophoresis and Gel Transfer Methods

The electrophoresis technique moves charged particles such as proteins through an electrically charged supporting medium. The negatively charged phosphate groups of DNA molecules migrate to the positive pole (anode) of the apparatus. **FIGURE 33.38** shows two ways of separating DNA fragments. The top example (A) shows cutting the same DNA molecule from the one (bacteriophage) genome with two different restriction endonucleases, *EcoR1* and *HindIII* (hundreds of other enzymes with distinct specificity have been isolated). Small fragments migrate faster than large fragments when they pass through the electric field from top (negative) to bottom (positive) through a slab of agarose gel. Heating the gel causes its protein fibers to congeal and form a grid through which DNA fragments pass. Separating DNA fragments by size in an electric field makes it relatively easy to

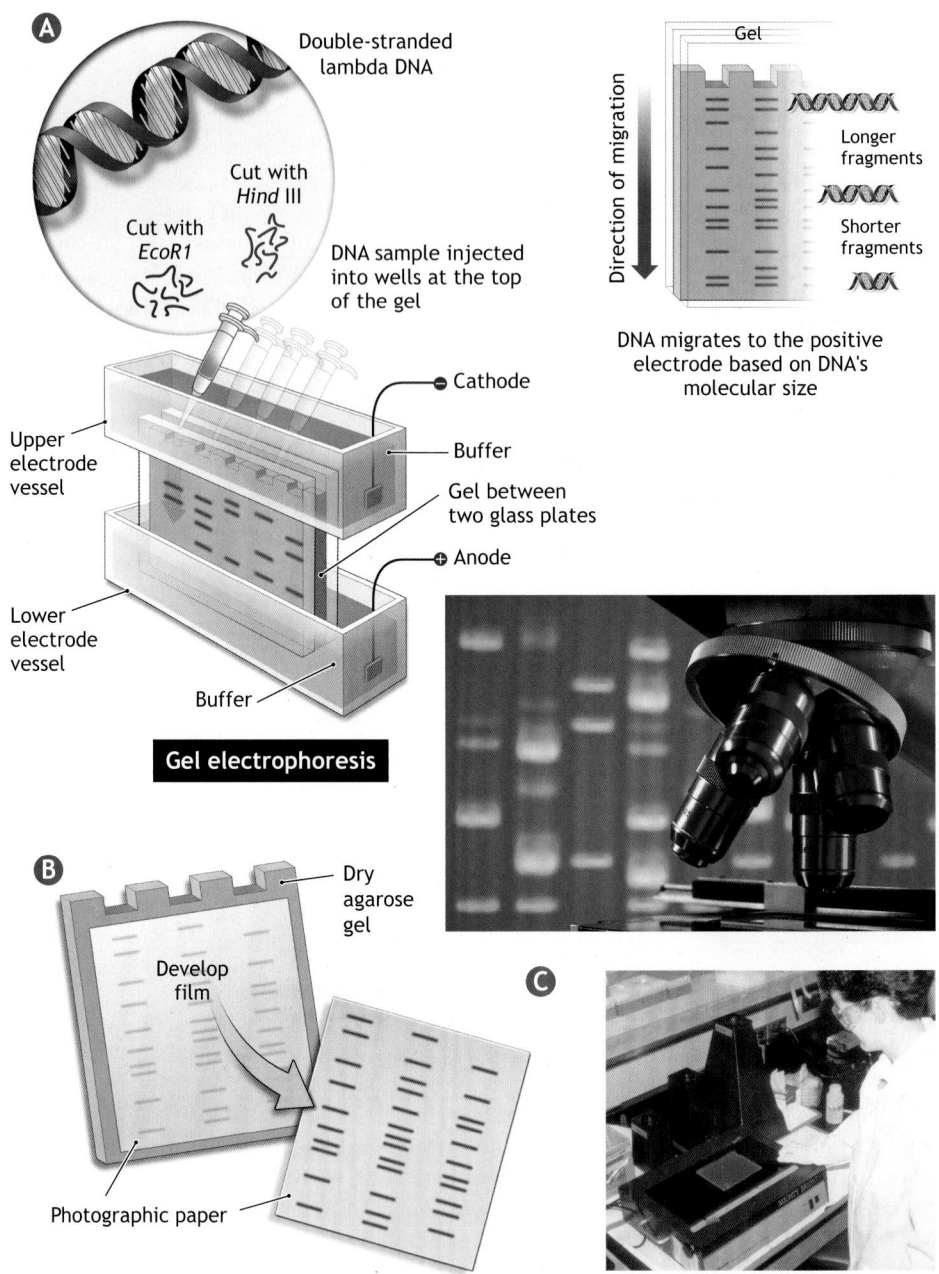

FIGURE 33.38 • Gel electrophoresis: separating DNA fragments by molecular size. **(A)** Two restriction endonucleases cleave DNA into two segments for placement at the top of a thin agarose gel slab supported in a vertical position. An electric current separates the DNA fragments as they pass through the hydrated gel according to their mobility; small fragments move more quickly through the electric current and fixate at the bottom of the gel at the positive electrode. Larger fragments settle nearer to the top. The *top right* photo reveals the DNA bands fluoresced under ultraviolet light. *Note*: The restriction enzyme takes the initials of the bacterial type and strain from its source; EcoR1 refers to *E. coli* strain RY13, and the 1 means this restriction enzyme was found first in the strain. The cleavage site is 5–GAATTC–3 and 3–CTTAAG–5; the HindIII source is *Haemophilus influenzae Rd*. The cleavage site is 5–AAGCTT–3 and 3–TTCGAA–5. **(B)** Autoradiography technique displays radioisotope ^{32}P-labeled DNA bands on exposed photographic paper placed over the agarose gel. **(C)** Dr. Kristin Stuempfle, Department of Health and Exercise Sciences, Gettysburg College, reviewing the film of a sequencing gel on a light box.

distinguish among DNA segments. Note the bands at the *lower right panel* of the gel. These represent smaller DNA fragments than the upper longer fragments. The DNA shows up clearly because soaking the medium with a DNA- or RNA-specific dye (ethidium bromide) stains DNA orange (pinkish in photo), which becomes clearly visible under **ultraviolet light**. Extraction of DNA provides samples of pure DNA fragments. Purified DNA can be used in cloning experiments or for matching in size to other DNA fragments.[79,151]

Figure 33.38B shows an alternative technique using the labeled **radioisotope** ^{32}P to expose DNA bands when photographic paper placed over the gel reveals particles emitted from the isotope. **FIGURE 33.39** illustrates three gel transfer methods to separate fragments of genetic material and proteins: **Southern blot**, **Northern blot**, and **Western blot** (www.biosynth.com/index.asp?topic_id=144).

DNA Amplification with the Polymerase Chain Reaction

The polymerase chain reaction (PCR) method, developed in 1987 by American biochemist Kary Banks Mullis 🔵 (1944– ; 1993 Nobel Prize in Chemistry [www.nobelprize.org/nobel_prizes/chemistry/laureates/1993/mullis-autobio.html]; invention of the PCR method),

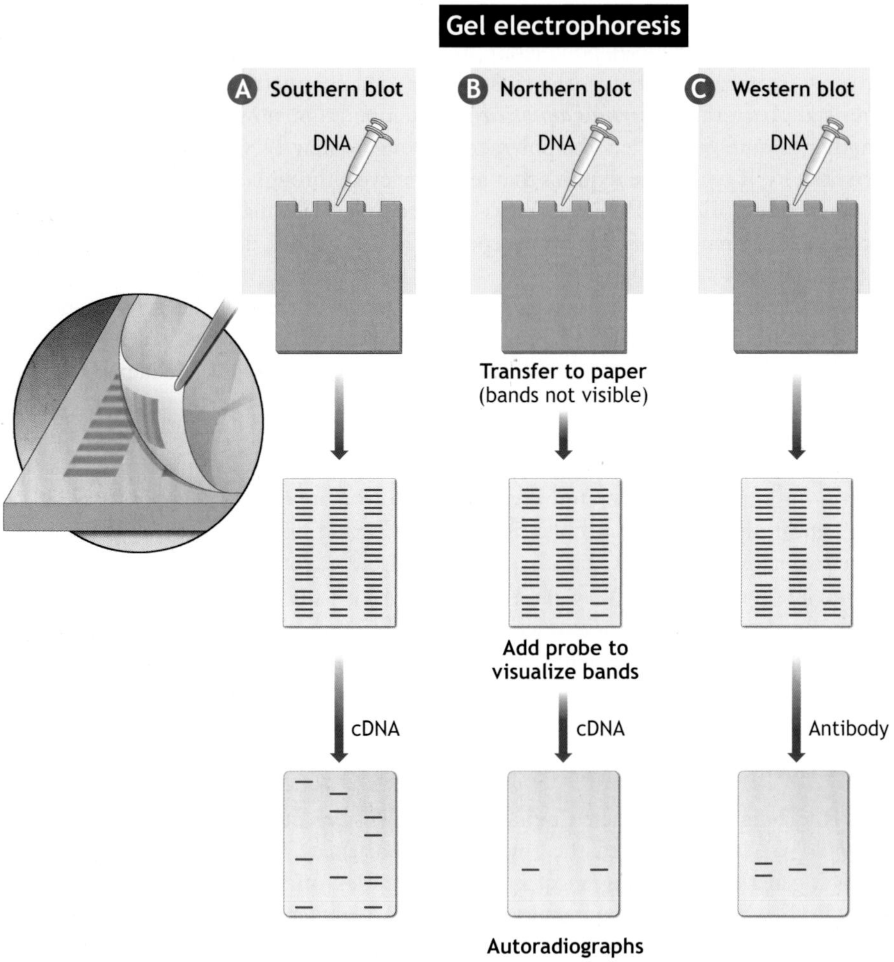

Ultraviolet light: electromagnetic rays at higher frequencies than the violet end of the visible spectrum

Radioisotope: isotope that becomes more stable by emitting radiation

Southern blotting: technique that detects single-stranded DNA from transferring DNA fragments to nylon paper with a DNA-binding probe

Northern blotting: hybridization technique that binds a DNA probe to a target RNA molecule; the technique detects a specific RNA sequence in a cell

Western blotting: technique for separating genetic fragments using a probe (usually an antibody) that binds to a target protein

FIGURE 33.39 • Identifying DNA sequences by three gel transfer methods. **(A)** Southern blot (named for Dr. E. M. Southern) produced when single-stranded DNA on a sheet of nitrocellulose is placed in a tray of buffer atop a sponge. The pattern on the gel is copied, or "blotted," to the radioactively labeled nucleic acids. This process produces radioactive bands, which means that nucleic acid bands hybridize with those labeled by radioactivity. **(B)** Northern blots are produced when RNA on a nitrocellulose blot hybridizes with a single-stranded DNA probe without using alkali (alkali hydrolyzes RNA). **(C)** Western blot gel electrophoresis separates proteins using antibody probes to target specific proteins.

In vitro: in an artificial environment such as a test tube or culture medium

Anneal: rejoining separated single complementary strands of DNA to form a double helix

Thermus aquaticus: thermally stable bacterium that survives at very high temperatures found in hot springs and geysers. The bacterium provides the important Taq DNA-replicating polymerase; voted 1989 "Molecule of the Year" by the prestigious journal *Science*

represents a milestone in molecular biology.[114] The PCR method, carried out *in vitro* without prior transfer in living cells, artificially amplifies an extremely small amount of DNA and rapidly creates billions of copies of a specific region of a single DNA molecule. FIGURE **33.40** illustrates the basic concept of the PCR, in which purified DNA polymerase copies a DNA template in three cycles of replication. In the first step of the initial cycle, a minute amount of double-stranded DNA is heated to about 94°C (201.2°F) for several minutes to denature (separate) the strands. Each strand has a known sequence of nucleotides on either side of the target nucleotides. Next, two short, specifically designed synthetic primers of known DNA sequence (shown in *green* and *red*) hybridize or anneal to one of the two separated strands at the exact beginning and ending position of the target DNA nucleotide sequence. In other words, only the target

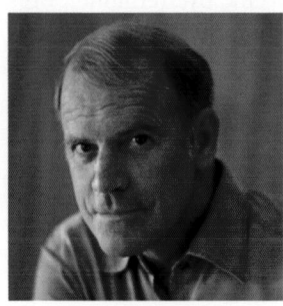

Kary Banks Mullis

sequence, bracketed by the primers, duplicates because no primers attach elsewhere along the DNA fragment.

The annealing process cannot withstand the initial high temperature required to separate the double helix, so it occurs at a lower 54°C (129.2°F). At this temperature, the single-stranded DNA fragments match complementary nucleotide sequences at the ends of the target DNA sequence. DNA synthesis would not proceed without appropriate primers. Adding a heat-resistant DNA polymerase to the reaction in step 3 synthesizes a new DNA strand, now creating two strands. The most widely used polymerase (Taq) is isolated from the heat-resistant bacterium *Thermus aquaticus*. The temperature, now increased to 70°C (158°F) for another minute or two, lets the polymerase elongate new DNA strands that begin at the primers. The PCR technique requires that reactants cycle through a varied temperature profile during incubation, and the PCR apparatus (thermocycler) automatically progresses through a preset thermal sequence. This first cycle, repeated 20 to 40 times, doubles the amount of DNA synthesized in each succeeding cycle.

The PCR method only clones DNA fragments with known beginning and ending sequences. With prior knowledge of the code, it takes only 20 repeat cycles to duplicate enough target DNA to produce 1,048,536 copies (2^{20}) of the original sequence. The second and third cycles displayed in Figure 33.40 show how the three different stages of the PCR method eventually copies millions or even billions of the original DNA sequence. Note the example for three cycles at the right of the figure. The second cycle repeats the first cycle. It progresses through each temperature change, first to separate strands at about 94°C (201.2°F), then to anneal the primers at a cooler 54°C (129.2°F), and finally through polymerase action to make two additional DNA strands at 72°C (161.6°F). Note that the third cycle produces eight double-stranded DNA molecules; after seven cycles, the newly created DNA consists of double strands with flush ends (same length) uniquely identical to the original target sequence. The next 17 cycles produce the additional 1,048,528 copies, and just 10 more cycles produce 1000 million more target molecules!

Applications of PCR

The PCR technique has impacted numerous fields besides molecular biology[69]; they include biotechnology, entomology and the environmental sciences, molecular epidemiology, forensic science, genetic engineering, most medical specialties, microbiology, proteomics, the food industry, and even apparel manufacturing. Fourteen years ago at the 2000 Sydney Olympic Games, a special ink containing a small DNA snippet from a saliva swab from two Australian athletes was affixed to labels, tags, pins, and stickers of official Olympic merchandise to thwart counterfeiters. An electronic scanner could check the invisible ink to verify an item's authenticity. The same DNA-marking strategy, impossible to reverse-engineer, can verify rare and one-of-a-kind objects from premium grade oil, diamonds and jewelry, to fine wine. The DNA-"tagging" was applied to items at the 2013 Super Bowl game (see "FYI: Thwarting Counterfeits at Major Sporting Events"). PCR also can identify diverse viruses and bacteria or any DNA extracted from a current or ancient plant or animal organism. It identifies the unique sequence of a miniscule amount of DNA nucleotide material, even in substances millions of years old.

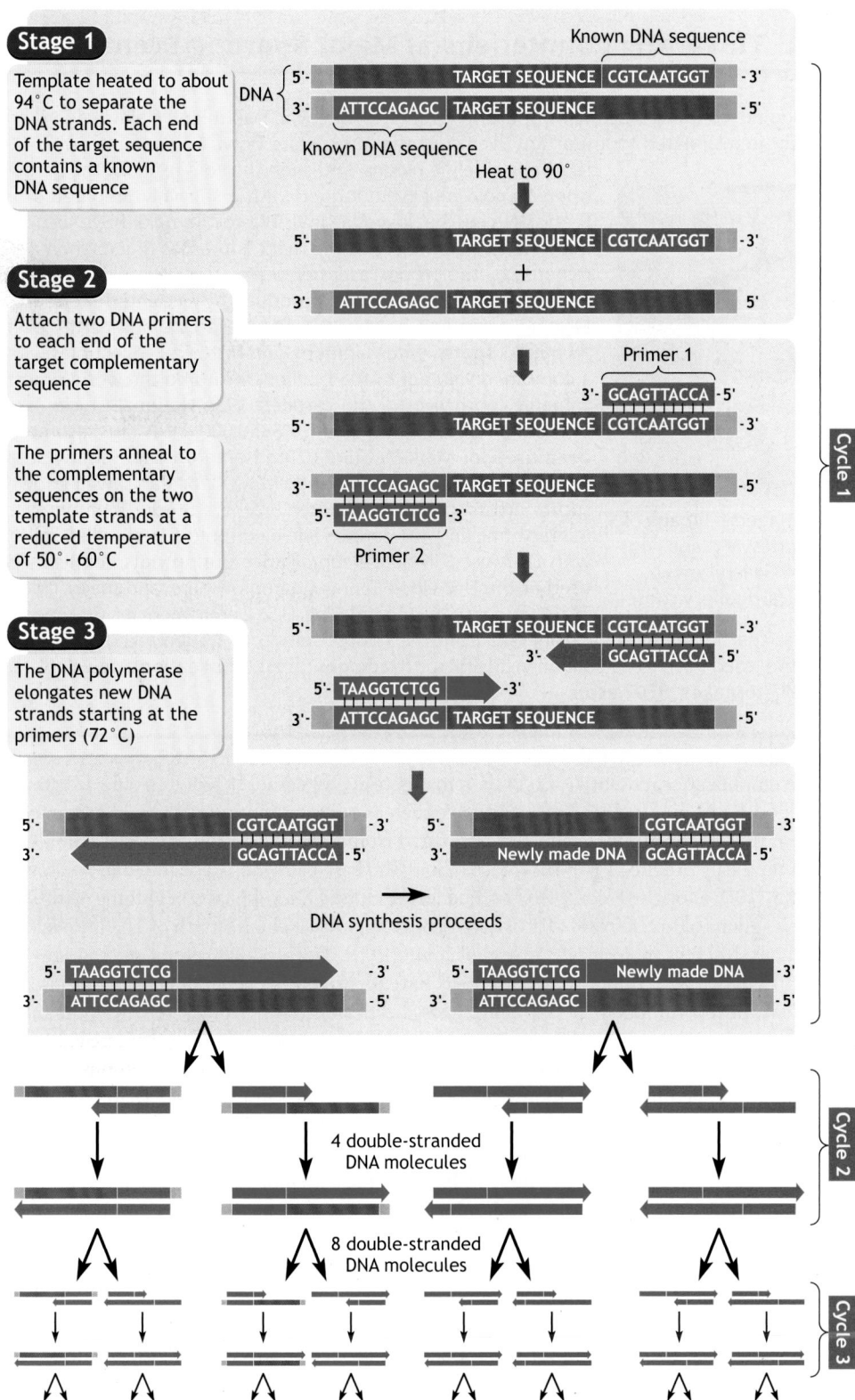

FIGURE 33.40 • Artificial DNA amplification using the PCR method. *Cycle 1.* Three stages during the first PCR cycle. *Cycle 2.* Second PCR cycle produces four double strands of DNA. *Cycle 3.* Third cycle produces eight double-stranded DNA molecules. Each succeeding cycle produces twice as much DNA as was produced in the previous cycle. Thirty cycles produce more than 1 billion DNA fragments. Several hours of production create hundreds of billions of copies. The thermocycler PCR apparatus controls reaction temperature to ensure that repeated replication cycles and separation occur systematically on a preset schedule.

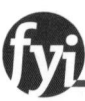

Thwarting Counterfeits at Major Sporting Events

DNA tagging continues at major sporting events to uncover fraudulent claims regarding important items related to important events. At the 2013 Super Bowl, for example, over 100

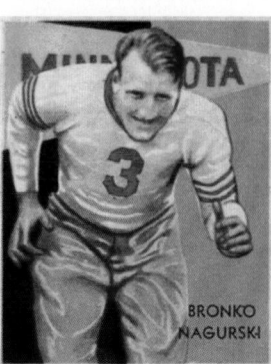

Bronco Nagerski (Image of card courtesy Vintage Football Card Gallery, **www. footballcardgallery.com**)

footballs, sideline pylons, and even the coin used for the game-opening coin toss were tagged with a specially prepared synthetic DNA ink that leaves an invisible-to-the-naked-eye security mark (**www.psadna.com**). The mark fluoresces green when illuminated by the proper laser frequency. The DNA ink has a 1-in-33 trillion chance of being reproduced by counterfeiters. This tagging procedure has been used to examine and certify over 18 million sports, entertainment, and historical collectibles with a combined value of over $1 billion, including the world's most valuable football card, the certified 1935 National Chicle card of Bronko Nagurski that sold for $350,000. DNA tags also have been used for Mark McGuire's 70th homerun ball, Sammy Sosa autographed baseballs, Super Bowl XXXV artifacts, well-known sports artists' paintings, Warner Brothers Studio memorabilia, military tracking for counterfeit electronic parts, pellets filled with DNA used in police surveillance during riots, tennis balls used at the U.S. Open Tennis Championships, and major clothing manufacturer apparel. The U.S. Department of Commerce estimates that losses to U.S. businesses from the counterfeiting of trademarked consumer products exceed $200 to 250 billion yearly (**http://trade.gov/press/publications/newsletters/ita_0507/stopfakes_0507.asp**).

The amplification potential for PCR remains truly awesome. It requires only 1/10th of one-millionth of a liter (0.1 μL) of a substance such as saliva or another body fluid or tissue to prove that the genetic sample's sequence originated from a specific person or species. The PCR method can easily produce 1 g of substance (about 500 base pairs long), equal to one-millionth of a gram (10^6), enough to completely sequence or clone DNA. In fact, beginning with less than a picogram (0.000 000 000 001 or 10^{12} g) of DNA with a chain length of 10,000 nucleotides (about 100,000 molecules), in several hours PCR can produce several micrograms of DNA (10^{11} molecules). Interestingly, scientists have identified the genetic blueprint of insects trapped within 80-million-year-old amber (fossilized pine resin) from a miniscule amount of DNA, using present-day insects to "match" the DNA sequences. In a controversial report published in *Nature* (October 2000), scientists reported reviving a bacterium (spore) from a drop of fluid trapped for 250 million years in a crystal of rock salt excavated 1850 feet below the earth's surface. In extinct fossils, on the other hand, not enough DNA sequences exist for cloning because the DNA decomposes significantly every 5000 years. Although some gene fragments may survive, cloning a "Jurassic Park" prehistoric monster falls outside the realm of possibility with today's available molecular paleoarcheology technologies. With the steps outlined in "FYI: Five Steps to Cloning an Extinct Mammal," advocates of cloning prehistoric or extinct animals believe the time will come when molecular techniques will be sufficiently advanced to accomplish what today is not possible.

In forensic medicine, a single hair salvaged from a crime scene can be matched for its DNA sequence to hair samples from a suspect or victim (**www.ncjrs.gov/pdffiles1/nij/bc000614.pdf**). When a PCR-generated DNA sequence matches the original DNA template strand sequence, chances of misidentifying the true suspect become almost infinitesimal against a coincidental DNA match. In fact, if an individual's known DNA profile matches the DNA profile from the crime scene, the probability is 82 billion to 1 that the crime scene DNA comes from that person!

Paternity cases routinely involve DNA analysis using PCR techniques such as DNA fingerprinting **autoradiography** to identify parental offspring correctly (**Fig. 33.41**). In the figure's example, the DNA from suspected fathers 1 and 2 did not match the known marker DNA from the child; thus father 3, with an exact banding match, was deemed the biologic

Paternity: fatherhood

Autoradiography: process that produces an image (autoradiograph) on a photographic film placed flat on an electrophoresis gel; shows the position of radioactive molecules "transferred" to the gel

father. The control DNA from a known source verifies the validity of the test procedures. The many variations of the PCR method allow researchers to produce hybrid genes with desirable (or undesirable) traits. Fusing DNA segments from different biologic specimens "transferred" to the gel opens a tremendous avenue to study genetic variation in cells and tissues. It also elucidates how "errors" in specific gene sequences relate to diseases and how genetic engineering can combat them.

Five Steps to Cloning an Extinct Mammal

In 1999, French polar explorers unearthed a 23,000-lb block of permafrost containing the remains of a woolly mammoth (*Mammuthus primigenius*) in Siberia. Nine years later, researchers sequenced the nuclear genome of an artist's rendering of this extinct mammoth (**www.nature. com/nature/journal/v456/n7220/abs/nature07446.html**). This possibility led a number of genetic research facilities worldwide to propose extracting DNA from the soft tissues of the extinct creature with the goal to clone it back to life if they could find sufficient DNA material

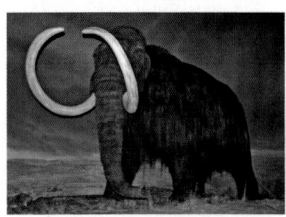 from the cell's nucleus for cloning. In 2012, a subsequent expedition uncovered the remains of another woolly mammoth at a depth of 5 to 6 m (16 to 20 ft) in a tunnel dug by locals searching for mammoth bones (**www.csmonitor.com/Science/2012/0912/ Pleistocene-Park-Scientists-edge-closer-to-cloning-woolly- mammoth**). Unfortunately, little soft tissue and bone remained (with too little quality DNA) to give cloning a chance for success. Nonetheless, had sufficient DNA been available, scientists most likely would have used the following five-step procedure to clone a 40,000-year-old late Pleistocene woolly mammoth from "de-extinction." (see Figure 33.44 for the steps used to clone Dolly the sheep [**www.animalresearch.info/en/medical-advances/151/ cloning-dolly-the-sheep/**]):

Step 1. *Obtain a DNA sample*: Find cells from the extinct animal's internal tissues, skin, bones, teeth, or hair, with sufficient, extractable "undegraded" DNA. This also might include DNA from stuffed museum specimens, or animals preserved in alcohol at the time of their death. For extinct animals, sufficient DNA material must be available from the cell's nucleus for analysis.

Step 2. *Rebuild genome*: Using the genome of a related living animal, reassemble the extinct animal's DNA.

Step 3. *Swap DNA*: Remove the ovarian eggs of the related animal and replace their nuclei with the restored genetic material from the extinct animal. The most difficult task requires finding well-preserved tissue with an undamaged gene.

Step 4. *Treat the eggs*: Fuse the nuclei with the eggs and trigger cell division by use of electric current or with chemicals.

Step 5. *Prepare for gestation by implanting the embryos*: Transfer the duplicating embryonic cells into the womb of the related animal for gestation until the surrogate mother gives birth to the previously extinct species.

Injection Experiments

Injection **transfection** performed in cultured cells refers to a microtechnique for introducing an outside (exogenous) DNA donor source into a recipient host. Injection of purified DNA with a known sequence of nucleotides for a particular gene presents a potentially desirable strategy to express an outcome trait in the host. Injection strategies have been useful in exercise physiology–related animal research. By injecting a gene with a particular trait into the egg of a mother, the new trait can be "turned on" in the offspring. This allows researchers to observe the effects of "knocking out" a section of one gene and replacing it with another segment to glean insight into the functional role of that gene product.

    Consider the example in **FIGURE 33.42** that illustrates the basic principle of microinjection applied to a mouse model. Immediately after the **gametes** join (one egg and one sperm), a microinjection technique using a thin glass needle inserts a target gene or **transgene** into the larger male **pronucleus** just before the cells fuse into a single egg. The egg is then surgically

Transfection: introduction of an external donor source of DNA into a recipient host

Gamete: egg or sperm

Transgene: genetic engineering technique that places a foreign gene in the cells of a different species

Pronucleus: fertilized egg containing the haploid egg or sperm nucleus

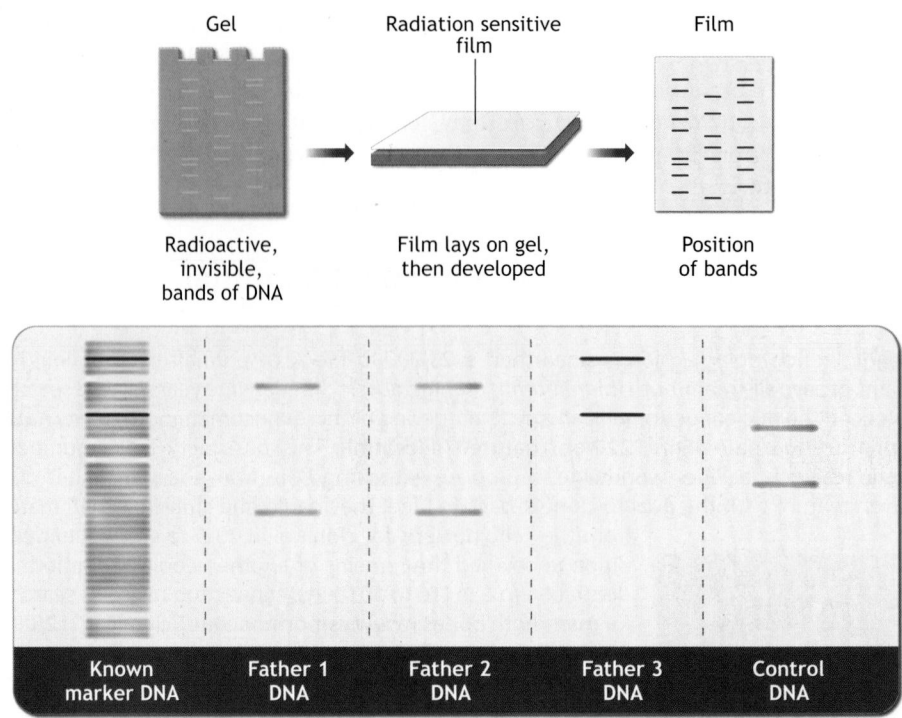

FIGURE 33.41 • DNA fingerprinting autoradiography compares DNA fragments after their separation by gel electrophoresis to identify the child's father. Matched patterns of DNA banding from different tissues or body fluids confirm the original DNA source. Specific restriction enzymes sever the DNA fragments at precise sites in the chain. Thus, snippets of DNA, known as RFLPs (restriction fragment-length polymorphisms), have different lengths and hence different molecular weights. A match between the known marker DNA and the sample (e.g., father 3) provides *prima facie* direct evidence that father 3 is the biologic father. As of July 2, 2009, 240 previously convicted criminals have been exonerated on the basis of DNA analysis of forensic evidence, often years following incarceration (**www.innocenceproject.org**). The Innocence Project, affiliated with the Benjamin N. Cardozo School of Law at Yeshiva University in New York, is a national litigation and public policy organization dedicated to exonerating wrongfully convicted people through DNA testing and reforming the criminal justice system to prevent future injustice. We recommend the following book for its riveting (but disturbing), frank discussion about the criminal justice system and the important role DNA fingerprinting should play to ensure that the accused have the opportunity to present objective evidence (data) about criminal wrongdoing: Scheck B, et al. *Actual Innocence: When Justice Goes Wrong and How to Make It Right*. New York: Doubleday, 2003.

Founder mice: original engineered mice (with one copy of a transgene) bred together to create transgenic animals

Heterozygous: having two different copies (alleles) of the same gene

Homozygous: having two identical copies (alleles) of the same gene

Knockin animal model: replacing a normal gene with a mutant gene (akin to "trading places" at a specific gene location or locus), and observing the effects on the offspring

Knockout animal model: specific gene(s) inactivated (disabled) by inserting a gene cassette that disrupts the coding sequence (or operation) linked to a specific target gene

harvested and implanted into the womb of a female rodent who serves as the "foster" mother. When the mother produces progeny, the newborns, referred to as **founder mice**, should carry a copy of the transgene on a single chromosome (i.e., be **heterozygous** for the transgene). When two founder mice breed, 25% of the progeny receive two copies of the transgene (i.e., are **homozygous** for the transgene), 50% have one transgene, and 25% have no transgenes. These percentages follow basic laws of inheritance discovered by geneticist Gregor Mendel. Researchers have used hundreds of strains of transgenic organisms created with the above procedures to study the metabolic and developmental characteristics of many diseases (**http://oba.od.nih.gov/oba/ibc/faqs/transgenicanimalfaqs-aug2011.pdf**).

Working with transgenic organisms has proved beneficial for experimenting with different genetic manipulations including mutated genes to shed light on possible mechanisms for disease conditions. Consider the following four ways researchers carry out such experiments:

1. Replacing a normal gene with a mutant gene ("trading places") and observing effects on the offspring (**knockin animal model**)
2. Inactivating or interrupting a normal gene's function and observing effects on the offspring (**knockout animal model**)

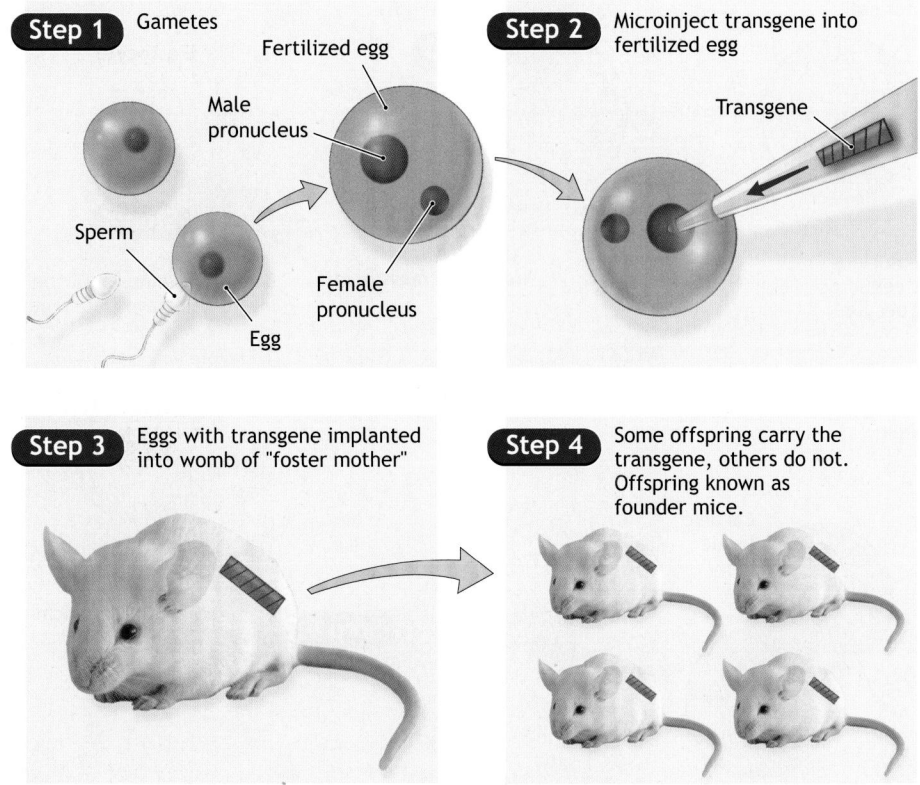

FIGURE 33.42 • Generalized procedure for creating transgenic offspring by injecting a target gene (transgene) into a fertilized egg. Some of the progeny, called founder mice, carry the transgene in their chromosomes, but the process may fail in others.

3. Adding a mutant gene and observing the combined effects of the mutant gene and normal gene on the offspring
4. Increasing the expression of a given protein by increasing the number of copies of a gene

Because of its relevance to exercise physiology, we take a closer look later in this chapter at strategies for disabling genes related to obesity using the elegant "knockout" or gene-targeting techniques. Similar techniques led to the 2007 Nobel Prize in Physiology or Medicine awarded to researchers Mario R. Capecchi 🖼 (1937–), Sir Martin J. Evans 🖼 (1941–), and Oliver Smithies 🖼 (1925–) for their groundbreaking advances related to powerful techniques for introducing specific gene modifications in mice by embryonic stem cells and DNA recombination in mammals (http://nobelprize.org/nobel_prizes/medicine/laureates/2007/press.html).

Cloning a Mammal

Genetics researchers use three methods to clone a mammal:

1. Somatic cell nuclear transfer (SCNT)
2. Roslin technique
3. Honolulu technique

SCNT Method. FIGURE 33.43 illustrates the eight-step SCNT technology, also called therapeutic cloning, to create stem cells from somatic cells (cells other than a sperm or egg cell). This modern technique had its genesis when experimental embryologist Hans Spemann 🖼 (1869–1938; 1935 Nobel Prize in Physiology or Medicine for discovering the "organizer effect" in embryonic development at the gastrula stage) with colleague Hilde Mangold (1898– 1924) pioneered microsurgical techniques while working with embryos (www.bioinfo.org. cn/book/Great%20Experiments/great30.htm; www.nature.com/nrm/journal/v7/n4/box/ nrm1855_BX1.html). Spemann and Mangold's histologic evidence from experiments with

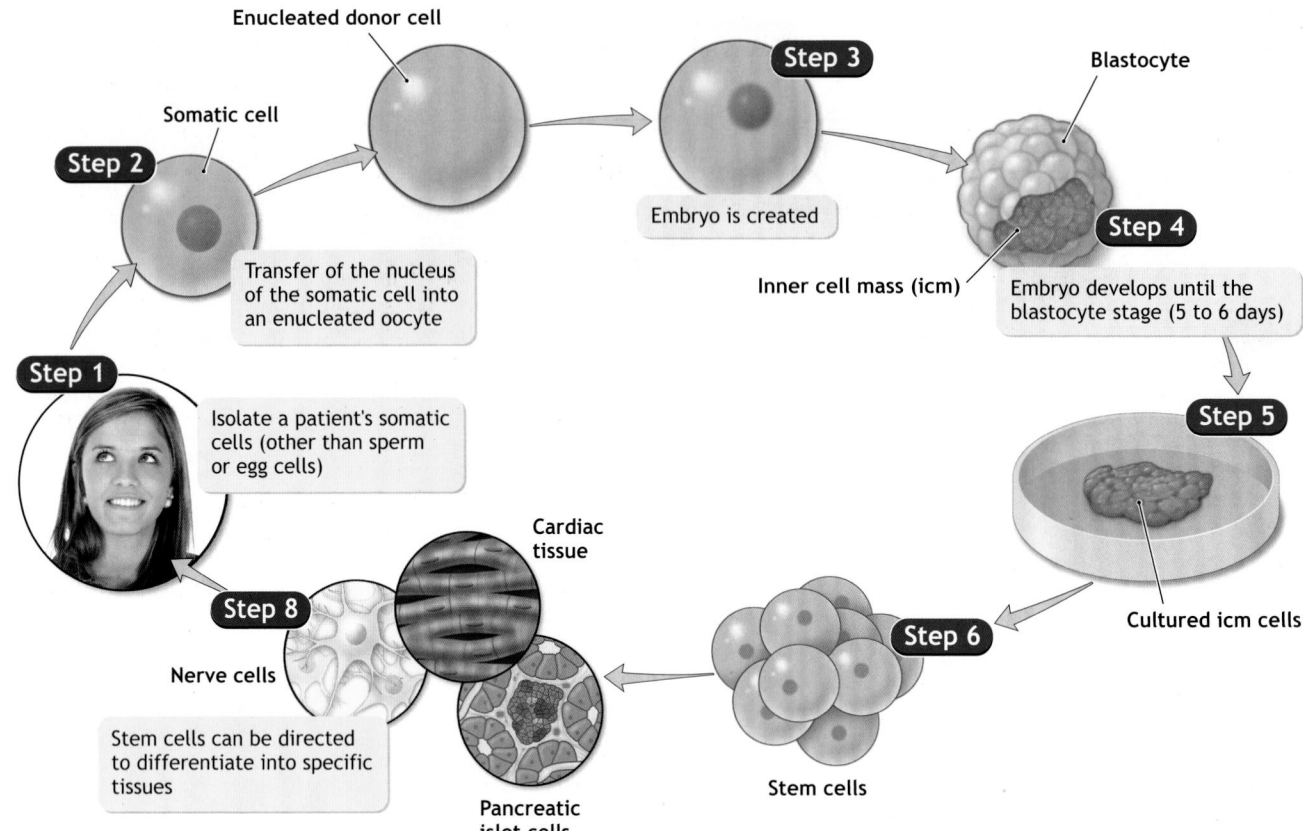

FIGURE 33.43 • Eight-step SCNT (somatic cell nuclear transfer) technology to create stem cells from somatic cells. Tissue rejection is eliminated with SCNT because the new grafts (tissues) are autologous (donor and host are the same individual). SCNT is not reproductive cloning because it uses only unfertilized egg cells to generate stem cells.[82] The International Society for Stem Cell Research provides additional details about SCNT (**www.isscr.org/public/therapeutic.htm**).

five manipulated embryos proved the reality of the concept of induction (interaction between two groups of cells in which one group directly influences the developmental fate of the other).

In the SCNT technique, two cells are required—a donor cell and an oocyte (an unfertilized egg cell early in development). Somatic cells are secured from the patient and prepared for the next step, the transfer of the nucleus of the cell with its DNA into an enucleated oocyte (not having a nucleus eliminates most of the genetic information). This process (step 3) prompts the cell to begin forming an embryo (a fertilized egg that can begin cell division). In step 4, the embryo undergoes cell division until it develops into the blastocyte stage, a mass of about 100 cells. At this stage of development, the mass remains a group of undifferentiated cells. The next phase of the process (step 5) separates the inner cell mass (ICM) from the cell by a microchemical technique called immunosurgery (using different chemicals to dislodge the ICM from the cell wall). The cultured ICMs produce pluripotent stem cells (step 6), the most versatile kinds of cells, with the potential to become different types of tissues (i.e., skin, brain, heart, muscle, kidney, bone, pancreas, intestine). In essence, stem cells are relatively unspecialized cells that have not yet differentiated into any specific type of tissue. Once the cells become differentiated (e.g., acquire the features of a specialized cell and develop into specific tissues), as shown in step 7, the new line of specialized cell types can be reintroduced into the patient. This begins the process of creating new tissues to replace or repopulate damaged or diseased tissues.

Roslin Method. In 1997, scientists at Edinburgh's Roslin Institute in Scotland (**www.roslin. ac.uk**) tapped the complete genetic library contained within the zygote (i.e., cell **totipotent** potentiality) to clone the Dorset sheep "Dolly." This milestone represented the first such viable intact donor derived from adult mammalian cells.[164] The researchers removed an unfertilized

Totipotent: the cell possesses the required genetic information or "blueprint" to form an intact organism

oocyte from an adult ewe and replaced its nucleus with the nucleus from a mammary gland cell of an adult sheep. They then implanted this egg in another ewe, producing the healthy offspring sheep. The idea behind the **nuclear transfer** experiment was to produce genetically engineered transgenic mammals inexpensively that could reliably produce large quantities of pharmaceuticals in their milk. A likely benefit would be large quantities of human proteins for drug synthesis to treat diseases such as cystic fibrosis, hemophilia, and emphysema, with potential benefits toward aging and cancer research. Milk produced from transgenic sheep, goats, and cattle can yield up to 40 g of protein per liter at relatively low cost. This circumvents the need to use purified, expensive blood to harvest protein, with risk of contamination from AIDS or hepatitis C. Proteins produced in human cell cultures have high cost and relatively low yields. Transgenetically produced proteins have application in the **nutraceutical** industry, **xenotransplantation**, animal models of disease, and cell therapy (www.sciencedirect.com/science/article/pii/S1359644605034525).

The first Dolly experiments represented a milestone in cloning technology, but not before unleashing a firestorm of criticism concerning ethical and scientific issues related to the possibilities of eventual experiments with human cloning. FIGURE **33.44** shows that Dolly possesses the same genes as the cells from the ewe's udder. The reproductive cell cycle developed normally following intermediate stages (keeping donor cells "**quiescent**" so that their DNA did not replicate or divide) until the early embryo developed. The researchers then transplanted the embryo into a receptive ewe. Following several hundred unsuccessful implants, Dolly was born from the implanted ewe and survived. Dolly subsequently gave birth through normal mating to produce six healthy lambs.

Honolulu Technique. This cloning technique, developed by researchers in Hawaii,[123] differs substantially from the SNCT and the Roslin methods (http://library.thinkquest.org/24355/data/details/media/honoluluanim.html). The Honolulu technique does not generate clones either by injection or fusion of embryonic or fetal cells or by fusion of adult cells (the technique used to create Dolly). In contrast, adult mouse cells created new mice genetically identical to the parent mouse. Using a special pipette, the donor nucleus was microinjected into an egg whose nucleus was previously removed. The resulting cells were cultured and placed into a surrogate mouse, allowing the clone to develop. By repeating the procedure, the team created second and third generations of cloned mice that genetically matched their sister/parent, sister/grandparent, and sister/great grandparent. The research succeeded in cloning mice from adult cells by using (1) a new method and (2) a new cell type able to repeat the procedure to produce clones of clones of clones—essentially creating identical mice born a generation or more apart. The Honolulu technique, in contrast to the SNCT and Roslyn methods, allows researchers to manipulate adult donor nuclei. The same Honolulu technique also produced three live male offspring from tail-tip cells. Two died shortly after birth, but the surviving clone developed normally and mated successfully, producing two healthy litters. The Honolulu technique shows that animals of either sex can be cloned with somatic cells used in the process.

Gene Knockout Technique

Mice provide a useful model to study genetic manipulations because of control afforded the experimental subjects and the environment, and the animal's shorter life span. For example, researchers can study a strain of normal-sized mice with black fur, obese mice with black fur, obese mice with white fur, and so on. Genetic "tampering" can verify whether the gene actually modulated the specific effect independent of its influence on fur color. Deactivating a gene(s) within the DNA known to produce an obese strain of mice should produce litters of normal-weight mice.

FIGURE **33.45** illustrates the five-step experimental strategy for creating a transgenic mouse with a knocked-out gene (www.princeton.edu/~achaney/tmve/wiki100k/docs/Gene_knockout.html).

Step 1. A DNA fragment receives a genetically modified gene (**gene cassette**, shown in purple), thus altering the target gene's usual nucleotide sequence.
Step 2. Growth of the cell culture produces one or more cell colonies containing the altered gene. Finding such a colony means the mutant gene altered the DNA fragment.

Nuclear transfer: DNA removed from an unfertilized egg and introduced into the nucleus of a specially prepared cell by an electrical pulse or chemical to fuse the two substances together to initiate their development

Nutraceutical: genetically engineered product that alters or modifies characteristics of a product or its byproduct

Xenotransplantation: transfer of organs or tissues from a donor of one species to a recipient of another; successful transplants require that the immune system of the recipient accept the donor organ successfully

Quiescent: having all but the most fundamental functions of a cell or group of cells stopped; in essence, with switched-off genes that define the special functions of the cell (i.e., restricting food supply or creating an unfavorable internal cellular environment)

Gene cassette: artificially constructed DNA segment containing a genetic marker with restriction sites at both ends of the nucleotide segment

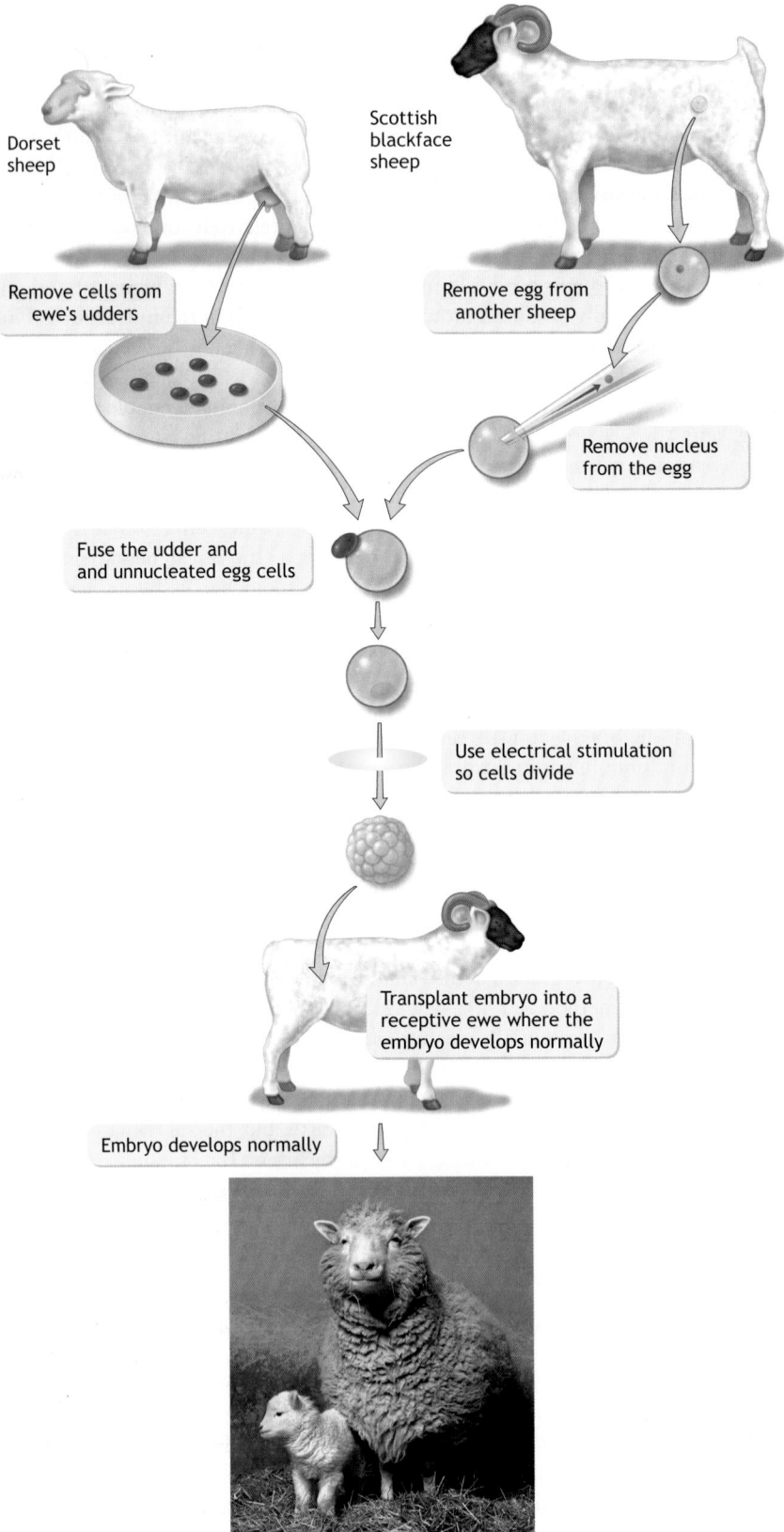

FIGURE 33.44 • Steps in cloning a mammal. Dorset sheep Dolly (*bottom photo*) has genes identical to those of the ewe that donated the original genes (Dorset sheep, *upper left*). Dolly, the first mammal to be cloned from adult DNA, was put down by lethal injection on February 14, 2003 (**www.ornl.gov/sci/techresources/Human_Genome/elsi/cloning.shtml**). Dolly suffered from lung cancer and crippling arthritis. The unnamed sheep from which Dolly was cloned died several years prior to Dolly's creation. (Photo of Dolly and her lamb Bonnie courtesy of The Roslin Institute, The University of Edinburgh).

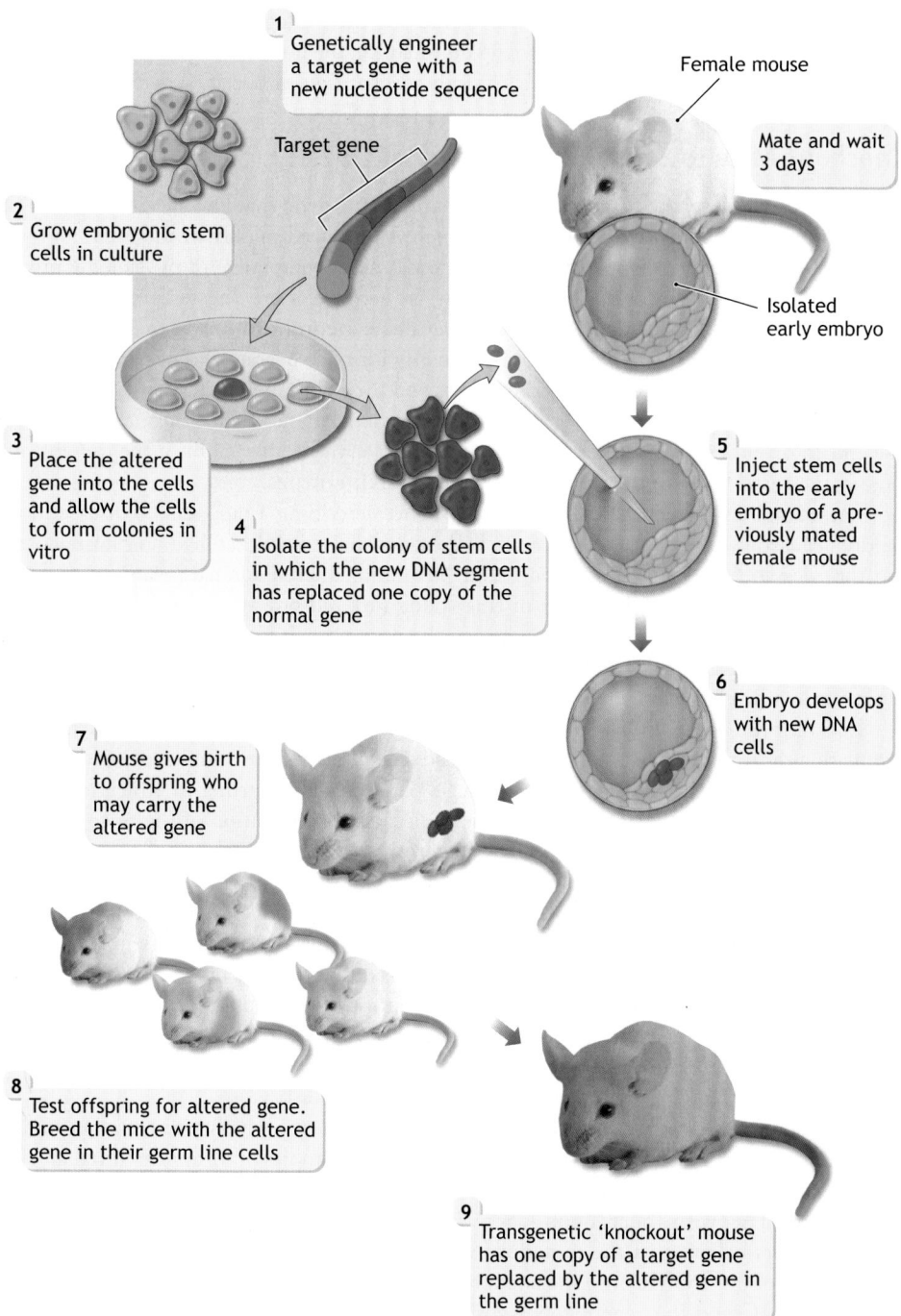

1 Genetically engineer a target gene with a new nucleotide sequence

Target gene

2 Grow embryonic stem cells in culture

3 Place the altered gene into the cells and allow the cells to form colonies in vitro

4 Isolate the colony of stem cells in which the new DNA segment has replaced one copy of the normal gene

Female mouse

Mate and wait 3 days

Isolated early embryo

5 Inject stem cells into the early embryo of a previously mated female mouse

6 Embryo develops with new DNA cells

7 Mouse gives birth to offspring who may carry the altered gene

8 Test offspring for altered gene. Breed the mice with the altered gene in their germ line cells

9 Transgenetic 'knockout' mouse has one copy of a target gene replaced by the altered gene in the germ line

FIGURE 33.45 • Creating a transgenic mouse with a knockout gene. Transgenic mice represent a unique tool for understanding how interactions between individual genes and environmental stressors affect human health and disease.

Step 3. Inject the genetically altered cells into the developing embryo of a previously mated female mouse.

Step 4. Place the developing embryo into a normal **pseudopregnant** mouse that gives birth to a litter in which most progeny possess cells with the altered gene.

Step 5. Mating two offspring with the mutant gene can produce an offspring with the mutant gene on each of two chromosomes. The grafted transgene also can be incorporated into the mice from another strain of mouse into a totally different organism.

Pseudopregnant: ovulation induced by sterile copulation

If the original gene alteration inactivated the function of one of the genes, then the transgenic mouse inherits the mutant gene that replaced or "knocked out" the primary target gene. This strain of mice can be reliably bred to produce progeny with the foreign gene now

Germ line: cell lineage consists of mature reproductive germ cells (sperm, egg)

permanently part of their **germ line** DNA. In studying the etiology of cancer, for example, two transplanted oncogenes (*ras* and *myc*) remain dominant in the host and always produce a mouse with cancer. The same strategy can apply to study mechanisms of obesity described below.

Knockout Mice to Study Mechanisms of Obesity

Proopiomelanocortin (POMC): precursor of neurotransmitters (endorphins) and hormones (melanocortin peptides), whose roles include pigmentation, adrenocortical function, food intake and fat storage, and immune and neural functions

Neurohormone: hormone formed by neurosecretory cells and liberated by nerve impulses (e.g., norepinephrine)

Researchers have developed transgenic mice that lack the gene that encodes for the complex molecule **proopiomelanocortin** (**POMC**), which is produced mainly in the brain and skin. POMC, a precursor of melanocortin peptides, possesses a wide range of physiologic properties that include roles in food intake and body fat accumulation. The researchers originally intended to study POMC-deficient mice to evaluate **neurohormone** signaling and CNS functioning. However, their strain of transgenic mutant mice overate and became obese, with altered pigmentation that produced yellowish fur on their abdomen instead of typical brownish-black fur. They also showed significantly less adrenal tissue than littermates of normal size and color. Figure 33.46A shows that by 2 mo of age, the body weight of the mutant mice steadily increased to twice the weight of their normal littermates.

These findings coincided with a previous report describing a rare genetic disease in two children caused by a mutant POMC gene.[84] These red-haired children had no melanocortins, and they developed severe obesity soon after birth and suffered adrenal insufficiency. Figure 33.46D shows the rapid weight gain of this young girl and boy, whose weight far exceeded typical age standards. The connection between the mice and children was striking; functional characteristics caused by the POMC gene mutation in humans paralleled those in the transgenic mice with yellow pigmentation and obesity.

Injecting the obese, POMC-deficient mice with the melanocortin peptide, melanocyte-stimulating–hormone agonist (–MSH) produced a significant body weight loss within 1 day; within 1 wk, body weight decreased by about 38% and declined further to 48% after the second week (Fig. 33.46B). A reversal also occurred in the pigmentation of the mice, and their fur lost its yellowish tinge. Within 10 days of terminating –MSH "therapy," the mice began to regain lost weight, reaching preinjection weight in another 14 days. Their yellow fur color in the ventral and dorsal sites also reappeared. In contrast, –MSH injections and subsequent cessation of treatment produced no effect on body mass or fur pigmentation in normal control littermates. The researchers explained that weight loss during treatment exceeded expectations from the energy-balance equation. This occurred, although the mutant mice ate significantly more food daily than the control mice (35.7 vs. 24.2 g; Fig. 33.46C). Because fat cells contain melanocortin receptors, and these receptors induce **lipolysis**, melanocortin-based drugs may eventually prove helpful as therapeutic agents to combat obesity.

Lipolysis: splitting up (hydrolysis) or chemical decomposition of triglyceride

Leptin: protein hormone involved with appetite and fat storage

Interestingly, injections of MSH analogues also reduced excess body fat in another strain of obese transgenic mice deficient in the hormone **leptin**.[63] In studies of 87 unrelated Italian obese children and adolescents, three new mutations were identified within the POMC signal peptide (substitution of Ser with Thr at codon 7; Ser with Leu at codon 9; Arg with Gly at codon 236).[41] The researchers believe that the mutations in codons 7 and 9 of the signal peptide alter the translocation of pre-POMC into the endoplasmic reticulum and, therefore, explain the linkage between POMC and the genetic predisposition to obesity, a view shared by others studying this association. Further studies of genetic variations in the POMC coding region provide new insights concerning the etiology of obesity.[13,46] Ongoing experiments with transgenic animal and human models help researchers understand the etiology of obesity and its treatment.[65]

Antisense RNA: RNA complementary in sequence to mRNA, thus capable of base pairing with it by using the nontemplate strand of DNA to transcribe RNA from it. Analogous to two original strands in DNA base pairing with each other. In practice, synthesis of an oligonucleotide hybridizes a mutant mRNA sequence, stopping its translation into protein

Extremes in obesity have been linked to DNA polymorphisms in the translated portion of the leptin (*LEP*) gene.[97] Leptin-regulated endocannabinoids (marijuana-like substances naturally produced in the brain) stimulate appetite and play a role in food regulation as a component in the leptin-signaling cascades.[42] In the not too distant future, excess body fat may provide a ready source of stem cells from which to create replacement tissues (e.g., bone, muscle, cartilage) for diseased or damaged ones.[171] Incorporating a person's own stem cells would avoid rejection of transplanted tissue and circumvent moral objections concerning the use of human embryonic stem cells.

Newer approaches also apply genetic techniques using **antisense RNA** to suppress expression of a target gene as a way to assess gene function. By incompletely blocking the function of knockout genes, researchers should be able to uncover unexpected roles for sequenced genes.[58,148,166]

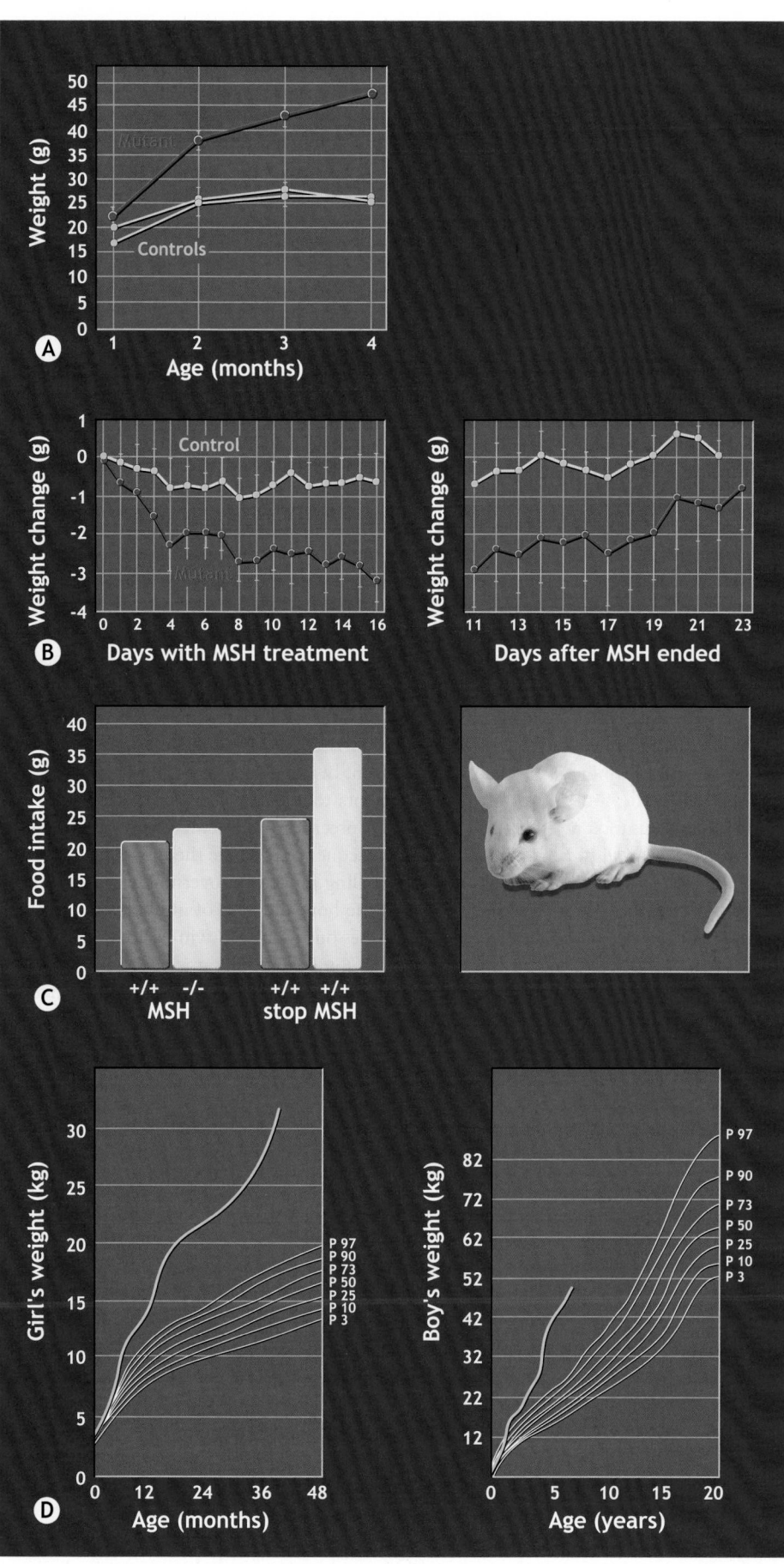

FIGURE 33.46 • POMC-deficient transgenic mice provide new clues to obesity. **(A)** Body weight gain in mutant and control mice. **(B)** Change in body weight with and without treatment. **(C)** Differences in food intake with and without treatment. **(D)** Extreme weight gain in a young boy and girl with the POMC mutation. The white lines represent growth curves for children representing the 3rd through 97th percentile (p). (Data from A, B, and C modified from Yaswen L, et al. Obesity in the mouse model of proopiomelanocortin deficiency responds to peripheral melanocortin. *Nat Med* 1999;5:1066. Data in D from Krude H, et al. Severe early-onset obesity, adrenal insufficiency and red hair pigmentation caused by POMC mutations in humans. *Nat Genet* 1998;19:155.)

The field of proteomics using sophisticated imaging software and molecular scanners integrated with protein chemistry techniques allows researchers to study how proteins expressed in a genome act in complex, biologic processes.[43,60]

For example, scientists have developed an ion channel "nanopore" technique (www.ncbi.nlm.nih.gov/pubmed/21138270) that discriminates among almost identical DNA molecules that differ by only one base pair or one nucleotide.[155] This level of differentiation permits highly accurate molecular identification to unscramble intricacies of gene expression and ultimately to develop strategies that target mutagens. Research with 380 Europeans with early-onset and morbid adult obesity and 1416 age-matched, normal-weight controls identified three new genetic loci for obesity (*NPC1*, endosomal/lysosomal Niemann-Pick C1 gene; near *MAF*, encoding the transcription factor c-MAF; near *PTER*, phosphotriesterase-related gene).[109]

HUMAN PERFORMANCE RESEARCH

Molecular biologists studying physical activity and exercise training seek to decipher signaling pathways by which genes transcribe the effects of a mechanical stressor and resultant phenotypic expression. For example, resistance training applies muscular overload of the biceps as a mechanical stressor, while increasing upper-arm strength and size represent expression of a phenotype characteristic. Crucial, unanswered questions concern "where" and "how" skeletal overload translates into newly acquired "strength" and muscle hypertrophy. The answers likely reside within signal transduction pathways leading from cell surface receptors to the nucleus, resulting in transcription of genes and subsequent protein synthesis. Scientists study the intricacies of how different signaling processes interact, integrate, and differentiate to produce function and consequences, and possibly even share common intermediates.[6]

Consider a seemingly simple series of movements such as releasing the bowstring when shooting an arrow and the highly complex maneuvers of a triple back somersault from a 10-m diving platform. The movement patterns of both activities require precise coordination and integration of neural stimulation and muscular action. In turn, each component of the movement demands specific timing and force requirements to achieve a desired outcome. At the molecular level, thousands of enzymes govern such precision requirements, each turning on and off at precisely the right time and in the correct sequence to make the movement successful (or unsuccessful). A better understanding of signaling processes governing enzyme activity between stressors and genes may someday explain the how and why of individual differences in human movement capacities. For example, why does one identical twin perform better than the other twin in a particular activity? Identical twins come from the same genetic pool, so one would expect few differences in performance between them, but this is not the case. Even if twins had identical experiences in mastering the mechanics of an activity, from practice time to coaching, their performance levels would differ. Fractions of a second or tenths of a centimeter often mean the difference between victory and second place—whether the performers are twins or Olympic-caliber athletes. A combination of biochemical individuality and known allelic variations should enable researchers to determine optimal nutritional profiles (i.e., targeted doses of vitamins, minerals, and other nutrients) to create personalized comprehensive lifestyle prescriptions tailored to the needs of each person.[48] A tremendous challenge also exists among the disciplines to determine the molecular basis of disease expression, as, for example, for type 2 diabetes or cardiovascular diseases.[3,59,86,111,152]

When reduced to the most fundamental level, all physical activities, or aspects of all life, ultimately depend on the multiplicity of molecular events that turn genes on and off. The new generation of molecular exercise scientists must expand research to uncover how different signaling mechanisms regulate transcriptional, translational, and posttranslational events. Elucidation of these mechanisms will enable scientists to manipulate experimental variables to answer questions related to our field. For example, how does long-term exercise intensity and duration alter levels of a specific mRNA or an upstream signaling molecule such as Ca^{2+}, an intermediary involved in multiple signal transduction cascades?[50] A simple muscle contraction corresponds to a 100-fold increase in intramuscular Ca^{2+} concentration (from 107 to 105 M). Some researchers believe that the huge Ca^{2+} influx, which coincides with myofilament cross-bridge cycling (see Chapter 18), serves as an important signaling messenger that links a muscle's function to transcriptional dynamics.[6] Other exercise-related physiologic regulators of transcription include hypoxia and cellular oxidative stress (or redox). The hypoxic state affects production of erythropoietin (*EPO* gene) and **glucose transporter-1** (**GLUT-1**). Understanding the functional characteristics of how genes operate under hypoxic conditions will provide key information about oxygen delivery to cells and ultimately its use via citric acid cycle reactions, electron transport, and ATP synthesis associated with oxidative energy transformations.[66]

Oxygen free radicals and reducing agents (i.e., antioxidants) also modulate transcription.[143] In Chapter 6, we discuss how the mitochondrion's reduction of oxygen to form water serves as the final common step in ATP synthesis. Imprecise coupling of this pathway forms free radicals of oxygen. Diverse antioxidants within skeletal muscle then scavenge and quench most of these **reactive oxygen species** (**ROS**).[25,132,136,140] However, during high-intensity endurance exercise when aerobic metabolism increases 15- to 20-fold, ROS form in greater numbers to possibly produce damaging effects similar to those produced by lipid peroxidation.[62,83,92,146]

The protein **thioredoxin** (reduces oxidized proteins) helps to balance a cell's redox state during energy metabolism and also appears to affect transcriptional activity.[67] Determining how ROS influence transcription will pave the way for improved understanding of long-term health effects (or potential risks) of aerobic-type activities. Researchers have discovered that endurance training nearly doubles mitochondrial protein and mitochondrial mass.[116] This means that having a robust experimental model (endurance exercise/training) from which to study gene expression will surely lead to important discoveries about the essence of endurance exercise effects and adaptations per se. In fact, experiments have already described alterations in mRNA gene expression with long-term electrical stimulation,[167] including exercise effects related to muscle mitochondria,[16,75] and molecular-related alterations in skeletal muscle and muscle fiber type.[52] Microgravity's effects on gene expression in skeletal muscle provide a fruitful area for further study.[9,72,100,102,137,146,168]

Studies of identical twins attempt to explain why one individual tends to participate regularly in sports and physical activities while the other twin shows little inclination to remain physically active. As part of the HERITAGEFamily Study,[32,76] a search for genes related to body composition changes following 20 wk of exercise training from 364 sib-pairs from 99 Caucasian families provided evidence of linkage of fat-free mass and insulin-like growth factor 1 genes, including gene sites for BMI and fat mass, and plasma leptin levels with the low-density lipoprotein receptor gene.

Three viable areas for application of molecular biology research to the sport sciences involve various gene therapy techniques (viral and nonviral delivery strategies):

1. To treat acute and chronic musculoskeletal injuries such as muscle tears, cartilage defects, and tendon ruptures
2. To reconstruct ligaments, osseous nonunions, and meniscus tears
3. To transplant tissue or genetic material

One hopes that inserting relevant genes directly into target tissues or systemically via vectors into the bloodstream will increase the probability of successful therapy and accelerated recuperation.[101] Researchers in the molecular biology sciences are just now beginning to track down the flaws in human DNA that cause debilitating musculoskeletal disease, as for example, those involved with lumbar disks.[5,99] One must temper such expectations by perhaps justifiable concerns that genetic engineering's potential benefits could also result in "tinkering" with issues related to doping and drug testing.

New techniques of molecular and cell biology—such as nuclear magnetic resonance–detected carbon-14, nitrogen-15, and hydrogen exchange—now make it possible to study aspects of protein structure and functions.[55] For example, the computer-generated structural model of a protein in **Figure 33.47** shows color-coded regions in a computer-generated model of high- and low-stability constants when binding to another molecule such as **monoclonal antibody** D1.3. The *red region* that interacts directly with D1.3 shows the highest stability; the *yellow* and *blue* regions remain unaffected by D1.3 binding. Thus, high and low regions of stability within a protein molecule may relate differently to its functional associations with other molecules. The important implication for a fusion product from a protein synthesis is that sites within the conformational structure of a molecule may serve dual functions for cancer cells and antibodies, depending on the molecule's configuration and structural residues.

Crucial questions concern what "signals" control cooperation among different molecules and whether changes occur selectively in some regions within the protein molecule proteins and not others. For example, the following question remains unanswered: What

Glucose transporter-1 (GLUT1): facilitates glucose transport across the plasma membrane independently of the hormone insulin

Reactive oxygen species (ROS): oxygen free radical formed from imprecise coupling during oxygen's reduction to water in the final stage of electron transport–oxidative phosphorylation

Thioredoxin: protein involved in oxidation–reduction reactions to balance the cell's redox state

Monoclonal antibody: pure antibody of a single type that only recognizes a single antigen; produced in cell culture

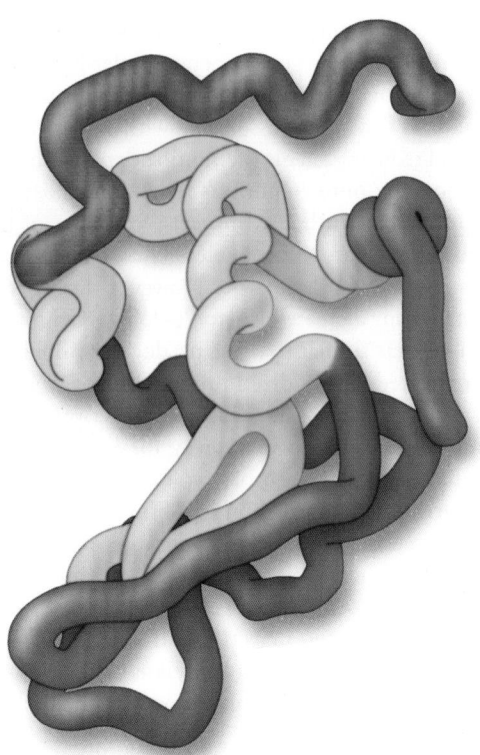

FIGURE 33.47 • Computer-generated model of hen egg white lysozyme (HEWL) color-coded to show regions of high (*red*) and lower (*blue* and *yellow*) stability constants when binding to monoclonal antibody D1.3 (along the red area). Lysozyme, discovered by Sir Alexander Fleming (1881–1955) 5 years before he discovered penicillin, protects against bacterial infection. This small enzyme, the first ever to have its structure solved, attacks the bacterial protective cell wall. Some bacteria build a protective outer layer of carbohydrate chains interlocked by short peptide strands, which brace their delicate plasma membranes against their high intracellular osmotic pressure. Lysozyme breaks these carbohydrate chains, destroying the cell membrane's structural integrity, and the bacteria burst under their own internal pressure. The lysozyme from hen egg whites protects proteins and fats that nourish the developing chick. (Figure constructed using GRASP software (**http://wiki.c2b2.columbia.edu/honiglab_public/index.php/Software:GRASP**). Dr. Ernesto Freire. Professor of Biology and Biophysics and Director of the Biocalorimetry Center, Johns Hopkins University, Baltimore.)

contributions do genetics and environmental factors make in affecting the complex etiology of many common and debilitating diseases?[23] The model describing gene–exercise interaction in **FIGURE 33.48** affects health status indirectly by altering gene expression that itself affects intermediate phenotypes and disease outcome.[147] In addition, increased physical activity through formal exercise and training influence health.[158] Often, indirect evidence can link a particular disease state with an outcome variable.

the**Point**   Appendix M, available online at http://thepoint.lww.com/mkk8e, contains a list of selected references for human and animal research and molecular biology from 2009 through 2013.

In the first comprehensive examination of strenuous physical activity and the risk of developing Parkinson's disease, Harvard researchers reported that men who exercised regularly and vigorously early in their adult life had a lower risk for developing Parkinson's disease than sedentary counterparts.[33] The most physically active men at the start of the study cut their risk of developing Parkinson's by 50% compared with male study participants who were the least physically active. Men who reported having regularly engaged in strenuous physical activity in early adult life cut their risk by 60% compared with those who did not. Among women, strenuous activity in the early adult years was linked to a lower risk of Parkinson's, but the relationship was not statistically significant, and no clear association existed between physical activity later in life and Parkinson risk.

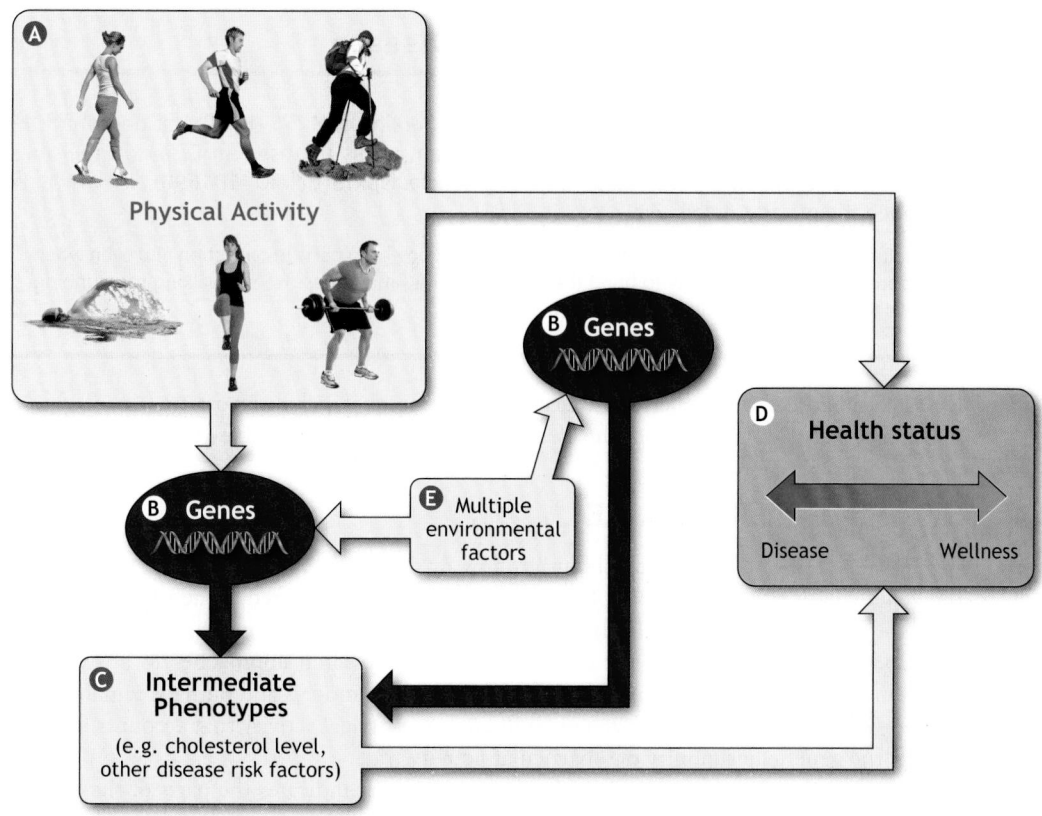

FIGURE 33.48 • Model of gene–exercise interaction, intermediate phenotype, and multiple environmental factor interactions in determining health status along the disease–wellness continuum. (Adapted from Bray MS. Genomics, genes, and environmental interaction: the role of exercise. *J Appl Physiol* 2000;88:788.) *Note*: The journal *Medicine & Science in Sports & Exercise* now publishes an annual update of the human gene map for performance- and health-related fitness phenotypes. The inaugural issue (Rankinen T, et al. *Med Sci Sports Exerc* 2001;33:855) contained specific reference to genes and their location published through December 2000; the most recent update highlights research through 2007 (Bray MS, et al. The human gene map for performance and health-related fitness phenotypes: the 2006–2007 update. *Med Sci Sports Exerc* 2009;41:35.)

A recent randomized control trial assessed the effects of progressive resistance exercise (PRE) on Parkinson's disease motor function scales.[37] The study compared 6-, 12-, 18-, and 24-mo outcomes of patients with Parkinson's disease who received either PRE only or a modified program (MP) of stretching, balance, and strengthening exercise. Pairs of patients matched by sex and off-medication scores on the motor subscale of the Unified Parkinson Disease Rating Scale (UPDRS-III) were randomly assigned to the two interventions. Patients exercised 2 days a week for 24 mo at a gym. A personal trainer directed both weekly sessions for the first 6 mo and 1 weekly session after 6 mo. The primary outcome was the off-medication UPDRS-III score. Of 51 patients, 20 in the PRE group and 18 in the MP group completed the trial. At 24 mo, the mean off-medication UPDRS-III score decreased significantly more with PRE than with MP (mean difference, −7.3 points; 95% confidence interval, −11.3 to −3.6; $p < 0.001$). PRE training statistically and clinically reduced UPDRS-III scores compared with MP training and is recommended as a useful adjunct therapy to improve Parkinsonian motor signs.

A crucial challenge to information generated from this type of research requires resolution: Scientists must connect the evidence about the interaction of the genes in Parkinson's with physical inactivity throughout life.[29,126] This is true for all of the other major diseases and the increasingly suggestive role for a genetic basis of physical activity.[53] A review of the topic posits that dopamine receptor 1 (*Drd1*; five different lines of research suggest *Drd1*'s involvement in physical activity regulation) and nescent helix loop helix (Nhlh2; through its effect on β-endorphin production and interaction with melanocortin-4 receptor) serve as excellent candidate genes for regulation of physical activity, and the scientific rush to understand inactivity-induced diseases.

 **Discoverer of Parkinson's Disease**

In 1817, British surgeon and paleontologist James Parkinson (1755–1824) first described this degenerative disorder of the central nervous system in his treatise, "An Essay on the Shaking Palsy" (**http://neuro.psychiatryonline.org/article.aspx?articleID=101698**), in which he described the malady as follows:

> Involuntary tremulous motion, with lessened muscular power, in parts not in action and even when supported; with a propensity to bend the trunk forwards, and to pass from a walking to a running pace: the senses and intellects being uninjured.

Research supports several other potential candidate genes that include myostatin (*Mstn*), glucose transporter 4 (*Slc2a4*), and 3-phosphoadenosine 5-phosphosulfate synthase (*Papss2*).

SHAPING THE FUTURE

A general systems genetics research design flow or schema has been proposed to determine the genetic basis of a phenotype.[90] Four questions must be answered sequentially in helping to shape the future of molecular biology research in kinesiology and the exercise sciences (**FIG. 33.49**). The box at the right illustrates different research approaches to answer each question of interest. For Question 1, research with mouse models and humans remains fairly robust—it supports a significant genetic influence on physical activity that accounts for 20 to 92% of the genetic heritability of a particular activity trait.

For Question 2, prior research with genome mapping indicates the parts of the genome associated with the particular trait investigated. These mapped genomic regions, known as quantitative trait loci (QTL), can narrow the focus of possible gene candidates related to physical activity. According to the author, QTL can be categorized as single-effect where the genetic factors arising from QTL act individually on physical activity, or as epistatic, where genetic factors in the QTL must work interactively with genetic factors in other genomic locations before they can have an effect on the phenotype. The answer to Question 3, the identification of the involved genes, has been more problematical. Only two genes have been positively identified with enough scientific support evidence from different lines of research related to physical activity (*Drd2* and *Nhlh2*, mentioned previously). The final question "How do the genes work to regulate the phenotype?" will require considerably more cooperative research from many disciplines before clear answers emerge.

To students with a keen interest in the genetics and molecular biology of physical activity (and inactivity), the future path to discovery remains wide open and should be pursued. The decade ahead is rich with topics for investigation, and we encourage faculty and their students to pursue similar lines of scientific investigation. We believe the kinesiological sciences have a shared responsibility with other basic and applied disciplines to contribute to our understanding of these exciting new areas of interest.

We anticipate that during the next decade, researchers from diverse disciplines will continue to cross boundaries to solve challenging questions in exercise physiology. We are encouraged that the University of Aberdeen in Scotland, to our knowledge, was the first program to offer an MSc in Molecular Exercise Physiology (**www.abdn.ac.uk/sms/postgraduate/molecular-exercise-physiology.shtml**), where the MSc program, including Diploma and Certificate programs, represented an important new subfield in sports science that focuses on genetics and signal transduction related to exercise. In this program, molecular exercise physiologists aim to identify the genetic determinants of human performance on a molecular level and characterize the mechanisms responsible for the adaptation of cells and organs to exercise. Students must complete a full-time original research project that covers topics from method optimization to mechanisms that regulate the adaptation to exercise. The University of Bedfordshire, England, also offers the MSc in Molecular and Cellular Exercise Physiology (**www.beds.ac.uk/howtoapply/courses/postgraduate/next-year/molecular-and-cellular-exercise-physiology**), and other universities and colleges in the United States are planning their own degree programs relating to molecular exercise physiology. We are heartened that

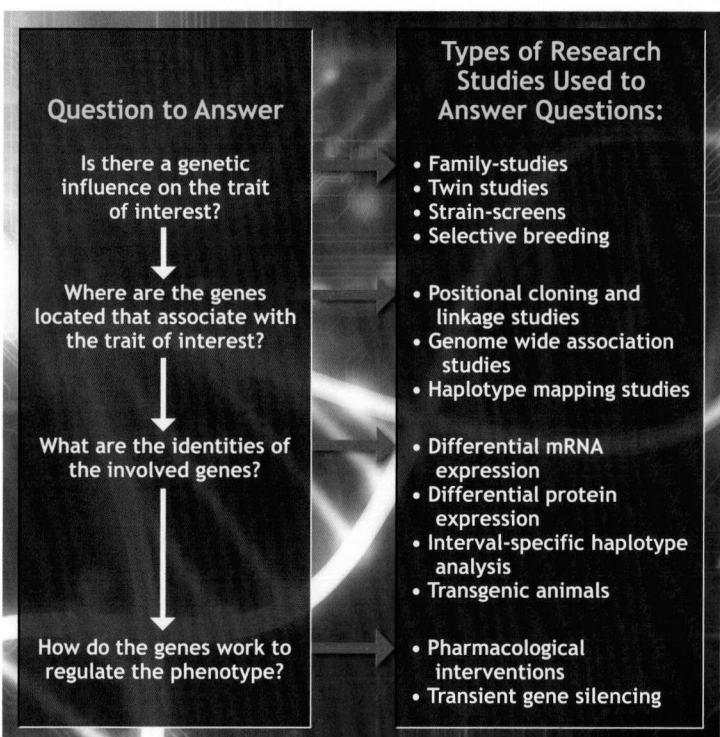

FIGURE 33.49 • Proposed research schema to determine the genetic basis of any physical activity trait of interest. Modified from Lightfoot JT. Current understanding of the genetic basis for physical activity. *J Nutr* 2011;141:526. The author cites 49 animal and human studies related to the genetics of physical activity, including different lines of evidence to support the first three questions posed in the figure.

other programs in kinesiology now give students the opportunity to complete coursework in molecular biology as part of the required core or elective curriculum, and offer interdisciplinary study in molecular biology, biochemistry, functional genomics, epigenomics, pharmacology, molecular and cellular neuroscience, and integrative physiology (http://www.sph.umd.edu/KNES/research/exphys.html; http://ki.se/ki/jsp/polopoly.jsp?d=39823&l=en; http://cms.skidmore.edu/exercisescience/molecular-exercise-physiology-laboratory.cfm). Working together, exercise physiologists trained in molecular biology (or molecular biologists with training in exercise physiology can profit from the insights of biologists, geneticists, pharmacologists, and chemists who study human physical activity at the molecular level. Their shared explorations will benefit all humanity.

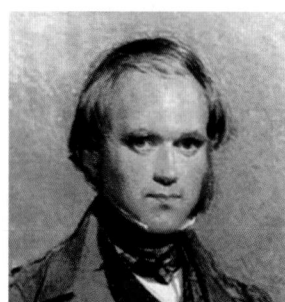

Charles Darwin

Each (organic being) at some period of life, during some season of the year, during each generation or at intervals, has to struggle for life, and to suggest great destruction. When we reflect on this struggle, we may console ourselves with the full belief that the war of nature is not incessant, that no fear is felt, that death is generally prompt, and that the vigorous, the healthy, and the happy survive and multiply.

Charles Darwin
The Origin of the Species

the**Point** References are available online at
http://thepoint.lww.com/mkk8e.

Index

Page numbers in italics denote figures. Those followed by (t) denote tables.

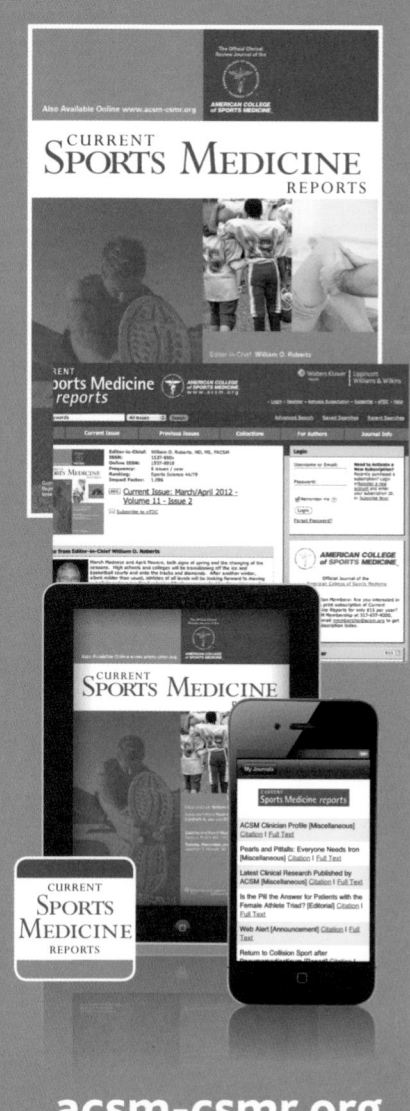

acsm-csmr.org

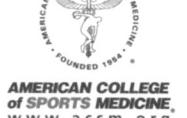

CURRENT SPORTS MEDICINE REPORTS

The Official Clinical Review Journal of the American College of Sports Medicine

AMERICAN COLLEGE of SPORTS MEDICINE
www.acsm.org

Submit your order today and save 20%!

Current Sports Medicine Reports helps keep physicians up to date with the expanding volume of information published in sports medicine. This bimonthly publication divides the field of sports medicine into 12 major categories. Each issue covers two areas in depth, providing a thorough review of the most current sports medicine literature published.

Categories include:

- Head, Neck, and Spine
- General Medical Conditions
- Chest and Abdominal Conditions
- Environmental Conditions
- Sideline and Event Management
- Training, Prevention, and Rehabilitation
- Nutrition and Ergogenic Aids
- Exercise is Medicine
- Extremity and Joint Conditions
- Sport-Specific Illness and Injury
- Competitive Sports
- Special Populations

ACSM Physician Member? Receive the journal in print for only $15!
Contact ACSM Membership at 317-637-9200, ext. 309 or email membership@acsm.org to order your subscription today.
Physician Members receive free online access to the journal.

Subscription Reply Form

Bimonthly • ISSN 1537-890X • acsm-csmr.org

CURRENT SPORTS MEDICINE REPORTS

❏ **YES!** Please start my subscription to **Current Sports Medicine Reports**.

	Individual	Student/Resident
In the U.S.	❏ $321.00 $256.80	❏ $147.00 $117.60
Outside the U.S.	❏ $377.00 $301.60	❏ $147.00 $117.60

PAYMENT OPTIONS
❏ Payment enclosed (make payable to Lippincott Williams & Wilkins)
❏ Order online at **LWW.com** Use Promo Code WDR425ZZ at checkout
❏ Call 1-800-638-3030 (US); 1-301-223-2300 (International)
❏ Charge my ❏ VISA ❏ MasterCard ❏ AMEX ❏ Discover ❏ Diners Card

Card #_____ Exp. Date _____

Signature _____

Prices are for individual subscriptions only. Prices are in U.S. funds. All shipping and handling charges are included. Air freight delivery charges apply to orders outside North America. Add states sales tax where applicable. In Canada, add GST. In EU, add VAT. Prices are subject to change. Individual and student/resident subscription rates include print and access to the online version.

Please print

Name _____

Institution _____

Address_____

City_____State_____Zip _____

Country _____

Phone _____

E-mail_____
Please provide your email for online access instructions, savings offers, and updates.

Wolters Kluwer Health | Lippincott Williams & Wilkins

PO Box 1600 • Hagerstown, MD 21741-1600 USA
Journal Orders & Requests • 250 Waterloo Road • London, UK SE1 8RD

MDR425ZZ

BUSINESS REPLY MAIL

FIRST-CLASS MAIL PERMIT NO. 31 HAGERSTOWN, MD

POSTAGE WILL BE PAID BY ADDRESSEE

NO POSTAGE
NECESSARY
IF MAILED
IN THE
UNITED STATES

CURRENT
SPORTS MEDICINE
REPORTS

PO BOX 1600
HAGERSTOWN MD 21741-9932